Merritt's Neurology

11th Edition

EDITED BY

Lewis P. Rowland, M.D.

Professor of Neurology
Columbia University College of Physicians and Surgeons
Neurological Institute
New York Presbyterian Hospital
Columbia University Medical Center
New York, New York

LIPPINCOTT WILLIAMS & WILKINS
A **Wolters Kluwer** Company

Philadelphia · Baltimore · New York · London
Buenos Aires · Hong Kong · Sydney · Tokyo

Acquisitions Editor: Anne M. Sydor
Developmental Editor: Joyce A. Murphy
Production Manager: Bridgett Dougherty
Senior Manufacturing Manager: Ben Rivera
Marketing Manager: Adam Glazer
Design Coordinator: Doug Smock
Production Service: TechBooks
Printer: Quebecor World/Taunton

Library of Congress Cataloging-in-Publication Data

Merritt's neurology.—11th ed./edited by Lewis P. Rowland.
  p. ; cm.
  Includes bibliographical references and index.
  ISBN 0-7817-5311-2
   1. Nervous system—Diseases. 2. Neurology. I. Rowland, Lewis P. II. Merritt, H.
Houston (Hiram Houston), 1902–1979. III. Title: Neurology.
  [DNLM: 1. Nervous System Diseases. WL 140 M572 2005]
RC346.M4 2005
616.8—dc22

2005003408

Care has been taken to confirm the accuracy of the information presented and to describe generally accepted practices. However, the authors, editors, and publisher are not responsible for errors or omissions or for any consequences from application of the information in this book and make no warranty, expressed or implied, with respect to the currency, completeness, or accuracy of the contents of the publication. Application of this information in a particular situation remains the professional responsibility of the practitioner.

The authors, editors, and publisher have exerted every effort to ensure that drug selection and dosage set forth in this text are in accordance with current recommendations and practice at the time of publication. However, in view of ongoing research, changes in government regulations, and the constant flow of information relating to drug therapy and drug reactions, the reader is urged to check the package insert for each drug for any change in indications and dosage and for added warnings and precautions. This is particularly important when the recommended agent is a new or infrequently employed drug.

Some drugs and medical devices presented in this publication have Food and Drug Administration (FDA) clearance for limited use in restricted research settings. It is the responsibility of the health care provider to ascertain the FDA status of each drug or device planned for use in their clinical practice.

10 9 8 7 6 5 4 3 2 1

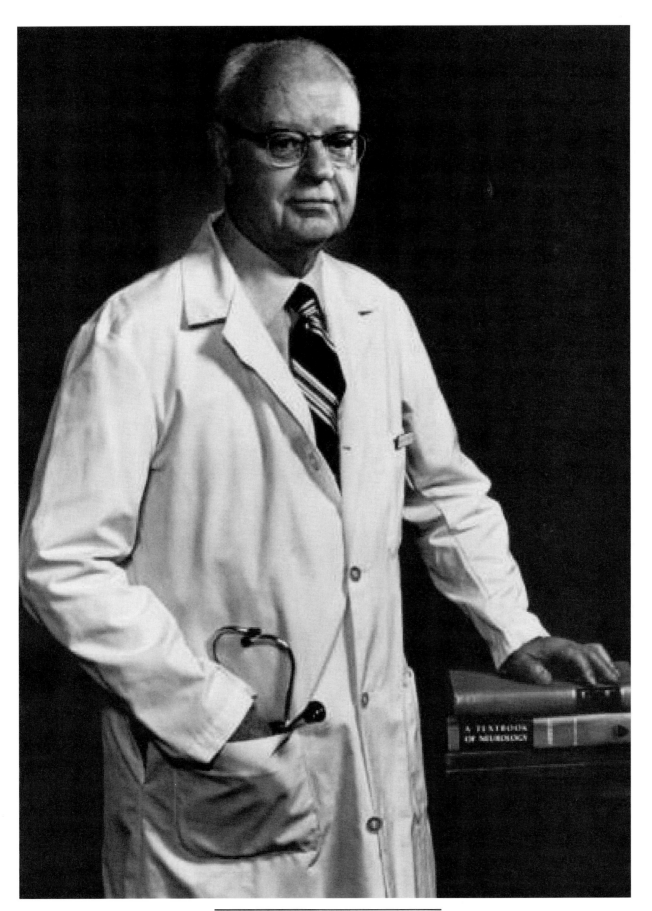

Dedicated to H. Houston Merritt (1902–1979)

CONTENTS

Contributing Authors *xi*
Preface *xxi*
Color tip

SECTION I: SYMPTOMS OF NEUROLOGIC DISORDERS 1

1. **Delirium and Dementia** *3*
   Scott A. Small and Richard Mayeux

2. **Aphasia, Apraxia, and Agnosia** *8*
   J. P. Mohr

3. **Syncope, Seizures and Their Mimics** *13*
   Lawrence J. Hirsch, Dewey K. Ziegler, and
   Timothy A. Pedley

4. **Coma** *20*
   John C. M. Brust

5. **Diagnosis of Pain and Paresthesias** *29*
   Lewis P. Rowland

6. **Dizziness and Hearing Loss** *32*
   Ian S. Storper

7. **Impaired Vision** *38*
   Myles M. Behrens

8. **Headache** *45*
   Neil H. Raskin and Mark W. Green

9. **Involuntary Movements** *48*
   Stanley Fahn

10. **Syndromes Caused by Weak Muscles** *52*
    Lewis P. Rowland

11. **Gait Disorders** *56*
    Sid Gilman

12. **Signs and Symptoms in Neurologic Diagnosis** *60*
    Lewis P. Rowland

SECTION II: HOW TO SELECT DIAGNOSTIC TESTS 65

13. **Computed Tomography and Magnetic Resonance Imaging** *67*
    Robert DeLaPaz

14. **Electroencephalography and Evoked Potentials** *79*
    Ronald G. Emerson, Thaddeus S. Walczak,
    and Timothy A. Pedley

15. **Electromyography, Nerve Conduction Studies, and Magnetic Stimulation** *89*
    Clifton L. Gooch and Seth Pullman

16. **Neurovascular Imaging** *100*
    J. P. Mohr and Robert DeLaPaz

17. **Endovascular Surgical Neuroradiology** *114*
    Philip M. Myers and Sean D. Lavine

18. **Lumbar Puncture and Cerebrospinal Fluid Examination** *123*
    Robert A. Fishman

19. **Muscle and Nerve Biopsy** *127*
    Arthur P. Hays and Michael D. Daras

20. **Neuropsychologic Evaluation** *130*
    Yaakov Stern

21. **DNA Diagnosis** *134*
    Lewis P. Rowland, Salvatore DiMauro,
    and Michio Hirano

SECTION III: INFECTIONS OF THE NERVOUS SYSTEM 137

22. **Bacterial Infections** *139*
    Burk Jubelt

23. **Focal Infections** *167*
    Gary L. Bernardini

24. **Viral Infections** *175*
    Burk Jubelt

25. **Acquired Immunodeficiency Syndrome (AIDS)** *211*
    Carolyn Barley Britton

26. **Fungal and Yeast Infections** *228*
    Leon D. Prockop

27. **Neurosarcoidosis** *232*
    John C. M. Brust

28. **Spirochete Infections: Neurosyphilis** *235*
    Leonidas Stefanis and Lewis P. Rowland

29. Spirochete Infections: Leptospirosis *243*
Burk Jubelt

30. Spirochete Infections: Lyme Disease *244*
Burk Jubelt

31. Parasitic Infections *246*
Burk Jubelt

32. Bacterial Toxins *259*
Burk Jubelt

33. Reye Syndrome *262*
Darryl C. De Vivo

34. Prion Diseases *264*
Burk Jubelt

35. Whipple Disease *270*
Elan D. Louis

SECTION IV: VASCULAR DISEASES *273*

36. Pathogenesis, Classification, and Epidemiology of Cerebrovascular Disease *275*
Ralph L. Sacco

37. Examination of the Patient with Cerebrovascular Disease *291*
Randolph S. Marshall

38. Transient Ischemic Attack *293*
John C. M. Brust

39. Cerebral Infarction *295*
John C. M. Brust

40. Cerebral and Cerebellar Hemorrhage *303*
J. P. Mohr and Christian Stapf

41. Genetics of Stroke *305*
Suh-Hang Hank Juo and Ralph L. Sacco

42. Other Cerebrovascular Syndromes *308*
Frank M. Yatsu

43. Differential Diagnosis of Stroke *312*
Mitchell S. V. Elkind and J. P. Mohr

44. Stroke in Children *315*
Arnold P. Gold and Marc C. Patterson

45. Treatment and Prevention of Strokes *324*
Frank M. Yatsu

46. Subarachnoid Hemorrhage *328*
Stephan A. Mayer, Gary L. Bernardini, Robert A. Solomon, and John C. M. Brust

47. Cerebral Veins and Sinuses *338*
Robert A. Fishman

48. Vascular Disease of the Spinal Cord *342*
Leon A. Weisberg

SECTION V: DISORDERS OF CEREBROSPINAL AND BRAIN FLUIDS *347*

49. Hydrocephalus *349*
Leon D. Prockop

50. Brain Edema and Disorders of Intracranial Pressure *357*
Robert A. Fishman

51. Superficial Siderosis of the Central Nervous System *365*
Robert A. Fishman

52. Hyperosmolar Hyperglycemic Nonketotic Syndrome *366*
Stephan A. Mayer and Leon D. Prockop

SECTION VI: TUMORS *369*

53. General Considerations *371*
Lisa M. DeAngelis

54. Tumors of the Skull and Cranial Nerves *378*
Lisa M. DeAngelis and Jeffrey N. Bruce

55. Tumors of the Meninges *386*
Lisa M. DeAngelis and Jeffrey N. Bruce

56. Gliomas *393*
Lisa M. DeAngelis

57. Lymphomas *406*
Lisa M. DeAngelis and Casilda M. Balmaceda

58. Pineal Region Tumors *414*
Lisa M. DeAngelis and Jeffrey N. Bruce

59. Tumors of the Pituitary Gland *420*
Lisa M. DeAngelis, Pamela U. Freda, and Jeffrey N. Bruce

60. Congenital and Childhood Central Nervous System Tumors *428*
James H. Garvin, Jr., Neil A. Feldstein, and Saadi Ghatan

61. Vascular Tumors and Malformations *449*
J. P. Mohr and John Pile-Spellman

62. **Metastatic Tumors** *459*
    Lisa M. DeAngelis

63. **Spinal Tumors** *470*
    Paul C. McCormick and Lewis P. Rowland

SECTION VII: TRAUMA *481*

64. **Head Injury** *483*
    Stephan A. Mayer

65. **Spinal Injury** *502*
    *Christopher Commichou, Joseph T. Marrotta,
    and Nazli Janjua*

66. **Intervertebral Disks and Radiculopathy** *510*
    Paul C. McCormick

67. **Cervical Spondylotic Myelopathy** *517*
    Lewis P. Rowland and Paul C. McCormick

68. **Lumbar Spondylosis** *521*
    Lewis P. Rowland and Paul C. McCormick

69. **Cranial and Peripheral Nerve Lesions** *523*
    *Clifton L. Gooch, Dale J. Lange, and
    Werner Trojaborg*

70. **Thoracic Outlet Syndrome** *543*
    Lewis P. Rowland and Louis H. Weimer

71. **Neuropathic Pain** *545*
    Clifton L. Gooch

72. **Radiation Injury** *551*
    *Steven R. Isaacson, Casilda Balmaceda,
    and Michael D. Daras*

73. **Electrical and Lightning Injury** *557*
    Lewis P. Rowland

74. **Decompression Sickness** *558*
    Leon D. Prockop

SECTION VIII: BIRTH INJURIES AND DEVELOPMENTAL ABNORMALITIES *561*

75. **Neonatal Neurology** *563*
    *M. Richard Koenigsberger, Ram Kairam,
    Douglas R. Nordli, Jr., and Timothy A. Pedley*

76. **Floppy Infant Syndrome** *573*
    Juan M. Pascual and Darryl C. De Vivo

77. **Static Disorders of Brain Development** *576*
    Isabelle Rapin

78. **Laurence-Moon-Biedl Syndrome** *586*
    Melvin Greer

79. **Structural Malformations** *587*
    Melvin Greer

80. **Marcus Gunn and Möbius Syndromes** *601*
    Lewis P. Rowland and Marc C. Patterson

SECTION IX: GENETIC DISEASES OF THE CENTRAL NERVOUS SYSTEM *605*

81. **Chromosomal Diseases** *607*
    Ching H. Wang and Marc C. Patterson

82. **Disorders of Amino Acid Metabolism** *611*
    John H. Menkes

83. **Disorders of Purine and Pyrimidine Metabolism** *620*
    Marc C. Patterson and Lewis P. Rowland

84. **Lysosomal and Other Storage Diseases** *622*
    Marc C. Patterson and William G. Johnson

85. **Disorders of Carbohydrate Metabolism** *641*
    Salvatore DiMauro

86. **Glucose Transporter Type 1 Deficiency Syndrome** *644*
    Darryl C. De Vivo, Juan M. Pascual, and Dong Wang

87. **Disorders of Deoxyribonucleic Acid (DNA) Maintenance, Transcription, and Translation** *646*
    Marc C. Patterson

88. **Hyperammonemia** *650*
    Marc C. Patterson

89. **Peroxisomal Diseases: Adrenoleukodystrophy, Zellweger Syndrome, and Refsum Disease** *653*
    Marc C. Patterson and Darryl C. De Vivo

90. **Organic Acidurias** *658*
    Stefano DiDonato and Graziella Uziel

91. **Disorders of Metal Metabolism** *660*
    John H. Menkes

92. **Acute Intermittent Porphyria** *668*
    Lewis P. Rowland

93. **Neurologic Syndromes With Acanthocytes** *671*
    *K-H. Christopher Min, Timothy A. Pedley,
    and Lewis P. Rowland*

94. **Cerebral Degenerations of Childhood** *675*
Eveline C. Traeger and Isabelle Rapin

95. **Diffuse Sclerosis** *682*
Marc C. Patterson and Lewis P. Rowland

96. **Differential Diagnosis** *684*
Eveline C. Traeger and Isabelle Rapin

SECTION X: DISORDERS OF MITOCHONDRIAL DNA *693*

97. **Mitochondrial Encephalomyopathies: Diseases of Mitochondrial DNA** *695*
Salvatore DiMauro, Eric A. Schon, Michio Hirano, and Lewis P. Rowland

98. **Leber Hereditary Optic Neuropathy** *702*
Michio Hirano and Myles M. Behrens

99. **Mitochondrial Diseases with Mutations of Nuclear DNA** *705*
Darryl C. De Vivo and Michio Hirano

SECTION XI: NEUROCUTANEOUS DISORDERS *711*

100. **Neurofibromatosis** *713*
Arnold P. Gold and Marc C. Patterson

101. **Encephalotrigeminal Angiomatosis** *718*
Arnold P. Gold and Marc C. Patterson

102. **Incontinentia Pigmenti** *722*
Arnold P. Gold and Marc C. Patterson

103. **Tuberous Sclerosis Complex** *724*
Arnold P. Gold and Marc C. Patterson

SECTION XII: PERIPHERAL NEUROPATHIES *733*

104. **General Considerations** *735*
Norman Latov

105. **Hereditary Neuropathies** *738*
Michael E. Shy

106. **Acquired Neuropathies** *748*
Thomas H. Brannagan III, Louis H. Weimer, and Norman Latov

SECTION XIII: DEMENTIAS *769*

107. **Alzheimer Disease and Related Dementias** *771*
Scott A. Small and Richard Mayeux

SECTION XIV: ATAXIAS *781*

108. **Hereditary Ataxias** *783*
Susan B. Bressman, Rachel J. Saunders-Pullman, and Roger N. Rosenberg

SECTION XV: MOVEMENT DISORDERS *801*

109. **Huntington Disease** *803*
Stanley Fahn

110. **Sydenham and Other Forms of Chorea** *807*
Stanley Fahn

111. **Myoclonus** *812*
Stanley Fahn

112. **Gilles de la Tourette Syndrome** *815*
Stanley Fahn

113. **Dystonia** *816*
Stanley Fahn and Susan B. Bressman

114. **Essential Tremor** *827*
Elan D. Louis

115. **Parkinsonism** *828*
Stanley Fahn and Serge Przedborski

116. **Progressive Supranuclear Palsy** *846*
Paul E. Greene

117. **Tardive Dyskinesia and Other Neuroleptic-induced Syndromes** *849*
Stanley Fahn and Robert E. Burke

SECTION XVI: SPINAL CORD DISEASES *853*

118. **Hereditary and Acquired Spastic Paraplegia** *855*
Lewis P. Rowland and Paul H. Gordon

119. **Hereditary and Acquired Motor Neuron Diseases** *861*
Lewis P. Rowland, Hiroshi Mitsumoto, and Darryl C. De Vivo

120. **Syringomyelia** *870*
Elliott L. Mancall

SECTION XVII: DISORDERS OF THE NEUROMUSCULAR JUNCTION *875*

121. **Myasthenia Gravis** *877*
Audrey S. Penn and Lewis P. Rowland

122. **Lambert-Eaton Syndrome** *885*
Audrey S. Penn

123. **Botulism and Antibiotic-induced Neuromuscular Disorders** *886*
Audrey S. Penn

124. **Acute Quadriplegic Myopathy** *888*
Michio Hirano and Louis H. Weimer

SECTION XVIII: MYOPATHIES *891*

125. **Identifying Disorders of the Motor Unit** *893*
Lewis P. Rowland

126. **Progressive Muscular Dystrophies** *895*
Petra Kaufmann, Louis H. Weimer, and Lewis P. Rowland

127. **Familial Periodic Paralysis** *911*
Lewis P. Rowland and Paul H. Gordon

128. **Congenital Disorders of Muscle** *915*
Olajide Williams

129. **Myoglobinuria** *921*
Lewis P. Rowland

130. **Muscle Cramps and Stiffness** *924*
Robert B. Layzer and Lewis P. Rowland

131. **Dermatomyositis** *929*
Lewis P. Rowland

132. **Polymyositis, Inclusion Body Myositis, and Related Myopathies** *932*
Lewis P. Rowland

133. **Myositis Ossificans** *937*
Lewis P. Rowland

SECTION XIX: DEMYELINATING DISEASES *939*

134. **Multiple Sclerosis** *941*
Saud A. Sadiq

135. **Marchiafava-Bignami Disease** *963*
Lewis P. Rowland

136. **Central Pontine Myelinolysis** *965*
Gary L. Bernadini and Elliott L. Mancall

SECTION XX: AUTONOMIC DISORDERS *969*

137. **Neurogenic Orthostatic Hypotension and Autonomic Failure** *971*
Louis H. Weimer

138. **Acute Autonomic Neuropathy** *974*
Louis H. Weimer

139. **Familial Dysautonomia** *976*
Alan M. Aron

SECTION XXI: PAROXYSMAL DISORDERS *979*

140. **Migraine and Other Headaches** *981*
Neil H. Raskin and Mark W. Green

141. **Epilepsy** *990*
Carl W. Bazil, Martha J. Morrell, and Timothy A. Pedley

142. **Febrile Seizures** *1015*
Linda D. Leary, Douglas R. Nordli, Jr., and Timothy A. Pedley

143. **Transient Global Amnesia** *1017*
John C. M. Brust

144. **Ménière Syndrome** *1018*
Ian S. Storper

145. **Sleep Disorders** *1022*
June M. Fry and Bradley V. Vaughn

SECTION XXII: SYSTEMIC DISEASES AND GENERAL MEDICINE *1031*

146. **Endocrine Diseases** *1033*
Gary M. Abrams and Earl A. Zimmerman

147. **Hematologic and Related Diseases** *1050*
Robert W. Pratt, David J. Adams, and Casilda M. Balmaceda

148. **Hepatic Disease** *1064*
Neil H. Raskin and Peter Y. Kim

149. Cerebral Complications of Cardiac Surgery *1067*
Mitchell S. V. Elkind and Eric J. Heyer

150. Bone Disease *1073*
Roger N. Rosenberg

151. Renal Disease *1079*
Neil H. Raskin and J. Kirk Roberts

152. Respiratory Support for Neurologic Diseases *1082*
Stephan A. Mayer and Matthew E. Fink

153. Paraneoplastic Syndromes *1087*
Lisa M. DeAngelis and Lewis P. Rowland

154. Nutritional Disorders: Malnutrition, Malabsorption, and B$_{12}$ and Other Deficiencies *1091*
Bradford B. Worrall and Lewis P. Rowland

155. Vasculitis Syndromes *1099*
Lewis P. Rowland and Marcelo R. Olarte

156. Hypertrophic Pachymeningitis *1111*
John C. M. Brust

157. Neurologic Disease During Pregnancy *1112*
Alison M. Pack and Martha J. Morrell

158. Hashimoto Encephalopathy *1120*
Ji Y. Chong

SECTION XXIII: PSYCHIATRY AND NEUROLOGY *1123*

159. Mood Disorders *1125*
Ralph N. Wharton

160. Anxiety Disorders *1132*
Ralph N. Wharton

161. Schizophrenia *1137*
Arielle D. Stanford, Cheryl Corcoran, and Dolores Malaspina

162. Somatoform Disorders *1142*
Daniel T. Williams

SECTION XXIV: ENVIRONMENTAL NEUROLOGY *1149*

163. Alcoholism *1151*
John C. M. Brust

164. Drug Dependence *1161*
John C. M. Brust

165. Iatrogenic Disease *1166*
Louis H. Weimer and Lewis P. Rowland

166. Complications of Cancer Chemotherapy *1168*
Lisa M. DeAngelis and Casilda M. Balmaceda

167. Occupational and Environmental Neurotoxicology *1173*
Leon D. Prockop and Lewis P. Rowland

168. HIV, Fetal Alcohol and Drug Effects, and the Battered Child *1185*
Claudia A. Chiriboga

169. Falls in the Elderly *1191*
Gary M. Abrams and Lewis P. Rowland

SECTION XXV: REHABILITATION *1193*

170. Neurologic Rehabilitation *1195*
Laura Lennihan and Glenn M. Seliger

SECTION XXVI: ETHICAL AND LEGAL GUIDELINES *1199*

171. End-of-Life Issues in Neurology *1201*
Lewis P. Rowland

Index *1205*

Gary M. Abrams, M.D.
Associate Professor
Department of Neurology
University of California
Chief, Department of Neurology/Rehabilitation
University of California, San Francisco/Mt. Zion Medical
    Center
San Francisco, California

David J. Adams, M.D.
Clinical Professor of Neurology
Department of Neurology
Columbia University College of Physicians
    and Surgeons
Attending Physician
Department of Neurology
New York Presbyterian Hospital
Columbia University Medical Center
New York, New York

Alan M. Aron, M.D.
Professor of Pediatrics and Clinical Neurology
Departments of Neurology and Pediatrics
Mount Sinai-New York University Medical Center
Director, Attending Neurologist, and
    Attending Pediatrician
Department of Pediatric Neurology
Mount Sinai Hospital
New York, New York

Casilda M. Balmaceda, M.D.
Assistant Professor of Neurology
Columbia University College of Physicians and Surgeons
Assistant Attending Neurologist
Neurological Institute
New York Presbyterian Hospital
Columbia University Medical Center
New York, New York

Carl W. Bazil, M.D., Ph.D.
Assistant Professor of Neurology
Columbia University College of Physicians
    and Surgeons
Attending Neurologist
Neurological Institute
New York Presbyterian Hospital
Columbia University Medical Center
New York, New York

Myles M. Behrens, M.D.
Professor of Clinical Ophthalmology
Columbia University College of Physicians and Surgeons
Attending Ophthalmologist
New York Presbyterian Hospital
Columbia University Medical Center
New York, New York

Gary L. Bernardini, M.D., Ph.D.
Associate Professor of Neurology
Albany Medical College
Director
Stroke and Neurocritical Care Unit
Albany Medical Center
Albany, New York

Thomas H. Brannagan III, M.D.
Associate Professor of Clinical Neurology
Department of Neurology and
    Neuroscience
Weill Medical College of Cornell University
Associate Attending Physician
Department of Neurology
New York Presbyterian Hospital
Columbia University Medical Center
New York, New York

Susan B. Bressman, M.D.
Chair
Department of Neurology
Phillips Ambulatory Care Center
Beth Israel Hospital
New York, New York

Carolyn Barley Britton, M.D., M.Sc.
Associate Professor of Clinical Neurology
Columbia University College of Physicians
    and Surgeons
Associate Attending Neurologist
Neurological Institute
New York Presbyterian Hospital
Columbia University Medical Center
New York, New York

Jeffrey N. Bruce, M.D.
Associate Professor of Neurological Surgery
Columbia University College of Physicians
    and Surgeons
Attending Neurological Surgeon
Neurological Institute
New York Presbyterian Hospital
Columbia University
    Medical Center
New York, New York

John C. M. Brust, M.D.
Professor of Clinical Neurology
Department of Neurology
Columbia University College of Physicians
    and Surgeons
Attending Neurologist
Neurological Institute
New York Presbyterian Hospital
Columbia University Medical Center
Director, Department of Neurology
Harlem Hospital Center
New York, New York

Robert E. Burke, M.D.
Professor of Neurology
Attending Neurologist
Columbia University College of Physicians
    and Surgeons
Attending Neurologist
Neurological Institute
New York Presbyterian Hospital
Columbia University Medical Center
New York, New York

Stephan Chan, M.D.
Assistant Professor of Radiology
Columbia University College of Physicians
    and Surgeons
Neuroradiologist
Neurological Institute
New York Presbyterian Hospital
Columbia University Medical Center
New York, New York

Ji Y. Chong, M.D.
Assistant Professor of Neurology
Stroke and Critical Care Division
Columbia University College of Physicians and Surgeons
Assistant Attending Physician
Neurological Institute
New York Presbyterian Hospital
Columbia University Medical Center
New York, New York

Claudia A. Chiriboga, M.D.
Associate Professor of Neurology and Clinical Pediatrics
Columbia University College of Physicians and Surgeons
Associate Attending Neurologist
Neurological Institute
New York Presbyterian Hospital
Columbia University Medical Center
New York, New York

Christopher Commichou, M.D.
Assistant Professor of Neurology
University of Vermont College of Medicine
Director, Neurocritical Care and Stroke
Fletcher Allen Health Care
Burlington, Vermont

Cheryl Corcoran, M.D.
Director of the Prodromal Schizophrenia Research Clinic
New York State Psychiatric Institute
Assistant Professor of Clinical Psychiatry
New York Presbyterian Hospital
Columbia University Medical Center
New York, New York

Michael D. Daras, M.D., Ph.D
Clinical Professor
Columbia University College of Physicians
    and Surgeons
Attending Neurologist
Neurological Institute
New York Presbyterian Hospital
Columbia University Medical Center
New York, New York

Lisa M. DeAngelis, M.D.
Professor of Neurology
Weill College of Medicine of Cornell University
Chairman
Department of Neurology
Memorial Hospital
New York, New York

Robert DeLaPaz, M.D.
Professor of Radiology
Columbia University College of Physicians and Surgeons
Attending Radiologist
Director, Division of Neuroradiology
New York Presbyterian Hospital
Columbia University Medical Center
New York, New York

Darryl C. De Vivo, M.D.
Sidney Carter Professor of Neurology
Professor of Pediatrics
Columbia University College of Physicians
    and Surgeons
Attending Neurologist and Pediatrician
Department of Neurology
Neurological Institute
New York Presbyterian Hospital
Columbia University Medical Center
New York, New York

Stefano DiDonato, M.D.
Chief
Department of Research
Istituto Nazionale Neurologico C. Besta
Milano, Italy

Salvatore DiMauro, M.D.
Lucy G. Moses Professor
Department of Neurology
Columbia University College of Physicians
    and Surgeons
New York, New York

Mitchell S. V. Elkind, M.D., M.S.
Assistant Professor of Neurology
Columbia University College of Physicians and Surgeons
Assistant Attending Neurologist
New York Presbyterian Hospital
Neurological Institute
Columbia University Medical Center
New York, New York

Ronald G. Emerson, M.D.
Professor of Clinical Neurology and Clinical Pediatrics
Columbia University College of Physicians and Surgeons
Attending Neurologist
Neurological Institute
New York Presbyterian Hospital
Columbia University Medical Center
New York, New York

Stanley Fahn, M.D.
H. Houston Merritt Professor of Neurology
Columbia University College of Physicians and Surgeons
Attending Neurologist
Neurological Institute
New York Presbyterian Hospital
Columbia University Medical Center
New York, New York

Neil A. Feldstein, M.D.
Assistant Professor of Neurological Surgery
Columbia University College of Physicians and Surgeons
Attending Neurosurgeon
Neurological Surgery Department
Children's Hospital of New York
New York, New York

Matthew E. Fink, M.D.
Professor
Department of Neurology and Medicine
Director
Division of Vascular and Critical Care Neurology
Albert Einstein College of Medicine
Beth Israel Medical Center and St. Luke's Roosevelt Hospital
  Center
New York, New York

Robert A. Fishman, M.D.
Professor Emeritus
Department of Neurology
University of California, San Francisco
Attending Neurologist
Department of Neurology
University of California, San Francisco Hospitals
San Francisco, California

Pamela U. Freda, M.D.
Associate Professor of Clinical Medicine
Department of Medicine
Columbia University College of Physicians and Surgeons

Assistant Attending Physician
Department of Medicine
New York Presbyterian Hospital
Columbia University Medical Center
New York, New York

June M. Fry, M.D., Ph.D.
Professor
Department of Neurology
Drexel University College of Medicine
Philadelphia, Pennsylvania
Director
Center for Sleep Medicine
Lafayette Hill, Pennsylvania

James H. Garvin, Jr., M.D., Ph.D.
Professor of Clinical Pediatrics
Columbia University College of Physicians and Surgeons
Attending Pediatrician
New York Presbyterian Hospital
Columbia University Medical Center
New York, New York

Sid Gilman, M.D.
William J. Herdman Professor
Department of Neurology
University of Michigan
Attending Neurologist
University of Michigan Health System
Ann Arbor, Michigan

Arnold P. Gold, M.D.
Professor of Clinical Neurology and Clinical Pediatrics
Columbia University College of Physicians and Surgeons
Attending Neurologist and Pediatrician
Neurological Institute
New York Presbyterian Hospital
Columbia University Medical Center
New York, New York

Clifton L. Gooch, M.D.
Associate Professor of Clinical Neurology
Columbia University College of Physicians and Surgeons
Director
Electromyography Laboratory
New York Presbyterian Hospital
Columbia University Medical Center
New York, New York

Paul H. Gordon, M.D.
Assistant Professor
Columbia University College of Physicians and Surgeons
Assistant Attending Physician
Department of Neurology
Neurological Institute
New York Presbyterian Hospital
Columbia University Medical Center
New York, New York

Mark W. Green, M.D.
Clinical Professor
Columbia University College of Physicians and Surgeons
Director
Columbia University Medical Center
Department of Neurology
New York, New York

Paul E. Greene, M.D.
Associate Professor of Neurology
Columbia University College of Physicians and Surgeons
Associate Attending Neurologist
Neurological Institute
New York Presbyterian Hospital
Columbia University Medical Center
New York, New York

Melvin Greer, M.D.
Professor and Chairman
Department of Neurology
University of Florida College of Medicine
Gainesville, Florida

Arthur P. Hays, M.D.
Associate Professor of Clinical Neuropathology
Department of Pathology
Columbia University College of Physicians and Surgeons
Associate Attending in Pathology
Department of Pathology
New York Presbyterian Hospital
Columbia University Medical Center
New York, New York

Eric J. Heyer, M.D.
Associate Professor of Clinical Anesthesiology
    and Clinical Neurology
Columbia University College of Physicians and Surgeons
Chief
Division of Neurosurgical Anesthesiology
Neurological Institute
New York Presbyterian Hospital
Columbia University Medical Center
New York, New York

Michio Hirano, M.D.
Associate Professor
Columbia University College of Physicians and Surgeons
Attending Physician
Neurological Institute
New York Presbyterian Hospital
Columbia University Medical Center
New York, New York

Lawrence Hirsch, M.D.
Associate Clinical Professor
Columbia University College of Physicians
    and Surgeons
Associate Neurologist
Neurological Institute

New York Presbyterian Hospital
Columbia University Medical Center
New York, New York

Stephen R. Isaacson
Associate Professor
Department of Radiation Oncology
Columbia University College of Physicians and Surgeons
New York, New York

William G. Johnson, M.D.
Professor of Neurology
University of Medicine and Dentistry of New Jersey
Robert Wood Johnson Medical School
Piscataway, New Jersey
Attending Neurologist
Robert Wood Johnson University Hospital
New Brunswick, New Jersey

Burk Jubelt, M.D.
Professor and Program Director
Department of Neurology
SUNY Upstate Medical University
Attending Neurologist
Department of Neurology
University Hospital
Syracuse, New York

Suh-Hang Hank Juo, M.D., Ph.D.
Assistant Professor
Genoma Center
Columbia University College of Physicians and Surgeons
New York, New York

Ram Kairam, M.D.
Chairman
Department of Pediatrics
Bronx Lebanon Hospital Center
Bronx, New York

Petra Kaufmann, M.D., M.Sc.
Florence Irving Assistant Professor of Neurology
Department of Neurology
Columbia University College of Physicians and Surgeons
Assistant Attending Neurologist
Neurological Institute
New York Presbyterian Hospital
Columbia University Medical Center
New York, New York

Peter Y. Kim, M.D., Ph.D.
Assistant Professor
Department of Neurology
Columbia University College of Physicians
    and Surgeons
Assistant Attending Neurologist
New York Presbyterian Hospital
New York, New York

M. Richard Koenigsberger, M.D.
Professor of Clinical Neurology and Pediatrics
Departments of Neurology, Pediatrics
Columbia University College of Physicians
    and Surgeons
Director
Child Neurology Clinic
New York Presbyterian Hospital
New York, New York

Dale J. Lange, M.D.
Associate Professor of Clinical Neurology
Associate Attending Neurologist
Neurological Institute
New York Presbyterian Hospital
Columbia University Medical Center
New York, New York

Norman Latov, M.D., Ph.D.
Professor of Neurology and Neurosciences
Weill Medical College of Cornell University
Professor
Neurological Institute
New York Presbyterian Hospital
Columbia University Medical Center
New York, New York

Sean D. Lavine, M.D.
Assistant Professor
Neurological Surgery and Radiology
Columbia University College of Physicians and Surgeons
Co-Director
Neuroendovascular Services
Neurological Institute
New York Presbyterian Hospital
Columbia University Medical Center
New York, New York

Robert B. Layzer, M.D.
Professor of Neurology Emeritus
University of California, San Francisco
San Francisco, California

Linda D. Leary, M.D.
Assistant Professor of Clinical Neurology and Pediatrics
Columbia University College of Physicians and Surgeons
Attending Physician
Pediatric Neurology and Epilepsy
Children's Hospital of New York Presbyterian Hospital
New York, New York

Laura Lennihan, M.D.
Associate Professor of Clinical Neurology
Department of Neurology
Columbia University College of Physicians
    and Surgeons
New York, New York
Chief, Department of Neurology
Helen Hayes Hospital
West Haverstown, New York

Elan D. Louis, M.D.
Associate Professor of Neurology
Columbia University College of Physicians
    and Surgeons
Assistant Attending Neurologist
New York Presbyterian Hospital
Columbia University Medical Center
New York, New York

Dolores Malaspina, M.D., M.P.H.
Director of Division of Clinical Neurobiology
New York State Psychiatric Institute
Professor of Clinical Psychiatry
New York Presbyterian Hospital
Columbia University Medical Center
New York, New York

Elliott L. Mancall, M.D.
Professor
Department of Neurology
Jefferson Medical College
Attending Neurologist
Jefferson Hospital for Neuroscience
Philadelphia, Pennsylvania

Joseph T. Marotta, M.D., F.R.C.P. (C)
Professor Emeritus of Neurology
Department of Neurological Sciences
University of Western Ontario
London Health Sciences Centre
London, Ontario
Canada

Randolph S. Marshall, M.D.
Associate Professor
Department of Neurology
Columbia University College of Physicians
    and Surgeons
New York, New York

Stephan A. Mayer, M.D.
Assistant Professor of Neurology
    (in Neurological Surgery)
Assistant Attending Neurologist
Director, Columbia-Presbyterian Neuro-Intensive Care Unit
Neurological Institute
New York Presbyterian Hospital
Columbia University Medical Center
New York, New York

Richard Mayeux, M.D.
Professor
Director, Sergievsky Center
Co-Director, Taub Institute
Columbia University College of Physicians
    and Surgeons
Attending Neurologist
Neurological Institute
New York Presbyterian Hospital
Columbia University Medical Center
New York, New York

Paul C. McCormick, M.D.
Professor of Clinical Neurology
Department of Neurology
Columbia University College of Physicians and Surgeons
Attending Neurologist
New York Presbyterian Hospital
New York, New York

John H. Menkes, M.D.
Professor Emeritus
Departments of Neurology and Pediatrics
University of California, Los Angeles
Director of Pediatric Neurology
Cedars Sinai Medical Center
Los Angeles, California

Philip M. Meyers, M.D.
Assistant Professor
Department of Radiology and Neurological Surgery
Columbia University College of Physicians and Surgeons
Clinical Director
Neuroendovascular Service
Department of Radiology and Neurological Surgery
New York Presbyterian Hospitals of Columbia
   and Cornell
New York, New York

K.-H. Christopher Min, M.D., Ph.D.
Assistant Professor of Neurology
Columbia University College of Physicians and Surgeons
Assistant Attending Neurologist
The Neurological Institute
New York Presbyterian Hospital
Columbia University Medical Center
New York, New York

Hiroshi Mitsumoto, M.D.
Wesley J. Howe Professor of Neurology
Director, Eleanor and Lou Gehrig MDA/ALS Research Center
Division Head, Neuromuscular Disease
New York Presbyterian Hospital
Columbia University Medical Center
New York, New York

J. P. Mohr, M.D.
Sciarra Professor of Clinical Neurology
Attending Neurologist
Director, Columbia University Stroke Unit
Neurological Institute
New York Presbyterian Hospital
Columbia University Medical Center
New York, New York

Martha J. Morrell, M.D.
Professor of Clinical Neurology
Stanford University
Chief Medical Officer

NeuroPace Inc.
Mountain View, California

Douglas R. Nordli, Jr., M.D.
Lorna S. and James P. Langdon Chair of Pediatric Epilepsy
Children's Memorial Hospital
Northwestern University
Chicago, Illinois

Marcelo R. Olarte, M.D.
Clinical Professor
Department of Neurology
Columbia University College of Physicians and Surgeons
Chief
Division of General Neurology and Attending Physician
New York Presbyterian Hospital
New York, New York

Alison M. Pack, M.D.
Assistant Professor of Clinical Neurology
Department of Neurology
Columbia University College of Physicians and Surgeons
New York, New York

Juan M. Pascual, M.D., Ph.D.
Colleen Giblin Research Laboratories
Columbia University College of Physicians and Surgeons
Children's Hospital of New York
Neurological Institute
Columbia University Medical Center
New York, New York

Marc C. Patterson, M.D.
Professor
Department of Neurology
Columbia University College of Physicians and Surgeons
Director
Division of Pediatric Neurology
Children's Hospital of New York-Presbyterian
New York, New York

Timothy A. Pedley, M.D.
Henry and Lucy Moses Professor of Neurology
Department of Neurology
Columbia University College of Physicians and Surgeons
Neurologist-in-Chief
Neurological Institute
New York Presbyterian Hospital
Columbia University Medical Center
New York, New York

Audrey S. Penn, M.D.
Deputy Director
National Institute of Neurological Disorders and Stroke
National Institute of Health
Bethesda, Maryland

John Pile-Spellman
Professor of Radiology, Neurology, Neurosurgery
Columbia University College of Physicians
    and Surgeons
Professor of Neurology
Department of Neurology
New York Presbyterian Hospital
Columbia University Medical Center
New York, New York

Robert W. Pratt, M.D.
Fellow in Clinical Neurophysiology and
    Neuromuscular Disease
Department of Neurology
The Neurological Institute
New York Presbyterian Hospital
Columbia University Medical Center
New York, New York

Leon D. Prockop, M.D.
Professor
Department of Neurology
College of Medicine, University of South Florida
Tampa, Florida

Peter Proctor, M.D.
Comprehensive Epilepsy Center
Neurological Institute
New York Presbyterian Hospital
Columbia University Medical Center
New York, New York

Serge Przedborski, M.D., Ph.D.
Professor
Department of Neurology
Columbia University College of Physicians
    and Surgeons
Attending Neurologist
New York Presbyterian Hospital
Columbia University Medical Center
New York, New York

Seth Pullman, M.D., FRCPC
Associate Professor
Department of Neurology
Columbia University College of Physicians
    and Surgeons
Director
Clinical Motor Physiology Laboratory
Neurological Institute
New York Presbyterian Hospital
Columbia University Medical Center
New York, New York

Isabelle Rapin, M.D.
Professor of Neurology and Pediatrics (Neurology)
Albert Einstein College of Medicine
Attending Neurologist
Jacob Medical Center

Montefiore Medical Center
Bronx, New York

Neil H. Raskin, M.D.
Professor
Department of Neurology
University of California, San Francisco
Attending Physician
Department of Neurology
Moffitt/Long Hospital
San Francisco, California

J. Kirk Roberts, M.D.
Assistant Professor of Clinical Neurology
Columbia University College of Physicians
    and Surgeons
Assistant Attending Physician
Neurological Institute
New York Presbyterian Hospital
Columbia University Medical Center
New York, New York

Roger N. Rosenberg, M.D.
Abe (Brunky), Morris and William Zale
    Distinguished Chair and Professor
Professor of Neurology
University of Texas Southwestern Medical Center
Dallas, Texas
Attending Neurologist
Zale-Lipsky University Hospital and Parkland Hospital
Dallas, Texas

Lewis P. Rowland, M.D.
Professor of Neurology
Columbia University College of Physicians
    and Surgeons
Attending Neurologist
Neurological Institute
New York Presbyterian Hospital
Columbia University Medical Center
New York, New York

Ralph L. Sacco, M.S., M.D.
Professor of Neurology and Epidemiology
Director, Division of Stroke and Critical Care
Associate Chair of Neurology
Attending Neurologist
Neurological Institute
New York Presbyterian Hospital
Columbia University Medical Center
New York, New York

Saud Sadiq, M.D.
Associate Professor
Albert Einstein College of Medicine
Yeshiva University
Chairman
Department of Neurology
St. Luke's-Roosevelt Hospital
New York, New York

Rachel J. Saunders-Pullman, M.D.
Assistant Professor, Albert Einstein College of Medicine
Yeshiva University
Bronx, New York
Attending Physician
Beth Israel Hospital
New York, New York

Eric A. Schon, Ph.D.
Lewis P. Rowland Professor of Neurology
Professor of Genetics and Development in Neurology
Columbia University College of Physicians and Surgeons
New York, New York

Glenn M. Seliger, M.D.
Assistant Professor of Neurology
Assistant Attending Neurologist
New York Presbyterian Hospital
New York, New York
Director of Head Injury Services
Helen Hayes Hospital
West Haverstraw, New York

Michael E. Shy, M.D.
Professor of Neurology and Molecular Medicine and Genetics
Wayne State University
Co-Director Neuromuscular Division
Director of Inherited Neuropathy Clinic
Co-Director of MDA Clinic
Detroit Medical Center
Detroit, Michigan

Michael B. Sisti, M.D.
Assistant Professor of Clinical Neurological Surgery
Columbia University College of Physicians and Surgeons
Assistant Attending Neurosurgeon
Neurological Institute
New York Presbyterian Hospital
Columbia University Medical Center
New York, New York

Scott A. Small, M.D.
Assistant Professor of Neurology
Columbia University College of Physicians
    and Surgeons
Assistant Attending Neurologist
New York Presbyterian Hospital
Neurological Institute
New York Presbyterian Hospital
Columbia University Medical Center
New York, New York

Robert A. Solomon
Byron Stookey Professor and Chairman
Department of Neurological Surgery
Columbia University College of Physicians and Surgeons
Chief of Neurosurgery
Neurological Institute
New York Presbyterian Hospital

Columbia University Medical Center
New York, New York

Arielle D. Stanford, M.D.
Postdoctoral Shizophrenia Research Fellow
Assistant in Clinical Psychiatry
New York Presbyterian Hospital
Columbia University Medical Center
New York, New York

Christian Stapf, M.D.
Assistant Professor of Neurology
Charité—Campus Benjamin Franklin
Freie Universitaet
Berlin, Germany
Research Scientist in Neurology
Columbia University College of Physicians and Surgeons
Stroke Center/The Neurological Institute
New York Presbyterian Hospital
Columbia University Medical Center
New York, New York
Attending Neurologist
Lariboisière Hospital
Paris, France

Leonidas Stefanis, M.D., Ph.D.
Senior Researcher
Department of Neurobiology
Foundation for Biomedical Research
Academy of Athens
Athens, Greece

Yaakov Stern, M.D.
Professor of Clinical Neuropsychology
Sergievsky Center and the Taub Institute
Columbia University College of Physicians and Surgeons
Professor of Clinical Neuropsychology
Neurological Institute
New York Presbyterian Hospital
Columbia University Medical Center
New York, New York

Ian S. Storper, M.D.
Assistant Professor of Clinical Otolaryngology
Department of Otolaryngology/Head and Neck Surgery
Columbia University College of Physicians and Surgeons
Assistant Attending Physician
Department of Otolaryngology/Head and Neck Surgery
New York Presbyterian Hospital
Columbia University Medical Center
New York, New York

Eveline C. Traeger, M.D.
Assistant Professor
Departments of Pediatrics and Neurology
Robert Wood Johnson School of Medicine
University of Medicine and Dentistry of New Jersey
Attending Physician
Robert Wood Johnson University Hospital
New Brunswick, New Jersey

Werner Trojaborg, M.D.
Professor
University Hospital, CPH, Denmark
Clinical Neurophysiology Department
Denmark

Graziella Uziel, M.D.
Assistant
Department of Pediatric Neurology
Istituto Nazionale Neurologico C. Besta
Milano, Italy

Bradley V. Vaughn, M.D.
Associate Professor of Neurology
Department of Neurology
University of North Carolina
Chapel Hill, North Carolina

Thaddeus S. Walczak, M.D.
Associate Clinical Professor of Neurology
University of Minnesota
Director of Clinical Neurophysiology
MINCEP Epilepsy Care
Minneapolis, Minnesota

Ching H. Wang, M.D., Ph.D.
Associate Professor
Department of Neurology and Biochemistry
Stanford University
Attending Physician
Department of Neurology and Pediatrics
Stanford University Medical Center
Stanford, California

Louis H. Weimer, M.D.
Associate Clinical Professor
Department of Neurology
Columbia University College of Physicians
    and Surgeons
Assistant Attending Neurologist
Neurological Institute
New York Presbyterian Hospital
Columbia University Medical Center
New York, New York

Leon A. Weisberg, M.D.
Professor of Neurology
Department of Psychiatry and Neurology
Tulane Health Science Center
Chief of Neuroscience
Charity Hospital
Chief of Neurology
Tulane Hospital
Tulane Health Science Center
New Orleans, Louisiana

Ralph N. Wharton, M.D.
Clinical Professor of Psychiatry
Columbia University College of Physicians and Surgeons
Attending Psychiatrist
New York Presbyterian Hospital
Columbia University Medical Center
New York, New York

Daniel T. Williams, M.D.
Clinical Professor
Department of Psychiatry
Columbia University College of Physicians
    and Surgeons
Attending Physician
Department of Psychiatry
New York Presbyterian Hospital
Columbia University Medical Center
New York, New York

Olajide Williams, M.D., M.S.
Assistant Professor
Department of Neurology
Columbia University College of Physicians
    and Surgeons
Attending Physician Department of Neurology
Harlem Hospital
New York, New York

Bradford P. Worrall, M.D., M.Sc.
Assistant Professor
Department of Neurology and Public
    Health Sciences
University of Virginia
Assistant Professor
Department of Neurology
University of Virginia Health System
Charlottesville, Virginia

Frank M. Yatsu, M.D.
Chairman Emeritus
Department of Neurology
University of Texas-Houston Medical Center
Neurologist
Department of Neurology
Hermann Hospital
Houston, Texas

Dewey K. Zeigler, M.D.
Professor Emeritus
Department of Neurology
University of Kansas Medical School
Staff Physician
Department of Neurology
Kansas University Medical Center
Kansas City, Kansas

Earl A. Zimmerman, M.D.
Professor
Department of Neurology
Albany Medical College
Attending Physician Department of Neurology
Albany Medical Center Albany, New York

PREFACE

When H. Houston Merritt first published this *Text-book of Neurology* in 1955, he was the sole author. The book became popular, and he revised it himself through the fourth edition. As the mass of information increased, he finally accepted contributions from colleagues for the fifth edition. Even then, he wrote most of the book himself, and he continued to do so for the sixth edition despite serious physical disability. He died in 1979, just as the sixth edition was released for distribution.

The seventh edition, published in 1984, was prepared by seventy of Merritt's students. Thirty of them headed neurology departments and others had become distinguished clinicians, teachers, and investigators. That edition was a landmark in the history of neurology. It documented the human legacy of a singular leader whose career set models for clinical investigation (when it was just beginning), clinical practice, teaching, editing books and journals, administering medical schools and departments, and commitment to national professional and voluntary health organizations.

We now provide the eleventh edition. The list of authors has changed progressively, as a dynamic book must do. Yet the ties to Merritt persist. Many of his personal students are still authors, and their students, Merritt's intellectual grandchildren, are appearing in increasing numbers.

Merritt's Neurology is intended for medical students, house officers, practicing neurologists, non-neurologist clinicians, nurses, and other healthcare workers. We hope it will be generally useful in providing the essential facts about common and rare diseases or conditions that are likely to be encountered.

We have tried to maintain Merritt's literary attributes: direct, clear, and succinct writing; emphasis on facts rather than unsupported opinion (now called "evidence-based medicine"); and ample use of illustrations and tables.

The book now faces competition from other books, including electronic textbooks, but its success is based on several attributes. A book, unlike a computer, can be taken and used almost anywhere. A one-volume textbook is handier, more mobile, and less expensive than the multivolume sets that now dot the scene. Briefer paperbacks provide less information and fewer references.

This edition includes comprehensive revisions demanded by the progress of research in every chapter listed in the table of contents. New chapters have been added on endovascular neurology, a major advance in diagnosis and treatment, and in psychiatric conditions—schizophrenia, mood disorders, anxiety, and somatoform disorders. Other new chapters cover diseases of DNA translation, pachymeningitis, and Hashimoto encephalopathy.

In almost every chapter, the impact of molecular genetics has required much updating. The progress of medical science has produced monographs on virtually all subjects. A challenge to our authors has been the need to transmit the essential information without unduly enlarging the textbook.

We have retained the general organization of previous editions, including arbitrary decisions about the placement of some subjects. Does the discussion of seizures or multiple sclerosis in pregnancy belong in chapters on pregnancy, epilepsy, or multiple sclerosis? Is the Lambert-Eaton syndrome best described in a chapter on neuromuscular disorders, or one on paraneoplastic syndromes? We have opted for redundancy on these issues. It makes the book a bit longer than it might be otherwise, but the reader does not have to keep flipping pages to find the information.

The impact of molecular genetics has left other marks. Do we continue to organize the book by clinical syndromes and diseases or do we group by the nature of the mutation? "Channelopathies" or "neuromuscular disease" for Lambert-Eaton disease? "Channelopathy" for familial hemiplegic migraine or a form of headache? "Nondystrophic myotonia" or periodic paralysis for the hyperkalemic type? Triplet repeat or ataxia or spinobulbar muscular atrophy? We have opted for the clinical classification while recognizing that we are on the verge of understanding the pathogenesis of these increasingly scrutable diseases.

Another uncertainty involves eponyms: use apostrophe or not? There is no consensus in medical publishing because not everyone recognizes there is a problem. English-language neurology journals and the influential *New England Journal of Medicine* have not changed, but journals devoted to genetics or radiology have dropped the apostrophe and so have the AMA journals. The Council of Biology Editors has taken a strong stand against the use of the possessive form.

It is not only the possessive inference that is objectionable. The legendary humorist A. J. Liebling once wrote: "I had Bright's disease and he had mine." In other usage, the nominal adjective is not the possessive; no one objects to Madison Avenue, Harvard University, Nobel Prize, or

Kennedy Center. And there are other challenges, including the grating sibilance of "Duchenne's dystrophy," and the inconsistency of people who use that term, sometimes with the apostrophe and sometimes without. In the neuromuscular community, "Duchenne dystrophy" is surely preferred. And consider our hapless heroes whose names end in an "s": Graves, Kufs, Gowers, Menkes and others become incorrectly singular when the apostrophe is inserted (creating the nonexistent "Kuf's disease"). If the possessive is added at the end, something sounds wrong in "Graves's disease."

We have therefore followed the general rules of Victor McKusick in dealing with eponyms, giving general preference to the nonpossessive form without being totally rigid about it. Often, an inserted "the" can smoothly precede the eponym, especially in hyphenated compounds such as "the Guillain-Barré syndrome." Nevertheless, as McKusick states: "some nonpossessive terms, because of long usage in the possessive, roll off the tongue awkwardly—e.g., the Huntington disease, the Wilson disease, the Hodgkin disease, etc." I myself have a hard time saying "Bell palsy." But Huntington disease, Alzheimer disease, Parkinson disease, and Hodgkin disease are heard with increasing frequency, even without a preceding "the." Once the nonpossessive form is used in conversation, it is more likely to sound natural.

In another tribute to the tremendous impact of Victor McKusick, we have retained the practice of giving his catalog numbers for genetic diseases. Readers can then find the history of the syndrome and current research data in the catalog, which is now online. In this day of gender-neutral writing, it is awkward to use the acronym MIM for *Mendelian Inheritance in Man*. It seems too late to change that historic title, but "Human Mendelian Inheritance" would be euphonic.

On the other hand, the stiff-man syndrome remains a problem. Papers entitled "stiff-man syndrome in a woman" or "in a boy" ought to be fixed and "stiff-person syndrome" is just plain awkward. My personal attempts to use the eponym, "Moersch-Woltman syndrome" have had zero success, partly because the names do not trip lightly off the lip, and reversing the order is no better.

We thank all the authors for their devoted and skillful work. In the editor's office, Hope Poulos has kept her head when I was losing mine, and she remained patient when I misplaced files. She has been remarkably patient in tracking correspondence. At Lippincott Williams & Wilkins, Joyce Murphy was patient with the dribbling appearance of chapters as e-mail attachments so that she could skillfully supervise editing. Production was supervised most skillfully by Stephanie Lentz at Techbooks.

We formally dedicate the book to H. Houston Merritt. I personally dedicate it also to all the spouses and children of all the contributors, especially to Esther E. Rowland; our children, Andrew, Steven, and Joy; and our grandchildren, Mikaela, Liam, Cameron Henry, Mariel, and Zuri. All of them, Rowlands and others, have suffered neglect because of the contributors' clinical research and writing assignments that provide the substance and content of this book.

REFERENCES

American Medical Association. *Manual of Style. A guide for authors and editors*, 9th ed. Chicago: American Medical Association, 1998:469–472.

McKusick VA. *Mendelian Inheritance in Man. A catalog of human genes and genetic disorders*. 12th ed. Baltimore, Johns Hopkins University Press, 1998.

McKusick VA. On the naming of clinical disorders, with particular reference to eponyms. *Medicine* 1998;77:1–2.

AIDS	Acquired immunodeficiency syndrome	**HIV**	Human immunodeficiency virus
C₃	A specific component of complement	**IVIG**	Intravenous immunoglobulin therapy
CBC	Complete blood count	**MELAS**	Mitochondrial encephalopathy with lactic acidosis and stroke
CNS	Central nervous system		
CSF	Cerebrospinal fluid	**MRA**	Magnetic resonance angiography
CT	Computed tomography	**MRI**	Magnetic resonance imaging
DNA	Deoxyribonucleic acid	**MS**	Multiple sclerosis
ECG	Electrocardiogram	**MTDNA**	Mitochondrial DNA
EEG	Electroenecephalography	**PET**	Positron emission tomography
EMG	Electromyography	**RNA**	Ribonucleic acid
ESR	Erythrocyte sedimentation rate	**SPECT**	Single-photon emission computed tomography
GM1	A specific neural ganglioside		
BUN	Blood urea nitrogen	**TIA**	Transient ischemic attack

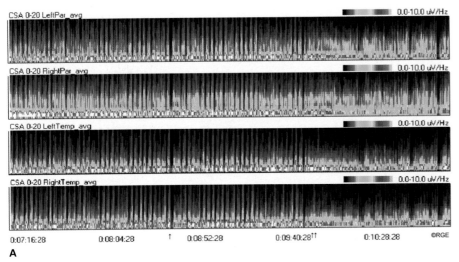

CSA 0-20 LeftPar_avg   0.0-10.0 uV/Hz

CSA 0-20 RightPar_avg   0.0-10.0 uV/Hz

CSA 0-20 LeftTemp_avg   0.0-10.0 uV/Hz

CSA 0-20 RightTemp_avg   0.0-10.0 uV/Hz

0:07:16:28   0:08:04:28   ↑   0:08:52:28   0:09:40:28††   0:10:28:28   ©RGE

A

FIGURE 14.8

B

FIGURE 149.1

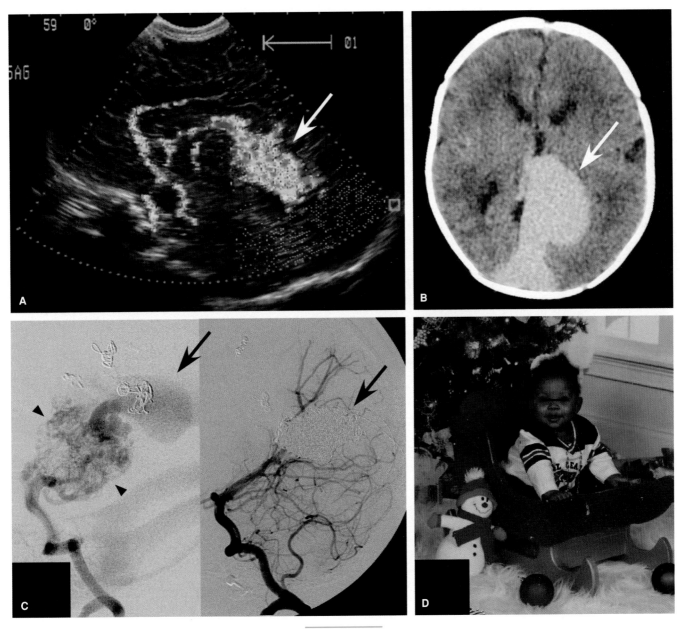

FIGURE 17.5

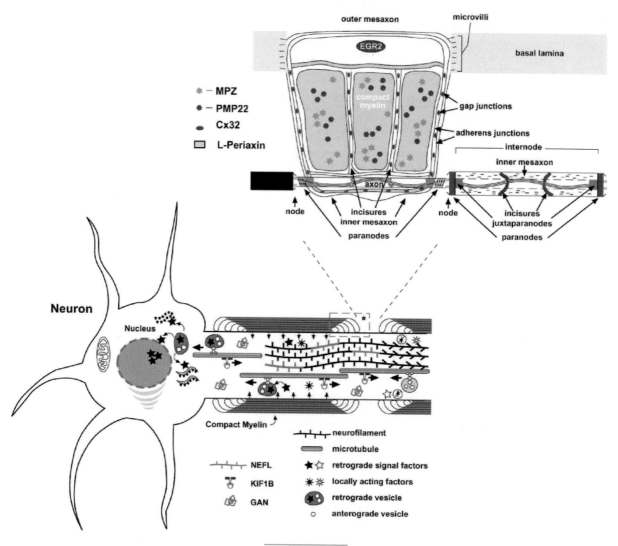

Schwann Cell

- * − MPZ
- ● − PMP22
- ◗ − Cx32
- ▢ − L-Periaxin

outer mesaxon

microvilli

basal lamina

EGR2

compact myelin

gap junctions

adherens junctions

internode

inner mesaxon

axon

node

incisures
inner mesaxon

paranodes

node

incisures
juxtaparanodes

paranodes

Neuron

Nucleus

Compact Myelin

neurofilament

microtubule

NEFL

KIF1B

GAN

★☆ retrograde signal factors

✳✴ locally acting factors

⬤ retrograde vesicle

○ anterograde vesicle

FIGURE 105.1

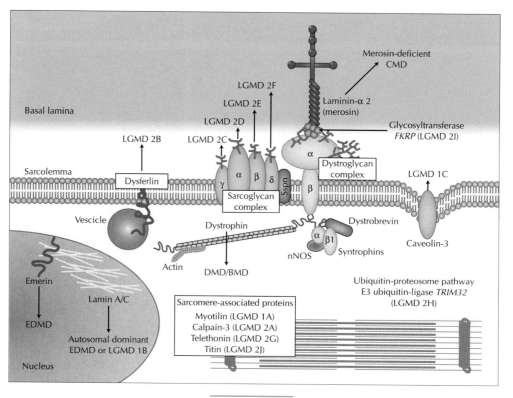

Merosin-deficient
CMD

LGMD 2F

LGMD 2E

Laminin-α 2
(merosin)

Glycosyltransferase
FKRP (LGMD 2I)

Basal lamina

LGMD 2D

LGMD 2B

LGMD 2C

α

Dystroglycan
complex

LGMD 1C

Sarcolemma

Dysferlin

γ α β δ

Sspn

β

Sarcoglycan
complex

Vescicle

Dystrophin

Dystrobrevin

Caveolin-3

α

β1

Actin

nNOS

Syntrophins

DMD/BMD

Emerin

Lamin A/C

EDMD

Autosomal dominant
EDMD or LGMD 1B

Nucleus

Ubiquitin-proteosome pathway
E3 ubiquitin-ligase *TRIM32*
(LGMD 2H)

Sarcomere-associated proteins
Myotilin (LGMD 1A)
Calpain-3 (LGMD 2A)
Telethonin (LGMD 2G)
Titin (LGMD 2J)

FIGURE 126.1

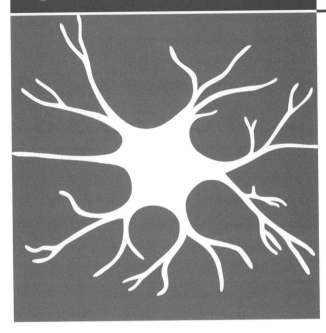

Symptoms of Neurologic Disorders

Delirium and Dementia

Scott A. Small and Richard Mayeux

Delirium and dementia are frequently encountered disorders in patients at any age, but they are most often found in the elderly. *Delirium* is a state of mental confusion that may be accompanied by fluctuations in consciousness, anxiety, hallucinations, illusions, and delusions. It may accompany infections, metabolic disorders, and other medical or neurologic diseases or may be related to substance use or withdrawal. *Dementia,* in contrast, is a condition in which memory and other cognitive functions are impaired to the extent that they interfere with normal social or occupational activities, in the absence of confusion or altered consciousness. Most often dementia is the result of a degenerative brain disease but stroke and infections may also cause dementia.

DELIRIUM

Hippocrates first described the features of delirium. Principal criteria for the diagnosis of delirium include a disturbance in consciousness and a change in cognitive function occurring over a short period of time, such as a few hours or a day. Associated features include: disruption of the sleep-wake cycle, drowsiness, restlessness, incoherence, irritability, emotional lability, perceptual misinterpretations (illusions), and hallucinations.

Manifestations of delirium often worsen at night. Rapid onset of impairment in memory and language, and disorientation not previously observed are indicative of delirium. Other characteristics include the presence of a medical or neurologic condition to which mental impairment is secondary and the disappearance of mental impairment if the primary medical or neurologic disorder is reversed.

Delirium may result from a number of general medical and neurologic conditions. Almost any severe acute medical or surgical condition, under the right circumstances, may cause delirium. Common causes may be divided into the categories of primary brain disorders and systemic illness. Primary brain disorders include head injury, stroke, raised intracranial pressure, infection, and epilepsy. Systemic illnesses may be infectious, cardiovascular, and endocrine. Substance intoxication including alcohol and drug abuse as well as withdrawal from such substances may lead to delirium.

Hospitalized individuals are at highest risk for delirium, which occurs in 10% to 20% of inpatients. The risk is higher for the older patient who stays in the hospital for a long time. Thus, predisposing factors include advanced age, the presence of dementia, and impaired physical or mental health. Elderly patients undergoing cardiovascular or orthopedic surgical procedures and those patients in intensive care or cancer treatment units have the highest incidence of delirium. Patients with limited hearing and vision deprived of hearing aids or glasses for prolonged periods are also at risk for delirium.

The following frequently used medications have been known to cause delirium:

Atropine and related anticholinergic compounds
Antipsychotics
Barbiturates
Benzodiazepines
Bromides
Chlordiazepoxide (Librium)
Chloral hydrate
Cimetidine and related compounds
Clonidine
Codeine
Cocaine
Digitalis
Dopamine agonists
Ethanol
Furosemide
Glutethimide (Doriden)
Haloperidol and other atypical neuroleptics
Lithium
Levodopa
Meprobamate
Mephenytoin
Methyldopa
Nifedipine

Opioids
Narcotics
Phencyclidine hydrochloride (PCP)
Phenytoin
Prednisone
Propranolol
Ranitidine
Theophylline
Tricyclic antidepressants

In elderly patients, anticholinergic and hypnotic agents are particularly common causes of drug-induced delirium.

Management of Delirium

Delirium is a medical emergency and prompt review of the precipitating factors is crucial because the disease or drug intoxication may be fatal if untreated. Four key steps in the management of delirium include: 1) identifying the cause, 2) controlling the behavior, 3) preventing complications, and 4) supporting functional needs. The occurrence of delirium may double the risk of death within hours or weeks. Successful treatment of delirium eliminates much of this increased mortality risk. The two best predictors of fatal outcome are advanced age and the presence of multiple physical diseases.

Diagnostic Evaluation for Delirium

The diagnostic evaluation is dictated by findings during the medical history and physical examination. First-line investigations include electrolytes, CBC, liver and thyroid function tests, ESR, toxicology screen, syphilis serology, blood cultures, urine culture, chest xray, and ECG. If the cause cannot be determined from these tests, additional investigations to consider include neuroimaging, CSF analysis, EEG, HIV antibody titer, cardiac enzymes, blood gases, and autoantibody screen.

The fluctuating state of awareness in delirium is accompanied by characteristic EEG changes. The varying levels of attention parallel the slowing of background EEG rhythms. Triphasic waves may be present as well. Appropriate treatment of the underlying disease improves both the mental state and the EEG of the patient.

The management of delirium may require symptomatic treatment of behavior associated with the delirium. Antipsychotic drugs are the most effective for behavior control in patients who are not experiencing withdrawal from alcohol or other substances. Haloperidol and atypical antipsychotics such as risperidone have been used with some success. Benzodiazepines remain the treatment of choice for delirium related to withdrawal from alcohol and drugs.

DEMENTIA

Dementia is characterized by progressive intellectual deterioration that interferes with daily social or occupational functions. Memory, orientation, abstraction, ability to learn, visuospatial perception, language function, constructional praxis, and higher executive functions such as planning, organizing, and sequencing activities, are all impaired in dementia. In contrast to patients with delirium, people with dementia are usually alert and aware until later in the course of the disease. While delirium is most often associated with intercurrent systemic diseases or drug intoxication, dementia is usually due to a primary degenerative or structural disease of the brain.

Alzheimer disease (see Part XIII, Dementias) is the most frequent form of dementia, accounting for over 50% of the total number of cases in both clinical and autopsy series (Table 1.1).

Cerebrovascular disease may also be a cause of dementia as well as a contributing risk factor. Vascular dementia may be defined as a clinical syndrome of acquired intellectual impairment resulting from brain injury, due to ischemic or hemorrhagic cerebrovascular disease or to hypoperfusion of brain structures. Of all cases of dementia, 15% to 20% are attributed to vascular disease. The diagnosis of vascular dementia is based on the presence of cognitive loss and cerebrovascular lesions demonstrated by brain imaging. Dementia may also occur in association with large-vessel disease with multiple strokes (multi-infarct dementia) or with a single stroke ("strategic stroke"), which may also occur in patients with Alzheimer disease. An essential requirement for the differentiation of vascular dementia is that the dementia and cerebrovascular disorder are temporally linked. Parkinsonism (see Chap. 115, Parkinsonism) is also frequently associated with dementia and some consider dementia with Lewy bodies (DLB) disease the second most frequent cause of dementia (see Chap. 107). Huntington disease (see Chap. 109, Huntington Disease) is much less common, but is still an important cause of dementia in the presenium. Less common degenerative diseases include the frontotemporal dementias (see Chap. 107), progressive supranuclear palsy (see Chap. 116, Progressive Supranuclear Palsy), and the hereditary ataxias (see Chap. 108).

Intracranial mass lesions, including brain tumors and subdural hematomas, cause dementia without focal neurologic signs in as many as 5% of the cases of dementia in some series. With the use of brain imaging, these patients are rapidly identified and treated.

The frequency of chronic communicating hydrocephalus (normal pressure hydrocephalus) as a cause of dementia in adults varies from 1% to 5% in different series. Diagnosis is usually straightforward when the hydrocephalus follows intracranial hemorrhage, head injury, or meningitis, but in idiopathic cases it is often difficult to

▶ TABLE 1.1 Diseases that Cause Dementia

	Number of Subjects	Clinical Series [a]	Autopsy Series [b]	Washington Heights Community Series [c]
Depressed; psychotic; no dementia	—	42	—	522
Patients with dementia	—	474	1000	514
Degenerative				
Alzheimer disease	267	56.3%	50.3%	54.6%
Vascular; multiinfarct	40	8.4	22.3	7.0
Mixed (Alzheimer with vascular/multiinfarct)	23	4.9	13.4	17.1
Other degenerative				
Huntington disease	26	5.5	—	0
Parkinson disease	7	1.5	1.0	5.6
Progressive supranuclear palsy	6	1.2	—	0.2
Amyotrophic lateral sclerosis with dementia	3	0.6	—	0
Progressive hemiatrophy	2	0.4	—	0
Pick disease	1	0.2	2.1	0
Olivopontocerebellar atrophy	—	—	0.5	0
Epilepsy	1	0.2	—	0
Metabolic; toxic; nutritional; alcoholism; Wernicke-Korsakoff	17	3.6	1.1	8.8
Drug toxicity	8	1.7	—	0
Metabolic				
(thyroid; B12; hepatic; hypercalcemia)	8	1.7	—	0
Infectious				
Creutzfeldt-Jakob disease	3	0.6	0.9	0
Acquired immunodeficiency syndrome	24	5.1	—	0
Other infections or inflammatory neurosyphilis; multiple sclerosis; encephalitis	2	0.4	1.3	0
Vasculitis	3	0.6	—	0
Hydrocephalus	8	3.8	1.1	0
Intracranial tumors	12	2.5	4.5	0
Posttraumatic; subdural	3	0.6	1.5	0
Cause undetermined	—	—	—	6.7

PA, pernicious anemia.
[a] Combined series. Data from Wells, 1977; Katzman R, personal series.
[b] Data from Jellinger, 1976.
[c] Data from Mayeux R, personal New York City community series, the Washington Heights-Inwood Community Aging Project, 1993.

differentiate communicating hydrocephalus from ventricular enlargement due to brain atrophy.

HIV-associated dementia is now among the most common of the infectious causes and is among the most common causes of dementia in young adults. Creutzfeldt-Jakob disease and other prion-related dementias are additional transmissible causes of dementia. Nonviral infections rarely present as chronic rather than acute encephalopathy. Fungal meningitis may occasionally present as dementia.

Nutritional, toxic, and metabolic causes of dementia remain important but are rare because they may be reversible. Vitamin B$_{12}$ deficiency occasionally causes dementia and may be seen without anemia or spinal cord disease. Among the metabolic disorders that may present as dementia, hypothyroidism is the most important. Inherited metabolic disorders that may lead to dementia in adults include Wilson disease, the adult form of ceroid lipo-fuscinosis (Kufs disease), cerebrotendinous xanthomatosis, metachromatic leukodystrophies, and mitochondrial disorders. Finally, prolonged administration of drugs or heavy-metal exposure may cause chronic intoxication due to the patient's inability to metabolize the drug or to idiosyncratic reactions and may be mistaken for dementia.

Differential Diagnosis

The first symptoms of dementia include occasional forgetfulness, misplacing objects, and word-finding difficulties. With aging a decline in memory is observed, and the making the distinction between cognitive decline in old age and early dementia may be difficult. Attempts have been made to better define cognitive changes associated with aging, and varying sets of criteria have produced multiple terms, including age-associated memory impairment (AAMI), age-related cognitive change (ARCD) and mild cognitive impairment (MCI). MCI is used as a clinical term to describe the transition between normal aging and Alzheimer disease or another dementia. Published criteria for MCI include the absence of dementia and complaints of memory impairment with general cognitive function and activities of daily living preserved. Follow-up examinations of individuals with MCI indicate that some, but not all, develop dementia over time. Therefore, it is likely that demonstrable changes in cognitive function are not an inevitable occurrence with age, and that early dementing illnesses are contributing causes. Although other, non-dementing etiologies may also cause cognitive decline, identifying different causes remains difficult.

The diagnosis in a patient with dementia and depression may sometimes be difficult. Depression may be an early manifestation of Alzheimer disease. In depression, memory loss typically declines as the mood worsens. The onset of the memory problems may be more abrupt than usually occurs in dementia and is often mild, tending to plateau. Neuropsychologic test results may be atypical for dementia.

The differential diagnosis of dementia requires an accurate history and neurologic and physical examination. The history of a typical patient with Alzheimer disease is one of an insidious onset and a slowly progressive but relentless course of decline in an otherwise healthy individual. The history of a patient with vascular dementia may include an abrupt onset of the disease, a history of an obvious stroke, or the presence of hypertension or cardiac disease. A history of alcoholism should raise suspicion of Korsakoff psychosis.

Examination of the patient with Alzheimer disease usually yields normal results except for the presence of extrapyramidal signs, such as rigidity, bradykinesia, change in posture, and primitive reflexes, such as the snout reflex. The vascular dementia patient, on the other hand, may have evidence of hemiparesis or other focal neurologic signs. Huntington disease is readily recognized by the chorea and dysarthria. Patients with Parkinson disease characteristically develop extrapyramidal signs. Symptoms and signs associated with the onset of dementia in Parkinson disease include depression, advanced age, and severe motor manifestations. Progressive supranuclear palsy is recognized by the limitation of vertical eye movements and extrapyramidal signs. Myoclonus occurs most often in Creutzfeldt-Jakob disease, but may be seen in the advanced stages of Alzheimer disease and other dementias. Unsteadiness of gait is a hallmark of communicating hydrocephalus, but is even more severe in Creutzfeldt-Jakob disease, in the hereditary ataxias, and sometimes in Korsakoff psychosis.

Neuropsychologic testing is an effective way to confirm the presence of dementia. Age, education, socioeconomic background, and premorbid abilities are usually considered in the interpretation of the test scores. Neuropsychologic testing is particularly helpful in differentiating dementia from age-related losses and depression. Such testing may also provide clues to the etiology of dementia. For example, Alzheimer disease most often affects memory performance, while cerebrovascular disease may impair executive functions, such as tasks that require timed decision-making.

Diagnostic tests to differentiate Alzheimer disease from other dementias have been developed, but lack sufficient accuracy to warrant their routine use. The pathologic constituents of amyloid-beta protein and tau protein have been measured in cerebrospinal fluid, and may help to identify patients with Alzheimer disease. Typically, amyloid beta protein declines as tau increases in the cerebrospinal fluid. While these tests definitely represent an advance over prior methods, none has yet been demonstrated to improve accuracy over the use of the NINCDS-ADRDA clinical criteria. Though several genes have been associated with certain forms of familial disease and a single gene with sporadic Alzheimer disease, screening for mutated gene variants, as a diagnostic test, is not recommended. The NINCDS-ADRDA are the standard clinical criteria for the diagnosis of Alzheimer disease and may be reasonably accurate and reliable indicators.

CT and MRI are important in order to identify tumor or stroke as possible causes of dementia. Atrophy, stroke, brain tumor, subdural hematoma, and hydrocephalus are readily diagnosed by current methods of neuroimaging. Changes in white matter intensity must be interpreted with caution. Intensity changes may be due to small vessel ischemic disease, normal aging, or dilated Virchow-Robin spaces from generalized atrophy in Alzheimer disease. Functional brain imaging with SPECT may also be helpful. Bilateral temporoparietal hypoperfusion, an indication of metabolic deficits, is suggestive of Alzheimer disease or idiopathic Parkinson disease with dementia. Bilateral frontal hypometabolism suggests frontotemporal dementia, progressive supranuclear palsy, or depression. Multiple hypometabolic zones throughout the brain suggest vascular dementia or HIV-associated dementia. Functional magnetic resonance imaging (fMRI) is a relatively new functional imaging modality but has not yet been perfected for diagnostic purposes. Also, the EEG is useful in identifying and differentiating Creutzfeldt-Jakob disease, which is characterized by periodic discharges as well as generalized slowing.

Blood tests are essential for diagnosis of dementia associated with endocrine disease and liver or kidney failure. It is also important to obtain thyroid function studies because hypothyroidism is a reversible cause of dementia. Vitamin B_{12} deficiency may be detected, even in patients who are not anemic, by determining serum vitamin B_{12} levels. Although neurosyphilis is rare today, it too is a reversible cause of dementia; a serologic test for syphilis is mandatory. Measurements of blood levels of drugs may detect intoxication. The ESR and screens for connective tissue disease (such as antinuclear antibodies and rheumatoid factor) should be performed if the clinical picture suggests evidence of vasculitis or arthritis. In any young adults with dementia, an HIV titer should be considered, and if an associated movement disorder is present, a test for ceruloplasmin should be performed.

Details of the differential diagnosis of diseases that cause dementia are provided in subsequent chapters. It is important to emphasize that an exhaustive evaluation of patients with dementia is warranted. Although effective treatment for the primary degenerative diseases is limited, many other disorders that cause dementia are amenable to treatment that may arrest, if not reverse, the cognitive decline.

MENTAL STATUS EXAMINATION

The mental status evaluation is an essential part of every neurologic examination. It includes evaluation of awareness and consciousness, behavior, emotional state, content and stream of thought, and sensory and intellectual capabilities. Intellectual impairment is obvious in such florid conditions as delirium tremens or advanced dementia, but a cognitive deficit may not be evident in early cases of delirium or dementia unless the physician specifically tests mental status.

Traditionally, mental status examinations test information (e.g., Where were you born? What is your mother's name? Who is the President? When did World War II occur?); orientation (e.g., What place is this? What is the date? What time of day is this?); concentration (tested by using serial reversals, e.g., Spell "world" backwards. Name the months of the year backwards, beginning with December.); calculation (e.g., doing simple arithmetic, making change, counting backwards by 3s or 7s); and reasoning, judgment, and memory (e.g., Identify these three objects, please try to remember their names. Please repeat a short story after me and try to remember it for a few minutes.).

The most important and sensitive items are probably orientation to time, serial reversals, and a memory phrase. The mini-mental status exam (MMSE) was introduced as a standard measure of cognitive function to be used for both research and clinical purposes. It is short, around 10 minutes, and relatively easy to administer even at the bedside. The scoring scheme is shown in Table 1.2, and the maximum score is 30 points. A score of less than 24 is considered consistent with dementia.

It is important to emphasize that the MMSE, like all brief mental status exams, is not precise. Some investigators use a score of 26 as a cutoff to include more mild forms of dementia and to improve specificity. The MMSE tends to underdiagnose dementia in the well-educated patient and to overdiagnose dementia in the poorly educated patient. Therefore, the MMSE should be used only as a first step, and should not replace a history or a more detailed examination of neuropsychologic function (see Chap. 20).

In addition to testing the mental status, it is necessary to test higher intellectual functions, including disorders

▶ **TABLE 1.2 Mini-mental Status Examination**

Cognitive Domain	Specific Questions	Scoring
Orientation	1. What is the (year) (day) (month) (date) (season)?	1. 1 point for each correct response (maximum 5 points)
	2. What is the (name of this place) (address) (floor) (city) (state)?	2. 1 point for each correct response (maximum 5 points)
Registration	Name three objects (Take 1 second to say each; then ask the patient to name all three after you have said them; then repeat them until all three are learned)	3 points if all three objects are repeated on first trial; deduct 1 point for each repetition required
Attention/calculation	Serial sevens, or spelling "word" backwards	1 point for each correct response (maximum 5 points)
Recall	Ask for the three objects repeated for registration	1 point for each correct response (maximum 3 points)
Language	1. Ask patient to name a pencil and a watch	1. 1 point for each correct response (maximum 2 points)
	2. Ask patient to repeat the following: "no ifs, ands, or buts"	2. 1 point for correct response
	3. Ask patient to "take a paper in your right hand, fold it in half, and put it on the floor"	3. 1 point for each correct response (maximum 3 points)
	4. Ask patient to read and obey the following: "close your eyes"	4. 1 point for correct response
Visuospatial	5. Ask patient to write a sentence	5. 1 point for correct response
	Copy a design	1 point for correct response

Modified from Folstein et al., 1975.

of language (dysphasias); constructional apraxia; and right-to-left disorientation; as well as testing the inability to carry out complex commands, especially those requiring crossing the midline (e.g., Touch your left ear with your right thumb.); inability to carry out imagined acts (ideomotor apraxia, e.g., Pretend that you have a book of matches and show me how you would light a match.); unilateral neglect; or inattention on double stimulation. These abnormalities are more often associated with focal brain lesions, but may also be impaired in delirium or dementia. Examination of aphasia, apraxia, and agnosia is described in detail in Chapter 2.

SUGGESTED READINGS

Burns A, Gallagley A, Byrne J. Delirium. *J Neurol Neurosurg Psychiatry.* 2004;75:362–367.

Casserly I, Topol E. Convergence of atherosclerosis and Alzheimer's disease: inflammation, cholesterol, and misfolded proteins. *Lancet.* 2004;363:1139–1146.

Clark CM, Xie S, Chittams J, Ewbank D, et al. Cerebrospinal fluid tau and beta-amyloid: how well do these biomarkers reflect autopsy-confirmed dementia diagnoses? *Arch Neurol.* 2003;60:1696–1702.

DeCarli C. Mild cognitive impairment: prevalence, prognosis, etiology and treatment. *Lancet Neurol.* 2003;2:15–21.

Devanand DP, Sano M, Tang M, et al. Depressed mood and the incidence of Alzheimer's Disease in the elderly living in the community. *Arch Gen Psych.* 1996;53:175–182.

American Psychiatric Association. *Diagnostic and Statistical Manual of Mental Disorders. DSM-IV TR,* 4th ed. Washington, DC: American Psychiatric Association; 2000.

Fick DM, Agostini JV, Inouye SK. Delirium superimposed on dementia: a systematic review. *J Am Geriatr Soc.* 2002;50:1723–1732.

Folstein MF, Folstein S, McHugh P. "Mini-mental state": a practical method for grading the cognitive state of patients for the clinician. *J Psychiatr Res.* 1975;12:189–198.

Katzman R, Brown T, Fuld P, et al. Validation of a short orientation-memory-concentration test of cognitive impairment. *Am J Psychiatry.* 1983;140:734–739.

Lee HB, Lyketsos CG. Depression in Alzheimer's disease: heterogeneity and related issues. *Biol Psychiatry.* 2003;54:353–362.

McKeith I, Mintzer J, Aarsland D, et al. Dementia with Lewy bodies. *Lancet Neurol.* 2004;3:19–28.

McKhann G, Drachman D, Folstein M, et al. Clinical diagnosis of Alzheimer's disease: report of the NINCDS-ADRDA Work Groups under the auspices of Department of Health and Human Services Task Force on Alzheimer's Disease. *Neurology.* 1984;34:939–944.

Panza F, D'Introno A, Colacicco AM, et al. Vascular risk and genetics of sporadic late-onset Alzheimer's disease. *J Neural Transm.* 2004;111:69–89.

Roman GC. Vascular dementia: distinguishing characteristics, treatment and prevention. *J Am Geriatr Soc.* 2003;51:296–304.

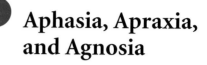

Aphasia, Apraxia, and Agnosia

J. P. Mohr

APHASIA

Judging from the clinical effects of an injury to the cerebrum on one side, over 95% of all people may be said to have left-hemisphere dominance for speech and language. This is true even in persons taken to be left-handed; in them, some disturbance in speech and language may occur from injury to either cerebral hemisphere. The most predictable sites for disturbances in speech and language are the regions in and bordering on the sylvian fissure. The farther away from this zone a brain injury occurs, the less likely is disturbance in speech and language. The clinical syndromes resulting from these lesions form a group of disorders known as the *aphasias.*

The long-standing, still popular classifications of aphasia are based on classic and now somewhat outmoded views that the front half of the brain performs motor or executive functions and the back half sensory or receptive functions, with the two regions connected by pathways in the white matter. Classically, frontal lesions have been inferred to cause *motor aphasia,* those affecting the posterior regions cause *sensory aphasia,* and those interrupting the pathways between the frontal and posterior regions cause *conduction aphasia.* This formulation posits an anatomic, functional loop. This loop includes an afferent portion from the eyes and ears connecting to the visual and auditory system, an intrahemispheral portion through the white matter connecting the temporal with the frontal lobes (the arcuate fasciculus), and an efferent portion from the frontal lobes to the mouth and hand permitting words heard to be repeated aloud and words seen to be copied manually.

Apart from the crude replication of sounds heard and shapes seen that even those ignorant of the language conveyed by the sounds or forms are capable of reproducing, meaning is thought to be assigned to these shapes and sounds by access of the perisylvian region to the rest of the brain through a broad range of intrahemispheral and transcallosal pathways. Interruption of these inferred linkage pathways outward from the auditory sensory regions around the Heschl transverse gyri is postulated to produce *transcortical sensory aphasia,* in which words heard are repeated aloud or copied without comprehension. Likewise, interruption of the inferred inward-directed pathways to the inferior frontal region for vocalizations would cause *transcortical motor aphasia,* in which words may be repeated and copied but no spontaneous communication by conversation or writing occurs. Other "disconnections" have also been proposed for pathways to or from the periphery, which presumably would be in the subcortical white matter. Disconnections of incoming pathways bearing visual lexical information yield *pure alexia;* those of pathways conveying auditory material cause *pure word deafness.* The combination of these two disconnections causes *subcortical sensory aphasia.* Disconnections of efferent pathways from the motor speech zones produce *pure word mutism* or *subcortical motor aphasia.*

Although these generalizations have held sway for almost 150 years, uncritical acceptance of the expected clinical effects of certain lesion locations or predictions of lesion locations by the clinical features have proved misleading for clinicians attempting to infer the site, size, and presumed cause of a brain lesion in a patient with acute impairment indicative of a clinical disorder of speech and language. Hoping to mitigate this problem, the author presents the material that follows to emphasize the clinical features that aid in local lesion diagnosis, with less reliance on the classical concepts.

Stroke is the most common cause of acute lesions. The arrangement of the individual branches of the upper division of the sylvian artery favors the wide variety of focal embolic obstructions that produce this remarkable array of syndromes. The more specific the speech abnormality is, the more limited the focal infarction. Because the sensorimotor cortex is part of the same arterial supply of the upper division of the middle cerebral artery, the larger infarcts and other disorders, such as basal ganglia hemorrhages, abscesses, large tumors, and acute encephalitis, usually cause accompanying contralateral hemiparesis and hemisensory syndromes, making the identification of perisylvian disease a fairly easy process. One disorder, known as *primary progressive aphasia,* appears to be an unusual form of atrophy, primarily causing a relentless decline in speech and language function without the accompanying motor, sensory, or visual impairment, or other clinical evidence of a large lesion affecting the main pathways serving these functions.

Clinical Features of the Motor Aphasias

For speech and language, the smaller and more superficial that the injury is, the briefer and less severe is the disruption. Rapid improvement occurs even when the lesion involves sites classically considered to cause permanent speech and language disturbances, such as with the foot of the third frontal gyrus (Broca area). The larger the

acute lesion, the more evident the dysphasia and the longer the delay before speech improves. In larger sylvian lesions, dysphasia is evident in disordered grammar, especially when tests involve single letters, spelling, and subtleties of syntax. Problems with syntax occur not only in speaking and writing but also in attempts to comprehend words heard or seen. For example, the word "ear" is responded to more reliably than is "are," "cat" more than "act," and "eye" more than "I." The language content of spontaneously uttered sentences is condensed, missing many of the filler words, causing *telegraphic speech,* or *agrammatism.* Agrammatism is an important sign of a major lesion of the operculum and insula.

When the causative lesion involves many gyri, as with large infarcts, hemorrhages, and neoplasms or abscesses large enough to produce unilateral weakness, the reduction of both speech and comprehension is profound and is called *total aphasia.* Within weeks or months in cases of infarction and hemorrhage, comprehension improves, especially with nongrammatic forms, and speaking and writing seem to be affected more than listening and reading. This last syndrome, in which dysphasia is most evident in speaking and writing, is known as *motor aphasia;* the eponym *Broca aphasia* is often used. This syndrome emerges from an initial total aphasia, as a late residual. It is not the more commonly seen acute syndrome of a circumscribed infarction, even when the lesion is confined to the pars opercularis of the inferior frontal gyrus (Broca area).

Any acute focal lesion roughly a gyrus in size, involving any portion of the insula or the individual gyrus forming the upper banks of the opercular cortex (from the anteroinferior frontal region to the anterior parietal), acutely disrupts the acquired skills involving the oropharyngeal, laryngeal, and respiratory systems that mediate speech, causing mutism at worse, and at best, effortful speaking with numerous hesitancies in uttered syllables. Writing may be preserved, although it is usually confined to a few simple words. Comprehension of words heard or seen is generally intact because these functions are largely subserved by posterior regions, provided the tests undertaken are not unusually complex (e.g., passive voice, double negatives). The speech that emerges from mutism within minutes, hours, or days of the onset of motor aphasia consists mostly of crude vowels (*dysphonia*) and poorly articulated consonants (*dysarthria*). Disturbed coordination (*dyspraxia*) of speaking and breathing alters the rhythm of speech (*dysprosody*). This faulty intonation, stress, and phrasing of words and sentences is known collectively as *speech dyspraxia.* The language conveyed through this speech is usually only slightly disturbed, but the grammatic forms used in speaking or writing are sometimes simplified.

The more anterior the lesion along the operculum, the more speech dyspraxia predominates, especially with involvement of the inferior frontal region (Broca area) located adjacent to the sensorimotor cortex. When the sensorimotor cortex itself is affected, dysarthria and dysphonia are more prominent than dysprosody and dyspraxia. The errors in pronunciation may make it impossible to understand the language being used by the patient, but strictly speaking the deficiencies are not a language disorder. Only rarely does this syndrome persist, and a large number of these patients seem normal months later, the acute syndrome all but forgotten despite the lesion found on later brain imaging.

When an acute lesion occurs more posteriorly along the sylvian operculum, the precise sensorimotor control over the positioning of the oropharynx may be impaired, causing unusual mispronunciations as well as mild dysphasia. The disturbed pronunciation is not simple dysarthria. Instead, the faulty oropharyngeal positionings yield sounds that differ from those intended (e.g., "dip" is said instead of "top"). The errors, analogous to the typing errors of a novice unfamiliar with the typewriter keyboard, are called *literal paraphasias*. The listener may mistake the utterances as language errors (*paraphasias*) or may be impressed with some of the genuine paraphasias and give the condition the name *conduction aphasia* (see the following). The patient's comprehension is usually intact despite the disordered pronunciation. The focus of the lesion may lie in the posterior insula, inferior parietal region, or even in the posterior superior temporal plane, the region inferred by former generations of neurologists to cause a more severe syndrome (Wernicke aphasia—see below).

Sensory Aphasias

A different set of acute symptoms results from acute focal lesions in the posterior half of the temporal lobe and the posterior parietal and lateral occipital regions. As in the motor aphasias, infarction is usually the cause of the discrete syndromes, while hemorrhage, epilepsy, and acute encephalitis may account for sudden major syndromes. Even large lesions in these areas are usually far removed enough from the sensorimotor cortex that hemiparesis and speech disturbances (e.g., dysprosody, dysarthria, or mutism) are only occasionally part of the clinical picture.

In many patients with large posterior lesions, the acute effects (lasting hours or days) may mimic those of large frontal lesions with mutism. For patients who may vocalize from the outset, the elements of the speech are almost the reverse of the insular-opercular syndromes: syntax is better preserved than semantics; speech is filled with small grammatic words, but the predicative words (i.e., words that contain the essence of the message) are omitted or distorted. Patients vocalize easily, engage in simple conversational exchanges, and even appear to be making an effort to communicate; however, little coordinated meaning is conveyed in the partial phrases, disjointed clauses, and incomplete sentences. In the most severe form, speech is incomprehensible gibberish. Errors take the form of words that fail to occur (*omissions*), are mispronounced as similar-sounding words (*literal paraphasias*), or are replaced by others that have a similar meaning (*verbal paraphasias*). A similar disturbance affects understanding words heard or seen. These language disturbances may require prolonged conversation to be revealed in mild cases. This disturbance in language contrasts with motor aphasia, and so is often labeled as sensory aphasia, or *Wernicke aphasia*, but neither syndrome is purely motor or sensory.

The posterior portions of the brain are more compact than the anterior portions. As a result, large infarctions or mass lesions from hemorrhage, abscess, encephalitis, or brain tumors in the posterior brain tend to cause similar clinical disorders with few variations in syndrome type. Contralateral hemianopia usually implies a deep lesion. When hemianopia persists for more than about 1 week, the aphasia is likely to persist.

Highly focal lesions are uncommon and when present, usually mean focal infarction. Lesions limited to the posterior temporal lobe usually produce only a part of the larger syndrome of sensory aphasia. Speech and language are only slightly disturbed, reading for comprehension may pass for normal, but auditory comprehension of language is grossly defective. This syndrome was classically known as *pure word deafness*. Patients with this disorder also usually reveal verbal paraphasias in spontaneous speech and disturbed silent reading comprehension. This syndrome might be better named the *auditory form of sensory aphasia*. It has a good prognosis, and useful clinical improvement occurs within weeks; some patients regain almost normal function.

A similarly restricted dysphasia may affect reading and writing to a greater degree, far more so than auditory comprehension, because of a more posteriorly placed focal lesion that damages the posterior parietal and lateral occipital regions. Testing is required to document this more complex impairment in reading and writing, which may not be readily discovered by conversational assessment. Reading comprehension and writing morphology are strikingly abnormal in these patients. This syndrome has traditionally been known as *alexia with agraphia*, but spoken language and auditory comprehension are also disturbed (although less than reading and writing). A better label might be the *visual form of sensory aphasia*. It also has a good prognosis.

The more limited auditory and visual forms of Wernicke's aphasia are rarely produced by mass lesions from any cause and tend to blend in larger lesions. Whether the major syndrome of sensory aphasia is a unified disturbance or a synergistic result of several separate disorders has not been determined.

Amnestic Aphasia

Anomia or its more limited form *dysnomia* is the term applied to errors in tests of naming. Detection of this syndrome requires special testing because naming errors are common in acutely ill patients, even in some patients with acute meningitis, and thus are of less diagnostic importance than is the type of errors made. In all major aphasic syndromes, errors in language production cause defective naming (dysnomia), taking the form of paraphasias of the literal (e.g., "flikt" for "flight") or verbal (e.g., "jump" for "flight") type. For this reason, it is not usually of diagnostic value to focus a clinical examination on dysnomias alone, because they have little value as signs of focal brain disease. However, in the pattern known as *amnestic dysnomia* patients act as though the name has been forgotten and may give functional descriptions instead. Invoking lame excuses, testimonials of prowess, claims of irrelevance, or impatience, patients seem unaware that the amnestic dysnomia is a sign of disease. The disturbance is common, to some degree in normal (healthy) individuals—especially among the elderly—but in those with disease it is prominent enough to interfere with conversation. Amnestic aphasia, when fully developed, is usually the result of disease of the deep temporal lobe gray and white matter. A frequent cause is Alzheimer disease, in which atrophy of the deep temporal lobe occurs early, and forgetfulness for names may be erroneously attributed to old age by the family. Identical symptoms may occur in the early stages of evolution of mass lesions from neoplasms or abscess but are rarely a sign of infarction in the deep temporal lobe. Other disturbances in language, such as those involving grammar, reading aloud, spelling, or writing, are usually absent at a time when the amnestic dysnomia is prominent, unless the responsible lesion encroaches on the adjacent temporal parietal or sylvian regions. When due to a mass lesion, the disturbance often evolves into the full syndrome of Wernicke aphasia. A gradual atrophy in the perisylvian regions may produce *primary progressive aphasia.*

An acute, deep lesion on the side of the dominant hemisphere may cause dysphasia if it involves the posterior thalamic nuclei that have reciprocal connections with the language zones. Large-mass lesions or slowly evolving thalamic tumors distort the whole hemisphere, producing symptoms that make it difficult to recognize the distinct components of the clinical picture. Small lesions are most often hematomas and are the usual cause of the sudden syndrome. As in delirium, consciousness fluctuates widely in this syndrome. As it fluctuates, language behavior varies from normal to spectacular usage. The syndrome may be mistaken for delirium stemming from metabolic causes (e.g., alcohol withdrawal). This is also important in the theory of language because the paraphasic errors are not due to a lesion that affects the cerebral surface, as was claimed traditionally. Prompt CT usually demonstrates the thalamic lesion.

APRAXIA

The term *apraxia* (properly known as *dyspraxia* because the disorder is rarely complete) refers to disturbances in the execution of learned movements, other than the disturbances caused by any coexisting weakness. These disorders are widely considered to be the body-movement equivalents of the dysphasias and like them, have been classified into motor, sensory, and conduction forms. Like the aphasias, these classifications are easier to conceptualize than to demonstrate in actual practice.

Limb-kinetic or Innervatory Dyspraxia

This motor form of dyspraxia occurs as part of the syndrome of paresis caused by a cerebral lesion. Attempts to use the involved limbs reveal a disturbance in movement beyond that simply accounted for by weakness. Patients appear clumsy or unfamiliar with the movements called for in such tasks as writing or using utensils because attempted movements are disorganized. Although difficult to demonstrate and easily overlooked in the presence of the more obvious weakness, innervatory dyspraxia is a useful sign to elicit because it indicates that the lesion causing the hemiparesis involves the cerebrum, presumably including the premotor region and other association systems. Dyspraxias of this type are thought to be caused by a lesion involving the cerebral surface or the immediately adjacent white matter; this type of disturbance is not seen in lesions that involve the internal capsule or lower parts of the neuraxis.

Ideational Dyspraxia

Ideational dyspraxia is a different type of disorder altogether. Movements of affected body parts appear to suffer from the absence of a basic plan, although many spontaneous actions are easily carried out. This disorder is believed to be analogous to sensory aphasia, which features a breakdown of language organization despite continued utterance of individual words. The term is apparently derived from the simplistic notion that the lesion disrupts the brain region containing the motor plans for the chain of individual movements involved in complex behaviors such as feeding, dressing, or bathing. To the observer, patients appear uncertain about what to do next and may be misdiagnosed as confused. The lesion causing ideational dyspraxia is usually in the posterior half of the dominant hemisphere. The coexisting sensory aphasia often directs diagnostic attention away from the dyspraxia, which like innervatory dyspraxia, is only rarely prominent enough to result in distinct clinical recognition. The symptoms are quite prominent in atrophic disorders such as Alzheimer disease, where it may prove difficult to separate ideational apraxia from the agnosias (see below).

Ideomotor Dyspraxia

This form of dyspraxia is frequently present, if infrequently pursued clinically. It was a primary syndrome to seek in the days before readily available brain imaging, since its presence was inferred to reflect a distinct lesion anatomy. The term derives from the notion that a lesion disrupts the connections between the regions of the brain containing ideas and that involved in the execution of movements.

The disturbance is analogous to conduction aphasia; motor behavior is intact when executed spontaneously, but faulty when attempted in response to verbal command. For movements to be executed by the nondominant hemisphere in response to dictated commands processed by the dominant hemisphere, the lesion could involve the presumed white-matter pathways through the dominant hemisphere to its motor cortex, the motor cortex itself, or the white matter connecting to the motor cortex of the nondominant hemisphere through the corpus callosum.

Ideomotor dyspraxia is a common finding when clinically sought in hemispheric lesions because so many presumed pathways are involved. The syndrome is most frequently encountered in the limbs served by the nondominant hemisphere when the lesion involves the convexity of the dominant hemisphere. Concomitant right hemiparesis and dysphasias, usually of the motor type, are often more readily apparent to the physician, so the ideomotor dyspraxia of the nondominant limbs may pass without notice. Dysphasia may make it impossible to determine whether ideomotor dyspraxia is present. When mild, dyspraxia may be demonstrated by showing that patients cannot make movements on command, although they may mimic the behavior demonstrated by the examiner and execute it spontaneously at other times. The disturbances are most apparent for movements that involve the appendages (e.g., fingers, hands) or oropharynx. Axial and trunk movements are often spared.

AGNOSIA

When patients with brain lesions respond to common environmental stimuli as if they had never encountered them previously, even though the primary neural pathways of sensation function normally, this disorder is called an agnosia. Because the disturbances seen in response to a few stimuli are assumed to apply to others with similar properties, agnosias embrace specific classes of stimuli (e.g., agnosia for colors) or more global disturbances for a form of sensation (e.g., visual or auditory agnosia).

Such sweeping categorizations are often faulty since careful examination often shows that the abnormality may be explained in some other way, including genuine unfamiliarity with the stimuli, faulty discrimination due to poor lighting, poor instructions from the examiner, or an overlooked end-organ failure (e.g., peripheral neuropathy, otosclerosis, cataracts). Faulty performance may also result from a dysphasia or dyspraxia. Errors arising from dysphasia are easily understood; dyspraxia may be more difficult to recognize. It is often unclear whether dyspraxia produces agnosia, or vice versa. Posterior parietal lesions arising from cardiac arrest, neoplasm, or infections may impair cerebral control of the precise eye movements required in the practiced exploration of a picture or other complex visual stimuli; the resulting chaotic but conjugate eye movements prevent the victim from naming or interacting properly with the stimuli. This abnormality seems to be a form of cerebral blindness (which patients may deny) and is an essential element of the *Balint syndrome* (i.e., biparietal lesions cause disordered ocular tracking, bilateral hemineglect, and difficulty deciphering complex thematic pictures). Similar disturbances in skilled manual manipulation of objects may be documented in anterior parietal lesions that interfere with the ability to name or use an object properly.

When all these variables have been taken into account, a small group of patients may remain for whom the term *agnosia* may apply. Some neurologists continue to deny that such a state exists, claiming that the functional errors presumably result from a combination of dementia and impaired primary sensory processing; others postulate anatomic disconnections due to lesions that lie between intact language areas and intact cerebral regions responsible for processing sensory input.

Two claimed clinical subtypes of visual agnosia embrace these differing theories of agnosia; *apperceptive agnosia* refers to abnormality in the discrimination process, and *associative agnosia* implies an inability to link the fully discriminated stimulus to prior experience in naming or matching the stimulus to others. Modern imaging has more accurately found the site and cause of the lesion, relieving the necessity for the time-consuming effort required to separate these two syndrome types. However, the occurrence of the two syndromes and their degree of distinction one from another bears on mechanisms of brain function and remains of keen interest to neurologists. Clinically, patients with apperceptive visual agnosia are said to fail tests of copying a stimulus or cross-matching a stimulus with others having the same properties (e.g., different views of a car), whereas patients with the associative form may not have difficulty copying and cross matching; neither type may name the stimulus, as such. Disturbances of the ability to respond to stimuli have been described for colors (*color agnosia*) and for faces (*prosopagnosia*). Although the definition of agnosia requires that a patient treat the stimuli as unfamiliar, the errors often pass almost unnoticed (e.g., dark colors are misnamed for other dark colors; names of famous people are mismatched with their pictures).

In the auditory system, a similar disturbance may occur with a normal audiogram in discrimination of sounds (cortical deafness or *auditory agnosia*), including words (*pure word deafness* or *auditory agnosia for speech*). A patient's inability to recognize familiar objects by touch while still being able to recognize them by sight is referred to as *tactile agnosia*.

In practical clinical terms, the clinical diagnosis of agnosia is justified when patients respond to familiar stimuli in an unusually unskillful manner, treat the stimuli as unfamiliar, or misname them for other stimuli having similar hue, shape, or weight. However, these patients may not show other signs of dysphasia or dyspraxia in other tests. The special testing is time consuming but may yield results diagnostic of a disorder arising from lesions of the corpus callosum, the deep white matter, or the cerebrum adjacent to the main sensory areas. The usual cause is atrophy or primary or metastatic tumor. When the disorder develops further, the more obvious defects occur in formal confrontation visual-field testing, and the "agnosia" is even more difficult to demonstrate.

SUGGESTED READINGS

Albert ML. Treatment of aphasia. *Arch Neurol.* 1998;55:1417–1419.

Alexander MP, Baker E, Naeser MA, et al. Neuropsychological and neuroanatomical dimensions of ideomotor apraxia. *Brain.* 1992;115:87–107.

Balint R. Seelenlähmung des "Schauens," optische Ataxia und räumlische Störung der Aufmerksamkeit. *Monatsschr Psychiatr Neurol.* 1909;25:51–81.

Binder JR, Mohr JP. The topography of callosal reading pathways: a case-control analysis. *Brain.* 1992;115:1807–1826.

Carlesimo GA, Casadio P, Sabbadini M, Caltagirone C. Associative visual agnosia resulting from a disconnection between intact visual memory and semantic systems. *Cortex.* 1998;34:563–576.

Geschwind N. Disconnexion syndromes in animals and man. *Brain.* 1965;88:237–294, 585–644.

Gorno-Tempini ML, Dronkers NF, Rankin KP, Ogar JM, Phengrasamy L, et al. Cognition and anatomy in three variants of primary progressive aphasia. *Ann Neurol.* 2004;55:335–346.

Karbe H, Thiel A, Weber-Luxenburger G, Herholz K, Kessler J, Heiss WD. Brain plasticity in poststroke aphasia: what is the contribution of the right hemisphere? *Brain Lang.* 1998;64:215–230.

Kertesz A, Hudson L, Mackenzie IR, Munoz DG. The pathology and nosology of primary progressive aphasia. *Neurology.* 1994;44:2065–2072.

Mesulam MM. Primary progressive aphasia—a language-based dementia. *N Engl J Med.* 2003;349:1535–1542.

Mohr JP, Pessin MS, Finkelstein S, et al. Broca aphasia: pathologic and clinical aspects. *Neurology.* 1978;28:311–324.

Peigneux P, Van der Linden M, Garraux G, Laureys S, Degueldre C, et al. Imaging a cognitive model of apraxia: the neural substrate of gesture-specific cognitive processes. *Hum Brain Mapp.* 2004;2:119–142.

Salvan CV, Ulmer JL, DeYoe EA, Wascher T, Mathews VP, et al. Visual object agnosia and pure word alexia: correlation of functional magnetic resonance imaging and lesion localization. *Comput Assist Tomogr.* 2004;28:63–67.

Tranel D. Neurology of language. *Curr Opin Neurol Neurosurg.* 1992;5:77–82.

Victor M, Angevine JB, Mancall EL, et al. Memory loss with lesions of the hippocampal formation. *Arch Neurol.* 1961;5:244–263.

Wu T, Kansaku K, Hallett M. How self-initiated memorized movements become automatic: a functional MRI study. *J Neurophysiol.* 2004;91:1690–1698.

Chapter 3

Syncope, Seizures and Their Mimics

Lawrence J. Hirsch, Dewey K. Ziegler, and Timothy A. Pedley

Unexplained loss of consciousness is a common clinical problem. Seizure and syncope are high on the list of diagnostic possibilities. Making the distinction may be critical to the patient's survival. This chapter includes information on the clinical features that help discriminate among causes of loss of consciousness and other episodic alterations of behavior and responsiveness.

SYNCOPE

Syncope is a transient alteration of consciousness and loss of muscular tone that results from an acute, reversible global reduction in cerebral blood flow. It is one of the most common causes of partial or complete loss of consciousness and accounts for 3% to 5% of visits to emergency rooms and 1% to 3% of hospital admissions. The prevalence of syncope was as high as 29% in young military pilots and is just as high in the elderly. Over a 10-year period, 16% to 23% of middle-aged or elderly adults experience syncope. In institutionalized elderly people, the annual rate is 6%.

In all forms of syncope, there are sudden decreases in cerebral perfusion. This occurs when systolic blood

▶ **TABLE 3.1 Classification and Causes of Syncope**

(Approximate frequency in parentheses, % of all cases of presumed syncope*)

I. Neurally-mediated reflex syncope (17–22%) ("neurocardiogenic" syncope)
   a. Vasovagal (14%)
   b. Situational (micturition, cough, etc)
   c. Carotid sinus hypersensitivity
II. Orthostatic hypotension (11%)
III. Cardiac (17%)
   a. Arrhythmia (14%)
   b. Structural
IV. Neurological (7%) (transient loss of consciousness mimicking syncope)
   a. Seizure
   b. TIA
   c. Subclavian steal
   d. Migraine
V. Unknown (39%)

*Relative frequencies extracted from Kapoor WN. Current evaluation and management of syncope. *Circulation* 2002;106:1606–1609.

pressure drops below 60 mmHg or when cerebral blood flow ceases for more than 6 to 10 seconds. The causes of syncope are diverse (Table 3.1) and there is no uniformly satisfactory classification.

A neurologic cause for syncope is found in fewer than 10% of cases, and the etiology cannot be determined in one-third of the cases. Brain imaging, vascular imaging, and EEG are unlikely to provide helpful information unless the history suggests seizures or there are focal neurologic signs or symptoms.

Although syncope is generally benign, nearly one-third of persons who experience syncope sustain injuries as a result, including hip or limb fractures. Additional morbidity may relate to the cause of syncope. The prognosis is excellent for those without cardiac disease. One-year mortality is nearly 0% in vasovagal syncope, 5% in syncope of unknown cause, and 18% to 33% in cardiac syncope. Overall, one-third of patients who experience syncope will have recurrence within 3 years.

Clinical Manifestations of Syncope

In reporting syncope, many patients say that they "passed out," "fainted," or "had a spell." Careful history taking, with attention to the meaning patients attach to words, is the cornerstone of differentiating syncope from other conditions (Tables 3.2 and 3.3). Three important, differential points for syncope include precipitating stimuli or situations, the character and evolution of prodromal symptoms, and the absence of a true postictal phase.

The following description is typical of most syncopal events. In the premonitory phase, the person feels lightheaded (impending faint) and is often apprehensive, with a strong but ill-defined sensation of malaise. Peripheral

vasoconstriction imparts a pale or ashen appearance to the skin. Profuse sweating occurs and is often accompanied by nausea and an urge to urinate or defecate. Vision blurs and characteristically fades or "grays out" before consciousness is lost. Attacks usually occur when the person is standing or sitting and may be aborted if the subject can lie down or lower the head below the level of the heart. If the attack proceeds, the patient loses muscle tone and falls as consciousness is lost. The period of unconsciousness is brief, lasting only seconds and rarely more than 30 seconds unless the patient is maintained upright or has a sustained arrhythmia. Brief tonic posturing is often seen for a few seconds, occasionally up to 10 to 20 seconds, and may resemble decerebrate or opisthotonic posturing. Even more common are the presence of a few clonic or myoclonic jerks ("convulsive syncope"), which were noted in 90% of young adults with videotaped self-induced syncope, and invariably occurred at least a few seconds after the loss of consciousness. This contrasts with a seizure, where movements may occur before, during or after loss of consciousness. Some patients recall the jerks, which probably originate in the lower brainstem. Although these involuntary movements may suggest a seizure, the absence of a typical tonic-clonic sequence (tonic phase of approximately 30 seconds followed by rhythmic clonic jerking for at least another 30 seconds), prompt recovery (within seconds rather than several minutes), and other features of the attack should lead to the correct diagnosis of syncope. Table 3.2 lists other helpful features for distinguishing between seizure and syncope.

The EEG during syncope shows diffuse rhythmic slowing, sometimes followed by flattening of the record if severe. Ictal patterns are not seen, including during tonic postures or myoclonic jerks.

Neurally Mediated Reflex Syncope

This type of syncope, also referred to as "neurocardiogenic," consists of a triggering stimulus that leads to bradycardia (cardioinhibitory response), decreased vascular tone (vasodepressor response), or both (mixed response, which is probably most common). Head-up tilt-table testing is useful for diagnosis and treatment in adults when syncope is recurrent and requires treatment.

In a typical protocol, patients are tilted to 60° to 70° for 20 to 45 minutes. In normal individuals, cerebral blood flow is maintained during upright tilting by means of vasoconstriction of systemic blood vessels that is mediated primarily by mechanoreceptors in the aortic arch and carotid sinus. A positive test is defined as induction of syncope, and is classified as cardioinhibitory, vasodepressive, or mixed. However, false positives occur in up to 10% of adult controls and are even more common if isoproterenol (up to 46%) or nitroglycerin is given. Therefore, tilt testing is definitive only when a positive response is

▶ **TABLE 3.2 Syncope vs. Seizure: Useful Distinguishing Features**

	Syncope	*Seizure*
Before spell		
Trigger (position, emotion, Valsalva)	Common	Rare
Sweating & nausea	Common	Rare
Aura (e.g., déjà vu, smell) or unilateral symptoms	Rare	Common
During spell (from eyewitness)		
Pallor	Common	Rare
Cyanosis	Rare	Common
Duration of LOC	<20 secs	>60 secs
Movements	A few clonic or myoclonic jerks; brief tonic posturing (few secs); duration <15 secs; always begin after LOC	Prolonged tonic phase, then prolonged rhythmic clonic movements; duration >1 min; may begin at onset of LOC or before; unilateral jerking (partial seizure)
Automatisms	Occasional	Common (in complex partial and secondarily generalized seizures)
Tongue biting, lateral	Rare	Occasional
Frothing/hypersalivation	Rare	Common
After spell		
Confusion/disorientation	Rare; <30 secs	Common; several mins or longer
Diffuse myalgias	Rare, brief, usually shoulders/chest	Common, hours-days
CK elevation	Rare	Common (esp. after 12 to 24 hrs)
Features that are not helpful for differentiating	Incontinence, prolactin level, dizziness, fear, injury other than lateral tongue biting, eye movements (rolling back), brief automatisms, vocalizations, visual or auditory hallucinations	Incontinence, prolactin level, dizziness, fear, injury other than lateral tongue biting, eye movements (rolling back), brief automatisms, vocalizations, visual or auditory hallucinations

CK = creatine kinase; Esp. = especially; GTC = generalized tonic-clonic; LOC = loss of consciousness; min = minute; sec = second; w/ = with; w/out = without.

obtained in conjunction with typical symptoms, preferably confirmed by a family member or other witness of the patient's spontaneous spells. A primarily cardioinhibitory response suggests that cardiac pacing will be of benefit, whereas a primarily vasodepressor response would not be helped by pacing.

The most common neurally mediated reflex syncope is *vasovagal*, which is also the most frequent cause of syncope in young people, although it is common at all ages. In vasovagal syncope, there is a provoking stimulus, such as pain, apprehension of pain, or sudden emotional shock. The likelihood of syncope is increased with fasting, hot overcrowded rooms, prolonged standing, and fatigue. Medications exacerbate all types of syncope, including antihypertensives, antipsychotics, antidepressants, anticholinergics, levodopa, dopamine agonists, other antiparkinsonian drugs, and medication for erectile dysfunction such as sildenafil.

Carotid sinus syncope, another type of neurally mediated reflex syncope, arises when the carotid sinus displays unusual sensitivity to normal pressure stimuli. This is a common cause of syncope and unexplained falls in older patients with atherosclerosis. Carotid sinus syncope is triggered by head-turning, tight collars, and shaving, situations that result in reflex cardioinhibition (including asystole), a vasodepressor response, or both. Carotid massage, including in an upright position, with ECG monitoring and appropriate supervision, has been recommended in the diagnostic evaluation of unexplained syncope in patients over age 45, but this is not usually performed by the neurologist, and it should be avoided if there is a bruit or known carotid disease. A positive response consists of reproducing typical symptoms associated with a ventricular pause of 3 seconds or more (cardioinhibitory; likely to respond to pacing) or a fall in blood pressure of 50 mmHg or more (vasodepressive; unlikely to respond to pacing) after 5 to 10 seconds of carotid sinus massage. Prolonged pauses of greater than 6 seconds predict occurrence of spontaneous asystolic episodes during 2 years follow-up examination.

Situational syncope refers to reflex syncope occurring with specific triggers such as micturition (most common in older men while standing after arising from bed), coughing, sneezing, trumpet playing, weightlifting, or after exercise. These syndromes usually involve a similar neurally mediated reflex bradycardia or vasodepressor response plus other superimposed exacerbating features such as decreased venous return due to Valsalva effect or orthostatic hypotension. Consciousness is regained as the patient becomes recumbent.

Orthostatic Hypotension and Syncope

A mild orthostatic fall in blood pressure often occurs in normal individuals without causing symptoms. However, syncope results when vascular reflexes that maintain vascular tone and cerebral blood flow with upright posture are impaired. Bilateral shoulder pain in a "coat hanger" distribution may occur just before the syncopal episode, presumably due to muscle ischemia from hypoperfusion. Causes are divided into primary autonomic failure, secondary autonomic failure, and drug-induced.

Primary disorders include multiple system atrophy, especially the Shy-Drager variant, and Parkinson disease with autonomic dysfunction. The most common secondary cause of autonomic neuropathy and orthostatic hypotension is diabetes, although amyloidosis, paraneoplastic disorders, and some hereditary or toxic neuropathies may also have prominent autonomic involvement. Autonomic neuropathy may occur alone or with polyneuropathy. Prescribed drugs are common exacerbating factors, especially in the elderly, but susceptibility varies markedly from one individual to another. Orthostatic hypotension may also follow prolonged standing or an illness that leads to prolonged bed rest. Conditions that cause debilitation or lower blood pressure, such as malnutrition, anemia, blood loss, or adrenal insufficiency, also predispose to orthostatic hypotension. Orthostatic hypotension is discussed in more detail in Chapter 137.

Cardiac Syncope

Cardiac syncope, due to arrhythmia or structural heart disease, occurs at all ages, but is especially frequent in the elderly. Diagnosis of a cardiac cause of syncope is particularly important, because the 5-year mortality rate may exceed 50% in this group of patients, and most causes are treatable.

Either tachyarrhythmias or bradyarrhythmias may cause syncope. The most commonly diagnosed arrhythmias are sinus node dysfunction (including bradycardia/tachycardia syndrome), atrioventricular conduction system disease, and paroxysmal supraventricular and ventricular tachycardias. Other cardiac conditions that may cause syncope include a failing myocardium from cardiomyopathy or multiple infarctions, valvular disease, myxoma, congenital heart disease, aortic dissection, pericardial tamponade, and pulmonary emboli.

Clues to a primary cardiac cause of syncope include lack of a clear trigger, absence of sweating and nausea before the spell, no relation to posture (the syncope may occur while supine), older age, palpitations preceding syncope, family history of sudden death, or underlying cardiac disease. In contrast, a cardiac cause is unlikely in younger patients who have a history consistent with neurally mediated reflex syncope and normal ECG. In older patients or those with non-specific cardiac abnormalities, the only way to make a definite diagnosis is by recording the ECG during a typical spell. The use of implantable (subcutaneous) loop recorders now enables prolonged monitoring (many months) in anyone with unexplained syncope, especially if recurrent or with risk factors for arrhythmia. For a select group of patients, exercise testing and intracardiac electrophysiologic recordings may be necessary for diagnosis. Invasive electrophysiologic testing is required when the conduction disturbance must be localized precisely for ablation or similar procedures.

Differential Diagnosis of Syncope

The most common neurologic spell that may be confused with syncope is *seizure*. Table 3.2 summarizes the most useful features that differentiate the two. Postictal lethargy and confusion suggest a generalized tonic-clonic seizure as do lateral tongue biting, frothing, cyanosis, and postictal diffuse myalgias. Features most suggestive of syncope are pre-ictal sweating and nausea, and lack of a postictal state.

"Drop seizures" may cause sudden falls with brief alteration of consciousness. Myoclonic, tonic and atonic drops have been described. Drop seizures almost always begin in childhood as one manifestation of severe epilepsy. Other seizure types and a static encephalopathy are usually present. On rare occasions, patients fall during complex partial seizures of frontal or temporal origin without secondary generalization. These patients almost always have a long history of epilepsy, making the diagnosis straightforward. To complicate matters further, seizures (especially those arising from the temporal lobe) occasionally cause significant arrhythmias, including bradycardia or asystole. Even more rarely, cerebral hypoxia may precipitate an epileptic seizure in patients with a latent seizure predisposition.

Other conditions may also have to considered in one differential diagnosis (Table 3.3). *Transient ischemic attack* (TIA) due to ischemia in the vertebrobasilar system is a rare cause of transient loss of consciousness. Episodic ischemia of the reticular formation of the brainstem is the presumptive cause. Vertebrobasilar TIAs causing loss of consciousness are virtually always associated with additional manifestations of brainstem, cerebellar, or occipital lobe dysfunction (e.g., cranial nerve palsies, ataxia, visual field deficits, nystagmus, hemianopia, and other focal findings).

In the *subclavian steal* syndrome, reversal of flow in the vertebral artery directs blood away from the brain to help supply an ischemic arm distal to the subclavian artery stenosis, usually on the left. Symptoms are triggered by arm exercise and may cause brief vertebrobasilar ischemia as above, often with dizziness or vertigo, and occasionally including loss of consciousness. *Basilar migraine* may include confusion or even loss of consciousness, but its slow evolution and associated symptoms make diagnosis fairly straightforward.

Treatment of Syncope

Treatment must be based on accurate diagnosis of the underlying cause of syncope. Isolated neurally mediated reflex syncopal episodes require no treatment other than reassurance. Refractory vasovagal syncope, confirmed by tilt-table testing, is typically treated with behavioral therapy, avoidance maneuvers, volume expansion, and occasionally with medications or cardiac pacing. Use of exacerbating drugs such as antihypertensives should be re-assessed. Behavioral therapy involves avoiding precipitants such as rapidly arising from bed, prolonged standing, hot environments, Valsalva maneuvers, dehydration, large carbohydrate meals, prolonged fasting, alcohol and the specific triggers of situational syncope. Sleeping with the head of the bed elevated at least 10 degrees may help, and repetitive tilt training or portable chairs may be tried. Syncope may often be aborted by avoidance maneuvers such as lowering the head, isometric muscular contraction including sustained bilateral handgrip to increase venous return, leg crossing, squatting, and similar maneuvers. Volume expansion is usually achieved using supplemental salt and the mineralocorticoid fludrocortisone, although the efficacy of this regimen has never been proved. Compression stockings that include abdominal support decrease venous pooling and may be helpful, but they are not well tolerated.

Beta-antagonists have been a traditional treatment for neurally mediated reflex syncope based on the theory that the initiating problem is inappropriate triggering of cardiac mechanoreceptors due to forceful contraction of an underfilled left ventricle, thus sending signals to the central nervous system of increased rather than decreased pressure. However, there is evidence that this is not the underlying mechanism in many or most cases, and randomized trials of beta-antagonists have failed to show benefit. Midodrine, an alpha-1 agonist, is effective for orthostatic hypotension and possibly for other forms of syncope with a prominent vasodepressor component. Nighttime doses and sleeping flat should be avoided, because supine hypertension is a common side effect. When spells are severe, recurrent, and primarily cardioinhibitory in nature, randomized trials have confirmed that cardiac pacing is effective in decreasing recurrence, both in carotid sinus syncope and vasovagal syncope. Other treatments that have been used but are unproven include selective serotonin reuptake inhibitors, disopyramide, anticholinergic medications, calcium-channel antagonists, central stimulants, alpha-2 agonists, nonsteroidal anti-inflammatory drugs, vasopressin analogues, octreotide for postprandial syncope, and erythropoietin if anemic.

SEIZURES AND MIMICS

Many nonepileptic events are mistaken for epileptic seizures, and some may be confused with syncope as well (Table 3.3). Approximately one-third of patients referred to tertiary centers for evaluation of intractable epileptic seizures have some other diagnosis, especially psychogenic seizures or syncope. Selected examples of seizure mimics are discussed below and in Table 3.3.

Infants and Young Children

In infants and young children, the following attacks may be misdiagnosed as epilepsy: apneic spells, benign infantile shuddering, hyperekplexia (exaggerated startle), esophageal reflux (Sandifer syndrome), self-stimulatory behaviors, tics and other paroxysmal movement disorders, basilar migraine, and breath-holding spells. Breath-holding spells are dramatic but benign events, usually beginning at 1–2 years of age, triggered by vigorous crying (cyanotic type) or minor trauma (pallid type) and may lead to loss of consciousness. Fortunately, children outgrow these spells by 5–6 years of age without specific treatment.

Panic Attacks and Hyperventilation

Panic attacks and anxiety attacks with hyperventilation are often unrecognized by neurologists. In both conditions, symptoms may mimic partial seizures with affective symptoms. In panic attacks, patients typically describe a suffocating sensation or "lack of oxygen," racing heart beat or palpitations, trembling or shaking, feelings of depersonalization or detachment, blurring of vision, gastrointestinal discomfort, and fear, especially of dying or "going crazy." Hyperventilation episodes may be similar, and the overbreathing may not be obvious unless specifically sought. The most common complaints with hyperventilation are dizziness, a sense of floating or levitation, feelings of anxiety, epigastric or substernal discomfort, carpopedal spasm, flushing or chills, and sometimes "feeling like my mind goes blank." Conversely, temporal lobe seizures with an aura of fear are sometimes misdiagnosed as panic attacks. A period of unresponsiveness, prominent automatisms, and shorter duration (less than 5 minutes) suggests an epileptic etiology.

Psychogenic Nonepileptic Seizures

Psychogenic nonepileptic seizures (PNES) are found in about 30% of the patients admitted to epilepsy-monitoring units. Definitive diagnosis of psychogenic seizures on the basis of history alone is usually not possible. However, the diagnosis may be suggested by a history of physical or sexual abuse, personal or family history of psychiatric disease, or atypical or variable attacks with precipitating factors that include strong emotional or psychologic

▶ **TABLE 3.3 Differential Diagnosis of Seizures and Syncope**

Diagnosis	May be Confused with: (Seizure, Syncope, or Both)	Clinical Features Suggestive of Diagnosis
Panic attack, hyperventilation	Seizure	Often with environmental trigger; severe fear; hyperventilation with perioral cyanosis, bilateral hand paresthesias, carpopedal spasm; no complete LOC; dyspnea; palpitations; >5 mins in duration (seizures are shorter); associated depression and phobias (95%), esp. agoraphobia; onset in young adulthood.
Cataplexy	Both	No LOC; other features of narcolepsy present (daytime somnolence, hypnagogic hallucinations, sleep paralysis); triggered by emotion, esp. laughter.
TIA, vertebrobasilar	Syncope	If transient loss of consciousness, virtually always accompanied by focal neurological features (e.g., dysarthria, dysphagia, vertigo, diplopia, ataxia, unilateral weakness or numbness)
TIA, limb-shaking	Seizure	Non-rhythmic, coarse, 3 Hz to 12 Hz shaking of arm and/or leg contralateral to severe carotid stenosis. Can mimic focal seizures; due to borderline perfusion; may occur upon standing
TIA with aphasia and other negative symptoms	Seizure	Recurrent isolated aphasia can be due to seizure ; if recurrent with no infarct on imaging, consider focal seizures. Similarly with other recurrent, stereotyped negative symptoms initially diagnosed as TIA, including unilateral weakness or numbness.
Subclavian steal	Syncope	Vertebrobasilar ischemia triggered by arm exercise; focal neurological symptoms, especially vertigo and other brainstem symptoms, with or without LOC.
Psychogenic (conversion disorder)	Both	Psychiatric history, esp. somatization; history of physical or sexual abuse; eyes closed and normal vital signs during spell; recurrent spells not responding to treatment; precipitation by hyperventilation or other suggestive techniques
Fugue attacks	Seizure	Can be difficult to distinguish from nonconvulsive status epilepticus without EEG
Migraine (esp. basilar)	Both	Slow march of neurological symptoms over >5 mins and prolonged duration (usually 20–60 mins); posterior circulation symptoms; scintillating scotomata; subsequent headache (may be absent)
Hypoglycemia	Both	Long prodrome; no rapid recovery unless treated.
Transient global amnesia	Seizure	Prolonged spell (hours) with normal behavior except for amnesia; personal identity always intact (if not, suspect psychogenic etiology)
Sleep disorders (somnambulism, night terrors, confusional arousals, enuresis, REM behavior disorder, hypnagogic hallucinations, periodic limb movements, paroxysmal nocturnal dystonia)	Seizure	Sometimes difficult to distinguish from seizures without video/EEG monitoring, polysomnography, or both, esp. if no reliable witness. Paroxysmal nocturnal dystonia is probably epilepsy in many or most cases. Slow wave sleep parasomnias are usually in first third of night.
Staring/behavioral spells in patients with static encephalopathy or dementia	Seizure	Sometimes difficult to distinguish from seizures without video/EEG monitoring
"Drop attacks"	Both	Can be due to cataplexy, cervical spine disease, basilar ischemia, vertigo attack (Meniere), seizures (myoclonic, tonic, atonic; rarely complex partial), or syncope (esp. cardiac)

Esp. = especially; LOC = loss of consciousness; REM = rapid eye movement; TIA = transient ischemic attack.

elements. Repeatedly normal interictal EEGs in the presence of medically refractory seizures also raise the possibility of the diagnosis of PNES. Incontinence and injuries are unusual but may occur with PNES.

Violent flailing or thrashing of arms and legs, side-to-side head movements, and pelvic thrusting are common in psychogenic nonepileptic seizures, although similar phenomena may be observed in partial seizures of frontal lobe origin. Preserved consciousness with sustained bilateral motor activity of the arms and legs is rare in epilepsy but may occur in frontal lobe seizures, especially those involving the supplementary motor area. Other features consistent with or suggestive of PNES include lack of spells arising from sleep, spells in the physician's office, prolonged spells, starting and stopping of symptoms or movements, variability from spell to spell, motionless state with eyes closed, lack of tachycardia, and a slow-motion, neurasthenic state with hypophonia during recovery. Even experienced observers may not always be able to distinguish epileptic seizures from psychogenic spells. Thus, a secure diagnosis of PNES may be made only by inpatient monitoring with simultaneous video-EEG recording. A negative ictal EEG alone does not prove a nonepileptic etiology as many simple partial seizures and a small portion of complex partial seizures (predominantly of extratemporal origin) show no definite scalp EEG correlate. In these cases, clinical semiology, stereotypy, and spells arising from EEG-documented sleep allow proper diagnosis. To complicate matters further, PNES and epileptic seizures frequently co-exist in the same patient. Therefore, recording nonepileptic attacks in a patient with uncontrolled seizures does not, by itself, prove that all the patient's seizures are psychogenic. Before reaching a final conclusion, one must verify with the patient and family that the recorded events are typical of the habitual spells experienced at home.

Serum prolactin measurements may help classify a convulsive spell with bilateral motor involvement for at least 30 seconds as psychogenic or epileptic. Prolactin should be drawn 10 to 30 minutes after the event and compared with interictal baseline prolactin levels drawn on a different day at the same time. With epileptic generalized tonic-clonic seizures, prolactin levels are elevated to at least 3 times baseline. An epileptic rather than psychogenic etiology is also more likely if there is a prominent but transient metabolic acidosis and elevated CK after 12 to 24 hours.

Sleep Disorders

Some sleep disorders mimic seizures. In children, the most common diagnostic problem is a *parasomnia:* sleep talking (somniloquy), somnambulism, night terrors, and enuresis. Confusion with complex partial seizures arises because these conditions are paroxysmal, may include automatic behavioral mannerisms, and tend to be recurrent. In ad-

dition, the patient is usually unresponsive during the attacks and amnesic for them afterward. Most parasomnias occur during the period of deepest slow-wave sleep, especially just before or during the transition into the first rapid eye movement period. They tend to occur in the early part of the night. Seizures are less predictable, although they tend to occur shortly after going to sleep or in the early morning. Finally, parasomnias lack the complex automatisms, stereotyped postures, and clonic movements typical of epileptic seizures.

Patients with narcolepsy may have periods with intermittent "microsleep" causing abnormal automatic behaviors. They also experience cataplexy, a sudden loss of tone (leading to head nodding, knee-buckling or falling) precipitated by emotions, especially laughter, but without loss of consciousness.

Migraine

Some migraine events may be mistaken for seizures, especially when the headache is mild or inconspicuous. *Basilar artery migraine* may include episodic confusion and disorientation, lethargy, mood changes, vertigo, ataxia, bilateral visual disturbances, and alterations in, or even loss of, consciousness. In children, migraine may occur as a confusional state that resembles nonconvulsive status epilepticus, or as paroxysms of cyclic vomiting with signs of vasomotor instability (flushing, pallor, mydriasis) and photophobia. Positive visual phenomena occur in either occipital seizures or migraine. Seizure is suggested by shorter duration of visual symptoms (usually less than 1 to 2 minutes vs. 5 to 60 minutes in migraine) and seeing colors, whereas migraine is suggested by prolonged symptoms with slow evolution, straight or jagged lines such as in fortification spectra, scintillations, and black and white phenomena. Occipital seizures may be followed by postictal migraine. Thus a stereotyped visual aura lasting less than 1 to 2 minutes is strongly suggestive of seizure, even if it is typically followed by a migraine headache.

Transient Ischemic Attack

TIAs are not usually confused with seizures. Diagnosis is occasionally difficult when a TIA is manifest by isolated aphasia or unilaterally disturbed sensation, or when muscle weakness results in a fall. In general, focal sensory symptoms associated with epilepsy show sequential Jacksonian spread from one body area to another and include positive phenomena (paresthesias), whereas ischemia usually causes numbness and lacks this type of spread. However, seizures sometimes cause strictly negative phenomena such as aphasia, weakness or numbness. When recurrent, stereotyped, and without imaging evidence of ischemia or acute infarct, seizure should be considered for these TIA- or stroke-like symptoms.

SUMMARY

A patient's transient loss of consciousness is a common reason practitioners seek consultation with a neurologist. Syncope and seizures are the most frequent causes, although the differential diagnosis is extensive. When evaluating syncope, a primary cardiac cause is the most important to diagnose and is suggested by underlying cardiac disease, abnormal EKG, older age, no relation to posture, and a lack of autonomic symptoms such as nausea and diaphoresis at the onset. Other common causes include neurally mediated reflex syncope (including vasovagal) and orthostatic hypotension. Although history may often lead to the proper diagnosis, definitive diagnosis of recurrent spells is best made by recording a *typical* spell, often requiring tilt-table testing, carotid massage, implantable loop recorders or video/EEG/ECG monitoring. Behavioral modification is usually adequate treatment. Medication is sometimes helpful. In severe and recurrent syncope that is primarily cardioinhibitory (bradycardia or asystole without a significant vasodepressor component), cardiac pacing may be effective.

SUGGESTED READINGS

Benditt DG, Ermis C, Pham S, et al. Implantable diagnostic monitoring devices for evaluation of syncope, and tachy- and brady-arrhythmias. *J Interv Card Electrophysiol* 2003;9:137–144.

Benbadis SR, Wolgamuth BR, Goren H, Brenere S, Fouad-Tarazi F. Value of tongue-biting in the diagnosis of seizures. *Arch Intern Med* 1995;155:2346–2349.

Benditt DG, van Dijk JG, Sutton R, et al. Syncope. *Curr Probl Cardiol* 2004;29(4):152–229.

Bergfeldt L. Differential diagnosis of cardiogenic syncope and seizure disorders. *Heart* 2003;89:353–358.

Brignole M. Randomized clinical trials of neurally mediated syncope. *J Cardiovasc Electrophysiol* 2003;14 (Suppl):S64–S69.

Brignole M, Albani P, Benditt D, et al. Task force report. Guidelines on management (diagnosis and treatment) of syncope. *Eur Heart J* 2001;22:1256–1306.

Chen-Scarabelli C, Scarabelli TM. Neurologic syncope. *BMJ* 2004; 329(7461):336–341.

Connolly SJ, Sheldon RS, Roberts RS, et al. The North American Vasovagal Pacemaker Study: a randomized trial of permanent cardiac pacing for the prevention of vasovagal syncope. *J Am Coll Cardiol* 1999;33: 16–20.

Devinsky O. Nonepileptic psychogenic seizures: quagmires of pathophysiology, diagnosis and treatment. *Epilepsia* 1998;39:458–462.

Gambardella A, Reutens DC, Andermann F. Late-onset drop attacks in temporal lobe epilepsy: a re-evaluation of the concept of temporal lobe syncope. *Neurology* 1994:1074–1078.

Gastaut H, Fischer-Williams M. Electro-encephalographic study of syncope: its differentiation from epilepsy. *Lancet* 1957;2:1018–1025.

Hoefnagels WA, Padberg GW, Overweg J, van der Velde EA, Roos RAC. Transient loss of consciousness: the value of the history for distinguishing seizure from syncope. *J Neurol* 1991;238:39–43.

Kapoor WN. Current evaluation and management of syncope. *Circulation* 2002;106:1606–1609.

Kapoor WN, Karpf M, Wieand S, et al. A prospective evaluation and follow-up of patients with syncope. *N Engl J Med* 1983;309:197–203.

Landau WM, Nelson DA. Clinical neuromythology XV. Feinting science: Neurocardiogenic syncope and collateral vasovagal confusion. *Neurology* 1996;46:609–618.

Lempert T, Bauer M, Schmidt D. Syncope: a videometric analysis of 56 episodes of transient cerebral hypoxia. *Ann Neurol* 1994;36:233–237.

Lusic I, Pintaric I, Hozo I, Boic L, Capkun V. Serum prolactin levels after seizure and syncopal attacks. *Seizure* 1999;8:218–222.

Luzza F, Di Rosa S, Pugliatti P, Ando G, Carerj S, Rizzo F. Syncope of psychiatric origin. *Clin Auton Res* 2004;14(1):26–29.

Maddens M. Tilt-table testing in patients with syncope: what does it really tell us? *J Am Geriatric Soc* 2002;50:1451–1453.

Moroney JT, Sacco RL. Cerebrovascular disorders. In: Engel J Jr, Pedley TA, eds. *Epilepsy: A comprehensive textbook.* Philadelphia: Lippincott-Raven 1997:2693–2704.

Neufeld MY, Treves TA, Chistik V, Korczyn AD. Sequential serum creatine kinase determination differentiates vaso-vagal syncope from generalized tonic-clonic seizures. *Acta Neurol Scand* 1997;95:137–139.

Oribe E, Amini R, Nissenbaum E, Boal B. Serum prolactin levels are elevated after syncope. *Neurology* 1996;47:60–62.

Passman R, Horvath G, Thomas J, et al. Clinical spectrum and prevalence of neurologic events provoked by tilt table testing. *Arch Intern Med* 2003;163:1945–1948.

Pritchard PB, Wannamaker BB, Sagel J, Daniel CM. Serum prolactin and cortisol levels in evaluation of pseudoepileptic seizures. *Ann Neurol* 1985;18:87–89.

Raj SR, Sheldon RS. Role of pacemakers in treating neurocardiogenic syncope. *Curr Opin Cardiol* 2003;18:47–52.

Saygi S, Katz A, Marks DA, Spencer S. Frontal lobe partial seizures and psychogenic seizure: comparison of clinical and ictal characteristics. *Neurology* 1992;43:1274–1277.

Sra JS, Mohammad RJ, Boaz A, et al. Comparison of cardiac pacing with drug therapy in the treatment of neurocardiogenic (vasovagal) syncope with bradycardia or asystole. *N Engl J Med* 1993;328:1085–1090.

Sturzenegger MH, Meienberg O. Basilar artery migraine: a follow-up study in 82 cases. *Headache* 1985;25:408–415.

Weimer LH, Williams O. Syncope and orthostatic intolerance. *Med Clin North Am* 2003;87:835–865.

Zaidi A, Clough P, Cooper P, et al. Misdiagnosis of epilepsy: many seizure-like attacks have a cardiovascular cause. *J Am Coll Cardiol* 2000;36:181–184.

Chapter 4

Coma

John C. M. Brust

Consciousness, the awareness of self and environment, requires both arousal and cognitive content; the anatomic substrate includes both reticular activating system and cerebral cortex. Coma is a state of unconsciousness that differs from syncope in being sustained and from sleep in being less easily reversed. Cerebral oxygen uptake (cerebral metabolic rate of oxygen [$CMRO_2$]) is normal in sleep or actually increases during the rapid eye movement stage, but $CMRO_2$ is abnormally reduced in coma.

Coma is clinically defined by the neurologic examination, especially responses to external stimuli. Terms such as *lethargy, obtundation, stupor,* and *coma* usually depend on the patient's response to normal verbal stimuli, shouting, shaking, or pain. These terms are not rigidly defined and it is useful to record both the response and the stimulus that elicited it. Occasionally, the true level of consciousness may be difficult or impossible to determine (e.g., when there is catatonia, severe depression, neuromuscular blockade, or akinesia plus aphasia).

Confusional state and *delirium* are terms that refer to a state of inattentiveness, altered cognitive content, and sometimes hyperactivity, rather than to a decreased level of arousal; these conditions may presage or alternate with obtundation, stupor, or coma.

EXAMINATION AND MAJOR DIAGNOSTIC PROCEDURES

In the assessment of a comatose patient, it is first necessary to detect and treat any immediately life-threatening condition: hemorrhage is stopped; the airway is protected with intubation when necessary (e.g., prevention of aspiration in a patient who is vomiting); circulation is supported; and an electrocardiogram is obtained to detect dangerous arrhythmia. If the diagnosis is unknown, blood is drawn for glucose determination, after which 50% dextrose is given intravenously with parenteral thiamine. (Administering glucose alone to a thiamine-deficient patient may precipitate Wernicke-Korsakoff syndrome.) When opiate overdose is a possibility, naloxone hydrochloride (Narcan®) is given. If trauma is suspected, damage to internal organs and cervical fracture should be considered until radiographs determine otherwise.

The next step is to ascertain the site and cause of the lesion. The incident or immediate history is obtained from whomever accompanies the patient, including ambulance drivers and police. Examination should include the following: skin, nails, and mucous membranes (for pallor, cherry redness, cyanosis, jaundice, sweating, uremic frost, myxedema, hypo- or hyperpigmentation, petechiae, dehydration, decubiti, or signs of trauma); the breath (for acetone, alcohol, or fetor hepaticus); and the fundi (for papilledema, hypertensive or diabetic retinopathy, retinal ischemia, Roth spots, granulomas, or subhyaloid hemorrhages). Fever may imply infection or heat stroke; hypothermia may occur with cold exposure (especially in patients with alcohol intoxication), hypothyroidism, hypoglycemia, sepsis, or infrequently, a primary brain lesion. Asymmetry of pulses may suggest dissecting aneurysm. Urinary or fecal incontinence may signify an unwitnessed or unidentified seizure, especially in patients who subsequently awaken spontaneously. The scalp should be inspected and palpated for signs of trauma (e.g., Battle sign), and the ears and nose are examined for blood or CSF. Resistance to passive neck flexion but not to turn-ing or tilting suggests meningitis, subarachnoid hemorrhage, or foramen magnum herniation, but may be absent early in the course of the disorder and in patients who are deeply comatose. Resistance to manipulation in all directions suggests bone or joint disease, including fracture.

In their classic monograph, Plum and Posner (1980) divided the causes of coma into supra- and infratentorial structural lesions and diffuse or metabolic diseases. By concentrating on motor responses to stimuli, respiratory patterns, pupils, and eye movements, the clinician can usually identify the category of coma.

Motor Responses

The patient is observed in order to assess respiration, limb position, and spontaneous movements. Myoclonus or seizures may be subtle (e.g., twitching of one or two fingers or the corner of the mouth). More florid movements, such as facial grimacing, jaw gyrations, tongue protrusion, or complex repetitive limb movements, may defy ready interpretation. Asymmetric movements or postures may signify either focal seizures or hemiparesis.

Asymmetry of muscle tone suggests a structural lesion, but it is not always clear which side is abnormal. *Gegenhalten,* or *paratonia,* is resistance to passive movement that in contrast to parkinsonian rigidity, increases with the velocity of the movement and unlike clasp-knife spasticity, continues through the full range of the movement; it is attributed to diffuse forebrain dysfunction and is often accompanied by a grasp reflex.

Motor responses to stimuli may be appropriate, inappropriate, or absent. Even when patients are not fully awake, they may be roused to follow simple commands. Some patients who respond only to noxious stimuli (e.g., pressure on the sternum or supraorbital bone, pinching the neck or limbs, or squeezing muscle, tendon, or nail beds) may make voluntary avoidance responses. The terms "decorticate" and "decerebrate" posturing are physiologic misnomers but refer to hypertonic flexion or extension in response to noxious stimuli. In *decorticate rigidity,* the arms are flexed, adducted, and internally rotated, and the legs are extended; in *decerebrate rigidity,* the arms and legs are all extended. These postures are most often associated with cerebral hemisphere disease, including metabolic encephalopathy, but may follow upper brainstem lesions or transtentorial herniation.

Flexor postures generally imply a more rostral lesion and have a better prognosis than extensor posturing, but the pattern of response may vary with different stimuli, or there may be flexion of one arm and extension of the other. When these postures seem to occur spontaneously, there may be an unrecognized stimulus (e.g., airway obstruction or bladder distention). With continuing rostrocaudal deterioration, there may be extension of the arms and flexion of the legs until, with lower brainstem destruction, there is flaccid unresponsiveness. However, lack of motor response to any stimulus should always raise the possibility of limb paralysis caused by cervical trauma, Guillain-Barré neuropathy, or the locked-in state.

Respiration

In Cheyne-Stokes respiration (CSR), periods of hyperventilation and apnea alternate in a crescendo-decrescendo fashion. The hyperpneic phase is usually longer than the apneic, so that arterial gases tend to show respiratory alkalosis; during periods of apnea, there may be decreased responsiveness, miosis, and reduced muscle tone. CSR occurs with bilateral cerebral disease, including impending transtentorial herniation, upper brainstem lesions, and metabolic encephalopathy. It usually signifies that the patient is not in imminent danger. Conversely, "short-cycle CSR" (*cluster breathing*) with less smooth waxing and waning is often an ominous sign of a posterior fossa lesion or dangerously elevated intracranial pressure.

Sustained hyperventilation is usually due to metabolic acidosis, pulmonary congestion, hepatic encephalopathy, or stimulation by analgesic drugs (Fig. 4.1). Rarely, it is the result of a lesion in the rostral brainstem. *Apneustic breathing,* consisting of inspiratory pauses, is seen with pontine lesions, especially infarction; it occurs infrequently with metabolic coma or transtentorial herniation.

Respiration having a variably irregular rate and amplitude (*ataxic breathing*) indicates medullary damage and may progress to apnea, which also occurs abruptly in acute posterior fossa lesions. Loss of automatic respiration with preserved voluntary breathing (*Ondine curse*) occurs with medullary lesions; as the patient becomes less alert, apnea may be fatal. Other ominous respiratory signs are end-expiratory pushing (e.g., coughing) and "fish-mouthing" (i.e., lower-jaw depression with inspiration). Stertorous breathing (i.e., inspiratory noise) is a sign of airway obstruction.

Pupils

Pupillary abnormalities in coma may reflect an imbalance between input from the parasympathetic and sympathetic nervous systems or lesions of both. Although many people have slight pupillary inequality, anisocoria should be considered pathologic in a comatose patient. Retinal or optic nerve damage does not cause anisocoria, even though there

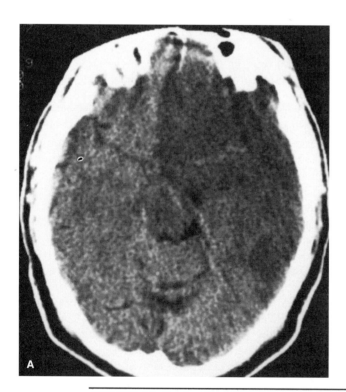 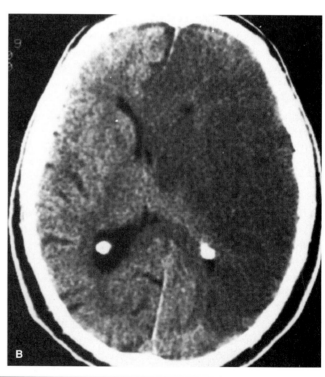

FIGURE 4.1. Cerebral herniation secondary to hemispheral infarction. Noncontrast axial CT demonstrates an extensive area of decreased density within the left frontal, temporal, and parietal lobes with relative sparing of the left thalamus and left occipital lobe. A dense left middle cerebral artery is seen, consistent with thrombosis. **A:** Obliteration of the suprasellar cistern by the medial left temporal lobe indicates uncal herniation. **B:** Left-to-right shift of the left frontal lobe, left caudate nucleus, and left internal capsule denote severe subfalcine herniation. (Courtesy of Dr. S. Chan, Columbia University College of Physicians and Surgeons, New York, NY, with permission.)

is an afferent pupillary defect. Parasympathetic lesions (e.g., oculomotor nerve compression in uncal herniation or after rupture of an internal carotid artery aneurysm) cause pupillary enlargement and ultimately full dilation with loss of reactivity to light. Sympathetic lesions, either intraparenchymal (e.g., hypothalamic injury or lateral medullary infarction) or extraparenchymal (e.g., invasion of the superior cervical ganglion by lung cancer), cause Horner syndrome with miosis. With involvement of both systems (e.g., midbrain destruction), one or both pupils are in midposition and are unreactive. Pinpoint but reactive pupils following pontine hemorrhage are probably the result of damage to descending intraaxial sympathetic pathways, as well as to a region of the reticular formation that normally inhibits the Edinger-Westphal nucleus.

With few exceptions, metabolic disease does not cause unequal or unreactive pupils. Fixed, dilated pupils after diffuse anoxia-ischemia denote a bad prognosis. Anticholinergic drugs, including glutethimide, amitriptyline, and antiparkinsonian agents, abolish pupillary reactivity. Hypothermia and severe barbiturate intoxication may cause not only fixed pupils but a reversible picture that mimics brain death. Bilateral or unilateral pupillary dilation and nonreactivity may accompany (or briefly follow) a seizure. In opiate overdose, miosis may be so severe that a very bright light and a magnifying glass are necessary to detect reactivity. Some pupillary abnormalities are local in origin (e.g., trauma or synechiae).

Eyelids and Eye Movements

Closed eyelids in a comatose patient mean that the lower pons is intact, and blinking means that reticular activity is taking place; however, blinking may occur with or without purposeful limb movements. Eyes that are conjugately deviated away from hemiparetic limbs indicate a destructive cerebral lesion on the side toward which the eyes are directed. Eyes turned toward paretic limbs may mean a pontine lesion, an adversive seizure, or the wrong-way gaze paresis of thalamic hemorrhage. Eyes that are dysconjugate while at rest may mean paresis of individual muscles, internuclear ophthalmoplegia, or preexisting tropia or phoria.

When the brainstem is intact, the eyes may rove irregularly from side to side with a slow, smooth velocity; jerky movements suggest saccades and relative wakefulness. Repetitive smooth excursions of the eyes first to one side and then to the other, with 2- to 3-second pauses in each direction (*periodic alternating* or *ping-pong gaze*), may follow bilateral cerebral infarction or cerebellar hemorrhage with an intact brainstem.

If cervical injury has been ruled out, oculocephalic testing (the *doll's-eye maneuver*) is performed by passively turning the head from side to side; with an intact reflex arc (vestibular–brainstem–eye muscles), the eyes move conjugately in the opposite direction. A more vigorous stimulus is produced by irrigating each ear with 30 mL to 100 mL of ice water. A normal, awake person with head elevated 30° has nystagmus with the fast component in the direction opposite the ear stimulated, but a comatose patient with an intact reflex arc has deviation of the eyes toward the stimulus, usually for several minutes. Simultaneous bilateral irrigation causes vertical deviation, upward after warm water and downward after cold water.

Oculocephalic or caloric testing may reveal intact eye movements, gaze palsy, individual muscle paresis, internuclear ophthalmoplegia, or no response. Cerebral gaze paresis may often be overcome by these maneuvers, but brainstem gaze palsies are usually fixed. Complete ophthalmoplegia may follow either extensive brainstem damage or metabolic coma, but except for barbiturate or phenytoin sodium (Dilantin) poisoning, eye movements are preserved early in metabolic encephalopathy. Unexplained disconjugate eyes indicate a brainstem or cranial nerve lesion (including abducens palsy due to increased intracranial pressure).

Downward deviation of the eyes occurs with lesions in the thalamus or midbrain pretectum and may be accompanied by pupils that do not react to light (*Parinaud syndrome*). Downward eye deviation also occurs in metabolic coma, especially in barbiturate poisoning and after a seizure. Skew deviation, or vertical divergence, follows lesions of the cerebellum or brainstem, especially the pontine tegmentum.

Retraction and convergence nystagmus may be seen with midbrain lesions, but spontaneous nystagmus is rare in coma. *Ocular bobbing* (i.e., conjugate brisk downward movements from the primary position) usually follows destructive lesions of the pontine tegmentum (when lateral eye movements are lost) but may occur with cerebellar hemorrhage, metabolic encephalopathy, or transtentorial herniation. Unilateral bobbing (i.e., nystagmoid jerking) signifies pontine disease.

DIAGNOSTIC TESTS

CT or MRI is promptly performed whenever coma is unexplained. Unless meningitis is suspected and the patient is clinically deteriorating, imaging should precede lumbar puncture. If imaging is not readily available, a spinal tap is cautiously performed with a 20-gauge or 22-gauge needle. If imaging reveals frank, transtentorial or foramen magnum herniation, the comparative risks of performing a lumbar puncture or of treating for meningitis without CSF confirmation must be weighed individually for each patient.

Other emergency laboratory studies include serum levels of glucose, sodium, calcium, and BUN or creatinine;

determination of arterial pH and partial pressures of oxygen (PO_2) and carbon dioxide (PCO_2); as well as blood or urine toxicology testing (including serum levels of sedative drugs and ethanol). Blood and CSF should be cultured, and liver function studies and other serum electrolyte levels determined. The use of coagulation studies and other metabolic tests is based on index of suspicion.

The EEG may distinguish coma from psychic unresponsiveness or locked-in state, although alpha-like activity in coma after brainstem infarction or cardiopulmonary arrest may make the distinction difficult. In metabolic coma, the EEG is always abnormal, and early in the course it may be a more sensitive indicator of abnormality than the clinical state of the patient. The EEG may also reveal asymmetries or evidence of clinically unsuspected seizure activity. Infrequently, patients without clinical seizures demonstrate repetitive electrographic seizures or continuous spike-and-wave activity; conversely, patients with subtle motor manifestations of seizures sometimes display only diffuse electrographic slowing. Distinguishing true status epilepticus from myoclonus (common after anoxic-ischemic brain damage) is often difficult, both clinically and electrographically; and if any doubt exists, anticonvulsant therapy should be instituted.

COMA PRESENTATIONS

Coma from Supratentorial Structural Lesions

Coma may result from bilateral cerebral damage or from sudden large unilateral lesions that functionally disrupt the contralateral hemisphere (*diaschisis*). CT studies indicate that with acute hemisphere masses, early depression of consciousness correlates more with lateral brain displacement than with transtentorial herniation. Eventually, however, downward brain displacement and rostrocaudal brainstem dysfunction ensue. Transtentorial herniation is divided into lateral (uncal) or central types. In *uncal herniation* (as in subdural hematoma), there is early compression of the oculomotor nerve by the inferomedial temporal lobe with ipsilateral pupillary enlargement. Alertness may not be altered until the pupil is dilated, at which point there may be an acceleration of signs with unilaterally and then bilaterally fixed pupils and oculomotor palsy, CSR followed by hyperventilation or ataxic breathing, flexor and then extensor posturing, and progressive unresponsiveness. Aqueduct obstruction and posterior cerebral artery compression may further raise supratentorial pressure. If the process is not halted, there is progression to deep coma, apnea, bilaterally unreactive pupils, ophthalmoplegia, and eventually circulatory collapse and death.

In *central transtentorial herniation* (as in thalamic hemorrhage), consciousness is rapidly impaired, pupils are of normal or small diameter and react to light, and eye movements are normal. CSR, gegenhalten, and flexor or extensor postures are also seen. As the disorder progresses, the pupils become fixed in mid position; this is followed by the same sequence of unresponsiveness, ophthalmoplegia, and respiratory and postural abnormalities as seen in uncal herniation. During the downward course of transtentorial herniation, there may be hemiparesis ipsilateral to the cerebral lesion, attributed to compression of the contralateral midbrain peduncle against the tentorial edge (*Kernohan notch*). The contralateral oculomotor nerve is occasionally compressed before the ipsilateral oculomotor nerve.

The major lesions causing transtentorial herniation are traumatic (e.g., epidural, subdural, or intraparenchymal hemorrhage), vascular (e.g., ischemic or hemorrhagic), infectious (e.g., abscess or granuloma, including lesions associated with acquired immunodeficiency syndrome), and neoplastic (primary or metastatic). CT or MRI locates and often defines the lesion.

Coma from Infratentorial Structural Lesions

Infratentorial structural lesions may compress or directly destroy the brainstem. Such lesions may also cause brain herniation, either transtentorially upward (with midbrain compression) or downward through the foramen magnum, with distortion of the medulla by the cerebellar tonsils. Abrupt tonsillar herniation causes apnea and circulatory collapse; coma is then secondary, for the medullary reticular formation has little direct role in arousal. In coma, *primary infratentorial structural lesions* are suggested by bilateral weakness or sensory loss, crossed cranial nerve and long tract signs, miosis, loss of lateral gaze with preserved vertical eye movements, dysconjugate gaze, ophthalmoplegia, short-cycle CSR, and apneustic or ataxic breathing. The clinical picture of pontine hemorrhage (i.e., sudden coma, pinpoint but reactive pupils, and no eye movement) is characteristic, but if the sequence of signs in a comatose patient is unknown, it may not be possible to tell whether the process began supratentorially or infratentorially without the use of imaging. Infrequent brainstem causes of coma include multiple sclerosis and central pontine myelinolysis.

Coma from Metabolic or Diffuse Brain Disease

In metabolic, diffuse, or multifocal encephalopathy, cognitive and respiratory abnormalities occur early; there is often tremor, asterixis, or multifocal myoclonus. Gegenhalten, frontal release signs (i.e., snout, suck, or grasp), and flexor or extensor posturing may occur. Except in anticholinergic intoxication, the pupils remain reactive. The eyes may be deviated downward, but the presence of sustained lateral deviation or disconjugate eyes argues against the diagnosis of a metabolic disturbance. Metabolic disease, however, may cause both focal seizures and lateralizing neurologic signs, often shifting but sometimes persisting (as in hypoglycemia and hyperglycemia).

Arterial gas determinations are especially useful in diagnosing metabolic coma. Of the diseases listed in Table 4.1,

▶ **TABLE 4.1 Causes of Abnormal Ventilation in Unresponsive Patients**

Hyperventilation
Metabolic acidosis
Anion gap
Diabetic ketoacidosis[a]
Diabetic hypoosmolar coma[a]
Lactic acidosis
Uremia[a]
Alcoholic ketoacidosis
Acidic poisons (ethylene glycol, methyl alcohol, paraldehyde)[a]
No anion gap
Diarrhea
Pancreatic drainage
Carbonic anhydrase inhibitors
NH_4Cl ingestion
Renal tubular acidosis
Ureteroenterostomy
Respiratory alkalosis
Hepatic failure[a]
Sepsis[a]
Pneumonia
Anxiety (hyperventilation syndrome)
Mixed acid–base disorders (metabolic acidosis and respiratory alkalosis)
Salicylism
Sepsis[a]
Hepatic failure[a]
Hypoventilation
Respiratory acidosis
Acute (uncompensated)
Sedative drugs[a]
Brainstem injury
Neuromuscular disorders
Chest injury
Acute pulmonary disease
Chronic pulmonary disease
Metabolic alkalosis
Vomiting or gastric drainage
Diuretic therapy
Adrenal steroid excess (Cushing syndrome)
Primary aldosteronism
Bartter syndrome

[a] Common causes of stupor or coma. From Plum and Posner, 1980, with Permission.

psychogenic hyperventilation is more likely to cause delirium than stupor, but may coexist with hysterical coma. Cognitive change associated with metabolic alkalosis is usually mild.

Metabolic and diffuse brain diseases causing coma are numerous but the diversity is not overwhelming. Most entities listed in Table 4.2 are described in other chapters.

HYSTERIA AND CATATONIA

Hysterical (conversion) unresponsiveness is rare and probably overdiagnosed. Indistinguishable clinically from malingering, it is usually associated with closed eyes, eupnea or tachypnea, and normal pupils. The eyelids may resist passive opening and when released, close abruptly or jerkily rather than with smooth descent; lightly stroking the eyelashes causes lid fluttering. The eyes do not slowly rove but move with saccadic jerks, and ice-water caloric testing causes nystagmus rather than sustained deviation. The limbs usually offer no resistance to passive movement yet demonstrate normal tone. Unless organic disease or drug effect is also present, the EEG pattern is one of normal wakefulness.

In catatonia (which may occur with schizophrenia, depression, toxic psychosis, or other brain diseases), there may be akinetic mutism, grimacing, rigidity, posturing, catalepsy, or excitement. Respirations are normal or rapid, pupils are large but reactive, and eye movements are normal. The EEG is usually normal.

LOCKED-IN SYNDROME

Infarction or central pontine myelinolysis may destroy the basis pontis, producing total paralysis of the lower cranial nerve and limb muscles with preserved alertness and respiration. At first glance, the patient appears unresponsive, but examination reveals voluntary vertical and sometimes horizontal eye movements, including blinking. (Even with facial paralysis, inhibition of the levator palpebrae may produce partial eye closure.) Communication is possible with the use of purposeful blinking or eye movements to indicate "yes," "no," or in response to letters.

VEGETATIVE STATE

The terms *akinetic mutism* and *coma vigil* have been used to describe a variety of states, including coma with preserved eye movements following midbrain lesions, psychomotor bradykinesia with frontal lobe disease, and isolated diencephalic and brainstem function after massive cerebral damage. For this last condition, the term

▶ **TABLE 4.2 Diffuse Brain Diseases or Metabolic Disorders That Cause Coma**

Deprivation of oxygen, substrate, or metabolic cofactor
  Hypoxia
  Diffuse ischemia (cardiac disease, decreased peripheral circulatory resistance, increased cerebrovascular resistance, widespread small vessel occlusion)
  Hypoglycemia
  Thiamine deficiency (Wernicke-Korsakoff syndrome)
Disease of organs other than brain
  Liver (hepatic coma)
  Kidney (uremia)
  Lung (carbon dioxide narcosis)
  Pancreas (diabetes, hypoglycemia, exocrine pancreatic encephalopathy)
  Pituitary (apoplexy, sedative hypersensitivity)
  Thyroid (myxedema, thyrotoxicosis)
  Parathyroid (hypo- and hyperparathyroidism)
  Adrenal (Addison or Cushing disease, pheochromocytoma)
  Other systemic disease (cancer, porphyria, sepsis)
Exogenous poisons
  Sedatives and narcotics
  Psychotropic drugs
  Acid poisons (e.g., methyl alcohol, ethylene glycol)
  Others (e.g., anticonvulsants, heavy metals, cyanide)
Abnormalities of ionic or acid–base environment of central nervous system
  Water and sodium (hypo- and hypernatremia)
  Acidosis
  Alkalosis
  Magnesium (hyper- and hypomagnesemia)
  Calcium (hyper- and hypocalcemia)
  Phosphorus (hypophosphatemia)
Disordered temperature regulation
  Hypothermia
  Heat stroke
Central nervous system inflammation or infiltration
  Leptomeningitis
  Encephalitis
  Acute toxic encephalopathy (e.g., Reye syndrome)
  Parainfectious encephalomyelitis
  Cerebral vasculitis
  Subarachnoid hemorrhage
  Carcinomatous meningitis
Primary neuronal or glial disorders
  Creutzfeldt-Jakob disease
  Marchiafava-Bignami disease
  Adrenoleukodystrophy
  Gliomatosis cerebri
  Progressive multifocal leukoencephalopathy
Seizure and postictal states

Modified from Plum and Posner, 1980.

vegetative state is preferred to refer to patients with sleep–wake cycles, intact cardiorespiratory function, and primitive responses to stimuli, but without evidence of inner or outer awareness (Table 4.3).

Patients who survive coma usually show varying degrees of recovery within 2 to 4 weeks; those who enter the

▶ **TABLE 4.3 Criteria for Determination of Vegetative State**

1. No evidence of awareness of self or surroundings. Reflex or spontaneous eye opening may occur.
2. No meaningful and consistent communication between examiner and patient, auditory or written. Target stimuli not usually followed visually, but sometimes visual tracking present. No emotional response to verbal stimuli.
3. No comprehensible speech or mouthing of words.
4. Smiling, frowning, or crying inconsistently related to any apparent stimulus.
5. Sleep–wake cycles present.
6. Brainstem and spinal reflexes variables, e.g., preservation of sucking, rooting, chewing, swallowing, pupillary reactivity to light, oculocephalic responses, and grasp or tendon reflexes.
7. No voluntary movements or behavior, no matter how rudimentary; no motor activity suggesting learned behavior; no mimicry. Withdrawal or posturing can occur with noxious stimuli.
8. Usually intact blood pressure control and cardiorespiratory function. Incontinence of bladder and bowel.

vegetative state may recover further, even fully. *Persistent vegetative state* (PVS) is defined as a vegetative state present for at least 1 month. With a high degree of probability, PVS in adults and children may be considered permanent 12 months after traumatic injury and 3 months after nontraumatic injury (usually following anoxic-ischemic brain damage).

Of patients comatose following head injury, after one year roughly one-third are dead, 15% are in PVS, 45% are moderately to severely disabled, and 7% have made good recovery. Of patients comatose following anoxic-ischemic injury, after one year 53% are dead, 32% are in PVS, and only 15% have awakened. The neurologic examination and physiologic testing may more readily predict bad than good outcome. In patients with anoxic-ischemic coma, absent motor response to pain or absent pupillary reaction to light on day 3 has a nearly 100% positive predictive value for death or PVS. Other neurologic signs are less predictive. The EEG in comatose patients may identify intermittent or non-convulsive seizures or reflect cerebral ischemia caused by sudden elevations of intracranial pressure. Particular EEG abnormalities (e.g., invariant frequencies and amplitudes unreactive to stimuli, generalized suppression, or burst-suppression) may predict poor outcome and may be difficult to interpret in the presence of sedative drugs. More reliable is evoked-response testing, which is not influenced by drugs. In both traumatic and anoxic-ischemic coma, bilateral absence of the cortical N2O response to median nerve stimulation is nearly 100% specific for death or PVS.

Most patients with PVS have extensive thalamic and subcortical white matter damage, with less consistent damage to the cerebral cortex. Functional imaging and

▶ TABLE 4.4 Criteria for Determination of Brain Death

I. A. Prerequisites
    1. Clinical or neuroimaging evidence of an acute CNS catastrophe that is compatible with the clinical diagnosis of brain death
    2. Exclusion of complicating medical conditions that may confound clinical assessment (no severe electrolyte, acid-base, or endocrine disturbance)
    3. No drug intoxication or poisoning
    4. Core temperature $\geq 32°C$ (90 °F)
  B. Cardinal findings
Coma—no cerebral motor response to pain in all extremities (nail-bed pressure and supraorbital)
    1. Absence of brainstem reflexes
      a. Pupils
        i. No response to bright light
        ii. Size: mid position (4 mm) to dilated (9 mm)
      b. Ocular movement
        (i) No oculocephalic reflex (testing only when no fracture or instability of the cervical spine is apparent)
        (ii) No deviation of the eyes to irrigation in each ear with 50 mL of cold water (allow 1 min after injection and at least 5 mins between testing on each side)
      c. Facial sensation and facial motor response
        (i) No corneal reflex to touch with a throat swab
        (ii) No jaw reflex
        (iii) No grimacing to deep pressure on nail bed, supraorbital ridge, or temporomandibular joint
      d. Pharyngeal and tracheal reflexes
        (i) No response after stimulation of the posterior pharynx with tongue blade
        (ii) No cough response to bronchial suctioning
    2. Apnea-testing performed as follows:
      a. Prerequisites
        (i) Core temperature $\geq 36.5°C$ or 97 °F
        (ii) Systolic blood pressure ≥ 90 mm Hg
        (iii) Euvolemia. Option: positive fluid balance in the previous 6 hours
        (iv) Normal arterial PO_2. Option: preoxygenation to obtain arterial $PO_2 \geq 200$ mm Hg
      b. Connect a pulse oximeter and disconnect the ventilator.
      c. Deliver 100% O_2, 6 L/min, into the trachea (option: place a cannula at the level of the carina).
      d. Look closely for respiratory movements (abdominal or chest excursions that produce adequate tidal volumes).
      e. Measure arterial PO_2, PCO_2, and pH after approximately 8 mins and reconnect the ventilator. (CO_2 partial pressure increases at a rate of approximately 3 mm Hg per min.)
      f. If respiratory movements are absent and arterial PCO_2 is ≥ 60 mm Hg (option: 20 mm Hg increase in PCO_2 over a baseline normal PCO_2), the apnea test result is positive (i.e., it supports the diagnosis of brain death).
      g. If respiratory movements are observed, the apnea test result is negative. If deoxygenation or cardiac arrhythmia require termination of apnea testing before $PaCO_2$ of 60 mm Hg is reached, the test is indeterminate and another confirmation test should be considered.
II. Pitfalls in the diagnosis of brain death
The following conditions may interfere with the clinical diagnosis of brain death, so that the diagnosis may not be made with certainty on clinical grounds alone. Confirmation tests are recommended.
  A. Severe facial trauma
  B. Preexisting pupillary abnormalities
  C. Toxic levels of any sedative drugs, aminoglycosides, tricyclic antidepressants, anticholinergics, antiepileptic drugs, chemotherapeutic agents, or neuromuscular blocking agents
  D. Sleep apnea or severe pulmonary disease resulting in chronic retention of CO_2
III. Clinical observations compatible with the diagnosis of brain death
These manifestations are occasionally seen and should not be misinterpreted as evidence for brainstem function.
  A. Tendon reflexes; superficial abdominal reflexes; triple flexion response
  B. Babinski reflex
  C. Respiratory-like movements (shoulder elevation and adduction, back arching, intercostals expansion without significant tidal volumes)
  D. Spontaneous movements of limbs other than pathologic flexion or extension. Responses including facial twitching, flexion at the waist, slow turning of the head, undulating movements of the toes, and shoulder adduction with arm flexion. Such movements sometimes occur during apnea testing or following pronunciation of brain death and disconnection from the ventilator ("Lazarus sign").
  E. Sweating, blushing, tachycardia
  F. Normal blood pressure without pharmacological support or sudden increases in blood pressure
  G. Absence of diabetes insipidus

(continued)

▶ **TABLE 4.4 Criteria for Determination of Brain Death (Continued)**

IV. Confirmation laboratory tests (Options)

    For subjects 1 yr old or more and for adults, a repeat examination should be performed 6 hrs later. For subjects with anoxic-ischemic brain damage the interval should be 24 hrs.

    For children under 2 mths old , the interval should be 12 hrs, and for those >1 year to <18 yrs old, it should be 12 hrs.

    Children less than 2 mths old should have two confirmation tests. Children >2 mths to <1 yr old should have one confirmation test. For children >1 yr old and adults, confirmation tests are optional.

    A. Conventional angiography. Response: no intracerebral filling at the level of the carotid bifurcation or circle of Willis. The external carotid circulation is patent, and filling of the superior longitudinal sinus may be delayed.

    B. Electroencephalography. Response: no electrical activity during at least 30 mins of recording.

    C. Transcranial Doppler ultrasonography

        1. Response: 10% of patients may not have temporal insonation windows. Therefore, the initial absence of Doppler signals cannot be interpreted as consistent with brain death.

        2. Response: small systolic peaks in early systole without diastolic flow or reverberating flow, indicating very high vascular resistance associated with greatly increased intracranial pressure.

    D. Technetium-99m hexamethylpropylene-amineoxime brain scan. Response: no isotope uptake in brain parenchyma ("hollow skull phenomenon").

    E. Somatosensory evoked potentials. Response: bilateral absence of N20-P22 response with median nerve stimulation.

magnetoencephalographic responses to sensory stimulation may identify residual cerebral activity in PVS patients, some of whom demonstrate behavioral fragments such as facial grimacing, single word utterances, or screaming. Such responses are considered compatible with nonawareness. Nonetheless, making the diagnosis of PVS may be problematic.

A proposed separate category of incomplete wakefulness, the *minimally conscious state*, describes patients with inconsistent but discernible evidence of awareness. That proposal has added controversy to the already intense ethical debate generated by the technologic feasibility of indefinitely prolonging life without consciousness.

BRAIN DEATH

Unlike the vegetative state in which the brainstem is intact, the term *brain death* means that neither the cerebrum nor the brainstem is functioning. The only spontaneous activity is cardiovascular, apnea persists in the presence of hypercarbia sufficient for respiratory drive, and the only reflexes present are those mediated by the spinal cord (Table 4.4). In adults, brain death rarely lasts more than a few days and is always followed by circulatory collapse. In the United States, brain death is equated with legal death. When criteria are met, artificial ventilation and blood pressure support are appropriately discontinued, regardless of whether or not organ harvesting is intended.

SUGGESTED READINGS

Banasiak KJ, Lister G: Brain death in children. *Curr Op Pediatr* 2003;15:288–293.

Bernat JL: Questions remaining about the minimally conscious state. *Neurology* 2002;58:337–338.

Bernat JL. On irreversibility as a prerequisite for brain death determination. *Adv Exp Med Biol* 2004;550:161–167.

Childs NL, Mercer WN. Late improvement in consciousness after posttraumatic vegetative state. *N Engl J Med* 1996;334:24–25.

Claassen J, Mayer SA: Continuous electroencephalographic monitoring in neurocritical care. *Curr Neurol Neurosci Rep* 2002;2:534–540.

Fisher CM. The neurological examination of the comatose patient. *Acta Neurol Scand* 1969;45[Suppl 36]:1–56.

Giacino JT, Ashwal S, Childs N, et al: The minimally conscious state. Definition and diagnostic criteria. *Neurology* 2002;58:349–353.

Goudreau JL, Wijdicks EFM, Emery SF: Complications during apnea testing in the determination of brain death: predisposing factors. *Neurology* 2000;55:1045–1048.

Michelson DJ, Ashwal S. Evaluation of coma and brain death. *Semin Pediatr Neurol* 2004;11(2):105–118.

Payne K, Taylor RM, Stocking C, et al. Physicians' attitudes about the care of patients in the persistent vegetative state: a national survey. *Ann Intern Med* 1996;125:104–110.

Plum F, Posner JB. *The diagnosis of stupor and coma*, 3rd ed. Philadelphia: FA Davis Co, 1980.

Report of the Quality Standards Subcommittee of the American Academy of Neurology: Practice parameters. *Neurology* 1995;45:1012–1014; 1015–1018.

Robinson LR, Mickleson PJ, Tirschwell DL, et al: Predictive value of somatosensory evoked potentials for awakening from coma. *Crit Care Med* 2003;31:960–967.

Saposnik G, Bueri JA, Maurino J, et al: Spontaneous and reflex movements in brain death. *Neurology* 2000;54:221.

Schiff ND, Ribary U, Rodriguez Moreno D, et al: Residual cerebral activity and behavioural fragments can remain in the persistently vegetative brain. *Brain* 2003;125:1210–1234.

Wijdicks EFM: The diagnosis of brain death. *N Engl J Med* 2001;344:1215–1221.

Young GB: The EEG in coma. *J Clin Neurophysiol* 2000;17:473–485.

Chapter 5

Diagnosis of Pain and Paresthesias

Lewis P. Rowland

All pain sensations are carried by nerves and therefore concern neurology. However, not all pain is relevant to neurologic diagnosis. Some authorities divide pain into two major categories. *Neuropathic pain* is caused by a lesion of the peripheral or CNS and is manifest by sensory symptoms and signs. *Somatic pain* arises from the stimulation of peripheral nerve endings by lesions in a ligament, joint capsule, muscle or bone.

The pain of any acute traumatic lesion is a separate concern and except for attacks of herpes zoster or diabetic radiculopathy, pain in the thorax or abdomen almost always implies a visceral disorder rather than one of the spinal cord or nerve roots. Headache and other head pains, in contrast, are a major neurologic concern (see Chapters 8 and 140). In this chapter we will consider pain in the neck, low back, and limbs.

Pain syndromes often include another sensory aberration, *paresthesia*, a spontaneous and abnormal sensation. The problem may arise from an abnormality anywhere along the sensory pathway from the peripheral nerves to the sensory cortex. Paresthesias are often described as *pins-and-needles sensations* and are recognizable by anyone who has ever had an injection of local anesthetic for dental repairs. CNS disorders may cause particular kinds of paresthesias, as follows: focal sensory seizures with cortical lesions, spontaneous pain in the thalamic syndrome, or bursts of paresthesias down the back or into the arms on flexing the neck (*Lhermitte symptoms*) in patients with multiple sclerosis or other disorders of the cervical spinal cord. Level lesions of the spinal cord may cause either a band sensation or a girdle sensation, a vague sense of awareness of altered sensation encircling the abdomen, or there may be a *sensory level* (i.e., altered sensation below the level of the spinal cord lesion). Nerve root lesions or isolated peripheral nerve lesions may also cause paresthesias, but the most intense and annoying paresthesia is due to multiple symmetric peripheral neuropathy (polyneuropathy). *Dysesthesia* or *allodynia* is the term for the disagreeably abnormal sensations evoked by ordinarily non-noxious stimuli. For instance, merely touching the skin in an area of abnormal sensation or even the pressure of bedclothes or a breeze may not be tolerable.

Allodynia may follow lesions of the thalamus or peripheral nerves.

Myofascial pain and *fibromyalgia* are syndromes of chronic pain that are attributed to "trigger point" stimulation, without objective evidence of neural injury, and may be laden with emotional content.

Medical students are often confused by a patient's reports of paresthesias when the review of systems is recorded or when, in the sensory examination, they find abnormalities that do not conform to normal anatomic patterns. Two general rules may help:

1. If paresthesias are not persistent, if instead they come and go, they are not likely to imply a neurologic lesion. For instance, pressure on a nerve commonly causes transient paresthesias in normal people who cross their legs, sit too long on a toilet seat, drape an arm over the back of a chair, or lean on one elbow while holding a newspaper in that hand. Many people have fleeting paresthesias of unknown cause and no diagnostic significance.

2. If paresthesias do persist and the examiner fails to find a corresponding neurologic abnormality to explain it, the patient should be reexamined. Persistent paresthesias reliably imply an abnormality of sensory pathways.

NECK PAIN

Most chronic neck pain is caused by bony abnormalities (e.g., cervical osteoarthritis or other forms of arthritis) or by local trauma. If pain remains local (i.e., does not radiate into the arms), it is rarely of neurologic significance is unless there are abnormal neurologic signs. It may be possible to demonstrate overactive tendon reflexes, clonus, or Babinski signs in a patient who has no symptoms other than neck pain. These signs could be evidence of compression of the cervical spinal cord and might be an indication for cervical MRI or myelography to determine whether the offending lesion is arthritis, tumor, or congenital malformation of the cervical spine. However, neck pain is rarely the sole symptom of a compressive lesion.

Neck pain of neurologic significance is usually accompanied by other symptoms and signs, depending on the location of the lesion: *radicular* pain is denoted by radiation down the medial (ulnar) or lateral (radial) aspect of the arm, sometimes down to the corresponding fingers. Cutaneous sensation is altered within the area innervated by the compromised root, or below the level of spinal end compression. The motor disorder may be evident by weakness and wasting of hand muscles innervated by the affected root, and the gait may be abnormal if there are corticospinal signs of cervical spinal cord compression. When autonomic fibers in the spinal cord are compromised, abnormal urinary frequency, urgency, or incontinence may occur; there may be bowel symptoms, and men may note sexual dysfunction. Cervical cord compression may lead to loss of tendon reflexes in the arms and overactive reflexes in the legs. Cervical pain of neurologic significance may be affected by movement of the head and neck, and it may be exaggerated by natural Valsalva maneuvers in coughing, sneezing, or straining during bowel movements.

Cervical spondylosis is a more common cause of neck pain than is spinal cord tumor, but it is probably not possible to make the diagnostic distinction without MRI or myelography because the pain may be similar in the two conditions. In patients younger than 40 years, neck pain is less likely to be caused by cervical spondylosis and more likely to originate with tumors, spinal arteriovenous malformations, or congenital anomalies of the cervicooccipital region.

LOW BACK PAIN

The most common cause of low back pain is herniated nucleus pulposus, but it is difficult to determine the exact frequency because acute attacks usually clear spontaneously and chronic low back pain is colored by psychologic factors. The pain of an acute herniation of a lumbar disc is characteristically abrupt in onset and brought on by heavy lifting, twisting, or Valsalva maneuvers (sneezing, coughing, or straining during bowel movements). The patient may not be able to stand erect because paraspinal muscles contract so vigorously, yet the pain may be relieved as soon as the patient lies down, only to return again on any attempt to stand. The pain may be restricted to the low back or may radiate into one or both buttocks or down the posterior aspect of the leg to the thigh, knee, or foot. The distribution of pain sometimes gives a precise delineation of the nerve root involved, but this is probably true in only a minority of cases. The pain of an acute lumbar disc herniation is so stereotyped that the diagnosis may be made even if there are no reflex, motor, or sensory changes.

Chronic low back pain is a different matter. If neurologic abnormalities are present on examination, MRI or myelography is often indicated to determine whether the problem is caused by tumor, lumbar spondylosis with or without spinal stenosis, or arachnoiditis. If there are no neurologic abnormalities or if the patient has already had a laminectomy, chronic low back pain may pose a diagnostic and therapeutic dilemma. This major public health problem is accountable in many of the patients who enroll in pain clinics.

ARM PAIN

Pain in the arms takes on a different significance when there is no neck pain. Local pain arises from musculoskele-

tal diseases (e.g., bursitis or arthritis), which are now common because of widespread participation in sports by people who are not properly prepared.

Chronic pain may arise from invasion of the brachial plexus by tumors that extend directly from lung or breast tissue or that metastasize from more remote areas. The brachial plexus may also be affected by a transient illness (e.g., brachial plexus neuritis) that includes arm pain that is often poorly localized. The combination of pain, weakness, and wasting has given rise to the name *neuralgic amyotrophy*. Amyotrophy is taken from Greek words meaning loss of nourishment to muscles; in practice, it implies the wasting of muscle that follows denervation rather than originating in primary diseases of muscle.

Thoracic outlet syndromes are another cause of arm pain that originates in the brachial plexus. The pain of a true thoracic outlet syndrome is usually brought on by particular positions of the arm and is a cause of diagnostic vexation because there may be no abnormality on examination (see Chapter 70, Thoracic Outlet Syndrome). In a true thoracic outlet syndrome, the neurologic problems are often caused by compressed and distended blood vessels that in turn, secondarily compress nerves or lead to ischemia of nerves.

Single nerves may be involved in *entrapment neuropathies* that cause pain in the hands. Carpal tunnel syndrome of the median nerve is the best known entrapment neuropathy. The ulnar nerve is more commonly affected at the elbow but may be subject to compression at the wrist. The paresthesias of entrapment neuropathies are restricted to the distribution of the affected nerve and differ from the paresthesias of areas innervated by nerve roots, although the distinction may be difficult to make if only a portion of the area supplied by a particular nerve root is affected.

Causalgia (see Chapter 71, Neuropathic Pain) is the name given to a constant, burning pain accompanied by trophic changes that include red glossy skin, sweating in the affected area, and abnormalities of hair and nails. The trophic changes are attributed to an autonomic disorder. Causalgia was described in the 19th century in a monograph by Mitchell, Morehouse, and Keen when they reviewed gunshot wounds and other nerve injuries of American Civil War veterans. The basic mechanisms of causalgia are still poorly understood. The traumatic lesions of peripheral nerves are usually incomplete, and several nerves are often involved simultaneously.

Causalgia usually follows high-velocity missile wounds (e.g., from bullets or shrapnel). It is less commonly caused by traction injury and is only rarely seen in inflammatory neuropathy or other types of peripheral nerve disease. The arms are more often involved than the legs, and the lesions are usually above the elbow or below the knee. Symptoms usually begin within the first few days following injury. Causalgic pain most often involves the hand. The shiny red skin, accompanied by fixed joints, is followed eventually by osteoporosis. Both physical and emotional factors seem to play a role. Causalgia may be relieved by sympathectomy early in the course of treatment and may be due to *ephaptic transmission* through connections between efferent autonomic fibers at the site of partial nerve injury. This concept of an "artificial synapse" following nerve injury has been widely accepted but there has been no convincing anatomic or physiologic corroboration.

Reflex sympathetic dystrophy (now called *"complex regional pain"*) refers to the local tissue swelling and bony changes that accompany causalgia. Similar changes may be encountered after minor trauma or arthritis of the wrist. In the shoulder–hand syndrome, inflammatory arthritis of the shoulder joint may be followed by painful swelling of the hand, with local vascular changes, disuse, and atrophy of muscle and bone. Sympathectomy has been recommended for relief.

A major problem in selecting appropriate management of causalgic syndromes is the lack of properly controlled comparisons of placebo with sympathetic blockade, as well as the difficulty in evaluating psychogenic factors, and the confusion caused by incomplete syndromes (with or without preceding trauma, with or without attendant vascular abnormalities, and with or without response to sympathetic block).

LEG PAIN AND PARESTHESIAS

Leg pain due to occlusive vascular disease, especially with diabetes, varies markedly in different series but seems to be related to the duration of the diabetes and shows increasing incidence with age. Pain may be a major symptom of diabetic peripheral neuropathy of the multiple symmetric type. Diabetic mononeuritis multiplex, attributed to infarcts of the lumbosacral plexus or a peripheral nerve, is a cause of more restricted pain, usually of abrupt onset. Diabetic mononeuropathy may be disabling and alarming at the onset, but both pain and motor findings improve in a few months to 1 or 2 years. Nutritional neuropathy is an important cause of limb pain, especially in the legs, in some parts of the world. This condition was striking in prisoner-of-war camps in World War II and has also been noted in patients on hemodialysis. Sudden fluid shifts may cause peripheral nerve disease symptoms for a time after dialysis.

Barring intraspinal disease, the most common neurologic cause of leg pain and paresthesias is probably multiple symmetric peripheral neuropathy. The paresthesias usually take on a glove-and-stocking distribution, presumably because the nerve fibers most remote from the perikaryon are most vulnerable, or there is a length-dependent neuropathy with the longest most likely to be affected by a dying back process. The feet are usually affected, sometimes alone or sometimes with the hands; the hands are rarely involved alone. Mixed sensorimotor neuropathies show motor abnormalities with weakness and wasting, as well as loss of tendon reflexes. Some neuropathies are purely sensory. Pain is characteristic of severe diabetic neuropathy, alcoholic neuropathy, amyloid neuropathy, and some carcinomatous neuropathies, but it is uncommon in inherited neuropathies or the Guillain-Barré syndrome. The pain of peripheral neuropathy, for unknown reasons, is likely to be more severe at night.

Entrapment neuropathy rarely affects the legs; however, diabetic mononeuropathy and, especially, diabetic femoral neuropathy may cause pain of restricted distribution and abrupt onset, with later improvement of the condition that may take months.

Another major cause of leg pain is invasion of the lumbosacral plexus by tumor, but this is rarely an isolated event and other signs of the tumor are usually evident. The problem of distinguishing between spinal and vascular claudication is discussed in Chapter 68, Lumbar Spondylosis.

Limb pain and paresthesias are important in neurologic diagnoses not just because they persist for prolonged periods. They also become the objects of symptomatic therapy with analgesics, tricyclic antidepressant drugs, and monoamine oxidase inhibitors (which may affect abnormal sensations by actions other than antidepressant effects), transcutaneous nerve stimulation, dorsal column stimulation, cordotomy, acupuncture, and other procedures. The long list of remedies attests to the limitations of each. Psychologic factors may not be ignored in assessing and managing chronic pain problems.

SUGGESTED READINGS

Bruera ED, Portenoy RK, eds. *Cancer Pain: Assessment and Management.* Cambridge: Cambridge University Press, 2003.

Devo RA, Weinstein JN. Low back pain. *N Engl J Med* 2001;344:363–370.

Deyo RA, Rainville J, Kent DL. What can the history and physical examination tell us about low back pain? *JAMA* 1992;268:760–765.

Dotson RM. Causalgia—reflex sympathetic dystrophy—sympathetically maintained pain: myth and reality. *Muscle Nerve* 1993;16:1049–1055.

Dworkin RH, Backonja M, Rowbotham MC, et al. Advances in neuropathic pain: diagnosis, mechanisms, and treatment recommendations. *Arch Neurol* 2003;60:1524–1534.

Dworkin RH, Breitbart WS, eds. Psychosocial aspects of pain: A handbook for health care providers. In: *Progress in Pain Research and Management,* vol. 27. Seattle WA: International Association for the Study of Pain, 2004.

Fields HL. *Pain Mechanisms and Management.* New York: McGraw-Hill, 1999.

Frank A. Low back pain. *BMJ* 1993;306:901–909.

Frymoyer JW. Back pain and sciatica. *N Engl J Med* 1988;318:291–300.

Grabow TS, Christo PJ, Raja SN. Complex regional pain syndrome: diagnostic controversies, psychological dysfunction, and emerging concepts. *Adv Psychosom Med* 2004;25:89–101.

Hansson P, Fields HL, Hill RG, Marchettini P, eds. Neuropathic pain: pathophysiology and treatment. In: *Progress in Pain Research and Management,* vol. 21. Seattle WA: International Association for the Study of Pain, 2001.

Hartvigsen J, Lings S, Leboeuf-Yde C, Bakketeig L. Psychosocial factors at work in relation to low back pain and consequences of low back pain; a systematic, critical review of prospective cohort studies. *Occup Environ Med* 2004 Jan;61(1):e2.

Livingston WK, Fields HL, ed. *Pain and Suffering.* Seattle, WA: International Association for the Study of Pain, 1998.

Mitchell SW, Morehouse GR, Keen WW. *Gunshot Wounds and Other Injuries of Nerves.* Philadelphia: JB Lippincott, 1864.

Payne R, Patt RB, Hill S, eds. *Assessment and Treatment of Cancer Pain.* Seattle, WA: International Association for the Study of Pain, 1998.

Rose S, Wall PD. *Pain.* New York NY: Columbia University Press, 2000.

Schwartzman RJ, Maleki J. Postinjury neuropathic pain syndromes. *Med Clin North Am* 1999;83:597–626.

Speed C. Low back pain. *BMJ* 2004 May 8;328(7448):1119–1121.

Wall PD, Melzack R, eds. *Textbook of Pain,* 4th ed. Edinburgh: Churchill Livingstone, 1999.

Woolf CJ, Mannion RJ. Neuropathic pain: aetiology, symptoms, mechanisms, and management. *Lancet* 1999;353:1959–1964.

Chapter 6

Dizziness and Hearing Loss

Ian S. Storper

ANATOMY OF THE EAR

The ear is divided into three parts: the outer ear, the middle ear, and the inner ear. The outer ear consists of the auricle, external auditory canal, and tympanic membrane. The middle ear is the cavity that connects the outer ear to the cochlea and vestibular system. It consists of the ossicles, the tympanic segment of the facial nerve, oval and round windows, lateral Eustachian tube, and tympanic plexus. The inner ear consists of the cochlea and the vestibular system. The cochlea is the snail-shaped organ that transduces sound pressure waves into electrical impulses on the eighth nerve. The vestibular system has five end organs: the three semicircular canals, the utricle and the saccule. The horizontal, superior and posterior semicircular canals are located orthogonally and sense angular acceleration in their respective plane. The utricle and saccule sense linear acceleration and head position. The superior vestibular nerve consists of afferents from the horizontal and superior semicircular canals and the utricle. The inferior vestibular nerve consists of afferents from the posterior semicircular canal and the saccule. The superior and inferior vestibular nerves join to form the vestibular nerve. The vestibular nerve joins the cochlear nerve, consisting of auditory afferents, to form the vestibulocochlear, or eighth cranial, nerve. From here, the nerve projects to the cochlear and vestibular nuclei, and eventually to the auditory and vestibular cortices.

In animal models, the peripheral portion of the system is caudal to the Scarpa ganglion; the central portion is rostral. In human beings, the peripheral portion of the system includes the eighth nerve and all structures caudal; the central portion includes all structures rostral. Hearing loss, tinnitus, or vertigo may result from lesions to structures along these pathways. Many diagnoses may be determined by taking an accurate history and performing a careful physical examination. In certain cases, laboratory tests may be necessary to achieve a diagnosis; here the history and physical dictate the tests that should be ordered.

TINNITUS

Tinnitus is defined as any abnormal sound in the head. Up to 40% of Americans experience it at some time. It may be classified as objective or subjective, continuous or pulsatile. *Objective tinnitus* is heard by the examiner as well as the patient; *subjective tinnitus* is heard only by the patient. Although objective tinnitus is rare, it is associated with serious conditions that mandate early diagnosis.

Pulsatile objective tinnitus may be caused by intravascular turbulence, increased blood flow, or movement in the Eustachian tube. Audible bruits from vascular turbulence may caused by temporal arteritis, atherosclerosis of the carotid or vertebral arteries, aortic stenosis, arteriovenous malformations of the head and neck, and vascular tumors (e.g., glomus jugulare, tympanicum, or vagale). A continuous hum may result from asymmetric enlargement of the sigmoid sinus or internal jugular vein. Nonpulsatile objective tinnitus may result from temporomandibular joint (TMJ) syndrome or palatal myoclonus.

Pulsatile subjective tinnitus may be caused by hypertension, hyperthyroidism, or increased intracranial pressure. In addition, intracranial aneurysms and atherosclerosis may cause this symptom. As part of the diagnostic evaluation of pulsatile tinnitus, the stethoscope should be used for auscultation of the ear, head, and neck in all patients who complain of noises in the head or ear. Patients with pulsatile tinnitus should also have their blood pressures checked and fundi examined.

Subjective tinnitus is usually caused by damage to the auditory system. The abnormality may be central or peripheral. While symmetrical, bilateral, longstanding tinnitus is usually caused by presbycusis and is innocuous, it may also be an early warning signal. For instance, tinnitus after exposure to loud noise is due to cochlear injury, usually resulting from a temporary threshold shift in hearing. Repeated exposure to noise may result in permanent cochlear damage and permanent hearing loss.

Unilateral tinnitus is an early symptom of acoustic neuroma and reflects hearing loss. Persistent tinnitus therefore requires otologic evaluation, including hearing tests. The basic hearing tests for evaluation of patients with tinnitus include pure tone and speech audiometry, as well as middle ear impedance measures of tympanometry and measurement of the threshold and decay of the stapedial reflex. If the audiogram does not show a clear explanation of the cause of the tinnitus, MRI is indicated to rule out central pathology.

HEARING LOSS

Hearing loss may be central or peripheral. Central hearing loss is rare. Typical symptoms include difficulty hearing despite normal audiogram or difficulty understanding words in complicated situations, such as background noise. Often, patients with central hearing loss are told by numerous physicians that their hearing is normal. For diagnosis, a central audiologic evaluation includes understanding words. If central hearing loss has been found, it is essential to check MRI to rule out the possibility of thalamic lesion. To remedy central hearing loss, listening therapy is ordered.

Hearing loss, as we usually think of it, is peripheral. It may be classified as conductive or sensorineural. When a patient with hearing loss is evaluated, history and physical examination are essential. The history should include degree of hearing loss, laterality, time course, types of sounds that appear to be deficient, whether there was an inciting event, and what the patient's own voice sounds like. Patients should be questioned as to whether there are associated symptoms, such as tinnitus, vertigo, or fullness in the ear. Family history should be discussed, because many causes of hearing loss are inherited. On physical examination, the auricle, external auditory canal and tympanic membranes are evaluated. Moreover, in the case of Eustachian tube dysfunction, nasopharyngeal examination should be performed to rule out tumor.

Diagnostic Testing

Diagnostic testing begins in the clinician's office with Weber and Rinne testing. The Weber test is performed by placing a 256 Hz tuning fork in the center of the patient's forehead and asking where it is heard. The Rinne test is performed by placing a 128 Hz tuning fork in the air in front of the ear and then on the bone behind the ear. The patient is asked which is perceived as louder. In normal ears and in those with sensorineural hearing loss, the sound is heard louder in front of the ear. If the tuning fork is heard louder behind an ear, there is conductive hearing loss of at least 30 decibels (dB) present. The Weber test lateralizes toward an ear with asymmetric, conductive loss

and away from an ear with an asymmetric, sensorineural loss.

The next test to be checked is the complete audiologic evaluation (CAE). This test consists of pure-tone audiometry, speech reception thresholds and discrimination, impedance testing, and acoustic reflexes. Additional diagnostic testing, outlined in the sections below, is ordered if the cause of the hearing loss is not apparent.

Conductive Hearing Loss

Conductive hearing loss occurs when there is a physical impediment to sound reaching the oval window. Most commonly, it is caused by blockage of the external auditory canal with cerumen. Other causes from the external ear include infection (by swelling of the skin or purulent drainage), stenosis due to trauma or bony overgrowth, and neoplasms such as squamous cell or basal cell carcinoma. Middle ear causes include tympanic membrane perforation, cholesteatoma, Eustachian tube dysfunction, ossicular fixation, ossicular discontinuity, tumors such as glomus tympanicum, and either acute or serous otitis media. Patients with conductive hearing loss often complain that they hear their own voice reverberate.

The cause of conductive hearing loss is usually determined by history and physical examination. Cerumen impaction, auditory canal or middle ear tumor, infection or fluid, Eustachian tube dysfunction, stenosis, tympanic membrane perforation, and cholesteatoma are all readily apparent on examination. Patients with ossicular discontinuity or otosclerosis often have normal examinations. However, the Weber test will lateralize to the affected ear and bone conduction will be heard louder than air conduction (termed negative) in the Rinne test.

Once conductive hearing loss is suspected, CAE is ordered unless a patient is acutely infected; in that instance, treatment is prescribed first. CAE will confirm whether conductive loss is indeed present. In addition, impedance testing will let the clinician know whether there is fluid in a middle ear, Eustachian tube dysfunction, unrecognized eardrum perforation, or normal pressures. A hypercompliant tympanic membrane may suggest ossicular discontinuity; a normal to stiff tympanic membrane may suggest otosclerosis, a condition where extra spongy bone grows around the edge of the stapes footplate, inhibiting sound transmission to the inner ear. If a tumor is suspected or a cholesteatoma—which appears as pearly white debris—is seen, the next diagnostic test to be checked is CT of the temporal bones. It will delineate the extent of the disease and help in determining appropriate management. If the hearing loss is purely conductive and the physical examination is normal, CT is unnecessary.

The treatment of conductive hearing loss is aimed at the underlying cause. Cerumen is removed. Infections are treated with oral and topical antibiotics.

Management of malignant tumor typically involves surgical resection and radiation therapy. Cholesteatomas and glomus tympanicum tumors are removed surgically. Chronic ear infections with tympanic membrane perforation, otosclerosis and ossicular discontinuity also may be successfully repaired with microsurgical techniques. In the absence of serious illness, or if there is persistent postoperative conductive hearing loss, hearing aids may be considered.

In children with conductive hearing loss due to serous otitis media, pressure equalization tubes may restore hearing to normal levels if the fluid does not respond to medical management. In all children with conductive hearing loss, either surgical restorative measures or amplification should be employed as soon as possible, as it is well known that speech and language delays may otherwise occur.

Sensorineural Hearing Loss

Sensorineural hearing loss occurs with defects in the cochlea, cochlear nerve, or the brainstem and cortical connections. Patients tend to speak with a loud voice, because they cannot hear their own voices well. Findings on physical examination are normal unless a middle ear disorder extends into the inner ear. In that case the hearing loss will be both conductive and sensorineural, or "mixed." In sensorineural hearing loss, tuning-fork tests show that air conduction exceeds bone conduction (positive Rinne test); in the Weber test, the tuning fork seems louder in the better ear.

History and thorough physical examination are crucial. As in conductive hearing loss, duration of symptoms, laterality, associated symptoms, inciting event, and family history are important. CAE is performed to determine the degree of the loss and may help determine the cause. Patients with cochlear damage may show low-frequency hearing loss, a flat audiometric configuration, or more commonly, high-frequency hearing loss. The most common cause is presbycusis, or age-related cochlear hair cell degeneration. Typically, symmetric high-frequency hearing loss is found. Other causes include noise exposure, ototoxic drugs, congenital cochlear defects, and viral or bacterial infections. Speech discrimination is less preserved, compared to the extent of pure-tone hearing loss. The stapedial reflex threshold, as determined by impedance measurements, is present.

Patients with damage to the cochlear nerve, such as the neural form of presbycusis or compression of the nerve by an acoustic neuroma, usually show high-frequency hearing loss, as do patients with cochlear lesions. In nerve lesions, however, speech discrimination tends to be more severely affected than pure-tone hearing loss. The stapedial reflex either is absent or shows abnormal adaptation or decay. The test is carried out as part of impedance audiometry and is useful in determining the site of the lesion.

In all cases of asymmetric sensorineural hearing loss, it is imperative to conduct an MRI of the brain and internal auditory canals with, and without, gadolinium. MRI has higher sensitivity and specificity than any other test in the diagnosis of cerebellopontine angle tumors, such as acoustic neuroma.

Central lesions, such as recurrent small strokes or multiple sclerosis, often cause no detectable pure-tone hearing loss because the central auditory pathways are bilateral. Some patients, however, do note hearing loss. MRI may show microvascular small-vessel ischemic disease or abnormalities consistent with multiple sclerosis. If MRI is normal, hearing should be evaluated by brainstem auditory evoked responses, which may show bilateral conduction delay despite normal pure-tone hearing. Central auditory testing may show abnormalities.

As in conductive hearing loss, it is important to determine the cause of the hearing loss. Determining the cause and its remediation may prevent progression of the hearing loss or the causative disease. Unfortunately, for chronic loss, hearing is not medically or surgically restorable. Most patients with sensorineural hearing loss, however, may be helped by amplification; hearing aids that are smaller and more effective than in the past are now available. The narrow range between speech and noise is being ameliorated by improved speech processing strategies. The latest in hearing aid technology, including digital programmable devices, allows individuals to change the hearing aid settings under different acoustic conditions for better hearing, particularly in environments with noisy backgrounds. Patients with profound bilateral sensorineural hearing loss that does not respond to hearing aids may be candidates for cochlear implantation.

DIZZINESS, DISEQUILIBRIUM AND VERTIGO

There are three symptoms that are often referred to as "dizziness" by patients: dizziness, disequilibrium, and vertigo. *Dizziness* is a nonspecific term that describes a sensation of altered spatial orientation. Some authors describe it as any sensation of discomfort in the head. Dizziness may also be called "lightheadedness" or "wooziness" by patients. It may be caused by circulatory, metabolic, endocrine, degenerative, or psychologic factors. Specific classifications include presyncopal lightheadedness, ocular dizziness, multisensory dizziness, physiologic dizziness and psychophysiologic dizziness. Peripheral vestibular and central lesions must be ruled out.

Vertigo may be defined as any abnormal sensation of motion between a patient and the surroundings. It is often a spinning sensation but may also be experienced as a feeling of linear motion or falling. Vertigo may be central or peripheral.

Disequilibrium is synonymous with "unsteadiness" or "imbalance." Patients may feel normal when they are stationary, but notice difficulty when they walk. Often, they have no symptoms of vertigo or dizziness. Disequilibrium suggests a central process, but it may be peripheral. Patients with severe, bilateral, peripheral vestibular loss may also note unsteady gait and oscillopsia, the symptom in which objects seem to be moving up and down while the patient is walking.

The sense of equilibrium and position in space is an integrated function of multiple peripheral sensory inputs into the brain, including the visual, vestibular, and proprioceptive systems. The vestibular system plays a dual role, responding to gravity and linear acceleration through the utricle and saccule, and to angular acceleration through the semicircular canals. The afferent nerves from the otoliths and semicircular canals maintain a balanced, tonic rate of firing into the vestibular nuclei. If insufficient or conflicting information between the left and right ears is delivered to the CNS, vertigo results. Damage to a semicircular canal or its afferent nerve results in a sensation of angular rotation in the plane of the canal; damage to an otolith organ or its afferent nerve results in a linear or tilting sensation. Most commonly, lesions involve the entire vestibular system or nerve on one side. In this case, a sensation of motion in the horizontal plane is generated, as the vertical components cancel out.

Typical features of peripheral vertigo include a short or episodic time course, a precipitating factor, and the presence of autonomic symptoms, including sweating, pallor, nausea or vomiting. There may be associated symptoms of tinnitus, hearing loss, auditory fullness, or facial nerve weakness. In patients with central vertigo, the autonomic symptoms are relatively less severe and associated hearing loss is unusual. Associated neurologic symptoms are different and may include: diplopia, hemianopsia, weakness, numbness, dysarthria, ataxia, and loss of consciousness. Oscillopsia may be severe.

COMMON CAUSES OF VERTIGO

Diagnosis

The history and physical examination are essential in determining the proper differential diagnosis for a dizzy patient. Table 6.1 and Table 6.2 contain lists of potential causes that differentiate between peripheral vertigo and central vertigo.

Points to address in the history include whether the symptom is that of vertigo, disequilibrium or dizziness. It is important to understand the nature of the symptom, as well as it may be communicated by a patient. Whether symptoms have an inciting factor, presence of autonomic or associated symptoms, duration, frequency, past history,

▶ **TABLE 6.1 Common Causes of Peripheral Vertigo**

Benign paroxysmal positional vertigo
Bacterial or viral infections
Vestibular neuritis
Ménière disease
Labyrinthine ischemia or hemorrhage
Tumor
Trauma
Temporal bone fracture
Labyrinthine concussion
Perilymphatic fistula (fistula may also be caused by cholesteatoma)
Metabolic disorders
Diabetes mellitus
Uremia
Hypothyroidism
Paget disease
Acute alcohol intoxication
Ototoxicity
Aminoglycosides
Cisplatin
Autoimmune inner ear disease

exacerbating maneuvers, and severity are all important. The sequence of events in an episode, such as whether an aura or a sensation of auditory fullness precedes an episode, or if symptoms are episodic, is crucial. If hearing loss, tinnitus or fullness in an ear is present, peripheral etiology is probable. If a patient loses consciousness or is disoriented, central etiology is probable. Also, if neurologic symptoms such as visual changes, hemiparesis, sensory changes, or headaches are present, a central etiology is probable.

The past medical history is also important. Many patients with vertigo have experienced it before. Family history is also relevant; numerous disorders causing such symptoms may be hereditary. A careful social history

▶ **TABLE 6.2 Common Causes of Central Vertigo**

Neurologic complications of ear infections
Epidural, subdural, intraparenchymal brain abscess
Meningitis
Vascular disease
Vertebrobasilar insufficiency
Brainstem or cerebellar hemorrhage or infarct
Migraine
Tumors
Trauma
Cerebellar degeneration syndromes
Alcoholic, familial, etc.
Disorders of the craniovertebral junction
Basilar impression
Atlantoaxial dislocations
Chiari malformations
Multiple sclerosis
Seizure

should be recorded, because alcohol, intoxicating drugs, and otosyphilis may contribute to symptoms. It is important to evaluate the possibility of mental illness, as 10% to 15% of patients with vertigo may have psychogenic cause.

The physical examination is crucial. Complete neuro-otologic and neurologic examinations are necessary. Cholesteatoma, infections, and middle ear tumors that extend medially may be seen on examination. The presence and character of nystagmus should be assessed. Gait and positional testing should be performed. Unless deemed medically unsafe, it should be determined whether vertigo may be induced on examination, and how the patient appears during the episode.

Necessity for diagnostic testing is considered next. If there is a possibility of associated hearing loss or tinnitus, CAE should be performed. Electronystagmography (ENG) may yield important information as to whether disease is central or peripheral, and occasionally yields a diagnosis. ENG should not be performed in the acutely vertiginous patient, as the induced symptoms may be unbearable.

MRI of the brain and internal auditory canals is performed to rule out intracranial pathology. The MRI should be done with and without gadolinium; diffusion-weighted images are used if stroke is being considered. MRI should be performed on all patients in whom the examiner suspects a central process, and in all patients who have had symptoms for two weeks or more. Cervical four-vessel and transcranial Doppler examinations are checked in people who are at risk for stroke. If a patient has an implanted metal device or if middle ear pathology, such as cholesteatoma, is seen on exam, CT of the temporal bones is the preferred test.

Treatment

Treatment of vertigo is aimed at its cause. The best prognostic indicator for recovery from vertigo is the proper identification of its etiology. For cases of peripheral vertigo, vestibular suppressants may be used to ameliorate the symptom, while the disease is managed. It is important to discontinue use as soon as possible, as long-term use may delay compensation.

There are three categories of vestibular suppressants. Anticholinergic drugs are thought to be effective by decreasing the rate of firing in the vestibular nuclei. The author prefers glycopyrrolate 2 mg po, twice daily as needed, provided that there are no medical contraindications. There is some sedating effect of this medication, but it is much less than with other drugs used to treat vertigo. Scopolamine, another drug in this class, is available in a patch preparation, which makes it ideal for treating motion sickness. Antihistamines are also used in the treatment of vertigo; the most commonly used of these is meclizine. These drugs are thought to affect this condition by their anticholinergic effects. While these drugs are use-

ful, they are much more sedating than pure anticholinergics. Benzodiazepines are also effective for vertigo control. However, the author prescribes them only for severe or refractory cases, owing to their habit-forming potential. For acute cases of severe peripheral vertigo, intramuscular promethazine or intravenous droperidol are beneficial.

For cases of persistent disequilibrium due to bilateral vestibular weakness or central vertigo, the gold standard is vestibular rehabilitation. This is administered by physical therapists with special training, on proper equipment.

COMMON CLINICAL ENTITIES CAUSING VERTIGO AND HEARING LOSS

Benign Positional Paroxysmal Vertigo (BPPV)

This condition is characterized by recurrent episodes of vertigo that are induced by changing head positions. Episodes last seconds at a time, and are usually first noticed after tossing in bed or reaching an item on a high shelf. There is a latency of a few seconds after the stimulating position is assumed. Most commonly, it occurs in the posterior semicircular canal and it is associated with torsional nystagmus, beating toward the floor if the patient is lying down with the head turned toward the offending ear. As the patient reverses position, a few beats of nystagmus are experienced, with the rapid phase toward the opposite side. To diagnose this condition, the patient is asked to lie down quickly from a sitting position, with the head extended and turned all the way to one side. This is called the Dix-Hallpike maneuver. If torsional nystagmus is induced, with latency and fatigability, BPPV is diagnosed. If no nystagmus is induced, the maneuver is repeated to the opposite side.

Histologic sections of temporal bones from some affected patients may demonstrate calcium carbonate crystals in the posterior semicircular canal ampulla; hence this disease is called cupulolithiasis. Fifty percent of the time, the case begins after head trauma because asymptomatic crystals, which have formed in the temporal bones on both sides, have probably jarred loose from one side.

BPPV is self limiting. Most patients are free of symptoms within a few months. Symptoms may be abolished by a variety of canalith repositioning maneuvers, the most reliable of which is the Epley index maneuver; it resolves the condition in about 95% of cases. However, symptoms may recur in the future. Labyrinthine suppressants may reduce the intensity of the vertigo. Avoiding the offending position is highly effective in avoiding the symptoms. If disabling positional vertigo persists despite canalith repositioning maneuvers and suppressant therapy, obliteration of the posterior semicircular canal through a transmastoid approach is highly effective in treating posterior canal BPPV. Hearing and the remainder of the vestibular function are preserved.

If symptoms do not respond to positional maneuvers or nystagmus is not as described above, the syndrome must be differentiated from endolymphatic hydrops with a positional component, a CNS process, or hysteria. Neurotologic evaluation including CAE, ENG, and MRI may be necessary.

Vestibular Neuritis

In this condition, vertigo occurs suddenly and severely with nausea, vomiting and nystagmus; it may last up to two weeks, and the patient may feel unsteady for several weeks afterward. There may be associated unilateral hearing loss, tinnitus and fullness. Caloric tests show a reduced response on the affected side. This syndrome occurs once; if it recurs, the diagnosis is Ménière disease. Fifty percent of the time, vestibular neuronitis follows a viral illness, leading many clinicians to believe that there is a postviral, autoimmune etiology. Vestibular suppressants prescribed only as necessary, followed by encouragement of physical activity is the recommended course of treatment.

Ménière Disease

This illness is characterized by recurrent attacks of vertigo, hearing loss, tinnitus, and aural fullness. As Ménière disease is caused by endolymphatic hydrops, management is with low-sodium diet and diuretics, with vestibular suppressants added for persistent vertigo. Chapter 144 is devoted to a discussion of this condition.

Perilymphatic Fistula

This is an abnormal communication between the perilymphatic space and endolymphatic space, or between the perilymphatic space and the middle ear, caused by rupture of inner ear membranes due to pressure trauma, such as may be experienced during scuba diving, weight lifting, or even forceful nose blowing. Sudden hearing loss and vertigo are the cardinal symptoms. Fistula may arise spontaneously in children with congenital defects of the inner ear. Prior inner ear surgery also increases the risk. Surgery to patch the fistula is necessary in select patients, in order to stop vertigo or progression of hearing loss.

Cerebellopontine Angle Tumors

The most common tumor involving the cerebellopontine angle is acoustic neuroma. The earliest symptoms are hearing loss and tinnitus; vertigo is also occasionally seen at initial presentation. This tumor therefore must be considered in the evaluation of a patient with asymmetric sensorineural hearing loss, unilateral tinnitus, or vertigo. Early diagnosis is important because microsurgical techniques have made it possible to remove the tumor completely without damaging the facial nerve, and even preserve hearing in certain conditions. Moreover, for small tumors, radiotherapy may provide a viable treatment option. All patients with asymmetric sensorineural hearing loss, unilateral tinnitus, or persistent vertigo for longer than two weeks should undergo MRI of the brain and internal auditory canals with and without gadolinium to rule out the possibility of this diagnosis. Other tumors of the cerebellopontine angle that may cause similar symptoms include meningioma, epidermoid, cholesterol granuloma, lipoma, hemangioma, and malignancy. Malignancies may include plasmacytoma, and metastases from breast, prostate, lung, renal and other carcinomas.

Drug Toxicity

Aminoglycosides, intravenous loop diuretics, intravenous erythromycin, intravenous vancomycin, intravenous cisplatin, anticonvulsants, and alcohol may cause dizziness in the form of vertigo, disequilibrium, and light-headedness. Hearing loss and tinnitus may also occur in any of the above, with the exception of alcohol intoxication. These symptoms are bilateral and are often accompanied by ataxic gait, as they variously affect the vestibular and cochlear apparatuses. Sedatives (e.g., diazepam, phenobarbital), antihistamines, mood elevators, and antidepressants may also cause light-headedness and disequilibrium. Intake of possibly toxic drugs should be reviewed with any patient complaining of "dizziness." Cessation of use of a drug usually causes clearing of the symptoms in a few days, although vestibular and cochlear damage due to aminoglycosides, intravenous loop diuretics, intravenous erythromycin, intravenous cisplatin and intravenous vancomycin may result in permanent ataxia or hearing loss. Vestibular rehabilitation and hearing aids may be of benefit. Intake of large amounts of salicylates causes reversible tinnitus and high-frequency sensorineural hearing loss.

Cardiac Arrhythmia

Cardiac arrhythmias sufficient to lower cardiac output may cause dizziness. The patient may not notice palpitations. If a cardiac arrhythmia is suspected, 24- to 48-hour continuous electrocardiograph monitoring (Holter monitor) may help establish the relationship of arrhythmias to episodes of dizziness.

Presbycusis and Presbyastasis

With the increase in life expectancy, many patients now reach ages at which degenerative losses cause disequilibrium. Above 50 years of age, there is an almost linear decline in the numbers of hair cells in the cochlea and vestibular system; age-related deterioration of vision and proprioception and loss of the ability to integrate information from those sensory systems also causes disequilibrium in older patients.

Presbycusis is the term for age-related hearing loss. It usually begins in the high frequencies and progresses to involve all frequencies. Hearing aids are the usual treatment; for extreme cases, cochlear implantation has been performed successfully.

Presbyastasis is the term for age-related loss of balance. This condition responds well to vestibular rehabilitation. It should be performed by physical therapists with special training, on special equipment. The goal is to teach patients alternative balance strategies, in an effort to prevent a fall.

Psychophysiologic Causes of Vertigo: Hyperventilation

Acute anxiety attacks or panic attacks may cause vertigo. It is not always easy to differentiate psychophysiologic cause and effect because vertigo may sometimes trigger acute anxiety or panic. Typically, the physical examination does not correlate to the history or suspected diagnosis. Laboratory tests including MRI are necessarily ordered when the symptoms are vague, as the physical examination is often unremarkable in patients with cerebellopontine angle pathology. Once the clinician is certain that anxiety is the cause of the patient's symptoms, evaluation by a psychiatrist should be requested. Patients with anxiety, depression, and panic attacks may respond to specific therapy and the appropriate psychopharmacologic agents.

SUGGESTED READINGS

Baloh RW, Honrubia V. *Clinical Neurophysiology of the Vestibular System, 2nd ed. Contemporary Neurology Series.* Philadelphia: FA Davis Co., 1990.

Baloh RW. Clinical practice. Vestibular neuritis. *N Engl J Med* 2003;248: 1027–1032.

Brackmann DE. Surgical treatment of vertigo. *J Laryngol Otol* 1990;104: 849–859.

Cohen HS, Kimball KT. Treatment variations on the Epley maneuver for benign paroxysmal positional vertigo. *Am J Otolaryngol* 2004 Jan–Feb;25(1):33–37.

El Kashlan HK, Telian SA. Diagnosis and initiating treatment for peripheral system disorders: imbalance and dizziness with normal hearing. *Otolaryngol Clin North Am* 2000;33:563–578.

Epley JM. The canalith repositioning maneuver for treatment of benign paroxysmal positional vertigo. *Otolaryngol Head Neck Surg* 1992;107:399–404.

Ménière P. Memoire sur des lesions de l'orielle interne donnant lieu a des symptoms de congestion cerebrale apoplectiforme. *Gaz Med Paris* 1861;16:597–601.

Minor LB. Labyrinthine fistulae: pathobiology and management. *Curr Opin Otolaryngol Head Neck Surg* 2003;11:340–346.

Newman AN, Storper IS, Wackym PA. Central representation of the eighth cranial nerve. In: Canalis RF, Lambert PR, eds. *The Ear: Comprehensive Otology.* Philadelphia: Lippincott Williams & Wilkins, 2000:141–156.

Schuknecht HF. Cupulolithiasis. *Arch Otolaryngol* 1969;90:113–126.

Schuknecht HF. *Pathology of the Ear,* 2nd ed. Philadelphia: Lea & Febiger, 1994.

Storper IS, Spitzer JB, Scanlan M. Use of glycopyrrolate in the treatment of Meniere's Disease. *Laryngoscope* 1998;108:1442–1445.

Wackym PA, Storper IS, Newman AN. Cochlear and vestibular ototoxicity. In: Canalis RF, Lambert PR, eds. *The Ear: Comprehensive Otology.* Philadelphia: Lippincott Williams & Wilkins, 2000:571–585.

Yueh B, Shapiro N, MacLean CH, et al. Screening and management of adult hearing loss in primary care: a scientific review. *JAMA* 2003;289:1976–1985.

Zadeh MH, Storper IS, Spitzer JB. Diagnosis and treatment of sudden-onset sensorineural hearing loss: a study of 51 patients. *Otolaryngol Head Neck Surg* 2003;128:92–98.

Chapter 7

Impaired Vision

Myles M. Behrens

Impaired vision may be due to a lesion in one or both eyes, in the retrobulbar visual pathway (including the optic nerve and optic chiasm), or in the retrochiasmal pathway. The retrochiasmal pathway includes the optic tract, geniculate body (where synapse occurs), the visual radiation through the parietal and temporal lobes, and the occipital cortex. The pattern of visual loss may identify the site of the lesion. The course and accompanying symptoms and signs may clarify its nature.

OCULAR LESIONS

Impaired vision of ocular origin may be caused by refractive error, opacity of the ocular media (which may be seen by external inspection or ophthalmoscopy), or a retinal abnormality (e.g., retinal detachment, inflammation, hemorrhage, vascular occlusion). There may be associated local symptoms or signs, such as pain or soft tissue swelling.

OPTIC NERVE LESIONS

A visual defect may originate in the optic nerve, particularly if the symptoms affect only one eye. The hallmarks of optic nerve dysfunction include blurred vision (indicated by decreased visual acuity), dimming or darkening of vision (usually with decreased color perception), and decreased pupillary reaction to light. This pupillary sign

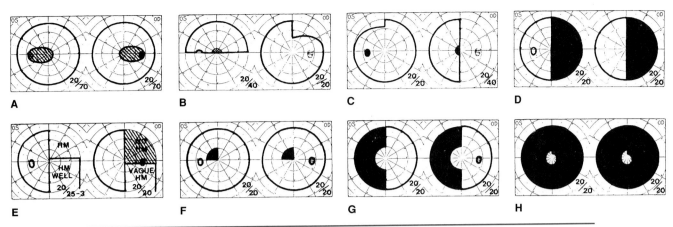

FIGURE 7.1. A: Bilateral centrocecal scotoma. **B:** Inferior altitudinal defect with central scotoma OS. (left eye) and upper temporal hemianopic (junctional) defect OD. (right eye). **C:** Bitemporal hemianopia. **D:** Total right homonymous hemianopia. **E:** Incongruous right homonymous hemianopia. **F:** Congruous left homonymous hemianopic scotoma. **G:** Left homonymous hemianopia with macular sparing. **H:** Bilateral congruous homonymous hemianopia.

is not seen if the problem is media opacity, minor retinal edema, or nonorganic visual loss. It may be present to a mild degree in simple amblyopia.

The *relative afferent pupillary defect* results from an optic nerve lesion in one eye; the sign is best shown by the swinging-flashlight test. A bright flashlight is swung from one eye to the other just below the visual axis, while the subject stares at a distant object in a dark room. Constriction of the pupils should be the same when either eye is illuminated. However, if an eye with optic nerve dysfunction is illuminated, the pupils constrict less quickly in response to the light, less completely, and less persistently than when the normal fellow eye is illuminated. If the expected constriction does not occur or if the pupils actually dilate after an initial constriction on stimulation of one eye, the test is positive. Both pupils are equal in size at all times in purely afferent defects because there is hemi-decussation of all afferent light input to the midbrain with equal efferent stimulation through both third cranial nerves. Therefore, if one pupil is fixed to light because of an efferent defect, the other one may be observed throughout the performance of this test.

The patient may be aware of, or the examiner may find, a *scotoma* (blind spot) in the visual field. This is often central or centrocecal (because the lesion affects the papillomacular bundle that contains the central fibers of the optic nerve), or altitudinal (because arcuate or nerve-fiber–bundle abnormalities respect the nasal horizontal line, corresponding to the separation of upper and lower nerve-fiber bundles by the horizontal raphe in the temporal portion of the retina). These abnormalities are often evident on confrontation tests of the visual fields.

In a central scotoma of retinal origin (e.g., macular edema affecting photoreceptors), the patient may report

that lines seem to be distorted (*metamorphopsia*) or objects may seem small (*micropsia*). Recovery of visual acuity may be delayed in comparison to a normal fellow eye, after photostress such as a flashlight stimulus for 10 seconds.

Bilateral optic nerve abnormalities, in particular those with centrocecal scotomas (Fig. 7.1A), suggest a hereditary, toxic, nutritional, or demyelinating disorder; unilateral optic nerve disease is usually ischemic, inflammatory, or compressive. The course and associated symptoms and signs help differentiate these possibilities.

Optic nerve infarction (anterior ischemic optic neuropathy) usually affects patients older than 50 years of age. The visual defect is usually primarily altitudinal, occasionally centrocecal, sudden in onset, and stable (occasionally progressive during the initial weeks). There is pallid swelling of the optic disc with adjacent superficial hemorrhages. The swelling resolves in 4 to 6 weeks, leaving optic atrophy and arteriolar narrowing on the disc (Fig. 7.2). The cause may be arteritis (e.g., giant cell or temporal arteritis, often with associated symptoms and signs) but is usually idiopathic, painless, and only rarely associated with carotid occlusive disease. In the idiopathic nonarteritic variety, the discs are characteristically crowded, with small if any, physiologic cup, thus suggesting structural susceptibility. The fellow eye is often similarly affected after months or years.

Optic neuritis usually affects young adults. It typically begins with a central or centrocecal scotoma and subacute progression of the defect, followed by a gradual resolution; there may be residual optic atrophy. Initially, the disc may be normal (retrobulbar neuritis) or swollen (papillitis). Local tenderness or pain on movement of the eye is usually present and suggests such an intraorbital inflammatory disorder. The *Pulfrich phenomenon* is a stereo

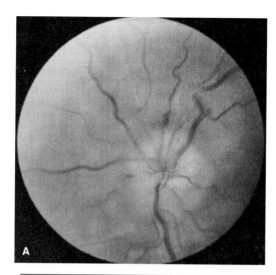 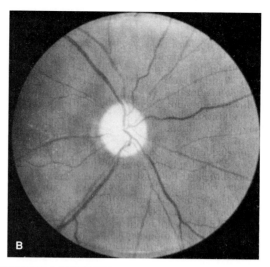

FIGURE 7.2. **A:** Pallid swelling of the disc with superficial hemorrhages in a patient with acute anterior ischemic optic neuropathy. **B:** Optic atrophy with arteriolar narrowing after anterior ischemic optic neuropathy.

illusion that may be caused by delayed conduction in one optic nerve, making it difficult to localize moving objects. This is not specific and may occur with retinal abnormality or media defect. The *Uhthoff symptom* is an exacerbation of a symptom after exercise or exposure to heat; it is not specific but occurs most often in demyelinating disorders. If in a case suggesting optic neuritis there is evidence of preexisting optic atrophy in either eye, or optic neuropathy in the fellow eye (e.g., if the degree of relative afferent pupillary defect is less than anticipated, suggesting subclinical involvement of the other eye), demyelinating disease is also suggested. While almost always demyelinating, optic neuritis may have some other etiology that may respond to steroid therapy, such as sarcoidosis, systemic lupus erythematosus, or focal inflammatory pseudotumor.

In *compressive optic neuropathy,* there is usually steady progression of visual defect, although it may be stepwise or even remitting. The disc may remain relatively normal in appearance for months before primary optic atrophy is indicated funduscopically by decrease in color of the disc, visible fine vessels on the disc, and peripapillary nerve fibers (best seen with a bright ophthalmoscope with red-free light). This form of optic atrophy must be distinguished from other specific types (e.g., glaucoma, in which the nerve head has an excavated or cupped appearance; postpapilledema [secondary] atrophy with narrowing and sheathing of vessels and often indistinct margins; retinal pigmentary degeneration with narrowed vessels, which may also be seen after central retinal artery occlusion or optic nerve infarction; and congenital defects, such as coloboma or hypoplasia of the disc, with a small nerve head and a peripapillary halo that corresponds to the expected normal size of the disc).

ELECTROPHYSIOLOGIC TESTING

Visual evoked potentials (VEP, Chapter 14) are elicited by stimulation of either eye by light or pattern reversal. They are recorded by scalp electrodes placed over the occiput, with computerized subtraction of baseline brain-electrical activity, to assess pathologic diminution of amplitude or, in demyelinating lesions, delay in conduction. Electroretinography (ERG) measures the change in electric potential of the retina in response to light, and is abnormal if there is a visual defect arising in the outer layer of the retina, but not from lesions in the ganglion cell or optic nerve. VEP and ERG may be recorded multifocally to provide retinotopic or topographic information; the novel complex stimuli are provided by multiple stimuli and mathematic adjustments to derive multiple individual responses. Multifocal VEP provides an objective perimetric assessment of the visual field, which may be compared to computerized threshold static perimetry (Fig 7.3) and analyzed to assess decreased amplitude and conduction delay. Multifocal ERG may determine if small scotomas (small areas of visual impairment) or decreased acuity arise in the outer retina or optic nerve.

Electrophysiologic testing helps to identify a retinal disorder causing visual impairment that is not evident by ophthalmoscopic appearance, as in *acute multifocal placoid-pigment epitheliopathy* (AMPPE) or discernable retinal arterial occlusion, which in combination with hearing loss and encephalopathy is called the *Susac syndrome* (i.e., microangiopathy of brain and retina). Electroretinographic analysis is sometimes the only way to identify central scotomas arising from cone dystrophy or acute zonal occult outer retinopathy (AZOOR), the so-called large blind spot syndrome. Retinopathy may also be paraneoplastic.

A. Humphrey Visual Fields

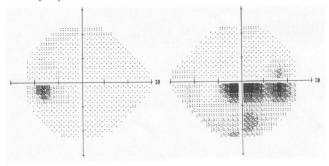

B. mfVEP

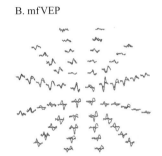

FIGURE 7.3. A: Computerized (Humphrey) perimetry in 52-year-old man with normal vision OS but with **B:** inferior altitudinal scotoma OD of sudden onset, painless, associated with optic disc swelling OD and underlying susceptible crowded small cup-type discs OU, attributed to anterior ischemic optic neuropathy with corroboratory multifocal VEP; normal OS and normal above OD but inferiorly diminished amplitude without evident conduction delay OD.

LESIONS OF THE OPTIC CHIASM

In a patient with optic neuropathy, recognition of an upper temporal hemianopic visual-field defect in the other eye (which may be asymptomatic) is evidence of a chiasmal lesion that affects the anteriorly crossing lower fibers (Fig. 7.1B). In contrast to optic nerve lesions, the majority of chiasmal lesions are compressive. The typical visual-field defect is bitemporal hemianopia (Fig. 7.1C). Because the macular fibers permeate the chiasm, any compressive lesion of the chiasm with a visual-field defect is accompanied by temporal hemianopic dimming of red objects of any size, in a pattern that respects the vertical line and permits secure confrontation testing.

RETROCHIASMAL LESIONS

Homonymous hemianopia results from a retrochiasmal lesion. There may be varying awareness of the defect. It may be mistakenly attributed to the eye on the side of the defect, or the patient may be aware only of bumping into things on that side or of trouble reading (i.e., slowness and difficulty seeing the next word with right homonymous hemianopia,

or difficulty finding the next line with left hemianopia). The patient may ignore that side of the visual acuity test chart that corresponds to the hemianopia, but may see 20/20 unless there is another defect (see Fig. 7.1D).

With subtotal lesions, the congruity of the visual-field defect in the two eyes helps in localization. Optic tract and geniculate lesions tend to have grossly incongruous visual-field defects (Fig. 7.1E). The farther posterior the lesion, the more congruous the defect because the fibers from corresponding retinal loci in the two eyes converge on the same occipital locus.

With optic tract lesions anterior to the geniculate synapse, *optic atrophy* may develop. The eye with a temporal field defect develops a bow-tie pattern of atrophy, which may also occur with chiasmal lesions. The nasal portion of the disc is pale due to loss of the nasal fibers; the usual mild temporal pallor is more evident due to loss of the nasal half of the papillomacular bundle. An imaginary vertical line through the macula corresponds to the vertical line that separates the nasal and temporal halves of the visual field. There is a relatively pink appearance above and below where fibers from the temporal retina reach the disc.

With optic tract lesions, afferent pupillary input is impaired. When the lesion is grossly incongruous, a relative afferent pupillary defect may occur on the side with the greater deficit. It is found in the eye with temporal hemianopia when homonymous hemianopia is total, because the temporal half-field is more extensive than the nasal half-field. The *Wernicke hemianopic pupillary phenomenon* may be difficult to elicit; pupillary constriction is more vigorous when the unaffected portion of the retina is stimulated. When an optic tract lesion is close to, and encroaches on the chiasm, visual acuity in the ipsilateral eye diminishes. There may be a relative afferent pupillary defect on that side, as well.

Retrogeniculate lesions are not accompanied by clinical impairment of pupillary reactivity or optic atrophy. The homonymous hemianopic visual-field defect tends to be superior when the temporal lobe radiations are affected, and the defect is denser below if the lesion is parietal. Occipital lesions result in precisely congruous defects, often scotomas with preserved peripheral vision (Fig. 7.1F). If the scotoma is large enough, the area of preserved peripheral vision may be present only in the eye with the loss of temporal field (a preserved temporal crescent). This corresponds to the most anterior portion of the occipital cortex. The central portion of the visual field is represented in the posterior striate cortex, a marginal perfusion zone of both posterior and middle cerebral arteries. When the posterior cerebral artery is occluded, collateral supply from the middle cerebral artery may allow gross *macular sparing* (Fig. 7.1G), preserving central vision. Homonymous hemianopia of occipital origin is often total. Isolated homonymous hemianopia is due to an infarct in 90% of patients. *Cerebral blindness* (bilateral homonymous hemianopia [Fig. 7.1H]) may require distinction from hysterical blindness; opticokinetic nystagmus (OKN) may be elicited in psychogenic disorders, but not after bilateral occipital lesions when they are complete.

Transient Visual Events

Irritative visual phenomena include formed visual hallucinations (usually of temporal lobe origin) and unformed hallucinations (usually of occipital origin), including the *scintillating homonymous scotoma* of migraine. *Amaurosis fugax* of one eye is occasionally due to vasospasm in migraine but is usually due to ophthalmic-carotid hypoperfusion or embolization, or cardiogenic emboli. A helpful clue is the ophthalmoscopic recognition of embolic fragments that have become impacted in retinal arterioles; these may be atheromatous (*Hollenhorst plaques*) or calcific. Transient visual obscurations that are fleeting, frequent, and often induced by change of position may be caused by hypoperfusion in severe papilledema. Formed or unformed hallucinations may be release phenomena when there is visual loss, owing to a lesion anywhere along the visual pathway. *Phosphenes* (light flashes) may occur in several kinds of optic nerve lesions, including demyelinating optic neuritis, or they may occur with movement of the eye. Vitreoretinal traction is a frequent and benign cause of light flashes, especially with advancing age, although a retinal tear premonitory to retinal detachment may occur and must be ruled out.

IMPAIRMENT OF OCULAR MOTILITY

Impairment of ocular motility is often a clue to diagnosis in many neurologic disorders. It may reflect a supra-, inter-, or infranuclear (e.g., fascicular or peripheral nerve) neurogenic lesion, neuromuscular transmission defect, myopathy, or mechanical restriction in the orbit. *Diplopia* (double vision) indicates malalignment of the visual axes if it is relieved by occlusion of either eye. Diplopia of monocular origin is psychogenic or due to a disturbance of the refractive media in the eye (e.g., astigmatism or opacity of the cornea or lens). Malalignment of the visual axes may occur in psychogenic convergence spasm, as suggested by associated miosis, due to the near response; in decompensation of strabismus, including convergence insufficiency, usually of no pathologic import; and less frequently, in divergence insufficiency, possibly due to bilateral sixth cranial nerve paresis, occasionally caused by increased intracranial pressure. The diplopia and malalignment of the visual axes in these cases are usually comitant, or equal in all directions of gaze. If strabismus begins in early childhood, there may be habitual suppression of the image of one eye, with impaired development of vision in that eye (*amblyopia*) rather than diplopia.

Incomitance, or inequality in the alignment of the visual axes in the direction of gaze, suggests limitation of action of one or more muscles. The deviation is generally greater if the paretic eye is fixing. The patient may use one eye or adopt a head-turn or tilt to avoid diplopia (e.g., turning to the right when the right lateral rectus is limited, or tilting to the left if the right superior oblique is affected, to avoid the need for the intortional effect of that muscle). The patient may not be aware of either the diplopia or these adaptations.

To determine which muscle is impaired, the examiner obtains information from the history and examination, including the use of a red glass. It is important to know whether the diplopia is vertical or horizontal, whether it is crossed (i.e., the visual axes are divergent) or uncrossed (i.e., convergent), whether greater with near vision (if adducting muscles are involved) or at a distance (if abducting muscles are involved), and the direction of the gaze in which the diplopia is maximal.

If the pattern of motility limitation conforms to muscles innervated by a single nerve, the lesion probably affects that nerve. With a third cranial nerve palsy there is ptosis, limitation of action of the medial, inferior, and superior rectus muscles and of the inferior oblique muscle; all the extraocular muscles are affected except the lateral rectus (sixth cranial nerve) and superior oblique (fourth cranial nerve). *Internal ophthalmoplegia* (i.e., pupillary enlargement with defective constriction and defective accommodation) may be evident. When the ptotic lid is lifted, the eye is abducted (unless the sixth cranial nerve is also affected), and on attempted downward gaze the globe may be seen to intort (i.e., as evidenced by observation of nasal episcleral vessels) if the fourth cranial nerve is intact. If more than one of these nerves is affected, the lesion is probably in the cavernous sinus, superior orbital fissure, or orbital apex. There may also be fifth cranial nerve (ophthalmic division) and oculosympathetic defect (*Horner syndrome*). The latter is indicated by relative miosis, mild ptosis, and incomplete and delayed dilation of the pupil. Such involvement is usually due to tumor, aneurysm, or inflammation, whereas isolated involvement of one of the ocular motor nerves may be ischemic in origin.

Mechanical limitation of ocular motility may occur with orbital lesions, such as thyroid ophthalmopathy, orbital fracture, or tumor. It is indicated by limitation on forced duction, such as an attempt to rotate the globe with forceps (traction test), or by elevation of intraocular pressure on the attempted movement with relatively intact velocity *saccades* (i.e., rapid eye movements). Other symptoms or signs of orbital lesions include proptosis (or enophthalmos in the case of fracture) beyond the acceptable normal asymmetry of 2 mm, resistance to retropulsion, vascular congestion, tenderness, and eyelid abnormality other than ptosis (e.g., retraction, lid-lag, swelling).

Myasthenia gravis (see Chapter 121) is suggested when affected muscles do not conform to the distribution of a single nerve, even though sometimes they may, and when symptoms vary, including diurnal fluctuation and fatigability. A demonstrable increase in paresis or a slowing of saccades may occur after sustained gaze or repetitive movement. Ptosis may similarly increase after sustained upward gaze, may lessen after rest in sustained eye closure, or a momentary lid twitch may be seen on return of gaze from downward to straight ahead. There is no clinical abnormality of the pupils in myasthenia gravis.

Analysis of saccadic function is of particular value in the analysis of supra- and internuclear ocular motility defects. The supranuclear control mechanisms of ocular movements include the following: the *saccadic system* of rapid conjugate eye movement of contralateral frontal lobe origin to achieve foveal fixation on a target (i.e., a combination of *pulse*, burst discharge in agonist with total inhibition of antagonist, and *step*, increased level of agonist and decreased level of antagonist discharge to maintain the new eccentric position); the *pursuit system* of slow, conjugate movement of ipsilateral occipital lobe origin to maintain foveal fixation on a slowly moving target; the *vestibular system* of slow conjugate movement to maintain stability of the retinal image if the head moves in relation to the environment; and the *vergence system* of dysconjugate slow movement to maintain alignment of the visual axes for binocular single vision. *Optokinetic nystagmus* (OKN) is the normal response to a sequence of objects moving slowly across the field of vision and may be considered a combination of pursuit and refixation saccades, which allows continuous pursuit, because vision is suppressed during the saccadic phase.

The polysynaptic saccadic pathway crosses at the level of the fourth cranial nerve nucleus to enter the *pontine paramedian reticular formation* (PPRF). This is where ipsilateral saccades and other horizontal movements are generated by stimulation of neurons in the sixth cranial nerve nucleus and also interneurons therein that travel up the opposite *medial longitudinal fasciculus* (MLF), to stimulate the contralateral subnucleus for the medial rectus in the third cranial nerve nucleus and assure normal, conjugate gaze. Pathways for vertical movement seem to require bilateral stimuli. The immediate supranuclear apparatus for generating vertical gaze is in the midbrain, the rostral interstitial nucleus of the MLF.

General dysfunction of saccades (i.e., with limitation, slowing, or hypometria) is seen in several disorders, including Huntington disease (see Chapter 109), hereditary ataxias (see Chapter 108), progressive supranuclear palsy (see Chapter 116), and Wilson disease (see Chapter 91). *Congenital ocular motor apraxia* is a benign abnormality of horizontal saccades that resolves with maturity. Infants with this abnormality are unable to perform horizontal saccades and substitute characteristic head thrusts past

the object of regard, achieving fixation by the contraversive vestibular doll's-head movement, and then maintaining it while slowly rotating the head back. Focal dysfunction of saccades is manifested by lateral gaze paresis after contralateral frontal or ipsilateral pontine lesions; vestibular stimuli may overcome frontal but not pontine gaze palsies

Internuclear ophthalmoplegia is the result of a lesion in the MLF that interrupts adduction in conjugate gaze, although convergence may be intact. Abduction nystagmus is seen in the contralateral eye. When the defect is partial, adducting saccades are slow, with resultant dissociation of nystagmus more marked in the abducting eye, as seen when OKN is elicited. When the lesion is unilateral, an ischemic lesion is likely; a bilateral syndrome suggests multiple sclerosis. Vertical gaze-evoked nystagmus and *skew deviation* (one eye higher than the other) may be seen. The latter is a supranuclear vertical divergence of the eyes, seen with brainstem or cerebellar lesions.

A unilateral pontine lesion that involves both the MLF and PPRF causes the combination of ipsilateral gaze palsy and internuclear ophthalmoplegia on contralateral gaze, a pattern called the *"one-and-a-half syndrome."* The only remaining horizontal movement is abduction of the contralateral eye. The eyes are straight or exodeviated, especially if there is gaze preference away from the side of the gaze palsy. Superimposed esodeviation with related diplopia may occur if there is sixth cranial nerve (fascicular) involvement, as well.

Vertical gaze disorders are seen with midbrain lesions (the *sylvian aqueduct syndrome*). Characteristic dyssynergia on attempted upward saccades is best demonstrated by the use of downward-moving OKN stimuli. Failure of inhibition leads to co-firing of oculomotor neurons with convergence-retraction nystagmus and related fleetingly blurred vision or diplopia. This may also occur to a lesser extent, with horizontal saccades, causing excessive adductor discharge and "pseudo sixth cranial nerve paresis." There is usually pupillary sluggishness in response to light (i.e., often with light-near dissociation) due to the interruption of the periaqueductal afferent light input to the third cranial nerve nuclei. Concomitant abnormalities may include lid retraction (*Collier sign*), defective or excess accommodation or convergence, and skew deviation or monocular elevator palsy.

Oscillopsia is a sensation of illusory movement of the environment that is unidirectional or oscillatory; it is seen with acquired nystagmus of various types. *Nystagmus* is an involuntary rhythmic oscillation of the eyes, generally conjugate and of equal amplitude, but occasionally dysconjugate as in the sylvian aqueduct syndrome, or dissociated in amplitude as in internuclear ophthalmoplegia. The oscillations may be pendular or jerk type; the latter is more common in acquired pathologic nystagmus. In jerk nystagmus, the slow phase is operative and the fast phase is a recovery movement. The amplitude usually increases on gaze in the direction of the fast phase.

Horizontal and upward gaze-evoked nystagmus may be due to sedative or anticonvulsant drugs. Otherwise, *vertical nystagmus* indicates posterior fossa disease. Extreme end-gaze physiologic nystagmus, which may be of greater amplitude in the abducting eye, must be distinguished. It occurs only horizontally. *Jerk nystagmus* in the primary position, or rotatory nystagmus, usually indicates a vestibular disorder that may be either central or peripheral. In a destructive peripheral lesion, the fast phase is away from the lesion; the same pattern is seen with a cold stimulus when the horizontal canals are oriented vertically (i.e., with the head elevated 30° in the supine position). *Downbeating nystagmus* in the primary position, often more marked on lateral gaze to either side, frequently indicates a lesion at the cervicomedullary junction. *Ocular bobbing* is usually associated with total, horizontal pontine gaze palsy. It is not rhythmic, is coarser than nystagmus, may vary in amplitude, and is occasionally asymmetric; the initial movement is downward with a slower return. *Upbeating nystagmus* in the primary position may indicate a lesion of the cerebellar vermis or medulla but is most commonly associated with lesions of the pons. *Seesaw nystagmus* is vertically dysconjugate with a rotary element, so that there is intortion of the elevating eye and simultaneous extortion of the falling eye. This pattern is often seen with parachiasmal lesions and is probably a form of alternating skew deviation due to involvement of vertical and tortional oculomotor control regions around the third ventricle. *Periodic alternating nystagmus* implies a non-sinister lesion of the lower brainstem; in effect, it is a gaze-evoked nystagmus to either side of a null point that cycles back and forth horizontally. In the primary position, there is nystagmus of periodically alternating direction. *Rebound nystagmus*, which may be confused with periodic alternating nystagmus, is a horizontal jerk nystagmus that is transiently present in the primary position after sustained gaze to the opposite side; it implies dysfunction of the cerebellar system.

Other ocular oscillations that follow cerebellar system lesions include *ocular dysmetria* where there is overshoot or terminal oscillation of saccades, *ocular flutter* or bursts of similar horizontal oscillation, actually back-to-back saccades without the usual latency, *opsoclonus* (i.e., chaotic multidirectional conjugate saccades), and *fixation instability*—square-wave jerks—in which small saccades interrupt fixation, with movement of the eye away from the primary position and then its return after appropriate latency for a saccade. *Ocular myoclonus* is a rhythmic ocular oscillation that often is vertical and associated with synchronous palatal myoclonus.

When oscillopsia is monocular, there may be dissociated pathologic nystagmus of posterior fossa origin, including the jellylike, primarily vertical, pendular nystagmus akin to myoclonus that is occasionally seen in multiple sclerosis. There may be benign myokymia of the superior oblique muscle, in which the patient is often aware of both a sensation of ocular movement and oscillopsia. Monocular nystagmus may also result from monocular visual loss in early childhood or from the insignificant and transient acquired entity of *spasmus nutans*, which is of uncertain etiology. It begins after 4 months of age and disappears within a few years. The nystagmus of spasmus nutans is asymmetric and rapid and may be accompanied by head nodding. It may be similar to congenital nystagmus. The latter begins at birth, is persistent and usually horizontal, either gaze-evoked or pendular, and is often seen with jerks to the sides. There may be a null point with head turn, adopted for maximal visual acuity. It originates in a motor disorder, although it may be mimicked by the nystagmus of early binocular visual deprivation.

SUGGESTED READINGS

Behrens MM. *Neuro-ophthalmic motility disorders.* American Academy of Ophthalmology and Otolaryngology CETV videotape, 1975;1(5).

Burde RM, Savino PJ, Trobe JD. *Clinical Decisions in Neuro-Ophthalmology*, 3rd ed. St. Louis, MO: CV Mosby, 2002.

Gass JD. The acute zonal retinopathies. *Am J Ophthalmol* 2000;130:655–657.

Glaser JS. *Neuro-ophthalmology*, 3rd ed. Philadelphia: JB Lippincott Co, 1999.

Hickman SJ, Dalton CM, Miller DH, Plant GT. Management of acute optic neuritis. *Lancet* 2002;360:1953–1962.

Hood DC, Odel JG, Wynn BJ. The multifocal visual evoked potential. *J Neuro-ophthalmol* 2003;23:279–289.

Hood DC, Odel JG, Chen CS, Wynn BJ. The multifocal electroretinogram. *J Neuro-ophthalmol* 2003;23:225–235.

Leigh RJ, Zee DS. *The Neurology of Eye Movements*, 3rd ed. Philadelphia: FA Davis Co, 1999.

Mizener JB, Kimura AE, Adamus G, et al. Autoimmune retinopathy in the absence of cancer. *Am J Ophthalmol* 1997;123:607–618.

Miller NR, Newman NJ. The essentials. *Walsh and Hoyt's Clinical Neuro-Ophthalmology*, 5th ed. Baltimore: Lippincott Williams & Wilkins, 1998.

Miller NR, Newman NJ, eds. *Walsh and Hoyt's Clinical Neuro-Ophthalmology*, 5th ed, vols. 1–5. Baltimore: Lippincott Williams & Wilkins, 1998.

O'Halloran HS, Berger JR, Lee WB, et al. Acute multifocal placoid pigment epitheliopathy and central nervous system involvement: nine new cases and a review of the literature. *Ophthalmology* 2001;108(5):861–868.

Sigelman J, Behrens MM, Hilal S. Acute posterior multifocal placoid pigment epitheliopathy associated with cerebral vasculitis and homonymous hemianopia. *Am J Ophthalmol* 1988;88(5):919–924.

Susac JO, Murtagh FR, Egan RA. MRI findings in Susac's syndrome. *Neurology* 2003;61:1783–1787.

Venkatramani J, Mitchell P. Ocular and systemic causes of retinopathy in patients without diabetes mellitus. *BMJ* 2004 Mar 13;328(7440):625–629.

Chapter 8

Headache

Neil H. Raskin and Mark W. Green

Nearly everyone is subject to headache from time to time; moreover, 40% of all people have severe headaches annually. The brain mechanism that generates headaches is activated by many factors. Genetic factors probably augment the system, so that some people are susceptible to more frequent or more severe head pain. The term *migraine* is used increasingly to refer to a mechanism of this kind, in contradistinction to prior usage of the term as an aggregation of certain symptoms. Even stress-related or *tension-type* headaches, perhaps the most common syndrome reported by patients, are an example of the expression of this mechanism when provoked by an adequate stimulus.

Headache is usually a benign symptom and only occasionally is a manifestation of a serious illness, such as brain tumor, aneurysmal rupture or giant cell arteritis. The first issue to resolve in the care of a patient with headache is to differentiate benign and more ominous causes. If the data supporting a benign process are strong enough, as reviewed in this chapter, neuroimaging may be deferred. If a benign diagnosis cannot be made, MRI is a better choice than CT for visualizing the posterior fossa; posterior fossa tumors are far more likely than forebrain tumors to cause headache as the sole symptom. Moreover, the Arnold-Chiari malformation, an important structural cause of headache, cannot be visualized adequately with CT.

GENERAL PRINCIPLES

The quality, location, duration, and time course of the headache and the conditions that produce, exacerbate, or relieve it should be elicited. It is important to determine an anchor in time for the onset of the attacks, and then determine whether there has been a characteristic frequency and pattern of symptoms.

Most headaches are dull, deeply located, and aching in quality. Superimposed on such nondescript pain may be other elements that have greater diagnostic value; for example, jabbing, brief, sharp pain, often occurring multifocally (*ice-pick-like* pain), is the signature of a benign disorder. A throbbing quality and tight muscles about the head, neck, and shoulder girdle are common nonspecific accompaniments of headache that suggest that intra- and extracranial arteries and skeletal muscles of the head and neck are activated by a generic mechanism that produces head pain. Tight, pressing "hat-band" headaches were once believed to indicate anxiety or depression, but studies have not supported this view.

Pain *intensity* seldom has diagnostic value and is quite subjective. Similarly, response to placebo medication does not provide useful information. Tension-type headaches are mild and few sufferers seek medical attention. More disabling tension-type headaches are almost always part of the spectrum of migraine and are treated as any other form of migraine. Administration of placebo simply identifies placebo responders, a group that includes about 30% of the population, or reflects the self-limited nature of many headaches. No evidence reveals that placebo responders have lower pain levels than non-responders or that they do not really have pain. Patients coming to an emergency department with the most severe headache of their lives usually have migraine. Meningitis, subarachnoid hemorrhage, and cluster headache also produce intense cranial pain. Contrary to common belief, the headache produced by a brain tumor is not usually severe.

Data about the *location* of the headache is occasionally informative. If the source is an extracranial structure, as in giant cell arteritis, correspondence with the site of pain is fairly precise. Inflammation of an extracranial artery causes scalp pain and extensive tenderness localized to the site of the vessel. Posterior fossa lesions cause pain that is usually occipitonuchal, at least early on, and supratentorial lesions most often induce frontotemporal pain. *Multifocality* alone is a strong indicator of benignity.

Time-intensity considerations are particularly useful. A ruptured aneurysm results in head pain that peaks in an instant, *thunderclap*-like manner; much less often, unruptured aneurysms or low volume hemorrhages may similarly signal their presence. Whether or not the attack is self-limited or responsive to medication is of no diagnostic value. Migraine attacks may also have an apoplectic onset. *Cluster headache* attacks peak over 3–5 minutes to 5 minutes, remain at maximal intensity for an hour or two, and then taper off. Most migraine attacks build up over hours, are maintained for several hours to days, and are characteristically relieved by sleep. Sleep disruption is characteristic of headaches produced by brain tumors, but is more commonly seen with migraine and cluster headache.

The relationship of a headache to specific biologic events or to physical environmental changes is essential information for triage of patients. The following exacerbating phenomena have high probability value in asserting that a headache syndrome is benign: provocation by red wine, sustained exertion, pungent odors, hunger, lack of sleep, weather change, or menses. Cessation or amelioration of headache during pregnancy, especially

▶ **TABLE 8.1 Studies Performed to Investigate Chronic Headache**

ERS
Antinuclear antibody titer
Thyroid microsomal antibody titer
Serum prolactin level
Lumbar puncture (pressure, malignant cells)
Neuroimaging
Temporal artery biopsy

in the second and third trimesters, is similarly pathognomonic of migraine. Patients with continuous benign headache often observe a pain-free interlude of several minutes on waking before the head pain begins once again. This phenomenon, wherein the cessation of sleep seems to unleash the headache mechanism, also occurs with other centrally mediated pain syndromes, such as thalamic pain, but does not occur among patients with somatic disease as the cause of pain.

A history of amenorrhea or galactorrhea leads to the possibility that the polycystic ovary syndrome or a prolactin-secreting pituitary adenoma is the source of headache (see Table 8.1). Headache arising *de novo* in a patient with a known malignancy suggests either cerebral metastasis or carcinomatous meningitis. When the pain is accentuated by eye movements, a systemic infection, particularly meningitis, should be considered. The eye itself is seldom the cause of acute orbital pain if the sclerae are white and non-injected; red eyes are generally a sign of ophthalmic disease. Head pain appearing abruptly after bending, lifting, or coughing may be a clue to a posterior fossa mass or the Arnold-Chiari malformation. Orthostatic headache arises after lumbar puncture or other causes of CSF leaks, and also occurs with subdural hematoma and benign intracranial hypertension. Similarly, acute sinusitis nearly always declares itself through a dark green, purulent nasal exudate, despite the fact that migraineurs often receive this diagnosis when nasal congestion and eye tearing accompany their attacks.

The analysis of facial pain requires a different approach. Trigeminal neuralgia, and less frequently glossopharyngeal neuralgia, are causes of facial pain. *Neuralgias* are painful disorders characterized by paroxysmal, fleeting, and often electric-shock—like episodes. These conditions are generally caused by demyelinating lesions, often at the nerve-root entry zones (the trigeminal or glossopharyngeal nerves in cranial neuralgia), activating a pain-generating mechanism in the brainstem. *Trigger* maneuvers characteristically provoke paroxysms of pain. However, the most common cause of facial pain by far is dental; provocation by hot, cold, or sweet foods is typical. Application of a cold stimulus repeatedly induces dental pain, whereas in neu-

ralgic disorders a refractory period usually occurs after the initial response so that pain cannot be induced repeatedly. The presence of refractory periods nearly always may be elicited in the history, thereby saving the patient from a painful testing experience.

Mealtimes offer the physician an opportunity to gain insight into the mechanism of a patient's facial pain. Does chewing, swallowing, or the taste of a food elicit pain? Activation of the pain by chewing points to trigeminal neuralgia, temporomandibular joint dysfunction, giant cell arteritis, or occasionally angina (*jaw claudication*), whereas the combination of swallowing *and* taste provocation points to glossopharyngeal neuralgia. Pain on swallowing is common among patients with *carotidynia* (facial migraine), because the inflamed, tender carotid artery abuts the esophagus during deglutition.

As in other painful conditions, many patients with facial pain do not describe stereotypic syndromes. These patients have sometimes had their syndromes categorized as "atypical facial pain," as though this were a well defined clinical entity. Only scant evidence shows that nondescript facial pain is caused by emotional distress, as is sometimes alleged. Vague, poorly localized, continuous facial pain is *characteristic* of the condition that may result from nasopharyngeal carcinoma and other somatic diseases; a burning, painful element often supervenes as deafferentation occurs and evidence of cranial neuropathy appears. Occasionally, the cause of a pain problem may not be promptly resolved, thus necessitating periodic follow-up examinations until further clues appear (and they usually do). *Facial pain of unknown cause* is a more reasonable tentative diagnosis than "atypical facial pain."

PAIN-SENSITIVE STRUCTURES OF THE HEAD

The most common type of pain results from activation of peripheral nociceptors in the presence of a normally functioning nervous system, as in the pain resulting from scalded skin or appendicitis. Another type of pain results from injury to or activation of the peripheral or central nervous system. Headache, formerly believed to originate peripherally, may originate from either mechanism. Headache may arise from dysfunction or displacement of, or encroachment on, pain-sensitive cranial structures. The following are sensitive to mechanical stimulation: the scalp and aponeurosis, middle meningeal artery, dural sinuses, falx cerebri, and the proximal segments of the large pial arteries. The ventricular ependyma, choroid plexus, pial veins, and much of the brain parenchyma are insensitive to pain. On the other hand, electrical stimulation near midbrain dorsal raphe cells may result in migraine like headaches. Thus, most of the brain is insensitive to electrode probing, but a particular midbrain site is nevertheless a putative locus for headache generation.

PET scanning in spontaneous migraine attacks has demonstrated that this region is activated. Sensory stimuli from the head are conveyed to the brain by the trigeminal nerves, particularly the first division, from structures above the tentorium in the anterior and middle fossae of the skull. The first three cervical nerves carry stimuli from the posterior fossa and infradural structures, explaining how neck pain is commonly a component of migraine. The ninth and tenth cranial nerves supply part of the posterior fossa and refer pain to the ear and throat.

Headache may occur as the result of the following:

1. Distention, traction, or dilation of intracranial or extracranial arteries;
2. Traction or displacement of large intracranial veins or their dural envelope;
3. Compression, traction, or inflammation of cranial and spinal nerves;
4. Spasm, inflammation, and trauma to cranial and cervical muscles;
5. Meningeal irritation and raised intracranial pressure; and
6. Perturbation of intracerebral serotonergic projections.

By and large, intracranial masses cause headache when they deform, displace, or exert traction on vessels, dural structures, or cranial nerves at the base of the brain; these changes often happen long before intracranial pressure rises. Such mechanical displacement mechanisms do not explain headaches resulting from cerebral ischemia, benign intracranial hypertension after reduction of the pressure, or febrile illnesses and systemic lupus erythematosus. Impaired central inhibition as a result of perturbation of intracerebral serotonergic projections has been postulated a possible mechanism for these phenomena, and for migraine as well.

APPROACH TO THE PATIENT WITH HEADACHE

The patient who has the first severe headache ever and the one who has had recurrent headaches for many years raise entirely different diagnostic possibilities. The probability of finding a potentially serious cause is considerably greater in patients with their first severe headache than in those with chronic recurrent headaches. Acute causes include meningitis, subarachnoid hemorrhage, epidural or subdural hematoma, glaucoma, and purulent sinusitis. In general, acute, severe headache with stiff neck and fever means meningitis, and without fever means subarachnoid hemorrhage. When the physician is confronted with such a patient, lumbar puncture is mandatory. Acute, persistent headache and fever are often manifestations of an acute systemic viral infection; if the neck is supple, lumbar puncture may be deferred. A first attack of migraine is always a possibility, but fever is rarely an associated feature.

Nearly all illnesses have been an occasional cause of headache; however, some illnesses are *characteristically* associated with headache. These include infectious mononucleosis, systemic lupus erythematosus, chronic pulmonary failure with hypercapnia, the sleep apnea syndrome (early morning headaches), Hashimoto thyroiditis, corticosteroid withdrawal, oral contraceptives, ovulation-promoting agents, inflammatory bowel disease, many illnesses associated with human immunodeficiency virus infection, and acute blood pressure elevation that occurs in pheochromocytoma and malignant hypertension. Pheochromocytoma and malignant hypertension are the exceptions to the generalization that hypertension *per se* is an uncommon cause of headache; a diastolic pressure of at least 120 mm Hg is requisite for hypertension to cause headache.

Adolescents with chronic daily frontal or holocephalic headache pose a special problem. Extensive diagnostic tests, including psychiatric assessment, are most often unrevealing. Fortunately, the headaches tend to stop after a few years, so that structured analgesic support may enable these teenagers to move through secondary school and enter college. By the time they reach their late teens, the cycle has usually ended.

The relationship of head pain to depression is not straightforward. Many patients in chronic daily pain cycles become depressed (a reasonable sequence of events); moreover, there is a greater-than-chance coincidence of migraine with both bipolar and unipolar depressive disorders. A bidirectional comorbidity of migraine and depression has been identified so it is more likely that both problems may arise out of a shared biochemical basis rather than either syndrome actually causing the other. The physician should be cautious about assigning depression as the cause of recurring headache; some drugs with antidepressant action are also effective in migraine apart from any antidepressant action.

Finally, note must be made of recurring headaches that may be pain-driven. As an example, *temporomandibular joint (TMJ) dysfunction* generally produces preauricular pain that is associated with chewing food. The pain may radiate to the head but is not easily confused with headache *per se*. Conversely, headache-prone patients may observe that headaches are more frequent and severe in the presence of a painful TMJ problem. Similarly, the pain attending otologic or endodontic surgical procedures may activate headache disorders. Treatment of such headaches is largely ineffectual until the cause of the primary pain is treated. Thus, pain about the head as a result of somatic disease or trauma may reawaken an otherwise quiescent migrainous mechanism.

SUGGESTED READINGS

Blumenthal HJ. Headaches and sinus disease. *Headache* 2001;41:883–888.

Breslau N, Rasmussen BK. The impact of migraine: epidemiology, risk factors, and co-morbidities. *Neurology* 2001;56(suppl 1):S4–S12.

Day JW, Raskin NH. Thunderclap headache: symptom of unruptured cerebral aneurysm. *Lancet* 1986;2:1247–1248.

International Headache Society Headache Classification Subcommittee. International Classification of Headache Disorders. *Cephalalgia* 2004:24(suppl 1):1–150.

Kaniecki R. Migraine and tension-type headache. An assessment of challenges in diagnosis. *Neurology* 2002;58(suppl 6):S15–S20.

Lance JW, Goadsby PJ. *Mechanism and Management of Headache,* 6th ed. London: Butterworth-Heineman, 1998.

Lipton R, Stewart WF, Cady R, Hall C, O'Quinn S, Kuhn T, Gutterman D. Sumatriptan for the range of headaches in migraine sufferers: results of the SPECTRUM study. *Headache* 2000;10:783–791.

Matharu MS, Bartsch T, Ward N, Frackowiak RS, Weiner R, Goadsby PJ. Central neuromodulation in chronic migraine patients with suboccipital stimulators: a PET study. *Brain* 2004;127(pt 1):220–230.

Moskowitz MA, Bolay H, Dalkara T. Deciphering migraine mechanisms: clues from familial hemiplegic migraine genotypes. *Ann Neurol* 2004;55(2):276–280.

Pietroban D, Striessnig J. Neurological diseases: neurobiology of migraine. *Nat Rev Neurosci* 2003:4:386–398.

Raskin NH. *Headache,* 2nd ed. New York: Churchill Livingstone, 1988.

Rasmussen BK, Olesen J. Symptomatic and nonsymptomatic headaches in a general population. *Neurology* 1992;42:1225–1231.

Silberstein S, Lipton R, Dalessio D. Wolff's Headache, 7th Ed. Oxford University Press, 2001.

Toth C. Medications and substances as a cause of headache: a systematic review of the literature. *Clin Neuropharmacol* 2003;26:122–136.

Chapter 9

Involuntary Movements

Stanley Fahn

Although convulsions, fasciculations, and myokymia are involuntary movements, these disorders have special characteristics and are not classified with the types of abnormal involuntary movements described in this chapter. The disorders commonly called abnormal involuntary move-

ments, or *dyskinesias*, are usually evident when a patient is at rest, are frequently increased by action, and disappear during sleep. There are exceptions to these generalizations. For example, palatal myoclonus may persist during sleep, and mild torsion dystonia may be present only during active voluntary movements (action dystonia), but not when the patient is at rest. The known dyskinesias are distinguished mainly by visual inspection of the patient. Electromyography may occasionally be helpful by determining the rate, rhythmicity, and synchrony of involuntary movements. The speed and duration of an individual contraction may often distinguish specific types of dyskinesias; for instance, differentiating an organic myoclonic jerk from a psychogenic one. Motor control physiology laboratories typically perform this service. Sometimes, patients have a dyskinesia that bridges the definitions of more than one disorder; this leads to compound terms such as choreoathetosis, which describes features of both chorea and athetosis. Most abnormal involuntary movements are continual or easily evoked, but some are intermittent or paroxysmal, such as tics, the *paroxysmal dyskinesias*, and *episodic ataxias*. Gross movements of joints are highly visible, unlike the restricted muscle twitching of fasciculation or myokymia.

TYPES OF DYSKINESIAS

Tremors are rhythmic oscillatory movements. They result from alternating contractions of opposing muscle groups (e.g., parkinsonian tremor at rest) or from simultaneous contractions of agonist and antagonist muscles (e.g., essential tremor). A useful way to differentiate tremor clinically is to determine whether the tremor is present under the following conditions: when the affected body part is at rest, as in parkinsonian disorders; when posture is maintained (e.g., with arms outstretched in front of the body or with elbows flexed with arms in a winged position), as in Wilson disease and essential tremor (see Chapter 114); when action is undertaken (e.g., writing or pouring water from a cup), as in essential tremor that increases with action; or when intention is present (e.g., finger-to-nose maneuver), as in cerebellar disease (see Chapter 108).

The term *myoclonus* (see Chapter 111) refers to ultrabrief, shocklike movements that may arise from contractions or inhibitions (negative myoclonus). *Chorea* delineates brief, irregular contractions that, although rapid, are not as lightning-like as myoclonic jerks. In classic choreic disorders, such as Huntington disease (see Chapter 109) and Sydenham chorea (see Chapter 110), the jerks affect individual muscles as random events that seem to flow from one muscle to another. They are not repetitive or rhythmic. *Ballism* is a form of chorea in which the choreic jerks are of large amplitude, producing flinging movements of the affected limbs. Chorea is presumably related to disorders of the caudate nucleus but sometimes involves other structures. Ballism is more often related to lesions of the subthalamic nucleus.

Dystonia (see Chapter 113) is a syndrome of sustained muscle contraction that frequently causes twisting and repetitive movements or abnormal postures. Dystonia is represented by the following presentations: (1) sustained contractions of both agonist and antagonist muscles, simultaneously and in the same muscle groups repeatedly ("patterning"), in contrast to the flowing of choreic movements; (2) an increase of these involuntary contractions when voluntary movement in other body parts is attempted ("overflow"); (3) rhythmic interruptions (*dystonic tremor*) of these involuntary, sustained contractions when the patient attempts to oppose them; (4) inappropriate or opposing contractions during specific voluntary motor actions (*action dystonia*); and (5) torsion spasms that may be as rapid as chorea but differ because the movements are continual, patterned, and of a twisting nature in contrast to the random and seemingly flowing movements of chorea. Torsion spasms may be misdiagnosed as chorea; the other characteristics frequently lead to the misdiagnosis of a conversion reaction.

Tics may be simple jerks or complex sequences of coordinated movements that appear suddenly and intermittently. When simple, the movements resemble a myoclonic jerk. Complex tics often include head-shaking, eye-blinking, sniffing, shoulder-shrugging, facial distortions, arm-waving, touching parts of the body, jumping movements, or making obscene gestures (*copropraxia*). Usually tics are rapid and brief, but occasionally they may be sustained motor contractions (i.e., dystonic). In addition to motor tics, vocalizations may be a manifestation of tics. These range from sounds, such as barking, throat-clearing, or squealing, to verbalization, including the utterance of obscenities (*coprolalia*) and the repetitions of one's own sounds (*palilalia*) or the sounds of others (*echolalia*). Motor and vocal tics are the essential features of the Tourette syndrome (see Chapter 112).

One feature of tics is the compelling need felt by the patient to make the motor or phonic tic, with the result that the tic movement brings relief from unpleasant sensations that develop in the involved body part. Tics may be voluntarily controlled for brief intervals, but such a conscious effort is usually followed by more intense and frequent contractions. The milder the disorder is, the more control the patient may exert over the tics. Tics may sometimes be suppressed in public. The spectrum of severity and persistence of tics is wide. Sometimes, tics are temporary, and sometimes they are permanent.

Many persons develop personalized mannerisms. These physiologic tics may persist after repeated performances of motor habits and have therefore been called *habit spasms*. As a result, unfortunately, all tics have been considered by some physicians as habit spasms of psychic origin. Today, however, the trend is to consider pathologic tics a neurologic disorder.

Stereotypic movements (*stereotypies*) may resemble tics, but these are usually encountered in persons with mental retardation, autism, or schizophrenia. However, bursts of stereotypic shaking movements, especially of the arms, may be encountered in otherwise normal children. Stereotypic movements are also encountered in the syndrome of drug-induced tardive dyskinesia (see Chapter 117) and refer to repetitive movements that most often affect the mouth; in *orobuccolingual dyskinesia*, there are constant chewing movements of the jaw, writhing and protrusion movements of the tongue, and puckering movements of the mouth. Other parts of the body may also be involved, particularly the trunk and the digits.

Athetosis is a continuous, slow, writhing movement of the limbs (distal and proximal), trunk, head, face, or tongue. When these movements are brief, they merge with chorea (*choreoathetosis*). When the movements are sustained at the peak of the contractions, they merge with dystonia, and the term *athetotic dystonia* may be applied.

Akathistic movements are those of restlessness. They commonly accompany the subjective symptom of *akathisia*, an inner feeling of motor restlessness or the need to move. Today, akathisia is most commonly seen as a side effect of antipsychotic drug therapy, either as acute akathisia or tardive akathisia, which often accompanies tardive dyskinesia. Akathistic movements (e.g., crossing and uncrossing the legs, caressing the scalp or face, pacing the floor, and squirming in a chair) may also be a reaction to stress, anxiety, boredom, or impatience; it may then be termed *physiologic* akathisia. Pathologic akathisia, in addition to that induced by antipsychotic drugs, may be seen in the encephalopathies of confusional states, in some dementias and in Parkinson disease. Picking at the bedclothes is a common manifestation of akathistic movements in bedridden patients.

Two other neurologic conditions in which there are subjective feelings of the need to move are *tics* and the *restless legs syndrome*. The latter is characterized by formication in the legs, particularly in the evening when the patient is relaxing and sitting or lying down and attempting to fall asleep. These sensations of ants crawling under the skin disappear when the patient walks around. This disorder is not understood but may respond to opioids, levodopa, and dopamine agonists.

Continued muscle stiffness due to continuous muscle firing may be the result of neuromyotonia, encephalomyelitis with rigidity and myoclonus (spinal interneuronitis), the stiff limb syndrome, and the stiff person syndrome (see Chapter 130). The last tends to involve axial and proximal limb muscles.

Paroxysmal movement disorders are syndromes in which the abnormal involuntary movements appear for

▶ **TABLE 9.1** **Clinical Features of PKD, PNKD, and PED**

Feature	**PKD**	**PNKD**	**PED**
Male:female	4:1	1.4:1	13:13 (N=26)
Inheritance	AD	AD	AD
Genetic mapping	1. 16p11.2–q12.1 (also designated as DYT10)	1. Mount-Reback syndrome 2q34 (FDP1) (also designated as DYT8)	With autosomal recessive rolandic epilepsy; 16p12-11.2
	2. 16q13–q22.1 possibly identical with ICCA and the sodium/glucose cotransporter gene (see #3 in PNKD)	2. With diplopia and spasticity (CSE); chromosome 1p21 (also designated as DYT9)	
		3. With familial infantile convulsions; ICCA, chromosome 16, pericentric, sodium/glucose cotransporter	
Age at onset			
Range (yrs):	<1–40	<1–30	2–30
Median (yrs):	12	12	11.5
Mean (yrs):	12	12	12
Attacks			
Duration	<5 min	2 min to 4 hrs	5 min to 2 hrs
Frequency	100/d to 1/mo	3 per days to 2 per year	1/d to 2/mo
Trigger	Sudden movement, startle, hyperventilation	Nil	Prolonged exercise; muscle vibration; nerve stimulation; transmagnetic stimulation (TMS) of motor
Precipitant	Stress	Stress, caffeine, fatigue	Stress
Movement pattern	Any combination of dystonic postures, chorea, athetosis, and ballism; unilateral or bilateral.	Any combination of dystonic postures, chorea, athetosis, and ballism; unilateral or bilateral.	Any combination of dystonic postures, chorea, athetosis, and ballism; unilateral or bilateral.
Treatment	Anticonvulsants	Clonazepam, benzodiazepines, acetazolamide, antimuscarinics	Acetazolamide, antimuscarinics, benzodiazepines

CSE, choreoathetosis/spasticity episodica; ICCA, infantile convulsions with choreoathetosis; TMS, transcranial magnetic stimulation.

brief periods out of a background of normal movement patterns. They may be divided into four distinct groups: (1) the *paroxysmal dyskinesias,* (2) *paroxysmal hypnogenic dyskinesias,* many of which are frontal lobe seizures, (3) *episodic ataxias,* and (4) *hyperekplexias.* The molecular genetics of the episodic ataxias implicate abnormalities of membrane ionic channels as underlying mechanisms for the paroxysmal movement disorders.

Three types of paroxysmal dyskinesias are recognized (see Table 9.1). All three consist of bouts of any combination of dystonic postures, chorea, athetosis, and ballism. They may be unilateral, always on one side, on either side, or bilateral. Unilateral episodes may be followed by a bilateral one. The attacks may be severe enough to cause a patient to fall down. Speech is often affected, with inability to speak due to dystonia, but there is never any alteration of consciousness. Very often, patients report variable sensations at the beginning of the paroxysms. *Paroxysmal kinesigenic dyskinesia* is the easiest to recognize. Attacks are very brief, usually lasting seconds, and always less than 5 minutes. They are induced by sud-

den movements, startle, or hyperventilation, and may occur many times a day; they respond to anticonvulsants. The primary forms of paroxysmal dyskinesias are inherited in an autosomal-dominant pattern, but secondary causes are common, particularly with multiple sclerosis. Attacks of *paroxysmal non-kinesigenic dyskinesia* last minutes to hours, and sometimes longer than a day. Usually, they range from 5 minutes to 4 hours. They are primed by consuming alcohol, coffee, or tea, as well as by psychologic stress, excitement, and fatigue. There are usually no more than three attacks per day, and often attacks may be months apart. No consistent response to therapeutic interventions is yet available. This form may sometimes be the major presentation of a psychogenic movement disorder. *Paroxysmal exertional dyskinesia* is triggered by prolonged exercise; attacks last from 5 minutes to 30 minutes. Four types of episodic ataxias have been distinguished (see Table 9.2).

Hyperekplexia (excessive startle syndrome) consists of dramatic, complex motor responses to a sudden tactile verbal stimulus. The syndrome was originally

TABLE 9.2 Clinical and Genetic Features of Episodic Ataxias

Type	Age at Onset (Yrs)	Clinical Presentation	Acetazolamide Response	Precipitant	Frequency/ Duration	Interictal	Gene
Myokymia, neuromyotonia (EA-1)	2–15	Aura of weightless or weak, then ataxia, dysarthria, tremor, facial twitching	In some kindreds; anticonvulsants may help	Startle, movement, exercise, excitement, fatigue	Up to 15 per day; usually one or less per day; seconds to minutes, usually 2 min to 10 min	Myokymia, shortened Achilles tendon; PKD	12p13, K+ channel, different point mutations in KCNA1
Vestibular (EA-2) channel	0–40, usually 5–15	Ataxia, vertigo, nystagmus, dysarthria, headache, ptosis, ocular palsy, vermis atrophy	Very effective	Stress, alcohol, fatigue, exercise, caffeine	Daily to q 2 mos; usually hours; 5 min to weeks	Nystagmus, mild ataxia, less common: dysarthria, and progressive cerebellar	19p13, Ca+ channel, CACNL1A4 familial hemiplegic migraine
Ocular (EA-3)	20–50	Ataxia, diplopia, vertigo, nausea	No response	Sudden change in head position	Daily to year; minutes to hours	Symptoms gradually become constant	Unknown
Tinnitus (EA-4)	1–41	Ataxia, tinnitus, falling, headache, blurred vision, vertigo, nausea	Effective	None	Daily; 10 min to 30 mins	Myokymia; some with ataxia	Unknown

described with local names, such as jumping Frenchmen of Maine, Myriachit, and Latah; these may reflect cultural patterns of behavior, and may incorporate echolalia and echopraxia. Hyperekplexia may be hereditary (glycine receptor on chromosome 5q) or sporadic. When it is severe, the patient's movements must be curtailed because a sudden attack may lead to injury from falling.

Although most of the involuntary movements described are the result of CNS disorders, particularly in the basal ganglia, some dyskinesias arise from the brainstem, spinal cord, or peripheral nervous system. Dyskinesias attributed to peripheral disorders are hemifacial spasm (see Chapter 69), painful legs–moving toes, jumpy stumps, belly-dancer's dyskinesia, and the sustained muscle contractions seen in reflex sympathetic dystrophy (see Chapter 71). Psychogenic movement disorders seem to be increasingly more common. Usually, they appear with a mixture of different types of movements, particularly shaking, paroxysmal disorders, fixed postures, or bizarre gaits. Careful evaluation for inconsistency, incongruity, false weakness or sensory changes, sudden onset, deliberate slowness, and the appearance of marked fatigue and exhaustion from the "involuntary" movements helps suggest the diagnosis, which is best established by relief of the signs and symptoms using psychotherapy, suggestion, and physiotherapy.

SUGGESTED READINGS

Baloh RW, Yue Q, Furman JM, Nelson SF. Familial episodic ataxia: clinical heterogeneity in four families linked to chromosome 19p. *Ann Neurol* 1997;41:8–16.

Bhatia KP, Bhatt MH, Marsden CD. The causalgia-dystonia syndrome. *Brain* 1993;116:843–851.

Bhatia KP, Griggs RC, Ptacek LJ. Episodic movement disorders as channelopathies. *Mov Disord* 2000;15(3):429–433.

Brown. Physiology of startle phenomena. In: Fahn S, Hallett M, Lüders HO, Marsden CD, eds. *Negative Motor Phenomena*. Advances in Neurology, vol 67. Philadelphia: Lippincott–Raven Publishers, 1995:273–287.

Demirkiran M, Jankovic J. Paroxysmal dyskinesias: Clinical features and classification. *Ann Neurol* 1995;38:571–579.

Dressler D, Thompson PD, Gledhill RF, Marsden CD. The syndrome of painful legs and moving toes: a review. *Mov Disord* 1994;9:13–21.

Fahn S. Motor and vocal tics. In: Kurlan R, ed. *Handbook of Tourette's Syndrome and Related Tic and Behavioral Disorders*. New York: Marcel Dekker, 1993:3–16.

Fahn S. Paroxysmal dyskinesias. In: Marsden CD, Fahn S, eds: *Movement Disorders*, 3rd ed. Oxford: Butterworth-Heinemann, 1994:310–345.

Fahn S. Psychogenic movement disorders. In: Marsden CD, Fahn S, eds. *Movement Disorders*, 3rd ed. London: Butterworth-Heineman, 1994:358–372.

Fahn S, Frucht SJ, Hallett M, Truong DD, eds. *Myoclonus and Paroxysmal Dyskinesias*. Advances in Neurology, vol. 89. Lippincott Williams & Wilkins, Philadelphia, 2002.

Garcia-Borreguero D, Odin P, Schwarz C. Restless legs syndrome: an overview of the current understanding and management. *Acta Neurol Scand* 2004 May;109(5):303–317.

Hening WA. Subjective and objective criteria in the diagnosis of the restless legs syndrome. *Sleep Med* 2004 May;5(3):285–292.

Iliceto G, Thompson PD, Day BL, et al. Diaphragmatic flutter, the moving umbilicus syndrome, and belly dancers' dyskinesia. *Mov Disord* 1990;5:15–22.

Jeste DV. Tardive dyskinesia rates with atypical antipsychotics in older adults. *J Clin Psychiatry* 2004;65(Suppl 9):21–24.

Kulisevsky J, Marti-Fabregas J, Grau JM. Spasms of amputation stumps. *J Neurol Neurosurg Psychiatry* 1992;55:626–627.

Marsden CD, Fahn S, eds. *Movement Disorders*. London: Butterworth-Heineman, 1982.

Marsden CD, Fahn S, eds. *Movement Disorders*, 2nd ed. London: Butterworth-Heineman, 1987.

Marsden CD, Fahn S, eds. *Movement Disorders*, 3rd ed. London: Butterworth-Heineman, 1994.

Steckley JL, Ebers GC, Cader MZ, McLachlan RS. An autosomal dominant disorder with episodic ataxia, vertigo, and tinnitus. *Neurology* 2001;57:1499–1502.

Tan A, Salgado M, Fahn S. The characterization and outcome of stereotypic movements in nonautistic children. *Mov Disord* 1997;12:47–52.

Walters AS, Wagner ML, Hening WA, et al. Successful treatment of the idiopathic restless legs syndrome in a randomized double-blind trial of oxycodone versus placebo. *Sleep* 1993;16:327–332.

Winkelmann J, Muller-Myhsok B, Wittchen HU, et al. Complex segregation analysis of restless legs syndrome provides evidence for an autosomal dominant mode of inheritance in early age at onset families. *Ann Neurol* 2002;52(3):297–302.

Chapter 10

Syndromes Caused by Weak Muscles

Lewis P. Rowland

Weakness implies that a muscle cannot exert normal force. Neurologists use the words *paralysis* or *plegia* to imply total loss of contractility; anything less than total loss is *paresis*. In practice, however, someone may mention a *partial hemiplegia*, which conveys the idea even if it is internally inconsistent. *Hemiplegia* implies weakness of an arm and leg on the same side. *Crossed hemiplegia* is a confusing term, generally implying unilateral cranial nerve signs and hemiplegia on the other side, a pattern seen with brainstem lesions above the decussation of the corticospinal tracts. *Monoplegia* is weakness of one limb; *paraplegia* means weakness of both legs.

This chapter describes syndromes that result from pathologically weak muscles, so that a student new to neurology may find the sections of the book that describe specific diseases. There is more than one approach to this problem because no single approach is completely satisfactory. Elaborate algorithms have been devised but the flowchart may be too complicated to be useful, unless it is run by a computer.

It may be simpler to determine first, whether there is pathologic weakness, then to find evidence of specific syndromes that depend on recognition of the following characteristics: distribution of weakness, associated neurologic abnormalities, tempo of disease, genetics, and age of the patient.

RECOGNITION OF WEAKNESS, PSEUDOWEAKNESS, OR FATIGUE

Patients with weak muscles do not often use the word "weakness" to describe their symptoms. Rather, they say they cannot climb stairs, rise from chairs, or run, or they note foot-drop (and may actually use that term). They may have difficulty buttoning or turning keys or doorknobs. If proximal arm muscles are affected, it may be difficult to lift packages, comb hair, or work overhead. Weakness of cranial muscles causes ptosis of the eyelids, diplopia, dysarthria, dysphagia, or the cosmetic distortion of facial paralysis. These specific symptoms will be analyzed later.

Some people use the word weakness when there is no neurologic abnormality. For instance, aging athletes may find that they can no longer match the achievements of youth, but that is not pathologic weakness. Weakness in a professional athlete causes the same symptoms that are recognized by other people when the disorder interferes with the conventional activities of daily life. Losing a championship race, running a mile in more than 4 minutes, or jogging only 5 miles instead of a customary 10 miles are not symptoms of diseased muscles.

Others who lack the specific symptoms of weakness may describe *chronic fatigue*. They cannot do housework; they have to lie down to rest after the briefest exertion. If they plan a social activity in the evening, they may spend the entire day resting in advance. Employment may be in jeopardy. Myalgia is a common component of this syndrome, and there is usually evidence of depression.

The chronic fatigue syndrome affects millions of people and is a major public health problem. Vast research investments have been made to evaluate possible viral, immune, endocrine, autonomic, metabolic, and other precipitating factors. None, however, seems as consistent as depression and psychosocial causes. It is not as some put it, a diagnosis of exclusion. Instead, the characteristic history is recognizable and on examination there is no limb weakness or reflex alteration.

Fatigue seems to be a special problem in multiple sclerosis. Because it affects most patients, is the prime cause of disability for many patients, and sometimes occurs in attacks as an isolated symptom; some authorities attribute fatigue in multiple sclerosis as a symptom of interruption of corticospinal transmission. Other possible causes to be considered are depression, deconditioning, drug therapy, or systemic illness.

Fading athletes and depressed, tired people with aching limbs have different emotional problems, but both groups lack the specific symptoms of muscle weakness, and they share two other characteristics: No abnormality appears on neurologic examination, and no true weakness is evident on manual muscle examination. That is, there is no weakness unless the examiner uses brute force. A vigorous young adult examiner may outwrestle a frail octogenarian, but that does not imply pathologic weakness in the latter. Students and residents must use reasonable force in tests of strength against resistance.

Fatigue and similar symptoms may sometimes be manifestations of systemic illness due to anemia, hypoventilation, congestive heart failure with hypoxemia and hypercapnia, cancer, or systemic infection. There is usually other evidence of the underlying disease, however, and that syndrome is almost never mistaken for a neurologic disorder.

Other patients have *pseudoweakness*. For instance, some patients attribute a gait disorder to weak legs, but it is immediately apparent on examination or even before formal examination that they have parkinsonism. Sometimes a patient with peripheral neuropathy may have difficulty with fine movements of the fingers, not because of weakness but owing to severe sensory loss. Another patient may have difficulty raising one or both arms due to limited range of motion from bursitis, not limb weakness. A patient with arthritis may be reluctant to move a painful joint. These circumstances are explained by findings on examination.

Examination may also resolve another problem in the evaluation of symptoms that might be due to weakness. Sometimes, when limb weakness is mild, it is difficult for the examiner to know how much resistance to apply to determine whether the apparent weakness is real. Then, the presence or absence of wasting, fasciculation, or altered tendon reflexes may give the crucial clues. Symptomatic weakness is usually accompanied by some abnormality on examination. Even in myasthenia gravis, symptoms may fluctuate in intensity, but there are always objective signs of abnormality on examination if the patient is currently having symptoms. There is a maxim; a normal neurologic examination is incompatible with the diagnosis of symptomatic myasthenia gravis.

Finally, examination may uncover patients with pseudoweakness that may actually be the result of deceit, deliberate or otherwise; for example, hysterical patients and Munchausen deceivers or other malingerers who feign weakness all lack specific symptoms. Patients may betray inconsistencies in the history because they may participate in some activities but not in others that involve the same muscles. On examination, their dress, cosmetic facial makeup, and behavior may be histrionic. In walking, they may stagger dramatically, but they do not fall or injure themselves by bumping into furniture. In manual muscle tests, they abruptly give way, or they shudder in tremor rather than apply constant pressure. Misdirection of effort is one way to describe that behavior. Some simply refuse to participate in the test. The extent of disorder may be surprising, however. Psychogenic breathing impairment may lead to the use of a mechanical ventilator.

PATTERNS OF WEAKNESS

In analyzing syndromes of weakness, the examiner uses several sources of information for the differential diagnosis. The pattern of weakness and associated neurologic signs define some of the anatomic possibilities, to answer the question of *where* the lesion is located. Patient age and the tempo of evolution aid in deciding *what* the lesion is.

The differential diagnosis of weakness encompasses much of clinical neurology, so the reader will be referred to other sections for some of the review. For instance, the first task in the analysis of a weak limb is to determine whether the condition is due to a lesion of the upper or lower motor neuron, a distinction that is made on the basis of clinical findings. Overactive tendon reflexes with clonus, Hoffmann signs, and Babinski signs denote an upper motor neuron disorder. Lower motor neuron signs include muscle weakness, wasting, and fasciculation, with loss of tendon reflexes. These distinctions may seem crude, but they have been considered reliable guides for generations of neurologists.

If the clinical signs imply a lower motor neuron disorder, the condition could be due to problems anywhere in the motor unit (e.g., motor neuron or axon, neuromuscular junction, or muscle). This determination is guided by principles stated in Chapter 125. Diseases of the motor unit are also covered in that chapter, so the following information will be concerned primarily (but not entirely) with central lesions.

Hemiparesis

If there is weakness of the arm and leg on the same side, and if upper motor neuron signs imply a central lesion, the lesion could be in the cervical spinal cord or in the brain. Pain in the neck or in the distribution of a cervical dermatome might be clues to the site of the lesion. Unilateral facial weakness may be ipsilateral to the hemiparesis, placing the lesion in the brain and above the nucleus of the seventh cranial nerve; a change in mentation or speech may indicate that the lesion is cerebral, not cervical. Sometimes, however, there are no definite clinical clues to the site of the lesion, and the examiner must rely on findings in MRI, CT, EEG, analysis of CSF, or myelography to determine the site and nature of the lesion together.

The course of hemiparesis gives clues to the nature of the disorder. The most common cause in adults is cerebral infarction or hemorrhage. Abrupt onset, prior transient ischemic attacks, and progression to maximal severity within 24 hours in a person with hypertension or advanced age are indications that a stroke has occurred. If no cerebral symptoms are present, conceivably, there could be transverse myelitis of the cervical spinal cord but that condition would be somewhat slower in evolution (days rather than hours) and would more likely involve all four limbs. Similarly, multiple sclerosis is more likely to be manifest as bilateral corticospinal signs than by a pure hemiplegia.

If hemiparesis of cerebral origin progresses for days or weeks, it is reasonable to suspect a cerebral mass lesion, whether the patient is an adult or a child. If the patient has had focal seizures, that possibility is the more likely. In addition to brain tumors, other possibilities include arteriovenous malformation, brain abscess, or other infections. Infectious or neoplastic complications of AIDS are constant considerations these days. Metabolic brain disease usually causes bilateral signs with mental obtundation and would be an unusual cause of hemiparesis, even in a child.

Hemiparesis of subacute evolution could arise in the cervical spinal cord if there were, for instance, a neurofibroma of a cervical root. That condition would be signified by local pain in most cases, and because there is so little room in the cervical spinal canal, bilateral corticospinal signs probably would be present.

In general, hemiparesis usually signifies a cerebral lesion rather than one in the neck, and the cause is likely to be denoted by the clinical course and by CT or MRI.

Paraparesis

Paresis means weakness and *paraparesis* is used to describe weakness of both legs. The term has also been extended, however, to include gait disorders caused by lesions of the upper motor neuron, even when there is no weakness on manual muscle examination. The disorder is then attributed to *spasticity* or the clumsiness induced by malfunction of the corticospinal tracts. In adults, the most common cause of that syndrome, *spastic paraparesis of middle life,* is multiple sclerosis. The differential diagnosis includes tumors in the region of the foramen magnum, Chiari malformation, cervical spondylosis, arteriovenous malformation, and primary lateral sclerosis (all described in other sections of this book). The diagnosis cannot be made on clinical grounds alone and requires information from CSF examination (protein, cells, gamma globulin, oligoclonal bands), evoked potentials, CT, MRI, and myelography.

When there are cerebellar or other signs in addition to bilateral corticospinal signs, the disorder may be multiple sclerosis or an inherited disease, such as olivopontocerebellar degeneration. The combination of lower motor neuron signs in the arms and upper motor neuron signs in the legs is characteristic of amyotrophic lateral sclerosis; the same syndrome has been attributed, without proof, to cervical spondylosis. That pattern may also be seen in syringomyelia but it is exceptional to find syringomyelia without typical patterns of sensory loss.

Other clues to the nature of spastic paraparesis include cervical or radicular pain in neurofibromas or other extra-axial mass lesions in the cervical spinal canal. There may be concomitant cerebellar signs or other indications of multiple sclerosis.

It is said that brain tumors in the parasagittal area may cause isolated spastic paraparesis by compressing the leg areas of the motor cortex in both hemispheres. This possibility seems more theoretic than real, however, because no well documented cases have been reported.

Chronic paraparesis may also be due to lower motor neuron disorders. Instead of upper motor neuron signs, there is flaccid paraparesis, with loss of tendon reflexes in the legs. This differential diagnosis includes motor neuron diseases, peripheral neuropathy, and myopathy as described in Chapter 125.

Paraparesis of acute onset (days rather than hours or weeks) presents a different problem in diagnosis. If there is back pain and tendon reflexes are preserved, or if there are frank upper motor neuron signs, a compressive lesion may be present. As the population ages, metastatic tumors increasingly become a more common cause. In children or young adults, the syndrome may be less ominous, even with pain, because the disorder is often due to acute transverse myelitis. This may be seen in children or adults, and in addition to the motor signs, a sensory level usually designates the site of the lesion. Spinal MRI or myelography is needed to make this differentiation. In elderly people, a rare cause of acute paraplegia is infarction of the spinal cord. That syndrome is sometimes also seen after surgical procedures that require clamping of the aorta.

If the tendon reflexes are lost and there is no sensory level on the trunk in a patient with an acute paraparesis, the most common cause is the Guillain-Barré syndrome, at any age from infancy to the senium. The presence of sensory loss may facilitate that diagnosis, but sometimes little or no sensory impairment occurs. Then, the diagnosis depends on examination of the CSF and EMG with nerve conduction studies. The Guillain-Barré syndrome, however, may also originate from diverse causes.

In developing countries, acute paralytic poliomyelitis is still an important cause of acute paraplegia. Rarely, an acute motor myelitis may be due to some other virus. In China, for instance, there have been summertime outbreaks of an acute motor axonopathy that differs in details from both Guillain-Barré syndrome and poliomyelitis but, like the other syndromes, causes paraparesis.

The opposite of paraplegia would be weakness of the arms with good function in the legs, or *bibrachial paresis*. Lower motor neuron syndromes of this nature are seen in some cases of amyotrophic lateral sclerosis (with or without upper motor neuron signs in the legs). The arms hang limply at the side while the patient walks with normal movements of the legs. Similar patterns may be seen in some patients with myopathy of unusual distribution. It is difficult to understand how a cerebral lesion could cause weakness of the arms without equally severe weakness of the legs, but this man-in-the-barrel syndrome is seen in comatose patients who survive a bout of severe hypotension. The site of the lesion is not known, but it could be bilateral and prerolandic.

Monomelic Paresis

If one leg or one arm is weak, pain in the low back or the neck may point to a compressive lesion. Whether acute or chronic, herniated nucleus pulposus is high on the list of possibilities if radicular pain is present. Acute brachial plexus neuritis (neuralgic amyotrophy) is another cause of weakness in one limb with pain; a corresponding syndrome of the lumbosacral plexus is much less common. Peripheral nerve entrapment syndromes may also cause monomelic weakness and pain, but the pain is local, not radicular. Mononeuritis multiplex may also cause local pain, paresthesia, and paresis.

In painless syndromes of isolated limb weakness in adults, motor neuron disease is an important consideration if there is no sensory loss. Sometimes, in evaluating a limb with weak, wasted, and fasciculating muscle, the examiner is surprised because tendon reflexes are preserved or even overactive, instead of being lost. This apparent paradox implies lesions of both upper and lower motor neurons; it is almost pathognomonic of amyotrophic lateral sclerosis. The signs may be asymmetric in early stages of the disease.

Although rare, it is possible for strokes or other cerebral lesions to cause monomelic weakness with upper motor neuron signs. Weakness stemming from a cerebral lesion may be more profound in the arm, but abnormal signs are almost always present in the leg, too; that is, the syndrome is really a hemiparesis.

Neck Weakness

Difficulty holding up the head is seen in some patients with diseases of the motor unit, although it is almost never seen in patients with upper motor neuron disorders. Usually, patients with neck weakness also have symptoms of disorder of the lower cranial nerves (dysarthria and dysphagia) and often also of adjacent cervical segments, as manifest by difficulty raising the arms. Amyotrophic lateral sclerosis and myasthenia gravis are probably the two most common causes.

Rarely, there is isolated weakness of neck muscles, with difficulty holding the head up, but no oropharyngeal or arm symptoms. This *floppy-head syndrome* or *dropped-head syndrome* is a disabling disorder usually due to one of three conditions: motor neuron disease, myasthenia gravis, or polymyositis. Some cases, however, are idiopathic. New terms have been introduced to explain this syndrome—the *bent spine syndrome* and *isolated myopathy of the cervical extensor muscles*—which may be variations of the same condition. EMG shows a myopathic pattern in affected paraspinal muscles, and MRI may show replacement of muscle tissue by fat in either the cervical or thoracic areas, or both.

Weakness of Cranial Muscles

The syndromes associated with weakness of cranial muscles are reviewed in Chapters 7 and 69. The major problems in achieving a differential diagnosis involve identifying the sites of local lesions that affect individual nerves of ocular movement, facial paralysis, or the vocal cords. Pseudobulbar palsy, precipitated by upper motor neuron lesions, must be distinguished from the bulbar palsy seen with lower motor neuron disease, and then delineated from a form of amyotrophic lateral sclerosis. This distinction depends on associated signs of upper or lower motor neuron lesions. Myasthenia gravis may affect the eyes, face, or oropharynx and only rarely, the vocal cords; in fact, the diagnosis of myasthenia gravis is doubtful if there are no cranial symptoms. Brainstem syndromes in the aging population may be due to stroke, meningeal carcinomatosis, or brainstem encephalitis.

SUGGESTED READINGS

Adams RW. The distribution of muscle weakness in upper motor neuron lesions affecting the lower limb. *Brain* 1990;113:1459–1476.

Asher R. Munchausen's syndrome. *Lancet* 1954;1:339–341.

Ashizawa T, Rolak LA, Hines M. Spastic pure motor monoparesis. *Ann Neurol* 1986;20:638–641.

Blackwood SK, MacHale SM, Power MJ, et al. Effects of exercise on cognitive and motor function in chronic fatigue syndrome and depression. *J Neurol Neurosurg Psychiatry* 1998;65:541–546.

Goshorn RK. Chronic fatigue syndrome: a review for clinicians. *Semin Neurol* 1998;18:237–242.

Hatcher S, House A. Life events, difficulties, and dilemmas in the onset of chronic fatigue syndrome. *Psychol Med* 2003;33(7):1185–1192.

Hopkins A, Clarke C. Pretended paralysis requiring artificial ventilation. *BMJ* 1987;294:961–962.

Knopman DS, Rubens AB. The value of CT findings for the localization of cerebral functions: the relationship between CT and hemiparesis. *Arch Neurol* 1986;43:328–332.

Lange DJ, Fetell MR, Lovelace RE, Rowland LP. The floppy-head syndrome. *Ann Neurol* 1986;20:133 [abstr].

Layzer RB. Asthenia and the chronic fatigue syndrome. *Muscle Nerve* 1998;21:1609–1611.

Mahjneh I, Marconi G, Paetay A, et al. Axial myopathy—an unrecognized entity. *J Neurol* 2002;249(6):730–734.

Marsden CD. Hysteria—a neurologist's view. *Psychol Med* 1986;16:277–288.

Maurice-Williams RS, Marsh H. Simulated paraplegia: an occasional problem for the neurosurgeon. *J Neurol Neurosurg Psychiatry* 1985;48:826–831.

Myer BV. Motor responses evoked by magnetic brain stimulation in psychogenic limb weakness: diagnostic value and limitations. *J Neurol* 1992;239:251–255.

Oerlemans WG, de Visser M. Dropped head syndrome and bent spine syndrome: two separate clinical entities or different manifestations of axial myopathy? *J Neurol Neurosurg Psychiatry* 1998;65:258–259.

Price JR, Couper J. Cognitive behaviour therapy for chronic fatigue syndrome in adults (Cochrane Review). In: *The Cochrane Library*, iss 1. Chichester, UK: John Wiley & Sons, Ltd, 2004.

Racke MK, Hawker K, Frohman EM. Fatigue in multiple sclerosis: is the picture getting simpler or more complex? *Arch Neurol.* 2004;61(2):201–207.

Rutherford OM. Long-lasting unilateral muscle wasting and weakness following injury and immobilization. *Scand J Rehabil Med* 1990;22:33–37.

Sabin TD. An approach to chronic fatigue syndrome in adults. *Neurologist* 2003;9(1):28–34.

Sage JI, Van Uitert RL. Man-in-the-barrel syndrome. *Neurology* 1986;36:1102–1103.

Serratrice G, Pouget J, Pellissier JF. Bent spine syndrome. *J Neurol Neurosurg Psychiatry* 1996;65:51–54.

Thijs RD, Notermans NC, Wokke JH, et al. Distribution of muscle weakness of central and peripheral origin. *J Neurol Neurosurg Psychiatry* 1998;65:794–796.

C h a p t e r   1 1

Gait Disorders

Sid Gilman

Observation of the stance and gait of patients with neurologic symptoms may provide important diagnostic information and may immediately suggest particular disorders of motor or sensory function, or even specific diseases. Some types of gait are so characteristic of certain diseases that the diagnosis may be obvious at the initial encounter with a patient. An example of this is the typical posture and gait associated with Parkinson disease.

In normal bipedal locomotion, one leg and then the other alternately supports the erect moving body. Each leg undergoes brief periods of acceleration and deceleration as body weight shifts from one foot to the other. As the moving body passes over the supporting leg, the other leg swings forward in preparation for its next support phase. One foot or the other is constantly in contact with the ground, and when support of the body is transferred from the trailing leg to the leading leg, both feet are on the ground momentarily.

Normal bipedal locomotion requires two processes: continuous ground reaction forces that support the body's center of gravity, and periodic movement of each foot from one position of support to the next in the direction of progression. As a consequence of these basic requirements, certain displacements of the body segments regularly occur in walking. To begin walking, a person raises one foot and accelerates the leg forward; this is the *swing phase* of walking. Muscle action in the supporting leg causes the center of gravity of the body to move forward, creating a horizontal reaction force at the foot. The greater this reaction force becomes, the greater the acceleration of the body, because the amount of force equals the body mass multiplied by the amount of acceleration.

The swing phase ends when the leg that has swung forward makes contact with the ground, which is when the *stance phase* of walking begins. During the stance phase, the body weight shifts to the opposite leg and another swing phase begins. The major muscle groups of the leg are active at the beginning and the end of the stance and swing phases. As the body passes over the weight-bearing leg, it tends to be displaced toward the weight-bearing side, causing a slight side-to-side movement. In addition, the body rises and falls with each step. The body rises to a maximum level during the swing phase and descends to a minimum level during the stance phase. As the body accelerates upward during the swing phase, the vertical floor reaction increases to a value that exceeds the body weight. The vertical floor reaction falls to a minimum during downward acceleration, reducing the total vertical reaction to a value less than the body weight.

EXAMINING STANCE AND GAIT

When examining patients' stances and gaits, the physician should observe them from the front, back, and sides. Patients should be asked to rise quickly from a chair, walk normally at a slow pace and then at a fast pace, and then turn around. They should walk successively on their toes, on their heels, and then in tandem (i.e., placing the heel of one foot immediately in front of the toes of the opposite foot and attempting to progress forward in a straight line). They should stand with their feet together and the head erect, first with open eyes and then with closed eyes, to determine whether they can maintain their balance.

When a person walks normally, the body should be held erect with the head straight and the arms hanging loosely at the sides, each moving rhythmically forward with the opposite leg. The shoulders and hips should be approximately level. The arms should swing equally. The steps should be straight and about equal in length. The head should not be tilted, and there should be no appreciable scoliosis or lordosis. With each step, the hip and knee should flex smoothly, and the ankle should dorsiflex with a barely perceptible elevation of the hips as the foot clears the ground. The heel should strike the ground first, and the weight of the body should be transferred successively onto the sole of the foot and then onto the toes. The head and then the body should rotate slightly with each step, without lurching or falling.

Although there are gross similarities in the way that normal people walk, each person walks in a distinctive fashion. The distinctions between people reflect both their individual physical characteristics and their personality traits. Among the variables that compose the physical characteristics are speed, stride length, positions of the feet (e.g., with the toes pointing outward or pointing inward), characteristics of the walking surface, and the type of footwear worn. Perhaps more important are the goals to be accomplished in walking, as well as the person's aspirations, motivations, and attitudes. For some situations, speed is the most important factor. In other situations, safe arrival or the minimal expenditure of energy may be more important. Some people learn to walk gracefully or in the least obtrusive manner possible and consequently may expend extra energy. Others learn to walk ungracefully but as effectively as possible for the amount of energy expended. The manner of walking may provide clues to personality traits (e.g., aggressiveness, timidity, self-confidence, aloofness).

Gait in Hemiparesis

Hemiparesis from an upper motor neuron lesion results in a characteristic posture and gait, owing to the combined effects of spasticity and weakness of the affected limbs. Patients with hemiparesis usually stand and walk with the affected arm flexed and the leg extended. In walking, they have difficulty flexing the hip and knee and dorsiflexing the ankle; the paretic leg swings outward at the hip to avoid scraping the foot on the floor. The leg maintains a stiff posture in extension and rotates in a semicircle, first away from and then toward the trunk, with a circumduction movement. Despite the circumduction, the foot may scrape the floor so that the toe and outer side of the sole of the shoe become worn first. The upper body often rocks slightly to the opposite side during the circumduction movement. The arm on the hemiparetic side usually moves little during walking, remaining adducted at the shoulder, flexed at the elbow, and partially flexed at the

wrist and fingers. In a person without a previous motor disorder, loss of the swinging motion of an arm may be the first sign of a progressive upper motor neuron lesion that will result in a hemiparesis.

Gait in Paraparesis

Paraparesis usually results from lesions of the thoracic portion of the spinal cord. The gait of these patients results from the combined effects of spasticity and weakness of the legs and consists of slow, stiff movements at the knees and hips with evidence of considerable effort. The legs are usually maintained extended or slightly flexed at the hips and knees and are often adducted at the hips. In some patients, particularly those with severe spasticity, each leg may cross in front of the other during the swing phase of walking, causing a *scissors gait*. The steps are short, and patients may move the trunk from side to side in attempts to compensate for the slow, stiff movements of the legs. The legs circumduct at the hips, and the feet scrape the floor, so that the soles of the shoes become worn at the toes.

Gait in Parkinsonism

The gait in Parkinson disease reflects a combination of akinesia (difficulty in initiating movement), dystonia (relatively fixed abnormal postures), rigidity, and tremor. These patients stand in a posture of general flexion, with the spine bent forward, the head bent downward, the arms moderately flexed at the elbows, and the legs slightly flexed. They stand immobile and rigid, with a paucity of automatic movements of the limbs and a masklike, fixed facial expression with infrequent blinking. Although the arms are held immobile, often a rest tremor involves the fingers and wrists at 4 to 5 cycles per second. When these patients walk, the trunk bends even farther forward; the arms remain immobile at the sides of the body or become further flexed and carried somewhat ahead of the body. The arms do not swing. As patients walk forward, the legs remain bent at the knees, hips, and ankles. The steps are short so that the feet barely clear the ground and the soles of the feet shuffle and scrape the floor. The gait, with characteristically small steps, is termed *marche à petits pas*. Forward locomotion may lead to successively more rapid steps, and the patient may fall unless assisted; this increasingly rapid walking is called *festination*. If patients are pushed forward or backward, they cannot compensate with flexion or extension movements of the trunk. The result is a series of propulsive or retropulsive steps. Parkinsonian patients may sometimes walk with surprising rapidity for brief intervals. These patients often have difficulty when they start to walk after standing still or sitting in a chair. They may take several very small steps that cover little distance before taking longer strides. The walking movements may stop involuntarily, and the patient may freeze on attempts to pass through a doorway or into an elevator.

Gait in Cerebellar Disease

Patients with disease of the cerebellum stand with their legs farther apart than normal and may develop *titubation*, a coarse fore-and-aft tremor of the trunk. Often, they cannot stand with their legs so close that the feet are touching; they sway or fall in attempts to do so, whether their eyes are opened or closed. They walk cautiously, taking steps of varying length, some shorter and others longer than usual. They may lurch from one side to another. Because of this unsteady or *ataxic gait,* that they usually attribute to poor balance, they fear walking without support and tend to hold onto objects in the room, such as a bed or a chair, moving cautiously between these objects. When gait ataxia is mild, it may be enhanced by asking the patient to attempt tandem walking in a straight line, successively placing the heel of one foot directly in front of the toes of the opposite foot. Patients commonly lose their balance during this task and must quickly place one foot to the side to avoid falling.

When disease is restricted to the vermal portions of the cerebellum, disorders of stance and gait may appear without other signs of cerebellar dysfunction, such as limb ataxia or nystagmus. This pattern is seen in alcoholic cerebellar degeneration. Diseases of the cerebellar hemispheres, unilateral or bilateral, may also affect gait. With a unilateral cerebellar-hemisphere lesion, ipsilateral disorders of posture and movement accompany the gait disorder. Patients usually stand with their shoulders on the sides of the lesion lower than the other; there is accompanying scoliosis. The limbs on the side of the cerebellar lesion show decreased resistance to passive manipulation (*hypotonia*). When these patients attempt to touch their noses and then the examiners' fingers (the finger-nose-finger test), they miss their targets and experience side-to-side tremors generated from the shoulder. When they attempt to touch the knee of one leg with the heel of the other leg and then move the heel smoothly down along the shin (the heel-knee-shin test), a side-to-side tremor of the moving leg develops, generated from the hip. On walking, patients with cerebellar disease show ataxia of the leg ipsilateral to the cerebellar lesion; consequently they stagger and progressively deviate to the affected side. This may be demonstrated by asking them to walk around a chair. As they rotate toward the affected side, they tend to fall into the chair; rotating toward the normal side, they move away from the chair in a spiral. Patients with bilateral cerebellar-hemisphere disease show a disturbance of gait similar to that seen in disease of the vermis, but signs of cerebellar dysfunction also appear in coordinated limb movements. Thus, these patients show abnormal finger-nose-finger and heel-knee-shin tests, bilaterally.

Gait in Sensory Ataxia

Another characteristic gait disorder results from loss of proprioceptive sensation in the legs, owing to lesions of the afferent fibers in peripheral nerves, dorsal roots, dorsal columns of the spinal cord, or medial lemnisci. Patients with such lesions are unaware of the position of the limbs and consequently have difficulty standing or walking. They usually stand with their legs spread widely apart. If asked to stand with their feet together and eyes open, they remain stable, but when they close their eyes, they sway and often fall (*Romberg sign*). They walk with their legs spread widely apart, watching the ground carefully. In stepping, they lift the legs higher than normal at the hips and fling them abruptly forward and outward. The steps vary in length and may cause a characteristic slapping sound as the feet contact the floor. They usually hold their bodies somewhat flexed, often using canes for support. If vision is impaired and these patients attempt to walk in the dark, the gait disturbance worsens.

Psychogenic Gait Disorders

Psychogenic disorders of gait often appear in association with many other neurologic complaints, including "dizziness," loss of balance, and weakness of both legs or the arm and leg on one side of the body. The gait is usually bizarre, easily recognized, and unlike any disorder of gait evoked by organic disease. In some patients, however, hysteric gait disorders may be difficult to identify. The key to the diagnosis is the demonstration that objective organic signs of disease are missing. In hysteric hemiplegia, patients drag the affected leg along the ground behind the body and do not circumduct the leg, scraping the sole of the foot on the floor, as in hemiplegia due to an organic lesion. At times, the hemiplegic leg may be pushed ahead of the patient and used mainly for support. The arm on the affected side does not develop the flexed posture commonly seen with hemiplegia from organic causes, and the hyperactive tendon reflexes and Babinski signs on the hemiplegic sides are missing.

Hysteric paraplegic patients usually walk with one or two crutches, or lie helplessly in bed, with the legs maintained in rigid postures or at times completely limp. The term *astasia-abasia* refers to patients who cannot stand or walk but who can carry out natural movements of the limbs while lying in bed. At times, patients with hysteric gait disorders walk only with seemingly great difficulty, but they show normal power and coordination when lying in bed. On walking, patients cling to the bed or objects in the room. If asked to walk without support, they may lurch dramatically while managing feats of extraordinary balance to avoid falling. They may fall, but only when a nearby physician or family member may catch them or when soft objects are available to cushion the fall. The gait disturbance is often dramatic, with the patient lurching wildly in many directions and finally falling, but only when other people are watching the performance. They often demonstrate remarkable agility in their rapid postural adjustments when they attempt to walk.

Gait in Cerebral Palsy

The term *cerebral palsy* includes several different motor abnormalities that usually result from perinatal injury. The severity of the gait disturbance varies, depending on the nature of the lesion. Mild limited lesions may result in exaggerated tendon reflexes and extensor-plantar responses with a slight degree of talipes equinovarus but no clear gait disorder. More severe and extensive lesions often result in bilateral hemiparesis; patients stand with the legs adducted and internally rotated at the hips, extended or slightly flexed at the knees, with plantar flexion at the ankles. The arms are held adducted at the shoulders and flexed at the elbows and wrists. Patients walk slowly and stiffly with plantar flexion of the feet, causing them to walk on the toes. Bilateral adduction of the hips causes the knees to rub together or to cross, causing a scissors gait.

The gait in patients with cerebral palsy may be altered by movement disorders. Athetosis is common and consists of slow, serpentine movements of the arms and legs between the extreme postures of flexion, with supination and extension with pronation. On walking, patients with athetotic cerebral palsy show involuntary limb movements that are accompanied by rotary movements of the neck and constant grimacing. The limbs usually show the bilateral hemiparetic posture described previously; however, superimposed on this posture may be partially fixed, asymmetric limb postures with for example, flexion with supination of one arm and extension with pronation of the other. Asymmetric limb postures commonly occur in association with rotated postures of the head, generally with extension of the arm on the side to which the chin rotates and flexion of the opposite arm.

Gait in Chorea

Chorea literally means "the dance" and refers to the gait disorder seen most often in children with Sydenham chorea or adults with Huntington disease. Both conditions are characterized by continuous and rapid movements of the face, trunk, and limbs. Flexion, extension, and rotary movements of the neck occur with grimacing movements of the face, twisting movements of the trunk and limbs, and rapid piano-playing movements of the digits. Walking generally accentuates these movements. In addition, sudden forward or sideward thrusting movements of the pelvis and rapid twisting movements of the trunk and limbs result in a gait resembling a series of dancing steps. With walking, patients speed up and slow down at unpredictable times, evoking a lurching gait.

Gait in Dystonia Musculorum Deformans

The first symptom of this disorder often consists of an abnormal gait resulting from inversion of one foot at the ankle. Patients walk initially on the lateral sides of the feet; as the disease progresses, this problem worsens and other postural abnormalities develop, including elevation of one shoulder and hip, and twisted postures of the trunk. Intermittent spasms of the trunk and limbs then interfere with walking. Eventually, there is torticollis, tortipelvis, lordosis, or scoliosis. Finally, patients may become unable to walk.

Gait in Muscular Dystrophy

In muscular dystrophy, weakness of the muscles of the trunk and the proximal parts of the legs produces a characteristic stance and gait. In attempting to rise from the seated position, patients flex the trunk at the hips, put their hands on their knees, and push the trunk upward by working their hands up the thighs. This sequence of movements is termed the *Gowers sign*. Patients stand with exaggerated lumbar lordosis and a protuberant abdomen because of weakness of the abdominal and paravertebral muscles. They walk with the legs spread widely apart, showing a characteristic waddling motion of the pelvis that results from weakness of the gluteal muscles. The shoulders often slope forward, and winging of the scapulae may be seen as the patients walk.

Senile Gait Disorders

Many disorders of gait have been observed in elderly persons, including those people who have overt neurologic disease.

Cautious Gait

This gait is often seen in normal (healthy) elderly people. It is characterized by a slightly widened base, shortened stride, slowness of walking, and turning in a block. There is no hesitancy in the initiation of gait and no shuffling or freezing. The rhythms of walking and foot clearance are normal. There is mild disequilibrium in response to a push and difficulty in balancing on one foot.

Subcortical Disequilibrium

This gait disorder is seen with progressive supranuclear palsy and multiinfarct dementia. Patients have marked difficulty maintaining the upright posture and show absent or poor postural adjustments in response to perturbations. Some patients hyperextend the trunk and neck and fall backward or forward, thus impairing locomotion. These patients commonly show ocular palsies, dysarthria, and the parkinsonian signs of rigidity, akinesia, and tremors.

Frontal Disequilibrium

Many patients with frontal disequilibrium cannot rise, stand, or walk; some can not even sit without support. Standing and walking are difficult or impossible. When they try to rise from a chair, they lean backward rather than forward, and they cannot bring their legs under their centers of gravity. When they attempt to step, their feet frequently cross and move in a direction that is inappropriate to their centers of gravity. Clinical examination usually reveals dementia, signs of frontal release (e.g., suck, snout, and grasp reflexes), motor perseveration, urinary incontinence, pseudobulbar palsy, exaggerated muscle stretch reflexes, and extensor-plantar responses.

Isolated Gait Ignition Failure

Patients with this disorder have difficulty starting to walk and continuing walking, even though they have no impairment of equilibrium, cognition, limb praxis, or extrapyramidal function. Once they start to walk, the steps are short and their feet barely clear the ground, thereby creating a shuffling appearance. With continued stepping, however, the stride lengthens, foot clearance is normal, and the arms swing normally. If their attention is diverted, their feet may freeze momentarily and shuffling may recur. Postural responses and stance base are normal, and falls are rare. The terms *magnetic gait* or *apraxia of gait* pertain to both isolated gait ignition failure and frontal gait disorder.

Frontal Gait Disorder

This disturbance is often seen with multiinfarct dementia or normal pressure hydrocephalus. Characteristically, these patients stand on wide bases (though sometimes narrow bases) and take short steps with shuffling, hesitate in starting to walk and in turning, and show moderate disequilibrium. Associated findings include cognitive impairment, pseudobulbar palsy with dysarthria, signs of frontal release (e.g., suck, snout, and grasping reflexes), paratonia, signs of corticospinal tract disease, and urinary dysfunction. In patients who have this gait disorder in association with normal pressure hydrocephalus, ventricular shunting may restore a normal gait.

Gait in Lower Motor Neuron Disorders

Diseases of the motor neurons or peripheral nerves characteristically cause distal weakness, and foot-drop is a common manifestation. In motor neuron disease and in the hereditary neuropathies (e.g., Charcot-Marie-Tooth disease), the disorder is likely to be bilateral. If the patient has a compressive lesion of one peroneal nerve, the process may be unilateral. In either case, patients can not dorsiflex the feet in walking, as would be normal each time the swinging leg begins to move. As a result, the toes are scuffed along the ground. To avoid this awkwardness, patients raise the knees higher than usual, resulting in a "steppage" gait. If the proximal muscles of the legs are affected (in addition to, or instead of distal muscles), the gait also has a waddling appearance.

SUGGESTED READINGS

Alexander NB. Differential diagnosis of gait disorders in older adults. *Clin Geriatr Med* 1996;12:689–703.

Dietz V. Physiology of human gait: neural processes. In: Růžička M, Hallett M, Jankovic J, eds. *Gait Disorders. Advances in Neurology,* vol. 87. Philadelphia: Lippincott Williams & Wilkins, 2001:53–63.

Dietz V. Gait disorder in spasticity and Parkinson's disease. In: Růžička M, Hallett M, Jankovic J, eds. *Gait Disorders. Advances in Neurology,* vol. 87. Philadelphia: Lippincott Williams & Wilkins, 2001: 143–154.

Hallett M. Cerebellar ataxic gait. In: Růžička M, Hallett M, Jankovic J, eds. *Gait Disorders. Advances in Neurology,* vol. 87. Philadelphia: Lippincott Williams & Wilkins, 2001:155–163.

Iansek R, Ismail NH, Bruce M, Huxham FE, Morris ME. Frontal gait apraxia: pathophysiological mechanisms and rehabilitation. In: Růžička M, Hallett M, Jankovic J, eds. *Gait Disorders. Advances in Neurology,* vol. 87. Philadelphia: Lippincott Williams & Wilkins, 2001:363–374363–374.

Jankovic J, Nutt JG, Sudarsky L. Classification, diagnosis, and etiology of gait disorders. In: Růžička M, Hallett M, Jankovic J, eds. *Gait Disorders. Advances in Neurology,* vol. 87. Philadelphia: Lippincott Williams & Wilkins, 2001:119–133.

Morris M, Iansek R, Matyas T, Summers J. Abnormalities in the stride length-cadence relation in parkinsonian gait. *Mov Disord* 1998;13: 61–69.

Ondo W. Gait and balance disorders. *Medical Clin N Am* 2003;87(4): 793–801.

Thach WT, Bastian AJ. Role of the cerebellum in the control and adaptation of gait in health and disease. *Progr Brain Res* 2004;143: 353–366.

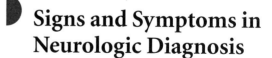

Chapter 12

Signs and Symptoms in Neurologic Diagnosis

Lewis P. Rowland

An anonymous sage said that 90% of the neurologic diagnosis depends on the patient's medical history and the remainder comes from the neurologic examination and laboratory tests. Sometimes, of course, findings in blood tests, MRI, or CT are pathognomonic, but students have to learn which tests are appropriate and when to order them. It is therefore necessary to know which diagnostic possibilities are reasonable considerations for a particular patient. In the consideration of these different diagnostic possibilities, specific symptoms are not the only ingredient in the analysis of a patient's history, as this chapter briefly reviews.

It is commonly taught that neurologic diagnosis depends on answers to two questions that are considered separately and in sequence:

1. *Where is the lesion?* Is it in the cerebrum, basal ganglia, brainstem, cerebellum, spinal cord, peripheral nerves, neuromuscular junction, or muscle?
2. *What is the nature of the disease?*

If the site of the lesion can be determined, the number of diagnostic possibilities is manageable. An experienced clinician, however, is likely to deal with both questions simultaneously; site and disease are identified at the same time. Sometimes, the process is reversed. To take an obvious example, if a patient suddenly becomes speechless or awakens with a hemiplegia, the diagnosis of stroke is presumed. The location is then deduced from findings on examination, and both site and process are ascertained by CT or MRI. If there are no surprises in the imaging study (e.g., demonstration of a tumor or vascular malformation), further laboratory tests might be considered to determine the cause of an ischemic infarct.

The specific nature of different symptoms and findings on examination are reviewed in preceding chapters and in teaching manuals on the neurologic examination. Other considerations that influence diagnosis are briefly described here.

AGE OF THE PATIENT

The symptoms and signs of a stroke may be virtually identical in a 10-year-old, a 25-year-old, and a 70-year-old patient, but the diagnostic implications are vastly different for each patient. Some brain tumors are more common in children, and others are more common in adults. Progressive paraparesis is more likely to be due to spinal cord tumor in a child, whereas in an adult it is more likely to be due to multiple sclerosis. Focal seizures are less likely to be fixed in pattern and are less likely to indicate a specific structural brain lesion in a child than in an adult. Myopathic weakness of the legs in childhood is more likely to be caused by muscular dystrophy than polymyositis; the reverse is true in patients older than 25 years. Muscular dystrophy rarely begins after age 35. Multiple sclerosis rarely starts after age 55. Hysteria is not a likely diagnosis when neurologic symptoms start after age 50. These ages are arbitrary, but the point is that age is a consideration in some diagnoses.

GENDER SPECIFICITY

Only a few diseases are gender-specific. X-linked diseases (e.g., Duchenne muscular dystrophy) occur only in boys or, rarely, in girls with chromosome disorders. Among young adults, autoimmune diseases are more likely to affect women, especially systemic lupus erythematosus and myasthenia gravis, although young men are also affected in some cases. Women are exposed to the neurologic complications of pregnancy and may be at increased risk of stroke because of oral contraceptives. Men are more often exposed to the possibility of head injury.

ETHNICITY

Stating the race of the patient in every case history is an anachronism of modern medical education. In neurology, race is important only when sickle cell disease is considered. Malignant hypertension and sarcoidosis may be more prevalent in blacks, but whites are also susceptible. Other ethnic groups, however, are more susceptible to particular diseases: Tay-Sachs disease, familial dysautonomia, and Gaucher disease in Ashkenazi Jews; familial inclusion; body myopathy in Iranian Jews; familial Creutzfeldt-Jakob disease in Libyan Jews; thyrotoxic periodic paralysis in Japanese and perhaps in other Asians; nasopharyngeal carcinoma in Chinese people; sickle cell disease in people of African descent; Marchiafava-Bignami disease in Italian wine drinkers (a myth?); and hemophilia in descendants of the Romanovs. Ethnicity is rarely important in diagnosis.

SOCIOECONOMIC CONSIDERATIONS

In general, social deprivation leads to increased mortality, and the reasons are not always clear. Ghetto dwellers, whatever their race, are prone to the ravages of alcoholism, drug addiction, and trauma. Impoverishment is also accompanied by malnutrition, infections, and the consequences of medical neglect. Within the ghetto and in other social strata, the HIV epidemic has generated concern about the risk factors for male homosexuals, intravenous drug users, prostitutes, and recipients of blood transfusions. For most other neurologic disorders, however, race, ethnicity, sex, sexual orientation, and socioeconomic status do not affect the incidence.

Inequities of access affect these conditions in the United States and, globally, poor countries suffer from tragedies of malnutrition, parasitic diseases, and AIDS. Embargos have become popular political weapons but impose punishment on innocent civilian adults and children. It is not just poverty that impedes access; rural areas in any continent may have limited access to imaging or advanced therapeutic technology (a problem that has generated helicopter transfer and telemedicine). The 40 million US citizens without health insurance have limited access.

TEMPO OF DISEASE

Seizures, strokes, and syncope are all abrupt in onset but differ in manifestations and duration. Syncope is the briefest. There are usually sensations that warn of the impending loss of consciousness. After fainting, the patient begins to recover consciousness in a minute or so. A seizure may or may not be preceded by warning symptoms. It may be brief or protracted and is manifested by alteration of consciousness or by repetitive movements, stereotypical behavior, or abnormal sensations. A stroke due to cerebral ischemia or hemorrhage strikes "out of the blue" and manifests as hemiparesis or other focal brain signs. The neurologic disorder that follows brain infarction may be permanent, or the patient may recover partially, or completely, in days or weeks. If the signs last less than 24 hours, the episode is called a transient ischemic attack (TIA). Sometimes, it is difficult to differentiate a TIA from the postictal hemiparesis of a focal motor seizure, especially if imaging shows no lesion and the seizure was not witnessed. Another syndrome of abrupt onset is subarachnoid hemorrhage, in which the patient is struck by a severe headache that is instantaneously severe, and that is sometimes followed by loss of consciousness.

Symptoms of less than apoplectic onset may progress for hours (intoxication, infection, or subdural hematoma), days (Guillain-Barré syndrome), or longer (most tumors of the brain or spinal cord). The acute symptoms of increased intracranial pressure or brain herniation are sometimes superimposed on the slower progression of a brain tumor. Progressive symptoms of brain tumor may be punctuated by seizures. Heritable or degenerative diseases tend to progress slowly, becoming most severe only after years of increasing disability (e.g., Parkinson disease or Alzheimer disease).

Remissions and exacerbations are characteristic of myasthenia gravis, multiple sclerosis, and some forms of peripheral neuropathy. Bouts of myasthenia tend to last for weeks at a time; episodes in multiple sclerosis may last only days in the first attacks and then tend to increase in duration and to leave more permanent residual neurologic disability. These diseases sometimes become progressively worse without remissions.

The symptoms of myasthenia gravis vary in a way that differs from any other disease. The severity of myasthenic symptoms may vary from minute to minute. More often, however, there are differences in the course of a day (usually worse in the evening than in the morning, but sometimes vice versa) or from day to day.

Some disorders characteristically occur in bouts that usually last minutes or hours, but rarely longer. Periodic paralysis, migraine headache, cluster headaches, and narcolepsy are in this category. To recognize the significance of these differences in tempo, it is necessary to have some knowledge of the clinical features of the several disorders.

DURATION OF SYMPTOMS

It may be of diagnostic importance to ask patients how long they have been having similar symptoms. Long-standing headache is more apt to be a migraine, tension, or vascular headache, but headache of recent onset is likely to imply intracranial structural disease and should never be underestimated. Similarly, a seizure or drastic personality change of recent onset implies the need for CT, MRI, and other studies to evaluate possible brain tumor or encephalopathy. If no such lesion is found or if seizures are uncontrolled for a long time, perhaps video-electroencephalographic monitoring should be carried out to determine the best drug therapy or surgical approach.

MEDICAL HISTORY

It is always important to know whether any systemic disease is in the patient's background. Common disorders, such as hypertensive vascular disease or diabetes mellitus, may be discovered for the first time when the patient is examined because of neurologic symptoms. Because they are common, these two disorders may be merely coincidental, but depending on the neurologic syndrome, either diabetes or hypertension may actually be involved in the pathogenesis of the neural signs. If the patient is known to have a carcinoma, metastatic disease is assumed to be the basis of neurologic symptoms until proved otherwise. If the patient is taking medication for any reason, the possibility of intoxication must be considered. Cutaneous signs may point to neurologic complications of von Recklinghausen disease or other phakomatoses or may suggest lupus erythematosus or some other systemic disease.

IDENTIFYING THE SITE OF DISORDER

Aspects of the history may suggest the nature of the disorder; specific symptoms and signs suggest the site of the disorder. *Cerebral disease* is implied by seizures or by focal signs that may be attributed to a particular area of the brain; hemiplegia, aphasia, or hemianopia are examples. Generalized manifestations of cerebral disease are seizures, delirium, and dementia. *Brainstem disease* is suggested by cranial nerve palsies, cerebellar signs of ataxia of gait or limbs, tremor, or dysarthria. Dysarthria may be to the result of incoordination in disorders of the cerebellum itself or its brainstem connections. Cranial nerve palsies or the neuromuscular disorder of myasthenia gravis may also impair speech. Ocular signs have special localizing value. Involuntary movements suggest *basal ganglia disease.*

Spinal cord disease is suggested by spastic gait disorder and bilateral corticospinal signs, with or without bladder symptoms. If there is neck or back pain, a compressive lesion should be suspected; if there is no pain, multiple sclerosis is likely. The level of a spinal compressive lesion is more likely to be indicated by cutaneous sensory loss than by motor signs. The lesion that causes spastic paraparesis may be anywhere above the lumbar segments.

Peripheral nerve disease usually causes both motor and sensory symptoms (e.g., weakness and loss of sensation). The weakness is likely to be more severe distally, and the sensory loss may affect only position or vibration sense. A more specific indication of peripheral neuropathy is loss of cutaneous sensation in a glove-and-stocking distribution.

Neuromuscular disorders and *diseases of muscle* cause limb or cranial muscle weakness without sensory symptoms. If limb weakness and loss of tendon jerks arethe only signs (with no sensory loss), electromyography and muscle biopsy are needed to determine whether the disor-

der is one of motor neurons, peripheral nerve, or muscle. The diseases that cause these symptoms and signs are described later in this volume.

SUGGESTED READINGS

Angel M. Privilege and health—what is the connection? *N Engl J Med* 1993;329:126–127.

Brust JCM. *Practice of Neural Science,* 2nd ed. New York: McGraw-Hill, in press.

DeMyer WE. *Technique of the Neurological Examination,* 5th ed. New York: McGraw-Hill, 2003.

Farmer P. *Pathologies of Power. Berkeley CA.* University of California Press, 2003.

Epstin AM. Health Care in America—still too separate, not yet equal. *N Engl J Med* 2004;6:603–605.

Fried R. *The Hyperventilation Syndrome: Research and Clinical Treatment.* Baltimore: Johns Hopkins University Press, 1987.

Haerer AF. *DeJong's the Neurologic Examination,* 5th ed. Philadelphia: JB Lippincott Co, 1992.

Navarro N. Race or class versus race and class: mortality differences in the United States. *Lancet* 1990;336:1238–1240.

Vastag B. Health disparities report. *JAMA* 2004;291(6):684 (Abstr); full report by US Department of Health and Human Services available at http://www.ahrq.gov/qual/nhdr03/nhdrsum03.htm.

Wang DZ. Telemedicine: the solution to provide rural stroke coverage and the answer to the shortage of stroke neurologists and radiologists. *Stroke* 2003;34(12):2951–2956.

Wiebers DO, ed. *Mayo Clinic Examinations in Neurology,* 7th ed. St. Louis, MO: Mosby-Year Book, 1998.

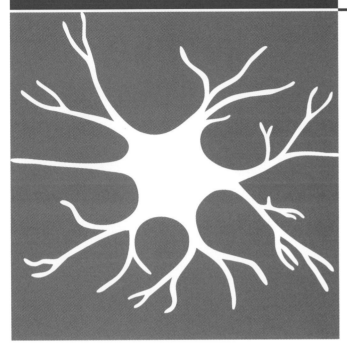

How to Select
Diagnostic Tests

Computed Tomography and Magnetic Resonance Imaging

Robert DeLaPaz

CT and MRI are the core imaging methods in neurodiagnosis. CT is often more accessible and less expensive, but MRI is the "gold standard" for detecting and delineating intracranial and spinal lesions. In the past, the major advantage of CT was the speed and simplicity of imaging, which reduced patient discomfort and motion artifact. Ultrafast MR methods such as echo-planar imaging (EPI) now allow similarly rapid imaging with MRI. CT technology has also advanced to allow acquisition of angiography (CTA) and dynamic physiologic imaging such as cerebral perfusion (CTP), comparable to MR angiography (MRA) and MR perfusion-weighted imaging (PWI). Although CT and MRI technologies are converging in some areas, there remain inherent advantages of MRI, based on its sensitivity to tissue physiology and biochemistry, such as with diffusion-weighted imaging (DWI) for cerebral ischemia, functional imaging (fMRI) for cerebral activation and spectroscopy (MRS) for specific diagnosis of metabolic and neoplastic disorders. Continued experience and advances in CT and MRI technology will likely lead to improved sensitivity and specificity of existing methods and development of unique and complementary neurodiagnostic applications in the future.

COMPUTED TOMOGRAPHY

CT is based on image reconstruction from sets of quantitative x-ray measurements through the head. A circular scanner gantry houses the x-ray source and detectors; the plane of the circle may be tilted to perform scans at a range of angles from axial to coronal, depending on head position, but not in the sagittal plane. A fan beam of xrays emitted from a single source passes through the head to an array of detectors. The x-ray source rotates around the patient's head, and the x-ray attenuation through the section plane is measured in compartments called voxels (a voxel is volume element similar to a picture element, or pixel, with the added dimension of the section thickness to create an image volume component). The computer reconstructs the image from about 800,000 measurements and assigns a number to each voxel according to its x-ray attenuation, which is proportional to tissue electron density averaged over the volume of the voxel. These values are displayed along a gray scale from black for low density (low attenuation), to white for high density.

In the head, CT differentiates CSF and brain as well as white and gray matter, shows the main divisions of the basal ganglia and thalamus, depicts the major arteries and veins and images the skull and skull base in detail. Iodinated water-soluble contrast agents, which have high x-ray density, may be given intravenously to enhance differences in tissue density, show vascular structures, or detect areas of blood–brain barrier breakdown. CT is especially useful for identifying acute hemorrhage, which appears as much higher density than normal brain or CSF and may have a variable or nonspecific appearance on MRI (Fig. 13.1).

The major limitation of CT is imaging the posterior fossa, where linear artifacts appear because bone selectively attenuates the low energy components of the x-ray beam; the resulting "beam hardening" creates dense or lucent streaks that project across the brainstem and may obscure underlying lesions.

CT technology has advanced beyond a simple, single section, static imaging method. Scan time-per-section may be shortened to less than 1 second to minimize motion artifact and multisection helical CT may now acquire contiguous thin sections to produce three-dimensional (3D)-data sets of an entire body part, such as the neck or head, in less than 1 minute. The increased speed of CT has also made it suitable for imaging dynamic processes, such as cerebral blood flow (CT perfusion, CTP) and for 3D depiction of vascular structures (CT angiography, CTA), which will be discussed in more detail later in this chapter.

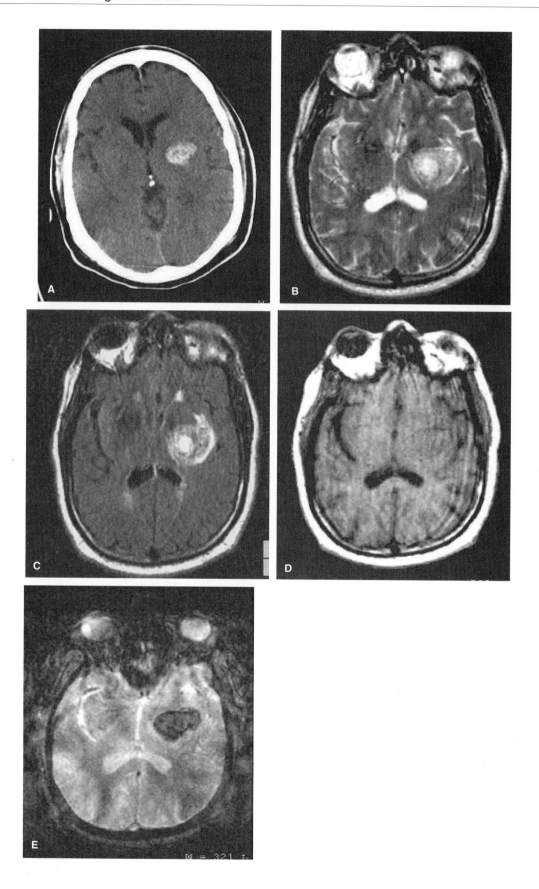

MAGNETIC RESONANCE IMAGING

Certain atomic nuclei, such as hydrogen protons, have "spin" properties that cause them to behave like microscopic bar magnets (magnetic dipoles) with a north and south pole. When placed in a strong, external magnetic field these nuclei tend to be in one of two states: a low energy state aligned with (parallel to) the magnetic field, or a high energy state aligned against (anti-parallel to) the magnetic field.

In proton-based MRI, radiowaves or radiofrequency (RF) pulses are applied at a frequency that resonates with the hydrogen nuclei in tissue water or lipid molecules, resulting in a shift of a small percentage of protons (a few per million) into higher energy states. This population of higher energy protons "line up" to create a momentary magnetic vector that is pointed away from the central axis (Z axis) of the main magnetic field. The RF pulses are described by the angle that they rotate or "flip" the magnetic vector off the Z axis, typically 90° or 180°. Following imposition of the radiofrequency pulse, "relaxation" of these protons back to their original lower energy state is accompanied by a reorientation and decay of the magnetic vector and emission of detectable radiowave signals that are characteristic of the water or fat in a particular tissue. Two tissue-specific relaxation-time constants are important in this process. Each describes an initially rapid, then slower, exponential rate of signal change. T1 is the longer time constant, generally from 500 milliseconds to 2,000 milliseconds in the brain, and is a measure of the rate of the proton magnetic vector reorientation back along the Z axis of the magnetic field. T2 is the shorter time constant, usually 40 milliseconds to 100 milliseconds in the brain, and is a measure of the rate of decay of the magnetic vector produced by interaction of protons during the relaxation process. The differences in tissue T1 and T2 relaxation times enable MRI to distinguish between fat, muscle, bone marrow, and gray or white matter of the brain. Most lesions in the brain prolong these relaxation times by increasing the volume or changing the magnetic properties of tissue water.

MR images are displayed as maps of signal intensity received from the tissue. Proton spatial location is achieved by applying a magnetic field gradient across the magnet bore, creating slight variations in proton resonance frequency across the object being imaged. The specific location of the radiowave emissions may be determined by measurement of the exact radiofrequency.

Factors that influence the appearance of MR images include (1) the imaging technique or pulse sequence (e.g., spin echo SE, gradient echo GRE, or inversion recovery IR), (2) the applied RF "flip" angle, (3) the repetition time (TR, the interval between repeated pulse sequences), (4) the echo time (TE, the interval between radiofrequency excitation and measurement of the radiowave emission signal), and (5) the timing, amplitude and duration of gradients applied during the pulse sequence. The most commonly used, basic MRI technique is the *spin-echo* (SE) pulse sequence, which repeats a sequence of 90° then 180° radiofrequency pulses and measures the signal after each 180° pulse within a TR time, typically between 500 milliseconds and 2000 milliseconds. The 90° pulse creates the radiowave perturbation of the tissue protons, and the following 180° pulse reinstitutes the phase or "refocuses" the emitted signal to produce an "echo" at the TE time which is the signal used for image reconstruction.

MR images may be acquired to emphasize or "weight" the differences between tissues, based on specific characteristics of the tissue, such as T1 or T2 relaxation, proton-density, magnetic susceptibility (i.e., the tendency

---

FIGURE 13.1. **Acute Intracerebral Hemorrhage on CT and MRI. A:** Noncontrast axial CT shows a left basal ganglia, hyperdense, acute hematoma. **B:** T2W MRI shows the hematoma to be hyperintense and surrounded by high signal edema. **C:** FLAIR image also shows the hematoma as a hyperintense lesion surrounded by high signal edema. **D:** Noncontrast T1W MRI shows the hematoma and edema to be slightly hypointense compared to normal brain. **E:** GRE MRI shows patchy low signal within the hematoma and a thin rim of low signal at its margin. The appearance of this acute hematoma is highly specific on the CT scan but is nonspecific on MRI. Without the CT for comparison, this lesion on MRI may be interpreted as a partially hemorrhagic or calcified mass, such as metastatic neoplasm. This pattern of signal on MRI is best explained by a predominance of nonparamagnetic (diamagnetic) oxyhemoglobin within intact red blood cells through most of the lesion so that the appearance is that of any lesion with high water content (hyperintense on T2W and FLAIR, hypointense on the T1W). There appears to be partial conversion to paramagnetic deoxyhemoglobin within some of the intact red blood cells creating local microscopic magnetic field gradients which explains the low signal on the GRE image. Further evolution of intracerebral hematomas results in formation of methemoglobin and lysis of RBCs, resulting in very short T1 relaxation time which produces hyperintensity on T1W, T2W, FLAIR and GRE images (T1 "shine through") in the subacute period, days to weeks after onset. This is followed by eventual degeneration to residual paramagnetic tissue hemosiderin and ferritin deposits with isointense signal on the T1W, isointense or low signal on the T2W and FLAIR images, and low signal on GRE images, months to years after onset. (Courtesy of Dr. R.L. DeLaPaz.)

to have magnetic properties), proton diffusion, tissue perfusion and vascular flow characteristics. T1-weighted images (T1W, using short TR and short TE) are most useful for depicting anatomy and show CSF and most lesions as low signal (dark), except for areas of fat, subacute hemorrhage, or gadolinium (Gd) enhancement, which appear as high signal (bright). T2-weighted images (T2W, using long TR and long TE) are more sensitive for lesion detection and show CSF and most lesions as high signal, except areas of hemorrhage or chronic hemosiderin deposits, which may appear as low signal. Proton-density or "balanced" images (PD, using long TR and short TE) show mixed contrast characteristics, reflecting both T1 and T2 weighting. The addition of an *inversion* 180° pulse before the 90° to180° pulse sequence, timed to suppress CSF signal, results in the fluid-attenuated inversion recovery (FLAIR) pulse sequence. FLAIR images are T2-weighted with low-signal CSF and display most lesions with higher conspicuity than T2W or PD images. Gradient-echo (GRE) images are created by using a single radiofrequency pulse with a flip angle of 90° or less, without the following 180° pulse; gradient switching refocuses the emitted radiowaves and generates the signal echoes. GRE imaging allows fast acquisition of 3D volume studies and is often the only method that will detect the low signal of subtle magnetic susceptibility variations around hemorrhage or calcium. GRE imaging may also be acquired with flow sensitivity to produce magnetic resonance angiograms (MRA) which show flowing blood in vascular structures as high signal. The static images produced by all of these methods usually show rapidly flowing blood, dense calcification, cortical bone, and air as black signal voids because of flow signal dephasing, absence of protons or local magnetic susceptibility differences.

Early MR imaging was very slow because only one "line" of each image was obtained with each TR cycle. Faster imaging has evolved by collecting more data in each TR cycle, beginning with double SE methods which acquire both PD and T2W images during the same TR time. Multi-echo or *"fast spin-echo"* (FSE) methods acquire even more echoes in each TR cycle, typically 8-16, which speeds data collection and has reduced acquisition times from 8 to 10 minutes to 2 to 3 minutes high-resolution images through the entire brain. This approach was extended to its end point with echo-planar imaging (EPI) where rapid, interleaved gradient switching is used to acquire an entire image in less than 100 milliseconds and a set of images through the entire brain in less than 1 second. EPI is the basis for most functional brain imaging such as diffusion and perfusion imaging (Fig. 13.2).

Diffusion-weighted images (DWI) are typically produced by adding specialized gradients to EPI SE pulse sequences, making them sensitive to molecular-level water motion. DWI shows areas of abnormally restricted water motion (e.g., acute cerebral infarct), as high signal. Perfusion-weighted images (PWI) are typically acquired using EPI GRE pulse sequences for rapid,

multi-slice imaging during the first pass of an intravascular bolus of gadolinium contrast agent. This produces a transient signal reduction curve in each voxel, whose shape reflects relative cerebral blood volume (rCBV) and mean transit time (MTT), which may be used to calculate relative cerebral blood flow (rCBF). CBF may also be imaged using a method called arterial-spin labeling (ASL), which detects the rate of arrival of arterial blood-water proton "spins" that are "labeled" noninvasively in the neck by a radiofrequency pulse, analogous to the injection of an intravascular contrast agent.

USES OF COMPUTED TOMOGRAPHY

For reasons of cost, speed, and availability, CT is still widely used for screening in the evaluation of acute stroke, head injury, or acute infections. It is especially useful for patients who are neurologically or medically unstable, uncooperative, or claustrophobic, as well as for patients with pacemakers or other metallic implants that may be contraindications for MRI. Most current CT scanners are capable of scan times of 1-second-per-image and a typical screening, noncontrast head study with patient handling and scanner set up takes 5 to 10 minutes. If a mechanical ventilator is being used, CT is often used for imaging because most respirators will not function in the high magnetic field of the MR scanner. Although some MR methods are sensitive to acute hemorrhage, the resulting appearance is variable and may be nonspecific (Fig. 13.1).

In daily clinical practice, CT is widely accepted as the more reliable and unambiguous method for detecting acute brain parenchymal or extra-axial hemorrhage, especially subarachnoid hemorrhage. CT is also superior for evaluating the bones of the skull and spine, although MRI is superior in studying invasive processes of the bone marrow.

Contrast-enhanced CT (CECT) is used to detect lesions that involve breakdown of the blood-brain barrier, such as brain or spinal tumors, infections, and other inflammatory conditions. CECT is often used to rule out cerebral metastases. However, it is less sensitive than Gd-enhanced MRI (Gd-MRI), which is also better for detection of other intracranial tumors and infections.

Intravenous CT contrast agents are based on iodine, and the older and cheaper agents are classified as high-osmolar contrast media (HOCM). Newer, nonionic agents, classified as low-osmolar contrast media (LOCM), are more expensive but less allergenic, and they cause less morbidity than do HOCM. LOCM are especially useful in patients at high risk for adverse reaction, such as those with severe heart disease, renal insufficiency, asthma, severe debilitation, or previous allergic reaction to iodinated contrast (HOCM).

Spiral or *helical* CT increases scanning speed and image acquisition to less than 1-second-per-section and

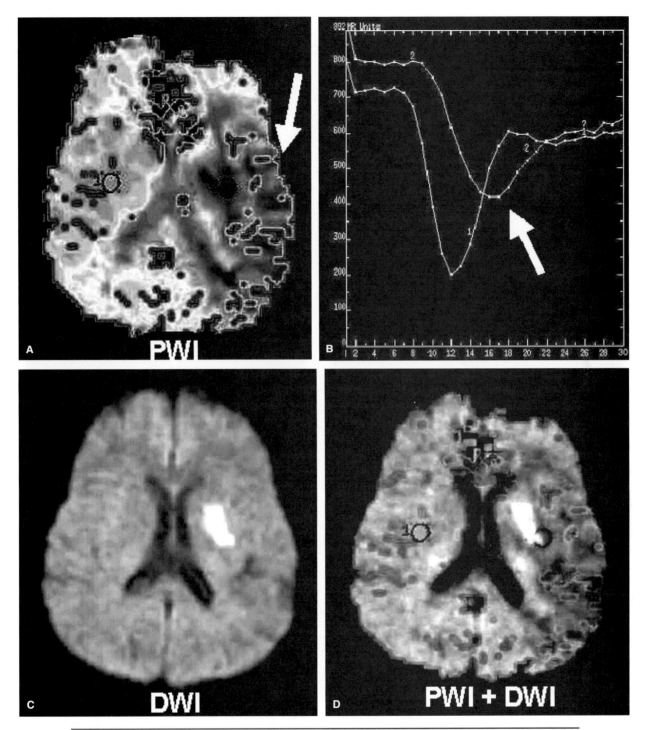

FIGURE 13.2. MR PWI-DWI Mismatch in Acute Stroke. A: Axial calculated MR PWI shows reduced blood flow as low signal in the left basal ganglia and middle cerebral artery territory (arrow). **B:** Time-intensity curves from the PWI source images, obtained at 2-second intervals (x-axis, left to right) during a bolus injection of Gd-chelate, show an inverted peak of signal as the bolus passes through brain tissue. The earlier, deeper peak is from the normal right hemisphere. The peak in the abnormal region on PWI is delayed by 10 seconds (arrow) and shows reduced blood volume (reduced peak area, CBV) which together indicate reduced blood flow (CBF). **C:** Axial MR DWI shows high signal in the left basal ganglia indicating restricted diffusion in infarcted tissue. **D:** Co-registered overlay of the PWI and DWI show a "mismatch" between the large area of reduced blood flow and the smaller infarct. The difference represents the "ischemic penumbra" of tissue that may be prevented from infarcting with restoration of normal blood flow. (Courtesy of Dr. R. L. DeLaPaz)

allows large-volume acquisitions that may be used for *three-dimensional* (3D) presentation of anatomic information. Single and multislice spiral scanning is now fast enough to allow acquisition of the entire neck or head during an intravenous infusion of contrast agent for 3D reconstruction of vascular anatomy, CT angiography (CTA). Maximum intensity projection (MIP) reformations or 3D renderings with surface shading may be used to display vascular abnormalities such as stenosis or aneurysm. Advantages of CTA over catheter angiography include more widely available technology, less specialized skill requirements, and less invasive intravenous administration of contrast material. However, the use of CTA has been growing slowly, owing to competition from existing MRA. In contrast to MRA, the iodinated contrast agent used is potentially more toxic because of the risk of allergic reactions and direct cardiac volume stress, as well as renal toxicity.

Another limitation of CTA is the time-consuming processing required to edit out bone and calcium and to generate 3D surface renderings, although this has improved recently with the availability of specialized software that partially automates this process. Rapid, multi-section CT is also used to generate brain perfusion studies by repeated imaging of the same brain region during a rapid intravenous bolus-contrast injection. This method suffers from limited volume coverage (a 2cm-thick multi-section slab; the width of the detector array) and the risks of iodinated contrast injection, in contrast to MRI perfusion methods where whole brain coverage is obtainable and risks of Gd-chelate contrast injection are negligible. However, recent studies have demonstrated semi-quantitative measures of cerebral blood volume (CBV), cerebral mean transit time (MTT, or a similar measure: time-to-peak, TTP) and cerebral blood flow (CBF) with CT perfusion (CTP) and clinical usefulness as a quick screening method for confirmation of acute cerebral ischemia in major vascular territories. Use of a noncontrast CT scan to exclude acute hemorrhage followed by CTA to confirm vascular stenosis or occlusion and CTP to confirm ischemia is becoming a popular initial workup for suspected cerebral ischemia prior to intravenous thrombolysis with recombinant tissue plasminogen activator (rtPA).

USES OF MAGNETIC RESONANCE IMAGING

MRI is the neuroimaging method of choice for most intracranial and intraspinal abnormalities. The technical advantages of MRI are threefold: (1) Greater soft tissue contrast provides better definition of anatomic structures and greater sensitivity to pathologic lesions; (2) multiplanar capability displays dimensional information and relationships that are not readily available on CT; and (3) MRI may

better demonstrate physiologic processes such as blood flow, CSF motion, and special properties of tissue, such as water diffusion or biochemical makeup (using MRS). Other advantages include better visualization of the posterior fossa, lack of ionizing radiation, and better visualization of intraspinal contents.

There are some disadvantages of MRI. The most practical problem is the need for cooperation from the patient because most individual MRI sequences require several minutes and a complete study lasts 20 minutes to 60 minutes. However, EPI and single-shot multi-echo methods (e.g. FSE) may acquire low-resolution images in as little as 75 milliseconds and whole brain studies in 30 seconds to 40 seconds. These may be used to salvage an adequate study for identifying or excluding major lesions in uncooperative patients.

In addition, about 5% of all persons are claustrophobic inside the conventional MR unit. Oral or intravenous sedation may be used to ensure cooperation, but closer patient monitoring is then required. Development of low-magnetic-field, "open" MRI systems has improved patient acceptance, but these systems sacrifice image quality because of the lower signal-to-noise ratio. Newer 1.5T and 3.0T clinical MRI systems have shorter bore lengths that reduce patient perception of a closed tube while maintaining full MR capabilities.

MRI is contraindicated in patients with some metallic implants, especially cardiac pacemakers, cochlear implants, older-generation aneurysm clips, metallic foreign bodies in the eye, and implanted neurostimulators. Patients who are not dependent on their cardiac pacemakers have been scanned under close supervision followed by reprogramming of the pacemaker after exposure to the high magnetic field. Newer aneurysm clips have been designed to be nonferromagnetic and nontorqueable at high-magnetic-field strengths, but the U.S. Food and Drug Administration (FDA) still urges caution in performing MRI in all patients with aneurysm clips, especially at field strengths above 1.5T. Individual clips may develop unpredictable magnetic properties during manufacture, and careful observation of initial images for magnetic artifacts should be used as an additional precaution, with slow removal of the patient if substantial artifact is seen. Published lists of MR-compatible clips and metallic objects provide advice about specific clip types and any unusual metallic implants.

Some authorities consider pregnancy (especially in the first trimester) a relative contraindication to MRI, primarily because safety data are incomplete. To date, no harmful effect of MRI has been demonstrated in pregnant women or fetuses. In fact, late-pregnancy fetal MRI, after approximately 18 weeks, is becoming a common imaging study. An additional unknown risk to the fetus is the effect of intravenous MR contrast agents such as Gd- and iron-based agents. The urgency, need, and benefits of the MRI study for the patient should be considered in relation to potential unknown risks to the fetus in early pregnancy.

Indications for Gadolinium-enhanced MRI

Most intravenous contrast agents for MRI are one of several chelates of gadolinium, a rare-earth heavy metal. These agents are water-soluble and cross the damaged blood-brain barrier in a manner similar to that of iodinated CT contrast media. The local extravascular accumulation of the Gd-chelate shortens both T1 and T2 relaxation times, an effect best seen as high signal on T1-weighted images. Comparison with precontrast images is needed to exclude preexisting high signal, such as hemorrhage, fat, and occasionally, calcification. Specialized MR methods may improve detection of Gd-chelate enhancement. For instance, magnetization transfer improves contrast enhancement by suppressing nonenhancing tissue signal, and fat suppression helps in the evaluation of the skull base and orbital regions. Unlike iodinated contrast material, Gd-chelate administration is associated with few adverse reactions.

Gd-MRI has been most useful in increasing sensitivity to neoplastic and inflammatory lesions. This high sensitivity may show brain tumors that are often difficult to detect on CT, such as small brain metastases, schwannomas (especially within the internal auditory canal), optic nerve or hypothalamic gliomas, and meningeal carcinomatosis. In addition, the multiplanar capability of Gd-MRI delineates the extent of neoplastic lesions so well that the images may be used directly to plan neurosurgery and radiation therapy.

Gd-MRI is superior to CECT in detecting cerebral metastases, but even Gd-MRI at standard dosages may miss metastatic lesions. Newer nonionic Gd-chelate contrast agents allow up to three times as much contrast agent to be used. In some cases, triple-dose Gd-MRI detects metastases not seen with the standard method. Similar high detection rates may be achieved with standard-dose Gd-chelate when it is combined with magnetization-transfer MRI. Maximizing lesion sensitivity is especially significant in patients with solitary metastases, for whom surgical resection is a therapeutic option, in contrast to multiple lesions, for which radiation or chemotherapy may be better options.

MRI is the imaging method of choice for detecting the demyelinating plaques of multiple sclerosis in both the brain and spinal cord. Multiple sclerosis plaques are characteristically seen on T2-weighted images as multifocal hyperintense lesions within the periventricular white matter and corpus callosum. They appear ovoid and oriented along medullary veins, perpendicular to the long axis of the lateral ventricles (*Dawson fingers*). Gd-MRI may identify active inflammation by contrast enhancement of acute demyelinating plaques and distinguish them from nonen-

hancing chronic lesions. Serial Gd-MRI studies allow the progress of the disease to be monitored. Magnetization-transfer imaging, without Gd contrast injection, has also been used to identify abnormal white-matter regions that appear normal on T2-weighted images.

Gd-MRI is vastly superior to CECT in the detection of meningitis, encephalitis (especially herpes simplex encephalitis and acute disseminated encephalomyelitis), and myelitis. Epidural abscess or empyema may also be better delineated on Gd-MRI. In AIDS, many kinds of lesions show increased signal intensity within the cerebral white matter on noncontrast T2-weighted images. These lesions may be further characterized by Gd-MRI. For example, if a single, large or dominant, homogeneously enhancing mass is seen on Gd-MRI, the favored diagnosis is cerebral lymphoma. If multiple, small ring-enhancing lesions are found, the probable diagnoses include cerebral toxoplasmosis, granulomas, or fungal infection. When no enhancement is present, the white-matter lesions may be the result of HIV encephalitis (if symmetric) or progressive multifocal leukoencephalopathy (if asymmetric). Thus, the presence or absence of contrast enhancement, the character of contrast enhancement, and the pattern of signal abnormality are all important features in the differential diagnosis.

Gd-MRI is also useful in evaluation of the spine. Herniated discs and degenerative spondylosis may well be evaluated on noncontrast MRI in the unoperated patient, but Gd-MRI is needed in patients with a "failed back syndrome," to separate nonenhancing recurrent disc herniation from enhancing postsurgical scarring or fibrosis. Identification and delineation of spinal tumors and infections are also improved with Gd-MRI. However, Gd enhancement of vertebral bone marrow metastases may make them isointense with normal fatty marrow on T1-weighted images without fat suppression. Screening precontrast T1-weighted images without fat suppression should always be obtained of the spine. MRI is much more sensitive to bone marrow metastases than conventional radionuclide bone scans.

Recently, DWI of the spine has been used to discriminate compression fractures associated with metastases, which show restricted diffusion (high signal on DWI) from benign, osteoporotic compressions that show normal to prolonged diffusion (normal to low signal on DWI). The emergency evaluation of spinal cord compression is also best done with pre- and postcontrast Gd-MRI because multilevel disease may be directly visualized and definitive characterization of lesions can be done immediately (i.e., intra- versus extramedullary, dural and spinal involvement). For these reasons, the indications for conventional and CT myelography are decreasing. Outside the spine, fat-suppressed MRI of spinal nerve roots and peripheral nerves, known as MR *neurography,* identifies compressive or traumatic nerve injuries.

Appropriate Utilization of Gadolinium-Enhanced MRI

Some experts have proposed universal administration of Gd for MRI. The use of Gd, however, adds to the direct costs of MRI and increases imaging time, as well as increasing patient discomfort from the intravenous needle placement. Others recommend that Gd-MRI should be restricted to specific clinical situations in which efficacy has been demonstrated (except when a significant abnormality on routine noncontrast MRI requires further characterization).

In some clinical situations, Gd-MRI is not very useful because relatively few contrast-enhancing lesions are typically found. These clinical situations include complex partial seizures, headache, dementia, head trauma, psychosis, low back or neck pain (in unoperated patients), and congenital craniospinal anomalies. MRI evaluation in many of these conditions would be improved by special MR pulse sequences directed to the structures of greatest interest. For example, patients with temporal lobe epilepsy or Alzheimer disease benefit most by high-resolution coronal imaging of the temporal lobes, for evidence of hippocampal atrophy or sclerosis. Patients who have experienced remote head trauma or child abuse might be best served by a T2-weighted GRE pulse sequence, which is more sensitive than the SE pulse sequence in detecting chronic blood products such as hemosiderin deposition that may be seen in brain parenchyma after axonal shear injuries, or on the subarachnoid pial surface after repeated subarachnoid hemorrhages.

Magnetic Resonance Angiography

On standard SE images, the major arteries and veins of the neck and brain are usually seen as areas of signal void, owing to relatively fast blood flow. A GRE pulse sequence may show flowing blood as areas of increased signal intensity known as *flow-related enhancement* (not to be confused with Gd contrast enhancement). In these images, the soft tissues appear relatively dark. After a series of contiguous thin sections is obtained with either two-dimensional (2D) or 3D GRE techniques, a map of the blood vessels is reconstructed as a set of *maximum intensity projection* (MIP) angiograms that may be viewed in any orientation and displayed with 3D surface shading. These MRA images, like a conventional angiogram, may show the vascular anatomy but also have the advantage of multiple viewing angles that provide oblique and other nonstandard angiographic views. MRA, like CTA, does not require specialized catheter skills and avoids the 0.5% to 3% risk of neurologic complications associated with arterial catheter angiography. An advantage of MRA over CTA is that it is completely noninvasive, requiring no contrast injection, although the quality may be improved if done during or following Gd injection.

In the evaluation of the carotid arteries in the neck or the arteries of the circle of Willis, the most commonly used MRA technique is the *time-of-flight* (TOF) method. TOF is sensitive to T1 relaxation effects and may produce false-positive or obscuring high-signal artifacts from orbital fat, hemorrhage, or areas of Gd enhancement. Another important MRA technique, the *phase-contrast* (PC) technique, depends on the phase (rather than magnitude) of the MR signal. PC technique shows the direction and velocity of blood flow, may be adjusted to low or high flow sensitivity, and is useful for evaluating altered hemodynamics, such as flow reversal after major vessel occlusion or stenosis. MRA during and following intravenous (IV) injection of Gd-chelate reduces flow-related artifact and allows separation of the arterial and venous blood flow phases. The improved signal-to-noise using parallel multichannel coil technology at 1.5T or imaging at 3.0T has also allowed higher spatial resolution and improved visualization of small, distal, intracranial vascular structures, with a result that rivals conventional catheter angiography.

MRA may overestimate cervical carotid stenosis because local high velocity or turbulent flow may cause signal loss, but it compares favorably with conventional angiography in detecting carotid stenosis. Conventional angiography is still the "gold standard" for cerebrovascular imaging, but extracranial carotid evaluation is now done primarily with ultrasound and MRA.

Indications for MRA include stroke, TIA, possible venous sinus thrombosis, arteriovenous malformation (AVM), and vascular tumors (for delineation of vascular supply and displacements). It is thought that MRA reliably detects aneurysms as small as 3 mm. Conventional angiography, however, is still the most sensitive examination for evaluation of intracranial aneurysms or AVMs, owing to its higher spatial resolution and ability to observe the rapid sequence of vascular filling, especially the early venous filling seem with AVMs.

Functional MRI

The term *functional* is used here in a broad sense, to encompass several MRI methods that are used to image physiologic processes such as tissue blood flow, water diffusion, and biochemical makeup (with MRS), as well as cerebral activation with sensory, motor, and cognitive tasks. Tissue blood flow is most commonly imaged with MRI using a *first-pass* or *bolus-tracking* method that records the signal changes occurring when rapidly repeated images are acquired during the first passage of an intravascular bolus of paramagnetic contrast material through the brain, usually Gd-chelate (Fig. 13.2). Using T2*- or T2-weighted EPI or fast GRE techniques, MR images are acquired every 1 second to 3 seconds over the whole brain, and the signal decreases that occur in cerebral tissue with passage of the contrast bolus are plotted against time. Based on the central volume theorem, the area under this time–intensity curve is proportional to cerebral blood volume (CBV), and other manipulations of the data may give CBF, MTT, and other measures of tissue perfusion. This method has been used most extensively with primary brain tumors, where CBV seems to correlate well with histologic tumor grade and demonstrates response to treatment of the tumor. The obvious application to cerebral ischemic disease has become more widespread, and measures of perfusion delay, such as MTT and TTP, are sensitive indicators of small reductions in cerebral perfusion. A second method of MR perfusion imaging is called *arterial spin labeling* (ASL) and, like TOF MRA, depends on T1 relaxation and flow phenomena, without the use of injected contrast agents. Hydrogen nuclei (protons) in intra-arterial water are "labeled" by RF exposure in the neck which alters their nuclear "spin" and the arrival of these "spin-labeled" protons in brain tissue is proportional to cerebral blood flow, analogous to the injection of an intra-arterial contrast agent. This method is currently less widely used than bolus tracking because it is more technically challenging but gives more quantitative CBF images.

A second important functional MRI technique is *diffusion-weighted imaging* (DWI). This is most commonly performed using an EPI SE pulse sequence with gradients added before and after the 180-degree pulse. The images produced are sensitive to cellular level motion of diffusing water protons. On DW images, areas with high diffusion rates show low signal, and those with low diffusion rates appear as high signal. Quantitative displays of diffusion rates, known as *apparent diffusion coefficient* (ADC) maps show diffusion rates with the opposite polarity: high ADC (high rate) as high signal and low ADC as low signal. Severe cerebral ischemia causes a rapid decrease in intracellular diffusion, and this restricted diffusion appears as high signal on DWI within minutes of cell injury (Fig. 13.2). After the initial reduction in diffusion, there is a gradual rise through normal to prolonged diffusion rates during the 1 week to 2 weeks after infarction, as cells disintegrate and freely diffusible water dominates the encephalomalacic tissue. A minor pitfall of DWI is called "T2 shine-through," where high signal on T2-weighted images may produce high signal on DWI, falsely indicating restricted diffusion. This error may be avoided by the use of calculated ADC maps which will show these regions as isointense to high signal, indicating normal or increased diffusion rates. DWI is an essential part of acute stroke imaging, takes less than 1 minute to acquire a whole-brain study, and is available on virtually all current high field MRI systems. DWI may be combined with perfusion imaging to identify the so-called *penumbra zone* of potentially salvageable tissue which lies within the area of reduced perfusion but outside the DWI high signal, which generally indicates infarcted tissue unlikely to recover.

Another functional technique, magnetic resonance spectroscopy (*MRS*) may be performed on most clinical high-field MR scanners (1.5T or 3.0T). Proton spectroscopy is more widely used than MRS of other nuclei, and produces semiquantitative spectra of common tissue metabolites, including *N*-acetylaspartate (NAA; a marker of healthy neurons and axons), creatine (the molecular storage depot for high-energy phosphates), choline (a component of cell membranes and myelin), and lactate (elevated with normal tissue energetic stress and in many pathologic tissues). Adequate proton spectra may be obtained from as little as 0.5 cc of tissue at 1.5 T and smaller volumes at 3.0T. MRS images (MRSI, metabolite maps) may be generated from the individual spectral peaks to show the distribution of a single metabolite over a 2D slice or in a 3D volume, albeit at lower spatial resolution than anatomic MR images. A widely accepted clinical use of proton MRS is the identification of brain neoplasms, which tend to show a characteristic but not completely specific pattern of elevated choline, reduced NAA, and elevated lactate (Fig. 13.3).

MRS is also used to characterize multiple sclerosis plaques, hippocampal seizure foci, degenerative diseases such as Alzheimer disease or amyotrophic lateral sclerosis (ALS), and metabolic disorders such as MELAS.

Using MRI to map cerebral activation is specifically called *functional MRI* (Fig. 13.4).

Although flow-sensitive techniques such as Gd-contrast bolus and ASL methods have been used to identify cerebral activation, the technique most widely used is the *blood-oxygen-level-dependent* (BOLD) method. This is based on local increases in CBF and CBV with the consequent intravascular shift from deoxyhemoglobin to oxyhemoglobin in areas of cerebral activation. With T2*- or T2-weighted EPI or fast GRE images and rapidly repeated acquisitions (every 1 to 3 seconds at each slice level), MR images show small increases in signal in areas of cerebral activation. BOLD fMRI has been used most extensively in research on motor, sensory, and cognitive activation. Growing clinical applications of fMRI include mapping of motor, sensory, and language function prior to surgery, radiation therapy, or embolization procedures; monitoring recovery of function after brain injury or stroke; and mapping specific cognitive changes in degenerative brain diseases.

PARADIGM: DIAGNOSTIC WORKUP FOR ACUTE STROKE

In the first evaluation of patients with acute stroke, both CT and MRI are being used. In many centers, non-noncontrast CT is the primary choice because of availability, immediate access, less need for patient cooperation, and lower cost. In addition, hemorrhage, calcification, and skull fracture are easy to recognize on CT, making it a useful comprehensive screening technique. However, static CT images prior to or following contrast injection have a sensitivity of about 50% compared to 90% to 100% for DWI in the detection

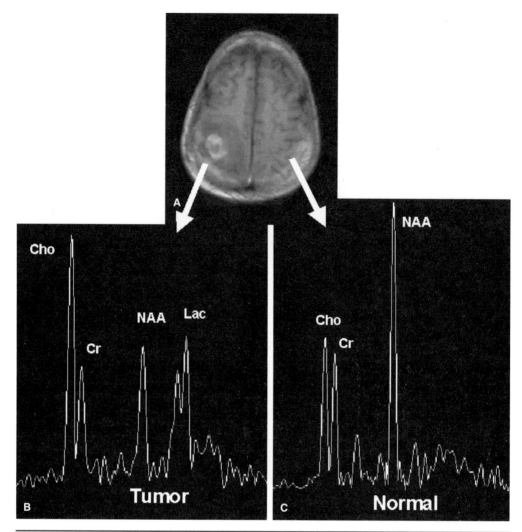

FIGURE 13.3. Proton MRS of recurrent glioblastoma. A: Axial contrast enhanced T1W MRI shows a round, enhancing lesion of recurrent glioblastoma in the right parietal lobe. **B:** MR spectrum from this lesion shows marked elevation of choline (Cho), slight reduction of creatine (Cr), marked reduction of N-acetylaspartate (NAA) and presence of a large lactate (Lac) concentration, typical of a rapidly growing neoplasm. **C:** MR spectrum of the contralateral normal brain shows normal Cho, Cr and NAA levels and no visible Lac. **D:** MR spectroscopic image (MRSI) of Cho concentration over an axial section of the brain shows the marked elevation in the region of the lesion (arrow). **E:** MRSI of Cr shows slight reduction in the lesion (arrow). **F:** MRSI of NAA show marked reduction in the lesion (arrow). **G:** MRSI of Lac shows its presence in the lesion (arrow) and absence from the rest of the brain (the high signal ring around the brain is skull and scalp lipid signal contamination). (Courtesy of Dr. R.L. DeLaPaz and Dr. D.C. Shungu)

of nonhemorrhagic infarction in the first 6 hours after the ictus. They are also insensitive to microhemorrhages in infarcts compared to GRE MRI. In addition, infarcts within the brainstem and cerebellum are usually better demonstrated by MRI because artifact frequently obscures these regions on CT.

The development of dynamic, multislice CT techniques, using intravenous contrast injections, have changed the role of CT in acute stroke. CT perfusion (CTP) images may be acquired during the first pass of an intravenous contrast bolus injection and CT angiography (CTA) may be acquired immediately afterward, during a continued, slow infusion.

These methods are used as a quick method of confirming early cerebral ischemia in major vascular territories and for confirming the presence of vascular occlusive disease.

However, there are several limitations of CTP and CTA. The volume of brain imaged with CTP is limited to an approximately 2-cm thick slab which must be placed through the suspect vascular territory, making this an inadequate tool for evaluating many motor and sensory deficits, which may be produced by lesions in different vascular territories from hemispheric cortex to lower brain stem. CTP discrimination of completed infarct from potentially salvageable

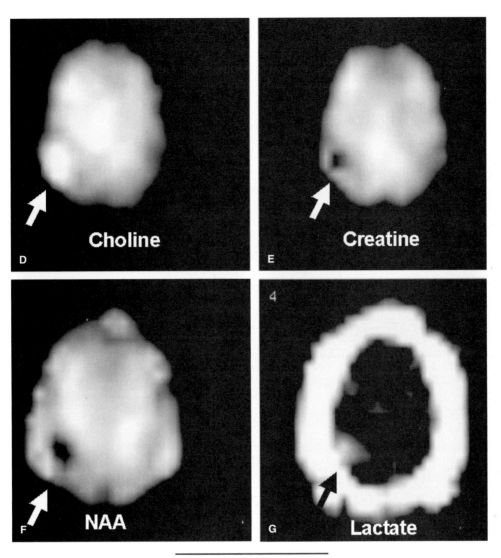

FIGURE 13.3. *(Continued)*

"penumbra" has proven problematic because it is dependent on quantitative thresholds of CBV or CBF to separate these regions, which are not highly reproducible due to the different post processing methods being used and the biologic variation of these measures from patient to patient. CTP is also relatively insensitive to small lacunar infarcts. High volumes of iodinated contrast, as much as 150cc, are needed for combined CTP and CTA which may be problematic in patients with compromised cardiac or renal function. The complex post processing needed for these studies also requires substantial time and personnel support.

MRI is the modality of choice for acute ischemic stroke evaluation because of the high sensitivity and specificity of DWI for cerebral ischemia, including small lacunar infarcts; the reliable identification of the ischemic penumbra with the DWI-PWI mismatch; the ability to acquire DWI and PWI over the whole brain; the detection of microhemorrhages with GRE images; and the capability to also acquire functional and metabolic information using fMRI and MRS.

As noted above, DWI may specifically identify cerebral infarction within minutes of onset, and when combined with quantitative ADC maps, may specify the age of a lesion to within a few hours, acutely, or a few days, subacutely. The use of the DWI-PWI mismatch to identify potentially salvageable tissue in the ischemic penumbra is currently undergoing clinical trials to test the hypothesis that the use of this "physiologic" definition of treatable tissue will allow thrombolytic agents to be given beyond the current limit of 3 hours post ictus while still minimizing the risk of hemorrhagic transformation. (Fig. 13.2) Use of the DWI-PWI mismatch has also been proposed for triage of patients to intra-arterial thrombolytic therapy as late as 8 hours after ictus, possibly performing the intra-arterial therapy within the MRI scanner, using MR-catheter tracking techniques, and monitoring therapy progress in real time with repeated DWI and PWI imaging.

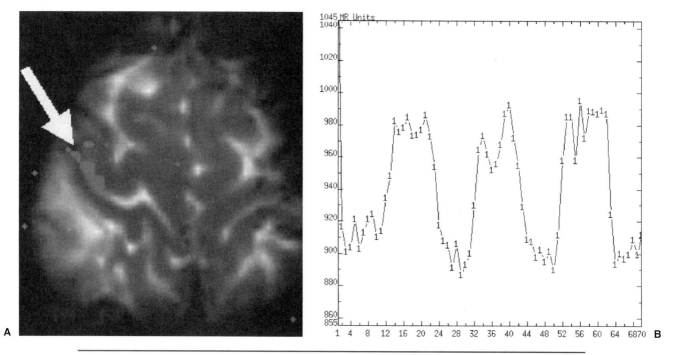

FIGURE 13.4. Functional MRI for Surgical Planning. A: Axial T2*-weighted EPI image acquired during a left-hand grasping task shows activation of the precentral gyrus *(arrow)* immediately anterior to a region of high-signal cortical dysplasia scheduled for surgical resection. **B:** Time–intensity curves show three phases of increased signal, each during a 30-sec period of repeated hand grasping separated by 30-sec periods of rest. The rise in signal is produced by the BOLD effect, as local increases in blood flow in areas of cortical activation produce increased levels of oxyhemoglobin (decreased levels of deoxyhemoglobin) in capillaries and venules. (Y-axis represents signal intensity; X-axis shows sequential image numbers, each separated by 3 secs. EPI GRE pulse sequence with TR 3000 ms, TE 90 ms, flip 90 degrees.) (Courtesy of Dr. R.L. DeLaPaz.)

MRA of the brain is often used with DWI and PWI in the acute stroke setting to determine patency of the vessels of the intracranial circulation. Acute occlusion of the major vessels of the circle of Willis or of the superior portions of the internal carotid arteries and basilar artery may be detected, but occlusion of small, distal branches is not as well demonstrated (Fig. 13.2); recent improvements in image quality using parallel multichannel coil technology at 1.5T and imaging at 3.0T are likely to reduce this limitation. Arterial and venous flow may be separated to identify venous occlusion, using flow velocity-sensitive and contrast-bolus timed acquisitions. MRA may also be used serially for evaluation of therapy, such as for intraarterial thrombolysis, and in the near future may compete with conventional angiography for diagnostic evaluation and guidance of intraarterial thrombolytic therapy.

MRA and duplex ultrasonography of the carotid arteries are the methods most commonly used to evaluate possible internal carotid-origin stenosis. If necessary, invasive angiography may corroborate the presence of carotid stenosis and may depict ulcerations that are not well seen on MRA or duplex ultrasonography.

FLAIR and T2W MR imaging also show high signal in acute infarcts and are usually sensitive to lesions after

about 6 hours to 12 hours. During the first 5 days after stroke onset, Gd enhancement may be seen within the small arteries of the ischemic vascular territory, with gyral cortical enhancement present 5 days to several months after onset. Focal reversible FLAIR, T2W and occasionally DWI lesions with TIAs may also be seen on MRI, and are rarely seen on CT.

SUGGESTED READINGS

Adamson AJ, Rand SD, Prost RW, Kim TA, Schultz C, Haughton VM. Focal brain lesions: effect of single-voxel proton MR spectroscopic findings on treatment decisions. *Radiology* 1998;209:73–78.

Akeson P, Larsson EM, Kristoffersen DT, Jonsson E, Holtas S. Brain metastases—comparison of gadodiamide injection-enhanced MR imaging at standard and high dose, contrast-enhanced CT and noncontrast-enhanced MR imaging. *Acta Radiol* 1995;36:300–306.

Anderson CM, Saloner D, Lee RE, et al. Assessment of carotid artery stenosis by MR angiography: comparison with x-ray angiography and color-coded Doppler ultrasound. *AJNR* 1992;13:989–1008.

Anzalone N, Scotti R, Riva R, Neuroradiologic differential diagnosis of cerebral intraparenchymal hemorrhage, *Neurol Sci.* 2004;25(suppl 1): S3–S5.

Atlas SW, Sheppard L, Goldberg HI, Hurst RW, Listerud J, Flamm E. Intracranial aneurysms: detection and characterization with MR angiography with use of an advanced postprocessing technique in a blinded-reader study. *Radiology* 1997;203:807–814.

Bammer R, Fazekas F, Diffusion imaging of the human spinal cord and the vertebral column. *Top Magn Reson Imaging.* 2003;14(6):461–476.

Barboriak DP, Provenzale JM, MR arteriography of intracranial circulation, *AJR Am J Roentgenol.* 1998;171(6):1469–1478.

Barkovich AJ, Atlas SW, Magnetic resonance imaging of intracranial hemorrhage, *Radiologic Clinics of North America* 1988;26:801–820.

Boska MD, Mosley RL, Nawab M, Nelson JA, Zelivyanskaya M, Poluektova L, Uberti M, Dou H, Lewis TB, Gendelman HE, Advances in neuroimaging for HIV-1 associated neurological dysfunction: clues to the diagnosis, pathogenesis and therapeutic monitoring *Curr HIV Res.* 2004;2(1):61–78.

Brant-Zawadzki M, Heiserman JE. The roles of MR angiography, CT angiography, and sonography in vascular imaging of the head and neck. *AJNR* 1997;18:1820–1825.

Carmody RF, Yang PJ, Seeley GW, et al. Spinal cord compression due to metastatic disease: diagnosis with MR imaging versus myelography. *Radiology* 1989;173:225–229.

Castillo M, Kwock L, Scatliff J, Mukherji SK. Proton MR spectroscopy in neoplastic and non-neoplastic brain disorders. *Magn Reson Imaging Clin N Am* 1998;6:1–20.

DeLaPaz RL. Echo planar imaging. *Radiographics* 1994;14:1045–1058.

Del Sole A, Gambini A, Falini A, Lecchi M, Lucignani G. In vivo neurochemistry with emission tomography and magnetic resonance spectroscopy: clinical applications. *Eur Radiology* 2002;12:2582–2599.

Di Costanzo A, Trojsi F, Tosetti M, et al. High-field proton MRS of human brain, *Eur J Radiol* 2003;48:146–153.

Duncan JS. Imaging and epilepsy. *Brain* 1997;120 (Pt 2):339–377.

Grossman RI, Gomori JM, Ramer KN, Lexa FJ, Schnall MD. Magnetization transfer: theory and clinical applications in neuroradiology. *Radiographics* 1994;14:279–290.

Hennig J, Speck O, Koch MA, Weiller C. Functional magnetic resonance imaging: a review of methodological aspects and clinical applications. *J Magn Reson Imaging* 2003;18:1–15.

Hoeffner EG, Case I, Jain R, et al. Cerebral perfusion CT: technique and clinical applications. *Radiology* 2004;231:632–644.

Jewells V, Castillo M. MR angiography of the extracranial circulation. *Magn Reson Imaging Clin N Am* 2003;11(4):585–597.

Kantarci K, Jack CR Jr. Neuroimaging in Alzheimer's disease: an evidence-based review. *Neuroimaging Clin N Am* 2003;13(2):197–209.

Lane B. Practical imaging of the spine and spinal cord. *Top Magn Reson Imaging* 2003;14(6):438–443.

Latchaw RE (Chair), Yonas H, Hunter GJ, et al. Guidelines and recommendations for perfusion imaging in cerebral ischemia: a scientific statement for healthcare professionals by the Writing Group on Perfusion Imaging, from the Council on Cardiovascular Radiology of the American Heart Association. *Stroke* 2003;34:1084–1104.

Ogawa S, Menon RS, Kim SG, Ugurbil K. On the characteristics of functional magnetic resonance imaging of the brain. *Annu Rev Biophys Biomol Struct* 1998;27:447–474.

Pretorius PM, Quaghebeur G. The role of MRI in the diagnosis of MS. *Clinical Radiol* 2003;58(6):434–448.

Provenzale JM, Jahan R, Naidich TP, Fox AJ. Assessment of the patient with hyperacute stroke: imaging and therapy. *Radiology* 2003;229(2):347–359.

Pruitt AA. Nervous system infections in patients with cancer. *Neurol Clin* 2003;21(1):193–219.

Ross JS, Masaryk TJ, Schrader M, et al. MR imaging of the postoperative lumbar spine: assessment with gadopentetate dimeglumine. *AJNR* 1990;11:771–776.

Rowley HA, Roberts TPL. Clinical perspectives in perfusion: neuroradiologic applications. *Topics in Magnetic Resonance Imaging* 2004;15:28–40.

Runge VM, Muroff LR, Jinkins JR. Central nervous system: review of clinical use of contrast media. *Top Magnet Resonan Imaging* 2001;12(4):231–263.

Schaefer PW, Budzik RF Jr, Gonzalez RG. Imaging of cerebral metastases. *Neurosurg Clin N Am.* 1996;7(3):393–423.

Schwartz RB, Tice HM, Hooten SM, Hsu L, Stieg PE. Evaluation of cerebral aneurysms with helical CT: correlation with conventional angiography and MR angiography. *Radiology* 1994;192:717–722.

Shellock FG. Reference Manual for Magnetic Resonance Safety, Implants and Devices, 2004 ed. Los Angeles CA: Biomedical Research Publishing Group, 2004.

Shellock FG, Magnetic Resonance Procedures: Health Effects and Safety. Boca Raton FL: CRC Press, 2001.

Sohn CH, Sevick RJ, Frayne R. Contrast-enhanced MR angiography of the intracranial circulation. *Magn Reson Imaging Clin N Am* 2003;11(4):599–614.

Sze G, Zimmerman RD. The magnetic resonance imaging of infectious and inflammatory diseases. *Radiol Clin North Am* 1988;26:839–885.

Tomandl BF, Klotz E, Handschu R, et al. Comprehensive imaging of ischemic stroke with multisection CT. *RadioGraphics* 2003;23:565–592.

Chapter 14

Electroencephalography and Evoked Potentials

Ronald G. Emerson, Thaddeus S. Walczak, and Timothy A. Pedley

Electroencephalography (EEG) and evoked potentials (EPs) are measures of brain electrical activity. The EEG displays spontaneous brain activity as a continuous graph of voltage and frequency changes occurring over time. In contrast, EPs reflect activity of the central nervous system in response to specific stimuli. Unlike anatomic imaging methods, such as CT and MRI that provide information about brain structure, EEG and EP studies are measures of brain function. Functional and structural investigations are often complementary. Electrophysiologic studies are especially important to the differential diagnosis when neurologic disorders are unaccompanied by detectable alterations in brain morphology. In this chapter is an overview of the current capabilities and limitations of these techniques in clinical practice.

THE NORMAL ADULT EEG

EEG activity is characterized by the frequency and voltage of the signals. A major feature of the EEG during wakefulness is the alpha rhythm, an 8- to 12-cycles-per-second (cps) pattern detected over the parietal and occipital regions, bilaterally (Fig. 14.1). The alpha rhythm is seen best when the patient is awake and relaxed with eyes closed.

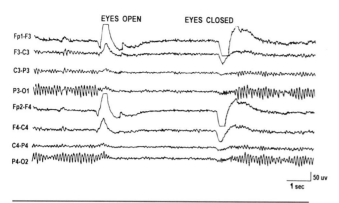

FIGURE 14.1. Normal EEG in an awake 28-year-old man.

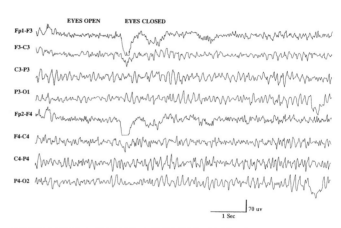

FIGURE 14.2. Diffuse slowing in a 67-year-old patient with dementia. Six-cps to seven-cps activity predominates over the parietooccipital regions. Although reactive to eye closure, the frequency of this rhythm is abnormally slow.

It attenuates when the eyes are opened, or the subject is alerted. Beta activity, between 13 cps and 25 cps, is usually maximal in the frontal and central regions. High-voltage, very rhythmic beta activity suggests the effect of sedative-hypnotic medications. A small amount of slower frequencies, usually in the theta (4 cps to 7 cps) range, may be seen diffusely, especially in children.

Sleep is divided into five stages, on the basis of the combinations of EEG patterns, eye movements, and axial EMG. Stage 1 is a transitional period between wakefulness and sleep. The alpha rhythm disappears during stage 1 and is replaced by low-voltage, slower activity. Vertex waves, high-voltage "sharp" transients, are recorded maximally at the vertex. Stage 2 sleep is characterized by sleep spindles (symmetric 12-cps to 14-cps sinusoidal waves). The EEG in stages 3 and 4 is composed of high-voltage, widely distributed, slow-wave activity. Rapid eye movement (REM) sleep is characterized by low-voltage, mixed-frequency activity, similar to that seen in early stage 1, together with REM and generalized atonia. REM occurs about 90 minutes after sleep onset in adults and is not usually seen in routine studies. The presence of REM in a daytime EEG suggests sleep deprivation, withdrawal from REM-suppressant drugs, alcohol withdrawal, or narcolepsy (Chapter 145).

COMMON EEG ABNORMALITIES

Diffuse slowing of background rhythms is the most common EEG abnormality (Fig. 14.2). This finding is etiologically nonspecific and occurs in patients with diffuse encephalopathies of diverse causes, including toxic, metabolic, anoxic, and degenerative conditions. Multiple structural abnormalities may also cause diffuse slowing.

Focal slowing suggests localized, parenchymal dysfunction (Fig. 14.3). Focal neuroradiologic abnormalities are found in 70% of patients with significant focal slowing and must always be suspected in this situation. Localized

slowing may also be seen in patients with focal seizure disorders, even when no lesions are found. Focal voltage attenuation usually indicates localized lesions of gray matter but may also be seen with subdural, epidural, or even subgaleal fluid collections (Fig. 14.3).

Triphasic waves are generalized bisynchronous waves occurring in brief runs (Fig. 14.4). As the name suggests, they typically have three phases; the second phase is positive and usually the most prominent. Approximately one-half the patients with triphasic waves have hepatic encephalopathy and the remainder have other toxic-metabolic encephalopathies.

Epileptiform discharges (EDs) are the interictal hallmark of epilepsy. They are strongly associated with seizure disorders and are uncommon in normal adults. The particular pattern of ED may suggest a specific epileptic syndrome, as follows.

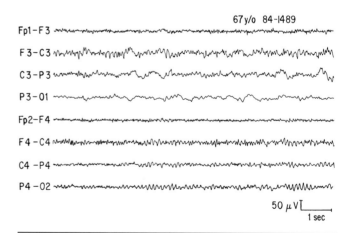

FIGURE 14.3. Focal slow activity with attenuation of the alpha rhythm over the left hemisphere in a 67-year-old patient with an acute left hemispheral infarction.

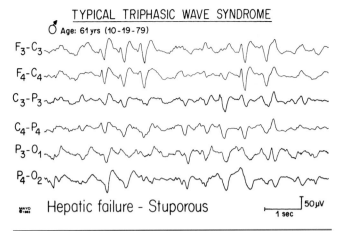

FIGURE 14.4. Triphasic waves in a 61-year-old patient with hepatic failure. (Courtesy of Bruce J. Fisch.)

Periodic lateralized epileptiform discharges (PLEDs) usually indicate the presence of an acute destructive cerebral lesion. Focal EDs recur at 1 cps to 2 cps in the setting of a focally slow or attenuated background activity (Fig. 14.5). In a study of nearly 600 patients with PLEDs, acute cerebral infarction had occurred in 35%, other mass lesions were shown to have caused an additional 26%, and cerebral abscess, anoxia, or various other causes comprised the remainder. Clinically, PLEDs are associated with seizures, obtundation, and focal neurologic signs.

Generalized periodic sharp waves typically recur at 0.5 cps to 1 cps on an attenuated background. This pattern is most commonly seen following cerebral anoxia. It

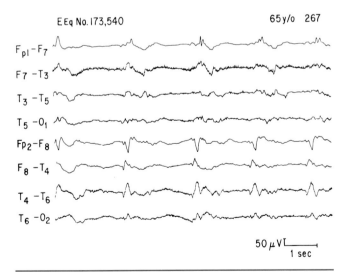

FIGURE 14.5. Right hemispheral PLEDs in a 65-year-old patient with herpes simplex encephalitis. (From Pedley TA, Emerson RG. Clinical neurophysiology. In: Bradley WG, Daroff RB, Fenichel GM, Marsden CD, eds. *Neurology in Clinical Practice*, 2nd ed. Boston: Butterworth-Heinemann, 1996:460; with permission.)

is also recorded in about 90% of patients with Creutzfeldt-Jakob disease.

CLINICAL UTILITY OF ELECTROENCEPHALOGRAPHY

Epilepsy

The EEG is the most useful laboratory test to help establish the diagnosis of epilepsy and assist in the accurate classification of seizures and specific epileptic syndromes. Characteristic interictal EDs strongly support the diagnosis of epilepsy, but absence of EDs does not exclude it. EDs are recorded on the first EEG in 30% to 50% of patients with epilepsy, and in 60% to 90% by the third EEG. Additional EEGs do not increase the yield further. Thus, 10% to 40% of patients with epilepsy will not have interictal discharges, even with repeated EEGs. Sleep, sleep deprivation, hyperventilation, and photic stimulation increase the yield of EDs in some patients.

Conversely, interictal EDs are infrequent in healthy normal subjects or patients without epilepsy. EDs occur in only 1.5% to 3.5% of normal children. Asymptomatic siblings of children with benign focal epilepsy or childhood absence epilepsy may have interictal EDs as a manifestation of a genetic trait. EDs occur in 2.7% of adult patients with various illnesses, including neurologic diseases, but without a history of seizures. The presence of EDs in an appropriate clinical context provides strong support for a diagnosis of epilepsy but does not establish it unequivocally.

The type of interictal ED, together with the patient's clinical features, often allow diagnosis of a specific epilepsy syndrome. Confident diagnosis of an epilepsy syndrome helps guide treatment and also provides information about prognosis. Table 14.1 summarizes specific characteristics of epileptiform abnormalities in some common epileptic syndromes. Clinical features of the syndromes are summarized in Chapter 141. A useful example is the distinction between generalized 3-cps spike-and-wave and temporal spike-and-wave discharges. The 3 cps spike-and-wave pattern is seen in childhood absence epilepsy, a syndrome with early age of onset, absence, tonic-clonic seizures, and a generally good prognosis (Fig. 14.6). Either ethosuximide or valproic acid is the medication of choice. In contrast, temporal lobe spikes are seen in complex partial seizures or complex partial seizures with secondary generalization (Fig. 14.7). Prognosis is poorer, and phenytoin sodium, carbamazepine, lamotrigine, or oxcarbazepine are medications of choice.

EEG results also help in the management of epilepsy. Finding interictal EDs after a single seizure increases the likelihood of seizure recurrence and therefore influences the decision about whether to treat with antiepileptic

▶ **TABLE 14.1   Epileptiform Abnormalities in the Common Epilepsy Syndromes**

Syndrome/Diagnosis	Findings
West syndrome (hypsarrhythmia)	No organized background rhythm
	Random high-voltage slow activity
	Multifocal epileptiform discharges
	Abrupt attenuation (infantile spasm)
Lennox-Gastaut syndrome	Slow generalized spike and wave (<2 cps)
	Significantly slowed background rhythm
Childhood absence epilepsy	Generalized spike and wave (>3 cps)
	Usually precipitated by hyperventilation
	Normal background rhythm
Benign rolandic epilepsy	Focal centrotemporal epileptiform discharge
	Normal background rhythm
Juvenile myoclonic epilepsy	Generalized polyspike wave (often >3 cps)
	May be precipitated by photic stimulation
	Normal background rhythm
Localization-related epilepsy (e.g., temporal lobe seizures)	Focal epileptiform discharges
	Occasional focal slowing
	Occasional mild slowing of background

drugs. Similarly, the presence of interictal EDs increases the likelihood of seizure recurrence when consideration is being given to discontinuing antiepileptic drugs after a period of seizure control.

Dementia and Diffuse Encephalopathies

The EEG provides useful clues in obtunded patients. Triphasic waves suggest a toxic-metabolic cause. High-voltage beta activity suggests the presence of sedative-hypnotic medications. Generalized voltage attenuation is seen in Huntington disease. Generalized periodic sharp waves are seen in about 90% of patients with Creutzfeldt-Jakob disease within 12 weeks of clinical onset. EEG is critical when spike-wave stupor is the cause of obtundation. EEG may be normal early in the course of Alzheimer disease, when cognitive changes are minor and the diagnosis is still uncertain. As moderate to severe symptoms appear, diffuse slowing is seen (Fig. 14.2). Almost all patients with biopsy-proven Alzheimer disease have unequivocal EEG abnormalities within 3 years of the onset of symptoms. Focal slowing is uncommon and if present, suggests multiinfarct dementia or another multifocal cause.

Focal Brain Lesions

As neuroimaging has become widely available, EEG has come to play a less important role in the diagnosis of structural lesions. EEG is necessary, however, to assess the

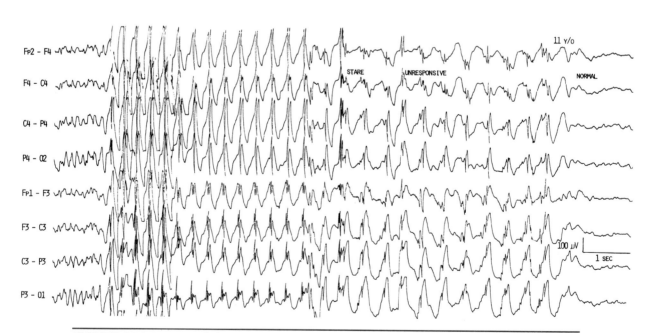

FIGURE 14.6. Ten-second absence seizure in an 11-year-old with staring spells. Three-cps to four-cps generalized spike wave is seen at the beginning of the seizure. The rate gradually slows toward the end of the seizure. Then patient was asked to follow a simple command 6 secs after seizure onset and was unable to do so.

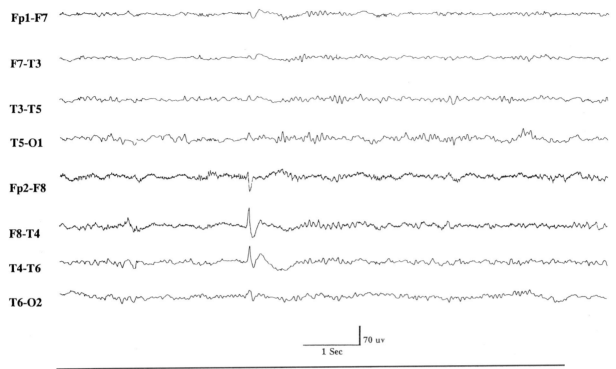

Fp1-F7

F7-T3

T3-T5

T5-O1

Fp2-F8

F8-T4

T4-T6

T6-O2

70 uv

1 Sec

FIGURE 14.7. Right anterior temporal epileptiform discharge in a 32-year-old patient with complex partial seizures emerging from the right temporal lobe.

epileptogenic potential of mass lesions. Focal EEG abnormalities accompany one-half of hemispheral transient ischemic attacks. Normal EEG in a patient with a neurologic deficit strongly suggests a lacunar infarction. EEG slowing in hemispheric infarcts gradually improves with time; in contrast, focal slowing in neoplasms remains the same or worsens. Recognizing this difference may be useful when neuroradiologic findings do not distinguish between semiacute infarction and neoplasm.

Cerebral Infections

Focal changes are noted in more than 80% of patients with herpes encephalitis, and PLEDs are seen in more than 70% (Fig. 14.5). PLEDs typically appear 2 to 15 days after onset of illness, but the interval may be as long as 1 month. Serial EEG is therefore useful if early studies are nonfocal. Early focal findings strongly suggest this diagnosis if the clinical picture is compatible, and may indicate the appropriate site for biopsy. Virtually diagnostic EEG changes are seen in subacute sclerosing panencephalitis, namely those of stereotyped bursts of high-voltage delta waves at regular intervals of 4 seconds to 10 seconds. Early in the disease, slow-wave bursts may be infrequent or confined to sleep, so serial EEG may be useful. EEG findings in patients infected with HIV are nonspecific. Diffuse slowing may precede clinical neurologic manifestations. The slowing becomes more persis-

tent in patients with dementia related to acquired immunodeficiency syndrome. Focal slowing suggests the presence of a superimposed cerebral lesion, such as lymphoma or toxoplasmosis.

LONG-TERM EEG MONITORING

Over the past decade, traditional EEG machines that wrote with mechanical pens onto fan-fold paper have given way to digital, computer-based systems. These systems facilitate interpretation by allowing the electroencephalographer to manipulate EEG data at the time of interpretation and to supplement standard visual analysis of EEG patterns with information provided by various signal-processing techniques. By eliminating what would previously have been stacks of paper, they also make recording and interpretation of EEG over a prolonged period of time practical.

In epilepsy monitoring units, EEG is recorded continuously, along with time-locked video and audio. For outpatient EEG monitoring, compact portable devices permit EEG to be recorded for days at time, while the patient maintains his or her daily routine. EEG data thus acquired is often processed by programs that automatically detect spikes and seizures although at present, available software produces frequent false-positive detections necessitating careful manual review of computer-detected events. Long-term EEG monitoring has improved

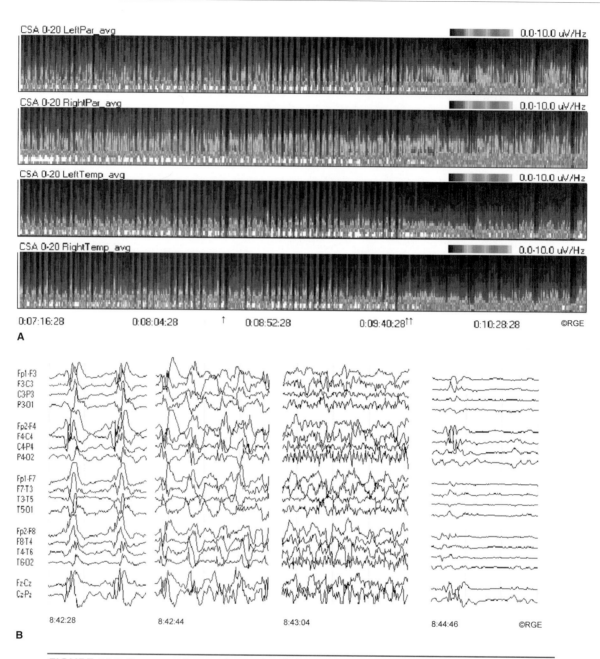

FIGURE 14.8. Compressed spectral array (CSA) depicting the voltage spectra derived from four channels of EEG in a patient in status epilepticus. Seizures recurred every several minutes for nearly 3 hrs, finally abating following an increase in the dose of pentobarbital (double arrow). The abscissa of each chart represents time as indicated, and the ordinate represents frequency from 0 Hz to 20 Hz. Voltage is encoded with use of a color scale, as illustrated. The accompanying EEG illustrates segments from a single seizure (single arrow). (See color insert).

diagnostic accuracy. For patients in whom the diagnosis of epilepsy is uncertain, the issue may often be resolved with monitoring. For patients with epilepsy, monitoring aids in determination of seizure type and epilepsy syndrome. With inpatient monitoring, antiepileptic medications can be discontinued increasing the likelihood that seizures will be recorded. Longer recording periods also increase the likelihood that interictal EDs will be recorded and the diagnosis of epilepsy further supported. Characteristic ictal EEG patterns are found in all tonic-clonic and almost all complex partial seizures allowing a secure diagnosis in these situations. However ictal EEG may remain normal in approximately half of simple partial seizures. In patients with medically refractory epilepsy undergoing evaluation for surgical treatment, video/EEG monitoring is often performed with intracranial electrodes to define precisely the seizure-onset zone.

In intensive care units (ICU), continuous EEG monitoring is becoming increasingly commonplace. In patients in whom sedation or pharmacologic paralysis limits the utility of the neurologic examination, continuous EEG monitoring may be a powerful tool for assessing neurologic condition in real time. Applications include management of seizures and status epilepticus (including nonconvulsive seizures), management of drug-induced coma for treatment of increased intracranial pressure, prognostication, and potentially the detection of cerebral ischemia. Nonconvulsive seizures are common in critically ill neurologic patients, present in 27% of 53 consecutive patients with altered mental status in one study, and may well go unnoticed without EEG monitoring. In the ICU, simultaneous video monitoring may be invaluable in characterizing movements thought possibly to be ictal, as well helping to identify various artifacts on the EEG. Automated seizure detection is also useful, as are color spectral displays based on fast Fourier transforms (FFT) of the EEG. The latter present quantitative data about the EEG frequencies present in an appealing and easily understood manner, and by summarizing many hours of EEG activity in a single screen, make it easy to recognize patterns that repeat or evolve over time (Fig. 14.8).

EVOKED POTENTIALS

Principles of Evoked Potential Recording

Visual, auditory, and somatosensory stimuli cause small electric signals to be produced by neural structures along the corresponding sensory pathways. These EPs are generally of much lower voltage than ongoing spontaneous cortical electric activity. They are usually not apparent in ordinary EEG recordings and are detected with the use of averaging techniques. Changes in EPs produced by disease states generally consist of delayed responses, reflecting conduction delays in responsible pathways, or attenuation or loss of component waveforms, resulting from conduction block or dysfunction of the responsible generator.

Clinically, EP tests are best viewed as an extension of the neurologic examination. Abnormalities identify dysfunction in specific sensory pathways and suggest the location of a responsible lesion. They are most useful when they identify abnormalities that are clinically inapparent or confirm abnormalities that correspond to vague or equivocal signs or symptoms.

Visual Evoked Potentials

The preferred stimulus for visual evoked potential (VEP) testing is a checkerboard pattern of black and white squares. Pattern reversal (i.e., change of the white squares to black and the black squares to white) produces an occipital positive signal, the P100, approximately 100 milliseconds after the stimulus. Because fibers arising from the nasal portion of each retina decussate at the optic chiasm (Fig. 14.9), an abnormality in the P100 response to stimulation of one eye necessarily implies dysfunction anterior to the optic chiasm on that side. Conversely, delayed P100 responses following stimulation of both eyes separately may result from bilateral abnormalities either anterior or posterior to the chiasm or at the chiasm. Unilateral hemispheral lesions do not alter the latency of the P100 component, as a result of the contribution of a normal response from the intact hemisphere.

Acute optic neuritis is accompanied by loss or severe attenuation of the VEP. Although the VEP returns, the latency of the P100 response almost always remains abnormally delayed, even if vision returns to normal (Fig. 14.10). Pattern-reversal VEPs (PRVEPs) are abnormal in nearly all patients with a definite history of optic neuritis. More important, PRVEPs are abnormal in about 70% of patients with definite multiple sclerosis who have no history of optic neuritis.

Despite the sensitivity of PRVEPs to demyelinating lesions of the optic nerve, the VEP changes produced by plaques are often not distinguishable from those produced by many other diseases that affect the visual system; these include ocular disease (major refractive error, media opacities, glaucoma, retinopathies), compressive lesions of the optic nerve (extrinsic tumors, optic nerve tumors), noncompressive optic nerve lesions (ischemic optic neuritis, nutritional and toxic amblyopias), and diseases affecting the nervous system diffusely (adrenoleukodystrophy, Pelizaeus-Merzbacher disease, spinocerebellar degenerations, Parkinson disease). VEPs may help distinguish blindness from hysteria and malingering. If a patient reports visual loss, a normal VEP strongly favors a psychogenic disorder.

Brainstem Auditory Evoked Potentials

Brainstem auditory evoked potentials (BAEPs) are generated by the auditory nerve and the brainstem in response to a "click" stimulus. The normal BAEP includes a series of signals that occurs within 7 milliseconds after the stimulus, comprising three components important to clinical interpretation (Fig. 14.11): wave I arising from the peripheral portion of the auditory nerve; wave III generated in the tegmentum of the caudal pons, most likely the superior olive or the trapezoid body; and wave V generated in the region of the inferior colliculus. Although brainstem auditory pathways decussate at multiple levels, unilateral abnormalities of waves III and V are most often associated with ipsilateral brainstem disease.

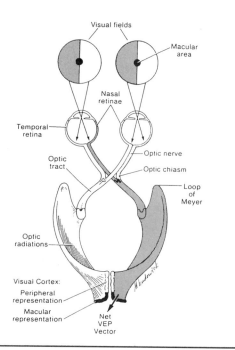

FIGURE 14.9. Primary visual pathways illustrating decussation of nasal retinal fibers at the optic chiasm and projections to the visual cortex. (From Epstein CM. Visual evoked potentials. In: Daly DD, Pedley TA, eds. *Current Practice of Clinical Electroencephalography*, 2nd ed. New York: Raven Press, 1997:565; with permission.)

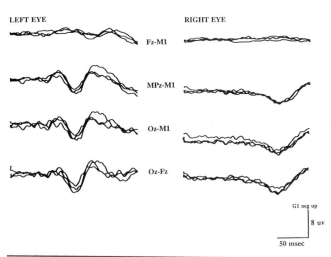

FIGURE 14.10. Pattern shift VEP in a patient with right optic neuritis. The response to left-eye stimulation is normal. Right-eye stimulation produces a marked delay of the P100 response. The relative preservation of waveform morphology despite pronounced latency prolongation is typical of demyelinating optic neuropathies. Unless otherwise specified, electrode positions are standard locations of the International 10–20 System. MPz corresponds to an electrode positioned mid-way between Oz and Pz. M1 is an electrode on the left mastoid process.

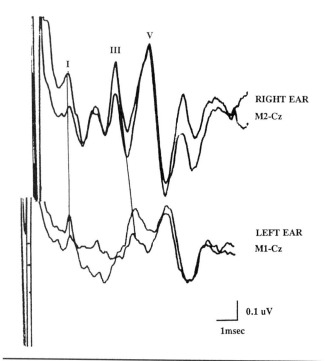

FIGURE 14.11. BAEP study in a patient with a left intracanalicular acoustic neuroma. The BAEP to right ear stimulation is normal. The I to III interpeak latency is prolonged following left-ear stimulation, reflecting delayed conduction between the distal eighth nerve and the lower pons.

BAEPs in Neurologic Disorders

The clinical utility of BAEPs derives from the close relationship of BAEP waveform abnormalities and structural pathology of their generators, and the resistance of BAEPs to alteration by systemic metabolic abnormalities or medications. BAEPs are often abnormal when structural brainstem lesions exist (Fig. 14.12). They are virtually always abnormal in patients with brainstem gliomas. Conversely, brainstem lesions that spare the auditory pathways, such as ventral pontine infarcts producing the locked-in syndrome or lateral medullary infarcts, do not produce abnormal BAEPs. Barbiturate levels high enough to produce an isoelectric EEG leave BAEPs unchanged, as do hepatic and renal failure. BAEPs are therefore useful for demonstrating brainstem integrity in toxic and metabolic perturbations that severely alter the EEG.

BAEPs are sensitive for detection of tumors of the eighth cranial nerve; abnormalities are demonstrated in more than 90% of patients with acoustic neuroma. BAEP abnormalities seen with acoustic neuromas and other cerebellopontine angle tumors range from prolongation of the I to III interpeak interval, thereby indicating a conduction delay between the distal eighth cranial nerve and lower pons (Fig. 14.11), to preservation of wave I with loss of subsequent components, to loss of all BAEP waveforms. The sensitivity of the BAEP to acoustic nerve lesions may be extended by decreasing the stimulus intensity over a prescribed range and evaluating the

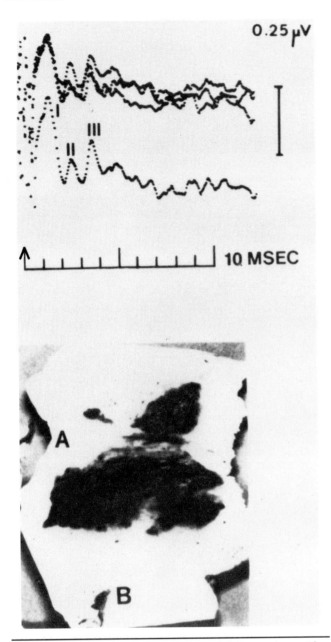

FIGURE 14.12. Abnormal BAEP recorded in a patient with a brainstem hemorrhage sparing the lower one-third of the pons. Waves IV and V are lost, but waves I, II, and III are preserved. (From Chiappa KH. Evoked potentials in clinical medicine. In: Baker AB, Baker LH, eds. *Clinical Neurology*. New York: Harper & Row, 1990:22; with permission.)

effects on the BAEP waveforms (latency-intensity function). Some patients with small intracanalicular tumors have normal standard BAEPs, and abnormality is revealed only by latency-intensity function testing.

BAEPs help establish the diagnosis of multiple sclerosis when they detect clinically unsuspected or equivocal brainstem lesions. BAEPs are abnormal in about 33% of patients with multiple sclerosis, including 20% of those who have no other signs or symptoms of brainstem lesions. The BAEP findings in multiple sclerosis consist of the absence or decreased amplitude of BAEP components, or an increase in the III to V interpeak latency.

BAEPs may be useful in demonstrating brainstem involvement in generalized diseases of myelin, such as metachromatic leukodystrophy, adrenoleukodystrophy, and Pelizaeus-Merzbacher disease. BAEP abnormalities may also be demonstrable in asymptomatic heterozygotes for adrenoleukodystrophy.

BAEPs are also used to evaluate hearing in infants and others who may not cooperate for standard audiologic tests. The latency-intensity test permits determination of the wave V threshold, as well as the relationship of wave V latency to stimulus intensity, and often allows characterization of hearing loss as sensorineural or conductive.

Somatosensory Evoked Potentials

Somatosensory evoked potentials (SSEPs) are generally elicited by electric stimulation of the median and posterior tibial nerves, and reflect sequential activation of structures along the afferent sensory pathways, principally the dorsal column-lemniscal system. The components of median-nerve SSEP testing that are important to clinical interpretation include: the Erb's point potential, recorded as the afferent volley traverses the brachial plexus; the N13, representing post-synaptic activity in the central gray matter of the cervical cord; the P14, arising in the lower brainstem, most likely in the caudal medial lemniscus; the N18, attributed to post-synaptic potentials generated in the rostral brainstem; and the N20, corresponding to activation of the primary cortical somatosensory receiving area (Fig. 14.13). The posterior-tibial SSEP is analogous to the median SSEP and includes components generated in the gray matter of the lumbar spinal cord, brainstem, and primary somatosensory cortex.

SSEPs are altered by diverse conditions that affect the somatosensory pathways, including focal lesions (e.g., strokes, tumors, cervical spondylosis, syringomyelia) or diffuse diseases (e.g., hereditary system degenerations, subacute combined degeneration, and vitamin E deficiency). Of patients with multiple sclerosis, 50% to 60% have SSEP abnormalities, even in the absence of clinical signs or symptoms. SSEP abnormalities are also produced by other diseases affecting myelin (adrenoleukodystrophy, adrenomyeloneuropathy, metachromatic leukodystrophy, Pelizaeus-Merzbacher disease). In adrenoleukodystrophy and adrenomyeloneuropathy, SSEP abnormalities may be present in asymptomatic heterozygotes. Abnormally large-amplitude SSEPs, reflecting enhanced cortical excitability, are seen in progressive myoclonus epilepsy, in some patients with photosensitive epilepsy, and in late-infantile ceroid lipofuscinosis.

SSEPs are commonly used to monitor the integrity of the spinal cord during neurosurgical, orthopedic, and vascular procedures where there is risk of injury; SSEPs may detect adverse changes before they become irreversible.

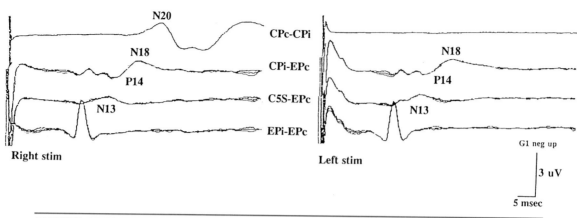

FIGURE 14.13. Median SSEPs in a patient with a right putamen hemorrhage. Following right median nerve stimulation, the SSEP is normal. Following left median nerve stimulation, the N20 cortical response is absent, while more caudally generated potentials are preserved.

Although SSEPs primarily reflect the function of the dorsal columns, they are generally sensitive to spinal cord damage produced by compression, mechanical distraction, or ischemia.

Motor-Evoked Potentials

It is possible to assess the descending motor pathways by motor-evoked potential (MEP) testing. MEP studies entail stimulation of the motor cortex and recording the compound muscle-action potential of appropriate target muscles. The cortex is stimulated either by direct passage of a brief high-voltage electric pulse through the scalp or by use of a time-varying magnetic field to induce an electric current within the brain. MEPs evaluate the integrity of the descending motor pathways, complementing data about sensory pathways provided by SSEPs, and providing information about diseases of the motor system. Intraoperative MEP monitoring is being used with increasing frequency, along with SSEP monitoring, during surgical procedures that place the spinal cord at risk.

SUGGESTED READINGS

Ajmone-Marsan C. Electroencephalographic studies in seizure disorders: additional considerations. *J Clin Neurophysiol* 1984;1:143–157.

American Electroencephalographic Society. Guidelines in electroencephalography, evoked potentials, and polysomnography. *J Clin Neurophysiol* 1994;11(1):1–147.

Chiappa KH. *Evoked Potentials in Clinical Medicine*, 3rd ed. Philadelphia: Lippincott-Raven Publishers, 1997.

Claassen J, Mayer SA, Kowalski RG, et al. Detection of electrographic seizures with continuous EEG monitoring in critically ill patients. *Neurology* 2004;62(10):1743–1748.

Devinsky O, Kelley K, Porter RJ, Theodore WH. Clinical and electroencephalographic features of simple partial seizures. *Neurology* 1988;38:1347-521347–1352.

Ebersole JS. Sublobar localization of temporal neocortical epileptogenic foci by source modeling. *Adv Neurol* 2000;84:353–363.

Eeg-Olofsson O, Petersen I, Sellden U. The development of the electroencephalogram in normal children from the age of one through fifteen years. *Neuropaediatrie* 1971;4:375–404.

Emerson RG and Adams DC. Intraoperative monitoring by evoked potential techniques. In: Aminoff MJ, ed. *Electrodiagnosis in Clinical Neurology*, 5th ed. New York: Churchill Livingstone, In press.

Fisch BJ, Klass DW. The diagnostic specificity of triphasic wave patterns. *Electroencephalogr Clin Neurophysiol* 1988;70:1–8.

Kellaway P. Orderly approach to visual analysis: characteristics of the normal EEG of adults and children. In: Ebersole JS, Pedley TA, eds. *Current Practice of Clinical Electroencephalography*, 3rd ed. New York: Lippincott Williams & Wilkins, 2003:100–159.

Hallett M. Transcranial magnetic stimulation and the human brain. *Nature* 2000;406:147–150.

Hirsch LJ, Claassen J, Mayer SA, et al. Stimulus-induced rhythmic, periodic, or ictal discharges (SIRPIDS): a common EEG phenomenon in the critically ill. *Epilepsia* 2004;45(2):109–123.

Lai CW, Gragasin ME. Electroencephalography in herpes simplex encephalitis. *J Gin Neurophysiol* 1988;5:87–103.

Lee EK, Seyal M. Generators of short latency human somatosensory evoked potentials recorded over the spine and scalp. *J Clin Neurophysiol* 1998;15:227–234.

Lerman P. Benign partial epilepsy with centro-temporal spikes. In: Roger J, Bureau M, Dravet C, et al, eds. *Epilepsy Syndromes in Infancy, Childhood, and Adolescence*, 2nd ed. London: John Libbey & Co, 1992:189–200.

Levy SR, Chiappa KH, Burke CJ, Young RR. Early evolution and incidence of electroencephalographic abnormalities in Creutzfeldt-Jakob disease. *J Clin Neurophysiol* 1986;3:1–21.

Mills KR. Magnetic brain stimulation: a review after 10 years experience. *Electroencephalogr Clin Neurophysiol* 1999;49(suppl):239–244.

Novotny EJ Jr. The role of clinical neurophysiology in the management of epilepsy. *J Clin Neurophysiol* 1998;15:96–108.

Pohlmann-Eden B, Hoch DB, Chiappa, KH. Periodic lateralized epileptiform discharges: a critical review. *J Clin Neurophysiol* 1996;13:519–530.

Pedley TA, Mendiratta A, Walczak TS. Seizures and Epilepsy. In Ebersole JS, Pedley TA, eds. *Current Practice of Clinical Electroencephalography*, 3rd ed. New York: Lippincott Williams & Wilkins, 2003:506–587.

Privitera M, Hoffman M, Moore JL, Jester D. EEG detection of nontonic-clonic status epilepticus in patients with altered consciousness. *Epilepsy Res* 1994;18:155–166.

Reeves AL, Westmoreland BE, Klass DW. Clinical accompaniments of the burst-suppression EEG pattern. *J Clin Neurophysiol* 1997;14:150–153.

Scheuer ML. Continuous EEG monitoring in the intensive care unit. *Epilepsia* 2002;43:114–127.

Salinsky M, Kanter R, Dasheiff RM. Effectiveness of multiple EEGs in supporting the diagnosis of epilepsy: an operational curve. *Epilepsia* 1987;28:331–334.

Zifkin BG, Cracco RQ. An orderly approach to the abnormal EEG. In: Ebersole JS, Pedley TA, eds. *Current Practice of Clinical Electroencephalography*, 3rd ed. New York: Lippincott Williams & Wilkins, 2003:288–302.

Chapter 15

Electromyography, Nerve Conduction Studies, and Magnetic Stimulation

Clifton L. Gooch and Seth Pullman

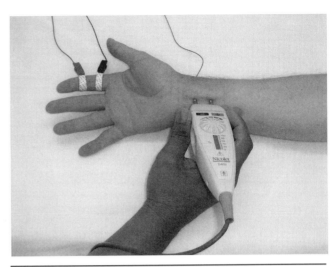

FIGURE 15.1. Set-up for sensory nerve conduction studies. A bipolar stimulator is placed over the median nerve at the wrist, and self-adhesive recording electrodes were placed over the pure sensory branches of the same nerve in the index finger (second digit), ensuring that only sensory nerve responses are recorded. The patient was grounded through a self-adhesive ground electrode placed over the dorsum of the hand.

Advances in electronics enabled clinical assessment of peripheral nerve and muscle physiology in the mid 20th century, spawning a new neurologic specialty. Electrodiagnostic techniques have become increasingly sophisticated in the digital age and are indispensable for the proper diagnosis and management of patients with neuromuscular disease. This chapter provides a brief overview of nerve conduction studies (NCS), needle EMG, special techniques for assessing neuromuscular junction function, and the emerging field of magnetic stimulation.

NERVE CONDUCTION STUDIES

Sensory and Motor Nerve Conduction Studies

Nerve conduction studies measure the speed and strength of an electrical impulse conducted along a peripheral nerve. Typically, the impulse is generated using a bipolar stimulator placed on the surface of the skin over the anatomic course of the nerve being tested. The intensity and duration of this transcutaneous stimulus is gradually increased until all of the axons within that nerve are depolarized, sparking an action potential that travels down the nerve to the recording site. For *sensory nerve conduction studies*, the recording electrodes are placed on the surface of the skin overlying the nerve (usually over a pure sensory branch) at some distance from the site of stimulation (Fig. 15.1).

When an action potential passes under these bipolar recording electrodes, a *sensory nerve action potential* (SNAP) waveform is recorded and displayed on the screen of the EMG system (Fig. 15.2).

Although modern equipment is computerized with digital processing and storage to capture and analyze the data, the waveform display owes its origins to the cathode ray oscilloscope. By convention, the X-axis of the tracing is the time base (or sweep speed) in milliseconds, while the Y-axis measures the strength of the impulse. The electrical

strength of the impulse is indicated by the *amplitude* of the waveform, measured either in microvolts (sensory waveforms) or millivolts (motor waveforms) and is represented on the tracing by the vertical height of the waveform. The time between delivery of the stimulus and the appearance

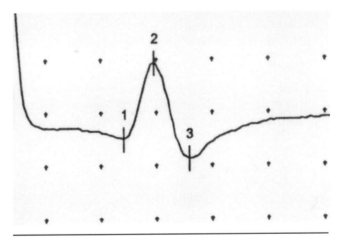

FIGURE 15.2. A sensory nerve action potential (SNAP), recorded using the set-up depicted in Fig. 15.1. The horizontal space between two dots, or graticules (one division), is assigned a specific value (the time base, or sweep speed, shown here as 1 millisecond per division) to enable time measurements. Vertical divisions are also assigned a specific value to enable measurement of stimulus strength (the gain, or sensitivity, shown here as 10 microvolts per division). The time between the stimulus artifact and the peak of this waveform (the sensory latency) is 2.75 milliseconds, and the peak-to-peak height of the waveform (the sensory amplitude) is 13.2 microvolts, within the normal range for control subjects.

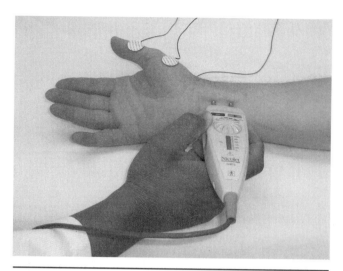

FIGURE 15.3. Set-up for motor nerve conduction studies. The bipolar stimulator is again placed over the median nerve at the wrist, but the recording electrodes are placed over the median-innervated muscles in the thenar eminence (principally the abductor pollicis brevis). Instead of recording neuronal depolarization, this set-up records the depolarization of an innervated muscle. The field strength of muscle depolarization is an order of magnitude stronger than that of a sensory nerve, and recordings are made with sensitivities set in the millivolt, rather than microvolt, range.

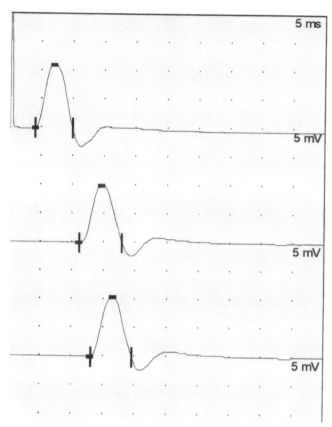

FIGURE 15.4. A compound motor action potential (CMAP). These three responses were recorded from the extensor digitorum brevis muscle of the foot following stimulation of the peroneal nerve at three different sites: the ankle (top waveform), below the knee at the fibular head (middle waveform) and above the knee (bottom waveform). The sensitivity was 5 millivolts/division and the sweep speed was 5 milliseconds/division for this tracing. These waveforms have onset latencies of 4.0 milliseconds, 11.1 milliseconds, and 13 milliseconds respectively, predictably increasing as the distance between the stimulating and recording electrodes increases. Calculated conduction velocities (using latency and inter-electrode distances measured on the patient) for both the proximal and distal segments is 46 meters/second. Amplitudes are 11.5 millivolts, 10.4 millivolts and 10.2 millivolts respectively, all within normal limits.

of the waveform at the recording site is a measure of the speed of nerve conduction and is known as the *latency*, measured in milliseconds and represented on the tracing by the horizontal distance from the initial stimulus artifact to the waveform captured at the recording site. Using this value and the distance between the stimulating and recording points measured on the patient, a *nerve conduction velocity* may be calculated.

Motor nerve conduction studies are performed similarly, except that the recording electrodes are placed over an innervated muscle, rather than over the nerve itself, to ensure a pure motor response is recorded. (Fig. 15.3).

The action potential passes down the nerve and across the neuromuscular junction into the muscle. The recording electrodes capture the electrical potential generated by depolarization of the innervated muscle, subsequently generating a waveform known as the *compound motor action potential* (CMAP) (Fig. 15.4).

As muscle tissue is much more electrically potent than nerve fibers, the CMAP is an order of magnitude larger than the SNAP and its amplitude is measured in millivolts, rather than microvolts. Otherwise, latency and amplitude measures are similar to those for the SNAP.

Both latency and conduction velocity depend on an intact, myelinated nerve, as myelin and the saltatory conduction it fosters are essential for fast-action potential propagation in normal subjects. In contrast, the amplitude of the waveform depends primarily on the number of axons

functioning within the nerve. Slowing of conduction velocity or prolongation of latency usually implies demyelinating injury, while loss of amplitude usually correlates with axonal loss or dysfunction. However, when demyelination is severe enough to cause complete block of transmission in most of the axons within a nerve at a specific point along its course, nerve conduction studies done on different segments of the same nerve may reveal a specific abnormality. With such focal demyelination, recordings made with the site of injury between the stimulating and recording electrodes produce waveforms having a much lower amplitude than those in recordings made with the stimulating and recording electrodes placed along a more normal segment

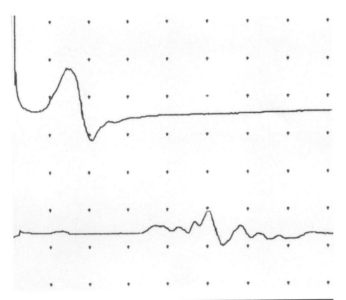

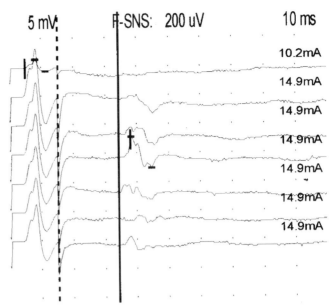

FIGURE 15.5. Conduction block with temporal dispersion. Two CMAPs recorded from the abductor hallucis muscle of the foot following stimulation of the tibial nerve at the ankle and the knee (top and bottom, respectively) in a patient with demyelinating neuropathy. The sensitivity was 1 millivolt/division, and the sweep speed was 5 milliseconds/division. When stimulation is moved from the ankle to the knee, the recorded waveform dramatically decreases in amplitude (from 1.1 millivolts to 0.5 millivolts, a 54% decline); its duration lengthens; and its morphology becomes irregular and complex. These findings suggest significant demyelination of the nerve segment between the stimulation sites, with axonal conduction block in the majority of motor axons, along with increasing variability in the range of axonal conduction times causing increased waveform duration (temporal dispersion).

FIGURE 15.6. A series of F waves recorded from the thenar eminence following repeated median nerve stimulation in a patient with cervical radiculopathy. The screen is split with lower sensitivity (5 millivolts/division) to the left of the dotted line, to show the full initial CMAPs generated by distal stimulation, and higher sensitivity (200 microvolts/division) to the right, to allow visualization of the much smaller F-wave responses. The sweep speed is 10 milliseconds per division. The dark vertical line is a marker placed to measure the latency to the earliest F-wave potential in the group (by convention). In this tracing, the F-wave responses were slightly prolonged at 34 milliseconds, due to a C-8 radiculopathy.

of the same nerve. When severe enough, this loss of waveform amplitude arising from focal nerve injury is known as a *conduction block* and is an important diagnostic feature of acquired demyelinating neuropathies (Fig. 15.5).

Late Responses

Routine nerve conduction studies are limited to accessible segments in the proximal and distal arms and legs. However, the nerve roots are not easily stimulated, and *long-latency reflex* tests are typically used to assess these most proximal segments. When a stimulus is delivered to the distal nerve, action potentials are propagated both proximally and distally. The impulse traveling up the motor axons (in a direction opposite to the normal flow or *antidromic*) eventually reaches the anterior-horn cells, depolarizing them. The anterior-horn cells then generate a second action potential that travels back down the axon into the muscle (in the direction paralleling the normal flow or *orthodromic*), where it is recorded as a much

smaller waveform known as the *F wave*, so named because it was originally recorded from the intrinsic muscles of the foot (Fig. 15.6).

The time required for this round trip up and down the motor nerve is measured as *the F-wave latency*. Although pathology at any point along the nerve may prolong the F-wave latency, if normal function of the distal nerve is documented by routine motor nerve conduction study, F-wave prolongation must be the result of slowing in the proximal segment.

A different long latency response, *the H reflex* (named after Hoffman, who first described it in 1918) may be elicited in the legs by electrical stimulation of the IA sensory nerve afferents in the tibial nerve at the knee. This is accomplished while recording the soleus muscle contraction resulting from activation of the same monosynaptic stretch-reflex pathway elicited by deep-tendon reflex testing during physical examination. The H reflex is the electrical equivalent of the ankle jerk, and aids primarily in the assessment of L5-S1 nerve root disease. By analyzing motor and sensory nerve conductions and long latency responses in multiple nerves, the nature of a given neuronal injury (axonal, demyelinating or both) and its geographic distribution may be identified, aiding in the diagnosis of radiculopathy, plexopathy, mononeuropathy, and polyneuropathy.

NEEDLE ELECTROMYOGRAPHY

Basic Concepts

After all indicated nerve conduction studies are performed, the next step of the electrodiagnostic evaluation is usually choosing which muscle or group of muscles should be tested by needle EMG. A needle-recording electrode is placed directly into the selected muscle, which is then activated by voluntary contraction rather than extrinsic electrical stimulation. Normal, full, voluntary muscle contraction requires activation of each motor axon within a given motor nerve at the level of the anterior-horn cell, with subsequent propagation of an action potential to the end of each axonal branch. Each of these activated terminal branches then initiate transmission across the neuromuscular junction, activating single muscle fibers. A single motor axon with all of its branches and innervated muscle fibers is known as a *motor unit*. The strength of a muscle contraction is determined primarily by how many motor units are simultaneously activated and by how fast they are firing. The recording characteristics of the EMG needle enable live recording and analysis of individual and aggregate motor unit waveforms.

Insertional and Spontaneous Activity

During needle EMG examination, at least five parameters are measured: *insertional activity*, *spontaneous activity*, *motor unit configuration*, *motor unit recruitment*, and the *interference pattern*. Different areas throughout the muscle are explored to insure a representative sample and to detect focal changes. Insertional activity is the brief burst of electrical activity recorded when the EMG needle is moved through the muscle, directly stimulating and injuring muscle fibers and generating a cluster of high frequency spikes lasting from 50 milliseconds to a few hundred milliseconds. In some nerve or muscle diseases, the insertional activity may be consistently prolonged with each movement of the needle. Such increased insertional activity suggests excessive irritability of the muscle fiber and is a hallmark of denervating disorders (diseases of the motor axon or cell body of the motor neuron), although it may also appear in inflammatory myopathy and some other primary muscle diseases. Once needle movement has ceased, no other electrical activity should normally appear as long as the muscle is at rest.

Muscle fibers that have lost innervation through motor-axon injury or which are irritated by myopathic disease or inflammation may periodically undergo spontaneous

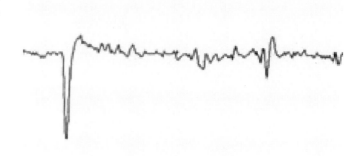

FIGURE 15.7. Spontaneous activity in a resting muscle. This tracing was recorded from the triceps muscle of a patient with cervical radiculopathy. A positive sharp wave, named for its sharp initial positive (downward) deflection, is seen on the left. On the right, a smaller triphasic fibrillation is seen. These potentials are markers of active denervation and result from the random, spontaneous depolarization of denervated single muscle fibers.

depolarization, generating brief spikes (*fibrillations*) and waves with a sharp positive component (*positive sharp waves*) in the resting muscle; sharp waves usually fire in a regular pattern with a frequency of 0.5 Hz to 15 Hz (Fig. 15.7).

This spontaneous activity is most strongly associated with denervating axonal injury at any point from the anterior horn to the nerve terminal (e.g. radiculopathy, plexopathy, axonal polyneuropathy, mononeuropathy), but may also be prominent in inflammatory myopathies, such as polymyositis or dermatomyositis. Lesser degrees of spontaneous activity may be observed in other myopathies (e.g. myotonic dystrophy, Duchenne muscular dystrophy) and in some toxic, metabolic, and infectious myopathies (e.g. myoglobinuria or rhabdomyolysis, hyperkalemic periodic paralysis, trichinosis). Some neuromuscular junction disorders, such as myasthenia gravis or botulism may also produce scattered spontaneous activity in a few muscles.

Other aberrant discharges may appear with neurogenic or myopathic disease, including fasciculations (e.g., motor neuron disease, benign fasciculation syndrome), complex repetitive discharges (e.g., denervation, inflammatory myopathy), myotonic discharges (e.g., myotonic dystrophy, myotonia congenital), myokymic discharges (e.g., radiation plexopathy, Guillain-Barré syndrome, multiple sclerosis), and neuromyotonic discharges (e.g., Isaacs syndrome).

Motor Unit Configuration

Assessment of the waveform generated by motor-unit activation (*the motor-unit action potential or* MUAP) yields important information (Fig. 15.8). MUAP parameters include waveform duration, amplitude and morphology (number of turns or baseline crossings). Because a muscle may contain hundreds of motor units, the EMG examination must include a representative sample of motor units collected at varying levels of voluntary contraction.

Diseases of the motor nerve and muscle alter these motor-unit parameters in characteristic ways. When motor axons begin to die, the muscle fibers supplied by them lose their innervation. However, other surviving motor axons in the same nerve branch to re-innervate these denervated muscle fibers in a process called *collateral reinnervation*. This compensatory repair gradually expands both the total number of muscle fibers innervated by surviving motor units, as well as the geographic territory within the muscle served by those units over several months. Reinnervated motor units produce abnormally enlarged MUAPs of long duration, high amplitude, and increased complexity (*neurogenic MUAPs*), which are markers of chronic motor axonal injury (Fig. 15. 9).

In contrast, myopathies destroy some of the muscle fibers in most or all of the motor units within a muscle, thereby reducing both the number and distribution of fibers within each unit, producing abnormally small MUAPs of short duration, low amplitude, and increased complexity (the *myopathic MUAP*, Fig. 15.10).

Disorders of the neuromuscular junction such as myasthenia gravis may also prevent activation of enough fibers, owing to cumulative neuromuscular junction blockade, to produce myopathic-appearing MUAPs; the earliest phases of collateral reinnervation and the latest phases of dener-

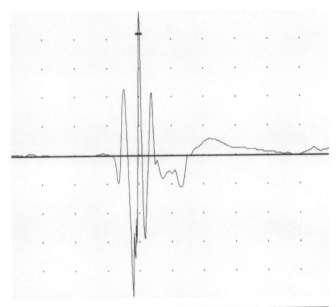

FIGURE 15.9. A neurogenic MUAP. This waveform was recorded during voluntary activation of the gastrocnemius muscle with a concentric needle electrode, in a patient with a distal, symmetric diabetic neuropathy. Sweep speed was 5 milliseconds/division and sensitivity was 1 millivolt/division. This waveform has a high amplitude of 10 millivolts, a significantly prolonged duration of 29 milliseconds, and is highly complex, with more than ten turns. As an individual motor axon dies during denervating injury, the muscle fibers it previously supplied lose all innervation. Surviving nearby axons subsequently branch to supply these muscle fibers, increasing their size and territory, resulting in increased MUAP size with higher amplitude, longer duration, and complex morphology.

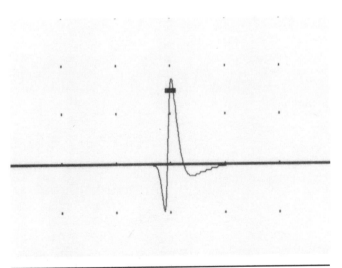

FIGURE 15.8. A normal motor unit action potential (MUAP). This waveform was recorded from the biceps muscle with a concentric needle electrode as the first potential recruited during minimal voluntary contraction in a normal subject. Sweep speed was 10 milliseconds/division and sensitivity was 500 microvolts/division. This waveform has an amplitude of 1.4 millivolts, a duration of 12.5 milliseconds, and a simple morphology with three turns.

vation during neurogenic atrophy may also produce short-duration motor units.

Recruitment and Interference Patterns

Needle EMG examination also enables assessment of motor-unit recruitment patterns. As a muscle begins to contract at the lowest force levels, the first recruited motor unit begins to fire repeatedly at a specific frequency. As demand for more strength increases, the firing frequency of the motor unit increases until a second motor unit is recruited. The specific firing frequency of the first recruited motor unit at the moment the second motor unit appears is *the recruitment frequency*. Abnormally high recruitment frequencies appear as motor units are lost, forcing surviving units to fire at faster and faster rates before additional units appear, a result of reductions in the number of motor units available for recruitment and for generation of force. In contrast, lower recruitment frequencies are seen in myopathies because most motor units are smaller and weaker, owing to loss of muscle fibers (*early recruitment*). Consequently, more motor units must be activated earlier than in normal subjects to generate the same levels of force.

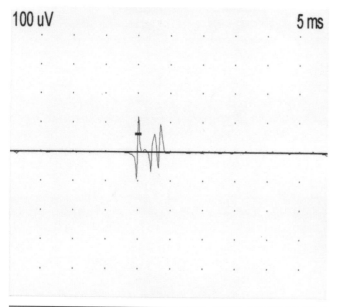

100 uV   5 ms

FIGURE 15.10. **A myopathic MUAP.** This waveform was recorded during voluntary activation of the vastus lateralis muscle with a concentric needle electrode in a patient with polymyositis. Sweep speed was 5 milliseconds/division and sensitivity was 100 microvolts/division. This waveform has a low amplitude of 210 microvolts, a low-normal duration of 7 milliseconds, and is complex with eight turns. As individual muscle fibers within a motor unit drop out during myopathic injury, the electric potential it generates when activated shrinks proportionately, resulting in decreased MUAP size with loss of amplitude and duration, and an increasingly complex morphology.

Following damage to the upper motor-neuron pathway, recruitment is disordered and motor units may fire at a slower than needed rate despite true maximal voluntary effort, as disrupted descending impulses improperly modulate firing frequency.

The *interference pattern* is the overlapping pattern generated by the simultaneous activation of large numbers of MUAPs during maximal contraction; it is assessed in terms of both spike density and the amplitude of the summated response. This response typically appears as a dense band of competing waveform activity at slow sweep speeds, which normally obscures the baseline tracing (Fig. 15.11).

Normal recruitment from low-, to intermediate-, to full contraction should produce a full interference pattern with a conical onset, as amplitudes increase progressively with the recruitment of larger and larger motor units to generate increasing force. *Incomplete or reduced interference patterns* (despite maximal contraction) are seen in advanced denervating disorders as more and more motor units drop out, ultimately leaving a "gap-toothed" or "picket-fence" pattern (Fig. 15.12).

Maximal voluntary effort must be elicited before interference patterns may be assessed accurately because poor volitional effort on the part of the patient may also result in an incomplete pattern; weakness due to central motor-neuron injury may also result in reduced recruitment. In contrast, full *interference patterns* appear early with myopathic disorders. A full pattern appears almost immediately with minimal effort, owing to the large numbers of weakened motor units that are required to generate even low levels of force. This pattern also has a lower envelope amplitude because the amplitude of the constituent motor units is low.

TESTS OF NEUROMUSCULAR TRANSMISSION

Repetitive Nerve Stimulation

Repetitive nerve stimulation (RNS) studies assess neuromuscular transmission, using a standard motor nerve-conduction setup (see "Nerve Conduction Studies" above) to deliver a series of supramaximal stimulations to a motor nerve at a specific frequency, while recording each generated CMAP. CMAP trains of four waveforms to ten

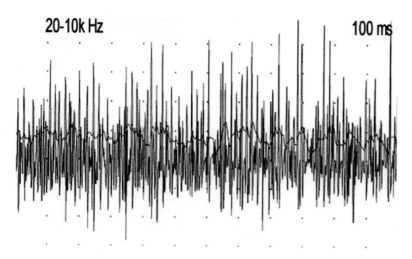

20-10k Hz   100 ms

FIGURE 15.11. **A normal interference pattern.** This dense, overlapping group of MUAP waveforms was recorded with a concentric needle electrode from the biceps muscle, during maximal voluntary contraction in a normal subject. It represents the simultaneous activation of all the functional motor units within that muscle. The sweep speed was 100 milliseconds/division and the sensitivity was 1 millivolt/division.

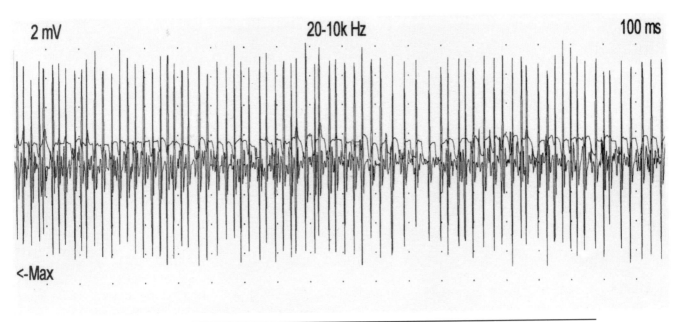

2 mV   20-10k Hz   100 ms

<-Max

FIGURE 15.12. A reduced interference pattern. This pattern of MUAP waveforms was recorded with a concentric needle electrode from the biceps muscle of a patient with amyotrophic lateral sclerosis, during maximal voluntary contraction. The sweep speed was 100 milliseconds/division and the sensitivity was 2 millivolts/division. Instead of the normal, dense band of overlapping MUAPs observed in the normal subject (Fig. 15.11), a "picket fence" pattern representing the activation of only a few motor units emerges because so many motor units have been lost. The MUAP amplitude of the most prominent surviving unit is increased (8 millivolts to 10 millivolts), consistent with collateral reinnervation, but the sweep speed is too low on this tracing to enable an assessment of duration or complexity.

waveforms are usually recorded at rates from 2 Hz to 5 Hz (low frequency stimulation). By convention, the waveforms within each train are displayed horizontally on the same baseline, from left to right, from first- to last stimulated (Fig. 15.13).

Trains are then evaluated either for decreases in consecutive CMAP size (as assessed by area or amplitude, from the first to a later potential and expressed as percent decrement) or for increases in size (usually expressed in percentage increments). Most protocols include one baseline train, followed by a brief period of voluntary exercise without stimulation, and then followed by one immediate, post-exercise train and several more trains, at intervals over the next 3 minutes to 5 minutes. The role of exercise is explained below. For high-frequency stimulation studies, either transcutaneous stimulation at rates of 10 Hz to 50 Hz or maximal voluntary contraction itself, which provides painless activation of the nerve at similar rates, is used. High frequency RNS studies are used in clinical practice almost exclusively to assess increments in CMAP amplitude of presynaptic disorders such as Lambert-Eaton myasthenic syndrome (as described below and in Chapter 122).

Post-synaptic Neuromuscular Junction Dysfunction

Patients with postsynaptic neuromuscular-junction dysfunction, most commonly caused by myasthenia gravis, may demonstrate decremental responses with low-frequency stimulation. During normal neuromuscular junction transmission, depolarization of the motor axon induces release of acetylcholine from the nerve terminal; the transmitter then diffuses across the synaptic cleft to

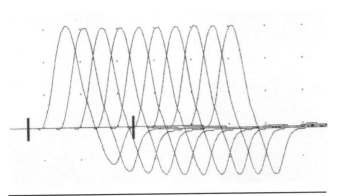

FIGURE 15.13. Repetitive nerve stimulation (RNS). A train of ten CMAPs recorded from the thenar eminence following repetitive nerve stimulation of the median nerve at a frequency of 3 Hz, arrayed in the order of their stimulation (left to right). Each individual CMAP is normal, and no significant change in CMAP amplitude or area is observed during repetitive stimulation.

activate a group of acetylcholine receptors on the muscle fiber, each of which generates a local depolarization. With summation, these local depolarizations ultimately reach threshold for the generation and propagation of a muscle-action potential, which then initiates muscle-fiber contraction. Declining acetylcholine release has been documented in normal subjects with stimulation at low frequencies, but these normal declines do not affect neuromuscular transmission because of the abundance of acetylcholine receptors at the post-synaptic muscle end plate, ensuring adequate muscle fiber depolarization despite the lower levels of acetylcholine released (the *safety margin* for neuromuscular transmission). However, in myasthenia and other post-synaptic disorders, the decline in acetylcholine release becomes critical because there are fewer functional acetylcholine receptors at the muscle end plate. The result is failure of neuromuscular transmission at increasing numbers of neuromuscular junctions with continued stimulation. As increasing numbers of muscle fibers drop out with successive stimulation, the size of the CMAP (the electrical signature of all of the muscle fibers firing after a single stimulation) also decreases (Fig. 15.14).

Additionally, the size (amplitude or area) of a single CMAP immediately after brief exercise, in myasthenia, may increase by 10% to 50% or more compared to the baseline (pre-exercise) CMAP. This phenomenon, known as *post-exercise facilitation* or *post-tetanic potentiation*, is attributed to a temporary increase in acetylcholine release after a brief maximal contraction. Post-exercise facilitation may be assessed by comparing the first CMAP in the first train acquired immediately after exercise to the amplitude of the first CMAP in the pre-exercise train. In addition to post-exercise facilitation of CMAP amplitude, any decrement in the baseline train may transiently improve in the train immediately after exercise (*decrement repair*).

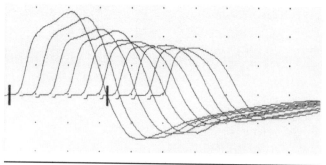

FIGURE 15.14. Decrement during repetitive nerve stimulation. Progressive decreases in the size of CMAPs were recorded from the thenar eminence during a train of RNS at 3 Hz, in a patient with myasthenia gravis. Losses in both amplitude and area of 40% to 50% appeared during RNS, owing to transmission failure at increasing numbers of neuromuscular junctions, which was consistent with significant neuromuscular junction dysfunction in the tested muscle.

However, after this transient repair, decrement typically worsens in trains recorded over the next 3 minutes to 4 minutes, often dipping below baseline (*post-activation exhaustion*) as reserve acetylcholine levels are exhausted. Decrement ultimately returns to pre-exercise levels within 10 minutes.

Pre-synaptic Neuromuscular Junction Dysfunction

In the presynaptic Lambert-Eaton myasthenic syndrome (LEMS), the CMAP amplitude may be low during routine nerve conduction studies, and low frequency RNS produces decrement similar to that seen in postsynaptic dysfunction. Both the low baseline CMAP and the decrement seen on low-frequency stimulation are the result of the combination of normal decline in acetylcholine release at low rates of stimulation superimposed on the diminished release of acetylcholine resulting from antibody blockade of the presynaptic voltage-gated calcium channel. High-frequency RNS, in contrast, characteristically leads to CMAP increment over 1 second to 2 seconds, usually exceeding 100%. The pain of high-frequency stimulation may be avoided by an alternative method of equal sensitivity. After acquisition of routine CMAP, the patient voluntarily contracts the muscle with maximum force for 10 seconds to 20 seconds, after which a second CMAP is obtained immediately; this "exercise test" shows post-exercise facilitation comparable in magnitude to the increment observed after high-frequency stimulation.

Single-Fiber Electromyography

Another test of the neuromuscular junction is single-fiber electromyography (SFEMG), in which a needle records the potentials generated by single muscle fibers. When an axon is selectively stimulated and a single muscle-fiber action potential is measured (*stimulated SFEMG*), the interval between stimulus and response varies with each stimulus. This normal variation results from the fluctuating time required for electrochemical transmission across the junction and is quantitated as *jitter*. *Volitional SFEMG* recordings are easier to perform, and measure jitter by assessing the differences between two voluntarily activated muscle fibers belonging to the same motor unit. With neuromuscular dysfunction, jitter increases and in severe cases, complete block of neuromuscular transmission may be documented. SFEMG is the single most sensitive assay of neuromuscular-junction dysfunction in myasthenia gravis, having a sensitivity of 95% when applied to a clinically affected muscle (Fig. 15.15A and Fig. 15.15B).

Though SFEMG is sensitive, it is not specific and may be increased in any condition causing damage to nerve or muscle. Consequently, it is essential to carry out appropriate nerve-conduction studies and standard EMG before

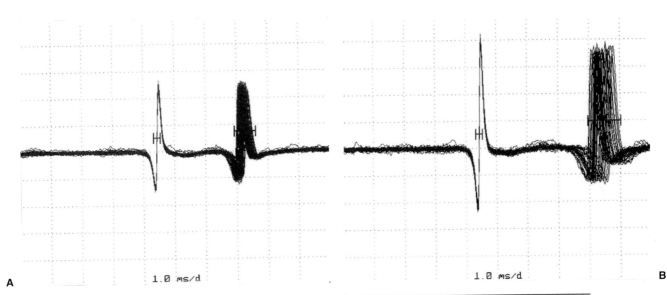

FIGURE 15.15. A: Single-fiber electromyography in a normal subject. In this tracing, 50 to 100 consecutive discharges generated by two single-muscle fibers, from the same motor unit, during voluntary activation of the frontalis muscle are superimposed. The tracings are arrayed so that the first (left) potential is superimposed in exactly the same place with each discharge. Consequently, the variability in the time between the firing of the first (left) and second (right) potential with each discharge (the interpotential interval) is illustrated solely in the varying position of the second waveform. This variability, quantitated as *jitter,* is due to the variability in the time required for neuromuscular transmission at the same neuromuscular junction from discharge to discharge. The jitter in this fiber pair was 51 microseconds, normal for the patient's age of 60 years. **B:** Single-fiber electromyography in a patient with myasthenia gravis. This recording of two single-muscle fiber discharges was also made during volitional activation of the frontalis muscle, using the same set up and recording methods described in Fig. 15.15-A. This tracing illustrates the increased variability in neuromuscular transmission time seen during neuromuscular junction dysfunction, and is clearly different from that of the normal subject above. The jitter in this fiber pair was 160 microseconds, well above the upper limits of the normal range.

considering SFEMG. SFEMG has many applications, but is most useful for confirming neuromuscular-junction dysfunction in suspected myasthenia gravis when other tests are equivocal or negative (Fig. 15.11).

TRANSCRANIAL MAGNETIC STIMULATION

Transcranial magnetic stimulation (TMS) evokes compound motor potentials through noninvasive stimulation of the cortex. Developed for clinical use 20 years ago, TMS has become an important method for studying the conductivity and excitability of the corticospinal system, abnormal cortical circuitry in neurologic diseases, and the reorganization of sensorimotor and visual systems after peripheral and central lesions. TMS is based on the principle that electromagnetic induction may stimulate neural tissue. TMS is accomplished through the generation of high intensity (5 kiloampere to 10 kiloampere) current stored in series capacitors and discharged as a quick pulse through wire coils placed on the surface of the head.

The coils induce a magnetic flux of short duration (100 microseconds to 200 microseconds) and high intensity (1 Tesla to 2 Tesla). The magnetic fields, in turn, induce electrical current in the underlying cerebral cortex. TMS delivery devices are embedded in a nonconductive plastic or rubber material and typically fashioned into figure eight, butterfly, or flat or concave circular shapes, and applied near the part of the brain under study. The various shapes and sizes are designed to distribute or focus the induced magnetic fields. Round coils generate more diffuse magnetic fields and figure-eight coils produce a narrower region of neural activation.

Stimulus intensity is expressed as a function of either the motor threshold or the percentage of machine output. TMS is much less painful than transcranial electrical stimulation (TES), which causes uncomfortable shocks in the underlying skin and muscle. Unlike transcranial electrical stimulation, which directly excites cortical long tracts, the induced electrical fields of TMS preferentially stimulate neural elements oriented parallel to the surface of the brain (i.e. primarily interneurons). TMS pulses are associated with benign acoustic clicks and mild scalp and facial muscle activation. A momentary sense of disorientation at maximal stimulation may be felt. However, there are virtually no clinical cognitive or sensory effects at low intensities of TMS stimulation. Waveform recordings are usually obtained from a contralateral distal limb muscle, the motor-evoked potential (MEP).

TMS may be delivered as a single pulse, in paired pulses, or as repetitive trains of stimulation (rTMS). Paired pulse and rTMS are powerful in studying human brain function, transiently stimulating or inhibiting different brain areas in awake and behaving subjects. Effects of rTMS on cortical excitability and inhibition outlast (for minutes to hours) the stimulation itself, a characteristic that could lead to therapeutic applications. Clinical trials have been conducted primarily in depression but also in Parkinson disease, epilepsy, obsessive-compulsive disorders and schizophrenia.

Single-pulse TMS

Following a single TMS, the MEP latency and amplitude measure the integrity of pathways and membrane excitability characteristics of the upper motor neuron. Central motor-conduction time is calculated by subtracting the peripheral MEP latency (i.e., cervical or lumbosacral proximal roots to distal limb muscles) from the total conduction latency (i.e., TMS to MEP onset of the same muscle) and is obtained with a single, maximal TMS over the primary motor cortex (Fig. 15.16).

Prolongation of the central motor-conduction time may originate with the loss of large myelinated motor axons subsequent to degeneration, and the test assesses upper motor neuron dysfunction. Central motor-conduction time is helpful in diagnosing and following progression in patients with upper motor neuron diseases, such as amyotrophic lateral sclerosis. However, central motor-conduction time may be of limited value when large diameter axons remain normal, or in diseases where long tract integrity is known to be normal, such as with Parkinson disease.

MEP amplitudes and latencies are influenced by multiple factors, including configuration and placement of the TMS coil, stimulus intensity, presence of conditioning pulses, muscle facilitation, and degree of phase cancellation. Suprasegmental modulation of MEPs may be inferred in several ways, including demonstration of relatively unchanged F-wave properties under the same stimulus conditions. Motor threshold is defined as the lowest stimulus intensity that evokes MEPs of 50 microvolts in amplitude in five of ten trials. Stimulus intensity is expressed as a percentage of the TMS device's maximum output. MEP amplitude is usually measured peak-to-peak, increases with stimulus intensity, and plateaus at 80% of the amplitude of the wave produced by peripheral stimulation.

Further assessment of the central motor circuitry may be obtained via peri-stimulus time histograms, using single-fiber EMG to record from a contralateral muscle after TMS. This method reveals multiple evoked responses that provide insight into upper motor-neuron pathophysiology. The first MEP or D-wave results from direct activation of the upper motor neuron and the subsequent I waves result from indirect excitation of upper motor neurons through cortical interneurons. Peri-stimulus time histograms may be used to evaluate upper motor-neuron dysfunction in amyotrophic lateral sclerosis, showing that the rising phase of the excitatory postsynaptic potential evoked in the anterior horn cell is abnormal in form and desynchronized.

Voluntary muscle activation during TMS lowers the motor threshold and increases the MEP amplitude. MEP facilitation by muscle activation is also associated with shorter latency. This facilitation may result from an increased number and synchronization of descending impulses from the motor cortex, or from reafferent facilitation at the spinal level. Recruitment is measured by plotting a stimulus-response curve of stimulus intensity versus MEP amplitude. The slope of this curve is normally increased by facilitation, as well as by maneuvers that enlarge cortical representation of muscles, such as highly skilled, fine-motor actions. Temporal summation may also follow repeated delivery of stimuli. In the first minutes following rTMS trains at low frequency (1 Hz), the amplitude of single-pulse MEP decreases. Conversely, high-frequency (greater than 10 Hz) stimulation increase the response; these patterns resemble long-term depression and facilitation.

Silent Period

The cortical or central silent period is measured from an actively contracting muscle, representing suppression of voluntary EMG activity for up to 300 milliseconds after a single TMS. The cortical silent period is an important method of assessing inhibitory mechanisms in neurologic disease. The silent period typically follows an MEP but may be induced by subthreshold stimuli that do not produce an MEP. This 'negative effect' is mechanistically distinct from the positive effect seen in MEP induction. Although the origin of the initial segments of the cortical silent period are controversial, the latter part of the silent period is modulated by central mechanisms.

Paired-pulse TMS

Paired pulses time-locked at precise interstimulus intervals (ISIs) may demonstrate changes in cortical excitability, specifically intracortical inhibition and facilitation. Changes in cortical modulation of inhibitory and excitatory processes provide a window on motor control as well

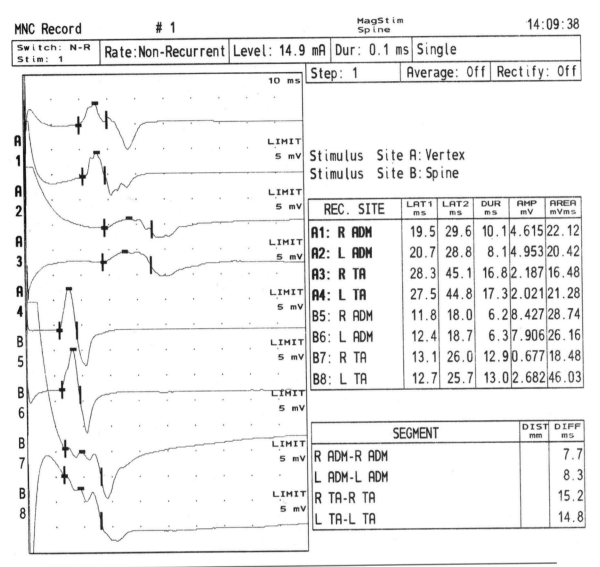

MNC Record   # 1   MagStim   14:09:38
                                                              Spine

Switch: N-R Stim: 1	Rate:Non-Recurrent	Level: 14.9 mA	Dur: 0.1 ms	Single

Step: 1	Average: Off	Rectify: Off

Stimulus   Site A: Vertex
Stimulus   Site B: Spine

REC. SITE	LAT1 ms	LAT2 ms	DUR ms	AMP mV	AREA mVms
A1: R ADM	19.5	29.6	10.1	4.615	22.12
A2: L ADM	20.7	28.8	8.1	4.953	20.42
A3: R TA	28.3	45.1	16.8	2.187	16.48
A4: L TA	27.5	44.8	17.3	2.021	21.28
B5: R ADM	11.8	18.0	6.2	8.427	28.74
B6: L ADM	12.4	18.7	6.3	7.906	26.16
B7: R TA	13.1	26.0	12.9	0.677	18.48
B8: L TA	12.7	25.7	13.0	2.682	46.03

SEGMENT	DIST mm	DIFF ms
R ADM-R ADM		7.7
L ADM-L ADM		8.3
R TA-R TA		15.2
L TA-L TA		14.8

FIGURE 15.16. **Transcranial magnetic stimulation (TMS) in a normal subject.** These tracings show the motor-evoked responses recorded from the right and left abductor digiti minimi (ADM) muscle of the hand and the right, and left tibialis anterior (TA) muscles, following stimulation of the cerebral cortex with the stimulator placed over the vertex of the skull (traces A1–A4), and following stimulation of the spine; cervical stimulation for the ADM and lumbosacral stimulation for the TA is shown in traces B5–B8. Latencies, in milliseconds, from stimulation to the onset of the waveform recorded from the muscle are shown in the first column (LAT 1). Central-conduction latency (i.e., time from cortex to spinal segment) is calculated by subtracting the peripheral-conduction latency (i.e., time from spine to muscle) from the total-conduction latency (i.e., time from cortex to muscle), and is shown in "SEGMENT" table, final column (DIFF).

as maturation in the nervous system. The first pulse, or conditioning stimulus, is generally just subthreshold compared to the second or test pulse in studies using short ISIs between 1 millisecond and 15 milliseconds. At ISIs up to 6 milliseconds, an inhibition of the test MEP amplitude is normally found, while facilitation of MEP amplitudes may occur at ISIs between 6 milliseconds and 15 milliseconds. Paired-pulse TMS at longer ISIs (100 milliseconds to 250 milliseconds), using suprathreshold stimuli for both conditioning and test pulses, has been used to investigate

longer term effects. Cortical inhibitory mechanisms underlying short- and long-interval ISIs appear to be distinct.

Repetitive TMS

The first TMS capacitors could recharge only after several seconds. With technical advances, rTMS output increased from just under 1 Hz to pulse trains up to 50 Hz. rTMS at frequencies greater than 20 Hz increases cerebral blood flow and neuronal excitability, while low-frequency rTMS (1 Hz to 2 Hz) has the opposite effect. The therapeutic potential of TMS has long been of interest because it could be a painless and safe alternative to electroshock therapy, which has lasting motor benefit in severe parkinsonism. Enhanced cortical excitability is suggested by increased MEP amplitude after rTMS and by persistent focal metabolic enhancement as demonstrated by PET. However, rTMS may have negative effects on the motor system, so the underlying mechanisms must be more fully understood before widespread use may be expected.

SUGGESTED READINGS

Nerve Conduction Studies and Electromyography

American Association of Electromyography and Electrodiagnosis Nomenclature Committee. Glossary of terms in clinical electromyography. *Muscle Nerve* 1987;10(8 Suppl):G1–G60.

Buchthal F. Electromyography in the evaluation of muscle diseases. *Neurological Clinics* 1985;3:573–598.

Cornblath DR, Sumner AJ, Daube J, et al. Conduction block in clinical practice. *Muscle Nerve* 1991;14:869–871.

Daube JR. Needle examination in clinical electromyography. *Muscle Nerve* 1991;14(8):685–700.

Dumitru D, Amato A, Zwarts M. Electrodiagnostic Medicine, 2nd Edition, 2002, New York.

Falck B, Stalberg E. Motor nerve conduction studies: measurement principles and interpretation of findings. *J Clin Neurophysiol* 1995;12:254–279.

Gutmann L. Pearls and pitfalls in the use of electromyography and nerve conduction studies. *Semin Neurol* 2003;23:77–82.

Kimura J, ed. Electrodiagnosis in Diseases of Nerve and Muscle, Principles and Practice, 3rd Edition, 2001, Oxford University Press.

Kimura J. Principles and pitfalls of nerve conduction studies. *Electroencephalogr Clin Neurophysiol Suppl* 1999;50:12–15.

Oh J, ed. Clinical Electromyography, Nerve Conduction Studies, 3rd Edition, 2003, Lippincott Williams & Wilkins, Philadelphia.

Wilbourn AJ, Aminoff M. AAEE minimonograph #32: the electrophysiologic examination in patients with radiculopathies. *Muscle Nerve* 1988;11(11):1099–1114.

Tests of Neuromuscular Transmission

Drachman DB. Myasthenia gravis. *N Engl J Med* 1994;330:1797–1810.

Howard JF, Sanders DB, Massey JM. The electrodiagnosis of myasthenia gravis and the Lambert-Eaton myasthenic syndrome. *Neurologic Clin N Amer* 1994;12:305–329.

Maselli RA. Pathophysiology of myasthenia gravis and Lambert-Eaton syndrome. *Neurologic Clin N Amer* 1994;12:387–399.

Oh SJ. Electromyography: Neuromuscular Transmission Studies. Baltimore MD, Williams & Wilkins, 1988.

Sanders DB. Clinical neurophysiology of disorders of the neuromuscular junction. *J Clin Neurophysiology* 1993;12:169–XX.

Sanders DB, Stalberg EV. Single fiber electromyography. *Muscle Nerve* 1996;19:1069–1083.

Tim RW, Sanders DB. Repetitive nerve stimulation studies in the Lambert-Eaton myasthenic syndrome. *Muscle Nerve* 1994;17:995–1001.

Vincent A, Lang B, Newsom-Davis J. Autoimmunity to the voltage-gated calcium channel underlies the Lambert-Eaton myasthenic syndrome, a paraneoplastic disorder. *Trends in Neuroscience* 1989;12:496–502.

Wilbourn AJ. Sensory nerve conduction studies. *J Clin Neurophysiol* 1994;11:584–601.

Transcortical Magnetic Stimulation

Amassian VE, Cracco RQ, Maccabee PJ. Focal stimulation of human cerebral cortex with the magnetic coil: a comparison with electrical stimulation. *Electroencephalogr Clin Neurophysiol* 1989;74:401–416.

Barker AT, Jalinous R, Freeston IL. Non-invasive magnetic stimulation of human cortex. *Lancet* 1985;1:1106–1107.

Eisen AA, Shtybel W. Clinical experience with transcranial magnetic stimulation. *Muscle Nerve* 1990;13:995–1011.

Fitzgerald PB, Brown TL, Daskalakis ZJ. The application of transcranial magnetic stimulation in psychiatry and neurosciences research. *Acta Psychiatr Scand* 2002;105:324–340.

Hallett M. Transcranial magnetic stimulation: a tool for mapping the central nervous system. *Electroencephalogr Clin Neurophysiol Suppl* 1996;46:43–51.

Kobayashi M, Pascual-Leone A. Transcranial magnetic stimulation in neurology. *Lancet Neurol* 2003;2:145–156.

Pascual-Leone A, Valls-Sole J, Wassermann EM, Hallett M. Responses to rapid-rate transcranial magnetic stimulation of the human motor cortex. *Brain* 1994;117:847–858.

Rothwell JC, Hallett M, Berardelli A, et al. Magnetic stimulation: motor evoked potentials. The International Federation of Clinical Neurophysiology. *Electroencephalogr Clin Neurophysiol Suppl* 1999;52:97–103.

Uncini A, Treviso M, Di Muzio A, Simone P, Pullman S. Physiological basis of voluntary activity inhibition induced by transcranial cortical stimulation. *Electroencephalogr Clin Neurophysiol* 1993;89:211–220.

Wassermann EM, Lisanby SH. Therapeutic application of repetitive transcranial magnetic stimulation: a review. *Clin Neurophysiol* 2001;112:1367–1377.

Chapter 16

▶ Neurovascular Imaging

J. P. Mohr and Robert DeLaPaz

Brain imaging plays a dominant role in the diagnosis, classification, and prognosis of stroke for those institutions with modern imaging equipment. *Plain skull x-ray films are rarely helpful in diagnosis and have receded into the background.* Noninvasive studies from Doppler insonation through CT and MRI continue to expand the scope of their clinical indications.

COMPUTED TOMOGRAPHY

CT is a computerized display of a larger range of attenuation of the x-ray energy passing through the nervous system from emitter to detector than may be resolved by the naked-eye inspection of a conventional head or spine x-ray. The resulting CT scan may be tuned to display those structures or disease conditions that excessively, or only slightly,

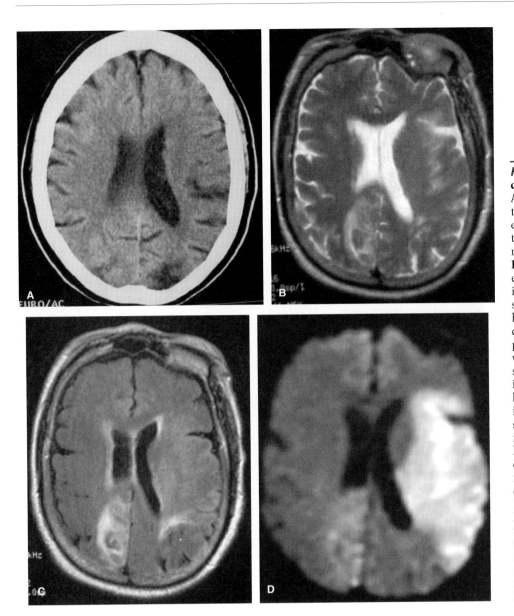

FIGURE 16.1. Hyperacute cerebral infarct (3 hours). A: Axial noncontrast computed tomography appears normal except for the low density in the left medial parietal cortex representing a chronic infarct. **B:** Axial T2-weighted fast spin echo magnetic resonance (MR) image shows slight elevation of signal in the left insular cortex, high curvilinear signal at the deep margin of the chronic left parietal infarct, and high signal with central low signal in a subacute hemorrhagic infarct in the medial right parietal lobe. **C:** Axial fluid, attenuated-inversion recovery MR image shows slightly increased signal in the left periventricular region, high signal at the margin of the chronic infarct, and mixed signal in the subacute infarct. **D:** Axial diffusion-weighted image (b = 1,000) shows a large region of high signal, representing low water-proton diffusion rates, in the large middle cerebral artery infarct, which was produced by carotid dissection 3 hours before the study. (Courtesy of Dr. R. L. DeLaPaz.)

absorb (attenuate) the x-ray signal. Leading among these is the characteristic high-density (high-attenuation) appearance (bright) on CT seen with an *acute hemorrhage mass* (*hematoma*). In the minutes, hours, and days up to the first week. This distinctive change allows clinicians to detect stroke caused by hematoma, separating it from the low-attenuation lesion (dark) typical of bland infarction (Figs. 16.1 and 16.2).

The presence as well as the volume of an acute parenchymatous hematoma may be estimated accurately, allowing serial studies to determine if there is further enlargement in the initial hours or days after a stroke. In the case of *hemorrhagic infarction* (not hematoma), the high density of the scattered-blood signals may mimic hematoma or may be reduced by the low-attenuation effect of the associated infarction; sometimes this actually creates an isodense effect that is indistinguishable from normal brain.

As the breakdown of hemoglobin causes the high signal of fresh blood to diminish over days or weeks (hemoglobin breakdown), the CT appearance evolves from initial hyperdensity, through an isodense (subacute) phase, to hypodensity in the chronic state (Fig. 16.1). In the subacute phase, contrast administration may result in ring enhancement around the hemorrhage (Fig. 16.3), a pattern different from the gyral enhancement typical of infarction (Fig. 16.1). This ring or rim enhancement may appear similar to that of a *tumor* or *abscess*, a pitfall that is especially misleading with isodense or hypodense images of late hematomas.

In the chronic state, the mass of the hematoma subsides, allowing the adjacent brain to be restored toward

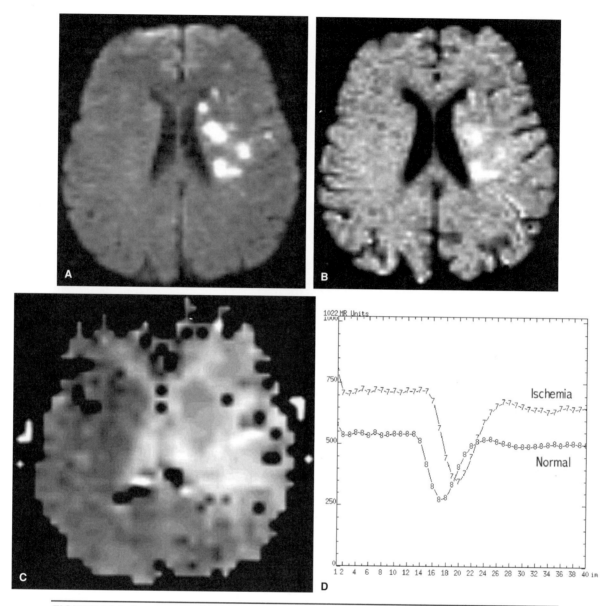

FIGURE 16.2. Acute cerebral infarct (24 hours). A: Axial diffusion-weighted image (DWI, b = 1,000) shows a patchy region of high signal, representing low water-proton diffusion rates, in an acute, deep, left-basal ganglia and corona radiata infarct. **B:** The exponential apparent-diffusion coefficient (ADC) map represents the ratio of signal on the DWI to the T2-weighted (b = 0) image. This map corrects for high signal on the DWI produced by high signal on the T2-weighted image, the T2 "shine through" effect. This acute infarct produces high signal on both the DWI and exponential ADC maps, confirming reduced tissue-water diffusion. **C:** This map of relative perfusion delay, time to peak, was produced by rapid scanning with T2*-weighted images during an intravenous gadolinium contrast bolus injection. The high signal area in the region of the left-sided infarct represents a large zone of relatively delayed arrival of the peak signal change produced by the gadolinium bolus as it passes through the tissue capillary bed. **D:** The time-intensity curves show the transient drop in signal on T2*-weighted images as the gadolinium bolus passes through and indicate a substantial delay in the left-sided ischemic zone (9-sec peak arrival delay; X axis is image number with TR = 3 secs and Y axis is signal intensity). **E:** Axial fluid attenuated-inversion recovery magnetic resonance (MR) image shows patchy increased signal in the infarct. The square outline represents the voxel used for proton MR spectroscopy. **F:** Proton MR spectrum (TR 2,000, TE 144) shows a slight elevation of choline (Cho), a slight decrease in *N*-acetylaspartate (NAA), and a marked elevation of lactate (peak inversion is due to J-coupling of lactate doublet). Peak areas represent relative concentrations of tissue metabolites. (Courtesy of Dr. R. L. DeLaPaz.)

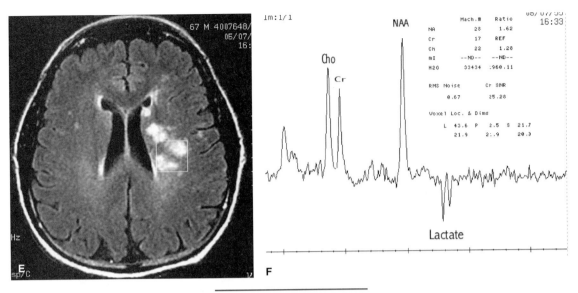

Im:1/1

FIGURE 16.2. *(Continued)*

its original shape and size, often reducing the hematoma to a slit-like cavity. Many smaller hematomas disappear without creating a cavity, leaving tissue isodense (with the same attenuation characteristics) as normal brain.

In *subarachnoid hemorrhage*, the usual diffuse spread of blood mixes with subarachnoid CSF and, unless it is associated with a large mass of hemorrhage, may have a more transient high-density appearance and may not even be visible; lumbar puncture may help make the diagnosis of subarachnoid bleeding in those patients with normal CTs.

With *nonhemorrhagic infarction*, CT may appear normal for several days after the infarction, especially if the edema component of the infarct is slight. Ischemic infarcts with little collateral flow or edema may remain isodense or may not enhance for days or weeks, later appearing only as focal atrophy. When there is collateral supply that allows reflow into the ischemic region, the attendant edema produces an appearance of hypodensity, usually allowing CT to be positive within 24 hours. Although CT may overestimate the size of deep lesions, it better approximates the volume of discrete surface infarcts, especially after several months when the acute effects of edema and necrotic tissue reabsorption have subsided (Fig. 16.4).

Within the brain, CT may differentiate abnormal from normal soft tissues, particularly after intravenous administration of iodinated contrast agents; abnormal enhancement implies a breakdown of the blood–brain barrier. The use of contrast agents may allow an enhanced signal, reflecting infarction to be seen within 1 week; the findings may persist for 2 weeks to 2 months. With contract agents, an enhancement pattern outlining the gyral surface of the brain (gyral enhancement) is often seen, but rarely encountered in hematoma.

Standard CT techniques still do not distinguish partial ischemia from actual infarction. In the early stages, relying on CT alone (with or without contrast) clinicians may be frustrated by the difficulty of determining how much tissue is viable and how much damage is permanent.

Types of CT

Spiral CT obtains serial scans during the first pass of an intravenous contrast bolus. The images may give relative measures of ischemia (i.e., diminished regional blood flow) from the derived blood-volume and perfusion-delay maps.

Stable xenon-enhanced CT may also be useful, also scanning the entire neck or head with a bolus intravenous infusion of contrast agent to create images of the vascular system, a process known as a CT angiogram (CTA). Using a special imaging display technique such as "maximum intensity projection reformation," often with three-dimensional (3D) surface shading, the vascular features displayed may allow detection and characterization of arterial stenosis or aneurysm. The advantages of CT angiography over conventional catheter angiography include its more widely available technology, fewer specialized skill requirements for the operator, and relatively noninvasive intravenous administration of contrast material. However, use of the CT angiogram has been slow to grow because of competition from magnetic resonance angiography (MRA) (see below). Further, in contrast to MRA, the iodinated contrast agent used in the CT angiogram is potentially more toxic, owing to its propensity for allergic reactions, direct cardiac volume stress, or renal toxicity. CT angiography also involves time-consuming post processing, which is

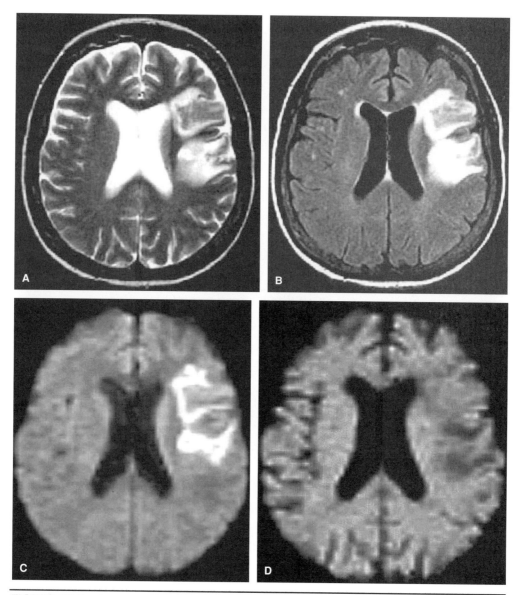

FIGURE 16.3. **Chronic cerebral infarct with T2 "shine through."** **A:** Axial T2-weighted fast-spin echo (FSE) MRI shows high signal in a chronic, left-middle cerebral artery (MCA) territory infarct. **B:** Axial fluid attenuated-inversion recovery (FLAIR) MR image also shows high signal in the chronic, left MCA territory infarct. **C:** Axial diffusion-weighted image (DWI, b = 1,000) shows a region of high signal corresponding to the MCA infarct and the high signal seen on the FSE and FLAIR images. **D:** The exponential apparent-diffusion coefficient (ADC) map represents the ratio of signal on the DWI to the T2-weighted (b = 0) image. This map corrects for high signal on the DWI produced by high signal on the T2-weighted image, the T2 "shine through" effect. The exponential ADC map shows low signal in the lesion, indicating high water-diffusion rates, as would be expected in a chronic infarct. Acute infarcts produce high signal on both the DWI and exponential ADC maps, indicating reduced tissue-water diffusion (Fig. 16.2). (Courtesy of Dr. R. L. DeLaPaz.)

required to edit out bone and calcium and to generate three-dimensional surface rendering. For institutions lacking MR, however, these techniques at least allow an expansion of the use of CT technology.

MRI is more sensitive than CT in demonstrating parenchymal abnormalities and may also be augmented by a contrast agent, gadolinium.

MAGNETIC RESONANCE IMAGING

In many institutions, MRI has taken over the imaging of both hemorrhagic and ischemic stroke. The physics of MRI are discussed in Chapter 13. Selection of the pulse sequence and plane of imaging is necessary to achieve the maximum utility of the technique. In order to diagnose and

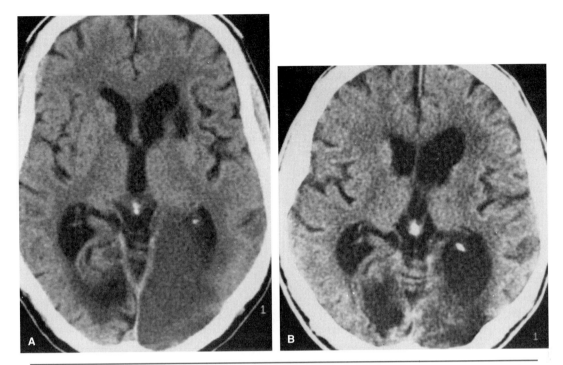

FIGURE 16.4. Cerebral infarction, acute and chronic phases. A: Axial noncontrast computed tomography reveals focal regions of discrete lucency in left basal ganglia and right occipital regions without mass effect, suggesting nonacute infarcts. A "fainter," less well-defined, left occipital lucency is also noted, with effacement of cortical sulci and the atrium of the ventricle, suggesting more recent infarction. **B:** Follow-up noncontrast scan 2 mos later demonstrates interval demarcation of the left occipital infarct with evidence of focal atrophy, and a "negative mass effect" on the atrium, which appears larger. Similar change is noted in left frontal horn. (Courtesy of Drs. J. A. Bello and S. K. Hilal.)

date hemorrhage, T1- and T2-weighted images are necessary (Fig. 13.1 in Chapter 13 and Fig. 16.5).

Compared with the simpler imaging issues for CT, the acute appearance of *parenchymal hemorrhage* on MRI is much more complicated, and varies as the hemorrhage evolves. Hyperacute hemorrhage, within the first 12 hours to 24 hours, often appears isointense (the same as normal brain) to slightly hypointense, not only on the commonly available T1-weighted technique but also on T2-weighted images, and in many instances on the more complex displays known as FLAIR (fluid-attenuated inversion recovery) or GE (gradient echo, also known as T2*). This pattern arises because the acute hematoma, actually a clot, is first composed of intact red blood cells with fully oxygenated hemoglobin, giving it the same MR signal characteristics as brain tissue. As deoxygenation occurs, the deoxyhemoglobin generated is paramagnetic and produces low signal on T2-weighted images (shortens T2 relaxation) but has little effect on T1-weighted images. Over days to a week, the hemoglobin within the red cells evolves further into methemoglobin, which has a stronger paramagnetic effect and produces high signal on T1-weighted images (shortens T1 relaxation), with persistent low signal on T2-weighted images.

As the red cells break down over days within the subacute hematoma, the distribution of methemoglobin becomes more uniform and the dominance of the shortened T1-relaxation time produces high signal on both T1-weighted and T2-weighted images. This appearance remains stable for weeks to months until the hemorrhagic debris is cleared by phagocytes, leaving only hemosiderin at the site of the hemorrhage. Similarly to the all-but-normal CT appearance of a late hematoma, MR imaging of the chronic hemorrhagic site is isointense on T1-weighted images and hypointense to isointense on T2-weighted images. However, GE images are especially sensitive to hemosiderin deposits and are now used to seek signs of chronic hemorrhage as low signal, even when both T1-weighted and T2-weighted images are isointense. As a consequence, GE images are particularly useful as a screen for occult, prior hemorrhage associated with suspected prior hematoma. This is including those from such varied causes as trauma, hypertensive hemorrhage, hemorrhage from anticoagulation or vascular malformations, and even the small arterial wall hemorrhages increasingly demonstrated by better MR techniques in a setting of amyloid angiopathy.

The appearance of *subarachnoid* and *other extra-axial hemorrhage* follows similar stages of signal change but may

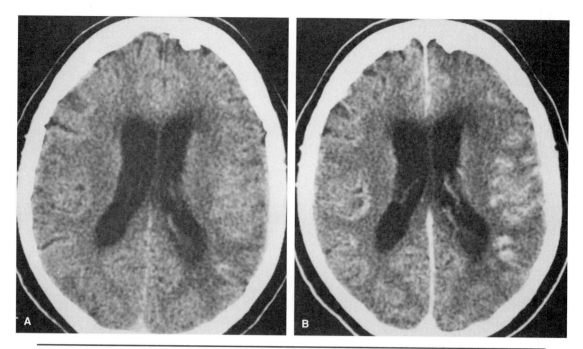

FIGURE 16.5. Hemorrhagic infarction. A: Axial precontrast computed tomography shows focal left-parietal gyral density consistent with hemorrhagic infarction. Note edema and sulcal effacement in left frontoparietal cortical region. **B:** Postcontrast enhancement in area of recent hemorrhagic infarction. (Courtesy of Drs. J. A. Bello and S. K. Hilal.)

evolve more rapidly or slowly, depending on location and the degree of cerebrospinal fluid-dilution effects. Although extensive experience has been accumulated with the CT scan diagnosis of acute subarachnoid hemorrhage, recent experience with FLAIR indicates a high sensitivity to subarachnoid hemorrhage. FLAIR may identify subarachnoid hemorrhage as an abnormal high signal in sulci that appear normal on CT. However, this high signal is less specific than high density on CT and may also represent cells or elevated protein content in CSF caused by infection or meningeal neoplasm. GE images are not sensitive for, or specific for, acute subarachnoid hemorrhage but may show signs of repeated prior subarachnoid hemorrhage as a low signal along the pial surface; this is caused by deposition of hemosiderin ("hemosiderosis"), a finding worth seeking in the lower subarachnoid spaces in the posterior fossa.

For the diagnosis of *acute brain ischemia and infarction*, MRI is unquestionably more sensitive and specific than CT. The multiplanar capability, lack of artifact from bone, and the greater sensitivity to tissue changes mean MRI has particular advantages over CT for imaging infarcts in the brainstem (Fig. 16.6).

Diffusion-weighted imaging (DWI), described in more detail in Chapter 13, has revolutionized acute infarct detection. Severe cerebral ischemia and infarction cause a rapid decrease in intracellular diffusion that consistently produces high signal on DWI, even within minutes of cell injury. T2-weighted and FLAIR images show high signal

in acute infarction only after a delay of 6 to 12 hours. DWI is also more specific for acute infarction. High-signal lesions on FLAIR or T2-weighted images may represent acute, subacute, or chronic infarction, whereas the DWI shows high signal only in acute lesions. After the initial reduction in diffusion, there is a gradual rise through normal to prolonged diffusion rates during the 1-week to 2-week period after infarction, as cells disintegrate and freely diffusible water dominates the infarcted tissue.

A minor pitfall of DWI in subacute infarcts is the phenomenon called "T2 shine through," where high signal on T2-weighted images may produce high signal on DWI, falsely indicating reduced diffusion. This pitfall may be avoided by the use of calculated apparent-diffusion coefficient maps. DWI has become an essential part of acute stroke imaging and because this method takes less than a minute to acquire a whole brain study, it is being used to screen a variety of clinical presentations for possible ischemic injury.

MRI methods for assessing *cerebral perfusion*, described in more detail in Chapter 13, have also transformed the evaluation of acute cerebral ischemia. Tissue blood flow is most commonly imaged with MRI using a "first pass" or "bolus tracking" method that records the signal changes occurring when rapidly repeated images are acquired during the first passage through the brain of an intravascular bolus of paramagnetic contrast material. The agent used is usually gadolinium-diethylene-triamine pentaacetic acid. This rapid imaging may be done during routine contrast

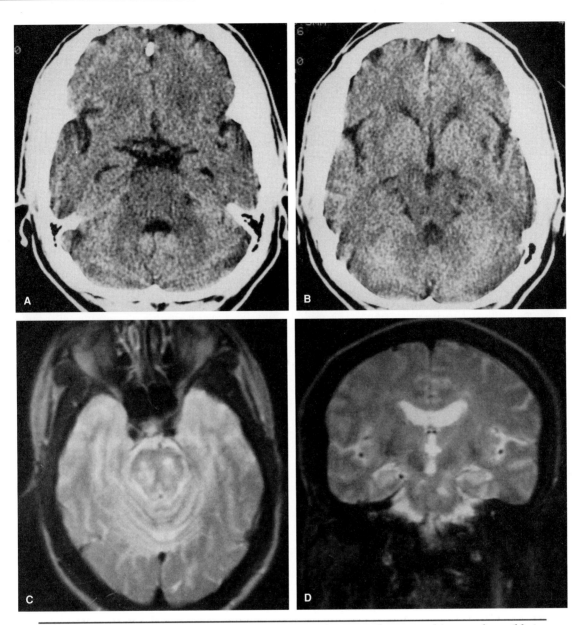

FIGURE 16.6. Brainstem infarction. Noncontrast axial computed tomographies reveal possible infarcts in left brachium pontis (**A**) and right midbrain (**B**). Axial (**C**) and coronal (**D**) T2-weighted magnetic resonance scans of the same patient clearly show these and additional small infarcts not seen on CT. (Courtesy of Drs. J. A. Bello and S. K. Hilal.)

administration, adding minimal time to the routine examination. It provides maps of relative cerebral blood volume (CBV), cerebral blood flow (CBF), bolus mean transit time or time to peak (MTTP), and any or all usable for estimations of impaired regional blood flow. Measures of perfusion delay such as mean transit time and time to peak are proving to be sensitive indicators of subtle reductions in cerebral perfusion. A second method of MR perfusion imaging is called "spin tagging" or "time of flight" imaging and, like time-of-flight MRA, depends on T1 relaxation and flow enhancement phenomena without the use of injected contrast agents. This method is less widely used than

bolus tracking but is capable of giving more quantitative cerebral blood flow measurements but with more limited coverage of the brain. These methods may be used to identify relatively underperfused brain regions distal to arterial stenoses or occlusions. They may also give an indication of the potentially salvageable "penumbra" of ischemic but not-yet-infarcted brain, adjacent to an infarction, as indicated by high signal on DWI.

Magnetic resonance spectroscopy (MRS—also described in Chapter 13), using either proton (^{1}H) or phosphorus (^{31}P), has limited application in the evaluation of acute ischemia. Although changes characteristic of injured or dead tissue may be seen, such as reduced *N*-acetylaspartate and elevated lactate, on proton MRS and reduced energy metabolites on phosphorus MRS, the long duration (3 minutes to 20 minutes) and low resolution (2 cm to 8 cm voxel size) of these methods limit practical application in the acute stroke patient. Proton MRS may be helpful with enhancing subacute infarction in deep, white matter where routine imaging may suggest primary brain tumor. Although both infarct and tumor may show reduced *N*-acetylaspartate and elevated lactate, a markedly elevated choline peak is strong evidence for tumor and against infarction. Adding DWI may also be helpful because diffusion rates are usually normal-to-prolonged in tumor (iso- to low-signal on DWI) in contrast to low-diffusion rates in acute to subacute infarction (high signal on DWI).

Efforts are being made to quantitate changes in perfusion that may be important in predicting the risk of infarction in zones inferred to have ischemia. The normal diffusion of water through tissue is thought to be disrupted (reduced) in ischemia, and may be calculated using perfusion-weight imaging as an apparent diffusion coefficient (ADC). It is presumed that the value observed represents a net shift of extracellular water into the intracellular compartment (cytotoxic edema), resulting in a reduction of free-water diffusion. The significance of the ADC remains a subject of intense research but if confirmed, could greatly improve the identification of tissue at risk for infarction, showing whether interventions assist or fail to modify the course of salvageable brain tissue.

MAGNETIC RESONANCE ANGIOGRAPHY

MRA, also described in Chapter 13, is widely used for screening the extracranial and intracranial vasculature. Used in conjunction with Doppler ultrasound, the combination in many centers is now the preferred noninvasive means of evaluating carotid bifurcation stenosis. Depending on the institution and interventionalists or surgeons, this combination may be the only preoperative imaging studies done. Although MRA and Doppler ultrasound generally depict a similar degree of stenosis, some artifacts on MRA may be misleading. High flow rates may produce signal loss within the lumen, usually exaggerating the degree of stenosis. In addition, turbulent flow may mimic complex plaque anatomy or ulceration. When the MRA and Doppler disagree substantially, catheter angiography may be required for definitive diagnosis.

MRA is also used for screening the intracranial circulation. Large vessels of the circle of Willis may be imaged effectively and rapidly, but current resolution precludes detailed observation of vessels more distal than the second-order branches of the middle cerebral artery. Despite these advantages, conventional angiography remains the gold standard for evaluation of subtle segmental stenoses produced by arteritis, especially in small distal branches. Although MRA images are not as sharp as those of conventional angiography, all vessels are visualized simultaneously and may be viewed from any angle; most important, MRA is completely safe, noninvasive, and may be added to the routine MRI examination. The use of MRA as a screening technique for intracranial aneurysms is also increasing. MRA may detect aneurysms as small as 3 mm under optimal conditions, but the current practical lower limit in clinical usage is probably 5 mm in diameter. Given the results of studies indicating the low risk of hemorrhage for aneurysms smaller than 5 mm to 7 mm, MRA may soon eclipse conventional angiography for all screening. A pitfall with time-of-flight MRA is the high signal produced by subacute parenchymal or subarachnoid hemorrhage that may mimic an aneurysm or AVM. Phase-contrast MRA may be a better choice in patients with known hemorrhage. Other indications for screening MRA include stroke, TIA, and possible venous sinus thrombosis.

CATHETER ANGIOGRAPHY

Analysis of cerebrovascular disease has become increasingly precise with newer, noninvasive technologies. At one time the only method, and then the mainstay of vascular imaging, conventional catheter angiography is now sharing preference with the newer technique cited above. In many centers today, conventional angiography is used only to study intracranial vascular disease that is not visualized by MRI, MRA, or Doppler techniques.

Catheter angiography involves the intra-arterial injection of water-soluble, iodinated contrast agents; transient opacification of the arterial lumen is filmed by conventional radiographic or digital-subtraction techniques. Angiography is unsurpassed in the detailed anatomic depiction of stenosis, occlusion, recanalization, ulceration, or dissection of large and small intra- and extracranial arteries (Fig. 16.7). It is expensive, requires specialized catheter skills, and carries a 0.5% to 3% risk of embolic stroke.

Despite the concerns cited, it still offers advantages in the diagnosis of ischemic stroke in the hyperacute phase. For a diagnosis of embolism, angiography should be carried out within hours of the ictus because the embolic particle may fragment early, changing the appearance of the affected vessel from occlusion, to stenosis or a normal lumen, depending on the delay time. When atheromatous stenosis of large arteries is suspected, preangiographic Doppler ultrasound (see the following) may help to tailor the angiographic study and enable the angiographer to concentrate on the major territories thought to be affected. Catheter angiography is the primary method

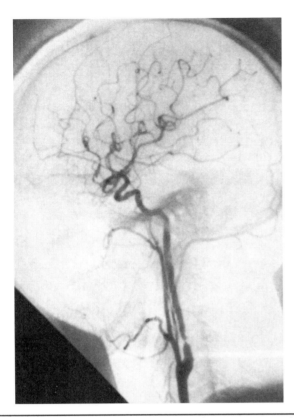

FIGURE 16.7. Proximal internal carotid stenosis. Lateral arteriogram of the common carotid shows an ulcerated plaque of the proximal internal carotid with hemodynamically significant stenosis. Anterior circulation failed to fill, and was cross-filled from the contralateral side. (Courtesy of Drs. J. A. Bello and S. K. Hilal.)

for preoperative evaluation of intracranial aneurysms and arteriovenous malformations, especially if interventional catheter therapies are being considered.

Catheter angiography techniques have become more sophisticated and now include interventional methods for the treatment of neurovascular disease. Thrombolytic agents may be delivered directly to intravascular clots, including higher order, intracranial vessel branches using *superselective microcatheter techniques* and to major dural sinuses using retrograde venous approaches, as described in Chapter 17. Arterial stenosis may be treated with angioplasty, which involves catheter placement of an intravascular balloon at the stenotic site and then balloon inflation to expand the vessel. *Angioplasty* is used mostly for atherosclerotic disease in the extracranial vessels, sometimes followed by placement of a wire-mesh stent to help keep the lumen patent. Increasingly, angioplasty is also used to expand the *symptomatic vasospasm-induced stenoses* with subarachnoid hemorrhage and for some instances of arterial dissections. Its use in *intracranial atheromatous* and *moyamoya* stenoses remains incompletely assessed.

Occlusion of abnormal vessels and aneurysms may also be performed using intravascular techniques. Arteriovenous malformations and fistulas may be treated by occlusion of the feeding arteries with coils (flexible metal, spiral coils that induce local thrombosis), and the AVM nidus may be occluded with bucrylate, a rapidly setting polymer glue. Trial results encourage the treatment of *intracranial aneurysms* by catheter placement of coils (less often by balloons) instead of traditional craniotomy-associated surgical clipping. Emergency arterial occlusions are also performed for uncontrollable *epistaxis* and *postoperative hemorrhage in the neck, paranasal sinus,* and *skull base regions.*

DOPPLER MEASUREMENTS

Although no longer used in most modern institutions, the simplest Doppler devices pass a high-frequency, continuous-wave, sound signal over the tissues in the neck, receive the reflected signal, and process them through a small speaker. Technicians using such *continuous-wave Doppler* devices listen with the human ear for the pitch of the sound. A rough judgment may be made of the degree of the Doppler shift to infer whether the blood is moving through an artery or vein beneath the probe, and whether the velocity is normal, decreased, or increased and if increased, whether blood flow is smooth or turbulent. Little experience is required to separate the high-frequency arterial signal from the low-frequency venous sound or to recognize the extremely high frequencies of severe stenosis. However, more effort is required to quantitate the signal, using techniques described below. More important, because the Doppler shift equation depends on the cosine of the beam versus the flowing blood within the artery, unintended or undetected errors in probe angulation may have major effects on signal production.

Extracranial Duplex Doppler Studies

To assist in proper probe angulation, *duplex Doppler* devices have two crystals, one atop the other (hence the term, duplex), in a single-probe head; one crystal handles the Doppler shift for spectral analysis and the other, the B-mode image of the vessel walls. Improvement in crystal designs continue to reduce the need for larger probe sizes, but even the most modern of them make it difficult to insonate the carotid artery above the mandible. The Doppler shift crystal has an adjustable-range gate to permit analysis of flow signals from specific depths in the tissues, eliminating conflicting signals where arteries and veins overlie one another. Some even have two range gates, providing an adjustable "volume" or "window" to insonate the moving blood column in an artery with volumes as small as 0.6 mm, the size of the tightest stenosis. The capacity to

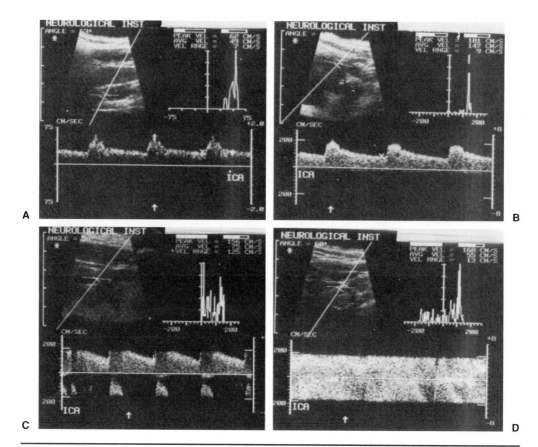

FIGURE 16.8. Four studies, each showing different degrees of stenosis of the extracranial internal carotid. The studies, obtained with the Diasonics DRF 400 instrument, image the carotid by B-mode ultrasound (upper left-hand corner of each of the four pictures) by passing the ultrasound beam through the tissues (*angled line*) and sampling the flow velocity at a point within the lumen of the vessel (*horizontal bracketed line*). From this sample, the device displays the waveforms representing the velocity profile, calculated from the Doppler shift (waveforms shown with velocity in cm/sec in each picture). The mean velocities are then calculated from a sample taken near the peak of each waveform (small *arrow* under each waveform line). The spectrum of velocities (i.e., degree of turbulence) is displayed as "peak vel" (i.e., velocity), "mean vel," and "vel range" (shown in graphic form in the upper right-hand corner of each picture). Examples of varying degrees of stenosis are shown: normal flow, left upper corner; moderate (60% to 80%) stenosis with moderate turbulence, right upper corner; severe (80% to 90%) stenosis with marked turbulence, left lower corner; extremely severe (90% to 99%) stenosis with extreme turbulence, right lower corner.

interrogate the flow pattern from wall to wall across the lumen has made this technique useful for detecting, measuring, and monitoring degrees of stenosis (Fig. 16.8).

Because duplex Doppler is sensitive to cross-sectional area and not to wall anatomy, it may actually exceed conventional angiography in estimating the degree of stenosis, compared with conventional two-dimensional (2D) angiography. B-mode vessel imaging is improving its ability to document most minor ulcerations, and controversies remain whether minor (even major) ulceration itself is an independent risk factor for stroke, requiring health risks like conventional angiography for its documentation.

As a separate issue, duplex Doppler methods may also be used to insonate the extracranial vertebral arteries as they pass through the intervertebral foramina. The limitations on diagnosis due to the small segments that may be

viewed should be obvious but occlusion above the site of the probe may be inferred by a high-resistance signal.

Intracranial Doppler Studies

Using a probe with great tissue-penetration properties, it is possible to insonate the major vessels of the circle of Willis, the distal intracranial segments of the vertebral arteries, and much of the length of the basilar artery. Current transcranial Doppler devices are range gated, and the latest models even give a color-coded and B-mode display of the major intracranial arteries (Fig. 16.9). The signals accurately document the direction and velocity of the arterial flow insonated by the narrow probe beam. Spectrum analysis of the signal allows estimation of the degree of stenosis, as does extracranial duplex Doppler.

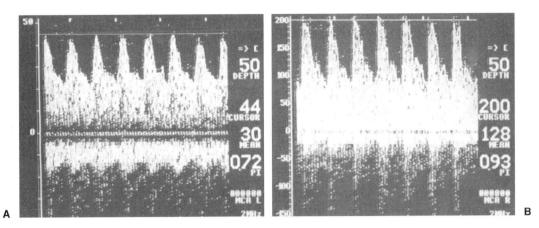

FIGURE 16.9. Two examples of transcranial Doppler insonations of the middle cerebral artery, obtained at a depth of 50 mm from the side of the head overlying the temporal bone, using the Carolina Medical Electronics TC-64B device. The velocity profile of the Doppler shift is insonated at this depth from the blood in the middle-cerebral artery flowing toward the probe (upper *arrow* directed to the right in each picture). The left picture shows a normal peak (cursor 44 [cm/sec], **left**) and mean (30) and pulsatility index (0.72 PI, i.e., the difference between the peak systolic velocity and the end diastolic velocity divided by the mean velocity). **Right:** The peak (200 cursor) and mean (128 mean) velocities and the pulsatility index (0.93) are higher, consistent with local stenosis at this point in the course of the middle cerebral artery.

Care must be taken to determine which artery is being insonated; the middle cerebral and posterior cerebral are often mis-insonated. The technique is user sensitive, requiring patience to detect the signal and then to find the best angle for insonation at a given depth. Minor anatomic variations may cause misleading changes in signal strength. Because the procedure is safe, fast, and uses a probe and microprocessor of tabletop size, the device may be taken to the bedside even in an intensive care unit, and may be used to diagnose developing vasospasm, collateral flow above occlusions, recanalization of an embolized artery, and the presence of important basilar or cerebral artery stenosis. When combined with MRI, it is possible to make a noninvasive diagnosis of stenosis of the basilar artery or of the stem of the middle cerebral artery.

Hemodynamically important extracranial stenosis may damp the waveform in the ipsilateral arteries above, allowing the effect of the extracranial disease to be measured and followed serially. A challenge test of contralateral compression may be done to determine whether the effects of unilateral extracranial stenosis are compensated or lack anatomic collaterals. Inhalation of 5% CO_2 with oxygen (O_2) has been introduced to determine if vasoreactivity of the cerebral-convexity arterial tree responds to the vasodilatory challenge of the CO_2. A healthy vasculature undergoes vasodilation in response to such a challenge and there is a measurable change of velocity profiles in the middle cerebral artery, as a result. If no changes in velocity profiles are seen, it is inferred that the vessels over the cerebral hemisphere of clinical interest have become fully dilated, in attempting to maintain collateral blood flow from adjacent vascular territories, and may be near a state of inadequate flow.

REGIONAL CEREBRAL BLOOD FLOW

This oldest and least expensive of the techniques uses ^{133}Xe, inhaled or injected, to generate precise measurements of cortical blood flow. This is one method that may be used at the bedside, in the operating room, or in the intensive care unit, but its spatial resolution is inferior to that of PET or SPECT and it provides no information about subcortical perfusion. It is commonly used with hypercapnia or hypotension to test the autoregulatory capacity of resistance vessels. For instance, focal failure of the vasodilatory response, if distributed in the territory of a major vessel, has been taken as evidence of maximal dilation and therefore of reduced perfusion pressure. This finding is correlated with measures of elevated cerebral blood volume by SPECT, and oxygen extraction fraction by PET, and may indicate hemodynamic insufficiency. This is the same vasodilatory response assessed by transcranial Doppler techniques described above.

STABLE-XENON COMPUTED TOMOGRAPHY

CT may measure changes in tissue density over a period of minutes when nonradioactive xenon gas (essentially a freely diffusible high-attenuation contrast agent) is inhaled and circulates through the capillary bed. This method measures flow in both deep- and surface structures at high resolution, and provides automatic registration to the anatomic information in the baseline CT. It is limited by problems of signal-to-noise ratio and also by

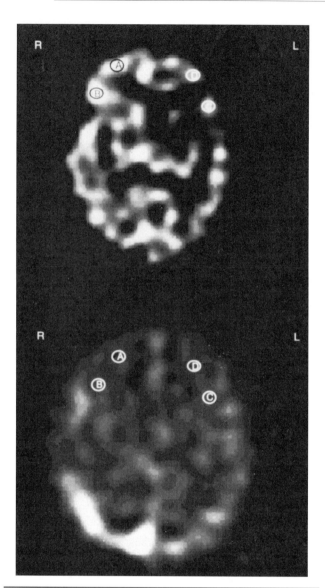

FIGURE 16.10. Single photon emission computed tomography (SPECT) study of a 64-year-old woman after 2 weeks of progressive saltatory aphasia and right hemiparesis. The syndrome was attributed to a distal field infarct in the left hemisphere, and the left internal carotid artery was occluded. SPECT simultaneously imaged cerebral blood flow (CBF) with ^{123}I-IMP and cerebral blood volume (CBV) with ^{99m}Tc-labeled red blood cells. **Top:** CBF; **bottom:** CBV. Four areas of interest (**A–D**) were selected on the CBF image and samples on the CBV image. In the frontal cortex, blood flow was reduced and volume was increased on the left. The CBV/CBF ratio was 0.76 for **A** and **D** and 0.66 for **B** and **C**, thus implying a lower perfusion pressure on the left. (As is conventional for computed tomography and magnetic resonance imaging figures, the left side of brain is on the right of the figure.)

the physiologic and anesthetic effects of the high xenon concentrations (approximately 30%).

SINGLE PHOTON EMISSION COMPUTED TOMOGRAPHY

Like PET, SPECT involves tomographic imaging of injected radioisotopes. However, these isotopes emit single photons rather than positrons, a difference that gives SPECT a more favorable cost-benefit ratio, makes it more widely available, and more clinically useful. However, SPECT is limited in application and is used widely only for imaging cerebral perfusion. Cerebral blood volume imaging is also available, and combined flow-and-volume scans are possible. Metabolic and receptor agents are being developed. SPECT imaging of infarction and ischemia appears to offer high sensitivity and early detection, but specificity is not yet established. In contrast to PET, SPECT may be used hours after an injection of the tracer; cerebral blood flow may be assessed under unique circumstances (e.g., during an epileptic seizure). Another promising use may be determination of cerebrovascular reserve through dilation challenge (CO_2 or acetazolamide) or combined flow-and-volume imaging (Fig. 16.10).

These techniques may identify the areas where blood flow is reduced owing to perfusion pressure, and would therefore possibly be of causal relevance, as opposed to the areas where flow is reduced as a result of diminished metabolic demand (e.g., due to infarction), therefore being of less therapeutic significance. Similarly to the methods used for cardiac procedures, these techniques may indicate regions of tissue viability.

POSITRON EMISSION TOMOGRAPHY (PET)

PET generates axial images using physical and mathematic principles similar to those used in CT, but the source of radiation is internal to the imaged organ, originating in injected or inhaled radioisotopes. The radioisotopes are short lived and require an adjacent cyclotron. The expense and technical complexity limit the availability of PET. On the other hand, the biochemical flexibility and sensitivity of PET are unparalleled. PET is superior to any other technique in imaging specific receptors or protein synthesis and turnover.

DISCUSSION

All these laboratory methods may be summarized with respect to their information content under four headings: vascular anatomy, tissue damage, hemodynamics, and biochemistry (Table 16.1).

▶ **TABLE 16.1 Predominant Applications of Neurovascular Imaging Techniques**

	Tissue Damage	Vascular Anatomy	Hemodynamics	Biochemistry
CT	✓			
MRI	✓		✓	
MR angiography		✓		
MR spectroscopy				✓
Positron emission tomography			✓	✓
^{133}Xe regional cerebral blood flow			✓	
Stable xenon CT			✓	
Single proton CT emission			✓	
Angiography		✓		
Doppler		✓	✓	

MR, CT.

Although most techniques provide information in many domains, Table 16.1 indicates only the predominant applications. All cerebrovascular laboratory techniques may be assigned to one or more of the four main categories, but overlap is common and the boundaries are sometimes blurred. For instance, tissue damage visualized by CT or MRI may be either hemorrhagic or ischemic infarction. Although the information may be useful in suggesting the more likely cause, vascular anatomy and local hemodynamics are usually more informative. For example, carotid occlusion or local absence of vascular reserve are two distinctly different causes of ischemic infarction and may lead to distinctly different treatment options. Finally, the assessment of local metabolism and biochemistry, best performed by PET and MRS, is not known to be useful clinically, but it is an area of active research.

SUGGESTED READINGS

Beauchamp NJ Jr, Ulug AM, Passe TJ, van Zijl PC. MR diffusion imaging in stroke: review and controversies. *Radiographics* 1998;18:1269–1283; discussion 1283–1285.

Brant-Zawadzki M, Heiserman JE. The roles of MR angiography, CT angiography, and sonography in vascular imaging of the head and neck. *AJNR Am J Neuroradiol* 1997;10:1820–1825.

Gonzalez RG, Schaefer PW, Buonanno FS, et al. Diffusion-weighted MR imaging: diagnostic accuracy in patients imaged within 6 hours of stroke symptom onset. *Radiology* 1999;210:155–162.

Hacke W, Warach S. Diffusion-weighted MRI as an evolving standard of care in acute stroke. *Neurology* 2000;54:1548–1549.

Hagen T, Bartylla K, Piepgras U. Correlation of regional cerebral blood flow measured by stable xenon CT and perfusion MRI. *J Comput Assist Tomogr* 1999;23:257–264.

Hunter GJ, Hamberg LM, Ponzo JA, et al. Assessment of cerebral perfusion and arterial anatomy in hyperacute stroke with three-dimensional functional CT: early clinical results. *AJNR Am J Neuroradiol* 1998;19:29–37.

Kaps M, Damian MS, Teschendorf U, Dorndorf W. Transcranial Doppler ultrasound findings in middle cerebral artery occlusion. *Stroke* 1990;21:532–537.

Koenig M, Klotz E, Luka B, Venderink DJ, Spittler JF, Heuser L. Perfusion CT of the brain: diagnostic approach for early detection of ischemic stroke. *Radiology* 1998;209:85–93.

Kushner MJ, Zanette EM, Bastianello S, et al. Transcranial Doppler in acute hemispheric brain infarction. *Neurology* 1990;41:109–113.

Lennihan L, Petty GW, Fink ME, et al. Transcranial Doppler detection of anterior cerebral artery vasospasm. *J Neurol Neurosurg Psychiatry* 1993;56(8):906–909.

Marshall RS, Rundek T, Sproule DM, Fitzsimmons BF, Schwartz S, Lazar RM. Monitoring of cerebral vasodilatory capacity with transcranial Doppler carbon dioxide inhalation in patients with severe carotid artery disease. *Stroke* 2003;34:945–949. (Epub)

Nussel F, Wegmuller H, Huber P. Comparison of magnetic resonance angiography, magnetic resonance imaging and conventional angiography in cerebral arteriovenous malformation. *Neuroradiology* 1991;33:56–61.

Patel SC, Levine SR, Tilley BC, et al. Lack of clinical significance of early ischemic changes on computed tomography in acute stroke. *JAMA* 2001;286:2830–2838.

Perren F, Horn P, Kern R, Bueltmann E, Hennerici M, Meairs S. A rapid noninvasive method to visualize ruptured aneurysms in the emergency room: three-dimensional power Doppler imaging. *J Neurosurg* 2004;100:619–622.

Ricci PE Jr. Proton MR spectroscopy in ischemic stroke and other vascular disorders. *Neuroimaging Clin N Am* 1998;8:881–900.

Saur D, Kucinski T, Grzyska U, et al. Sensitivity and interrater agreement of CT and diffusion-weighted MR imaging in hyperacute stroke. *AJNR* 2003;24(5):878–885.

Schwartz RB, Tice HM, Hooten SM, Hsu L, Stieg PE. Evaluation of cerebral aneurysms with helical CT: correlation with conventional angiography and MR angiography. *Radiology* 1994;192:717–722.

Schellinger PD, Bryan RN, Caplan LN, et al. The role of diffusion and perfusion weighted MR imaging for the diagnosis of acute ischemic stroke. Report of the Therapeutics and Technology Assessment Subcommittee of the American Academy of Neurology. *Neurology* 2004; In press.

Singer MB, Atlas SW, Drayer BP. Subarachnoid space disease: diagnosis with fluid-attenuated inversion-recovery MR imaging and comparison with gadolinium-enhanced spin-echo MR imaging—blinded reader study. *Radiology* 1998;208:417–422.

Sorensen AG, Copen WA, Ostergaard L, et al. Hyperacute stroke: simultaneous measurement of relative cerebral blood volume, relative cerebral blood flow, and mean tissue transit time. *Radiology* 1999;210:519–527.

Steinke W, Hennerici M, Rautenberg W, Mohr JP. Symptomatic and asymptomatic high-grade carotid stenosis in Doppler color flow imaging. *Neurology* 1992;42:131–138.

von Kummer R, Bourquain H, Bastianello S, et al. Early prediction of irreversible brain damage after ischemic stroke at CT. *Radiology* 2001;219:95–100.

Warach S. Stroke neuroimaging. *Stroke* 2003;34(2):345–347.

Chapter 17

Endovascular Surgical Neuroradiology

Philip M. Meyers and Sean D. Lavine

The science of endovascular surgical neuroradiology (ESNR), the treatment of cerebrovascular diseases using minimally invasive intravascular techniques, has made tremendous strides in the past decade. Based largely on developments in computer-aided imaging and microcatheter design, navigation of the cerebral and spinal vasculature is now reliable, facilitating the safety and efficacy of endovascular techniques for treatment of cerebrovascular diseases. In this chapter, we highlight areas in which endovascular therapies demonstrate the promise of better patient care.

CEREBRAL ANEURYSMS

The treatment of cerebral aneurysms is one of the proving grounds for ESNR, and it is highly controversial in the United States. Although cerebral aneurysms affect relatively few Americans each year (6 per 100,000 to 16 per 100,000), clinicians are concerned about the high morbidity and mortality of subarachnoid hemorrhage. Five percent to 15% of all strokes are the result of ruptured saccular aneurysms, and more than half of these patients die within the first 30 days. In the 1960s, it was demonstrated that the benefits of craniotomy and surgical clipping of cerebral aneurysms outweighed the risks of treating without surgery, depending on the location of the aneurysm. Nevertheless, only 20% to 30% of the patients survive the event without disabling neurologic or cognitive deficits.

In 1990, the Guglielmi Detachable Coil (GDC) was introduced into clinical use for the treatment of cerebral aneurysms. Initially an experimental device, the GDC was approved by the FDA in 1995 for the treatment of aneurysms for which surgical clipping was not an option. The coils work by filling the blood space within the aneurysm, inducing local thrombosis that later heals. Now, "biologically-active" coil technology helps to induce healing and improves the efficacy and durability of endovascular treatment (Fig. 17.1).

To aid coil occlusion of wide-neck aneurysms, balloon-remodeling or stent-assisted coil occlusion is used. With these techniques, a second device—either a temporary balloon or permanent endovascular stent—is used to keep coils in the aneurysm from falling back into the main artery. In September 2002, the FDA approved Neuroform, the first cerebrovascular stent device, for wide-necked cerebral aneurysms. Later, GDC received FDA approval for the treatment of all aneurysms. The need for evidence-based outcomes research is apparent but technology advances faster than the time required to perform clinical trials. Answers to many current questions remain elusive.

The International Subarachnoid Aneurysm Trial (ISAT) compared endovascular occlusion and surgical clipping of ruptured cerebral aneurysms, aiming to determine whether coils resulted in fewer dead or "dependent patients," defined by modified Rankin score of 3–6 (see Table 17.1 for explanation of modified Rankin Scale). This study enrolled 2,143 patients, mostly in Europe. Eighty-eight percent of patients were in good neurologic condition following their hemorrhages, and 92% of the aneurysms were less than 11 mm in diameter. Enrollment of patients with subarachnoid hemorrhage depended on agreement by the neurosurgeon and the endovascular specialist that the aneurysm could reasonably be treated by either method. Enrollment commenced in 1994 and was halted in 2003 when it became clear that coil occlusion resulted in better outcomes than neurosurgical clipping. In terms of patient survival free of disability at 1 year, coiling had a 22.6% superiority over surgical clipping, with an absolute risk reduction of 6.9% (p = 0.00082). Recurrent hemorrhages were not significantly different in the two groups. At 2 years, the gap widened to 26.8% relative risk reduction, and 8.7% absolute risk reduction.

For unruptured aneurysms, management remains controversial. The International Study of Unruptured Intracranial Aneurysms (ISUIA) is assessing the natural history of unruptured aneurysms and also the risks of treatment. From 1991 to 1998, 4,060 patients were enrolled: 1,692 subjects with 2,686 aneurysms did not receive treatment; 1,917 patients underwent craniotomy, and 451 received coil therapy. For patients who did not receive any intervention, the risk of hemorrhage was 0% to 40% in the anterior cerebral circulation depending predominantly on aneurysm size and 2.5% to 50% in the posterior circulation. Surgical morbidity and mortality was 10.1% to 12.6% at 1 year, while endovascular morbidity and mortality ranged from 7.1% to 9.8%, and varied according to patient age, aneurysm size, and location. Because the endovascular treatment cohort was small, wide confidence intervals limited comparability with the surgical cohort.

ISUIA raises concerns about the natural history of intracranial aneurysms. Fifty-one (3%) patients in the untreated cohort had a subarachnoid hemorrhage during the study period, and nearly all hemorrhages occurred within 5 years of diagnosis. For patients with aneurysms less than 7-mm diameter in the anterior cerebral circulation, the risk

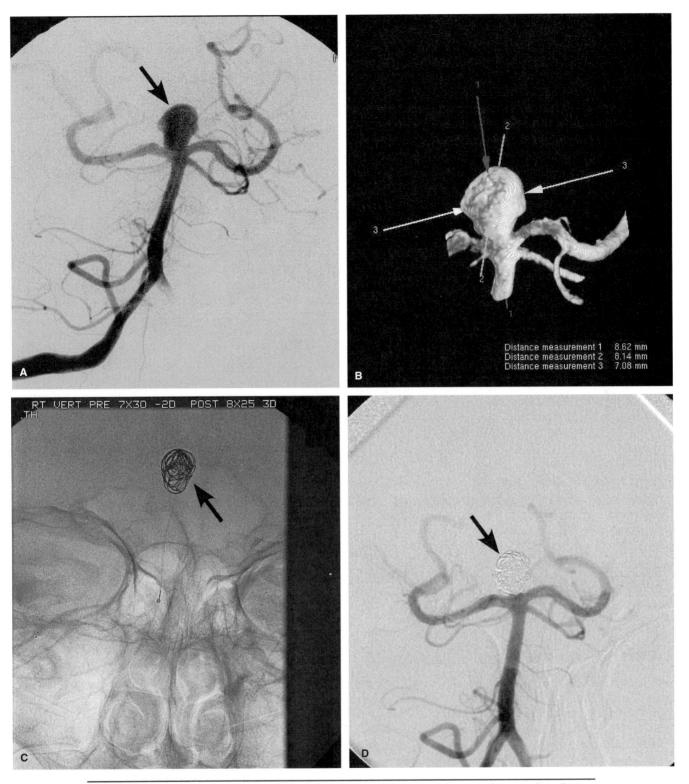

FIGURE 17.1. A: 58-yr-old woman with chronic hypertension, sinusitis, and a long smoking history developed worsening headaches and was found to harbor an 11 mm aneurysm of the basilar artery terminus (*arrow*). **B:** arteriographic evaluation including rotational arteriography with 3-dimensional reconstructions permits preoperative endovascular treatment planning. In a multi-disciplinary team paradigm, treatment options including craniotomy with surgical clipping or endovascular coil occlusion were discussed with the patient. **C:** Under general anesthesia, a microcatheter measuring 0.67 mm diameter is guided into the aneurysm from the femoral artery using high resolution roadmap imaging and the aneurysm is progressively occluded using special aneurysm coils (*arrow*), in this case a combination of GDC and "second generation" biologically active coils were used. **D:** Surveillance arteriography at 6 mos demonstrates complete occlusion of the aneurysm (*arrow*) and no new aneurysm in other aspects of the cerebral circulation.

▶ **TABLE 17.1** **Modified Rankin Scale to Assess Functional Clinical Outcomes**

Modified Rankin Scale	Clinical Description
0	Normal, No symptoms at all
1	No significant disability despite symptoms; able to carry out all usual duties and activities
2	Slight disability; unable to carry out all previous activities, but able to look after own affairs without assistance
3	Moderate disability; requiring some help, but able to walk without assistance
4	Moderately severe disability; unable to walk without assistance and unable to attend to own bodily needs without assistance
5	Severe disability; bedridden, incontinent and requiring constant nursing care and attention
6	Dead

of rupture was only 0.1% per year, which compared favorably with greater risks with either treatment. Patients under 50 years with asymptomatic aneurysms had the lowest surgical morbidity and mortality (5% to 6% at 1 year). Meanwhile, older age, although it does not affect the risk of aneurysmal hemorrhage, increased the risk of surgical morbidity and mortality. Although endovascular aneurysm treatment in the patients over 50 years appears safer than craniotomy and clipping, the long-term risks and durability of endovascular aneurysm occlusion remain to be proven.

ENDOVASCULAR REVASCULARIZATION USING STENT-ANGIOPLASTY

Extracranial Carotid Revascularization

Seven hundred and fifty thousand people have strokes each year, at an estimated cost of $45 billion in treatment and lost productivity. Carotid occlusive disease is responsible for 25% of these strokes. Large population-based studies indicate that the prevalence of carotid stenosis is about 0.5% after age 60 but increases to 10% after age 80. The majority of cases are asymptomatic. Surgical carotid endarterectomy is the accepted standard of treatment for revascularization of extracranial carotid occlusive disease. This has been validated by multiple, randomized, controlled trials that demonstrated better results over best medical therapy. However, carotid artery stenting has emerged as a new alternative (Fig. 17.2).

The proposed benefit of endovascular treatment of carotid stenosis centers on reduction of operative risks related to endarterectomy: concomitant cardiac morbidity, contralateral carotid occlusion, cranial nerve injury, and inaccessibility of the stenotic vessel behind the mandible. Stent angioplasty is currently used for patients with medical contraindications to surgery, restenosis after endarterectomy, radiation-induced stenosis, high cervical stenosis, or contralateral carotid occlusion.

The first carotid angioplasty was performed in 1980, and the technique has improved with the development of metallic stents and vascular filtration devices. A *stent* is a mesh device that holds the walls of a narrowed blood vessel open with or without angioplasty. A *vascular filtration device* is used to prevent strokes at the time of stent-angioplasty; a semi-permeable membrane traps particles of atherosclerotic plaque or blood clots that might arise from the vessel wall during the procedure. In nonrandomized trials, balloon angioplasty showed a technical success rate of 92% to 96%, acceptable morbidity rates of 2.0% to 7.9% and mortality rates of 0% to 2.0%. These early results compared favorably with the morbidity and mortality of previous surgical trials. In general, stent-assisted angioplasty achieved better results than simple balloon angioplasty, in terms of event-free survival and rates of early restenosis. Consequently, stent augmentation is performed over simple angioplasty in most circumstances.

Only one large, randomized trial directly compared carotid surgery with stent-angioplasty, enrolling 504 patients with symptomatic carotid stenosis (at least 30% luminal diameter reduction) and considered suitable for either endarterectomy (253 patients) or stent-angioplasty (251 patients, with 26% receiving stents at the discretion of the treating physician). Patients not suitable for endarterectomy were randomized either to stent-angioplasty or medical treatment. There were no significant outcome differences between endarterectomy and stent angioplasty at 30 days (death: 3% stent-angioplasty vs. 2% surgery; disabling stroke 4% for both; and nondisabling stroke 4% for both). Complications were more numerous than in some previous reports but not significantly different from others. Analysis of long-term survival demonstrated no differences between stenting and endarterectomy in the rate of ipsilateral stroke or any disabling stroke, in up to 3 years of follow-up examinations.

The use of a distal protection filter during stent-angioplasty may render endovascular revascularization techniques preferable to surgery. The first trial randomized 307 high risk patients to endarterectomy or to stent-angioplasty with distal protection. The patients had congestive heart failure, needed open heart surgery within 6 weeks, or had a recent myocardial infarction or unstable angina. Perioperative stroke and death rates were 7.3% for surgery versus 4.4% for stenting. Rates of myocardial infarction were 7.3% for surgery vs. 2.6% for stenting. Results are awaited from CREST, the Carotid Revascularization Endarterectomy versus Stent Trial, a randomized, controlled trial comparing stent-supported angioplasty with endarterectomy in patients with symptomatic stenosis of 50% or more.

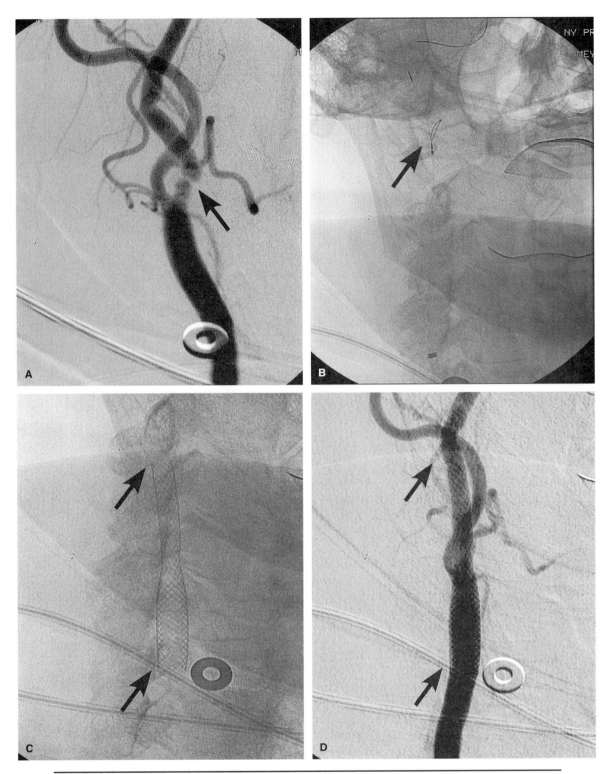

FIGURE 17.2. **82-year-old, right-handed woman with hypertension, hyperlipidemia, coronary artery disease and progressive right internal carotid artery stenosis despite aggressive medical therapy with anti-platelet and statin medications. A:** Right common carotid arteriography demonstrates severe (greater than 90%) stenosis of the proximal right internal carotid artery (*arrow*). **B:** Fluororadiograph demonstrates placement of a vascular filtration device across the site of stenosis prior to stent-angioplasty (*arrow*). **C** and **D:** Fluororadiograph and right common carotid arteriogram demonstrate placement of the endovascular stent with restoration of normal blood flow in the right carotid artery (*arrows*). The patient tolerated the procedure very well and was discharged the following morning.

▶ **TABLE 17.2** Annual Death and Stroke Rates
                According to the Distribution
                of Stenosis

Disease Distribution	Death Rate, %/year	Any Stroke, %/year	Ipsilateral Stroke, %/year
Carotid	9.5–17.2	3.9–11.7	3.1–8.1
Middle Cerebral	3.3–7.7	2.8–4.2	4.7
Vertebrobasilar	6.1–9.7	2.4–13.1	0–8.7

Intracranial Cerebral Revascularization

Intracranial atherosclerosis accounts for about 10% of all ischemic strokes or 40,000 annually in the United States. Besides race and ethnicity, risk factors include insulin-dependent diabetes mellitus, hypercholesterolemia, cigarette smoking and hypertension. Intracranial stenosis is usually detected when a patient has had an acute stroke. Most published data on the natural history of intracranial atherosclerosis came from patients examined by conventional angiography or transcranial Doppler sonography. The natural history remains elusive; intracranial stenosis may progress, regress, or remain stable. Current imaging does not predict the course of a given lesion, or the precise composition of the lesion (e.g., local intravascular thrombosis or stenotic atherosclerosis).

Prognosis after stroke with intracranial stenosis may depend on the location and extent of the lesion. Most information about prognosis in intracranial atherosclerosis has been based on retrospective analysis (see Table 17.2).

The successful use of balloon angioplasty for the treatment of intracranial atherosclerosis has been increasingly reported but the procedure is technically demanding and carries substantial risk. Most practitioners reserve endovascular revascularization for patients who are refractory to maximal medical therapy, a somewhat undefined term indicating that the physician has treated the patient with some regimen of anticoagulant or antiaggregating (antiplatelet) medication. In the vertebrobasilar circulation, the risk of a major complication with revascularization approaches 28% in one series, but was 12% in another trial with the most flexible balloon-mounted stents. However, in neurologically unstable patients, with crescendo TIAs or stroke in progress, the risk of major morbidity or death from therapeutic revascularization may approach 50%.

ACUTE STROKE THERAPY

Stroke is the third leading cause of death and the leading cause of disability in industrialized nations with 750,000 new strokes each year and more than 200,000 deaths per year in the United States at a cost of more than $45 billion. Eighty percent of strokes are ischemic. Intravenous administration of recombinant tissue plasminogen activator (r-tPA), a thrombolytic agent is the only treatment that improves outcomes after acute ischemic stroke. Among myriad stroke trials, only two were successful and resulted in FDA approval for intravenous administration of r-tPA for ischemic stroke within zero hours to 3 hours of stroke onset. Meanwhile, intra-arterial thrombolysis using the plasminogen activator urokinase remains unproven but has become the *de facto* community standard for stroke treatment outside the time frame for intravenous thrombolysis but within 3 hours to 6 hours after stroke onset. Although intra-arterial therapies using thrombolytic agents or mechanical thrombectomy devices remain unproven, there is tremendous interest in these techniques and the possibility of near-term medical advancement (Fig. 17.3).

Intra-arterial administration of thrombolytics may be more effective, and at lower dosages, than intravenous injections. Recanalization rates for major cerebrovascular occlusions using intra-arterial therapy approach 70%, compared to 34% for intravenous thrombolysis. Recanalization safety and efficacy has been demonstrated for intra-arterial administration of recombinant pro-urokinase for middle cerebral artery occlusion of less than 6 hours duration.

ARTERIOVENOUS MALFORMATIONS (AVM) AND DURAL FISTULAS

Evaluation and treatment of AVMs are controversial because information remains incomplete on the etiology, prevalence, incidence, and risk of these lesions, without or with treatment. The current treatment paradigm generally involves surgical resection of the AVM, and surgical morbidity may be mitigated by preoperative endovascular embolization (Fig. 17.4).

Among patients at Columbia including 545 procedures, preoperative embolization was performed with a 2% risk of permanent, disabling neurologic injury. The annual incidence of these malformations is about 1.5 per 100,000 population, with prevalence rates of 10.3 per 100,000 to 52.1 per 100,000 population. Symptomatic lesions account for 12% or 1.2 per 100,000 person years in patients aged 20 years to 40 years. The annual risk of hemorrhage has been estimated at 2% to 4%. In the only prospective determination of hemorrhage risk, the annual risk was 2% for AVMs for those without hemorrhage, but for patients with prior hemorrhage the risk increased to 32.9% in the first year, and 11.3% annually, thereafter.

Dural arteriovenous fistulae are acquired artery-to-vein shunts within dural mater, often without a distinctive vascular nidus. They constitute 10% to 15% of all

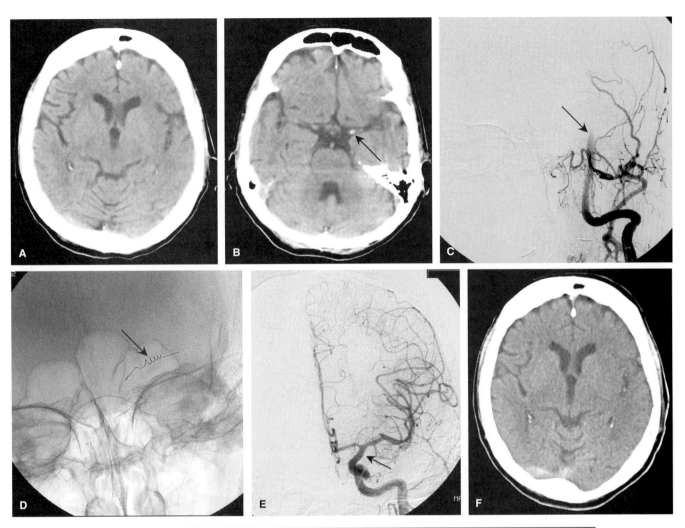

FIGURE 17.3. **75-year-old, right-handed woman with new-onset atrial fibrillation developed sudden right hemiplegia, neglect, and global aphasia during evaluation for cardioversion in the hospital facility.** **A** and **B:** nonenhanced CT brain scan demonstrates asymmetric density in the left carotid terminus (*arrow*) but no evidence of stroke or hemorrhage. Because of the likelihood of a carotid "T" occlusion and low likelihood of flow restoration at this location with intravenous thrombolytic therapy, the patient was immediately referred for intra-arterial treatment. **C:** Left carotid arteriography shows opacification of the left external carotid artery branches but intracranial occlusion of the left internal carotid artery (*arrow*). **D:** a mechanical thrombectomy device, in this case the Concentric Merci X-series device and one of a number of stroke now undergoing clinical testing, was deployed through a microcatheter using standard transfemoral catheterization technique across the site of the occlusion in the left carotid terminus and proximal left middle cerebral artery (*arrow*). **E.** left carotid arteriography immediately following thrombectomy demonstrates complete restoration of flow in the left anterior circulation (*arrow*) without the use of thrombolytic agents and the attendant risks of intracranial hemorrhage. **F:** CT brain scan following treatment demonstrates to reperfusion hemorrhage and the patient made an excellent neurologic recovery. At 30-day follow-up, she was able to sign the research consent for her original thrombectomy procedure.

intracranial AVMs. Symptoms depend on the location of the fistula and include pulse-synchronous tinnitus, exophthalmos, cranial nerve syndromes, dementia, venous infarcts, and intracranial hemorrhage. Unlike "true" AVMs of the brain parenchyma, dural fistulas are amenable to curative endovascular treatment with transvenous embolization (Fig. 17.5).

Similarly, pediatric fistulas including the vein of Galen malformation may be curable with endovascular treatment. Compared with reports of surgical series in which 90% of children with vein of Galen malformations died at surgery and 10% were severely disabled, up to 80% may be palliated or cured by endovascular techniques, with good to excellent functional outcomes.

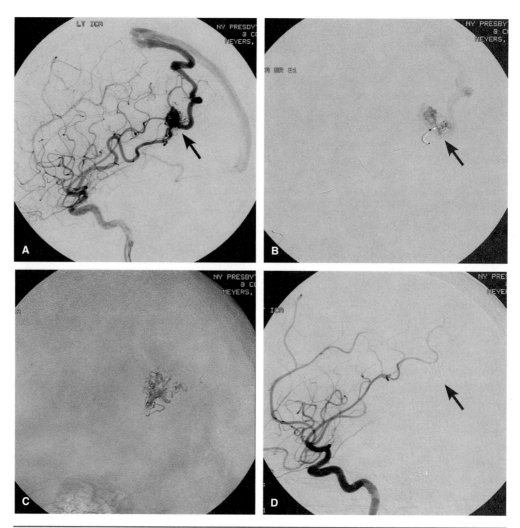

FIGURE 17.4. **32-year-old woman with seizures and left hemicranial headaches was found to harbor a subcortical arteriovenous malformation in the left parietal lobe. A:** Left carotid arteriography confirmed the presence of the AVM with multiple nidal aneurysms (*arrow*). **B:** Under local anesthesia only, a 0.5 mm diameter microcatheter is placed in close proximity to the arteriovenous malformation for injection of anesthetic agents, amobarbital and lidocaine, for purposes of provocative neurologic testing (*arrow*). Testing is performed in conjunction with members of the Neuropsychology service both to determine the risk of causing neurologic deficits at embolization and surgical resection. In this case, no changes in neurologic function were identified. **C:** Fluoro-radiography of the cranium following occlusion of the AVM with n-butyl-cyanoacrylate (NBCA "glue") shows radio-opaque glue filling of the sinusoids within the AVM nidus (*arrow*). **D:** Control arteriography following occlusion of the AVM shows complete obliteration of the AVM nidus and no other branch vessel occlusion (*arrow*). The patient tolerated embolization and resection without any complication and returned to work in nine days.

PERCUTANEOUS SPINAL INTERVENTION—VERTEBROPLASTY

Back pain is a common and costly problem in Western countries. It is estimated that back pain periodically incapacitates up to 20% of the American workforce at an annual cost of more than $24 billion in lost productivity and treatment. Pain of spinal origin has a lifetime prevalence of greater than 60% and an annual incidence of 5%.

Percutaneous treatment is used for two common causes of spinal pain: facet joint arthropathy and osteoporotic vertebral compression fractures. Vertebroplasty, the use of cement to stabilize vertebral fracture fragments to palliate spinal pain, may become the new standard of care for management of pain and disability due to either osteoporotic or neoplastic compression fractures. Vertebral collapse most commonly occurs during normal exertion and loading forces in elderly persons with osteoporosis. One and one-half million osteoporotic fractures occur each

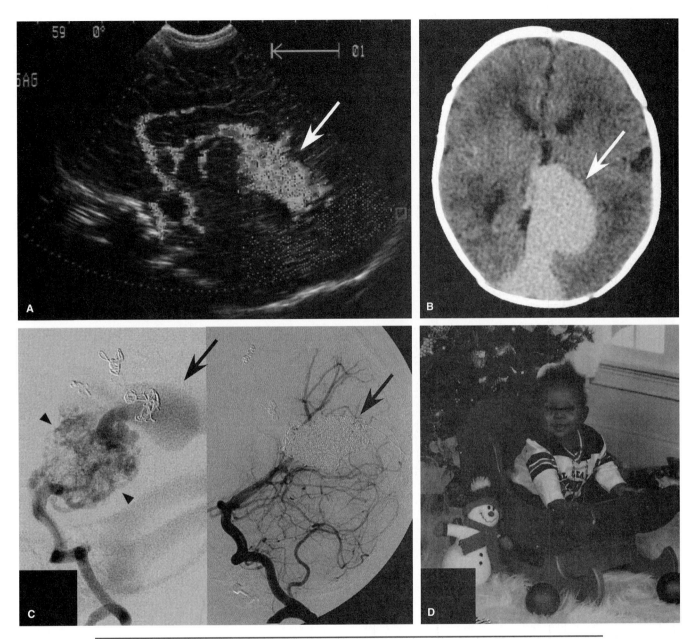

FIGURE 17.5. **Classical presentation of a choroidal-type vein of Galen malformation: neonate presents with severe congestive heart failure difficult to control medically and has a loud cranial bruit. A:** Transcranial color Doppler ultrasonography demonstrates an abnormally large high-flow midline vascular structure (*white arrow*). **B:** CT brain scan confirms the presence of an enlarged midline vascular structure that is highly suspicious for a vein of Galen malformation in the neonate with high-output cardiac failure (*white arrow*). **C:** A combination of trans-arterial and trans-venous techniques are used to completely occlude this type of congenital fistula with aneurysmal dilatation of the median prosencephalic vein of Markowski (*black arrows*). **D:** Because there was no pre-existing brain atrophy, this child made a complete and full recovery following treatment and remains neurologically normal several years following curative embolization. (See color insert).

year, including 700,000 vertebral fractures. The lifetime risk of symptomatic vertebral compression fractures is 16% for white women and 5% for white men. Vertebral compression fractures are defined by 15% loss of vertebral height and classified by morphologic deformity. The most commonly compressed vertebral bodies are T8, T12, L1, and L4. Symptomatic fractures cause severe pain and hospitalization in 8%, and prolonged nursing care in 2%. The result may be life-threatening pneumonia, immobilization and deep venous thrombosis, loss of independence, and depression. Mortality rates are 1.23 times higher in women with compression fractures than in age-matched controls.

Percutaneous vertebroplasty is a minimally invasive, radiologically guided procedure to treat the pain caused by vertebral compression fractures and symptomatic spinal tumors. Pain control and functional improvement are the proximate goals of the procedure. Under conscious sedation and local anesthesia, an 11-gauge to 13-gauge bone-biopsy needle is guided through one or both pedicles of the affected vertebra and into the vertebral body, under CT or fluoroscopic guidance. Polymethyl-methacrylate (PMMA), a cement commonly used in orthopedic procedures, is opacified with barium or tungsten powder, then injected into the vertebral body under fluoroscopic guidance. Intraosseous venography confirms the appropriate position of the needle before the cement is deposited. Care is taken to avoid injections into local veins. Overall, the morbidity risk of vertebroplasty is 1% to 2%, with mostly minor complications.

No comprehensive, prospective, randomized trial has been completed on percutaneous vertebroplasty. In retrospective case series, immediate pain relief was achieved in 70% to 90% with complication rates less than 1%. In one series, 12% of treated patients developed additional fractures requiring intervention, but there was no increased risk of new spinal compression fractures in treated patients. In a small prospective trial, 21 patients had vertebroplasty and 19 had medical therapy; early results suggested a benefit to vertebroplasty. However, placebo responses were not eliminated. Trials comparing vertebroplasty to a sham intervention may be required to prove the efficacy of the procedure.

SUGGESTED READINGS

Berman MF, Solomon RA, Mayer SA, Johnston SC, and Yung PP. Impact of hospital-related factors on outcome after treatment of cerebral aneurysms. *Stroke* 2003;34(9):2200–2207.

Cross DT 3rd, Tirschwell DL, Clark MA, et al. Mortality rates after subarachnoid hemorrhage: variations according to hospital case volume in 18 states. *J Neurosurg* 2003;99(5):810–817.

CAVATAS investigators: Endovascular versus surgical treatment in patients with carotid stenosis in the Carotid and Vertebral Artery Transluminal Angioplasty Study (CAVATAS): a randomised trial. *Lancet* 2001;357:1729–1737.

ISAT Collaborative Group. International Subarachnoid Aneurysm Trial (ISAT) of neurosurgical clipping versus endovascular coiling in 2143 patients with ruptured intracranial aneurysms: a randomized trial. *Lancet.* 2002;360:1267–1274.

Hartmann A, Pile-Spellman J, Stapf C, et al. Risk of endovascular treatment of brain arteriovenous malformations. *Stroke.* 2002;33:1816–1820.

Higashida RT, Hopkins LN, Berenstein A, Halbach VV, Kerber C. Program requirements for residency/fellowship education in neuroendovascular surgery/interventional neuroradiology: a special report on graduate medical education. *AJNR Am J Neuroradiol* 2000;21:1153–1159.

Furlan AJ, Higashida R, Wechsler L, et al. Intra-arterial prourokinase for acute ischemic stroke: the PROACT II study: a randomized controlled trial. *JAMA* 1999;282:2003–2011.

Gupta R, Schumacher HC, Mangla S, et al. Urgent endovascular revascularization for symptomatic intracranial atherosclerotic stenosis. *Neurology* 2003;61(12):1729–1735.

Higashida RT, Meyers PM, Phatouros CC, et al. Technology Assessment Committees of the American Society of Interventional. Therapeutic Neuroradiology and the Society of Interventional Radiology. Reporting Standards for Carotid artery angioplasty and stent placement. *Stroke* 2004;35(5):e112–e134.

Johnston SC, Wilson CB, Halbach VV, et al. Endovascular and surgical treatment of unruptured cerebral aneurysms: comparison of risks. *Ann Neurol* 2000;48(1):11–19.

Johnston SC, Dudley RA, Gress DR, and Ono L. Surgical and endovascular treatment of unruptured cerebral aneurysms at university hospitals. *Neurology* 1999;52(9):1799–1805.

Johnston SC, Gress DR, and Kahn JG. Which unruptured cerebral aneurysms should be treated? A cost-utility analysis. *Neurology* 1999; 52(9):1806–1815.

Kado DM, Browner WS, Palermo L, et al. Vertebral fractures and mortality in older women: a prospective study. Study of Osteoporotic Fractures Research Group. *Arch Int Med* 1999;159:1215–1220.

Lempert T, Malek AM, Halbach VV, et al. Endovascular treatment of ruptured posterior circulation cerebral aneurysms. Clinical and angiographic outcomes. *Stroke* 2000;31:100–110.

Malek AM, Halbach VV, Higashida RT, et al. Treatment of dural arteriovenous malformations and fistulas. *Neurosurg Clin North Am* 2000;11:85–99.

Meyers PM, Halbach VV, Malek AM, et al. Dural carotid cavernous fistula: definitive endovascular management and long-term follow-up. *Amer J Ophthalmol* 2002;134:85–92.

Meyers PM, Halbach VV, Barkovich AJ. Endovascular surgical approaches to anomalies of cerebral vasculature. In: *Pediatric Neuroimaging*, 3rd ed. Philadelphia: Lippincott-Raven, 1999.

Powell J, Kitchen N, Heslin J, Greenwood R. Psychosocial outcomes at three and nine months after good neurological recovery from aneurysmal subarachnoid hemorrhage: predictors and prognosis. *J Neurol Neurosurg Psychiatry* 2002;72:772–781.

Roubin GS, New G, Iyer SS, et al.: Immediate and late clinical outcomes of carotid artery stenting in patients with symptomatic and asymptomatic carotid artery stenosis: a 5-year prospective analysis. *Circulation* 2001;103:532–537.

Schumacher HC, Khaw AV, Meyers PM, Gupta R, et al. Intracranial angioplasty and stent placement for cerebral atherosclerosis. *J Vasc Intervent Radiol* 2004;15(1 Pt 2):S123–S132.

Wholey MH, Wholey M, Mathias K, et al.: Global experience in cervical carotid artery stent placement. *Catheter Cardiovasc Interv* 2000;50:160–167.

Chapter 18

Lumbar Puncture and Cerebrospinal Fluid Examination

Robert A. Fishman

INDICATIONS

Lumbar puncture (LP) should be performed only after clinical evaluation of the patient and consideration of the potential value and hazards of the procedure. CSF findings are important in the differential diagnosis of the gamut of CNS infections, including meningitis and encephalitis, as well as subarachnoid hemorrhage, confusion states, acute stroke, status epilepticus, meningeal malignancies, demyelinating diseases, and CNS vasculitis. CSF examination usually is necessary in patients with suspected intracranial bleeding to establish the diagnosis, although CT, when available, may be more valuable. For example, primary intracerebral hemorrhage or posttraumatic hemorrhage is often readily observed with CT, thus making LP an unnecessary hazard. However, in primary subarachnoid hemorrhage, LP may establish the diagnosis when CT is falsely negative. LP may ascertain whether the CSF is free of blood before anticoagulant therapy for stroke is begun. Extensive subarachnoid or epidural bleeding is a rare complication of heparin anticoagulation that starts several hours after a traumatic bloody tap; therefore, heparin therapy should not commence for at least 1 hour after a bloody LP. LP has limited therapeutic usefulness (e.g., intrathecal therapy in meningeal malignancies and fungal meningitis).

CONTRAINDICATIONS

LP is contraindicated in the presence of infection in skin overlying the spine. A serious complication of LP is the possibility of aggravating a preexisting, often unrecognized brain herniation syndrome (e.g., uncal, cerebellar, or cingulate herniation) associated with intracranial hypertension. This hazard is the basis for considering papilledema to be a relative contraindication to LP. The availability of CT has simplified the management of patients with papilledema. If CT reveals no evidence of a mass lesion or edema, then LP is usually needed in the presence of papilledema to establish the diagnosis of pseudotumor cerebri and to exclude meningeal inflammation or malignancy.

Hazards of Bleeding Disorders

Thrombocytopenia and other bleeding diatheses predispose patients to needle-induced subarachnoid, subdural, and epidural hemorrhage. LP should be undertaken only for urgent clinical indications when the platelet count is depressed to about 50,000/mm^3 or below. Platelet transfusion just before the puncture is recommended if the count is below 20,000/mm^3 or dropping rapidly. The administration of protamine to patients on heparin, and vitamin K or fresh frozen plasma to those receiving warfarin, is recommended before LP to minimize the hazard of the procedure.

COMPLICATIONS

Complications of LP include worsening of brain herniation or spinal cord compression, headache, subarachnoid bleeding, diplopia, backache, and radicular symptoms. Postprocedural headache is the most common complication of LP, occurring in about 25% of patients and usually lasting 2 days to 8 days. It results from low CSF pressures caused by persistent fluid leakage through the dural hole. Characteristically, the head pain is present in the upright position, may be promptly relieved by having the patient assume the supine position, and is aggravated by coughing or straining. Aching of the neck and low back, nausea, vomiting, and tinnitus are common complaints. Postprocedural headache is avoided when a small-gauge stiletted needle is used and if multiple puncture holes are not made. The bevel of the spinal needle should be inserted parallel to the longitudinal axis to minimize transection of the longitudinal fibers of the dura.

The management of the problem depends on strict bedrest in the horizontal position, adequate hydration, and simple analgesics. If conservative measures fail, the use of a "blood patch" is indicated. The technique uses the epidural injection of autologous blood close to site of the dural puncture to form a fibrinous tamponade that apparently seals the dural hole.

CEREBROSPINAL FLUID PRESSURE

The CSF pressure should be measured routinely. The pressure within the right atrium is the reference zero level with the patient in the lateral decubitus position. The normal lumbar CSF pressure ranges between 60 mm and 200 mm water (and as high as 250 mm in extremely obese subjects). In recent years, pressures have been recorded in centimeters (cm) rather than millimeters (mm) because the disposable manometers now are so marked. Thus, the normal CSF pressure is 7 cm to 20 cm. With the use of the clinical manometer, the arterial pulsatile-pressure waves are obscured, but respiratory pressure waves reflecting changes in central venous pressures are visible.

Low pressures may occur after a previous LP, with dehydration, spinal subarachnoid block, or in the presence of CSF fistulas. Intracranial hypotension may be a technical artifact when the needle is not properly inserted in the subarachnoid space. Increased pressures occur in patients with brain edema, intracranial mass lesions, infections, acute stroke, cerebral venous occlusions, congestive heart failure, pulmonary insufficiency, and hepatic failure. Low CSF pressures may result from CSF leakage due to a dural fistula. They are also low when assessed below a spinal subarachnoid block. Benign intracranial hypertension (pseudotumor cerebri) and spontaneous intracranial hypotension (SIH) are discussed elsewhere in this book.

CEREBROSPINAL FLUID CELLS

Normal CSF contains no more than 5 lymphocytes or mononuclear cells/mm^3. A higher white cell count is pathognomonic of disease in the CNS or meninges. A stained smear of the sediment must be prepared to obtain an accurate differential cell count. Various centrifugal and sedimentation techniques have been used. A pleocytosis occurs with the gamut of inflammatory disorders. The changes characteristic of the various meningitides are listed in Table 18.1.

The heterogeneous manifestations of neuro-AIDS are associated with a wide range of cellular responses. Other disorders associated with a pleocytosis include brain infarct, subarachnoid bleeding, cerebral vasculitis, acute demyelination, and brain tumors. Eosinophilia most often accompanies parasitic infections, such as cysticercosis, and may reflect blood eosinophilia. Cytologic studies for malignant cells are rewarding with some CNS neoplasms.

Bloody CSF due to needle trauma contains increased numbers of white cells contributed by the blood. A useful approximation of a true white cell count may be obtained by the following correction for the presence of the added blood: If the patient has a normal hemogram, subtract from the total white cell count (cells/mm^3) one white cell for each 1,000 red blood cells present. Thus, if bloody fluid contains 10,000 red cells/mm^3 and 100 white cells/mm^3, 10 white cells would be accounted for by the added blood and the corrected leukocyte count would be 90/mm^3. If the patient's hemogram reveals significant anemia or leukocytosis, the following formula may be used to determine more accurately the number of white cells (WBC) in the spinal fluid corrected for the bloody tap.

$$WBC_{CSF} = \frac{WBC_{BL} \times RBC_{CSF}}{RBC_{BL}}$$

The presence of blood in the subarachnoid space produces a secondary inflammatory response that leads to a disproportionate increase in the number of white cells. After an acute subarachnoid hemorrhage, this elevation in the white cell count is most marked about 48 hours after onset, when meningeal signs are most striking.

To correct CSF protein values for the presence of added blood resulting from needle trauma, subtract 1 mg for every 1,000 red blood cells. Thus, if the red cell count is 10,000/mm^3 and the total protein is 110 mg/dL, the corrected protein level would be about 100 mg/dL. The corrections are reliable only if the cell count and total protein are both made on the same tube of fluid.

BLOOD IN THE CEREBROSPINAL FLUID: DIFFERENTIAL DIAGNOSIS AND THE THREE-TUBE TEST

To differentiate between a traumatic spinal puncture and preexisting subarachnoid hemorrhage, the fluid should be collected in at least three separate tubes (the "three-tube test"). In traumatic punctures, the fluid generally clears between the first and the third collections. This change is detectable by the naked eye and should be confirmed by cell count. In subarachnoid bleeding, the blood is generally evenly mixed in the three tubes. A sample of the bloody fluid should be centrifuged and the supernatant fluid compared with tap water to exclude the presence of pigment. The supernatant fluid is crystal clear if the red count is less than about 100,000 cells/mm^3. With bloody contamination of greater magnitude, plasma proteins may be sufficient to cause minimal CSF xanthochromia, an effect that requires enough serum to raise the CSF protein concentration to about 150 mg/dL.

After an acute subarachnoid hemorrhage, the supernatant fluid usually remains clear for 2 hours to 4 hours or even longer, after the onset. The clear supernatant may mislead the physician to conclude erroneously that the observed blood is the result of needle trauma in patients who have had an LP within 4 hours of aneurysmal rupture. After an especially traumatic puncture, some blood and xanthochromia may be present for as long as 2 days to 5 days. In pathologic states associated with a CSF protein content exceeding 150 mg/dL and in the absence of bleeding, faint xanthochromia may be detected. When the protein is elevated to much higher levels, as would be the case in spinal block, polyneuritis, or meningitis, the xanthochromia may be considerable. A xanthochromic fluid with a normal protein level, or a minor elevation to less than

▶ **TABLE 18.1 Cerebrospinal Fluid Findings in Meningitis**

Meningitis	Pressure (cm H₂O)	Leukocytes (mm³)	Protein (mg/dL)	Glucose (mg/dL)
Acute bacterial	Usually elevated	Several hundred to more than 60,000; usually few thousand; occasionally less than 100 (especially meningococcal or early in disease); polymorphonuclear leukocytes predominate	Usually 100–500, occasionally more than 1,000	5–40 in most cases (in absence of hyperglycemia)
Tuberculous	Usually elevated; may be low with dynamic block in advanced stages	Usually 25–100; rarely more than 500; lymphocytes predominate except in early stages when polymorphonuclear leukocytes may account for 80% of cells	Nearly always elevated, usually 100–200; may be much higher if dynamic block	Usually reduced; less than 45 in 75% of cases
Cryptococcal	Usually elevated	0–800; average 50; lymphocytes predominate	Usually 20–500; average 100	Reduced in most cases; average 30 (in absence of hyperglycemia)
Viral	Normal to moderately elevated	5 to a few hundred but may be more than 1,000, particularly with lymphocytic choriomeningitis; lymphocytes predominate but may be more than 80% polymorphonuclear leukocytes in first few days	Frequently normal or slightly elevated; less than 100; may show greater elevation in severe cases	Normal (reduced in 25% of cases of mumps and herpes simplex)
Syphilitic (acute)	Usually elevated	Average 500; usually lymphocytes; rarely polymorphonuclear leukocytes	Average 100	Normal (rarely reduced)
Cysticercosis	Often increased; low with dynamic block	Increased mononuclear and polymorphonuclear leukocytes with 2–7% eosinophilia in about 50% of cases	Usually 50–200	Reduced in 20% of cases
Sarcoid	Normal to considerably elevated	0 to less than 100 mononuclear cells	Slight to moderate elevation	Reduced in 50% of cases
Tumor	Normal or elevated	0 to several hundred mononuclear leukocytes plus malignant cells	Elevated, often to high levels	Normal or greatly reduced (low in 75% of carcinomatous meningitis cases)

CSF immunoglobulins are commonly increased in all described conditions (including carcinomatous meningitis) and in multiple sclerosis.

$$\frac{\text{IgG(CSF)} \times \text{albumin(serum)}}{\text{IgG(serum)} \times \text{albumin (CSF)}}$$

The normal index is less than about 0.65. The presence of multiple oligoclonal bands (with gel electrophoresis) is also a measure of abnormally increased CSF immunoglobulins.

150 mg/dL, usually indicates a previous subarachnoid or intracerebral hemorrhage. Xanthochromia may be caused by severe jaundice, carotenemia, or rifampin therapy.

CHARACTERISTICS OF CSF

Pigments

The two major pigments derived from red cells that may be observed in CSF are oxyhemoglobin and bilirubin. Methemoglobin is seen only spectrophotometrically. Oxyhemoglobin, released with lysis of red cells, may be detected in the supernatant fluid within 2 hours after subarachnoid hemorrhage. It reaches a maximum in about the first 36 hours and gradually disappears over the next 7 days to 10 days. Bilirubin is produced in vivo by leptomeningeal cells after red cell hemolysis. Bilirubin is first detected about 10 hours after the onset of subarachnoid bleeding. It reaches a maximum at 48 hours, and may persist for 2 weeks to 4 weeks after extensive bleeding. The severity of the meningeal signs associated with subarachnoid bleeding correlates with the inflammatory response (i.e., the severity of the leukocytic pleocytosis).

Total Protein

The normal total protein level of CSF ranges between 15 mg/dL and 50 mg/dL. Although an elevated protein level lacks specificity, it is an index of neurologic disease reflecting a pathologic increase in endothelial cell permeability. Greatly increased protein levels, 500 mg/dL and above, are seen in meningitis, bloody fluids, or spinal cord tumor with spinal block. Polyneuritis (Guillain-Barré syndrome), diabetic radiculoneuropathy, and myxedema also may increase the level to 100 to 300 mg/dL. Low protein levels, below 15 mg/dL, occur most often with CSF leaks caused by a previous LP or traumatic dural fistula, and uncommonly in pseudotumor cerebri.

Immunoglobulins

Although many proteins may be measured in CSF, only an increase in immunoglobulins is of diagnostic importance. Such increases are indicative of an inflammatory response in the CNS and occur with immunologic disorders and infectious diseases (e.g., bacterial, viral, spirochetal, and fungal). Immunoglobulin assays are most useful in the diagnosis of multiple sclerosis, other demyelinating diseases, and CNS vasculitis. The CSF level is corrected for the entry of immunoglobulins from the serum by calculating the IgG index (Table 18.1). More than one oligoclonal band in CSF, noted with gel electrophoresis (and absent in serum) is also abnormal, occurring in 90% of multiple sclerosis cases and in the gamut of inflammatory diseases.

Glucose

The CSF glucose concentration depends on the blood level. The normal range of CSF is between 45 mg/dL and 80 mg/dL, in patients with blood glucose between 70 mg/dL and 120 mg/dL (i.e., 60% to 80% of the normal blood level). CSF values between 40 mg/dL and 45 mg/dL are usually abnormal, and values below 40 mg/dL are invariably so. Hyperglycemia during the 4 hours before LP results in a parallel increase in CSF glucose. The CSF glucose approaches a maximum, and the CSF-to-blood ratio may be as low as 0.35 in the presence of a greatly elevated blood glucose level and in the absence of any neurologic disease. An increase in CSF glucose is of no diagnostic significance apart from reflecting hyperglycemia within the 4 hours before LP.

The CSF glucose level is abnormally low (*hypoglycorrhachia*) in several diseases of the nervous system, apart from hypoglycemia. It is characteristic of acute purulent meningitis and is a usual finding in tuberculous and fun-

gal meningitis. CSF glucose levels are usually normal in viral meningitis, although reduced in about 25% of mumps cases and in some cases of herpes simplex and zoster meningoencephalitis. The CSF glucose may be reduced in other inflammatory meningitides, including cysticercosis, amebic meningitis (*Naegleria*), acute syphilitic meningitis, sarcoidosis, granulomatous arteritis, and other vasculitides. The glucose level is also reduced in the chemical meningitis that follows intrathecal injections and in subarachnoid hemorrhage, usually 4 days to 8 days after the onset of bleeding. The major factor responsible for the depressed glucose levels is increased anaerobic glycolysis in adjacent neural tissues, and to a lesser degree, by a polymorphonuclear leukocytosis. Thus, the decrease in CSF glucose level is characteristically accompanied by an inverse increase in CSF lactate level. A low CSF glucose with a decreased lactate level indicates impairment of the glucose transporter responsible for the transfer of glucose across the blood–brain barrier.

MICROBIOLOGIC AND SEROLOGIC REACTIONS

The use of appropriate stains and cultures is essential in cases of suspected infection. Tests for specific bacterial and fungal antigens and countercurrent immunoelectrophoresis are useful in establishing a specific cause. DNA amplification techniques using the polymerase chain reaction have improved diagnostic sensitivity. Serologic tests for syphilis on CSF include the reagin antibody tests and specific treponemal antibody tests. The former are particularly useful in evaluating CSF because positive results occur even in the presence of a negative blood serology. There is no logical basis for applying specific treponemal antibody tests to CSF because these antibodies are derived from the plasma, where they are present in greater concentration.

SUGGESTED READINGS

Fishman RA. *Cerebrospinal Fluid in Diseases of the Nervous System,* 2nd ed. Philadelphia: WB Saunders, 1992.

Oliver WJ, Shope TC, Kuhns LR. Fatal lumbar puncture: fact versus fiction—an approach to a clinical dilemma. *Pediatrics* 2003;112 (3 Pt 1):174–176.

Roos KL. Lumbar puncture. *Semin Neurol* 2003;23(1):105–114.

Chapter 19

Muscle and Nerve Biopsy

Arthur P. Hays and Michael D. Daras

Biopsy of skeletal muscle or peripheral nerve is performed in patients with neuromuscular disorders, myopathy or peripheral neuropathy, if the diagnosis cannot be established with other methods. At the least, the findings may indicate whether a syndrome of limb weakness is neurogenic or myopathic. This determination is made in conjunction with the findings on EMG and nerve conduction studies; the interpretations based on biopsy and electrophysiologic studies are usually congruent with each other and with clinical data from the history and examination. At best, the biopsy of muscle and nerve may give a specific tissue diagnosis. Sometimes, however, the findings are not diagnostic because the defining lesion has been missed in the biopsy, which is only a tiny sample of a voluminous tissue, and the lesions may be present in one area but not in another. Also, the pathologic changes may be too mild to distinguish from normal or too advanced to draw conclusions, as in "end-stage" muscle.

The yield of a specific diagnosis is relatively low, but has been increasing steadily through technologic innovations. In myopathies, histochemical and immunohistochemical stains applied to frozen tissue sections and biochemical analysis of enzymes, structural proteins, or DNA have transformed the prospects of tissue-based diagnosis. Precise diagnoses in peripheral nerve disorders often require immunohistochemical stains to localize human antigens, resin histology (semithin plastic sections), electron microscopy, and teased preparations of myelinated nerve fibers.

DIAGNOSTIC TESTING: MAKING THE DECISION

The performance and analysis of a muscle and nerve biopsy are time-consuming and expensive. Therefore, the decision for biopsy is made only after a thorough evaluation that includes the patient's history, family history, neurologic examination, laboratory tests, cerebrospinal fluid examination, and electrodiagnostic studies. These investigations obviate the need for biopsy in typical cases of myasthenia gravis, myotonic dystrophy, amyotrophic lat-

eral sclerosis, Guillain-Barré syndrome, diabetic neuropathy, or any defined toxic neuropathy. Additionally, a rapidly expanding number of diseases can be diagnosed by DNA analysis of blood leukocytes without recourse to tissue analysis (e.g., McArdle disease, mitochondrial disorders, Charcot-Marie-Tooth disease type IA and Duchenne or Becker muscular dystrophy, as described in Chapters 85, 98, 106, and 127).

If a biopsy is deemed necessary, the neurologist formulates a preliminary diagnosis and informs the pathologist to direct evaluation of the specimen most efficiently. The surgical procedure should be performed by an experienced neurologist or surgeon, identifying the tissue correctly and avoiding mechanically induced artifacts or insufficient quantity for examination. If special methods are not available locally, the service usually may be provided by a regional research center.

SKELETAL MUSCLE BIOPSY

Muscle biopsy may be conducted through an incision (open biopsy) or with a needle (percutaneous biopsy). The advantages of needle biopsy include a nearly invisible scar and the ability to sample multiple sites. However, the disadvantages of smaller specimens are poor myofiber orientation and quality of specimen, which make the open approach preferable. The final decision is made based on the experience of the physician who performs the biopsy and the preference of the laboratory. For an open biopsy, the skin and subcutaneous tissue are anesthetized (lidocaine 2%), carefully avoiding muscle infiltration. In children, sedation is required. A small incision is then made away from the myotendinous region, along the axis of the muscle, and extended to include the fascia. Four samples are collected for histopathology (i.e., fixed in formalin), histochemistry and immunohistochemistry (i.e., frozen in isopentane-liquid nitrogen), biochemistry (i.e., frozen in liquid nitrogen) and electron microscopy (i.e., fixed in glutaraldehyde).

Muscle biopsy is indicated in patients with limb weakness, infantile hypotonia, exercise intolerance, myoglobinuria, or cramps. A biopsy is also important in the final assessment of patients with a presumptive diagnosis of a muscular dystrophy, polymyositis, inclusion body myositis, congenital myopathy, glycolytic or oxidative enzyme defect, or myopathies associated with alcoholism, electrolyte disturbance, drug toxicity, carcinoma, endocrine disorders, or long-term treatment with steroids. It is also justified in polymyalgia rheumatica and eosinophilic fasciitis. In conjunction with sural nerve biopsy, it may demonstrate the extent of denervation in a peripheral neuropathy

Muscles preferred for biopsy are the vastus lateralis or biceps in disorders of proximal limb weakness and the gastrocnemius, tibialis anterior, or peroneus brevis in conditions affecting distal muscles. The muscle should be affected clinically and electrophysiologically. A clinically normal muscle may not be involved pathologically. Severely affected muscle should also be avoided, as it may show only end-stage changes, such as atrophy, fibrosis and fat deposition. Muscles subject to the trauma of intramuscular injections, EMG needles, or acupuncture must be avoided. The deltoid muscle should not be biopsied because the sample might include an intramuscular injection granuloma.

Routine histology of muscle may demonstrate groups of atrophic myofibers in a neurogenic disorder, or myopathic features that include necrotic fibers, regenerating fibers, excessive sarcoplasmic glycogen, or centrally located myonuclei. Lymphocytic infiltration of connective tissue is seen in dermatomyositis, polymyositis, and inclusion body myositis. The diagnosis of vasculitis or amyloidosis is occasionally established by finding changes in the muscle biopsy.

Histochemical techniques applied to cryosections of muscle permit the recognition of fiber-type grouping; target fibers; fiber-type predominance; selective fiber atrophy; central cores; nemaline rods; excessive sarcoplasmic glycogen, lipid, or mitochondria (ragged red fibers); deficiency of phosphorylase, phosphofructokinase, adenylate deaminase, or cytochrome *c* oxidase activity; and other structurally specific abnormalities that are not visible by conventional light microscopy of paraffin-embedded tissue. An example is provided by the finding of rimmed vacuoles and the intracellular amyloid inclusions of inclusion body myositis.

Biochemical assays of muscle may detect a quantitative reduction of enzymes of intermediary metabolism, including enzymes of the glycolytic pathway, acid maltase, adenylate deaminase, and enzymes of mitochondria (carnitine palmitoyl transferase, enzymes of the citric acid cycle, and electron transport chain).

Immunohistochemical stains may detect the absence of dystrophin in Duchenne muscular dystrophy and a mosaic pattern of dystrophin in female carriers of the mutation. Discontinuities of sarcolemmal dystrophin are found in Becker dystrophy. These dystrophinopathies may be detected by DNA analysis of blood leukocytes or by electrophoresis of a muscle homogenate (Western blot), to show quantitative or qualitative abnormalities of the protein. Dystrophin analysis is indicated in any patient with possible limb-girdle dystrophy, polymyositis, inclusion body myositis, myoglobinuria, myalgia, hyperCKemia or spinal muscular atrophy. Genetic lack of sarcoglycan proteins, merosin, dysferlin, calpain 3, emerin, or other proteins may be demonstrated by immunohistochemistry or immunoblot in the appropriate muscular dystrophies and confirmed by DNA analysis. Evaluation of mitochondrial DNA of muscle or blood may detect deletions in

Kearns-Sayre syndrome and point to mutations in other mitochondrial encephalomyopathies.

PERIPHERAL NERVE BIOPSY

Nerve biopsy is indicated in patients with peripheral neuropathy when additional information about the nature and severity of the disorder is needed. The biopsy is most likely helpful in mononeuritis multiplex or in patients with palpably enlarged nerves; biopsy is often uninformative in distal symmetric axonal neuropathies. In children, the pathologic features in nerve cells may be diagnostic in three diseases (metachromatic leukodystrophy, adrenoleukodystrophy, and Krabbe disease), but the biopsy may usually be avoided by making a diagnosis with blood analysis. Nerve biopsy also provides a diagnosis in giant axonal neuropathy. Several other central nervous system disorders are expressed pathologically in nerve: neuronal ceroid lipofuscinosis, Lafora disease, infantile neuroaxonal dystrophy, and lysosomal storage diseases. The best source of tissue for analysis in these cases, however, is not a nerve but rather skin and conjunctiva, because electron microscopic examination may show distinctive features in terminal nerve fibers and skin appendages.

The human sural nerve is the most widely studied nerve in health and disease, and it is most frequently recommended for biopsy. If mononeuritis multiplex spares the sural nerve, other cutaneous nerves may be selected (e.g., a branch of the superficial peroneal nerve at the head of the fibula or the radial sensory nerve at the wrist). Motor nerve fibers may be examined specifically in a nerve that supplies a superfluous or accessory muscle, such as the gracilis muscle in the medial thigh. Neurologists often choose simultaneous biopsy of both sural nerve and gastrocnemius muscle in patients with neuropathy because vasculitis, amyloidosis, sarcoid, lymphoma, and other systemic disorders are focal and lesions may be encountered in either tissue. The muscle also may demonstrate the degree of denervation.

Diagnosis may often be established by microscopic examination of paraffin-embedded tissue in nine conditions: vasculitis, amyloidosis, leprosy, sensory perineuritis, cholesterol emboli, infiltration of nerve by leukemic or lymphoma cells, malignant angioendotheliomatosis (intravascular lymphoma), giant axonal neuropathy, or adult polyglucosan body disease. Amyloid deposits in plasma cell dyscrasia may be identified by antibodies to immunoglobulin light chains. Amyloid deposits in the familial neuropathy resulting from transthyretin mutations may be distinguished by antibodies to the mutant protein. Small cell lymphoma and chronic lymphocytic leukemia may be separated from inflammatory reactions by application of lymphocyte markers.

Most neuropathies do not have distinctive pathologic findings and usually require examination of semithin sections of epoxy–resin-embedded tissue. Teased nerve fibers and electron microscopy are necessary to identify the focal thickening of myelin sheaths (*tomacula*) of hereditary neuropathy with liability to pressure palsy, and they may detect subtle degrees of demyelination, remyelination, or axonal degeneration and regeneration. These features occur in normal nerves with increasing age, and evaluation may require formal, quantitative study (morphometry). Electron microscopy also demonstrates accumulation of neurofilaments, widened myelin lamellae, and various intracellular inclusions in neuropathies, and is needed to assess unmyelinated nerve fibers.

Axonal neuropathy is recognized by marked depletion of fibers and interstitial fibrosis, with or without myelin debris or regeneration of axons. It is most likely caused by a toxic or metabolic disorder, such as alcoholism or diabetes. Other axonopathies include vasculitis, amyloidosis, paraneoplastic syndromes, and infection (including the distal symmetric neuropathy of AIDS). Segmental demyelination and remyelination, recognized by thinly myelinated fibers and onion bulbs, are most often the result of an immunologically mediated or hereditary neuropathy. If demyelination is not pronounced in semithin plastic sections, it may be proved by electron microscopy or analysis of teased, myelinated nerve fibers.

Sural nerve biopsy is recommended in patients with suspected chronic inflammatory demyelinating polyneuropathy but who have atypical clinical features or equivocal electrodiagnostic findings, before commencing therapy with intravenous gamma globulin, plasmapheresis, or steroids. The pathologic findings do not distinguish chronic inflammatory demyelinating polyneuropathy from Charcot-Marie-Tooth disease type I, but an acquired myelinopathy is favored by finding prominent variability of abnormalities among nerve fascicles, inflammatory infiltrates, and endoneurial edema. The neuropathies associated with IgM paraproteinemia and antibody-to-myelin associated glycoprotein resemble chronic inflammatory demyelinating polyneuropathy, both clinically and pathologically; deposits of the C3 component of complement may be seen along the periphery of myelin sheaths, usually with IgM located at the same site. Other demyelinative neuropathies include diphtheria, hereditary disorders other than Charcot-Marie-Tooth disease type I, Guillain-Barré syndrome, and acute or chronic inflammatory neuropathies in the early phase of human immunodeficiency virus infection. The inflammatory neuropathies are multifocal, and the sural nerve may be normal or show only axonal degeneration.

Complications of sural nerve involvement include permanent loss of discriminative sensation in the lateral border of the foot extending to the fifth toe, heel, and lateral malleolus, as well as neuropathic pain and paresthesias, such as causalgia in about 5% of patients or twinges of pain for several days when bending forward, caused by stretching of the nerve. In weeks or months, however, the sensory symptoms may subside completely or decrease to a tolerable level.

SKIN PUNCH BIOPSY

Skin punch biopsy is used to assess the extensive cutaneous network of sensory and autonomic nerves. The procedure is particularly useful in assessing small, unmyelinated fibers in patients with painful or other small-fiber neuropathy. It is simple and minimally invasive. As many neuropathies begin at the terminus of the longest nerve fibers and "die back" gradually toward the nerve cell, proximally, they may be detected first as a loss of the nerve endings in the epidermis. Skin biopsy is minimally invasive, and multiple samples may be obtained to compare proximal and distal sites in the same limb. In practice, axons are visualized by immunohistochemistry using the panaxonal marker PGP9.5 (a ubiquitin hydrolase). Nerve fibers are counted in a given length of the epidermis (epidermal nerve fiber density), to demonstrate a quantitative reduction from normal values. Potentially, other fibers may be evaluated, such as the sympathetic innervation of sweat glands and blood vessels, although no published analytic methods and normative values are available yet. The procedure may assess the course and special distribution of involvement in peripheral nerve disease. However, the pure sensory fiber neuropathy (usually manifest by burning feet and painful paresthesias) and toxic neuropathies are specific indications.

SUGGESTED READINGS

Dubowitz V. *Muscle Biopsy. A Practical Approach.* London: Churchill Livingstone, 1984.

Dubowitz V. *Muscle Disorders in Childhood,* 2nd ed. Philadelphia: WB Saunders, 1995.

Engel AG, Franzini Armstrong C. *Myology,* 3rd ed. New York: McGraw-Hill, 2004.

Graham DI, Lanatos PI. *Greenfield's Neuropathology,* 6th ed. London: Hodder & Stoughton Educational, 2002.

Griffin JW, Mc Arthur JC, Polydefkis M. Assessment of cutaneous innervation by skin biopsies. *Curr Op Neurol* 2001;14(5):655–659.

Lacomis D. The utility of muscle biopsy. *Curr Neurol Neurosci Rep* 2004;4(1):81–86.

Mendell JR, Kissel JT, Cornblath DR. *Diagnosis and Management of Peripheral Nerve Disorders.* New York: Oxford University Press, 2001.

Midroni G, Bilbao JM. *Biopsy Diagnosis of Peripheral Neuropathy.* Boston: Butterworth-Heinemann, 1995.

Said G. Indications and usefulness of nerve biopsy. *Arch Neurol* 2002; 59(10):1532–1535.

Chapter 20

Neuropsychologic Evaluation

Yaakov Stern

Neuropsychologic testing is a valuable adjunct to neurologic evaluation, especially to help make the diagnosis of such conditions as dementia, and to evaluate or quantify cognition and behavior in brain diseases. The tests are important in research as well.

STRATEGY OF NEUROPSYCHOLOGIC TESTING

Conditions that affect the brain often cause cognitive, motor, or behavioral impairment that may be detected by appropriately designed tests. Defective performance on a test may suggest specific pathology. Alternately, patients with known brain changes may be assessed to determine how the damaged brain areas affect specific cognitive functions. Before relating test performance to brain dysfunction, however, other factors that may affect test performance must be considered.

Typically, test performance is compared with values derived from populations similar to the patient in age, education, socioeconomic background, and other variables. Scores significantly below mean expected values imply impaired performance. Performance sometimes may be evaluated by assumptions about what may be expected from the average person (e.g., repeating simple sentences or simple learning and remembering).

Comparable data may not exist for the patient being tested. This problem is common in older populations or for those with language and cultural differences. This situation may be addressed by collecting local normal characteristics that are more descriptive of the served clinical population or by evaluating the cognitive areas that remain intact. In this way, the patient guides the clinician in terms of the level of performance that should be expected in possibly affected domains. Other factors that also influence test performance must be considered, including depression or other psychiatric disorders, medication, and the patient's motivation to participate fully.

Patterns of performance, such as strengths in some cognitive domains and weaknesses in others, have been associated with specific conditions, based on empiric observation and knowledge of the brain pathology associated with those conditions. Observation of these patterns may aid in diagnosis.

TEST SELECTION

Neuropsychologic tests in an assessment battery come from many sources. Some were developed for academic purposes (e.g., intelligence tests), and others from experimental psychology. The typical clinical battery consists of a series of standard tests that have been proved useful and are selected for the referral issue. These tests should have established reliability and validity. A trade-off exists between the breadth of application and ease of interpretation, available from standard batteries, and the ability to pinpoint specific or subtle disorders, offered by more experimental tasks that are useful in research but have not yet been standardized.

Most tests are intended to measure performance in specific cognitive or motor domains, such as memory, spatial ability, language function, or motor agility. These domains may be subdivided (e.g., memory may be considered verbal or nonverbal; immediate, short-term, long-term, or remote; semantic or episodic; public or autobiographic; or implicit or explicit). No matter how focused a test is, however, multiple cognitive processes are likely to be invoked. An ostensibly simple task, such as the Wechsler Adult Intelligence Scale Digit Symbol–Coding subtest (using a table of nine digit–symbol pairs to fill in the proper symbols for a series of numbers), assesses learning and memory, visuospatial abilities, motor abilities, attention, and speeded performance. In addition, tests may be failed for more than one reason: Patients may draw poorly because they may not appreciate spatial relationships or because they plan the construction process poorly. Relying solely on test scores may lead to spurious conclusions.

TESTS USED IN A NEUROPSYCHOLOGIC EVALUATION

Intellectual Ability

Typically, a test such as the Wechsler Adult Intelligence Scale-III (WAIS-III) or the Wechsler Intelligence Scale for Children-III (WISC-III) is used to assess the present level of intellectual function. These tests yield a global intelligence quotient (IQ) score, and verbal and performance IQ scores that are standardized, so that 100 is the mean expected value at any age (with a standard deviation of 15). The WAIS-III also groups some of the subtests, based on "more refined domains of cognitive functioning," into four index scales: Verbal Comprehension, Perceptual Organization, Working Memory, and Processing Speed. The index scales have the same psychometric properties as the traditional IQ scores.

▶ **TABLE 20.1 Subtests of the Wechsler Adult Intelligence Scale-III**

Verbal subsets	
Vocabulary	Defining 33 words. Typically represents "premorbid" level of ability.
Similarities	Deriving relevant superordinate category or similarity for 19 word pairs. Assesses abstract reasoning.
Arithmetic	20 verbal arithmetic problems.
Digit span	Standardized assessment of digits forward and backward. Primarily assesses attention and working memory.
Information	28 general information items. Assesses "old stores" of information.
Comprehension	18 items assessing appreciation of social norms and standards and proverb interpretation.
Letter-number sequencing[a]	New. Listening to a combination of numbers and letters and recalling the numbers first in ascending order and then the letters alphabetical order. Assesses working memory.
Performance subtests	
Picture completion	Determining the missing feature in 25 pictures.
Digit symbol-coding	Using a table of nine digit-symbol pairs to fill in the proper symbols for a series of numbers. Taps new learning, visuospatial abilities, and speeded performance.
Block design	Arranging blocks with red, white, and half-red and half-white sides to form 14 designs. A complex visuospatial task.
Matrix reasoning	New. Identifying the picture that completes a pattern, using pattern completion, classification, analogy, or serial reasoning. A nonverbal intelligence test.
Picture arrangement	Arranging sets of comic-strip pictures so that they tell a coherent story.
Symbol search[a]	New. Visually scanning a target group of items (composed of two symbols) and a search group (composed of five symbols) and indicating whether either of the target symbols match any of the symbols in the search group.
Object assembly	Assembling five jigsaw puzzles.

[a] Contributes to index scores but not to intelligence quotient scores.

The WAIS-III consists of seven verbal and seven performance subtests. Scaled scores range from 1 to 19, with a mean of 10 and a standard deviation of 3; the average range for subtest scaled scores is from 7 to 13 (Table 20.1).

The overall, Verbal IQ and Performance IQ scores supply information about the level of general intelligence, but the neuropsychologist is usually more interested in the "scatter" of subtest scores, which indicates strengths and weaknesses. The subtests are better considered as separate

▶ **TABLE 20.2 Typical Subclassifications of Memory Addressed by Neuropsychologic Tests**

Verbal and nonverbal	Memory for material that is or is not verbally encoded.
Immediate, short-term, long-term, and remote	Length of time between exposure to material and recall. The length of time has implications for how the memory may be stored and retrieved.
Semantic and episodic	Memory for encodeable knowledge, such as vocabulary or facts about the world, as opposed to memory for events.
Public and autobiographic	Memory for public commonly known events versus events that occurred in one's own life.
Implicit and explicit	Memory tested on tasks that do not require conscious explicit recollection of recent exposures (such as motor skills, procedural skills, classical conditioning, or priming) versus tasks that demand explicit recall of prior information (such as recall or recognition tasks).
Working	Similar to what in the past has been called short-term memory, working memory provides a buffer for briefly holding on to information, such as a telephone number or the name of a newly met person. It is also important for tasks that require mental manipulation of information, such as multistep arithmetic problems. For many theorists, working memory also has a more important role as the work space where recalled information is actually used, manipulated, and related to other information, allowing complex cognitive processes such as comprehension learning and reasoning to take place.

tests, each assessing specific areas of cognitive function. There are many other tests of general intelligence, including some that are nonverbal.

Memory

The subclassifications of memory have evolved from clinical observation and experimentation; most are important to the assessment (Table 20.2).

For example, preservation of remote memories, despite the inability to store and recall new information, is the hallmark of specific amnestic disorders. Other subclassifications are used to evaluate different clinical syndromes.

Construction

Construction, typically assessed by drawing or assembly tasks, requires both accurate spatial perception and an organized motor response. The Block Design and Object

Assembly subtests of the WAIS-R are examples of assembly tasks. In the Rey Osterrieth Complex Figure, the patient is asked to copy a figure that contains many details embedded within an organizing framework. In addition to the scores these tests yield, the clinician attends to the patient's construction performance to determine factors that may underlie poor performance (e.g., a disorganized impulsive strategy may be more related to anterior brain lesions, whereas difficulty aligning angles may arise in parietal lobe injury).

Language

"Mapping" of different aphasic disorders to specific brain structures was one of the early accomplishments of behavioral neurology. In neuropsychologic assessment, this model is often followed. Comprehension, fluency, repetition, and naming are assessed in spoken or written language.

Perceptual

Neuropsychologists may provide a standardized version of the neurologists' perceptual tasks: double (simultaneous) stimulation in touch, hearing, or sight; stereognosis; graphesthesia; spatial perception; or auditory discrimination.

Executive

The ability to plan, sequence, and monitor behavior has been called "executive function." These functions, linked to the prefrontal cortex, rely on and organize other intact cognitive functions that are required components for performance. Formal tests of executive function may be divided into set switching and set maintenance. For set switching, the Wisconsin Card Sort uses symbols that may be sorted by color, number, or shape. Based only on feedback about whether each card was or was not correctly placed, the subject must infer an initial sort rule. At intervals, the sort rule is changed without the subject's knowledge; subjects must switch based only on their own observation that the current rule is no longer effective.

The Stroop Color-Word Test assesses set maintenance. The subject is given a series of color names printed in contrasting ink colors (e.g., the word "blue" printed in red ink) and is asked to name the color of the ink. The response set must be maintained while the subject suppresses the alternate (and more standard) inclination to read words without regard to the color of the print.

Certain working memory tasks, such as the Number Letter Ordering Subtest of the WAIS-III, require patients to manipulate retained information and are also considered to have an executive component that assesses prefrontal cortex function.

Motor and Praxis

Tests of motor strength, such as grip strength, and of motor speed and agility, such as assessing speed and peg placement, establish lateral dominance and focal point of impairment. In some diseases, such as the dementia of AIDS, reduced motor agility is part of the diagnosis. Higher order motor tasks, such as double-alternating movements or triple sequences, are used to assess motor sequencing or programming, as opposed to pure strength or speed.

Attention

The ability to sustain attention is often tested by cancellation tasks, in which the patient must detect and mark targets embedded in distractors, or by reaction-time tasks. Speed and accuracy are the outcome measures. Mental tracking tasks such as Digit Span Forward may also be included in this category.

Concept Formation and Reasoning

Brain damage is often associated with concrete reasoning. Tests of concept formation include verbal tasks, such as proverb interpretation, and nonverbal tasks, where underlying concepts must be extracted from visual displays. Tests of abstract reasoning include the Similarities subtest of the WAIS-III, where the subject must explain how two words are alike. The quality of the response is judged. A general classification response that is pertinent to both words receives a higher score than a specific property or function that is relevant to both.

Personality and Emotional Status

Mood may affect test performance. At minimum, the neuropsychologist notes the psychiatric history and probes for current psychiatric symptoms. Standardized mood rating scales are also available. Many neurophysiologists use standardized personality scales to aid in diagnosis and test interpretation.

CLINICAL OBSERVATION

Along with the formal scores, the intake interview and testing period afford an extensive period to observe the patient under controlled conditions. These clinical observations are valuable for diagnosis. Formal test scores capture only certain aspects of performance. The patient's problem-solving approach or the nature of the errors made may be telling. Also important in timed tasks is determining whether the patient may complete them with additional time or is actually incapable of solving them. Another important dimension of assessment is the patient's ability to learn and follow directions, for the many tests.

More subtle aspects of behavior include responses or coping abilities when confronted with difficult tasks, the ability to remain socially appropriate as the session progresses, and the subjects' appreciation of their own capacities.

REFERRAL ISSUES

Neuropsychologic testing is useful for the diagnosis of some conditions and is a tool for evaluating or quantifying the effects of disease on cognition and behavior. The tests may assess the beneficial or adverse effects of drug therapy, radiation, or surgery. Serial evaluations give quantitative results that may change with time. In temporal lobectomy for intractable epilepsy, tests that help identify the location of dysfunction are required in presurgical evaluation in order to minimize the possibility of adverse effects. Specific referral issues are summarized in the following paragraphs.

Dementia

Testing may detect early dementing changes and discriminate them from "normal" performance or obtain information contributing to differential diagnosis either between dementia and nondementing illness, such as depression versus dementia, or between alternate forms of dementia (e.g., Alzheimer disease, dementia with Lewy bodies, or vascular dementia). Test results may also confirm or quantify disease progression and measure efficacy of clinical interventions.

Other Brain Disease

The effects on cognitive function of stroke, cancer, head trauma, Parkinson disease, Huntington disease, multiple sclerosis, brain infection or other conditions may be investigated. Testing may be prompted by the patient's complaints. The evaluation helps to clarify the cause or extent of the condition.

Epilepsy

Testing is needed for presurgical evaluation, because determining the lateral dominance of memory and language, as well as the focal point of cognitive impairments, are important concerns. Pre- and postoperative evaluations after other types of neurosurgery are also common.

Toxic Exposure

Testing may evaluate consequences of toxic or potentially toxic exposures, either on an individual basis or for particular exposed groups (e.g., factory workers). Ex-

posures may include metals, solvents, pesticides, alcohol and drugs, or any other compounds that may affect the brain.

Medication

The potential effect of medications on the central nervous system may be evaluated in therapeutic trials or clinical practice. For example, in trials of agents to treat Alzheimer disease, neuropsychologic tests are typically primary measures of drug efficacy. In clinical practice, adverse or therapeutic effects of newly introduced medications may be evaluated.

Psychiatric Disorders

Testing may help in the differential diagnosis of psychiatric and neurologic disorders, especially affective disorders and schizophrenia. It may also assess cognition and areas of competence in patients with these conditions.

Learning Disability

Testing will evaluate learning disabilities and the residuals of these disabilities in later life. Behavioral disorders, attention deficit disorder, autism, dyslexia, and learning problems are common referral issues.

EXPECTATIONS FROM A NEUROPSYCHOLOGIC EVALUATION

The minimum that a neuropsychologic evaluation yields is an extensive investigation of the abilities of the patient. In these cases, although the studies do not lead to a definite diagnosis, they help to determine the patient's capacities, establish a baseline from which to track the future, and advise the patient and family.

Sometimes the evaluation suggests that additional diagnostic tests would be useful. For example, if a patient's pattern of performance deviates substantially from that typically expected at the current stage of dementia, a vascular contribution may be considered. Similarly, evaluation may suggest the value of psychiatric consultation or more intensive electroencephalographic recordings.

Many times the neuropsychologist may offer a tentative diagnosis or discuss the possible diagnoses compatible with the test findings. Neuropsychologic evaluation may not yield a diagnosis without appropriate clinical and historic information. In the context of a multidisciplinary testing, however, it may provide evidence to confirm or refute a specific diagnosis. Testing might best be considered an additional source of information to be used by the clinician for diagnosis in conjunction with the neurologic examination and laboratory tests.

HOW TO REFER

The more information the examiner has at the start, the more directly the issues may be addressed. For example, if magnetic resonance imaging has revealed a particular lesion, tests may be tailored specifically. The examination is not an exploration of the ability to detect a lesion, but is a contribution to understanding the implications of the lesion. Similarly, the more explicit the referral question, the more likely the evaluation may yield useful information. Besides providing the relevant history, a useful referral describes the problem to be assessed. This is often a statement of the differential diagnosis being entertained. Alternately, the neurologist or the family may simply want to document the current condition or explore some specific aspect of performance, such as language.

SUGGESTED READINGS

Caccappolo-vanVliet E, Manly J, Tang MX, et al. The neuropsychological profiles of mild Alzheimer's disease and questionable dementia as compared to age-related cognitive decline. *J Int Neuropsych Soc* 2003;9:720–732.

Lezak MD. *Neuropsychological Assessment,* 3rd ed. New York: Oxford University Press, 1995.

Ron MA, Toone BK, Garralda ME, Lishman WA. Diagnostic accuracy in presenile dementia. *Br J Psychiatry* 1979;134:161–168.

Wechsler D. *Wechsler Intelligence Scale for Children,* 3rd ed. San Antonio, TX: The Psychological Corp., 1991.

Wechsler D. *Wechsler Adult Intelligence Scale,* 3rd ed. San Antonio, TX: The Psychological Corp., 1997.

Chapter 21

DNA Diagnosis

Lewis P. Rowland, Salvatore DiMauro, and Michio Hirano

Molecular genetics has revolutionized clinical medicine. Before 1980, diagnosis of an inherited disease depended primarily on clinical recognition. For some diseases, biochemical tests identified the disease by the excretion or storage of an abnormal metabolite or, best of all, by finding decreased activity of the responsible enzyme.

That was the era of biochemical genetics, and one of the clinical lessons we learned was the recognition of phenotypic heterogeneity. The same enzyme abnormality might be associated with totally different clinical manifestations. For instance, the original clinical concept of muscle phosphorylase deficiency was a syndrome of muscle cramps and myoglobinuria induced by exertion, usually starting in adolescence. Later, however, we recognized totally different disorders as manifestations of phosphorylase deficiency. Infantile and late-onset forms have symptoms of limb weakness but no myoglobinuria. Biochemical analysis in these diseases, as described in the chapters on metabolic diseases, is still important.

The molecular genetic era of neurology began in 1983 with linkage of Huntington disease to the short arm of chromosome 4. Four years later, identification of mutations in the gene for the protein dystrophin as the cause of Duchenne muscular dystrophy demonstrated the capacity of positional cloning (isolating genes within a chromosomal locus) to reveal the cause of monogenic disorders (inherited diseases due to mutations in single genes). Since then, about 500 chromosomal loci and more than 250 causative genes have been linked to human neurologic diseases. The process of gene hunting (identification of disease-causing genes) has been greatly accelerated by two draft sequences of the human genome; these sequences have largely eliminated positional cloning by allowing investigators to identify candidate genes and pathogenic mutations within chromosomal loci linked to diseases. In addition to diseases of the nuclear genome, more than 150 point mutations and large-scale rearrangements of the mitochondrial genome have been recognized as causes of neurologic diseases.

▶ TABLE 21.1 DNA Diagnosis in Neurologic Disease

Amino acid metabolism defects: glutaric acidurias; 4-hydroxybutyric aciduria; phenylketonuria; nonketotic hyperglycinemia; maple-syrup urine disease

Ataxias: SCA, FA, MJD, AT, EA, AVED, abetalipoproteinemia, AVED, ARSA, AOA

Congenital disorders of glycosylation

Dementia: Alzheimer disease, Pick disease, FTD tauopathy

Epilepsy: PME1, BFNC, GEFS+, SMEI, GEFS+/Absence, JME, Lafora disease, Unverricht-Lundborg disease; ADNFLE, Partial epilepsy with auditory features

Episodic ataxia

Glucose transporter defects: Glut 1 deficiency syndrome

Hemiplegic migraine

Huntington disease

Inclusion body myopathy

Headaches: hemiplegic migraine

Leukodystrophies: ALD, Alexander disease, benign megalencephaly with leukodystrophy, Canavan disease, Krabbe disease, MLD, vacuolating leukoencephalopathy

Lipid metabolism disorders: long-chain fatty acid oxidation defects (CPT I and II deficiencies, CACT); beta-oxidation defects; multiple acyl-CoA dehydrogenation defects

Lysosomal disorders: beta-galactosidase deficiency, disorders of glycoprotein degradation, Fabry disease, Farber disease, Gaucher disease, GM2 gangliosidoses, MLD, MSD, Krabbe disease, LAMP-2 deficiency, mucopolysaccharidoses, mucolipidoses, NCL, Niemann-Pick diseases, Pompe disease, Schindler disease

Mental retardation, developmental disorders: Down syndrome, fragile X, Williams syndrome, Angelman syndrome, Prader-Willi syndrome

Metabolic myopathies: Acid maltase deficiency; carnitine palmityl transferase II (CPT II) deficiency; phosphorylase deficiency (McArdle disease) phosphofructokinase deficiency (Tarui disease), PGK deficiency, PGAM deficiency; LDH deficiency; beta-enolase deficiency

Mitochondrial encephalomyopathies: KSS, PEO, MELAS, MERRF, NARP, LHON, MNGIE, Leigh syndrome

Motor neuron diseases: FALS (SOD1, alsin, SMA, XSBMA)

Movement disorders: DRPLA, DYT, Huntington disease, Menkes disease, Wilson disease

Muscular dystrophies: DMD, BMD, DM, EDMD, FSHD, LGMD, congenital, distal forms

Myasthenia gravis: congenital

Myopathies: OPMD, congenital myopathies, distal myopathies, HIBM

Myotonia congenita; nondystrophic myotonias

Myotonic muscular dystrophies: DM, PROMM

Parkinson disease: Juvenile PD/Parkin, SNCA, UCHL1

Periodic paralysis: HoPP, HyPP, Andersen syndrome

Peripheral neuropathies: CMT, DSS, FAP, HMN, HNPP, HSAN, HSMN, CCFDN

Peroxisomal disorders: Zellweger syndrome, RCDP, X-ALD, Refsum disease, D-bifunctional deficiency, Acyl-CoA deficiency, racemase deficiency

Phakomatoses: NF1, NF2, tuberous sclerosis, VHL, xeroderma pigmentosum

Prion diseases: CJD, GSS, FFI

Spastic paraplegia: hereditary spastic paraplegias

Stroke syndromes: activated protein C resistance (Leiden factor V mutation), CADASIL, DCH, homocystinuria, protein C deficiency, protein S deficiency

Tumor syndromes: phakomatoses, retinoblastoma, Turcot syndrome

ADNFLE, autosomal dominant nocturnal frontal lobe epilepsy; ALD, adrenoleukodystrophy; AT; ataxia-telangiectasia; AOA, ataxia with oculomotor apraxia; ARSA, autosomal recessive spastic ataxia; AVED, ataxia with vitamin E deficiency; BFNC, benign familial neonatal convulsions; BMD, Becker muscular dystrophy; CACT, carnitine acyl-carnitine deficiency; CADASIL, cerebral autosomal dominant arteriopathy with subcortical infarcts and leucoencephalopathy; CCFDN, congenital cataracts, facial dysmorphism and neuropathy; CJD, Creutzfeldt-Jakob disease; CMT, Charcot-Marie-Tooth; DCH, Dutch cerebral hemorrhage; DM, myotonic muscular dystrophy (dystrophia myotonica); DMD, Duchenne muscular dystrophy; DRPLA, dentato-rubro-pallido-luysian atrophy; DSS, Dejerine-Sottas syndrome; DYT, dystonia; EA, episodic ataxia; EDMD, Emery-Dreifuss muscular dystrophy; FA, Friedreich ataxia; FAD, familial Alzheimer disease; FALS, familial amyotrophic lateral sclerosis; FAP, familial amyloidotic polyneuropathy; FFI, familial fatal insomnia; FSHMD, facioscapulohumeral muscular dystrophy; FTD, frontotemporal dementia (familial tauopathy, Wilhelmsen-Lynch disease); JME, juvenile myoclonic epilepsy; GEFS+, generalized epilepsy with febrile seizures plus; GEFS+/Absence, generalized epilepsy with febrile seizures and absence; GSS, Gerstmann-Sträussler-Scheinker disease; HIBM, hereditary inclusion body myopathy; HNPP, hereditary neuropathy with liability to pressure palsies; HoPP, hypokalemic periodic paralysis; HMN, hereditary motor neuropathies; HSAN, hereditary sensory and autonomic neuropathies; HyPP, hyperkalemic periodic paralysis; KSS, Kearns-Sayre syndrome; LDH, lactate dehydrogenase; LGMD, limb-girdle muscular dystrophy; LHON, Leber hereditary optic atrophy; MELAS, mitochondrial encephalomyelopathy, lactic acidosis, and stroke; MERRF, myoclonus epilepsy and ragged red fibers; MJD, Machado Joseph disease; MLD, metachromatic leukodystrophy; MSD, multiple sulfatase deficiency; MNGIE, mitochondrial neurogastrointestinal encephalomyopathy; NARP, neuropathy, ataxia, retinitis pigmentosa; NCL, neuronal ceroid lipofuscinosis; NF1, neurofibromatosis type 1 (von Recklinghausen disease); NF2, neurofibromatosis type 2, familial acoustic neuroma; OPMD, oculopharyngeal muscular dystrophy; PEO, progressive external ophthalmoplegia; PGK, phosphoglycerate kinase; PGAM, phosphoglycerate mutase; PME, progressive myoclonus epilepsy; PROMM, proximal myotonic myopathy (Ricker syndrome); RCDP, rhizomelic chondrodysplasia punctata; SCA, spinocerebellar atrophy; SMA, spinal muscular atrophy (Werdnig-Hoffmann, Kugelberg-Welander syndromes); SMEI, severe myoclonic epilepsy of infancy; SNCA, synuclein alpha; UCHL1, ubiquitin carboxy terminal hydrolase L1X-ALD; VHL, Von Hippel-Lindau; XSBMA, X-linked spinobulbar muscular atrophy (Kennedy syndrome).

DNA ANALYSIS: NOMENCLATURE

We can now diagnose genetic diseases by DNA analysis. Currently, several hundred individual diseases are amenable to DNA diagnosis, and it would take a booklet to tabulate them one by one. Instead, they may be grouped into 29 broad clinical categories (Table 21.1).

For some conditions, we are in the peculiar position of trying to decide whether the disease should be named according to the change in DNA or, as in the past, by the clinical features. The dilemma arises because of three kinds of genetic heterogeneity (Table 21.2).

One is called *allelic heterogeneity*, in which different mutations in the same gene locus cause one phenotype. By contrast, *allelic affinity* refers to different mutations in the same gene producing different phenotypes As a result, more than one clinical syndrome may be caused by mutations in the same gene (one gene: multiple phenotypes). For example, duplication of the *PMP22* gene causes Charcot-Marie-Tooth disease 1A while deletion of the same gene causes hereditary neuropathy with liability to pressure palsy (HNPP). Those clinical differences might be related to the dosage of the mutated gene, which differs as a result of a deletion or a duplication. More mysterious are conditions associated with mutations in lamin A/C, which have been associated with seven different phenotypes: autosomal dominant Emery-Dreifuss muscular dystrophy, limb-girdle muscular dystrophy 1B, Charcot-Marie Tooth disease 2C, familial partial lipodystrophy, cardiomyopathy, mandibuloacral dysplasia, and progeria. How this multiplicity arises is uncertain; modifying actions of other genes or environmental factors may play a role.

Conversely, the third type is *locus heterogeneity*, that is, the same clinical syndrome may be caused by mutations in different genes on different chromosomes, as exemplified by limb-girdle muscular dystrophy that has been subclassified into 17 genetically distinct forms, and by spinocerebellar ataxia (SCA) that has been molecularly delineated into SCA 1 through SCA 22 (one phenotype: multiple genes). It is difficult for clinicians to communicate about numeric names like these, but no alternative is in sight unless distinctive clinical manifestations emerge to provide old-fashioned names for diseases (i.e., in plain words).

Another problem of nomenclature arises from the diverse clinical syndromes caused by similar mutations, such as expansion of trinucleotide repeats or mutations in ion channel genes. Genetic diseases are often grouped according to etiologic categories, as in the case of diseases arising from ion channel mutations, and these disorders are often described as channelopathies. Although the molecular changes are similar, there is little clinical similarity, for instance, between hemiplegic migraine and periodic paralysis (except that they are intermittent disorders).

▶ **TABLE 21.2 Genetic Terms**

allelic heterogeneity: Different mutations in the same gene at the same chromosomal locus cause a single phenotype, the same disease or syndrome.

allelic affinity: Different mutations in the same gene at the same chromosomal locus cause more than one phenotype, different diseases or syndromes.

locus heterogeneity: Mutations in genes at different chromosomal loci cause the same phenotype, disease or syndrome.

GENE IDENTIFICATION: MULTIPURPOSE ANALYSIS

Identification of disease genes has more than diagnostic value; for many of these disorders, the functions of candidate gene products was known and provided pathogenic insights, which led to more rational therapeutic approaches. For example, pathogenic human SOD1 gene mutations that cause familial ALS have been expressed in transgenic mice, which have been valuable models to use in the study of pathogenic mechanisms and to identify potential therapeutic drugs such as minocycline.

At present, there are still major impediments to widespread applicability of DNA analysis for diagnosis. First, reimbursement for mutation screening is not established in many parts of the United States or elsewhere. Second, as a result, a systematic development of diagnostic laboratories has not yet emerged, not even commercially. Consequently, testing is often left to research laboratories, which is an inefficient use of resources. A nonprofit web site (http://www.genetests.org) lists laboratories that perform genetic tests and serves as an online textbook of human genetics.

SUGGESTED READINGS

DiMauro S, Schon EA. Mitochondrial respiratory chain diseases. *N Engl J Med* 2003;348:2656–2668.

GeneTests: Medical Genetics Information Resource (database online). Seattle: University of Washington and Children's Health System, 1993–2004. Updated weekly. Available at *http://www.genetests.org*

Harding AE. The DNA laboratory and neurological practice. *J Neurol Neurosurg Psychiatry* 1993;56:229–233.

McKusick VA. *Mendelian Inheritance in Man*, 12th ed. Baltimore: Johns Hopkins University Press, 1998.

Online Mendelian Inheritance in Man, OMIM™. Baltimore: Johns Hopkins University and Bethesda: National Center for Biotechnology Information, National Library of Medicine. Available at *http://www.ncbi.nlm.nih.gov/omim*

Pulst SM. *Neurogenetics*. New York: Oxford Press, 2000.

Rosenberg RN, Prusiner SB, DiMauro S, et al. *The Molecular and Genetic Basis of Neurological Disease*, 3rd ed. Boston: Butterworth-Heinemann, 2003.

Rowland LP. The first decade of molecular genetics in neurology; changing clinical thought and practice. *Ann Neurol* 1992;32:207–214.

Rowland LP. Molecular basis of genetic heterogeneity: role of the clinical neurologist. *J Child Neurol* 1998;13:122–132.

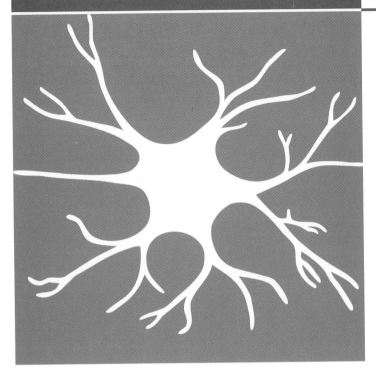

Infections of the
Nervous System

Chapter 22

Bacterial Infections

Burk Jubelt

The parenchyma, coverings, and blood vessels of the nervous system may be invaded by virtually any pathogenic microorganism. It is customary, for convenience of description, to divide the syndromes produced according to the major site of involvement. This division is arbitrary because the inflammatory process frequently involves more than one of these structures.

Involvement of the meninges by pathogenic microorganisms is known as *leptomeningitis,* because the infection and inflammatory response are generally confined to the subarachnoid space and the arachnoid and pia. Cases are divided into acute, subacute, and chronic meningitis, according to the rapidity with which the inflammatory process develops. This rate of development, in part, is related to the nature of the infecting organism.

ACUTE PURULENT MENINGITIS

Bacteria may gain access to the ventriculo-subarachnoid space by way of the blood, in the course of septicemia or as a metastasis from infection of the heart, lung, or other viscera. The meninges may also be invaded by direct extension, from a septic focus in the skull, spine, or parenchyma of the nervous system (e.g., sinusitis, otitis, osteomyelitis, and brain abscess). Organisms may gain entrance to the subarachnoid space through compound fractures of the skull and fractures through the nasal sinuses or mastoid, or after neurosurgical procedures. Pathogen introduction by lumbar puncture is rare. The pathologic background, symptoms, and clinical course of most patients with acute purulent meningitis are similar, regardless of the causative organisms. The diagnosis and therapy depend on the isolation and identification of the organisms and the determination of the source of the infection.

Acute purulent meningitis may be the result of infection with almost any pathogenic bacteria. Isolated examples of infection by the uncommon forms are recorded in the literature. In the United States, *Streptococcus pneumoniae* now accounts for about one-half of cases when the infecting organism is identified, and *Neisseria meningitidis* accounts for about one-fourth of the cases (Table 22.1).

In recent years, there has been an increase in the incidence of cases in which no organism may be isolated. These patients now make up the third major category of purulent meningitis. This may be due to the administration of therapy before admission to the hospital and the performance of lumbar puncture. In the neonatal period, group B streptococci and *Escherichia coli* are the most common causative agents. Approximately 60% of the postneonatal bacterial meningitis of children used to be caused by *Hemophilus influenzae.* The impact of *H. influenzae B* vaccine has been dramatic. In the past decade there has been a 100-fold decrease in incidence. In 1997 there were less that 300 cases reported. Overall fatality rate from bacterial meningitis is now 10% or less. Many deaths occur during the first 48 hours of hospitalization.

For convenience, special features of the common forms of acute purulent meningitis are described separately. Neonatal infections are reviewed in Chapter 75.

Meningococcal Meningitis

Meningococcal meningitis was described by Vieusseux in 1805, and the causative organism was identified by Weichselbaum in 1887. It occurs in sporadic form and at irregular intervals in epidemics. Epidemics are especially likely to occur during large shifts in population, as in time of war.

Pathogenesis

Meningococci *(N. meningitidis)* may occasionally gain access to the meninges directly from the nasopharynx through the cribriform plate. The bacteria, however, usually are recovered from blood or cutaneous lesions before the meningitis, thus indicating that spread to the nervous system is hematogenous in most instances. The ventricular

▶ **TABLE 22.1** Causes of 248 Cases of Bacterial Meningitis in 1995 and Overall Fatality Rate According to Organism

Organism	No. of Cases Reported	Percentage of Total[a]	Incidence[b]	Case Fatality Rate (%)[c]
Hemophilus influenzae	18	7	0.2	6
Streptococcus pneumoniae	117	47	1.1	21
Neisseria meningitidis	62	26	0.6	3
Group B streptococcus	31	12	0.3	7
Listeria monocytogenes	20	8	0.2	15

[a]Because of rounding, the percentages do not total 100.
[b]The incidence is the number of cases per 100,000 population.
[c]Outcome data were missing for 11 cases of meningitis (4%). The fatality rates are based on cases with known outcome.
From Schuchat A, Robinson K, Werger J, et al., 1997.

fluid may be teeming with organisms before the meninges become inflamed.

Recent studies have defined more clearly the role of bacterial elements in the initiation of meningitis with meningococcus and other bacteria. The bacterial capsule appears most important in the attachment and penetration to gain access to the body. Elements in the bacterial cell wall appear critical in penetration into the CSF space through vascular endothelium and the induction of the inflammatory response.

Pathology

In acute fulminating cases, death may occur before there are any significant pathologic changes in the nervous system. In the usual case, when death does not occur for several days after the onset of the disease, an intense inflammatory reaction occurs in the meninges. The inflammatory reaction is especially severe in the subarachnoid spaces over the convexity of the brain and around the cisterns at the base of the brain. It may extend a short distance along the perivascular spaces into the substance of the brain and spinal cord but rarely breaks into the parenchyma. Meningococci, both intra- and extracellular, are found in the meninges and CSF. With progress of the infection, the pia-arachnoid becomes thickened, and adhesions may form. Adhesions at the base may interfere with the flow of CSF from the fourth ventricle and may produce hydrocephalus. Inflammatory reaction and fibrosis of the meninges along the roots of the cranial nerves are thought to be the cause of the cranial nerve palsies that are seen occasionally.

Damage to the auditory nerve often occurs suddenly, and the auditory defect is usually permanent. Such damage may result from extension of the infection to the inner ear or thrombosis of the nutrient artery. Facial paralysis frequently occurs after the meningeal reaction has subsided. Signs and symptoms of parenchymal damage (e.g., hemiplegia, aphasia, and cerebellar signs) are infrequent

and are probably due to infarcts as the result of thrombosis of inflamed arteries or veins.

With effective treatment, and in some cases without treatment, the inflammatory reaction in the meninges subsides, and no evidence of the infection may be found at autopsy in patients who die months or years later.

In the past, the inflammation in meningitis had been attributed mainly to the toxic effects of the bacteria. In all types of meningitis, the contribution to the inflammatory process of various cytokines released by phagocytic and immuno-active cells, particularly interleukin 1 and tumor necrosis factor, has been recognized. These studies have formed the basis for the use of antiinflammatory corticosteroids in the treatment of meningitis. Several studies in both *H. influenzae* and *S. pneumonia* meningitis have suggested an improved outcome with the use of corticosteroids, particularly if the steroids are given shortly before the initiation of antibiotics. Treatment usually continues for 4 days. Corticosteroids are beneficial in the treatment of children with acute bacterial meningitis. The data in adults are too limited to make a definite recommendation but favor steroid therapy.

Epidemiology

Meningococcus is the causative organism in about 25% of all cases of bacterial meningitis in the United States. Serogroup B is now the most commonly reported causative type (50%). Although both the sporadic and the epidemic forms of the disease may attack individuals of all ages, children and young adults are predominantly affected. The normal habitat of the meningococcus is the nasopharynx, and the disease is spread by carriers or by individuals with the disease. A polysaccharide vaccine for groups A, C, Y, and W-135 meningococci has reduced the incidence of meningococcal infection among military recruits. The vaccine also has been used for control of serogroup C outbreaks in schools and on college campuses.

Symptoms

The onset of meningococcal meningitis is similar to that of other forms of meningitis, and is accompanied by chills and fever, headache, nausea and vomiting, pain in the back, stiffness of the neck, and prostration. The occurrence of herpes labialis, conjunctivitis, and a petechial or hemorrhagic skin rash is common with meningococcal infections. At the onset, the patient is irritable. In children, there is frequently a characteristic sharp, shrill cry (meningeal cry). With progress of the disease, the sensorium becomes clouded and stupor or coma may develop. Occasionally, the onset may be fulminant and accompanied by deep coma. Convulsive seizures are often an early symptom, especially in children, but focal neurologic signs are uncommon. Acute fulminating cases with severe circulatory collapse are relatively rare.

Signs

The patient appears acutely ill and may be confused, stuporous, or semicomatose. The temperature is elevated at 101°F to 103°F, but it may occasionally be normal at the onset. The pulse is usually rapid and the respiratory rate is increased. Blood pressure is normal except in acute fulminating cases when there may be profound hypotension. A petechial rash may be found in the skin, mucous membranes, or conjunctiva but never in the nail beds. It usually fades in 3 days or 4 days. There is rigidity of the neck with positive Kernig and Brudzinski signs. These signs may be absent in newborn, elderly, or comatose patients. Increased intracranial pressure causes bulging of an unclosed anterior fontanelle and periodic respiration. The reflexes are often decreased but occasionally may be increased. Cranial nerve palsies and focal neurologic signs are uncommon and usually do not develop until several days after the onset of the infection. The optic disks are normal, but papilledema may develop if the meningitis persists for more than a week.

Laboratory Data

The blood white cell count is increased, usually in the range of 10,000/mm^3 to 30,000/mm^3, but occasionally may be normal or higher than 40,000/mm^3. The urine may contain albumin, casts, and red blood cells. Meningococci may be cultured from the nasopharynx in most cases, from the blood in more than 50% of the cases in the early stages, and from the skin lesions when these are present.

The CSF is under increased pressure, usually between 200 mm H$_2$O and 500 mm H$_2$O. The CSF is cloudy (purulent) because it contains a large number of cells, predominantly polymorphonuclear leukocytes. The cell count in the fluid is usually between 2,000/mm^3 and 10,000/mm^3.

Occasionally, it may be less than 100/mm^3 and infrequently more than 20,000/mm^3. The protein content is increased. The sugar content is decreased, usually to levels below 20 mg/dL. Gram-negative diplococci may be seen intra- and extracellularly in stained smears of the fluid, and meningococci may be cultured in more than 90% of untreated patients. Particle agglutination may rapidly identify bacterial antigens in the CSF. It may not be relied on for definite diagnosis, however, because of relatively low specificity and sensitivity. For meningococcus, the capsular polysaccharide is the antigen detected. In unusual instances, the CSF may demonstrate minimal or no increase in cell count and no bacteria on the Gram stain, but *N. meningitidis* may be isolated. Clear CSF in a patient with suspected bacterial meningitis must be cultured carefully.

Complications and Sequelae

The complications and sequelae include those commonly associated with an inflammatory process in the meninges and its blood vessels (i.e., convulsions, cranial nerve palsies, focal cerebral lesions, damage to the spinal cord or nerve roots, hydrocephalus) and those that are due to involvement of other portions of the body by meningococci (e.g., panophthalmitis and other types of ocular infection, arthritis, purpura, pericarditis, endocarditis, myocarditis, pleurisy, orchitis, epididymitis, albuminuria or hematuria, adrenal hemorrhage). Disseminated intravascular coagulation may complicate the meningitis. Complications may also arise from intercurrent infection of the upper respiratory tract, middle ear, and lungs. Any of these complications may leave permanent residua, but the most common sequelae are due to injury of the nervous system. These include deafness, ocular palsies, blindness, changes in mentality, convulsions, and hydrocephalus. With the available methods of treatment, complications and sequelae of the meningeal infection are rare, and the complications due to the involvement of other parts of the body by the meningococci or other intercurrent infections are more readily controlled.

Diagnosis

Meningococcal meningitis may be diagnosed with certainty only by the isolation of the organism from the CSF. The diagnosis may be made, however, with relative certainty before the organisms are isolated in a patient with headache, vomiting, chills and fever, neck stiffness, and a petechial cutaneous rash, especially if there is an epidemic of meningococcal meningitis or if there has been exposure to a known case of meningococcal meningitis.

To establish the diagnosis of meningococcal meningitis, cultures should be made of the skin lesions, nasopharyngeal secretions, blood, and CSF. The diagnosis may be established in many cases by examination of smears of the sediment of the CSF after application of the Gram stain.

Prognosis

The mortality rate of untreated meningococcal meningitis varied widely in different epidemics but was usually between 50% and 90%. With present-day therapy, however, the overall mortality rate is about 10%, and the incidence of complications and sequelae is low.

Features of the disease that influence the mortality rate are the age of the patient, bacteremia, rapidity of treatment, complications, and general condition of the individual. The lowest fatality rates are seen in patients between the ages of 5 years and 10 years. The highest mortality rates occur in infants, in elderly debilitated individuals, and in those with extensive hemorrhages into the adrenal gland.

Treatment

Antibiotic therapy for bacterial meningitis usually commences before the nature of the organism is assured. Therefore, the initial regimen should be appropriate for most likely organisms, the determination of which depends to some extent on the patient's age and the locale. Third-generation cephalosporins, usually ceftriaxone or cefotaxime, have become the first choice of treatment for bacterial meningitis. Their spectrum is broad, and they have become particularly useful since the occurrence of *H. influenzae* and *S. pneumoniae* strains that are resistant to penicillin or ampicillin and amoxicillin. They also require less frequent administration than the penicillins. In circumstances when *S. pneumoniae* resistance to cephalosporin is an issue, vancomycin should be added. If the Gram stain or epidemic setting clearly suggests that meningococcus is the infectious organism, penicillin or ampicillin may be used. Chloramphenicol remains an acceptable choice if allergy to the penicillins and cephalosporins is a problem. Unless a dramatic response to therapy occurs, the CSF should be examined 24 hours to 48 hours after the initiation of treatment, to assess the effectiveness of the medication. Posttreatment examination of the CSF is not a meaningful criterion of recovery, and the CSF does not need to be reexamined if the patient is clinically well.

Dehydration is common in this condition, and fluid balance should be monitored carefully to avoid hypovolemic shock. Hyponatremia frequently occurs and may be caused either by overzealous free-water replacement or inappropriate antidiuretic hormone secretion. Heparinization should be considered if disseminated intravascular coagulation occurs.

Anticonvulsants should be used to control recurrent seizures. Cerebral edema may require the use of osmotic diuretics or the administration of corticosteroids, but only if early or impending cerebral herniation is evident. Persons who have had intimate contact with patients with meningococcal meningitis may be given rifampin as a prophylactic measure.

Hemophilus influenzae Meningitis

Infections of the meninges by *H. influenzae* were reported as early as 1899. In the United States and other countries where *H. influenzae* B vaccination is widespread, the incidence of meningitis is now negligible. It remains an important disease elsewhere, however. Where it is still prevalent, *H. influenzae* meningitis is predominantly a disease of infancy and early childhood; more than 50% of the cases occur within the first 2 years of life and 90% before the age of 5. In the United States, *H. influenzae* meningitis is now more common in adults. Serotype B is the most common.

In adults, *H. influenzae* meningitis is more commonly secondary to acute sinusitis, otitis media, or fracture of the skull. It is associated with CSF rhinorrhea, immunologic deficiency, diabetes mellitus, and alcoholism. Currently, cases tend to occur in the autumn and spring, with fewest occurring in the summer months.

The pathology of *H. influenzae* meningitis does not differ from that of other forms of acute purulent meningitis. In patients with a protracted course, localized pockets of infection in the meninges or cortex, internal hydrocephalus, degeneration of cranial nerves, and focal loss of cerebral substance secondary to thrombosis of vessels may be found.

The symptoms and physical signs of *H. influenzae* meningitis are similar to those of other forms of acute bacterial meningitis. The disease usually lasts 10 days to 20 days. It may occasionally be fulminating, and frequently it is protracted and extends over several weeks or months.

The CSF changes are similar to those described for the other acute meningitides. The organisms may be cultured from the CSF. Blood cultures are often positive early in the illness.

The mortality rate in untreated cases of *H. influenzae* meningitis, in infants, is greater than 90%. The prognosis is not so grave in adults, in whom spontaneous recovery is more frequent. Adequate treatment has reduced the mortality rate to about 10%, but sequelae are not uncommon. These include paralysis of extraocular muscles, deafness, blindness, hemiplegia, recurrent convulsions, and mental deficiency. Recent studies have indicated that treatment with antiinflammatory corticosteroids reduces the frequency of the sequelae, particularly if started just before the initiation of antibiotic treatment.

The diagnosis of *H. influenzae* meningitis is based on isolation of the organisms from the CSF and blood.

H. influenzae capsular antigens may be detected in the CSF by particle agglutination, which may provide information rapidly, but is less sensitive and specific than is culture identification.

Because of resistance to ampicillin, third-generation cephalosporins are commonly used in initial therapy of meningitis and are effective.

Subdural effusion, which may occur in infants with any form of meningitis, is most commonly seen in connection with *H. influenzae* meningitis. Persistent vomiting, bulging fontanelles, convulsion, focal neurologic signs, and persistent fever should lead to consideration of this complication. Prompt relief of the symptoms usually follows evacuation of the effusion by tapping the subdural space through the fontanelles. Persistent or secondary fever without worsening of meningeal signs may be due to an extracranial focus of infection, such as a contaminated urinary or venous catheter, or to drug administration.

Pneumococcal Meningitis

Pneumococcus *(S. pneumoniae)* is about equal in frequency to meningococcus as a cause of meningitis, except that it is seen more frequently in the elderly population. Meningeal infection is usually a complication of otitis media, mastoiditis, sinusitis, fractures of the skull, upper respiratory infections, and infections of the lung. Alcoholism, asplenism, and sickle cell disease predispose patients to developing pneumococcal meningitis. The infection may occur at any age, but more than 50% of the patients are younger than 1 year of age or older than 50 years of age.

The clinical symptoms, physical signs, and laboratory findings in pneumococcal meningitis are the same as those in other forms of acute purulent meningitis. The diagnosis is usually made without difficulty because the CSF contains many of the organisms. When Gram-positive diplococci are seen in smears of the CSF or its sediment, a positive quellung reaction serves to identify both the pneumococcus and its type. Particle agglutination of CSF and serum may be helpful in demonstrating pneumococcal antigen.

Before the introduction of sulfonamides, the mortality rate in pneumococcal meningitis was almost 100%. It is now approximately 20% to 30%. The prognosis for recovery is best in cases that follow fractures of the skull and those with no known source of infection. About 30% of survivors have permanent sequelae. The mortality rate is especially high when the meningitis follows pneumonia, empyema, or lung abscess or when a persisting bacteremia indicates the presence of an endocarditis. The triad syndrome of pneumococcal meningitis, pneumonia, and endocarditis (Austrian syndrome) has a particularly high fatality rate.

The prevalence of penicillin-resistant *S. pneumoniae* in the United States has made a third-generation cephalosporin the initial treatment for *S. pneumoniae*, until sensitivities are established. Because some strains also may be relatively resistant to the cephalosporins, vancomycin is often used initially as well. The treatment should be continued for 12 days to 15 days. Chloramphenicol is an alternative drug for adults who are sensitive to the penicillins or cephalosporins. Any primary focus of infection should be eradicated by surgery if necessary. Persistent CSF fistulas after fractures of the skull must be closed by craniotomy and suturing of the dura. Otherwise, the meningitis will almost certainly recur.

Staphylococcal Meningitis

Staphylococci (*S. aureus* and *S. epidermidis*) are a relatively infrequent cause of meningitis. Meningitis may develop as a result of spread from furuncles on the face or from staphylococcal infections elsewhere in the body. It is sometimes a complication of cavernous sinus thrombosis, epidural or subdural abscess, and neurosurgical procedures involving shunting to relieve hydrocephalus. Endocarditis may be found in association with staphylococcal meningitis. Intravenous treatment with a penicillinase-resistant penicillin (nafcillin) is the preferred treatment. Therapy must be continued for 2 weeks to 4 weeks. In nosocomial infections or other situations in which resistance to nafcillin is likely, treatment with vancomycin is appropriate. Complications, such as ventriculitis, arachnoiditis, and hydrocephalus, may occur. The original focus of infection should be eradicated. Laminectomy should be performed immediately when a spinal epidural abscess is present, and cranial subdural abscess should be drained through craniotomy openings.

Streptococcal Meningitis

Infection with streptococcus accounts for less than 5% of all cases of meningitis. The symptoms are not distinguished from other forms of meningitis. Members of other organism groups may occasionally be isolated from CSF. It is always secondary to some septic focus, most commonly in the mastoid or nasal sinuses. Treatment is the same as outlined for the treatment of pneumococcal meningitis, together with surgical eradication of the primary focus.

Meningitis Caused by Other Bacteria

Meningitis in the newborn infant is most often caused by group B hemolytic streptococci. Coliform gram-negative bacilli, especially *Escherichia coli* (*E. coli*) are also common. It often accompanies septicemia and may show none of the typical signs of meningitis in children and adults. Instead, the infant shows irritability, lethargy, anorexia, and bulging fontanelles. Meningitis caused by Gram-negative enteric bacteria also occurs frequently in immunosuppressed or chronically ill, hospitalized adult patients, and in persons with penetrating head injuries, neurosurgical procedures, congenital defects, or diabetes mellitus. In these circumstances, meningitis may be difficult to recognize because of altered consciousness related to the underlying illness.

A third-generation cephalosporin and an aminoglycoside are currently used for treatment of Gram-negative meningitides. If *Pseudomonas aeruginosa* is present or suspected, ceftazidime is preferred. If initial response is poor, intraventricular administration of the aminoglycoside may be considered. Care also must be taken to ensure that the organism is sensitive to the agents chosen; if not, some other antibiotic should be selected. Gram-negative bacillary meningitis has a high mortality rate (40% to 70%) and a high morbidity rate.

Meningitis caused by *Listeria monocytogenes* may occur in adults with chronic diseases (e.g., renal disease with dialysis or transplantation, cancer, connective tissue disorders, chronic alcoholism) and in infants. It may occur, however, without any predisposing factor and the incidence of such appears to be increasing. The highest incidence occurs in neonates and adults over 60 years of age. Occasionally, *L. monocytogenes* meningitis occurs with prominent brainstem findings (rhombencephalitis). A laboratory report of "diphtheroids" seen on Gram stain or isolated in culture should suggest the possible presence of *L. monocytogenes*. *Listeria* septicemia occurs in about 65% of patients, and the organism may be isolated from blood cultures even when not recoverable from the CSF. The treatment of choice for *L. monocytogenes* meningitis is ampicillin. If *Listeria* is considered a reasonable possibility, ampicillin should be added to initial therapy, because the bacterium is resistant to cephalosporins. Trimethoprim/sulfasoxazole is an acceptable alternative. The illness has a mortality rate of 30% to 60%, with the highest fatality rate among elderly patients with malignancies.

Acute Purulent Meningitis of Unknown Cause

Patients may have clinical symptoms indicative of an acute purulent meningitis but with atypical CSF findings. These patients have usually manifested nonspecific symptoms and have often been treated for several days with some form of antimicrobial therapy in dosages sufficient to modify the CSF abnormalities but not sufficient to eradicate the infection. Their symptoms are of longer duration, and the patients have less marked alterations of mental status and die later in their hospitalization than do patients with proven bacterial meningitis. In these cases, the CSF pleocytosis is usually only moderate (500 cells/mm^3 to 1,000 cells/mm^3 with predominance of polymorphonuclear leukocytes), and the sugar content is normal or only slightly decreased. Organisms are not seen on stained smears and are cultured with difficulty. Repeated lumbar puncture may be helpful in arriving at the correct diagnosis.

Antibiotics should be selected on the basis of epidemiologic or clinical factors. The age of the patient and the setting in which the infection occurred are the primary considerations. In patients with partially treated meningitis and in those with meningitis of unknown etiology, third-generation cephalosporins and vancomycin are now considered the antibiotics of choice for initial therapy. Ampicillin should be added in neonates or if *L. monocytogenes* is considered. Therapy should be modified if an organism different from that originally suspected is isolated or if the clinical response is less than optimal. The mortality and frequency of neurologic complications of these patients are similar to those of patients in whom the responsible bacteria have been identified.

Recurrent Bacterial Meningitis

Repeated episodes of bacterial meningitis signal a host defect, either in local anatomy or in antibacterial and immunologic defenses. They usually follow trauma; several years may pass between the trauma and the first bout of meningitis. *S. pneumoniae* is the most common pathogen, accounting for about a third of cases. Bacteria may enter the subarachnoid space through the cribiform plate, a basilar skull fracture, erosive bony changes in the mastoid, congenital dermal defects along the craniospinal axis, penetrating head injuries, or neurosurgical procedures. CSF rhinorrhea or otorrhea is often present but may be transient. It may be detected by testing for a significant concentration of glucose in nasal or aural secretions. Cryptic CSF leaks may be demonstrated by polytomography of the frontal and mastoid regions, by monitoring the course of radioiodine-labeled albumin instilled intrathecally or by CT after intrathecal injection of water-soluble contrast material.

Treatment of recurrent meningitis is similar to that for first bouts. Patients with recurrent pneumococcal meningitis should be vaccinated with pneumococcal vaccine. Long-term prophylactic treatment with penicillin should be considered. Surgical closure of CSF fistulas is indicated to prevent further episodes of meningitis.

SUBACUTE MENINGITIS

Subacute meningitis is usually due to infection with tubercle bacilli or mycotic organisms. The clinical syndrome differs from that of acute purulent meningitis in that the onset of symptoms is usually less acute, the degree of inflammatory reaction less severe, and the course more prolonged.

Tuberculous Meningitis

Tuberculous meningitis differs from that caused by most other common bacteria in that the course is more prolonged, the mortality rate is higher, the CSF changes are acutely less severe, and treatment is less effective in preventing sequelae.

Pathogenesis

Tuberculous meningitis is always secondary to tuberculosis elsewhere in the body (Figs. 22.1 and 22.2).

The primary focus of infection is usually in the lungs but may be in the lymph glands, bones, nasal sinuses, gastrointestinal tract, or any organ in the body. The onset of meningeal symptoms may coincide with signs of acute miliary dissemination, or there may be clinical evidence of activity in the primary focus; however, meningitis is often the only manifestation of the disease.

Tubercular meningitis usually occurs after the rupture of a meningeal or parenchymal tubercle into the ventricular or subarachnoid space. Tubercles in the nervous system of any appreciable size are rare in the United States, but dissemination may be from minute or microscopic granulomas near the meningeal surfaces. When meningitis is a manifestation of miliary dissemination, it suggests that the meningitis stems from bacteria lodging directly in the choroid plexus or meningeal vessels.

Pathology

In tubercular meningitis, the meninges over the surface of the brain and the spinal cord are cloudy and thickened, but the process is usually most intense at the base of the brain. A thick collar of fibrosis may form around the optic nerves, cerebral peduncles, and basilar surface of the pons and midbrain. The ventricles are moderately dilated and the ependymal lining is covered with exudate or appears roughened (granular ependymitis). Minute tubercles may be visible in the meninges, choroid plexus, and cerebral parenchyma.

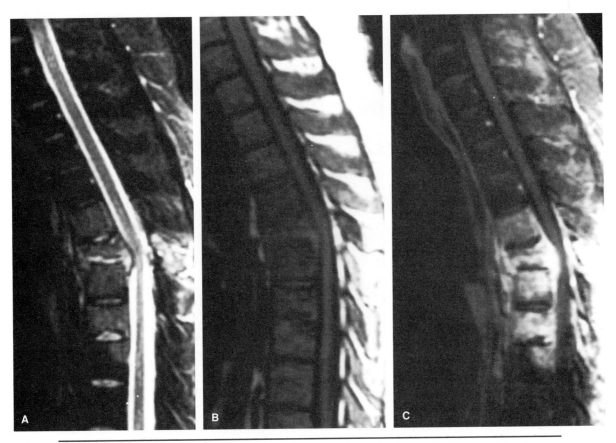

FIGURE 22.1. Potts disease (spinal tuberculosis). A: T2-weighted sagittal MR scan of the thoracic spine shows abnormally increased signal intensity within four to five consecutive vertebral bodies of the lower thoracic spine. Also evident is a compression fracture of one of the thoracic vertebral bodies with apparent impingement upon the lower thoracic spinal cord. **B and C:** T1-weighted sagittal MR scans of thoracic spine, before and after gadolinium enhancement, show marked enhancement of affected thoracic vertebral bodies with mild epidural extension, especially at the level of the compression fracture. (Courtesy of Dr. S. Chan.)

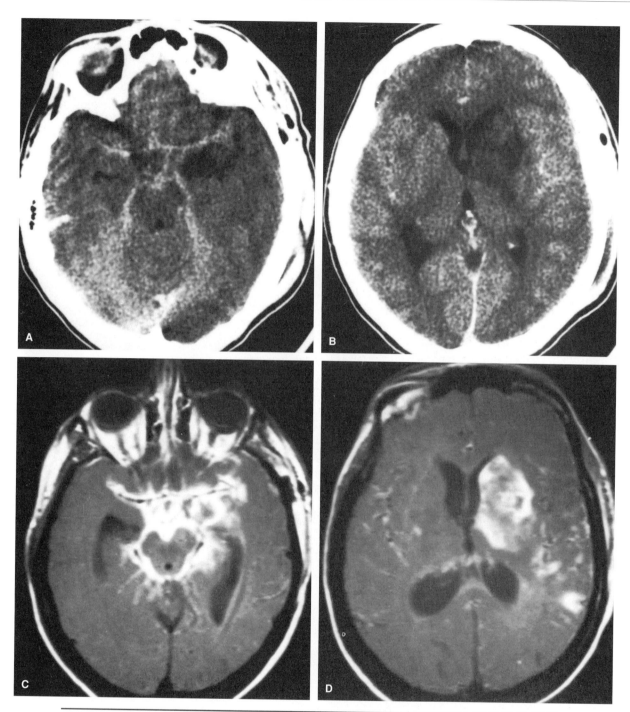

FIGURE 22.2. **Tuberculous meningitis. A and B:** Contrast-enhanced axial CTs demonstrate large nonenhancing hypodense lesion in the left temporal lobe **(A)** and left basal ganglia **(B)** most consistent with infarcts. Significant cisternal enhancement is seen consistent with meningitis. **C and D:** T1-weighted axial magnetic resonance scans after gadolinium enhancement show florid contrast enhancement within basal cisterns most consistent with exudative meningitis of tuberculosis. Enhancement of the left temporal lobe and left basal ganglia lesions suggests persistent inflammation within these infarcts. (Courtesy of Dr. S. Chan.)

On microscopic examination, the exudate in the thickened meninges is chiefly composed of mononuclear cells, lymphocytes, plasma cells, macrophages, and fibroblasts with an occasional giant cell. The inflammatory process may extend for a short distance into the cerebral substance where microscopic granulomas may also be found. Proliferative changes are frequently seen in the inflamed vessels of the meninges, producing a panarteritis that may lead to thrombosis and cerebral infarcts.

Incidence

Until the 1980s, the incidence of tuberculosis and tubercular meningitis had been declining steadily in the United States, owing to hygienic improvements and, later, the development of antibiotic therapy. The incidence, however, is now slowly increasing in part, a result of the propensity of HIV-infected individuals to develop tuberculosis, and in part because of the increased immigration from Asian, Latin American, and African countries, which are known to have a high incidence of the disease. Although tuberculous meningitis may occur at any age, it is most common in childhood and early adult life. In areas with a high incidence of tuberculosis, tuberculous meningitis is seen most commonly in infants and young children. In areas of low incidence, such as the United States, tuberculous meningitis is more common in adults. Until recently, adult cases occurred mainly over the age of 40 years. With the increased incidence of tuberculosis, however, younger adults are again developing the illness.

Symptoms

The onset is usually subacute, with headache, vomiting, fever, bursts of irritability, and nocturnal wakefulness as the most prominent symptoms. Anorexia, loss of weight, and abdominal pain may be present. The prodromal stage lasts for 2 weeks to 3 months in most cases. In young children, a history of close contact with a person known to have tuberculosis is a diagnostic help. Stiffness of the neck and vomiting become evident within a few days. Convulsive seizures are not uncommon in children during the first days of the disease. The headache becomes progressively more severe; there is bulging of the fontanelles in infants. The pain often causes the infant to emit a peculiarly shrill cry (meningeal cry). With progress of the disease, patients become stuporous or comatose. Blindness and signs of damage to other cranial nerves may appear, or there may be convulsive seizures or focal neurologic signs.

Physical Findings

The physical findings in the early stages are those associated with meningeal infection (i.e., fever, irritability, stiffness of the neck, and Kernig and Brudzinski signs). Tendon reflexes may be exaggerated or depressed. Signs of increased intracranial pressure and focal brain damage are rarely present at the onset. The initial irritability is gradually replaced by apathy, confusion, lethargy, and stupor. Papilledema, cranial nerve palsies, and focal neurologic signs are common in the late stages of the disease. There may be external ophthalmoplegia, usually incomplete, unilateral, and involving chiefly the oculomotor nerve. Ophthalmoscopy may demonstrate choroid tubercles. Clinical evidence of tuberculosis elsewhere in the body is usually present. Convulsions, coma, and hemiplegia occur as the disease advances. The temperature is only moderately elevated ($100°F$ to $102°F$) in the early stages, but rises to high levels before death. The respiratory and pulse rates are increased. In the terminal stages, respirations become irregular and of the Cheyne-Stokes type.

Diagnosis

The diagnosis of tuberculous meningitis may be established by recovery of the organisms from the CSF. The CSF findings are, however, quite characteristic and a presumptive diagnosis may be made when the typical abnormalities are present. These include increased pressure; slightly cloudy or ground-glass appearance of the CSF, with formation of a pellicle on top and a fibrin web or clot at the bottom on standing; moderate pleocytosis of 25 cells/mm^3 to 500 cells/mm^3, with lymphocytes as the predominating cell type; increased protein content; decreased sugar content with values in the range of 20 mg/dL to 40 mg/dL; a negative serologic test for syphilis or cryptococcal antigen; and absence of growth when the CSF is inoculated on routine culture media. In about 25% of patients, a neutrophilic predominance may initially be seen with a shift to lymphocytes over the next 24 hours to 48 hours. Although none of these abnormalities is diagnostic, their occurrence in combination is usually pathognomonic, and is sufficient evidence to warrant intensive therapy until the diagnosis may be confirmed; confirmation is by stained smears of the sediment or pellicle, by culture of the CSF, or by detection of mycobacterial DNA in the CSF by polymeric chain reaction (PCR). PCR is highly sensitive, specific and rapid, being completed in 24 hours to 48 hours. It is not, however, foolproof. Smears of the CSF sediment demonstrate acid-fast bacilli in 20% to 30% of patients, on single examination; with repeated examinations, the yield of positive smears increases to 75%. The yield is probably lower in HIV-infected patients, because the illness tends to be more indolent. Diagnosis is ultimately based on the recovery of the mycobacterium from culture, which may require several weeks.

Other diagnostic aids include a thorough search for a primary focus, including radiographs of the chest and tuberculin skin tests. Patients with tuberculous meningitis may have hyponatremia caused by inappropriate secretion of antidiuretic hormone. CT or MRI of the brain in tuberculous meningitis may disclose enhancing exudates in the subarachnoid cisterns, hydrocephalus, areas of infarction, and associated tuberculomas.

Tuberculous meningitis must be differentiated from other forms of acute and subacute meningitis, viral infections, and meningeal reactions to septic foci in the skull or spine. Acute purulent meningitis is characterized by a high cell count and the presence of the causative organisms in the CSF. Preliminary antibiotic therapy of purulent meningitis may cause the CSF findings to mimic those of tuberculous meningitis.

The CSF in syphilitic meningitis may show changes similar to those of tuberculous meningitis. The normal or relatively normal sugar content and the positive serologic reactions make the diagnosis of syphilitic meningitis relatively easy.

The clinical picture and CSF findings in cryptococcus meningitis may be identical with those of tuberculous meningitis. The differential diagnosis may be made by finding the budding yeast organisms in the counting chamber or in stained smears, by detecting cryptococcal antigen in CSF by the latex agglutination test, and by obtaining a culture of the fungus. Much less frequently, other mycotic infections may involve the meninges.

Meningeal involvement in the course of viral infections, such as mumps, lymphocytic choriomeningitis, or other forms of viral encephalitis, may give a clinical picture somewhat similar to that of tuberculous meningitis. In these cases, the CSF sugar content is usually normal or only minimally depressed.

Diffuse involvement of the meninges by metastatic tumors (carcinoma or sarcoma) or by gliomas may produce meningeal signs. The CSF may contain numerous lymphocytes and polymorphonuclear leukocytes and a reduced-sugar content. The triad of mental clarity, lack of fever, and hyporeflexia suggests neoplastic meningitis. A protracted course or the finding of neoplastic cells in the CSF excludes the diagnosis of tuberculous meningitis.

CNS sarcoidosis may also cause meningitis with CSF changes similar to those of tuberculous meningitis. Failure to detect microbes by smear or culture, and a protracted course are clues to the diagnosis of sarcoidosis. The angiotension converting enzyme (ACE) assay may be positive in the serum or CSF. Rarely, leptomeningeal biopsy may be needed to establish the diagnosis, but most patients show systemic signs of sarcoidosis in lymph nodes, liver, lung, or muscle (see Chapter 27).

Prognosis and Course

The natural course of the disease is death in 6 weeks to 8 weeks. With early diagnosis and appropriate treatment, the recovery rate approaches 90%. Delay in diagnosis is associated with rapid progression of neurologic deficits and a poorer prognosis. Prognosis is worst at the extremes of life, particularly in the elderly person. The presence

of cranial-nerve abnormalities on admission, confusion, lethargy, and elevated CSF-protein concentration are associated with a poor prognosis. The presence of active tuberculosis in other organs, or of miliary tuberculosis, does not significantly affect the prognosis if antitubercular therapy is given. Relapses occasionally occur after months or even years in apparently cured patients.

Sequelae

Minor or major sequelae occur in about 25% of the patients who recover. These vary from minimal degree of facial weakness to severe intellectual and physical disorganization. Physical defects include deafness, convulsive seizures, blindness, hemiplegia, paraplegia, and quadriplegia. Intracranial calcifications may appear 2 years to 3 years after the onset of the disease.

Treatment

Treatment should be started immediately without waiting for bacteriologic confirmation of the diagnosis in a patient with the characteristic clinical symptoms and CSF findings. It is generally agreed that the prognosis for recovery and freedom from sequelae are directly related to the promptness of therapy initiation. Concomitant with the resurgence of tuberculosis in the United States has been the emergence of multidrug-resistant organisms. Treatment is now commonly started with four drugs, usually isoniazid, rifampin, pyrazinamide, and ethambutol; streptomycin is an alternative if one of the preferred antibiotics may not be used. Other second-line drugs may be substituted if absolutely necessary. The regimen later may be modified, and the number of agents reduced, if the sensitivities of the isolated bacterium allow. Treatment is usually for 18 months to 24 months. Corticosteroids may prove beneficial in the early phases of the disease when there is evidence of subarachnoid block or impending cerebral herniation. Peripheral neuropathy secondary to isoniazid treatment may be prevented by giving pyridoxine. Intrathecal therapy is not indicated.

In association with the HIV epidemic has been an increased incidence of infection with nontubercular mycobacteria, particularly of the avium-intracellulare group. Although these organisms are occasionally isolated from the CSF, the meningeal reaction related to their presence is a mild and indolent process. Treatment of these infections is difficult.

SUBDURAL AND EPIDURAL INFECTIONS

Cerebral Subdural Empyema

A collection of pus in the preformed space between the inner surface of the dura and the outer surface of the arachnoid of the brain is known as *subdural empyema*.

Etiology

Subdural empyema may result from the direct extension of infection from the middle ear, the nasal sinuses, or the meninges. It may develop as a complication of compound fractures of the skull or in the course of septicemia. An acute attack of sinusitis just before the development of subdural empyema is common. The mechanism of the formation of subdural empyema after compound fractures of the skull is easily understood, but the factors that lead to subdural infection rather than leptomeningitis or cerebral abscess in patients with infections of the nasal sinuses or mastoids are less clear. Chronic infection of the mastoid or paranasal sinuses, with thrombophlebitis of the venous sinuses or osteomyelitis and necrosis of the cranial vault, commonly precedes the development of the subdural infection.

The infection is most often cause by streptococcus. Other bacteria frequently recovered from subdural pus are staphylococci and gram-negative enteric organisms.

Pathology

The pathologic findings depend on the mode of entry of the infection into the subdural space. In traumatic cases, there may be osteomyelitis of the overlying skull, with or without accompanying foreign bodies. When the empyema is secondary to infection of the nasal sinuses or middle ear, thrombophlebitis of the venous sinuses or osteomyelitis of the frontal or temporal bone is a common finding. Dorsolateral and interhemispheric collections of pus are common; collections beneath the cerebral hemispheres are uncommon. After paranasal infections, subdural pus forms at the frontal poles and extends posteriorly over the convexity of the frontal lobe. Following ear infection, the subdural pus passes posteriorly and medially over the falx to the tentorium and occipital poles. The brain beneath the pus is molded in a manner similar to that seen in cases of subdural hematoma. Thrombosis or thrombophlebitis of the superficial cortical veins, especially in the frontal region, is common and produces a hemorrhagic softening of the gray and white matter drained by the thrombosed vessels. The subarachnoid spaces beneath the subdural empyema are filled with a purulent exudate, but there is no generalized leptomeningitis in the initial stage.

Incidence

Subdural empyema is a relatively rare form of intracranial infection, occurring less than half as frequently as brain abscess. It may develop at any age but is most common in children and young adults. Males are more frequently affected than females.

Symptoms and Signs

Symptoms include those associated with the focus or origin of the infection and those cause by the intracranial

extension. Local pain and tenderness are present in the region of the infected nasal sinus or ear. Orbital swelling is usually present when the injection is secondary to frontal sinus disease. Chills, fever, and severe headache are common initial symptoms of the intracranial involvement. Neck stiffness and Kernig sign are present. With progression of the infection, the patient lapses into a confused, somnolent, or comatose state. Thrombophlebitis of the cortical veins is manifested by jacksonian or generalized convulsions and by the appearance of focal neurologic signs (e.g., hemiplegia, aphasia, paralysis of conjugate deviation of the eyes, cortical sensory loss). In the late stages, the intracranial pressure is increased and papilledema may occur. The entire clinical picture may evolve in as little as a few hours or as long as 10 days.

Laboratory Data

A marked peripheral leukocytosis is usually present. Radiographs of the skull may show evidence of infection of the mastoid or nasal sinuses or of osteomyelitis of the skull. The CSF is under increased pressure. It is usually clear and colorless, and there is a moderate pleocytosis, varying from 25 cells/mm^3 to 500 cells/mm^3, with 10% to 80% polymorphonuclear leukocytes. In some patients, the CSF cellular response may chiefly be composed of lymphocytes or mononuclear cells. Rarely, CSF pleocytosis may be absent. The protein content is increased, with values commonly in the range of 75 mg/dL to 150 mg/dL. The sugar content is normal, and the CSF is sterile unless the subdural infection is secondary to a purulent leptomeningitis. Spinal puncture should be done with caution; instances of transtentorial herniation within 8 hours after lumbar puncture have been described in this condition. Lumbar puncture should be avoided if the diagnosis may be established in other ways.

CT of the head characteristically demonstrates a crescent-shaped area of hypodensity at the periphery of the brain and mass displacement of the cerebral ventricles and midline structures. Usually, there is contrast enhancement between the empyema and cerebral cortex. CT may fail to define the pus collection in some patients with typical clinical manifestations, however; for these patients MRI seems to be more sensitive.

Diagnosis

The diagnosis of subdural empyema should be considered whenever meningeal symptoms or focal neurologic signs develop in patients presenting evidence of a suppurative process in nasal sinuses, mastoid process, or other cranial structures.

Subdural empyema must be differentiated from other intracranial complications of infections in the ear or nasal sinus. These include epidural abscess, sinus thrombosis, and brain abscess. The presence of focal neurologic signs and neck stiffness is against the diagnosis of epidural abscess.

Making the differential diagnosis between subdural empyema and septic thrombosis of the superior longitudinal sinus is difficult because focal neurologic signs and convulsive seizures are common to both conditions. In fact, thrombosis of the sinus or its tributaries is a frequent complication of subdural empyema. Factors in favor of the diagnosis of sinus thrombosis are a septic temperature and the absence of signs of meningeal irritation. Subdural empyema may also be confused with viral encephalitis or various types of meningitis. The diagnosis may be obscured by early antibiotic therapy. Brain abscess may be distinguished by its relatively insidious onset and protracted course.

Clinical Course

The mortality rate is high (25% to 40%), in part because of failure to make an early diagnosis. If the disorder is untreated, death commonly follows the onset of focal neurologic signs, occurring within 6 days. Uncontrollable cerebral edema contributes to a lethal outcome. The causes of death are dural venous sinus thrombosis, fulminant meningitis, and multiple intracerebral abscesses. With prompt evacuation of the pus, and chemotherapy, recovery is possible even after focal neurologic signs have appeared. Gradual improvement of the focal neurologic signs may occur after recovery from the infection. Seizures, hemiparesis, and other focal deficits may be long-term sequelae, however.

Treatment

The treatment of subdural empyema is prompt surgical evacuation of the pus through trephine operation, carefully avoiding passage through the infected nasal sinuses. Systemic antibiotic therapy should commence before surgery and should be tailored to any suspected organism. If *S. aureus* is suspected, penicillin G and metronidazole with vancomycin are suitable as broad-spectrum treatment, before culture reports are available. Otherwise, a third-generation cephalosporin should be substituted for penicillin. Treatment duration is usually 3 weeks to 4 weeks. Instillation of antibiotics into the subdural space during surgery is of uncertain efficacy but commonly is done. Treatment of cerebral edema is also a necessity in the management of subdural empyema.

Intracranial Epidural Abscess

Abscesses confined to the epidural space are frequent and are almost always associated with overlying infection in the cranial bones. Penetration from chronic sinusitis or mastoiditis is most common, but infection after head trauma or neurosurgery may also cause this problem. Occasionally, no source is apparent. Frequently, intracranial epidural abscess is associated with deeper penetration of the infection and subdural empyema, meningitis, or intraparenchymal abscess. Severe headache, fever, malaise, and findings referable to the initial site of infection are the features of isolated, intracranial epidural abscess. Focal neurologic findings are rarely present. Diagnosis is made most conveniently by CT or MRI, which usually demonstrates a characteristic extradural defect (Fig. 22.3).

MRI appears to be more sensitive when the lesion is small. If no abnormality is detected, repeat scanning should be performed when headache persists after antibiotic treatment of an infected sinus or other focus. Evaluation of CSF is not of great help. The protein may be modestly elevated and a mild pleocytosis may be present, but organisms are not seen on Gram stain and cultures are routinely negative. Lumbar puncture is certainly discouraged until after scanning has established that significant mass effect is not present. As with most abscesses, surgical drainage is usually necessary to ensure cure. If, however, the scan and lack of neurologic findings suggest that the infection is confined to the epidural space, trephination may suffice and a craniotomy may be avoided. Appropriate antibiotic treatment is the same as that for subdural empyema because the sources of infection are similar. It is not clear whether irrigation of the epidural space with antibiotic is useful.

Spinal Epidural Abscess

Spinal epidural abscess is a collection of purulent material located outside the dura mater within the spinal canal. Infections of the spinal epidural space are accompanied by fever, headache, pain in the back, weakness of the lower extremities, and finally, complete paraplegia.

Etiology

Infections may reach the fatty tissue in the spinal epidural space by one of three routes: direct extension from inflammatory processes in adjacent tissues (e.g., decubitus ulcers, carbuncles, or perinephric abscesses); metastasis through the blood from infections elsewhere in the body; and invasion (e.g., perforating wounds, spinal surgery, or lumbar puncture). The first route of infection accounts for most cases. The primary site of infection is most often a furuncle on the skin. Septic foci in the tonsils, teeth, lungs, heart, uterus, or other organ may metastasize to the epidural fat. Chronic debilitating diseases, diabetes mellitus, immunosuppressive therapy, and heroin abuse are also contributing factors.

S. aureus accounts for 50% to 60% of epidural abscesses. Other bacteria responsible include *E. coli*, other

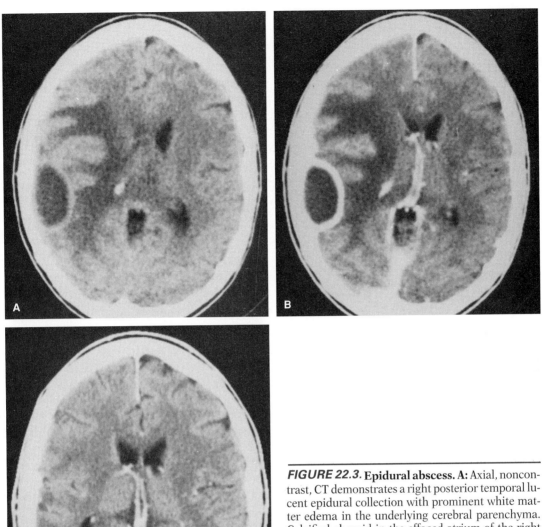

FIGURE 22.3. Epidural abscess. **A:** Axial, noncontrast, CT demonstrates a right posterior temporal lucent epidural collection with prominent white matter edema in the underlying cerebral parenchyma. Calcified choroid in the effaced atrium of the right lateral ventricle is shifted anteromedially. **B:** Post-contrast scan at this same level demonstrates abnormal dural enhancement and shift of the internal cerebral veins, owing to the mass effect. **C:** A contrast-enhanced scan after surgical drainage demonstrates resolution of the abscess, edema, mass effect, and shift. (Courtesy of Drs. J. A. Bello and S. K. Hilal.)

gram-negative organisms, and hemolytic and anaerobic streptococci.

Pathology

No region of the spine is immune to infection, but the midthoracic vertebrae are most frequently affected. The character of the osteomyelitis in the vertebra is similar to that encountered in other bones of the body. The laminae are most commonly involved, but any part of the vertebra, including the body, may be the seat of the infection. The infection in the epidural space may be acute or chronic.

In acute cases, which are by far the most common, a purulent necrosis of the epidural fat extends over several segments but may extend over many segments of the cord. The pus is usually posterior to the spinal cord but may be on the anterior surface. When the infecting organism is of low virulence, the infection may localize and assume a granulomatous nature.

The lesions in the spinal cord depend on the extent to which the infection has progressed before treatment is begun. Necrosis in the periphery of the cord may result from pressure of the abscess, or myelomalacia of one or several segments may occur when the veins or arteries are thrombosed. There is ascending degeneration and descending degeneration flanking the level of the necrotic lesion. The substance of the spinal cord occasionally may be infected by extension through the meninges, with the formation of a spinal cord abscess.

Incidence

Spinal epidural abscesses account for approximately 1 admission of every 20,000 admissions to hospitals in the United States. They may occur at all ages; 60% affect adults between 20 years of age and 50 years of age.

Symptoms and Signs

The symptoms of acute spinal epidural abscess develop suddenly, several days or weeks after an infection of the skin or other parts of the body. The preceding infection occasionally may be so slight that it is overlooked. Severe back pain is usually the presenting symptom (Stage I—localized manifestations). Malaise, fever, neck stiffness, and headache may be present or follow in a few days. Usually within hours, but sometimes not for several weeks, initial symptoms are followed by radicular pain (Stage II—radicular manifestations). If the abscess is untreated, muscular weakness and paralysis of the legs may develop suddenly (Stage III—cord compression).

Fever and malaise are usually present in the early phase; lethargy or irritability develops as the disease progresses. There is neck stiffness and a Kernig sign. Local percussion tenderness over the spine is an important diagnostic sign. Tendon reflexes may be increased or decreased, and the plantar responses may be extensor. With thrombosis of the spinal vessels, a flaccid paraplegia occurs with complete loss of sensation below the level of the lesion and paralysis of the bladder or rectum. Immediately after the onset of paraplegia, tendon reflexes are absent in the paralyzed extremities. There is often erythema and swelling in the area of back pain.

In chronic cases in which the infection is localized and there is granuloma formation, the neurologic signs are similar to those seen with other types of extradural tumors. Fever is rare; weakness and paralysis may not develop for weeks or months.

Laboratory Data

In acute cases, leukocytosis is present in the blood. The erythrocyte sedimentation rate is usually elevated. Radiographs of the spine are usually normal but may show osteomyelitis or a contiguous abscess (Fig. 22.4).

Myelography is almost invariably abnormal. Complete extradural block is found in 80% of patients; the others demonstrate partial block. It is critically important to consider the possibility of epidural abscess in any case of acute

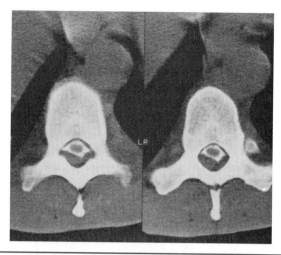

FIGURE 22.4. Epidural abscess. Axial CT myelography demonstrates abnormal epidural soft-tissue density posterior to and deforming the thecal sac, with anterior displacement of the cord at this lower thoracic level. (Courtesy of Dr. S. K. Hilal.)

or subacute myelopathy, because lumbar puncture may penetrate the pus and carry infection into the subarachnoid space. When complete block or a lower thoracic-lumbar abscess is suspected, myelography should be performed by cervical puncture. The needle should be advanced slowly and suction applied with a syringe as the epidural space is approached. If the abscess has extended to the level of the puncture, pus may be withdrawn for culture and the procedure terminated.

Epidural abscesses may be demonstrated by spinal CT, with or without use of intravenous contrast material. MRI, especially with gadolinium enhancement, is even more sensitive (Fig. 22.5). When lesions are clearly defined by either of these techniques, myelography is not necessary.

CSF pressure is normal or increased and there is complete or almost complete subarachnoid block. The CSF is xanthochromic or cloudy in appearance. There is usually a slight or moderate pleocytosis in the CSF, varying from a few to several hundred cells per cubic millimeter. If the process is acute, neutrophils usually predominate; if chronic, lymphocytes predominate. Rarely, no cells may be present. The protein content is increased with values commonly between 100 mg/dL and 1,500 mg/dL. The CSF sugar content is normal, and CSF cultures are sterile unless meningitis has developed.

Diagnosis

A presumptive diagnosis may be made when subarachnoid block is found in a patient with back and leg pain of acute onset with back tenderness and signs of meningeal irritation. This is true when there is a history of recent pyogenic infection. The diagnosis should be made before signs of cord compression appear.

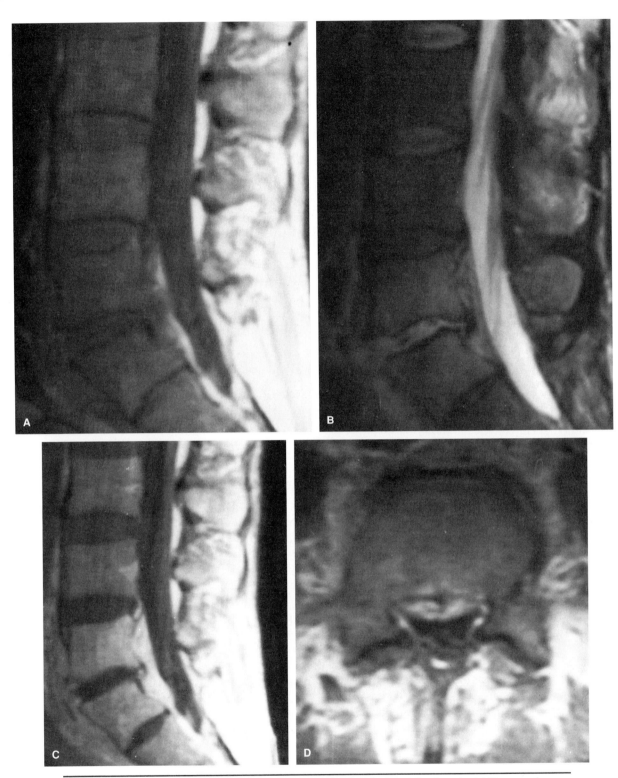

FIGURE 22.5. **Epidural abscess. A and B:** T1-weighted and T2-weighted sagittal MR scans demonstrate a vague area of mixed signal intensity within the anterior epidural space extending from the top of the L5 vertebral level down to the S1 level, suggestive of an underlying epidural process. Also noted is mild increased signal intensity within the L5 and S1 vertebral bodies on the T2-weighted images suggestive of adjacent vertebral inflammation or degeneration. (Degenerative disc disease is present at the L4-L5 disc space.) **C and D:** T1-weighted sagittal and axial MR scans demonstrate significant contrast enhancement within the anterior epidural space between L5 and S1 levels, consistent with epidural infection. Axial view shows compression upon spinal sac anteriorly. Patient had known *Staphylococcus aureus* sepsis; epidural abscess receded with intravenous antibiotics. (Courtesy of Dr. S. Chan.)

Acute spinal epidural abscess must be differentiated from acute or subacute meningitis, acute poliomyelitis, infectious polyneuritis, acute transverse myelitis, multiple sclerosis, and epidural hematoma. The clinical, CSF, and MRI findings are sufficient to differentiate these conditions. Chronic epidural abscess may be confused with chronic adhesive arachnoiditis or tumors in the epidural space.

The diagnosis of granulomatous infection is rarely made before operation. The signs are those of chronic cord compression. Operation is indicated by the presence of these signs and evidence of spinal subarachnoid block.

Course and Prognosis

If treatment is delayed in acute spinal epidural abscess, complete or incomplete compression syndrome almost invariably develops. Flaccid paraplegia, sphincter paralysis, and sensory loss below the level of the lesion persist throughout the life of the individual.

The mortality rate is approximately 30% in the acute cases and 10% in the chronic cases. Death may occur in acute cases as a direct result of the infection or secondary to complications. Total recovery may occur in patients who do not have total paralysis or who have weakness lasting less than 36 hours. Of patients paralyzed for 48 hours or more, 50% progress to permanent paralysis and death.

Treatment

The treatment of spinal epidural abscess is prompt surgical drainage by laminectomy. Antibiotics should be administered before and after the operation, and should include a third-generation cephalosporin and vancomycin. If the abscess is due to local extension, then metronidazole should be added for anaerobes. Aerobic and anaerobic cultures should be obtained at operation. The area of suppuration should be irrigated with an antibiotic solution. Delay in draining the abscess may result in permanent paralysis. Little improvement may be expected in acute cases with signs of transection if the operation is performed after they occur because these signs are caused by softening of the spinal cord secondary to thrombosis of the spinal vessels. In chronic cases where compression of the cord plays a role in the production of the signs, considerable improvement in the neurologic symptoms and signs may be expected after the operation.

When there is back pain with minimal or no neurologic abnormality, surgery may not be needed, but epidural aspiration for culture is used to guide antibiotic therapy, followed by MRI monitoring of the course. This is potentially perilous because progression of neurologic dysfunction may be rapid and irreversible. Close observation and immediate surgical drainage are necessary if neurologic deterioration occurs.

Infective Endocarditis

Etiology

The etiology of infective endocarditis has changed remarkably in the antibiotic era. Rheumatic heart disease now accounts for fewer than 25% of cases, whereas it once accounted for nearly 75%. Endocarditis secondary to prosthetic valves or other intravascular devices, intravenous drug addiction, and degenerative cardiac disease related to aging has become more prominent. Congenital heart abnormalities remain an important cause, especially in children. Unfortunately, morbidity and mortality rates have not been affected much by these etiologic changes and the use of antibiotics, thus probably reflecting more severe infections associated with these newer causes. In the past, the terms acute or subacute were used to describe infective endocarditis. These subdivisions, however, are artificial; the underlying cause of the endocarditis and the specific organism involved are more useful considerations when determining prognosis and treatment.

Signs and Symptoms

Neurologic complications of infective endocarditis are important because of their frequency and severity. They may be the first manifestation of the underlying intracardiac infection. Cerebral infarcts, either bland or less often hemorrhagic, are most common. Infarcts of cranial or peripheral nerves and of the spinal cord rarely occur. Intracranial hemorrhage caused by mycotic aneurysms, brain abscess, and meningitis also are frequent. These complications presumably result from emboli of infective material from the heart. Inflammatory arteritis also has been implicated as a cause, particularly of intracranial hemorrhage when no mycotic aneurysm is apparent. An encephalopathy sometimes with prominent psychiatric features may occur and may be related to microemboli, with or without microabscess formation, vasculitis, toxic effects of medications, or metabolic derangements associated with the illness occurring either individually or concurrently. Seizures may occur in association with any of the cerebral complications.

Infective endocarditis always should be considered in sudden neurologic vascular events, particularly when known predisposing factors exist, such as cardiac disease, drug addiction, fever, or infection elsewhere in the body. The frequency of neurologic events is between 20% and 40% in most reported series of endocarditis. They appear to occur more frequently in the elderly patient. As might be anticipated, neurologic complications are more frequent in endocarditis that affects the left side of the heart. Right-sided lesions usually cause meningitis, intracerebral abscesses, or encephalopathy rather than embolic-related events, although these still rarely occur. The type of organism is also important in determining the frequency of neurologic events. *S. aureus* and *S. pneumoniae* in particular are associated with a high risk of nervous system complications.

Testing and Diagnosis

Diagnostic evaluation of neurologic events depends in part on whether the presence of infective endocarditis already has been established. Imaging studies are important to define the nature of lesions that have focal neurologic findings. Differentiation of infarcts from hemorrhages or abscesses may be accomplished by either CT or MRI. On occasion, both techniques may be necessary to define clearly the nature of the lesion. Analysis of the CSF is mandatory in cases of meningitis, regardless of whether the diagnosis of infective endocarditis already has been made. Such analysis also is useful in encephalopathic conditions to evaluate for low-grade meningitic infection. Lumbar puncture also should be considered strongly in stroke associated with fever even if endocarditis is not yet documented. Lumbar puncture is probably not useful in known cases of infective endocarditis with focal CNS presentations where a clearly defined lesion has been identified with imaging studies. Demonstration of suspected mycotic aneurysms may be made by arteriography. The usefulness of magnetic resonance angiography has not been established yet. Some practitioners have advocated arteriography in all cases of infective endocarditis. No controlled studies have been done to determine the indications for arteriography, and indications for surgical treatment of detected aneurysms also are uncertain.

Treatment

Treatment of infective endocarditis with nervous system complications is primarily treatment of the cardiac lesion. Prolonged antibiotic treatment is required, and surgical replacement of infected valves may be appropriate. In most instances, treatment of nervous system events is nonspecific and supportive. Brain abscesses that do not resolve rapidly with systemic antibiotics should be drained. As noted, indications for surgical management of mycotic aneurysms is uncertain and must be decided on an individual basis. The aneurysms usually do not have a neck and may not be conveniently clipped. Sacrifice of the distal vessel usually is necessary, and further cerebral damage is possible.

Leprosy

Leprosy (Hansen disease) is a chronic disease due to infection by *Mycobacterium leprae*, which has a predilection for the skin and the peripheral nerves. The bacillus has this predilection for mucous membranes and skin, including superficial nerves, because these are the cooler areas of the body where the temperature is ideal for bacillary multiplication. Two major clinical types are recognized:

lepromatous and tuberculoid. The type that predominates appears to depend on the nature of the immunologic response to the organism.

Etiology

M. leprae is an acid-fast, rod-shaped organism morphologically similar to the tubercle bacillus. The organism may be demonstrated in the cutaneous lesion and is sometimes present in the blood of lepromatous patients. The disease is transmitted by direct contact, which must be intimate and prolonged because the contagion virulence is low. The portal of entry is probably through abrasions in the skin or mucous membranes of the upper respiratory tract. The incubation period is long, averaging 3 years to 4 years in children and longer in adults. Transmission from patients with tuberculoid leprosy is rare.

Pathology

The affected nerve trunks are diffusely thickened or are studded with nodular swellings. There is an overgrowth of connective tissue with degeneration of the axon and myelin sheath. Bacilli are present in the perineurium and endoneural septa. They also have been found in dorsal root ganglia, spinal cord, and brain, but they do not produce any significant lesions within the CNS. Degenerative changes in the posterior funiculi of the cord that are found in some cases may be attributed to the peripheral neuritis.

Epidemiology

Leprosy is most common in tropical and subtropical climates, and it is estimated that 10 million to 20 million people are infected. The disease is prevalent in South and Central America, China, India, and Africa. It is uncommon in Europe or North America. In the United States, the disease is mostly confined to Louisiana, Texas, Florida, Southern California, Hawaii, and New York. The number of new cases in the United States has increased in recent years as a result of immigration from endemic areas.

Children are especially susceptible to the disease, but it may occur in adults. In childhood, the disease is evenly distributed between the two sexes but among adults, men are more frequently affected than women.

Symptoms and Signs

In most cases, a mixture of cutaneous and peripheral nerve lesions occurs. Neurologic involvement is more frequent and occurs early in the tuberculoid form. The earliest manifestation of neural leprosy is an erythematous macule, the lepride. This lesion grows by peripheral extension to form an annular macule. The macule has an atrophic depigmented center that is partially or completely anesthetic. These lesions may attain an enormous size and cover the major portion of one extremity or the torso. Infection of the nerve may result in the formation of nodules or fusiform swelling along its course. Although any of the peripheral nerves may be affected, the disease has a predilection for the ulnar, great auricular, posterior tibial, common peroneal, and cranial nerves V and VII. These nerves are involved at locations where their course is superficial. Repeated attacks of neuralgic pains often precede the onset of weakness or sensory loss.

Cranial Nerves

Involvement of cranial nerve V is evident by the presence of patches of anesthesia on the face. Involvement of the entire sensory distribution of the nerve or its motor division is rare. Keratitis, ulceration, and blindness may ensue as results of injury to the anesthetic cornea. Complete paralysis of the facial nerve is rare, but weakness of a portion of one or several muscles is common. The muscles of the upper half of the face are most severely affected. Partial paralysis of the orbicularis oculi and other facial muscles may result in lagophthalmos, ectropion, and facial asymmetry. Involvement of the oculomotor or other cranial nerves is rare.

Motor System

Weakness and atrophy develop in the muscles innervated by the affected nerves. There is wasting of the small muscles of the hands and feet, with later extension to the forearm and leg, but the proximal muscles usually are spared. Clawing of the hands or feet is common, but wrist drop and foot drop are late manifestations. Fasciculations may occur and contractures may develop.

Sensory System

Cutaneous sensation is impaired or lost in the distribution of the affected nerves in a somewhat irregular or patchy fashion. Various types of dissociated sensory impairment are seen. The sensory impairment may be of a nerve or root distribution but more commonly it is of a glove-and-stocking type. Deep sensation, pressure pain, the appreciation of vibration, and position sense usually are spared or are affected less severely than is superficial cutaneous sensation.

Reflexes

Tendon reflexes are usually preserved until late, advanced stages of nerve damage, when they are reduced or lost. The abdominal skin reflexes and plantar responses are normal.

Other Signs

Vasomotor and trophic disturbances are usually present. Anhydrosis and cyanosis of the hands and feet are common. Trophic ulcers develop on the knuckles and on the plantar surface of the feet. There may be various arthropathies and resorption of the bones of the fingers, starting in the terminal phalanges and progressing upward. The skin shrinks as digits become shorter, and finally the nail may be attached to a small stump.

Laboratory Data

There are no diagnostic changes in the blood, although mild anemia and an increased erythrocyte sedimentation rate may be seen. As many as 33% of lepromatous patients have false-positive serologic tests for syphilis. The only CSF abnormality is a slight increase in the protein content.

Diagnosis

The diagnosis of leprosy is made without difficulty from the characteristic skin and neuritis lesions. The clinical picture occasionally may have a superficial similarity to that of syringomyelia, hypertrophic interstitial neuritis, or von Recklinghausen disease. The correct diagnosis usually is not difficult if the possibility of leprosy is kept in mind and scrapings from cutaneous lesions and nerve biopsy specimens are examined for acid-fast bacilli.

Course and Prognosis

The prognosis in the neural form (primarily tuberculoid) of the disease is less grave than that in the cutaneous form (primarily lepromatous), in which death ensues within 10 years to 20 years. Neural leprosy is not necessarily fatal. The progress of the neuritis is slow, and the disease may come to a spontaneous arrest or may be controlled by therapy. Incapacitation may result from the paralyses and disfigurement.

Treatment

Dapsone (4,4-diamino-diphenylsulphone), a folate antagonist, is the primary drug for treatment, supplemented by a single dose of rifampin once per month for the tuberculoid form. Treatment continues for at least 6 months. For the lepromatous form, dapsone and rifampin are supplemented with clofazimine, and treatment continues for at least 2 years.

RICKETTSIAL INFECTIONS

Rickettsiae are obligate intracellular parasites about the size of bacteria. They are visible in microscopic preparations as pleomorphic coccobacilli. Each rickettsiae pathogenic for humans is capable of multiplying in arthropods and in animals and humans. They have a gram-negative–like cell wall and an internal structure similar to that of bacteria (i.e., with a prokaryotic DNA arrangement and ribosomes). Diseases due to rickettsiae are divided into five groups on the basis of their biologic properties and epidemiologic features: typhus, spotted fever, scrub typhus, Q fever, and trench fever. Invasion of the nervous system is common only in infections with organisms of the first three groups. Infection with Rocky Mountain spotted fever is the most important rickettsial infection currently in the United States. A sixth group of rickettsiae in the genus *Ehrlichia* have come to be recognized as significant pathogens in humans in the past 10 years. Ehrlichial infections have also been associated with CNS symptoms, but the frequency of nervous system infection is still not certain.

Rocky Mountain Spotted Fever

Rocky Mountain spotted fever is an acute endemic febrile disease produced by infection with the *Rickettsia rickettsii*. It is transmitted to humans by various ticks, the most common of which are the *Dermacentor andersoni* (wood tick) in the Rocky Mountain and Pacific Coast states and the *Dermacentor variabilis* (dog tick) in the East and South. Rabbits, squirrels, and other small rodents serve as hosts for the ticks and are responsible for maintaining the infection in nature. Diseases of the Rocky Mountain spotted fever group are present throughout the world.

Pathology

The pathologic changes are most severe in the skin, but the heart, lungs, and CNS also are involved. The brain is edematous, and minute petechial hemorrhages are present. The characteristic microscopic lesions are small round nodules composed of elongated microglia, lymphocytes, and endothelial cells. These are scattered diffusely through the nervous system in close relation to small vessels. Vessels in the center of the lesions show severe degeneration. The endothelial cells are swollen, and the lumen may be occluded. Minute areas of focal necrosis are common as the result of thrombosis of small arterioles. Some degree of perivascular infiltration without the presence of nodules may be seen in both the meninges and the brain parenchyma.

Epidemiology

The disease has been reported from almost all states and from Canada, Mexico, and South America. Approximately 1,000 cases are reported annually in the United States, mostly from rural areas. Most cases are seen during the period of maximal tick activity—the late spring and early summer months.

Symptoms and Signs

A history of tick bite is elicited in 80% of affected patients. The incubation period varies from 3 days to 12 days. The onset is usually abrupt, with severe headache, fever, chills, myalgias, arthralgias, restlessness, prostration, and, at times, delirium and coma. A rose-red maculopapular rash appears between the second and sixth day (usually on the fourth febrile day) on the wrists, ankles, palms, soles, and forearms. The rash rapidly spreads to the legs, arms, and chest. The rash becomes petechial and fails to fade on pressure by about the fourth day.

Neurologic symptoms occur early and are frequently a prominent feature. Headache, restlessness, insomnia, and back stiffness are common. Delirium or coma alternating with restlessness is present during the height of the fever. Tremors, athetoid movements, convulsions, opisthotonos, and muscular rigidity may occur. Retinal venous engorgement, retinal edema, papilledema, retinal exudates, and choroiditis may occur. Deafness, visual disturbances, slurred speech, and mental confusion may be present and may persist for a few weeks following recovery.

Laboratory Data

The white cell count is either normal or mildly elevated. Proteinuria, hematuria, and oliguria commonly occur. CSF pressure and glucose are usually normal. The CSF is clear, but a slight lymphocytic pleocytosis and protein elevation may occur. Eosinophilic meningitis has been reported.

Diagnosis

The diagnosis is made on the basis of the development of the characteristic rash and other symptoms of the disease after exposure to ticks. Clinical distinction from typhus fever may be impossible. The onset of the rash in distal parts of the limbs favors a diagnosis of Rocky Mountain spotted fever. In rare instances, however, neurologic signs may occur before the rash appears. A rise in antibody titer during the second week of illness may be detected by specific complement fixation, immunofluorescence and microagglutination tests, or by the Weil-Felix reaction with *Proteus* OX-19 and OX-2.

Course and Prognosis

In patients who recover, the fever falls at about the end of the third week, although mild cases may become afebrile before the end of the second week. Convalescence may be slow, and residuals of damage to the nervous system may persist for several months.

In untreated cases, the overall case fatality is about 20%. Prognosis depends on the severity of the infection, host factors (e.g., age, the presence of other illness), and the promptness with which antimicrobial treatment is started.

Treatment

Control measures include personal care and vaccination. Tick-infested areas should be avoided. If exposure is necessary, high boots, leggings, or socks should be worn outside the trouser legs. Body and clothing should be inspected after exposure, and attached ticks should be removed with tweezers. The hands should be carefully washed after handling the ticks. Workers whose occupations require constant exposure to tick-infested regions should be vaccinated yearly, just before the advent of the tick season.

The treatment of Rocky Mountain spotted fever is the prompt administration of doxycycline or tetracycline. In children, chloramphenicol is the alternative to doxycycline to avoid the tooth discoloration caused by tetracycline. Any patient seriously considered to have Rocky Mountain spotted fever should be treated promptly while diagnostic tests proceed.

The other rickettsial infections that may affect the nervous system directly either are rare or do not occur in the United States. Except for some variation in their incubation times, the pathology and clinical picture are similar to those of Rocky Mountain spotted fever and are not described again. All such infections respond to tetracyclines or chloramphenicol.

Typhus Fever

Three types of infection with rickettsiae of the typhus group are recognized: primary louse-borne epidemic typhus; its recrudescent form, Brill-Zinsser disease; and flea-borne endemic murine typhus.

Epidemiology

Since its recognition in the 16th century, typhus has been known as one of the great epidemic diseases of the world. It is especially prevalent in war times or whenever there is a massing of people in camps, prisons, or ships.

Epidemic typhus (caused by *R. prowazekii*) is spread among humans by the human body louse (*Pediculus humanus corporis*). Outbreaks of epidemic typhus last occurred in the United States in the 19th century. Freedom of the population from lice explains the absence of epidemics in the United States. Sporadic cases in the United States have been associated with flying squirrel contact. The location of the disease is now limited to the Balkans and Middle East, North Africa, Asia, Mexico, and the Andes. In the epidemic form, all age groups are affected.

Rickettsiae may remain viable for as long as 20 years in the tissues of recovered patients without manifest symptoms. Brill-Zinsser disease is a recrudescence of epidemic typhus that occurs years after the initial attack and may cause a new epidemic.

Murine typhus (*R. typhi*) is worldwide in distribution and is distributed to humans by fleas. The disease is most prevalent in southeastern and Gulf Coast states and among individuals whose occupations bring them into rat-infested areas. The disease is most common in the late summer and fall months.

Diagnosis

A presumptive diagnosis of typhus fever may be made on the basis of the characteristic skin rash and signs of involvement of the nervous system. The diagnosis is established by the Weil-Felix reaction, which becomes positive in the fifth to eighth day of the disease. The titer rises in the first few weeks of the convalescence and then falls. Antibodies to specific rickettsiae may be demonstrated by complement fixation, microagglutination, or immunofluorescence reactions.

Course and Prognosis

The course of typhus fever usually extends over 2 weeks to 3 weeks. Death from epidemic typhus usually occurs between the ninth and eighteenth day of illness. In patients who recover, the temperature begins to fall after 14 days to 18 days and reaches normal levels in 2 days to 4 days. Complications include bronchitis and bronchopneumonia, myocardial degeneration, gangrene of the skin or limbs, and thrombosis of large abdominal, pulmonary, or cerebral vessels.

The prognosis of epidemic typhus depends on the patient's age and immunization status. The disease is usually mild in children younger than 10 years of age. After the third decade, mortality increases steadily with each decade. Death is usually due to the development of pneumonia, circulatory collapse, and renal failure. The mortality rate for murine typhus in the United States is low (less than 1%). There are no neurologic residua in patients who recover. Treatment is with doxycycline or chloramphenicol, as in Rocky Mountain spotted fever.

Scrub Typhus

Scrub typhus is an infectious disease caused by *R. tsutsugamushi* (*R. orientalis*), which is transmitted to humans by the bite of larval trombiculid mites (chiggers). It resembles the other rickettsial diseases and is characterized by sudden onset of fever, cutaneous eruption, and the presence of an ulcerative lesion (eschar) at the site of attachment of the chigger.

Epidemiology

The disease is limited to eastern and southeastern Asia, India, and northern Australia and adjacent islands.

Symptoms and Signs

The disease begins abruptly, after an incubation period of 10 days to 12 days, with fever, chills, and headache. The headache increases in intensity and may become severe. Conjunctival congestion, moderate generalized lymphadenopathy, deafness, apathy, and anorexia are common symptoms. Delirium, coma, restlessness, and muscular twitchings are present in severe cases. A primary lesion (the eschar) is seen in nearly all cases and represents the former site of attachment of the infected mite. There may be multiple eschars. The cutaneous rash appears between the fifth and eighth day of the disease. The eruption is macular or maculopapular and nonhemorrhagic. The trunk is involved first with later extension to the limbs.

Diagnosis

The diagnosis is made on the basis of the development of typical symptoms, the presence of the characteristic eschar, and a rising titer to *Proteus* OXK in the Weil-Felix test during the second week of illness. Immunofluorescence testing with specific antigens may be diagnostic.

Course, Prognosis and Treatment

In fatal cases, death usually occurs in the second or third week as a result of pneumonia, cardiac failure, or cerebral involvement. In the preantibiotic era, mortality could reach 60%, depending on geographic locale and virulence of the strain. Deaths are rare with appropriate antibiotic treatment, which is similar to treatment used for Rocky Mountain spotted fever.

In patients who recover, the temperature begins to fall at the end of the second or third week. Permanent residua are not common, but the period of convalescence may extend over several months.

Human Ehrlichiosis

The nature and extent of infections in humans with rickettsia of the genus *Ehrlichia* is still not fully determined. These organisms appear to infect leukocytes. Two forms of human infection have been identified. One species, *E. chaffeensis*, is associated with HME and the organism may be preferentially found in these cells. The causative organism of HGE has not yet been assigned a species. Serologically it cross-reacts with *E. equus*, but it is not clear if it is the same species. Both human infections are detectable in the appropriate cells as coccobacillary forms. It has become possible to cultivate the organ-

isms, and PCR reactions are also coming into use to detect infection. Most studies still rely on antibody detection. *E. chaffeensis* appears to be transmitted by *Amblyomma americanum* (lone star tick) and possibly by *D. variabilis*, whereas the human granulocytic ehrlichiosis agent is transmitted by *Ixodid* ticks and probably *Dermacentor andersonii*.

Epidemiology

The epidemiologic range for both agents appears to be extending. Whether this is an actual phenomenon or due to an heightened awareness of the infection is still unclear. HME is more common in the South and Southeast, whereas HGE was first found in the Midwest. Now cases have been reported from New England and New York State, in keeping with the distribution of *Ixodes scapularis*. Coinfection of HGE with *Borrelia burgdorferi* and HME with Rocky Mountain spotted fever has been reported.

Symptoms and Signs

Infection of both organisms usually presents as a febrile systemic process often associated with myalgia and headache. Changes in mental status and ataxia have also been noted and are correlated with more serious illness. Rashes have been reported in about 20% of cases. This makes it difficult to distinguish the illness from Rocky Mountain spotted fever, whose distribution overlaps with *E. chaffeensis*. CSF pleocytosis and elevated proteins have been reported and appear to correlate with altered mental status.

Diagnosis

Because of the nonspecific nature of the symptoms and signs, a high index of suspicion is required. A history of exposure to ticks may be helpful, but epidemiologic studies have shown serologic evidence of infection usually is not correlated with known tick bites. As might be anticipated, lymphopenia is often a feature of *E. chaffeensis* infection, whereas granulocytopenia is usually noted with the HGE infection. Elevated hepatic enzymes are usually present. The rickettsiae may often be found in infected leukocytes. Confirmation of the diagnosis is by antibody titers or immunofluorescent detection of the intracellular organisms. PCR detection of the organisms' DNA, when it is more widely available, will be an important diagnostic technique because of its sensitivity and rapidity. Culturing of the causative organisms is now also possible but is not as sensitive as PCR.

Course, Prognosis, and Treatment

A complete understanding of the course of both HME and HGE has yet to be determined. Initially, a high proportion of reported cases was fatal in both HME and HGE. However, serologic studies indicate asymptomatic or minor infections are common. Clinically, it has also been found that some cases may be self-limited, even without treatment. Treatment with doxycycline results in rapid improvement. Therefore, prognosis appears to be good, if the diagnosis is promptly made and treatment started. Whether chloramphenicol will be an acceptable alternative antibiotic has yet to be established.

OTHER BACTERIAL INFECTIONS

Brucellosis

Brucellosis (undulant fever) is a disease with protean manifestation due to infection with short, slender, rod-shaped, gram-negative microorganisms of the genus *Brucella*. The infection is transmitted to humans from animals, usually cattle or swine. The illness is prone to occur in slaughterhouse workers, livestock producers, veterinarians, and persons who ingest unpasteurized milk or milk products. An acute febrile illness is characteristic of the early stages of the disease. The common symptoms include chilly sensations, sweats, fever, weakness, and generalized malaise; 70% of patients experience body aches and nearly 50% complain of headache. Physical signs of lymphadenopathy, splenomegaly, hepatomegaly, and tenderness of the spine, however, are infrequent, occurring in less than 25% of cases. The early constitutional symptoms are followed by the subacute and chronic stages in about 15% to 20% of patients with localized infection of the bones, joints, lungs, kidneys, liver, lymph nodes, and other organs.

Involvement of the nervous system is not common. Cases have been reported with meningitis and sometimes with accompanying cranial nerve paresis, meningoencephalitis, meningomyelitis, optic neuritis, and peripheral neuritis. Brain abscesses also have been reported.

The CSF in reported cases is under increased pressure, with a lymphocytic pleocytosis varying from a few to several hundred cells. The protein content is moderately to greatly increased, and the sugar content is decreased. The CSF has increased gamma globulin levels and often contains *Brucella*-agglutinating antibodies.

In the few patients with CNS involvement who came to autopsy, there was a subacute meningitis with perivascular infiltrations, thickening of the vessels in the brain and spinal cord, and degenerative changes in the white and gray matter. Organisms have been cultured from the CSF of a few patients.

The diagnosis is made from a history of symptoms of the disease, culture of the organisms from the blood or CSF, and serologic testing. Treatment is with doxycycline or other tetracycline plus an aminoglycoside. Trimethoprim/sulfoxazole is an alternative to the tetracycline.

Behçet Syndrome

An inflammatory disorder of unknown cause, characterized by the occurrence of relapsing uveitis and recurrent genital and oral ulcers, was described by Behçet in 1937. The disease may involve the nervous system, skin, joints, peripheral blood vessels, and other organs. Evidence of CNS involvement is present in 25% to 30% of patients. Neurologic symptoms antedate the more diagnostic criteria of aphthous stomatitis, genital ulcerations, and uveitis, in only 5% of cases. Pathologic confirmation of cerebral involvement has been obtained in a few cases. The disease appears to have a predilection for young adult men.

Etiology and Pathology

The cause of Behçet syndrome is unknown. No infectious organism has been isolated consistently, although there have been several reports of a virus having been recovered from patients with the disease. Circulating immune complexes of the IgA and IgG variety may be detected in patients' serums. The disease is associated with HLA-B5 tissue type in Japan and the Mediterranean nations.

In patients studied at necropsy, there was a mild inflammatory reaction in the meninges and in the perivascular spaces of the cerebrum, basal ganglia, brainstem, and cerebellum and degenerative changes in the ganglion cells. Inflammatory changes were also found in the iris, choroid, retina, and optic nerve.

Epidemiology

The disease is common in northern Japan, Turkey, and Israel; the incidence in Japan is 1 in 10,000 population. The syndrome is seen less commonly in the United States. An annual incidence of 1 in 300,000 population was determined for Olmstead County, Minnesota. The age at onset is in the third and fourth decades of life; men are more frequently affected than women. The exact incidence of neurologic symptoms is not known, but it approximates 10% of affected individuals.

Symptoms and Signs

The ocular signs include keratoconjunctivitis, iritis, hypopyon, uveitis, and hemorrhage into the vitreous. Ocular symptoms occur in 90% of patients and may progress to total blindness in one or both eyes. The cutaneous lesions are in the nature of painful recurrent and indolent ulcers, most commonly found on the genitalia or the buccal mucosa. Virtually all patients have recurrent oral aphthous ulcers. Arthritis occurs in about 50% of patients. Furunculosis, erythema nodosum, thrombophlebitis, and nonspecific skin sensitivity are also common. Patients with Behçet syndrome often develop a pustule surrounded by erythema at the site of a needle puncture; when present, the finding is considered virtually pathognomonic.

Any portion of the nervous system may be affected. Cranial nerve palsies are common. Other symptoms and signs include papilledema, convulsions, mental confusion, coma, aphasia, hemiparesis, quadriparesis, pseudobulbar palsy, and evidence of involvement of the basal ganglia, cerebellum, or spinal cord.

Laboratory Data

A low-grade fever is common during the acute exacerbations of the disease. Fever may be accompanied by an elevation of the sedimentation rate, anemia, and a slight leukocytosis in the blood. A polyclonal increase in serum gamma globulin may be present. Coagulation profile may disclose elevated levels of fibrinogen and factor VIII.

The CSF pressure may be slightly increased. There is a pleocytosis of a mild or moderate degree. Either lymphocytes or neutrophils may predominate. There is a moderate increase in the protein content. CSF sugar, when reported, has been normal. The serologic tests for syphilis are negative in the blood and CSF. Elevation of the CSF gamma globulin content has been reported. CSF cultures have been negative. Mild diffuse abnormalities may be found on the electroencephalogram. CT may demonstrate lesions of decreased density that may be contrast enhancing. On MRI, T2-weighted high-signal white matter lesions are often seen.

Diagnosis

The diagnosis is based on the occurrence of signs of a meningoencephalitis in combination with the characteristic cutaneous and ocular lesions. The disease may simulate multiple sclerosis with multifocal involvement of the nervous system, including the brainstem, cerebellum, and corticospinal tract. Syphilis is excluded by the negative serologic tests. Sarcoidosis is excluded by the absence of other characteristic clinical signs of this disease; lack of diagnostic changes in biopsied lymph nodes, liver, or other tissues; and the presence of serum ACE.

Course

The course of the disease is characterized by a series of remissions and exacerbations extending over several years. During the period of remission, all symptoms may improve greatly. Unilateral amblyopia or complete blindness may result from the ocular lesions. Residuals of the neurologic lesions are not uncommon.

Neurologic and posterior uveal tract lesions indicate a poor prognosis. Death has occurred from the disease, chiefly when the CNS became involved. Permanent remission of symptoms has not been reported.

Treatment

Various antibiotics, chemotherapy, and corticosteroids have been used in the treatment, but there is no evidence that any of these forms of therapy have any effect on the course of the disease. When the neurologic components of the disease are life threatening, immunosuppressive therapy may be considered. Therapy is difficult to assess because of the variable natural course of the disease.

Vogt-Koyanagi-Harada Syndrome

This rare disease, characterized by uveitis, retinal hemorrhages and detachment, depigmentation of the skin and hair, and signs of involvement of the nervous system, was reported by Vogt, Koyanagi, and Harada in the 1920s. The dermatologic signs include poliosis and canities (i.e., patchy whitening of eyelashes, eyebrows, and scalp hair), alopecia (i.e., patchy loss of hair), and vitiligo (i.e., patchy depigmentation of skin).

The nervous system is affected in practically all cases. The neurologic symptoms are caused by an inflammatory adhesive arachnoiditis. The most common patient complaint is headache, sometimes accompanied by dizziness, fatigue, and somnolence. Neurosensory deafness, hemiplegia, ocular palsies, psychotic manifestations, and meningeal signs may occur. The CSF is under increased pressure. There is a moderate degree of lymphocytic pleocytosis. The CSF protein content is normal or slightly elevated; an elevated gamma globulin has been reported. The CSF glucose level is normal. The period of activity of the process lasts for 6 months to 12 months and is followed by a recrudescence of the ophthalmic and neurologic signs.

The cause of the disease is unknown. It has been suggested that it is caused by a viral infection, but proof for this is lacking. The eye lesions are similar to those of sympathetic ophthalmia. There is no specific therapy, but some reports suggest that administration of corticosteroids may be of value.

Mollaret Meningitis

Patients with recurrent episodes of benign, aseptic meningitis were first described by Mollaret in 1944.

Symptoms and Signs

The disease is characterized by repeated, short-lived, spontaneous, remitting attacks of headache and by nuchal rigidity. Between attacks, the patient enjoys good health. The meningitic episodes usually last 2 days or 3 days. Most are characterized by a mild meningitis without associated neurologic abnormalities. Transient neurologic disturbances (i.e., coma, seizures, syncope, diplopia, dysarthria, disequilibrium, facial paralysis, anisocoria, and extensor plantar responses) have been reported. The patient's body temperature is moderately elevated with a maximum of 104°F (40°C). Neck stiffness and the signs of meningeal irritation are present. The first attack may appear at any age between childhood and late adult years. Both sexes are equally affected. The episodes usually last for 3 years to 5 years.

Laboratory Data

During the attacks, there is a CSF pleocytosis and a slight elevation of the protein content. The CSF sugar content is normal. The cell counts range from 200 to several thousand/mm³; most cells are mononuclear. Large fragile endothelial cells are found in the CSF in the early phases of the disease; their presence is variable and is not considered essential for the diagnosis.

Etiology

Proposed etiologic agents in individual cases have included herpes simplex type I, epidermoid cyst, and histoplasmosis, but none has been found with consistency. In recent years, detection of herpes simplex type II genome by PCR has been regularly, but not uniformly, reported in recurrent aseptic meningitis to which the name Mollaret meningitis is often applied. It is uncertain whether this constitutes a dilution of the eponym. It is therefore still not possible to determine whether Mollaret meningitis is a syndrome of multiple etiologies or a disease that excludes known causes.

Diagnosis and Treatment

The differential diagnosis of the condition includes recurrent bacterial meningitis, recurrent viral meningitis, sarcoidosis, hydatid cyst, fungal meningitis, intracranial tumors, Behçet syndrome, and the Vogt-Koyanagi-Harada syndrome. The latter two conditions may be differentiated by eye and skin lesions and associated findings.

Patients with Mollaret meningitis always recover rapidly and spontaneously without specific therapy. There is no effective therapy for shortening the attack or preventing fresh attacks.

Aseptic Meningeal Reaction

Aseptic meningeal reaction (sympathetic meningitis, meningitis serosa) refers to those cases with evidence of a meningeal reaction in the CSF in the absence of any infecting organism. Four general classes of cases fall into this category: those in which the meningeal reaction is caused by a septic or necrotic focus within the skull or spinal canal (e.g., parameningeal infection); those in which the meningeal reaction is stems from the introduction of foreign substances (e.g., air, dyes, drugs, blood) into the

subarachnoid space; those in association with connective tissue disorders; and those associated with systemically administered medications (e.g., trimethoprim/sulfoxazole or nonsteroidal antiinflammatory agents).

The symptoms present in the patients in the first group are associated with the infection or morbid process in the skull or spinal cavity. Only occasionally are there any symptoms and signs of meningeal irritation.

In the second group of patients, where the meningeal reaction is to the result of the introduction of foreign substances into the subarachnoid space, fever, headache, and stiffness of the neck may occur. The appearance of these symptoms leads to the suspicion that an actual infection of the meninges has been produced by the inadvertent introduction of pathogenic organisms. The normal sugar content of the CSF and the absence of organisms on culture establish the nature of the meningeal reaction.

An aseptic meningeal reaction may complicate the course of systemic lupus erythematosus and other collagen vascular diseases. In certain instances, the meningeal reaction in patients with systemic lupus erythematosus may be induced by nonsteroidal antiinflammatory drugs or azathioprine.

The findings in the CSF characteristic of an aseptic meningeal reaction are an increase in pressure, a varying degree of pleocytosis (10 cell/mm³ to 4,000 cell/mm³), a slight or moderate increase in the protein content, a normal sugar content, and the absence of organisms on culture. Exceptionally, and without explanation, the aseptic meningeal reaction of systemic lupus erythematosus may be accompanied by low CSF sugar values. With a severe degree of meningeal reaction, the CSF may be purulent in appearance and may contain several thousand cells per cubic mm³ with a predominance of polymorphonuclear leukocytes. With a lesser degree of meningeal reaction, the CSF may be normal in appearance or only slightly cloudy and may contain a moderate number of cells (10 cell/mm³ to several hundred/mm³), with lymphocytes being the predominating cell type in the CSF.

The pathogenesis of the changes in the CSF is not clearly understood. The septic foci in the head more commonly associated with an aseptic meningeal reaction are septic thrombosis of the intracranial venous sinuses; osteomyelitis of the spine or skull; extradural, subdural, or intracerebral abscesses; or septic cerebral emboli. Nonseptic foci of necrosis are accompanied only rarely by an aseptic meningeal reaction. Occasionally, patients with an intracerebral tumor or cerebral hemorrhage located near the ventricular walls may show similar changes in the CSF.

The diagnosis of an aseptic meningeal reaction in patients with a septic or necrotic focus in the skull or spinal cord is important, in that it directs attention to the presence of this focus and the necessity for appropriate surgical and medical therapy before the meninges are actually invaded by the infectious process, or before other cerebral or spinal complications develop.

Meningism

Coincidental with the onset of acute infectious diseases in childhood or young adult life there may be headache, stiffness of the neck, Kernig sign, and, rarely, delirium, convulsions, or coma. The appearance of these symptoms may lead to the tentative diagnosis of an acute meningitis or encephalitis.

Meningism refers to the syndrome of headache and signs of meningeal irritation in patients with an acute febrile illness, usually of a viral nature, in whom the CSF is commonly under increased pressure but normal in other respects. The condition may prove diagnostically confusing.

There is no completely satisfactory explanation for the syndrome. Acute hypotonicity of the patient's serum, inappropriate secretion of antidiuretic hormone, and an increased formation of CSF have been considered as possible causes. The characteristic findings on lumbar puncture are a slight or moderate increase in pressure, a clear colorless CSF that contains no cells, and a moderate reduction in the protein content of the CSF.

The condition is brief in duration. Spinal puncture, usually performed as a diagnostic measure in these cases, is the only therapy necessary for the relief of the symptoms. The reduction of pressure by the removal of CSF results in the disappearance of symptoms. Rarely is more than one puncture necessary.

Mycoplasma pneumoniae Infection

Mycoplasmas, originally called pleuropneumonia-like organisms, lack a cell wall. Individual mycoplasmas are bounded by a unit membrane that encloses the cytoplasm, DNA, RNA, and other cellular components. They are the smallest of free-living organisms and are resistant to penicillin and other cell wall-active antimicrobials.

Of mycoplasmas that infect humans, *M. pneumoniae* is the only species that has been clearly shown to be a significant cause of disease. It is a major cause of acute respiratory disease, including pneumonia. A variety of neurologic conditions have been described in association with *M. pneumoniae* infection: meningitis, encephalitis, postinfectious leukoencephalitis, acute cerebellar ataxia, transverse myelitis, ascending polyneuritis, radiculopathy, cranial neuropathy, and acute psychosis. The most common neurologic condition appears to be meningitis or meningoencephalitis with alterations in mental status. The neurologic features associated with *M. pneumoniae* infection, however, are so diverse that the correct diagnosis may not be made on clinical grounds, alone. The CSF usually contains polymorphonuclear leukocytes and mononuclear cells in varying proportions. The CSF has a normal or mildly elevated protein content and a normal glucose level. Bacterial, viral, and mycoplasma cultures of the CSF are usually sterile. How-

ever, detection of mycoplasma in tissue or CSF has been accomplished.

Retrospective diagnosis may be made by cold isohemagglutinins for human type O erythrocytes. These may be detected in about 50% of patients during the second week of illness; they are the first antibodies to disappear. Specific antibodies may also be demonstrated. PCR is now being used to detect mycoplasma in the blood and CSF.

Doxycycline and erythromycin are the drugs of choice for *M. pneumoniae* infections. It is not known if the postinfectious neurologic complications benefit from antimicrobial treatment.

Legionella pneumophila Infection

L. pneumophila is a poorly staining gram-negative bacterium that either does not grow or grows very slowly on most artificial media. The organism was first isolated from fatal cases of pneumonia among persons attending an American Legion Convention in Philadelphia in 1976. The bacterium is acquired by inhalation of contaminated aerosols or dust from air-conditioning systems, water, or soil.

Symptoms and Signs

Pneumonia is the most typical systemic manifestation of infection. Upper respiratory infection, a severe influenza-like syndrome (Pontiac fever), and gastrointestinal disease may also occur.

Several neurologic conditions have been described in association with *L. pneumophila* infection (Legionnaires' disease, legionellosis): acute encephalomyelitis, severe cerebellar ataxia, chorea, and peripheral neuropathy. Confusion, delirium, and hallucinations are common symptoms. The pathophysiology of these syndromes is unclear because bacteria rarely have been demonstrated in the CNS. Myoglobinuria and elevated serum creatine kinase levels also have been reported.

Laboratory Data

L. pneumophila is rarely recovered from pleural fluid, sputum, or blood; it frequently may be isolated from respiratory secretions by transtracheal aspiration or bronchoalveolar lavage and lung biopsy tissue. A retrospective diagnosis may be made by a significant rise in specific serum antibodies detected by immunofluorescence.

Treatment

The treatment of choice is azithromycin or erythromycin. Relapses are uncommon if treatment is continued for 14 days. When relapses occur, they usually respond to a second course of the antibiotic.

The true incidence of neurologic involvement in Legionnaires' disease is still unknown. The neurologic deficit is known to be reversible, but little exact information about recovery is available.

SUGGESTED READINGS
Acute Bacterial Meningitis

Bashir E, Laundy M, Booy R. Diagnosis and treatment of bacterial meningitis. *Arch Dis Child* 2003;88:615–620.

van de Beek D, de Gans J, McIntyre P, Prasad K. Corticosteroids in acute bacterial meningitis. *The Cochrane Database of Systematic Reviews.* 2003;1:CD004305.

Benson CA, Harris AA. Acute neurologic infections. *Med Clin North Am* 1986;70:987–1011.

Carter JA, Neville BGR, Newton CRJC. Neuro-cognitive impairment following acquired central nervous system infections in childhood: a systematic review. *Brain Res Rev* 2003;43:57–69.

Centers for Disease Control and Prevention. *Prevention and control of meningococcal disease. Recommendations of the Advisory Committee on Immunization Practices (ACIP). MMWR* 2000;49:1–10.

Dunne DW, Quagliarello V. Group B streptococcal meningitis in adults. *Medicine (Baltimore)* 1993;72:1–10.

de Gans J, van de Beek D. Dexamethasone in adults with bacterial meningitis. *N Engl J Med* 2002;347:1549–1556.

Gilbert D, Moellering RJ, Sande M. eds. *The Sanford Guide to Antimicrobial Therapy,* 34th ed. Vienna: Antimicrobial Therapy Inc., 2004.

Holt DE, Halket S, de Louvois J, Harvey D. Neonatal meningitis in England and Wales: 10 years on. *Arch Dis Child* 2001;84:F85–F89.

Mancebo J, Domingo P, Blanch L, et al. Post-neurosurgical and spontaneous gram-negative bacillary meningitis in adults. *Scand J Infect Dis* 1986;18:533–538.

Mylonakis E, Hohmann EL, Calderwood SB. Central nervous system infection with *Listeria monocytogenes.* 33 years' experience at a general hospital and review of 776 episodes from the literature. *Medicine (Baltimore)* 1998;77:313–336.

Pruitt AA. Infections of the nervous system. *Neurol Clin* 1998;16:419–447.

Qayyum Q, Scerpella E, Moreno J, Fischl M. Report of 24 cases of Listeria monocytogenes infection at the University of Miami Medical Center. *Rev Invest Clin* 1997;49:265–270.

Quagliarello V, Scheld W. Treatment of bacterial meningitis. *N Engl J Med* 1997;336:708–716.

Roos K. Acute bacterial meningitis. *Semin Neurol* 2000;20:293–306.

Schuchat A, Robinson K, Wenger J, et al. Bacterial meningitis in the United States in 1995. *N Engl J Med* 1997;337:970–976.

Zangwill KM, Schuchat A, Riedo FX, et al. School-based clusters of meningococcal disease in the United States. Descriptive epidemiology and a case-control analysis. *JAMA* 1997;277:389–395.

Subacute Meningitis
Tuberculous Meningitis

Bernaerts A, Vanhoenacker FM, Parizel PM, et al. Tuberculosis of the central nervous system: overview of neuroradiological findings. *Eur Radiol* 2003;13:1876–1890.

Garcia-Monco JC. Central nervous system tuberculosis. *Neurol Clin* 1999;17:737–759.

Hosoglu S, Geyik MF, Balik I, et al. Predictors of outcome in patients with tuberculous meningitis. *Int J Tuberc Lung Dis* 2002;6:64–70.

Hosoglu S, Ayaz C, Geyik MF, Kokoglu OF, Ceviz A. Tuberculous meningitis in adults: an eleven-year review. *Int J Tuberc Lung Dis* 1998;2:553–557.

Kashyap RS, Kainthla RP, Satpute RM, Agarwal NP, Chandak NH, Purohit HJ, Taori GM, Daginawala HF. Differential diagnosis of tuberculous meningitis from partially-treated pyogenic meningitis by cell ELISA. *BMC Neurol* 2004; Oct 22;4(1):16.

Pai M, Flores LL, Pai N, et al. Diagnostic accuracy of nucleic acid amplification tests for tuberculous meningitis: a systematic review and meta-analysis. *Lancet* 2003;3:633–643.

Quagliarello V. Adjunctive steroids for tuberculous meningitis—more evidence, more questions. *N Engl J Med* 2004; Oct 21;351(17):1792–1794.

Schoeman J, Wait J, Burger M, et al. Long-term follow up of childhood tuberculous meningitis. *Devel Med & Child Neurol* 2002;44:522–526.

Thwaites G, Chau TTH, Mai NTH, et al. Tuberculous meningitis. *J Neurol Neurosurg Psychiatry* 2000;68:289–299.

Zuger A, Lowy FD. Tuberculosis. In: Scheld WM, Whitley RJ, Durack DT, eds. *Infections of the central nervous system.* Philadelphia: Lippincott-Raven, 1997:417–443.

Subdural and Epidural Infections
Cerebral Subdural Empyema

Baum PA, Dillon WP. Utility of magnetic resonance imaging in the detection of subdural empyema. *Ann Otol Rhinol Laryngol* 1992;101:876–878.

Bernardini GL. Diagnosis and management of brain abscess and subdural empyema. *Curr Neurol Neurosci Rep* 2004; Nov; 4(6):448–456.

Helfgott DC, Weingarten K, Hartman BJ. Subdural empyema. In: Scheld WM, Whitley RJ, Durack DT, eds. *Infections of the Central Nervous System.* Philadelphia: Lippincott-Raven, 1997:495–505.

Kaufman DM, Litman N, Miller MH. Sinusitis: induced subdural empyema. *Neurology* 1983;33:123–132.

Kaufman DM, Miller MH, Steigbigel NH. Subdural empyema: analysis of 17 recent cases and review of the literature. *Medicine (Baltimore)* 1975;54:485–498.

Tsuchiya K, Osawa A, Katase S, et al. Diffusion-weighted MRI of subdural and epidural empyemas. *Neuroradiology* 2003;45:220–223.

Intracranial Epidural Abscess

Gellin BG, Weingarten K, Gamache FWJ, Hartman BJ. Epidural abscess. In: Scheld WM, Whitley RJ, Durack DT, eds. *Infections of the Central Nervous System.* Philadelphia: Lippincott-Raven, 1997:507–522.

Helfgott DC, Weingarten K, Hartman BJ. Subdural empyema. In: Scheld WM, Whitley RJ, Durack DT, eds. *Infections of the Central Nervous System,* 2nd ed. Philadelphia: Lippincott-Raven, 1997:495–505.

Tsai Y-D, Chang W-N, Shen C-C, et al. Intracranial suppuration: a clinical comparison of subdural empyemas and epidural abscesses. *Surg Neurol* 2003;59:191–196.

Weingarten K, Zimmerman RD, Becker RD, et al. Subdural and epidural empyemas: MR imaging. *AJR Am J Roentgenol* 1989;152:615–621.

Spinal Epidural Abscess

Darouiche RO, Hamill RJ, Greenberg SB, et al. Bacterial spinal epidural abscess. Review of 43 cases and literature survey. *Medicine (Baltimore)* 1992;71:369–385.

Hooten WM, Kinney MO, Huntoon MA. Epidural abscess and meningitis after epidural corticosteroid injection. *Mayo Clin Proceed* 2004;79(5):682–686.

Joshi SM, Hatfield RH, Martin J, Taylor W. Spinal epidural abscess: a diagnostic challenge. *Brit J Neurosurg* 2003;17:160–163.

Khan S-NH, Hussain MS, Griebel RW, Hatting S. Title comparison of primary and secondary spinal epidural abscesses: a retrospective analysis of 29 cases. *Surg Neurol* 2003;59:28–33.

Lu C-H, Chang W-N, Lui C-C, Lee P-Y, Chang H-W. Adult spinal epidural abscess: clinical features and prognostic factors. *Clin Neurol Neurosurg* 2002;104:306–310.

Reihsaus E, Waldbaur H, Seeling W. Spinal epidural abscess: a meta-analysis of 915 patients. *Neurosurg Rev* 2000;23:175–204.

Soehle M, Wallenfang T. Spinal epidural abscesses: clinical manifestations, prognostic factors, and outcomes. *Neurosurgery* 2002;51:79–87.

Infective Endocarditis

Bertorini TE, Gelfand M. Neurological complications of bacterial endocarditis. *Compr Ther* 1990;16:47–55.

Brust J, Dickinson P, Hughes J, Holtzmann R. The diagnosis and treatment of cerebral mycotic aneurysms. *Ann Neurol* 1990;27:238–246.

Calza L, Manfredi R, Chiodo F. Infective endocarditis: a review of the best treatment options. *Expert Opin Pharmacother* 2004 Sep;5(9):1899–1916.

Francioli P. Complications of infective endocarditis. In: Scheld WM, Whitley RJ, Durack DT, eds. *Infections of the Central Nervous System.* Philadelphia: Lippincott-Raven, 1997:523–553.

Garvey GJ, Neu HC. Infective endocarditis—an evolving disease. A review of endocarditis at the Columbia-Presbyterian Medical Center 1968–1973. *Medicine (Baltimore)* 1978;57:105–127.

Heimberger TS, Duma RJ. Infections of prosthetic heart valves and cardiac pacemakers. *Infect Dis Clin North Am* 1989;3:221–245.

Gregoratos G. Infective endocarditis in the elderly: diagnosis and management. *Am J Geriatric Cardiology* 2003;12:183–189.

Millar BC, Moore JE. Current trends in the molecular diagnosis of infective endocarditis. *Europ J Clin Microbiol Infect Dis* 2004;23(5):353–365.

Mourvillier B, Trouillet JL, Timsit JF, Baudot J, Chastre J, Regnier B, Gibert C, Wolff M. Infective endocarditis in the intensive care unit: clinical spectrum and prognostic factors in 228 consecutive patients. *Intensive Care Med* 2004 Nov;30(11):2046–2052. Epub 2004 Sep 15.

Prendergast BD. Diagnostic criteria and problems in infective endocarditis. *Heart* (British Cardiac Society) 2004;90(6):611–613.

Salgado AV, Furlan AJ, Keys TF, et al. Neurologic complications of endocarditis. A 12-year experience. *Neurology* 1989;39:173–178.

Tunkel AR, Pradhan SK. Central nervous system infections in injection drug users. *Infect Dis Clin N Am* 2002;16:589–605.

Valencia E, Miro J. Endocarditis in the setting of HIV infection. *Mayo Clin Proceed* 2004;79(5):682–686.

Leprosy

Chad DA, Hedley-Whyte ET. Case 1-2004: a 49-year-old woman with asymmetric painful neuropathy. *N Engl J Med* 2004;350:166–176.

Browne SG. Leprosy—clinical aspects of nerve involvement. In: Hornabrook RW, ed. *Topics on Tropical Neurology.* Philadelphia: FA Davis, 1975:1–6.

Charosky CB, Gatti JC, Cardama JE. Neuropathies in Hansen's disease. *Int J Lepr Other Mycobact Dis* 1983;51:576–586.

Nations SP, Katz JS, Lyde CB, Barohn RJ. Leprous neuropathy: an American perspective. *Semin Neurol* 1998;18:113–124.

Ooi WW, Srinivasan J. Leprosy and the peripheral nervous system: basic and clinical aspects. *Muscle Nerve* 2004 Oct;30(4):393–409.

Pedley JC, Harman DJ, Waudby H, McDougall AC. Leprosy in peripheral nerves: histopathological findings in 119 untreated patients in Nepal. *J Neurol Neurosurg Psychiatry* 1980;43:198–204.

Porichha D, Mukherjee A, Ramu G. Neural pathology in leprosy during treatment and surveillance. *Lepr Rev* 2004 Sep;75(3):233–241.

Sabin TD, Swift TR, Jacobson RR. Leprosy. In: Dyck PJ, Thomas PK, Griffin JW, Low PA, Poduslo JF, eds. *Peripheral Neuropathy,* 3rd ed, vol. 2. Philadelphia: WB Saunders, 1993:1354–1379.

Turkof E, Richard B, Assadian O, et al. Leprosy affects facial nerves in a scattered distribution from the main trunk to all peripheral branches and neurolysis improves muscle function of the face. *Am J Trop Med Hyg* 2003;68:81–88.

Rickettsial Infections

Bleck TP. Central nervous system involvement in rickettsial diseases. *Neurol Clin* 1999;17:801–812.

Kim JH, Durack DT. Rickettsiae. In: Scheld WM, Whitley RJ, Durack DT, eds. *Infections of the central nervous system.* Philadelphia: Lippincott-Raven, 1997:403–416.

Marrie TJ, Raoult D. Rickettsial infections of the central nervous system. *Semin Neurol* 1992;12:213–224.

Rizzo M, Mansueto P, DiLorenzo G, et al. Rickettsial disease: Classical and modern aspects. *New Microbiologica* 2004;27(1):87–103.

Shaked Y. Rickettsial infection of the central nervous system: the role of prompt antimicrobial therapy. *Q J Med* 1991;79:301–306.

Spach DH, Liles WC, Campbell GL, et al. Tick-borne diseases in the United States. *N Engl J Med* 1993;329:936–947.

Rocky Mountain Spotted Fever

Bell WE, Lascari AD. Rocky Mountain spotted fever. Neurological symptoms in the acute phase. *Neurology* 1970;20:841–847.

Case records of the Massachusetts General Hospital. Weekly clinico-pathological exercises. Case 32-1997. A 43-year-old woman with rapidly changing pulmonary infiltrates and markedly increased intracranial pressure. *N Engl J Med* 1997;337:1149–1156.

Latham RH, Schaffner W. Rocky Mountain spotted (and spotless) fever. *Compr Ther* 1992;18:18–21.

Massey EW, Thames T, Coffey CE, Gallis HA. Neurologic complications of Rocky Mountain spotted fever. *South Med J* 1985;78:1288–1290, 1303.

Masters EJ, Olson GS, Weiner SJ, Paddock CD. Rocky mountain spotted fever. *Arch Intern Med* 2003;163:769–774.

Sexton DJ, Kaye KS. Rocky mountain spotted fever. *Med Clin N Amer* 2002;86:351–360.

Thorner AR, Walker DH, Petri WA Jr. Rocky mountain spotted fever. *Clin Infect Dis* 1998;27:1353–1359.

Typhus Fever

Herman E. Neurological syndromes in typhus fever. *J Nerv Ment Dis* 1949;109:25–36.

Scrub Typhus

Lee HC, Ko WC, Lee HL, Chen HY. Clinical manifestations and complications of rickettsiosis in southern Taiwan. *J Form Med Assoc* 2002;101:385–392.

Ripley MS. Neuropsychiatric observations on tsutsugamushi (scrub typhus). *Arch Neurol Psychiatry* 1946;56:42–54.

Ehrlichiosis

Dumler JS, Bakken JS. Human ehrlichioses: newly recognized infections transmitted by ticks. *Annu Rev Med* 1998;49:201–213.

Gardner SL, Holman RC, Krebs JW, Berkelman R, Childs JE. National surveillance for the human ehrlichioses in the United States, 1997–2001, and proposed methods for evaluation of data quality. *Ann NY Acad Sci* 2003;990:80–89.

Horowitz HW, Aguero-Rosenfeld ME, McKenna DF, et al. Clinical and laboratory spectrum of culture-proven human granulocytic ehrlichiosis: comparison with culture-negative cases. *Clin Infect Dis* 1998;27:1314–1317.

Lee MS, Goslee TE, Lessell S. Ehrlichiosis optic neuritis. *Am J Ophthalmology* 2003;135:412–413.

Nadelman RB, Horowitz HW, Hsieh TC, et al. Simultaneous human granulocytic ehrlichiosis and Lyme borreliosis. *N Engl J Med* 1997;337:27–30.

Parola P. Tick-borne rickettsial diseases: emerging risks in Europe. *Comp Immunol Microbiol Infect Dis* 2004;27(5):297–304.

Ratnasamy N, Everett ED, Roland WE, McDonald G, Caldwell CW. Central nervous system manifestations of human ehrlichiosis. *Clin Infect Dis* 1996;23:314–319.

Sexton DJ, Corey GR, Carpenter C, et al. Dual infection with Ehrlichia chaffeensis and a spotted fever group rickettsia: a case report. *Emerg Infect Dis* 1998;4:311–316.

Stone JH, Dierberg K, Aram G, Dumler JS. Human monocytic ehrlichiosis. *JAMA* 2004 Nov 10;292(18):2263–2270.

Other Bacterial Infections

Brucellosis

Bahemuka M, Babiker MA, Wright SG, et al. The pattern of infection of the nervous system in Riyadh: a review of 121 cases. *Q J Med* 1988;68:517–524.

Bodur H, Erbay A, Akinci E, et al. Neurobrucellosis in an endemic area of brucellosis. *Scand J Infect Dis* 2003;35:94–97.

McLean DR, Russell N, Khan MY. Neurobrucellosis: clinical and therapeutic features. *Clin Infect Dis* 1992;15:582–590.

Memish ZA, Balkhy HH. Brucellosis and international travel. *J Travel Med* 2004;11(1):49–55.

Mousa AR, Koshy TS, Araj GF, et al. *Brucella* meningitis: presentation, diagnosis and treatment—a prospective study of ten cases. *Q J Med* 1986;60:873–885.

Seidel G, Pardo CA, Newman-Toker D, Olivi A, Eberhart CG. Neurobrucellosis presenting a leukoencephalopathy. The role of cytotoxic T lymphocytes. *Arch Pathol Lab Med* 2003;127:e374–e377.

Shakir RA, Al-Din AS, Araj GF, et al. Clinical categories of neurobrucellosis. A report on 19 cases. *Brain* 1987;110:213–223.

Behçet Syndrome

Al-Kawi MZ, Bohlega S, Banna M. MRI findings in neuro-Behçet's disease. *Neurology* 1991;41:405–408.

Banna M, el-Ramahl K. Neurologic involvement in Behçet disease: imaging findings in 16 patients. *AJNR Am J Neuroradiol* 1991;12:791–796.

Behçet H. Uber rezidivierende Aphthose durch ein Virusverursachte Geschwur am Mund, am Auge und an den Genitalien. *Dermatol Monatsschr* 1937;105:1152–1157.

Inaba G. Behçet's disease. In: Vinken PJ, Bruyn GW, Klawans HL, McKendall RR, eds. *Handbook of Clinical Neurology*. Vol. 56. New York: Elsevier Science Publishing Co., Inc., 1989:593–610.

Namer IJ, Karabudak R, Zileli T, et al. Peripheral nervous system involvement in Behçet's disease. Case report and review of the literature. *Eur Neurol* 1987;26:235–240.

Kural-Seyahi E, Fresko I, Seyahi N, et al. The long-term mortality and morbidity of Behcet syndrome: a 2-decade outcome survey of 387 patients followed at a dedicated center. *Medicine* 2003;82:60–76.

Serdaroglu P, Yazici H, Ozdemir C, et al. Neurologic involvement in Behçet's syndrome. A prospective study. *Arch Neurol* 1989;46:265–269.

Wechsler B, Vidailhet M, Piette JC, et al. Cerebral venous thrombosis in Behçet's disease: clinical study and long-term follow-up of 25 cases. *Neurology* 1992;42:614–618.

Yazici H, Barnes CG. Practical treatment recommendations for pharmacotherapy of Behçet's syndrome. *Drugs* 1991;425:796–804.

Vogt-Koyanagi-Harada Syndrome

Hormigo A, Bravo-Marques JM, Souza-Ramalho P, et al. Uveomeningoencephalitis in a human immunodeficiency virus type 2–seropositive patient. *Ann Neurol* 1988;23:308–310.

Inomata H, Kato M. Vogt-Koyanagi-Harada disease. In: Vinken PJ, Bruyn GW, Klawans HL, McKendall RR, eds. *Handbook of Clinical Neurology*, vol. 56. New York: Elsevier Science Publishing Co, Inc., 1989: 611–626.

Pattison EM. Uveomeningoencephalitic syndrome (Vogt-Koyanagi-Harada). *Arch Neurol* 1965;12:197–205.

Riehl J-L, Andrews JM. Uveomeningoencephalitic syndrome. *Neurology* 1966;16:603–609.

Solaro C, Messmer Uccelli M. Intravenous methylprednisolone for aseptic meningitis in Vogt-Koyanagi-Harada syndrome. *Eur Neurol* 2000;44:129–130.

Mollaret Meningitis

Achard JM, Lallement PY, Veyssier P. Recurrent aseptic meningitis secondary to intracranial epidermoid cyst and Mollaret's meningitis: two distinct entities or a single disease? A case report and a nosologic discussion. *Am J Med* 1990;89:807–810.

Frederiks JAM, Bruyn GW. Mollaret's meningitis. In: Vinken PJ, Bruyn GW, Klawans HL, McKendall RR, eds. *Handbook of Clinical Neurology*, vol. 56. New York: Elsevier Science Publishing Co. Inc., 1989:627–635.

Jensenius M, Myrvang B, Storvold G, Bucher A, Hellum KB, Bruu AL. Herpes simplex virus type 2 DNA detected in cerebrospinal fluid of 9 patients with Mollaret's meningitis. *Acta Neurol Scand* 1998;98: 209–212.

Mollaret P. La méningite endothélio-leucocytaire multirecurrente bénigne. Syndrome nouveau ou maladie nouvelle? *Rev Neurol (Paris)* 1944;76:57–76.

Aseptic Meningeal Reaction

Alexander EL, Alexander GE. Aseptic meningoencephalitis in primary Sjögren's syndrome. *Neurology* 1983;33:593–598.

Canoso JJ, Cohen AS. Aseptic meningitis in systemic lupus erythematosus. *Arthritis Rheum* 1975;18:369–374.

Roos KL. Mycobacterium tuberculosis meningitis and other etiologies of the aseptic meningitis syndrome. *Sem Neurol* 2000;20:329–335.

Meningism

Fishman RA. *Cerebrospinal Fluid in Diseases of the Nervous System*, 2nd ed. Philadelphia: WB Saunders, 1992.

Mycoplasma pneumoniae Infection

Behan PO, Feldman RG, Segerra JM, Draper IT. Neurological aspects of mycoplasmal infection. *Acta Neurol Scand* 1986;74:314–322.

Bitnum A, Ford-Jones EL, Petric M, et al. Acute childhood encephalitis and mycoplasma pneumoniae. *Clin Infect Dis* 2001;32:1674–1684.

Francis DA, Brown A, Miller DH, et al. MRI appearances of the CNS manifestations of *Mycoplasma pneumoniae*: a report of two cases. *J Neurol* 1988;235:441–443.

Ieven M, Demey H, Ursi D, et al. Fatal encephalitis caused by *Mycoplasma pneumoniae* diagnosed by the polymerase chain reaction. *Clin Infect Dis* 1998;27:1552–1553.

Pellegrini M, O'Brien TJ, Hoy J, Sedal L. *Mycoplasma pneumoniae* infection associated with an acute brainstem syndrome. *Acta Neurol Scand* 1996;93:203–206.

Socan M, Ravnik I, Bencina D, et al. Neurological symptoms in patients whose cerebrospinal fluid is culture and/or polymerase chain reaction-positive for mycoplasma pneumoniae. *Clin Infect Dis* 2001;32:e31–e35.

Sotgiu S, Pugliatti M, Rosati G, Deiana GA, Sechi GP. Neurological disorders associated with mycoplasma pneumoniae infection. *Eur J Neurol* 2003;10:165–168.

Legionella pneumophila Infection

Andersen BB, Sogaard I. Legionnaires' disease and brain abscess. *Neurology* 1987;37:333–334.

Heath PD, Booth L, Leigh PN, Turner AM. Legionella brain stem encephalopathy and peripheral neuropathy without preceding pneumonia [letter]. *J Neurol Neurosurg Psychiatry* 1986;49:216–218.

Johnson JD, Raff MJ, Van Arsdall JA. Neurologic manifestations of Legionnaires disease. *Medicine (Baltimore)* 1984;63:303–310.

Pendelbury WW, Perl DP, Winn WC Jr, McQuillen JB. Neuropathologic evaluation of 40 confirmed cases of "Legionella" pneumonia. *Neurology* 1983;33:1340–1344.

Sommer JB, Erbguth FJ, Neundorf B. Acute disseminated encephalomyelitis following Legionella pneumophila infection. *Eur Neurol* 2000;44:182–184.

Weir AI, Bone I, Kennedy DH. Neurological involvement in legionellosis. *J Neurol Neurosurg Psychiatry* 1982;45:604–608.

Chapter 23

Focal Infections

Gary L. Bernardini

MALIGNANT EXTERNAL OTITIS AND OSTEOMYELITIS OF THE BASE OF THE SKULL

Malignant external otitis is an invasive infection of the external auditory canal; it penetrates the epithelium and spreads to the surrounding soft tissue to cause cellulitis and abscess. If untreated, the infection may extend to the temporomandibular joint, mastoid, or more commonly to soft tissues below the temporal bone. The syndrome is most frequently observed in elderly diabetic patients and in immunocompromised people (e.g., patients with HIV chemotherapy, or organ transplantation).

Owing to its anatomic location in the temporal bone, the facial nerve may be affected as the first symptom in up to 30% of patients. Other common symptoms are severe otalgia that worsens at night, purulent otorrhea, and painful swelling of surrounding tissues. Conductive hearing loss may result from obstruction of the external auditory canal. Trismus may indicate irritation of the masseter muscles or involvement of the temporomandibular joint. Rarely, dysphagia results from lesions of cranial nerves IX through XII, and the findings may be mistaken for laryngeal carcinoma. Fever and weight loss are uncommon. Mastoid tenderness is evident on examination. The diagnostic finding of granulation tissue, stemming from extension of infection to the cartilaginous portion of the ear canal, may be seen on otoscopic examination.

Laboratory testing includes erythrocyte sedimentation rate (ESR), white blood cell count (WBC), red blood cell count (RBC), glucose and creatinine levels, and culture of ear secretions. There may be a mildly elevated or normal white blood cell count but the ESR is almost always elevated (greater than 50 mm/h). CT is most useful in showing location and extent of disease and evaluating evidence of bony erosion, but films may appear normal early in the illness. MRI with and without gadolinium, is the study of choice but MRI is not useful in detecting bony changes. Isotope bone scans are sensitive but not specific. Newer techniques using technetium (^{99m}Tc) methylene diphosphonate and gallium-67 single photon emission CT may be more sensitive and accurate in early detection of malignant external otitis, sensitive in measuring ongoing infectious process, and beneficial in monitoring response to therapy.

In most cases, *Pseudomonas aeruginosa* is the causative organism. In HIV-positive individuals or in AIDS, either *P. aeruginosa* or the fungus *Aspergillus fumigatus* may be isolated. In some patients with AIDS, *Streptococcus*, *Staphylococcus*, and *Proteus* species may be isolated as mixed or sole pathogens. Broad-spectrum antibiotics instead of antipseudomonal agents are used in these cases. In the preantibiotic era, mortality rates were greater than 50% and surgical debridement was the treatment of choice. Standard treatment with intravenous antibiotics consisted of an antipseudomonal penicillin for 4 weeks to 8 weeks, combined with an aminoglycoside for at least 2 weeks, or if tolerated, 4 weeks to 6 weeks. Current successful treatment is based on single-drug therapy with either the antipseudomonal, third-generation cephalosporin ceftazidime, or the fluoroquinolone ciprofloxacin, in patients with limited external otitis (i.e., without bony erosion or cranial neuropathy). Double-antibiotic therapy is considered with more extensive lesions. Drug-resistant strains have been found for both ceftazidime and ciprofloxacin. In one study, resistance to ciprofloxacin in patients with malignant otitis externa increased over time. In drug-resistant cases, third-generation cephalosporins and antipseudomonal penicillins in combination with debridement may be necessary. Despite these new treatments, the mortality rate is still 10% to 20% and may be as high as 50% if cranial nerves are involved. If untreated or inadequately treated, malignant external otitis may result in osteomyelitis of the base of the skull, sigmoid sinus thrombosis, abscess formation, meningitis, and death.

Osteomyelitis of the base of the skull is a rare complication of malignant external otitis, chronic mastoiditis, or paranasal sinus infection. As with malignant otitis, the patients are usually elderly, diabetic, or immunocompromised. Particularly in the diabetic patient with microangiopathy, local trauma as a result of external auditory canal irrigation with tap water contaminated with *P. aeruginosa*, may penetrate the skin of the canal leading to osteomyelitis. Symptoms include headache, otalgia, hearing loss, and otorrhea, but patients are frequently without fever. Osteomyelitis may occur in conjunction with otitis but usually appears weeks or months after starting antibiotics. As the process spreads, cranial nerves may be affected, especially the VII and VIII nerves. Extension of skull-base osteomyelitis to the jugular foramen or hypoglossal canal may affect cranial nerves IX through XII, leading to dysphagia. In advanced cases, spread to the petrous pyramid may affect III, IV, V, and VI cranial nerves, to cause ocular palsies or trigeminal neuralgia.

Laboratory abnormalities include a normal or slightly elevated white blood cell count and a high erythrocyte sedimentation rate. In general, leukocytosis is not common and not useful to diagnosis and management. The use of thin-cut CT sections through the skull base and temporal bones to visualize bony involvement plays an important role in the diagnosis of osteomyelitis and in assessing the extent of disease. Carcinoma of the ear canal may cause similar clinical and radiographic findings, and bone biopsy may be needed if there is no response to appropriate antibiotic therapy.

MRI is useful in delineating soft tissue involvement but has not proved beneficial for initial diagnosis or determining efficacy of treatment for skull base osteomyelitis. Technetium bone scanning is a sensitive indicator of osteomyelitis but is not helpful in determining resolution of disease. Technetium uptake is nonspecific and may be seen in a number of conditions such as infection, trauma, neoplasm, and postoperatively. Gallium-67 scans may be useful in tracking resolution of disease over time. Neither bone nor gallium scans are useful in determining the exact extent of the infection. *P. aeruginosa* is the typical causative organism, but *Staphylococcus aureus* or other organisms such as *Staphylococcus epidermidis*, *Proteus*, *Salmonella*, *Mycobacterium*, *Aspergillus*, and *Candida* have been implicated, rarely.

Therapy for osteomyelitis consists of intravenous administration of antibiotics, usually a combination of a antipseudomonal penicillin or cephalosporin with an aminoglycoside, to provide synergy and to prevent the emergence of drug-resistant bacteria. Peak and trough levels of the aminoglycosides must be watched carefully to avoid potential ototoxicity and nephrotoxicity, particularly in elderly patients with renal insufficiency. Ciprofloxacin has been effective when used alone or with other antibiotics. Ceftazidime has bactericidal activity against *Pseudomonas* and may be used as monotherapy. The disease is usually extensive, and conservative management of skull base osteomyelitis is still an extended course of two-drug therapy. Monthly gallium scans may help to determine the response and duration of antibiotic therapy. In refractory cases, hyperbaric oxygen has been used as adjuvant therapy. Antibiotics should be continued for at least 1 week after the gallium scan becomes normal. Follow-up gallium scans may be performed 1 week after completion of antibiotic therapy to detect early recurrence and at 3 months for late recurrence. Mortality rates of 40% have been reported, but with prolonged antibiotic therapy, complete cure may be achieved. Poor prognostic indicators include cranial nerve involvement or intracranial extension. Recurrences may manifest up to one year later; true cure is considered when the patient is disease free for a year after treatment is begun.

BRAIN ABSCESS AND SUBDURAL EMPYEMA

Brain Abscess

Encapsulated or free pus in the substance of the brain after an acute focal purulent infection is known as brain abscess. Abscesses vary in size from a microscopic collection of inflammatory cells to an area of purulent necrosis, involving the major part of one hemisphere. Abscess of the brain has been known for over 200 years, and surgical treatment started with Macewen in 1880.

Advances in the diagnosis and treatment of brain abscesses have been achieved with the use of CT, MRI, MR spectroscopy, stereotactic brain biopsy and aspiration, and new antimicrobials.

Etiology

Brain abscesses are classified on the basis of the likely entry point of the infection. For example, brain abscesses arise most commonly from direct extension of cranial infections (mastoid, teeth, paranasal sinuses, ear, or osteomyelitis of the skull), infections after fracture of the skull or neurosurgical procedures, spread via intracerebral veins, or as hematogenous metastases from infection elsewhere in the body. Brain abscess is almost never a consequence of bacterial meningitis, except in infants.

Infections in the middle ear or mastoid may spread to the cerebellum or temporal lobe through involvement of the bone and meninges or by seeding of bacteria through valveless emissary and sinus veins that drain these regions, with or without extradural or subdural infection or thrombosis of the transverse sinus. An abscess in one hemisphere may follow infection in the contralateral mastoid, presumably by hematogenous spread of the organism. Infection in the frontal, ethmoid, or rarely, the maxillary sinuses spreads to the frontal lobes through erosion of the skull. Subdural or extradural infection or thrombosis of the venous sinuses may also be present. Twenty percent to 30% of brain abscesses have no obvious source.

Metastatic seeding from a remote site may cause brain abscess (e.g., arising in the lungs, by bronchiectasis or lung abscess) or less frequently from bacterial endocarditis. Other sources include the tonsils, abscessed teeth, and upper respiratory tract, from which the infection may reach the brain along the carotid sheath, or after urinary tract or intra-abdominal or -pelvic infections. With metastatic spread, the cerebral lesions are found in the distal territories of the middle cerebral artery and frequently are multiple. Congenital cardiac defects and pulmonary arteriovenous malformations (as in hereditary hemorrhagic telangiectasia) predispose to brain abscess. In these two

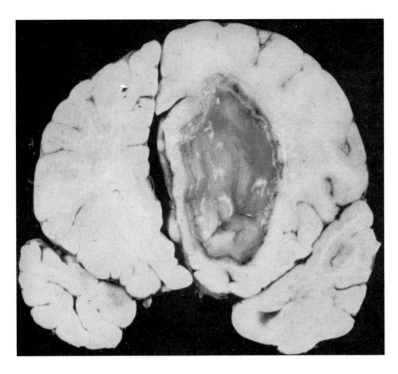

FIGURE 23.1. Brain abscess. Fresh abscess in frontal lobe, secondary to pulmonary infection. (Courtesy of Dr. Abner Wolf.)

disorders, infected emboli bypass the pulmonary filtration system and gain access to the cerebral arterial system.

The occurrence of abscesses of the brain after penetrating brain injury is low, although entry of bacteria into the brain is common after such injuries with the introduction of infected missiles or tissues into the brain through compound fractures of the skull. In children, penetration of a lead pencil tip through the thin squamous portion of the temporal bone has resulted in abscess around the foreign material in the frontal lobe.

The infecting organism may be any of the common pyogenic bacteria depending on the site of entry; the most common are *S. aureus*, streptococci (anaerobic, aerobic, or microaerophilic species), *Enterobacteriaceae*, *Pseudomonas*, and anaerobes such as *Bacteroides*. In infants, gram-negative organisms are the most frequent isolates. After penetrating head injury, abscess formation is usually due to *S. aureus*, streptococci, *Enterobacteriaceae*, or *Clostridium* species; *S. epidermidis* infection follows neurosurgical procedures. In the immunocompromised host, *Toxoplasma*, fungi, *Nocardia*, and *Enterobacteriaceae* are frequently found. Pneumococci, meningococci, and *Hemophilus influenzae* are major causes of bacterial meningitis but are rarely recovered from a brain abscess. Brain abscess is an infrequent complication of parasitic infection such as *Entamoeba histolytica*. Cultures may be sterile in patients who have received antimicrobial therapy before biopsy, but any material obtained should be sent to the laboratory. A positive Gram stain may guide therapy even when the culture is negative. In a study of 90 patients with a diagnosis of brain abscess, microbiologic diagnosis was obtained in 83%. More than one pathogen was found in 23% of the cases, and blood cultures were positive in only 30%.

Pathology

The pathologic changes in brain abscesses are similar regardless of the origin: direct extension to the brain from epidural or subdural infection, retrograde thrombosis of veins, or hematogenous metastasis (Fig. 23.1).

Four stages of maturation of brain abscess are recognized: (1) within the first 3 days, suppurative inflammation of brain tissue is characterized by early cerebritis, appearing as either patchy or nonenhancing hypodensity on CT or MRI, (2) late cerebritis (with an area of central necrosis, edema, and ring enhancement on CT and MRI), (3) early capsule formation, and (4) final maturation of the capsule that takes about 2 weeks. When host defenses control the spread of the infection, macroglia and fibroblasts proliferate in an attempt to surround the infected and necrotic tissue, and granulation tissue and fibrous encapsulation develops. The microglia produce a wide variety of chemokines that initiate or promote the inflammatory process in the brain parenchyma and are responsible for recruitment of peripheral immune cells into the CNS. The capsule formed by the inflammatory response is thicker on the cortical surface than on the ventricular side. If the capsule ruptures, purulent material is released into the ventricular system, a process associated with a high mortality rate. Edema of adjacent cerebrum or the entire hemisphere is common (Fig. 23.2).

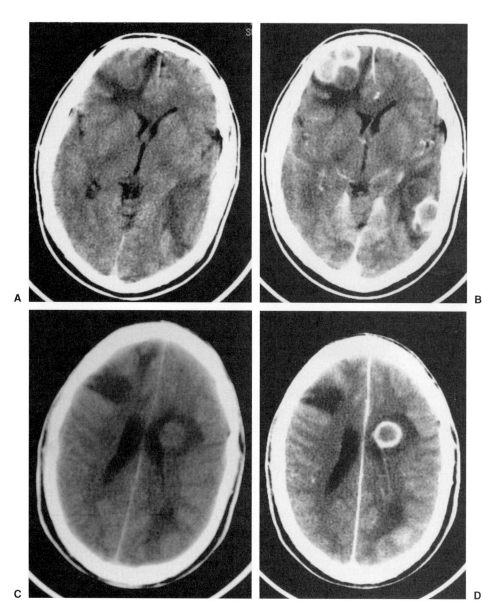

FIGURE 23.2. Multiple brain abscesses. A: and B: Multiple brain abscesses seen on CT both before and after intravenous contrast. Symptoms started 2 weeks after dental cleaning, presenting as severe headache and drowsiness; isolates from an abscess revealed *Streptococcus viridans* sp. Note characteristic ring enhancement **(B)** and marked edema with midline shift **(A and B)** around three abscesses in the right frontal lobe; a daughter abscess shows less ring enhancement and is directed inward. In addition, there is a left temporoparietal ring-enhancing lesion, with possible adjacent early cerebritis lesion, with surrounding edema. **C: and D:** A periventricular abscess in the same patient seen on a higher cut CT, with and without contrast; note ependymal enhancement after the administration of contrast, indicating extension of the abscess into the left lateral ventricle. (Courtesy of Dr. L. Fontana.)

Incidence

Brain abscesses were common in the first half of the 20th century, but the introduction of effective therapy for purulent infection of the mastoid process and nasal sinuses has greatly reduced the incidence of all intracranial complications of these infections, including brain abscess. Over the past 30 years, advances in the management of brain abscesses have resulted in a significant decline in mortality from between 30% and 50% before 1980, to 4% to 20% today. Brain abscesses constitute less than 2% of all intracranial surgery. Brain abscess may occur at any age but is still encountered in the first to third decades of life, as a result of the high incidence of mastoid and nasal sinus disease during those years. Up to 25% of all cases affect children less than 15 years old, with a cluster in the 4-year-

old to 7-year-old age group, usually the result of cyanotic congenital heart disease or an otic source.

Symptoms and Signs

The symptoms of brain abscess are those of any expanding lesion in the brain, and a nonlocalizing headache is the most common symptom. Fever is present in less than 50% of patients; many are afebrile. Edema of surrounding brain tissue may rapidly increase intracranial pressure so that worsening headache, nausea, and vomiting are early symptoms. Sudden worsening of preexisting headache with new onset of nuchal rigidity often heralds rupture of brain abscess into the ventricular space. Abrupt onset of a severe headache is less common with abscess and is more often associated with acute bacterial meningitis or subarachnoid hemorrhage. Seizures, focal or generalized, are common with abscess.

Focal signs, including altered mental status and hemiparesis, are seen in approximately 50% of patients, depending on abscess location. Hemiparesis may be seen with lesions of the cerebral hemispheres. Apathy and mental confusion have been linked with abscesses in the frontal lobe. Hemianopia and aphasia, particularly anomia, are found when the temporal or parietooccipital lobes are involved. Ataxia, intention tremor, nystagmus, and other classic symptoms may be seen with cerebellar abscess. Frequently, however, the signs of an abscess in the cerebrum or cerebellum are related solely to that of increased intracranial pressure (nausea, vomiting, and headache). Abscesses in the brainstem are rare. The classic findings of a brainstem syndrome are often lacking because the abscess tends to expand longitudinally along fiber tracts rather than transversely. Overall, papilledema is present in only about 25% of all patients. Signs of injury to the third or sixth cranial nerve are sometimes the result of increased intracranial pressure.

Subdural or, rarely, epidural infections in the frontal regions may give the same signs and symptoms as those of an abscess in the frontal lobe. Fever and focal seizures favor the diagnosis of subdural rather than intraparenchymal abscess.

Thrombosis of the lateral (transverse) sinus often follows middle ear or mastoid infection and may be accompanied by seizures and signs of increased intracranial pressure, making the clinical differentiation between this condition and abscess of the temporal lobe or cerebrum difficult. With lateral sinus thrombosis, papilledema may be due to interference of venous drainage from the brain. Focal neurologic signs favor the diagnosis of abscess.

Diagnostic Tests

Brain abscess may be suspected clinically when seizures, focal neurologic signs, or increased intracranial pressure develop in a patient with congenital heart disease or with a known acute or chronic infection in the middle ear, mastoid, nasal sinuses, heart, or lungs. The diagnosis is supported by CT or MRI (Figs. 23.2 and 23.3).

Elevated white blood cell count or erythrocyte sedimentation rate is not reliably present with brain abscess. Blood cultures are positive in only 10% of patients but should always be obtained with suspected brain abscess, even in the absence of fever. Lumbar puncture is contraindicated in patients suspected of having a brain abscess because of the clear risk of transtentorial herniation. In early studies, CSF examination reported elevated opening pressures and results consistent with aseptic meningitis. In the series of Merritt and Fremont-Smith, opening pressures were elevated to well over 200 mm H_2O in 70% of the cases. The

CSF is usually clear but may be cloudy or turbid. The CSF cell count varies from normal to 1,000 cells/mm^3, or more. In unencapsulated abscesses near the ventricular or subarachnoid spaces, the cell count is high, with a high percentage of polymorphonuclear leukocytes. The cell count may be normal or only slightly increased when the abscess is firmly encapsulated. The cell count in 34 patients at various stages of the disease varied between 4 cells/mm^3 and 800 cells/mm^3 with an average of 135 cells/mm^3, protein content was between 45 mg/dL and 200 mg/dL, and CSF glucose was normal.

Extension of the abscess to the meninges or ventricles is accompanied by an increase in the CSF cell count and other findings associated with acute meningitis or ventriculitis. Rupture of an abscess into the ventricles is signaled by a sudden rise of intracranial pressure and the presence of free pus, with marked increases in CSF cell count 20,000/mm^3 to 50,000/mm^3. A decrease in glucose content below 40 mg/dL indicates that the meninges have been invaded by bacteria. Only rarely are CSF cultures positive.

MRI and CT are the studies of choice, both for diagnosis and treatment of brain abscess. Plain radiographs of the skull may show separation of sutures in infants or children and an increase in the convolution markings. CT permits accurate localization of cerebritis or abscess and serial assessment of the size of the lesion, its demarcation, the extent of surrounding edema, and total mass effect. MRI with gadolinium is more sensitive and specific than contrast CT in diagnosing early cerebritis. MR spectroscopy may differentiate anaerobic from aerobic or sterile brain abscesses on the basis of metabolic patterns of lactate, amino acids, or acetate. With a mature encapsulated abscess, both contrast CT and MRI with gadolinium reveal the ring-enhancing mass with surrounding vasogenic edema.

The differential diagnosis, based on the appearance of lesions seen on neuroimaging, includes glioblastoma, metastatic tumor, infarct, arteriovenous malformation, resolving hematoma, and granuloma. Features supporting the diagnosis of brain abscess include gas within the center of a ring-enhancing lesion, a thinner rim (less than 5 mm) than with brain tumors, and ependymal enhancement associated with ventriculitis or ventricular rupture (Fig. 23.2D). MRI with DWI and calculation of the ADC may aid in differentiating tumor from abscess. The signal is hyperintense on DWI MRI with brain abscess. Thallium-201 brain SPECT may differentiate intracerebral lymphoma from Toxoplasma encephalitis in patients with AIDS. Unlike pyogenic brain abscesses, the signal of Toxoplasma abscesses may not be hyperintense on DWI MRI.

Either CT or MRI may distinguish abscess from mycotic aneurysms or herpes encephalitis, each of which may cause similar symptoms and signs. Mycotic aneurysm, usually in the distribution of the middle cerebral arteries, may be accompanied by aseptic meningitis in bacterial

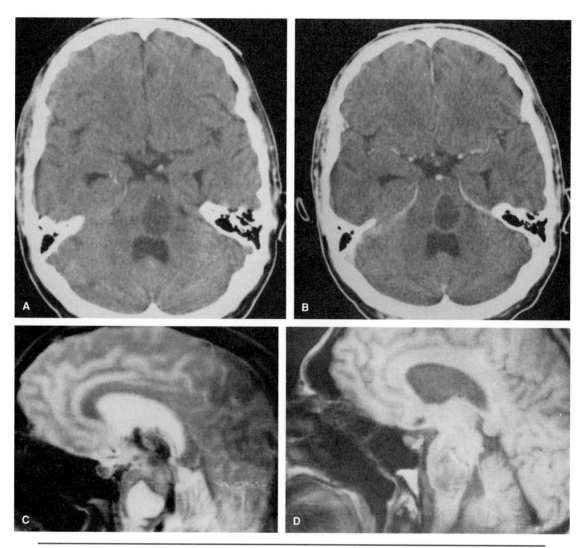

FIGURE 23.3. Brainstem abscess. A: Axial noncontrast computed tomography demonstrates a round, low-density, left-pontine lesion with mass effect on the fourth ventricle. **B:** Ring enhancement of the lesion after contrast is typical of an abscess. Sagittal T2-weighted **(C)** and sagittal T1-weighted **(D)** MRIs demonstrate the lesion to be cystic and isointense to cerebrospinal fluid signal (compare with signal within the lateral ventricle). Note definition of the abscess rim in **D**. The sagittal MRIs are useful in planning a surgical approach through the fourth ventricle. (Courtesy of Drs. J. A. Bello and S. K. Hilal.)

endocarditis. CT or MRI may exclude abscess, but angiography may be necessary to identify the aneurysm before rupture. Herpes simplex encephalitis is manifest by headache, fever, and an acute temporal lobe or frontal lobe syndrome. On CT or MRI, the temporal lobe is swollen, with irregular lucency and patchy contrast enhancement.

Treatment

Before CT, the treatment of brain abscess was surgical, including incision and drainage through a burr hole, or open craniotomy with marsupialization, packing the cavity, and complete extirpation. The introduction of CT revolutionized the management of brain abscess. CT made it possible to diagnose and localize cerebritis or abscess, dictate choice of treatment, and monitor patient response. The current recommended treatment for most brain abscesses is CT-guided stereotactic or free-hand needle aspiration, therapeutic drainage, and obtaining diagnostic specimens for culture and special studies, along with appropriate antimicrobial therapy. Stereotactic aspiration is the treatment of choice for most abscesses except for those that are very superficial or large. Based on Gram-stain results and presumptive source of the abscess, empiric antimicrobial therapy may be started. Early surgery is recommended, especially for abscesses close to the ventricles into which the lesion may rupture. Nonoperative treatment may be appropriate for some patients who are clinically stable but poor surgical candidates, or in those with surgically inaccessible lesions.

Open craniotomy is now performed infrequently and is reserved for patients with multiloculated abscesses that require complete excision or those with more resistant pathogens such as fungi or *Norcardia*.

Choosing the appropriate antimicrobial therapy depends on the ability of the drug to penetrate the abscess cavity and its activity against the suspected pathogen. Chloramphenicol was the standard therapy for brain abscesses at one time, but it lacks bactericidal activity, side effects are serious, and it is rarely used today. Brain abscesses that arise from intracranial extension of sinus infection, with usual isolates of microaerophilic streptococci and anaerobic organisms, may be treated with intravenous high-dose penicillin G (10 million units per day to 20 million units per day) and metronidazole. Combination therapy with cefotaxime or other cephalosporins, in combination with metronidazole, appears to be highly effective for empiric treatment of brain abscesses. Additional antibiotic coverage may be needed for some organisms (e.g., *Actinomyces* species) when the abscess is secondary to dental procedures or dental abscess. Special consideration of antimicrobial coverage for *Enterobacteriaceae* and *P. aeruginosa* should be made when an otogenic source of brain abscess is suspected. Vancomycin may be given initially in cases of brain abscess from neurosurgical procedures, likely due to *S. epidermidis*, while awaiting final culture results. It is generally recommended that parenteral antibiotics should be given for a total of 6 weeks to 8 weeks, followed by an additional 2-month to 3-month course of oral antibiotic therapy.

Clinical and CT or MRI responses are monitored to assess the effectiveness of antibiotic treatment or the need for repeated surgery. Follow-up CT may show a small area of residual enhancement even after adequate antimicrobial therapy. Occasionally, a previous ring-enhancing lesion on CT disappears with medical management, suggesting that these reversible lesions are forms of suppurative cerebritis.

Seizures may occur in up to 50% of patients with brain abscess, early in the course. However, one large retrospective study found seizures in only of patients with brain abscess.. Anticonvulsants such as phenytoin or carbamazepine may be administered for prophylaxis or to prevent the recurrence of seizures. Generally, these agents are given for at least 3 months after surgery for abscess.

The use of corticosteroids for these patients is controversial. In patients with life-threatening cerebral edema or impending herniation, a short course of high-dose corticosteroids may be appropriate. Further deterioration with severe brain edema may require intubation with hyperventilation and the administration of intravenous mannitol to control elevated intracranial pressures. Hemicraniectomy may be considered for cases of increased intracranial pressure refractory to medical therapy. Prolonged use of corticosteroids is not recommended because the steroids may interfere with granulation tissue formation and reduce the concentration of antibiotics within the infected tissue.

Prognosis

The outcome of untreated brain abscess is, with rare exceptions, death. Mortality in pre-CT series varied from 35% to 55%. In the era of advanced neuroimaging with CT or MRI, the mortality rate of brain abscesses is 0% to 30%. Overall morbidity and mortality of brain abscess is related to the rapidity of onset of symptoms and diagnosis, the primary source of infection, the presence of single or multiple abscesses, and the patients neurologic status at the time of diagnosis. Patients with depressed level of consciousness on admission tend to do poorly. In a univariate analysis of mortality, a Glasgow Coma Scale score on admission of less than or equal to 9 was an independent predictor of in-hospital mortality in one study.

Immunocompromised individuals have worse outcomes and higher mortality rates. The highest death rate is found when the primary infection is in the lungs. Intraventricular rupture of a brain abscess is associated with mortality rates exceeding 80%.

Sequelae of brain abscess include recurrence of the abscess or the development of new abscesses if the primary focus persists. Residual neurologic sequelae with hemiparesis, seizures, or intellectual or behavioral impairment is seen in 30% to 56% of patients.

Subdural Empyema

Subdural empyema is a collection of loculated pus in the subdural space. Symptoms are similar to those of brain abscess. Subdural infection in adults usually arises from contiguous spread of infection; paranasal sinusitis is the most common source. Otitis, head trauma, and neurosurgical procedures are other causes. The most common pathogen in subdural empyema are anaerobic and microaerophilic streptococci, particularly those of the *Streptococcus milleri* group. In a minority of cases, *Staphylococcus aureus* and multiple organisms, including Gram-negative organisms such as *Escherichia coli*, and anaerobic organisms, such as *Bacteroides*, may be present. *Pseudomonas aeruginosa* or *Staphylococcus epidermidis* may be found in cases following neurosurgical procedures. In patients with advanced AIDS, *Salmonella* species have been detected as a causative agent.

The infection spreads to the subdural space through retrograde thrombophlebitis via the venous sinuses, or as direct extension through bone and dura. Once the infection develops, it may spread over the convexities and along the falx, although characteristic loculation is common. Associated complications include septic cortical-vein thrombosis, brain or epidural abscess, and meningitis. The syndrome typically presents with an initial focal headache, fever, and, in 80% to 90% of patients, focal neurologic signs. The combination of fever, a rapid progressive neurologic deterioration, and focal seizures is particularly suggestive of this disorder. Symptoms of subdural empyema may begin 1 week to 2 weeks after a sinus infection.

Lumbar puncture is contraindicated because of the mass effect. CT scan reveals a crescent-shaped area of hypodensity over a hemisphere, along the dura, or adjoining the falx, with enhancement of the margins around the empyema after administration of contrast. However, the diagnostic test of choice is MRI with gadolinium enhancement, for the delineation of the presence and extent of the subdural empyema, and to identify concurrent intracranial infections. CT may miss some lesions that can be detected by MRI.

Treatment of nearly all cases of subdural empyema involves prompt surgical drainage and antibiotic therapy. Intravenous antibiotics are given depending on the organism identified or if unknown, empiric treatment with antibiotics similar to those used in brain abscess. Anticonvulsants are frequently required. There is controversy about which type of neurosurgical technique is used for drainage of subdural empyema. CT accurately localizes the pus collection, and some advocate drainage through selective burr holes. Others prefer craniotomy for more complete removal of the infection, especially when the empyema is loculated. Limited craniotomy is also used for placement of a drain into the subdural space and for local infusion of appropriate antibiotics. Use of either burr hole or craniotomy for drainage of subdural empyema is individualized. In cases of fulminant subdural empyema, decompressive craniectomy, irrigation of the empyema, and subdural drainage may be required. The recommended duration of antibiotic therapy is 3 weeks to 4 weeks after surgical drainage.

SUGGESTED READINGS

Osteomyelitis and Malignant External Otitis

Berenholz L, Katzenell U, Harell M. Evolving resistant pseudomonas to ciprofloxacin in malignant otitis externa. *Laryngoscope* 2002;112:1619–1622.

Chandler JR. Malignant external otitis and osteomyelitis of the base of the skull. *Am J Otol* 1989;10:108–110.

Damiani JM, Damiani KK, Kinney SE. Malignant external otitis with multiple cranial nerve involvement. *Am J Otol* 1979;1:115–120.

Dinapoli RP, Thomas JE. Neurologic aspects of malignant external otitis: report of three cases. *Mayo Clin Proc* 1971;46:339–344.

Grandis JR, Curtin HD, Yu VL. Necrotizing (malignant) external otitis: prospective comparison of CT and MRI in diagnosis and follow-up. *Radiology* 1995;196:499–504.

Hern JD, Almeyda J, Thomas DM, et al. Malignant otitis externa in HIV and AIDS. *J Laryngol Otol* 1996;110:770–775.

Karantanas AH, Karantzas G, Katsiva V, et al. CT and MRI in malignant external otitis: a report of four cases. *Comput Med Imaging Graph* 2003;27:27–34.

Mardinger O, Rosen D, Minkow B, et al. Temporomandibular joint involvement in malignant external otitis. *Oral Surg Med Oral Pathol Radiol Endod* 2003;96:398–403.

Meyers BR, Mendelson MH, Parisier SC, Hirschman SZ. Malignant external otitis. Comparison of monotherapy vs combination therapy. *Arch Otolaryngol Head Neck Surg* 1987;113:974–978.

Murray ME, Britton J. Osteomyelitis of the skull base: the role of high resolution CT in diagnosis. *Clin Radiol* 1994;49:408–411.

Paramsothy M, Khanijow V, Ong TO. Use of gallium-67 in the assessment of response to antibiotic therapy in malignant otitis externa—a case report. *Singapore Med J* 1997;38:347–349.

Ress BD, Luntz M, Telischi FF, et al. Necrotizing external otitis in patients with AIDS. *Laryngoscope* 1997;107:456–460.

Rubin GJ, Bransteeter BF IVth, Yu VL. The changing face of malignant (necrotizing) external otitis: clinical, radiological, and anatomic correlations. *Lancet Infect Dis* 2004;4:34–39.

Sreepada GS, Gangadhar S, Kwartler JA. Skull base osteomyelitis secondary to malignant otitis externa. *Curr Opin Otolaryngol Head Neck Surg* 2003;11:316–323.

Slattery WH, Brackmann DE. Skull base osteomyelitis. Malignant external otitis. *Otolaryngol Clin North Am* 1996;29:795–806.

Tierney MR, Baker AS. Infections of the head and neck in diabetes mellitus. *Infect Dis Clin North Am* 1995;9:195–216.

Brain Abscess and Subdural Empyema

Alderson D, Strong AJ, Ingham HR, Selkon JB. Fifteen-year review of the mortality of brain abscess. *Neurosurgery* 1981;8:1–6.

Bernardini GL. Diagnosis and management of brain abscess and subdural empyema. *Curr Neurol Neurosci Rep* 2004;4(6):448–456.

Chong-Han CH, Cortez SC, Tung GA. Diffusion-weighted MRI of cerebral toxoplasma abscess. *AJR* 2003;181:1711–1714.

Clark DB. Brain abscess and congenital heart disease. *Clin Neurosurg* 1966;14:274–287.

Courville CB, Nielsen JM. Fatal complications of otitis media: with particular reference to intracranial lesions in a series of 10,000 autopsies. *Arch Otolaryngol* 1934;19:451–501.

Curless RG. Neonatal intracranial abscess: two cases caused by Citrobacter and a literature review. *Ann Neurol* 1980;8:269–272.

de Falco R, Scarano E, Cigliano A, et al. Surgical treatment of subdural empyema: a critical review. *J Neurosurg Sci* 1996;40:53–58.

Dill ST, Cobbs CG, McDonald CK. Subdural empyema: analysis of 32 cases and review. *Clin Infect Dis* 1995;20:372–386.

Garg M, Gupta RK, Husain M, et al. Brain abscesses: etiologic categorization with in vivo proton MR spectroscopy. *Radiology* 2004;230:519–527.

Greenlee JE. Subdural empyema. *Curr Treat Options Neurol* 2003;5:13–22.

Guzman R, Barth A, Lovblad KO, et al. Use of diffusion-weighted magnetic resonance imaging in differentiating purulent brain processes from cystic brain tumors. *J Neurosurg* 2002;97:1101–1107.

Harvey FH, Carlow TJ. Brainstem abscess and the syndrome of acute tegmental encephalitis. *Ann Neurol* 1980;7:371–376.

Heilpern KL, Lorber B. Focal intracranial infections. *Infect Dis Clin North Am* 1996;10:879–898.

Kagawa M, Takeshita M, Yato S, Kitamura K. Brain abscess in congenital cyanotic heart disease. *J Neurosurg* 1983;58:913–917.

Kielian T. Microglia and chemokines in infectious diseases of the nervous system. Views and reviews. *Front Biosci* 2004;9:732–750.

Jansson AK, Enblad P, Sjolin J. Efficacy and safety of cefotaxime in combination with metronidazole for empirical treatment of brain abscesses in clinical practice: a retrospective study of 66 consecutive cases. *Eur J Clin Microbiol Infect Dis* 2004;23:7–14.

Loeser E Jr, Scheinberg L. Brain abscesses: a review of ninety-nine cases. *Neurology* 1957;7:601–609.

Macewen W. *Pyogenic Infective Diseases of the Brain and Spinal Cord: Meningitis, Abscess of Brain, Infective Sinus Thrombosis.* Glasgow UK: James Maclehose & Son, 1893.

Mathisen GE, Johnson JP. Brain abscess. *Clin Infect Dis* 1997;25:763–779.

Merritt HH, Fremont Smith F. *The Cerebrospinal Fluid.* Philadelphia: WB Saunders, 1938.

Pfister HW, Feiden W, Einhaupl KM. Spectrum of complications during bacterial meningitis in adults. Results of a prospective clinical study. *Arch Neurol* 1993;50:575–581.

Rosenblum ML, Hoff JT, Norman D, et al. Decreased mortality from brain abscesses since the advent of computerized tomography. *J Neurosurg* 1978;49:658–668.

Seydoux C, Francioli P. Bacterial brain abscesses: factors influencing mortality and sequelae. *Clin Infect Dis* 1992;15:394–401.

Shaw MDM, Russell JA. Cerebellar abscess: a review of 47 cases. *J Neurol Neurosurg Psychiatry* 1975;38:429–435.

Smith HP, Hendricks EB. Subdural empyema and epidural abscess in children. *J Neurosurg* 1983;58:392–397.

Tattevin P, Bruneel F, Clair B, et al. Bacterial brain abscesses: a retrospective study of 94 patients admitted to an intensive care unit (1980 to 1999). *Am J Med* 2003;115:143–146.

Wada Y, Kubo T, Asano T, et al. Fulminant subdural empyema treated with a wide decompressive craniectomy and continuous irrigation—case report. *Neurol Med Chir* 2002;42:414–416.

Weingarten K, Zimmerman RD, Becker RD, Heier LA, Haimes AB, Deck MD. Subdural and epidural empyemas: MR imaging. *AJR Am J Roentgenol* 1989;152:615–621.

Weisberg LA. Nonsurgical management of focal intracranial infection. *Neurology* 1981;31:575–580.

Wispelwey B, Dacey RG Jr, Scheld WM: Brain abscess. In: Scheld WM, Whitley RJ, Durack DT, eds. *Infections of the Central Nervous System.* New York: Raven Press, 1991.

Zimmerman RA. Imaging of intracranial infections. In: Scheld WM, Whitley RJ, Durack DT, eds. *Infections of the Central Nervous System.* New York: Raven Press, 1991.

Chapter 24

▶ Viral Infections

Burk Jubelt

Although rabies has been known since ancient times and acute anterior poliomyelitis was recognized in 1840, our knowledge of the role of viruses in the production of neurologic disease is of recent origin. In 1804, Zinke showed that rabies could be produced in a normal dog by inoculation of saliva from a rabid animal, but the filterable nature of rabies virus was not demonstrated until 1903. In 1908, Landsteiner and Popper produced a flaccid paralysis in monkeys by the injection of an emulsion of spinal cord from a fatal case of poliomyelitis. In the 1930s, filterable viruses were recovered from patients with epidemic encephalitis (arboviruses) and aseptic meningitis (lymphocytic choriomeningitis virus). With the use of electron microscopic, tissue culture, and immunologic techniques, many additional viruses that infect the nervous system have been recovered and characterized.

Although the list of viruses that cause human disease in epidemic or sporadic forms is extensive, most viral infections of the CNS are uncommon complications of systemic illnesses caused by common human pathogens. After viral multiplication in extraneural tissues, dissemination to the CNS occurs by the hematogenous route or by spread along nerve fibers.

Viruses are *classified* according to their nucleic acid type, size, sensitivity to lipid solvents (enveloped versus nonenveloped), morphology, and mode of development in cells. The principal division is made according to whether the virus contains RNA or DNA. RNA viruses usually replicate within the cytoplasm of infected cells, whereas DNA viruses replicate in the nucleus. Members of almost every major animal virus group have been implicated in the production of neurologic illness in animals or humans (Table 24.1).

The nature of the lesions produced varies with the virus and the conditions of infection. They may include neoplastic transformation, system degeneration, or congenital defects, such as cerebellar agenesis and aqueductal stenosis, as well as the inflammatory and destructive changes often considered typical of viral infection. In addition, the concept that a viral infection causes only an acute illness quickly following an infection of the host has been altered. It has been demonstrated that in slow-onset viral infections, illness may not appear until many years after exposure to the pathogenic agent.

ACUTE VIRAL INFECTIONS

CNS Viral Syndromes

Acute viral infections of the nervous system may manifest clinically in three forms: viral (aseptic) meningitis, encephalitis, or myelitis, the latter of which is infrequent (Table 24.2).

Viral *meningitis* is usually a self-limited illness characterized by signs of meningeal irritation, such as headache, photophobia, and neck stiffness. *Encephalitis* entails involvement of parenchymal brain tissue, as indicated by convulsive seizures, alterations in the state of consciousness, and focal neurologic abnormalities. When both meningeal and encephalitic findings are present, the term *meningoencephalitis* may be used. Viral infections may also localize to the parenchyma of the spinal cord, resulting in *myelitis*. Myelitis may occur from infection of spinal motor neurons (paralytic disease or poliomyelitis), sensory neurons, autonomic neurons (bladder paralysis), or demyelination of white matter (transverse myelitis). When both encephalitis and myelitis occur, the term *encephalomyelitis* is used. The CSF findings in these three acute viral syndromes are usually similar, consisting of an increase in pressure, pleocytosis (most often lymphocytic) of varying

▶ **TABLE 24.1** Viral Infection of the Nervous System

Virus Type	Representative Viruses Responsible for Neurologic Disease
RNA viruses	
Picornavirus family	Poliovirus
Enterovirus genus	Coxsackievirus
	Echovirus
	Enteroviruses 70 and 71
Hepatovirus genus	Hepatitis A virus
Togavirus family	
Alphavirus genus (arbovirus)	Equine encephalitis (eastern, western, Venezuela)
Flavivirus family and genus (arbovirus)	St. Louis encephalitis
	Japanese encephalitis
	Tick-borne encephalitis
	West Nile Virus
Bunyavirus family (arbovirus)	California encephalitis
Reovirus family	Colorado tick fever (coltivirus)
Togavirus family	
Rubivirus genus	Rubella virus
Orthomyxovirus family	Influenza A and B viruses
Paramyxovirus family	Measles and subacute sclerosing panencephalitis
	Mumps
Arenavirus family and genus	Lymphocytic choriomeningitis
Rhabdovirus family	Rabies
Retrovirus family	Human immunodeficiency virus, acquired immunodeficiency syndrome (AIDS)
	Human T-cell lymphotrophic virus (HAM/TSP)
DNA viruses	
Herpesvirus family	Herpes simplex virus
	Varicella-zoster (virus)
	Cytomegalovirus
	Epstein-Barr virus, infectious mononucleosis
	Human herpesvirus 6–8
Papovavirus family	Progressive multifocal leukencephalopathy
Poxvirus family	Vaccinia virus
Adenovirus family	Adenovirus

▶ **TABLE 24.2** Relative Frequency of Meningitis and Encephalitis of Known Viral Etiology (Number of Patients)

	Aseptic Meningitis	Encephalitis	Paralytic Disease	Total
Mumps	28	11	1	40
Lymphocytic choriomeningitis	7	0	0	7
Herpes simplex virus	2	7	0	9
Poliovirus	18	5	66	89
Coxsackievirus A	18	1	0	19
Coxsackievirus B	71	4	0	75
Echovirus	55	3	1	59
Arbovirus	3	5	0	8

From Buescher, et al. Central nervous system infections of viral etiology: the changing pattern. *Res Publ Assoc Res Nerv Ment Dis* 1968;44:147–163; with permission.

degree, a moderate protein content elevation, and a normal sugar content.

Pathology and Pathogenesis

Common biologic properties of members of a specific virus group may dictate how they attack the CNS and the type of disease they produce. For example, individual picornaviruses, such as poliovirus and echovirus, may cause similar clinical syndromes. Members of specific virus groups also show different predilections for cell types or regions of the nervous system. Thus, members of the myxovirus group attack ependymal cells, and herpes simplex virus (HSV) shows preference for frontal and temporal lobes.

The tendency for a disease to appear in an epidemic or sporadic form may also be related to the biologic properties of the virus. Most epidemic forms of meningitis, encephalitis, or myelitis are caused by infection with enteroviruses or arboviruses (togaviruses, flaviviruses, bunyaviruses). The enteroviruses (picornaviruses) are relatively acid- and heat resistant, allowing for fecal-hand-oral transmission during the hotter months of the year. Arboviruses require a multiplication phase in mosquitoes or ticks before they may infect people; human epidemics occur when climatic and other conditions favor a large population of infected insect vectors. Neurologic diseases caused by members of other virus groups usually occur sporadically or as isolated complications of viral infections of other organs or systems.

Diagnosis

The methods used for detecting a specific infective agent are dictated by an assessment of (1) occurrence of illness in an epidemic or endemic setting, and (2) seasonal occurrence of the various acute viral infections. Infection with the picornaviruses or arboviruses tends to occur in the summer and early fall; other viruses, such as mumps, occur in late winter or spring.

The diagnosis may be made by a combination of virus isolation (inoculation of blood, nasopharyngeal washings, feces, CSF, or tissue suspensions into susceptible animals or tissue culture systems), serologic tests, and amplification of viral nucleic acids. Infectious virus particles in human fluids and tissues are usually few in number, and many viruses are easily disrupted and inactivated even at room temperature. Tissues and fluids to be used for virus isolation studies should therefore be frozen unless they can be immediately transferred to the laboratory in appropriate transport media.

The ability to recover virus from the CSF varies according to the nature of the agent. Some viruses, such as mumps virus, may frequently be isolated from the CSF, whereas other viruses, such as poliovirus and HSV type 1, are rarely recovered.

Serologic tests are applicable to all known acute viral diseases of the nervous system. Serum should be frozen and kept at a low temperature until the tests are done. The diagnosis of an acute viral infection and the establishment of the type of virus rest on the development of antibodies to the infection, traditionally a four-fold antibody rise. It is therefore necessary to show that antibodies are not present or are present only in low titer in the early stages of the illness and that they are present in high titer at a proper interval after the onset of symptoms. Several to many days are usually required for antibody development; serum removed in the first few days of the illness may therefore serve as the control (acute-phase serum). Serum withdrawn in the convalescent stage, 3 to 5 weeks after the onset of the illness, may be used to determine whether antibodies have developed (convalescent-phase serum). When there is no change in titer, positive tests merely indicate that the individual has at some time in the past had an infection with this type of virus and that it probably is not the cause of the present illness.

If brain tissue from a patient is available in fatal cases or by brain biopsy, further studies may define the responsible virus. Brain sections may be analyzed by immunostaining techniques (immunofluorescence, immunoperoxidase) to determine whether specific viral antigens are present. Electron microscopy may indicate the presence of virus particles or components of specific morphology. Suspensions of brain and spinal cord may be injected into susceptible animals and tissue culture cell lines. In special instances, tissue cultures are initiated from brain tissue itself. Such brain cell cultures may then be examined for the presence of viral antigens or infective virus. If an agent is recovered, final identification may be made by neutralization with known specific antiserum.

Any material used for viral isolation may also be used for amplification of viral nucleic acid by the PCR. Identification is then made by the use of complimentary probes (hybridization).

Treatment

Antiviral chemotherapeutic agents are now available for several viruses: acyclovir for HSV; acyclovir, famciclovir, and foscarnet for varicella-zoster virus (VZV); ganciclovir and foscarnet for cytomegalovirus (CMV), and reverse transcriptase and protease inhibitors for HIV.

Immunization procedures with either live-attenuated vaccines or inactivated virus are readily available for rabies, poliomyelitis, hepatitis A and B, mumps, influenza, rubella, measles, chickenpox (varicella), and vaccinia. Immunization against the arboviruses is used mainly to protect laboratory workers and military personnel.

Although additional antiviral chemotherapeutic agents will likely become available in the future, vector control and mass immunization now seem to be the most practical means of effective prevention.

ENTEROVIRUS (PICORNAVIRUS) INFECTIONS

Picornaviruses are small, nonenveloped RNA viruses that multiply in the cytoplasm of cells. They are the smallest RNA viruses, hence the name "pico (small) RNA virus." Human picornaviruses may be divided into three subgroups: enteroviruses, found primarily in the gastrointestinal tract; rhinoviruses, found in the nasopharynx; and hepatitis A viruses (hepatoviruses). The enteroviruses comprise the *polioviruses, coxsackieviruses,* and *echoviruses,* all of which are capable of producing inflammation in the CNS. Some enteroviruses are considered *unclassified enteroviruses 68 to 71;* CNS disease has occurred with enteroviruses 70 and 71, as well as with hepatitis A virus.

The enteroviruses are resistant to the acid and bile of intestinal contents and may survive for long periods in sewage or water. They grow only in primate cells and are highly cytocidal. Virus particles may form crystalline arrays in the cytoplasm of cells, which are recognized as acidophilic inclusions in histologic preparations.

Poliomyelitis

Acute anterior poliomyelitis (infantile paralysis, Heine-Medin disease) is an acute, generalized disease caused by poliovirus infection. It is characterized by destruction of motor neurons in the spinal cord, brain, and brainstem and by the appearance of a flaccid paralysis of the muscles innervated by the affected neurons. Although the disease has probably occurred for many centuries, the first clear description was given by Jacob Heine in 1840, and the foundation of our knowledge of the epidemiology of the disease was laid by Medin in 1890. The studies of Landsteiner, Popper, Flexner, Lewis, and others in the first decade of the 20th century proved that the disease was caused by a virus.

Pathology and Pathogenesis

Invasion of the nervous system occurs as a relatively late and infrequent manifestation. Orally ingested virus multiplies in the pharynx and ileum and probably in lymphoid tissue of the tonsils and Peyer patches. The virus then spreads to cervical and mesenteric lymph nodes and may be detected in the blood shortly thereafter. Viremia is accompanied by no symptoms or by a brief minor illness (fever, chills). It is still not definitely known how the virus gains access to the nervous system in paralytic cases. The most likely possibility is by direct spread from the blood at defective areas of the blood–brain barrier. Less likely is neural spread from the intestine or from neuromuscular junctions.

The virus has a predilection for the large-motor cells, causing chromatolysis with acidophilic inclusions and necrosis of the cells. Degeneration of the neurons is accompanied by an inflammatory reaction in the adjacent meninges and the perivascular spaces, and by secondary proliferation of the microglia. Recovery may occur in partially damaged cells but the severely damaged cells are phagocytized and removed. The degenerative changes are most intense in the ventral-horn cells and the motor cells in the medulla; however, neurons in the posterior horn, the posterior-root ganglion, and elsewhere in the CNS are occasionally involved. Rarely, inflammation is also present in the white matter. Although the pathologic changes are most intense in the spinal cord, medulla, and motor areas of the cerebral cortex, any portion of the nervous system may be affected, including the midbrain, pons, cerebellum, basal ganglia, and nonmotor cerebral cortex.

Epidemiology

Acute anterior poliomyelitis is worldwide in distribution but is more prevalent in temperate climates. It may occur in sporadic, endemic, or epidemic form at any time of the year, but it is most common in late summer and early fall. Acute anterior poliomyelitis was formerly the most common form of viral infection of the nervous system. Before 1956, between 25,000 and 50,000 cases occurred annually in the United States.

Since the advent of effective vaccines, the incidence of the disease has dramatically decreased in the United States, as well as in other developed countries. In fact, in these countries, paralytic poliomyelitis is becoming a clinical rarity, except for isolated cases and small epidemics in areas where the population has not been vaccinated. In the United States, in the 1980s and 1990s fewer than 10 cases of paralytic poliomyelitis occurred each year, with most being vaccine-associated. Since switching to an all inactivated poliovirus vaccine (IPV) schedule in 2000, no indigenous cases have occurred. Paralytic poliomyelitis, however, is still a health problem in six developing countries of the world. Worldwide in 2003, only 682 cases of paralytic poliomyelitis were reported to the WHO.

Three antigenically distinct types of poliovirus have been defined. All three types may cause paralytic po-

liomyelitis or viral meningitis, but type I seems to be the one most often associated with paralytic disease.

The disease may occur at any age. It is rare before age 6 months. In the late 19th and early 20th centuries, poliomyelitis changed from an endemic to an epidemic disease. In the early epidemics, 90% of paralytic cases occurred in persons younger than 5 years of age. As epidemics recurred, there was a shift of paralytic cases to older individuals, so that the majority of cases occurred in children older than 5 years of age and in teenagers. Paralysis was also seen more frequently in young adults.

Prophylaxis

Oral poliomyelitis vaccination (OPV) with live attenuated virus is effective in the prevention of paralytic infections. Antibody response depends on multiplication of attenuated virus in the gastrointestinal tract. Significant antibody levels develop more rapidly and persist longer than those that follow intramuscular immunization with formalized polioviruses (IPV). OPV is also capable of spreading and thus immunizing contacts of vaccinated individuals, but it may also cause vaccine-associated poliomyelitis. Because of this, the recommendations for vaccination in the United States were changed to an all-IPV schedule. However, in endemic areas of the world, OPV is still preferred.

Symptoms

The symptoms at the onset of poliomyelitis are similar to those of any acute infection (fever, chills, nausea, prostration). In about 25% of the patients, these initial symptoms subside in 36 hours to 48 hours, and patients are apparently well for 2 days to 3 days until there is a secondary rise in temperature (dromedary type) accompanied by symptoms of meningeal irritation. In most patients, this second phase of the illness directly follows the first, without any intervening period of freedom from symptoms. The headache increases in severity and muscle soreness appears, most commonly in the neck and back. Drowsiness or stupor occasionally develops, but patients are irritable and apprehensive, when aroused. Convulsions are occasionally seen at this stage, in infants.

When it occurs, paralysis usually develops between the second and fifth day, after the onset of signs of nervous system involvement; it may be the initial symptom or in rare instances, may be delayed for as long as 2 weeks to 3 weeks. After the onset of paralysis, there may be extension of the motor loss for 3 days to 5 days. Further progress of signs and symptoms rarely occurs after this time. The fever lasts for 4 days to 7 days and subsides gradually. The temperature may return to normal before the paralysis develops or while the paralysis is advancing. Limb muscles are usually involved, but in severe cases respiratory and cardiac muscles may be affected. Acute cerebellar ataxia, isolated facial nerve palsies, and transverse myelitis have been observed in poliovirus-infected individuals.

Laboratory Data

Leukocytosis is present in the blood. CSF pressure may be increased. A CSF pleocytosis develops in the period before the onset of the paralysis. Initially, polymorphonuclear (PMN) leukocytes predominate, but a shift to lymphocytes occurs within several days. The CSF protein content is slightly elevated, except in patients with a severe degree of paralysis, when it may be elevated to 100 mg/dL to 300 mg/dL and may persist for several weeks.

Diagnosis

Acute anterior poliomyelitis may be diagnosed without difficulty, in most patients, when there is acute development of asymmetric flaccid paralysis, accompanied by the characteristic changes in the CSF. A presumptive diagnosis may be made in the preparalytic stage and in nonparalytic cases during an epidemic. The diagnosis may be suspected in patients who have not been vaccinated or who have defects in their immune response. The diagnosis of poliovirus infection may be established by recovery of the virus from stool (usually lasts 2 weeks to 3 weeks), throat washings (during the first week), or rarely, from CSF or blood. Recovery of virus from the throat or feces and the additional demonstration of a four-fold rise in the patient's antibody titer are required before a specific viral diagnosis may be made. Polymerase chain reaction (PCR) genomic amplification testing of the CSF is usually positive. Recent generation MRI may show inflammation localized to the spinal cord anterior horns.

Prognosis

Fewer than 10% of patients die from the acute disease. Death is usually the result of respiratory failure or pulmonary complications. The mortality rate is highest in the bulbar form of the disease, where the rate is often greater than 50%. The prognosis is poor when paralysis is extensive or when there is slow progress of paralysis, with exacerbations and involvement of new muscles over a period of days. The prognosis with regard to return of function depends on age (infants and children have more recovery) and the extent of paralysis, as muscle groups only partially paralyzed are more likely to recover.

New symptoms develop in about 50% of patients 30 years to 40 years after the acute poliomyelitis. These new symptoms have been collectively called the *postpolio syndrome*. In some of these patients, a slowly progressive weakness with atrophy and fasciculations develops and has been referred to as *postpolio progressive muscular atrophy* (see Chapter 120).

Treatment

Treatment is essentially supportive. Attention should be given to respiration, swallowing, and bladder and bowel functions.

Treatment of patients with paralysis of respiratory muscles or bulbar involvement requires great care. They should be watched carefully for signs of respiratory embarrassment, and as soon as these become apparent, mechanical respiratory assistance should immediately be given. The development of anxiety in a previously calm patient is a serious warning of either cerebral anoxia or hypercarbia and may precede labored breathing or cyanosis. Treatment in the convalescent stage, and thereafter, consists of physiotherapy, muscle reeducation, application of appropriate corrective appliances, and orthopedic surgery.

Coxsackievirus Infections

In 1948, Dalldorf and Sickles inoculated specimens obtained from patients with suspected poliomyelitis into the brains of newborn mice and discovered the coxsackieviruses, which were named for a town in upstate New York where there was an outbreak. Two subgroups, A and B, may be distinguished by their effects on suckling mice. In mice, group A viruses cause myositis leading to flaccid paralysis and death. Group B viruses cause encephalitis, myocarditis, pancreatitis, and necrosis of brown fat. Animals experience tremors, spasms, and paralysis before death. Twenty-three group A and six group B serotypes are currently recognized.

In humans, both group A and group B coxsackieviruses usually cause aseptic meningitis, a sign of nervous system involvement. When enteroviral meningitis occurs in infants, residual cognitive, language, and developmental abnormalities may occur. Occasionally, coxsackievirus infection causes encephalitis and rarely, paralytic disease or acute cerebellar ataxia are seen. Classic extraneural manifestations caused by group A coxsackieviruses are herpangina, hand-foot-and-mouth disease, and other rashes. Group B coxsackieviruses usually cause pericarditis, myocarditis, and epidemic myalgia (pleurodynia, Bornholm disease). They may also cause disseminated infection with severe encephalitis in newborns and may cause congenital anomalies if infection of the mother occurs in early pregnancy.

Signs and Symptoms

The symptoms and signs of meningeal involvement caused by coxsackieviruses are similar to those that follow infection with other viruses that cause aseptic meningitis. The onset may be acute or subacute with fever, headache, malaise, nausea, and abdominal pain. Stiffness of the neck and vomiting usually begin 24 hours to 48 hours after the initial symptoms. There is a mild or moderate fever. Muscular paralysis, sensory disturbances, and reflex changes are rare. Paralysis, when present, is mild and transient. Meningeal symptoms occasionally occur in combination with myalgia, pleurodynia, or herpangina.

The CSF pressure is normal or slightly increased. There is a mild or moderate pleocytosis in the CSF, ranging from $25/mm^3$ to $250/mm^3$ with 10% to 50% PMN cells. The protein content is normal or slightly increased, and the sugar content is normal.

Diagnosis

The diagnosis of coxsackievirus infection may be established by recovering the virus from the feces, throat washings, or CSF, and by demonstrating an increase in viral antibodies in the serum. Viral genomic amplification (PCR technique) is also being used for diagnosis. Meningitis caused by a coxsackievirus may not be distinguished from aseptic meningitis caused by other viral agents, except by laboratory studies. It is differentiated from meningitis caused by pyogenic bacteria and yeast by the relatively low cell count and the normal sugar content in the CSF. Differentiation must also be made from other diseases associated with lymphocytic pleocytosis in the CSF, including: tuberculous, fungal, or syphilitic meningitis; leptospirosis; Lyme disease; *Listeria monocytogenes, Mycoplasma,* or *Rickettsia* infections; toxoplasmosis; meningitis caused by other viruses; or parameningeal infections. Compared with these pathogenic entities, coxsackievirus infections are more benign, and the CSF sugar content is normal.

Treatment

Treatment during the acute stage of the infection is supportive. However, for containment of outbreaks, good hygiene with careful hand washing techniques may be preventive. The broad-spectrum, antipiconaviral agent pleconaril, currently under development, has activity against coxsackieviruses.

Echovirus Infections

This group of enteroviruses was originally isolated in cell culture from the feces of apparently normal persons. They were considered "orphans" because at the time, it was thought they did not cause disease. The designation "echo" is an acronym derived from the first letters of the term *enteric cytopathogenic human orphans.* Thirty-two serotypes are now recognized. Many strains cause hemagglutination of human type-O erythrocytes.

The echoviruses cause gastroenteritis, macular exanthems, and upper respiratory infections. Echovirus-9 in-

fections may cause a petechial rash that may be confused with meningococcemia. When the nervous system is infected, the syndrome of aseptic meningitis usually results.

Signs and Symptoms

The clinical picture of infection with the echoviruses is similar to that of other enterovirus infections. Children are affected more frequently than adults. The main features are fever, coryza, sore throat, vomiting, and diarrhea. A rubelliform rash is often present. Headache, neck stiffness, lethargy, and irritability indicate involvement of the nervous system. The disease usually runs a benign course that subsides in 1 week or 2 weeks, but complications similar to those seen with coxsackievirus infections may occur.

Cerebellar ataxia has been reported in children as the result of echovirus infection. The onset of ataxia is acute; the course is benign with remission of symptoms within a few weeks. Pupil-sparing oculomotor nerve paralysis and other cranial nerve palsies have rarely been observed. Echoviruses may cause a persistent CNS infection in children with agammaglobulinemia; this is an echovirus-induced meningoencephalitis often associated with a dermatomyositis-like syndrome. It may respond to treatment with immune globulin.

Diagnosis and Treatment

The CSF pleocytosis may vary from several hundred to a thousand or more cells per cubic millimeter, but it is usually less than $500/mm^3$. Early in the infection, there may be as many as 90% PMN leukocytes; within 48 hours of onset, however, the response becomes completely mononuclear. The CSF protein content is normal or slightly elevated; the sugar content remains normal.

The echoviruses are commonly recovered from feces, throat swabs, and CSF. Virus typing is carried out by antibody testing. Viral genomic amplification is also being used for diagnosis. The differential diagnosis of echovirus meningitis is similar to that of coxsackievirus infections. Treatment is similar to that for coxsackieviruses.

Infections with EV 70 and 71 and Hepatitis A Virus

Newly recognized enteroviruses are now named as *unclassified enteroviruses* (EV). Several of these new enteroviruses have caused CNS infections.

Epidemiology

EV70 has caused epidemics of acute hemorrhagic conjunctivitis (AHC), which initially occurred in Africa and Asia. Neurologic abnormality occurs in about 1 in 10,000 or 1 in 15,000 cases of AHC, and primarily in adults. Outbreaks of AHC have recently occurred in Latin America and the southeastern United States, but these manifestations were without any neurologic disease. The most common neurologic picture is a polio-like syndrome of flaccid, asymmetric, and proximal paralysis of the legs accompanied by severe radicular pain. Paralysis is permanent in more than 50% of patients. Isolated cranial nerve palsies (primary facial nerve), pyramidal tract signs, bladder paralysis, vertigo, and sensory loss have been reported. Because neurologic involvement usually occurs about 2 weeks after the onset of AHC, it may be difficult to isolate the virus at the time when neurologic signs are seen. Thus, diagnosis often depends on serologic studies. The neurologic disorder has rarely been seen without its preceding conjunctivitis.

EV71 has been recognized as causing outbreaks of hand-foot-and-mouth disease (HFMD). Upper respiratory infections and gastroenteritis also occur. Neurologic involvement may occur in up to 25% of patients, with children and teenagers primarily affected. Neurologic manifestations include aseptic meningitis, cerebellar ataxia, and various forms of poliomyelitis (flaccid monoparesis, or bulbar polio). Most of these paralytic cases have occurred in Europe and Asia. Two cases of transient paralysis were seen in an outbreak in New York. In 1997, an epidemic of EV 71 with HFMD, brain stem encephalitis (rhombencephalitis) and pulmonary edema began to occur in the Asian-Pacific region. The largest epidemic occurred in Taiwan in 1998, where the fatality rate for patients with neurologic involvement was 11%. Manifestations included myoclonic jerks, tremors, ataxia, cranial nerve palsies, coma, and respiratory failure. Most of the patients had MRI T2-weighted high intensity lesions in the brain stem. Polio-like flaccid paralysis occurred in about 10% of patients. Diagnosis may be made by virus isolation from throat, feces, or vesicles and by antibody studies. Viral genomic amplification has been used but is not yet generally available.

Hepatitis A virus has apparently caused encephalitis as a distinct entity, although hepatic encephalopathy is obviously more common. It has also been associated with transverse myelitis.

Arbovirus Infections

The arboviruses (*ar*thropod-*bo*rne) are small, spherical, ether-sensitive (enveloped) viruses that contain RNA. More than 400 serologically distinct arboviruses are currently recognized. Although the term *arbovirus* is no longer an official taxonomic term, it is still useful to designate viruses transmitted by vectors. Arboviruses include the alphaviruses (formerly group A arboviruses), flaviviruses (formerly group B arboviruses), bunyaviruses, and some reoviruses (Table 24.1).

The alphaviruses are one genus in the togavirus family; the other genus comprises the rubiviruses (rubella viruses). The equine encephalitides are caused by alphaviruses. The flavivirus family is composed of more than 60 viruses, including the viruses that cause yellow fever, St. Louis, Japanese, and West Nile encephalitides. The bunyaviruses include the California encephalitis group. The reovirus family includes the virus causing Colorado tick fever. St. Louis and California encephalitides have been the most common arboviral encephalitides in the United States until the recent appearance of West Nile virus infections.

Epidemiology

Arboviruses multiply in a blood-sucking arthropod vector. In their natural environment, transmission alternates between the invertebrate vector and a mammal. Mosquitoes and ticks are the most common vectors. Birds seem to be the principal natural hosts, but wild snakes and some rodents are probably a secondary reservoir. People and horses are usually incidental hosts, and human or horse infection in most arbovirus infections terminates the chain of infection (dead-end hosts).

Arbovirus infection of the nervous system may result in viral meningitis but more frequently, results in moderate or severe encephalitis. Diseases caused by arboviruses typically occur in late summer and early fall.

Clinical Syndromes

Approximately 80 arboviruses are known to cause human disease. The spectrum of disease produced is broad, ranging from hemorrhagic fevers (yellow fever) to arthralgia, rashes, and encephalitis.

Diagnosis

Arboviruses are difficult to isolate in the laboratory. The virus may be recovered from blood during the early phases (2 days to 4 days) of the illness. In nonfatal cases, the diagnosis usually depends on the demonstration of a four-fold rise in antibodies during the course of the illness. The virus may be isolated from the tissues at necropsy by the intracerebral inoculation of infant mice and susceptible tissue culture cells. Genomic amplification is available through some state health departments as a diagnostic test for the more common arbovirus infections.

Equine Encephalitis

Three distinct types of equine encephalitis occur in the United States: Eastern equine encephalitis (EEE), Western equine encephalitis (WEE), and Venezuelan equine encephalitis (VEE). They are to the result of infection from three serologically distinct alphaviruses. Infection with these viruses was thought to be limited to horses, until 1932, when Meyer reported an unusual type of encephalitis in three men who were working in close contact with affected animals. The first cases in which EEE virus was recovered from human brain tissue were reported in Massachusetts in 1938 by Fothergill and coworkers. Many arboviruses take their name from the location in which they were first isolated; they are not confined, however, by specific geographic boundaries. EEE is usually localized to the Atlantic and Gulf coasts and the Great Lakes areas. Infrequently, cases of EEE have been reported in regions west of the Mississippi River, as well as in Central and South America and the Philippines. WEE virus infection is now known to occur in all parts of the United States, although most frequently in the western two-thirds of the country. VEE occurs in Central and South America and the southern half of the United States, but is a rare cause of encephalitis.

Pathology

In EEE, the brain is markedly congested, and there are widespread degenerative changes in nerve cells. The meninges and perivascular spaces of the brain are intensely infiltrated with PMN leukocytes and round cells. Focal vasculitic lesions, often with thrombus formation, may occur. Destruction of myelin is prominent only near the necrotic foci. Lesions are found in both the white and gray matter and are most intensive in the cerebrum and brainstem, but they may also be present in the cerebellum and spinal cord.

In contrast to EEE, the pathology of WEE is less intense and is characterized by less inflammation (primarily mononuclear) and a paucity of nerve cell changes.

Incidence

Equine encephalitis is a rare human infection, tending to occur as isolated cases or in small epidemics. Epizootics in horses may precede the human cases by several weeks. Equine encephalitis mainly affects infants, children, and adults older than 50 years of age. Inapparent infection is common in all age groups.

Symptoms

Infection with the EEE virus begins with a short prodrome (approximately 5 days) of fever, headache, malaise, and nausea and vomiting. This is followed by the rapid onset of neurologic manifestations: confusion, drowsiness, stupor, or coma with convulsive seizures and neck stiffness. Cranial nerve palsies, hemiplegia, and other focal neurologic signs are common.

The symptoms of WEE and VEE are less severe. Onset is acute, with general malaise and headache, occasionally followed by convulsions and nausea and vomiting. There is moderate fever and neck stiffness. The headaches increase in severity and there is drowsiness, lethargy, or coma. Paresis and cranial nerve palsies may occur.

Laboratory Data

Leukocytosis may occur in the blood, especially in EEE; white blood cell counts as high as $35,000/mm^3$ have been reported. CSF changes are greatest in EEE, in which the pressure is always moderately or greatly increased. The CSF is cloudy or purulent, containing 500 cells/mm^3 to 3,000 cells/mm^3. Initially, a predominance of PMN leukocytes usually occurs. The protein content is increased, but the sugar content is normal. With abatement of the acute stage, the cell count drops, and lymphocytes become the predominating cell type, although PMN cells persist as a significant fraction.

The CSF changes in the WEE and VEE are less severe. The pressure is usually normal, and the cellular increase is moderate, with counts varying from normal to 500 cells/mm^3, with mononuclear cells as the predominating cell type.

Diagnosis

Isolation of equine encephalitis viruses from blood and CSF is infrequent but should be attempted. Most arboviral infections are diagnosed serologically, with IgM assays available for rapid diagnosis. Genomic amplification is available for EEE.

MRI may reveal focal lesions in the basal ganglia, thalami, and brainstem in about 50% of patients with EEE (Fig. 24.1). CT is less sensitive. A similar distribution of lesions on MRI has been seen in several other arboviral encephalitides (Japanese encephalitis, Central European tick-borne encephalitis).

Equine encephalitis must be differentiated from other acute infections of the CNS. These include postinfectious encephalomyelitis (i.e., exanthems, occurrence usually in the late fall and winter, abnormal MRI), advanced bacterial and tuberculous meningitis with parenchymal involvement (i.e., low CSF sugar content, positive cultures), brain abscess (i.e., abnormal imaging), parasitic encephalitis (detected by serology), and other viral infections. Differentiation from other viral encephalitides, except that caused by HSV, may be made only by viral diagnostic testing.

Course and Prognosis

The average mortality rate in EEE is about 50%. The duration of the disease varies from less than 1 day in fulminating cases, to more than 4 weeks in less severe cases. In patients who recover, sequelae such as mental deficiency, cranial nerve palsies, hemiplegia, aphasia, and convulsions are common. Children younger than 10 years are more

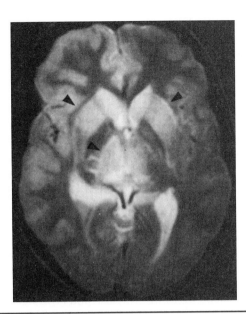

FIGURE 24.1. **Eastern equine encephalitis.** Proton-density MR image 3 days after the onset of neurologic symptoms revealed large, bilateral, asymmetric lesions of the caudate, putamen, and thalamus *(arrowheads)*. Less frequently, lesions may also be seen in the cortex, primarily in the medial temporal cortex and insula (not shown). (From Deresiewicz RL, et al., 1997; with permission. Copyright © 1997 Massachusetts Medical Society. All rights reserved.)

likely to survive the acute infection, but they also have the greatest chance of being left with severe neurologic disability.

The fatality rate in WEE is about 10%. Sequelae among young infants are frequent and severe but sequelae are uncommon in adults. The mortality rate in VEE is less than 0.5%; nearly all deaths have occurred in young children.

Treatment

Treatment in the acute stage of equine encephalitis is entirely supportive. Vaccines against the causative viruses have been produced, but their use should be confined to laboratory workers and others who are subject to unusually high levels of exposure to the viruses. Vaccination in a large-scale community program is not indicated because of the low incidence of the disease. EEE and WEE have been prevented by controlling the vector (i.e., the use of large-scale insecticide spraying). However, the key to prevention is avoiding contact with mosquitoes, avoiding endemic areas, wearing appropriate clothing, and using mosquito repellents.

St. Louis Encephalitis

The first outbreak of acute encephalitis in which a virus was definitely established as the causative agent was an epidemic that occurred in St. Louis in 1933. This type of encephalitis probably existed in this area before 1933, as cases of encephalitis had occurred in St. Louis during the previous 14 years. Since 1933, repeated outbreaks have occurred in the United States with increasing frequency and widening geographic distribution.

The virus responsible for St. Louis encephalitis (SLE) is a mosquito-transmitted flavivirus. Epidemics follow two epidemiologic patterns: rural and urban. Rural epidemics tend to occur in the western United States. The rural cycle involves birds as the intermediate host, similar to WEE. Urban epidemics occur primarily in the midwestern United States, the Mississippi River Valley, and the eastern United States. Urban outbreaks may be abrupt and extensive because the virus may replicate in urban mosquitoes. SLE primarily affects the elderly population. As with other arboviruses, disease in humans usually appears in midsummer to early fall.

Pathology

Grossly, there is a mild degree of vascular congestion and occasional petechial hemorrhages. Microscopic changes include a mild infiltration of mononuclear cells in the meninges and blood vessels of the brain; mononuclear-, microglial-, and glial-cell accumulation in the parenchyma of both the gray and white matter; and degenerative changes in neurons. The nuclear masses of the thalamus and midbrain are affected more often than the cortex.

Symptoms and Signs

Infection with the SLE virus usually results in inapparent infection. About 75% of patients with clinical manifestations have encephalitis; the others have aseptic meningitis or nonspecific illness. SLE is a disease of older adults. Encephalitic signs and symptoms develop in almost all patients older than 40 years of age. The onset of neurologic symptoms may be abrupt or may be preceded by a prodromal illness of 3 days' or 4 days' duration, and are characterized by headache, myalgia, fever, sore throat, and nausea and vomiting. The headache increases in severity and neck stiffness develops. Other common signs include pathologic reflexes, intention tremors, ataxia, cranial nerve abnormalities and confusion. In more severe cases, there may be delirium, coma or stupor, focal neurologic signs, and infrequently, seizures, which is considered a poor prognostic sign.

Laboratory Data

A mild to moderate leukocytosis occurs in the blood. The CSF is usually abnormal, with a mild pleocytosis in most patients that averages approximately 100 cells/mm^3. Counts as high as 500 cells/mm^3 or higher have been reported. Lymphocytes are the predominating cell type, although predominance of PMN cells may be found early in the disease. The sugar content is normal. Hyponatremia arising from inappropriate secretion of antidiuretic hormone occurs in 25% to 33% of patients.

Diagnosis

The SLE virus is rarely isolated from the blood or CSF, and diagnosis depends on serologic testing. An immunoglobulin M (IgM) assay is available for rapid diagnosis. Genomic amplification assays are now available for diagnosis. MRI may reveal T2-weighted hyperintensities in the substantia nigra. The differential diagnosis is similar to that of the equine encephalitides.

Course and Prognosis

The disease runs an acute course in most patients and usually results in death or recovery within 2 weeks to 3 weeks. Mortality has varied from 2% to 20%. The most common sequelae of SLE are headaches, insomnia, easy fatigability, irritability, and memory loss, and these usually clear in several years. About 25% of survivors have permanent neurologic sequelae of cranial nerve palsies, hemiplegia, gait disorders, and aphasia.

Treatment

There is no specific treatment or a vaccine for SLE. Supportive care is essential. Vector control and avoidance of contact is preventive.

West Nile Virus Encephalitis

In the summer of 1999, an outbreak of encephalitis suddenly appeared in New York City. As was later determined, this was the first appearance of West Nile virus (WNV) in the Western Hemisphere. New York was the only site of reported cases of human encephalitis, although bird deaths and infected mosquitoes were also found in Connecticut and New Jersey. In the first half of the 19th century WNV was found in Africa and the Middle East. In the 1960s, it spread to Asia, and in the 1980s to Eastern Europe. Over the last 4 years, WNV has spread to all of the continental United States except two Western states. In 2002, there were about 3,000 cases of WNV encephalitis/meningitis; in 2003 there were about 2,000 cases.

WNV is a mosquito-transmitted flavivirus similar to SLE virus. Because of serologic cross reactivity with SLE, the initial outbreak in NYC was thought to be caused by SLE. However, the death of avian hosts, which does not occur with SLE, distinguished the infection from SLE. Genomic sequencing of the isolates revealed that the outbreak was caused by WNV. Crows are the most commonly involved birds. Similar to SLE, WNV primarily affects el-

derly humans. Similar to other arbovirus infections, disease occurs in midsummer to early fall.

Pathology

Maximum neuropathologic changes usually occur in the brain stem, cranial nerves and anterior horns of the spinal cord. Less frequently the basal ganglia may be involved. The inflammation is more intense than that seen in SLE. Pathologic findings include neuronal necrosis, neuronophagia, and the formation of microglial nodules.

Symptoms and Signs

Similar to SLE, most infections are inapparent. It has been estimated that less than 1% of those infected develop encephalitis. The illness usually begins abruptly with fever, headache, vomiting, myalgia and arthralgia. A maculopapular rash may be seen. This is followed by involvement of the brain stem and, about 10% of the time, the spinal cord. Three syndromes are recognized to occur after the initial phase: meningitis, encephalitis, and poliomyelitis-like paralysis. Encephalitis may manifest as confusion, seizures, and altered level of consciousness including coma, respiratory failure and cranial nerve palsies. Less frequently, tremors and parkinsonian features may be seen.

Laboratory Data

The white blood cell count is usually normal but may be mildly increased or decreased. Similar to SLE, hyponatremia resulting from the syndrome of inappropriate secretion of antidiuretic hormone (SIADH) secretion may be seen. The CSF reveals a lymphocytic pleocytosis up to 1500 cells/mm^3 although a majority of PMN cells may seen early. The protein is usually elevated. CSF glucose is normal. The EEG may reveal diffuse slowing, and CT is usually normal. MRI may reveal meningeal and spinal cord parenchymal enhancement. Less frequently, T2 hyperintensities in the brain and spinal cord have been noted.

Diagnosis

WNV is not usually isolated from either the blood or CSF. Rapid diagnosis depends on detecting WNV-specific IgM in the serum or CSF. PCR testing for WNV sequences in the CSF may also be diagnostic.

Course and Prognosis

WNV encephalitis has an acute course over 2 weeks to 3 weeks. Poor prognostic factors include advanced age of 75 years or older and having diabetes mellitus. In the New York city epidemic, the death rate was 12%. One year after infection, only about 40% had made full recovery. Dementia and paralysis were the most frequent residuae.

Treatment and Prevention

There is no specific treatment for WNV encephalitis. Supportive care is the mainstay of management, especially for respiratory failure. Vector control, spraying, repellent use, and protective clothing are important for controlling the disease.

Japanese Encephalitis

Epidemiology

Japanese encephalitis (JE) was first identified as a distinct disease after a large epidemic in 1924, although a form of the encephalitis had been recognized as early as 1871. The causative agent is a mosquito-transmitted flavivirus. Occurrence may be endemic (tropical areas) or epidemic (temperate zones). JE remains a major medical problem throughout Asia, with as many as 10,000 cases annually. The pathologic changes seen with JE are much more intense than those of SLE. In addition to infiltration with lymphocytes, monocytes, and microglial cells, severe neuronal necrosis occurs with neuronophagia in the entire cerebral cortex, basal ganglia, cerebellum, and spinal cord. The disease is most common in children, and the mortality rate in some epidemics has been as high as 50%. This figure is undoubtedly skewed because most mild cases of JE are not admitted to hospitals. Severe neurologic residual effects and mental defects are common, especially in the young.

Symptoms

The clinical picture in JE is different than that of SLE. Seizures, focal neurologic deficits and movement disorders occur in 50% to 70% of patients. Dystonia and parkinsonian features are the common movement disorders. Similar to WNV, but seen less frequently, acute flaccid paralysis may occur in JE.

Diagnosis

The diagnosis may be established by isolation of the virus from the blood, CSF, or cerebral tissue and by appropriate antibody tests. Neuroimaging studies have revealed findings similar to those reported for EEE (i.e., lesions of the thalami, basal ganglia, and brainstem).

Treatment

There is no specific treatment. Vector control and vaccination are preventive. An inactivated-virus vaccine is routinely used in Japan, China, and Korea and is available for residents of the United States who are traveling to endemic or epidemic areas of Asia.

California (La Crosse) Encephalitis

Human neurologic disease associated with infection by the California encephalitis virus was first recognized in the early 1960s. Subsequently, La Crosse virus, also a member of the California virus serogroup, has been shown to cause most of these infections. The California virus serogroup is now classified among the bunyaviruses, a group of enveloped viruses with segmented, helical, circular ribonucleoproteins.

Epidemiology

Infection most frequently occurs in the upper midwestern United States, but it is found throughout the eastern half of the continental United States. These viruses are now known to be among the more important causes of encephalitis in the United States; fortunately, the encephalitis is usually mild.

The virus is transmitted by woodland mosquitoes. Its cycle involves small woodland animals as intermediate hosts, but not birds. Consequently, rural endemic rather than epidemic disease usually occurs.

The disease occurs in the late summer and early fall, and nearly all patients are children. Infants younger than 1 year of age and adults are rarely affected.

Symptoms and Signs

Headache, fever, nausea and vomiting, changes in sensorium, meningeal irritation, seizures and upper motor neuron signs commonly have been reported.

Diagnosis

Unlike most other viral infections, in cases of infection with California virus serogroup agents, the peripheral blood count is often quite elevated (20,000 cells/mm^3 to 30,000 cells/mm^3). The CSF contains an increased number of lymphocytes and shows the other findings typical of viral meningitis or encephalitis. The diagnosis may be established by serologic tests and genomic amplification.

Course, Prognosis, and Treatment

The case fatality is low (less than 1%). Recovery usually occurs within 7 days to 10 days. Emotional liability, learning difficulties, and recurrent seizures have been reported as sequelae. Treatment is supportive.

Other Arbovirus Encephalitides

Colorado Tick Fever

Colorado tick fever (CTF) is caused by a coltivirus (reovirus family) transmitted by wood ticks with small animals as intermediate hosts. CTF is confined to the geographic area of the tick in the Rocky Mountains. Infection often involves hikers, foresters, or vacationers, and is seen most often in the spring and summer. Three days to 6 days after a tick bite, an abrupt febrile illness develops with headache, myalgia, retroorbital pain, and photophobia. About 50% of patients have a biphasic fever pattern. Peripheral leukopenia and thrombocytopenia are common. Aseptic meningitis occurs in about 20% of patients. This is a benign disease; encephalitis and permanent sequelae are almost never seen. Diagnosis may readily be made by virus isolation from the blood or by serology.

Tick-borne Encephalitis

Tick-borne encephalitis (TBE) viruses are closely related flaviviruses transmitted by wood ticks. Disease is seen primarily in the northern latitude woodlands of Siberia and Europe. The Siberian strains cause a severe encephalitis (Russian spring–summer encephalitis virus). The European and Scandinavian strains (Central European encephalitis) tend to cause a milder encephalitis that may present as a biphasic illness, with recrudescence several weeks after the initial influenza-like illness. A case of TBE has been seen in Ohio after foreign tick exposure. Powassan virus, a member of the TBE complex, has been isolated from a few patients with severe encephalitis in the Northeastern United States and Canada. A related virus, louping ill, causes a sporadic, mild encephalitis in the British Isles.

Other arboviruses that have occasionally caused epidemics of encephalitis include Rift Valley fever in Africa and Murray Valley encephalitis in Australia.

Rubella

Rubella virus is not an arbovirus but it is now classified as a togavirus. It is an enveloped RNA virus that causes rubella (German measles), an exanthematous, respiratory spread disease that may produce marked neurologic damage in the unborn child of a mother infected during pregnancy (congenital rubella syndrome [CRS]). Gregg, an Australian ophthalmologist, was the first to correlate the occurrence of congenital cataracts among newborn babies with maternal rubella infection during the first trimester of pregnancy. CRS is now known to produce a variety of defects, including deafness, mental retardation, and cardiac abnormalities. The frequency of congenital defects is highest in the first trimester of pregnancy and falls as gestation advances. Rubella virus induces a chronic, persistent infection in the fetus. For a long time after birth, infants may shed virus from the nasopharynx, eye, or CSF. Virus production continues despite the development of neutralizing and hemagglutinating antibodies by the infected child.

Pathology

The lesions in the nervous system are those of a chronic leptomeningitis with infiltration of mononuclear cells, lymphocytes, and plasma cells. Small areas of necrosis and glial cell proliferation are seen in the basal ganglia, midbrain, pons, and spinal cord. Microscopic vasculitis and perivascular calcification may also occur.

Symptoms and Signs

The infant with rubella encephalitis is usually lethargic, hypotonic, or inactive at birth or within the first few days or weeks after birth. Within the next several months, restlessness, head retraction, opisthotonic posturing, and rigidity may develop. Seizures and a meningitis-like illness may occur. The anterior fontanelle is usually large; microcephaly occurs infrequently. The child may have other associated defects, such as deafness, cardiovascular anomalies, congestive heart failure, cataracts, thrombocytopenia, and areas of hyperpigmentation about the navel, forehead, and cheeks. Improvement of varying degrees may be noted after the first 6 months to 12 months of life.

Laboratory Data

The CSF contains an increased number of cells (lymphocytes), as well as a moderately increased protein content. Rubella virus can be recovered from the CSF of approximately 25% of patients and may persist in the CSF for more than 1 year after birth.

Diagnosis

Specific diagnosis may be made by recovery of the virus from throat swab, urine, CSF, leukocytes, bone marrow, or conjunctivae, or by serologic tests. A rubella-specific IgM serologic test may be used for diagnosis in the newborn.

Treatment

The primary method of treatment is prevention of fetal infection. Live rubella virus vaccine should be given to all children between 1 year of age and puberty. Adolescent girls and nonpregnant women should be given vaccine if they are shown by serologic testing to be susceptible to rubella virus. Prevention has been highly effective. In the

United States since 1980, fewer than 10 cases per year of CRS have been reported.

Other Rubella Diseases

Rubella virus also has caused postinfectious encephalomyelitis with acquired rubella and rarely, a chronic or slow viral infection termed *progressive rubella panencephalitis* (see below).

MYXOVIRUS INFECTIONS

Mumps Meningitis and Encephalomyelitis

Mumps is a disease caused by a paramyxovirus that has predilection for the salivary glands, mature gonads, pancreas, breast, and the nervous system. It is spread via respiratory droplets. There is only one serotype. Like other paramyxoviruses, mumps is an enveloped virus that develops from the cell surface by a budding process.

Clinical evidence of involvement of the nervous system occurs in the form of a mild meningitis or encephalitis in a small percentage of patients. Other neurologic complications of mumps include encephalomyelitis, myelitis, and peripheral neuritis. During mumps meningitis, virus replicates in choroidal and ependymal cells. It is not clear, however, if the encephalitis results from direct action of the virus or from immune-mediated demyelination (postinfectious encephalomyelitis).

Pathology

The pathology of mumps meningitis and encephalitis has not been clearly elucidated because the low mortality rate reduces the emergent need for definition. The pathologic changes are limited to infiltration of the meninges and cerebral blood vessels with lymphocytes and mononuclear cells. The morbid changes in patients with encephalomyelitis include perivenous demyelination with infiltration by lymphocytes and phagocytic microglia. Although pathologic changes are more prominent in white matter, focal areas of neuronal destruction may be seen.

Epidemiology

The incidence of neurologic complications of mumps varies greatly in different epidemics, ranging from a low of less than 1% to a high of about 70%. About two-thirds of patients with mumps parotitis have CSF pleocytosis, but only 50% of those with pleocytosis have CNS symptoms. Conversely, only about 50% of patients with CNS manifestations have parotitis.

Although the two sexes are equally susceptible to mumps, neurologic complications are three times more frequent in males. Children are commonly affected, but epidemics may occur in young adults living under community conditions, such as army camps. Most cases of mumps encephalitis in the United States appear to occur in the late winter and early spring. Only several hundred cases of mumps occur annually in the United States.

Symptoms and Signs

In most patients, the symptoms of involvement of the nervous system are those of meningitis (i.e., headache, drowsiness, neck stiffness). These symptoms commonly appear 2 days to 10 days after the onset of the parotitis; they occasionally precede the onset of swelling of the salivary glands. These symptoms are benign and disappear within a few days. When encephalitis occurs, it is usually mild.

Complications

Deafness is the most common sequela of mumps. Hearing loss, which is unilateral in more than 65% of patients, may develop gradually or it may have an abrupt onset accompanied by vertigo and tinnitus. The deafness that follows mumps seems to be the result of damage to the membranous labyrinth. Orchitis, oophoritis, pancreatitis, and thyroiditis may also occur. Severe myelitis, polyneuritis, encephalitis, optic neuritis, and other cranial nerve palsies may develop 7 days to 15 days after the onset of parotitis, presumably from immune-mediated postinfectious encephalomyelitis.

A few cases of hydrocephalus have been reported in children who have had mumps virus infections. The hydrocephalus seems to stem from aqueductal stenosis induced by mumps virus, replication in aqueductal ependymal cells, and subsequent gliosis.

Laboratory Data

In mumps meningitis, the blood usually shows a relative lymphocytosis and a slight leukopenia. The CSF is under slightly increased pressure. The cell count is increased, usually in the range of 25 cells/mm^3 to 500 cells/mm^3, but occasionally the counts may be as high as 3,000 cells/mm^3. Lymphocytes usually constitute 90% to 96% of the total, even in CSF with a high cell count, but PMN leukocytes occasionally predominate in the early stages. The degree of pleocytosis is not related to the severity of symptoms, and it may persist for 30 days to 60 days. Inclusions of viral nucleocapsid-like material have been recognized by electron microscopic observation of CSF cells from patients with mumps meningitis. The protein content is normal or moderately increased, and mumps-specific oligoclonal immunoglobulin G (IgG) may be present. The sugar content is usually normal but may show a moderate reduction in 5% to 10% of patients. Mumps virus may be recovered from the CSF in a significant number of cases.

Diagnosis

Mumps meningitis is diagnosed on the basis of meningeal symptoms and CSF pleocytosis in a patient with mumps. In patients in whom neurologic symptoms develop during an epidemic of mumps, and there is no evidence of involvement of the salivary glands, the diagnosis may not be made with certainty unless the virus may be recovered from the CSF or there is a significant increase in antibodies in the serum. The presence of specific IgM antibody in the CSF is diagnostic. Virus may usually be recovered from the saliva, throat, urine, and CSF.

Mumps meningitis must be differentiated from other forms of meningitis, especially tuberculous and fungal, if the CSF glucose is low. A normal sugar content and the absence of organisms in the CSF are important in excluding acute purulent, tuberculous, or fungal meningitis.

Treatment

Since licensure of the live-attenuated mumps vaccine in 1967, the incidence of mumps has decreased to less than 5% of the prevaccine level. CNS complications (primarily meningitis) from the vaccine, if they occur at all, are rare.

Subacute Measles Encephalitis

Measles virus causes a wide spectrum of neurologic disease ranging from subclinical involvement and acute measles encephalitis (see "Postinfectious Encephalomyelitis," below), within days after the onset of a measles exanthem, to chronic subacute sclerosing panencephalitis (see below). Toxic encephalopathy and acute infantile hemiplegia rarely occur with measles infections; these seem to be complications of severe febrile illnesses of childhood and are not specific syndromes caused by measles.

Subacute measles encephalitis (e.g., measles inclusion-body encephalitis, immunosuppressive measles encephalitis) occurs as an opportunistic infection in immunosuppressed or immunodeficient patients. Most cases have occurred in children, but a few have occurred in adults. Several cases have been reported in patients with no obvious immune defects. A history of measles exposure 1 month to 6 months before the onset of neurologic disease may usually be obtained.

Symptoms and Signs

The disease is characterized by generalized and focal seizures, including epilepsia partialis continua, occasional focal deficits, and a progressive deterioration of mental function leading to coma and death in several weeks to 4 months or 5 months.

Diagnosis and Treatment

Routine CSF tests are normal. Diagnosis may be difficult because there may not be a history of a rash or even obvious exposure. At the time of presentation, measles antibody may not be present in the serum or CSF. Brain biopsy may be required. Pathology reveals numerous inclusions in neurons and glia with microglial activation, but minimal perivascular inflammation. The role of postexposure immunoglobulin prophylaxis is unclear. In several patients, intravenous ribavirin treatment has resulted in temporary improvement.

RHABDOVIRUS INFECTION

Rabies

Rabies (i.e., hydrophobia, lyssa, rage) is an acute viral disease of the CNS that is transmitted to humans by the bite of an infected (rabid) animal. It is characterized by a variable incubation period, restlessness, hyperesthesia, convulsions, laryngeal spasms, widespread paralysis, and almost invariably death.

Etiology

Rabies virus is an enveloped bullet-shaped virus that contains single-stranded RNA. Because of its characteristic morphology, rabies has been classified among the *rhabdo* (rod-shaped) viruses. The virus appears capable of infecting every warm-blooded animal. Rabies virus is present in the saliva of infected animals and is transmitted to humans by bites or abrasions of the skin. The bite of a rabid dog or exposure to bats is the usual circumstance, but the disease may be transmitted by cats, wolves, foxes, raccoons, skunks, and other domestic or wild animals. After inoculation, the virus replicates in muscle cells and then travels to the CNS by way of both sensory and motor nerves by axonal transport. After CNS invasion, dissemination of virus is rapid, with early selective involvement of limbic system neurons.

Several cases of airborne transmission of rabies have occurred in spelunkers of bat-infested caves and in laboratory workers. Unusual human-to-human transmission has occurred in two patients who were recipients of corneal transplants.

The incubation period usually varies between 1 month and 3 months, with the extremes of 10 days and more than 1 year. In general, the incubation period is directly related to the severity of the bite or bites and their location. The period is shortest when the wound is on the face and longest when on the leg.

Pathology

The pathology of rabies is that of a generalized encephalitis and myelitis. There is perivascular infiltration of the entire CNS with lymphocytes and, to a lesser extent, PMN leukocytes and plasma cells. The perivascular infiltration is usually mild and may be focal or diffuse. Diffuse degenerative changes occur in the neurons. Pathognomonic of the disease is the presence of cytoplasmic eosinophilic inclusions, with central basophilic granules that are found in neurons (Negri bodies) (Fig. 24.2).

These are usually found in pyramidal cells of the hippocampus and cerebellar Purkinje cells, but they may be seen in neurons of the cortex and other regions of the CNS, as well as in the spinal ganglia. These inclusions contain rabies virus antigen, as demonstrated by immunofluorescence. Rabies virus nucleocapsids have been found in electron microscopic studies of the inclusions. These inclusion bodies are occasionally absent. There is proliferation of microglia with the formation of rod cells, that may be collected into small nodules (Babès nodules). In cases with a long incubation period, the degenerative changes in neurons may be quite severe, with little or no inflammatory reaction.

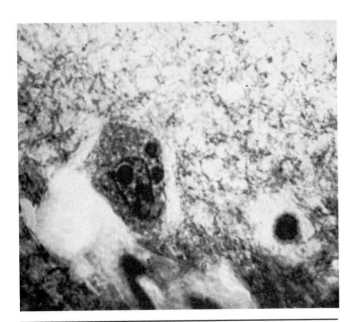

FIGURE 24.2. Rabies. Inclusion bodies (Negri bodies) in cytoplasm of a ganglion cell of cerebral cortex.

Incidence

The incidence of rabies is inversely proportional to the control of rabid animals. Wildlife rabies has become an increasingly serious problem in the United States during the 1990s. However, the disease in wildlife is almost nonexistent in Great Britain, where strict animal regulations are enforced. Human rabies is a clinical rarity in the United States and most of the countries of central Europe, but it is still common in southeastern Europe and Asia. Usually, two to three cases of human rabies occur annually in the United States.

The incidence of the disease in individuals who have been bitten by rabid dogs is low (15%), but it is high (40%) when the bite is inflicted by a rabid wolf. The incidence is highest when the wounds are severe and near the head. It is low when the bite is inflicted through clothing, the process of which cleans some or most of the infecting saliva from the teeth.

Symptoms

Onset is denoted by pain or numbness in the region of the bite in about 50% of patients. Other initial symptoms include fever, apathy, drowsiness, headache, and anorexia. This period of lethargy passes rapidly into a state of excitability in which all external stimuli are apt to cause localized twitching or generalized convulsions. There may be delirium with hallucinations and bizarre behavior (thrashing, biting, severe anxiety). A profuse flow of saliva occurs; spasmodic contractions of the pharynx and larynx are precipitated by any attempt to consume liquid or solid food. As a result, the patient violently refuses to accept any liquids, hence, the name hydrophobia. The body temperature is usually elevated and may reach 105°F to 107°F (40.6°C to 41.7°C) in the terminal stages. The stage of hyperirritability gradually passes into a state of generalized paralysis and coma. Death results from paralysis of respiration.

The disease occasionally begins with paralysis (paralytic form or dumb rabies) without convulsive phenomena or laryngeal spasm. The paralysis is a flaccid type and may start in one limb and spread rapidly to involve the others. The paralysis is more often symmetric than asymmetric. Symptoms and signs of a transverse myelitis may develop.

Laboratory Data

Leukocytosis occurs in the blood, and albumin may be present in the urine. The CSF is under normal pressure, and a lymphocytic pleocytosis is present, varying from 5 cells/mm^3 to several hundred cells/mm^3 in only about 50% of patients. The protein content is usually increased.

Diagnosis

Rabies is often diagnosed from the appearance of the characteristic symptoms after the bite of a rabid animal. The diagnosis may occasionally be made by fluorescent antibody staining of corneal smears or skin biopsies from the back of the neck, although both false-negative and false-positive results occur. Serum and CSF should also be tested for rabies antibodies. However, negative results for these tests do not rule out the possibility of rabies. The presence of rabies antibodies in the CSF is diagnostic. Virus isolation from the saliva, throat, tears, and CSF should also be attempted, although this is rarely successful. With the recent introduction of PCR techniques, virus detection in these specimens appears to be more successful. The only sure way of making the diagnosis while the patient is alive is by brain biopsy. The differential diagnosis includes all forms of encephalitis and, for the paralytic form of rabies includes differentiating those viruses causing lower motor neuron paralysis.

Course and Prognosis

The disease is almost always fatal and usually runs its course in 2 days to 10 days. Death within 24 hours of the onset of symptoms has been reported. Several cases with recovery have been reported.

Treatment

There is no specific antiviral therapy. Treatment during the encephalitic phase is supportive and, as noted, rarely successful. Specific treatment is entirely prophylactic and includes both passive antibody and vaccine. Passive immunization is by use of human rabies immune globulin. Immune globulin is infiltrated into the wound and given intramuscularly. A full course of active immunization with rabies vaccine should be given.

ARENAVIRUS INFECTIONS

Lymphocytic Choriomeningitis (LCM)

LCM is a relatively benign viral infection of the meninges and CNS. The clinical features of the disease were described by Wallgren in 1925 (under the term *aseptic meningitis*). The disease is of historic importance because it was the first in which a virus was proved to be the cause of a benign meningitis with a predominance of lymphocytes in the CSF. The role of the virus in human disease was established by Rivers and Scott in 1935, when they isolated it from the CSF of two patients with the clinical syndrome described by Wallgren.

LCM virus is an enveloped RNA virus. It causes less than 0.5% of cases of viral meningitis. Neurologic disease develops in only about 15% of those infected. Mice are the major

reservoir of the virus and are implicated as the intermediate host. Both pet and laboratory hamsters have also been a source of infection. Ingestion of food contaminated by animal excreta and wound exposure to contaminated dirt are thought to be the modes of transmission. Human-to-human transmission does not occur. The disease is most common in the winter, when mice move indoors.

Symptoms and Signs

Onset of the infection is characterized by fever, headache, malaise, myalgia, and symptoms of upper respiratory infection or pneumonia. In a few patients, meningeal symptoms develop within 1 week after the onset. Occasionally, there is a remission in the prodromal symptoms, and the patient is apparently in good health when meningeal symptoms develop. Severe headache, nausea, and vomiting mark the beginning of neurologic involvement, most often aseptic meningitis. The temperature is moderately elevated (99° to 104°F [37.2° to 40.0°C]). The usual signs of meningitis (stiff neck, Kernig and Brudzinski signs) are present. The parenchyma is occasionally involved (encephalitic or meningoencephalitic forms), but good restoration of function usually occurs. Fewer than 12 deaths have been reported.

Laboratory Data

In the early influenza-like stages, leukopenia and thrombocytopenia may be seen. Later, the leukocyte count may be elevated with a predominance of PMN leukocytes. The CSF findings are similar to those of other viral causes of meningitis.

Diagnosis, Prognosis, and Treatment

A definitive viral diagnosis may be made by recovery of the virus from blood or CSF, but in most patients the diagnosis is made by serology. The differential diagnosis is similar to that of enterovirus infection, the most common cause of viral meningitis.

The duration of the meningeal symptoms varies from 1 to 4 weeks with an average of 3 weeks. The mortality rate is low, and complete recovery is the rule, except in the rare patients with encephalitis in whom residuals of focal lesions in the brain or spinal cord may be present. There is no specific treatment.

Other Arenavirus Infections

Junin (Argentinian hemorrhagic fever) and Machupo (Bolivian hemorrhagic fever) viruses and Lassa fever virus of Africa cause severe hemorrhagic fevers. Although hemorrhage and shock are the usual causes of death from these severe systemic infections, neurologic involvement is not unusual.

ADENOVIRUS INFECTIONS

Adenoviruses are nonenveloped (ether-resistant), icosahedral DNA containing viruses of which there are more than 30 serotypes. These viruses were not discovered until 1953 when they were isolated from tissue culture of surgically removed tonsils and adenoids, thus the name.

Symptoms and Signs

Adenoviruses may be spread by both respiratory and gastrointestinal routes and cause a variety of clinical syndromes. Respiratory infection is most often seen, manifested by coryza, pharyngitis, and, at times, pneumonia. Pharyngoconjunctival fever, epidemic keratoconjunctivitis, pertussis-like syndrome, and hemorrhagic cystitis are other manifestations. Most infections occur in children; about 50% of these infections are asymptomatic. Epidemics of respiratory diseases have occurred among military personnel. Opportunistic infections have occurred in both adults and children. Neurologic involvement has occurred mostly in children as an encephalitis or meningoencephalitis and is quite rare. Encephalopathy has also been reported.

Diagnosis and Treatment

Only a few pathologic studies have been performed, and the encephalitis appears to be of the primary type with virus invasion of the brain. Histologic changes include perivascular cuffing and mononuclear cell parenchyma infiltrates, but in some patients, little or no inflammation is seen. Virus has been isolated from the brain and CSF in several patients. The encephalitis is usually of moderate to severe intensity with meningism, lethargy, confusion, coma, and convulsions. Ataxia has also been reported. Death occurs in up to 30% of patients. CSF pleocytosis often, but not always, occurs and may be PMN or mononuclear. The protein content may be normal or elevated. Diagnosis may be made by serology or by isolation of virus from the CSF, throat, respiratory secretions, and feces. There is no specific treatment.

HERPESVIRUS INFECTIONS

The herpesvirus group is composed of DNA-containing viruses that have a lipid envelope and multiply in the cell nucleus. Members of this group share the common feature of establishing latent infections. Herpesviruses may remain quiescent for long periods of time, being demonstrable only sporadically or not at all until a stimulus triggers reactivated infection. Within cells, accumulations of virus particles may often be recognized in the nucleus in the form of acidophilic inclusion bodies. There are now eight recognized members of the human herpesvirus family: HSV types 1 and 2, VZV, Epstein-Barr virus (EBV), CMV, human herpes virus-6 (HHV-6), human herpes virus-7 (HHV-7), and human herpes virus-8 (HHV-8) (Kaposi sarcoma herpesvirus). All of these viruses are capable of causing neurologic disease, but only a few cases have been reported in association with HHV-7 and HHV-8.

Herpes Simplex Encephalitis

Encephalitis caused by HSV is the single most important cause of fatal sporadic encephalitis in the United States. Early diagnosis is crucial because there is effective antiviral treatment.

Etiology

Two antigenic types of HSV are distinguished by serologic testing. Type 1 strains (HSV-1) are responsible for almost all cases of HSV encephalitis in adults and cause oral herpes. Type 2 strains (HSV-2) cause genital disease. In the neonatal period, HSV-2 encephalitis occurs as part of a disseminated infection or as localized disease acquired during delivery. In adults, HSV-2 is spread by venereal transmission and causes aseptic meningitis.

Pathogenesis

HSV-1 is transmitted by respiratory or salivary contact. Primary infection usually occurs in childhood or adolescence. It is usually subclinical or may cause stomatitis, pharyngitis, or respiratory disease. About 50% of the population has antibody to HSV-1 by age 15 years, whereas 50% to 90% of adults have antibody, depending on socioeconomic status. HSV-1 encephalitis may occur at any age, but more than 50% of cases occur in patients older than 20 years of age. This finding suggests that encephalitis most often occurs from endogenous reactivation of virus rather than from primary infection. Neurologic involvement is a rare complication of reactivation. During the primary infection, virus becomes latent in the trigeminal ganglia. Years later, nonspecific stimuli cause reactivation that is usually manifested as herpes labialis (cold sores). Presumably, virus may reach the brain through branches of the trigeminal nerve to the basal meninges, resulting in localization of the encephalitis to the temporal and orbital frontal lobes. Alternatively, serologic studies suggest that about 25% of cases of HSV-1 encephalitis occur as part of a primary infection. Experimental studies indicate that this could occur by spread of virus across the olfactory bulbs to the orbital frontal lobes and subsequently the temporal lobes. The encephalitis is sporadic without seasonal variations. HSV-1 encephalitis rarely occurs as an opportunistic infection in immunocompromised hosts.

Except when infantile infection occurs at delivery, HSV-2 is spread by sexual contact. Thus, primary infection usually occurs during the late teenage or early adult years. As noted previously, HSV-2 causes aseptic meningitis in adults, that probably occurs as part of the primary infection. As with HSV-1, opportunistic infections may also occur in immunocompromised patients.

Pathology

In fatal cases, intense meningitis and widespread destructive changes occur in the brain parenchyma. Necrotic, inflammatory, or hemorrhagic lesions may be found. These lesions are maximal, most often in the frontal and temporal lobes. There is often an unusual degree of cerebral edema accompanying the necrotic lesions. Eosinophilic intranuclear inclusion bodies (i.e., Cowdry type A inclusions) are present in neurons. These inclusions containing herpesvirus particles are recognized on electron microscopic examination.

Symptoms and Signs

The most common early manifestations are fever, headache, and altered consciousness and personality (Table 24.3). Onset is most often abrupt and may be ushered in by major motor or focal seizures. The encephalitis may evolve more slowly, however, with aphasia or mental changes preceding more severe neurologic signs. Most patients have a temperature between 101°F and 104°F (38.4°C and 40.0°C) at the time of admission. Nuchal rigidity or other signs of meningeal irritation are often found. Mental deficits include confusion and personality changes varying from withdrawal to agitation with hallucinations.

A progressive course ensues within hours to several days, with an increasing impairment of consciousness and the development of focal neurologic signs. Rarely, the course may be subacute or chronic, lasting several months. Focal signs, such as hemiplegia, hemisensory loss, focal seizures, and ataxia, are considered distinguishing features of herpes encephalitis but are seen in less than 50% of affected patients on initial examination. Herpetic skin lesions are seen in only a few patients but are also seen with other diseases. A history of cold sores is not helpful in making the differential diagnosis because the incidence is similar to that of the general population.

Laboratory Data

There is a moderate leukocytosis in the blood. The CSF pressure may be moderately or greatly increased. Pleocytosis in the CSF varies from less than 10 cells/mm³ to 1,000 cells/mm³; lymphocytes usually predominate, but occasionally PMN leukocytes may predominate early in the infection, followed by a shift to lymphocytes. Red blood

▶ **TABLE 24.3 Manifestations of Herpes Simplex Encephalitis at Presentation**

	NIAID Collaborative Study[a]	Swedish Study[b]
Symptoms		
Altered consciousness	97% (109/112)	100% (53/53)
Fever	90% (101/112)	100% (53/53)
Headache	81% (89/110)	74% (39/53)
Seizures	67% (73/109)	—
Vomiting	46% (51/111)	38% (20/53)
Hemiparesis	33% (33/100)	—
Memory loss	24% (14/59)	—
Signs		
Fever	92% (101/110)	—
Personality alteration (confusion, disorientation)	85% (69/81)	57% (30/53)
Dysphasia	76% (58/76)	36% (19/53)
Autonomic dysfunction	60% (54/88)	—
Ataxia	40% (22/55)	—
Hemiparesis	38% (41/107)	40% (21/33)
Seizures	38% (43/112)	62% (33/53)
Focal	(28/43)	—
Generalized	(10/43)	—
Both	(5/43)	—
Cranial nerve deficits	32% (34/105)	—
Papilledema	14% (16/111)	—

[a]Data from Whitley, et al. Herpes simplex encephalitis: vidarabine versus acyclovir therapy. *N Engl J Med* 1986;314:144–149.
[b]Data from Skoldenberg, et al. Acyclovir vs. vidarobine in herpes simplex encephalitis: randomised multicentre study in consecutive Swedish patients. *Lancet* 1984;2:707–711.

cells are frequently seen, but their presence or absence is not diagnostic. The CSF sugar content is usually normal but may be low. Virus is rarely recovered from the CSF. In 5% to 10% of patients, the initial CSF examination is normal.

EEG and MRI are the most likely diagnostic studies to be abnormal at onset and during the first week of infection. The EEG is usually abnormal (about 80% in biopsy-proven cases) with diffuse slowing or focal changes over temporal areas; periodic complexes against a slow-wave background may be seen. CT may demonstrate low-density abnormality, mass effect, or linear enhancement in more than 90% of patients, but it is often normal during the first week (Fig. 24.3). Thus, CT cannot be relied on for early diagnosis. MRI often reveals focal lesions in the first week of disease when the CT scan is normal (Fig. 24.4).

Diagnosis

Because HSV encephalitis has a high mortality rate and the outcome of therapy is affected by the patient's level of consciousness and neurologic deficits, diagnostic

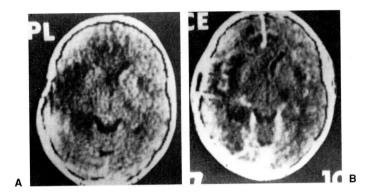

A **B**

FIGURE 24.3. Herpes simplex encephalitis. A: Axial CT on day 10 shows a low-density lesion in the right-temporal and basal-frontal lobes. **B:** Corresponding contrast-enhanced CT shows gyral enhancement in the sylvian fissure and insular regions that is greater on the right. An abnormal CT is not usually seen until day 6 or day 7 after the onset of manifestations. Eventually, a majority of scans show gyral enhancement in the sylvian fissure area. These findings should raise the suspicion of an underlying infectious lesion such as herpes, early infarction from emboli or vasculitis, or metastatic tumors. (From Davis JM, et al. Computed tomography of herpes simplex encephalitis with clinicopathological correlation. *Radiology* 1978;129:409–417; with permission.)

measures leading to a presumptive diagnosis should be initiated as soon as possible. Presumptive diagnosis for treatment may be based on clinical, CT, CSF, EEG, and MRI findings. Definite diagnosis may be established only by recovery of virus from the CSF (rare) or brain, demonstration of viral DNA in the CSF or brain by PCR, or finding of viral antigen in the brain. Because patients may show a rise in antibody titer with recurrent HSV cutaneous lesions or with inapparent infection, a four-fold rise in the serum antibody titer to herpesvirus may occur in patients with encephalitis from other causes. The appearance of herpes antibodies in the CSF is a useful retrospective diagnostic test, but these antibodies occur too late in the disease to aid in therapy selection.

The differential diagnosis of HSV-1 encephalitis includes other viral and postinfectious encephalitides; bacterial, fungal, and parasitic infections; and tumors. Brain abscess is often the most difficult diagnosis to exclude. Before the advent of MRI, about 25% of biopsy-negative patients had another treatable disease.

Prognosis and Treatment

Without treatment, the disease is fatal in about 70% to 80% of patients, and patients who survive the acute disease are usually left with severe neurologic residuals. Measures to decrease life-threatening brain edema, including the administration of corticosteroids, are indicated.

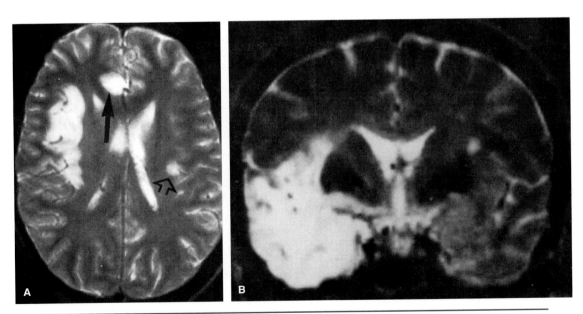

A **B**

FIGURE 24.4. Herpes simplex encephalitis. A: T2-weighted axial MRI reveals high-signal intensity in the right insular cortex, medial-right frontal cortex *(solid arrow)*, and left insular cortex *(open arrow)*. (From Runge VM. *Magnetic Resaonance Imaging of the Brain.* Philadelphia: JB Lippincott Co, 1994:190; with permission.) **B:** T2-weighted coronal MRI shows increased signal in the left temporal lobe and early involvement of the right side. (From Schroth et al., 1987; with permission.) An abnormal MR image is usually seen by day 1 or day 2 after the onset of manifestations. Coronal images are the most useful for detecting the herpes simplex lesions.

Vidarabine, a DNA polymerase inhibitor, decreased mortality to 44% at 6 months, compared to 70% for patients receiving placebo. Subsequently, acyclovir was demonstrated to be more efficacious than vidarabine in two controlled trials. In the National Institute of Allergy and Infectious Disease study, acyclovir reduced mortality to 28% compared to 55% for vidarabine at 18 months. Acyclovir selectively inhibits virus-specific polymerase, has less toxicity than vidarabine, and is now the drug of choice. Outcome depends on patient age, level of consciousness, and the rapidity with which treatment is instituted. After presumptive diagnosis, acyclovir treatment should be instituted even if MRI cannot be performed until the next day. If deterioration in the clinical course occurs over the next 48 hours to 72 hours, brain biopsy is indicated. Relapses have occurred after a 10-day treatment regimen; hence, a 14-day course is now recommended.

Herpes Zoster

Herpes zoster (shingles) is a viral disease that produces inflammatory lesions in the posterior root ganglia and is characterized clinically by pain and a skin eruption in the distribution of the affected ganglia. Involvement of motor roots or the CNS occurs in a small percentage of patients.

Etiology

The virus of herpes zoster is VZV, the causative agent of chickenpox (varicella). VZV is a large, enveloped, DNA-containing virus that has the same structure as that of other herpesviruses. Children may catch chickenpox from exposure to adults with shingles, but adults are subject to herpes zoster only if they have had chickenpox earlier in life. The CNS complications (acute cerebellar ataxia, encephalitis, myelitis, meningitis) of varicella are thought to occur by a postinfectious autoimmune mechanism (see "Acute Disseminated Encephalomyelitis" below), although direct viral invasion may occur less frequently. Epidemiologic considerations led Hope-Simpson to speculate that zoster infection is a reactivation of latent VZV originally acquired in a childhood attack of chickenpox. Herpes zoster frequently occurs in connection with other systemic infections, immunosuppressive therapy, and localized lesions of the spine or nerve roots (e.g., acute meningitides, tuberculosis, Hodgkin disease, metastatic carcinoma, trauma to the spine).

Pathology

Although symptoms are usually confined to the distribution of one or two sensory roots, the pathologic changes are usually more widespread. The affected ganglia of the spinal or cranial nerve roots are swollen and inflamed. The inflammatory reaction is chiefly one of a lymphocytic nature, but a few PMN leukocytes or plasma cells may also be present. The inflammatory process commonly extends to the meninges and into the root entry zone (posterior poliomyelitis). Not infrequently, some inflammatory reaction occurs in the ventral horn and in the perivascular space of the white matter of the spinal cord. The pathologic changes in the ganglia of the cranial nerves and in the brainstem are similar to those in the spinal root and spinal cord.

Incidence

Herpes zoster is a relatively common disease with an incidence that varies from 1 case to 5 cases per 1,000 people each year. Rates are higher in patients with malignancies and in those receiving immunosuppressive therapy. Symptoms of involvement of the nervous system, with the exception of pain, are rare, only occurring in about 10% of patients. Zoster is more common in middle or later life.

Symptoms and Signs

The initial symptom is usually a neuralgic pain or dysesthesia in the distribution of the affected root. The pain is followed in 3 days to 4 days by reddening of the skin and the appearance of clusters of vesicles in part of the area supplied by the affected roots. These vesicles that contain clear fluid may be discrete or may coalesce. Within 10 days to 2 weeks, the vesicles are covered with a scab which, after desquamation, leaves a pigmented scar. These scars are usually replaced by normally colored skin in the ensuing months. Permanent scarring may occur if there is ulceration or secondary infection of the vesicles. Coincidental to the eruption is adenopathy that is usually painless.

Herpes zoster is primarily an infection of the spinal ganglia, but the cranial ganglia are affected in about 20% of patients. The thoracic, lumbar, cervical, and sacral segments are involved in descending order of frequency. Involvement is almost always unilateral.

Among the less common symptoms are impairment of cutaneous sensation and muscle weakness in the distribution of the affected root, malaise, fever, headache, neck stiffness, and confusion. The latter symptoms indicate involvement of the meninges. Involvement of the cervical or lumbar segments may be accompanied by weakness and occasionally, subsequent atrophy of isolated muscle groups in the arm or leg (zoster paresis). The rare involvement of sacral segments may result in bladder paralysis with urinary retention or incontinence. Oculomotor palsies may also occur.

Ophthalmic Zoster

Involvement of the trigeminal ganglion occurs in about 20% of patients. Any division of the ganglion may be involved, but the first division (ophthalmic) is by far the most commonly affected. The seriousness of the involvement of this ganglion is attributed to the changes that develop in the eyes secondary to panophthalmitis or scarring of the cornea. There may be a temporary or permanent paresis of the muscles supplied by the oculomotor nerves, as a complication of ophthalmic zoster.

Geniculate Herpes

Otic zoster with involvement of the geniculate ganglion (Ramsay Hunt syndrome), although rare, assumes prominence because of paralysis of the facial muscles. The rash is usually confined to the tympanic membrane and the external auditory canal. It may spread to involve the outer surface of the lobe of the ear, and when it is combined with cervical involvement, vesicles are found on portions of the neck. Loss of taste over the anterior two-thirds of the tongue occurs in more than 50% of patients. Partial or complete recovery is the rule. Involvement of the ganglia of Corti and Scarpa is accompanied by tinnitus, vertigo, nausea, and loss of hearing.

Complications

Although the CSF shows a lymphocytic pleocytosis, meningeal symptoms are uncommon. Signs of involvement of the tracts of the spinal cord in the form of a Brown-Séquard syndrome or a transverse or ascending *myelitis* have occurred. Mental confusion, ataxia, and focal cerebral symptoms have been attributed to involvement of the brain by VZV (herpes zoster *encephalitis*). *Polyneuritis* of the so-called infectious or Guillain-Barré type has been reported as a sequela of herpes zoster. Involvement of the anterior roots may result in zoster paresis. A more recently recognized complication of ophthalmic zoster is acute contralateral hemiplegia and at times other ipsilateral hemisphere signs, such as aphasia, that occur weeks or months later (herpes zoster ophthalmicus with delayed contralateral hemiparesis). An *arteritis*, apparently with viral invasion, develops in the carotid and other vessels ipsilateral to the zoster ophthalmicus, resulting in hemispheric infarction.

Postherpetic neuralgia is most common in elderly debilitated patients and chiefly affects the ophthalmic or intercostal nerves. The pains are persistent, sharp, and shooting in nature. The skin is sensitive to touch. These pains may persist for months or years and are often refractory to all forms of treatment.

Laboratory Data

The abnormalities in the laboratory findings are confined to the CSF. Even in uncomplicated herpes zoster, there is an inconstant lymphocytic pleocytosis that may be found before the onset of the rash. The CSF may be normal in patients with symptoms of involvement of only one thoracic segment, but it is usually abnormal when the cranial ganglia are involved or when paralysis or other neurologic signs is present. The cell count varies from 10 cells/mm^3 to several hundred cells/mm^3, with lymphocytes as the predominating cell type. The protein content is normal or moderately increased; the sugar content is normal.

Diagnosis

Herpes zoster is diagnosed without difficulty when the characteristic rash is present. In the preeruptive stage, the pain may lead to the erroneous diagnosis of disease of the abdominal or thoracic viscera. The possibility of herpes zoster should be considered in all patients with root pains of sudden onset that have existed for less than 4 days. Difficulties in diagnosis may also be encountered when the vesicles are widespread or when they are scant or entirely absent (zoster sine herpete). It is possible that herpes zoster may cause intercostal neuralgia or facial palsy without any readily apparent cutaneous eruption, but a careful search usually reveals a few vesicles.

If necessary, VZV may be cultured from vesicular fluid, detected by electron microscopic examination of vesicular fluid, and identified by immunohistochemical staining of cells from vesicular scrapings. PCR amplification techniques may be used to detect viral DNA in vesicular fluid and CSF.

Treatment

There is still no effective means of preventing herpes zoster. Treatment of uncomplicated zoster includes only the use of analgesics and nonspecific topical medications for the rash. Use of topical antiviral agents is of questionable benefit. Although antibiotics have no effect on the virus, they may be indicated to control secondary infection. Systemic acyclovir (oral or intravenous) has been the agent of choice for the treatment of acute herpes zoster. Several new antiviral agents (valacyclovir, famciclovir) also to decrease pain, virus shedding, and healing time of acute herpes zoster. In addition, famciclovir significantly reduces the duration of postherpetic neuralgia. All of these agents decrease viral dissemination and its complications. For this reason, they are indicated for systemic complications, especially in immunosuppressed patients, and for zoster encephalomyelitis and arteritis. Because the arteritis may develop from an allergic response, it has been treated with a combination of corticosteroids and an antiviral agent. Zoster immune globulin is useful in prophylaxis of varicella in immunosuppressed children, but it is not helpful for zoster.

Postherpetic neuralgia is difficult to treat. It is refractory to the usual analgesics. Sectioning the affected posterior roots is usually not successful in relieving pain. The efficacy of corticosteroids is minimal (decreases in duration of acute neuritis and time to healing, but not in the incidence or duration of postherpetic neuralgia). Their use would seem risky because of immunosuppression and possible virus dissemination. Amitriptyline, other tricyclic antidepressants, and anticonvulsants (carbamazepine, phenytoin sodium, gabapentin) are the mainstays of therapy.

Cytomegalovirus (CMV) Infection

Cytomegalic inclusion body disease is an infection that occurs *in utero* by transplacental transmission. The responsible agent is CMV, a member of the herpesvirus family. CMV infection results in the appearance of large, swollen cells that often contain large eosinophilic intranuclear and cytoplasmic inclusions.

Signs and Symptoms

Intrauterine infection of the nervous system may result in stillbirth or prematurity. The cerebrum is affected by a granulomatous encephalitis with extensive subependymal calcification. Hydrocephalus, hydranencephaly, microcephaly, cerebellar hypoplasia, or other types of developmental defects of the brain may be found. Convulsive seizures, focal neurologic signs, and mental retardation are common in infants who survive (Table 24.4).

Jaundice with hepatosplenomegaly, purpura, and hemolytic anemia may be present. Periventricular calcification is often seen in radiographs of the skull. Many affected infants succumb in the neonatal period, but prolonged periods of survival are possible. Subclinical or silent congenital infections may result in deafness and developmental abnormalities. There may also be progressive CNS damage and, presumably, a persistent infection for months after birth.

CMV infections may also occur in adults (Table 24.4), producing a mononucleosis-like syndrome, but involvement of the nervous system is uncommon in this acute adult form of the disease. CNS infection in immunodeficient patients, including those with AIDS, is probably more frequent, however. CNS involvement in immunocompromised patients is often asymptomatic, although fatal encephalitis may occur. The encephalitis has a subacute or chronic course and is clinically indistinguishable from HIV encephalitis (HIV dementia). MRI demonstrates either diffuse or focal white matter abnormalities in about 25% of patients. CMV infection also causes subacute polyradiculomyelopathy in AIDS patients. The polyradiculomyelopathy has a subacute onset of leg weakness and numbness leading to a flaccid paraplegia.

▶ **TABLE 24.4** Cytomegalovirus Neurologic Infections

Diseases and Features	Host and Frequency

Cytomegalic inclusion body disease
Encephalitis
  Microcephaly
  Seizures
  Mental retardation
  Periventricular calcifications
  Disseminated disease
	Neonates, congenital disease; rare

Encephalitis/ventriculitis
  Subacute course
  Progressive mental status changes
  Disseminated disease in immunocompromised-compromised patients
  MRI: periventricular hyperintensities, meningeal enhancement
	Immunocompromised patients (described primarily in AIDS patients); uncommon
	Immunocompetent patients; rare

Polyradiculitis/polyradiculomyelitis
  Pain and paresthesia in legs and perineum
  Sacral hypesthesia
  Urinary retention
  Subacute ascending hypotonic paraparesis
  Eventually ascends to cause myelitis
  CSF: pleocytosis (PMNs > lymphocytes), low glucose, high protein level,
  CMV positive by culture or PCR
  Usually disseminated disease
  MRI: lumbosacral leptomengeal enhancement
	Immunocompromised patients (described only in AIDS patients); common

Multifocal neuropathy
  Markedly asymmetric
  Numbness, painfull paresthesia for months, followed by sensorimotor neuropathy
  Usually disseminated disease
  CMV positive in CSF by culture or PCR
	Immunocompromised patients (described only in AIDS); uncommon

From Jubelt B. Ropka S. Infectious diseases of the nervous system. In: Rosenberg RN, ed., *Atlas of Clinical Neurology.*, 2nd ed. Philadelphia: Current Medicine, 2003;403–475; with permission.

Diagnosis and Treatment

For cytomegalic inclusion body disease, CMV may be recovered from urine, saliva, or liver biopsy specimens. Complement-fixation and neutralization tests are available. A presumptive diagnosis may be made by finding typical cytomegalic cells in stained preparations of urinary sediment or saliva.

In adult infections, virus may be cultured from extraneural sites. Antibody testing is usually not helpful in immunodeficient patients. CMV may not be cultured from the CSF; PCR amplification is the best microbiologic test. In polyradiculomyelopathy, PMN cells are often seen in the CSF, and there may be meningeal enhancement on MRI.

Both ganciclovir and foscarnet have been reported to be beneficial for some postnatally acquired infections. Some patients respond to treatment with cidofovir.

Epstein-Barr Virus Infection

Infectious mononucleosis (glandular fever) is a systemic disease of viral origin with involvement of the lymph nodes, spleen, liver, skin, and, occasionally, the CNS. It occurs sporadically and in small epidemics. It is most common in children and young adults.

Signs and Symptoms

The usual symptoms and signs are headache, malaise, sore throat, fever, enlargement of the lymph nodes in the cervical region, occasionally enlargement of the spleen, and changes in the blood. Unusual manifestations include a cutaneous rash, jaundice, and symptoms of involvement of the nervous system.

Although neurologic complications rank first as a cause of death, there have been few autopsy studies of the brain in fatal cases of infectious mononucleosis. Acute cortical inflammation similar to that seen in other viral infections has been observed. Atypical cells, probably lymphocytes, have been found in the inflammatory exudate.

The exact incidence of involvement of the nervous system is unknown, but it is probably less than 1%. A lymphocytic pleocytosis in the CSF may be found in the absence of any neurologic symptoms or signs. Severe headache and neck stiffness may be the initial or only symptoms of cerebral involvement (aseptic meningitis). Signs of encephalitis (delirium, convulsions, coma, and focal deficits) are rare manifestations. Optic neuritis, paralysis of the facial and other cranial nerves, acute autonomic neuropathy, infectious polyneuritis (Guillain-Barré syndrome), and transverse myelitis have been reported in a few patients. Acute cerebellar ataxia has also been associated with infectious mononucleosis.

CNS manifestations may appear early in the course of the disease in the absence of any other findings, but usually occur 1 week to 3 weeks after onset. The prognosis for EBV encephalitis is excellent with few fatalities and minimal residua.

Laboratory Data

In the laboratory examination, the important findings are leukocytosis in the blood, with an increase in lymphocytes and the appearance of abnormal mononuclear cells (atypical lymphocytes). Liver function tests are often abnormal, and heterophil antibody is present in 90% of patients. With involvement of the meninges, the CSF shows a lymphocytic pleocytosis (10 cells/mm^3 to 600 cells/mm^3) with or without a slight increase in protein content. The sugar content is normal, and CSF serologic tests for syphilis are negative. False-positive tests for syphilis are occasionally obtained on the serum.

Diagnosis and Treatment

The diagnosis is established by the appearance of neurologic symptoms in patients with other manifestations of the disease. The differential diagnosis includes other viral diseases that cause a lymphocytic meningeal reaction. The diagnosis may be made by a study of the blood, the heterophil antibody reaction, and measurement of specific antibodies to EBV antigens. At times, EBV may be isolated from the oropharynx. PCR amplification is also available for diagnosis. MRI abnormalities have been reported, with both gray and white matter lesions, in about 25% of patients.

There is no specific therapy. Treatment with steroids may be indicated in certain patients with severe pharyngotonsillitis or other complications.

Human Herpesvirus-6 Infection

Human Herpesvirus-6 (HHV-6) was first isolated from AIDS patients in 1986. Two years later it was shown to be the etiologic agent for roseola infantum (exanthema subitum, sixth disease). HHV-6 has also been found to cause opportunistic CNS disease in immunocompromised individuals.

Symptoms and Signs

Roseola is an acute, self-limited disease of infants and children. It is caused by an HHV-6 primary infection. It begins with abrupt onset of high fever, lasting 3 days to 4 days. Febrile convulsions commonly occur with a high fever. As the temperature rapidly falls, a transient maculopapular rash appears on the neck and trunk. The rash fades in 1 day to 3 days. Other physical findings are minimal but include mild injection of the pharynx and tympanic membranes and postoccipital and postauricular lymphadenopathy.

Complications

The most common CNS complications of roseola are febrile seizures, which occur in up to one-third of patients. Several studies suggest that recurrent seizures may develop in a small percentage of these patients. Meningoencephalitis has also occurred as a complication of roseola. Manifestations include persistent fever, a depressed level of consciousness, and seizures. The prognosis is variable. There is usually a mild mononuclear pleocytosis in the CSF. Less frequently, encephalopathy (no CSF pleocytosis) and demyelination have been reported.

Recurrent HHV-6 infections have been associated with a range of illnesses (pneumonia, bone marrow suppression, possibly lymphoma and encephalitis) in immunocompromised patients. The encephalitis occurring in these patients is usually more severe than that seen during roseola, and is more likely to result in death.

Diagnosis

During roseola, initially the peripheral white blood cell count may be slightly elevated but with disease progression, leukopenia is invariably present. This finding, along with the characteristic presentation and course, makes a presumptive diagnosis of roseola. Diagnosis is confirmed by isolation of virus (throat, saliva, blood) and seroconversion. Since HHV-6 appears to be latent in the brain, it is not clear what role CSF PCR amplification and CSF antibody assays will have in diagnosis. The diagnosis of reactivated infection is also confirmed by virus isolation and, at times, with a concomitant four-fold rise in IgG titer.

Treatment

For treatment of roseola, antipyretics are important for controlling the fever, which should decrease the incidence of febrile seizures. Anticonvulsants may be needed to treat recurrent seizures. Systemic antiviral agents should be used for CNS or systemic disease occurrence with roseola or with reactivation. In vitro, HHV-6 resembles CMV in its antiviral susceptibilities. It is apparently resistant to acyclovir but susceptible to ganciclovir and foscarnet. No clinical trials have been undertaken.

ACUTE DISSEMINATED ENCEPHALOMYELITIS

Acute disseminated encephalomyelitis (ADE) may occur in the course of various infections, particularly the acute exanthematous diseases of childhood, and following vaccinations; thus, ADE is also known by the terms *post-* or postinfectious encephalomyelitis (PIE) and *postvaccinal encephalomyelitis*. The clinical symptoms and the pathologic changes are similar in all of these cases, regardless of the nature of the precipitating infection or vaccination.

Etiology and Pathogenesis

The list of diseases that may be accompanied or followed by signs and symptoms of an encephalomyelitis is probably not yet complete, but it includes measles, rubella, varicella, smallpox, mumps, influenza, parainfluenza, infectious mononucleosis, typhoid, mycoplasmal infections, and upper respiratory and other obscure febrile diseases. Additionally, vaccination against measles, mumps, rubella, influenza, and rabies may trigger these signs and symptoms. Neurologic reactions may also follow inoculations with typhoid vaccine or with serum, particularly inoculations against tetanus. In these latter conditions, the clinical picture is more likely to be that of a mononeuritis or generalized polyneuritis.

The pathogenesis of ADE is not known. Virus is not usually isolated from the nervous system, so an allergic or autoimmune reaction appears to be the most likely cause. Presumably, the virus triggers an immune-mediated reaction against CNS myelin, causing a disease similar to experimental allergic encephalomyelitis. This could possibly involve an extraneural interaction of a virus with the immune system without viral invasion of the CNS.

Pathology

Little or no change occurs in the external appearance of the brain or spinal cord. On sectioning, many small yellowish-red lesions are present in the white matter of the cerebrum, cerebellum, brainstem, and spinal cord. The characteristic feature of these lesions is a loss of myelin, with relative sparing of the axis cylinders. Brain lesions are oval or round and usually surround a distended vein. Lesions are usually found in large numbers in almost all parts of the CNS, but in some cases they may be concentrated in the white matter of the cerebrum, while in others the cerebellum, brainstem, or spinal cord may be most severely affected. On microscopic examination, there is perivenular lymphocytic and mononuclear cell infiltration and demyelination. On myelin-stained specimens, there is destruction of myelin sheaths within the lesions, with a fairly sharp margin between the affected and normal areas. Axis cylinders are affected secondarily to a much lesser extent than the myelin sheaths. Phagocytic microglial cells may also be found within lesions and in perivascular spaces of adjacent vessels. Although lesions are concentrated in the white matter, a few patches may be found in the gray matter. Occasionally, nerve cells in these areas may be destroyed or may show various degenerative changes. ADE and PIE are monophasic diseases, as the lesions have a similar age of onset. *Acute hemorrhagic leukoencephalitis* appears to be a fulminant form of ADE or PIE. Pathologic lesions are similar to those of ADE, with the addition of microscopic hemorrhages and perivascular PMN-cell infiltrates.

Epidemiology

Previously, smallpox vaccination (vaccinia virus) was one of the more frequent causes of PIE or postvaccinal encephalomyelitis. The exact frequency has not been accurately established because of the wide range reported, varying from more than 1 case per 100 vaccinees to less than 1 case per 100,000 vaccinees. Because smallpox has apparently been eradicated as a natural disease, vaccination is no longer recommended. Thus, vaccinia virus is no longer a common cause of PIE. The smallpox virus (variola virus) also probably caused this syndrome in the past.

The incidence of encephalomyelitis following vaccination against rabies with the old nerve-tissue-prepared vaccines ranged as high as 1 in 600 persons, with a mortality rate of 10% to 25%. With the duck-embryo vaccine, this complication has decreased to approximately 1 in 33,000 recipients. This complication rarely has been reported with the new human diploid-cell vaccine (several cases); there have also been a few cases of associated Guillain-Barré syndrome.

Damage to the nervous system with the acute exanthems occurs most commonly following measles, for which the incidence is approximately 1 in 1,000 persons. In countries using measles vaccination, however, measles is no longer a common cause of PIE. The incidence following measles vaccine is only about 1 in 1 million recipients. PIE followed rubella or mumps much less frequently than it did after natural measles, but even this occurrence has decreased with vaccination. VZV infections are now probably the more common single cause of PIE, although the exact incidence is not known. Nonspecific upper respiratory infections are probably the most common overall cause.

Symptoms and Signs

The symptoms and signs of ADE or PIE are related to the portion of the nervous system that is most severely damaged. Because any portion of the nervous system may be affected, it is not surprising that variable clinical syndromes may occur. In some cases, there are signs and symptoms of generalized involvement (ADE), but one or more portions of the neuraxis may suffer the brunt of the damage, resulting in various clear-cut clinical syndromes: meningeal, encephalitic, brainstem, cerebellar, spinal cord, or neuritic.

Symptoms of involvement of the meninges (headaches, neck stiffness) are common early in the course of all types. In some cases, no further symptoms are present. In others, these initial symptoms and signs may be followed by evidence of damage to the cerebrum. In this *encephalitic form*, there may be convulsions, stupor, coma, hemiplegia, aphasia, or other signs of focal cerebral involvement. Cranial nerve palsies, especially *optic neuritis*, or signs and symptoms of cerebellar dysfunction predominate in a few cases. *Acute cerebellar ataxia* constitutes about 50% of cases of PIE following varicella, whereas cerebral and spinal involvement are more common with measles and vaccinia.

Overall, spinal cord involvement is more common than involvement of either the brainstem or cerebellum. This may be disseminated in the cord or, more commonly, may take the form of an *acute transverse myelitis* or ATM, a syndrome of multiple causes. It may be acute, developing over hours to several days, or subacute, developing over 1 week to 2 weeks. The most common picture is a transverse myelitis interrupting both motor and sensory tracts at one level, usually thoracic. It usually begins with localized back or radicular pain followed by abrupt onset of bilateral paresthesia in the legs, an ascending sensory level, and a paraparesis that often progresses to paraplegia. Urinary bladder and bowel involvement occurs early and is prominent.

In general, patients with rapid progression and flaccidity below the level of the lesion have the worst prognosis. The syndrome may also take the form of an ascending myelitis, a diffuse or patchy myelitis, or a partial myelitis (Brown-Séquard syndrome, anterior spinal artery distribution lesion, posterior column myelopathy). Only about 25% to 33% of cases of ATM are caused by viral infections or vaccinations, via a demyelinating process. Less frequently, a complete transverse myelitis may result from direct virus invasion of the cord (e.g., poliovirus or herpesviruses). Other less frequent causes of ATM include systemic lupus erythematosus, other vasculitides, other causes of spinal cord infarction, multiple sclerosis, and trauma. Idiopathic ATM is most frequent. Obviously, it is important to exclude cord compression by epidural abscess or tumor, intrinsic cord bacterial or fungal infections, tumors, and treatable vascular diseases in making the differential diagnosis.

Other parainfectious syndromes may also be seen. Acute toxic encephalopathy and Reye syndrome are seen more frequently after varicella, influenza, and rubella. Peripheral nerve involvement with an acute ascending paralysis of the Guillain-Barré type is more frequent with rabies vaccine, especially with the older brain-derived preparations, and after influenza and upper respiratory infections. Brachial neuritis is the usual neurologic complication of antitetanus vaccine.

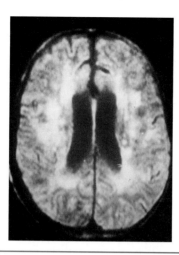

FIGURE 24.5. Postinfectious encephalitis. Proton-density MR image shows a lesion that began 2 weeks after a nonspecific upper respiratory tract infection. There is prominent diffuse cerebral white matter disease. (From Jubelt B, Ropka S. Infectious diseases of the nervous system. In: Rosenberg RN, ed., *Atlas of Clinical Neurology.* Philadelphia: Current Medicine, 1998:12.1–12.71; with permission.)

Laboratory Studies

The CSF pressure may be slightly elevated. There is a mild to moderate increase in white cells (15 cells/mm^3 to 250 cells/mm^3), with lymphocytes as the predominating cell type. The protein content is normal or slightly elevated (35 mg/dL to 150 mg/dL); the sugar content is normal. The CSF myelin basic protein level is usually increased. The EEG is abnormal in most patients, usually with slow frequency of 4 Hz to 6 Hz and high voltage. The abnormalities are usually generalized and symmetric, but focal or unilateral changes may be found. The abnormalities persist for several weeks after apparent clinical recovery. Persisting abnormalities correlate well with permanent neurologic damage or convulsive disorders. After several days, CT may show diffuse or scattered low-density lesions in the white matter, some of which may enhance with contrast. MRI usually reveals an increased signal intensity on T2-weighted images (Fig. 24.5).

Diagnosis

Because there is no specific diagnostic test, the diagnosis of PIE or postvaccinal encephalomyelitis should be considered when neurologic signs develop 4 days to 21 days following onset of acute exanthems, an upper respiratory tract infection, or after vaccination. The differential diagnosis includes practically all of the acute infectious diseases of the nervous system, particularly acute or subacute encephalitis, and acute diffuse multiple sclerosis.

Prognosis and Course

The mortality rate is high (10% to 30%) in patients with severe involvement of the cerebrum in measles or rubella, or after rabies vaccination with the old brain-derived vaccine. It is low in patients with acute cerebellar ataxia or involvement only of the peripheral nerves. Death may occur as a result of cerebral damage in the acute stage or following intercurrent infections, bed sores, or urinary sepsis in late stages. In patients who survive, the neurologic signs usually improve considerably, with about 90% having complete recovery. The exception is measles, in which sequelae may occur in 20% to 50% of patients. Sequelae include seizures, mental syndromes, and hemiparesis. Delayed postencephalitic sequelae, such as parkinsonism, do not occur; as a rule, there are no new symptoms after recovery from an acute attack.

Treatment

The administration of ACTH or high-dose intravenous corticosteroids reduces and sometimes reverses the severity of the neurologic defects. Several reports suggest that some patients who fail steroid treatment may respond to either IV Ig or plasmapheresis.

CHRONIC VIRAL INFECTIONS

Chronic or slow viral infections that result in chronic neurologic disease are caused by both conventional viruses and the unconventional transmissible spongiform encephalopathy agents. However, the transmissible spongiform encephalopathy agents, or prions, as presently understood, are not true viruses (see Chapter 34).

Conventional agents cause chronic inflammatory or demyelinating disease; in humans, these include subacute sclerosing panencephalitis (SSPE), progressive rubella panencephalitis (PRP), progressive multifocal leukoencephalopathy (PML), human T-cell lymphotropic virus (HTLV)-associated myelopathy (HAM)/tropical spastic paraparesis (TSP), and AIDS.

In SSPE, a chronic inflammatory disease is caused by a defect in the production of measles virus, that results in a cell-associated infection. With PRP, both inflammation and demyelination may be seen. The pathogenic mechanisms have not yet been defined, but the virus does not appear to be defective. PML is a noninflammatory demyelinating disease that occurs in immunocompromised hosts; it is caused by an opportunistic papovavirus infection. HAM/TSP is an inflammatory demyelinating disease caused by HTLV, a retrovirus. AIDS is reviewed in Chapter 25. Other conventional viruses (enteroviruses, HSV, VZV, CMV, measles virus, adenovirus) may cause chronic opportunistic infections in immunocompromised patients.

Subacute Sclerosing Panencephalitis

SSPE (Dawson disease or subacute inclusion body encephalitis) is a disease caused by a defective measles virus. It is characterized by progressive dementia, incoordination, ataxia, myoclonic jerks, and other focal neurologic signs. First described by Dawson in 1933 and 1934 as "subacute inclusion encephalitis," it was thought to be of viral origin because of the presence of type A intranuclear inclusions. Numerous cases have since been reported, but recovery of a viral agent was not possible until the advent of specialized techniques of viral isolation by co-cultivation of brain cells with extraneural cells capable of replicating fully infectious virus. The cases reported by Pette and Doring in 1939 as "nodular panencephalitis" and by Van Bogaert in 1945 as "subacute sclerosing leukoencephalitis" appear to be the same disease. The name of this disease reflects a combination of the three terms.

Pathology

In severe, long-standing cases, the brain may feel unduly hard. A perivascular infiltration occurs in the cortex and white matter with plasma and other mononuclear cells. Patchy areas of demyelination and gliosis occur in the white matter and deeper layers of the cortex. The neurons of the cortex, basal ganglia, pons, and inferior olives show degenerative changes. Intranuclear and intracytoplasmic eosinophilic inclusion bodies are found in neurons and glial cells. When examined with the electron microscope, these inclusions are seen to be composed of hollow tubules similar to the nucleocapsids of paramyxoviruses. Fluorescent antibody staining of inclusions shows that they are positive for measles virus.

Incidence

Children younger than 12 years are predominantly affected, although a few cases occur in adults. Boys are more often affected than girls, and more cases have occurred in rural than in urban settings. The incidence of SSPE has decreased markedly in the United States since the introduction of the live-attenuated measles vaccine. After natural measles infection, the incidence of SSPE is 5 cases to 10 cases per 1 million clinical measles infections. After vaccine, the rate is less than 1 case per 1 million vaccine recipients. Only about a half-dozen cases now occur annually in the United States.

Symptoms

SSPE has a gradual onset without fever. Forgetfulness, inability to keep up with schoolwork, and restlessness are common early symptoms. These are followed in the course of weeks or months by incoordination, ataxia, myoclonic jerks of the trunk and limbs (often noise-induced), apraxia, and loss of speech; seizures and dystonic posturing may occur. Vision and hearing are preserved until the terminal stage, in which there is a rigid quadriplegia simulating complete decortication.

Laboratory Data and Diagnosis

Elevated levels of measles antibody may be found in serum and CSF. The CSF is under normal pressure, and the cell count is normal or, rarely, only slightly increased. The protein content is normal, but a striking increase in the CSF immunoglobulin content is found, even in an otherwise normal fluid. Oligoclonal IgG bands, representing measles virus-specific antibodies, may be demonstrated by agarose electrophoresis of CSF. CSF PCR genomic amplification has only been used in a few cases and was positive. The EEG often shows a widespread abnormality of the cortical activity, with a "burst suppression" pattern of high-amplitude slow-wave (or spike and slow-wave) complexes occurring at a rate of every 4 seconds to 20 seconds, either synchronous with or independent of the myoclonic jerks. CT may show cortical atrophy and focal or multifocal low-density lesions of the white matter. MRI may reveal periventricular white-matter changes on T2-weighted images.

Pathogenesis

A defect in measles virus production seems to occur because the viral M (membrane) protein may not be found in the brain tissue of affected patients. The M protein is necessary for alignment of nucleocapsids under viral proteins in the cell membrane so that budding of virus may take place. Thus, in SSPE there is no budding and no release of extracellular virus. There is accumulation of measles virus nucleocapsids within cells (cell-associated infection), and virus spread occurs by cell fusion. Brain cells may be incapable of synthesizing the M protein, or selective antibody pressure might cause a restricted cell-associated infection, because more than 50% of patients with SSPE have had an acute measles infection before reaching 2 years of age, when maternal antibody may still have been present.

Course, Prognosis, and Treatment

The course is prolonged, usually lasting several years. Both rapidly progressive disease, leading to death in several months, and protracted disease lasting more than 10 years, have occurred. Spontaneous long-term improvement or stabilization occurs in about 10% of patients. Intraventricular interferon alfa with intravenous or intraventricular ribavirin has resulted in clinical improvement or stopped progression in some cases. No controlled studies have been performed.

Progressive Rubella Panencephalitis

Rubella virus, like measles virus, has been recognized to cause slowly progressive rubella panencephalitis. This is a rare disease of children and young adults. Fewer than two dozen cases have been reported. Most cases have occurred in patients with the congenital rubella syndrome, but several cases have appeared following postnatally acquired rubella. None have been ascribed to rubella vaccine.

Pathology and Pathogenesis

There does not appear to be a defect in rubella virus production, as occurs in SSPE. Unlike measles virus, rubella virus does not have an M protein. Because of the recognition that immune complexes are in the serum and CSF, it is thought that immune complex deposition in vascular endothelium results in vasculitis.

The pathologic condition is characterized by inflammation and demyelination. The inflammation consists of lymphocytic and plasma cell infiltration of the meninges and perivascular spaces of the gray and white matter. Extensive demyelination with atrophy and gliosis of the white matter is usually seen, together with vasculitis involving arterioles with fibrinoid degeneration and mineral deposition. Arterioles may be thrombosed, and there are adjacent microinfarcts. IgG deposits have been demonstrated in vessels.

Symptoms and Signs

PRP usually occurs in the second decade of life, beginning with dementia similar to that of SSPE. Cerebellar ataxia, however, is more prominent. Gait ataxia is initially seen, but the arms subsequently become involved. Later, pyramidal tract involvement is seen. Optic atrophy and retinopathy similar to those seen in congenital rubella occur. Seizures and myoclonus are not prominent. Symptoms and signs suggestive of infection (headache, fever, nuchal rigidity) are not seen.

Laboratory Data

Routine blood tests are normal. The EEG reveals diffuse slowing; periodicity is rare. CT may demonstrate ventricular enlargement, that is most prominent in the fourth ventricle and cisterna magna because of cerebellar atrophy. The CSF is under normal pressure. There is usually a lymphocytic pleocytosis with up to 40 cells/mm^3, but the fluid is occasionally acellular. The protein is increased in the range of 60 mg/dL to 150 mg/dL, with the IgG fraction being up to 50% of this. Most of the IgG is composed of oligoclonal bands directed against rubella virus. Conventional

serologic techniques demonstrate elevated serum and CSF antibody titers against rubella virus. Recovery of the virus is difficult and requires co-cultivation.

Diagnosis and Treatment

The diagnosis may easily be made in a patient with the congenital rubella syndrome. In postnatally acquired cases, SSPE is the other major diagnostic consideration. Other dementing illnesses of childhood should be considered; however, the combined data of the clinical picture (especially when ataxia ensues), the CSF findings, and serology should be diagnostic. The course is protracted over 8 years to 10 years. There is no specific treatment.

RETROVIRUS INFECTIONS

HIV Infection

See Chapter 25.

HTLV-associated Myelopathy/ Tropical Spastic Paraparesis

Etiology

HTLV is a retrovirus that causes adult T-cell leukemia and a chronic progressive myelopathy (for hereditary and acquired spastic paraplegia see Chapter 118). Chronic HAM has been referred to as TSP in tropical areas, hence the abbreviation HAM/TSP. Of the two serotypes of HTLV, more cases of HAM/TSP are caused by HTLV-I.

Pathology and Pathogenesis

Patients have a mild chronic meningoencephalomyelitis with mononuclear infiltrates of the meninges and perivascular cuffing primarily in the spinal cord. In addition, there are proliferation of smaller parenchymal vessels, thickening of the meninges, and a reactive astrocytic gliosis. A second prominent feature is demyelination in the pyramidal tracts and posterior columns.

Like HIV, HTLV apparently enters the CNS via infected peripheral blood mononuclear cells, thereby causing secondary infection of glial cells. Demyelination may be caused by an immune-mediated cytotoxic T cells or antibody response rather than by direct infection with HTLV.

Epidemiology

TSP occurs in tropical islands (including the Caribbean), as well as in tropical areas of the United States, Central and South America, India, and Africa. The prevalence is quite variable, ranging from 12 cases to 128 cases per 100,000 population. HAM is found on the southwestern and northern islands of Japan; the prevalence is not known. The temporal behavior of HAM/TSP reflects an endemic myelopathy. Most cases occur after age 30 years, but childhood cases have been reported. There is a female preponderance.

More cases of HAM/TSP are being recognized throughout the United States, in both immigrants and native residents. As in HIV infection, exposure is related to intravenous drug use, sexual transmission, and blood transfusions.

Symptoms and Signs

Onset is usually gradual, with weakness of one leg followed in several months by weakness of the other leg. Other complaints include numbness and dysesthesia, bladder dysfunction, and impotence. Infrequently, more abrupt onset may occur. Examination reveals spastic paraparesis with overactive tendon reflexes (legs more than arms) and Babinski signs. Posterior column dysfunction is common, and hypesthesia is often noted diffusely below the midthoracic level. Less frequently, a distinct sensory level or peripheral neuropathy (25%) is found. Cerebral involvement caused by white matter disease and made evident by encephalopathy and seizures has been described in several patients. Neurogenic muscular atrophy and polymyositis occur rarely.

Laboratory Studies

CSF examination may be entirely normal, but a mild lymphocytic pleocytosis may be seen. About 50% of patients have an elevated CSF protein content in the 50-mg/dL to 90-mg/dL range. Increased CSF IgG levels and oligoclonal bands are found in most patients. Antibodies to HTLV are increased in both serum and CSF. The ratio of helper to suppressor T cells is increased. MRI may show white matter lesions in the brain, even in asymptomatic patients. High T2 signals may also be seen in the spinal cord.

Diagnosis

Diagnosis depends on the appropriate clinical and CSF manifestations and a positive antibody response in the serum and CSF. PCR amplification methodology is becoming commercially available. The differential diagnosis includes other causes of spastic paraparesis, including multiple sclerosis (see Chapters 118 and 134).

Course, Prognosis, and Treatment

Most patients progress slowly, over months to a few years, and may stabilize. Responses to corticosteroids and danazol have been reported in uncontrolled studies. In a recent double-blind, controlled trial, two-thirds of patients reported benefit from interferon alfa.

Progressive Multifocal Leukoencephalopathy

Progressive multifocal leukoencephalopathy (PML) is a rare subacute demyelinating disease caused by an opportunistic papovavirus. The disease occurs in patients with defective cell-mediated immunity. Cases have occurred primarily in patients with reticuloendothelial diseases, such as Hodgkin disease, other lymphomas, and leukemia before the AIDS epidemic. Cases have also occurred in patients with carcinoma or sarcoidosis and in those immunosuppressed therapeutically. In most of these disorders, PML is a rare complication; it occurs in 2% to 5% of AIDS patients. A few cases have occurred in the apparent absence of an underlying disease.

Pathology

The condition is characterized by the presence of multiple, partly confluent areas of demyelination in various parts of the nervous system, accompanied at times by a mild degree of perivascular infiltration. These multifocal areas of demyelination are most prominent in the subcortical white matter, whereas involvement of cerebellar, brainstem, or spinal cord white matter is less common. As the disease progresses, the demyelinated areas coalesce to form large lesions. Hyperplasia of astrocytes into bizarre giant forms that may resemble neoplastic cells is found. There is loss of oligodendroglia with relative sparing of axons in the lesions. Neurons are not infected. Eosinophilic intranuclear inclusions are seen in oligodendroglial cells at the periphery of the lesions. Electron microscopic studies have shown that these inclusions are composed of papovavirus particles (Fig. 24.6).

It is presumed that the demyelination is caused by destruction of oligodendroglia by the virus. Most cases have been caused by the JC strain and possibly several by the SV-40 strain. Isolation of these agents requires special techniques of co-cultivating brain cultures from patients with permissive cell lines; human fetal brain tissue could also be used to induce virus replication.

Symptoms and Signs

The clinical manifestations are diverse and are related to the location and number of lesions. Onset is subacute to chronic with focal or multifocal signs (hemiplegia, sensory abnormalities, field cuts, and other focal signs of lesions in the cerebral hemispheres). Cranial nerve palsies, ataxia, and spinal cord involvement are less common. As the number of lesions increases, dementia ensues.

Laboratory Data and Diagnosis

A definite diagnosis of PML may be made by pathologic investigation (brain biopsy). However, PCR amplification of JC virus RNA in the CSF usually obviates biopsy. The

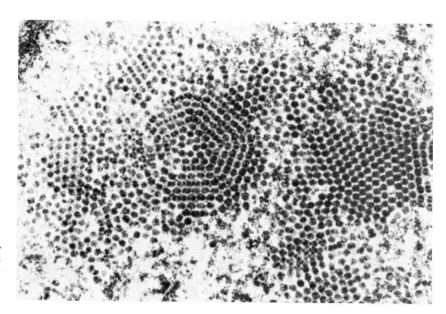

FIGURE 24.6. Progressive multifocal leukoencephalopathy. Papovavirus-like particles are present in a glial nucleus (×65,000). (Courtesy of Dr. G. M. Zu Rhein.)

CSF is usually normal. The EEG often demonstrates nonspecific diffuse or focal slowing. CT reveals nonenhancing multiple lucencies in the white matter. MRI may demonstrate additional white matter abnormalities (Fig. 24.7).

Serology is not helpful to the diagnosis because most people have been exposed to the JC strain in the first two decades of their lives. A presumptive diagnosis may be made on the basis of the clinical presentation and the appropriate CT findings in an immune-compromised patient.

Pathogenesis

Apparently, the virus is latent in the kidney and in B lymphocytes and enters the CNS in activated B lymphocytes. Once virus enters the brain, glial cells (astrocytes and oligodendroglia) support virus replication because viral transcription factors are selectively expressed in these cells.

Course, Prognosis, and Treatment

The course usually lasts months with 80% of patients dying within 9 months. Rarely, the course may last several years, with the longest verified course recorded at 6 years. In most patients with AIDS, the inflammatory response has been prominent and the course longer than that noted with other underlying disease. If possible, treatment should include an attempt to improve immune function. There is no specific treatment. Spontaneous improvement has been reported.

Encephalitis Lethargica

Encephalitis lethargica (sleeping sickness, von Economo disease) is a disease of unknown cause that occurred in epidemic form from 1917 to 1928. Clinically, the disease was characterized by signs and symptoms of diffuse involvement of the brain and the development of various sequelae in a large percentage of recovered patients. Although the disease spread rapidly over the entire world, the epidemic form is apparently extinct. It may now occur as very rare, isolated cases. Encephalitis lethargica affected patients of all ages and both sexes equally, including people of all races and occupations.

Etiology

The etiology of encephalitis lethargica is unknown. It is presumed that the disease was caused by a virus, but proof is lacking. Because of the concurrence of encephalitis lethargica and the pandemic of influenza beginning in 1918, there has been speculation about a common etiology; this has not been resolved but is probably unlikely.

Pathology and Pathogenesis

The pathologic lesions in the subacute stages were similar to those of other encephalitides, with inflammation in the meninges, around blood vessels, and in the parenchyma (both gray and white matter) of the brain and spinal cord. Acute degenerative changes of neurons also occurred.

Symptoms and Signs

The symptoms and signs were usually of acute or subacute onset. Fever was usually present at the outset and was usually mild. In fatal cases, a rise to 107°F (41.7°C) or higher, in the terminal stages, occurred often. Headache and lethargy were common early symptoms. Disorders of eye movements were present in about 75% of patients. An acute organic psychosis was not uncommon. The most frequent motor symptoms were all categories of basal ganglia disease.

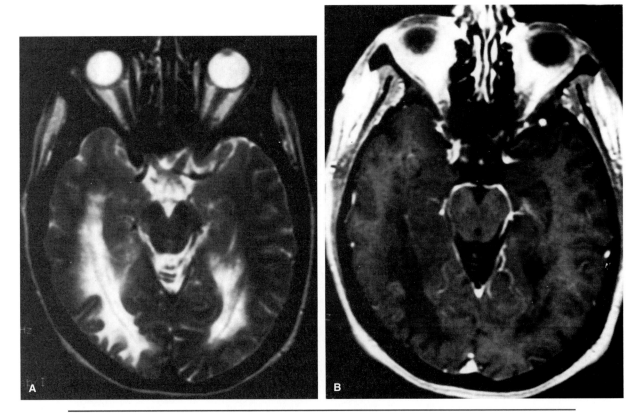

FIGURE 24.7. Progressive multifocal leukoencephalopathy. A: T2-weighted, spin-echo, axial MR image shows increased signal intensity of the temporooccipital white matter that is greater on the right than the left. Relative cortical sparing is seen. **B:** T1-weighted, gradient-echo, axial MR image after gadolinium administration shows decreased signal intensity in the same areas, with no evidence of abnormal enhancement. Note the normal enhancement of both internal carotid arteries and posterior cerebral arteries on the gradient-echo enhanced images. (Courtesy of Dr. S. Chan, Columbia University College of Physicians and Surgeons, New York, NY)

Laboratory Studies and Diagnosis

Pertinent laboratory studies showed a lymphocytic pleocytosis in the CSF and an elevated CSF protein in about 50% of patients.

The diagnosis of encephalitis lethargica may be justified in any patient with signs and symptoms of encephalitis, along with special features of disturbed sleep rhythm and diplopia in the acute stage, and the development of signs of injury of the basal ganglia at that time or in subsequent years.

Course and Complications

The duration of the acute stage was about 4 weeks and merged gradually into the so-called postencephalitic phase of the disease. The mortality rate was about 25% and was highest among infants and elderly persons.

The frequency of sequelae is unknown. In some instances, symptoms were merely a continuation of those present in the acute stage. In others, the symptoms developed after an interval of several months or many years, during which the patient was apparently well. The parkinsonian syndrome that develops after encephalitis lethargica may often be distinguished from idiopathic parkinsonism because of an early age of onset and unusual features, such as grimaces, torticollis, torsion spasms, myoclonus, oculogyric crises, facial and respiratory tics, and bizarre postures and gaits. Behavior disorders and emotional instability without evidence of intellectual impairment were common sequelae in children.

SUGGESTED READINGS

General

Evans AS, Kaslow RA, eds. *Viral Infections of Humans,* 4th ed. New York: Plenum Publishing, 1997.

Fields BN, Knipe PM, Howley PM, Griffin DE, eds. *Virology,* 4th ed. Philadelphia: Lippincott-Raven Publishers, 2001.

Johnson RT. *Viral Infections of the Nervous System,* 2nd ed. New York: Lippincott-Raven Publishers, 1998.

Koskiniemi M, Korppi M, Mustonen K, et al. Epidemiology of encephalitis in children: a prospective multicentre study. *Eur J Pediatr* 1997;156:541–545.

Koskiniemi M, Rautonen J, Lehtokoski-Lehtiniemi E, Vaheri A. Epidemiology of encephalitis in children: a 20-year survey. *Ann Neurol* 1991;29:429–497.

Lennette EH, Lennette DA, Lennette ET, eds. *Diagnostic Procedures for Viral, Rickettsial and Chlamydial Infections*, 7th ed. Washington, DC: American Public Health Association, 1995.

McKendall RR, Stroop WC, eds. *Handbook of Neurovirology*. New York: Marcel Dekker, 1994.

Nathanson N, ed. *Viral Pathogenesis*. Philadelphia: Lippincott-Raven Publishers, 1997.

Nath A, Berger JR, eds. *Clinical Neurovirology*. New York: Marcel Dekker, Inc., 2003.

Roos, KL. Encephalitis. *Neurol Clinics* 1999;17:813–833.

Scheld WM, Whitley RJ, Durack DT, eds. *Infections of the Central Nervous System*, 2nd ed. Philadelphia: Lippincott-Raven Publishers, 1997.

Thomson Jr, RB, Bertram H. Laboratory diagnosis of central nervous system infections. *Infect Dis Clinics N America* 2001;15:1047–1071.

Tyler KL, Martin JB, eds. *Infectious Diseases of the Central Nervous System*. Philadelphia: FA Davis Co, 1993.

Vinken PJ, Bruyn GW, Klawans HL, McKendall RR, eds. *Viral Disease. Handbook of Clinical Neurology*, vol 56. New York: Elsevier Science, 1989.

Enterovirus (Picornavirus) Infections

Baker RC, Kummer AW, Schultz JR, Ho M, Gonzalez del Rey J. Neurodevelopmental outcome of infants with viral meningitis in the first three months of life. *Clin Pediatr (Phila)* 1996;35:295–301.

Berlin LE, Rorabaugh ML, Heldrich F, et al. Aseptic meningitis in infants less than 2 years of age: diagnosis and etiology. *J Infect Dis* 1993;168:888–892.

Ropka SL, Jubelt B. Enteroviruses. In: Nath A, Berger JR, eds. *Clinical Neurovirology*. New York: Marcel Dekker, Inc., 2003:359–377.

Sawyer MH, Holland D, Aintablian N. Diagnosis of enteroviral central nervous system infection by polymerase chain reaction during a large community outbreak. *Pediatr Infect Dis J* 1994;13:177–182.

Poliomyelitis

Centers for Disease Control and Prevention. Poliomyelitis prevention in the United States: updated recommendations of the Advisory Committee on Immunization Practices. *MMWR* 2000;(Suppl RR5):1–22.

Centers for Disease Control and Prevention. Global polio eradication initiative: strategic plan 2004. *MMWR* 2004;53:107–108.

Davis LE, Bodian D, Price D, et al. Chronic progressive poliomyelitis secondary to vaccination of an immunodeficient child. *N Engl J Med* 1977;297:241–245.

Jubelt B, Drucker JS. Poliomyelitis and the postpolio syndrome. In: Younger DS, ed. *The Motor Disorders Textbook*. Philadelphia: Lippincott-Raven Publishers, 1998:381–395.

Kornreich L, Dagan O, Grunebaum M. MRI in acute poliomyelitis. *Neuroradiology* 1996;38:371–372.

Patriarca PA, Sutter RW, Oostvogel PM. Outbreaks of paralytic poliomyelitis, 1976–1995. *J Infect Dis* 1997;175[Suppl 1]:S165–S172.

Price RW, Plum F. Poliomyelitis. In: Vinken PJ, Bruyn GW, Klawans HL, eds. *Infections of the Nervous System. Handbook of Clinical Neurology*, vol 34. New York: Elsevier/North-Holland, 1978:93–132.

Wyatt HV. Poliomyelitis in hypogammaglobulinemics. *J Infect Dis* 1972;128:802–806.

Coxsackievirus Infections

Cree BC, Bernardini GL, Hays AP, Lowe G. A fatal case of coxsackievirus B4 meningoencephalitis. *Arch Neurology* 2003;60:107–112.

Farmer K, MacArthur BA, Clay MM. A follow-up study of 15 cases of neonatal meningoencephalitis due to coxsackie virus B5. *J Pediatr* 1975;87:568–571.

Kaplan MH, Klein SW, McPhee J, Harper RG. Group B coxsackievirus infections in infants younger than three months of age: a serious illness. *Rev Infect Dis* 1983;5:1019–1032.

Medlin JF, Dagan R, Berlin LE, et al. Focal encephalitis with enterovirus infections. *Pediatrics* 1991;88:841–845.

Echovirus Infections

McKinney RE, Katz SL, Wilfert CM. Chronic enteroviral meningoencephalitis in agammaglobulinemic patients. *Rev Infect Dis* 1987;9:334–356.

Modlin JF. Perinatal echovirus infection: insights from a literature review of 61 cases of serious infection and 16 outbreaks in nurseries. *Rev Infect Dis* 1986;8:918–926.

Centers for Disease Control and Prevention. Outbreaks of aseptic meningitis associated with echoviruses 9 and 30 and preliminary surveillance reports on enterovirus activity—United States, 2003. *MMWR* 2003;52:761–764.

Enteroviruses 70 and 71 Infections

Hayward JC, Gillespie SM, Kaplan KM, et al. Outbreak of poliomyelitis-like paralysis associated with enterovirus 71. *Pediatr Infect Dis J* 1989;8:611–616.

Huang C-C, Liu C-C, Chang Y-C et al. Neurologic complications in children with enterovirus 71 infection. *N Engl J Med* 1999;341:936–942.

Nolan MA, Craig ME, Lahra MM et al. Survival after pulmonary edema due to enterovirus 71 encephalitis. *Neurology* 2003;60:1651–1656.

Vejjajiva A. Acute hemorrhagic conjunctivitis with nervous system complications. In: Vinken PJ, Bruyn GW, Klawans HL, McKendall RR, eds. *Viral Disease. Handbook of Clinical Neurology*, vol 56. New York: Elsevier Science, 1989:349–354.

Arbovirus Infections

Aguilar MJ, Calanchini PR, Finley KH. Perinatal arbovirus encephalitis and its sequelae. *Res Publ Assoc Nerv Ment Dis* 1968;44:216–235.

Booss J, Karabatsos N. Arthropod-borne virus encephalitis. In: Nath A, Berger JR, eds. *Clinical Neurovirology*. New York: Marcel Dekker, Inc., 2003:327–357.

Centers for Disease Control and Prevention. Arboviral infections of the central nervous system—United States, 1996–1997. *MMWR* 1998;47:517–522.

Lowry PW. Arbovirus encephalitis in the United States and Asia. *J Lab Clin Med* 1997;129:405–411.

Equine Encephalitides

Deresiewicz RL, Thaler SJ, Hsu L, Zamani AA. Clinical and neuroradiographic manifestations of eastern equine encephalitis. *N Engl J Med* 1997;336:1867–1874.

Earnest MP, Goolishian HA, Calverley JR, et al. Neurologic, intellectual, and psychologic sequelae following western encephalitis. *Neurology* 1971;21:969–974.

Ehrenkranz NJ, Ventura AK. Venezuelan equine encephalitis virus infection in man. *Annu Rev Med* 1974;25:9–14.

Przelomski MM, O'Rourke E, Grady GF, et al. Eastern equine encephalitis in Massachusetts: a report of 16 cases: 1970–1984. *Neurology* 1988;38:736–739.

Rozdilsky B, Robertson HE, Charney J. Western encephalitis: report of eight fatal cases, Saskatchewan epidemic, 1965. *Can Med Assoc J* 1968;98:79–86.

St. Louis Encephalitis

Jones SC, Morris J, Hill G, Alderman M, Ratard RC. St. Louis encephalitis outbreak in Louisiana in 2001. *J Louisiana State Med Soc* 2002;154:303–306.

Marfin AA, Bleed DM, Lofgren JP, et al. Epidemiologic aspects of a St. Louis encephalitis epidemic in Jefferson County, Arkansas, 1991. *Am J Trop Med Hyg* 1993;49:30–37.

Monath TP, Tsai TF. St. Louis encephalitis: lessons from the last decade. *Am J Trop Med Hyg* 1987;37[Suppl]:S40–S59.

Waysay M, Diaz-Arrastia R, Suss RA, Kojan S, Haq A, et al. St. Louis encephalitis: a review of 11 cases in a 1995 Dallas, Tex, epidemic. *Arch Neurol* 2000;57:114–118.

West Nile Virus Encephalitis

Agamanolis DP, Leslie MJ, Caveny EA, et al. Neuropathological findings in West Nile virus encephalitis: a case report. *Ann Neurol* 2003;54:547–551.

Jeha LE, Sila CA, Lederman RJ, et al. West Nile virus infection: a new acute paralytic illness. *Neurology* 2003;61:55–59.

Johnson RT, Cornblath DR. Poliomyelitis and flaviviruses. *Ann Neurol* 2003;53:691–692.

Johnson RT, Irani DN. West Nile encephalitis in the United States. *Curr Neurol Neurosci Rep* 2002;2:496–500.

Kleinschmidt-DeMasters BK, Marder BA, Levi ME, et al. Naturally acquired West Nile virus encephalomyelitis in transplant recipients: clinical, laboratory, diagnostic, and neuropathological features. *Arch Neural* 2004;61(8):1210–1220.

Li J, Loeb JA, Shy ME, et al. Asymmetric flaccid paralysis: a neuromuscular presentation of West Nile virus infection. *Ann Neurol* 2003;53:703–710.

Nash D, Mostashari F, Fine A, et al. The outbreak of West Nile virus infection in the New York City area in 1999. *N Engl J Med* 2001;344:1807–1814.

Sejvar JJ, Haddad MB, Tierney BC, et al. Neurologic manifestations and outcome of West Nile virus infection. *JAMA* 2003;290:511–515.

Tyler KL. West Nile virus infection in the United States. *Arch Neurol* 2004;61:1190–1195.

Japanese Encephalitis

Centers for Disease Control and Prevention. Inactivated Japanese encephalitis virus vaccine. Recommendations of the Advisory Committee on Immunization Practices. *MMWR* 1993;42(RR-1):1–15.

Kalita J, Misra UK, Pandey S, Khole TN. A comparison of clinical and radiological findings in adults and children with Japanese encephalitis. *Arch Neurol* 2003;61:1760–1764.

Kumar S, Misra UK, Kalita J, et al. MRI in Japanese encephalitis. *Neuroradiology* 1997;39:180–184.

Murgod UA, Muthane UB, Ravi V, Radhesh S, Desai A. Persistent movement disorders following Japanese encephalitis. *Neurology* 2001;57:2313–2315.

Richter RW, Shimpjyo S. Neurologic sequelae of Japanese B encephalitis. *Neurology* 1961;11:553–559.

Solomon T, Dung NM, Kneen R, et al. Seizures and raised intracranial pressure in Vietnamese patients with Japanese encephalitis. *Brain* 2002;125:1084–1093.

Solomon T, Kneen R, Dung NM, et al. Poliomyelitis-like illness due to Japanese encephalitis virus. *Lancet* 1998;351:1094–1097.

California (La Crosse) Encephalitis

Centers for Disease Control. La Crosse encephalitis in West Virginia. *MMWR* 1988;37:79–82.

Chun RWM, Thompson WH, Grabow JD, Mathews CG. California arbovirus encephalitis in children. *Neurology* 1968;18:369–375.

Clark GG, Pretula HL, Langkop CW, Martin RJ, Calisher CH. Occurrence of La Crosse (California serogroup) encephalitis viral infections in Illinois. *Am J Trop Med Hyg* 1983;32:838–843.

Demikhov VG, Chaitsev VG, Butenko AM, et al. California serogroup virus infections in the Ryazan region of the USSR. *Am J Trop Med Hyg* 1991;45:371–376.

Eldridge BF, Glaser C, Pedrin RE, Chiles RE. The first reported case of California encephalitis in more than 50 years. *Emerg Infect Dis* 2001;7:451–452.

McJunkin JE, De Los Reyes EC, Irazuzta JE, et al. La Crosse encephalitis in children. *N Engl J Med* 2001;344:801–807.

Other Arbovirus Encephalitides

Bennett NM. Murray Valley encephalitis, 1974: clinical features. *Med J Aust* 1976;2:446–450.

Centers for Disease Control and Prevention. Outbreak of Powassan encephalitis—Maine and Vermont, 1999–2001. *MMWR* 2001;50:761–764.

Embil JA, Camfield P, Artsob H, Chase DP. Powassan virus encephalitis resembling herpes simplex encephalitis. *Arch Intern Med* 1983;143:341–343.

Goodpasture HC, Poland JD, Francy DB, et al. Colorado tick fever: clinical, epidemiologic, and laboratory aspects of 228 cases in Colorado in 1973–1974. *Ann Intern Med* 1978;88:303–310.

Meegen JM, Niklasson B, Bengtsson E. Spread of Rift Valley fever virus from continental Africa. *Lancet* 1979;2:1184–1185.

Schellinger, PD, Schmutzhard E, Fiebach JB, et al. Poliomyelitic-like illness in Central European encephalitis. *Neurology* 2000;55:299–302.

Rubella

Centers for Disease Control and Prevention. Rubella and congenital rubella syndrome—United States, 1994–1997. *MMWR* 1997;46:350–354.

Desmond MM, Wilson GS, Melnick JL, et al. Congenital rubella encephalitis. *J Pediatr* 1967;71:311–331.

Miller E, Cradock-Watson JE, Pollock TM. Consequence of confirmed maternal rubella at successive stages of pregnancy. *Lancet* 1982;2:781–784.

Numazaki K, Fujikawa T. Intracranial calcification with congenital rubella syndrome in a mother with serologic immunity. *J Child Neurol* 2003;18:296–297.

Waxham NR, Wolinsky JS. Rubella virus and its effects on the central nervous system. *Neurol Clin* 1984;2:367–385.

Mumps, Meningitis, and Encephalomyelitis

Black S, Shinefield H, Ray P, et al. Risk of hospitalization because of aseptic meningitis after measles-mumps-rubella vaccination in one- to two-year-old children: an analysis of the Vaccine Safety Datalink (VSD) Project. *Pediatr Infect Dis J* 1997;16:500–503.

Koyama S, Morita K, Yamaguchi S, et al. An adult case of mumps brain stem encephalitis. *Intern Med* 2000;39:499–502.

Johnstone JA, Ross CAC, Dunn M. Meningitis and encephalitis associated with mumps infection: a 10-year study. *Arch Dis Child* 1972;47:647–651.

Jubelt B. Enterovirus and mumps virus infections of the nervous system. *Neurol Clin* 1984;2:187–213.

Koskiniemi M, Donner M, Pettay O. Clinical appearance and outcome in mumps encephalitis in children. *Acta Paediatr Scand* 1983;72:603–609.

Levitt LP, Rich RA, Kinde SW, et al. Central nervous system mumps: a review of 64 cases. *Neurology* 1970;20:829–834.

Thompson JA. Mumps: a cause of acquired aqueductal stenosis. *J Pediatr* 1979;94:923–924.

Subacute Measles Encephalitis

Croxson MC, Anderson NE, Vaughan AA, et al. Subacute measles encephalitis in an immunocompetent adult. *J Clin Neurosci* 2002;9:600–604.

Gazzola P, Cocito L, Capello E, et al. Subacute measles encephalitis in a young man immunosuppressed for ankylosing spondylitis. *Neurology* 1999;52:1074–1077.

Hughes I, Jenney MEM, Newton RW, et al. Measles encephalitis during immunosuppressive treatment for acute lymphoblastic leukaemia. *Arch Dis Child* 1993;68:775–778.

Mustafa MM, Weitman SD, Winick NJ, et al. Subacute measles encephalitis in the young immunocompromised host: report of two cases diagnosed by polymerase chain reaction and treated with ribavirin, and review of the literature. *Clin Infect Dis* 1993;16:654–660.

Rabies

Baer GM, Shaddock JH, Houff SA, et al. Human rabies transmitted by corneal transplant. *Arch Neurol* 1982;39:103–107.

Centers for Disease Control and Prevention. Human death associated with bat rabies—California, 2003. *MMWR* 2004;53:33–35.

Centers for Disease Control and Prevention. First human death associated with raccoon rabies–Virginia. *MMWR* 2003;52:1102–1103.

Chopra JS, Banerjee AK, Murthy JMK, Pal SR. Paralytic rabies: a clinicopathological study. *Brain* 1980;103:789–802.

Dupont JR, Earle KM. Human rabies encephalitis: a study of forty-nine fatal cases with a review of the literature. *Neurology* 1965;15:1023–1034.

Fishbein DB, Robinson LE. Rabies. *N Engl J Med* 1993;329:1632–1638.

Jackson AC, Warrell MJ, Rupprecht CE, et al. Management of rabies in humans. *Clin Infect Dis* 2003;36:60–63.

Mani J, Reddy BC, Borgohain R, et al. Magnetic resonance imaging in rabies. *Postgrad Med J* 2003;79:352–354.

Lymphocytic Choriomeningitis

Barton LL, Mets MB. Congenital lymphocytic choriomeningitis virus infection: decade of rediscovery. *Clin Infect Dis* 2001;33:370–374.

Biggar RJ, Woodall JP, Walter PD, Haughie GE. Lymphocytic choriomeningitis outbreak associated with pet hamsters: fifty-seven cases from New York State. *JAMA* 1975;232:494–500.

Chesney PJ, Katcher ML, Nelson DB, Horowitz SD. CSF eosinophilia and chronic lymphocytic choriomeningitis virus meningitis. *J Pediatr* 1979;94:750–752.

Lehmann-Grube F. Diseases of the nervous system caused by lymphocytic choriomeningitis virus and other arenaviruses. In: Vinken PJ, Bruyn GW, Klawans HL, McKendall RR, eds. *Viral Disease. Handbook of Clinical Neurology*, vol 56. New York: Elsevier Science, 1989:355–381.

Rousseau MC, Saron MF, Brouqui P, Bourgeade A. Lymphocytic choriomeningitis virus in southern France: four case reports and a review of the literature. *Eur J Epidemiol* 1997;13:817–823.

Adenovirus Infections

Anders KH, Park CS, Cornford ME, Vinters HV. Adenovirus encephalitis and widespread ependymitis in a child with AIDS. *Pediatr Neurosurg* 1990–1991;16:316–320.

Davis D, Henslee J, Markesbery WR. Fatal adenovirus meningoencephalitis in a bone marrow transplant patient. *Ann Neurol* 1988;23:385–389.

Kelsey SD. Adenovirus meningoencephalitis. *Pediatrics* 1978;61:291–293.

Roos R. Adenovirus. In: Vinken PJ, Bruyn GW, Klawans HL, McKendall RR, eds. *Viral Disease. Handbook of Clinical Neurology*, vol 56. New York: Elsevier Science, 1989:281–293.

Straussberg R, Harel L, Levy Y, Amir J. A syndrome of transient encephalopathy associated with adenovirus infection. *Pediatrics* 2001;107(5):E69.

Herpes Simplex Encephalitis

Britton CB, Mesa-Tejada R, Fenoglio CM, et al. A new complication of AIDS: thoracic myelitis caused by herpes simplex virus. *Neurology* 1985;35:1071–1074.

Cinque P, Cleator GM, Weber T, et al. The role of laboratory investigation in the diagnosis and management of patients with suspected herpes simplex encephalitis: a consensus report. The EU Concerted Action on Virus Meningitis and Encephalitis. *J Neurol Neurosurg Psychiatry* 1996;61:339–345.

Dennett C, Cleator GM, Klapper PE. HSV-1 and HSV-2 in herpes simplex encephalitis: a study of sixty-four cases in the United Kingdom. *J Med Virol* 1997;53:1–3.

Dix RD, Waitzman DM, Follansbee S, et al. Herpes simplex virus type 2 encephalitis in two homosexual men with persistent lymphadenopathy. *Ann Neurol* 1985;17:203–206.

McKendall RR. Herpes simplex. In: Vinken PJ, Bruyn GW, Klawans HL, McKendall RR, eds. *Viral Disease. Handbook of Clinical Neurology*, vol 56. New York: Elsevier Science, 1989:207–227.

Raschilas F, Wolff M, Delatour F, Chaffaut C, De Broucker T, et al. Outcome of and prognostic factors for herpes simplex encephalitis in adult patients: results of a multicenter study. *Clin Infect Dis* 2002;35:254–260.

Sage, JI, Weinstein MP, Miller DC. Chronic encephalitis possibly due to herpes simplex virus: two cases. *Neurology* 1985;35:1470–1472.

Schlageter N, Jubelt B, Vick NA. Herpes simplex encephalitis without CSF leukocytosis. *Arch Neurol* 1984;41:1007–1008.

Schroth G, Gawehn J, Thron A, et al. Early diagnosis of herpes simplex encephalitis by MRI. *Neurology* 1987;37:179–183.

Steiner I. Herpes simplex viruses. In: Nath A, Berger JR, eds. *Clin Neurovirology*. New York: Marcel Dekker, Inc., 2003:109–128.

De Tiege X, Heron B, Lebon P, Ponsot G, Rozenberg F. Limits of early diagnosis of herpes simplex encephalitis in children: a retrospective study of 38 cases. *Clin Infect Dis* 2003;36:1335–1339.

Whitley RJ, Cobbs CG, Alford CA Jr, et al. Diseases that mimic herpes simplex encephalitis: diagnosis, presentation, and outcome. *JAMA* 1989;262:234–239.

Herpes Zoster

Berrettini S, Bianchi MC, Segnini G, Sellari-Franceschini S, Bruschini P, Montanaro D. Herpes zoster oticus: correlations between clinical and MRI findings. *Eur Neurol* 1998;39:26–31.

deSilva SM, Mark AS, Gilden DH, et al. Zoster myelitis: improvement with antiviral therapy in two cases. *Neurology* 1996;47:929–931.

Eidelberg D, Sotrel A, Horoupian S, et al. Thrombotic cerebral vasculopathy associated with herpes zoster. *Ann Neurol* 1986;19:7–14.

Gnann Jr JW, Whitley RJ. Herpes zoster. *New Engl J Med* 2002;347:340–346.

Gilden DH. Varicella-zoster virus infections. In: Vinken PJ, Bruyn GW, Klawans HL, McKendall RR, eds. *Viral Disease. Handbook of Clinical Neurology*, vol 56. New York: Elsevier Science, 1989:229–247.

Gilden DH, Wright RR, Schneck SA, et al. Zoster sine herpete: a clinical variant. *Ann Neurol* 1994;35:530–533.

Hope-Simpson RE. The nature of herpes zoster: a long-term study and a new hypothesis. *Proc R Soc Med* 1965;58:9–20.

Jemsek J, Greenberg SB, Tabor L, et al. Herpes zoster-associated encephalitis: clinicopathologic report of 12 cases and review of the literature. *Medicine* 1983;62:81–97.

Johnson RW, Whitton TL. Management of herpes zoster (shingles) and post herpetic neuralgia. *Exp Op Pharmacother* 2004;5(3):551–559.

Jubelt B. Clinical trials report: valacyclovir and famiciclovir therapy for herpes zoster. *Curr Neurol* 2002;2:477–478.

Mulder RR, Lumish RM, Corsello GR. Myelopathy after herpes zoster. *Arch Neurol* 1983;40:445–446.

Pappagallo M, Haldey EJ. Pharmacological management of postherpetic neuralgia. *CNS Drugs* 2003;17:771–780.

Ryder JW, Croen K, Kleinschmidt-DeMasters BK, et al. Progressive encephalitis three months after resolution of cutaneous zoster in a patient with AIDS. *Ann Neurol* 1986;19:182–188.

Thomas JE, Howard FM Jr. Segmental zoster paresis: a disease profile. *Neurology* 1972;22:459–466.

Whitley RJ, Weiss H, Gnann JW Jr, et al. Acyclovir with and without prednisone for the treatment of herpes zoster: a randomized, placebo-controlled trail. The National Institute of Allergy and Infectious Diseases Collaborative Antiviral Study Group. *Ann Intern Med* 1996;125:376–383.

Cytomegalovirus Infection

Arribas JR, Storch GA, Clifford DB, Tselis AC. Cytomegalovirus encephalitis. *Ann Intern Med* 1996;125:577–587.

Cohen BA. Prognosis and response to therapy of cytomegalovirus encephalitis and meningomyelitis in AIDS. *Neurology* 1996;46:444–450.

Cohen BA, McArthur JC, Grohman S, et al. Neurologic prognosis of cytomegalovirus polyradiculomyelopathy in AIDS. *Neurology* 1993;43:493–499.

Miller RF, Lucas SB, HallCraggs MA, et al. Comparison of magnetic resonance imaging with neuropathological findings in the diagnosis of HIV- and CMV-associated CNS disease in AIDS. *J Neurol Neurosurg Psychiatry* 1997;62:346–351.

Modlin JF, Grant PE, Makar RS, Roberts DJ, Krishnamoorthy KS. Case 25-2003: a newborn boy with petechiae and thrombocytopenia. *New Engl J Med* 2003;349:691–700.

Perlman JM, Argyle C. Lethal cytomegalovirus infection in preterm infants: clinical, radiological, and neuropathological findings. *Ann Neurol* 1992;31:64–68.

Pierelli F, Tilia G, Damiani A, et al. Brainstem CMV encephalitis in AIDS: clinical case and MRI features. *Neurology* 1997;48:529–530.

Pomeroy C, Ribes JA. Cytomegalovirus. In: Nath A, Berger JR, eds. *Clinical Neurovirology* New York: Marcel Dekker, Inc., 2003:177–205.

Talpos D, Tien RD, Hesselink JR. Magnetic resonance imaging of AIDS-related polyradiculopathy. *Neurology* 1991;41:1995–1997.

Wildemann B, Haas J, Lynen N, et al. Diagnosis of cytomegalovirus encephalitis in patients with AIDS by quantitation of cytomegalovirus genomes in cells of cerebrospinal fluids. *Neurology* 1998;50:693–697.

Epstein-Barr Virus Infection

Bray PF, Culp KW, McFarlin DE, et al. Demyelinating disease after neurologically complicated primary Epstein-Barr virus infection. *Neurology* 1992;42:278–282.

Domachowske JB, Cunningham CK, Cummings DL, et al. Acute manifestations and neurologic sequelae of Epstein-Barr virus encephalitis in children. *Pediatr Infect Dis J* 1996;15:871–875.

Erzurum S, Kalavsky SM, Watanakanakorn C. Acute cerebellar ataxia and hearing loss as initial symptoms of infectious mononucleosis. *Arch Neurol* 1983;40:760–762.

Portegies P, Corssmit N. Epstein-Barr virus and the nervous system. *Curr Opin Neurol* 2000;13:301–304.

Russell J, Fisher M, Zivin JA, et al. Status epilepticus and Epstein-Barr virus encephalopathy. *Arch Neurol* 1985;42:789–792.

Silverstein A, Steinberg G, Nathanson M. Nervous system involvement in infectious mononucleosis: the heralding and/or major manifestation. *Arch Neurol* 1972;26:353–358.

Tselis A. Epstein-Barr virus and the nervous system. In: Nath A, Berger JR, eds. *Clinical Neurovirology* New York: Marcel Dekker, Inc. 2003:155–176.

Human Herpesvirus-6 Infection

Carrigan DR, Harrington D, Knox KK. Subacute leukoencephalitis caused by CNS infection with human herpesvirus-6 manifesting as acute multiple sclerosis. *Neurology* 1996;47:145–148.

Kamei A, Ichinohe S, Onoma R, Hiraga S, Fujiwara T. Acute disseminated demyelination due to primary human herpesvirus-6 infection *Eur J Pediatr* 1997;56:709–712.

Knox KK, Carrigan DR. Active human herpesvirus (HHV-6) infection of the central nervous system in patients with AIDS. *J Acquir Immune Defic Syndr Hum Retrovirol* 1995;9:69–73.

McCullers JA, Lakeman FD, Whitley RJ. Human herpesvirus 6 is associated with focal encephalitis. *Clin Infect Dis* 1995;21:571–576.

Mookerjee BP, Vogelsang G. Human herpesvirus-6 encephalitis after bone marrow transplantation: successful treatment with ganciclovir. *Bone Marrow Transplant* 1997;20:905–906.

Sing N, Carrigan DR. Human herpesvirus-6 in transplantation: an emerging pathogen. *Ann Intern Med* 1996;124:1065–1071.

Yoshikawa T, Asano Y. Central nervous system complications in human herpesvirus-6 infection. *Brain & Develop* 2002;22:307–314.

Acute Disseminated Encephalomyelitis

Arnason BGW. Neuroimmunology. *N Engl J Med* 1987;316:406–408.

Case records of the Massachusetts General Hospital. Case 37-1995. *N Engl J Med* 1995;333:1485–1493.

Cohen O, Steiner-Birmanns B, Biran I, et al. Recurrence of acute disseminated encephalomyelitis at the previously affected brain site. *Arch Neurol* 2001;58:797–801.

Dale RC, de Sousa C, Chong WK, et al. Acute disseminated encephalomyelitis, multiphasic disseminated encephalomyelitis and multiple sclerosis in children. *Brain* 2000;123:2407–2422.

Fenichel GM. Neurological complications of immunization. *Ann Neurol* 1982;12:119–128.

Jeffrey DR, Mandler RN, Davis LE. Transverse myelitis: retrospective analysis of 33 cases, with differentiation of cases associated with multiple sclerosis and parainfectious events. *Arch Neurol* 1993;50:532–535.

Johnson RT, Griffin DE, Hirsch RL, et al. Measles encephalitis: clinical and immunological studies. *N Engl J Med* 1984;310:137–141.

Kepes JJ. Large focal tumor-like demyelinating lesions of the brain: intermediate entity between multiple sclerosis and acute disseminated encephalomyelitis? A study of 31 patients. *Ann Neurol* 1993;33:18–27.

Kesselring J, Miller DH, Robb SA, et al. Acute disseminated encephalomyelitis: MRI findings and the distinction from multiple sclerosis. *Brain* 1990;113:291–302.

Marchioni E, Marinou-Aktipi K, Uggetti C, et al. Effectiveness of intravenous immunoglobulin treatment in adult patients with steroid-resistant monophasic or recurrent acute disseminated encephalomyelitis. *J Neurol* 2002;249:100–104.

Miravalle A, Roos KL. Encephalitis complicating smallpox vaccination. *Arch Neurol* 2003;60:925–928.

Pellegrini M, O'Brien TJ, Hoy J, Sedal L. *Mycoplasma pneumoniae* infection associated with an acute brainstem syndrome. *Acta Neurol Scand* 1996;93:203–206.

Straub J, Chofflon M, Delavalle J. Early high-dose intravenous methylprenisolone in acute disseminated encephalitis: a successful recovery. *Neurology* 1997;49:1145–1147.

Tenembaum S, Chamoles N, Fejerman N. Acute disseminated encephalomyelitis: a long-term follow-up study of 84 pediatric patients. *Neurology* 2002;59:1224–1231.

Ziegler DK. Acute disseminated encephalitis: some therapeutic and diagnostic considerations. *Arch Neurol* 1966;14:476–488.

Wingerchuk DM. Postinfectious encephalomyelitis. *Curr Neurol Neurosci Reports* 2003;3:256–264.

Subacute Sclerosing Panencephalitis

Dyke PR. Neuroprogressive disease of postinfectious origin: a review of a resurging subacute sclerosing panencephalitis (SSPE). *MRDD Res Reviews* 2001;7:217–225.

Gagnon A, Bouchard RW. Fulminating adult-onset subacute sclerosing panencephalitis in a 49-year-old man. *Arch Neurol* 2003;60:1160–1161.

Garg RK. Subacute aclerosing panencephalitis. *Postgrad Med J* 2002; 78:63–70.

Freeman JM. The clinical spectrum and early diagnosis of Dawson's encephalitis. *J Pediatr* 1969;75:590–603.

Mawrin C, Lins H, Koenig B, et al. Spatial and temporal disease progression of adult-onset subacute sclerosing panencephalitis. *Neurology* 2002;58:1568–1571.

Ozturk A, Gurses C, Baykan B, et al. Subacute sclerosing panencephalitis: clinical and magnetic resonance imaging evaluation of 36 patients. *J Child Neurol* 2002;17:25–29.

Risk WS, Haddad FS. The variable natural history of subacute sclerosing panencephalitis: a study of 118 cases from the Middle East. *Arch Neurol* 1979;36:610–614.

Tomoda A, Nomura K, Shiraishi S, et al. Trial of intraventricular ribavirin therapy for subacute sclerosing panencephalitis in Japan. *Brain & Develop* 2003;27:514–517.

Progressive Rubella Panencephalitis

Frey TK. Neurological aspects of rubella virus infection. *Intervirology* 1997;40:167–175.

Guizzaro A, Volpe E, Lus G, et al. Progressive rubella panencephalitis: follow-up EEG study of a case. *Acta Neurol (Napoli)* 1992;14:485–492.

Townsend JJ, Stroop WG, Baringer JR, et al. Neuropathology of progressive rubella panencephalitis after childhood rubella. *Neurology* 1982;32:185–190.

Wolinsky JS. Progressive rubella panencephalitis. In: Vinken PJ, Bruyn GW, Klawans HL, McKendall RR, eds. *Viral Disease. Handbook of Clinical Neurology,* vol 56. New York: Elsevier Science, 1989:405–446.

HTLV-associated Myelopathy/Tropical Spastic Paraparesis

Dover AG, Pringle E, Guberman A. Human T-cell lymphotropic virus type 1 myositis, peripheral neuropathy, and cerebral white matter lesions in the absence of spastic paraparesis. *Arch Neurol* 1997;54:896–900.

Feng J, Misu T, Fujihara K, et al. Interferon-α significantly reduces cerebrospinal fluid CD4 cell subsets in HAM/TSP. *J Neuroimmunology* 2003;141:170–173.

Izumo S, Goto MD, Itoyama MD, et al. Interferon-alpha is effective in HTLV-I-associated myelopathy: a multicenter, randomized, double-blind, controlled trial. *Neurology* 1996;46:1016–1021.

Jacobson S. Immunopathogenesis of human T cell lymphotropic virus type I-associated neurological disease. *J Infect Dis* 2002;186:S187–S192.

Janssen RS, Kaplan JE, Khabbaz RF, et al. HTLV-I-associated myelopathy/tropical spastic paraparesis in the United States. *Neurology* 1991;41:1355–1357.

Jernigan M, Morcos Y, Lee SM, et al. IgG in brain correlates with clinicopathological damage in HTLV-1 associated neurologic disease. *Neurology* 2003;60:1320–1327.

Kasahata N, Shiota J, Miyazawa Y, Nakano I, Murayama S. Acute human T-lymphotropic virus type 1-associated myelopathy. *Arch Neurol* 2003;60:873–876.

Lehky TJ, Flerlage N, Katz D, et al. Human T-cell lymphotropic virus type II-associated myelopathy: clinical and immunologic profiles. *Ann Neurol* 1996;40:714–723.

McKendall RR, Oas J, Lairmore MD. HTLV-I-associated myelopathy endemic in Texas-born residents and isolation of virus from CSF cells. *Neurology* 1991;41:831–836.

Nagai M, Yamano Y, Brennan MB, Mora CA, Jacobson S. Increased HTLV-I proviral load and preferential expansion of HTLV-I tax-specific CD8[+] T cells in cerebrospinal fluid from patients with HAM/TSP. *Ann Neurol* 2001;50:807–812.

Orland JR, Engstrom J, Fridey J, et al. Prevalence and clinical features of HTLV neurologic disease in the HTLV outcomes study. *Neurology* 2003;61:1588–1594.

Progressive Multifocal Leukoencephalopathy

Bergui M, Bradac GB, Oquz KK, Boghi A, et al. Progressive multifocal leukoencephalopathy: diffusion-weighted imaging and pathological correlations. *Neuroradiology* 2004;46(1):22–25.

Brooks BR, Walker DL. Progressive multifocal leukoencephalopathy. *Neurol Clin* 1984;2:299–313.

Cinque P, Bossolasco S, Brambilla AM, et al. The effect of highly active antiretroviral therapy-induced immune reconstitution on development and outcome of progressive multifocal leukoencephalopathy: study of 43 cases with review of the literature. *J Neurovirology* 2003;9(Suppl 1):73–80.

Dworkin MS. A review of progressive multifocal leukoencephalopathy in persons with and without AIDS. *Curr Clin Topics Infect Dis* 2002;22:181–195.

Gasnault J, Kahraman M, de Goër de Herve MG, et al. Critical role of JC virus-specific CD4 T-cell responses in preventing progressive multifocal leukoencephalopathy. *AIDS* 2003;17:1443–1449.

Gillespie SM, Chang Y, Lemp G, et al. Progressive multifocal leukoencephalopathy in persons infected with human immunodeficiency virus, San Francisco, 1981–1989. *Ann Neurol* 1991;30:597–604.

Hall CD, Dafni U, Simpson D, et al. Failure of cytarabine in progressive multifocal leukoencephalopathy associated with human immunodeficiency virus infection. AIDS Clinical Trials Group 243 Team. *N Engl J Med* 1998;338:1345–1351.

Holman RC, Janssen RS, Buehler JW, et al. Epidemiology of progressive multifocal leukoencephalopathy in the United States: analysis of mortality and AIDS surveillance data. *Neurology* 1991;41:1733–1736.

Koralnik IJ. New insights into progressive multifocal leukoencephalopathy. *Curr Op Neurol* 2004;17(3):365–370.

Marra CM, Rajicic N, Barker DE, et al. A pilot study of cidofovir for progressive multifocal leukoencephalopathy in AIDS. *AIDS* 2002;16:1791–1797.

Richardson Y Jr. Progressive multifocal leukoencephalopathy 30 years later. *N Engl J Med* 1988;318:315–317.

Encephalitis Lethargica

Blunt SB, Lane RJ, Turjanski N, Perkin GD. Clinical features and management of two cases of encephalitis lethargica. *Mov Disord* 1997;12:354–359.

Calne DB, Lees AJ. Late progression of postencephalitic Parkinson's syndrome. *Can J Neurol Sci* 1988;15:135–138.

Cree BC, Bernardini GL, Hays AP, Lowe G. A fatal case of coxsackievirus B4 meningoencephalitis. *Arch Neurol* 2003;60:107–112.

Dickman MS. von Economo encephalitis. *Arch Neurol* 2001;58:1696–1698.

Howard RS, Lees AJ. Encephalitis lethargica: a report of four recent cases. *Brain* 1987;110:19–33.

McCall S, Henry JM, Reid AN, Taubenberger JK. Influenza RNA not detected in archival brain tissues from acute encephalitis lethargica cases or in postencephalitic Parkinson cases. *J Neuropath Exper Neurology* 2001;60:696–704.

Ward CD. Neuropsychiatric interpretations of postencephalitic movement disorders. *Mov Disord* 2003;18:623–630.

Yahr MD. Encephalitis lethargica (von Economo's disease, epidemic encephalitis). In: Vinken PJ. Bruyn GW. Klawans HL, eds. *Infections of the Nervous System. Handbook of Clinical Neurology,* vol 34. New York: Elsevier/North-Holland, 1978:451–457.

Chapter 25

Acquired Immunodeficiency Syndrome (AIDS)

Carolyn Barley Britton

HISTORY

AIDS is the most important pandemic of the 20th and early 21st centuries. The first clinical description in 1981 was soon followed by epidemiologic surveillance criteria proposed by the Centers for Disease Control (CDC) in 1982. AIDS was the occurrence of unusual opportunistic infections or malignancies indicative of a defect in cell-mediated immunity without a known cause.

In 1983, HIV-I, the retrovirus that causes AIDS, was isolated from human peripheral-blood lymphocytes. An explosive pace of research followed. The virus was sequenced and its structure elucidated by x-ray crystallography. There were rapid advances in understanding the viral life cycle, mechanisms of human infection and pathogenesis, and development of successful drug therapies. HIV infection of the CD4 (T4 helper) lymphocytes caused the cellular immune defect of AIDS. Soon after infection, HIV replicates vigorously in peripheral-blood lymphocytes and lymphoid tissues throughout the body, including gut-associated lymphoid, and brain microglial and macrophage cells. Disseminated viral infection caused systemic and neurologic disorders, such as the wasting syndrome and dementia, which are now recognized as AIDS-defining illnesses even in the absence of opportunistic infections or neoplasia.

Serologic studies showed that there may be a latency of several years between HIV infection and AIDS, the latter indicative of advanced immunosuppression. Direct viral nucleic acid detection (viral load) and viral replication assays showed that there is no virologic latency after initial infection. Despite ongoing viral replication, most infected people are asymptomatic or experience transient self-limited illnesses. Some have chronic lymphadenopathy or the AIDS-RC of adenopathy, weight loss, fever, and diarrhea.

CLASSIFICATION OF HIV DISEASE

The CDC proposed staging criteria for HIV infection in 1986, and modified them in 1987 to include the neurologic syndromes of AIDS dementia and myelopathy, among 23 AIDS defining illnesses (Table 25.1).

Future revisions were anticipated based on improved understanding of HIV biology. The 1993 revisions added three laboratory categories that are stratified by CD4-cell numbers and three clinical categories (Table 25.2).

AIDS-defining illnesses were expanded to include positive HIV serology and pulmonary tuberculosis, recurrent bacterial pneumonia, invasive cervical carcinoma, or a CD4 lymphocyte count less than 200 cells/mm^3. The revisions define the end stage of HIV infection and clarify the relationship of specific clinical syndromes that are not diagnostic of AIDS, especially those of neurologic disease, to advanced immunosuppression.

The classification system guides medical management of HIV infected persons. The Walter Reed classification system has not gained wide acceptance.

HIV replication (viral load) is the determining factor for progression to clinical endpoints, such as AIDS or death. Viral load assays have supplanted staging criteria for decisions about antiretroviral therapy. Staging is still useful for prognosis and decisions about opportunistic infection prophylaxis.

Epidemiology

HIV infection is a worldwide pandemic affecting virtually all population groups, with especially rapid spread in developing countries, where more than 95% of new cases occur. Transmission occurs through homosexual or

▶ TABLE 25.1 Classification of HIV Infections

Group I
  Acute infection (transient symptoms with seroconversion)
Group II
  Asymptomatic infection (seropositive only)
Group III
  Persistent generalized lymphadenopathy
Group IV
  Other disease
  Subgroup A
    Chronic constitutional disease
  Subgroup B
    Neurologic disease
  Subgroup C
    Specified secondary infections
    Category C–1
      Diseases listed in the CDC definition for AIDS
    Category C–2
      Other specified secondary infections
  Subgroup D
    Specified secondary cancers (includes cancers fulfilling CDC definition of AIDS)
  Subgroup E
    Other conditions

From Centers for Disease Control. *MMWR* 1986;35:334–339.

▶ **TABLE 25.2 1992 CDC Classification of HIV Infection**

Laboratory Categories
Category 1–CD4 lymphocyte count >500 cells/mm³
Category 2–CD4 lymphocyte count from 200 cells/mm³ through 499 cells/mm³
Category 3–CD4 lymphocyte count <200 cells/mm³
Clinical Categories
Category A–asymptomatic infection, persistent generalized lymphadenopathy, and acute primary HIV infection
Category B–symptomatic conditions not included in the CDC 1987 surveillance case definition of AIDS that are judged by a physician to be HIV-related or where medical management is complicated by HIV infection (e.g., sepsis, bacterial endocarditis, pulmonary tuberculosis, cervical dysplasia or carcinoma, vulvovaginal candidiasis)
Category C–any of the 23 conditions listed in CDC 1987 case definition for AIDS

Adapted from US Congress. CDC Case Definition of AIDS: Implications of the Proposed Revisions-Background Paper. OTA-BP- H-89, Washington, D.C.: US Government Printing Office, 1992.

heterosexual contact, exposure to contaminated blood or blood products, or perinatally. Worldwide, heterosexual activity is the most common mode of transmission. In the United States, homosexual activity is slightly more frequent than injection drug use (IDU) as the most common exposure, but seroconversions are more common in IDU. In Western Europe, IDU accounts for slightly more cases than homosexual activity.

Retrospective analysis of banked blood showed that HIV was present in the United States in the 1970s. From 1981 to 2001, the CDC estimates 1.3 million to 1.4 million persons in the U.S. were infected with HIV. There were 816,149 cases of AIDS and 467,910 deaths reported to the CDC. Five states reported 64% of cases: New York, Florida, New Jersey, California, and Puerto Rico. Eighty per cent of cases were in the Northeast (44%) and the South (36%). A transmission risk is identified for more than 90% of cases. Recipients of blood products or clotting factor for hemophilia, or other coagulation/blood disorders, account for less than 1% of adult AIDS cases. Routine testing of blood products has largely eliminated this source of infection in the United States.

The introduction of highly active antiretroviral therapy (HAART) profoundly changed HIV/AIDS epidemiology in the U.S. and other developed countries, was responsible for a 38% decline in incident AIDS cases, and was associated with a 67% decline in deaths from AIDS in the U.S. Since 1998, the annual number of AIDS cases and deaths has been stable at 40,000 and 16,000, respectively. Other developed countries have experienced a similar decline in AIDS cases and deaths. Tragically, for developing countries, the limited access to effective public health campaigns and

to medical treatment has resulted in a rapidly expanding pandemic.

Occupational exposure with documented transmission and seroconversion has occurred in 57 health care workers as of December, 2001. Percutaneous exposure was the most common risk, but mucocutaneous exposure, alone or with percutaneous exposure, also occurred. Most exposures were to blood or bloody fluid. Possible occupational transmission has occurred in 138 additional health care workers who were exposed to HIV-contaminated blood, body fluids, or laboratory solutions, but HIV seroconversion after a specific occupational exposure was not documented. Prospective studies of known exposures estimate the average risk for HIV transmission after a percutaneous exposure to HIV-infected blood as approximately 0.3% and after mucous membrane exposure, 0.09%. Although there were documented cases of seroconversion after broken skin exposure, the average risk is not precisely quantified but is expected to be less than the mucocutaneous exposure risk. The transmission risk for percutaneous exposure is increased by exposure to a large quantity of blood from the source contact, (e.g., by visibly blood-contaminated devices, large-bore needles from a vein or artery, deep injury, and by exposure to a contact with advanced disease and high viral load).

The progress of the AIDS epidemic in the U.S. and its subsequent stabilization shows the rapidity of expansion of the virus within a population, and the effectiveness of aggressive public health strategies and treatment. AIDS incidence increased throughout the 1980s and began to decline in the mid-1990s. The first 100,000 AIDS cases were reported in the first 8 years of surveillance; more than 500,000 cases were reported in the second 8-year period. The cumulative number of AIDS cases through 2002 of 859,000 indicates a stabilized epidemic (Table 25.3).

However, a 2% increase in incidence in 2002 over 2001 underscores the need for continued vigilance. Changes in the case definition were responsible for a transient increase in AIDS cases after 1993. HIV/AIDS name-based reporting is now required in most states. Dual reporting allows accurate assessment of the scope and demographics of the epidemic, appropriate funding initiatives, and identification of persons for counseling about treatment. The CDC has proposed more aggressive identification measures for certain populations (i.e., routine testing of persons in medical settings of high HIV prevalence, pregnant women, children, and partners of those testing positive for HIV), through intensive partner notification measures.

The fastest-growing populations with AIDS in the United States are women, African-American and Hispanic minorities, and intravenous drug users (Table 25.3).

A rise in seroconversion among some young homosexual male populations implies a need for continued

> **TABLE 25.3** **Epidemiology of HIV/AIDS: United States and Global Data, 2002 and 2003**

United States—Through December, 2002	
Adults/adolescents	849,780
Pediatric (under age 13)	9,220
Total	859,000
Demographics-Adult	
Race	
African-American	42 %
Non-Hispanic white	37 %
Hispanic	20 %
Gender	
Men	77 %
Women	23 %
Global—2003	
Total cases through 2003	37,800,000
Sub-Saharan Africa	25,000,000
South and Southeast Asia	6,500,000
Number of new HIV infections in 2003	4,800,000
Deaths due to AIDS in 2003	2,900,000
Children with AIDS (<15) through 2003	2,100,000

Adapted from: Centers for Disease Control and Prevention (CDC) (*www.cdc.gov*) 2004 Report on the global AIDS epidemic. Geneva; Joint United Nations Program on HIV/AIDS, July 2004

vigilance in targeted education and is a reminder that identification of infected persons without ongoing educational efforts is not an adequate prevention strategy.

In 2000, AIDS became the leading cause of death among African American men ages 35 years to 44 years and women ages 25 years to 34 years. The disproportionate representation of African American and Hispanic men is related to intravenous drug use. Minority women are also directly or indirectly affected by drug use but unprotected heterosexual activity has become the predominant transmission risk for this group.

HIV infection has been reported in virtually every country and in some, with devastating impact. In developing countries, rapid spread is related to inadequate public health and health-care infrastructures. The World Health Organization (WHO) estimated that 37.8 million people worldwide were infected by the end of 2003, and approximately 20 million had died. There are an estimated 2.1 million infected children under 15 years of age, most of whom are in sub-Saharan Africa. There were an estimated 3.1 million deaths due to HIV/AIDS-associated illness. Globally, there are an estimated 14,000 new cases of HIV infection daily, and nearly 3 million annual deaths by 2003. Although unprotected heterosexual activity is the predominant transmission risk, there are substantial risks in health-care settings due to contaminated blood or needles. Seventy percent of the HIV/AIDS cases are in sub-Saharan Africa, and 17% are in Asia.

AIDS IN CHILDREN

By the end of 2002, nearly 10,000 children in the U.S. under age 13 years were reported to the CDC, comprising slightly more than 1% of all AIDS cases, and most were infected perinatally. Perinatal infection disproportionately affects African Americans and Hispanics, a measure of their disproportionate number among seropositive women. Since 1992, perinatal transmission in the United States has declined dramatically from a peak of 1000 cases to 2000 cases annually, to 100 cases annually in 2001, as a result of successful implementation of CDC guidelines for maternal counseling, testing, and zidovudine treatment.

Worldwide, perinatal transmission unfortunately continues because treatment is not widely available. An estimated 650,000 children died of HIV/AIDS in 2002. Millions of uninfected children will be orphaned by the loss of both parents to AIDS.

Etiology

Virologic, serologic, and epidemiologic data support the conclusion that AIDS is caused by HIV infection. HIV is an enveloped RNA virus. It contains an RNA-dependent, DNA polymerase (reverse transcriptase) that produces a provirus capable of integrating into host-cell DNA. In the target cell, the virus exists in both free and integrated states. It is a lentivirus. The best-known of this family is the visna virus, which is similar to HIV in that it demonstrates cellular tropism, establishes persistent infection, and after long, clinical latency establishes a slowly progressive demyelinating disease in ovines.

Human HIV infection is considered a cross-species (zoonotic) infection, arising from monkeys infected with simion immunodeficiency virus (SIV) through multiple independent transmissions. Of the two recognized viral species, HIV-1 is found worldwide and is more prevalent, whereas HIV-2 is found in Western Africa and in Europe among African immigrants and their sexual partners. Sporadic cases of HIV-2 occur in the United States. HIV-2 less frequently causes immunodeficiency and AIDS than HIV-1. Three phylogenetic groups of HIV-1 (M, N, and O) and each comprises several viral strains. Group M (the main group) is responsible for the global epidemic. Group O (the outlier) is found in Cameroon, Gabon and Equatorial Guinea. Group N (non-M/non-O) was isolated from two individuals in Cameroon. SIV was isolated first from macaque monkeys in captivity and later found in African green monkeys. The sooty mangabey is the primate host suspected of transmitting HIV-2. This subspecies is infected with a strain of SIV that is genomically and phylogenetically related to HIV-2. Its natural habitat is the epicenter of the HIV-2 epidemic and large numbers of wild animals are infected. The chimpanzee seems to be the primate host for HIV-1.

The recognition of HIV infection as a zoonosis raises concern for animal-to-human transmission of other potentially pathogenic retroviruses.

Although scientific data overwhelmingly support the view that HIV is the cause of AIDS, other theories have been proposed, including toxic drug exposure or an as-yet-unidentified agent. In 1992, 35 cases of HIV-negative CD4 cell lymphopenia or AIDS were reported from the United States and six other countries. Some cases had risk factors associated with HIV; others had no reported risk factors. Alternative theories of infection lack substantial scientific support.

Pathogenesis

Infection of CD4 lymphocytes by HIV, mediated by viral attachment to the cell surface CD4 receptor, leads to cell death. In humans, the CD4 receptor is expressed on several cell types, including neurons and glia in the brain, yet there is no evidence of viral replication in cells other than lymphocytes, macrophages, monocytes, and their derivatives. A co-receptor necessary for viral entry into cells was identified in 1996 as a chemokine receptor. In acute and early HIV infection, a macrophage-tropic viral strain predominates and uses the chemokine receptor CCR5 (R5 virus). In chronic infection, T-cell tropic strains predominate and use the receptor CXCR4 (X4 virus). Other chemokine receptors are sometimes used, especially by HIV-2. Genetic variation in the chemokine receptor may affect susceptibility to HIV infection. Relative resistance to infection is observed in people who are homozygous for a 32 base-pair deletion in CCR5. Progression rates in AIDS may be affected by changes in the presentation by infected cells of viral epitopes to cytotoxic T lymphocytes, the HLA-I. Accelerated progression to AIDS is associated with a single amino acid substitution in the HLA-B35 allele (HLA-B*35-Px). However, the predictive value of observations about the effect of HLA polymorphisms on disease progression may be restricted to specific populations. Primary HIV infection may be asymptomatic or in 50% to 70% of the cases, result in an acute, self-limited mononucleosis-like illness with fever, headaches, myalgia, malaise, lethargy, sore throat, lymphadenopathy, and maculopapular rash. Painful ulceration of the buccal mucosa may impede swallowing (odynophagia).

Acute infection is characterized by viremia, high viral replication rates, ease of viral isolation from peripheral blood lymphocytes, and high serum levels of a viral-core antigen, p24. Initial viral load in acute infection may be as high as 1 million RNA molecules per milliliter. Cytotoxic lymphocytes and soluble factors from CD8 lymphocytes are effective in reducing viral load to a set point that differs for each individual. Despite the effective early immune response, there is almost simultaneous immune dysfunction. Neutralizing antibodies of the IgM- and later the IgG type

appear in 2 to 6 weeks, resulting in clearance of viremia and a decrease in serum p24 levels. Rarely, antibodies do not appear for several months and exceptionally not at all.

Adverse immunologic effects occur early and are more severe in symptomatic persons. An early absolute lymphopenia affects both CD4 helper and CD8 suppressor cells with lymphocyte hyporesponsiveness to mitogens and antigens and thrombocytopenia. Lymphocytosis usually follows, especially of CD8 lymphocytes, with inversion of the CD4/CD8 ratio. Atypical lymphocytes are sometimes seen. Early changes in the CD4/CD8 ratio are usually transient with reversion to more normal values but with persistent functional abnormalities. Cutaneous anergy is a direct result of the viral effects on CD4 cells.

After acute infection and seroconversion, clinical latency may last several years before the onset of symptoms of secondary infection, malignancy, or neurologic disease appear. There is no biologic latency, however; HIV infection is a chronic, persistent infection of variable viral replication rate.

The viral load set point after acute infection correlates with rate of progression to symptomatic infection or AIDS. Several proprietary assays provide quantitative measurement of plasma HIV-RNA. The branched (b)DNA assay detects as few as 20 copies to 50 copies per milliliter. Recognition of acute infection is important because early antiretroviral treatment may prevent the extensive seeding of lymphoid tissues or eliminate infection. Without treatment, viral replication is robust.

It is estimated that 10 billion virions enter plasma daily in untreated people. Productively infected, peripheral blood lymphocytes turn over rapidly with a half life of 1.6 days. Most of the total viral load is in tissues, not plasma. In lymphoid tissue, virus is contained in two compartments: CD4+ lymphocytes or macrophages; and follicular dendritic cells within germinal centers, where virus is passively adherent. The total lymphoid viral burden is three times that of plasma, the majority in follicular dendritic cells. The total body viral load is 100 billion HIV-RNA copies. Approximately 10% of latently infected cells contain replication-competent provirus. Cellular destruction of lymphoid tissue is mediated by direct HIV cytopathic effects, autoimmunity, and other mechanisms. Eventually the lymphoid system is overwhelmed by the viral burden, which increases with advancing disease and culminates in AIDS.

Other factors that may augment HIV replication and the onset of symptoms are as follows: the biologic variability of HIV and the appearance of increasingly virulent strains; host immunogenetics; interaction with concomitant infection by cytomegalovirus, herpes simplex virus, hepatitis B and c viruses, human herpes virus-6, human T-lymphotropic virus type 1, or malaria that upregulate expression of HIV; and up regulation of infection and cell-killing ability by cytokines. Cytokines are released by immune cells in response to infection and may up regulate or down regulate viral replication.

Other immunologic abnormalities in AIDS are caused by effects of HIV on immune cells other than the CD4 lymphocyte, such as B cells or macrophages, which result in hypergammaglobulinemia, impaired antibody responses to new antigens (including encapsulated bacteria), and increased levels of immune complexes. Antibodies to platelets may cause thrombocytopenia. Loss of cellular immune function and impairment of B-cell and macrophage function increase susceptibility to some bacterial infections, opportunistic organisms, and rare neoplasms.

HAART and specific prophylaxis have reduced the incidence of AIDS-related opportunistic infections and neoplasms in the United States and other countries where treatment is readily available. The types of infections or neoplasms that complicate HIV infection have not changed, and are similar worldwide. In untreated HIV infection, pneumocystis carini pneumonia (PCP) is the most common opportunistic pathogen. Other opportunistic infections are often multiple: fungal (candidiasis, cryptococcosis, aspergillosis, histoplasmosis, coccidioidomycosis, and others); viral cytomegalovirus (CMV), disseminated herpes simplex (HSV), varicella zoster (VZV) or parasitic (toxoplasmosis, cryptosporidiosis, strongyloidiasis, isosporiasis, and Acanthamoeba infection). Mycobacteria (tuberculosis and atypical forms), Salmonella, *Treponema pallidum,* and *Staphylococcus aureus* are common causes of pulmonary and systemic bacterial infections. Many of these infections involve the CNS, secondarily in most cases, but sometimes as the primary infection. The papovavirus that causes progressive multifocal leukoencephalopathy (PML) causes a primary brain infection. Pathogens that are common in developing countries, such as Trypanosomiasis, are sometimes seen in recent immigrants to the United States. Hepatitis B and hepatitis C infections are important comorbid conditions, especially common among those who acquire HIV from injection drug use. Kaposi sarcoma, Hodgkin lymphoma, and non-Hodgkin lymphoma are the most commonly encountered neoplasms.

CNS Pathogenesis

HIV enters the CNS at the time of primary infection and may result in no apparent disease, in acute self-limited syndromes, or in chronic disorders. These are caused by HIV itself, secondary opportunistic infections or neoplasia, metabolic abnormalities, medical treatment, or nutritional disorders. Neurologic disorders are found in up to 70% of patients in clinical series of AIDS and more than 80% of autopsy series. In 10% to 20%, the neurologic disorder is the first manifestation of AIDS. Uncommonly a neurologic disorder is the sole evidence of chronic HIV in-

fection and the cause of death. Early, effective, antiretroviral treatment has decreased the incidence of secondary opportunistic infections and neoplasms of the nervous system and the incidence of primary HIV-related syndromes. However, autopsy series of HAART-treated patients who died of AIDS or unrelated causes show abnormalities in most brains, which in some cases were the cause of death.

Evidence of early CNS invasion includes isolation of virus from CSF or neural tissues (brain, spinal cord, peripheral nerve) and intrathecal production of antibodies to HIV. How HIV enters the CNS is not known. Possible mechanisms include intracellular transport across the blood-brain barrier within infected macrophages, as free-virus seeding the leptomeninges, or as free virus after replication within the choroid plexus or vascular epithelium. In the brain, viral infection is detected only in microglial cells or macrophages by in situ hybridization techniques; it is not found in neurons or glial cells, even though these cells have CD4 and chemokine receptors.

The high frequency of neurologic disorders in HIV infection has led to the designation of HIV as a *neurotropic virus.* The term neurotropic implies selective vulnerability and homing of the virus to neurons. Alternatively the high frequency of neurologic disorders may be explained by the chronicity of infection that results in continued seeding of the CNS. Specific neurotropism is not needed for continued accrual of neurologic damage. It has been difficult to establish correlation of neurologic syndromes with productive viral replication in the affected tissue. There is an increase, however, in the viral burden or viral load with advancing disease that parallels dementia and other neurologic syndromes.

The mechanism of neurologic injury is believed to be indirect. Potential mechanisms include immune-mediated indirect injury; restricted persistent cellular infection; cellular injury due to cytokines released by infected monocytes and macrophages; excitotoxic amino-acid injury; voltage-mediated increase of intracellular calcium; free-radical damage; potentiation of inflammatory damage by chemokines and lipid inflammatory mediators (arachidonic acid and platelet activating factor); direct cellular toxicity of HIV gene products, such as the envelope gp 120, tat and gp41; and cross-reacting antibody to an HIV glycoprotein binding a cell membrane epitope, resulting in cell receptor blockade. More than one mechanism may be important. Genetic changes in the virus in the host may result in noncytopathic CNS virus with enhanced replicative capacity in monocytes and macrophages, leading to a greater viral burden in the CNS than is apparent in the periphery. Phenotypic and viral load discordance are documented in several studies of plasma and CSF.

This compartmentalization of virus may explain the occurrence of neurologic syndromes when peripheral viral replication appears well controlled.

CLINICAL SYNDROMES

HIV-Related Syndromes

Neurologic disorders may occur at any stage from first infection and seroconversion to AIDS. Even without other manifestations of HIV infection, some are diagnostic of AIDS (dementia and myelopathy). All levels of the neuraxis may be affected, including multisystem disorders. Neurologic disorders are likely to be transient in early HIV infection; in chronic infection, neurologic disorders are more prevalent and more often chronic or progressive.

The neurologic syndromes in early HIV infection are indistinguishable from disorders that occur with infection by other viruses (Table 25.4).

These include aseptic meningitis, reversible encephalopathy, leukoencephalitis, seizures, transverse myelitis, cranial and peripheral neuropathy (Bell palsy, Guillian-Barré syndrome), polymyositis, and myoglobinuria. Brachial neuritis and ganglioneuritis are rarely reported. The course is typically self-limited and patients often experience full neurologic recovery.

CSF abnormalities (pleocytosis up to 200 cells/mm^3 and oligoclonal bands) differentiate HIV syndromes from postinfectious disorders. Tests for HIV antibody may be negative because these syndromes may precede or accompany seroconversion, and the tests must be repeated in several weeks. If acute HIV infection is strongly suspected, p24 antigen and viral load assay should be considered if serology is negative. Hepatitis B and hepatitis C serology should be determined in all HIV seropositives. Early antiretroviral therapy may be offered to decrease the high viral load typical of acute infection quickly, thereby lowering the viral-load set point. No specific treatment is indicated for these self-limited disorders except that plasmapheresis or immune globulin is used for the Guillain-Barré syndrome and steroids for polymyositis.

▶ **TABLE 25.4 Primary HIV-Related Neurologic Syndromes: Acute Infection**

Acute aseptic meningitis
Acute encephalopathy
Leukoencephalitis
Seizures, generalized or focal
Transverse myelitis
Cranial and peripheral neuropathy
Bell's palsy
Acute inflammatory demyelinating polyneuropathy of the Guillain-Barré type
Polymyositis
Myoglobinuria

From Britton CB. In: Rowland LP, ed. *Merritt's Textbook of Neurology.* Update 11. Philadelphia: Lea & Febiger, 1992.

▶ **TABLE 25.5 Primary HIV-Related Neurologic Syndromes: Chronic Infection**

Persistent or recurrent meningeal pleocytosis with or without meningeal symptoms
Organic brain syndromes
Dementia, static or progressive with or without motor signs
Mild cognitive impairment, neuropsychologic test criteria only
Organic psychiatric disorder
Cerebrovascular syndromes
Cerebellar ataxia
Seizure disorder
Multisystem degeneration
Chronic progressive myelopathy
Anterior horn cell disease
Cranial and peripheral neuropathy
Bell's palsy
Hearing loss
Phrenic nerve paralysis
Lateral femoral cutaneous nerve
Chronic inflammatory demyelinating polyneuropathy
Distal symmetric sensory neuropathy
Mononeuritis multiplex
Autonomic neuropathy
Myopathy

Partially adapted from Britton CB. In: Rowland LP, ed. *Merritt's Textbook of Neurology.* Update 11. Philadelphia: Lea & Febiger, 1992.

In chronic HIV infection, neurologic disorders may accompany systemic HIV disease or secondary disorders (Table 25.5).

Chronic or recurrent meningeal pleocytosis may occur sometimes with meningeal symptoms but often asymptomatic. Chronic pleocytosis does not predict any specific neurologic complication. Ascribing CSF pleocytosis to HIV infection requires exclusion of secondary pathogens or tumor.

Cognitive impairment is a well recognized complication of chronic HIV infection and may be mild or severe (Table 25.6).

Mild cognitive impairment, detected by neuropsychologic tests, does not significantly impair daily function.

▶ **TABLE 25.6 HIV-1-Associated Cognitive/Motor Complex AIDS Dementia Complex**

Severe manifestations
HIV-1–associated dementia complex
HIV-1–associated myelopathy
Mild manifestations
HIV-1–associated minor cognitive/motor disorder

From American Academy of Neurology AIDS Task Force. Nomenclature and research case definitions for neurologic manifestations of human immunodeficiency virus-type 1 (HIV-1) infection. *Neurology* 1991;41(6):778–785.

Minor motor signs, usually motor slowness, may be present. Severe dementia, HIV-1 associated dementia complex [HIV-1-associated dementia (HAD), HIV-1-associated dementia complex (HADC) or HIV dementia (HIV-D)] or AIDS dementia complex (ADC) is diagnostic of AIDS. Other designations are subacute encephalitis, subacute encephalopathy or HIV encephalitis. The word complex is used to denote the association of dementia with motor and behavioral signs. Myelopathy and peripheral neuropathy coexist in 25% of patients. Hepatitis C coinfection, common in injection drug users, may contribute to cognitive impairment but does not appear to impact HIV disease progression or response to antiretroviral therapy.

HAD or ADC is an insidiously progressive subcortical dementia. Early symptoms include apathy, social withdrawal, diminished libido, slow thinking, poor concentration, and forgetfulness. Psychiatric syndromes are sometimes profound and may be the first manifestation of HIV infection, expressed as psychosis, depression, or mania. Motor signs include slow movements, leg weakness, and gait ataxia. There may be headache, tremor, seizures, parkinsonian features, or frontal release signs. Although the disorder is usually progressive, some patients develop a static level of disability, and some improve in response to medical treatment for HIV or complicating disorders. When progressive, the disease culminates in akinetic mutism, an immobile bedridden state with global cognitive impairment and urinary incontinence.

In children, there may be a similar static or progressive encephalopathy. Most affected children meet criteria for AIDS, but progressive encephalopathy may occur before immunologic dysfunction is severe, as in adults. Neurologic findings include intellectual deterioration, microcephaly, loss of developmental milestones, and progressive motor impairment that may culminate in spastic quadriparesis and pseudobulbar palsy. Seizures are usually due to fever. Myoclonus and extrapyramidal rigidity are rare.

The CSF is usually normal or shows mild pleocytosis, protein elevation, and oligoclonal bands. CSF gamma globulin content is increased owing to intrathecal synthesis of antibody to HIV antigens. Virus may be cultured from CSF. Both CSF and plasma viral load correlate with dementia occurrence but may be discordant in some cases where CSF is greater than plasma. Phenotypic discordance is also observed, sometimes causing different patterns of drug resistance. CSF markers of immune activation may correlate with severity of dementia and include HIV p24 antigen, β-microglobulin, tumor necrosis factor, and antimyelin basic protein. None of these is predictive of or specific for dementia. Other CSF and serum markers also lack predictive value or specificity but may correlate with severity of dementia; the list includes serum neopterin and tryptophan levels, CSF tryptophan and serotonin metabolites, and CSF quinolinic acid levels.

In adults, CT or MRI may show cortical atrophy and ventricular dilatation, sometimes with white matter changes. On CT, there is attenuation of white matter; MRI shows hyperintense white matter lesions on T2-weighted and proton density scans, ranging from discrete foci to large confluent periventricular lesions (Fig. 25.1).

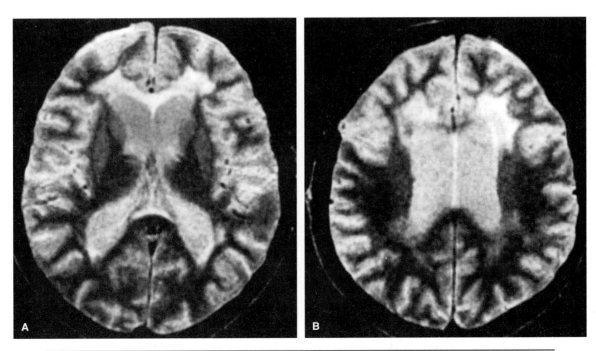

FIGURE 25.1. A and **B**: T_2-weighted MRI scan from patient with progressive dementia showing ventricular dilatation, cortical atrophy, and periventricular frontal lobe white matter hyperintensity.

CT in children shows basal ganglia calcification and cerebral atrophy. MRI white matter changes may not correlate with dementia and may disappear spontaneously or with antiretroviral therapy.

Abnormalities in functional neuroimaging are detected in HIV-infected people, whether with and without dementia. The abnormalities become worse or change with progressive cognitive impairment. Fluorodeoxyglucose-positron emission tomography (FDG-PET) shows relative hypermetabolism in the thalamus and basal ganglia in HIV-infected people. Progressive dementia is accompanied by cortical and subcortical hypometabolism. SPECT shows multifocal cortical perfusion deficits in the frontal lobes, worse in those with dementia. Cerebral metabolite abnormalities demonstrated by magnetic resonance spectroscopy (MRS) include elevated myoinositol and choline levels in frontal white matter indicative of glial proliferation in patients with mild cognitive impairment. Severe dementia is associated with decreased levels of N-acetyl aspartate, a neuronal marker. Dynamic cerebral blood volume (CBV) studies by functional MRI (fMRI) show increased CBV in deep and cortical gray matter in HIV-positive people and even greater increases in deep gray matter of those with dementia. Abnormalities may improve with antiretroviral treatment.

Pathologic abnormalities in brain include microglial nodules, giant cells, focal perivascular demyelination and gliosis, and neuronal loss in frontal cortex. Although there is often no correlation between the severity of these pathologic changes and the severity of dementia, recent studies suggest that neuronal injury may be missed by standard pathologic survey techniques. In a prospective study, severity of neurocognitive impairment was correlated with microneuro-anatomic injury to dendritic structures that resulted in dendritic simplification, and not to viral burden or presence of microglial nodules and multinucleated giant cells. Astrocyte cell death through apoptotic mechanisms may reduce the neuroprotective functions of this cellular population. In vitro studies show that soluble Fas ligand (sFasL) from HIV-infected macrophages triggers apoptosis of uninfected astrocytes. A study of pre-HAART HIV infected patients with dementia showed elevated CSF sFasL levels in this group compared to HIV negative controls and HIV positive nondemented patients. More prospective data is needed to understand the role of apoptosis in HIV dementia, and the utility of markers for apoptosis as predictors of dementia.

The incidence of AIDS dementia is less than the frequency of pathologic abnormalities. The CDC reported a prevalence of 7.3% for the diagnosis of HIV encephalopathy in 1987 through 1991. The Multicenter AIDS Cohort Study Group reported a 4% prevalence of dementia diagnosis with a 7% annual rate and 15% overall probability of dementia before death. There are increased mortality rates among demented patients.

The diagnosis of HAD or ADC requires exclusion of secondary opportunistic infections or neoplasms. Other confounding variables include drug use, vitamin B_{12} deficiency, metabolic disorders and an aging HIV-infected population due to successful antiretroviral treatment. Older survivors of HIV are at risk for vascular disease and Alzheimer disease as well as degenerative disorders associated with dementia. In most studies, HAART reduces the incidence and mortality of AIDS dementia. An Australian study is a notable exception where dementia accounted for a greater proportion of AIDS defining illnesses after HAART, but with longer survival after diagnosis. In general, the prevalence of dementia in HIV is expected to increase with longer survival. Clinical trials of selegeline, a monoamine oxidase-type B inhibitor, and nimodipine suggest a trend for improvement in cognitive impairment. Antioxidants and agents that block gp120 are ineffective. Memantine and selegiline studies are ongoing.

Longitudinal cohort studies have shown no neuropsychologic deterioration in asymptomatic people who are HIV positive. Neuropsychologic test abnormalities do accrue with advancing disease but not necessarily with overt dementia. Those showing a decline in neuropsychologic test performance, however, have an increased risk of death. In early studies, the strongest predictors of significant dementia identified in a multiinstitution study of 19,462 HIV-infected persons are CD4+ T-lymphocyte counts of less than 100 cells/μL, anemia and an AIDS defining infection or neoplasm (18.6% to 24.9% risk in 2 years). In the post-HAART era, dementia is often independent of advanced immunosuppression.

Several studies have evaluated the CSF viral load as a predictor of future dementia. A prospective study found that high CSF HIV-1 RNA levels at baseline, but not plasma levels, predicted neuropsychologic impairment after a median follow-up of one year. Other cross-sectional studies also show correlation of higher CSF HIV-1 RNA viral levels with dementia severity, but also find high levels in other CNS infections. There is no consensus that CSF HIV-1 RNA levels may be used as a predictor of dementia in an individual but they are useful for the symptomatic patient. Viral genotyping and drug resistance testing for plasma and CSF isolates are necessary for the symptomatic patient. Antiretroviral therapy that includes drugs with good CNS penetration may benefit the symptomatic patient with CNS virologic escape.

Stroke syndromes occur in 0.5% to 8% of patients in clinical studies, and infarcts are more frequent at autopsy. Stroke syndromes may be follow secondary infections or neoplasms, such as cryptococcus or other fungi, toxoplasmosis, tuberculosis, herpes zoster, cytomegalovirus, syphilis, or Kaposi sarcoma. Other causes include HIV-related vasculitis, cardiogenic emboli, thrombogenic conditions such as hyperviscosity, disseminated intravascular coagulopathy, and lupus anticoagulant. Cerebral hemorrhage may follow HIV-associated thrombocytopenia or toxoplasmosis. Lipid abnormalities due to HIV, prolonged inflammatory states or to antiretroviral treatment may increase stroke risk, especially in long survivors. Impaired glucose metabolism due to antiretroviral therapy may also add to stroke risk. A retrospective study of the risk of cardiovascular and cerebrovascular disease among 36,766 HIV infected patients cared for at Veterans Affairs facilities between January 1993 and June 2001 did not show an increase in stroke or myocardial infarction diagnoses. A prospective study is necessary.

Evaluation of cerebrovascular syndromes includes imaging; CSF examination; cultures for viruses, bacteria, mycobacteria, and fungi; serum and CSF antibodies for cryptococcus, syphilis, and toxoplasmosis; plasma and CSF HIV viral load; polymerase chain reaction (PCR) of CSF for suspect pathogens; echocardiography; Doppler; lipid profiles; coagulation profiles; platelet count; and determination of procoagulants. If vasculitis is suspected, angiography or brain or meningeal biopsy may be useful. Management is directed to the underlying mechanism and may include a change in antiretroviral therapy.

Seizures may occur at any stage of HIV infection and may be focal or generalized. The incidence is uncertain, but in one study of 100 consecutive cases, secondary pathogens were identified in 53% and HIV encephalopathy in 24%; there was no identified cause in 23%. All patients with seizures should be evaluated for other pathogens or tumor.

Leukoencephalopathies in acute or chronic HIV infection include acute fulminating and fatal leukoencephalitis; multifocal vacuolar leukoencephalopathy presenting as rapid dementia; and a relapsing-remitting leukoencephalitis that may simulate multiple sclerosis. The pathogenesis of these syndromes is uncertain. A severe demyelinating leukoencephalopathy with intense perivascular infiltration by HIV-gp41 immunoreactive monocytes/macrophages and lymphocytes is described in patients who failed HAART treatment despite good virologic response in one case. Some speculate this illness is a form of immune reconstitution disease.

Chronic progressive myelopathy, an AIDS-defining illness, is characterized by progressive spastic, ataxic paraparesis with bowel and bladder disorders. Although most patients rapidly become wheelchair bound, others progress indolently for years. Subclinical myelopathy may be detected by electrophysiologic studies in otherwise asymptomatic subjects. Pathologic findings are similar to those of subacute combined degeneration owing to vitamin B_{12} deficiency and include vacuolar change with intramyelin swelling or demyelination that is most severe in the lateral and posterior columns. Microglial nodules and giant cells are sometimes seen, and HIV may be detected by hybridization techniques or cultured. Pathologic abnormalities are more commonly detected than clinical symptoms. The diagnosis of HIV myelopathy requires exclusion of cord compression, cord ischemia, secondary infections, and nutritional deficiency. MRI may show gadolinium-enhanced lesions of myelitis.

No specific treatment is available for myelopathy. Improvement on azidothymidine (AZT) therapy has been reported, but the drug is generally ineffective. The impact of protease inhibitors and HAART is unknown.

Amyotrophic lateral sclerosis-like (ALS) illness is reported in several cases as an initial illness in unrecognized HIV infection, and with varying degrees of immunosuppression from profoundly reduced to near normal CD 4 lymphocyte levels. EMO features were consistent with ALS in one series of six patients. Patients were distinguished from classic sporadic ALS by young age, rapid clinical progression, co-occurrence of dementia in two cases with imaging abnormalities and improvement with antiretroviral therapy. Complete recovery is reported with virologic control of HIV, suggesting a direct pathogenetic role of the virus in the illness. Autopsy of two cases disclosed motor neuron loss in one.

Peripheral and autonomic neuropathy occur in otherwise asymptomatic HIV-infected subjects, especially with advancing disease. Clinical syndromes include mononeuritis multiplex, chronic inflammatory demyelinating polyneuropathy (CIDP), distal symmetric polyneuropathy, and ganglioneuritis.

CIDP is distinguished from Guillain-Barré syndrome by a subacute or progressive course and variable response to steroids or plasmapheresis. Electrodiagnostic studies show demyelination with variable axonal damage. Histopathologic studies reveal epineurial inflammatory cell infiltrates and primary demyelination with variable axonal degeneration. HIV is sometimes cultured from nerve. CSF findings are nondiagnostic, although pleocytosis is sometimes found.

Distal sensorimotor neuropathy is the most common peripheral nerve disorder of AIDS, increasing in frequency with advancing disease. The incidence of neuropathy is also increasing because of longer survival of HIV infected people. Symptoms include painful, burning dysesthesias that are often confined to the soles of the feet. Signs include stocking-glove sensory loss, mild muscle wasting and weakness, and loss of ankle jerks. Conduction studies show sensorimotor neuropathy with mixed axonal and demyelinating features.

Pathologic findings include axonal degeneration, loss of large myelinated fibers, and variable inflammatory cell infiltration. Vasculitis is sometimes found. CSF may be normal or show mild pleocytosis and elevated protein content. HIV may be cultured from nerve, but the cellular localization of the virus is not known. The neuropathy may be mediated by the binding of gp120 envelope viral glycoprotein to sensory ganglion cells.

The pain syndrome may be disabling, sometimes responsive to tricyclic antidepressants, anticonvulsants, and nonsteroidal or narcotic analgesia. Pain control may be difficult. Peptide T was ineffective in clinical trials. Immune globulin is sometimes used in refractory cases with anecdotal reports of success. Vasculitis may respond to prednisone. Clinical trials show that lamotrigine and recombinant human nerve growth factor are effective treatments. The latter is currently unavailable.

Myopathy is uncommon, characterized by proximal limb weakness, mild creatine kinase elevation, and myopathic features on EMG. Pathologic findings include muscle fiber degeneration with or without inflammatory cell infiltrates. An HIV-related cause is suspected after exclusion of other causes. AZT causes a clinically similar myopathy related to effects on mitochondria, with ragged red fibers. Cytochrome oxidase is deficient in AZT and not in HIV myopathy. Some patients respond well to steroid therapy without accelerated progression of HIV disease.

OPPORTUNISTIC INFECTIONS AND NEOPLASMS

Secondary opportunistic infections and neoplasia are diagnostic of AIDS (Table 25.7).

Their incidence and severity have declined since 1996 because of potent combination antiretroviral regimens that include protease inhibitors. Even before the use of potent drug regimens for HIV, prophylactic therapy had decreased the incidence of many infections.

Meningitis may be due to viruses (herpes group [HSV, VZV, CMV, and Epstein-Barr virus (EBV)], hepatitis B and C), fungi (cryptococcus, Histoplasma, Coccidioides, Candida) bacteria (Listeria, Treponema pallidum, pyogenic bacteria, Salmonella, Staphylococcus aureus, atypical or conventional mycobacteria), and neoplasm (lymphoma). Cryptococcal infection, the most common cause of meningitis in AIDS, reported in 6% to 11% of patients in older clinical series, has declined in incidence due to HAART and prophylactic therapy. There are no specific distinguishing features except that meningeal signs may be mild or absent. The diagnosis is made by detecting cryptococcal antigen in serum and CSF or by CSF culture. CSF cell count and chemistries may be normal or nondiagnostic when antigen is present. Stains of centrifuged CSF sediment may be more sensitive than antigen detection or India ink stains. CT may show normal patterns, atrophy, mass lesion (cryptococcoma), hydrocephalus, or diffuse edema.

Treatment is discussed in Chapter 26. Oral agents (fluconazole and itraconazole) have generally replaced amphotericin B in management. Oral prophylaxis in late-stage HIV may prevent most fungal infections. Chronic suppressive therapy, once thought necessary for life, may be discontinued in accordance with CDC guidelines for successful immune reconstitution (CD 4+ T lymphocyte counts greater than 100 cells/μL to 200 cells/μL for longer than 6 months). Relapses may occur but are uncommon. Prophylaxis must be resumed if CD 4 counts decline below 100 cells/μL.

The clinical course of neurosyphilis may be altered by concomitant HIV infection. Occasionally, CSF Venereal Disease Research Laboratory (VDRL) test is nonreactive, and baseline CSF abnormalities render interpretation of CSF data difficult when the diagnosis is suspected. A study of neurosyphilis during the AIDS epidemic in San Francisco found 117 cases of neurosyphilis in an 8-year period, with 3,827 cases of early syphilis reported for the same period. Only 44 of these cases had neurologic syndromes clearly attributable to syphilis. Syndromes of early neurosyphilis (meningitis, meningovascular syndromes, uveitis with meningitis) were more common than late syndromes (general paresis and tabes dorsalis). Intravenous penicillin therapy is required for documented neurosyphilis. Relapse is more common in HIV-infected people, and follow-up is needed after cessation of therapy. Serology is tested monthly for 3 months and at 3-month intervals thereafter. If serologic titers rise, re-treatment is indicated.

The best treatment for late lues in dually affected patients is controversial. Some argue that intravenous therapy should be used in all dually infected patients even when the CSF is normal. We reserve intravenous therapy for symptomatic patients with positive serum and CSF serology and monitor those who do not meet criteria for neurosyphilis, as discussed in Chapter 28.

Tuberculous meningitis, atypical mycobacterial infection of brain, and tuberculomas are risks in HIV-infected persons. Conventional antituberculous therapy is usually effective for conventional mycobacteria. Prophylaxis with clarithromycin or azithromycin is reasonably effective for infections by atypical organisms, which otherwise require multidrug regimens. The incidence of tuberculous disease and drug resistance in AIDS has declined dramatically due to effective treatment strategies that include directly observed therapy. Atypical organisms are less common because of potent HIV therapy. Prophylaxis for atypical organisms may be discontinued for HAART-treated patients when CD 4 counts are greater than 100 cells/μL for longer than 3 months, and should be resumed when they decline to less than 100 cells/μL.

Viral encephalitis may be due to the herpes group, CMV most commonly, and HSV and VZV infrequently. Hepatitis C is an important co-morbid infection in HIV and may cause encephalopathy. Mycobacterium avium- intracellulare, toxoplasmosis, and lymphoma may also cause diffuse encephalopathy.

Focal brain syndromes are caused by toxoplasmosis, PML, abscesses owing to Nocardia, Listeria, Trypanosoma cruzi, Taenia solium, Candida, Cryptococcus,

▶ **TABLE 25.7 Secondary Neurologic Syndromes in HIV Infection and AIDS:
                 Opportunistic Infections and Neoplasms**

Leptomeninges
Viral
   CMV, HSV, VZV, EBV, hepatitis B and C
Fungal
   Cryptococcus, Histoplasma, Coccidioides, Candida
Bacterial
   Listeria, T. pallidum, pyogenic bacteria (Salmonella,
      Staphylococcus aureus) atypical or conventional
      mycobacteria
Neoplasm
   Lymphoma
Cerebral Syndromes
Diffuse Encephalopathy or Encephalitis
Viral
   CMV, HSV, VZV, hepatitis C
Bacterial
   Atypical mycobacterium
Parasitic
   Acanthamoeba, toxoplasmosis
Neoplasm
   Lymphoma
Focal Cerebral Syndromes
Viral
   HSV, VZV, PML
Fungal
   Abscess due to Cryptococcus, Candida, Zygomycetes,
      Histoplasma, Aspergillus
Bacterial
   Abscess due to pyogenic bacteria, mycobacteria
      (tuberculoma), Listeria, Nocardia
Parasitic
   Trypanosoma cruzi, Taenia solium, toxoplasmosis
Neoplasm
   Primary or metastatic lymphoma, glioma, metastatic Kaposi
      sarcoma
Cerebrovascular Syndromes and Seizures
Viral
   VZV, HSV, rarely PML
Fungal
   Cryptococcus or other fungi
Bacterial
   T. pallidum, M. tuberculosis

Parasitic
   Toxoplasmosis
Neoplasm
   Lymphoma, lymphomatoid granulomatosis, metastatic Kaposi
      sarcoma
Other
   Cerebral hemorrhage, cardiac emboli, vasculitis
Movement Disorders
Viral
   Progressive multifocal leukoencephalopathy; HIV
Bacterial
   CNS Whipple disease
Parasitic
   Toxoplasmosis
Spinal Cord Syndromes
Viral
   VZV, CMV, HSV, HTLV 1
Fungal
   Cryptococcus, *Sporotrichum schenckii*
Bacterial
   Mycobacteria
   Pyogenic bacteria
   Syphilis
Parasitic
   Toxoplasmosis
Neoplasm
   Lymphoma
   Kaposi sarcoma
Cranial and Peripheral Neuropathy
Viral
   CMV (retinitis, polyradiculitis, mononeuritis multiplex)
Bacterial
   Syphilis (uveitis, retinitis)
Fungal
   Candida (retinitis)
Parasitic
   Toxoplasmosis (retinitis)
Myositis
Bacterial
   S. aureus, mycobacteria
Parasitic
   Toxoplasmosis

Histoplasma, Aspergillosis, Coccidioides, Mycobacterium tuberculosis, atypical mycobacteria, and pyogenic bacteria.

Toxoplasmosis, the most common cause of intracranial mass lesions in AIDS, typically causes chronic, progressive focal signs and seizures. In some cases, the clinical disorder is one of subacute encephalopathy. CT or MRI discloses enhancing lesions with mass effect, typically involving the basal ganglia (Fig. 25.2).

Although the radiographic findings are not diagnostic, multiple lesions in the basal ganglia in patients with antitoxoplasma antibodies are presumptive evidence. CSF is nondiagnostic; highly specific polymerase chain reaction may detect toxoplasma DNA but is insensitive with case detection rates of 40% to 80%. Toxoplasmosis antibodies are found in more than 95% of patients. Seronegative toxoplasmosis is rare. Differential diagnosis is mainly lymphoma or, rarely, pyogenic abscess. Toxoplasmosis is treated in patients at risk for HIV, multiple lesions, and antibodies to the organism. Biopsy is reserved for those who show no clinical or radiographic response after a week of therapy.

Both prophylactic therapy and HAART have dramatically reduced the incidence of toxoplasmosis. Suppressive

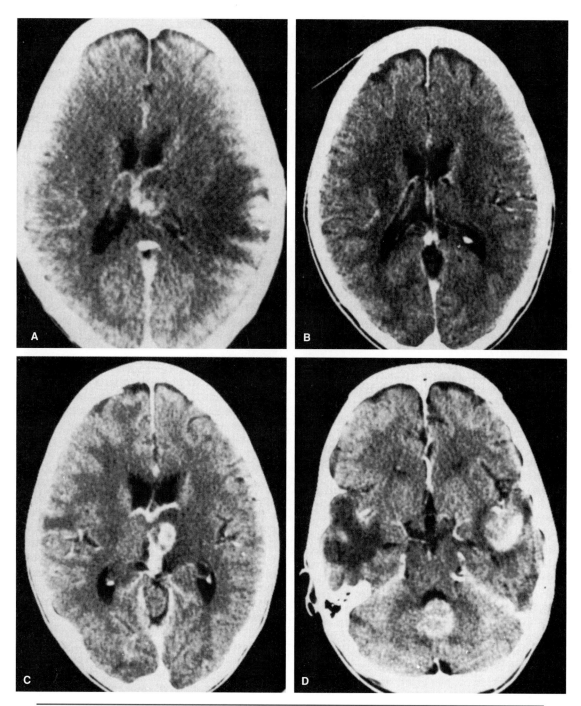

FIGURE 25.2. AIDS, toxoplasmosis. **A:** A contrast-enhanced axial CT scan shows left thalamic parietal and nodular enhancing lesions with adjacent edema and mass effect consistent with toxoplasmosis. **B:** A follow-up contrast-enhanced scan 6 weeks later demonstrates resolution of the lesions and mass effect with therapy. **C** and **D:** Contrast-enhanced axial CT scans obtained at the same (C), and lower (D) levels 11 weeks later demonstrate recurrent nodular and ring enhancement in the left thalamus with adjacent edema and mass effect. The edema in the right frontal and temporal regions, in (C) and (D), is related to another lesion. Additional enhancing lesions are present in the left temporal region and vermis (D). (Courtesy of Drs. J. A. Bello and S. K. Hilal.)

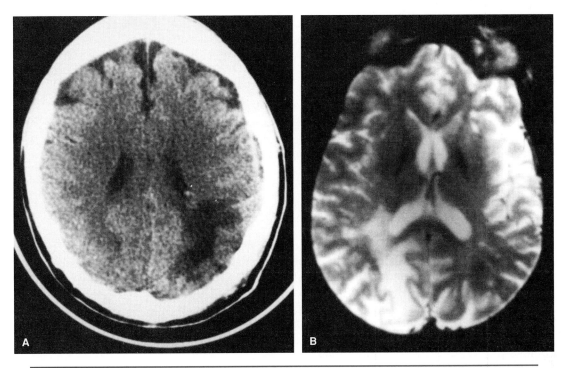

FIGURE 25.3. A: CT scan from a patient with biopsy-proven PML showing hypointense parieto-occipital lesion without mast effect. **B:** T2-weighted MRI scan from patient with biopsy-proven PML showing hyperintense parieto-occipital lesion.

therapy may be discontinued for those with successful reconstitution on HAART, CD4 counts of greater than 200 cells/μL for longer than 6 months, and resumed for CD 4 counts less than 200 cells/μL.

PML, before AIDS, was a rare infection seen in immunosuppressed people. After PML was recognized as a complication of AIDS in 1982, the death rate increased in the general population from 1.5 cases to 6.1 cases per 10 million population. The reported incidence in AIDS is 1.0% to 5.3%. Lytic viral infection of oligodendrocytes causes demyelination and progressive focal signs. Localization is hemispheric in 85% to 90% of cases; the posterior fossa is affected in the remainder. Focal or generalized seizures occur in 6% of patients.

PML may be the first AIDS-defining illness and may occur when immunosuppression is not severe. Prognosis is generally poor with death in 4 months to 6 months. The diagnosis may be suspected in a patient with focal signs, hypodense nonenhancing lesions on CT, and no mass effect. MRI is more sensitive, with high signal intensity lesions on T2-weighted studies without mass effect or enhancement (Fig. 25.3). The causative virus may be detected in CSF by PCR but a negative study does not exclude the diagnosis. Diagnosis requires brain biopsy in those who are CSF-PCR negative because imaging abnormalities may overlap those of toxoplasmosis, fungal infection, and lymphoma.

There may be spontaneous stabilization of PML lesions in HIV infection, and there may be a response to HAART. Clinical trials failed to show beneficial effect of intravenous or intrathecal cytosine arabinoside, topotecan, and cidofovir despite anecdotal reports of efficacy. HAART-immune reconstitution favorably impacts the clinical course of some, but not all patients with PML. This may be explained by a selective loss of JCV-specific CD4 cells. An improved prognosis is also associated with PML as the AIDS-defining illness, with CD4 cell counts greater than 300 cells/μL, evidence of inflammatory response indicated by gadolinium enhancement on MRI, and a low number or reduction in the JCV viral load in CSF. The impact of HAART on PML incidence is uncertain.

Lymphoma incidence is profoundly reduced from a range of 0.6% to 3% of patients in pre-HAART clinical series, to rare or no occurrence in post-HAART series. Clinical signs are nonspecific and include focal neurologic signs, seizures, cranial neuropathy, and headache. CT may be normal or may show hypodense lesions and single or multiple lesions with patchy or nodular enhancement. Epstein Barr virus DNA is found in PCR studies of CSF. Brain biopsy is required for diagnosis. Response to therapy with radiation and chemotherapy is improved by HAART, with longer survivals and reports of complete tumor regression. Opportunistic infections may coexist with tumor and should be excluded by appropriate studies.

Other neoplasms reported in AIDS include metastatic Kaposi sarcoma and rarely, primary glial tumors. Like lymphoma, the incidence of Kaposi sarcoma is dramatically decreased by effective immune reconstitution with HAART.

Movement disorders in patients with HIV infection are usually symptomatic of underlying cerebral infection, with toxoplasmosis most commonly seen. Dystonia is reported as a result of PML, toxoplasmosis, and neuroleptic sensitivity. Cerebellar syndromes are reported due to HIV alone or secondary opportunistic infection or tumor.

Infection of the spinal cord has been reported with the herpes group viruses, including HSV, CMV, and VZV; mycobacteria; pyogenic bacteria; fungus; and toxoplasmosis. Spinal-cord biopsy is necessary for definitive diagnosis and may be considered if systemic infection suggests metastatic foci in spinal cord. Metastatic non-Hodgkin lymphoma, primary lymphoma and Kaposi are reported in spinal cord, cauda equina, or vertebral bodies.

Infectious retinopathy may be caused by syphilis, toxoplasmosis, CMV, or Candida. *Cranial neuropathy* may complicate meningitis. Polyradiculopathy or cauda equina syndrome may be due to CMV infection. The diagnosis may be suspected, clinically, in patients with disseminated CMV and may respond to ganciclovir and foscarnet. Antiviral therapy may be given to patients with an otherwise typical syndrome even before CMV infection is confirmed. PCR studies of CSF are helpful if they produce positive results but negative studies do not exclude the diagnosis. Quantitative plasma PCR may identify persons at risk for CMV disease. Without treatment, the syndrome is progressive and fatal. Both the incidence and severity of CMV disease are lessened by potent antiretroviral therapy for HIV. There are CDC criteria for discontinuing prophylaxis for CMV retinitis but not for other neurologic syndromes. *Pyomyositis* may be caused by infection with *Staphylococcus aureus*, toxoplasmosis, or atypical mycobacteria.

DRUG-INDUCED SYNDROMES

The nucleoside analogs used to treat HIV infection cause dose-related and duration-related neurologic complications. Chronic zidovudine therapy may cause myopathy with ragged red fibers. Symptoms usually improve following cessation of the drug. The nucleoside antiretrovirals didanosine, zalcitabine, stavudine, and lamivudine may cause severe, dose-related, painful sensory neuropathy that is clinically indistinguishable from HIV neuropathy; it often improves after dose reduction or drug withdrawal. Failure to improve may indicate the comorbid occurrence of HIV-related neuropathy.

Patients with HIV infection experience hypersensitivity to many drugs, among them the neuroleptics, which may cause secondary parkinsonism or the neuroleptic malignant syndrome. *Nutritional deficiency* may include thiamine, vitamin B_{12}, folic acid, and glutathione, the lack of which may lead to encephalopathy, dementia, neuropathy, or spinal cord disorders. Metabolic abnormalities often occur in late-stage disease and are reversible causes

of encephalopathy. Testosterone deficiency in increasingly recognized in long survivors and may contribute to encephalopathy.

Diagnostic Evaluation

The diagnostic evaluation of patients with a suspected HIV-related illness includes an enzyme-linked immunosorbent assay (ELISA) for HIV serology. Positive results are confirmed by Western blot. Depending on local laws, serologic tests may require informed consent and counseling. In patients with otherwise typical viral syndromes, such as aseptic meningitis or transverse myelitis, HIV infection must be suspected even in the absence of known high-risk behavior. Absence of antibodies during the acute illness does not negate the diagnosis because these disorders typically occur with seroconversion. A convalescent titer should be obtained at least 6 weeks later and possibly again at 3 months and 6 months, to ensure true seronegativity. Rarely, patients may be seronegative for prolonged periods. Repeat testing or studies to detect viral antigen or nucleic acid are warranted in the presence of high-risk behavior or other indicative clinical information.

Other diagnostic studies include determination of CD-lymphocyte subset ratio, plasma HIV viral load, serum protein electrophoresis, quantitative immunoglobulins, and enumerated platelets. Baseline CSF HIV-1 RNA levels are not standard practice at this time. An anergy panel may assess deficient functional immune status.

Evaluation for specific neurologic syndromes should be preceded by a general physical examination, to exclude opportunistic infections or tumor. Evaluation may include biopsy of skin, lymph nodes, or bone marrow as well as chest radiography. Blood culture for viruses and fungi may be necessary.

Accurate neurologic diagnosis requires systematic evaluation, including assessment for the possibility of multiple diseases. EEG may show evidence of a focal lesion when scans are still nondiagnostic. CSF is most helpful in syphilis and fungal or tuberculous infection. In lymphoma meningitis, tumor cells are rarely recognized by cytologic studies. Viruses are infrequently cultured from CSF; HIV may be detected but may be a copassenger and not responsible for the disorder in question. HIV-1 RNA levels should be determined when lumbar puncture is performed, as CNS virologic escape is a risk for HIV-related syndromes such as dementia.

If hepatitis C coinfection is present, RNA levels in plasma and CSF should be assessed, as is the case for HIV. CMV may be cultured in CMV-related polyradiculopathy. Polymerase chain reaction of CSF may be helpful for pathogenic diagnosis of HSV, VZV, CMV, toxoplasma and PML, but negative results do not exclude the infection. CSF abnormalities are common in asymptomatic HIV infection and must be interpreted with caution in considering other possible conditions. CT or MRI is useful in distinguishing focal from diffuse brain lesions. Magnetic resonance spectroscopy (MRS) and thallium-SPECT may distinguish tumor from infection. Brain biopsy may be required for differential diagnosis. Stereotactic biopsy is a low-risk procedure in experienced hands. For solitary lesions, it is reasonable to treat for toxoplasmosis when serology or PCR is positive; biopsy is reserved for failure to respond to treatment and for PCR and seronegative cases.

Myelopathy is evaluated by MRI with gadolinium. CSF may be helpful in evaluating peripheral neuropathies, especially CMV polyneuropathy. EMG and nerve conduction studies are useful in evaluating myelopathy, anterior-horn cell disease, peripheral neuropathy, and myopathy. Nerve or muscle biopsy may be required.

Treatment, Course, and Prognosis

Potent combination antiretroviral therapy has transformed the course of AIDS from a fatal disease to a chronic illness. In the U.S., AIDS diagnosis and AIDS deaths have declined since 1996. Even before potent drug therapy for HIV, prophylactic therapy of common opportunistic infections reduced the incidence of AIDS and AIDS deaths. Improved medical care has reduced the need for hospital admissions in this population.

Antiretroviral drugs improve morbidity, owing to HIV and extended survival. Nineteen drugs in four classes have been approved for use, and more are in clinical trials or development, as follows: nucleoside reverse transcriptase (nRTI) inhibitor; nonnucleoside reverse transcriptase inhibitor (NNRTI); nucleotide RT inhibitor (ntRTI); and protease inhibitor (PI); fusion inhibitors. Nucleoside RT inhibitors block viral replication by incorporation into the DNA copy of the RNA genome and termination of the DNA synthesis. Included are 3'-azido-3-deoxythymidine (zidovudine), the dideoxy-nucleosides, dideoxyinosine and dideoxycytidine, lamivudine, stavudine, zalcitabine, and abacavir. Nonnucleoside RT inhibitors include nevirapine, delavirdine and efavirenz. Adefovir dipivoxil is the sole nucleotide-analog RT inhibitor. Protease inhibitors include ritonavir, saquinavir, indinavir, nelfinavir, amprenavir, lopinavir, fosamprenavir and atazanavir. Enfuvirtide, an HIV fusion inhibitor, is well tolerated and effective for treatment of resistant infection. Combination drug therapy that includes a protease inhibitor is recommended. New drugs are in development that target various phases of the viral cycle, and include attachment inhibitors, chemokine receptor inhibitors, HIV fusion inhibitors, and HIV integrase inhibitors. Despite improved therapy, HIV infection is a serious diagnosis and rapidly fatal in developing countries, there is no access to effective treatment. There are efforts by the World Health Organization and developed nations to address the dire need of developing countries but for many these efforts may be too little and too late. There are some successes in stabilization of the epidemic in developing countries with aggressive public health and treatment campaigns, such as Uganda and Brazil. However, therapy does not eliminate latent provirus and may fail if resistant mutants arise. There are ongoing efforts to develop an effective vaccine. Candidate vaccines are in clinical trials in areas of high seroprevalence and seroconversion. The complex biology of the virus and the host immunogenetic response to infection pose significant challenges to successful vaccine development.

PRECAUTIONS FOR CLINICAL AND LABORATORY SERVICES

Strict observation of contamination management procedures or universal precautions is mandatory. The hospital patient with known or suspected HIV infection is not isolated unless there is a respiratory infection, such as tuberculosis, or severe neutropenia. Strict precautions should be observed in the handling of all waste, body fluids, and surgical specimens. Gloves are worn to prevent skin and mucocutaneous contact with blood, excretions, secretions, and tissues of infected patients. Goggles or glasses should be used if heavy aerosol contamination with blood or other secretions is anticipated (e.g., in the operating room). Masks are not needed unless the patient requires respiratory isolation for other reasons. Needles and other sharp instruments in contact with infected blood should be disposed of in proper safety containers. Health-care workers should not recap needles to avoid needle-stick injury.

The risks to health-care workers are small but real. At least 57 people have been documented with HIV seroconversion following needle-stick injury or mucocutaneous exposure. The converse risk to patients from infected workers is exceedingly small, but HIV-positive workers should not engage in invasive procedures in which cuts may occur. Postexposure prophylaxis is recommended with two drugs for HIV exposure through percutaneous or mucosal routes and with three drugs for significant blood exposure, i.e. visibly contaminated needle or device with deep penetration. HIV, hepatitis B and C serologies are immediately determined. Problems encountered with postexposure prophylaxis include side effects of therapy, lack of efficacy, and false-positive HIV tests on rapid screening assays. Postexposure treatment is estimated to reduce HIV transmission risk by 80%.

HIV is readily inactivated by heat and standard sterilization solutions, including 70% alcohol. Special sterilization procedures may not be necessary but are often used.

HIV-infected patients in treatment may survive more than 20 years and may die of HIV infection, causes unrelated to HIV infection, or of complications related to treatment. The patients need rigorous evaluation for systemic and neurologic syndromes at all stages of infection, owing to the risk for multiple, coexistent, or sequential problems.

SUGGESTED READINGS

Albrecht H, Hoffmann C, Degen O, et al. Highly active antiretroviral therapy significantly improves the prognosis of patients with HIV-associated progressive multifocal leukoencephalopathy. *AIDS* 1998;12:1149–1154.

Ameisen JC, Lelievre JD, Pleskoff O. HIV/host interactions: new lessons from the Red Queen's country. *AIDS* 2002;16 (suppl 4):S25–S31.

American Academy of AIDS Task Force. Nomenclature and research case definition for neurologic manifestations of human immunodeficiency virus-type (HIV-1) infection. *Neurology* 1991;41:778–785.

Antinori A, Ammassari A, De Luca A, et al. Diagnosis of AIDS-related focal brain lesions: A decision-making analysis based on clinical and neuroradiologic characteristics combined with polymerase chain reaction assays in CSF. *Neurology* 1997;48:687–694.

Behar R, Wiley C, McCutchan JA. Cytomegalovirus polyradiculoneuropathy in acquired immune deficiency syndrome. *Neurology* 1987;37:557–561.

Bencherif B, Rottenberg DA. Neuroimaging of the AIDS dementia complex. *AIDS* 1998;12:233–244.

Berger JR, Tornatore C, Major EO, et al. Relapsing and remitting human immunodeficiency virus-associated leukoencephalomyelopathy. *Ann Neurol* 1992;31:34–38.

Bossolasco S, Marenzi R, Dahl H, et al. Human herpesvirus 6 in cerebrospinal fluid of patients infected with HIV: frequency and clinical significance. *J Neurol Neurosurg Psychiatry* 1999;67:789–792.

Bozzette SA, Ake CF, Tam HK, et al. Cardiovascular and cerebrovascular events in patients treated for human immunodeficiency virus infection. *N Engl J Med* 2003;348:702–710.

Brander C, Riviere Y. Early and late cytotoxic T lymphocyte responses in HIV infection. *AIDS* 2002;16(suppl 4):S97–S103.

Brew BJ, Pemberton L, Cunningham P, Law MG. Levels of human immunodeficiency virus type I RNA I cerebrospinal fluid correlate with AIDS dementia stage. *J Infect Dis* 1997;175:963–966.

Britton CB, Mesa-Tejada R, Fenoglio CM, et al. A new complication of AIDS: thoracic myelitis caused by herpes simplex virus. *Neurology* 1985;35:1071–1074.

Buchacz KA, Wilkinson DA, Krowka JF, et al. Genetic and immunological host factors associated with susceptibility to HIV-1 infection. *AIDS* 1998;12(suppl A):S87–S94.

Centers for Disease Control and Prevention. 1993 Revised classification system for HIV infection and expanded surveillance case definition for AIDS among adolescents and adults. *MMWR* 1992;41(RR-17): 1–19.

Centers for Disease Control and Prevention. Advancing HIV prevention: new strategies for a changing epidemic—United States, 2003. *MMWR* 2003;52:329–332.

Chalmers AC, Greco CM, Miller RG. Prognosis in AZT myopathy. *Neurology* 1991;41:1181–1184.

Centers for Disease Control and Prevention. Guidelines for preventing opportunistic infections among HIV-infected persons-2002. Recommendations of the U.S. Public Health Service and the Infectious Diseases Society of America. *MMWR* 2002;51(RR-6):1–26.

Centers for Disease Control and Prevention. Updated U.S. Public Health Service guidelines for the management of occupational exposures to HBV, HCV and HIV and recommendations for postexposure prophylaxis. *MMWR* 2001;50(RR-11):1–52.

Chang L, Ernst T, Leonido-Yee M, et al. Cerebral metabolite abnormalities correlate with clinical severity of HIV-1 cognitive motor complex. *Neurology* 1999;52:100–108.

Cinque P, Vago L, Ceresa D, et al. Cerebrospinal fluid HIV-1 RNA levels: correlation with HIV encephalitis. *AIDS* 1998;12:389–394.

Cornblath DR, McArthur JC, Kennedy PG, et al. Inflammatory demyelinating peripheral neuropathies associated with human T-cell lymphotrophic virus type III infection. *Ann Neurol* 1987;21:32–40.

The Dana Consortium on the Therapy of HIV Dementia and Related Cognitive Disorders. A randomized, double-blind, placebo-controlled trial of deprenyl and thioctic acid in human immunodeficiency virus-associated cognitive impairment. *Neurology* 1998;50:645–651.

De Luca A, Ciancio BC, Larussa D, et al. Correlates of independent HIV-1 replication in the CNS and of its control by antiretrovirals. *Neurology* 2002;59:342–347.

Dore GJ, McDonald A, Yueming L, et al. Marked improvement in survival following AIDS dementia complex in the era of highly active antiretroviral therapy. *AIDS* 2003;17:1539–1545.

Eidelberg D, Sotrel A, Vogel H, et al. Progressive polyradiculopathy in acquired immunodeficiency syndrome. *Neurology* 1986;36:912–916.

Eilbott DJ, Peress N, Burger H, et al. Human immunodeficiency virus type 1 in spinal cords of acquired immunodeficiency syndrome patients with myelopathy: Expression and replication in macrophages. *Proc Natl Acad Sci USA* 1989;86:3337–3341.

Ellis RJ, Moore DJ, Childers ME, et al. Progression to neuropsychological impairment in human immunodeficiency virus infection predicted by elevated cerebrospinal fluid levels of human immunodeficiency virus RNA. *Arch Neurol* 2002;58:923–928.

Epstein LG, Gendelman HE. Human immunodeficiency virus type 1 infection of the nervous system: pathogenetic mechanisms. *Ann Neurol* 1993;33:429–436.

Epstein LG, Sharer LR, Oleske JM, et al. Neurologic manifestations of human immunodeficiency virus infection in children. *Pediatrics* 1986;78:678–687.

Factor SA, Troche-Panetto M, Weaver SA. Dystonia in AIDS: report of four cases. *Mov Disord* 2003;18:1492–1498.

Flexner C. HIV-protease inhibitors. *N Engl J Med* 1998;338:1281–1292.

Flood JM, Weinstock HS, Guroy ME, et al. Neurosyphilis during the AIDS epidemic, San Francisco, 1985–1992. *J Infect Dis* 1998;177:931–940.

Gao F, Bailes E, Robertson DL, et al. Origin of HIV-1 in the chimpanzee Pan troglodytes. *Nature* 1999;397:436–441.

Gao X, Nelson GW, Karacki P, et al. Effect of a single amino acid change in MHC class I molecules on the rate of progression to AIDS. *N Engl J Med* 2001;344:1668–1675.

Geberding JL. Occupational exposure to HIV in health care settings. *N Engl J Med* 2003;348:826–833.

Goldstein JD, Dickson DW, Moser FG, et al. Primary central nervous system lymphoma in acquired immune deficiency syndrome. A clinical and pathologic study with results of treatment with radiation. *Cancer* 1991;67:2755–2765.

Gray F, Chretien F, Vallat Decouvelaere V, Scaravilli F. The changing pattern of HIV neuropathology in the HAART era. *J Neuropathol Exp Neurol* 2003;62:429–440.

Haase AT, Henry K, Zupancic M, et al. Quantitative tissue analysis of HIV-1 infection in lymphoid tissue. *Science* 1996;274:985–989.

Hall CD, Dafni U, Simpson D, et al. Failure of cytarabine in progressive multifocal leukoencephalopathy associated with human immunodeficiency virus infection. *N Engl J Med* 1998;338:1345–1351.

Hengge UR, Brockmeyer NH, Esser S, et al. HIV-1 RNA levels in cerebrospinal fluid and plasma correlate with AIDS dementia. *AIDS* 1998;12:818–820.

Ho DD, Rota TR, Schooley RT, et al. Isolation of HTLV-III from cerebrospinal fluid and neural tissues of patients with neurologic syndromes related to the acquired immunodeficiency syndrome. *N Engl J Med* 1985;313:1493–1497.

Hoffman TL, Doms RW. Chemokines and coreceptors in HIV/SIV-host interactions. *AIDS* 1998;12(suppl A):S17–S26.

Hollander H, Stringari S. Human immunodeficiency virus-associated meningitis. Clinical course and complications. *Am J Med* 1987;83:813–816.

Holtzman DM, Kaku DA, So YT. New onset seizures associated with human immunodeficiency virus infection: causation and clinical features in 100 cases. *Am J Med* 1989;87:173–177.

Husstedt IW, Grotemeyer KH, Busch H, et al. Progression of distal-symmetric polyneuropathy in HIV infection: a prospective study. *AIDS* 1993;7:1069–1073.

Jacobson MA, French M. Altered natural history of AIDS-related opportunistic infections in the era of potent combination antiretroviral therapy. *AIDS* 1998;12(suppl A):S157–S163.

Julander I, Martin C, Lappalainen M, et al. Polymerase chain reaction for diagnosis of cerebral toxoplasmosis in cerebrospinal fluid in HIV-positive patients. *Scand J Infect Dis* 2001;33:538–541.

Kahn JO, Walker BD. Acute human immunodeficiency virus type 1 infection. *N Engl J Med* 1998;339:33–39.

Kilby JM, Eron JJ. Novel therapies based on mechanisms of HIV-1 cell entry. *N Engl J Med* 2003;348:2228–2238.

Langford TD, Letendre SL, Marcotte TD, et al. Severe demyelinating leukoencephalopathy in AIDS patients on antiretroviral therapy. *AIDS* 2002;16:1019–1029.

Lascaux AS, Lesprit P, Deforges L, et al. Late cerebral relapse of a Mycobacterium avium complex disseminated infection in an HIV-infected patient after cessation of antiretroviral therapy. *AIDS* 2003;17:1410–1411.

Luft BJ, Haffner R, Korzun AH, et al. Toxoplasmic encephalitis in patients with the acquired immunodeficiency syndrome. *N Engl J Med* 1993;329:995–1000.

MacGowan DJL, Scelsa SN, Waldron M. An ALS-like syndrome with new HIV infection and complete response to antiretroviral therapy. *Neurology* 2001;57:1094–1097.

Mahe A, Bruet A, Chabin E, et al. Acute rhabdomyolysis coincident with primary HIV infection (Letter). *Lancet* 1989;2:1454–1455.

Marra CM, Rajicic N, Barker DE, et al. A pilot study of cidofovir for progressive multifocal leukoencephalopathy in AIDS. *AIDS* 2002;16:1791–1797.

Martin-Garcia, Kolson DL, Gonzalez-Scarano G. Chemokine receptors in the brain: their role in HIV infection and pathogenesis. *AIDS* 2002;16:1709–1730.

Maschke M, Kastrup O, Esser S, et al. Incidence and prevalence of neurological disorders associated with HIV since the introduction of highly active antiretroviral therapy (HAART). *J Neurol Neurosurg Psychiatry* 2000;69:376–380.

Mayeux R, Stern Y, Tang M-X, et al. Mortality risks in gay men with human immunodeficiency virus infection and cognitive impairment. *Neurology* 1993;43:176–182.

McArthur JC, Hoover DR, Bacellar H, et al. Dementia in AIDS patients: Incidence and risk factors. *Neurology* 1993;38:2245–2252.

McGowan JP, Shah S. Long-term remission of AIDS-related primary central nervous lymphoma associated with highly active antiretroviral therapy (letter). *AIDS* 1998;12:952–954.

Mellors JW, Rinaldo Jr CR, Gupta P, et al. Prognosis in HIV-1 infection predicted by the quantity of virus in plasma. *Science* 1996;272:1167–1170.

Michelet C, Arvieux C, Francois C, et al. Opportunistic infections occurring during highly active antiretroviral treatment. *AIDS* 1998;12:1815–1822.

Miller EN, Selnes OA, McArthur JC, et al. Neuropsychological performance in HIV-1-infected homosexual men: the Multicenter AIDS Cohort Study (MACS). *Neurology* 1990;40:197–203.

Miller JR, Barrett RE, Britton CB, et al. Progressive multifocal leukoencephalopathy in a male homosexual with T-cell immune deficiency. *N Engl J Med* 1982;307:1436–1438.

Morner A, Thomas JA, Bjorling, et al. Productive HIV-2 infection in the brain is restricted to macrophages/microglia. *AIDS* 2003;17:1451–1455.

Moulignier A, Moulonguet A, Pialoux G, Rozenbaum W. Reversible ALS-like disorder in HIV infection. *Neurology* 2001;57:995–1001.

Nath A, Jankovic J, Pettigrew LC. Movement disorders and AIDS. *Neurology* 1987;37:37–41.

Navia BA, Cho ES, Petito CK, et al. The AIDS dementia complex: Part II. Neuropathology. *Ann Neurol* 1986;19:525–535.

Navia BA, Jordan BD, Price RW. The AIDS dementia complex: Part I. Clinical features. *Ann Neurol* 1986;19:517–526.

Navia BA, Price RW. The acquired immunodeficiency syndrome dementia complex as the presenting or sole manifestation of human immunodeficiency virus infection. *Arch Neurol* 1987;44:65–69.

Pantaleo G, Gruziosi C, Fauci AS. Mechanisms of disease: The immunopathogenesis of human immunodeficiency virus infection. *N Engl J Med* 1993;328:327–335.

Petito CK, Navia BA, Cho ES, et al. Vacuolar myelopathy pathologically resembling subacute combined degeneration in patients with the acquired immunodeficiency syndrome. *N Engl J Med* 1985;312:874–879.

Phimister EG. In search of a better HIV vaccine-the heat is on. *N Engl J Med* 2003;348:643–644.

Portegeis P, Enting RH, deGans J, et al. Presentation and course of AIDS dementia complex: 10 years of follow-up in Amsterdam, the Netherlands. *AIDS* 1993;7:669–675.

Qureshi AI, Hanson DL, Jones JL, et al. Estimation of the temporal probability of human immunodeficiency virus (HIV) dementia after risk stratification for HIV-infected persons. *Neurology* 1998;50:392–397.

Redfield RR, Wright DC, Tramont EC. The Walter Reed staging classification for HTLV-III/LAV infection. *N Engl J Med* 1986;314:131–132.

Rostasy K, Monti L, Yiannoutsos C, et al. Human immunodeficiency virus infection, inducible nitric oxide synthase expression, and microglial activation: pathogenetic relationship to the acquired immunodeficiency syndrome dementia complex. *Ann Neurol* 1999;46:207–216.

Sacktor N, Lyles RH, Skolasky R, et al. HIV-associated neurologic disease incidence changes: Multicenter AIDS Cohort Study, 1990–1998. *Neurology* 2001;56:257–260.

Sacktor N, Skolasky RL, Tarwater PM, et al. Response to systemic HIV viral load suppression correlates with psychomotor speed performance. *Neurology* 2003;61:567–569.

San-Andres FJ, Rubio R, Castilla J, et al. Incidence of acquired immunodeficiency syndrome-associated opportunistic diseases and the effect of treatment on a cohort of 1115 patients infected with human immunodeficiency virus, 1989–1997. *Clin Infec Dis* 2003;36:1177–1185.

Sato Y, Osabe S, Kuno H, et al. Rapid diagnosis of cryptococcal meningitis by microscopic examination of centrifuged cerebrospinal fluid sediment. *J Neurol Sci* 1999;164:72–75.

Schiffito G, McDermott MP, McArthur JC, et al. Incidence and risk factors for HIV-associated distal sensory polyneuropathy. *Neurology* 2002;58:1764–1768.

Selnes OA, Galai N, McArthur JC, et al. HIV infection and cognition in intravenous drug users: long-term follow-up. *Neurology* 1997;48:223–230.

Simpson DM, Bender AN. Human immunodeficiency virus-associated myopathy: analysis of 11 patients. *Ann Neurol* 1988;24:79–84.

Simpson DM, McArthur JC, Olney R, et al. Lamotrigine for HIV-associated painful sensory neuropathies. A placebo-controlled trial. *Neurology* 2003;60:1508–1514.

So YT, Olney RK. Acute lumbosacral polyradiculopathy in acquired immunodeficiency syndrome: experience in 23 patients. *Ann Neurol* 1994;35:53–58.

Steinbrook R. The AIDS epidemic in 2004. *N Engl J Med* 2004;351:115–117.

Steinman RM, Germain RN. Antigen presentation and related immunological aspects of HIV-1 vaccines. *AIDS* 1998;12 (suppl A):S97–S112.

Taber KH, Hayman LA, Shandera WX, et al. Spinal disease in neurologically symptomatic HIV-positive patients. *Neuroradiol* 1999;41:360–368.

Telzak EE, Zweig-Greenberg MS, Harrison J, et al. Syphilis treatment response in HIV-infected individuals. *AIDS* 1991;5:591–595.

Thurnher MM, Post JD, Rieger A, et al. Initial and follow-up MR imaging findings in AIDS-related progressive multifocal leukoencephalopathy treated with highly active antiretroviral therapy. *AJNR* 2001;22:977–984.

Towfighi A, Skolasky RL, St. Hillaire C, Conant K, McArthur JC. CSF soluble Fas correlates with the severity of HIV-associated dementia. *Neurology* 2004;62:654–656.

Valcour VG, Shikuma CM, Watters MR, Sacktor NC. Cognitive impairment in older HIV-1 seropositive individuals: prevalence and potential mechanisms. *AIDS* 2004;18 (suppl 1):S79–S86.

Von Giesen H-J, Antke C, Hefter H, et al. Potential time course of human immunodeficiency virus type 1-associated minor motor deficits. *Arch Neurol* 2000;57:1601–1607.

Von Giesen H-J, Heintges T, Abbasi-Boroudjeni N, et al. Psychomotor slowing in Hepatitis C and HIV infection. *J Acquir Immune Defic Syndr* 2004;35:131–137.

Wildemann B, Haas J, Lynen N, et al. Diagnosis of cytomegalovirus encephalitis in patients with AIDS by quantitation of cytomegalovirus genomes in cells of cerebrospinal fluid. *Neurology* 1998;50:693–697.

Wiley CA, Masliah E, Morey M, et al. Neocortical damage during HIV infection. *Ann Neurol* 1991;29:651–657.

Wiley CA, Schrier RD, Nelson JA, et al. Cellular localization of human immunodeficiency virus infection within the brains of acquired immune deficiency syndrome patients. *Proc Natl Acad Sci USA* 1986;83:7089–7093.

Yankner BA, Sklonik PR, Shoukimas GM, et al. Cerebral granulomatous angiitis associated with isolation of human T- lymphotropic virus type III from the central nervous system. *Ann Neurol* 1986;20:362–364.

Yebra M, Garcia-Merino A, Albarran F, Varela JM, Echevarria JM. Cerebellar disease without dementia and infection with the human immunodeficiency virus (HIV). *Ann Intern Med* 1988;108:310–311.

Chapter 2 6

Fungal and Yeast Infections

Leon D. Prockop

CNS EFFECTS OF FUNGAL INFECTIONS

Fungal infection (mycosis) of the CNS results in one or more of the following tissue reactions: meningitis, meningoencephalitis, abscess or granuloma formation, or arterial thrombosis. Subacute or chronic meningitis and meningoencephalitis are most common, but granulomatous lesions and abscesses typify the response to some fungi. Thrombotic occlusions occur with other fungal infections. The lungs, skin, and hair are usually the primary sites of involvement by fungi.

Fungi exist in two forms, molds and yeasts. *Molds* are composed of tubular filaments called hyphae that are sometimes branched. *Yeasts* are unicellular organisms that have a thick cell wall surrounded by a well-defined capsule. Infecting fungi comprise two groups, pathogenic and opportunistic.

Pathogenesis and Pathology: Fungal Infections

The *pathogenic* fungi are those few species that may infect a normal (healthy) host after inhalation or implantation of the spores. Naturally, chronically ill or other immunologically compromised people are more susceptible to infection than normal (healthy) people. The compromised immune system in patients with AIDS has become a major contributing factor in the propagation of fungal infections. In nature, fungi grow as saprophytic, soil-inhabiting, mycelial units that bear spores. During infection, spores adapt to the higher temperatures and lower oxidation-reduction potentials of tissues. They also overcome host defenses by increased growth rates and by relative insensitivity to host-defense mechanisms (e.g., phagocytosis).

The pathogenic fungi cause histoplasmosis, blastomycosis, coccidioidomycosis, and paracoccidioidomycosis. The first three are endemic to some areas of North America, and the last is endemic to areas of Central and South America. Neurologic disorders are rare in patients with systemic North American blastomycosis or histoplasmosis. Coccidioidomycosis is a more common disease, especially in Arizona and California; meningitis is a dreaded and often fatal complication.

The second group of systemically infecting fungi, the *opportunistic* organisms, is not thought to incite infection in the normal host. Diseases include aspergillosis, candidiasis, cryptococcosis, mucormycosis (phycomycosis), nocardiosis, and even rarer fungal diseases. With some of these fungi, minor changes in host defenses may cause disease (e.g., candidal overgrowth in mucous membranes). With most opportunistic fungi, the CNS is infected only after major changes have occurred in the host. Factors that may foster fungal infection are those of: extensive use of antimicrobial agents that destroy normal (nonpathogenic) bacterial flora; administration of immunosuppressive agents or corticosteroids that lower host resistance; and the existence of systemic illnesses such as Hodgkin disease, leukemia, diabetes mellitus, AIDS, or other diseases that interfere with immune responses of the host. Prolonged therapeutic use of deep venous lines also seems to be a contributing factor.

Human mortality rates approach 95% with invasive CNS aspergillosis, which is seen with increased frequency in immunosuppressed patients (e.g., in bone marrow transplantation recipients). Although clinically apparent meningeal infection with candida is rare, candidiasis has become an increasingly common postmortem brain finding. In autopsy studies, candidiasis occurs in compromised patients and produces intracerebral microabscesses and noncaseating granulomas without diffuse leptomeningitis. In contrast to most mycoses in which neurologic disease is secondary to systemic involvement, cryptococcal meningitis may be a primary infection. Although this fungus is considered opportunistic, the factors that predispose to cryptococcal infection in some apparently normal individuals are unknown.

In mucormycosis, primary infections of the nasal sinuses and eye often extend to the brain or cranial nerves in the compromised patient. Rare fungal causes of neurologic disorders include allescheriosis, alternariasis, cephalosporiosis, cladosporiosis, diplorhinotrichosis, drechsleriasis, fonsecaeasis, madurellosis, paeciloycosis, penicilliosis, sporotrichosis, streptomycosis, torulopsosis, trichophytosis, and ustilago mycosis.

Diagnosis: Fungal Infections

Diagnosis of fungal infections is often difficult and depends on the alertness of the physician. The identification of characteristic findings in radiographs of the lungs and other organs, skin tests, antibody tests of serum and CSF, and isolation of organisms from lesions and CSF, are important diagnostic aids. Serial monitoring of serum antigen (e.g., *Aspergillus*) shows promise in early diagnosis. Brain CT and MRI may document mass lesions caused by granulomas or abscesses. Likewise, CT or MRI may demonstrate obliteration of subarachnoid spaces or hydrocephalus, findings that are useful in determining the management and prognosis for patients with meningitis.

Treatment: Fungal Infections

Treatment of human fungal infections is, at best, unsatisfactory. Penicillin and other commonly used antimicrobial agents are useless and may lead to spread of the infection, except in actinomycosis or nocardiosis. Actinomycosis is curable by either tetracycline antibiotics or penicillin, and nocardiosis responds to sulfonamides. Amphotericin B is the most effective therapy for most neurologic fungal disease. It may be combined with lipid preparations to increase solubility, minimize toxicity, and enhance drug delivery. Three lipid formulations are approved for use in the United States: amphotericin B colloidal dispersion, amphotericin B lipid complex, and liposomal amphotericin B. Important roles for other agents are being recognized, including: flucytosine, ketoconazole, fluconazole, itraconazole, and caspofungin.

CRYPTOCOCCOSIS

Cryptococcosis is the most common mycotic infection that directly involves the CNS and is a major cause of morbidity and mortality among immunosuppressed patients. The disease may simulate tuberculous meningitis, brain tumor, encephalitis, or psychosis.

Pathogenesis

Cryptococcus neoformans (*Torula histolytica* or *Torulopsis neoformans*) is a fungus found throughout the world. Infections by the small yeastlike spherule have been described under various terms such as torulosis, yeast meningitis, and European blastomycosis. Although the skin and mucous membranes may be the primary sites of infection, the respiratory tract is usually the portal of entry. The organism has been recovered in fruit, milk, soil, wasps' nests, some grasses and plants, human skin and mucous membranes, and the manure of pigeons and other birds. The manure serves as a reservoir from which human infection may occur.

In 30% to 60% of reported cases, cryptococcosis is associated with debilitating diseases, such as AIDS, lymphosarcoma, reticulum-cell sarcoma, leukemia, Hodgkin disease, multiple myeloma, sarcoidosis, tuberculosis, diabetes mellitus, renal disease, and lupus erythematosus. CNS infection may occur independently of, or in association with, systemic disease. By the time the diagnosis of systemic cryptococcosis is firmly established however, 70% of the patients have been found to have neurologic abnormalities.

Pathology

The changes in the nervous system include infiltration of the meninges by mononuclear cells and cryptococcal organisms. The organisms may be scattered diffusely throughout the parenchyma of the brain, with little or no local inflammatory reaction. Occasionally, an abscess or small granulomas form in the meninges of the brain or spinal cord.

Symptoms and Signs

Symptomatic onset of nervous system involvement is subacute. Meningeal symptoms usually predominate, but occasionally focal neurologic signs or mental symptoms are in the foreground. The usual clinical picture is that of subacute meningitis or encephalitis. The diagnosis of tuberculous meningitis is often entertained until the correct diagnosis is revealed by the peculiar appearance of some of the organism cells in the CSF. The diagnosis of yeast meningitis may be established by culture of the organism on Sabouraud medium.

Large granulomas in the cerebrum, cerebellum, or brainstem cause the same clinical syndromes as do other expanding lesions in these sites. Before the availability of CT and MRI, the diagnosis of a granuloma was rarely made before operation. Nonetheless, a definite diagnosis may be made only when meningeal involvement is also present and organisms are recovered from the CSF.

Laboratory Data

The CSF findings in infections with cryptococci are similar to those of tuberculous meningitis. The CSF is usually under increased pressure. There is a slight or moderate pleocytosis of 10 cells/mm^3 to 500 cells/mm^3. The protein content is increased. The sugar content is decreased, with values commonly between 15 mg/dL and 35 mg/dL. The diagnosis is made by finding the organisms in the counting-chamber centrifuge sediment of the fluid (Fig. 26.1), by growth on Sabouraud medium, or by the results of animal inoculation.

The organisms also may be cultured from the urine, blood, stool, sputum, and bone marrow. They are usually visible on smear or growth in cultures. Diagnosis may be established by the detection of cryptococcal antigen in serum and CSF.

Course

The disease in untreated patients is usually fatal within a few months, but occasionally it persists for several years with recurrent remissions and exacerbations (Fig. 26.2). Occasionally, yeast organisms in the CSF have been noted

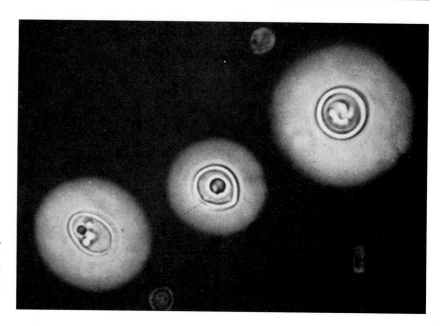

FIGURE 26.1. *Cryptococcus neoformans* meningitis. Fresh preparation of sediment from CSF stained with India ink. The capsule is three times the diameter of the cell. (Courtesy of Dr. Margarita Silva.)

for 3 years or longer. Spontaneous cure has been reported in a few cases.

Treatment

Treatment with amphotericin B has a definite beneficial effect. Butler and associates reported improvement in 31 of 36 treated patients. Of the 31 patients who showed

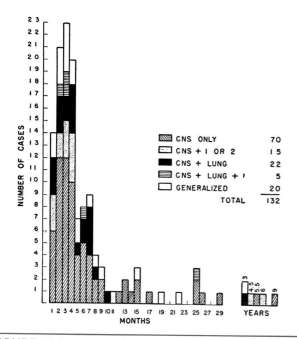

FIGURE 26.2. Duration of life (in months) for 132 patients with untreated cryptococcal meningitis, from onset to death. *Stippled areas 1* and *2* indicate cases in which skin or bones were also involved. (Courtesy of Dr. Charles Carton.)

improvement, 17 patients remained well, three patients died of unrelated causes, and 11 patients had one or more relapses of meningitis. In this era of epidemic AIDS, cryptococcosis is reported even more frequently than in previous years. Many authorities now consider fluconazole the drug of choice for AIDS-associated cryptococcal infection. Fluconazole should be continued for 3 months after the CSF is sterilized. Suppressive therapy with 200 mg orally, once daily, is employed in relapsing cases. Liver function studies must be monitored if phenytoin sodium is given concomitantly.

Alternative therapy employs amphotericin B and flucytosine. Combined treatment may be used to prevent failure resulting from the emergence of flucytosine resistance. Amphotericin B has sometimes been given by cisternal injection or by administration into the lateral ventricle through an Ommaya reservoir. Sterility of the CSF is probably the best monitoring endpoint of successful treatment. The course of treatment should be repeated if a relapse occurs.

Side effects of amphotericin B include thrombophlebitis, nausea and vomiting, fever, anemia, hypokalemia, and elevation of the blood urea level. Aspirin and antihistamines, blood transfusions, and temporary reduction in the drug dosage are of value in control of side effects.

MUCORMYCOSIS

Cerebral mucormycosis (phycomycosis) is an acute, rarely curable disease caused by fungi of the class *Phycomycetes*, especially of the genus *Rhizopus*. A common contaminant seen in laboratory cultures of serum, it is not ordinarily pathogenic. Cases have been reported in all parts of the United States, in Canada, and in England. The disease probably exists worldwide. It usually occurs as a complication of diabetes mellitus or a blood dyscrasia, particularly leukemia. Use of antibiotics and adrenocortical steroids may also predispose patients to mucormycosis.

The fungi enter the nose and in susceptible persons, cause sinusitis and orbital cellulitis. Subsequently, they may penetrate arteries to produce thrombosis of the ophthalmic and internal carotid arteries, and may later invade veins and lymphatics. Ocular, cerebral, pulmonary, intestinal, and disseminated forms of the disease exist.

Proptosis, ocular palsies, and hemiplegia are common neurologic signs associated with the fungal involvement of the orbital and internal carotid arteries. The organisms may invade the meninges, causing meningitis, or may extend into the brain to produce mycotic encephalitis.

Diagnosis is made by examination of the sputum, CSF, or exudate of tissue from the nasal sinuses. Culture of *Rhizopus* is corroborative but not diagnostic because it is a common contaminant.

A dramatic improvement in prognosis for these patients has been noted in recent years, with a 73% survival rate for patients diagnosed since 1970, compared to a 6% survival rate before 1970. Treatment consists of the administration of amphotericin B and control of predisposing factors (e.g., diabetes). Local drainage and early surgery (debridement) of the necrotic tissue should be performed to prevent spread of the disease.

SUGGESTED READINGS

General

Baddour LM, Gorbach SL. *Therapy of Infectious Diseases.* Philadelphia: WB Saunders, 2003.

Chandler FW, Watts JC. *Pathologic Diagnosis of Fungal Infections.* Chicago: American Society for Clinical Pathology Press, 1987.

Chimelli L, Rosemberg S, Hahn MD, et al. Pathology of the central nervous system in patients infected with the human immunodeficiency virus (HIV): a report of 252 autopsy cases from Brazil. *Neuropathol Appl Neurobiol* 1992;18:478–488.

Georgiev VS. *Opportunistic Infections: Treatment and Prophylaxis.* Totowa, NJ: Humana Press, 2003.

Khanna N, Chandramuki A, Desai A, Ravi V. Cryptococcal infections of the central nervous system: an analysis of predisposing factors, laboratory findings and outcome in patients from South India with special reference to HIV infection. *J Med Microbiol* 1996;45:376–379.

Kurstak E, Marquis G. *Immunology of Fungal Diseases.* New York: Marcel Dekker, 1989.

Malik R, Malhortra V, Gondal R, et al. Mycopathology of cerebral mycosis. *Acta Neurochir (Wien)* 1985;78:161–163.

Mori T, Ebe T. Analysis of cases of central nervous system fungal infections reported in Japan between January 1979 and June 1989. *Intern Med* 1992;31:174–179.

Ostrow TD, Hudgins PA. Magnetic resonance imaging of intracranial fungal infections. *Top Magn Reson Imaging* 1994;6:22–31.

Rippon JW. Mycosis. In: Vinken PH, Bruyn GW, Klawans HL, eds. *Infections of the Nervous System. Handbook of Clinical Neurology,* vol 35. Amsterdam: Elsevier/North-Holland, 1978.

Treseler CB, Suga AM. Fungal meningitis. *Infect Dis Clin North Am* 1990;4:789–808.

Verweij PE, Dompeling EC, Donnelly JP, Schattenberg AV, Meis JF. Serial monitoring of *Aspergillus* antigen in the early diagnosis of invasive aspergillosis: preliminary investigation with two examples. *Infection* 1997;25:86–89.

Walsh TJ, Hier DB, Caplan LR. Fungal infections of the central nervous system: comparative analysis of risk factors and clinical signs in 57 patients. *Neurology* 1985;35:1654–1657.

Wang F, So Y, Vittinghoff E, et al. Incidence proportion of and risk factors for AIDS patients diagnosed with HIV dementia, central nervous system toxoplasmosis, and cryptococcal meningitis. *J Acquir Immune Defic Syndr Hum Retrovirol* 1995;8:75–82.

Actinomycosis

Dailey AT, LeRoux PD, Grady MS. Resolution of an actinomycotic abscess with nonsurgical treatment. *Neurosurgery* 1993;31:134–136.

Funaki B, Rosenblum JD. MR of central nervous system actinomycosis. *AJNR Am J Neuroradiol* 1995;16(5):1179–1180.

Smego RA Jr. Actinomycosis of the central nervous system. *Rev Infect Dis* 1987;9:855–865.

Aspergillosis

Ashdown BC, Tien RD, Felsberg GJ. Aspergillosis of the brain and paranasal sinuses in immunocompromised patients: CT and MR imaging findings. *AJR* 1994;162:155–159.

Endo T, Tominaga T, Konno H, Yoshimoto T. Fatal subarachnoid hemorrhage, with brainstem and cerebellar infarction, caused by Aspergillus infection after cerebral aneurysm surgery: case report. *Neurosurgery* 2002;50(5):1147–1150.

Guermazi A, Gluckman E, Tabti B, Miaux Y. Invasive central nervous system aspergillosis in bone marrow transplantation recipients: an overview. *Eur Radiol* 2003;13(2):377–388.

Mikolich DJ, Kinsella LJ, Skowron G, Friedman J, Sugar AM. *Aspergillus* meningitis in an immunocompetent adult successfully treated with itraconazole. *Clin Infect Dis* 1996;23:1318–1319.

Murthy JM, Sundaram C, Prasad VS, et al. Aspergillosis of central nervous system: a study of 21 patients seen in a university hospital in south India. *J Assoc Physicians India* 2000;48(7):677–681.

Ng A, Gadong N, Kelsey A, et al. Successful treatment of aspergillus brain abscess in a child with acute lymphoblastic leukemia. *Pediatr Hematol Oncol* 2000;17(6):497–504.

Rhine WD, Arvin AM, Stevenson DK. Neonatal aspergillosis. *Clin Pediatr* 1986;25:400–403.

Walsh TJ, Hier DB, Caplan LR. Aspergillosis of the central nervous system: clinicopathological analysis of 17 patients. *Ann Neurol* 1985;18:574–582.

Blastomycosis

Friedman JA, Wijdicks EF, Fulgham JR, Wright AJ. Meningoencephalitis due to *Blastomyces dermatitidis*: case report and literature review. *Mayo Clin Proc* 2000;75(4):403–408.

Taillan B, Ferrari E, Cosnefroy JY, et al. Favourable outcome of blastomycosis of the brain stem with fluconazole and flucytosine treatment. *Ann Med* 1992;24:71–72.

Candida (Moniliasis)

Benjamin DK Jr, Poole C, Steinbach WJ, Rowen JO, Walsh TJ. Neonatal candidemia and end-organ damage: a critical appraisal of the literature using meta-analytic techniques. *Pediatrics* 2003;112(3 Pt 1):634–640.

de Medicos BC, de Medicos CR, Werner B, et al. Central nervous system infections following bone marrow transplantation: an autopsy report of 27 cases. *J Hematother Stem Cell Res* 2000;9:535–540.

Grouhi M, Dalal I, Nisbet-Brown E, Roifman CM. Cerebral vasculitis associated with chronic mucocutaneous candidiasis. *J Pediatr* 1998;133(4):571–574.

Parker JC, McCloskey JJ, Lee RS. Human cerebral candidosis: a postmortem evaluation of 19 patients. *Hum Pathol* 1981;12:23–28.

Coccidioidomycosis

Banuelos AF, Williams PL, Johnson RH, et al.. Central nervous system abscesses due to Coccidioides species. *Clin Infect Dis* 1996;22(2):240–250.

Erly WK, Bellon RJ, Seeger JF, Carmody RF. MR imaging of acute coccidioidal meningitis. *AJNR Am J Neuroradiol* 1999;20(3):509–514.

Herron LD, Kissel P, Smilovitz D. Treatment of coccidioidal spinal infection: experience in 16 cases. *J Spinal Disord* 1997;10(3):215-22215–222.

Williams PL, Johnson R, Pappagianis D, et al. Vasculitic and encephalitic complications associated with *Coccidioides immitis* infection of the central nervous system in humans: report of 10 cases and review. *Clin Infect Dis* 1992;14:673–682.

Histoplasmosis

Bradsher RW. Histoplasmosis and blastomycosis. *Clin Infect Dis* 1996; 22(suppl 2):S102–S111.

Paphitou NI, Barnett BJ. Solitary parietal lobe histoplasmoma mimicking a brain tumor. *Scan J Infect Dis* 2002;34(3):229–232.

Rivera IV, Curless RG, Indacochea FJ, Scott GB. Chronic progressive CNS histoplasmosis presenting in childhood: response to fluconazole therapy. *Pediatr Neurol* 1992;8:151–153.

Nocardiosis

Barnicoat MJ, Wierzbicki AS, Norman PM. Cerebral nocardiosis in immunosuppressed patients: five cases. *Q J Med* 1989;72:689–698.

Bross JE, Gordon G. Nocardial meningitis: case reports and review. *Rev Infect Dis* 1991;13:160–165.

Fleetwood IG, Embil JM, Ross IB. Nocardia asteroides cerebral abscess in immunocompetent hosts: report of three cases and review of surgical recommendations. *Surg Neurol* 2000;53(6):605–610.

Paracoccidioidomycosis

De Freitas MR, Nascimento OJ, Chimelli L. Tapia's syndrome caused by *Paracoccidioidis brasiliensis. J Neurol Sci* 1991;103:179–181.

Gasparetto EL, Liu CB, de Carvalho Neto A, Rogacheski E. Central nervous system paracoccidioidomycosis: imaging findings in 17 cases. *J Comput Assist Tomog* 2003;27(1):12–17.

Uncommon Fungal Diseases

Fetter BF, Klintworth GK.Uncommon fungal diseases of the nervous system. In: Vinken PH, Bruyn GW, Klawans HL, eds. *Infections of the Nervous System. Handbook of Clinical Neurology,* vol 35. Amsterdam: Elsevier/North-Holland, 1978.

Cryptococcosis

Adeyemi OM, Pulvirenti J, Perumal S, et al. Cryptococcosis in HIV-infected individuals. *AIDS* 2004;18(16):2218–2219.

Bozzette SA, Larsen RA, Chiu J, et al. A placebo-controlled trial of maintenance therapy with fluconazole after treatment of cryptococcal meningitis in the acquired immunodeficiency syndrome. California Collaborative Treatment Group. *N Engl J Med* 1991;324:580–584.

Brown RW, Clarke RJ, Gonzales MF. Cytologic detection of *Cryptococcus neoformans* in cerebrospinal fluid. *Acta Cytol* 1985;29:151–153.

Chen SC, Miller M, Zhou JZ, Wright LC, Sorrell TC. Phospholipase activity in *Cryptococcus neoformans:* a new virulence factor? *J Infect Dis* 1997;175:414–420.

De Wytt CN, Dickson PL, Holt GW. Cryptococcal meningitis: a review of 32 years' experience. *J Neurol Sci* 1982;53:283–292.

Dromer F, Mathoulin-Pelissier S, Fontanet A, et al. Epidemiology of HIV-associated cryptococcosis in France (1985–2001): comparison of the pre- and post- HAART eras. *AIDS* 2004;18(3):555–562.

Kavoor JM, Mhadevan A, Narayan JP, et al. Cryptococcal choroid plexitis as a mass lesion: MR imaging and histopathological correlation. *AJNR Am J Neuroradiol* 2002;23(2):273–276.

Lees SC, Dickson DW, Casadevall A. Pathology of cryptococcal meningoencephalitis: analysis of 27 patients with pathogenic implications. *Hum Pathol* 1996;27:839–847.

Ruiz A, Post MJ, Bundschu CC. Dentate nuclei involvement in AIDS patients with CNS cryptococcosis: imaging findings with pathologic correlation. *J Comput Assist Tomogr* 1997;21(2):175–182.

Sanchez-Portocarrero J, Perez-Cecilia E. Intracerebral mass lesions in patients with human immunodeficiency virus infection and cryptococcal meningitis. *Diagn Microbial Infect Dis* 1997;29(3):193-8193–198.

Speed B, Dunt D. Clinical and host differences between infections with the two varieties of *Cryptococcus neoformans. Clin Infect Dis* 1995;21:28–34.

Mucormycosis

Abril V, Ortega E, Segarra P, et al. Rhinocerebral mucormycosis in a patient with AIDS: a complication of diabetic ketoacidosis following pentamidine therapy. *Clin Infect Dis* 1996;23:845–946.

Anand VK, Alemar G, Griswold JA Jr. Intracranial complications of mucormycosis: an experimental model and clinical review. *Laryngoscope* 1992;102:656–662.

Hamilton JF, Bartkowski HB, Rock JP. Management of CNS mucormycosis in the pediatric patient. *Pediatr Neurosurg* 2003;38(4):212-5212–215.

McLean FM, Ginsberg LE, Stanton CA. Perineural spread of rhinocerebral mucormycosis. *AJNR Am J Neuroradiol* 1996;17:114–116.

Siegal JA, Cacayoring ED, Nassif AS, et al. Cerebral mucormycosis: proton MR spectroscopy and MR imaging. *Magn Reson Imaging* 2000;18(7):915-20915–920.

Talmi YP, Goldschmied-Reouven A, Bakon M, et al. Rhino-orbital and rhino-orbital-cerebral mucormycosis. *Otolaryngol Head Neck Surg* 2002;127(1):22–31.

Chapter 27

Neurosarcoidosis

John C. M. Brust

Sarcoidosis is a multisystem, granulomatous disease of unknown cause. Sarcoid granulomas resemble those of tuberculosis but lack tubercle bacilli or caseation, although central necrosis is sometimes seen. Active lesions contain epithelioid and multinucleate giant cells; such lesions may resolve but more often become fibrotic.

EPIDEMIOLOGY

Sarcoidosis occurs worldwide, with estimated prevalence ranging from 3 cases to 50 cases per 100,000 population. In the United States, it occurs more frequently in Black patients. Susceptibility to sarcoidosis is polygenetically influenced, and different polymorphisms involving the major histocompatibility complex predict the severity of disease. Onset is most often in the fourth or fifth decade, but the disease also affects children and the elderly. Sarcoid granulomas are attributed to immune responses to unidentified exogenous antigens. An infectious cause remains elusive.

PATHOLOGY

The disorder is mediated primarily by CD4+ T-helper 1 (Th1) cells and mononuclear phagocytes, with participation of numerous cytokines and chemokines that include interleukins, adhesion molecules, interferon-gamma, tumor necrosis factor-alpha (TNFα), and transforming growth factor-beta. Lesions may affect any organ, especially lung, lymph nodes, skin, bone, eyes, and salivary glands. The nervous system is involved clinically in about 5% of patients; half of them have central or peripheral nervous system symptoms. Although nearly 20% of these patients have only neurologic symptoms or signs, workup reveals systemic disease in as many as 97%. When nervous system disease complicates systemic sarcoidosis, it usually does so within 2 years of onset.

In the CNS sarcoid granulomas most often involve the meninges, especially at the base of the brain, with secondary infiltration of cranial nerves and obstruction of CSF flow. Lesions tend to be perivascular and thereby may spread intraparenchymally, frequently affecting the hypothalamus and less often other CNS structures, including the spinal cord. Granulomas also occur in peripheral nerves and muscle.

PRESENTATION: SIGNS AND SYMPTOMS

Given the unpredictable dispersal of lesions, sarcoidosis is a clinically protean disease, systemically and neurologically. Nearly 50% of patients with neurosarcoidosis have more than one neurologic complication, with relative frequencies varying among different clinical series (Table 27.1).

Although any cranial nerve may be affected, the most frequently affected is the seventh, sometimes in association with uveitis and parotitis (uveoparotid fever) but usually alone, thus suggesting Bell palsy. Facial weakness may be bilateral and either simultaneous or sequential, and may recur after recovery. Optic nerve involvement causes papillitis or retrobulbar neuritis and eventually optic atrophy. Trigeminal nerve involvement causes either sen-

▶ **TABLE 27.1 Symptoms and Signs in Neurosarcoidosis**

Signs and Symptoms	Mean (%) Incidence
Cranial neuropathy	53% (range, 37% to 73%)
CNS parenchymal disease	48% (range, 14% to 100%)
Aseptic meningitis	22% (range, 8% to 40%)
Peripheral neuropathy	17% (range, 6% to 40%)
Myopathy	15% (range, 7% to 26%)
Hydrocephalus	7% (range, 0% to 14%)

sory loss or neuralgia, and eighth cranial nerve lesions produce auditory and vestibular symptoms.

Granulomas involve the hypothalamus more often than the pituitary, thereby producing combinations of endocrinologic and nonendocrinologic symptoms that include diabetes insipidus, decreased libido, galactorrhea, amenorrhea, abnormal sleep patterns, altered appetite, temperature dysregulation, and abnormal behavior. Cerebral granulomas may be scattered diffusely, some too small to be detected on CT or MRI, or they may consist of one or more large masses that mimic a brain neoplasm. Seizures are common in such patients. Symptomatic subdural granulomas have occurred. Rarely, sarcoid vasculitis causes cerebral infarction in a pattern clinically and pathologically indistinguishable from what is commonly called granulomatous angiitis of the nervous system. Autoantibodies to endothelial cells have been identified in patients with neurosarcoid.

Meningeal infiltration may be asymptomatic or produce symptomatic aseptic meningitis. Complications include cauda equina signs, hydrocephalus, and ependymitis with encephalopathy.

Peripheral nerve lesions cause mononeuropathy, mononeuropathy multiplex, and sensory, motor, or sensorimotor polyneuropathy, either chronically progressive or resembling Guillain-Barré neuropathy. A positive muscle biopsy has been reported in as many as 75% of patients with sarcoidosis, and muscle granulomas may be seen on MRI. Muscle granulomas are usually asymptomatic, although they sometimes cause palpable nodules or progressive diffuse polymyositis.

DIAGNOSIS: LABORATORY DATA

In patients known to have sarcoidosis, the appearance of neurologic symptoms usually poses no diagnostic problem, but alternative possibilities must be kept in mind. Altered mental status could be caused by hypercalcemia, corticosteroid effects, or systemic organ involvement and metabolic derangement. Patients with neurologic symptoms require both systemic and neurologic investigation. CNS granulomas, symptomatic or asymptomatic, are apparent on either T2-weighted MRI or contrast-enhanced CT; they are sometimes calcified. Leptomeningeal CT enhancement is common, and imaging may reveal hydrocephalus and spinal cord, cauda equina, or optic nerve involvement.

Multiple periventricular and white matter lesions on T-2 and fluid-attenuated inversion recovery (FLAIR) MRI may suggest multiple sclerosis. MS plaques do not enhance with gadolinium beyond the acute inflammatory stage, but sarcoid granulomas may not enhance in patients receiving corticosteroids. These lesions might represent either granulomas or small infarcts secondary to granulomatous vasculitis. Consistent with the latter is occasional contrast enhancement along nearby blood vessels. The CSF may contain as many as a few thousand white cells (usually with lymphocytic preponderance), as well as elevated protein levels, low sugar content, elevated IgG and IgG index, oligoclonal bands, elevated angiotensin-converting enzyme (ACE) levels (also found in infection and malignancy), and an elevated CD4:CD8 cell ratio.

Other studies, tailored to need with individual patients, include chest radiographs (revealing either asymptomatic hilar adenopathy or more ominously, fibronodular disease), pulmonary function studies, bronchiolar lavage for lymphocytes, serum calcium (elevated in about 20% of patients with sarcoidosis), urinary calcium (elevated in 50% of patients), serum ACE (elevated in 65% of patients), serum gamma globulin (elevated in 50% of patients), serum sodium, and endocrinologic studies (thyroid function tests, cortisol, gonadotropins, testosterone or estradiol, and prolactin). About two-thirds of patients are anergic to tuberculin-purified protein derivative, mumps, and other antigens, and those who are positive are usually only weakly so. Ophthalmologic or otolaryngologic consultation may disclose unsuspected lesions. Systemic or brain gallium scanning may be positive but is nonspecific. Whole-body 2-fluoro-1-deoxyglucose PET may identify sites of inflammation not seen on MRI or with gallium scanning.

Diagnosis ultimately depends on histology; biopsy sites include lymph nodes (including transbronchial), salivary glands, conjunctiva, skin, liver, and as a last resort, meninges or brain. Kveim testing may be diagnostic, but the antigen is no longer generally available.

COURSE AND TREATMENT

About two-thirds of patients with neurosarcoidosis have a self-limited monophasic illness; the rest have a chronic, remitting-relapsing course. With treatment, death from neurologic disease is unusual. Although controlled studies are lacking, corticosteroids appear to reduce symptoms and size of granulomas; it is unclear whether they affect the natural history. Their use depends on the clinical setting. Short-term therapy may be given to patients with aseptic meningitis or isolated facial palsy. Long-term treatment is often necessary for intraparenchymal lesions, hydrocephalus, optic or other cranial nerve involvement,

peripheral neuropathy, or symptomatic myopathy. Prednisone 40 mg to 80 mg, daily, may be given for a few weeks and then slowly tapered either to a lowest possible maintenance dose or if possible, to discontinuation. Higher initial doses may be necessary in some patients. Adjunctive immunosuppressive treatment for refractory patients includes azathioprine, methotrexate, cyclophosphamide, and cyclosporine (ineffective in pulmonary sarcoidosis, but effective in neurosarcoidosis, even in some patients refractory to corticosteroids). Also useful in selected patients with neurosarcoidosis are chloroquine and hydroxychloroquine, which inhibit antigen presentation to T cells. Anecdotal reports also describe benefit from agents that inhibit TNFα, including pentoxifilline, thalidomide, etanercept, and infliximab. Radiation therapy has been used but with uncertain benefit.

SUGGESTED READINGS

Barnard J, Newman LS. Sarcoidosis: immunology, rheumatic involvement, and therapeutics. *Curr Op Rheumatol* 2001;13:84–91.

Berger C, Sommer C, Meinck HM. Isolated sarcoid myopathy. *Muscle Nerve* 2002;26:553–556.

Brust JCM, Rhee RS, Plank CR, et al. Sarcoidosis, galactorrhea, and amenorrhea: two autopsy cases, one with Chiari-Frommel syndrome. *Ann Neurol* 1977;2:130–137.

Challenor Y, Brust JCM, Felton C. Electrodiagnostic studies in sarcoidosis. *J Neurol Neurosurg Psychiatry* 1984;46:1219–1222.

Colover JJ. Sarcoidosis with involvement of the nervous system. *Brain* 1948;71:451–455.

Cordingley G, Navarro C, Brust JCM, Healton EB. Sarcoidosis presenting as senile dementia. *Neurology* 1981;31:1148–1151.

Gullapalli D, Phillips LH. Neurologic manifestations of sarcoidosis. *Neurol Clin* 2002;20:59–83.

Gullapalli D, Phillips LH. Neurosarcoidosis. *Curr Neurol Neurosci Rep* 2004;4(6):441–447.

Healton EB, Zito G, Chauhan P, Brust JCM. Subdural sarcoid granuloma. *J Neurosurg* 1982;32:776–778.

Hoitsma E, Faber CG, Drent M, Sharma OP. Neurosarcoidosis: a clinical dilemma. *Lancet Neurology* 2004;3(7):397–407.

Krumholz A, Stern BJ, Stern EG. Clinical implications of seizures in neurosarcoidosis. *Arch Neurol* 1991;48:842–844.

Maroun FB, O'Dea FJ, Mathieson G, et al. Sarcoidosis presenting as an intramedullary spinal cord lesion. *Can J Neurol Sci* 2001;28:163–166.

Miller DH, Kendall BE, Barter S, et al. Magnetic resonance imaging in central nervous system sarcoidosis. *Neurology* 1988;38:378–383.

Moller DR. Treatment of sarcoidosis–from a basic science point of view. *J Intern Med* 2003;353:31–40.

Newman LS, Rose CS, Maier LA. Sarcoidosis. *N Engl J Med* 1997;336:1224–1234.

Nowak DA, Widenka DC. Neurosarcoidosis: a review of its intracranial manifestation. *J Neurol* 2001;248:363–372.

Quinones-Hinojosa A, Chang EF, Khan SA, et al. Isolated trigeminal nerve sarcoid granuloma mimicking trigeminal schwannoma: case report. *Neurosurgery* 2003;52:700–705.

Said G, Lacroix C, Plante-Bordneure V, et al. Nerve granulomas and vasculitis in sarcoid peripheral neuropathy: a clinicopathological study of 11 patients. *Brain* 2002;125:264–275.

Stern BJ. Neurological complications of sarcoidosis. *Curr Op Neurol* 2004;17(3):311–316.

Tobias S, Prayson RA, Lee JH. Necrotizing neurosarcoidosis of the cranial base resembling an *en plaque* sphenoid wing meningioma: case report. *Neurosurgery* 2002;51:1290–1294.

Tsukada N, Yanegisawa N, Mochizuki I. Endothelial cell damage in sarcoidosis and neurosarcoidosis: autoantibodies to endothelial cells. *Eur Neurol* 1995;35:108–112.

Von Brevern M, Lempert T, Bronstein AM, et al. Selective vestibular damage in neurosarcoidosis. *Ann Neurol* 1997;42:117–120.

Chapter 28

Spirochete Infections: Neurosyphilis

Leonidas Stefanis and Lewis P. Rowland

DEFINITION

Neurosyphilis comprises several different syndromes that result from infection of the brain, meninges, or spinal cord by *Treponema pallidum* (Table 28.1). It is not known how much damage is caused by direct effects of the organism and how much by autoimmune mechanisms.

A clinical definition must include the results of diagnostic laboratory tests. Accordingly, neurosyphilis is defined by three findings: a syndrome consistent with neurosyphilis, abnormal blood titer of a treponemal antibody test, and positive nontreponemal antibody test in the CSF. All three must be present.

HISTORY

Neurosyphilis, recognized for about 100 years, has played an important role in the evolution of modern neurology. Paretic neurosyphilis was the first "mental disorder" for which specific cerebral pathology was found. Erb described spinal syphilis (tabes dorsalis) in 1892. Quincke introduced lumbar puncture, and CSF examination was used to diagnose infection, even in asymptomatic people. The organism was identified in the brain by Noguchi and Moore in 1913. The first effective treatment came in 1918 when Wagner-Jaurregg gave fever therapy for paresis. He was the first neurologist to win the Nobel Prize. Then came arsenical chemotherapy, the first planned use of a drug that would attack the organism without harming host tissues; this was Ehrlich's concept of "the magic bullet." Safer and more effective therapy came in 1945 with the introduction of penicillin, which has been used since.

Syphilis was also important in the evolution of this textbook. The subject has been allotted many pages because the disease was a major research interest of Houston Merritt and it was still prevalent when he wrote the first edition. His chapters were revised only slightly in subsequent editions, but now neurosyphilis is inextricably linked to HIV infection and AIDS. Classic clinical syndromes are now exceptional, and both diagnosis and ther-

apy have become more complicated; these changes require a recasting of the description.

EPIDEMIOLOGY

Following the introduction of penicillin in the 1940s and 50s, the incidence of neurosyphilis declined for two main reasons: (1) fewer people spread the disease because those affected were being identified and treated, and (2) many neurosyphilitic infections were prevented because penicillin was being used to treat gonorrhea and other infections. For instance, the frequency of neurosyphilis as a cause of first admission to a psychiatric hospital plummeted from 5.9 cases per 100,000 population in 1942 to 0.1 cases per 100,000 in 1965. New cases became so rare that many hospitals discarded routine testing to detect syphilis.

During the next few decades, some investigators detected a shift in the clinical patterns, but this finding was debated. The segment of the population with the highest incidence was young homosexual men. Then, in 1981, came AIDS. The incidence of primary and secondary syphilis rose from 13.7 cases per 100,000 in 1981 to 18.4 cases per 100,000 in 1989, an increase of 34%. In the ensuing years, the incidence of syphilis declined. In 1997, fewer than 8,000 cases of early syphilis were reported in the United States, the lowest rate in 38 years and a six-fold decline from 1990. This progress prompted proposals to eradicate syphilis in the United States. However, since the year 2000, there has been an unexpected increase in new cases of primary and secondary syphilis recorded in the United States. Trends in Western Europe and Canada were similar, presumably because of a resurgence of unsafe sexual practices, especially among homosexual men.

In addition to this alarming increase in the incidence of syphilis in industrialized countries, syphilis, like HIV, is an enormous health problem in developing countries. For instance, syphilis seropositivity among pregnant women in Sub-Saharan Africa may be higher than 10%.

Neurosyphilis ultimately develops in about 10% of untreated persons with early syphilis. Among those infected with HIV, about 15% have serologic evidence of syphilis, and about 1% have neurosyphilis.

Even before the HIV era, there had been a shift in clinical manifestations because of the widespread use of antibiotics. Previously common parenchymal forms became rare, while the incidence of meningeal and vascular syndromes rose (Table 28.2).

The diagnosis of neurosyphilis is often delayed because there are other, more common causes of stroke and meningitis. From 1985 to 1992 in San Francisco, parenchymal forms of neurosyphilis accounted for only 5% of 117 cases. Parenchymal forms of syphilis are now so rare that in the absence of a relevant symptoms or signs on neurological examination, testing for nontreponemal antibodies is no longer recommended in the evaluation of dementia.

▶ **TABLE 28.1** Classification of Neurosyphilis

Type	Clinical Symptoms	Pathology	CSF WBC	Brain CT or MRI
I. Asymptomatic	No symptoms; CSF abnormal	Various. Chiefly, leptomeningitis; arteritis or encephalitis may be present	<5 >5	Normal Meningeal enhancement
II. Meningeal and vascular Cerebral meningeal Diffuse	Increased intracranial pressure; cranial nerve palsies	Leptomeningitis with hydrocephalus; degeneration of cranial nerves; arteritis	≥5	Meningeal enhancement
Focal	Increased intracranial pressure; focal cerebral symptoms and signs of slow onset	Grnuoma formation (gumma)	Any	Mass lesion
Cerebrovascular	Focal cerebral symptoms and signs of sudden onset	Endarteritis with infarcts	Any	Subcortical or cortical infarct
Spinal meningeal and vascular	Paresthesias, weakness, atrophy, and sensory loss in limbs and trunk	Admixture of endarteritis and meningeal infiltration and thickening with degeneration of nerve roots and substance of the cord (myelomalacia)	Any	NA
III. Parenchymatous Tabetic	Pain, paresthesia, crises, ataxia, impairment of pupillary reflexes, loss of tendon reflexes impaired proprioceptive sensation, and trophic changes	Leptomeningitis and degenerative changes in posterior roots, dorsal funiculi, and brainstem	Any	NA
Paretic	Personality changes, convulsions, and dementia	Meningoencephalitis	Any	Optic atrophy
Optic atrophy[a]	Loss of vision, pallor of optic discs	Leptomeningitis and atrophy of optic nerves	Any	NA

NA, not applicable.
[a]Rarely occurs alone; usually found in tabetic or paretic neurosyphilis.
Data from Merritt et al., 1946; and Katz et al., 1993.

▶ **TABLE 28.2** Frequency of Different Forms of Symptomatic Neurosyphilis

	Preantibiotic Era (%)			Antibiotic Era (%)		AIDS Era (%)	
						HIV (−)	HIV (+) or AIDS
	1	2	3	4	5	6	7
Tabetic	45	48	45	15	11	5	0
Paretic	17	18	8	12	4	9	4
Taboparetic	4	7	9	23	23	—	—
Vascular	15	19	9	19	61	41	38
Meningeal	8	8	19	23	0	23	46
Optic neuritis	4	—	—	—	—	14	42
Spinal cord	4	—	10	8	—	—	—

1. Merritt et al., 1946 (457 patients).
2. Kierland et al. symptomatic neurosyphilis. *Ven Dis Inform* 1994;22:350–377 (2,019 patients).
3. Wolters, 1987 (518 patients, 1930–1940).
4. Wolters, 1987 (121 patients, 1970–1984).
5. Burke and Schaberg, 1985 (26 patients).
6. and 7. Katz et al., 1993 (HIV negative, 22 patients; HIV positive and AIDS, 24 patients).

PATHOLOGY

In early neurosyphilis, lymphocytes and other mononuclear cells infiltrate the meninges. The inflammatory reaction also involves the cranial nerves and provokes axonal degeneration. When the inflammation affects small meningeal vessels, occlusion due to endothelial proliferation may lead to ischemic necrosis of the brain and spinal cord. This process may cause demyelination, myelomalacia at the periphery of the cord, or transverse myelitis.

The pathology of dementia paralytica develops slowly. After an inflammatory meningeal reaction, lymphocytes and plasma cells infiltrate small cortical vessels and sometimes extend into the cortex, itself. The cortical inflammatory response provokes loss of cortical neurons and glial proliferation. Spirochetes may be demonstrated in the cortex in dementia paralytica, but only rarely in other forms of neurosyphilis.

In tabes dorsalis, the mononuclear inflammation of meninges and blood vessels is followed by insidious degeneration of the posterior roots and posterior fiber columns of the spinal cord (Fig. 28.1), as well as the cranial nerves occasionally.

CLINICAL DIAGNOSIS

The three most common forms of neurosyphilis are asymptomatic, meningeal, and vascular. Often, the meninges and cerebral vessels are affected together, in meningovascular neurosyphilis. The once prominent parenchymal forms, including general paresis (dementia paralytica) and tabes dorsalis, are rarely seen now. The major clinical syndromes are differentiated from other causes of the same manifestations only by finding blood and CSF changes indicative of syphilis. Of course, the patient with serologic evidence of syphilis and concomitant HIV or other viral meningitis poses a diagnostic dilemma. Therefore, the efficacy of diagnostic tests must be considered.

Serology

Isolation of *Treponema pallidum* (*T. pallidum*) is difficult and impractical for clinical diagnosis; instead, diagnosis rests on two categories of antibodies that are used as serologic tests for syphilis (STS). *Nontreponemal* antibodies react with reagin, a complex of cardiolipin, lecithin, and cholesterol. This complex was the basis for the original complement-fixation Wasserman test, for the more

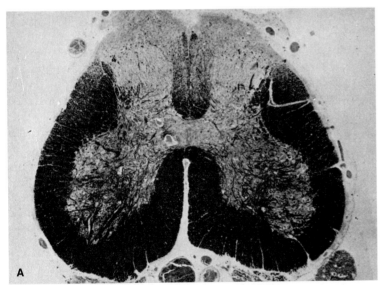

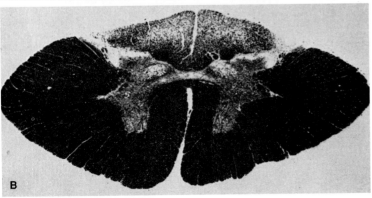

FIGURE 28.1. **Tabes dorsalis.** Degeneration of the posterior column in the sacral and thoracic cord (myelin sheath stain). (From Merritt et al., 1946.)

sensitive Kolmer test, and then for the Venereal Disease Research Laboratory (VDRL) test and a variation called the rapid plasma-reagin (RPR) test, a flocculation test macroscopically visible on a glass slide. The RPR test is not suitable for testing CSF.

The CSF VDRL test is highly specific, but false-positive reactions may result from contamination of CSF by blood, high CSF-protein content, or the presence of paraproteinemia or autoimmune disease. Some clinicians believe that the CSF VDRL test may be negative in some cases of neurosyphilis but if so, the clinical syndrome of neurosyphilis would then be difficult to prove, especially if the manifestations were not typical. Although accurate in diagnosis, the CSF VDRL test is not as reliable in following treatment (because the titer may not change); CSF pleocytosis is a more useful guide for monitoring treatment effects.

Even more specific is the fluorescent treponemal antibody (FTA) test. The antigen is prepared from the spirochete and may be absorbed (FTA-ABS) to remove sources of nonspecific and false reactions. A positive FTA-ABS test in plasma has high specificity for diagnosis but not for activity, because it may remain positive for years after successful treatment. In addition, the test is so sensitive that it may not be used on CSF because as little as 0.8 μL blood in 1 mL CSF may give a positive reaction. A diagnosis of syphilis requires a high titer in the blood on the VDRL test, ascertained by a positive FTA-ABS. In some centers, a variation of the FTA is the *microhemagglutination test* for *T. pallidum*.

Problems arise when specific treponemal tests designed for serum use are applied to CSF. They lack specificity because positive results appear with minor contamination by blood or with diffusion of serum immunoglobulins into CSF. Attempts to increase the reliability have included indices of intrathecal production (intrathecal *T. pallidum* antibody and *T. pallidum* hemagglutination assay); still it is difficult to be confident of the diagnosis of neurosyphilis if other CSF measures are normal. The specific treponemal antibody tests for CSF are more reliable in excluding neurosyphilis than in confirming it.

Another promising diagnostic technique is the polymerase chain reaction (PCR), which amplifies treponemal deoxyribonucleic or ribonucleic acid in CSF. This test is, in general, in good agreement with the rabbit inoculation test (RIT), which is performed only in specialized research centers. However, use of the PCR test is not yet fully developed.

Therefore, the diagnosis of neurosyphilis requires appropriate blood serology and a reactive CSF VDRL test. A reactive FTA-ABS in the blood indicates that the CSF VDRL result is not a false-positive response.

CSF Abnormalities

CSF pleocytosis is the best measure of disease activity, and the number of cells is roughly proportionate to the clinical syndrome. In an untreated patient, the CSF white blood cell (WBC) count should be at least 5 cells/mm^3 for secure diagnosis. The pleocytosis should respond to penicillin therapy within 12 weeks. The CSF protein content is usually increased, and the sugar content may be low or normal. The CSF content of gamma globulin may be increased and oligoclonal bands may be present, but these findings are nonspecific.

CLINICAL SYNDROMES

In the following discussion of clinical syndromes, we assume positive VDRL or FTA-ABS in serum, positive CSF VDRL, and CSF pleocytosis. These findings constitute the *modern diagnostic triad of neurosyphilis*, even in HIV-positive patients.

Asymptomatic Neurosyphilis

This diagnosis depends entirely on the serologic findings in blood and CSF. If the WBC count is more than 5 cells/mm^3, the disorder could be called "asymptomatic meningeal syphilis," and there may be meningeal enhancement on MRI.

Meningeal Neurosyphilis

This syndrome is seen within a year of the primary infection. The clinical manifestations are those of any acute viral or aseptic meningitis: malaise, fever, stiff neck, and headache. The CSF cell count may rise to several hundred per cm^3, CSF pressure may be increased, and CSF glucose may be low but is usually greater than 25 mg/dL. The protein content may exceed 100 mg/dL. The syndrome may subside spontaneously and is recognized by positive blood and CSF STS reactions.

Signs may not appear on examination, or there may be cranial nerve abnormalities, with facial diplegia or hearing loss. Occlusion of CSF pathways may cause obstructive or communicating hydrocephalus, and the course may be punctuated by cerebral infarction (meningovascular lues).

Cerebrovascular Neurosyphilis

Cerebral infarct syndromes of syphilis are similar to those of other more common causes; the diagnosis rests on typical findings in blood and CSF. Patients are younger than those with atherosclerosis and are more likely to have risk factors for venereal disease. Clinical evidence may imply concomitant meningeal disease (meningovascular disease), with a prodromal syndrome of headache or personality change for weeks before the ictus, and signs may progress for several days. MRI may show meningeal enhancement. Symptoms usually appear 5 years to 30 years after the primary infection, but manifestations may be seen earlier, especially in HIV-positive individuals.

Meningovascular Syphilis of the Spinal Cord

Conventional symptoms and signs of transverse myelitis (meningomyelitis) usually affect both sensory and motor pathways, as well as bladder control. The syndrome must be differentiated from tabes, a parenchymal infection. Syphilis has not been implicated, reliably, as a cause of amyotrophic lateral sclerosis (with both upper and lower motor neuron signs). However, a subacute syndrome of amyotrophy may be seen with appropriate serology and CSF pleocytosis. It is doubted that syphilis causes the "spastic paraplegia of Erb," an anterior spinal artery syndrome.

Gumma

This mass lesion, avascular granuloma, is now rarely seen but was found attached to the dura and was considered a localized form of meningeal syphilis.

Paretic Neurosyphilis

This form of neurosyphilis has also been called dementia paralytica, general paresis of the insane, or syphilitic meningoencephalitis. Spirochetes cause the chronic meningoencephalitis. The leptomeninges are opalescent to opaque, thickened, and adherent to the cortex; the cortical gyri are atrophic (Fig. 28.2). The sulci are widened and filled with CSF.

When the brain is sectioned, the ventricles are enlarged. The walls are covered with sandlike granulations termed *granular ependymitis* (Fig. 28.3).

Behavioral changes may suggest a psychosis but the most common problem is dementia, with loss of memory, poor judgment, and emotional lability. In the final stages, dementia and quadriparesis are severe (general paresis of the insane). Seizures may occur.

If untreated, paretic neurosyphilis is fatal in 3 to 5 years. Penicillin is an effective treatment, but ultimately clinical results depend on the nature and extent of neuropathology when treatment is started. If inflammatory reaction is the only cause of the cerebral dysfunction, cure is likely. If spirochetal infection has already destroyed significant numbers of cerebral neurons, the infection may be arrested, but cerebral functions will not be restored.

Tabes Dorsalis

Tabes dorsalis, also called progressive locomotor ataxia, is manifested by lancinating or lightning-like pains, progressive ataxia, loss of tendon reflexes, loss of proprioception, dysfunction of sphincters, and impaired sexual function in men. The chief signs are loss of tendon reflexes at the

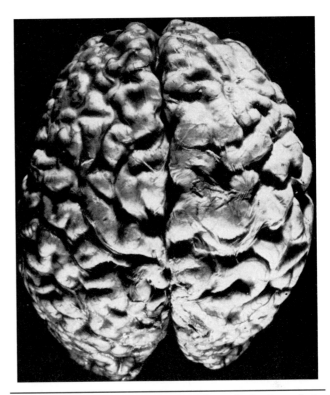

FIGURE 28.2. Paretic neurosyphilis. Thickening of the meninges and atrophy of the cerebral convolutions. (From Merritt et al., 1946.)

knees and ankles, impaired vibratory and position sense in the legs, and abnormal pupils (Table 28.3).

In 94% of patients with tabes dorsalis, the pupils are irregular or unequal, or show impaired responses to light. In 48%, Argyll-Robertson pupils are present, with loss of

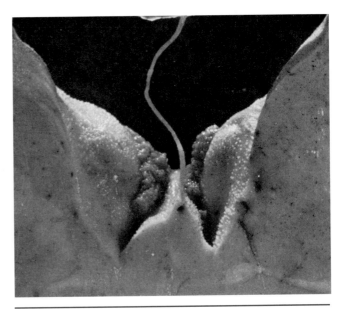

FIGURE 28.3. Paretic neurosyphilis. Granular ependymitis of the floor of lateral ventricles. (From Merritt et al., 1946.)

▶ **TABLE 28.3** Symptoms and Signs in Tabetic Neurosyphilis: Analysis of 150 Cases

Symptoms	%	Signs	%
Lancinating pains	75	Abnormal pupils	94
Ataxia	42	Argyll-Robertson	48
Bladder disturbance	33	Other abnormalities	64
Paresthesia	24	Reflex abnormalities	
Gastric or visceral crises	18	Absent ankle jerks	94
Visual loss	16	Absent knee jerks	81
Rectal incontinence	14	Absent reflexes	11
Deafness	7	Romberg sign	55
Impotence	4	Impaired sensation	
		Impaired vibratory sense	52
		Impaired vision	43
		Impaired touch and pain	13
		Optic atrophy	20
		Ocular palsy	10
		Charcot joints	7

From Merritt et al., 1946.

the light reaction but with preservation of pupillary constriction in accommodation. Other findings include impaired superficial and deep sensation; weakness, wasting, and hypotonia of muscles; optic atrophy with visual loss; other cranial nerve palsies; and trophic changes, including Charcot joints or "mal perforant." Dysfunction of bowel, bladder, or genitals is also frequent.

Tabes dorsalis is seldom fatal. Ataxia or blindness may be incapacitating. Atonic bladder may lead to urinary tract infection and death. Progression may be arrested spontaneously or with treatment, but the lancinating pains and ataxia often continue.

Congenital Neurosyphilis

Congenital syphilis has been recognized since the sixteenth century. The spirochete is transmitted from the mother to the fetus between the fourth and seventh months of pregnancy. Mothers who have had syphilis for longer than 7 months are less likely to give birth to an infected infant. The clinical types are similar to those in adults except that tabes dorsalis is uncommon. Additional features of congenital neurosyphilis are hydrocephalus and the Hutchinson triad (interstitial keratitis, deformed teeth, and hearing loss). Among babies born to infected mothers, conventional clinical, radiographic, and serological tests were good predictors of CNS invasion by the spirochete. Immunoblotting for specific immunoglobulin M (IgM) antibodies in serum identified all cases with CNS invasion. The penicillin treatment schedule for infants is similar to that used in adults. Although the infection may be arrested, preexisting damage and neurologic signs may persist.

TREATMENT

Early Syphilis

The treatment of neurosyphilis begins with the treatment of early syphilis, and the standard treatment has been a single, intramuscular (IM) injection of 2.4 million USP units of penicillin G benzathine (Table 28.4 and Table 28.5).

In early studies, the failure rate was about 4%. Doxycycline, 100 mg twice a day for 14 days may be used when there is allergy to penicillin. Azithromycin, an antibiotic with a long half life, has been proposed as an alternative, but its effectiveness is not yet certain. It may be administered as a single, oral dose of 2 g, thus combining ease of administration and compliance.

There is no prompt and reliable way to determine the adequacy of treatment. Instead, patients must return for repeat testing at 3 months, 6 months, and 12 months, or until serologic tests give negative results. The Centers for Disease Control and Prevention criterion for retreatment is failure of the VDRL titer to drop by a factor of 4 within 6 months to 12 months.

The occasional failure of this regimen has been documented when symptoms of neurosyphilis appeared after a few patients had received the standard dose of penicillin G benzathine. To avoid this problem, a fourth criterion for retreatment is being considered: a four-fold drop in VDRL

▶ **TABLE 28.4** Centers for Disease Control and Prevention Recommended Treatments for Syphilis[27]

Primary, secondary, or early latent syphilis*
Recommended: benzathine penicillin G, 2.4 million units in a single dose, intramuscularly
Penicillin allergy: doxycycline, 100 mg by mouth twice daily for 14 days

Late latent syphilis, syphilis of unkown duration, tertiary syphilis
Recommended: benzathine penicillin G, 2.4 million units weekly for 3 weeks, intramuscularly
Penicillin allergy: doxycycline, 100 mg by mouth twice daily for 28 days

Neurosyphilis, syphilitic eye disease, syphilitic auditory disease
Recommended: Aqueous crystalline penicillin G, 18–24 million units per day administered as 3–4 million units intravenously every 4 hours or continuous infusion for 10–14 days
Alternative: procaine penicillin 2.4 million units intramuscularly once daily plus probenecid 500 mg by mouth 4 times a day, both for 10–14 days[†]

*Latent syphilis is defined as seroreactivity without other evidence of disease. Early latent syphilis is diagnosed in patients infected within the preceding year as defined by 1 of the following (1) a documented seroconversion; (2) unequivocal symptoms of primary or secondry syphilis; or (3) a sex partner documented to have primary, secondary, or early latent syphilis. Pregnant women should not be treated with doxycycline.

[†]Patients with non-life threatening allergies to penicillin should ideally be desensitized. Patients with serious allergies to sulfonamides should not be treated with probenecid-containing regiments.

Table reproduced from Golden et al (2003) and Centers for Disease Control and Prevention (2002).

▶ **TABLE 28.5 Recommendations for use of Diagnostic Tests for Syphilis**

Immediate Diagnostic or Therapeutic Action	Further Investigation or Action
Primary syphilis	
Dark-field or direct fluorescent test	VDRL titer for follow-up
Secondary syphilis	
VDRL titer	VDRL titer for follow-up
Selected asymptomatic persons[a]	
VDRL titer	FTA-ABS if VDRL positive
Adequancy of treatment for early or late syphilis	
VDRL titer 3, 6, 12 mo after treatment	Retreate if high titer does not fall by 12 mo or if titer increases after initial fall
Seropositive persons[b]	
CSF VDRL, CSF cell count	Treat for neurosyphilis if CSF VDRL positive or pleocytosis
Follow-up after treatment for asymptomatic neurosyphilis	
CSF cell count 6 wks, 3 mo, and 6 mo after treatment	CSF cell count at 12 mo, 24 mo if normal at 6 mo
Suspected syphilis[c]	
Treat as for early syphilis	VDLR titer 1, 3, and 6 mo after treatment

[a]Includes all-pregnant women, proven contacts of people with infectious syphilis, and people in high-risk groups.
[b]Includes people with neurologic abnormalities, before treatment with nonpenicillin regimens, before retreatment after treatment failure.
[c]Includes women with newly discovered syphilis seropositivity late in pregnancy, infants of mothers with inadequately treated syphilis, proven contacts of those with infectious syphilis.
From Hart, 1986; with permission.

titer at 3 months and an eight-fold drop at 6 months. The general belief is that neurosyphilis may be prevented only if CSF is normal 2 years after treatment of early syphilis.

Neurosyphilis

Penicillin G benzathine does not provide therapeutic levels of the drug in CSF. Therefore, the recommended therapy for established neurosyphilis is: intravenous (IV) administration of aqueous penicillin G, 12 million United States Pharmacopeia (USP) units to 24 million USP units, daily, for 10 days to 14 days; or intramuscular (IM) aqueous penicillin G, 2.4 million USP units daily, with probenecid (Benemid), 2 g given orally each day. Probenecid enhances serum levels of penicillin by reducing renal excretion.

Penicillin may provoke allergic reactions of rash or anaphylaxis. The Jarisch-Herxheimer fever reaction may occur with any form of antisyphilitic treatment but seems to be less common in neurosyphilis. Intravenous ceftriaxone has been proposed as an alternative, but there are not enough data to recommend its routine use.

Gummas have responded to treatment with penicillin alone, penicillin plus steroids, and even steroids alone. If the clinical circumstances make that diagnosis likely, and if the clinical condition of the patient permits, a trial of conservative treatment is warranted. If the diagnosis is doubtful, or if the circumstances dictate more immediate attention, biopsy and excision may be appropriate. For patients with both AIDS and any form of syphilis, some authorities advocate treatment with a regimen recommended for neurosyphilis.

After a course of therapy, quantitative blood serology is determined at 3-month intervals and usually shows a decline in titer if it had previously been elevated. Clinical neurologic examination should be performed regularly. The CSF is examined at 6 months and 12 months. If not normal, CSF is reexamined in 2 years. After 3 years, if the patient has improved and is clinically stable, and if the CSF and serologic tests are normal, neurologic and CSF examinations are discontinued.

Retreatment is recommended with high doses of intravenous penicillin G in the following situations: if the clinical neurologic findings progress without the discovery of another cause, especially if CSF pleocytosis persists; if the CSF cell count is not normal at 6 months; if the VDRL test in serum or CSF fails to shows a decline or shows a four-fold increase; or if the first course of treatment was suboptimal.

Neurosyphilis and AIDS

Neurosyphilis now probably occurs more often in HIV-positive persons than in those not HIV-infected. About 15% of HIV-infected persons are coinfected with *T. pallidum*. How HIV infection affects neurosyphilis is a matter of debate, but suspicions abound about concomitant HIV infection. For example, some authorities state that immunodeficiency reduces resistance to acquisition of syphilis, thereby allowing the disease to be more aggressive, with more frequent and more rapid progression to neurosyphilis; with the increased severity, there is less response to therapy, and more frequent relapse. In one series, 20% of penicillin-treated patients had rising STS titers or new clinical signs. Some authors state that current treatment recommendations may be inadequate. Ophthalmic syphilis is more frequent. CSF cell counts and protein levels are higher, and the incidence of luetic meningitis has increased.

These views, however, are virtually all subjects of argument. The frequency of neurosyphilis in an HIV-positive population is probably less than 2%. In addition, *T. pallidum* is not more likely to invade the CNS or to remain present in the CSF following standard treatment. Postmortem examination showed no pathologic differences in neurosyphilis, regardless of whether or not the subjects were HIV-infected. There is no major difference in the clinical syndromes of neurosyphilis, and claims about more aggressive disease have been difficult to substantiate. Serologic responses to syphilis seem undiminished, and the infections respond to treatment, as well. HIV-infected patients may show a lower rate of serologic response to penicillin therapy, but the clinical significance of this is uncertain.

The practical question is whether special syphilis treatment schedules are required for HIV-infected patients. A large trial of enhanced treatment of early syphilis included the addition of amoxicillin and probenecid to the conventional regimen; there was no decrease in the rate of treatment failure.

There are no substantiated data to warrant enhanced treatment regimens for syphilis in HIV-infected people. The questions, however, reinforce the need for careful evaluation and follow-up examination after treatment, so that retreatment may be given when needed. Serum RPR titers greater or equal to 1:32 and peripheral blood CD4+ T cell counts less than 350 cells/μL are risk factors for the development of neurosyphilis, and patients fulfilling these criteria should be evaluated and followed up aggressively. For patients who seem unlikely to comply, intravenous penicillin therapy (10 million USP units to 20 million USP units daily for 10 days to 14 days) is an option.

SUGGESTED READINGS

Adie WJ. Argyll-Robertson pupils, true and false. *BMJ* 1931;2:136–138.

Argyll-Robertson D. Four cases of spinal miosis with remarks on the action of light on the pupil. *Edinburgh Med J* 1869;15:487–493.

Augenbraun MH. Treatment of syphilis 2001: non-pregnant adults. *Clin Inf Dis* 2002;35:S187–S190.

Berger JR. Neurosyphilis in HIV-I seropositive individuals: a prospective study. *Arch Neurol* 1991;48:700–702.

Berry CD, Hooton TM, Collier AC, Lukehart SA. Neurologic relapse after benzathine penicillin therapy for secondary syphilis in a patient with HIV infection. *N Engl J Med* 1987;316:1587–1589.

Brandon WR, Boulos LM, Morse A. Determining the prevalence of neurosyphilis in a cohort co-infected with HIV. *Int J STD AIDS* 1993;4:99–101.

Burke JM, Schaberg DR. Neurosyphilis in the antibiotic era. *Neurology* 1985;35:1368–1371.

Dans PE, Cafferty L, Otter SE, Johnson RJ. Inappropriate use of the CSF VDRL test to exclude neurosyphilis. *Ann Intern Med* 1986;104:86–89.

Dowell ME, Ross PG, Musher DM, et al. Response of latent syphilis or neurosyphilis to ceftriaxone therapy in persons infected with HIV. *Am J Med* 1992;93:481–488.

Etgen T, Bischoff C, Resch M, Winbeck K, Conrad B, Sander D. Obstacles to the diagnosis and treatment of syphilitic amyotrophy. *Neurology* 2003;60:509–511.

Fleet WS, Watson RT, Ballinger WE. Resolution of a gumma with steroid therapy. *Neurology* 1986;36:1104–1107.

Flood JM, Weinstock HS, Guroy ME, et al. Neurosyphilis during the AIDS epidemic, San Francisco, 1985–1992. *J Infect Dis* 1998;177:931–940.

Golden MR, Marra CM, Holmes KK. Update on syphilis: Resurgence of an old problem. *JAMA* 2003;11:1510–1514.

Gourevich MN, Selwyn PA, Davenny K, et al. Effects of HIV infection on the serologic manifestations and response to treatment of syphilis in intravenous drug users. *Ann Intern Med* 1993;118:350–355.

Guinam ME. Treatment of primary and secondary syphilis: defining failure at 3- and 6-month follow-up. *JAMA* 1987;257:359–360.

Hahn RD, Cutler JC, Curtis AC, et al. Penicillin treatment of asymptomatic central nervous system syphilis. I. Probability of progression to symptomatic neurosyphilis. *Arch Dermatol* 1956;74:355–366.

Harrigan EP, MacLaughlin TJ, Feldman RG. Transverse myelitis due to meningovascular syphilis. *Arch Neurol* 1984;41:337–338.

Hart G. Syphilis tests in diagnostic and therapeutic decision making. *Ann Intern Med* 1986;104:368–376.

Heffelfinger JD, Weinstock HS, Berman SM, Swint EB. Primary and secondary syphilis-United States, 2000–2001. *JAMA* 2002;288:2963–2965.

Holmes MD, Brant-Zawadzki MM, Simon RP. Clinical features of meningovascular syphilis. *Neurology* 1984;34:553–556.

Hook EW III. Management of syphilis in HIV-infected individuals. *Am J Med* 1992;93:477–479.

Hook EW. Editorial response: diagnosing neurosyphilis. *Clin Infect Dis* 1994;18:295–297.

Hook EW, Marra CM. Acquired syphilis in adults. *N Engl J Med* 1992;326:1060–1069.

Jaffe HW, Kabins SA. Examination of CSF in patients with syphilis. *Rev Infect Dis* 1982;4(suppl):S842–S847.

Johns DR, Tierney M, Felsenstein D. Alteration in the natural history of neurosyphilis by concurrent infection with HIV. *N Engl J Med* 1987;316:1569–1572.

Katz DA, Berger JR, Duncan RC. Neurosyphilis: a comparative study of the effects of infection with human immunodeficiency virus. *Arch Neurol* 1993;50:243–249.

Knopman DS, Dekosky ST, Cummings JL, et al. Practice parameter: Diagnosis of dementia (an evidence-based review). *Neurology* 2001;56:1143–1153.

Lukehart SA, Hook EW III, Baker-Zander SA, et al. Invasion of the CNS by *Treponema pallidum*: implications for diagnosis and treatment. *Ann Intern Med* 1988;113:872–881.

Marra CM. Neurosyphilis. *Curr Neurol Neurosci Rep* 2004;Nov 4(6):435–440.

Marra CM, Boutin P, McArthur JC, et al. A pilot study evaluating ceftriaxone and penicillin G as treatment agents for neurosyphilis in human immunodeficiency virus-infected individuals. *Clin Inf Dis* 2000;30(3):540–544.

Marra CM, Crithlow CW, Hook EW, et al. Cerebrospinal fluid treponemal antibodies in untreated early syphilis. *Arch Neurol* 1995;52:68–72.

Marra CM, Gary DW, Kuypers J, Jacobson MA. Diagnosis of neurosyphilis in patients infected with HIV type 1. *J Infect Dis* 1996;174:219–221.

Marra CM, Longstreth WT, Maxwell CL, Lukeheart SA. Resolution of serum and cerebrospinal fluid abnormalities after treatment of neurosyphilis. *Sex Transm Dis* 1996;23:184–189.

Marra CM, Maxwell CL, Smith SL, Lukehart SA, et al. Cerebrospinal fluid abnormalities in patients with syphilis: association with clinical and laboratory features. *J Infect Dis* 2004;189(3):369–376.

Marra CM, Maxwell CL, Tantalo L, Eaton M, et al. Normalization of cerebrospinal fluid abnormalities after neurosyphilis therapy: does HIV status matter? *Clin Infect Dis* 2004;38(7):1001–1006.

Merritt HH, Adams RD, Solomon HC. *Neurosyphilis.* New York: Oxford University Press, 1946.

Michelow IC, Wendel GD, Norgard MV, Fiker Z, et al. Central nervous system infection in congenital syphilis. *New Engl J Med* 2002;346(23):1792–1798.

Musher DM, Hammill RJ, Baughn RE. Syphilis, the response to penicillin therapy, neurosyphilis, and the human immunodeficiency virus. *Ann Intern Med* 1990;113:872–881.

Noguchi H, Moore JW. A demonstration of *Treponema pallidum* in the brain of general paresis. *J Exp Med* 1913;17:232–238.

Rolfs RT, Joesoef MR, Hendershot EF, et al. A randomized trial of enhanced therapy for early syphilis in patients with and without human immunodeficiency virus infection. *N Engl J Med* 1997;337:307–314.

Rompalo AM, Joesoef MR, O'Donnell JA, et al. Clinical manifestations of early syphilis by HIV status and gender: results of the syphilis and HIV study. *Sex Transm Dis* 2001;28:158–165.

Centers for Disease Control and Prevention. Sexually transmitted disease treatment guidelines 2002:. *MMWR Recomm Rep* 2002;51(RR-6):1–78.

Simon RP. Neurosyphilis. *Neurology* 1994;44:2228–2230.

Tomberlin MG, Holton PD, Owens JL, Larsen RA. Evaluation of neurosyphilis in HIV-infected individuals. *Clin Infect Dis* 1994;18:288–294.

Timmermans M, Carr J. Neurosyphilis in the modern era. *J Neurol Neurosurg Psychiatry* 2004;75(12):1727–1730.

Walker DG, Walker GJ. Forgotten, but not gone: the continuing scourge of congenital syphilis. *Lancet Inf Dis* 2002;2(7):432–436.

Wagner-Jauregg J. Über die Einwirkung der Malaria auf die progressive Paralyse. *Psychiatr Neurol Wochenschr* 1918–1919;20:132–151.

Spirochete Infections: Leptospirosis

Burk Jubelt

Leptospirosis is caused by a group of closely related spirochetes belonging to the genus *Leptospira*. The organisms that cause human disease are now thought to belong to a single species, *L. interrogans*, with subtypes such as *canicola, pomona,* and *icterohaemorrhagiae* recognized serologically. More than 200 serovariants are arranged in 23 serologic groups.

Originally, specific serovariants were linked with particular clinical syndromes. Different serovariants, however, have been associated with the same or different clinical manifestations. Humans are incidental hosts for these spirochetes, which are enzootic in both wild and domestic animals, including cats, dogs, and cattle. Animals may become sick, clinically, and asymptomatic carriers may excrete the spirochete in urine for months or years.

Human infection comes from contact with infested animal tissue or urine, or from exposure to contaminated groundwater, soil, or vegetation. Leptospira may survive for prolonged periods outside of hosts in appropriate environmental conditions. The spirochete is thought to enter humans through mucocutaneous abrasions; it is not known whether the organism may penetrate intact skin.

Infection is not limited to specific human populations. Leptospirosis was once considered an occupational disease of people working with animal tissue, such as slaughterhouse employees, farmers, biologic laboratory workers, and those who prepare food products. With vigilance in protective measures, the incidence has decreased in these groups. In developed countries, more cases occur now in association with swimming or other recreational activities involving immersion in water and with living in slums, as well.

SYMPTOMS AND SIGNS

Symptoms usually appear abruptly 1 to 2 weeks after exposure and include: chills, fever, myalgia, headache, meningismus, and confusion ("clouded sensorium"). Gastrointestinal symptoms include nausea, emesis, anorexia, and diarrhea. There may be cough and chest pain. Cardiac manifestations, including bradycardia and hypoten-

sion, may be severe. Conjunctival suffusion is typical but not constant. There may be pharyngeal injection, cutaneous hemorrhages, or maculopapular rash. Hepatosplenomegaly and lymphadenopathy may occur. Acute renal failure is also seen. In this acute first phase, there is septicemia, and the organism may be isolated from CSF.

A second wave of symptoms may appear after the acute illness has apparently resolved. Original symptoms recur, sometimes with meningeal signs. Rarely, encephalitis, intracerebral hemorrhage, myelitis, optic neuritis, or peripheral neuritis develops. Mononeuritis or a Guillain-Barré-like picture may be seen. During the second phase of illness, immunoglobulin M (IgM) antibody to the *Leptospira* microorganisms and immune complexes may be found. Because the spirochete may no longer be isolated at this time, it is thought that the clinical symptoms seen during this phase of the disease are immune mediated. The ESR rate and liver function tests are usually abnormal. Urinalysis may reveal proteinuria, pyuria and microscopic hematuria.

DIAGNOSIS

Leptospiral infection may manifest clinically as aseptic meningitis. Although the agent may be recovered early in the syndrome, CSF pleocytosis is found infrequently in the first phase, but is prominent in the second. Usually, cell counts are in the range of 10 cells/mm^3 to several hundred cells per cm^3, but they may be higher. Neutrophils may be present early, but mononuclear cells usually predominate from the outset. Unlike most forms of viral meningitis, CSF protein content may exceed 100 mg/dL. The CSF glucose value is usually normal. It is likely that all pathogenic serovariants (*canicola, icterohaemorrhagiae,* and *pomona*) may cause aseptic meningitis.

Culture of the organism is possible if special facilities are available but results are slow to come. Dark-field examination of blood, urine, or CSF is unreliable. Serologic studies usually confirm the clinical diagnosis, but the antibody is not detected until the second phase of the illness, with the exception of IgM antibodies that may occasionally be detected earlier, at the end of the first week of illness. Genomic amplification techniques are still experimental. MRI may reveal enhancing, multiple, small cortical to cortical-subcortical lesions.

TREATMENT AND PROGNOSIS

Various antibiotics may treat leptospiral infection effectively. They must be administered early in the illness. High-dose penicillin is most generally used; doxycycline is the alternative for those who are allergic to penicillin. Spontaneous recovery is the rule for younger patients who are without other illnesses. Mortality is greater than 50% after 50 years of age, and is usually associated with severe liver disease and jaundice.

SUGGESTED READINGS

Bharti AR, Nally JE, Ricaldi JN, et al. Leptospirosis: a zoonotic disease of global importance. *Lancet Infect* 2003;3:757–771.

Centers for Disease Control and Prevention. Update: leptospirosis and unexplained acute febrile illness among athletes participating in triathlons—Illinois and Wisconsin, 1998. *JAMA* 1998;280:1474–1475.

Coyle PK, Dattwyler R. Spirochetal infection of the central nervous system. *Infect Dis Clin North Am* 1990;4:731–746.

Dimopoulou I, Politis P, Panagyiotakopoulos G, et al. Leptospirosis presenting with encephalitis-induced coma. *Intensive Care Med* 2002;28:1682.

Edwards GA, Domm BM. Human leptospirosis. *Medicine* 1960;39:117–156.

Farr RW. Leptospirosis. *Clin Infect Dis* 1995;21:1–6.

Gollop JH, Katz AR, Rudoy RC, et al. Rat-bite leptospirosis. *West J Med* 1993;159:76–77.

Jackson LA, Kaufmann AF, Adams WG, et al. Outbreak of leptospirosis associated with swimming. *Pediatr Infect Dis J* 1993;12:48–54.

Panicker JN, Mammachan R, Jayakumar RV. Primary neuroleptospirosis. *Postgrad Med J* 2001;77:589–590.

Theilen HJ, Luck C, Hanisch U, Ragaller M. Fatal intracerebral hemorrhage due to leptospirosis. *Infection* 2002;30:109–112.

Chapter 30

Spirochete Infections: Lyme Disease

Burk Jubelt

In 1975, a cluster of arthritis cases in children was recognized in Old Lyme, Connecticut. Many patients had had a migratory rash called erythema chronicum migrans (ECM), and some had neurologic or myocardial dysfunction. Affected adults also were seen. The syndrome was subsequently found to be caused by a previously unrecognized spirochete transmitted to humans by ixodid ticks. The spirochete has some characteristics of treponemes, but it is classified among the Borreliae (*Borrelia burgdorferi*). In the northeastern United States, the vector, *Ixodes scapularis*, regularly infests deer and mice. Other animals are also hosts for the tick.

EPIDEMIOLOGY

The disease occurs throughout the United States in regions where ixodid ticks are found, although all ixodid populations do not appear to be equal in supporting the presence of the spirochete. The United States has three main foci: the Northeast coastal states from Maryland to Maine, the upper Midwest (Minnesota and Wisconsin), and the Pacific coast (California and Oregon). The extent of human infection is unknown, but in the Lyme area antibodies are found in 4% of the population. The disease primarily occurs from May through September in temperate climates. About 20,000 Lyme cases are reported yearly in the United States. In Europe, a *B. burgdorferi* strain is associated with a similar clinical disorder called *Bannwarth syndrome* or tick-borne *meningopolyneuritis* (Garin-Bujadoux, Bannwarth). Although the manifestations of the disease were described in Europe earlier in the century and were associated with ixodid ticks, the nature of the infection was determined only after the spirochete was identified in North America.

Genetic variations of the spirochete probably account for differences between the syndromes described in Europe and in the United States. In the narrow sense, *B. burgdorferi* refers to the American isolate but broadly, it represents a more inclusive term, referring to all the variants that cause similar syndromes. The worldwide distribution of the spirochetes and associated illnesses is still being defined, but symptomatic infection seems to occur throughout the world wherever appropriate ticks reside. *Neuroborreliosis* is sometimes used synonymously with Lyme disease. However, other Borreliae that cause relapsing fever may also cause similar neurologic manifestations.

SIGNS AND SYMPTOMS

B. burgdorferi is most frequently transmitted to humans by the nymph stage of the tick, which is active in early summer, but transmission earlier or later may occur from contact with the adult arthropod. The organism may also be isolated from the tick larva, but it is difficult to recover from infected humans.

The course of infection in humans varies. It has been divided into three stages, but overlaps in symptoms and in timing are common. During the first stage (i.e., stage I, acute, localized infection, rash), usually a migrating ECM develops 3 days to 30 days after exposure. The center of the "bull's eye" rash is at the site of the tick bite. Smaller secondary rings, whose centers are less indurated than that of the primary lesion, often appear later. The CNS may be involved during local infection due to premeningitic seeding. Headache, myalgia, stiff neck, and even cranial nerve palsies (almost invariably the seventh nerve) may occur, but CSF is usually normal. The ECM usually resolves in 3 to 4 weeks, although transitory erythematous blotches and rings that do not migrate may occur later.

Prominent neurologic and cardiac manifestations are seen in the second stage (i.e., stage II, subacute stage, early disseminated disease, early neurologic), several weeks after the onset of ECM. Heart problems are usually confined to conduction defects but there may be myopericarditis with left ventricular dysfunction. Meningeal symptoms and signs constitute the major features of the neurologic illness, with headache and stiff neck principal. Fever is not a regular feature. Radiculitis or radiculoneuritis, multiple or isolated, is common and may cause severe root pain, or focal or generalized weakness. Radiculoneuritis may take the form of a Guillain-Barré-like syndrome, but the CSF shows pleocytosis. In Europe it is referred to as lymphocytic meningoradiculitis (Bannwarth syndrome).

Cranial nerves (usually the seventh nerve) are frequently involved. The facial palsy is usually bilateral. Both sides of the face may become paralyzed simultaneously or sequentially. Polyneuritis or mononeuritis multiplex may also occur. Identifying the cause requires a sensitive index of suspicion in areas where the disease is endemic. Neurologic disease may also occur without previous ECM or recognized tick bite. Occasionally, mild meningoencephalitis, along with irritability, emotional lability, decreased concentration and memory, and sleep abnormalities may occur.

The third stage (i.e., stage III, chronic, late neurologic) is characterized by chronic or late persistent infection of the nervous system. It usually occurs months after the original infection, but it may overlap with the subacute "early neurologic" disease of Stage II. Syndromes included in this stage are encephalopathy, encephalomyelopathy, and polyneuropathy. The encephalopathy is characterized by memory and other cognitive dysfunction. The encephalomyelopathy is characterized by signs of encephalopathy combined with progressive, long-tract signs that may involve the optic nerve and sphincters. White matter lesions may be visible on MRI of the brain. Usually there are elevated Lyme-antibody titers in the blood and CSF. Response to antibiotic treatment has been variable. The late polyneuropathy is primarily sensory. Patients complain of acral dysesthesia. Electrophysiologic evidence reveals a neuropathic process, and the sensory symptoms respond to appropriate antibiotic therapy. Chronic arthritis also occurs in stage III.

DIAGNOSIS

The combination of meningitis, radiculitis, and neuritis without fever occurs in virtually no other circumstance. If the appropriate history of tick exposure and ECM is obtained, the diagnosis is assured. Partial syndromes and

▶ **TABLE 30.1 CSF Analysis in Lyme Disease Encephalomyelitis**

Test	CSF
Opening pressure[a]	Normal
Total white cells/mm^3	166 (15–700)[b]
Lymphocytes (%)	93 (40–100)
Glucose (mg/dL)[c]	49 (33–61)
Protein (mg/dL)	79 (8–400)
IgG/albumin ratio (n = 20)	0.18 (0.9–0.44)
Oligoclonal bands (n = 4)	Present
Myelin basic protein (n = 5)	Absent
VDRL (n = 20)	Negative

[a]n = 38 except where noted
[b]Median (range)
[c]Serum glucose = 95 mg/dL (87 mg/dL to 113 mg/dL)
From Pachner and Steere, 1985; with permission.

absence of appropriate early findings, however, might require differentiation from a wide variety of illnesses, ranging from herniated disc to other causes of acute aseptic or subacute meningitis. Brain MRI and CT are normal, except in Stage III, and the EEG is usually normal or nonspecific.

CSF pressure is normal. Abnormalities in the CSF formula are usually, but not always, present (Table 30.1).

Oligoclonal bands are often present. *B. burgdorferi* has been isolated (cultured) from the CSF, a rare technical feat that may not be relied on for routine diagnosis. Demonstration of elevated levels of spirochete-specific immunoglobulin M (IgM) or IgG, in the serum or CSF as identified by enzyme-linked immunosorbent assay (ELISA), or less reliably by immunofluorescence antibody test (IFA), constitutes the basis of diagnosis in clinically appropriate circumstances. Specific confirmation of elevated titers is needed by Western blot reaction to spirochete proteins. The procedure is complicated by frequent cross-reactions with other proteins, and strict criteria of interpretation are required for the test results to be useful.

The diagnosis of Lyme disease, particularly chronic encephalomyelopathy, is complicated by vagaries of the immune response and the indefinite clinical picture. Rapid treatment of Lyme disease in the early stages, or perhaps even intercurrent use of antibiotics for other purposes, may result in the absence of agent-specific antibody response when the more chronic syndromes become apparent. In addition, antibody carriers in endemic areas may be asymptomatic, making the presence of antibodies inconclusive in questionable cases.

Brain SPECT has been suggested as a method for determining abnormality when other imaging procedures are normal. The specificity of the abnormalities for Lyme disease, as opposed to other encephalopathies however, is not yet determined. The ambiguities in the diagnosis of chronic encephalomyelopathy have led to a generous use of prolonged antibiotic treatment in doubtful circumstances, even sometimes when other neurologic problems such as multiple sclerosis, are clearly the cause. Polymerase chain reaction (PMR) technology and sensitive immunoassays have been applied to the detection of *B. burgdorferi* DNA and antigens in the CSF, but their usefulness is still undetermined.

TREATMENT

Oral doxycycline and amoxicillin have become the common medications for treatment of Lyme disease during early stage I, as characterized by ECM. In allergic patients, cefuroxime axetil or erythromycin may be used. Doxycycline should not be used during pregnancy or in children under 8 years of age. These agents usually prevent the development of subsequent stages.

Intravenously administered, third-generation cephalosporins, usually ceftriaxone, cefotaxime, or cefuroxime axetil, are now generally employed for treatment of neurologic symptoms. Before antibiotic therapy, the second-stage neurologic syndrome lasted for a mean of 30 weeks, although the intensity fluctuated. Intravenous antibiotics usually cause acute symptoms to resolve as the agents are being given. Motor signs last a mean of 7 to 8 weeks, irrespective of the use of antibiotics.

Even with mild CNS involvement, a prolonged period of subtle to moderate memory, emotional, and cognitive problems may follow successful treatment. In the best-documented late encephalomyelopathy cases, several months were required after treatment before clinical improvement was noted. The proper length of treatment is uncertain. For most cases, 4 weeks of treatment are required. As more chronic and less well documented cases have been treated, the tendency is to treat longer, even up to several months. The efficacy of prolonged treatment has not been established, however. Oral antibiotic doses appropriate for ECM therapy are sufficient to treat isolated nerve palsies associated with elevated spirochete-antibody levels.

The U.S. FDA approved the use of a vaccine constituted against the spirochete's Outer-surface protein A (OspA). However, in 2002 the vaccine was removed from the market because of poor public acceptance and reactions to the vaccine. Protective measures for the prevention of Lyme borreliosis may include the avoidance of tick-infested areas, the use of protective clothing, repellents, acaricides, tick checks, and modifications of landscapes in or near residential areas.

SUGGESTED READINGS

Benke T, Gasse T, Hittmair-Delazer M, Schmutzhard E. Lyme encephalopathy: long-term neuropsychological deficits years after acute neuroborreliosis. *Acta Neurol Scand* 1995;91:353–357.

Bloom BJ, Wyckoff PM, Meissner HC, Steere AC. Neurocognitive abnormalities in children after classic manifestations of Lyme disease. *Pediatr Infect Dis J* 1998;17:189–196.

Cadavid D, Barbour AG. Neuroborreliosis during relapsing fever: review of the clinical manifestations, pathology, and treatment of infections in humans and experimental animals. *Clin Infect Dis* 1998;26: 151–164.

Coyle PK. Lyme disease. *Curr Neurol Neurosci Reports* 2002;2:479–487.

Eskow E, Rao R-VS, Mordechai E. Concurrent infection of the central nervous system by *Borrelia burgdorferi* and *Bartonella henselae*. *Arch Neurol* 2001;58:1357–1363.

Halperin JJ. Nervous system Lyme disease. *J Neurol Sci* 1998;153: 182–191.

Halperin JJ. Lyme disease and the peripheral nervous system. *Muscle Nerve* 2003;28:133–143.

Halperin JJ, Logigian EL, Finkel MF, Pearl RA. Practice parameters for the diagnosis of patients with nervous system Lyme borreliosis (Lyme disease). Quality Standards Subcommittee of the American Academy of Neurology. *Neurology* 1996;46:619–627.

Hubalek Z, Halouzka J. Distribution of *Borrelia burgdorferi sensu lato* genomic groups in Europe: a review. *Eur J Epidemiol* 1997;13: 951–957.

Nachman SA, Pontrelli L. Central nervous system Lyme disease. *Sem Pedr Infect Dis* 2003;14:123–130.

Nowakowski J, Schwartz I, Nadelman RB, et al. Culture-confirmed infection and reinfection with *Borrelia burgdorferi*. *Ann Intern Med* 1997;127:130–132.

Oksi J, Kalimo H, Marttila RJ, et al. Inflammatory brain changes in Lyme borreliosis: a report on three patients and review of literature. *Brain* 1996;119:2143–2154.

Pachner AR, Steere AC. The triad of neurologic manifestations of Lyme disease: meningitis, cranial neuritis and radiculoneuritis. *Neurology* 1985;35:47–53.

Pacuzzi RM, Younger DS, eds. Lyme disease issue. *Semin Neurol* 1997;17(1):

Schmidt BL. PCR in laboratory diagnosis of human *Borrelia burgdorferi* infections. *Clin Microbiol Rev* 1997;10:185–201.

Stanek G, Strle F. Lyme borreliosis. *Lancet* 2003;362:1639–1647.

Chapter 31

▶ Parasitic Infections

Burk Jubelt

Disease caused by parasites is uncommon in developed countries. In tropical and less developed areas, however, parasitic infections exact a heavy toll on society. Poverty and poor living conditions play a significant role in the pathogenesis of these infections, but an appropriate climate for vectors to facilitate transmission is also necessary. The combination of increased international travel to and immigration from endemic areas has increased the likelihood of encountering tropical parasitic infections in the United States. Indigenous parasites are being encountered more frequently because of long-term survival of immunosuppressed patients who have increased susceptibility to infection. Parasitic infections may be divided into two categories: those caused by worms (helminths) and those caused by protozoa.

HELMINTHIC INFECTION

Helminths are large complex organisms that frequently elicit systemic allergic responses (eosinophilia) and more often cause focal, rather than diffuse, involvement of the nervous system. Helminths are divided into tapeworms (cestodes), flukes (trematodes), and roundworms (nematodes) (Table 31.1).

Cysticercosis

Cysticercosis is the result of encystment of the larvae of *Taenia solium*, the pork tapeworm, in the tissues. The infestation is acquired by ingestion of the ova usually by fecal contamination of food or less often by autoinfection via anal-oral transfer or reverse peristalsis of proglottids

▶ TABLE 31.1 Common Helminthic Infections of the Nervous System

Disease/Parasite	Geographic Location
Cestodes (tapeworms)	
Cysticercosis	Asia, Africa, Central and South
Taenia solium	America, Eastern and Central Europe, Southwest U.S.
Echinococcosis (hydatid cyst disease)	Worldwide
Trematodes (flukes)	
Schistosomiasis	
S. japonicum	Far East
S. mansoni	South America, Caribbean, Africa, and Middle East
S. haematobium	Africa, Middle East
Paragonimiasis	Asia, South Pacific, Central Africa, Central and South America
Nematodes (roundworms)	
Trichinosis	Worldwide
Eosinophilic meningitis	Southeast Asia, Pacific Islands,
Angiostrongylus cantonensis	Hawaii, Caribbean, and Africa
Africa	
Gnathostoma spinigerum	
Toxocariasis (visceral larva migrans)	Worldwide
Strongyloidiasis	Tropical and Subtropical regions, including United States

into the stomach. The larvae are not acquired by eating infected pork, and cysticercosis regularly occurs in vegetarians in endemic areas. Ingestion of infected pork results in the adult tapeworm infection.

Epidemiology

CNS involvement occurs in 50% to 70% of all cases. Virtually all symptomatic patients have CNS involvement. It is the most common parasitic infection of the CNS. Cerebral cysticercosis is common in Mexico, Central and South America, Southeast Asia, China, India, Central and Eastern Europe and Sub-Saharan Africa. It is now endemic in the southwestern United States. The disease has again become relatively common in the United States because of immigration from Mexico. The disease may occur in other areas where a reservoir of infected pigs exists. In Mexico, cerebral cysticercosis is found in 2% to 4% of the population in unselected autopsy studies.

Pathology

Typical cysts measure 5 to 10 mm and may be discrete and encapsulated, or delicate, thin-walled, and multicystic. The miliary form with hundreds of cysticerci is most common in children. Meningeal cysts cause a CSF pleocytosis. Live encysted larvae in the parenchyma cause little inflammation. Inflammation occurs when the larvae die, usually years after ingestion, which often correlates with the onset of symptoms.

Symptoms and Signs

Clinical manifestations may be divided into four basic types, depending on anatomic site: parenchymal, subarachnoid (or meningitic), intraventricular, and spinal. The most common presenting manifestations are seizures, increased intracranial pressure with headaches and papilledema, and meningitis.

In the parenchymal form, symptoms are related to the site of encystment. Cortical cysts frequently give rise to focal or generalized seizures. Other focal deficits may appear suddenly or may be more chronic. Signs include hemiparesis, sensory loss, hemianopsia, aphasia, or ataxia from cerebellar cysts. Stroke, which occurs secondary to vessel involvement, and dementia are occasionally seen. Rarely, an acute diffuse encephalitis, with confusion to coma, is seen at the time of the initial infection (miliary form).

The subarachnoid form may be the result of the rupture or death of an arachnoidal cyst or its transformation into the racemose form of the organism, which may enlarge within the basal cisterns and cause obstructive hydrocephalus. Symptoms of meningeal involvement vary from mild headache to a syndrome of chronic meningitis with meningism and communicating hydrocephalus. Spinal involvement may occur and may evolve into arachnoiditis and complete spinal subarachnoid block.

Cysts in the third ventricle or fourth ventricle (intraventricular form) obstruct the flow of CSF and may result in obstructive hydrocephalus. The cyst may move within the ventricular cavity and produce a "ball-valve" effect, resulting in intermittent symptoms. Sudden death may occur in these patients, occasionally without prior symptoms. This form frequently occurs in conjunction with the subarachnoid form.

The spinal form is rare. Extramedullary intradural lesions, which are usually cervical, and intramedullary lesions, which are usually thoracic, may be present.

Laboratory Data and Diagnosis

The diagnosis of cysticercosis should be considered in all patients who have ever resided in endemic areas and who have epilepsy, meningitis, or increased intracranial pressure. CT and MRI are useful in evaluating such patients. Hydrocephalus may be observed and the exact site of obstruction determined. Intravenous (IV) contrast may demonstrate intraventricular cysts. Parenchymal cysts may calcify, revealing single or multiple punctate calcifications on CT. On CT and MRI, viable cysts appear as small lucent areas that may enhance either diffusely or in a ring pattern (Fig. 31.1). Surrounding edema may also be seen.

Most patients have multiple cysts. CSF findings may be normal or may reveal a moderate pleocytosis and elevated pressure. In more severe meningitis, the CSF may contain several hundred to several thousand white blood cells (usually mononuclear), elevated protein content, and low glucose, presenting a clinical picture similar to that for fungal or tuberculous meningitis. Eosinophilic meningitis is occasionally seen but is uncommon. The presence of eosinophilia in the blood suggests another parasitic infestation and does not occur in pure neurocysticercosis. CSF or serum antibody tests are usually positive.

Treatment

Ventricular shunting is usually adequate for treatment of hydrocephalic forms of this disorder. Seizures may be controlled with anticonvulsants. Intractable seizures may develop, and surgical removal of cysts may be beneficial. Corticosteroids have been used to relieve the meningitic symptoms, but their value has not been established. Praziquantel, effective in stopping the progression of the parenchymal form of cysticercosis, was the first drug used successfully against the cysts. It is less effective for subarachnoid cysts or the chronic meningitic form with arachnoiditis. Albendazole has greater anticysticercal activity

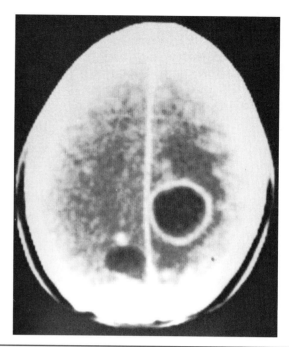

FIGURE 31.1. Cerebral cysticercosis: CT. Patient with partial seizures and normal examination. A large lucent lesion with rim enhancement is seen on the left. A nonenhancing lucency with small calcification appears in the right parietal region. Other small lesions are seen bilaterally. (Courtesy of Drs. Verity Grinnell and Mark A. Goldberg.)

and is now the drug of choice. Concomitant use of corticosteroids may be required to prevent severe inflammatory reactions and edema in response to the dying cysticerci.

Echinococcosis (Hydatid Cysts)

Epidemiology

Echinococcosis is a tissue infection of humans caused by the larvae of *Echinococcus species*. Two main forms of echinococcus occur, cystic hydatid disease caused by *E. granulosus*, and alveolar hydatid disease caused by *E. multilocularis*. *E. granulosus* is a tapeworm parasite of the dog family. There is an intermediate phase of development with hydatid cyst formation in other mammals. Sheep and cattle are usually the intermediate hosts, but humans may be infected as dead end hosts, especially by ova shed in dog feces. The disease is most common in countries where herd dogs assist with sheep and cattle raising. It is rare in the United States. The infestation may occur at any age but is most common in children living in rural areas.

E. multilocularis infections are perpetuated in a sylvatic cycle with wild carnivores. Red and arctic foxes are the most important definitive hosts. Much less frequently, domestic dogs may be the definitive host. *E. multilocularis* has a much wider geographic distribution than was previously thought. It is endemic in the northern hemisphere with cases occurring around the world including Alaska. The peak age for *E. multilocularis* is from 50 to 70 years.

The cysts are most commonly found in the liver and the lungs. If the embryos pass the pulmonary barrier, cyst formation may occur in any organ. The brain is involved in about 2% of the cases, and neurologic symptoms may develop in patients with cysts in the skull or spine. Cystic lesions caused by *E. granulosus* are usually large, spherical and single. They are most common in the cerebral hemispheres but may develop in the ventricles, subarachnoid and epidural spaces, cerebellum and spinal cord. In contrast, cysts caused by *E. multilocularis* are small, group in clusters and are usually located in the brain parenchyma. Hydatid disease of the heart may result in embolic cerebral infarcts.

Signs and Symptoms

The signs and symptoms that develop with enlarging cysts in the brain are similar to those of tumor in the affected region. Seizures and increased intracranial pressure may also occur. Involvement of the spine may result in radicular manifestations and spinal cord compression. Disease caused by *E. multilocularis* is more severe and more rapidly progressive.

Diagnosis

The diagnosis of hydatid cyst as the cause of symptoms is rarely made before operation. CT and MRI should be used to localize the lesions. *E. granulosus* cysts are usually single, nonenhancing, and of CSF density. Cysts in the subarachnoid space may be multiple and confluent. Cysts in both locations may have a multilocular appearance. Needle biopsy usually is precluded, because rupture of a cyst results in allergic manifestations, including anaphylaxis. In spinal disease, vertebral collapse is common and is evident on x-rays. Cysts formed as a result of *E. multilocularis* infection tend to be multiple, surrounded by edema and show ring-like enhancement. Eosinophilia is uncommon except after cyst rupture. Liver enzymes are usually normal. Serologic tests are positive in 60% to 90% of infected individuals but the results are not an accurate assessment, owing to cross-reactions with other parasitic diseases.

Treatment

Treatment is complete surgical removal without rupturing the cyst that occurs in about 25% of cases. Drug treatment with albendazole may decrease the size of cysts and prevent allergic reactions and secondary hydatidosis at the time of surgery. Chemotherapy alone may destroy the cysts.

Schistosomiasis (Bilharziasis)

Involvement of the nervous system by the ova of trematodes is rare. In most reported cases, the lesions were associated with infection with *Schistosoma japonicum*, but isolated cases of *S. haematobium* and *S. mansoni* have also been recorded. *S. japonicum* has a predilection for the cerebral hemispheres; *S. haematobium* and *S. mansoni* more frequently affect the spinal cord. These predilections appear to relate to the location of the adult worms from where ova are released. *S. japonicum* resides in superior mesenteric venules, but the occurrence of ectopic worms in cerebral venules may explain in part the high incidence of cerebral involvement. *S. mansoni* primarily resides in the inferior mesenteric venules, whereas *S. haematobium* is found in the vesical plexus.

Pathology

The presence of the ova in the nervous system causes an inflammatory exudate containing eosinophils and giant cells (granulomas), necrosis of the parenchyma, and deposition of calcium.

Epidemiology

Schistosomiasis is one of the most important worldwide parasitic diseases, occurring in over 200 million people. *S. japonicum* occurs mainly in Asia and in the Pacific tropics. *S. mansoni* is prevalent in the Caribbean, South America, Africa, and the Middle East. *S. haematobium* occurs in Africa and the Middle East. Symptoms may occur within a few months of exposure or may be delayed for 1 to 2 years. Relapses may occur several or many years after the original infection. The CNS is involved in 3% to 5% of the patients with *S. japonicum* but in fewer patients with other species.

Clinical Manifestations

Schistosomiasis occurs in three phases. The first, or cercarial dermatitis, is an acute reaction to the penetration of the skin by cercariae. The second is a serum sickness reaction, Katayama fever, which occurs 6 to 8 weeks after exposure and manifests as fever, urticaria, abdominal pain, diarrhea, and muscle pain. The third stage is a chronic infection of most internal organs (liver, spleen, bladder, heart, lungs). Cerebral schistosomiasis may be acute during Katayama fever or chronic with the third phase. Acute cases usually present as a diffuse fulminating meningoencephalitis with fever, headache, confusion, lethargy, and coma. Focal or generalized seizures, hemiplegia, and other focal neurologic signs are common. The chronic cerebral form usually simulates the clinical picture of a tumor with localizing signs and increased intracranial pressure with papilledema. Intracranial hemorrhages may also occur. Granulomatous masses in the spinal cord almost always present acutely with signs and symptoms of an incomplete transverse lesion, with or without spinal subarachnoid block, depending on the size of the lesion. The conus is the most common site of spinal cord involvement. Granulomatous root involvement may also occur. Clinical manifestations may include sphincter dysfunction, flaccid paraplegia, and sensory loss.

Laboratory Data

There is leukocytosis with an increase in eosinophils in the blood, although this may not be the case with the chronic cerebral form. The CSF pressure may be increased with large intracerebral lesions and partial or incomplete subarachnoid block with spinal lesions. A slight or moderate mononuclear pleocytosis in the CSF (sometimes with eosinophils) and an increased protein content may occur. Cerebral enhancing lesions may be seen with CT or MRI. Enlargement of the lower spinal cord may be demonstrated in some cases of spinal schistosomiasis by myelography, CT, or MRI (Fig. 31.2).

Diagnosis

The diagnosis is established from the history of gastrointestinal upset, eosinophilia in the blood, and the presence of ova in the stool or urine. The absence of ova in the stool and urine does not exclude the diagnoses. Serologic tests

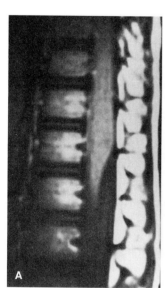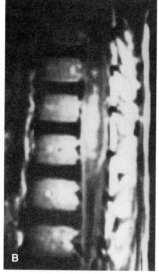

FIGURE 31.2. Spinal cord schistosomiasis: sagittal T1-weighted MRIs. A: Without contrast demonstrates markedly enlarged conus medullaris. **B:** With contrast demonstrates prominent regions of enhancement within the enlarged conus. [From Selwa et al. (1991, with permission).]

and biopsy of the rectal mucosa are also of value in the establishment of the diagnosis.

Treatment

The broad-spectrum drug praziquantel is the drug of choice. It is effective against all three human schistosomes. Because of the emergence of praziquantel-resistant strains of *S. mansoni* in some areas, oxamniquine is frequently added to the regimen for this schistosome. Oral steroids may decrease swelling. Anticonvulsive drugs should be given to control seizures. Surgical excision of the large granulomatous lesions may be required. Steroids and decompressive laminectomy may be needed when subarachnoid block is present.

Paragonimiasis

Paragonimiasis is the disease caused by the lung flukes *Paragonimus westermani* and *P. mexicanus*. Other *Paragonimus* species may rarely infect humans.

Epidemiology

These trematodes commonly infect humans in China, Korea, Japan, Southeast Asia, South Pacific areas, Africa, India, and Central and South America. Infection occurs by eating uncooked or poorly cooked freshwater crustaceans. Immature flukes exist in the intestines and spread through the body, occasionally reaching the brain and spinal cord.

Signs and Symptoms

Pulmonary and intestinal symptoms are the most common. Pulmonary involvement includes chronic cough, hemoptysis, and cavitary lesions on chest radiographs, thus simulating tuberculosis.

CNS involvement occurs in 10% to 15% of affected patients. Symptoms and signs of cerebral involvement include fever, headache, meningoencephalitis, focal and generalized seizures, dementia, hemiparesis, visual disturbances, and other focal manifestations. Various syndromes have been recognized: acute meningitis, chronic meningitis, acute purulent meningoencephalitis, infarction, epilepsy, subacute progressive encephalopathy, chronic granulomatous disease (tumorous form), and late inactive forms (chronic brain syndrome).

Laboratory Data

The CSF may be under increased pressure. The pleocytosis is primarily polymorphonuclear in acute forms and lymphocytic in more chronic forms. Eosinophils are occasionally present, and many red blood cells are occasionally seen in the acute cases. The protein content and gamma globulins are usually increased. The glucose content may be decreased.

Diagnosis

Diagnosis is most often made by detecting ova in the sputum and stool. Peripheral anemia, eosinophilia, leukocytosis, and elevated erythrocyte sedimentation rate and gamma globulins may occur. Serologic and skin tests are available. Positive CSF antibody tests are diagnostic but not very sensitive. CT and MRI may also be of assistance in diagnosis, revealing grape-like clusters of ring-enhancing lesions, with surrounding edema during acute disease, and ventricular dilatation and intracranial calcifications, including the characteristic "soap bubble" calcifications during chronic disease. During the early progressive course, mortality may reach 5% to 10%. The later chronic granulomatous state tends to be benign.

Treatment

Therapy includes praziquantel as the drug of choice (an alternative is bithionol) for the acute to subacute meningoencephalitis and surgical treatment for the chronic tumorous form.

Trichinosis (Trichinellosis)

Trichinosis is an acute infection caused by the roundworm *Trichinella spiralis* and less frequently by other *Trichinella* species.. Infection is acquired by eating larvae (in cysts) in raw or undercooked pork. Bear and other wild game meats have also been implicated.

Pathology

The pathologic changes in the nervous system include the presence of filiform larvae in the cerebral capillaries and in the parenchyma, perivascular inflammation, petechial hemorrhages, and granulomatous nodules.

Symptoms and Signs

Trichinosis manifests as a systemic infection stemming from larval migration (larviposition) with fever, headache, muscle pain and tenderness (muscle invasion), periorbital edema, facial edema, subconjunctival hemorrhages, and myocardial involvement. Gastrointestinal symptoms are less frequent, occurring in about 25% of symptomatic cases. Neurologic involvement occurs in 10% to 25% of symptomatic infections and develops any time within the first few weeks of the infection. There may be a severe diffuse encephalitis or meningoencephalitis with confusion, delirium, coma, seizures, and evidence of focal damage to the cerebrum, brainstem, or cerebellum. Edema of the optic nerve, meningeal signs, spinal cord syndromes, and neuropathies may also occur.

Laboratory Data

The most important laboratory findings are leukocytosis and eosinophilia in the blood. Muscle enzymes may be increased. The CSF is abnormal in about one-third of cases. There may be a slight lymphocyte pleocytosis, but eosinophilia is rare. The protein content and pressure are often elevated. The parasites are found in the CSF of approximately 30% of patients. CT and MRI may reveal single or multiple small hypodensities in the white matter or cortex in about three-fourths of cases, with about half of these lesions enhancing with contrast.

Diagnosis

The diagnosis is usually not difficult when neurologic symptoms appear in a group of individuals who have eaten infected pork and show the other manifestations of the disease (gastrointestinal symptoms, tenderness of the muscles, and edema of the eyelids). Difficulty is encountered in isolated cases when infection results from ingestion of meat other than pork or where the other manifestations of the infection are lacking. Trichinosis should be considered an etiologic factor in all patients with encephalitis of obscure nature. Repeated examination of the blood for eosinophilia and elevated muscle enzymes, biopsy of the muscles, and serologic tests should establish the diagnosis.

Prognosis

Recovery within a few days or weeks is the rule except when there is profound coma or evidence of severe damage to the cerebrum. For those with CNS involvement, mortality is 10% to 20%. Recovery is usually accompanied by complete or almost complete remission of the neurologic signs. Recurrent convulsive seizures have been reported as a late sequel. The CT and MRI lesions usually resolve in 4 to 8 weeks with treatment.

Treatment

Mebendazole or albendazole are used to treat tissue larvae. Corticosteroids are given to reduce inflammation and cerebral edema.

Eosinophilic Meningitis

The human nervous system may be invaded by the nematode rat lungworm, *Angiostrongylus cantonensis*, which uses a molluscan intermediate host and invades the domestic rat and other rodents in the course of its life cycle.

Infection in humans (accidental hosts) usually arises from the ingestion of raw snails, shrimp, crabs, and fish, which are the intermediate hosts. It is now endemic throughout Southeast Asia, the Pacific Islands, including Hawaii Africa and the Caribbean. Sporadic cases have been reported in many other regions.

Signs and Symptoms

Involvement of the human nervous system is usually characterized by acute meningitis (headache 90%, nuchal rigidity 60%, fever 50%), but less frequently there may be encephalitis, encephalomyelitis, radiculomyeloencephalitis, or involvement of cranial nerves (especially VI and VII). Onset occurs 2 to 45 days after the ingestion of the raw intermediate host, with an average of 10 to 16 days. Paresthesias and severe dysesthetic pains, probably from posterior root inflammation, occur in about 50% of the patients. The infection is most common in children. Nervous system lesions are the result of destruction of tissue by the parasite and to necrosis and aneurysmal dilatation of cerebral vessels, resulting in small or large hemorrhages.

Diagnosis and Treatment

A CSF pleocytosis of 100 to 1000 cells/mm^3 with many eosinophils is characteristic. However, the absence of CSF eosinophilia does not exclude the diagnosis. A peripheral blood eosinophilia is almost always seen. CT is usually normal. MRI may reveal: (1) increased signal intensity on T1 imaging in the globus pallidus and cerebral peduncle, (2) meningeal enhancement and cerebral and cerebellar punctate enhancement with contrast, (3) hyperintense signal in these areas on T2 images, and (4) ventriculomegaly. Serologic tests are available but are neither specific nor sensitive. Usually, the disease is self-limited. In severe cases, rarely, death may be the result of small or large hemorrhagic lesions in the brain. There is no specific therapy.

Other Eosinophilic Meningitis

Not all cases of eosinophilic meningitis are caused by *A. cantonensis* infestation; other parasitic infections (cysticercosis, schistosomiasis, paragonimiasis), coccidioidomycosis, foreign bodies, drug allergies, and neoplasms may also cause this syndrome but less frequently. Another nematode of the Far East, *Gnathostoma spinigerum*, usually causes eosinophilic meningitis when it invades the CNS; such invasion occurs much less frequently with *G. spinigerum* than with *A. cantonensis*. It has also caused the clinical syndromes of cranial nerve palsy, radiculomyelitis, encephalitis, and subarachnoid and intracranial hemorrhage. When the CNS is involved, the symptoms are more severe and the mortality is higher with

G. spinigerum, probably because of its larger size, than with *A. cantonensis* infection. Also, with *G. spinigerum*, CT and MRI are usually abnormal because parenchymal disease (brain and spinal cord) is more common. Because of immigration, *G. spinigerum* has become an emerging infection. Cases are being reported in Europe, Mexico and Central America.

Toxocariasis

In toxocariasis, visceral larva migrans is a syndrome of pulmonary symptoms, hepatomegaly, and chronic eosinophilia caused by the larvae of the dog and cat ascarids (roundworms) *Toxocara canis* and *T. cati*. Eggs from the animals' feces may be ingested, especially by children playing with infected dogs or contaminated soil. Although visceral larva migrans is uncommon and nervous system involvement is rare, the disease is always a potential threat owing to the ubiquitous infections of domestic animals.

Signs and Symptoms

Neurologic signs are most often manifest by focal deficits, especially hemiparesis. Encephalopathy and seizures also have occurred. Ocular involvement is more common than CNS disease.

Diagnosis

Eosinophils are infrequently seen in the CSF but are common in the periphery.

CT may reveal single or multiple low density lesions. MRI may reveal single or multiple relatively large cerebral white matter lesions. On T1 images the lesions may be either hypo- or hyperintense. T2 images are hyperintense. Most lesions have prominent T1-contrast enhancement. Meningeal enhancement may also be seen. Serology is helpful for diagnosis, and hypergammaglobulinemia is common. Larvae may be identified in the sputum or in tissue granulomas from biopsy.

Treatment

Albendazole is the drug of choice. Thiabendazole and mebendazole are alternative agents. Corticosteroids are used to suppress the intense inflammation that occurs with this infection. An association of toxocariasis with pica and lead encephalopathy has been noted. Another ascarid, *Ascaris lumbricoides*, has been reported to cause a similar neurologic syndrome.

Strongyloidiasis

Strongyloidiasis is an intestinal infection of humans caused by the nematode *Strongyloides stercoralis*. This infection occurs in tropical and subtropical regions throughout the world but also occurs in most areas of the United States. In the usual infection, the CNS is spared.

Signs and Symptoms

Disseminated strongyloidiasis (hyperinfection syndrome), however, is not an infrequent complication in the immunosuppressed or immunodeficient host. CNS involvement occurs as part of this disseminated infection. Neurologic signs include meningitis, altered mental states (encephalopathy to coma), seizures, and focal deficits from mass lesions or infarction.

Diagnosis and Treatment

CSF examination may be normal or may reveal a neutrophilic pleocytosis and an increased protein. Eosinophilia is infrequent. The glucose is normal. Diagnosis is usually made by finding the larvae in stool, sputum, duodenal aspirates or the CSF. Peripheral eosinophilia is not always present. With parenchymal involvement, CT and MRI may reveal ring-enhancing lesions or small cortical infarcts. Another clue to the diagnosis is the occurrence in the immunocompromised patient of an unexplained Gram-negative bacteremia and meningitis, a frequent accompaniment of disseminated strongyloidiasis. Mortality from disseminated disease is high. Thiabendazole and ivermectin are the drugs of choice. Corticosteroids may cause dissemination and should not be used.

PROTOZOAN INFECTION

Protozoa are small (microbial size) single-cell organisms that more frequently cause diffuse encephalitic, as opposed to focal, involvement of the nervous system. Protozoa do not elicit allergic reactions or cause eosinophilia.

Toxoplasmosis

Toxoplasmosis is the infection of humans by the protozoan organism *Toxoplasma gondii*. The infection, which has a predilection for the CNS and the eye, may be congenital with encephalitis and chorioretinitis; may cause meningoencephalitis during acquired primary infection in the immunocompetent host; and may cause mass lesions (granulomas, abscesses), encephalitis, and chorioretinitis in the immunocompromised host. Toxoplasmosis is especially prevalent in those with AIDS (see Chapter 25).

Etiology and Pathology

The toxoplasma are minute (about 2 to 3 mm), oval, pyriform, rounded, or elongated protoplasmic masses with a central nucleus. The important animal host for this organism is the cat. Infection is acquired by ingestion of oocysts from cat feces or contaminated soil. Infection may also occur by eating unwashed vegetables or undercooked meat. The organisms invade the walls of blood vessels in the nervous system and produce an inflammatory reaction. Miliary granulomas are formed. They may become calcified or undergo necrosis. The granulomatous lesions are scattered throughout the CNS and may be found in the meninges and ependyma. Hydrocephalus may develop from occlusion of the aqueduct of Sylvius by the resulting ependymitis. The microorganisms are present in the epithelioid cells of the granulomas, endothelial cells of blood vessels, and nerve cells. Lesions in the retina are common; occasionally, they are also present in the lungs, kidneys, liver, spleen, or skin.

Clinical Manifestations

In the congenital form, the symptoms are usually evident in the first few days of life. Rarely, congenital infections may not manifest for several years. The common manifestations are inanition, microcephaly, seizures, mental retardation, spasticity, opisthotonos, chorioretinitis, microphthalmos, or other congenital defects in development of the eye. Optic atrophy is common, and there may be an internal hydrocephalus. Depending on the extent of systemic disease, the liver and spleen may be enlarged with elevated bilirubin; fever, rash, and pneumonitis may also be present. The presence of calcified nodules in the brain may be demonstrated by CT or radiographs of the skull. Symptoms in the infantile form are similar to those of the congenital form but may not make their appearance until the third or fifth year of life. Cerebral calcifications are not found in postnatally acquired infections.

Acquired toxoplasmosis is most often asymptomatic in the normal host ($\approx$90%). In the remaining 10%, an infectious mononucleosis-like picture may be seen with lymphadenopathy and fever. Although atypical lymphocytes may be present in the peripheral blood, serologic tests for Epstein-Barr virus are negative. Rarely, meningoencephalitis with headache, confusion, delirium, drowsiness, and coma with seizures may be seen. Signs of meningeal irritation are uncommon.

Severe infections are more likely to occur in immunocompromised patients, and most are due to reactivation rather than to newly acquired infection. Extraneural manifestations may include pneumonitis, myocarditis, myositis, and chorioretinitis. Neurologic involvement may take one of several forms: subacute to chronic encephalopathic picture with confusion, delirium, obtundation, and coma, occasionally accompanied by seizures; acute meningoencephalitis with headache, fever, nuchal rigidity, and focal or generalized seizures, leading to status epilepticus and coma; and focal signs (hemiparesis, ataxia, or aphasia) resulting from single or multiple mass lesions (toxoplasmic abscess), probably the most common form and tends to be chronic. A combination of these three types of neurologic involvement is often seen.

Toxoplasmosis as a complication of neoplastic disease is relatively infrequent. Toxoplasmosis, however, is one of the most frequent CNS opportunistic infection of AIDS patients, accounting for about one-third of all CNS complications.

Laboratory Data

A moderate or severe anemia and a mild leukocytosis or leukopenia may be present. The CSF may be under increased pressure. The protein content is generally increased, and there is an inconstant pleocytosis. Cell counts as high as several thousand per cubic millimeter, mostly lymphocytes, have been recorded. The CSF glucose is normal or mildly reduced. CT may reveal calcifications in congenital infections. Low-density focal lesions may be seen. With contrast, these lesions usually show ring enhancement similar to a brain abscess or, less frequently, diffuse or no enhancement. Often, the lesions are multiple. MRI is more sensitive for demonstrating these lesions (Fig. 31.3).

Diagnosis

The diagnosis of congenital toxoplasmosis is usually considered in the newborn with chorioretinitis, microcephaly, seizures, mental retardation, cerebral calcifications, and

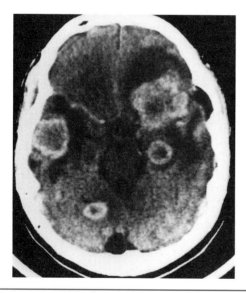

FIGURE 31.3. Cerebral toxoplasmosis. Enhanced axial CT demonstrates multiple, bilateral, ring-enhancing hypodense lesions of both temporal, right occipital and left frontal lobes with surrounding edema. (From Farrar WE, Wood MJ, Innes JA, Tubbs H. *Infectious Diseases: Text and Color Atlas*, 2nd ed. London: Gowers Medical Publishers, 1992:3.30, with permission.)

evidence of systemic infection. The diagnosis is more difficult to make in older children and adults with either acquired disease or reactivation of a latent infection. Toxoplasma may occasionally be demonstrated in CSF sediment with Wright or Giemsa stain. The organism rarely may be cultivated from CSF sediment by inoculation of laboratory mice.

Although a definite diagnosis may be made only by isolation of the organism from biopsy of brain or other tissues, a presumptive diagnosis may be made by using readily available serologic tests. Demonstration of immunoglobulin M (IgM) antibodies by enzyme-linked immunosorbent assay (ELISA) or indirect fluorescent antibody is particularly helpful for diagnosis of a congenital or an acute acquired infection. Polymeric chain reaction (PCR) detection of the organism in the CSF is specific but not very sensitive. In AIDS patients and in most immunocompromised patients, serum immunoglobulin G (IgG) antibody is usually positive, although a fourfold rise is infrequent. Serum IgM antibody is not usually detected. The presence of CSF antibodies may be a sensitive indicator of CNS infection.

Course, Prognosis, and Treatment

Prognosis is poor in the congenital form; more than 50% of affected infants die within a few weeks after birth. Mental and neurologic defects are present in the infants who survive. The mortality rate is also high in the infantile form of encephalitis. Most acquired infections in the immunocompetent patient are self-limited and do not require treatment. The severe, acquired or reactivated infections, which occur more commonly in immunocompromised patients, frequently result in death. These severe infections may at times be treated successfully with pyrimethamine and sulfadiazine. In AIDS patients, if a tissue diagnosis cannot be made but serum IgG titers are positive and the characteristic neuroradiologic abnormalities are present, empiric therapy should be instituted. Indefinite suppression therapy is frequently required for AIDS patients.

Cerebral Malaria

Malaria is the most common human parasitic disease, with 300 million to 500 million infected individuals in the world and about 2 million deaths each year. This disease is endemic in tropical and subtropical areas of Africa, Asia, and Central and South America. The disease may be seen almost anywhere, however, as a result of international travel. Malaria is transmitted by mosquitoes.

Involvement of the nervous system occurs in about 2% of affected patients and is most common in infections of the malignant tertian form, almost always caused by *Plasmodium falciparum*.

Pathology and Pathogenesis

The neurologic symptoms are effects of congestion or occlusion of capillaries and venules with pigment-laden parasitized erythrocytes and to the presence of multiple petechial hemorrhages. Apparently, parasitized erythrocytes adhere to vascular endothelial cells, thereby obstructing blood flow and causing anoxia. Lymphocytic and mononuclear perivascular inflammation and a microglial cell response may be seen, at times resulting in cerebral edema. Thrombotic occlusion of vessels and large intracranial hemorrhages are rare. It is probable that the pathologic changes in the nervous system are reversible.

Symptoms and Signs

The symptoms and signs are primarily those of an acute diffuse encephalopathy. Spinal cord lesions and a polyneuritis of the Guillain-Barré type have rarely been seen. The neurologic symptoms usually appear in the second or third week of the illness but may be the initial manifestation. The onset of cerebral symptoms has no relationship to the height of the fever. Headache, photophobia, vertigo, seizures, confusion, delirium, and coma are the most common symptoms. There may be neck stiffness. Focal signs, such as transient hemiparesis, aphasia, hemianopia, and cerebellar ataxia, are uncommon. Myoclonus, chorea, and intention tremors have been observed. Cranial nerve palsies and papilledema are rarely seen, although retinal hemorrhages are common. Psychic manifestations, such as delirium, disorientation, amnesia, or combativeness, are present in a large percentage of the patients. In severe malaria, pulmonary edema, renal failure, metabolic acidosis, hepatic failure, and gastrointestinal symptoms occur.

Laboratory Data

Laboratory findings include anemia and the presence in the red blood cells of many parasites. In most cases, the CSF is entirely normal. Elevated pressure, slight xanthochromia, a small or moderate number of lymphocytes, and a moderately increased protein content may be seen. CSF sugar content is normal. CT is usually normal in patients with mild cerebral disease. With moderate disease diffuse cerebral edema is usually seen. With severe disease, additional low density lesions may be seen in the thalamus and cerebellum.

Diagnosis

Cerebral malaria is diagnosed from the appearance of cerebral symptoms and the findings of the organisms of *P. falciparum* by microscopic examination of blood smears. ELISA kits for serologic diagnosis are available. Delirium, seizures, or coma, probably because of high fever, may occur as symptoms of general infection in patients with

P. vivax in the absence of cerebral involvement. The symptoms in these cases are transient and respond readily to antimalarial therapy.

Prognosis

The mortality rate is 20% to 40% in cases of cerebral malaria. It is highest (80%) when there is a combination of coma and convulsions. There are few or no residua in the patients who recover.

Treatment

Cerebral malaria is a true medical emergency. Because of resistance, chloroquine may no longer be relied upon in most areas. In critically ill patients, treatment includes quinidine or quinine given intravenously. Oral treatment should be substituted when the patient is able to swallow. Quinine or quinidine plus pyrimethamine-sulfadoxine (Fansidar), doxycycline, tetracycline or clindamycin should be used. In Southeast Asia, where multiple drug resistance occurs, various regimens include quinine plus tetracycline, quinine plus doxycycline, quinine plus mefloquine, artesunate (or artemether) plus mefloquine, and mefloquine plus doxycycline. Anticonvulsants should be given to control seizures. Transfusions of whole blood or plasma may be required. Other supportive measures include reduction of fever, fluid and glucose replacement, and respiratory support. Sedation may be necessary in excited or delirious patients. The use of dexamethasone is deleterious in the treatment of cerebral malaria. Mannitol should be used for life-threatening cerebral edema. An infrequent possibly corticosteroid-responsive postmalarial encephalopathy has been described.

Trypanosomiasis

Two distinct varieties of infection with trypanosomes are recognized: the African form (sleeping sickness), which is caused by infection with *Trypanosoma brucei*, and the South American form (Chagas disease), which is endemic in South America, Central America, and Mexico and is caused by infection by *T. cruzi*. Chagas disease occurs as far north as southern Texas.

Etiology and Pathology

In the African form of the disease, the organisms retain their trypanosome form and multiply by longitudinal fission. They are transmitted from person to person by the tsetse fly, occasionally by other flies or insects, and by mechanical contact. There are two variants of the species: *T. brucei gambiense* (mid and west Africa) and *T. brucei rhodesiense* (east Africa). The pathologic changes are those of a chronic meningoencephalitis.

The organisms of South American trypanosomiasis, when found in the blood, have an ordinary trypanosome structure. They do not, however, reproduce in the blood but invade tissues and are transformed into typical leishmania parasites. These may later assume the trypanosome form and reenter the blood. The infection is transmitted from an animal host (e.g., rodents, cats, opossum, armadillo) to humans by a blood-sucking reduviid bug known as the "kissing bug."

The pathologic lesion in the nervous system is a meningoencephalitis consisting of miliary granulomas composed of proliferated microglial cells, with lymphocytic-plasmocytic perivascular and meningeal infiltrates. The organisms are present in glial and some nerve cells. The lesions are diffusely scattered throughout the nervous system and are accompanied by a patchy reaction in the meninges and parenchyma.

Symptoms and Signs

African trypanosomiasis (sleeping sickness) evolves through two indistinct stages: febrile (hemolymphatic) and lethargic (meningoencephalitic). The incubation period is variable. In some cases, symptoms may have their onset within 2 weeks of the infection. In others, it may be delayed for months or years. The Rhodesian (East African) form usually has an acute to subacute course, whereas the Gambian (West African) disease is usually chronic.

The first stage of the disease is characterized by a remitting fever, exanthems, lymphadenitis, splenomegaly, arthralgia, myalgia, and asthenia. During this stage, which may last for several months or years, the organisms are present in the blood. The first stage may pass imperceptibly into the second stage, where the previous symptoms are exaggerated and nervous system involvement is evident in the form of tremors, incoordination, convulsions, paralysis, confusion, headaches, apathy, insomnia or somnolence, and finally, coma. There is progressive weakness with loss of weight. If the condition is untreated, death usually ensues within a year after the appearance of cerebral symptoms. Death from intercurrent infection is common.

In South American trypanosomiasis, the acute stage generally lasts about 1 month and is characterized by fever; conjunctivitis; palpebral and facial edema; enlargement of the lymph nodes, liver, and spleen; and, rarely, an acute encephalitis. During this stage, trypanosomes are present in the blood, and the leishmaniform bodies are seen in the tissue. The chronic stage is characterized by evidence of involvement of the viscera, particularly the heart and gastrointestinal tract. Neurologic involvement is rare and may be diffuse (mental alterations, seizures, choreoathetosis) or focal (hemiplegia, ataxia, aphasia). The disease is slowly progressive, with occasional acute exacerbations associated with fever. Death usually ensues within a few months or years.

Laboratory Data

Some degree of anemia is common in all forms of trypanosomiasis. The ESR, liver function tests, serum globulin fraction, and serum IgM may be increased. There is a lymphocytic pleocytosis in the CSF, increased protein content, increased gamma globulin fraction, and increased IgM, probably the most sensitive test.

Diagnosis

The diagnosis depends on the development of characteristic symptoms in residents of regions in which forms of the disease are endemic. The diagnosis is established by the demonstration of organisms in the blood or CSF, in material obtained from a biopsied lymph node, or by the inoculation of these substances into susceptible animals. Serologic and CSF antibody tests may also be diagnostic.

Treatment

Melarsoprol, an organic arsenical, is effective in the treatment of *T. brucei* infections of the nervous system (second stage). Suramin, pentamidine, or eflornithine are the drugs of choice for the acute first stage. Alternative medications for the second stage are eflornithine and nifurtimox. No drug treatment is established as safe and effective in chronic Chagas disease including the CNS component. Nifurtimox or benznidazole are usually effective, however, in the acute stage of infection.

Primary Amebic Meningoencephalitis

It has been known for many years that amebae (*Entamoeba histolytica*) may rarely invade the brain and produce circumscribed abscesses. However, free-living amebae are the species primarily causing meningoencephalitis. *Naegleria fowleri* causes an acute meningoencephalitis, primary amebic meningoencephalitis, whereas *Acanthamoeba* species may cause both acute and granulomatous amebic meningoencephalitis. Another species, *Leptomyxid amebae*, has caused a few cases. Amebic meningoencephalitis is rare but probably has a worldwide distribution. Most cases in the United States are reported from the Southeast.

Naegleria Infections

These infections usually occur in children or young adults who have been swimming in freshwater lakes or ponds. Inhalation of dustborne cysts may also occur in arid regions. Interestingly, the organism apparently invades the nervous system through the olfactory nerves and does not cause a systemic infection. The incubation period is several days to a week. The onset of symptoms of primary amebic meningoencephalitis is abrupt. Mild symptoms of an upper respiratory infection may occur. Fever, headache, and stiff neck are followed within 1 or 2 days by nausea and vomiting, lethargy, disorientation, seizures, increased intracranial pressure, coma, and then death.

The CSF picture is similar to that of an acute bacterial meningitis, with increased pressure, several hundred to thousands of white blood cells per cm^3 (primarily neutrophils), as many as several thousand red blood cells, an elevated protein content, decreased glucose, and negative Gram stain. Trophozoites may be recognized in a wet preparation of noncentrifuged CSF or with Wright or Giemsa stains. The organism may be cultured on special media or by mouse inoculation. A serologic test is available at the Centers for Disease Control and Prevention. The disease is rapidly fatal, but recovery with treatment has been reported in some cases. Amphotericin B has been used effectively alone or in combination with several drugs (rifampin, chloramphenicol, ketoconazole).

Acanthamoeba Infections

Acanthamoeba is a ubiquitous organism that may cause a subacute or chronic granulomatous amebic encephalitis as an opportunistic infection in alcoholic and immunocompromised patients. The organism probably causes a systemic infection through the respiratory tract and then seeds the brain by hematogenous spread. The meningoencephalitis may present with chronic fever and headache, followed by the gradual onset of focal neurologic signs (e.g., hemiparesis, aphasia, seizures with focal signature, ataxia) and abnormalities of mentation. Other signs include skin lesions, corneal ulcerations, uveitis, and pneumonitis.

There is CSF pleocytosis that is more often lymphocytic than polymorphonuclear. Protein is usually elevated, and glucose is normal or slightly decreased. Organisms occasionally may be recognized on wet preparations but have never been cultured from CSF. CT and MRI may reveal focal lesions. Biopsy is usually required for diagnosis. Several cases of acute meningoencephalitis, similar to those caused by *Naegleria*, have been reported. The disease is usually fatal. *In vitro*, the organism is usually sensitive to pentamidine, ketoconazole, flucytosine, and less so to amphotericin B.

SUGGESTED READINGS

General

The Medical Letter on Drugs and Therapeutics. Drugs for parasitic infections. *Handbook of Antimicrobial Therapy,* 16th ed. New Rochelle, New York, 2002:120–143.

Hughes AJ, Biggs BA. Parasitic worms of the central nervous system: an Australian perspective. *Internal Med J* 2002;32:541–553.
Lowichik A, Siegel JD. Parasitic infections of the central nervous system. *J Child Neurol* 1995;10:4–17 (Part I), 77–87 (Part II), 177–190 (Part III).
Scheld WM, Whitle RJ, Durack DT, eds. *Infections of the Central Nervous System,* 3rd ed. Philadelphia: Lippincott, Williams & Wilkins, 2004 (in press).
Strickland GT, ed. *Hunter's Tropical Medicine and Emerging Infectious Diseases,* 8th ed. Philadelphia: W.B. Saunders, 2000.
Warren KS, Mahmound AAF, eds. *Tropical and Geographic Medicine,* 2nd ed. New York: McGraw-Hill, 1990.

Helminthic Infection

Cysticercosis

Barinagarrementeria F, Cantu C. Frequency of cerebral arteritis in subarachnoid cysticercosis: an angiographic study. *Stroke* 1998;29:123–125.
Cantu C, Barinagarrementeria F. Cerebrovascular complications of neurocysticercosis. *Arch Neurol* 1996;53:233–239.
Carpio A, Hauser WA. Prognosis for seizure recurrence in patients with newly diagnosed neurocysticercosis. *Neurology* 2002;59:1730–1734.
Del Brutto OH. Albendazole therapy for subarachnoid cysticerci: clinical and neuroimaging analysis of inpatients. *J Neurol Neurosurg Psychiatry* 1997;62:659–661.
Del Brutto OH, Rajshekhar V, White AC Jr., et al. Proposed diagnostic criteria for neurocysticercosis. *Neurology* 2001;57:177–183.
Garcia HH, Del Brutto OH. Imaging findings in neurocysticercosis. *Acta Tropica* 2003;87:71–78.
Garcia HH, Gonzalez AE, Gilman RH et al. Diagnosis, treatment and control of *Taenia solium* cysticercosis. *Curr Opinion Infect Dis* 2003;16:411–419.
Garcia HH, Pretell EJ, Gilman RH et al. A trial of antiparasitic treatment to reduce the rate of seizures due to cerebral cysticercosis. *N Engl J Med* 2004;350:249–258.
Gilman RH, Del Brutto OH, Garcia HH et al. Prevalence of taeniasis among patients with neurocysticercosis is related to severity of infection. *Neurology* 2000;55:1062.
Martinez HR, Rangel-Guerra R, Arredondo-Estrada JH, Marfil A, Onofre J. Medical and surgical treatment in neurocysticercosis: a magnetic resonance study of 161 cases. *J Neurol Sci* 1995;130:25–34.
Mohanty A, Venkatrama SK, Das S, et al. . Spinal intramedullary cysticercosis. *Neurosurgery* 1997;40:82–87.
Parmar H, Shah J, Patwardhan V et al. MR imaging in intramedullary cysticercosis. *Neuroradiology* 2001;43:961–967.
Rosenfeld EA, Byrd SE, Shulman ST. Neurocysticercosis among children in Chicago. *Clin Infect Dis* 1996;23:101–113.

Echinococcosis

Algros M-P, Majo F, Bresson-Hadni S, et al. Intracerebral alveolar echinococcosis. *Infection* 2003;31:63–65.
Ciurea AV, Valisescu G, Nuteanu L, Carp N. Cerebral hydatid disease in children. Experience of 27 cases. *Child's Nerv Syst* 1995;11:679–686.
Khazim R, Fares Y, Heras-Palou C, Barnes PR. Posterior decompression of spinal hydatidosis: long term results. Fundacion Jimenez Diaz, Madrid, Spain. *Clin Neurol Neurosurg* 2003;105:209–214.
McManus DP, Zhang W, Li J, Bartley PB. Echinococcosis. *Lancet* 2003;362:1295–1304.
Peter J, Domingo Z, Sinclair-Smith C, de Villiers J. Hydatid infestation of the brain: difficulties with computed tomography diagnosis and surgical treatment. *Pediatr Neurosurg* 1994;20:78–83.

Schistosomiasis

Blunt SB, Boulton J, Wise R. MRI in schistosomiasis of conus medullaris and lumbar spinal cord. *Lancet* 1993;341:557.
Labeodan OA, Sur M. Intramedullary schistosomiasis. *Pediatr Neurosurg* 2003;39:14–16.

Liu LX. Spinal and cerebral schistosomiasis. *Semin Neurol* 1993;13: 189–200.

Moreno-Carvalho OA, Nascimento-Carvalho CM, da Silva Bacelar A, et al. Clinical and cerebrospinal fluid (CSF) profile and CSF criteria for the diagnosis of spinal cord schistosomiasis. *Arq Neuropsiquiatr* 2003;61(2-B):353–358.

Preidler KW, Riepl T, Szolar D, Ranner G. Cerebral schistosomiasis: MR and CT appearance. *Am J Neuroradiol* 1996;17:1598–1600.

Scrimgeour EM, Gajdusek DC. Involvement of the central nervous system in *Schistosoma mansoni* and *S. haematobium* infection. *Brain* 1985;108:1023–1038.

Paragonimiasis

Cha SH, Chang KH, Cho SY, et al. Cerebral paragonimiasis in early active stage: CT and MR features. *AJR Am J Roentgenol* 1994;162: 141–145.

Choo JD, Suh BS, Lee HS, et al. Chronic cerebral paragonimiasis combined with aneurismal subarachnoid hemorrhage. *Am J Trop Med Hyg* 2003;69:466–469.

Im JG, Chang KH, Reeder MM. Current diagnostic imaging of pulmonary and cerebral paragonimiasis, with pathological correlation. *Semin Roentgenol* 1997;32:301–324.

Kusner DJ, King CH. Cerebral paragonimiasis. *Semin Neurol* 1993; 13:201–208.

Trichinosis

Dupouy-Camet J, Kociecka W, Bruschi F, et al. Opinion on the diagnosis and treatment of human trichinellosis. *Expert Opin Pharmacother* 2002;3:1117–1130.

Ellrodt A, Lalfon P, LeBras P, et al. Multifocal central nervous system lesions in three patients with trichinosis. *Arch Neurol* 1987;44:432–434.

Feydy E, Touze E, Miaux Y, et al. MRI in a case of neurotrichinosis. *Neuroradiology* 1996;38:S80–S82.

Fourestie V, Douceron H, Brugieres P, et al. Neurotrichinosis: a cerebrovascular disease associated with myocardial injury and hypereosinophilia. *Brain* 1993;116:603–616.

Mawhorter SD, Kazura JW. Trichinosis of the central nervous system. *Semin Neurol* 1993;13:148–152.

Merritt HH, Rosenbaum M. Involvement of the nervous system in trichinosis. *JAMA* 1936;106:1646–1649.

Eosinophilic Meningitis

Koo J, Pien F, Kliks MM. *Angiostrongylus (Parastrongylus)* eosinophilic meningitis. *Rev Infect Dis* 1988;10:1155–1162.

Kuberski T, Wallace GD. Clinical manifestations of eosinophilic meningitis due to *Angiostrongylus cantonensis*. *Neurology* 1979;29: 1566–1570.

Lo Re V III, Gluckman SJ. Eosinophilic Meningitis. *Am J Med* 2003; 114:217–223.

Moore DAJ, McCroddan J, Dekumyoy P, Chiodin PL. Gnathostomiasis: an emerging imported disease. *Emerg Infect Dis* 2003;9:647–650.

Petjom S, Chaiwun B, Settakorn J, et al. *Angiostrongylus cantonensis* infection mimicking a spinal cord tumor. *Ann Neurol* 2002;52: 99–102.

Punyagupta S, Bunnag T, Juttijudata P. Eosinophilic meningitis in Thailand. Clinical and epidemiological characteristics of 162 patients with myeloencephalitis probably caused by *Gnathostoma spinigerum*. *J Neurol Sci* 1990;96:241–256.

Slom TJ, Cortese MM, Gerber SI, et al. An outbreak of eosinophilic meningitis caused by *Angiostrongylus Cantonensis* in travelers returning from the Caribbean. *N Engl J Med* 2002;346:688–675.

Tsai H-C, Liu Y-C, Kunin CM, et al. Eosinophilic meningitis caused by *Angiostrongylus Cantonensis* associated with eating raw snails: correlation of brain magnetic resonance imaging scans with clinical findings. *Am J Trop Med Hyg* 2003;68:281–285.

Toxocariasis (Visceral Larva Migrans)

Duprez TP, Bigaignon G, Delgrange E, et al. MRI of cervical cord lesions and their resolution in toxocara caris myelopathy. *Neuroradiology* 1996;38:792–795.

Gould IM, Newell S, Green SH, George RH. Toxocariasis and eosinophilic meningitis. *Br Med J* 1985;291:1239–1240.

Vidal JE, Sztajnbok J, Seguro AC. Eosinophilic meningoencephalitis due to *Toxocara Canis*: case report and review of the literature. *Am J Trop Med Hyg* 2003;69:341–343.

King TD, Moncrief JA, Vingiello R. Hemiparesis and *Ascaris lumbricoides* infection. *J La State Med Soc* 1979;131:5–7.

Xinou E, Lefkopoulos A, Gelagoti M, et al. CT and MR imaging findings in cerebral toxocaral disease. *Am J Neuroradiol* 2003;24:714–718.

Strongyloidiasis

Adedayo O, Grell G, Bellot P. Hyperinfective strongyloidiasis in the medical ward: review of 27 cases in 5 years. *Southern Med J* 2002;95: 711–716.

Capello M, Hotez P. Disseminated strongyloidiasis. *Semin Neurol* 1993; 13:169–174.

Masdeu JC, Tantulavanich S, Gorelick PP, et al. Brain abscess caused by *Strongyloides stercoralis*. *Arch Neurol* 1982;39:62–63.

Takayanagui OM, Lofrano MM, Araugo MB, Chimelli L. Detection of strongyloides stercoralis in the cerebrospinal fluid of a patient with acquired immunodeficiency syndrome. *Neurology* 1995;45:193–194.

Wachter RM, Burke AM, MacGregor RR. *Strongyloides stercoralis* hyperinfection masquerading as cerebral vasculitis. *Arch Neurol* 1984;41:1213–1216.

Other Helminths

Jeong SC, Bae JC, Hwang SH, Kim HC, Lee BC. Cerebral sparganosis with intracerebral hemorrhage: a case report. *Neurology* 1998;50:503–506.

Pau A, Perria C, Turtas S, et al. Long-term follow-up of the surgical treatment of intracranial coenurosis. *Br J Neurosurg* 1990;4:39–43.

Protozoan Infection

Toxoplasmosis

American Academy of Neurology. Evaluation and management of intracranial mass lesions in AIDS. Report of the Quality Standards Subcommittee of the American Academy of Neurology. *Neurology* 1998;50:21–26.

Barkovich AJ, Girard N. Fetal brain infections. *Childs Nerv Syst* 2003; 19:501–507.

Chong-Han CH, Cortez SC, Tung GA. Diffusion-weighted MRI of cerebral toxoplasma abscess. *American J Roentgenology* 2003;181:1711–1714.

Collazos J. Opportunistic infections of the CNS in patients with AIDS. *CNS Drugs* 2003;17:869–887.

Gherardi R, Baudriment M, Lionnet F, et al. Skeletal muscle toxoplasmosis in patients with acquired immunodeficiency syndrome: a clinical and pathological study. *Ann Neurol* 1992;32:535–542.

Mitchell CD, Erlich SS, Mastrucci MT, et al. Congenital toxoplasmosis occurring in infants perinatally infected with human immunodeficiency virus 1. *Pediatr Infect Dis J* 1990;9:512–518.

Navia BA, Petito CK, Gold JWM, et al. Cerebral toxoplasmosis complicating the acquired immune deficiency syndrome: clinical and neuropathological findings in 27 patients. *Ann Neurol* 1986;19:224–238.

Porter SB, Sande MA. Toxoplasmosis of the central nervous system in the acquired immunodeficiency syndrome. *N Engl J Med* 1992;327: 1643–1648.

Raffi F, Aboulker JP, Michelet C, et al. A prospective study of criteria for the diagnosis of toxoplasmic encephalitis in 186 AIDS patients. *AIDS* 1997;11:177–184.

Strittmatter C, Lang W, Wiestler OD, Kleihues P. The changing pattern of human immunodeficiency virus-associated cerebral toxoplasmosis: a study of 46 postmortem cases. *Acta Neuropathol* 1992;83:475–481.

Townsend JJ, Wolinsky JS, Baringer JR, Johnson PC. Acquired toxoplasmosis: a neglected cause of treatable nervous system disease. *Arch Neurol* 1975;32:335–343.

Cerebral Malaria

Bondi FS. The incidence and outcome of neurological abnormalities in childhood cerebral malaria: a long-term follow-up of 62 survivors. *Trans R Soc Trop Med Hyg* 1992;86:17–19.

Centers for Disease Control and Prevention. Availability and use of parenteral quinidine gluconate for severe or complicated malaria. *MMWR* 2000;49:1138–1140.

Mai NTH, Day NPJ, Chueng LV, et al. Post-malaria neurologic syndrome. *Lancet* 1996;348:917–921.

Mturi N, Musumba CO, Wamola BM, et al. Cerebral malaria: optimizing management. *CNS Drugs* 2003;17:153–165.

Newton CRJC, Hien TT, White N. Cerebral malaria. *J Neurol Neurosurg Psychiatry* 2000;69:433–441.

Newton CRJC, Warrell DA. Neurological manifestations of falciparum malaria. *Ann Neurol* 1998;43:695–702.

Patankar TF, Karnad DR, Shetty PG, et al. Adult cerebral malaria: prognostic importance of imaging findings and correlation with postmortem findings. *Radiology* 2002;224:811–816.

Schnorf H, Diserens K, Schnyder H, et al. Corticosteroid-responsive post-malaria encephalopathy characterized by motor aphasia, myoclonus, and postural tremor. *Arch Neurol* 1998;55:417–420.

van Hensbroek MB, Palmer A, Jaffar S, Schneider G, Kwiatkowski D. Residual neurologic sequelae after childhood cerebral malaria. *J Pediatr* 1997;131:125–129.

Trypanosomiasis

Barrett MP, Burchmore RJS, Stich A, et al. The trypanosomiases. *Lancet* 2003;362:1469–1480.

Carod-Artal FJ, Vargas AP, Melo M, Horan TA. American trypanosomiasis (Chagas' disease): an unrecognized cause of stroke. *J Neurol Neurosurg Psychiatry* 2003;74:516–518.

Hunter CA, Jennings FW, Adams JH, et al. Subcurative chemotherapy and fatal post-treatment encephalopathies in African trypanosomiasis. *Lancet* 1992;339:956–958.

Lejon V, Reiber H, Legros D, et al. Intrathecal immune response pattern for improved diagnosis of central nervous system involvement in trypanosomiasis. *J Infectious Dis* 2003;187:1475–1483.

Metzek K, Maciel JA Jr. AIDS and Chagas' disease. *Neurology* 1993;43:447–448.

Urbina JA. Specific treatment of Chagas disease: current status and new developments. *Curr Opinion Infect Dis* 2001;14:733–741.

Villanueva MS. Trypanosomiasis of the central nervous system. *Semin Neurol* 1993;13:209–218.

Primary Amebic Meningoencephalitis

Anonymous. Primary amebic meningoencephalitis—North Carolina, 1991. *MMWR* 1992;41:437–440.

Centers for Disease Control and Prevention. Primary amebic meningoencephalitis—Georgia, 2002. *MMWR* 2003;52:962–964.

Clavel A, Franco L, Letona S, et al. Primary amebic meningoencephalitis in a patient with AIDS: unusual protozoological findings. *Clin Infect Dis* 1996;23:1314–1315.

Gardner HAR, Martinez AJ, Visvesvara GS, Sotrel A. Granulomatous amebic encephalitis in an AIDS patient. *Neurology* 1991;41:1993–1995.

Gordon SM, Steinberg JP, DuPuis MH, et al. Culture isolation of *Acanthamoeba* species and leptomyxid amebas from patients with amebic meningoencephalitis, including two patients with AIDS. *Clin Infect Dis* 1992;15:1024–1030.

Grunnert ML, Cannon GH, Kushner JP. Fulminant amebic meningoencephalitis due to *Acanthamoeba*. *Neurology* 1981;31:174–177.

Martinez AJ, Visvesvara GS. Free-living, amphizoic and opportunistic amebas. *Brain Pathol* 1997;7(1):583–598.

Seidel JS, Harmatz P, Visvesvara GS, et al. Successful treatment of primary amebic meningoencephalitis. *N Engl J Med* 1982;306:346–348.

Chapter 32

▶ Bacterial Toxins

Burk Jubelt

The toxins elaborated by several pathogenic bacteria have a special predilection for the nervous system. The exotoxin of the diphtheria bacillus chiefly affects the peripheral nerves, tetanus affects the activity of the neurons in the CNS, and botulism interferes with conduction at the myoneural junction.

DIPHTHERIA

The exotoxin of *Corynebacterium diphtheriae* is a 62,000-Dalton polypeptide that inhibits protein synthesis in mammalian cells by inactivation of transfer RNA (tRNA) translocase (elongation factor 2). It is composed of two segments: one necessary for binding to the cell and a shorter portion that then is cleaved and enters the cell. The specificity of the exotoxin for heart and peripheral nerve is attributed to receptor binding affinity at the cell surface. The exotoxin is produced by a phage; strains of the bacterium that do not contain the phage are not pathogenic. The development of neuropathy is proportional to the severity of the primary infection. In pharyngeal infections, palatal and pharyngo-laryngo-esophageal paralysis are early and prominent features. The resistance of the other cranial nerves and brain to these effects is unexplained.

The symptoms and course of diphtheritic neuritis are considered in Chapter 106.

TETANUS

Tetanus (lockjaw) causes localized or generalized spasms of muscles resulting from tetanospasmin, a toxin produced by the bacterium *Clostridium tetani*.

Etiology

C. tetani is commonly shed in the excreta of humans and other animals. Its spores are ubiquitous in the environment. They enter the body through puncture wounds, compound fractures, or wounds from blank cartridges and fireworks. Infection has been reported from contamination of operative wounds, burns, parenteral injections (particularly in heroin addicts), and through the umbilicus of the newborn. The mere deposition of spores of the organism is not sufficient for infection. Necrotic tissue and an associated pyogenic infection are necessary for germination of the bacteria and production of tetanospasmin.

Prevention of tetanus is accomplished by immunization with toxoid (denatured toxin). Children should be immunized routinely and booster doses given every 10 years. Immediate booster immunization should be given to patients with penetrating wounds, unless a recent immunization may be documented. Immunity is not conferred by the disease, and patients should receive the toxoid and human tetanus immune globulin (HTIG), but at a different site.

Pathogenesis

Tetanospasmin is a single polypeptide chain of 1,315 amino acids, synthesized by a large bacterial plasmid. The toxin becomes active when nicked by a serine protease into small and large chains held together by a disulfide bridge. The large chain also contains an internal disulfide bridge, which appears to be necessary for penetration into the nerve cell. The small chain is responsible for toxin activity.

Tetanospasmin prevents synaptic vesicles from fusing with the cell membrane and prevents the release of neurotransmitters. It appears to bind to synaptobrevin, a protein involved in the fusion process. Tetanospasmin is active at the neuromuscular junction, autonomic terminals, and most importantly in inhibitory neurons in the CNS, inhibiting the release of gamma-aminobutyric acid (GABA) and glycine. The central effects usually overwhelm the peripheral effects, although autonomic dysfunction may become evident, clinically. Access to the CNS is by retrograde transport in alpha-motor neurons. Hematogenous spread of the toxin before neuronal transport probably accounts for generalized tetanus.

Pathology

No pathologic changes occur in the central or peripheral nervous system except those caused secondarily by anoxia or other metabolic derangement.

Incidence

The disease is found throughout the world where it most commonly is found in puncture-wound infections of the extremities caused by nails or splinters.

The incidence in developed countries has been dramatically reduced by immunization with denatured toxin (tetanus toxoid). In the United States about 50 cases per year are reported to the CDC. Worldwide, about 1 million cases occur; 50% are encountered in neonates because of nonsterile birthing technique. In the United States now, the infection is most common in narcotic addicts. The narcotic is "cut" by admixing with quinine, a substance that favors the growth of the organisms at the site of the injection.

Symptoms

The incubation period is usually between 5 and 10 days. It may be as short as 3 days or as long as 3 weeks. The severity of the disease usually is greater when the incubation period is short.

The symptoms may be localized or generalized. In the localized form, the spasms are confined to the injured limbs. This form is rare and is most commonly seen in patients who have been partially protected by prophylactic doses of antitetanic serum. When the portal of entrance is in the head (e.g., face, ear, tonsils), symptoms may be localized there (cephalic tetanus), with trismus, facial paralysis, and ophthalmoplegia.

In the generalized form, a prominent symptom is stiffness of the jaw (trismus, lockjaw). This is followed by stiffness of the neck, irritability, and restlessness. As the disease progresses, stiffness of the muscles becomes generalized. Rigidity of the back muscles may become so extreme that the patient assumes the position of opisthotonos. Rigidity of the facial muscles gives a characteristic facial expression, the so-called risus sardonicus. Added to the stiffness of the muscles are paroxysmal tonic spasms that may occur spontaneously or may be precipitated by an external stimulus. Dysphagia may develop from spasm of the pharyngeal muscles; cyanosis and asphyxia may result from spasm of the glottis or respiratory muscles. Seizures may occur and are probably secondary to anoxia caused by the spasms. Temperature may be normal but more commonly is elevated to 101°F to 103°F.

Laboratory Data

No specific changes are found in blood, urine, or CSF. There is no specific laboratory test of confirmation.

Diagnosis

The diagnosis of tetanus is made by the characteristic signs (e.g., trismus, risus sardonicus, tonic spasms) in a patient with a wound of the skin and deeper tissues. Occasionally, however, a history of an antecedent wound is denied.

The symptoms of strychnine poisoning differ from those of tetanus in that the muscles are relaxed between spasms and the jaw muscles are rarely involved. Other differential entities include black widow-spider bite, dystonic reactions, drug withdrawal, hypocalcemic tetany, stiff-man syndrome, status epilepticus, and rabies.

Course and Prognosis

The outlook is grave in all cases of generalized tetanus. The mortality rate is over 50%. Prognosis is best when the incubation period is long. The mortality rate is reduced by the prompt administration of serum and aggressive management of pulmonary and autonomic dysfunction. In fatal cases, death usually occurs in 3 to 10 days. Death is most commonly caused by respiratory compromise. In the patients who recover, there is a gradual reduction in the frequency and severity of spasms.

Treatment

The patient should be treated in an intensive care unit. The wound should be surgically cleaned. Antiserum does not neutralize toxins that have been fixed in the nervous system, but it is administered to neutralize toxin that has not yet entered the nervous system. It is customary to administer HTIG in a dose of 3000 U to 6000 U, intramuscularly, as soon as the diagnosis is made, although as little as 500 U may be equally effective. Intrathecal HTIG therapy has been reported to decrease mortality. However, a meta-analysis concluded that intrathecal administration was not more effective than parenteral administration

Penicillin G has been the antibiotic of choice for inhibiting further growth of the organisms. However, penicillin is a GABA antagonist. Metronidazole is therefore becoming the antibiotic of choice. Dirty wounds should be surgically debrided and cleaned. Tracheostomy should be performed to ensure adequate ventilation. Benzodiazepines are used commonly to control muscle spasms; high doses may be required. Benzodiazepines are also useful for immediate control of convulsions, but phenytoin or other suitable long-lasting anticonvulsant should be added if seizures occur. In severe cases, neuromuscular blockade may be necessary, in conjunction with the use of positive-pressure ventilation. Low dose anticoagulation with heparin then should be considered because the risk of pulmonary embolism is high in patients treated with blockade. For prevention, active immunization with tetanus toxoid should be given in infancy, with boosters at school entry about 7 years later, and then about every 10 years.

BOTULISM

Botulism is a poisoning by a toxin elaborated by *Clostridium botulinum*, a bacterium widely distributed in soil. Botulinum toxin impairs release of acetylcholine at all peripheral synapses, with resultant weakness of striated and smooth muscles and autonomic dysfunction (see also Chapter 123).

Pathogenesis

Botulinum toxin is a 150-kilodalton polypeptide with structure and major sequence homologies similar to those of tetanospasmin. It is also activated by nicking of the polypeptide into a larger and smaller chain held together by a disulfide bond. After synthesis, botulinum toxin exists in a macromolecular complex that resembles other bacteria-elaborated proteins. This complex appears necessary for pathogenicity, because the toxin alone is digested in the stomach. After absorption from the gastrointestinal tract, the toxin spreads hematogenously to peripheral presynaptic terminals, where it blocks the release of acetylcholine. As with tetanus toxin, botulinum toxin appears to interfere with synaptic-vesicle fusion to the presynaptic membrane. Different immune types (see below) bind to different proteins at the fusion site.

There are three forms of human botulism: food-borne (classic), wound, and intestinal (especially in infants, infantile botulism). Classic food-borne botulism is caused by toxin ingested after being produced in inadequately sterilized canned or prepared food. Home-canned or -cured foods are particularly at risk, although commercial products are occasionally implicated. *C. botulinum* growth is inhibited by other common bacteria. Methods of processing that kill those bacteria, but not the resistant *Clostridium* spores, favor germination and growth of the botulinum organism. Wound botulism results from contamination of wounds with bacteria and bacterial spores that multiply and locally produce toxin. Infantile botulism is caused by toxin produced by bacteria growing in the intestine.

Seven immunologic types of *C. botulinum* toxin have been identified. Types A, B, E and F cause human disease. The same types have been implicated in infantile botulism. Type E is associated with fish and marine-mammal products. Only types A and B have so far been found in wound botulism.

The toxin is thermolabile and is easily destroyed by heat. Botulism usually occurs when the preserved food is served uncooked and the rancid taste is obscured by acid dressings.

Symptoms and Signs

The symptoms of poisoning by the toxin appear 6 to 48 hours after the ingestion of contaminated food, and may or may not be preceded by nausea, vomiting, or diarrhea. The initial symptom is usually difficulty in convergence of the eyes, soon followed by ptosis and paralysis of the extraocular muscles. The pupils are dilated and may not react to light. The ocular symptoms are followed by weakness of the jaw muscles, dysphagia, and dysarthria. The weakness spreads to involve muscles of the trunk and limbs. Smooth muscle of the intestines and bladder is occasionally affected, with resulting constipation and retention of urine. Mentation is usually preserved, but convulsions and coma may develop, terminally. Blood and CSF are normal. In severe cases, symptoms may be those of cardiac or respiratory failure.

Infantile botulism occurs in the first year of life, with a peak incidence at 2 to 4 months of age. About 30% of infantile botulism in the United States appears to follow the ingestion of honey. A period of constipation of about 3 days is followed by the acute onset of hypotonia, weakness, dysphagia, poor sucking, and ptosis. It is estimated that 5% of cases of sudden infant death syndrome are caused by botulism, although the true frequency is unknown.

Diagnosis

The diagnosis is not difficult when several members of one household are affected, or if samples of the contaminated food may be obtained to test for the toxin. Bulbar palsy in acute anterior poliomyelitis may be excluded by the finding of normal CSF. Myasthenia gravis (MG) may be simulated, especially if the pupils are not clearly affected in a sporadic case of botulism. In MG, there is a decremental electromyographic response to repetitive stimulation of nerve, but in botulism there is an increasing response that resembles the Lambert-Eaton syndrome. The Miller-Fisher variant of the Guillain-Barré syndrome is also part of the differential, but in that disease ataxia is prominent.

Course

The course depends on the amount of toxin absorbed from the gut. The symptoms are mild and recovery is complete if only a small amount is absorbed. When large amounts are absorbed, death usually occurs within 4 to 8 days, primarily the result of circulatory failure, respiratory paralysis, or the development of pulmonary complications.

Treatment

Botulism may be prevented by taking proper precautions in the preparation of canned foods and discarding (without sampling) any canned food with a rancid odor or any in which gas has formed. The toxin is destroyed by cooking. There are no established means of preventing infant botulism, although honey should not be given in the first year of life.

Patients should be given botulinum antitoxin. In the United States, trivalent (A, B, E) antitoxin is available from the Centers for Disease Control and Prevention or some state health departments. The stomach should be lavaged gently and the lower gastrointestinal tract thoroughly cleansed by enemas and cathartics not containing magnesium. Respiratory assistance may be required. Feedings should be via enteral tube. Some beneficial effects on weakness have been reported with the use of guanidine, but the evidence is conflicting. There is also use of 2,4-Diaminopyridine.

SUGGESTED READINGS

Abrutyn E, Berlin JA. Intrathecal therapy in tetanus. *JAMA* 1991;266: 2262–2267.

Arnon SS, Schechter R, Inglesby TV, et al. Botulinum toxin as a biological weapon: medical and public health management. *JAMA* 2001;285:1059–1070.

Bleck TP, Brauner J.Tetanus. In: Scheld WM, Whitley RJ, Durack DT, eds. *Infections of the Central Nervous System*, 2nd ed. Philadelphia: Lippincott-Raven, 1997:629–653.

Centers for Disease Control and Prevention. Infant botulism—New York City, 2001-2002. *MMWR* 2003;52:21–24.

Centers for Disease Control and Prevention. Wound botulism among black tar heroin users-Washington, 2003. *MMWR* 2003;52:885–886.

Cherington M. Clinical spectrum of botulism. *Muscle Nerve* 1998;21: 701–710.

Cook TM, Protheroe RT, Handel JM. Tetanus: a review of the literature. *Brit J Anaesthesia* 2001;87:477–487.

Hughes JM, Hatheway C, Ostroff S. Botulism. In: Scheld WM, Whitley RJ, Durack DT, eds. *Infections of The Central Nervous System*, 2nd ed. Philadelphia: Lippincott-Raven, 1997:615–628.

Ijichi T, Yamada T, Yoneda S, et al. Brain lesions in the course of generalized tetanus. *J Neurol Neurosurg Psychiatry* 2003;74:1432–1434.

Maselli RA, Bakshi N. Botulism. *Muscle Nerve* 2000;23:1137–1144.

Robinson RF, Nahata MC. Management of botulism. *Ann Pharmacother* 2003;37:127–131.

Shapiro RL, Hatheway C, Swerdlow DL. Botulism in the United States: a clinical and epidemiologic review. *Ann Intern Med* 1998;129:221–228.

Chapter 33

Reye Syndrome

Darryl C. De Vivo

In 1963, Reye et al. reported clinical and pathologic observations in 21 children with encephalopathy and fatty changes in the viscera. Subsequently, the number of reported cases of Reye syndrome increased all over the world, with unexplained fluctuations in incidence from decade to decade. The disorder also affects infants and adults, although rarely. White children in suburban or rural environments seem to be more susceptible than urban black children.

CLINICAL PRESENTATION

Reye syndrome is usually associated with influenza B epidemics or sporadic cases of influenza A and varicella. Characteristically, the encephalopathy develops 4 to 7 days after the onset of the viral illness. It is invariably heralded by recurrent vomiting and often followed by somnolence, confusion, delirium, or coma. These children have frequently been treated with antiemetics, aspirin, or acetaminophen. Epidemiologic studies have shown a statistical association between the ingestion of aspirin-containing compounds and the development of Reye syndrome. These studies, however, do not prove a causal relationship.

PATHOLOGY AND PATHOGENESIS

Pathologic and metabolic observations suggest a primary injury to mitochondria throughout the body, with prominent involvement of the liver and brain. The primary injury may be compounded by many associated insults, including hyperpyrexia, hypoglycemia, hypoxia, hyperammonemia, free fatty acidemia, systemic hypotension, and intracranial hypertension.

DIAGNOSIS

An appropriate clinical history, characteristic neurologic findings, absence of any other explanation for the non-inflammatory encephalopathy, and distinctive laboratory abnormalities are usually sufficient for establishing the diagnosis. Important laboratory abnormalities include elevations of blood ammonia, lactate, and serum transaminases, and prolongation of the prothrombin time. CSF examination is normal or reflects the metabolic abnormalities. The CSF glucose content may be low, with hypoglycemia, and the CSF amino acids may be abnormal, with hyperammonemia. Brain imaging is often normal but may show cerebral edema. The EEG is diffusely abnormal, occasionally displaying paroxysmal, epileptiform activity in the more severely ill patients.

Many other conditions may cause a similar clinical picture. The differential diagnosis includes bacterial meningitis, viral encephalitis, drug intoxication (e.g., aspirin, valproic acid, and amphetamines), and other metabolic disorders (e.g., inherited defects of fatty-acid oxidation, branched-chain amino acid metabolism, and the Krebs-Henseleit urea cycle). Recurrent attacks of Reye-like syndrome imply an underlying metabolic disorder.

TREATMENT

The current mainstay of treatment is intensive supportive care and the administration of hypertonic glucose to promote an anabolic state. Most patients recover completely within a week after onset.

SUGGESTED READINGS

Arcinue EL, Mitchell RA, Sarnaik AP, et al. The metabolic course of Reye's syndrome: distinction between survivors and nonsurvivors. *Neurology* 1986;36:435–438.

Belay ED, Birsee JS, Holman RC, et al. Reye's syndrome in the United States from 1981 through 1997. *N Engl J Med* 1999;340:1377–1382.

Brown RE, Forman DT. The biochemistry of Reye's syndrome. *CRC Crit Rev Clin Lab Sci* 1982;17:247–297.

Bhutta AT, Van Savell H, Schexnayder SM. Reye's syndrome: down but not out. *South Med J.* 2003;96(1):43–45.

Consensus Conference. Diagnosis and treatment of Reye's syndrome. *JAMA* 1981;246:2441–2444.

Corkey BE, Hale DE, Glennon MC, et al. Relationship between unusual hepatic acyl coenzyme A profiles and the pathogenesis of Reye syndrome. *J Clin Invest* 1988;82:782–788.

De Vivo DC. Reye syndrome: a metabolic response to an acute mitochondrial insult? *Neurology.* 1978;28:105–108.

De Vivo DC. How common is Reye's syndrome? *N Engl J Med* 1983;309:179–180.

Di Donato S, Taroni F. Disorders of lipid metabolism. In: Rosenberg R, Prusiner S, DiMauro S, Barchi R, Nestler E, eds. *The Molecular and Genetic Basis of Neurologic and Psychiatric Disease,* 3rd ed. Philadelphia: Butterworth-Heinemann, 2003.

Glasgow JF, Middleton B. Reye syndrome—insights on causation and prognosis. *Arch Dis Child.* 2001;85:351–353.

Haymond MW, Karl I, Keating JP, DeVivo DC. Metabolic response to hypertonic glucose administration in Reye syndrome. *Ann Neurol* 1978;3:207–215.

Heubi JE, Daugherty CC, Partin JS, et al. Grade I Reye's syndrome outcome and predictors of progression to deeper coma grades. *N Engl J Med* 1984;311:1539–1542.

Hou JW, Chou SP, Wang TR. Metabolic function and liver histopathology in Reye-like illnesses. *Acta Paediatr* 1996;85:1053–1057.

Hurwitz ES, Barrett MJ, Bregman D, et al. Public health service study on Reye's syndrome and medications: report of the pilot phase. *N Engl J Med* 1985;313:849–857.

Hurwitz ES, Barrett MJ, Bregman D, et al. Public Health Service study of Reye's syndrome and medications. *JAMA* 1987;257:1905–1911.

Lichtenstein PK, Heubi JE, Daugherty CC, et al. Grade I Reye's syndrome. A frequent cause of vomiting and liver dysfunction after varicella and upper-respiratory-tract infection. *N Engl J Med.* 1983;309:133–139.

Lyon G, Dodge PR, Adams RD. The acute encephalopathies of obscure origin in infants and children. *Brain* 1961;84:680–708.

Monto AS. The disappearance of Reye's syndrome—a public health triumph. *N Engl J Med* 1999;340:1423–1424.

Partin JS, McAdams AJ, Partin JC, et al. Brain ultrastructure in Reye's disease. II. Acute injury and recovery process in three children. *J Neuropathol Exp Neurol* 1978;37:796–819.

Pranzatelli MR, De Vivo DC. The pharmacology of Reye syndrome. *Clin Neuropharmacol* 1987;10:96–125.

Reye BDK, Morgan G, Baral J. Encephalopathy and fatty degeneration of the viscera: a disease entity in childhood. *Lancet* 1963;2:749–752.

Stanley CA. New genetic defects in mitochondrial fatty acid oxidation and carnitine deficiency. *Adv Pediatr* 1987;34:59–88.

Stumpf DA. Reye syndrome: an international perspective. *Brain Dev* 1995;17[Suppl]:77–78.

Sullivan-Bolyai JZ, Corey L. Epidemiology of Reye's syndrome. *Epidemiol Rev* 1981;3:1–26.

Van Coster RN, De Vivo DC, Blake D, et al. Adult Reye's syndrome: a review with new evidence for a generalized defect in intramitochondrial enzyme processing. *Neurology* 1991;41:1815–1821.

You KS. Salicylate and mitochondrial injury in Reye's syndrome. *Science* 1983;221:163–165.

Chapter 34

Prion Diseases

Burk Jubelt

Prion diseases or the transmissible spongiform encephalopathies include several human diseases: kuru, Creutzfeldt-Jakob disease (CJD), new variant CJD (nvCJD), Gerstmann-Sträussler syndrome (GSS), and fatal familial insomnia (FFI), as well as diseases of animals (sheep scrapie, bovine spongiform encephalopathy, chronic wasting disease, and others). All these conditions are rare, but among them, CJD is the most common (Table 34.1). All have characteristic pathologic changes that led to the early designation of *spongiform encephalopathy*.

PATHOGENESIS

Like viruses, prions are transmissible. However, they differ from any known virus because the molecule does not include any detectable nucleic acid. It is resistant to heat, ultraviolet light, and ionizing radiation, which modify nucleic acids. However, the infectivity of the agent is susceptible to treatments that denature proteins (sodium dodecyl sulfate, phenol). The neologism "prion" was taken from the two key features of the agent, protein and infectious. (The preferred pronunciation is "pree-on.")

The human prion protein is encoded by a gene currently designated *PRNP* on the short arm of chromosome 20. The prion protein (PrP) is found in two isoforms. One is the normal cellular form (PrP^C). The other form differs only in physical characteristics and is found in scrapie (PrP^{SC}) and other animal prion diseases and in the human prion diseases. PrP^C is an intracellular membrane bound protein. Its normal biological function is unknown. PrP^{SC} is found not only intracellular but also extracellular in amyloid filaments and amyloid plaques. Delineation of the nature of this new agent gained a Nobel Prize for Stanley Prusiner.

The animal prion diseases include scrapie of sheep, transmissible mink encephalopathy, chronic wasting disease of elk and mule deer, and bovine spongiform encephalopathy (BSE). Scrapie was recognized in ancient times and was considered transmissible or infectious in the 1930s. Scrapie occurs primarily in Europe but has occurred in the United States. In the last decade the prion diseases have become a public health problem because of the epidemic of BSE ("mad cow" disease) in Great Britain. BSE occurred because cattle were fed scrapie-contaminated meat-and-bone meal. This same mechanism has caused a disease in domestic cats (feline spongiform encephalopathy) and felines in zoos. In addition, atypical CJD ("new variant" or CVJD) has affected young adults in Great Britain, Europe, and recently North America who were infected with the BSE agent.

TABLE 34.1 Relative Frequency of Human Prion Disease: Tissues Referred for Transmission to Primates

Syndrome	Number of Patients
Creutzfeldt-Jakob disease	278
Sporadic	234
Familial	36
Iatrogenic	8
Kuru	18
Gerstmann-Sträussler-Scheinker syndrome	2

Modified from Brown P, Gibbs CJ Jr, Rodgers-Johnson P, et al. Human spongiform encephalopathy: the NIH series of 300 cases of experimentally transmitted disease. *Ann Neurol* 1994;35:513–529.

EPIDEMIOLOGY OF HUMAN DISEASE

The human diseases may be sporadic, infectious, or genetic; 80% to 90% of CJD cases are sporadic. Iatrogenic CJD and familial CJD (autosomal dominant) each account for 5% to 10% of CJD cases. GSS and FFI are also genetic and rare (Table 34.1). Sporadic CJD is not spread like an ordinary infection because the agent has low infectivity. People with prior head and neck trauma and medical personnel may be at higher risk because of increased exposure to the agent. CJD has been transmitted by implanting electrodes or transplanting corneas from affected patients. Iatrogenic disease has also occurred with dura mater grafts and administration of growth hormone extract prepared from pooled human pituitary glands. Gajdusek and colleagues found that all these diseases may be transmitted to chimpanzees or guinea pigs (Brown et al., 1994; see Table 34.1). In that sense the diseases are infectious. Mutations in the *PrP* gene cause the inherited diseases, which are therefore both heritable and transmissible.

There is now debate about nomenclature, whether we should continue to refer to the diseases by the original clinicopathologic designations or whether they should all be lumped together as "prion disease" and identified by the specific mutation identified. The latter group points to people in the same family who have different clinical syndromes. PrP mutations have also been identified in atypical syndromes, such as dementia resembling Alzheimer disease, or spastic paraplegia.

▶ **TABLE 34.2** Mutations in the Prion Protein Gene Associated with Familial Prion Diseases[a]

Codon No.	Normal Amino Acids (s)	Mutant Amino Acid (s)	Familial Prion Disease
51–91	5 octa repeats	Additional 2–9 octa repeats	CJD
178	Asp	Asn	CJD
180	Val	Ile	CJD
183	Thr	Ala	CJD
196	Glu	Lys	CJD
200	Glu	Lys	CJD
203	Val	Ileu	CJD
208	Arg	His	CJD
210	Val	Ile	CJD
211	Glu	Gln	CJD
232	Met	Arg	CJD
102	Pro	Leu	GSS
105	Pro	Leu	GSS
117	Ala	Val	GSS
131	Tyr	Val	GSS
145	Tyr	Stop	GSS
198	Phe	Ser	GSS
202	Asp	Asn	GSS
212	Gln	Pro	GSS
217	Glu	Arg	GSS
232	Met	Thr	GSS
129	Val or Met	Val	178[Asn] CJD
		Met	178[Asn] FFI

[a]Other mutations have been described but only in single cases. CJD; Creutzfeldt-Jakob disease; GSS; Gerstmann-Sträussler-Scheinker syndrome; FFI; Familial Fatal Insomnia.

The former group, on the other hand, points to a strong tendency for specific mutations to be associated with specific clinical syndromes (Table 34.2) and to differences in transmissibility of the different clinical syndromes. For instance, Brown and colleagues (1994) found that all iatrogenic cases were transmitted to chimpanzees, as were 90% of sporadic CJD, but only 68% of the familial cases; 95% of the cases of kuru were transmitted, but only two of four cases of GSS were transmitted.

Additional molecular techniques may be useful for categorizing the prion diseases. Proteinase K digestion of CJD brain homogenates followed by Western blot analysis has demonstrated the presence of protease-resistant prion proteins (PrP[res]) of different patterns (based on the size and ratio of differently glycosylated isoforms). Thus far, four distinct patterns have been recognized: types 1 and 2, primarily in sporadic CJD; type 3, iatrogenic CJD; type 4, new variant. CJD may be further classified according to the three genotypes of methionine (M)/valine (V) polymorphism at codon 129 of the PrP gene (MM, MV and

VV). Homozygosity at codon 129 is over represented in individuals with sporadic or iatrogenic CJD. Even more intriguing is that all identified cases of nvCJD are homozygous for M. The prion proteins of the other prion diseases have not as yet been adequately analyzed by these techniques.

KURU

This progressive and fatal disorder occurs exclusively among natives (Fore people) of the New Guinea Highlands. It is manifested by incoordination of gait, severe trunk and limb ataxia, abnormal involuntary movements resembling myoclonus or chorea, convergent strabismus, and, later in the disease, dementia. The illness terminates fatally in 4 to 24 months. Cannibalism is considered the principal mode of transmission, affecting children, adolescents, and adult women. Since this practice was eliminated in the 1950s, the disease now is rare and affects only older adults of both sexes. Neuropathologic changes include widespread neuronal loss, neuronal and astrocytic vacuolization, and astrocytic proliferation. Amyloid plaques containing the abnormal prion protein (PrP) were first described in kuru, and called kuru plaques. These pathologic changes are most prominent in the cerebellum, where gross atrophy may be seen. The cerebrum and brainstem are involved to a lesser degree.

The similarity between the clinical and neuropathologic manifestations of kuru and those seen in scrapie-afflicted sheep led Gajdusek and Gibbs to infect higher primates with brain suspensions. Inoculation of chimpanzees was followed by the appearance of a kuru-like disease 14 months to several years later. Kuru was the first human-transmissible spongiform encephalopathy (prion disease) to be recognized. Gajdusek was awarded a Nobel Prize for this work.

CREUTZFELDT-JAKOB DISEASE

In 1920 and 1921, Creutzfeldt and Jakob described a progressive disease of the cortex, basal ganglia, and spinal cord that developed in middle-aged and elderly adults. CJD (i.e., spastic pseudosclerosis, corticostriatospinal degeneration) was the second human prion disease to be recognized. CJD occurs throughout the world but is relatively rare, with an incidence of about 1 case per 1 million people annually. This incidence is the same throughout the world except for the high incidence among Libyan Jews in Israel, and in a few populations elsewhere. The disease affects mainly middle-aged and older individuals, with an average age at onset of about 60 years.

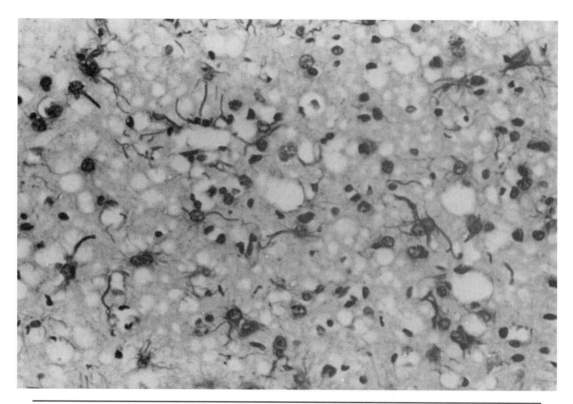

FIGURE 34.1. Creutzfeldt-Jakob disease. Section from cortex showing status spongiosis of the neuropil, loss of neurons, and prominent astrocytosis. Phosphotungstic acid hematoxylin stain, X 120. (Courtesy of Dr. Mauro C. Dal Canto.)

Pathology

The pathologic condition is essentially degenerative with grossly evident cerebral atrophy. Microscopic findings are similar to other prion diseases with neuronal loss, astrocytosis, and the development of cytoplasmic vacuoles in neurons and astrocytes (status spongiosis, Fig. 34.1).

Amyloid plaques that contain the abnormal PrP are found in the areas of infected tissue in most cases. There is no inflammation. The cortex and basal ganglia are most affected, but all parts of the neuraxis may be involved. Early lesions are more severe in the gray matter.

Symptoms and Signs

The clinical features include the gradual onset of dementia in middle or late life, but occasionally in young adults. Vague, prodromal symptoms of anxiety, fatigue, dizziness, headache, impaired judgment, and unusual behavior may occur. Once memory loss starts, it progresses rapidly, and other characteristic signs appear, sometimes abruptly. The most frequently seen signs, aside from dementia, are those of pyramidal tract disease (i.e., weakness and stiffness of the limbs with accompanying reflex changes), extrapyramidal signs (i.e., tremors, rigidity, dysarthria, and slowness of movements), and myoclonus, which is often stimulus sensitive. Other signs include amyotrophy, cortical blindness, seizures, and those of cerebellar dysfunction

(Table 34.3). None of the usual signs of an infection is seen.

Laboratory Data

Routine blood counts and chemistries are within normal limits. Routine CSF tests are usually within normal limits, although the protein content may rarely be elevated. In 1986, Harrington et al. described two abnormal proteins in the CSF of CJD patients on two-dimensional (2D) gel electrophoresis. These proteins were also found in acute herpes simplex encephalitis. This assay did not become used in general practice because of its procedural difficulty. Ten years later, studies from the same laboratory reported that the sequence of these two proteins matched that of brain proteins known as 14-3-3 neuronal proteins, which may play a role in conformational stabilization of other proteins. An immunoassay for the 14-3-3 protein was positive in 96% of CJD CSF samples. The assay was also positive in other diseases with acute massive neuronal dysfunction, especially herpes simplex encephalitis and acute infarction. Still, in the appropriate clinical setting, the immunoassay for the 14-3-3 protein is a highly supportive diagnostic test. However, at times the sensitivity of the test may only be 50% (e.g., owing to slower disease, variation between laboratories). Thus, a negative test does not exclude the diagnosis. The EEG may also be of diagnostic value because periodic complexes of spike or

> **TABLE 34.3** 232 Experimentally Transmitted Cases of Sporadic Creutzfeldt-Jakob Disease

	Percentage of Patients	
	At Onset	Later
Mental deterioration	69	100
Memory loss	48	100
Behavioral change	29	57
Aphasia, agnosia	16	73
Cerebellar signs	33	71
Visual, oculomotor signs	19	42
Headache	11	18
Sensory change	6	11
Involuntary movements	4	91
Myoclonus	1	78
Tremor, other	3	36
Pyramidal signs	2	62
Extrapyramidal signs	0.5	56
Lower motor neuron signs	0.5	12
Seizures	0	19
Pseudobulbar signs	0.5	7
Periodic electroencephalogram	0	60

Modified from Brown P, Gibbs CJ Jr, Rodgers-Johnson P, et al. Human spongiform encephalopathy: the NIH series of 300 cases of experimentally transmitted disease. *Ann Neurol* 1994;35:513–529.

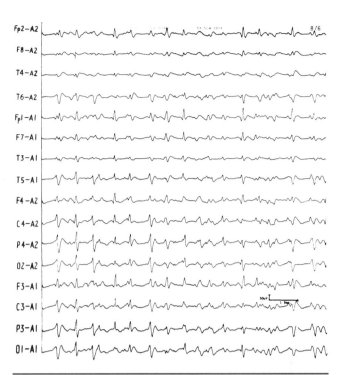

FIGURE 34.2. Creutzfeldt-Jakob disease. Record of a 65-year-old man shows spikes of sharp waves at intervals of 0.7 sec throughout the recording. Such periodicity with 0.5-sec to 2.0-sec intervals occurs in the middle and late stages and may be absent in the early stages of the disease.

slow-wave activity, at intervals of 0.5 second to 2.0 seconds, are characteristic in the middle and late stages of the disease (Fig. 34.2).

Increased signal intensity on T2-weighted, fluid-attenuated inversion recovery (FLAIR) and diffusion weighted (DWI) magnetic resonance imaging has been seen primarily in the basal ganglia, in a diffuse pattern, and occasionally in the cortex and cerebellum along the corticol ribbon (gyriform pattern). In a few cases, the thalamus has also been involved. DWI appears to be more sensitive than either T2 or FLAIR imaging, approaching 90–100% as compared to about 50%. CT and MRI may reveal cerebral atrophy late in the course of the disease.

Diagnosis and Differential Diagnosis

A definite diagnosis of CJD may only be made by neuropathologic, immunologic, or biochemical examination of the brain. In typical cases (e.g., dementia, myoclonus, periodic EEG), the diagnosis may be made clinically. However, the diagnosis is difficult to make in atypical cases (i.e., no myoclonus, absence of periodic EEG). In the atypical cases, the diagnosis of Alzheimer disease is often made. Other degenerative diseases, such as Pick disease, corticobasal ganglionic degeneration, familial myoclonic dementia, multisystem atrophy, and lithium toxicity may also be considered. The CSF test for the 14-3-3 protein may clarify the atypical cases. If not, brain biopsy is needed for evaluation of pathology or demonstration of protease-resistant PrP. In 2003 prions were found in olfactory mucosa and skeletal muscle, more readily available tissues for biopsy.

Course and Prognosis

The disease is fatal within 1 year in 90% of patients. Rarely, the course may be prolonged over several years. There is no specific treatment.

Transmissibility and Biohazard Potential

As with kuru, neurologic illness may be produced in primates by the inoculation of brain suspensions prepared from the brains of CJD patients. The mode of transmission of sporadic CJD is unknown. The agent has been detected in most internal organs (lung, liver, kidney, spleen, and lymph nodes), cornea, and blood but has not been detected in saliva or feces. One isolation from urine may have been a contaminant. These findings suggest a lack of significant spread by respiratory, enteric, or sexual contact. Failure to find an increased incidence in spouses also suggests that these usual modes of transmission of infections are not of major importance.

Isolation of Creutzfeldt-Jakob patients does not seem necessary except for precautions with internal body fluids, as in the precautions taken for serum hepatitis. Human-to-human transmission has been reported after corneal transplantation, use of inadequately sterilized stereotactic brain electrodes, parenteral administration of human growth hormone preparations, and the use of human dura mater grafts. Caution must be exercised in operating rooms and pathology laboratories and in the preparation of brain-derived biologicals. Medical personnel should avoid contact of open sores or conjunctiva with these tissues. Caution should be taken to avoid accidental, percutaneous exposure to CSF, blood, or tissue. Because the prion agents are highly resistant to ordinary physical or chemical treatment (routine autoclaving or formalin), special autoclaving procedures or special inactivating agents, including sodium hypochlorite (household bleach), are required. Disposable surgical instruments are recommended.

NEW VARIANT CREUTZFELDT-JAKOB DISEASE

In 1996, 10 cases of "new variant" CJD (nvCJD) were reported in Great Britain. These cases were unusual both clinically and pathologically in that they shared many characteristics normally associated with kuru. Symptoms started before age 40; several cases occurred in teenagers. Clinical manifestations included behavioral changes, sensory complaints and ataxia. Myoclonic jerks and the characteristic EEG abnormalities were not seen. Eventually involuntary movements and dementia occurred in most cases. The course was slower than conventional CJD, lasting up to 22 months. About 150 cases have now been reported, including two in North America. The pathologic changes were also unusual with minimal spongiosis but prominent plaque formation in the cerebellum and cerebrum. Transmission experiments of both BSE and new variant CJD brain tissue to animals confirmed the similar strain characteristics. Molecular analysis (proteinase K digestion) of brain homogenates from these new variant CJD cases revealed a Western blot pattern similar to that of BSE (type 4) rather than that of sporadic CJD (types 1 and 2). The diagnosis of nvCJD is more difficult to ascertain than that of sCJD. The periodic EEG is not seen, and the 14-3-3 protein is found in only about a third of the patients. Magnetic resonance imaging has revealed hyperintensity of the pulvinar on T2, FLAIR, and DW images in a high percentage of cases.

GERSTMANN-STRÄUSSLER-SCHEINKER DISEASE

GSS disease is the third human disease caused by a prion agent. It has also been referred to as the Gerstmann-Sträussler syndrome. GSS is an autosomal dominant familial disease (Table 34.2).

The age of onset varies from the 20s into the 70s but is greatest in the 40s and 50s. It has a lengthy course with a range of 2 to 10 years. Clinically, it begins with ataxia; dementia eventually supervenes. Brainstem involvement leads to symptoms suggesting olivopontocerebellar degeneration. Less common are the "telencephalic" form with dementia, parkinsonism, and pyramidal tract signs and also a form with neurofibrillary tangles. Pathologically, there is usually spongiform change and prominent amyloid plaque deposition in the cerebellum, cerebrum, and basal ganglia. There is also degeneration of the spinocerebellar and corticospinal tracts. The EEG usually shows diffuse slowing; only occasionally is periodicity seen. MRI reveals cerebral and cerebellar atrophy. The 14-3-3 protein is not found. As with CJD, there is no treatment.

FATAL FAMILIAL INSOMNIA

FFI is an autosomal-dominant disease with a course of 7 to 36 months, and an age at onset of between 18 to 61 years. Familial thalamic dementia or degeneration appears to be the same disease. The patients have progressive insomnia and dysautonomia (hyperhidrosis, tachycardia, tachypnea, hyperthermia, hypertension) and may develop pyramidal and cerebellar signs, dementia, and myoclonus. However, there may be diverse phenotypic expression of the disease, even among members of the same family. Some patients do not develop insomnia until later stages. Other patients may present with clinical features of CJD. The EEG usually shows diffuse slowing; periodicity has been described only rarely and then, only late in the disease. Magnetic resonance imaging is usually within normal limits and the 14-3-3 protein is not found.

These patients have a mutation of the *PrP* gene at codon 178, coupled with a methionine at codon 129 (Table 34.2). Patients who are homozygous for methionine at codon 129 have a much more rapid course than those who are heterozygous. Pathologically, there is prominent neuronal loss and gliosis in the thalamus, with little to no spongiform change. Patients with long duration or atypical presentations are more likely to have widespread lesions in the cerebral cortex, basal ganglia, brainstem, and cerebellum. Because the clinical manifestations of FFI vary, genotyping is crucial for confirming the diagnosis. There is no specific treatment.

SUGGESTED READINGS

General

Brown DR. Molecular advances in understanding inherited diseases. *Molec Neurobiol* 2002;25:287–302.

Brown P, Gibbs CJ Jr, Rodgers-Johnson P, et al. Human spongiform encephalopathy: the NIH series of 300 cases of experimentally transmitted disease. *Ann Neurol* 1994;35:513–529.

Kovacs GG. Mutations of the prion protein gene. Phenotypic spectrum. *J Neurol* 2002;249:1567–1582.

McKintosh E, Tabrizi SJ, Collinge J. Prion diseases. *J NeuroVirol* 2003;9:183–193.

Otvos L Jr, Cudic M. Post-translational modifications in prion proteins. *Curr Prot Peptide Sci* 2002;3:643–652.

Prusiner SM, Scott MR. Genetics of prions. *Annu Rev Genet* 1997;31:139–175.

Kuru

Gajdusek DC. Unconventional viruses and the origin and disappearance of kuru. *Science* 1977;197:943–960.

Goldfarb LG. Kuru: the old epidemic in a new mirror. *Microbes & Infect* 2002;4:875–882.

Hornabrook RW. Kuru—a subacute cerebellar degeneration: the natural history and clinical features. *Brain* 1968;91:53–74.

Lee HS, Brown P, Cervenakova L et al. Increased susceptibility to Kuru of carriers of PRNP 120 methionine/methionine genotype. *J Infect Dis* 2001;183:192–196.

Liberski PP, Gajdusek DC. Kuru: forty years later, a historical note. *Brain Pathol* 1997;7:555–560.

Prusiner SB, Gajdusek DC, Alpers MP. Kuru with incubation periods exceeding two decades. *Ann Neurol* 1982;12:1–9.

Creutzfeldt-Jakob Disease

General

Johnson RT, Gibbs CJ Jr. Creutzfeldt-Jakob disease and related transmissible spongiform encephalopathies. *N Engl J Med* 1998;339:1994–2004.

Louie JK, Gavali SS, Belay ED, et al. Barriers to Creutzfeldt-Jakob disease autopsies. California. *Emerg Infect Dis* 2004 Sep;10(9):1677–1680.

Mallucci G, Collinge J. Update on Creutzfeldt-Jakob disease. *Curr Opin Neurol* 2004 Dec;17(6):641–647.

Clinical and Epidemiologic

Brown P, Gibbs CJ Jr, Rodgers-Johnson P, et al. Human spongiform encephalopathy: the NIH series of 300 cases of experimentally transmitted disease. *Ann Neurol* 1994;35:513–529.

Centers for Disease Control and Prevention. Update: Creutzfeldt-Jakob disease associated with cadaveric dura mater grafts—Japan, 1979–2003. *MMWR* 2003;52:1179–1181.

Cousens SN, Zeidler M, Esmonde TF, et al. Sporadic Creutzfeldt-Jakob disease in the United Kingdom: analysis of epidemiological surveillance data for 1970–96. *BMJ* 1997;315:389–395.

Meissner B, Kortner K, Bartl M, et al. Sporadic Creutzfeldt-Jakob disease: magnetic resonance imaging and clinical findings. *Neurology* 2004 Aug 10;63(3):450–456.

Otto M, Cepek L, Ratzka P, et al. Efficacy of flupirtine on cognitive function in patients with CJD. A double-blind study. *Neurology* 2004;62:714–718.

Pocchiari M, Puopolo M, Croes EA, et al. Predictors of survival in sporadic Creutzfeldt-Jakob disease and other human transmissible spongiform encephalopathies. *Brain* 2004 Oct;127(Pt10):2348–2359.

Rabinstein AA, Whiteman ML, Shebert RT. Abnormal diffusion-weighted magnetic resonance imaging in Creutzfeldt-Jakob disease following corneal transplantations. *Arch Neurol* 2002;59:637–639.

Will RG, Alperovitch A, Poser S, et al. Descriptive epidemiology of Creutzfeldt-Jakob disease in six European countries, 1993–1995. *Ann Neurol* 1998;43:763–767.

Laboratory Diagnosis

Fukushima R, Shiga Y, Nakamura M, et al. MRI characteristics of sporadic CJD with valine homozygosity at codon 129 of the prion protein gene and PrpSC type 2 in Japan. *J Neurol Neurosurg Psychiatry* 2004;75:485–487.

Geschwind MD, Martindale J, Miller D, et al. Challenging the clinical utility of the 14-3-3 protein for the diagnosis of sporadic Creutzfeldt-Jakob disease. *Arch Neurol* 2003;60:813–816.

Kretzschmar HA, Ironside JM, DeArmond SJ, Tateishi J. Diagnostic criteria for sporadic Creutzfeldt-Jakob disease. *Arch Neurol* 1996;53:913–920.

Mendes OE, Shang J, Jungreis CA, Kaufer DI. Diffusion-weighted MRI in Creutzfeld-Jakob disease: a better diagnostic marker than CSF protein 14-3-3? *J Neuroimaging* 2003;13:147–151.

Steinhoff BJ, Räcker S, Herrendorf G, et al. Accuracy and reliability of periodic sharp wave complexes in Creutzfeldt-Jakob disease. *Arch Neurol* 1996;53:162–166.

Worrall BB, Rowland LP, Chin SS, Mastrianni JA. Amyotrophy in prion disease. *Arch Neurol* 2000;57:33–38.

Zerr I, Bodemer M, Gefeller O, et al. Detection of 14-3-3 protein in the cerebrospinal fluid supports the diagnosis of Creutzfeldt-Jakob disease. *Ann Neurol* 1998;43:32–40.

Familial CJD and Genetics

Campbell TA, Palmer MS, Will RG, et al. A prion disease with a novel 96base pair insertional mutation in the prion protein gene. *Neurology* 1996;46:761–766.

Chapman J, Arlazoroff A, Goldfarb LG, et al. Fatal insomnia in a case of familial Creutzfeldt-Jakob disease with the codon 200 (Lys) mutation. *Neurology* 1996;46:758–761.

Cochran EJ, Bennett DA, Cervenakova L, et al. Familial Creutzfeldt-Jakob disease with a five-repeat octapeptide insert mutation. *Neurology* 1996;47:727–733.

Prusiher SM, Scott MR. Genetics of prions. *Annu Rev Genet* 1997;31:139–175.

Molecular Basis, Phenotype, and Pathogenesis

Glatzel M, Abela E, Maissen M, Aguzzi A. Extraneural pathologic prion protein in sporadic Creutzfeldt-Jakob disease. *N Engl J Med* 2003;349:1812–1820.

Hill AF, Joiner S, Wadsworth JDF, et al. Molecular classification of sporadic Creutzfeldt-Jakob disease. *Brain* 2003;126:1333–1346.

Pietrini V, Puoti G, Limido L, et al. Creutzfeldt-Jakob disease with a novel extra-repeat insertional mutation in *PRNP* gene. *Neurology* 2003;61:1288–1291.

Zanusso G, Ferrari S, Cardone F, et al. Detection of pathologic prion protein in the olfactory epithelium in sporadic Creutzfeldt-Jakob disease. *N Engl J Med* 2003;348:711–719.

Transmissibility and Tissue Handling

Budka H, Aguzzi A, Brown P, et al. Tissue handling in suspected Creutzfeldt-Jakob disease (CJD) and other human spongiform encephalopathies (prion diseases). *Brain Pathol* 1995;5:319–322.

Committee on Health Care Issues, American Neurological Association. Precautions in handling tissues, fluids, and other contaminated materials from patients with documented or suspected Creutzfeldt-Jakob disease. *Ann Neurol* 1986;19:75–77.

Manuelidis L. Decontamination of Creutzfeldt-Jakob disease and other transmissible agents. *J Neuro Virol* 1997;3:62–65.

New Variant CJD

Bruce ME, Will RG, Ironside JW, et al. Transmissions to mice indicate that 'new variant' CJD is caused by the BSE agent. *Nature* 1997;389:498–501.

Collie D, Summers DM, Sellar RJ, et al. Diagnosing variant Creutzfeldt-Jakob disease with the pulvinar sign: MR imaging findings in 86 neuropathologically confirmed cases. *Am J Neuroradiol* 2003;24:1560–1569.

Epstein LG, Brown P. Bovine spongiform encephalopathy and a new variant of Creutzfeldt-Jakob disease. *Neurology* 1997;48:569–571.

Hill AF, Desbruslais M, Joiner S, et al. The same prion strain causes vCJD and BSE. *Nature* 1997;389:448–450.

Irani DN, Johnson RT. Diagnosis and prevention of bovine spongiform encephalopathy and variant Creutzfeldt-Jakob disease. *Annu Rev Med* 2003;54:305–319.

Zeidler M, Stewart GE, Barraclovah CR, et al. New variant Creutzfeldt-Jakob disease: neurological features and diagnostic tests. *Lancet* 1997;350:903–907.

Gerstmann-Sträussler-Scheinker Disease

Barbanti P, Fabbrini G, Salvatore M, et al. Polymorphism at codon 129 or codon 219 of PRNP and clinical heterogeneity in a previously unreported family with Gerstmann-Sträussler-Scheinker disease (PrP-P102L mutation). *Neurology* 1996;47:734–741.

Collins S, McLean CA, Master CL. Gerstmann-Strausster-Scheinker syndrome, fatal familial insomnia, and kuru: a review of these less common human transmissible spongiform encephalopathies. *J Clin Neurosci* 2001;8:387–397.

DeMichele G, Pocchiari M, Petraroli R, et al. Variable phenotype in a P102L Gerstmann-Strausster-Scheinker Italian family. *Can J Neurol Sci* 2003;30:233–236.

Majtenvi C, Brown P, Cervenakova L, Goldfarb LG, Tateishi J. A three-sister sibship of Gerstmann-Strausster-Scheinker disease with a CJD phenotype. *Neurology* 2000;54:2133–2137.

Parchi P, Chen SG, Brown P, et al. Different patterns of truncated prion protein fragments correlate with distance phenotypes in P102L Gerstmann-Strausster-Scheinker disease. *Proc Natl Acad Sci USA* 1998;95:8322–8327.

Fatal Familial Insomnia

Gambetti P, Parchi P, Chen SG. Hereditary Creutzfeldt-Jakob disease and fatal familial insomnia. *Clin Lab Med* 2003;23:43–64.

Johnson MD, Vnencak-Jones CL, McLean MJ. Fatal familial insomnia: clinical and pathologic heterogeneity in genetic half brothers. *Neurology* 1998;51:1715–1717.

McLean CA, Storey E, Gardner RJ, et al. The D178N (cis-129M) "fatal familial insomnia" mutation associated with diverse clinicopathologic phenotypes in an Australian kindred. *Neurology* 1997;49:552–558.

Padovani A, D'Alessandro M, Parchi P, et al. Fatal familial insomnia in a new Italian kindred. *Neurology* 1998;51:1491–1494.

Scaravilli F, Cordery RJ, Kretzschmar H, et al. Sporadic fatal insomnia: a case study. *Ann Neurol* 2000;48:665–668.

Tabernero C, Polo JM, Sevillano MD, et al. Fatal familial insomnia: clinical, neuropathological, and genetic description of a Spanish family [short report]. *J Neurol Neurosurg Psychiatry* 2000;68:774–777.

Wanschitz J, Kloppel S, Jarius C, et al. Alteration of the serotonergic nervous system in fatal familial insomnia. *Ann Neurol* 2000;48:788–791.

Zerr I, Giese A, Windl O, et al. Phenotypic variability in fatal familial insomnia (D178-129M) genotype. *Neurology* 1998;51:1398–1405.

Chapter 35

▶ Whipple Disease

Elan D. Louis

Whipple disease was originally described as a gastrointestinal disorder with arthralgia. It is caused by a bacterium, and infection is evident in many organs, including but not limited to the intestinal tract, heart, lungs, liver, kidneys, and brain. Polymerase chain reaction (PCR) analysis of DNA coding for bacterial RNA has led to classification of the Whipple organism. The organism, *Tropheryma whippelii*, belongs to the soil-derived *Actinomycetaceae* family of bacteria; and six strains of the organism have been identified. Although difficult to culture, the organism has been propagated *in vitro* in macrophages deactivated by interleukin-4 and in a human fibroblast cell line. Whipple disease has not been reproduced in animals.

The bacillus is rod shaped, 1.0 μm to 2.0 μm long, and weakly Gram positive, with a thick wall. It is large enough to be seen under light microscopy. The organism produces a cellular rather than a humoral immune response, and this is predominated by macrophage recruitment. Infected macrophages stain strongly with the periodic acid–Schiff (PAS) reaction. Examination by electron microscopy of these macrophages demonstrates that the areas of intense PAS staining are packed with bacilli. These areas usually have a distinctive sickle shape, and the macrophages are often referred to as sickle-form, particle-containing cells.

EPIDEMIOLOGY

Whipple disease is rare. Approximately 1,000 cases have been reported and the ratio of published to unpublished cases has been estimated to be 1:3. Most reported cases arose in North America or Europe, especially among white men. Among the nearly 700 patients analyzed by Dobbins (1987), 86.4% were male and 97.8% were white. People who worked with soil or animals accounted for two of every three cases. DNA of the organism was detected in five different sewage treatment plants in Germany, providing the first documented encounter with the organism outside of the human body and implicating an environmental source of infection. The route of infection is not known, although given the frequency of gastrointestinal symptoms, oral ingestion is suspected. Clusters of affected individuals within families include three pairs of siblings and a father-daughter pair.

SYSTEMIC DISEASE

Variability in bacterial strains as well as differences in host immunity may each play a role in development of disease in the setting of infection. Symptoms include weight loss (i.e., usually 20 to 30 pounds, occasionally as much as 100 pounds), abdominal pain (i.e., often nondescript epigastric pain), diarrhea (i.e., often with steatorrhea), and arthritis (i.e., often migratory and involving large joints). In 50% of patients, arthritis precedes the intestinal manifestations by 10 to 30 years. Other systemic manifestations include low-grade fever, lymphadenopathy, and increased skin pigmentation.

In systemic disease, blood studies may reveal anemia and hypoalbuminemia. Intestinal absorption studies often reveal steatorrhea and malabsorption. Diagnosis, however, is usually made by small-intestine biopsy, to demonstrate the PAS-staining macrophages. Because PAS-positive macrophages may be found in other diseases and in other tissues of apparently normal people, confirmation of the diagnosis is facilitated by detection of the actual bacillus, with the use of electron microscopy or by PCR analysis of infected tissue. If intestinal biopsy is PAS-negative, multiple biopsies with electron microscopic examination may be required to establish the diagnosis.

NEUROLOGIC MANIFESTATIONS

The proportion of patients with asymptomatic CNS infection is thought to be high; in one report 70% of Whipple disease patients without neurologic symptoms or signs had CSF findings consistent with *T. whippelii* infection. It is therefore important to include CSF examination even for patients who do not have neurologic symptoms. In 5% of patients with Whipple disease, the first symptoms are neurologic, but CNS symptoms may eventually occur in 6% to 43% of cases. In some cases, CNS disease may occur without evidence of infection elsewhere. The CNS is also involved frequently when systemic disease relapses after a course of antibiotics; these patients may then respond poorly to antibiotics.

Neurologic symptoms and signs are protean. Louis et al. (1996) reviewed reports of 84 cases of CNS Whipple disease. The following signs were most prevalent: cognitive changes (i.e., abnormalities of orientation, memory, or reasoning, 71%), supranuclear gaze palsy (i.e., more often vertical than horizontal, 51%), altered level of consciousness (i.e., somnolence, lethargy, stupor, or coma, 50%), psychiatric signs (i.e., depression, euphoria, anxiety, psychosis, or personality change, 44%), upper motor neuron signs (37%), and hypothalamic manifestations (i.e., polydipsia, hyperphagia, change in libido, amenorrhea, changes in sleep-wake cycle, insomnia, 31%). Other signs in 20% to 25% of cases included cranial nerve abnormalities, myoclonus, seizures, and ataxia (Table 35.1).

The combination of pendular vergence oscillations of the eyes in synchrony with masticatory myorhythmia (rhythmic myoclonic jerks) has been termed "oculomasticatory myorhythmia." When there is myorhythmia of skeletal muscles as well, the term "oculofacial-skeletal myorhythmia" has been used. Although these forms of myorhythmia are pathognomonic of CNS Whipple disease, they were noted in only 20% of patients. The classic triad

▶ **TABLE 35.1 Neurologic Signs in 84 Cases of CNS Whipple Disease**

Signs	Percent
Cognitive change	71
Supranuclear gaze palsy	51
Altered level of consciousness	50
Psychiatric signs	44
Upper motor neuron signs	37
Hypothalamic manifestations	31
Cranial nerve abnormalities	25
Myoclonus	25
Seizures	23
Ataxia	20
Oculomasticatory myorhythmia or oculo-facial-skeletal myorhythmia	20
Sensory deficits	12

of dementia, supranuclear gaze palsy, and myoclonus was noted in only 15% of cases.

LABORATORY DATA

In CNS Whipple disease, over half of the patients show a focal abnormality on CT or MRI, ranging from a small, focal lesion without mass effect, to large numbers of enhancing lesions with mass effect. However, these abnormalities are not specific. A low-level CSF pleocytosis (mean, 91 leukocytes (cells)/μL; range, 5 cells/μL to 900 cells/μL) is found in half the patients with the CNS disorder, and CSF protein content is high in half (mean, 75 mg/dL; range, 47 mg/dL to 158 mg/dL). When CNS Whipple disease is suspected clinically, the diagnosis may be confirmed by biopsy of any infected tissue, for identification of bacteria by light microscopy, electron microscopy, or PCR. In the Louis et al. review, biopsy was a sensitive technique; 70% of intestinal biopsies and 89% of all tissue biopsies (i.e., small bowel, brain, lymph node, vitreous fluid) were positive. Factors that contributed to a negative small-bowel biopsy included absence of chronic diarrhea, lack of endoscopic guidance, specimens not examined by electron microscopy, and biopsy not repeated at least once if initially negative. PCR has high sensitivity (87% to 97%) and specificity (100%) for Whipple disease in cases with biopsy proven disease.

TREATMENT

Given the rare nature of this illness, there have been no randomized, double-blind trials of antibiotic agents. If untreated, CNS disease may have a fulminant course, and may be fatal within 1 month. Even when treated, the prognosis is uncertain. Many antibiotics have been used with variable success. The most commonly used agents have been tetracycline, penicillin, and trimethoprim-sulfamethoxazole (TMP-SMX). A treatment regimen that has been proposed is ceftriaxone (2 g, IV bid) for 14 to 30 days, followed by either TMP-SMX (160mg/800mg po bid) or cefixime (400 mg/day) for one year. Interferon-γ may play a role in the treatment of Whipple disease. Serial lumbar puncture may be used to monitor response to treatment. There are few data on the appropriate time to terminate antibiotic therapy, although at least 1-year duration is considered necessary, given the propensity for recurrence.

SUGGESTED READINGS

Anderson M. Neurology of Whipple's disease. *J Neurol Neurosurg Psychiatry* 2000;68:2–5.

Dobbins WO III, ed. *Whipple's Disease.* Springfield, IL: Charles C Thomas, 1987.

Dykman DD, Cuccherini BA, Fuss IJ, et al. Whipple's disease in a father-daughter pair. *Digest Dis Sci* 1999;44:2542–2544.

Galldiks N, Burghaus L, Vollmar S, et al. Novel neuroimaging findings in a patient with Cerebral Whipple's disease: a magnetic resonance imaging and positron emission tomography study. *J Neuroimaging* 2004 Oct;14(4):372–376.

Louis ED, Lynch T, Kaufmann P, Fahn S, Odel J. Diagnostic guidelines in central nervous system Whipple's disease. *Ann Neurol* 1996;40:561–568.

Maiwald M, Schuhmacher F, Ditton H-J, von Herbay A. Environmental occurrence of Whipple's disease bacterium (*Tropheryma whippelii*). *Appl Environ Microbiol* 1998;64:760–762.

Marth T, Neurath M, Cuccherini BA, Strober W. Defects in monocyte interleukin-12 production and humeral immunity in Whipple's disease. *Gastroenterology* 1997;113:442–448.

Ramzan NN, Loftus E, Burgart LJ, et al. Diagnosis and monitoring of Whipple's disease by polymerase chain reaction. *Ann Intern Med* 1997;126:520–527.

Raoult D, Birg ML, La Scola B, et al. Cultivation of the bacillus of Whipple's disease. *N Eng J Med* 2000;342:620–625.

Relman DA, Schmidt TM, MacDermott RP, Falkow S. Identification of the uncultured bacillus of Whipple's disease. *N Engl J Med* 1992;327:293–301.

Schnider PJ, Reisinger EC, Berger T, et al. Treatment guidelines in central nervous system Whipple's disease. *Ann Neurol* 1997;41:561–562.

Schneider T, Stallmach A, Von Herbay A, et al. Treatment of refractory Whipple's disease with interferon-γ. *Ann Intern Med* 1998;129:875–877.

Schoedon G, Goldenberger D, Forrer R, et al. Deactivation of macrophages with IL-4 is the key to the isolation of *Tropheryma whippelii.* *J Infect Dis* 1997;176:672–677.

von Herbay A, Otto HF, Stolte M, et al. Epidemiology of Whipple's disease in Germany. *Scand J Gastroenterol* 1997;32:52–57.

von Herbay A, Ditton HJ, Schumacher F, Maiwald M. Whipple's disease: staging and monitoring by cytology and polymerase chain reaction analysis of cerebrospinal fluid. *Gastroenterology* 1997;113:434–441.

Whipple GH. A hitherto undescribed disease characterized anatomically by deposits of fat and fatty acids in the intestinal and mesenteric lymphatic tissues. *Johns Hopkins Hosp Bull* 1907;18:382–391.

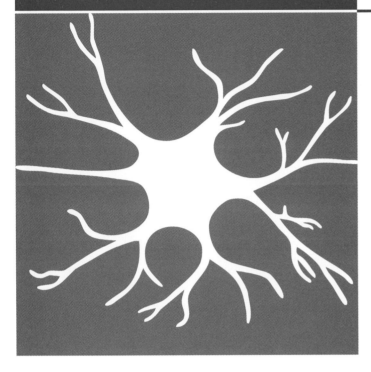

Vascular Diseases

Pathogenesis, Classification, and Epidemiology of Cerebrovascular Disease

Ralph L. Sacco

Stroke continues to be a major public health problem that ranks in the top four causes of death in most countries and is responsible for a large proportion of the burden of neurologic disorders. More often disabling than fatal, stroke is the leading cause of severe neurologic disability and results in enormous costs measured in both health-care dollars and lost productivity. Major strides have been made in understanding the epidemiology, etiology, and pathogenesis of cerebrovascular disease and have led to new approaches to diagnosis and treatment.

DEFINITION AND NOSOLOGY

In the broadest sense, the World Health Organization has defined stroke as "rapidly developing clinical signs of focal (at times global) disturbance of cerebral function, lasting more than 24 hours or leading to death with no apparent cause other than that of vascular origin." By conventional clinical definitions, if the neurologic symptoms continue for more than 24 hours, a person is diagnosed with stroke; otherwise, a focal neurologic deficit lasting less than 24 hours is defined as a transient ischemic attack (TIA). Such terms defined by the duration of neurologic symptoms are being redefined with the more widespread use of sensitive brain imaging, such as diffusion-weighted MRI. Patients with symptoms lasting less than 24 hours, but with an infarction imaged by MRI, have been reclassified as having a stroke instead of TIA. The most recent definition of stroke for clinical trials has required either symptoms lasting more than 24 hours or imaging of an acute clinically relevant brain lesion in patients with rapidly vanishing symptoms. The duration and severity of the syndrome then may be used to classify patients as those with minor or major stroke. The use of the term "brain attack," which may lack specificity, has been championed by the educational campaigns of national health organizations to help inform the public about the urgency of stroke. The proposed new definition of TIA is a "brief episode of neurologic dysfunction caused by a focal disturbance of brain or retinal ischemia, with clinical symptoms typically lasting less than one hour, and without evidence of infarction."

In addition to duration, stroke is classified by the pathology of the underlying focal brain injury, as being either an infarction or a hemorrhage. Intracranial hemorrhage may be subdivided into two distinct types, based on the site and vascular origin of the blood: subarachnoid, when the bleeding originates in the subarachnoid spaces surrounding the brain; and intracerebral, when the hemorrhage is into the substance or parenchyma of the brain. Ischemic infarction may be classified into various subgroups, based on the mechanism of the ischemia and the type and localization of the vascular lesion.

The cardinal feature of stroke is the sudden onset of neurologic symptoms. "Silent infarcts" may occur without apparent clinical manifestations, however, either because the patient and family are unaware of minor symptoms or a so-called "silent" area of brain has been affected. Premonitory stroke symptoms are not always found; fewer than 20% of stroke patients have a prior TIA. Focal premonitory symptoms, when present, usually predate infarction rather than hemorrhage. When they occur, they may be so nonspecific that they are not recognized as signs of an impending stroke. Within 90 days after a TIA, the risk of stroke has been reported to be as high as 10% to 20%, and nearly half of these patients will have their stroke in the first 1 day to 2 days after the TIA.

The neurologic symptoms often reflect the location and size of stroke, but they usually are not useful in differentiating the type of stroke. When headache, vomiting, seizures, or coma occur, hemorrhage is a more likely source than infarction. Specific neurologic symptoms that may occur in isolation or in various combinations include: loss of vision (hemianopia), double vision, weakness or sensory loss on one side of the body, dysarthria, alteration in higher cognitive functions (e.g., dysphasia, confusion, spatial disorientation, neglect, memory difficulties), difficulty walking, headache, or unilateral deafness. Part of the challenge is to differentiate precisely the affected anatomic region and the corresponding vascular territory, based on the clinical symptoms and signs. This step is reviewed in Chapter 38 in connection with the syndromes of specific cerebral arteries. A prerequisite, however, is a sound understanding of the anatomy of the vascular supply of the brain.

VASCULAR ANATOMY

The brain is perfused by the carotid and vertebral arteries, which begin as extracranial arteries leading from the aorta or other great vessels and course through the neck and base of the skull to reach the intracranial cavity (Fig. 36.1). The carotid and its branches are referred to as the anterior circulation and the vertebrobasilar as the posterior circulation.

The right common carotid originates from the bifurcation of the innominate, whereas the left originates directly from the aortic arch. The internal carotid arteries stem from the common carotid, usually at the level of the upper border of the thyroid cartilage, at the fourth cervical vertebrae; they give no branches in the neck and face, and enter the cranium through the carotid canal. The four main segments of the internal carotid are cervical, petrous, cavernous, and supraclinoid. The siphon is the term used to describe the series of turns made by the cavernous and supraclinoid segments. The internal carotid ends by dividing into the middle and anterior cerebral arteries, after giving off the ophthalmic, superior hypophyseal, posterior communicating, and anterior choroidal arteries. The carotid system therefore supplies the optic nerves and retina, plus the anterior portion of the cerebral hemisphere, which comprises the frontal, parietal, and anterior temporal lobes. In as many as 15% of adults, the posterior cerebral artery also arises directly from the internal carotid artery, so that the entire cerebral hemisphere (including the occipital lobe) is supplied by the

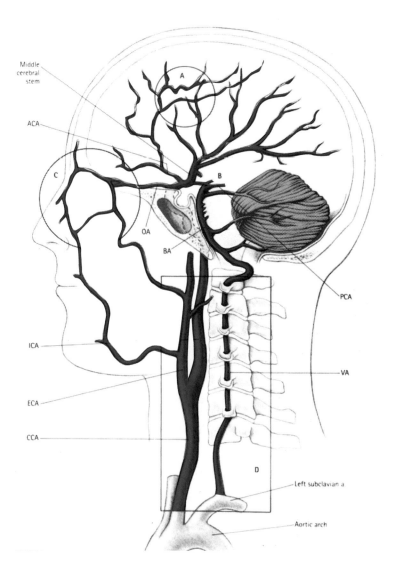

FIGURE 36.1. Arterial supply to the brain with enlarged detail of the sites of anastomosis in the cerebral circulation. A: Over the convexity, subarachnoid interarterial anastomoses link the middle (MCA), anterior (ACA), and posterior cerebral arteries (PCA) through the border zone. **B:** The circle of Willis provides communication between the anterior and posterior cerebral circulation via the anterior and posterior communicating arteries. **C:** Through the orbit, anastomoses occur between the external (ECA) and internal carotid arteries (ICA). **D:** Extracranial anastomoses connect the muscular branches of the cervical arteries to the vertebral arteries (VAs) and the ECAs. OA, ophthalmic artery; BA, basilar artery; CCA, common carotid artery.

internal carotid artery. The anterior choroidal artery supplies a number of structures in addition to the choroids plexus including: the inferior portion of the posterior limb of the internal capsule; the hippocampus; and portions of the globus pallidus, posterior putamen, the lateral geniculate, amygdala, and ventrolateral thalamus.

The middle cerebral artery is the largest branch of the internal carotid artery and appears almost as a direct continuation. It begins as a single trunk (stem or M1 segment) passing laterally to the sylvian fissure, where it becomes the M2 or insular segment, from which the 12 cerebral surface branches originate. The stem usually ends in either a bifurcation into the upper and lower division, or a trifurcation into three major trunks (upper, middle, and lower divisions). The cortical divisions supply almost the entire cortical surface of the brain, including insula, operculum, as well as the frontal, parietal, temporal, and occipital cortices; the frontal pole, the superior and extreme posterior rim of the convex surface, and medial cortical surfaces are not supplied by the middle cerebral artery.

The middle cerebral artery stem gives rise to the medial and lateral lenticulostriates, which supply the extreme capsule, claustrum, putamen, most of the globus pallidus, part of the head, and the entire body of the caudate, as well as the superior portions of the anterior and posterior limbs of the internal capsule. The upper division usually gives rise to the lateral orbitofrontal, ascending frontal, precentral (prerolandic), central (rolandic), and anterior parietal branches, whereas the lower division usually comprises the temporal polar, temporooccipital, anterior, middle, and posterior temporal branches. The posterior parietal and angular branches are more variable with respect to their origin from the MCA.

The anterior cerebral artery begins as a medial branch of the internal carotid artery, forming the proximal or A1 segment to the junction of the anterior communicating artery, where it continues as the distal or A2 segment. The largest branch is known as the recurrent artery of Heubner, and several cortical branches supply the medial and orbital surfaces of the frontal lobe.

The vertebral artery usually arises from the subclavian artery, courses through the transverse foramina, pierces the dura, and enters the cranial cavity to join the contralateral vertebral artery. The anterior and posterior spinal arteries and posterior inferior cerebellar artery, which supplies the inferior surface of the cerebellum, arise from the distal segments of the vertebrals. The lateral medulla, site of the focal injury in the Wallenberg syndrome, is supplied by the multiple, perforating branches of the posterior-inferior cerebellar artery or the direct medullary branches of the vertebral artery.

The basilar artery originates as the merger of the right and left vertebral arteries, usually at the level of the pontomedullary junction (Fig. 36.2).

Paramedian penetrators (i.e., short and long lateral circumferential penetrators), originate from the basilar

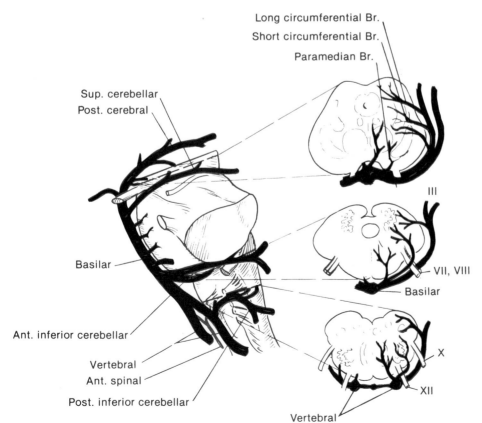

FIGURE 36.2. Vascular supply of the brainstem.

artery to supply the brainstem. The anterior inferior cerebellar and superior cerebellar arteries perfuse the ventrolateral aspect of the cerebellar cortex, and the internal auditory (labyrinthine) artery arises either directly from the basilar, or from the anterior cerebellar artery to supply the cochlea, labyrinth, and part of the facial nerve.

The basilar artery usually terminates into the right and left posterior cerebral arteries. A series of penetrators (i.e., posteromedial, thalamoperforates, thalamogeniculate, tuberothalamic) arises from the posterior communicating and posterior cerebral artery to supply the hypothalamus, dorsolateral midbrain, lateral geniculate, and thalamus. The posterior cerebral artery supplies the inferior surface of the temporal lobe, and medial and inferior surfaces of the occipital lobe, including the lingual and fusiform gyri.

A rich anastomotic network includes various extracranial intercommunicating systems, intracranial connections through the circle of Willis, and distal intracranial connections through meningeal anastomoses that traverse throughout the border zones, over the cortical and cerebellar surfaces. These networks protect the brain by providing alternate routes to circumvent obstructions in the main arteries. Obstruction of the extracranial internal carotid may remain asymptomatic if there is adequate perfusion made available through a variety of collateral pathways, including: the external carotid to the ophthalmic to the intracranial internal carotid, the contralateral carotid to the anterior cerebral artery and across the circle of Willis through the anterior communicating artery, the vertebrobasilar to the posterior cerebral artery and anterior through the posterior communicating artery, and distal interconnections between the distal middle cerebral artery and to branches of the posterior and anterior cerebral arteries. The small arteries and arterioles (100 μm or less in diameter) that arise from the surface arteries and penetrate the brain parenchyma function as end arteries with few interconnections.

PHYSIOLOGY

The adult brain, which weighs about 1500 g or 2% of the total body weight, requires an uninterrupted supply of about 150 g of glucose and 72 L of oxygen every 24 hours, accounting for 20% of the total body oxygen consumption. As the brain does not store these substances, dysfunction results after only a few minutes of deprivation when either the oxygen or the glucose content is reduced below critical levels. In the resting state, each cardiac contraction delivers about 70 mL of blood into the ascending aorta; 10 to 15 mL are allocated to the brain. Every minute, about 350 mL flows through each internal carotid artery, and 100 to 200 mL through the vertebrobasilar system, to provide a normal total cerebral blood flow of 50 mL/min per 100 g.

To ensure constant perfusion pressure and blood flow to the brain over a range of systemic blood pressures (cerebral autoregulation), the major cerebral arteries have a well developed muscular coat that allows constriction in response to increased blood pressure, and dilation with hypotension. The arterioles are exquisitely sensitive to changes in peripheral artery carbon dioxide ($PaCO_2$) and peripheral artery oxygen (PaO_2). When the partial pressure of CO_2 increases, the arterioles dilate and cerebral blood flow increases. When CO_2 tension is reduced such as after hyperventilation, the arterioles constrict and blood flow is reduced. Changes in the partial pressure of O_2 have the opposite effect. In normal subjects, cerebral autoregulation allows for a constant cerebral blood flow over a range of mean arterial pressures of 60 to 140 mm Hg. Focal cerebral activity, such as occurs when moving a limb, is accompanied by accelerated metabolism in the appropriate region, and is accommodated by increases in local blood flow and oxygen delivery. In patients with cerebrovascular disease, this compensatory mechanism may be destroyed.

PATHOGENESIS AND CLASSIFICATION

Brain Infarction

Brain or neuronal dysfunction occurs at cerebral blood flow levels of below 50 mg/dL, and irreversible neuronal injury is initiated at levels below 30 mg/dL. Both the degree and duration of reductions in cerebral blood flow are related to the likelihood of sustained neuronal injury. When blood supply is completely interrupted for 30 seconds, brain metabolism is altered. After 1 minute, neuronal function may cease. After 5 minutes of interruption, anoxia initiates a chain of events that may result in cerebral infarction; however, if oxygenated blood flow is restored quickly enough, the damage may be reversible, as with a TIA.

The following steps occur in the evolution of an infarct: (1) local vasodilatation and (2) stasis of the blood column, with segmentation of the red cells, are followed by (3) edema and (4) necrosis of brain tissue. The earliest ischemic changes are visualized by increased water content in diffusion-weighted MRI while with time, an infarct is well delineated by fluid-attenuated inversion recovery (FLAIR) and T2-weighted changes on MRI. (Fig. 36.4).

Exciting research into the cellular consequences of ischemia has led to the elucidation of the ischemic cascade. A chain of events at the neuronal level leads to cellular dysfunction and death starting with the failure of the sodium/potassium (Na/K) pump, the depolarization of the neuronal membrane, the release of excitatory neurotransmitters, and the opening of calcium channels. The influx of calcium is at the root of further neuronal injury, with damage to organelles and further destabilization of neuronal metabolism and normal function resulting. Calcium may enter the neuron through various voltage-sensitive and receptor-mediated channels (i.e., the N-methyl-d-aspartate

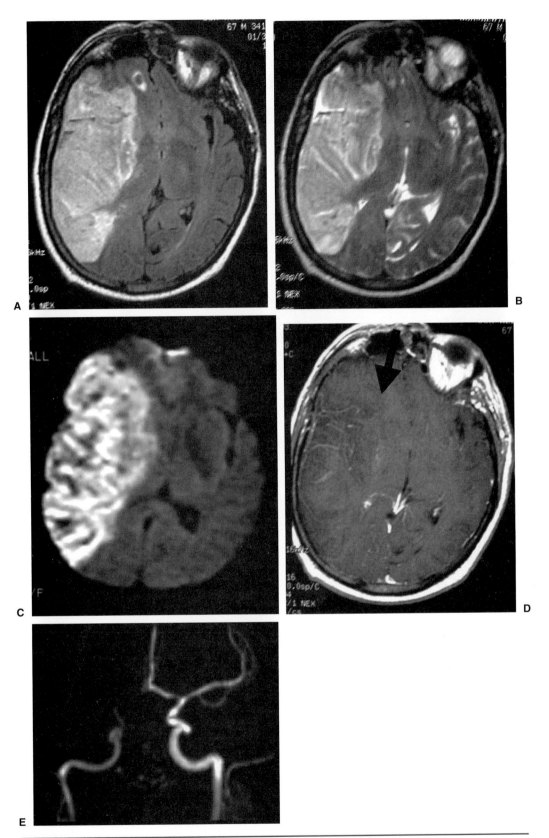

FIGURE 36.3. Acute cortical infarction. A and **B:** Proton-density and T2-weighted axial magnetic resonance scans show increased signal intensity within the medial cortex of left frontal and parietal lobes. Note the swelling of gray matter and prominence of blood vessels within this lesion. **C** and **D:** T1-weighted axial magnetic resonance scans, before and after gadolinium administration, demonstrate several linear foci of contrast enhancement within the area of infarction in the left frontal and parietal lobes, most consistent with enhancing arterial branches. Contrast enhancement of arterial branches is consistent with static blood flow within the infarct and generally is seen only within the first few hours to 5 days after the onset of acute infarction. **E:** MRA demonstrates occlusion of the distal ICA with non-visualization of the MCA and ACA. (Courtesy of Dr. S. Chan.)

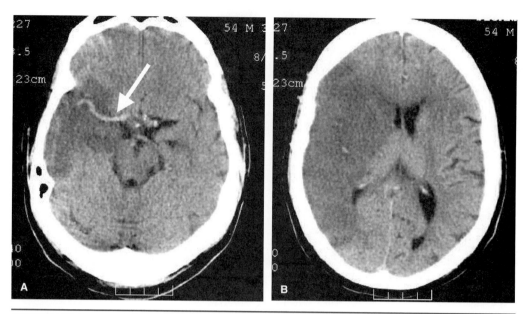

FIGURE 36.4. Acute infarct, right middle cerebral artery distribution. Noncontrast axial CT shows right frontal and temporal hypodensity, including cortex, and edema producing ventricular effacement and midline shift. Right anterior and posterior cerebral artery territories are spared. Similar appearance could result from occlusion of right internal carotid artery with competent circle of Willis. Arrow demonstrates R MCA density consistent with an acute occlusion. (Courtesy of Drs. J. A. Bello and S. K. Hilal.)

receptor). Excitatory neurotransmitters such as glutamate and glycine may lead to the further influx of calcium through these channels. These events may lead to delayed neuronal death and are the main target of various neuroprotective strategies. The ischemic penumbra has been defined as the region of the brain surrounding the core of an infarct, in which neuronal function is deranged but potentially salvageable. A diffusion-perfusion mismatch defined by MRI has been cited as a possible measure of the ischemic penumbra and a potential marker of patients likely to benefit from reperfusion strategies.

Persistently reduced perfusion and the consequences of the ischemic cascade may lead to extension of the core of the infarct to encompass the ischemic penumbra. If the interruption in blood flow is sufficiently prolonged and infarction results, the brain tissue first softens and then liquefies; a cavity finally forms when the debris is removed by the phagocytic microglia. In attempts to fill the defect, astroglia in the surrounding brain proliferate and invade the softened area, and new capillaries are formed.

Although most infarcts are bland, occasionally a hemorrhagic infarct is caused by local hemorrhage into the necrotic tissue, which may be petechial or confluent. Hemorrhagic infarct may occur when the occluding clot or embolus breaks up and migrates, thereby restoring flow through the infarcted area. More widespread use of MRI has shown that petechial hemorrhagic infarction is more frequent than originally suspected, and is related to the size of the infarct and the elevation of blood pressure.

Infarction may be confined to a single, vascular territory when the occlusion involves a small penetrant end-artery or distal intracranial branch. If the occlusion is more proximal in the arterial tree, ischemia may be more widespread and may involve more than one vascular territory or border zone; ischemia may result with limited infarction in the distal fields of the vascular supply. Intracranial proximal occlusions may result in both penetrant-artery ischemia and coexisting surface-branch territory infarction (Fig. 36.3).

Multiple mechanisms may lead to brain ischemia. Hemodynamic infarction originates as a result of an impediment to normal perfusion that usually is caused by a severe arterial stenosis or occlusion arising from atherosclerosis and coexisting thrombosis. Embolism occurs when a particle of thrombus originating from a more proximal source (e.g., arterial, cardiac, or transcardiac) travels through the vascular system and leads to an arterial occlusion. Small-vessel disease occurs when lipohyalinosis or local atherosclerotic disease leads to an occlusion of a penetrant artery. Less frequent conditions that lead to reductions in cerebral perfusion and result in infarction include: arterial dissection, primary or secondary vasculitis (e.g., meningitis caused by tuberculosis or syphilis), hypercoagulable states, vasospasm, systemic hypotension, hyperviscosity (e.g., polycythemia, dysproteinemia, or thrombocytosis), moyamoya disease, fibromuscular dysplasia, extrinsic compression of the major arteries by tumor, and occlusion of the veins that drain the

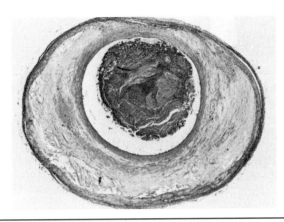

FIGURE 36.5. Carotid artery in cross-section. Note atherosclerotic changes and intraluminal thrombus.

brain. The four most frequent subtypes of cerebral infarction are large-vessel atherosclerotic, cardioembolic, small vessel (lacunar), and cryptogenic.

Large-vessel Atherosclerotic Infarction

Atherosclerotic plaque at a bifurcation or curve in one of the larger vessels leads to progressive stenosis, with the final large-artery occlusion caused by thrombosis of the narrowed lumen (Fig. 36.5).

Arteriosclerotic plaques may develop at any point along the carotid artery and the vertebrobasilar system, but the most common sites are the bifurcation of the common carotid artery into the external and internal carotid arteries, the origins of the middle and anterior cerebral arteries, and the origins of the vertebral from the subclavian arteries.

Ischemia is attributed to perfusion failure distal to the site of severe stenosis or occlusion of the major vessel. The site of infarction depends on the collateral flow but is usually in the distal fields or border zones. Specifying the degree of stenosis that will lead to perfusion difficulty depends on multiple factors and often is not defined easily. Classification schemes have relied on stenosis greater than 70% to 80% as being more reliably predictive of impending hemodynamic compromise. (Table 36.1)

An atherosclerotic stenosis or occlusion may also lead to a cerebral infarction through an embolic mechanism. In this case, emboli arising from the proximally situated atheromatous lesions occlude otherwise healthy branches located more distally in the arterial tree (Fig. 36.6).

Embolic fragments may arise from extracranial arteries affected by stenosis or ulcer, stenosis of any major cerebral artery stem, the stump of the occluded internal carotid artery, and even from intracranial tail of the anterograde thrombus atop an occluded carotid. The constituents of the offending embolism have earned the labels of "red" (thrombus) and "white" (platelet) clots, but it is nearly impossible to discriminate these based on clinical findings.

▶ **TABLE 36.1 Frequency of Extracranial Duplex Doppler and Transcranial Doppler Findings Among 105 Patients with Large Artery Atherosclerotic Infarction (Extracranial or Intracranial) Within the Northern Manhattan Stroke Study**

Finding	Left n (%)	Right n (%)
Extracranial internal carotid artery*		
Normal	17 (18%)	30 (32%)
Plaque and <40% stenosis	50 (53%)	37 (39%)
40%–79% stenosis	9 (10%)	7 (7%)
>80% stenosis	7 (7%)	7 (7%)
Occlusion	12 (13%)	13 (14%)
Extracranial vertebral artery**		
Normal	77 (85%)	80 (90%)
Proximal occlusion	10 (11%)	3 (3%)
Distal occlusion	4 (4%)	5 (6%)
Middle cerebral artery* **		
Normal	37 (50%)	35 (47%)
Accelerated velocities	19 (26%)	15 (21%)
Reduced velocities	8 (11%)	9 (12%)
Unable to insonnate	10 (14%)	15 (20%)

*Results not available for 10 L carotids and 11 R carotids.
**Results not available for 14 L vertebral and 16 R vertebrals
*** Results not available for 31 L MCAs and 31 R MCAs.

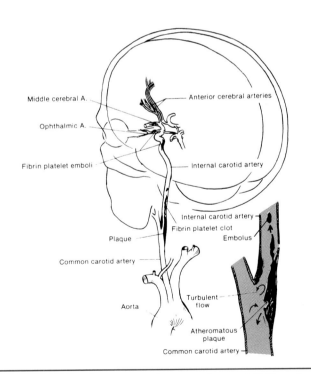

FIGURE 36.6. Atheromatous plaques at the carotid bifurcation may be a source of retinal and cerebral emboli.

Cardiac Embolism

Many strokes caused by embolism originate from a cardiac source of thrombus. A small particle of thrombus breaks off from the source and is carried through the bloodstream until it lodges in an artery too small to allow it to pass, usually a distal intracranial branch. In addition to thrombus, other types of particles that may embolize include: neoplasm, fat, air, or other foreign substances. Air emboli usually follow injuries or surgical procedures involving the lungs, the dural sinuses, or jugular veins. They also may be caused by the release of nitrogen bubbles into the general circulation after a rapid reduction in barometric pressure. Fat embolism is rare and almost always arises from a bone fracture. Most emboli are sterile, but some may contain bacteria if emboli arise, secondarily, from subacute or acute bacterial endocarditis. The most common sources of cardiac embolism include: valvular heart disease (e.g., mitral stenosis, mitral regurgitation, rheumatic heart disease); intracardiac thrombus, particularly along the left ventricular wall (mural thrombus) after anterior myocardial infarction, or in the left atrial appendage in patients with atrial fibrillation; ventricular or septal aneurysm; and cardiomyopathies leading to stagnation of blood flow and an increased propensity for the formation of intracardiac thrombus. A paradoxic embolus occurs when a thrombus crosses from the venous circulation to the left side of the heart, most often through a patent foramen ovale. Other possible causes of cerebral embolism are atrial myxoma, marantic endocarditis, and severe prolapse of the mitral valve.

Embolism is inferred when the brain image demonstrates an infarction confined to the cerebral-surface territory of a single branch, combinations of infarcts involving branches of different divisions of major cerebral arteries, or hemorrhagic infarction. The presenting syndrome usually reflects hemispheral dysfunction and a cortical rather than subcortical vascular territory (Table 36.2).

The difficult problem in arriving at a diagnosis of embolism is identifying the occluding particle and the source. Mural thrombi and platelet aggregates are remarkably evanescent, as has been inferred by findings on angiography. Embolic fragments are found in more than 75% of patients who undergo angiography within 48 hours of onset of the stroke, and are then gone when angiogram is repeated later. Embolism is demonstrated in only 11% of clinically similar cases, when angiogram is delayed beyond 48 hours from clinical onset of the stroke.

Persistence of embolic occlusion is the exception rather than the rule. Embolic obstruction of an arterial lumen is cleared most commonly by recanalization and fibrinolysis. During this process, the lumen may appear stenotic. The evanescent quality of emboli may explain the wide variation in the frequency with which this subtype is diagnosed in retrospective or prospective studies of stroke.

▶ **TABLE 36.2** **Primary Brain Site, Vascular Territory, and Syndrome Among 143 Cases of Cardiac Embolism Within the Northern Manhattan Stroke Study**

Characteristic	*N*	*Percent*
Site of infarction		
Cortical (Frontal, Parietal, Temporal, Occipital or combinations)	92	64%
Subcortical (Internal capsule, Corona Radiata, Basal Ganglia)	19	14%
Brainstem or Cerebellum	24	17%
Undetermined	8	5%
Vascular territory		
Middle Cerebral Artery	41	29%
Middle Cerebral Artery Branch	36	25%
Middle Cerebral Artery Stem	24	17%
Posterior Cerebral Artery	13	9%
Vertebrobasilar Arteries	20	14%
Undetermined	9	6%
Presenting syndrome		
Large Dominant	31	22%
Large Nondominant	39	27%
Small Hemispheral	19	13%
Posterior Cerebral	9	6%
Lacunar syndrome	24	17%
Brainstem or Cerebellar	18	13%
Undetermined	3	2%

More recently, the improved sensitivities of cerebral and cardiac imaging have led to better detection of sources of thrombi.

Small-Vessel Lacunar Infarction

These strokes have distinctive clinical syndromes, with a small zone of ischemia confined to the territory of a single vessel. They are understood to reflect arterial disease of the vessels penetrating the brain that supply the internal capsule, basal ganglia, thalamus, corona radiata, and paramedian regions of the brainstem (Fig. 36.7).

Disagreements abound about the pathogenesis of lacunar infarcts; some authors favor the use of the term lacune to describe size and location, without indicating a specific pathology. The pathologies of only a handful of such infarcts have been studied by serial section, and only a few of those studies have documented a tiny focus of microatheroma or lipohyalinosis stenosing one of the deep penetrating arteries. The arterial damage is usually the result of long-standing hypertension or diabetes mellitus. Rare causes include stenosis of the middle cerebral artery stem or microembolization to penetrant arterial territories. As defined radiologically, most small, deep infarcts do not have significant large-artery atherosclerosis, lack

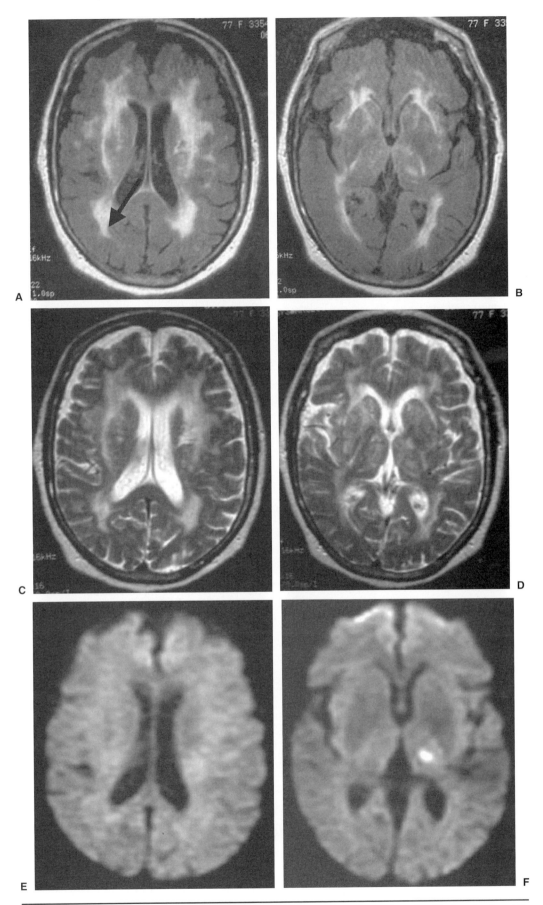

FIGURE 36.7. Axial MRI sequences demonstrating evidence of small vessel cerebral ischemia. **A** and **B:** FLAIR sequence showing bilateral periventricular white matter disease (arrow). **C** and **D:** T$_2$ sequence showing white matter disease and multiple lacunar infarctions. **E** and **F:** DWI sequence showing an acute L thalamic lacunar infarct.

▶ **TABLE 36.3** Primary Presenting Syndrome and Vascular Territory Among 172 Lacunar Infarcts in the Northern Manhattan Stroke Study

Characteristic	N	Percent
Presenting Syndrome		
Pure Motor Hemiparesis	67	39%
Sensorimotor Syndrome	42	24%
Ataxic Hemiparesis	27	16%
Pure Sensory Syndrome	14	8%
Brainstem Syndrome	10	6%
Lacunar, other	9	5%
Undetermined	3	2%
Vascular Territory		
Middle Cerebral Artery penetrant	85	49%
Posterior Cerebral Artery penetrant	31	18%
Vertebral or Basilar penetrant	39	23%
Undetermined	17	10%

even a potential cardiac source of embolism, and occur in vascular territories less likely to be occluded by emboli.

Many lacunar strokes are diagnosed by clinical characteristics alone. Clinical syndromes include pure motor hemiparesis, pure sensory syndrome, clumsy hand dysarthria, ataxic hemiparesis, and sensorimotor syndrome (Table 36.3).

When brain imaging is positive, it usually means that a strategically placed, small deep infarct is found. As the vascular lesion lies within vessels some 200 to 400 micrometers in diameter, cerebral angiography understandably may have normal findings. Incidental large vessel disease may be found in some angiographic series, but whether or not it is etiologically related to the site of infarction is often unclear.

Cryptogenic Infarction

Despite efforts to arrive at a diagnosis, the cause of infarction in a discouragingly large number of cases, remains undetermined. Some cases may be unexplained because appropriate laboratory studies are not performed, whereas others remain undetermined as a result of improper timing for the appropriate laboratory studies. The most frequent circumstances, however, are when normal or ambiguous findings are reached despite appropriate laboratory studies performed at the appropriate time.

Results from hospital- and community-based stroke studies indicated (1) that large artery atherosclerotic occlusive disease was a less frequent cause of stroke, (2) that small vessel or lacunar and cardioembolic infarction were relatively frequent, and (3) that the cause for most cases of infarction could not be easily classified

into these traditional diagnostic categories. This conclusion forced the creation of a separate diagnostic category name for cases whose mechanisms of infarction remained unproven, known as "infarct of undetermined cause" or "cryptogenic infarction."

Cases categorized as cryptogenic infarction have no bruit or TIA ipsilateral to the hemisphere affected by stroke, no obvious history suggestive of a definite cardiac embolism, and usually do not present with a lacunar syndrome. Brain imaging usually shows an infarct limited to a surface-branch territory, or may show a large zone of infarction affecting regions larger than that accounted for by a single penetrant-arterial territory. Noninvasive vascular imaging fails to demonstrate an underlying large vessel occlusion or stenosis. No definite cardiac source of embolism is uncovered by echocardiography, electrocardiography, or Holter monitor. If an angiogram is performed, the study results may be normal, may show a distal branch occlusion, or may show occlusion of a major cerebral artery stem or of the top of the basilar artery. As these latter occlusions may arise from embolus or thrombosis of an atherosclerotic vessel, their demonstration does not answer the question of source mechanism.

Many of these patients have a hemisphere syndrome, a surface infarction revealed by CT or MRI, and a corresponding branch occlusion documented by angiography or normal angiogram. This constellation of findings has been considered suggestive of embolism. Ample evidence exists for many occult sources of emboli; the difficulty is in proving their existences and their roles in the first or succeeding ischemic strokes. Emerging technologies have led to the suggestion that some cryptogenic infarcts may be explained by hematologic disorders causing hypercoagulable states (e.g., antiphospholipid antibody abnormalities). Others have implicated paradoxic emboli through a patent foramen ovale and an aortic arch atherosclerosis. Rather than reclassifying these cases into that of an embolism as the inferred mechanism, such cases should be labeled as cryptogenic until the mechanism, source, and determinants of these unexplained infarcts are clarified.

Intracranial Hemorrhage

Intracranial hemorrhage results from the rupture of a vessel anywhere within the cranial cavity. Intracranial hemorrhages are classified according to location (e.g., extradural, subdural, subarachnoid, intracerebral, intraventricular), according to the nature of the ruptured vessel or vessels (e.g., arterial, capillary, venous), or according to cause (e.g., primary, secondary). Trauma is often involved in the generation of extradural hematoma from laceration of the middle meningeal artery or vein, and subdural hematomas from traumatic rupture of veins that traverse the subdural space.

Intracerebral Hemorrhage

Intracerebral hemorrhage is characterized by bleeding into the substance of the brain, usually originating from a small penetrating artery. Hypertension has been implicated as the cause of weakening in the walls of arterioles and the formation of microaneurysms (Charcot-Brouchard). Among elderly, nonhypertensive patients with recurrent lobar hemorrhages, amyloid angiopathy has been implicated as an important cause. Other causes include arteriovenous malformations, aneurysms, moya-moya disease, bleeding disorders or anticoagulation, trauma, tumors, cavernous angiomas, and illicit-drug abuse. In blood dyscrasias (e.g., acute leukemia, aplastic anemia, polycythemia, thrombocytopenic purpura, scurvy), the hemorrhages may be multiple and of varied size.

The arterial blood ruptures under pressure and destroys or displaces brain tissue. If the hemorrhage is large, the ruptured vessel is often impossible to find at autopsy. The most common sites for arterial hemorrhage are the putamen, caudate, pons, cerebellum, thalamus, or deep white matter. Basal ganglia hemorrhages often extend to involve the internal capsule and sometimes rupture into the lateral ventricle, spreading through the ventricular system into the subarachnoid space (Fig. 36.8).

Intraventricular extension increases the likelihood of a fatal outcome. Bleeding into one lobe of the cerebral hemisphere or cerebellum usually remains confined within brain parenchyma. An inferior cerebellar hemorrhage is a neurologic emergency that needs to be diagnosed promptly, because early surgical evacuation of those hemorrhages of greater than 3 centimeters in diameter may prevent tonsillar herniation and apnea.

If the patient survives an intracerebral hemorrhage, blood and necrotic brain tissue are removed by phagocytes. The destroyed brain tissue is partially replaced by connective tissue, glia, and newly formed blood vessels, thus leaving a shrunken fluid-filled cavity. Less frequently, the blood clot is treated as a foreign body, calcifies, and is surrounded by a thick glial membrane.

Clinical Manifestations

The clinical picture is dictated by the location and size of the hematoma. It is characterized by headache, vomiting, and the evolution of focal motor or sensory signs over a period of minutes to hours. Among the moderate and large hematomas, consciousness is sometimes impaired at the start, and often becomes a prominent feature in the first 24 to 48 hours. Patients with intracerebral hemorrhage are often younger than stereotypic stroke patients, and in some series the condition was seen more frequently in men. The diagnosis and localization are established easily with CT, which shows the high density of acute blood.

Subarachnoid Hemorrhage

Subarachnoid hemorrhage occurs when the blood is localized to the surrounding membranes and cerebrospinal fluid. It is most frequently caused by leakage of blood from a cerebral aneurysm. The combination of congenital and acquired factors leads to a degeneration of the arterial wall and the release of blood, under arterial pressures, into the subarachnoid space and cerebrospinal fluid. Aneurysms may be distributed at different sites throughout the base of the brain, particularly at the origin or bifurcations of arteries at the circle of Willis. Other secondary causes that may lead to subarachnoid hemorrhage include arteriovenous malformations, bleeding disorders or anticoagulation, trauma, amyloid angiopathy, or central sinus thrombosis. Signs and symptoms include the abrupt onset of severe headache (a.k.a. "the worst headache of my life"), vomiting, altered consciousness, and sometimes coma; these characteristics often occur in the absence of focal localizing signs.

Subarachnoid hemorrhage affects younger patients than is typical for stroke, and is seen in women more often than in men. Hypertension, oral contraceptive use, and cigarette smoking are some of the known factors associated with this type of stroke. Fatalities are high, ranging from 30% to 70%, and depend on the severity of the initial presentation. Among those who survive, early rebleeding and delayed ischemic neurologic deficits from vasospasm may cause serious morbidity.

Frequency of Stroke Subtypes

Overall, ischemic stroke is 3 to four 4 times as frequent as hemorrhagic stroke, accounting for 70% to 80% of all strokes. Intracerebral hemorrhage usually accounts for 10% to 30% of the cases, depending on the geographic origin of the patients, with greater relative frequencies reported in Chinese and Japanese series. Frequency of subarachnoid hemorrhage is usually one-third to one-half that of intracerebral hemorrhage. Frequency of infarct subtypes depend on the sample from which cases are drawn (hospital- or population-based), the geographic region of the study, and the design of investigator-driven diagnostic algorithms. Cardioembolism as the source occurs in 15% to 30% of the cases, large vessel atherosclerotic infarction varies from 14% to 40%, and small-vessel lacunar infarcts account for 15% to 30%. Stroke from other determined causes, such as arteritis or dissection, usually accounts for a small percentage (less than 5%) of the cases. Infarcts of undetermined cause may account for as many as 40% of ischemic infarcts (Fig. 36.9).

Clinical features observed at stroke onset may help to distinguish cerebral infarction subtypes but are not reliable enough to lead to a definite determination of infarct subtype without confirmatory laboratory data.

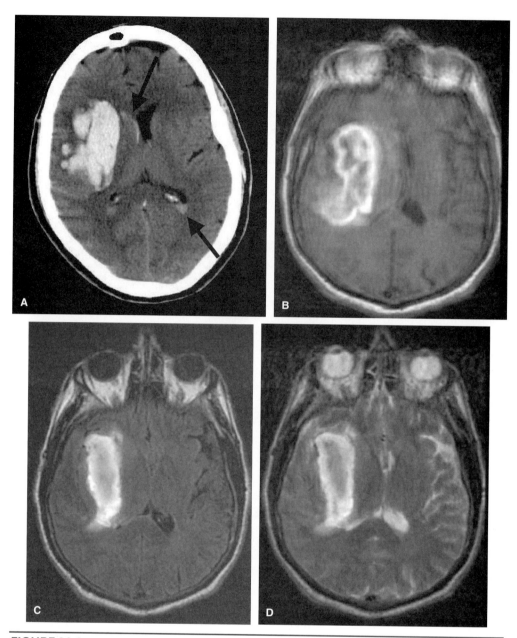

FIGURE 36.8. Large R basal ganglia intracerebral hemorrhage. **A:** CT shows blood in R basal ganglia and blood in the ventricles (arrows). **B:** ? gradient-echo sequence more sensitive for hemorrhage. **C:** T_1 MRI sequence showing increased signal consistent with acute blood. **D:** T_2 MRI sequence showing increased signal consistent with hemorrhage.

STROKE EPIDEMIOLOGY

Incidence, Prevalence, and Mortality

The magnitude of stroke impact is measured in public health terms by stroke-specific incidence, prevalence, and mortality. Stroke incidence is determined by the number of first cases of stroke, over a defined time interval in a defined population, whereas stroke prevalence measures the total number of cases (new and old), at a particular time also in a defined population. Both indices depend on the accurate and complete enumeration of cases and adequate knowledge of the underlying population at risk. Stroke incidence may be viewed as the sum of hospitalized, sudden fatal, and nonhospitalized stroke. The American Heart Association estimates that in the United States, there are almost 4.7 million stroke survivors (prevalence) and approximately 700,000 new or recurrent strokes occur per year. Overall, age-adjusted incidence rates range between 100 and 300 cases per 100,000 population per year,

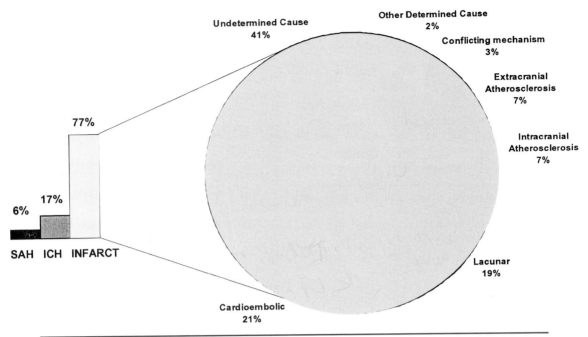

FIGURE 36.9. Frequency of stroke and first-choice infarct subtypes in the Northern Manhattan Stroke Study, 1993–1997.

and depend on the study methodology, country of origin, and population demographics. The age-adjusted stroke incidence rates (per 100,000) are 167 for white men and 138 for white women, while black patients have nearly twice the risk, with incidence rates (per 100,000) at 323 for men and 260 for women.

Mortality data are readily available but may underestimate the magnitude of stroke because not all patients with stroke die. Overall, stroke accounts for about 10% of all deaths in most industrialized countries, and most of these deaths are among persons over the age of 65. Stroke-related death rates are greatest in Japan and China. In the United States, at least 167,800 annual stroke-related deaths are recorded, with the average age-adjusted stroke mortality at 50 to 100 deaths per 100,000 population per year.

Stroke mortality in the US has been decreasing since the early 1900s. The rate of decline was constant 1% per year until 1969, when it accelerated to nearly 5% per year. From 1990 to 2000, although the stroke death rate fell 12.3%, the actual number of stroke deaths, given the aging of our population, rose 9.9%. The greatest declines in stroke death rates have been in the older age groups. The reasons for this mortality trend remain a subject of controversy. Epidemiologic data support various possibilities, including declining stroke incidence, improved survival, reduction in the severity of stroke, changing diagnostic criteria, and better stroke risk-factor control. Convincing evidence from National Hospital Discharge Surveys is accumulating in favor of improved survival rather than of declining incidence, as the explanation for the drop in stroke mortality. Recent

statistics have suggested that the decline in stroke mortality has ceased (reached a plateau).

Determinants of Stroke

Nonmodifiable Risk Factors

Although cerebrovascular disorders may occur at any age, at any time, in either sex, in all families, and in all races, each of these nonmodifiable factors affects the incidence of stroke. The strongest determinant of stroke is age. Although stroke is less common before the age of 40 years, stroke in young adults is of growing concern because of the impact of early disability. As our population ages, the prevalence and public health impact of stroke will undoubtedly increase.

Stroke incidence is greater among men, among those with a family history of stroke, and among certain race-ethnic groups (Fig. 36.10). In a hospital- and community-based cohort study of all cases of first stroke in northern Manhattan, black patients had an overall age-adjusted annual stroke incidence rate 2.4 times that of white patients; Hispanic patients, predominately from the Dominican Republic, had an incidence rate 1.6 times that of white patients.

In Japan, stroke is the leading cause of death in adults, and hemorrhagic stroke is more common than atherothrombosis. The predilection of atherosclerosis for the extracranial or intracranial circulation differs by race-ethnic group. Extracranial lesions are seen more frequently in white patients, whereas intracranial lesions are

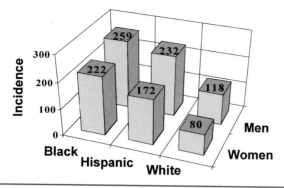

FIGURE 36.10. Average age-adjusted incidence rates of stroke (per 100,000 population) among persons aged 20 years in northern Manhattan, as occur in white, black, and Hispanic women. (Adapted from Sacco RL, Boden-Abdalla B, Gan R, et al., 1998.)

more common in black patients, Hispanic patients, and Asian patients. The reasons for these differences have yet to be explained adequately.

Modifiable Risk Factors

Nothing is accidental about stroke, even though it is implied by the misnomer of cerebral vascular accident (CVA). Instead, stroke is usually the result of predisposing conditions that originated years before the ictus. Epidemiologic investigations, such as prospective cohort and case-control studies, are continuing to identify numerous stroke risk factors. Current modifiable components of the stroke-prone profile include hypertension, cardiac disease (particularly atrial fibrillation), diabetes, hypercholesterolemia, physical inactivity, cigarette use, alcohol abuse, asymptomatic carotid stenosis, and a history of TIAs (Table 36.4).

▶ **TABLE 36.4 Modifiable Risk Factors That May Increase the Probability of Stroke**

Risk Factors	Modification
Hypertension	Antihypertensives, diet
Heart disease	Antiplatelets
Atrial fibrillation	Anticoagulants, antiarrhythmics
Diabetes mellitus	Glucose and blood pressure control
Hypercholesterolemia	Diet, lipid-lowering medication
Physical inactivity	Routine exercise
Smoking	Cessation
Heavy alcohol use	Quantity reduction
Asymptomatic carotid stenosis	Antiplatelets, endarterectomy, angioplasty
Transient ischemic attack	Antiplatelets, endarterectomy

After age, hypertension is the second most powerful, modifiable, stroke risk factor. It is prevalent in the population of the United States in both men and women and is of greater significance in black patients. The risk of stroke rises proportionately with increasing blood pressure. In Framingham, the relative risk of stroke for a 10-mmHg increase in systolic blood pressure was 1.9 for men and 1.7 for women, after controlling for other known stroke risk factors. Elevated systolic or diastolic blood pressure (or both) increases stroke risk by accelerating the progression of atherosclerosis and predisposing to small-vessel disease.

Cardiac disease clearly has been associated with an increased risk of ischemic stroke, in particular atrial fibrillation (AF), valvular heart disease, myocardial infarction (MI), coronary artery disease (CAD), congestive heart failure (CHF), electrocardiographic evidence of left-ventricular hypertrophy, and perhaps mitral-valve prolapse.

Chronic AF affects more than 2 million Americans and becomes more frequent with age. In the Framingham Study, AF was a strong predictor of stroke, with a nearly five-fold increased risk of stroke among those with nonvalvular AF. In those with coronary heart disease or cardiac failure, AF doubled the stroke risk in men and tripled the risk in women. With coexisting valvular disease, AF had an even greater impact on the relative risk of stroke. Left ventricular dysfunction and left atrial size, as determined by echocardiography, were also predictors of increased thromboembolic risk. Stroke risk is substantially reduced among those AF subjects treated with oral anticoagulant medicines.

Stroke risk nearly doubles in those with antecedent coronary artery disease and nearly quadruples in subjects with cardiac failure. Even after adjusting for the presence of other risk factors, left ventricular hypertrophy increased the risk of stroke by 2.3 in both men and women, and mitral annular calcification was associated with a relative risk of stroke of 2.1. Improved cardiac imaging has led to increases in the detection of such potential stroke risk factors as patent foramen ovale, aortic arch atherosclerotic disease, atrial septal aneurysms, valvular strands, and spontaneous echo contrast (i.e., a smokelike appearance in the left cardiac chambers visualized on transesophageal echocardiography).

Diabetes mellitus also has been associated with increased stroke risk, with relative risks ranging from 1.5 to 3.0, depending on the type and severity. The effect was found in both men and women, did not diminish with age, and was independent of coexisting hypertension.

Abnormalities of serum lipids (e.g., triglyceride, cholesterol, low-density lipoprotein (LDL), high-density lipoprotein (HDL)) are regarded as risk factors, more for CAD than for cerebrovascular disease. Older meta-analyses of prospective cohort studies among somewhat younger populations have failed to verify an independent relationship between stroke and elevated cholesterol. Part of this is explained by the recognition that not all strokes are due to atherosclerosis. More recent studies have found a protective effect of HDL for stroke, an association between carotid plaque or intima-media thickness and lipoprotein fractions, and a significant reduction in stroke risk among persons treated with the newest class of cholesterol-reducing medicines, statins.

Physical inactivity is a definite predictor of cardiac death, and evidence is accumulating regarding the beneficial effects of physical activity for stroke prevention. In the Northern Manhattan Stroke Study, leisure-time physical activity was found to be significantly associated with a reduced risk of stroke among men and women, young and old, and white, black, and Hispanic patients. Although a dose-response relationship was found, such that heavier (more strenuous) activity and longer duration of activity were more beneficial, even light activities in which elderly individuals may engage, such as walking, conferred a significant protective effect.

Cigarette smoking has been established clearly as a biologically plausible independent determinant of stroke. After controlling for other cardiovascular risk factors, cigarette smoking has been associated with relative risks of brain infarction of 1.7. Stroke risk was greatest in heavy smokers and reduced within 5 years among those who quit. It was an independent determinant of carotid-artery plaque thickness. The association of smoking and subarachnoid hemorrhage is particularly striking. A population-based, case-control study in Kings County, Washington, demonstrated an odds ratio of 11.1 for heavy smokers (i.e., smoking more than one pack per day) and 4.1 for light smokers (i.e., smoking no more than one pack per day) compared with nonsmokers. Overall, the stroke risk attributed to cigarette smoking is greatest for subarachnoid hemorrhage; intermediate for cerebral infarction, for which atherosclerotic stroke may be the most related; and lowest for cerebral hemorrhage.

The role of alcohol as a stroke risk factor depends on stroke subtype and dose. Excess drinking has been shown to be a risk factor for both intracerebral and subarachnoid hemorrhage, whereas the nature of a relationship between alcohol and cerebral infarction has been a more controversial subject. Study results include a definite, independent effect in both men and women, an effect only in men, and no effect after controlling for other confounding risk factors, such as cigarette smoking. A J-shaped relationship between alcohol and ischemic stroke has been noted in a few epidemiologic studies. The relative risk of stroke increased with heavy alcohol consumption (five or more drinks per day) and decreased with light to moderate drinking when compared with nondrinkers. In northern Manhattan, drinking up to two drinks per day was significantly protective for ischemic stroke compared with nondrinkers among old and young subjects,

both men and women, and in white, black, and Hispanic patients.

Asymptomatic carotid artery disease, which includes nonstenosing plaque or carotid stenosis, has been found to be associated with an increased stroke risk, particularly among those patients with more than 75% stenosis. The annual stroke risk was 1.3% in those with no more than 75% stenosis and 3.3% in those with more than 75% stenosis, with an ipsilateral stroke risk of 2.5%. The combined TIA and stroke risk was 10.5% per year in those with more than 75% carotid stenosis. Among persons with asymptomatic carotid artery disease, the occurrence of symptoms may depend on the severity and progression of the stenosis, the adequacy of collateral circulation, the character of the atherosclerotic plaque, and the propensity to form thrombus at the site of the stenosis.

TIAs are a strong predictor of subsequent stroke, with annual stroke risks ranging from 1% to 15%. The first 90 days after a TIA have the greatest stroke risk, with recent series demonstrating a 10% risk of stroke in that period. Amaurosis fugax or transient monocular blindness appears to have a better outcome than hemispheric ischemic attacks. TIAs, however, precede cerebral infarction in fewer than 20% of patients. The stroke risk after TIA probably depends on the presence and severity of underlying atherosclerotic disease, vascular distribution, adequacy of collateral perfusion, and distribution of confounding risk factors. These variables must be considered before comparing different studies or extrapolating results with the individual patient.

Potential Risk Factors

Other potential stroke risk factors identified by some studies need to be confirmed and clarified in further epidemiologic investigations. Migraine, oral contraceptive use, drug abuse, and snoring have been associated with a higher stroke risk. Various laboratory test result abnormalities, often reflecting an underlying metabolic-, coagulation-, or inflammatory disturbance, have been associated with stroke and identified as possible stroke precursors. These include hematocrit, polycythemia, sickle cell anemia, white blood count, C-reactive protein, fibrinogen, hyperuricemia, hyperhomocysteinemia, protein C and free protein S deficiencies, lupus anticoagulant, and anticardiolipin antibodies. Some are clear stroke risk factors, whereas others require further epidemiologic investigations.

Outcome

The immediate period after an ischemic stroke carries the greatest risk of death, with fatality rates ranging from 8% to 20% in the first 30 days. Case fatality rates are worse for hemorrhagic strokes, ranging from 30% to 80% for intracerebral and 20% to 50% for subarachnoid hemorrhage.

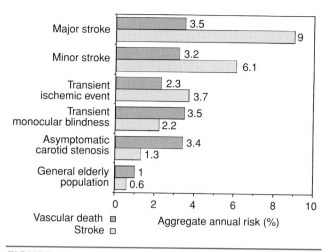

FIGURE 36.11. Aggregate estimates of annual vascular events in various subgroups. (Adapted from Wilterdink et al., 1992)

Characteristics that may be determined at the onset of stroke and used by the clinician to predict early mortality include impaired consciousness, severity of the initial clinical syndrome, hyperglycemia, and age.

Stroke survivors continue to have a three- to five-fold increased risk of death, compared with the age-matched general population. Annual aggregate estimates of death have been 5% for minor stroke and 8% for major stroke. Survival is influenced by age, hypertension, cardiac disease (e.g., MI, AF, CHF), and diabetes. Moreover, patients with lacunar infarcts appear to have a better long-term survival than do those with the other infarct subtypes.

Recurrent stroke is frequent and is responsible for major stroke morbidity and mortality. The immediate period after a stroke carries the greatest risk for early recurrence; rates range from 3% to 10% during the first 30 days. Early stroke recurrence is no trivial matter because of significant worsening of neurologic disability, an increased risk of mortality, and clearly a longer hospital stay. Thirty-day recurrence risks varied by infarct subtypes; the greatest rates were found in patients with atherosclerotic infarction and the lowest rates in patients with lacunes. After the early phase, the risk of stroke recurrence continues to threaten the quality of life of a stroke survivor. Long-term stroke recurrence rates range in different studies from 4% to 14% per year, with aggregate annual estimates of 6% for minor stroke and 9% for major stroke (Fig. 36.11).

Universal agreement has not been reached on the predictors of stroke recurrence. Although age is an important predictor of survival after stroke, both young and old are at risk for stroke recurrence. Some studies have found no effect of hypertension and cardiac disease, whereas others have suggested that these factors increased recurrence after stroke. Valvular disease, congestive heart failure, and atrial fibrillation have been found to be determinants of recurrent stroke. In northern Manhattan, hyperglycemia and ethanol abuse, were identified as predictors of stroke recurrence within 5 years. Further studies are required to clarify the predictors of stroke recurrences, and more rigorous control of vascular risk factors are needed to reduce the threat of a stroke recurrence among the increasing number of stroke survivors in our communities.

SUGGESTED READINGS

Albers GW, Caplan LR, Easton JD, et al. Transient ischemic attack—proposal for a new definition. *N Engl J Med* 2002;347:1713–1716.

American Heart Association. *Heart Disease and Stroke Statistics—2003 Update.* Dallas, TX.: American Heart Association, 2002.

Benavente O, Eliasziw M, Streifler JY, et al. Prognosis after transient monocular blindness associated with carotid-artery stenosis. *N Engl J Med* 2001;345:1084–1090.

Broderick J, Brott T, Kothari R, et al. The Greater Cincinnati/Northern Kentucky Stroke Study: preliminary, first-ever and total incidence rates of stroke among blacks. *Stroke* 1998;29:415–421.

Gan R, Sacco RL, Gu Q, et al. Lacunes, lacunar syndromes, and the lacunar hypothesis: the Northern Manhattan Stroke Study experience. *Neurology* 1997;48:1204–1211.

Goldstein LB, Adams R, Becker K, et al. Primary prevention of ischemic stroke : a statement for healthcare professionals from the Stroke Council of the American Heart Association. *Stroke* 2001;32:280–299.

Gorelick PB, Sacco RL, Smith DB, et al. Prevention of a first stroke: a review of guidelines and a multidisciplinary consensus statement from the National Stroke Association. *JAMA* 1999;281:1112–1120.

Hu FB, Stampher MJ, Colditz G, et al. Physical activity and risk of stroke in women. *JAMA* 2000;283:2961–2967.

Johnson SC, Gress DR, Browner WS, Sidney S. Short-term prognosis after emergency department diagnosis of TIA. *JAMA* 2000;284:2901–2906.

Law MR, Wald NJ, Rudnicka AR. Quantifying effect of statins on low density lipoprotein cholesterol, ischaemic heart disease, and stroke: systematic review and meta-analysis. *BMJ* 2003;326:1423.

Lawes CM, Bennett DA, Feigin VL, Rodgers A. Blood pressure and stroke: an overview of published reviews. *Stroke* 2004;35:776–785.

Sacco RL, Boden-Albala B, Gan R, et al. Stroke incidence among white, black, and Hispanic residents of an urban community. *Am J Epidemiol* 1998;147:259–268.

Sacco RL, Elkind M, Boden-Albala B, et al. The protective effect of moderate alcohol consumption on ischemic stroke. *JAMA* 1999;281:53–60.

Sacco RL, Shi T, Zamanillo MC, Kargman D. Predictors of mortality and recurrence after hospitalized cerebral infarction in an urban community: the Northern Manhattan Stroke Study. *Neurology* 1994;44:626–634.

Sacco RL, Benson RT, Kargman DE, et al. High-density lipoprotein cholesterol and ischemic stroke in the elderly The Northern Manhattan Stroke Study. *JAMA* 2001;285:2729–2735.

Wilterdink JL, Easton JD. Vascular event rates in patients with atherosclerotic cerebrovascular disease. *Arch Neurol* 1992;49:857–863.

Wolf PA, D'Agostino RB, Belanger AJ, Kannel WB. Probability of stroke: a risk profile from the Framingham Study. *Stroke* 1991;22:312–318.

Chapter 37

Examination of the Patient with Cerebrovascular Disease

Randolph S. Marshall

The goal of the examination of a patient suspected of having a stroke is to gain immediate information about the probable size, location, and etiology of the stroke. Successful treatment of ischemic stroke depends on starting within a few hours after the onset. MRI may detect ischemia within minutes to hours after symptoms begin; CT is commonly used as a diagnostic tool for stroke patients seen in the emergency department, to rule out hemorrhage before thrombolytic treatment is considered. The examining physician has the responsibility to identify the symptoms and signs that guide subsequent therapy. For patients who arrive too late—beyond the time window for acute treatment—the neurologic examination is the first step in the diagnostic workup, to establish stroke etiology and to start proper treatment aimed at preventing recurrence of stroke. Stroke scales such as the Glasgow Coma Scale and the NIH Stroke scale combine elements of the examination items discussed here to help predict early and late outcomes.

GENERAL EXAMINATION

Evaluation of the patient who has a suspected stroke of large size must first address the level of consciousness and cardiopulmonary status. Emergency signs of irregular or labored breathing and a decreased level of consciousness, particularly if accompanied by gaze deviation, hemiparesis, or unequal pupils, may indicate the need for immediate intubation in order to treat impending herniation from massive infarction. Reduced alertness is a sign of either extensive hemispheral injury or a sign of involvement of the brainstem reticular activating system, the latter of which could result from brainstem infarction or from compression on the brainstem by the herniating uncus of the temporal lobe. Alternatively, the patient may be in a postictal state from seizure caused by the ischemic injury.

The terms lethargic and stuporous are often used to describe levels of decreased consciousness, but it is most useful to describe alertness in terms of the minimal stimulus required for a given response (e.g., opens eyes in response to voice, or semipurposeful withdrawal in response to moderately noxious stimulus). More subtle impairment of attention and concentration is tested by asking the patient to count backward from 20 down to 1, or say the months of the year backward. The level of alertness may fluctuate after injury to the thalamus; thalamic injury is often a hemorrhage.

Coexisting metabolic derangement, such as drug toxicity or hyperglycemia, must be ruled out with appropriate laboratory tests. Papilledema is an additional sign of increased intracranial pressure that may contribute to decreased consciousness. Cheyne-Stokes respiration in conjunction with normal levels of consciousness may be associated with a smaller territory infarction that involves the insula. Cardiac conduction defects, arrhythmias, subendothelial myocardial infarction, and neurogenic pulmonary edema may occur as a consequence of subarachnoid hemorrhage or large territory infarction, presumably emanating from a centrally mediated increase in sympathetic neurotransmitter release. The blood pressure rises acutely in 70% to 80% of stroke patients, as a consequence of the infarction or hemorrhage, and then returns to baseline spontaneously over the course of a few days. Except for malignant hypertension with encephalopathy or hypertensive cerebral hematoma identified on brain CT, blood pressure is not treated acutely. Nuchal rigidity is often present in subarachnoid hemorrhage. Rarely, fever may be caused by brainstem infarction or subarachnoid hemorrhage. A systemic etiology must be sought and treated, however, because fever may exacerbate ischemic brain injury.

Beyond the examination required for emergency management of acute stroke, the general examination should focus on the cardiovascular system to seek a likely stroke etiology. Examination of the neck includes auscultation for carotid bruits, which result from turbulent flow in an artery narrowed by atherosclerotic plaque. Auscultation of bruits may be misleading if the sound arises from stenosis of the unimportant external carotid artery, or if the degree of stenosis in the internal carotid artery is great enough to dampen flow velocity below that which produces an audible bruit. Doppler ultrasound or MRA of the neck is needed if carotid stenosis is suspected. Fundoscopy may show retinal arterial narrowing, subhyloid hemorrhages, or cotton-wool spots (i.e., systemic signs of hypertension or diabetes).

The presence of murmurs or arrhythmia on cardiac examination suggests valvular disease or atrial fibrillation, both of which are independent risk factors and indications for anticoagulation therapy to prevent recurrence of stroke. The presence of fever with a cardiac murmur requires blood culture to rule out bacterial endocarditis. Auscultation of the lungs is important as a means of identifying signs of aspiration pneumonia or pulmonary edema caused by congestive heart failure.

NEUROLOGIC EVALUATION

The neurologic examination may provide valuable clues to the size, location, and etiology of the stroke. A few syndromes are predictive of specific stroke etiologies. For example, Wernicke aphasia, homonymous hemianopia, and the top-of-the-basilar syndrome of cortical blindness, agitation, ocular dysmotility, and amnesia are nearly always caused by embolism from a proximal arterial or cardiac source. The Wallenberg syndrome arises from infarction of the dorsolateral medulla, and is typically caused by thrombosis of the vertebral artery. The lacunar syndromes (see below) nearly always result from lipohyalinosis and fibrinoid necrosis of small, penetrating arterioles arising from the middle cerebral artery stems, the basilar artery, or the first portion of the posterior cerebral arteries.

The severity of the clinical syndrome at onset is correlated with the ultimate functional outcome. Level of alertness, ocular motility, motor power, and higher cerebral function are the keys to initial assessment. The most common sign of large stroke is the combination of gaze deviation, hemiparesis, and altered mentation. Hyperhydrosis, or excessive sweating, sometimes unilateral, may also occur in brainstem hemorrhage or large hemisphere stroke. In a comatose patient, asymmetry of tendon reflexes supports a diagnosis of unilateral brain injury when motor and sensory testing are not possible to obtain. Hypotonia may occur early after stroke, whereas tone often increases only after several days.

Even if fully alert, patients with gaze deviation and hemiparesis who are within the first several hours after stroke onset are at high risk for profound clinical worsening, owing to an edema-related mass effect that may peak as late as 3 to 5 days after stroke onset. Gaze palsies often occur with infarction involving the dorsolateral frontal lobes, producing gaze deviation to the opposite side of the hemiparesis.

Infarction of the lateral pons, on the other hand, produces hemiparesis on the same side as the direction of forced gaze. Other ocular dysmotility syndromes, including internuclear ophthalmoplegia, vertical gaze palsies, and nystagmus, may also occur with smaller infarcts in the brainstem. Visual fields should be tested by asking the patient to count fingers held at a distance or to identify the position of a moving finger in each of four visual quadrants. Homonymous hemianopia may be the only sign of a large, posterior, cerebral artery territory in-farction. An upper or lower homonymous quadrantanopia is produced by infarction involving the optic radiations hugging the lateral ventricular wall in the temporal or parietal lobe, respectively. A sectoranopia may be produced by injury to the lateral geniculate body of the thalamus, stemming from an anterior choroidal artery embolism.

Cortical involvement is suggested when aphasia or hemineglect are present. As a sign of dominant hemisphere injury, aphasia may involve abnormal responses in naming, fluency, comprehension, repetition, reading, or writing. Dysfluency predominates with frontal lobe injury, whereas comprehension deficits predominate with posterior temporal and parietal injury.

Severe Wernicke aphasia is characterized by poor auditory and reading comprehension, and fluent speech littered with paraphasic errors; the syndrome may be misdiagnosed as delirium, in the emergency room. Hemineglect, produced most often by nondominant parietal or frontal lobe injury, may be identified by unilateral extinction of visual or tactile stimuli when bilateral stimuli are presented. Rightward deviation on a line bisection test and failure to identify stimuli on the left side of an array of stimuli are also reliable signs of left hemineglect.

Short-term verbal memory may be acutely affected by stroke when one or both anteromedial thalami or medial temporal lobes are involved. Short-term memory is easily tested by asking the patient to recall three objects after a 5-minute delay. Long-term memory impairment may appear as disorientation or dementia in a patient with multiple prior strokes in both hemispheres.

Unilateral weakness is typical of stroke effects. A complete characterization of the motor loss is important because the distribution and time course of weakness will differ by stroke location and etiology. Proximal and distal upper and lower limbs should be assessed independently, on a five-point scale of power. Subtle weakness may be apparent only by the presence of a flattened nasolabial fold or widened palpebral fissure on one side of the face, or a unilateral pronator drift when the patient is asked to hold the arms outstretched with palms up. Slowed or clumsy fine movements of one hand or ataxic dysmetria on finger-nose-finger trial may follow a stroke involving either the contralateral corticospinal tract or the ipsilateral cerebellum or cerebellar connections to the brainstem.

Weakness affecting the face, arm, and leg equally in a fully awake patient implies a small infarct in a deep brain region such as the posterior limb of the internal capsule, where the fibers of the corticospinal tract converge into a small anatomic area. This pure, motor hemiparesis is one of four classic lacunar syndromes caused by small, deep infarcts in the capsule, basal ganglia, thalamus, or pons. Hemisensory loss is the syndrome associated with a thalamic lacunae. Clumsy-hand dysarthria, or ataxic hemiparesis, may result from injury to the lacunes in the corticospinal tract at any level, from the corona radiata to the pons.

The presence of dysphagia suggests brainstem injury. Fractionated hemiparesis (e.g., facio-linguo-brachial paresis with little or no leg weakness) suggests cortical involvement of the perisylvian region, as a result of embolic occlusion of a branch of the middle cerebral artery. An even smaller middle cerebral artery branch occlusion may produce isolated hand weakness, mimicking an ulnar or median neuropathy. Weakness that affects the leg suggests a paramedian infarction caused by embolic occlusion of the anterior cerebral artery. Arm and face weakness from anterior cerebral artery infarction may be the result of motor neglect as a consequence of injury to the paramedian supplementary motor area and cingulate gyrus.

Weakness of the proximal arm and leg but sparing facial and lingual function, is the most common result of the border-zone ischemia seen with hemodynamic failure from high-grade internal carotid artery stenosis. In patients with severe carotid occlusive disease, an attack of unilateral tremor or limb shaking may be precipitated by standing, a rarely seen sign that may be mistaken for focal seizure. Weakness caused by hemodynamic failure from large vessel atherostenosis may fluctuate before becoming a fixed hemiparesis. Stroke syndromes arising from embolic arterial occlusion are usually maximal at onset. Weakness caused by lacunar disease may sometimes have a stuttering, step-wise worsening course over several days.

SUGGESTED READINGS

Barnett HJM, Mohr JP, Stein BM, Yatsu FM, eds. *Stroke: Pathophysiology, Diagnosis and Management,* 3rd ed. New York: Churchill Livingstone, 1998.

Binder JR, Marshall R, Lazar RM, Benjamin JL, Mohr JP. Distinct syndromes of hemineglect. *Arch Neurol* 1992;49:1187–1194.

Chamorro A, Marshall RS, Valls-Solé J, Tolosa E, Mohr JP. Motor behavior in stroke patients with isolated medial frontal ischemic infarction. *Stroke* 1997;28:1755–1760.

Chimowitz MI, Furlan AJ, Sila CA, et al. Etiology of motor or sensory stroke: a prospective study of the predictive value of clinical and radiological features. *Ann Neurol* 1991;30:519–525.

Fisher CM. Lacunar infarcts. A review. *Cerebrovasc Dis* 1991;1:311–320.

Ginsberg MD, Busto R. Combating hyperthermia in acute stroke: a significant clinical concern. *Stroke* 1998;29:529–534.

Johnston KC, Connors AF Jr, Wagner DP, Haley EC Jr. Predicting outcome in ischemic stroke: external validation of predictive risk models. *Stroke* 2003;34:200–202.

Mayer SA, LiMandri G, Sherman D, et al. Electrocardiographic markers of abnormal left ventricular wall motion in acute subarachnoid hemorrhage. *J Neurosurg* 1995;83:889–896.

Mohr JP, Foulkes MA, Plois AT, et al. Infarct topography and hemiparesis profiles with cerebral convexity infarction: the Stroke Data Bank. *J Neurol Neurosurg Psychiatry* 1993;56:344–351.

Tatemichi TK, Young WL, Prohovnik I, et al. Perfusion insufficiency in limb-shaking transient ischemic attacks. *Stroke* 1990;21:341–347.

Tijssen CC, van Gisbergen JAM, Schulte BPM. Conjugate eye deviation: side, site, and size of the hemispheric lesion. *Neurology* 1991;41:846–850.

Uhl E, Kreth FW, Elias B, et al. Outcome and prognostic factors of hemicraniectomy for space occupying cerebral infarction. *J Neurol Neurosurg Psychiatry* 2004;75(2):270–274.

Chapter 38

Transient Ischemic Attack

John C. M. Brust

Transient ischemic attack (TIA) describes neurologic symptoms of ischemic origin that last less than 24 hours. In fact, most attacks last only a few minutes to an hour. TIAs have more than one mechanism. When severe major carotid or vertebrobasilar stenosis is present, transient thrombosis could be operative; such TIAs tend to be brief. Attacks without severe stenosis tend to last longer and often are associated with distal branch occlusion, suggesting embolism from an ulcerated plaque or a more proximal source. Some TIAs, especially vertebrobasilar, may have a hemodynamic basis, including transient hypotension and cardiac arrhythmia, and TIAs responsive to calcium-channel blockers suggest a vasospasm basis.

In the *subclavian steal syndrome*, stenosis of the left subclavian artery proximal to the origin of the vertebral artery leads to brainstem, cerebellar, or even cerebral symptoms, often manifested during exertion and accompanied by symptoms of left-arm claudication. Other TIAs may be a consequence of primary, intraparenchymal vascular disease. Unusual associated pathologies include fibromuscular dysplasia of the basilar artery and dissection of the middle cerebral artery. TIAs have also been associated with anemia, polycythemia, hyperviscosity, thrombocythemia, cerebral venous thrombosis, bacterial endocarditis, and temporal arteritis, and may clear with correction of the underlying disorder.

SIGNS AND SYMPTOMS

Symptoms vary with the arterial territory involved. *Transient monocular blindness (amaurosis fugax),* reflecting ischemia in the territory of the central retinal artery—a branch of the ophthalmic artery and ultimately the internal carotid artery—consists of blurring or darkening of vision, peaking within a few seconds (sometimes as if a curtain had descended), and usually clearing within minutes. In some patients, embolic particles (Hollenhorst plaques) are seen in retinal artery branches; in others, spasm of the central retinal artery and its branches is observed. Carotid territory TIAs that involve the brain produce varying combinations of limb weakness and sensory loss, aphasia, hemineglect, and homonymous hemianopia.

Posterior circulation TIAs cause symptoms referable to the cerebrum (visual field loss or cortical blindness), brainstem (cranial nerve and long tract symptoms, sometimes crossed or bilateral), and cerebellum. Some TIAs consist of pure hemiparesis or pure hemisensory loss, suggesting intrinsic disease of small, intraparenchymal penetrating vessels. TIAs may cause paroxysmal dyskinesias, including tremor, ataxia, limb dystonia, and myoclonic jerking. Coarse irregular shaking of an arm or leg lasting seconds to a minute, and sometimes precipitated by a change in posture, is often associated with carotid artery occlusion. Recurrent TIAs of the same type are more likely to be the result of critical narrowing of the involved artery than of embolism.

DIAGNOSIS

The diagnosis of TIA may be difficult to ascertain when symptoms are ambiguous (e.g., staggering or "drop attacks;" dizziness, light-headedness, or syncope; vertigo; fleeting diplopia; transient amnesia; atypical visual disturbance in one or both eyes such as flashes, distortions, or tunnel vision; a heavy sensation or "tiredness" in one or more limbs; and paresthesias in an area of fixed sensory loss or briefly affecting only one limb). The differential diagnosis of TIAs includes migraine, cardiac arrhythmia, seizures, hypoglycemia, compressive neuropathy, conversion, and neurosis.

Although TIAs are defined in terms of their clinical reversibility, and are presumed to signify ischemia too brief or incomplete to cause infarction, imaging frequently demonstrates appropriately located infarcts. Up to two-thirds of patients with TIA studied with diffusion-weighted MRI (DWI) have lesions consistent with acute ischemic injury, and in many of these patients follow-up imaging reveals infarction. DWI-detected abnormalities are especially likely when symptoms last more than an hour. Some investigators therefore believe that the definition of TIA should be changed to indicate brief episodes—typically less than one hour—without evidence at imaging of acute infarction.

TIA SIGNIFICANCE

The major significance of TIAs is prognostic. Fifteen percent of ischemic strokes are preceded by a TIA. After a first, non-retinal TIA, 10% to 20% of patients have a stroke within the next 90 days, and in half of them, the stroke occurs within the first 48 hours after the TIA. Retinal TIAs experience about half of this rate of risk. Crescendo TIAs—two or more attacks within 24 hours—are considered a medical emergency (see chapter 45). Asymptomatic coronary artery disease is especially common in patients with carotid stenosis. The overall risk of stroke, myocardial infarction, and vascular death remains high for at least 10 to 15 years in patients with TIA history. The treatment of TIAs and the prevention of stroke are discussed in Chapter 45.

SUGGESTED READINGS

Adams RJ, Chimowitz MI, Alpert JS, et al. Coronary risk evaluation in patients with transient ischemic attack and ischemic stroke: a scientific statement for healthcare professionals from the Stroke Council and the Council on Clinical Cardiology of the American Heart Association/American Stroke Association. *Stroke* 2003;34:2310–2322.

Albers GW, Caplan LR, Easton JD, et al. Transient ischemic attack—proposal for a new definition. *N Engl J Med* 2002;347:1713–1716.

Alvarez-Sabin J, Lozano M, Sastre-Garriga J, et al. Transient ischemic attack: a common initial manifestation of cardiac myxomas. *Eur Neurol* 2001;45:165–170.

Benavente O, Eliasziw M, Streifler JY, et al. Prognosis after transient monocular blindness associated with carotid artery stenosis. *N Engl J Med* 2001;345:1084–1090.

Blaser T, Hofmann K, Buerger T, et al. Risk of stroke, transient ischemic attack, and vessel occlusion before endarterectomy in patients with symptomatic severe carotid stenosis. *Stroke* 2002;33:1057–1062.

Clark TG, Murphy MF, Rothwell PM. Long-term risks of stroke, myocardial infarction, and vascular death in "low risk" patients with a non-recent transient ischemic attack. *J Neurol Neurosurg Psychiatry* 2003;74:577–580.

Crisostomo RA, Garcia MM, Tong DC. Detection of diffusion-weighted MRI abnormalities in patients with transient ischemic attack; correlation with clinical characteristics. *Stroke* 2003;34:932–937.

Demirkaya S, Topcuoglu MA, Vural D. Fibromuscular dysplasia of the basilar artery: a case presenting with vertebrobasilar TIAs. *Eur J Neurol* 2001;8:89–90.

Galvez-Jimenez N, Hanson MR, Hargreave MJ, et al. Transient ischemic attacks and paroxysmal dyskinesias: an under-recognized association. *Adv Neurol* 2002;89:421–432.

Iwamuro Y, Jito J, Shirahata M, et al. Transient ischemic attack due to dissection of the middle cerebral artery – case report. *Neurol Med-Chirurg* 2001;41:399–401.

Johnston CS, Sidney S, Bernstein AL, et al. A comparison of risk factors for recurrent TIA and stroke in patients diagnosed with TIA. *Neurology* 2003;60:280–285.

Johnston SC, Gress DR, Browner WS, et al. Short-term prognosis after emergency department diagnosis of TIA. *JAMA* 2000;284:2901–2906.

Klempen NL, Janardhan V, Schwartz RB, et al. Shaking limb transient ischemic attacks: unusual presentation of carotid artery occlusive disease. Report of two cases. *Neurosurgery* 2002;51:483–487.

Lovett JK, Dennis MS, Sandercock PAG, et al. Very early risk of stroke after a first transient ischemic attack. *Stroke* 2003;34(suppl):e138–e140.

Petzold A, Islam N, Plant GT. Video reconstruction of vasospastic transient monocular blindness. *N Engl J Med* 2003;348:1609–1610.

Rovira A, Rovira-Gols A, Pedraza S, et al. Diffusion-weighted MR imaging in the acute phase of transient ischemic attacks. *Am J Neuroradiol* 2002;23:77–83.

Wilkinson CC, Multani J, Bailes JE. Chronic subdural hematoma presenting with symptoms of transient ischemic attack (TIA): a case report. *W Virginia Med J* 2001;97:194–196.

Chapter 39

Cerebral Infarction

John C. M. Brust

Ischemic syndromes of specific vessels depend not only on the site of the occlusion but on the presence of previous brain damage, collateral circulation, and variations in the region supplied by a particular artery, including aberrations in the circle of Willis (e.g., if both anterior cerebral arteries arise from a common trunk, carotid artery occlusion may cause bilateral leg weakness; if one or both posterior cerebral arteries arise from the internal carotid, occlusion of the basilar artery is less likely to cause visual symptoms).

Syndromes of specific vessels do not always define the site or the nature of the occlusion (e.g., infarction in the region of the middle cerebral artery is often the result of thrombotic occlusion of the internal carotid artery; occlusion of the middle cerebral artery or its branches is usually embolic). Nonetheless, knowledge of individual artery syndromes helps the clinician to localize a lesion and to determine whether or not it is vascular in origin (Figs. 39.1 to 39.5) (Table 39.1).

SPECIFIC VESSEL OCCLUSIONS

Middle Cerebral Artery

Infarction in the region of the middle cerebral artery causes contralateral weakness, sensory loss, homonymous hemianopia, and depending on the hemisphere involved, either language disturbance or impaired spatial percep-

tion. If the main trunk of the artery is occluded, infarction affects the cerebral convexity and deep structures, including not only the motor and sensory cortices over the cerebral convexity, but also the posterior limb of the internal capsule; the face, arm, and leg are equally affected by weakness and sensory loss. If infarction spares the diencephalon after occlusion of the upper division, weakness and sensory loss are greater in the face and arm than in the leg. When infarction is limited to the region of the rolandic branch, such weakness and sensory loss may be the only signs. A small infarct or lacune in the internal capsule (from occlusion of a penetrating lenticulostriate branch of the proximal middle cerebral artery) may cause a syndrome of pure hemiparesis affecting face, arm, and leg but with no other symptoms.

With cerebral lesions, motor and sensory loss tend to be greatest distally, perhaps because the proximal limbs and the trunk are more likely to be represented in both hemispheres. Paraspinal muscles, for example, are rarely weak in unilateral cerebral disease, which also usually spares muscles of the forehead, pharynx, and jaw. Tongue weakness is variable, and small infarcts involving the motor cortex near the sylvian fissure may cause dysarthria without evident tongue or face weakness. If weakness is severe, muscle tone usually decreases initially and then gradually increases over days or weeks to spasticity with hyperactive tendon reflexes. A Babinski sign is usually present from the outset. When weakness is mild, or during recovery, there is more clumsiness and incoordination than loss of strength.

There is often paresis of contralateral conjugate gaze after an acute lesion in the so-called frontal-gaze center anterior to the prerolandic motor cortex or in its subcortical connections; the gaze palsy usually lasts only 1 day or 2 days, even when other signs remain severe. Sensory loss tends to involve discriminative and proprioceptive modalities. Pain and temperature sensation may be impaired but are seldom lost. Joint position sense, however, may be severely disturbed, causing limb ataxia or pseudoathetosis, and there may be loss of two-point discrimination, astereognosis, or failure to appreciate a touch stimulus if another is delivered simultaneously to the normal side of the body ("extinction"). Homonymous hemianopia is the result of damage to the optic radiations. If the lesion is primarily parietal, the field cut may be an inferior quadrantanopia; with temporal lesions, quadrantanopia is superior.

A lesion of the left opercular (perisylvian) cortex is likely to cause aphasia; when damage is widespread, the aphasia is global, causing muteness or nonfluent and amelodic speech and severe impairment of speech comprehension, writing, and reading abilities.

Restricted damage from branch occlusions may cause an aphasic syndrome. Frontal opercular lesions tend to cause Broca aphasia, with impaired speaking and writing

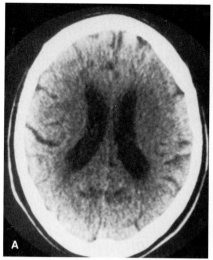
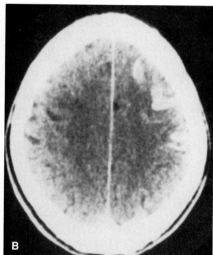

FIGURE 39.1. Cerebral infarction, 1 week after stroke. A: Before injection of contrast material, CT was normal. **B:** After injection of contrast material, there was gyral enhancement in a pattern conforming to the distribution of the middle cerebral artery. (Courtesy of Drs. S. K. Hilal and S. R. Ganti.)

ability but with relative preservation of comprehension. The relative contributions of cortical and white matter damage to this type of aphasia are the subjects of controversy. With posterior periopercular lesions, fluency and prosody are preserved, but paraphasia may reduce speech output to jargon; there may be impairment of speech comprehension, naming, repetition, reading, and writing abilities in different combinations.

When aphasia is severe, there is usually some impairment of nonlanguage cognitive functions; when aphasia is global, dementia is obvious. With Broca or global aphasia, hemiparesis is usually severe. When aphasia is the result of a restricted posterior lesion, hemiparesis is mild. Aphasia in left-handed patients, regardless of the hemisphere involved, tends to be milder and resolves more rapidly than in right-handed patients with left hemisphere injury.

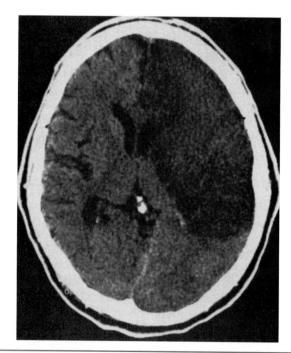

FIGURE 39.2. Subacute infarct, anterior and middle cerebral artery distributions. Noncontrast axial CT demonstrates radiolucency in the left basal ganglia and frontal and temporal opercula extending through the cortex. Note sulcal effacement and mild shift resulting from recent infarction involving the left anterior and middle cerebral artery territories; the left posterior cerebral artery territory is spared. (Courtesy of Drs. J. A. Bello and S. K. Hilal.)

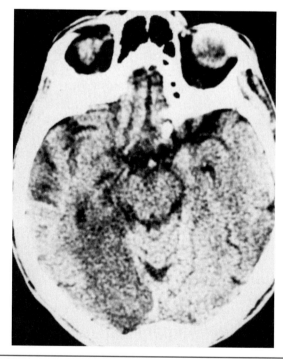

FIGURE 39.3. Acute posterior cerebral infarct. Noncontrast axial CT shows right occipital lucency, corresponding to posterior cerebral vascular distribution with mild mass effect (sulcal effacement) caused by acute infarction and edema. (Courtesy of Drs. J. A. Bello and S. K. Hilal.)

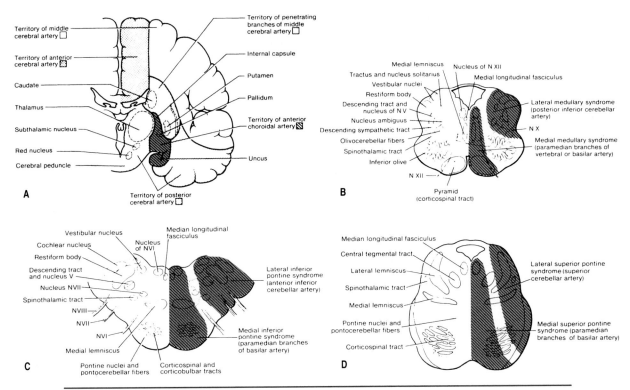

FIGURE 39.4. A: Arterial territories of the cerebrum. **B:** Arterial territories of the medulla. **C:** Arterial territories of the lower pons. **D:** Arterial territories of the upper pons.

Left hemisphere convexity lesions, especially parietal, may cause bilateral ideomotor apraxia, in which the patient may not perform learned motor acts on command but may describe the act and perform it when the setting is altered (e.g., after the examiner has given the patient an object, the use of which the patient could not imitate). Buccolingual apraxia often accompanies Broca aphasia. Ideational apraxia (loss of understanding of the purpose of actions and difficulty manipulating objects) follows bilateral hemisphere damage and associated dementia. Infarction of the angular or supramarginal gyri of the dominant hemisphere may cause Gerstmann syndrome (i.e., agraphia, acalculia, left-right confusion, and finger agnosia).

Right hemisphere convexity infarction, especially parietal, causes disturbances of spatial perception; the patient has difficulty copying simple pictures or diagrams (*constructional apraxia* or *apractagnosia*), interpreting maps, maintaining physical orientation (*topographagnosia*), or putting on clothing (dressing apraxia). Difficulty recognizing faces (*prosopagnosia*) is attributed to bilateral temporooccipital lesions. Hemineglect, a tendency to ignore the contralateral half of one's body or of external space, follows damage to the parietal lobe (or rarely, the diencephalon), right more often than left. Patients may not recognize the hemiplegia (*anosognosia*), their arm (*asomatognosia*), or any external object to the left of their own midline. These phenomena may occur without vi-

sual field defects in patients who are otherwise mentally intact.

Patients with right hemisphere convexity damage may have difficulty expressing or recognizing nonpropositional aspects of speech (pragmatics), such as emotional tone, sarcasm, or jokes. Right hemisphere lesions may also produce an acute confusional state.

Anterior Cerebral Artery

Infarction in the area of the anterior cerebral artery causes weakness, clumsiness, and sensory loss affecting mainly the distal contralateral leg. There may be urinary incontinence. Damage to the supplementary motor area may cause a speech disturbance that is considered aphasic by some physicians and defined as a kind of motor inertia by others. There may be motor neglect, an apparent disinclination to use the contralateral limbs despite little or no weakness. Involvement of the anterior corpus callosum may cause tactile anomia or ideomotor apraxia of the left limbs, which is attributed to the disconnection of the left language-dominant hemisphere from the right motor or sensory cortex. If the damage includes the territory supplied by the major diencephalic branch (recurrent artery of Heubner), the anterior limb of the internal capsule is affected and the face or even the arm is also weak. Infarction restricted to structures supplied by the artery of Heubner (i.e., head of caudate nucleus and, variably,

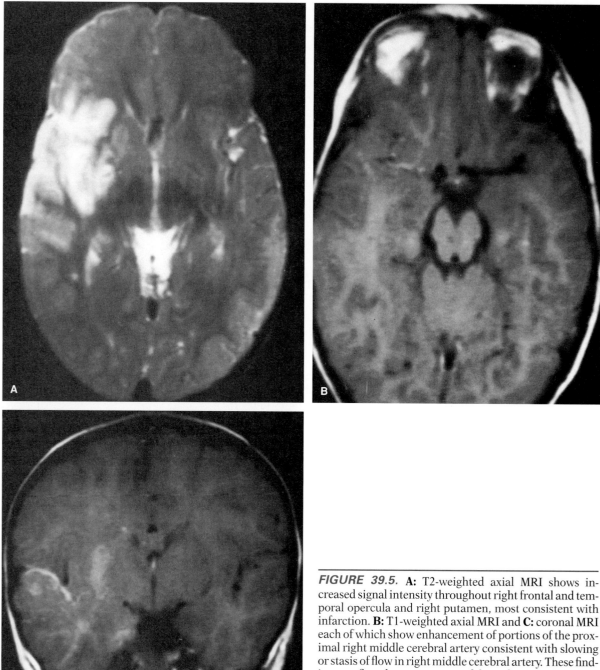

FIGURE 39.5. **A:** T2-weighted axial MRI shows increased signal intensity throughout right frontal and temporal opercula and right putamen, most consistent with infarction. **B:** T1-weighted axial MRI and **C:** coronal MRI each of which show enhancement of portions of the proximal right middle cerebral artery consistent with slowing or stasis of flow in right middle cerebral artery. These findings confirm the acute nature of this infarction. (Courtesy of Dr. S. Chan.)

putamen and anterior limb of internal capsule) causes unpredictable combinations of dysarthria, abulia, agitation, contralateral neglect, and language disturbance.

Bilateral infarction in the anterior cerebral artery region may cause a severe behavior disturbance, with apathy (*abulia*), motor inertia, muteness, incontinence, suck and grasp reflexes, and diffuse rigidity (*Gegenhalten*) or total unresponsiveness with open eyes (*akinetic mutism*). Symptoms and signs are attributed to destruction of the or-

bitofrontal cortex, deep limbic structures, supplementary motor area, or cingulate gyri.

Posterior Cerebral Artery

Occlusion of the posterior cerebral artery most often causes contralateral homonymous hemianopia by destroying the calcarine cortex. Macular (central) vision tends to be spared because the occipital pole receives a collateral blood supply from the middle cerebral artery.

▶ **TABLE 39.1 Syndromes of Cerebral Infarction**

Artery Occluded	*Syndrome*
Common carotid	Asymptomatic
Internal carotid	Ipsilateral blindness
	Contralateral hemiparesis and hemianesthesia
	Hemianopia
	Aphasia or denial and hemineglect
Middle cerebral	
Main trunk	Hemiplegia
	Hemianesthesia
	Hemianopia
	Aphasia or denial and hemineglect
Upper division	Hemiparesis and sensory loss (arm and face more affected than leg)
	Broca aphasia or denial and hemineglect
Lower division	Wernicke aphasia or nondominant behavior disorder without hemiparesis
Penetrating artery	Pure motor hemiparesis
Anterior cerebral	Hemiparesis and sensory loss affect leg more than arm
	Impaired responsiveness ("abulia" or "akinetic mutism"), especially if bilateral infarction
	Left-sided ideomotor apraxia or tactile anomia
Posterior cerebral	Cortical, unilateral: isolated hemianopia (or quadrantic field cut); alexia or color anomia
	Cortical, bilateral: cerebral blindness, with or without macular sparing
	Thalamic: pure sensory stroke; may leave anesthesia dolorosa with "spontaneous pain"
	Subthalamic nucleus: hemiballism
	Bilateral inferior temporal lobe: amnesia
	Midbrain: oculomotor palsy and other eye-movement abnormalities

Unilateral lesions are sometimes associated with visual perseveration (*palinopsia*) or release hallucinations in the blind field.

If the lesion affects the dominant hemisphere and includes the posterior corpus callosum, there may be *alexia* (without aphasia or agraphia) attributed to disconnection of the right occipital cortex (vision) from the left hemisphere (language). Such patients often have *anomia* for colors.

When infarction is bilateral, there may be cortical blindness, and sometimes the patient does not recognize or admit the loss of vision (Anton syndrome). Macular sparing, on the other hand, may produce tunnel vision. Other unusual phenomena of bilateral occipital injury are simultanagnosia (inability to synthesize the parts of what is seen into a whole), poor eye-hand coordination, difficulty coordinating gaze, *metamorphopsia* (distortion of what is seen, associated especially with occipitotemporal lesions), and visual agnosia.

Bilateral (and rarely unilateral) infarction in the posterior cerebral artery supply to the inferomedial temporal lobe or medial thalamus causes memory disturbance, sometimes so severe and lasting as to resemble Korsakoff syndrome. It is possible that some cases of transient global amnesia represent transient ischemic attacks of this region. Patients with bilateral lesions affecting both the occipital and temporal lobes may present with agitated delirium.

If posterior cerebral artery occlusion is proximal, the lesions may include the thalamus or midbrain, which are supplied by interpeduncular, paramedian, thalamoperforating, and thalamogeniculate branches. Infarction of the ventral posterior nucleus causes severe loss of all sensory modalities on the opposite side or sometimes dissociated sensory loss with relative preservation of touch, proprioception, and discriminative modalities or conversely of pain and temperature sensation. As sensation returns, there may be intractable persistent pain and *hyperpathia* on the affected side (e.g., thalamic pain, *analgesia dolorosa*, or Roussy-Dejerine syndrome). A lesion of the subthalamic nucleus causes contralateral hemiballism.

Several abnormal eye signs may be found when posterior cerebral artery disease affects the midbrain: bilateral (or less often, unilateral) loss of vertical gaze, convergence spasm, retractatory nystagmus, lid retraction (Collier sign), oculomotor palsy, internuclear ophthalmoplegia, decreased pupillary reactivity, and corectopia (eccentrically positioned pupil). Lethargy or coma follows damage to the reticular activating system. Peduncular hallucinosis, often consisting of formed and vivid hallucinations, may occur with infarcts restricted to either the thalamus or the pars reticulata of the substantia nigra. Posterior cerebral artery occlusion may cause contralateral hemiparesis by damaging the midbrain peduncle; it also causes contralateral ataxia by affecting the superior cerebellar outflow above its decussation.

An ipsilateral Horner syndrome may occur in thalamic infarcts that extend to sympathetic projections from the hypothalamus. Horner syndrome may also be the result of carotid artery dissection and damage to peripheral sympathetic projections from the superior cervical ganglion.

Anterior Choroidal Artery

Infarction in the area of the anterior choroidal artery produces inconsistent deficits, with varying combinations of contralateral hemiplegia, sensory loss, and homonymous hemianopia that sometimes spares a beak-like zone horizontally (upper and lower *homonymous sectoranopia*). Responsible structures include the midbrain peduncle or posterior limb of the internal capsule and the lateral geniculate body or early optic radiations. Symptoms are often incomplete and temporary.

Internal Carotid Artery

Internal carotid occlusion may be clinically silent or may cause massive cerebral infarction. Damage occurs most often in the territory of the middle cerebral artery or, depending on collateral circulation, of one of its branches, with syndromes of varying severity. When the anterior communicating artery is not present, infarction may include the territory of the anterior cerebral artery. Internal carotid artery occlusion (or abrupt hypotension in someone with tight stenosis) may also cause infarction in the border zones (watersheds) between the middle, anterior, and posterior cerebral arteries; syncope at onset, focal seizures, and transcortical aphasia (relatively preserved repetition) are often seen with such lesions. When the posterior cerebral artery arises directly from the internal carotid, there may be symptoms referable to the visual cortex, thalamus, inferior temporal lobe, or upper brainstem. Infrequently, carotid artery disease causes vertebrobasilar TIAs.

Emboli dislodged from atherosclerotic plaques in the internal carotid artery reach the retina through the ophthalmic and central retinal arteries, to cause partial or complete visual loss. Platelet-fibrin or cholesterol emboli may sometimes be seen ophthalmoscopically in retinal artery branches.

Bilateral border zone infarction after severe hypotension may cause cortical blindness (from parietooccipital damage at the common border zone between the three major arterial territories) or bibrachial palsy (from bilateral rolandic damage at the border zone of the anterior and middle cerebral arteries).

Vertebrobasilar Arteries

Several eponyms have been applied to brainstem syndromes, but except for the lateral medullary syndrome of Wallenberg, most original descriptions concerned patients with neoplasms. Brainstem infarction is more often the result of occlusion of the vertebral or basilar arteries than of their paramedian or lateral branches; classic medial or lateral brainstem syndromes are encountered less often than incomplete or mixed clinical pictures (Table 39.1).

That an infarct involves posterior fossa structures is suggested by bilateral long tract motor or sensory signs; crossed (e.g., left face and right limb) motor or sensory signs; dissociated sensory loss on one half of the body, with pain and temperature sensation more involved than proprioception; cerebellar signs; stupor or coma; dysconjugate eye movements or nystagmus, including internuclear ophthalmoplegia; Horner syndrome; and involvement of cranial nerves not usually affected by single hemispheric infarcts (e.g., unilateral deafness or pharyngeal weakness).

Brainstem infarction may cause only unilateral weakness indistinguishable from that seen with lacunes in the internal capsule.

SYNDROMES OF INFARCTION

Lateral Medullary Infarction

This infarction usually follows occlusion of the vertebral artery or less often, the posterior inferior cerebellar artery (Fig. 39.6).

Manifestations include vertigo, nausea, vomiting and nystagmus (involvement of the vestibular nuclei); gait and ipsilateral limb ataxia (cerebellum or inferior cerebellar peduncle); impaired pain and temperature sensation on the ipsilateral face (spinal tract and nucleus of the trigeminal nerve) and the contralateral body (spinothalamic tract); dysphagia, hoarseness, and ipsilateral weakness of the palate and vocal cords and decrease of the gag reflex (nucleus ambiguus, or ninth- and tenth-nerve outflow tracts); and ipsilateral Horner syndrome (descending sympathetic fibers). There may be hiccup and, if the nucleus or tractus solitarius is affected, ipsilateral loss of taste. Some patients have loss of pain and temperature sensation

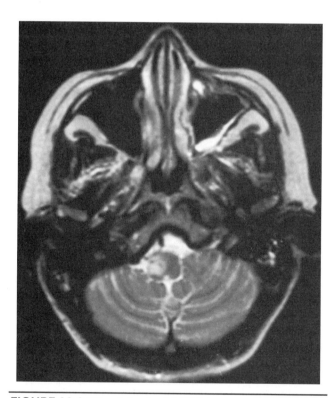

FIGURE 39.6. T2-weighted axial MRI demonstrates a single focus of increased signal intensity within the posterior aspect of the right medulla, consistent with an early infarct. This infarct accounted for the patient's acute presentation with the lateral medullary syndrome of Wallenberg, secondary to occlusion of a branch of the vertebral artery. (Courtesy of Dr. S. Chan.)

▶ **TABLE 39.2 Signs That Indicate the Level of Brainstem Vascular Syndromes**

Syndrome	Artery Affected	Structure Involved	Manifestations
Medial syndromes			
Medulla	Paramedian branches	Emerging fibers of 12th nerve	Ipsilateral hemiparalysis of tongue
Inferior pons	Paramedian branches	Pontine gaze center, near or in nucleus of 6th nerve	Paralysis of gaze to side of lesion
		Emerging fibers of 6th nerve	Ipsilateral abduction paralysis
Superior pons	Paramedian branches	Medial longitudinal fasciculus	Internuclear ophthalmoplegia
Lateral syndromes			
Medulla	Posterior inferior cerebellar or vertebral artery branches	Emerging fibers of 9th and 10th nerves	Dysphagia, hoarseness, ipsilateral paralysis of vocal cord; ipsilateral loss of pharyngeal reflex
		Vestibular nuclei	Vertigo, nystagmus
		Descending tract and nucleus of fifth nerve	Ipsilateral facial analgesia
		Solitary nucleus and tract	Taste loss on ipsilateral half of tongue posteriorly
Inferior pons	Anterior inferior cerebellar	Emerging fibers of seventh nerve	Ipsilateral facial paralysis
		Solitary nucleus and tract	Taste loss on ipsilateral half of tongue anteriorly
		Cochlear nuclei	Deafness, tinnitus
Mid-pons		Motor nucleus of fifth nerve	Ipsilateral jaw weakness
		Emerging sensory fibers of fifth nerve	Ipsilateral facial numbness

Modified from Rowland LP. In: Kandel ER, Schwartz JH, eds. *Principles of neural science.* New York: Elsevier, 1991.

over the contralateral and ipsilateral face, stemming from involvement of the crossed ascending ventral trigemino-thalamic tract, and some develop chronic pain, similar to thalamic pain, in the ipsilateral face or contralateral limbs (Table 39.2).

Infarction of Medial Medulla

An infarction of the medial medulla usually follows an occlusion of a vertebral artery or a branch of the lower basilar artery and involves the pyramidal tract, medial lemniscus, and hypoglossal nucleus or outflow tract. There is ipsilateral tongue weakness with deviation toward the paretic side, and contralateral hemiparesis and impaired proprioception, but cutaneous sensation is spared.

Lateral Pontine Infarction

This may affect caudal structures when there is occlusion of the anterior inferior cerebellar artery or rostral structures after occlusion of the superior cerebellar artery. The caudal syndrome resembles that of lateral medullary infarction, with vertigo, nystagmus, ataxia, Horner syndrome, and crossed face-and-body pain and temperature loss. There is ipsilateral deafness and tinnitus from involvement of the cochlear nuclei; if damage includes more medial structures, there is ipsilateral gaze paresis or facial weakness. Rostral, lateral pontine infarction causes the same constellation of symptoms except that the seventh and eighth cranial nerves are spared and there is ipsilateral paresis of the jaw muscles.

Medial Pontine Infarction Syndromes

These syndromes occur after occlusion of paramedian branches of the basilar artery and depend on whether the lesion is caudal or rostral. A constant feature is contralateral hemiparesis. When the lesion includes the nucleus of the seventh cranial nerve, there is ipsilateral facial weakness; when damage is more rostral, facial paresis is contralateral. There also may be dysarthria (corticobulbar projections to the hypoglossal nucleus), ipsilateral gaze palsy (abducens nucleus or paramedian reticular formation), abducens palsy (sixth nerve outflow tract), internuclear ophthalmoplegia (median longitudinal fasciculus), and limb or gait ataxia. Caudal lesions may cause contralateral loss of proprioception. Palatal myoclonus is attributed to involvement of the central tegmental tract and may be accompanied by rhythmic movements of the pharynx, larynx, face, eyes, or respiratory muscles.

Other Posterior Fossa Syndromes

A small infarct in the paramedian basis pontis affecting the pyramidal tract, nuclei of the basis pontis, and crossing pontocerebellar fibers may cause either ataxic hemiparesis, with contralateral weakness and cerebellar ataxia, or dysarthria clumsy-hand syndrome, with dysarthria and contralateral upper limb ataxia.

Symptoms resembling acute labyrinthitis, with vertigo, nausea, vomiting, and nystagmus, may accompany either infarction of the inferior cerebellum or occlusion of the internal auditory artery, which arises from the basilar or anterior inferior cerebellar arteries, with resulting infarction of the inner ear. Large cerebellar infarcts may mimic cerebellar hemorrhage, with headache, dizziness, ataxia, and if there is brainstem compression, abducens or gaze palsy with progression to coma and death.

Drop attacks are caused by fleeting loss of strength or muscle tone without loss of consciousness; bilateral ischemia of the pontine or medullary pyramidal tract is the explanation in some cases. Infarction of the corticobulbar and corticospinal tracts in the basis pontis (sparing the tegmentum) causes the locked-in syndrome, with paralysis of limbs and lower cranial nerves; communication using preserved eye movements reveals that consciousness is intact.

Midbrain Infarction

Midbrain infarction follows occlusion of the posterior cerebral artery, but the classic mesencephalic syndromes (oculomotor palsy with contralateral hemiparesis, the Weber syndrome, or crossed hemiataxia and chorea, the Benedikt syndrome) are infrequently the result of stroke.

Bilateral Upper Brainstem Infarction

Infarction at this site causes coma by destroying the reticular activating system. When the level is pontine, signs mimic those caused by hemorrhage, with reactive miotic pupils and loss of eye movements. When damage is mesencephalic, ophthalmoplegia is accompanied by midposition unreactive pupils. Rostral midbrain lesions cause different kinds of supranuclear vertical gaze palsy—upward, downward, bilateral, or monocular. If there is only partial loss of consciousness, bilateral, long-tract motor and sensory signs or cerebellar ataxia may be detected.

Pseudobulbar Palsy

This syndrome follows at least two major cerebral infarcts on different sides of the brain (which may occur at different times) or numerous lacunes on both sides. The bilateral hemisphere lesions cause bilateral corticospinal reflex signs (with or without major bilateral hemiparesis), supranuclear dysarthria and dysphagia (with impaired volitional movements but exaggerated reflex movement of the soft palate and pharynx), and emotional incontinence with exaggerated crying (or less often, laughing) that is attributed to release of limbic functions. Other causes of pseudobulbar palsy are multiple sclerosis and amyotrophic lateral sclerosis.

▶ **TABLE 39.3 Proposed Mechanisms of Vascular Dementia**

1. Critically located single infarcts.
   a. Severe aphasia with additional cognitive impairment (middle cerebral artery).
   b. Amnesia with bilateral inferomesial temporal or thalamic damage (posterior cerebral artery).
   c. Abulia, memory impairment, or language disturbance with inferomedial frontal damage (anterior cerebral artery).
   d. Acute confusion or psychosis with nonlanguage dominant parietal lobe damage (middle cerebral artery).
2. Multiinfarct dementia: Multiple large infarcts not necessarily in eloquent locations but usually destroying at least 100 mL of brain volume.
3. Small-vessel disease: Ranging from multiple small deep infarcts (lacunes) to more widespread patchy or diffuse ischemic lesions of the deep cerebral white matter. The latter condition, Binswanger disease, when severe produces abulia, abnormal behavior, pseudobulbar palsy, pyramidal signs, disturbed gait, and urinary incontinence. CT shows periventricular lucencies ("leukoaraiosis") and MRI reveals similarly located signal alterations. Such findings, however, are specific for neither cerebrovascular disease nor dementia.

Vascular Dementia

Cerebral infarction causes dementia by several mechanisms (Table 39.3).

Dementia also may follow hemorrhagic stroke, and its frequent occurrence in patients with cerebral amyloid angiopathy suggests possible overlap between that condition and Alzheimer disease. Although some workers have proposed chronic potentially reversible cerebral hypoperfusion as a cause of dementia, most reject such a mechanism.

The diagnosis of vascular dementia is problematic because the presence, as revealed clinically or by imaging studies, of one or more strokes hardly proves causality and coexisting Alzheimer disease may be excluded only pathologically.

SUGGESTED READINGS

Amarenco P, Hauw JJ. Cerebellar infarction in the territory of the superior cerebellar artery. A clinicopathologic study of 33 cases. *Neurology* 1990;40:1383–1390.

Amarenco P, Rosengart A, DeWitt D, et al. Anterior inferior cerebellar artery territory infarcts. Mechanisms and clinical features. *Arch Neurol* 1993;50:154–161.

Barth A, Bogousslavsky J, Regli F. The clinical and topographic spectrum of cerebellar infarcts: a clinical-magnetic resonance imaging correlation study. *Ann Neurol* 1993;33:451–456.

Bassetti C, Bogousslavsky J, Mattle H, et al. Medial medullary stroke: report of seven patients and review of the literature. *Neurology* 1997;48:882–890.

Bogousslavsky J, Regli F. Anterior cerebral artery territory infarction in the Lausanne Stroke Registry. Clinical and etiologic patterns. *Arch Neurol* 1990;47:144–150.

Bogousslavsky J, Regli F. Capsular genu syndrome. *Neurology* 1990;40:1499–1502.

Brust JCM. Vascular dementia is overdiagnosed. *Arch Neurol* 1988;45:799–801.

Brust JCM, Behrens MM. "Release hallucinations" as the major symptoms of posterior cerebral artery occlusion: a report of 2 cases. *Ann Neurol* 1977;2:432–436.

Brust JCM, Plank C, Burke A, et al. Language disorder in a right-hander after occlusion of the right anterior cerebral artery. *Neurology* 1982;32:492–497.

Brust JCM, Plank CR, Healton EB, Sanchez GF. The pathology of drop attacks: a case report. *Neurology* 1979;29:786–790.

Caplan LR. "Top of the basilar" syndrome. *Neurology* 1980;30:72–79.

Caplan LR, DeWitt LD, Pessin MS, et al. Lateral thalamic infarcts. *Arch Neurol* 1988;45:959–965.

Caplan LR, Schmahmann JD, Kase CS, et al. Caudate infarcts. *Arch Neurol* 1990;47:133–143.

Castaigne P, Lhermitte F, Buge A, et al. Paramedian thalamic and midbrain infarcts: clinical and neuropathological study. *Ann Neurol* 1981;10:127–148.

Damasio AR, Damasio H, Van Hoesen GW. Prosopagnosia: anatomic basis and behavioral mechanisms. *Neurology* 1982;32:331–341.

Devinsky O, Beard D, Volpe BT. Confusional states following posterior cerebral artery infarction. *Arch Neurol* 1988;45:160–163.

Erkinjuntti T, Roman G, Gauthier S, et al. Emerging therapies for vascular dementia and vascular cognitive impairment. *Stoke* 2004;35(4):1010–1017.

Feinberg WM, Rapcsak SZ. "Peduncular hallucinosis" following paramedian thalamic infarction. *Neurology* 1989;39:1535–1536.

Glass JD, Levey AI, Rothstein JD. The dysarthria-clumsy hand syndrome: a distinct clinical entity related to pontine infarction. *Ann Neurol* 1990;27:487–494.

Ghika JA, Bogousslavsky J, Regli F. Deep perforators from the carotid system. Template of the vascular territories. *Arch Neurol* 1990;47:1097–1100.

Graham NL, Emery T, Hodges JR. Distinctive cognitive profiles in Alzheimer's disease and subcortical vascular dementia. *J Neurol Neurosurg Psychiatry* 2004;75(1):61–71.

Hommel M, Bogousslavsky J. The spectrum of vertical gaze palsy following unilateral brain stem stroke. *Neurology* 1991;41:1229–1234.

Howard R, Trend P, Russell RW. Clinical features of ischemia in cerebral arterial border zones after periods of reduced cerebral blood flow. *Arch Neurol* 1987;44:934–940.

Hupperts RMM, Lodder J, Heuts-van Raak EPM, et al. Infarcts in the anterior choroidal artery territory. Anatomical distribution, clinical syndromes, presumed pathogenesis, and early outcome. *Brain* 1994;117:825–834.

Kataoka S, Hori A, Shirakawa T, et al. Paramedian pontine infarction. Neurological/topographical correlation. *Stroke* 1997;28:809–815.

Kim JS, Lee JH, Lee MC. Pattern of sensory dysfunction in lateral medullary infarction. Clinical-MRI correlation. *Neurology* 1997;49:1557–1563.

Kim JS, Sun SU, Lee TG. Pure dysarthria due to a small cortical stroke. *Neurology* 2003;60:1178–1180.

Kim JS. Pure lateral medullary infarction: clinical–radiological correlation of 130 acute, consecutive patients. *Brain* 2003;126:1864–1872.

Kubik CS, Adams RD. Occlusion of the basilar artery—clinical and pathological study. *Brain* 1946;69:73–121.

Lopez OL, Kuller LH, Becker JT. Diagnosis, risk factors, and treatment of vascular dementia. *Curr Neurol Neurosci Rep* 2004;4(5):358–367.

McKee AC, Levine DN, Kowall NW, Richardson EP Jr. Peduncular hallucinosis associated with isolated infarction of the substantia nigra pars reticulata. *Ann Neurol* 1990;27:500–504.

Mehler MF. The neuro-ophthalmologic spectrum of the rostral basilar artery syndrome. *Arch Neurol* 1988;45:966–972.

Melo TP, Bogousslavsky J, van Melle G, Regli F. Pure motor stroke: a reappraisal. *Neurology* 1992;42:789–798.

Naeser M, Palumbo CL, Helm-Estabrooks N, et al. Severe nonfluency in aphasia. Role of the medial subcallosal fasciculus and other white matter pathways in recovery of spontaneous speech. *Brain* 1989;112:1–38.

O'Brien MD. Vascular dementia is underdiagnosed. *Arch Neurol* 1988;45:797–798.

Pantoni L, Garcia JH. Pathogenesis of leukoaraiosis. A review. *Stroke* 1997;28:652–659.

Roman GC, Tatemichi TK, Erkinjuntii T, et al. Vascular dementia: diagnostic criteria for research studies. Report of the NINDS-AIREN International Workshop. *Neurology* 1993;43:250–260.

Rosetti AO, Reichhart MD, Bogousslavsky J: Central Horner's syndrome with contralateral ataxic hemiparesis. A diencephalic alternate syndrome. *Neurology* 2003;61:334–338.

Sacco RL, Bello JA, Traub R, Brust JCM. Selective proprioceptive loss from a thalamic lacunar stroke. *Stroke* 1987;18:1160–1163.

Schmahmann JD, Ko R, MacMore J. The human basis pontis: motor syndromes and topographic organization. *Brain* 2004;127:1269–1291.

Tatemichi TK. How acute brain failure becomes chronic. A view of the mechanisms of dementia related to stroke. *Neurology* 1990;40:1652–1659.

Tatu L, Moulin T, Bogousslavsky J, et al. Arterial territories of the human brain. Cerebral hemispheres. *Neurology* 1998;50:1699–1708.

Tijssen CC, van Gisbergen JAM, Schulte BPM. Conjugate eye deviation;side, site, and size of the hemispheric lesion. *Neurology* 1991;41:846–850.

van der Zwan A, Hillen B. Review of the variability of the territories of the major cerebral arteries. *Stroke* 1991;22:1078–1084.

Weiller C, Ringelstein EB, Reiche W, et al. The large striatocapsular infarct. A clinical and pathophysiological entity. *Arch Neurol* 1990;47:1085–1091.

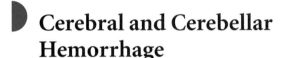

Chapter 40

Cerebral and Cerebellar Hemorrhage

J. P. Mohr and Christian Stapf

INTRACEREBRAL HEMORRHAGE

Most hemorrhages in the brain parenchyma arise in the region of the small arteries that serve the basal ganglia, thalamus, and brainstem and are caused by an arteriopathy of chronic hypertension or microatheroma. This disorder, often referred to as arteriolosclerosis, causes either occlusions with lacunar infarction or leakages that are brain hemorrhages. Small leakages or microbleeds may precede larger hemorrhage from small arteries and may be detected on gradient echo MRI.

Other well established risk factors for intracerebral hemorrhage include increasing age, cigarette smoking, alcohol consumption, and low serum cholesterol. Individuals of African, Hispanic, or Asian heritage show a higher incidence of brain hemorrhage than do whites. A few hemorrhages arise from congophilic amyloid angiopathy, a degenerative disorder affecting the media of the smaller arteries, mainly that of the cerebral gray matter, and seen

▶ **TABLE 40.1 Etiologic Factors for Intracerebral Hemorrhage**

Demographic
Age
Race/Ethnicity

Vascular Risk Factors
Chronic Hypertension (small vessel disease)
Alcohol
Smoking
Low Cholesterol

Vascular Pathology
Amyloid angiopathy (including hereditary forms)
Hemorrhagic transformation of subacute ischemic lesion
Cerebral venous/sinus thrombosis

Pre-existing Vascular Lesions
Cavernoma
Arteriovenous malformation

Malignant
Brain tumor
Cerebral metastasis

Inflammatory
Vasculitis (cerebral, systemic)
Endocarditis (mycotic aneurysm)

Hematologic
Coagulopathy
Thrombocytopenia

Iatrogenic
Anticoagulants
Fibrinolysis

Toxic
Cocaine
Amphetamines

in elderly individuals. Brain tumors, sympathomimetic drugs, coagulopathies, cavernomas and arteriovenous malformations also cause brain hemorrhages. Further differential diagnoses of underlying pathologies are summarized in Table 40.1.

Although treatment with anticoagulants or fibrinolytic agents entails a higher risk of hemorrhage with increasing doses, the role of aspirin intake in this context is controversial. The detection of microbleeds in gradient echo MR implies that aspirin is a risk factor for hemorrhage in patients on anticoagulant therapy; MRI evidence of microhemorrhages should prompt reconsideration of the indications for anticoagulation.

Because most spontaneous hemorrhages arise from tiny vessels, the accumulation of a hematoma takes time and explains the smooth onset of the clinical syndrome over minutes or hours. Compared with the violence of hemorrhage from aneurysm, terms like rupture rarely apply. The progressive course, frequent vomiting, and headache are major points that help to differentiate hem-

orrhage from infarction. Hemorrhage usually stops spontaneously by 30 minutes but in fatal cases, continues until death is caused by brain compression or by disruption of vital structures.

The *putamen* is the site most frequently affected. When the expanding hematoma involves the adjacent internal capsule, there is a contralateral hemiparesis, usually with hemianesthesia and hemianopia and in large hematomas, aphasia or impaired awareness of the disorder. However, small self-limiting hematomas close to the capsular region may occasionally mimic lacunar syndromes featuring pure motor or sensory deficits. When the hemorrhage arises in the *thalamus*, hemianesthesia precedes the hemiparesis. Once contralateral motor, sensory, and visual field signs are established, the main points that distinguish the two sites are (1) conjugate horizontal ocular deviation in putaminal hemorrhage and (2) impaired upward gaze in thalamic hemorrhage. *Pontine* hemorrhage usually plunges the patient into coma with quadriparesis and grossly disconjugate ocular motility disorders, although small hemorrhages may mimic syndromes of infarction. Primary spontaneous hemorrhages within the *mesencephalon* or the *medulla* remain objects of debate and are rare curiosities. When they occur, the anatomic involvement is usually secondary to hemorrhage originating in neighboring diencephalic, cerebellar, or pontine regions. In the *cerebral lobes*, there is an as-yet-unexplained predilection for hemorrhages to occur within the posterior two-thirds of the brain. When they affect one or more cerebral lobes, the syndrome is difficult to distinguish, clinically, from infarction because progressive evolution and vomiting are much less frequent in infarction; also, lobar white matter hematomas often result from arteriovenous malformations, amyloid angiopathy, tumors, or other causes that only uncommonly affect the basal ganglia, thalamus, and pons.

Cerebellar hemorrhage warrants separate description because the mode of onset differs from that of cerebral hemorrhage and because it often necessitates surgical evacuation. The syndrome usually begins abruptly with vomiting and severe ataxia (which usually prevents standing and walking); it is occasionally accompanied by dysarthria, adjacent cranial nerve (mostly sixth and seventh) affection, and paralysis of conjugate lateral gaze to one side, findings that may mislead clinicians into thinking the disease is primarily in the brainstem. However, a cerebellar origin is suggested by the lack of changes in the level of consciousness and lack of focal weakness or sensory loss.

Enlargement of the mass does not change the clinical picture until there is enough brainstem compression to precipitate coma, at which point it is too late for surgical evacuation of the hemorrhage to reverse the disorder. This small margin of time between an alert state and an irreversible coma makes it imperative to consider the diagnosis in all patients with this clinical syndrome and is a reason to have patients who present in the emergency room with vomiting of undetermined origin attempt to stand and walk. CT or MRI should be carried out promptly, and surgery should be performed within hours on all the larger hemorrhages, generally defined as those seen on three CT sections or those of a mass larger than 3 cm.

Treatment

Acute treatment of intracerebral hemorrhage includes airway protection, adequate ventilation, and blood pressure levels below a mean arterial pressure of 130 mmHg. Fluid balance and body temperature should be maintained at normal levels. Increased intracranial pressure may require osmotherapy, controlled hyperventilation, or barbiturate-induced coma. The administration of corticosteroids is generally avoided. Apart from cases suffering cerebellar hemorrhage, any decision on whether, how, and when to intervene neurosurgically after intracerebral hemorrhage is subject to current debates and awaits data from ongoing prospective trials. To date all clinical trial attempts have failed to show a superiority of hematoma evacuation over medical therapy, save for cerebellar hemorrhage, where surgery for the larger masses may be lifesaving and may be followed by satisfactory clinical outcomes.

SUGGESTED READINGS

Aring CD, Merritt HH. Differential diagnosis between cerebral hemorrhage and cerebral thrombosis. *Arch Intern Med* 1935;56:435–456.

Broderick JP, Adams HP, Barsan W, et al. Guidelines for the management of spontaneous intracerebral hemorrhage. A statement for healthcare professionals from a special writing group of the Stroke Council, American Heart Association. *Stroke* 1999;30:905–915.

Brott T, Broderick J, Kothari R, et al. Early hemorrhage growth in patients with intracerebral hemorrhage. *Stroke* 1997;28:1–5.

Greenberg SM. Cerebral amyloid angiopathy: prospects for clinical diagnosis and treatment. *Neurology* 1998;51:690–694.

Inaji M, Tomita H, Tone O, et al. Chronological changes of perihematomal edema of human intracerebral hematoma. *Acta Neurochir Suppl.* 2003;86:445–448.

Kase CS, Mohr JP, Caplan LR. Intracerebral hemorrhage. In: Barnett HJM, Mohr JP, Stein BM, Yatsu FM, eds. Stroke. *Pathophysiology, Diagnosis, and Management,* 3rd ed. New York: Churchill Livingstone, 1998:649–700.

Kandzari DE, Granger CB, Simoons ML, et al. Global Utilization of Streptokinase and tPA for Occluded Arteries-I Investigators. Risk factors for intracranial hemorrhage and nonhemorrhagic stroke after fibrinolytic therapy (from the GUSTO-I trial). *Am J Cardiol* 2004;93:458–461.

Lee SH, Bae HJ, Kwon SJ, et al. Cerebral microbleeds are regionally associated with intracerebral hemorrhage. *Neurology* 2004;62:72–76.

Mendelow AD, Teasdale GM, Barer D, et al. Outcome assignment in the International Surgical Trial of Intracerebral Hemorrhage. *Acta Neurochir* 2003;145:679–681.

Ng SC, Poon WS, Chan MT. The role of haematoma aspiration in the management of patients with thalamic haemorrhage: a pilot study with continuous compliance monitoring. *Acta Neurochir Suppl* 2003;86:469–471.

NINDS t-PA Stroke Study Group. Intracerebral hemorrhage after intravenous t-PA therapy for ischemic stroke. *Stroke* 1997;28:2109–2118.

Ott KH, Kase CS, Ojemann RG, Mohr JP. Cerebellar hemorrhage: diagnosis and treatment. *Arch Neurol* 1974;31:160–167.

Stapf C, Labowitz DL, Sciacca RR, et al. Incidence of adult brain arteriovenous malformation hemorrhage in a prospective population-based stroke survey. *Cerebrovasc Dis* 2002;13:43–46.

Wessels T, Moller-Hartmann W, Noth J, Klotzsch C. CT findings and clinical features as markers for patient outcome in primary pontine hemorrhage. *Am J Neuroradiol* 2004;25:257–260.

Chapter 41

Genetics of Stroke

Suh-Hang Hank Juo and Ralph L. Sacco

Numerous single-gene mutations of autosomal or mitochondrial DNA cause ischemic or hemorrhagic stroke. For example, mutations in the NOTCH3 gene are linked to cerebral autosomal dominant arteriopathy with subcentral infarcts and leucocephalopathy (CADASIL), and a point mutation in mitochondrial DNA causes MELAS. However, these Mendelian forms of stroke disorders are rare and account for only a tiny proportion of all strokes. With the advance of genomic technologies and the completion of the human genome sequence, a current goal is to identify susceptibility genes for common forms of stroke other than these rare syndromes. Linkage and association gene mapping are two approaches that may be applied to either stroke per se or stroke risk factors.

Stroke is a heterogeneous disease with multiple risk factors, which may increase the complexity of the gene mapping task. Many of the risk factors have been documented to have strong genetic components. The underlying genetic mechanism for stroke is likely to influence factors that lead to the increased risk of stroke. Therefore, to study genetics of stroke risk factors may reduce the complexity of genotype-phenotype relationship and so provide a better power to detect the genes conferring susceptibility.

ISCHEMIC STROKES

Twin and family studies suggest a genetic contribution to ischemic stroke. Using the isolated Icelandic population, linkage studies indicate that two genes, the phosphodiesterase 4D (PDE4D) and 5-lipoxygenase activating protein (FLAP) genes, may increase the risk of ischemic stroke by approximately two-fold. However, more studies are needed to confirm the results. Large-scale genetic studies of ischemic stroke are still lacking but two association studies of myocardial infarction (MI) demonstrated that is it possible to use genetic polymorphisms to elucidate its relationship to the disease. Unlike genome-wide linkage studies, where no particular candidate genes are hypothesized, the two association studies screened many polymorphisms as possible candidate genes, based on biological properties that might contribute to myocardial infarction (MI). These association studies suggest that genetic polymorphisms in genes for lymphotoxin-α, connexin 37, plasminogen-activator inhibitor type 1, and stromelysin-1 were associated with MI.

In addition to mapping susceptibility genes, an alternative approach is to investigate recognized stroke risk factors, such as hypertension, diabetes, or hyperlipidemia. These risk factors have strong heritability and may be measured in quantity. Using these quantitative risk factors as intermediate phenotypes may provide information on closer links between genotypes and phenotypes than using stroke as the outcome of interest. Although these studies may not provide a direct link between susceptibility genes and stroke, the susceptibility genes could be used as markers for early detection, prevention, intervention, and therapeutic drug targets. For example, the APOE gene is related to cholesterol levels, the ACE gene is related to hypertension, and the CAPN10 gene is related to type 2 diabetes. Like other human epidemiologic studies, the results of these genetic studies remain to be confirmed. It is likely that some of the susceptibility genes will be used in assessing patients' risks, in the future clinical practice.

Several Mendelian genetic disorders are associated with ischemic stroke (Table 41.1), including vasculopathies, metabolic or connective tissue diseases, and disorders of coagulation.

Common polymorphisms in genes, where rare mutations cause severe Mendelian forms of stroke, may also confer low risk for common forms of stroke. For example, patients with homocystinuria have severe homocystinemia (plasma level greater than 100 μmol/L) and elevated levels of homocysteine may be detected in urine. Patients' clinical symptoms may indicate a progression to severe neurologic deterioration and stroke. Some patients with homocystinuria show severe deficiency of methylene tetrahydrofolate reductase (MTHFR) caused by rare mutations in the MTHFR gene. A more common C-to-T

▶ **TABLE 41.1 Mendelian Type Disorders with Ischemic Stroke**

Disorder	Genetic Mechanism	Disease Gene
Coagulation disorders		
Protein C deficiency (MIM 176860)	AD inheritance	Protein C gene at 2q13–14
Protein S deficiency (MIM 176880)	AD inheritance	Protein S gene at 3p11.1–q11.2
Active protein C resistance Leiden type (MIM 227400.0001)	AD inheritance	Factor V gene at 1q23
Antithrombin III deficiency (MIM 107300)	AD inheritance	Antithrombin III gene at 1q23–25
Sickle cell disease (MIM 603903)	AR inheritance	Hemoglobin beta chain gene at 11p15.5
Connective tissue disorders		
Neurofibromatosis type I (MIM 162200)	AD inheritance	Neurofibromatosis type I gene at 17q11.2
Ehlers-Danlos syndrome type IV (MIM 130050)	AD inheritance	Type III collagen gene at 2q31
Marfan syndrome (MIM 154700)	AD inheritance	Fibrillin gene at 15q21.1
Vasculopathies		
Familial moyamoya disease (MIM 252350)	Unknown	Disease genes are mapped to 3p24.2–p26 and 17q25 but are not cloned.
Metabolic disorders		
Fabry disease (MIM 301500)	XR inheritance	A-galactosidase gene at Xq21.3–q22
MELAS (MIM 540000)	AD inheritance	Mitochondrial DNA
Homocysteinuria (MIM 236250)	AR inheritance	MTHFR gene at 1p36.3 or cystathionine B synthase at 21q22.3

AD, autosomal dominant; AR, autosomal recessive; XR, X-linked recessive.

polymorphism at nucleotide 677 (C677T) of the MTHFR gene generates only a minor risk of stroke. However, this C677T polymorphism is common and it may affect more people.

CEREBRAL AUTOSOMAL DOMINANT ARTERIOPATHY WITH SUBCENTRAL INFARCTS AND LEUCOCEPHALOPATHY (CADASIL)

CADASIL is characterized by recurrent episodes of subcortical infarcts or transient ischemic attacks, and a conspicuous absence of common stroke risk factors, such as hypertension. Symptoms start between ages 30 and 50 years. The variable clinical manifestations include dementia, pseudobulbar palsy, and migraine. There is no specific treatment, and the mean survival time is 20 years from onset of symptoms.

CADASIL is caused by mutations in the NOTCH3 gene on chromosome 19. The encoded NOTCH3 protein is a large transmembrane receptor with different functional domains. Numerous disease-associated mutations are distributed throughout the 34 EGFRs that make up the extracellular domain of the NOTCH3 receptor. All of the mutations lead to loss or gain of a cysteine residue and, therefore, to an unpaired cysteine residue within a given EGF domain. Most of the causative mutations are clustered within exons 3 and 4, encoding the first five EGF-like repeats. A genetic test may routinely detect 70% of the clustering mutations causing the disease. For the mutations outside the clustering region, skin biopsy with immunostaining for the NOTCH3 protein is particularly useful. A phenotypic variant of CADASIL was identified by familial clustering of hemiplegic migraine and labeled CADASILM ("M" for migraine).

INTRACEREBRAL HEMORRHAGE

Intracerebral hemorrhage (ICH) is more deadly than ischemic stroke, but it is rarer and hard to study. Two forms of inherited ICH with cerebral amyloid angiopathy have been described in Dutch and Icelandic populations. The Dutch form involves mutations in the amyloid precursor protein gene, and the Icelandic form is caused by a deletion mutation in the cystatin C gene on chromosome 20. Both autosomal-dominant diseases are characterized by lobar hemorrhages and premature death in young adults, without other cause of hemorrhage.

In contrast, the genetics of spontaneous ICH has received little attention. In a population-based study, being a first-degree relative of someone with ICH seemed to be a strong, independent risk factor. A meta-analysis reported other risk factors for ICH, including hypertension, alcohol abuse, older age, and male sex. Genetic studies have investigated the possible link between the APOE gene and ICH.

The APOE epsilon2 and epsilon4 alleles may be directly associated with cerebral amyloid angiopathy, with increased risk for and earlier age at first hemorrhage.

Vascular malformations are another common cause of ICH, including cerebral cavernous malformation (CCM) and arteriovenous malformation (AVM). CCMs are found in 0.1% to 0.5% of the population. They arise sporadically or may be dominantly inherited with incomplete clinical penetrance. Three CCM loci have been mapped: CCM1 on 7q21-q22 accounts for 40% of the cases, CCM2 on 7p13-p15 for 20% of cases, and CCM3 at 3q25.2-q27 for the remaining 40% of cases. So far, only one gene has been identified, *Krit1*, for CCM1.

Cerebral AVMs are typically solitary lesions, except in hereditary hemorrhagic telangiectasia (HHT) disease. HHT is an autosomal-dominant disorder characterized by mucocutaneous telangiectasias, frequent epistaxis, and gastrointestinal hemorrhage. AVMs in HHT affect the lung, brain, liver and, even more rarely, the spinal cord. Two genes have been identified for HHT: the ENODOGLIN, and ALK-1. Most AVMs are thought to be congenital and familial occurrence of cerebral AVM is rare. The preponderance of AVMs among Asian-heritage patients compared with whites suggests a genetic predisposition.

SUBARACHNOID HEMORRHAGE

Most spontaneous subarachnoid hemorrhages (SAH) are due to ruptured saccular aneurysms. Familial aggregation of SAH has been found even after adjusting for confounding factors, such as hypertension. The risk of SAH increases by three- to five-fold when there is a first-degree relative with SAH. An increased incidence of saccular aneurysm is seen in some families with polycystic kidney disease and other connective tissue disorders, such as the Marfan syndrome. Several genes have been implicated for SAH, and most of them are related to structural anomalies of the vessel wall. However, no risk genes have been identified.

SUGGESTED READINGS

Ariesen MJ, Claus SP, Rinkel GJ, Algra A. Risk factors for intracerebral hemorrhage in the general population: a systematic review. *Stroke* 2003;34:2060–2065.

Brass LM, Isaacsohn JI, Merikangas KR, Robinette CD. A study of twins and stroke. *Stroke* 1992;23:221–223.

Bromberg JEC, Rinkel GJE, Algra A, et al. Subarachnoid hemorrhage in first and second degree relatives of patients with subarachnoid hemorrhage. *BMJ* 1995;311:228–229.

Chabriat H, Vahedi K, Iba-Zazen MT, et al. The clinical spectrum of CADASIL, cerebral autosomal dominant inherited arteriopathy with subcortical infarcts and leukoencephalopathy. *Lancet* 1995;346:934–939.

Flossmann E, Schulz UG, Rothwell PM. Systematic review of methods and results of studies of the genetic epidemiology of ischemic stroke. *Stroke* 2004;35:212–227.

Hademenos GJ, Alberts MJ, Awad I, et al. Advances in the genetics of cerebrovascular disease and stroke. *Neurology* 2001;56:997–1008.

Humphries SE, Morgan L. Genetic risk factors for stroke and carotid atherosclerosis: insights into pathophysiology from candidate gene approaches. *Lancet Neurol* 2004;3(4):227–235.

Peters N, Herzog J, Op herk C, Dichgans M. A two-year clinical follow-up study in 80 CADASIL subjects: progression patterns and implications for clinical trials. *Stroke* 2004;35(7):1603–1608.

Rosand J, Altshuler D. Human genome sequence variation and the search for genes influencing stroke. *Stroke* 2003;34:2512–2516.

Singhal S, Bevan S, Barrick T, et al. The influence of genetic and cardiovascular risk factors on the CADASIL phenotype. *Brain* 2004;127 (Pt9):2031–2038.

Woo D, Sauerbeck LR, Kissela BM, et al. Genetic and environmental risk factors for intracerebral hemorrhage: preliminary results of a population-based study. *Stroke* 2002;33:1190–1195.

Zhang B, Fugleholm K, Day LB, et al. Molecular pathogenesis of subarachnoid haemorrhage. *Int J Biochem Cell Biol* 2003;35:1341–1360.

C h a p t e r 4 2

Other Cerebrovascular Syndromes

Frank M. Yatsu

LACUNAR STROKES

Lacunar strokes are syndromes associated with discrete occlusion of penetrating arterioles (less than 500 μm diameter), most frequently due to sustained hypertension and causing cystic degeneration of brain due to tissue infarction. The symptoms depend on the location of the small infarcts, but may be "silent" with no meaningful symptoms. The pathology from sustained hypertension is defined as lipohyalinosis, although the pathophysiology is uncertain. The most common lacunar syndromes are the following: pure motor hemiplegia, usually involving face and limbs on the side opposite the infarct; pure hemisensory stroke, usually in the same pattern as the pure motor lacunar stroke; ipsilateral ataxia and hemiparesis; and the dysarthria-clumsy-hand syndrome. The syndrome had originally been described in the late 19th century in France, but modern interest was generated by C. Miller Fisher, who has described more than 20 separate syndromes.

Pure motor hemiplegia occurs in varying combinations of face, arm, and leg weakness and the syndrome is seen with infarcts involving the corticospinal tracts in the internal capsule or the pons. Corresponding involvement of the ascending sensory fibers results in varying combinations

of pure hemisensory stroke, but a common site involves sensory nuclei of the thalamus.

Usually, the prognosis for the lacunar syndrome is good, provided the expected hypertension is controlled. However, multiple lacunar infarcts, whether symptomatic or "silent," correlate with diabetes mellitus, leukoaraiosis, impaired outcome with recurrences and mild cognitive impairment or dementia. The most common causes of "silent" or "preclinical" infarcts are atrial fibrillation and carotid stenosis. Wardlaw, et al. postulated a provocative, but untested hypothesis of blood-brain barrier dysfunction to account for lacunar strokes, leukoaraiosis, and dementia.

HYPERTENSIVE ENCEPHALOPATHY

This condition, like so-called malignant hypertension, is a medical emergency requiring immediate hypotensive therapy (rapid acting agents preferably, such as intravenous labetalol, nicardipine, sodium nitroprusside, hydralazine, and sometimes angiotensin converting enzyme (ACE) inhibitors) to minimize serious neurological complications such as strokes, but care must be made not to reduce the mean arterial pressure (MAP) below the level of autoregulation or as an initial mean arterial pressure (MAP) reduction by 15% to 20%. Otherwise, "watershed" or border-zone infarcts may result because flow is dependent upon pressure alone. As originally described in 1928 by Oppenheim and Fishberg, patients with hypertensive encephalopathy usually have diastolic blood pressures of greater than 140 mmHg (except in toxemia/eclampsia and in children with initial blood pressure usually much lower than adult men); the patients display encephalopathic symptoms such as confusion, drowsiness, seizures, as well as blurring of vision and headache, but no focal neurologic signs. Fundi frequently show hemorrhages, exudates and disc edema, and Grade IV Keith-Wagner changes. Brain MRI may show posterior leukoencephalopathy with decreased T1- and increased T2-white matter signal because of "breakthrough" which causes diapedesis of serum through the blood brain barrier. With reduction of MAP, the patient's sensorium frequently clears, a sign that is diagnostic for hypertensive encephalopathy.

FIBROMUSCULAR HYPERPLASIA

Fibromuscular bands of uncertain etiology form segmental narrowing of large arteries such as the carotid artery, and the bands may provoke platelet adhesion and thereby cause transient ischemic attacks or infrequently thromboembolic strokes. Most frequently they present with asymptomatic carotid bruits or are seen incidentally, during a cerebral angiogram and has the appearance of a "string of pearls." If the renal artery is involved, patients may develop hypertension; bruits may be heard over the renal artery. Antiplatelet drugs, anticoagulation, and angioplasty have been reported to reduce the frequency of TIAs in patients presenting with them.

MULTI-INFARCT OR VASCULAR DEMENTIA

This condition is discussed in Chapter 39.

CEREBRAL AMYLOID ANGIOPATHY

This disorder, also known as *congophilic angiopathy*, is considered to occur infrequently but the incidence is increasing in the aging population. Symptoms begin after the middle years of life, with intracerebral hemorrhage, usually lobar; multiple hemorrhages may occur simultaneously. Recurrences may occur within months or years. With multiple hemorrhages, cognitive impairment and dementia follow. Indications for surgical evacuation are similar to those from other causes of intracerebral hemorrhages: size with mass effect, location, and declining sensorium. Hereditary Dutch and Icelandic forms are discussed in Chapter 41. Cerebral amyloid angiopathy is also seen with prion disease, but intracerebral hemorrhage does not occur in that condition.

ANTIPHOSPHOLIPID SYNDROME (LUPUS ANTICOAGULANT AND ANTICARDIOLIPIN ANTIBODY SYNDROMES)

The antiphospholipid syndrome includes patients with either or both the lupus anticoagulant and anticardiolipin syndromes. Originally, the syndrome was described in patients with lupus erythematosus, whose blood had prolonged clotting time that was not corrected by adding normal plasma. It was concluded that the patients had a circulating anticoagulant, which proved to be IgG, IgM or IgA antibodies against the Factor Xa complex, and particularly against the cofactor, a phospholipid, or to the complex phospholipid called cardiolipin, antibodies to which account for a false-positive VDRL or RPR tests for syphilis (see Chapter 28). The immunoglobulins seem directed primarily against a beta-2-glycoprotein.

Three antiphospholipid syndromes exist. The *primary antiphospholipid syndrome* is characterized by recurrent fetal loss, mild thrombocytopenia, and false-positive VDRL or RPR. The *secondary antiphospholipid syndrome* may occur with lupus erythematosus and other immune-complex diseases, or may be associated with cancer and some drug reactions. The most common neurologic manifestations are: migraine-like headaches, strokes (either arterial or venous), encephalopathy with confusion or seizures, and retinopathy with amaurosis fugax and acute ischemic neuropathy. Paradoxically, these patients are prothrombotic, and they should be treated with long-term anticoagulation therapy. On the basis of retrospective studies, particularly from the Graham Hughes group in London, the optimal International Normalized Ratio (INR) prothrombin time to avert thrombosis was believed to be greater than 3.0. However, the only prospective study was carried out by Crowther et al., who found that high levels of INR (greater than 3.1 to 4.0) were not more beneficial than INR levels of 2.0 to 3.0. While treatment based upon these data is justified with an INR between 2.0 to 3.0, this issue remains controversial. This syndrome is known eponymously as the *Graham syndrome*, or as an *annexinopathy*. The Sneddon syndrome is the antiphospholipid syndrome plus livedo reticularis.

HYPERHOMOCYSTEINEMIA

This condition may result from low dietary folate intake, renal diseases, or inborn errors of metabolism, such as the impaired conversion of homocysteine to cystathionine by cystathionine-β-synthase due to a gene mutation; this enzyme has an obligate requirement for pyridoxine (B_6). Impaired remethylation of homocysteine to methylmalonic acid may occur because of mutations in the tetrahydrofolate reductase gene or in B_{12}-related enzyme activity. A number of retrospective studies have implicated hyperhomocystinemia with ischemic strokes and coronary artery disease. However, only the Vitamins Intervention for Stroke Prevention (VISP) study, involving 3,680 ischemic-stroke patients, a prospective, randomized, double-blind study for subjects suffering from ischemic strokes and having elevated homocysteine, who were treated with folate (2.5 mg), pyridoxine (25 mg) and vitamin B_{12} (400 μg) daily, showed no reduction in recurrent strokes over an average of 2 years with homocysteine reduction. A longer follow-up monitoring might have shown a difference, but on the basis of their data, the current status is that treatment of hyperhomocystinemia will not reduce stroke recurrence, myocardial infarction, or death.

STROKE IN YOUNG ADULTS

Stroke in young adults is usually defined as those occurring before age 40 to 45 years, and the causes differ from patients older than 65 years of age. Approximately 25% of all strokes occur before age 65 years, and 5% to 10% occur in subjects younger than 40 to 45 years old. Follow-up examination of young adults by Leys et al (2002), for a mean of 3 years, shows that the disease is not benign because it is associated with a 4.5% mortality rate during the first year, dropping to 1.6% thereafter, and a stroke recurrence rate of 1.4% during the first year.

Strokes in young adults involve a wide variety of disorders that are less commonly seen in older adults, and

▶ **TABLE 42.1 Differential Diagnosis of Stroke in Young Adults**

Vascular diseases

Atherosclerosis

Arteritis: isolated angiitis of the CNS; lupus erythematosus; polyarteritis nodosa; Sjögren syndrome; Behçet disease; lymphomatoid granulomatosis; drug abuse (heroin, "crack cocaine," amphetamine and related compounds such as ephedra and phenylpropanolamine); secondary to chronic meningitis; Takayasu arteritis; HIV infections and AIDS (may have nonbacterial thrombotic endocarditis also)

Arteriovenous or cryptic venous malformations, telangiectasias, and cavernous angiomas

Berry or Congenital aneurysms

CADASIL – Cerebral Autosomal Dominant Arteriopathy with Subcortical Infarcts and Leukoencephalopathy

Dissection (traumatic or spontaneous)

Fibromuscular Dysplasia

Migraine

MELAS – mitochondrial encephalopathy with lactic acidosis and stroke-like events

Moyamoya syndrome

Oral contraceptive use, including low-dose estradiol pills

Venous occlusive diseases

Cardiogenic emboli

Anatomic abnormalities and atherosclerosis patent foramen ovale (PFO); mitral valve prolapse, with redundancy of the mitral leaflet; valvular replacement; & cardiomyopathies—post-myocardial infarction, and alcoholic; endocardial fibrosis; aortic atheromas—$\geq$4 mm without calcification)

Arrhythmias (especially atrial fibrillation and sick-sinus syndrome)

Immunecomplex disorders and paraneoplastic syndromes (Libman-Sacks Syndrome with systemic lupus erythematosus; nonbacterial thrombotic endocarditis or marantic endocarditis, seen in AIDS and with neoplasms, occult and otherwise)

Infections (bacterial endocarditis; viral cardiomyopathy; rheumatic heart disease

Tumors (atrial myxoma)

Blood elements

Erythrocytes (sickle cell disease; polycythemia vera)

Platelets (thrombocytosis, usually >1 million/cmm; thrombotic thrombocytopenia purpura)

Proteins (resistance to protein C activation, Factor V Leiden; antiphospholipid syndrome, Sneddon syndrome; Waldenström macroglobulinemia)

Coagulation defects (deficiency of protein C, S and Antithrombin III, alcohol-induced prothrombotic state; paroxysmal nocturnal hemoglobinuria; plasminogen-activator inhibitor-1, PAI-1 polymorphism; prothrombin polymorphism –G20210A & 20209)

that also include the three major categories of vascular diseases: atherosclerosis; cardioembolic causes; and blood element abnormalities involving erythrocytes, platelets and proteins. Tables 42.1 and 42.2 list the various etiologies.

VASCULAR DISORDERS

Migraine, dissection, and premature atherosclerosis are prominent vascular diseases causing strokes in young adults. Complicated migraine with focal neurologic findings should not be treated with vasoconstrictive drugs, such as triptans or ergot derivatives, and should be treated with prophylactic medications, such as beta-blockers, calcium channel blockers or other vasodilators. If complicated migraine is associated with oral contraceptive use, the hormones should be discontinued. Dissection of an arterial wall should be treated with anticoagulation un-

til recanalization occurs or until occlusion is deemed permanent. Premature atherosclerosis as occurs with familial hyperlipidemia, diabetes mellitus, and hypertension is treated similarly to that occurring in older adults, such as with carotid endarterectomy, when indicated, and antiatherosclerosis measures.

Arteritis and strokes resulting from immune-complex diseases and drug abuse are more common in young adults; arteritis from immune-complex disease is usually symptomatic with strokes after systemic manifestations of the disease, such as polyarteritis nodosa, Sjögren disease and lupus erythematosus. "*Isolated angiitis* of the CNS" is unusual in frequently showing few, if any, peripheral evidences of immune-complex disorders; the cerebral angiogram results may be within normal limits, although sausage-shaped changes may be seen. Isolated angiitis of the CNS should be suspected in individuals with multifocal neurologic deficits, severe headache, and obtundation with

▌ **TABLE 42.2 Causes of Ischemic Strokes in Young Adults**

Cases	%
Atherosclerosis (esp. types II a & b, III & IV familial hypercholesterolemia; hypertensive, diabetic subjects)	20
Cardioembolic (PFO, arrhythmias, rheumatic heart disease, etc.)	20
Non-atherosclerotic arteriopathy (Migraine; dissection; etc.)	20
Prothrombotic states (Resistance to Protein C Activation, anti-phospholipid Syndrome, Protein C, S and AT III deficiency)	10
Peripartum (eclampsia, pre- & post-partum)	5
Uncertain causes	25

Modified from Leys D, et al. (2002); Hart RG, Miller VT (1983).

no discernible cause. To establish the diagnosis, a brain and leptomeningeal biopsy may be necessary, as described in Chapter 155. Treatment includes long-term steroids and occasionally, immunosuppressive drugs.

Intravenous drug abuse may lead to strokes due to arteritis or occlusive disease. Intracerebral hemorrhage may occur with drugs that raise arterial pressure, such as amphetamines and their derivatives (e.g., phenylpropanolamine and ephedra) as well as cocaine. Intravenous drug use may cause bacterial endocarditis with associated bacterial/fibrin emboli leading to mycotic aneurysms, which may rupture and cause subarachnoid hemorrhage. For drug-related strokes, the clinical history and drug screening are essential to establishing the diagnosis.

CARDIOGENIC EMBOLI

Arrhythmias, especially atrial fibrillation and sick-sinus syndrome, mitral-valve prolapse, and patent foramen ovale (PFO) are the most common cardiogenic causes of strokes in young adults. Mitral-valve prolapse is found in 15% or more of the population, detected clinically by a midsystolic click on auscultation and by mitral-leaflet billowing on 2D echocardiography. Transesophageal echocardiography may be needed to supplement transthoracic echocardiography, since this approach visualizes the posterior mitral leaflet more definitively.

Risks for embolization, congestive heart failure, and cardiac arrest are increased in the presence of leaflet redundancy; without these risks, mitral valve prolapse is relatively benign, except perhaps for tachycardia, which may be controlled with beta-antagonists. With leaflet redundancy, treatment includes antiplatelet drugs and, on occasion, anticoagulation to prevent embolization. With PFO, mechanical patency at autopsy is present in about one-fourth of the population. Paradoxic embolism

with right-to-left shunting of venous emboli occurs with larger PFOs and associated interatrial septal aneurysms. The appearance of echogenic bubbles (greater than 25) in the left atrium, after injection of vigorously shaken saline and the Valsalva maneuver, is diagnostic of PFO. Transcranial Doppler studies may detect these emboli in the middle-cerebral or carotid arteries, which is also considered diagnostic.

BLOOD ELEMENT ABNORMALITIES

Each constituent of blood may be a cause of strokes in young adults, and include erythrocytes, platelets and proteins. Erythrocyte disorders most commonly associated with strokes are sickle-cell anemia and polycythemia vera. Sickle-cell anemia is associated with a hyperviscosity state that provokes both larger arterial atherosclerosis and watershed infarcts, but subarachnoid hemorrhage may also occur. Blood transfusions and hydroxyurea to increase synthesis of fetal hemoglobin may reduce these complications. Polycythemia vera also causes vascular or stroke-like symptoms, such as TIAs, because of associated hyperviscosity. Thrombocytosis, particularly over 1 million cells/mm^3, is associated with TIAs; hyperviscosity may be treated effectively with aspirin to reduce platelet aggregation. It should be kept in mind that thrombocytosis (greater than 500,000 cells/mm^3) may be a harbinger of malignancies, such as leukemia. Other more drastic measures to reduce platelet counts if aspirin fails are: plateletpheresis, hydroxyurea, and recombinant interferon-α. Abnormalities in serum proteins also cause strokes and stroke-like symptoms by hyperviscosity but also by being prothrombotic. As shown in Table 42.1, diverse coagulation defects are associated with ischemic strokes or cortical-vein thrombosis; the most common is resistance to protein C activation, and in approximately 90% of these cases, it is due to a mutation in factor V, factor V-Leiden, in which arginine (R) is substituted by glutamine (Q) at position 506, written as R506Q. The antiphospholipid syndrome, perhaps the second most common protein abnormality causing a prothrombotic state, is as discussed above.

SUGGESTED READING

Arauz A, Murillo L, Cantú C, et al. Prospective study of single and multiple lacunar infarcts using magnetic resonance imaging. *Stroke* 2003;34:2453–2458.

Barnett HJM, Mohr JP, Stein BM, Yatsu FM. *Stroke: Pathophysiology, Diagnosis & Management,* 3rd ed. New York, Churchill-Livingstone, Inc., 1998.

Berlit P. The spectrum of vasculopathies in the differential diagnosis of vasculitis. *Semin Neurol* 1994;14:370–379.

Bogousslavsky J, Pierre P: Ischemic stroke in patients under age 45. *Neurol Clin* 1992;10:113–124.

Crowther MA, Ginsberg JS, Julian J, et al. A comparison of two intensities of warfarin for the prevention of recurrent thrombosis in patients with the antiphospholipid antibody syndrome. *N Engl J Med* 2003;349(12):1133–1138.

The French Study on Aortic Plaques in Stroke Group. Atherosclerotic disease of the aortic arch as a risk factor for recurrent ischemic stroke. *N Engl J Med* 1996;334:1216–1221.

Homma S, Sacco RL, Di Tullio MR, et al. for PFO in Cryptogenic Stroke Study (PICSS) Investigators. Effect of medical treatment in stroke patients with patent foramen ovale: PFO in Cryptogenic Stroke Study. *Circulation* 2002;105:2625–2631.

Horton SC, Bunch TJ. Patent foramen ovale and stroke. *Mayo Clinic Proceedings* 2004;79(1):79–88.

Lovett JK, Dennis MS, Sandercock PA, et al. Very early risk of stroke after a first transient ischemic attack. *Stroke* 2003;34(8):138–140.

Nguyen-Huynh MN, Fayad P, Gorelick PB, Johnston SC. Knowledge and management of transient ischemic attacks among US primary care physicians. *Neurology* 2003;61(10):1455–1456.

Rand J. The antiphospholipid syndrome. *Ann Rev Med* 2003;54:409.

Robinson RG. Neuropsychiatric consequences of stroke. *Annual Rev Med* 1997;48:217–229.

Schwartz RB. Hyperfusion encephalopathy: hypertensive encephalopathy and related conditions. *Neurologist* 2002;8(1):22–34.

Slovut DP, Olin JW. Current concepts: fibromuscular dysplasia. *N Engl J Med* 2004;350(18):1862–1871.

Toole JF, Malinow MR, Chambless LE, et al. Lowering homocysteine in patients with ischemic stroke to prevent recurrent stroke, myocardial infarction, and death: the Vitamin Intervention for Stroke Prevention (VISP) randomized controlled trial. *JAMA* 2004;291(5):565–575.

Vinters HV, Farag ES. Amyloidosis of cerebral arteries. *Adv Neurol* 2003;92:105–112.

Williams O, Brust, JCM. Hypertensive encephalopathy. *Curr Treat Options Cardiovasc Med* 2004;6(3):209–216.

Zöller B, Hillurp A, Berntorp E, Dahlbäck B. Activated protein C resistance due to a common factor V gene mutation is a major risk for venous thrombosis. *Annual Rev Med* 1997;48:45–48.

Chapter 43

Differential Diagnosis of Stroke

Mitchell S. V. Elkind and J. P. Mohr

The advent of thrombolytic therapy for acute ischemic stroke makes it urgent to differentiate cerebral infarction from hemorrhage or other causes of sudden neurologic symptoms. As treatment must be initiated within 3 hours of onset of symptoms, the diagnosis must be made rapidly. Libman et al. studied 411 patients who were diagnosed with stroke in an emergency room. Of those, a full 19% were determined to have one of several stroke "mimics." The most frequent diagnostic errors included seizures, systemic infection, brain tumor, and toxic-metabolic encephalopathy. Less frequent sources of misdiagnosis were positional vertigo, cardiac events, syncope, trauma,

subdural hematoma, herpes simplex virus encephalitis, transient global amnesia, dementia, demyelinating disease, cervical spine fracture, myasthenia gravis, parkinsonism, hypertensive encephalopathy, and conversion disorder. In multivariate analysis, factors that predicted a "true stroke" were the presence of angina and absence of loss of consciousness.

TYPES OF STROKE

Within the category of cerebral infarction, the diagnosis of *cerebral embolism* is suggested by sudden onset and a syndrome of circumscribed focal signs attributable to cerebral surface infarction, such as pure aphasia or pure hemianopia. A diagnosis of embolism is important because the risk of recurrence is high. The source of the embolus may be found in atrial fibrillation, acute or chronic endocarditis, recent myocardial infarction, or paradoxic embolism via a patent foramen ovale. Atrial fibrillation accounts for up to 24% of cerebral infarction in the elderly.

The brain is the first site of symptoms in most cases of systemic embolism; clinically recognized embolization at other anatomic sites is rare. When the source of embolization is not obvious on hospital admission, useful procedures include routine blood cultures, EEG monitoring, and echocardiography. The size of the embolic material sufficient to cause a focal stroke is often too small to detect the exact source and all too often eludes diagnosis. The cause of the embolus may not be determined in a third or more of cases, despite full use of laboratory investigations. When conducted within 24 hours of stroke onset, angiography usually demonstrates a pattern of arterial occlusion that is typical of embolus and permits diagnosis, but angiography is infrequently used. CT or MRI shows focal infarction and allows inference of the size of the occluded artery. CT and MRI show infarction within 24 hours if the occluded artery supplies a brain region large enough to cause a deficit that persists for several days.

A diagnosis of thrombosis is considered first when the stroke has been preceded by TIAs. When the syndrome is of sudden onset, thrombus is clinically inseparable from embolus. Thrombosis leading to stroke may occur in the extracranial cervical vessels, the intracranial arteries of the circle of Willis, or in the small vessels arising from the circle of Willis. The clinical syndrome associated with large artery thrombosis may be indistinguishable from that caused by embolism. Small penetrating-vessel infarcts, however, or "lacunar infarcts," usually spare cortical functions such as language and cognition. Instead, they tend to cause loss of elementary neurologic function. Symptoms include weakness, sensory loss, or ataxia affecting half of the body. Up to 25% of patients with lacunar infarcts have large-vessel disease or a cardioembolic source, so it is important to carry out a complete etiologic evaluation in all stroke patients.

Hemorrhage has a characteristically smooth onset, a helpful historical point in differential diagnosis. When the syndrome develops to an advanced stage within minutes or is halted at an early stage with only minor signs, the smooth evolution may not be apparent, and the clinical picture may then be inseparable from that of infarction. The hyperdense signal of blood on CT may immediately separate the clinically inobvious hemorrhage from infarct, and thus CT should be used whenever treatment with anticoagulants is planned. Exceptional cases have been reported in which the typical hyperdensity of intracerebral hemorrhage was absent, owing to severe anemia, but this is unlikely to cause problems clinically. There are no reliable CT findings to distinguish hemorrhagic infarction and frank hematoma. The greater sensitivity to blood signal of MRI shows hemorrhagic infarction more frequently than CT does.

The sudden onset and the focal signs give these syndromes the popular term, stroke, and distinguish cerebrovascular disease from other neurologic disorders. Hypertension, cardiac disease, arteriosclerosis, or other evidence of vascular disease are commonly present with cerebrovascular disease, unlike other neurologic causes of focal cerebral disorders.

THE DISTINCTION BETWEEN STROKE AND TRANSIENT ISCHEMIC ATTACK (TIA)

As described also in Chapter 38, the definition of TIA has been revised in the past decade. The distinction between TIA and completed stroke has, in general, been rendered less important for several reasons. First, MRI detects small, fixed lesions that would have been missed previously. The traditional definition of TIA as a focal deficit lasting up to 24 hours exaggerates the time needed for infarction to appear on MRI. Up to 50% of patients with transient deficits lasting less than 24 hours have evidence of ischemia on diffusion-weighted (DWI) and 50% of those with DWI abnormalities have evidence of fixed infarction on subsequent T2-weighted images. Similar results have been seen in large multicenter trials using both CT and MRI. In fact, one-third of all patients with symptoms lasting less than an hour show abnormalities on DWI.

Second, Johnston et al. found that the risk of stroke and other vascular events is as high or higher after TIA as after completed stroke, casting doubt on the justification for a more leisurely approach to the evaluation and treatment of patients with TIA. The risk of stroke after TIA is approximately 10% at 90 days; half of these occur within the first 2 days. An impressive 25% of TIA patients suffer stroke or another adverse vascular outcome in 90 days.

Five risk factors independently predict patients who are at highest risk for stroke after TIA: age over 60 years, diabetes mellitus, symptom duration more than 10 minutes, and residual weakness or speech disturbance. Further evidence from retrospective analyses of clinical trial databases (Johnston 2003) also suggests that patients who show substantial recovery from acute ischemic stroke, including TIA patients, have a greater risk of subsequent neurologic deterioration than patients with less recovery, possibly because an unstable vascular lesion is responsible.

For these and other reasons, it is clear that TIA is not as previously assumed, a benign condition. Some authorities have advised a change in the definition that emphasizes the presence or absence of biologic injury, rather than symptom duration, as the basis for diagnosis. The proposed new definition (Albers 2002) states that TIA is a "brief episode of neurologic dysfunction caused by focal brain or retinal ischemia, with clinical symptoms typically lasting less than one hour, and without evidence of acute infarction." It is hoped that this new concept of TIA will encourage more aggressive and expeditious treatment for TIA and facilitate better outcomes.

PEELING THE ONION

In patients who have experienced a prior infarct or hemorrhage, subsequent metabolic derangements or infections may precipitate a recrudescence of the original stroke syndrome. Hypoglycemia, hyponatremia, urinary tract infection, pneumonia, and starting new anxiolytic or other psychotropic medications are common precipitants of this phenomenon. The patient quickly returns to normal when the insult is reversed. This phenomenon has been labeled "peeling the onion," to reflect the way in which the layers of function are removed. Therefore, it is clinically important to carry out a thorough evaluation of possible metabolic and infectious causes of neurologic deterioration in all patients with a history of earlier brain injury, before seeking to diagnose a new neurologic event.

Lazar et al. reproduced this phenomenon experimentally by injecting a short-acting benzodiazepine (midazolam), suggesting that this reversal in function may be mediated through GABAergic mechanisms. They also demonstrated in a small number of patients with TIA without any imaged evidence of structural brain injury that the same recurrence of symptoms followed with midazolam challenge. This suggests that TIA may be associated with changes in brain function even when structural injury is not seen by MRI, again broadening of the definition of TIA.

NONVASCULAR DISORDERS IN THE DIFFERENTIAL DIAGNOSIS OF STROKE

Sudden neurologic symptom onset also characterizes trauma, epilepsy, and migraine. External signs usually indicate trauma but when absent, diagnosis depends on a history that is not always easily obtained. Signs of external trauma need not be present for acceleration-deceleration forces to cause focal traumatic injury. The most frequent sites of brain contusions are the frontal and temporal poles, but these lesions neither produce an easily recognized clinical picture nor one often encountered in cases of stroke; however, traumatic epidural and subdural hematomas may mimic stroke. Although the trauma itself is sudden, the accumulation of the hematoma takes time: minutes or hours for epidural hemorrhage, and as long as weeks for subdural hemorrhage.

Epidural hemorrhage is arterial in origin and usually produces a blood mass large enough to displace the brain and cause coma within hours after the injury. Apart from slower evolution, the clinical picture is otherwise similar to that of putaminal hemorrhage. Radiographs of the skull may reveal a fracture line that passes through the groove of the middle meningeal artery, which is usually a laceration. CT is the most helpful radiologic test, demonstrating the position of the hematoma in all cases and giving the diagnosis even in comatose patients, when the fine points of clinical examination may not be used. Surgical evacuation of the hematoma is usually appropriate even with severe brain injury because the dysfunction is due primarily to compression and the syndrome may be reversible when pressure from the hematoma is relieved.

Subdural hematoma is typically venous in origin. The bleeding may be recurrent. The precipitating trauma may have been trivial or forgotten by the patient, and the blood may have been present long enough (over a week) to become isodense (radiographically inapparent) on CT or MRI. Fluctuating and false localizing signs are frequent. Further, a clot may be found on both sides. These common features often make subdural hematoma difficult to diagnose. Lumbar puncture shows a range of findings from normal to the extremes of xanthochromic CSF under high pressure, with increased protein content. MRI has displaced angiography as the best way to show displacement of the brain away from the skull.

As a sign of acute stroke, *seizures* are rare except in cases of lobar hemorrhage. The immediate postictal deficit mimics that caused by major stroke. Only the obtundation and amnestic state, or evidence of tongue-biting, help suggest prior seizure. In a few cases, seizures develop months or years after a large infarct or hemorrhage. In these, the postictal state is often a relapse of the original stroke syndrome, which usually resolves toward the chronic preictal state after a few days. Without a proper history, it may be impossible to rule out new stroke. Rarely, seizures in a patient with a prior stroke appear to have caused a long-lasting or permanent worsening or intensification of the prior deficit, without evidence of recurrent infarction. It is not known how this unusual event occurs.

Migraine is increasingly appreciated as a major source of difficulty in the diagnosis of TIA. Migraine may begin in middle age; the aura alone, without headache, is commonly experienced by those who suffer chronic migraine. When symptoms are visual and a diagnosis of transient monocular blindness is considered, the differential diagnosis from migraine is the easiest; migraine typically produces a visual disorder that marches across the vision of both eyes as an advancing, thin, scintillating line that takes 5 to 15 minutes to pass out of vision. Subsequent unilateral, pounding headache may not occur but makes the diagnosis certain, when it does. It is difficult to diagnose migraine as a cause of symptoms of hemisphere dysfunction because the auras of classic migraine only rarely include motor, sensory, language, or behavioral elements. TIA rarely goes from one limb to another in a manner like the visual disorder of migraine. A diagnosis of migraine probably should not be considered as an explanation for transient hemisphere attacks unless the patient is young, has repeated attacks, experiences classic visual migraine auras at other times, and has a pounding headache contralateral to the sensory or motor symptoms in the hours after the attack. Studies of conditions long recognized clinically, such as familial hemiplegic migraine and the familial periodic ataxias, have demonstrated mutations in ion channel genes as the cause of some cases of transient strokelike deficits. Familial hemiplegic migraine, for example, is caused by a mutation in a calcium-channel gene on chromosome 19. These syndromes are generally recognized by the recurrence of stereotyped episodes throughout life, in people with an appropriate family history. Occasionally, sporadic cases may be seen in which the diagnosis of TIA has been entertained for years.

As indicated above, brain tumor and abscess may mimic TIA or stroke. Both usually evolve in days or weeks, which is longer than stroke, but may start with acute transient symptoms. It is commonly thought but rarely proven that intratumoral hemorrhage or focal seizure is responsible for many of these cases. One helpful historic point is that seizures often occur before focal signs are evident, a sequence that is rare in stroke. CT in tumor or abscess usually demonstrates an enhancing mass even when symptoms are mild. In contrast, CT in ischemic stroke is often negative in the first few days; contrast enhancement may not occur, and there are signs of a mass only when the syndrome is severe.

In parenchymatous hemorrhage, the areas around the hematoma do not usually enhance with contrast material, but contrast enhancement is common when hemorrhage has occurred into a tumor. If the CSF is examined, increased pressure and clear or slightly cloudy fluid are encountered equally in tumors, early abscesses, and large infarcts. The CSF usually shows mild or moderate pleocytosis in abscess, but the same findings may be present in large infarcts.

When coma is present, other diagnoses that must be considered include: metabolic alterations of glucose, renal function, electrolytes, alcohol, and drugs. The odor of acetone on the breath and the presence of sugar in the urine favor a diagnosis of diabetes mellitus. Transient mild glycosuria and hyperglycemia often follow cerebral hemorrhage or infarction but do not approach the elevations seen in diabetic coma. In renal failure, high levels of blood urea nitrogen (BUN) and creatinine often cause coma. Focal signs occasionally occur, and then remit when the cause is reversed, often accompanying unrecognized infection or severe disturbances in electrolyte balance.

Not uncommonly, however, focal deficits do not reverse immediately, particularly when the metabolic derangement, such as hypoglycemia, has been profound. An alcoholic odor to the breath, normal blood pressure, no evidence of hemiplegia, and a normal CSF are characteristic findings in cases of coma due to acute alcoholism. In barbiturate intoxication, the coma may feature total paralysis of ocular motility and flaccid paralysis of the limbs with preserved pupillary reactions, which is a rare combination in stroke. The CSF pressure may be slightly elevated (200 mm H_2O to 300 mm H_2O) in any form of coma due to hypoventilation and CO_2 retention. Because alcoholics and drug abusers are prone to head injuries, the diagnosis of subdural hematoma should always be considered and excluded with appropriate imaging tests.

SUGGESTED READINGS

Albers GW, Caplan LR, Easton JD, et al. Transient ischemic attack—proposal for a new definition. *N Engl J Med* 2002;347:1713–1716.

Bogousslavsky J, Martin R, Regli F, et al. Persistent worsening of stroke sequelae after delayed seizures. *Arch Neurol* 1992;49:385–388.

Caplan LR. "Top of the basilar" syndrome. *Neurology* 1980;30:72–79.

Gan R, Sacco RL, Kargman DE, et al. Testing the validity of the lacunar hypothesis: the Northern Manhattan Stroke Study experience. *Neurology* 1997;48:1204–1211.

Homma S, Di Tullio MR, Sacco RL, et al. Characteristics of patent foramen ovale associated with cryptogenic stroke. *Stroke* 1994;25:582–586.

Johnston SC, Gress DR, Browner WS, Sidney S. et al. Short-term prognosis after emergency department diagnosis of TIA. *JAMA* 2000;284:2901–2906.

Johnston SC, Leira EC, Hansen MD, Adams HP Jr. Early recovery after cerebral ischemia risk of subsequent neurological deterioration. *Ann Neurol* 2003;54:439–444.

Kasdon DL, Scott RM, Adelman LS, et al. Cerebellar hemorrhage with decreased absorption values on computed tomography: a case report. *Neuroradiology* 1977;13:265–266.

Kidwell CS, Alger JR, Di Salle F, Starkman S, Villablanca P, Bentson J, Saver JL. Diffusion MRI in patients with transient ischemic attacks. *Stroke* 1999;30:1174–1180.

Labovitz DL, Hauser WA, Sacco RL. Prevalence and predictors of early seizure and status epilepticus after first stroke. *Neurology* 2001;57:200–206.

Lazar RM, Fitzsimmons BF, Marshall RS, et al. Reemergence of stroke deficits with midazolam challenge. *Stroke* 2002;33:283–285.

Lazar RM, Fitzsimmons BF, Marshall RS, et al. Midazolam challenge reinduces neurological deficits after transient ischemic attack. *Stroke* 2003;34:794–796.

Libman RB, Wirkowski E, Alvir J, Rao TH. Conditions that mimic stroke in the ED. *Arch Neurol* 1995;52:1119–1122.

Mohr JP, Thompson JLP, Lazar RM, et al. A comparison of warfarin and aspirin for the prevention of recurrent ischemic stroke. *N Engl J Med* 2001;345:1444–1451.

Ophoff RA, Terwindt GM, Vergouwe MN. Familial hemiplegic migraine and episodic ataxia type-2 are caused by mutations in the Ca^{2+} channel gene CACNL1A4. *Cell* 1996;87:543–552.

Rogers LR, Cho ES, Kempin S, Posner JB. Cerebral infarction from nonbacterial thrombotic endocarditis. Clinical and pathological study including the effects of anticoagulation. *Am J Med* 1987;83:746–756.

Terwindt GM, Ophoff RA, Haan J, et al. Variable clinical expression of mutations in the P/Q-type calcium channel gene in familial hemiplegic migraine. Dutch Migraine Genetics Research Group. *Neurology* 1998;50:1105–1110.

Warach S, Kidwell CS. The redefinition of TIA: the uses and limitations of DWI in acute ischemic cerebrovascular syndromes. *Neurology* 2004;62:359–360.

Wijman CAC, Wolf PA, Kase CS, Kelly-Hayes M, Beiser AS. Migrainous visual accompaniments are not rare in late life. The Framingham Study. *Stroke* 1998;29:1539–1543.

Wolf PA, Abbott RD, and Kannel WB. Atrial fibrillation as an independent risk factor for stroke: the Framingham Study. *Stroke* 1991;22:983–988.

Chapter 4 4

▶ Stroke in Children

Arnold P. Gold and Marc C. Patterson

Children are not "small adults" when it comes to the diagnosis of stroke. In contrast to adults, the brain of the fetus or child is rapidly changing in organization and chemical composition. Neurologic functions change with neurologic maturation. The nervous system of a nonverbal, relatively spastic newborn is different from that of a school-aged child who has mastered language skills and has purposeful locomotion and prehension.

STROKE IN CHILDREN

Strokes in children differ from those in adults in three important ways: predisposing factors, clinical evolution, and anatomic site of pathology.

Cyanotic heart disease is one of the most common childhood conditions that predisposes to cerebral arterial or venous thrombosis. Leukemia commonly leads to cerebral hemorrhage. In contrast, diabetes, atherosclerosis, and hypertension predispose to stroke in adults.

Most stroke-prone children do not die as a direct result of stroke; they often improve much more than an adult with a comparable lesion because of the abundant collateral circulation or because of the differences in response of the immature brain to the lesion. The infant or young child with a new hemiplegia usually recovers to the point of being able to walk. Even though the outcome of a stroke is better in children than in adults, as many as half of all children with stroke have lifelong disability, and a third have recurrent strokes. In contrast to earlier reports, new studies suggest that children younger than 5 years old experience as many, if not more, difficulties with language acquisition after hemispheric stroke as do older children. Cognitive and social impairments are also frequent sequelae of stroke in early childhood.

The anatomic site of the stroke lesion also differs in children. For example, affected children commonly show occlusion of the intracranial portion of the internal carotid artery and its branches, whereas adults more frequently show extracranial occlusions of the internal carotid. Cerebral aneurysms in children usually occur at the peripheral bifurcations of cerebral arteries; in adults, cerebral aneurysms usually occur near the circle of Willis.

INCIDENCE

In a well-defined pediatric population in Rochester, Minnesota, the annual incidence of cerebrovascular disease was 2.52 cases per 100,000 children, or about 50% of the incidence of primary intracranial neoplasm. This figure did not include conditions associated with birth, infection, or trauma, and there were few African American children in the study. Sickle cell disease (SCD) is an important risk factor for stroke in children of African descent. A newborn inception cohort of 711 children with SCD from Dallas, Texas had a stroke incidence of 85 per 100 patient-years, with an 88.5% stroke-free survival to 18 years. Premature infants weighing less than 1500 g, who require intensive care for more than 24 hours, have a 50% incidence of complicating subependymal hemorrhage or intraventricular hemorrhage. Intracranial infections, viral or bacterial, may also precipitate vascular complications. Craniocerebral trauma occurs in 3% of children during the first 7 years of life and cerebrovascular complications are common. Sonography, MRI, MRA and CT (Figs. 44.1 through 44.4) have changed concepts of the incidence of these disorders in children.

CLINICAL EVALUATION

A variety of studies should be considered in the evaluation of a child with stroke (Table 44.1). Selection of tests is guided by the clinical situation.

Coagulopathy should be excluded as the cause of vasoocclusive or hemorrhagic infarctions in the newborn and young infant. Tissue injury occurs much more frequently from hypoxia and ischemia in the asphyxiated newborn. Vasculitis is an uncommon cause of stroke in

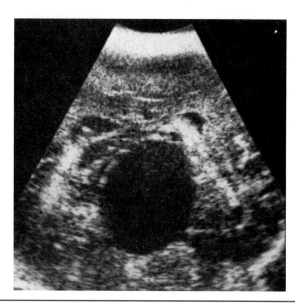

FIGURE 44-1. Coronal cranial sonogram of newborn demonstrates aneurysmal dilatation of vein of Galen due to deep midline vascular malformation.

young children. The possibility of embolic phenomena is increased with cardiac anomaly, particularly in the presence of a midline defect, which acts as a portal for paradoxic emboli. Older infants and children are susceptible to stroke events when there is a coagulopathy, but they also are more susceptible to vasculitis, which may result from immunologic or infectious causes.

ETIOLOGY

More than 100 risk factors for stroke have been identified in children, but the etiology remains obscure in at least half of the cases in large series. A rigid classification of childhood stroke is not possible because a specific cause (e.g., SCD) may cause hemorrhage in one child, and thrombosis in another. Nevertheless, the following list is a clinically useful classification, and includes occlusive vascular disease caused by thrombus or embolus, congenital anomalies (especially aneurysm or vascular malformation), hemorrhage, blood dyscrasias, and disorders that alter the permeability of the vascular wall:

Dural sinus and cerebral venous thrombosis
    Infections—face, ears, paranasal sinuses, meninges
    Dehydration and debilitating states
    Blood dyscrasias—sickle cell, leukemia, thrombotic
        thrombocytopenia
    Neoplasms (neuroblastoma)
    Sturge-Weber-Dimitri (trigeminal encephaloangiomatosis)
    Lead encephalopathy
    Vein of Galen malformation

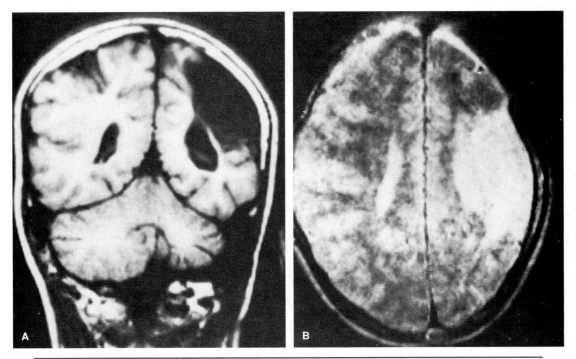

FIGURE 44-2. **MRI of a child with middle cerebral artery thrombosis and resultant hemiplegia with ischemic infarct. A:** T1-weighted coronal image. **B:** Axial T2-weighted image of left middle cerebral artery ischemic infarct.

Arterial thrombosis
  Idiopathic
  Dissecting cerebral aneurysm
  Arteriosclerosis—progeria
  Cyanotic heart disease
  Cerebral arteritis

Collagen disease—lupus erythematosus, periarteritis nodosa, Takayasu, Kawasaki
Trauma to cervical carotid or cerebral arteries
Inflammatory bowel disease
Delayed radiation
SCD
Extra-arterial disorders—craniometaphyseal dysplasia, mucormycosis, tumors of the base of the skull
Metabolic
  Diabetes mellitus

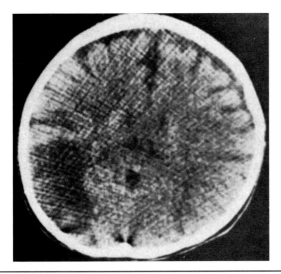

FIGURE 44-3. **Middle cerebral artery thrombosis of 24-hour duration.** CT reveals inhomogeneous hypodensity with hazy margins in the parietooccipital region (early scanner, right and left reversed).

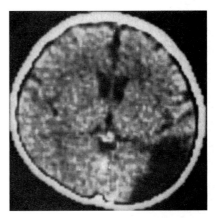

FIGURE 44-4. **Middle cerebral artery thrombosis, 3-week duration.** CT (same child as in Fig. 44.3 but with different scanner) shows homogeneous lucency with sharp well-defined margins.

▶ **TABLE 44.1** **Studies in the Evaluation of a Child with Stroke**

LABORATORY STUDIES	URINALYSIS
BLOOD SCREEN	Amino Acids
Coagulation Profile	Organic Acids
Fibrinogen	Homocysteine
Plasma-phase factors	
Factor V Leiden	CEREBROSPINAL FLUID ASSAY
Prothrombin 20210A	Chemistries (glucose, protein)
Lipoprotein (a)	Cell count and differential
Antithrombin III	Lactate
Protein C	Cultures
Protein S	
Plasminogen activator	**RADIOLOGIC STUDIES**
inhibitor –	CT, head
	MRI head
Anticardiolipin	MR angiogram/MR venogram
Antibody	Cerebral angiogram
Lipid Profile	
Homocysteine	**ULTRASOUND STUDIES**
	Carotid artery Doppler
Antinuclear Antibody	Vertebral artery Doppler
Lupus erythematosus	Transcranial Doppler
preparation	Echocardiogram
Erythrocyte	
sedimentation rate	**NUCLEAR MEDICINE STUDIES**
Amino acids	SPECT
Organic acids	
Blood cultures	**ELECTRICAL STUDIES**
Toxicology screen	EEG
Sickle-cell Preparation	
Mitochondrial DNA	
studies	

Hyperlipidemia
Homocysteinuria
CDG 1a (phosphomannomutase deficiency)
Sulfite oxidase deficiency
Molybdenum cofactor deficiency
Oral contraceptives
Drug abuse
Arterial embolism
    Air—complications of cardiac, neck, or thoracic surgery
    Fat-complications of long-bone fracture
    Septic complications of endocarditis, pneumonia, lung
      abscess
    Arrhythmias
    Complications of umbilical vein catheterization
Intracranial hemorrhage
    Neonatal
    Premature—subependymal and intraventricular
    Full term—subdural
    Vascular malformation
    Aneurysm
Blood dyscrasias
Trauma
Vitamin-deficiency syndromes
Hepatic disease

Hypertension
Complications of immunosuppressants and anticoagulants
Mitochondrial disease
MELAS
Migraine

ARTERIAL THROMBOSIS

Cerebral arterial thrombosis in children usually involves the intracranial area of the internal carotid artery, although the cervical portion of the internal carotid artery or a spinal artery may be occluded. Neurologic manifestations vary according to the area involved.

As in adults, systemic diseases, including collagen-vascular diseases and arteritis, may cause cerebral thrombosis in children. Cerebral arteritis usually results from bacterial infections, but other infections may also involve cerebral arteries. Herpes zoster ophthalmica and rarely chickenpox may have complicating vasculitis that causes delayed-onset hemiparesis. Bacterial pharyngitis, cervical adenitis, sinusitis, or pneumonitis may lead to cerebral arteritis. Mucormycosis infection associated with uncontrolled diabetes may extend from the paranasal sinuses to the arteries in the frontal lobe. Both syphilis and tuberculosis may result in cerebral thrombosis in children and adults.

Extrinsic conditions may traumatize or compress the cerebral arteries. Most of these occlusions in children affect the anterior circulation. Vertebrobasilar occlusion may follow cervical dislocations and occlusion of the vertebral artery at the C2 level. Tumors of the base of the skull, craniometaphyseal dysplasia, and retropharyngeal abscesses may compress cerebral arteries.

Sickle cell disease (SCD) commonly causes thrombosis of large or small arteries; less commonly, it results in dural-sinus thrombosis. 7% to 11% of patients with SCD have stroke before the age of 20 years. Large, cerebral artery thrombosis with telangiectasia (moyamoya) results in acute hemiplegia or alternating hemiplegia (Fig. 44.5).

Small arterial thrombosis may produce an altered state of consciousness, convulsions, or visual disturbances. About 65% of untreated children have repeated thromboses with additional impairment of motor and intellectual functions. Radiographic progression in the absence of clinically overt deficits suggests an increase in the stroke risk with time, and underscores the importance of treatment. Cerebrovascular complications are less common in children with sickle hemoglobin C disease and rarely occur in sickle cell trait. MRI, magnetic resonance angiography (MRA), and diffusion-weighted imaging (DWI) have become invaluable tools in defining stroke events in children, and transcranial Doppler is a useful adjunct for follow-up examination and screening.

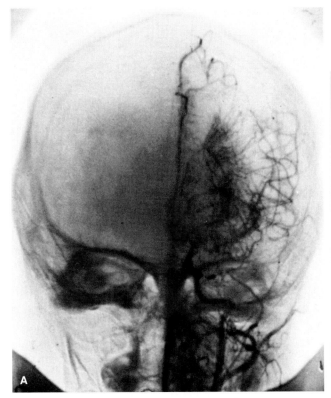
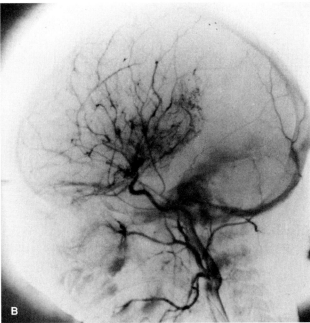

FIGURE 44-5. Moyamoya syndrome. Anteroposterior **(A)** and lateral **(B)** views from arterial phase of left common carotid arteriogram demonstrate multiple enlarged and serpentine lenticulostriate arteries, which have a "puff of smoke" appearance. Note occlusions of the proximal segments of the anterior and middle cerebral arteries.

Migraine may be manifested by hemiplegia or visual field defects. MRI changes are nonspecific, but punctate periventricular white matter changes are often attributed to migraine. MELAS should be considered when stroke accompanies migraine in a child.

Inflammatory bowel disease may lead to a hypercoagulable state with or without thrombocytosis. Delayed radiation vasculopathy, juvenile diabetes mellitus, homocystinuria, hyperlipidemia, drug abuse, and oral contraceptives result in acute hemiplegia.

Malignancies, most commonly lymphoreticular tumors, may be complicated by a cerebral infarct. Most often this is a complication of disseminated vascular occlusion or chemotherapy. Stroke may also result from direct metastatic spread or a complicating thrombocytopenia or fungal infection.

Coagulopathies may become evident with a thrombotic event. Protein C and protein S deficiencies increase the risk of stroke in childhood. Factor V-Leiden deficiency also predisposes to cerebral vessel thrombosis.

Many children with cerebral arterial thrombosis are healthy before the vascular occlusion occurs, and there is no apparent predisposing factor. A dissecting aneurysm arising from a congenital defect of the arterial wall has been implicated in some of these idiopathic cases.

Signs and Symptoms

Depending on the predisposing factor, the child with arterial thrombosis has specific clinical signs of the underlying disorder plus neurologic signs of the occluded cerebral artery that are usually found in the anterior circulation. A previously healthy child usually has an acute hemiplegia that is preceded by focal or generalized convulsions, fever, and altered consciousness; less commonly, a series of TIAs eventually results in a completed stroke. Acute hemiplegia is the typical neurologic finding, but hemisensory loss, visual field defects, and aphasia may be seen. The disorder maximally involves the hand; if it persists, the involved limbs are spastic, short, and atrophic. Seizures, focal or generalized, are often refractory to anticonvulsants.

The hemiplegia is usually an isolated episode. Bilateral carotid-artery thrombosis with telangiectasia typically presents with headaches before the hemiplegia, and recurrences or alternating hemiplegia is characteristic.

Laboratory Data

Blood count, erthrocyte sedimentation rate (ESR), and urinalysis are within normal limits at the time of thrombosis. The CSF is normal at first, and a mild leukocyte pleocytosis may occur a few weeks later. The EEG often reveals a slow-wave focus over the involved area. Although skull radiographs are within normal limits when thrombosis occurs, after several years they may show signs of cerebral atrophy, with thickening of calvarium, enlargement of the frontal and ethmoid sinuses, and elevation of the petrous pyramid of the temporal bone on the involved side.

CT supplies information about the site and age of the infarct. Within 24 hours there is a nonhomogeneous decreased-density lesion, secondary to edema (Fig. 44.3). By the end of the first week, liquefaction necrosis develops, and the infarct becomes homogeneous with defined margins (Fig. 44.4). At 3 months, the necrotic infarct is replaced by a cystic, fluid-containing cavity, and the lesion with sharp margins has the homogeneous density of CSF.

Sonography is invaluable in defining cerebral anatomy and hemorrhagic complications in the infant, especially in the premature infant (Fig. 44.1). MRI is an important diagnostic tool in the early diagnosis of ischemic lesions (Fig. 44.2). MRA is useful in defining the major portions of large- and medium-sized vessels of the intracranial circulation. Magnetic resonance venography is helpful in the diagnosis of venous sinus thrombosis if there are changes in vascular outflow. DWI (MR) is gaining prominence in diagnostic evaluation. Echo-planar DWI reveals acute and hyperacute ischemia not seen on conventional spin-echo imaging.

Arteriography, when performed early, may demonstrate the thrombosed cerebral artery; later there may be a recanalized vessel or evidence of collateral circulation. Cerebral angiography may usually be performed safely in children of all ages. Patency of other cerebral arteries and the ample collateral circulation in children contrast with the status of the cerebral arteries and collateral circulation in adult stroke patients. Children with SCD are at greater risk if the hemoglobin S is not maintained at a level below 20%, by exchange transfusion.

The following practical angiographic classification was formulated by Hilal et al. in 1971, to supply diagnostic and prognostic information for the following patterns.

Extracranial Occlusion

Trauma is the most common cause of thrombosis of the cervical portion of the internal carotid artery. Blunt trauma in the paratonsillar area of the oropharynx, or direct impact of the carotid artery against the transverse process of the second cervical segment, may cause occlusion. Characteristically, about 24 hours lapse between the traumatic incident and clinical manifestations. Nontraumatic conditions are usually infectious in origin.

Basal Occlusion Disease Without Telangiectasia

The thrombotic lesion involves the arteries of the base of the brain, as follows: supraclinoid area of the internal carotid artery, proximal segments of anterior or middle cerebral artery, or basilar artery. The condition is unilateral and does not recur.

Basal Occlusive Disease with Telangiectasia (Moyamoya)

This condition involves the arteries at the base of the brain, is often bilateral, and is associated with prominent telangiectasia, especially in the region of the basal ganglia (Fig. 44.5). Of varied etiology, it may complicate SCD, bacterial or tuberculous meningitis, or neurofibromatosis; it may also complicate the treatment plans of radiotherapy. Recurrent episodes of thrombosis are common and may result in alternating hemiplegia, epilepsy, and learning disabilities. Neuropsychologic testing has demonstrated the benefit of surgical intervention in preventing further deterioration of function.

Peripheral Leptomeningeal Artery Occlusions

Branch occlusions of the distal leptomeningeal arteries may occur with diabetes mellitus, SCD, trauma, infection, tumor encasement, or neurocutaneous syndromes. The excellent collateral circulation in children usually results in rapid recovery from the acute hemiplegia.

Perforating Artery Occlusion

Involvement of the small perforating arteries, most commonly the striate arteries, is seen in children with homocysteinuria or periarteritis nodosa. Episodes recur, causing a progressive neurologic deficit with alternating hemiparesis or quadriparesis, subarachnoid hemorrhage, or death.

Treatment

Therapeutic measures may include parenteral fluids, antibiotics when indicated, anticonvulsants, anticoagulants to prevent extension of the thrombus, and variations of the agents to control increased intracranial pressure. Revascularization procedures called *synangiosis* are used to enhance circulation to ischemic areas of the brain in moyamoya. Anastomoses of external carotid to internal carotid arteries are not feasible because the arteries leading to a child's brain are too narrow. Instead, the superficial temporal artery is attached to the surface of the brain, allowing the formation of a rich collateral network that supplies parts of the brain that would otherwise be ischemic.

Anticoagulants are rarely indicated, except in the older child and adolescent, or when a stroke is in progress.

Rarely does arterial thrombosis result in sufficiently increased pressure to require intracranial pressure monitoring or measures to reduce intracranial pressure. Bilateral cervical sympathectomies to increase regional blood flow and anastomosis of the external and internal carotid arteries have been of dubious value.

Sickle cell disease is treated by repeated blood transfusions. The risk of future strokes is reduced by a long-term transfusion program, to maintain hemoglobin S at a level below 20%. This has been documented in clinical trials that tracked cumulative neurologic deficits and imaging evidence of ischemic injury.

CEREBRAL EMBOLISM

In cerebral embolism, an artery may be occluded by air, fat, tumor, bacteria, parasites, foreign body, or a fragment from an organized thrombus. The middle cerebral artery, or its branches, are most commonly involved.

Cerebral embolism in childhood is usually cardiogenic, especially after cardiac catheterization or open heart surgery but is also seen with cardiac arrhythmias resulting from cyanotic congenital heart disease or rheumatic valvular disease, bacterial endocarditis, or atrial myxoma. Septic embolism from pulmonary inflammatory disease or bacterial endocarditis may result in brain abscesses or mycotic aneurysms. Fat embolism is an unusual complication of long-bone fractures.

Signs and Symptoms

The focal neurologic signs vary according to the artery occluded; manifestations are complete within seconds or minutes. There are also signs and symptoms of the causal disorder: transient blindness with air embolism; petechiae and hematuria with septic emboli; cutaneous petechiae, urinary free fat, and fat in the retinal vessels, with fat emboli caused by long-bone fracture or intravenous fat infusions.

Fat embolism has a characteristic clinical picture. A lucid interval of 12 to 48 hours occurs after a long-bone fracture. The child then becomes febrile with pulmonary symptoms that include dyspnea, cyanosis, and blood-tinged sputum. Within a few hours, there is an acute encephalopathy that may include focal neurologic signs, diabetes insipidus, seizures, delirium, stupor, or coma.

Laboratory Data

Routine laboratory studies after cerebral embolism are often within normal limits, but a moderate polymorphonuclear leukocytosis may be present. The CSF is usually normal, but there may be a mild elevation of the protein content. Septic embolism in bacterial endocarditis may cause an elevated CSF protein content and pleocytosis.

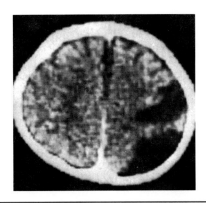

FIGURE 44-6. Cerebral embolism. CT 3 months after cerebral embolism shows multiple infarcts. Sharp margins have density of CSF.

Atrial myxomas commonly show peripheral blood leukocytosis, anemia, and an elevated ESR. The electroencephalogram characteristically shows a slow-wave abnormality in the areas supplied by the occluded vessel.

Transthoracic echocardiogram or the more sensitive transesophageal echocardiogram should be performed on all children to exclude underlying cardiac disease. MRI is often characteristic in showing multiple infarcts, some of which are hemorrhagic (Fig. 44.6).

The lesions become lucent, with sharp margins, 2 to 3 months later. DWI and fluid attenuated inversion recovery (FLAIR) MRI studies assist the rapid detection of stroke events. Lesions that conform to a territorial distribution are the sequelae of embolic strokes. Cerebral angiography should be performed in all children with septic emboli. It delineates the occluded artery and may demonstrate mycotic aneurysm.

Treatment

Management of cerebral embolism is primarily symptomatic, including anticonvulsants for seizures. Anticoagulants are rarely used in children, except for patients who are older. Corticosteroids, in dosages used in the management of cerebral edema, are effective in reversing the pulmonary symptoms of fat embolism.

INTRACRANIAL HEMORRHAGE

Hemorrhagic stroke in children usually results from trauma or bleeding disorders. When these conditions are excluded, intracranial hemorrhage is caused by an arteriovenous malformation or aneurysm.

Signs and Symptoms

The child with subarachnoid hemorrhage usually presents with acute onset of headache, vomiting, stupor or coma, and convulsions. Findings include stiff neck, Brudzinski and Kernig signs. Extensor-plantar responses and

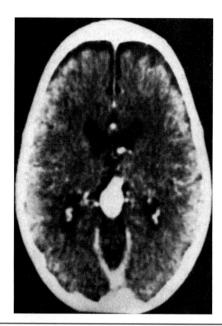

FIGURE 44-7. **Arteriovenous malformation.** CT shows aneurysmal dilatation of vein of Galen due to large, deep malformation. Note enlargement of draining sinuses and mild hydrocephalus with ventricular enlargement.

subhyaloid hemorrhages on funduscopic examination are often noted early. Fever and systemic hypertension are nonspecific findings. Ruptured cerebral aneurysm frequently presents with a catastrophic clinical picture. Bleeding from an arteriovenous malformation is less dramatic and is often associated with focal signs.

Laboratory Data

Blood dyscrasias are identified by appropriate blood studies. Children with bleeding from other causes have polymorphonuclear leukocytosis, normal or moderately elevated ESR, and transient albuminuria and glycosuria.

CSF analysis and CT document subarachnoid hemorrhage. Sonography in the infant with an open fontanelle and CT at any age are invaluable in the diagnosis of intracranial hemorrhage and its complications. CT may demonstrate arteriovenous malformation (Fig. 44.7) or giant cerebral arterial aneurysm.

MRI and MRA are often informative. Cerebral angiography is the definitive diagnostic technique for these conditions.

Treatment

The management of intracranial hemorrhage varies with the cause of the hemorrhage. Repeated lumbar punctures, mannitol, and corticosteroids are often used, but their effectiveness is controversial. Ruptured intracranial aneurysms require good nursing care, and unless the child is comatose or there is a medical contraindica-

tion, surgical extirpation offers the best prognosis. Except in cases of mycotic aneurysms, the occurrence of a second hemorrhage, shortly after the initial hemorrhage, is uncommon in children. Arteriovenous malformations should be surgically removed whenever possible. Embolization may be used preoperatively to reduce the size of the malformation or to treat inaccessible lesions. Traumatic arteriovenous fistulas are treated by ligation of the fistula, embolization, or the implantation of detachable balloons.

METABOLIC DISORDERS

MELAS is a mitochondrial disorder associated with two identifiable mitochondrial DNA mutations. MELAS is characterized by four criteria: a strokelike episode before age 40 years; encephalopathy characterized by seizures, dementia, or both; lactic acidosis; and ragged red fibers in the muscle biopsy (Chapter 97). Some patients with MELAS have features of other mitochondrial disorders.

Congenital disorder of glycosylation 1a is a multisystem disease resulting from deficiency of phosphomannomutase (PMM), an enzyme crucial in *n*-linked glycosylation, a ubiquitous process essential for the normal function of most proteins. The findings may mimic those of mitochondrial cytopathies, including stroke-like episodes, seizures, episodes of coma, and peripheral neuropathy. Blood tests may show elevated transaminases and creatine kinase, with low levels of albumen, cholesterol, and coagulations factors. Carbohydrate-deficient transferrin should be assayed in suspected cases. The diagnosis is confirmed by measurement of PMM activity. Homocystinuria (cystathionine beta-synthetase deficiency) is an autosomal-recessive inherited disorder featuring elevated serum methionine and homocystine concentrations, and excessive urinary excretion of homocystine. Subluxation of the ocular lens is characteristic. Mental retardation is common. Cerebral-arterial occlusive disease and venous thrombosis occur often, resulting in death. The elevated homocystine is responsive to high-dose pyridoxine.

SUGGESTED READINGS

Adams RJ, McKie VC, Hsu L, et al. Prevention of a first stroke by transfusions in children with sickle cell anemia and abnormal results on transcranial doppler ultrasonography. *N Engl J Med* 1998;339:5–11.

Barreirinho S, Ferro A, Santos M, et al. Inherited and acquired risk factors and their combined effects in pediatric stroke. *Pediatr Neurol* 2003;28(2):134–138.

Carter S, Gold AP. Acute infantile hemiplegia. *Pediatr Clin North Am* 1964;14:851–864.

deVeber G, Roach ES, Riela AR, Wiznitzer M. Stroke in children: recognition, treatment and future directions. *Semin Pediatr Neurol* 2000;7:309–317.

Devilat M, Toso M, Morales M. Childhood stroke associated with protein C or S deficiency and primary antiphospholipid syndrome. *Pediatr Neurol* 1993;9:67–70.

Eeg-Olofsson O, Ringheim Y. Stroke in children. Clinical characteristics and prognosis. *Acta Paediatr Scand* 1983;72:391–396.

Fisher M, Sotak CH, Minematsu K, et al. New magnetic resonance techniques for evaluating cerebrovascular disease. *Ann Neurol* 1992;32:115–122.

Fullerton HJ, Wu YW, Zhao S, Johnston SC. Risk of stroke in children: ethnic and gender disparities. *Neurology* 2003;61(2):189–194.

Ganesan V, Prengler M, McShane MA, Wade AM, Kirkham FJ. Investigation of risk factors in children with arterial ischemic stroke. *Ann Neurol* 2003;53(2):167–173.

Ganesan V, Savvy L, Chong WK, et al. Conventional cerebral angiography in children with ischemic stroke. *Pediatr Neurol* 1999;20:38–42.

Gold AP, Challenor YB, Gilles FH, et al. IX Strokes in children. *Stroke* 1973;4:835–894, 1009–1052.

Gold AP, Ransohoff J, Carter S. Arteriovenous malformation of the vein of Galen in children. *Acta Neurol Scand* 1964;40[suppl 11]:1–31.

Golomb MR, MacGregor DL, Domi T, et al. Presumed pre or perinatal arterial ischemic stroke: risk factors and outcomes. *Ann Neurol* 2001;50:163–168.

Gruppo R, DeGrauw A, Fogelson H, et al. Protein C deficiency related to valproic acid therapy; a possible association with childhood stroke. *J Pediatr* 2000;137:714–718.

Gunther G, Junker R, Strater R, et al. Symptomatic ischemic stroke in full term neonates: role of acquired and genetic prothrombotic risk factors. *Stroke* 2000;31:2437–2441.

Hilal SK, Solomon GE, Gold AP, et al. Primary cerebral arterial occlusive disease in children. II. Neurocutaneous syndromes. *Radiology* 1971;99:71–87.

Hirano M, Ricci E, Koenigsberger MR, et al. MELAS: an original case and clinical criteria for diagnosis. *Neuromusc Disord* 1992;2:125–135.

Humphreys RP. Complications of hemorrhagic stroke in children. *Pediatr Neurosurg* 1991;17:163–168.

Johnson AJ, Lee BCP, Lin W. Echoplanar diffusion-weighted imaging in neonates and infants with suspected hypoxic-ischemic injury: correlation with patient outcome. *AJR Am J Roentgenol* 1999;172:219–226.

Kamholz J, Tremblay G. Chickenpox with delayed contralateral hemiparesis caused by cerebral angiitis. *Ann Neurol* 1985;18:358–360.

Kenet G. Sadetzki S, Murad H, et al. Factor V Leiden and antiphospholipid antibodies are significant risk factors for ischemic stroke in children. *Stroke* 2000;31:1283–1288.

Kinugasa K, Mandai S, Kamata I, et al. Surgical treatment of moyamoya disease. Operative technique for encephalo-duro-arterio-myosynangiosis: follow-up, clinical results, and angiograms. *Neurosurgery* 1993;32:527–531.

Lacey DJ, Terplan K. Intraventricular hemorrhage in full-term neonates. *Dev Med Child Neurol* 1982;14:332–337.

Laxer RM, Dunn HG, Flodmark O. Acute hemiplegia in Kawasaki disease and infantile polyarteritis nodosa. *Dev Med Child Neurol* 1984;26:814–821.

Limbord TG, Ruderman RJ. Fat embolism in children. *Clin Orthop* 1978;136:267–269.

Lynch, JK. Cerebrovascular disorders in children. *Curr Neuro Neurosci Rep* 2004;2:129–138.

Martinowitz U, Heim M, Tadmor R, et al. Intracranial hemorrhage in patients with hemophilia. *Neurosurgery* 1986;18:538–540.

Matsushima Y, Aoyagi M, Niimi Y, et al. Symptoms and their pattern of progression in childhood moyamoya disease. *Brain Dev* 1990;12:784–789.

Michiels JJ, Stibbe J, Bertina R, et al. Effectiveness of long term oral anticoagulation treatment in preventing venous thrombosis in hereditary protein S deficiency. *Br Med J* 1987;295:641–643.

Nass RD, Trauner D. Social and affective impairments are important in recovery after acquired stroke in childhood. *CNS Spectr* 2004;9(6):420–434.

Nestoride E, Buoanno FS, Ferdinando S, Jones RM, et al. Arterial ischemic stroke in childhood: role of plasma-phase risk factors. *Curr Opinion in Neurol* 2000;15:139–144.

Ozduman K, Pober BR, Barnes P, et al. Fetal stroke. *Pediatr Neurol.* 2004;30(3):151–62.

Packer RJ, Rorke LB, Lange BJ, et al. Cerebrovascular accidents in children with cancer. *Pediatrics* 1985;76:194–201.

Paradis K, Bernstein ML, Adelson JW. Thrombosis as a complication of inflammatory bowel disease in children: a report of four cases. *J Pediatr Gastroenterol Nutr* 1985;4:659–662.

Patterson MC. Congenital disorders of glycosylation. In: Rosenberg RN, Prusiner SB, Di Mauro S, Barchi RL, Nestler EJ, eds. *The Molecular and Genetic Basis of Neurological and Psychiatric Disease,* 3rd ed. Philadelphia: Butterworth Heinemann, 2003:643–649.

Pavlakis S, et al. Brain infarction in sickle cell anemia: MRI correlates. *Ann Neurol* 1988;23:125–130.

Punt J. Surgical management of paediatric stroke. *Pediatr Radiol* 2004 Jan;34(1):16–23.

Quinn CT, Rogers ZR, Buchanan GR. Survival of children with sickle cell disease. *Blood* 2004;103(11):4023–4027.

Ribai P, Liesnard C, Rodesch G, et al. Transient cerebral arteriopathy in infancy associated with enteroviral infection. *Eur J Paediatr Neurol* 2003;7(2):73–75.

Sandok BA, von Estorff I, Giuliani ER. CNS embolism due to atrial myxoma—clinical features and diagnosis. *Arch Neurol* 1980;37:485–488.

Seibert JJ, Glasier CM, Kirby RS, et al. Transcranial Doppler, MRA, and MRI as a screening examination for cerebrovascular disease in patients with sickle cell anemia: an 8-year study. *Pediatr Radiol* 1998;28:138–142.

Shahar E, Gilday DL, Hwang PA, et al. Pediatric cerebrovascular disease: alterations of regional cerebral blood flow detected by Tc 99m-HMPAO SPECT. *Arch Neurol* 1990;47:578–584.

Shields WD, Manger MN. Ultrasound evaluation of neonatal intraventricular hemorrhage. I. Anatomy. *Perinatol Neonatol* 1983;75:19–25.

Shields WD, Manger MN. Ultrasound evaluation of neonatal intraventricular hemorrhage. II. Pathology. *Perinatol Neonatol* 1983;76:28–35.

Solomon GE, Hilal SK, Gold AP, et al. Natural history of acute hemiplegia of childhood. *Brain* 1970;93:107–120.

Stein BM, Wolpert SM. Arteriovenous malformations of the brain. Current concepts and treatment. *Arch Neurol* 1980;37:1–5, 69—75.

Thorarensen O, Ryan S, Hunter J, Younkin DP. Factor V Leiden mutation: an unrecognized cause of hemiplegic cerebral palsy, neonatal stroke, and placental thrombosis. *Ann Neurol* 1997;42:372–375.

Ueki K, Meyer FB, Mellinger JF. Moyamoya disease: the disorder and surgical treatment. *Mayo Clin Proc* 1994;69:749–759.

Van Beynum IM, Smeitink JA, den Heijer M, et al. Hyperhomocysteinemia: a risk factor for ischemic stroke in children. *Circulation* 1999;99:2040–2072.

Volpe JJ. Neonatal periventricular hemorrhage: past, present, and future. *J Pediatr* 1978;92:693–696.

Whitlock JA, Janco RL, Phillips JA. Inherited hypercoagulable states in children. *Am J Pediatr Hematol Oncol* 1989;11:170–173.

Yoffe G, Buchanan GR. Intracranial hemorrhage in newborn and young infants with hemophilia. *J Pediatr* 1988;113:333–336.

Chapter 45

▶ Treatment and Prevention of Strokes

Frank M. Yatsu

Therapies for stroke management and prevention are designed to (1) minimize or prevent stroke occurrence, (2) optimize functional recovery following strokes, and (3) avert stroke recurrences. Specific measures for treatment and prevention depend upon the stroke syndrome being considered.

Stroke syndromes are conveniently divided by neuroimaging findings and are classified as either ischemic or hemorrhagic. With ischemic strokes, the primary causes are atherothrombotic, with artery-to-artery thromboembolism and cardioembolic strokes with other causes from prothrombotic conditions noted above. Treatment and prevention will be directed primarily to atherothrombotic brain infarction (ABI) and cardioembolic strokes. Hemorrhagic strokes are categorized as: subarachnoid hemorrhages, primarily arising from berry or congenital aneurysms but may also be the result of a variety of arteriovenous malformations; and intracerebral hemorrhage, most commonly caused by sustained hypertension, but may occur with hypocoagulable states as well as either primary or metastatic tumors in the brain. Emphasis in this chapter will be on subarachnoid hemorrhage (SAH) and primary hypertensive intracerebral hemorrhage (ICH).

ATHEROTHROMBOTIC STROKES AND TIAS

ABI, usually with artery-to-artery thromboembolism, is the most common stroke syndrome; it results from atherosclerotic lesions that are primarily extracranial in white populations, while primarily intracranial in African American and Asian people. The syndromes of ABI form a continuum from TIAs to completed infarction with fixed neurologic deficits. Whether an intermediate condition of stroke-in-evolution or progressing stroke exists is controversial. Thrombosis on an atherosclerotic plaque may occur for several pathologic reasons. The first of these, and most common, is rupture of the plaque that stems from a high concentration of cholesterol-esters, foam cells, and inflammatory constituents that make the plaque unstable.

The complex process of atherosclerosis in which elevated low-density lipoprotein (LDL) and vascular smooth muscle proliferation play key roles is complicated by a number of inflammatory factors, such as vascular cell adhesion molecule-1 (VCAM-1) and monocyte chemo-attractant protein-1 (MCP-1), upregulated by NFκ-B, plus transcription factors affecting foam cells and other functions, such as peroxisomal proliferators-activated receptor-γ. Second, hemorrhage occurs into neovascularized tissue around the plaque, provoked by an upregulation of vascular endothelial growth factor (VEGF); and third, desquamation or denudation of the plaque surface occurs which exposes connective tissue elements leading to platelet adhesion, platelet "release reaction," recruitment of more platelets and prothrombotic activity with thrombus formation. Depending upon the size, character and tempo of the thrombus formation, the patients will experience either TIAs, believed to be primarily composed of platelet aggregates which disaggregate after causing temporary arteriolar occlusion, or a fixed neurologic deficit with a thrombus of fibrin plus platelets.

TIAs are brief neurologic events, customarily stated to last less than 24 hours, but most frequently persist for minutes to hours, in either the carotid or vertebrobasilar circulations, and the symptoms correspond to the temporarily occluded vessel, such as temporary blindness or amaurosis fugax if the ophthalmic artery is involved; aphasia, such as Broca aphasia, if the dominant operculofrontal artery is temporarily occluded; or contralateral hemiparesis if the sulcal branch of the middle cerebral artery is affected.

Since symptoms of TIA may be caused by conditions other than vessel occlusion from thromboemboli, it is crucial that a differential diagnosis be considered in patients with TIAs. For example, hemodynamic changes with reduced perfusion pressure, prothrombotic and hyperviscosity states, emboli, seizures and mass lesions, such as meningiomas and subdural hematomas, plus other conditions may cause temporary and recurrent stereotyped, neurologic deficits. For hemodynamic causes from cardiac arrhythmias, Holter monitoring may be needed to document the type of arrhythmia.

For TIAs caused by carotid stenosis of equal to or greater than 70% by diameter, carotid endarterectomy (CEA) by a skilled surgeon with an acceptable track record is the treatment of choice over medical therapy, in good surgical candidates, as demonstrated by three prospective studies: the North American Symptomatic Carotid Endarterectomy Trial (NASCET), the European Carotid Surgery Trial (ECST), and the U.S. Veterans Affairs Cooperative Study on CEA, all published in 1991. Efforts to determine the value of angioplasty and stents is being investigated, both for extra- and intracranial stenosis.

To prevent TIA recurrence and the potentials for a completed stroke in subjects with TIAs or minor strokes caused by extra- or intracranial occlusive disease, antiplatelet drugs such as aspirin have been effective. Meta-analyses on the benefits of aspirin show a reduction of strokes by approximately 25%. The optimum dose of daily aspirin, whether ultra-low doses at 30 to 75 or 80 mg to high doses of 1,300 mg remains controversial, but low doses appear effective and have less side effects such as gastrointestinal bleeding. The action of aspirin is to acetylate irreversibly and inhibit platelets' cyclooxygenase I, which thereby stops synthesis of the powerful platelet aggregant thromboxane A_2 (TXA2). Lower doses of aspirin have the advantage of minimizing inhibition of endothelial cells' production of prostacyclin (PGI2), the powerful platelet antiaggregant. The concept of a balance between TXA2 and PGI2 in the normal circulation without aggregate formation won Sir John Vane a Nobel Prize.

Newer anti-platelet drugs, which blunt the GP IIbIIIa receptor which is involved in platelet adhesion, appear to operate synergistically with aspirin in potentiating aspirin's anti-aggregant effects; these drugs are ticlopidine and clopidogrel and dipyridamole in combination with aspirin. Clopidogrel, an analog of ticlopidine, has fewer side effects such as diarrhea, bruising and leucopenia which require frequent monitoring when using ticlopidine. Dipyridamole plus aspirin may be the best combination to reduced recurrent TIAs or ischemic strokes following TIAs. Aspirin and clopidogrel increases bleeding so this combination should be avoided for chronic therapy.

Short-term subcutaneous heparin is not effective in preventing stroke recurrences compared to aspirin, according to the International Stroke Trial (IST) with nearly 20,000 ischemic stroke patients; similar findings were seen in the Chinese Acute Stroke Trial with nearly the same number of patients as the IST study. Whether anticoagulation will avert recurrent strokes in patients with intracranial stenoses only is currently being investigated, but since anticoagulation may not convey any benefits if the Warfarin-Aspirin Recurrent Stroke Study results are to be applied, aside from concerns of unwanted bleeding, use of antiplatelet agents is warranted until the above studies are completed.

COMPLETED STROKES WITH FIXED NEUROLOGIC DEFICITS

For patients with ischemic strokes caused by ABI or cardiogenic emboli, who had a negative CT or MRI of brain for bleeding and minimal infarction, and who were seen within 3 hours of onset of symptoms, the thrombolytic agent, tissue plasminogen activator (tPA), was found beneficial in the cooperative National Institutes of Neurological Diseases and Stroke (NINDS) study published in 1995. tPA was approved for patient use by the FDA in 1996. In the 624 ischemic stroke patients treated within three hours and assessed at three months, improvement of neurologic scores for tPA treated patients ranged from 33% to 55%

or an absolute difference between 11% to 13%. Thus, for every 100 patients treated with tPA, 11-13 would benefit with little or no neurologic deficits. However, tPA patients had a 6.0% incidence of intracerebral hemorrhage compared to 0.6% in placebo treated (P<0.01). Intracerebral hemorrhage did not worsen the neurologic status in the majority of these patients. Nonetheless, it remains a concern for many physicians, neurologists included, in not using tPA, particularly if urgent neurosurgical intervention for decompressive surgery is not available. Despite this worry, tPA should be used because it does offer the ischemic stroke patient a reasonable chance for substantial neurologic improvement. Specific guidelines for inclusion and exclusion must, of course, be met when using tPA (see Table 45.1). Randomized educational programs have been successful in increasing the use of tPA with good outcomes (Morgenstern, et al., 2003). Research is being conducted on the pathophysiologic mechanisms of intracerebral hemorrhage resulting from tPA treatment, and one line of investigation is on blunting the effects of the various matrix metalloproteinases (MMPs) that are upregulated by ischemic tissue, causing tissue breakdown, but which may be blocked experimentally. tPA is "toxic" to clone endothelial cells so that less "toxic" mutational forms of tPA, may be associated with less frequent intracerebral hemorrhages (Yatsu et al., 1995). Further, techniques using MRI for diffusion and perfusion weighted images and "mismatch" and the apparent diffusion coefficient (ADC) are being investigated in the hopes identifying definitively ischemically viable tissue, which may respond to revascularization, as opposed to necrotic areas. In addition, a variety of intraarterial devices to extract the thrombus are being studied as are the use of intraarterial, intrathrombus, thrombolytic agents.

▶ **TABLE 45.1 Tissue Plasminogen Activator (tPA) Exclusion Criteria**

Stroke or head trauma within the preceding 3 mths
Major surgery within the preceding 2 wks
History of intracerebral hemorrhage
Systolic blood pressure >185 mmHg
Diastolic blood pressure >110 mmHg
Rapidly improving or minor neurologic symptoms & signs
Evidences for subarachnoid hemorrhage
Gastrointestinal or urinary tract bleeding within 3 wks
Arterial puncture at a noncompressible site within 1 wk
Seizure at stroke onset
Prothrombin time >15 seconds
Heparin therapy within 2 days and elevated partial thromboplastin time
Platelet count <100,000/mm³
Blood glucose <30 mg/dL (2.7 mmol/L)
Blood glucose >400 mg/dL (21.6 mmol/L)
Patients requiring very aggressive therapy attempts for blood pressure reduction

The benefits conveyed with tPA in recanalizing occluded vessels has ignited renewed interest in neuroprotective agents. The general principle behind the rationale of using agents to preserve ischemically impaired tissue is the success in vitro of reversing the untoward effects of excitotoxic amino acids such as glutamate that are released during ischemia. For example, experimental animals stroke studies have shown beneficial effects of a variety of agents, such as N-Methyl-D-Aspartate (NMDA)-receptor antagonists (e.g., selfotel, Cerestat, and MK-801), as well as agents inhibiting glutamate secretion, (e.g., lubeluzole); calcium uptake; adhesion molecules; free radical trapping; and inflammatory cytokines, (e.g., intercellular adhesion molecule (ICAM-1) antibodies). Unfortunately, these and other promising neuroprotective agents in animal stroke models have been singularly unsuccessful in humans. Despite these setbacks, ongoing research in neuroprotection suggests that agents to convey benefit will be available in strokes, possibly inhibitors of c-Jun Kinase (JUNK) or free radical scavengers.

EMBOLIC STROKES OF CARDIAC AND AORTIC ORIGIN

Treatment of cardiogenic emboli depends on the offending pathology: infected prosthetic valves need replacement, and myxomatous emboli require surgical removal of the tumor. The most common cause of cardiogenic emboli (more than 50% of cases) is from arrhythmias, particularly atrial fibrillation, with or without mitral pathology, and recent myocardial infarction (MI). Post-MI emboli occur with large, anterior or septal infarcts, particularly those with akinetic segments, as detected by 2D echocardiography. Mitral valve prolapse and patent foramen ovale (PFO), both discussed above, occur more commonly in young adults.

In embolic strokes caused by atrial fibrillation, anticoagulation to reduce embolization is indicated with an international normalized ratio (INR) between 2.0 and 3.0. In the Stroke Prevention in Atrial Fibrillation (SPAF) study, anticoagulation reduced stroke recurrence substantially, even in patients over the age of 75 years. Chances of embolization are associated with the following risk factors: previous embolization, left ventricular hypertrophy with reduced ejection fraction, sustained hypertension, and congestive failure. In some series, women over the age of 75 years are at increased risk. Patients with atrial fibrillation and no risk factors, as seen in patients with hyperthyroidism and occasionally those with coronary artery disease (CAD), have a 1.5% risk of embolization, per year. With one risk factor, the percentage rises to approximately 7% per year, and with two or more, it is approximately 17% per year.

Aortic atheromas measuring at least 4 mm or more, without calcification, are considered thrombogenic, and anticoagulation to prevent embolization is being investigated for these patients.

INTRACEREBRAL HEMORRHAGE

Intracerebral hemorrhage is most commonly associated with long-standing hypertension and pathologic findings of Charcot-Bourchard aneurysm, which may be the site of hemorrhage. Five brain sites most commonly receiving the brunt of hemorrhage are: putamen, the most common site in Western Civilization populations; polar or white matter; thalamus; pons; and cerebellum. Massive intracerebral hemorrhages of more than 80 mL in volume are usually lethal because vital structures are irreversibly damaged. Smaller hemorrhages may be treated with supportive care, although preliminary studies on the potential benefits of infusing Factor VII as a prothrombogenic agent show promise and are being investigated prospectively. Large-polar or white-matter hemorrhages that cause herniation and decreasing sensorium may be amenable to surgical evacuation and have been investigated in a large international study—the 2002 International Surgical Trial in Intracerebral Hemorrhage (ISTICH) Preliminary results of that study, not yet published as of this writing, with over 1,000 subjects randomized to surgical or medical therapy appears to show no differences between the two methods of treatment.

For cerebellar hemorrhages, surgical decompression may be life saving, and clinicians must recognize the signs and symptoms of incipient brain-stem compression and herniation. Clinically, these patients present with headache (occipital), vertigo, nausea, vomiting and truncal ataxia without focal weakness, and may begin to develop declining sensorium and gaze-palsy. Accompanying neuroimaging studies indicating the need for surgical decompression include fourth ventricular shift, cisternal obliteration and ventricular enlargement. Lumbar puncture is contraindicated with intracerebral hemorrhage, particularly with cerebellar hemorrhages, since life-threatening tonsillar herniation may occur. Great caution must be taken in these patients subjected to ventriculostomy for the purposes of reducing intracranial pressure because upward cerebellar herniation may occur.

SUBARACHNOID HEMORRHAGE (SAH) FROM CONGENITAL OR BERRY ANEURYSM

Extirpation of the aneurysm is the definitive therapy for aneurysms causing SAH and may be accomplished surgically or with balloons and coagulation techniques, such as with coils deposited in the aneurysm. Following SAH and prior to surgery, patients should be sedated and kept in a quiet environment to prevent elevations of blood pressure that may provoke rebleeding, which is a major complication of SAH, along with vasospasm, ventricular dilatation, and Syndromes of Inappropriate ADH Secretions (SIADH). Antifibrinolytic agents, such as epsilon-amino-caproic acid, used to preserve the thrombus around an aneurysm thereby preventing rebleeding, have been unsuccessful. Vasospasm may be minimized with the calcium channel antagonist, nimodipine, which crosses the blood-brain barrier; intrathecal thrombolytic therapy may be useful in reducing vasospasm. Hydrocephalus may require ventricular shunting. Assessment of nitric oxide synthase (eNOS) polymorphism may be of value in predicting whether or not asymptomatic aneurysms are more likely to bleed.

STROKE REHABILITATION

A team approach for stroke rehabilitation, starting from a stroke recovery unit with experienced physiatrists and physical therapists, has proven beneficial for the optimum recovery of patients. This approach is particularly helpful in averting various complications from strokes, such as infections, contractures, and decubiti, and in maximizing independence for patients with hemiplegia/paresis by teaching them to transfer effectively from bed to wheelchair. Activities of daily living (ADLs) may be optimized for personal hygiene, dressing, and feeding, as well. Depression is a frequent accompaniment of strokes, partially because the reality of a physical disability exists but also because there is altered brain chemistry, which may respond well to selective serotonin-reuptake inhibitors (SSRIs) and tricyclic antidepressants. Speech and occupational therapists should be consulted to help patients improve their communication skills and ADL skills.

STROKE PREVENTION

Stroke prevention depends upon the stroke syndrome and its pathology, such as atherosclerosis, arteritis, cardiac diseases, dissection, and so on, but since atherosclerosis is the most common cause of ischemic strokes, the primary stroke syndrome, only interventions to prevent atherosclerosis will be reviewed here.

The risk factors for atherosclerosis are well known and require the active involvement of the physician to help patients develop motivational drives to control or stop these risk factors, which include hypertension, smoking, diabetes mellitus, elevated cholesterol, or more correctly, increased low-density lipoprotein (LDL), obesity, sedentary life, and negative stress levels. For hypertension, clinicians should familiarize themselves with the report of the Joint National Commission on Hypertension Prevention and Treatment VII (JNC7), published in 2003, which makes recommendations on optimal blood pressure goals, along with life-style changes to assist in this process. The

JNC7 notes that for each 10 mmHg elevation of systolic or diastolic blood pressure above 115/75, a 10% increase in vascular risks for coronary artery disease, strokes, and peripheral vascular disease occurs. Although no consensus exists, the ALLHAT study (Antihypertensive & Lipid Lowering Therapies for Heart Attack Treatment), which was primarily a North American study of over 42,000 subjects with moderate hypertension, who were aged 55 years and older and had one other risk factor for coronary artery disease, were randomly selected for treatment with a diuretic, an angiotensin converting enzyme (ACE) inhibitor and a calcium channel inhibitor, (respectively, chlorthaladone, lisinopril and amlodipine). The diuretic was as effective or more so than the other two medications in preventing vascular complications including strokes, although to achieve optimum blood pressure, most patients required treatment with 2 or more antihypertensive agents. Nonetheless, the ALLHAT study concluded that diuretics are not only the least expensive, but also as effective as any of the others. Clinicians must, of course, be comfortable with the drugs prescribed and be particularly vigilant regarding drug interactions and other complications related to medications. It should be kept in mind that reducing daily salt intake to 2 grams is equivalent in outcome to any one of the antihypertensive agents. Smoking is addictive, but efforts to have patients stop must be made and may necessitate psychologic counseling and medical aids, such as nicotine patches.

Diabetes control with hemoglobin A1c near 6% will reduce the occurrences of microangiopathy, such as diabetic retinopathy and renal nephropathy, but these patients frequently have elevated cholesterol and triglycerides plus hypertension or insulin resistance with what is called the metabolic syndrome, and attention must be given to other risks, not simply to tight glucose control. Elevated cholesterol, or more correctly increased LDL or reduced high-density lipoprotein (HDL) are atherogenic, although this issue had been controversial for many years because elderly stroke patients display total cholesterol in the "normal" range. However, LDL- and HDL-turnover studies and lipoprotein polymorphisms indicate a link between lipoprotein patterns and atherothrombotic strokes. Furthermore, use of statin drugs to reduce cholesterol in subjects with coronary heart disease is associated with reduction in primary and secondary endpoints for coronary artery disease as well as in ischemic strokes. The first such study is the 4S, or Scandinavian Simvastatin Survival Study, of 4,444 subjects with coronary artery disease. Subsequently, a number of such studies have verified these initial findings, which support the conclusion of the role of cholesterol in atherothrombotic strokes, with the additional benefits of the antiinflammatory role, the upregulation eNOS, and other actions of statins. Optimal LDL levels for ischemic stroke patients should be similar to those for patients with coronary artery disease, namely, reduction of LDL to less than 100 mg/dL. Since HDL is important for reverse cholesterol transport in taking cholesterol from plaques and delivering it to the liver for bile production, low levels (less than 35 mg/dL) should be increased with drugs such as niacin or fibric acid derivatives. Since fibric acid drugs and statins increase the risk of myoglobinuria, they should be used with care, but certain fibric acid derivatives appear to have a low risk of this complication. Fibric acid drugs increase levels of Peroxisomal Proliferator Activated Receptor (PPAR-γ), and this increases apo-AI synthesis, the major lipoprotein associated with HDL, thus increasing HDL levels, plus paroxonase, which is associated with HDL and prevents oxidation of LDL, the highly atherogenic form of LDL. Efforts to inhibit smooth-muscle cell proliferation may have clinical relevance in reducing atherosclerosis but needs *in vivo* proof.

Obesity, sedentary life style, and stress are factors which treating physicians may likely need consultative assistance from health-care specialists who possess expertise in these areas. Morbid obesity may require surgical intervention, such as gastric reconstruction. Developing coping skills for stress may require psychiatric or psychologic consultation.

SUGGESTED READINGS

Furlan A, Higashida M, Wechsler L, et al. Intra-arterial prourokinase for acute ischemic stroke. The PROACT II. Study. A randomized controlled trial. Prolyse in acute cerebral thromboembolism. *JAMA* 1999;282:2003–2011.

Grotta JC. tPA – the best current option for most patients. *N Engl J Med* 1997;337:1311–1313.

Hacke W, Kaste M, Fieschi C, et al. Intravenous thrombolysis with recombinant tissue plasminogen activator for acute hemispheric stroke. The European Cooperative Acute Stroke Study (ECASS). *JAMA* 1995;274:1017–1025.

Hill MD, Yiannakoulias N, Jeerakathil T, et al. The high risk of stroke immediately after transient ischemic attack: a population based study. *Neurology* 2004;62(11):2015–2020.

International T, et al. Stroke Trial (IST): randomized trial of aspirin, subcutaneous heparin, both, or neither among 19,435 patients with acute ischaemic stroke. International Stroke Trial Collaborative Group. *Lancet* 1997;349:1569—1581.

Chobanian AV, Bakris GL, Black HR, et al. The Seventh Report of the Joint National Committee on Prevention, Detection, Evaluation, and Treatment of High Blood Pressure: the JNC7 Report. *JAMA* 2003;289(19):2560–2572.

Lovett JK, Coull AJ, Rothwell PM. Early risk of recurrence by subtype of ischemic stroke in population-based incidence studies. *Neurology* 2004;62(4):569–573.

Mayberg MR, Wilson SE, Yatsu FM, et al. Carotid endarterectomy and prevention of cerebral ischemia in symptomatic carotid stenosis. Veterans Affairs Cooperative Studies Program 309 Trialist Group. *JAMA* 1991;266:3289–3294.

Miller VT, Pearce LA, Feinberg WM, et al. Differential effect of aspirin versus warfarin on clinical stroke types in patients with atrial fibrillation. Stroke Prevention in Atrial Fibrillation Investigators. *Neurology* 1996;46:238–240.

Mohr JP, Thompson JL, Lazar RM, et al. A comparison of warfarin and aspirin for the prevention of recurrent ischemic stroke. *N Engl J Med* 2001;345:1444–1451.

Third Report of the National Cholesterol Education Program (NCEP) Expert Panel on Detection, Evaluation, and Treatment of High Blood Cholesterol in Adults (Adult Treatment Panel III). Bethesda MD: National Cholesterol Education Program, National Heart, Lung, and Blood Institute, National Institutes of Health, September 2002:1–284. NIH Publication No. 02-5215. Available at http://www.nhlbi.nih.gov/guidelines/cholesterol/atp3full.pdf

NINDS tPA Stroke Study Group. Generalized efficacy of tPA for acute stroke. Subgroup analysis of the NINDS t-PA Stroke Trial. *Stroke* 1997;28:2119–2125.

North American Symptomatic Carotid Endarterectomy Trial Collaborators. Beneficial effect of carotid endarterectomy in symptomatic patients with high-grade carotid stenosis. *N Engl J Med* 1991;325:445–453.

Olsson SB, Executive Steering Committee on behalf of the SPORTIF III. Investigators. Stroke prevention with the oral direct thrombin inhibitor ximelagatran compared with warfarin in patients with non-valvular atrial fibrillation (SPORTIF III): randomised controlled trial. *Lancet* 2003;362(9397):1691–1698.

PROGRESS Collaborative Group. Randomized trial of a perindopril-based blood pressure-lowering regimen among 6,105 individuals with previous stroke or transient ischemic attacks. *Lancet* 2001;332:912–917.

Sivenius J, Cunha L, Diener HC, et al. Second European Stroke Prevention Study: antiplatelet therapy is effective regardless of age. ESPS2 Working Group. *Acta Neurol Scand* 1999;99(1):54–60.

The National Institute of Neurological Disorders and Stroke rt-PA Stroke Study Group. Tissue plasminogen activator for acute ischemic stroke. *N Engl J Med* 1995;333:1581–1587.

Yatsu FM, Zivin J. Hypertension in acute ischemic strokes. Not to treat. *Arch Neurol* 1985;42(10):999–1000.

Zöller B, Hillurp A, Berntorp E, Dahlbäck B. Activated protein C resistance due to a common factor V gene mutation is a major risk for venous thrombosis. *Annual Rev Med* 1997;48:45–48.

Chapter 46

Subarachnoid Hemorrhage

Stephan A. Mayer, Gary L. Bernardini, Robert A. Solomon, and John C. M. Brust

Subarachnoid hemorrhage (SAH) accounts for 5% of all strokes; it affects nearly 30,000 individuals per year in the United States, with an annual incidence of 1 per 10,000 population. Saccular (or berry) aneurysms at the base of the brain cause 80% of all cases of SAH. Nonaneurysmal causes of SAH are listed in Table 46.1. SAH most frequently occurs between ages 40 and 60 years, and women are affected more often than men.

SAH due to the rupture of an intracranial aneurysm is a devastating event; approximately 12% of patients die before receiving medical attention, and another 20% die after admission to the hospital. Of the two-thirds of patients who survive, approximately one-half remain permanently

▶ **TABLE 46.1 Nonaneurysmal Causes of SAH**

Trauma
Idiopathic perimesencephalic SAH
Arteriovenous malformation
Intracranial arterial dissection
Cocaine and amphetamine use
Mycotic aneurysm
Pituitary apoplexy
Moyamoya disease
CNS vasculitis
Sickle cell disease
Coagulation disorders
Primary or metastatic neoplasm

disabled, primarily as a result of neurocognitive deficits and depression. Advances in neurosurgery and intensive care, including an emphasis on early aneurysm clip application and aggressive therapy for vasospasm, have led to improved survival over the last three decades, with a reduction in overall case fatality from approximately 50% to 33%.

PATHOLOGY AND EPIDEMIOLOGY OF INTRACRANIAL ANEURYSMS

Saccular aneurysms most often occur at the circle of Willis or its major branches, especially at bifurcations. They arise where the arterial elastic lamina and tunica media are defective, and tend to enlarge with age. The typical aneurysm wall is composed only of intima and adventitia and may become paper thin. Many aneurysms, particularly those that rupture, are irregular and multilobulated, and larger aneurysms may be partially or completely filled with an organized clot that occasionally is calcified. The point of rupture is usually through the dome of the aneurysm.

Eighty-five percent to 90% of intracranial aneurysms are located in the anterior circulation, with the three most common sites being the junction of the posterior communicating and internal carotid artery (approximately 40%), the anterior communicating artery complex (approximately 30%), and the middle cerebral artery at the first major branch point in the sylvian fissure (approximately 20%). Posterior circulation aneurysms most often occur at the apex of the basilar artery or at the junction of the vertebral and posteroinferior cerebellar artery. Saccular aneurysms of the distal cerebral arterial tree are rare. Nearly 20% of patients have two or more aneurysms; many of these are "mirror" aneurysms on the same vessel, contralaterally.

Intracranial aneurysms are uncommon in children but occur with a frequency of 2% in adults, so that 2 million to 3 million Americans have aneurysms. However, more than 90% of these aneurysms are small (less than 10 mm) and remain asymptomatic throughout the patient's life. The annual risk of rupture of an asymptomatic intracranial aneurysm is approximately 0.7%. Important risk factors for the initial rupture of an aneurysm include increasing size, prior SAH from a separate aneurysm, and basilar apex and posterior communicating artery location (Table 46.2).

The most powerful of these risk factors is size; for example, internal carotid artery aneurysms of less than 7 mm in diameter bleed at a rate of approximately 0.1% per year, compared to an annual rate of 8% for those greater than 25 mm in size. Other risk factors for aneurysm rupture in approximate order of importance include: cigarette smoking, aneurysm-related headache or cranial nerve compression, heavy alcohol use, a family history of SAH, female gender (especially when postmenopausal), multiple aneurysms, hypertension, and exposure to cocaine or other sympathomimetic agents. In deciding whether to treat a patient with an unruptured intracranial aneurysm, the risks associated with repair should always be balanced against the patient's estimated lifetime risk of hemorrhage without repair.

The prevalence of aneurysms increases with age and is higher in patients with atherosclerosis, a family history of intracranial aneurysm, or autosomal-dominant polycystic kidney disease (PCKD). Intracranial aneurysms have also been associated with Ehlers-Danlos syndrome, Marfan syndrome, pseudoxanthoma elasticum, and coarctation of the aorta. Screening for unruptured intracranial

▶ **TABLE 46.2 5-Year Cumulative Hemorrhage Rates of Unruptured Aneurysms According to Size and Location**

| Primary Diagnosis (N) | <7 mm | | 8–12 mm | 13–25 mm | ≥25 mm |
	No Prior SAH	Prior SAH*			
Cavernous carotid artery (n = 210)	0	0	0	3.0%	6.4%
ACA, MCA, & ICA (not intracavernous) (n = 1037)	0	1.5%	2.6%	14.5%	40%
Post P-comm (n = 445)	2.5%	3.4%	14.5%	18.4%	50%

ACA, anterior communicating or anterior cerebral artery; ICA, internal carotid artery; MCA, middle cerebral artery; Post P-comm, vertebrobasilar, posterior cerebral arterial system, or the posterior communicating artery.
* Refers to prior subarachnoid hemorrhage from a separate intracranial aneurysm.
From: International Study of Unruptured Intracranial Aneurysms Investigators. *Lancet* 2003;362:103–110, with permission.

▶ TABLE 46.3 Hunt & Hess Grading Scale for Aneurysmal SAH

Grade	Clinical Findings	Hospital Mortality (%)*	
		1968	2002
I	Asymptomatic or mild headache	11	7
II	Moderate to severe headache, or oculomotor palsy	26	2
III	Confused, drowsy, or mild focal signs	37	10
IV	Stupor (localizes to pain)	71	35
V	Coma (posturing or no motor response to pain)	100	65
TOTAL		35	20

* Data from 275 patients reported by Hunt and Hess in 1968, and 404 patients treated at Columbia University Medical Center between 2000 and 2002.

aneurysms with magnetic resonance angiography (MRA) or CT angiography is indicated in patients with polycystic kidney disease (PCKD), and in family members who have two or more first-degree relatives with intracranial aneurysms; testing will be positive in approximately 10% of these individuals. Otherwise, routine screening of family members of SAH patients is not recommended.

CLINICAL MANIFESTATIONS

SAH usually commences with an explosive "thunderclap" headache followed by neck stiffness. Patients often describe the pain as "the worst headache of my life." The headache is usually generalized, but focal pain may refer to the site of aneurysmal rupture (e.g., periorbital pain related to an ophthalmic artery aneurysm). Common associated symptoms include loss of consciousness, nausea and vomiting, back or leg pain, and photophobia. In patients who lose consciousness, tonic posturing may occur and may be difficult to differentiate from a seizure. Although aneurysmal rupture often occurs during periods of exercise or physical stress, SAH may occur at any time, including during sleep.

More than one-third of SAH patients give a history of suspicious symptoms days or weeks earlier, including headache, stiff neck, nausea and vomiting, syncope, or disturbed vision. These prodromal symptoms are often due to minor leaking of blood from the aneurysm, and are therefore referred to as warning leaks or sentinel headaches. Initial misdiagnosis of SAH occurs in approximately 15% of patients, and those with the mildest symptoms are at greatest risk for being misdiagnosed. This often leads to delayed treatment after rebleeding or neurologic deterioration has occurred, resulting in increased morbidity and mortality.

Neck stiffness and the Kernig sign are hallmarks of SAH. However, these signs are not invariably present, and confusion and low back pain are sometimes more prominent than headache. Preretinal or subhyaloid hemorrhages—large, smooth-bordered, and on the retinal surface—occur in up to 25% of patients and are practically pathognomonic of SAH.

The most important determinant of outcome after SAH is the patient's neurologic condition on arrival at the hospital. Alterations in mental status are the most common abnormality. Some patients remain alert and lucid; others are confused, delirious, amnesic, lethargic, stuporous, or comatose. The modified Hunt and Hess grading scale serves as a means of risk stratification for SAH, based on the first neurologic examination (Table 46.3).

Patients classified as grade I or grade II SAH have a relatively good prognosis; grade III carries an intermediate prognosis, and grades IV and V have a poor prognosis. Focal neurologic signs occur in a minority of patients but may point to the site of bleeding; hemiparesis or aphasia suggests a middle cerebral artery aneurysm, and paraparesis or abulia (lack of ability to act or to make decisions) suggests an aneurysm of the proximal anterior cerebral artery. These focal signs are sometimes the result of a large focal hematoma, which may require emergency evacuation.

In 10% of patients with nontraumatic SAH and in two-thirds of those with negative angiography, CT reveals blood confined to the perimesencephalic cisterns, with the center of bleeding adjacent to the midbrain and pons. Most of these patients with perimesencephalic SAH may have a normal neurologic examination and a benign clinical course; rebleeding and symptomatic vasospasm or hydrocephalus almost never occur. The source of hemorrhage in these patients is presumably venous.

Symptoms and signs of an unruptured intracranial aneurysm may result from compression of adjacent neural structures or thromboembolism. These aneurysms are often, but not always, large or giant (greater than 25 mm). Aneurysms of the posterior communicating artery frequently compress the oculomotor nerve (almost always affecting the pupil). Aneurysms of the intracavernous segment of the internal carotid artery may damage the third, fourth, fifth, or sixth cranial nerves, and their rupture may lead to formation of a carotid cavernous fistula. Less often, large aneurysms compress the cortex or brainstem, causing focal neurologic signs or seizures. Thrombosis within the aneurysmal sac occasionally sends emboli to the distal territory of the artery, causing TIAs or infarction. In the absence of SAH, some patients experience sudden, severe headache without nuchal rigidity, perhaps related to aneurysmal enlargement, thrombosis, or meningeal irritation; these symptoms may clear with aneurysm clip application.

DIAGNOSTIC STUDIES

Computed Tomography

CT should be the first diagnostic study for establishing the diagnosis of SAH, owing to its ready availability and ease of interpretation. When SAH is misdiagnosed, the most common diagnostic error is failure to obtain a CT scan. CT most commonly demonstrates diffuse blood in the basal cisterns (Fig. 46.1); with more severe hemorrhages, blood extends into the sylvian and interhemispheral fissures, ventricular system, and over the convexities.

The distribution of blood may provide important clues regarding the location of the ruptured aneurysm. CT may also demonstrate a focal intraparenchymal or subdural hemorrhage, ventricular enlargement, a large thrombosed aneurysm, or infarction due to vasospasm. The sensitivity of CT for SAH is 90% to 95% within 24 hours, 80% at 3 days, and 50% at 1 week. Accordingly, a normal CT never rules out SAH; a lumbar puncture should always be performed in patients with suspected SAH and normal CT. MRI may also be used to make the initial diagnosis of SAH, or may be used to detect a completely thrombosed aneurysm when the initial angiogram is negative.

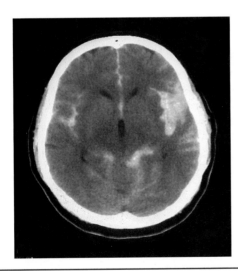

FIGURE 46-1. A: Noncontrast CT demonstrating hyperdensity within the lateral sylvian, anterior interhemispheric, and quadrigeminal cisterns, characteristic of acute aneurysmal subarachnoid hemorrhage. The predominance of blood in the left sylvian fissure is characteristic of a middle cerebral artery aneurysm in that region.

Lumbar Puncture

The CSF is usually grossly bloody. SAH may be differentiated from a traumatic tap by a xanthochromic (yellow-tinged) appearance of the centrifuged supernatant; however, xanthochromia may take up to 12 hours to appear. CSF pressure is nearly always high and the protein elevated. Initially, the proportion of CSF leukocytes to erythrocytes is that of the peripheral blood, with a usual ratio of 1:700; after several days a reactive pleocytosis and low-glucose levels may develop from sterile chemical meningitis caused by the blood. Red blood cells and xanthochromia disappear in about 2 weeks, unless hemorrhage recurs.

Angiography

Cerebral angiography is the definitive diagnostic procedure for detecting intracranial aneurysms and defining their anatomy (Fig. 46.2).

Although the increasing availability and image quality of CT and MRA has allowed some centers to use these tests to make the initial diagnosis, a four-vessel angiogram involving bilateral internal carotid and vertebral artery injections is mandatory when these tests are negative. Moreover, angiography performed either during coil insertion or after surgical clip application is generally advisable, to evaluate the adequacy of aneurysm repair and to screen for smaller secondary aneurysms that may be missed by CT or MR. Vasospasm, local thrombosis, or poor technique may lead to a false-negative angiogram. For this reason, patients with a negative angiogram at first screening should have a follow-up study 1 to 2 weeks later; an aneurysm will be demonstrated in about 5% of these cases. The exception to this rule is patients with perimesencephalic SAH, who usually do not require follow-up angiography.

COMPLICATIONS OF ANEURYSMAL SUBARACHNOID HEMORRHAGE

Rebleeding

Aneurysmal rebleeding is a dreaded complication of SAH. The risk of rebleeding is highest within the first 24 hours after the initial aneurysmal rupture (4%), and remains elevated (approximately 1% to 2% per day) for the next 4 weeks (Fig. 46.3).

The cumulative risk of rebleeding in untreated patients is 20% at 2 weeks, 30% at 1 month, and 40% at 6 months. After the first 6 months, the risk of rebleeding is 2% to 4% annually. Poor clinical grade and large aneurysm size are the strongest risk factors for in-hospital rebleeding. The prognosis of patients who rebleed is poor; approximately 50% die immediately, while another 30% die from subsequent complications. Although rebleeding is often attributed to uncontrolled hypertension, vascular-shear stress and endogenous fibrinolysis of clot around

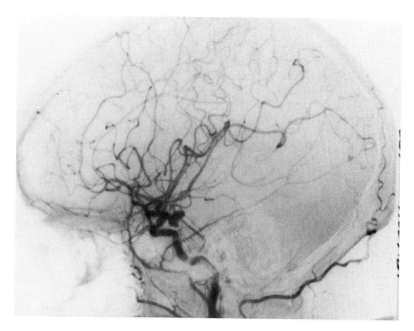

FIGURE 46.2. Lateral view of a left common carotid angiogram demonstrates a bilobed aneurysm of the left internal carotid artery at the level of the posterior communicating artery. (Courtesy Dr. S. Chan.)

the rupture point of the aneurysm may be more important causative mechanisms.

Vasospasm

Delayed cerebral ischemia from vasospasm accounts for a large proportion of morbidity and mortality after SAH. Progressive arterial narrowing develops after SAH in approximately 70% of patients, but delayed ischemic deficits develop in only 20% to 30%. The process begins 3 to 5 days after the hemorrhage, becomes maximal at 5 to 14 days, and gradually resolves over 2 to 4 weeks. Accordingly, deterioration attributable to vasospasm never occurs before the third day after SAH, and occurs with peak frequency between 5 and 7 days (Fig. 45.3). There is a strong relationship between the presence of thick, cisternal blood seen on initial CT and the development of symptomatic vasospasm. For reasons that are incompletely understood, the presence of large amounts of blood in the lateral ventricles adds to this risk (Table 46.4).

Symptomatic vasospasm usually involves a decrease in level of consciousness, hemiparesis, or both, and the process is usually most severe in the immediate vicinity of the aneurysm. In more severe cases, the symptoms develop earlier after aneurysm rupture, and multiple vascular territories are involved.

Although thick, subarachnoid blood is the principal precipitating factor, the precise cause of arterial narrowing after SAH is poorly understood. Vasospasm is not simply due to vascular smooth-muscle contraction; arteriopathic changes are seen in the vessel wall, including subintimal edema and infiltration of leukocytes. The prevailing view is that substances released from the blood clot interact with the vessel wall to cause inflammatory arterial spasm. Putative mediators include oxyhemoglobin (with its intrinsic vasoconstrictive properties), hydroperoxides and leukotrienes, free radicals, prostaglandins, thromboxane A_2 (TXA$_2$), serotonin, endothelin, platelet-derived growth factor, and other inflammatory mediators.

Hydrocephalus

Acute hydrocephalus occurs in 15% to 20% of patients with SAH and is primarily related to the volume of intraventricular and subarachnoid blood. In mild cases, hydrocephalus causes lethargy, psychomotor slowing, and impaired short-term memory. Additional findings may include limitation of upward gaze, sixth cranial nerve palsies, and lower extremity hyperreflexia. In more severe cases, acute obstructive hydrocephalus leads to elevated

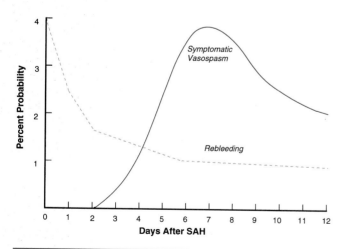

FIGURE 46.3. The daily percentage probability for the development of symptomatic vasospasm *(solid line)* or rebleeding *(dashed line)* after SAH. Day 0 denotes day of onset of SAH.

▶ **TABLE 46.4** Modified Fisher CT Rating Scale for the Prediction of Symptomatic Vasospasm

Grade	Criteria	Percentage of Patients	Frequency of DCI	Frequency of Infarction
0	No SAH or IVH	5%	0%	0%
1	Minimal/thin SAH, no biventricular IVH	30%	12%	6%
2	Minimal/thin SAH, *with* biventricular IVH	5%	21%	14%
3	Thick SAH, no biventricular IVH	43%	19%	12%
4	Thick SAH, *with* biventricular IVH	17%	40%	28%
	All patients	100%	20%	12%

Thick SAH refers to subarachnoid clot >5 mm in width completely fills at least one cistern or fissure. DCI, delayed cerebral ischemia (defined as symptomatic deterioration, cerebral infarction, or both resulting from vasospasm).
Data are based on a prospectively studied cohort of 276 patients at Columbia University Medical Center. From Claassen, et al, *Stroke* 2001;32:2012–2020, with permission.

intracranial pressure. Affected patients are stuporous or comatose, and progressive brain-stem herniation eventually results from continued CSF production, unless a ventricular catheter is inserted.

Delayed hydrocephalus may develop in from 3 to 21 days after SAH. The clinical syndrome is that of normal pressure hydrocephalus, with failure to fully recover and prominent symptoms of dementia, gait disturbance, and urinary incontinence. The clinical response to ventriculoperitoneal shunting is usually excellent. Overall, 20% of SAH survivors require shunting for chronic hydrocephalus.

Cerebral Edema

Brain swelling may occur after SAH, and in poor-grade patients, edema may contribute to increased intracranial pressure (ICP) or herniation syndromes. Global brain edema after SAH, which may be related to autoregulatory breakthrough in the setting of hypertension, is associated with loss of consciousness at ictus, and is a powerful predictor of poor outcome (Figure 46.4). Focal brain edema occurs most often in association with large hematomas, and may contribute to subfalcine herniation.

Seizures

Seizures occur in 5% to 10% of SAH patients during hospitalization, and in another 10% during the first year after discharge. Seizures after SAH are related primarily to focal pathology: large subarachnoid clots; subdural hematoma; or cerebral infarction. Ictal events at the onset of bleeding do not portend an increased risk of late seizures. With continuous electroencephalographic monitoring, nonconvulsive status epilepticus has become increasingly recognized as a cause of otherwise unexplained clinical deterioration after SAH, with ominous implications for prognosis.

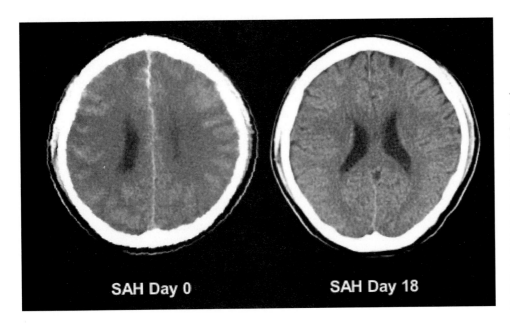

SAH Day 0   **SAH Day 18**

FIGURE 46-4. Global edema on the admission CT scan (SAH day 0) in a 55-year-old man with a Hunt-Hess Grade V SAH, showing effacement of the hemispheric sulci and disruption of the gray-white matter junction due to diffuse peripheral "finger-like" extension of the normal demarcation between gray and white matter. A follow-up CT scan on SAH day 18 shows complete normalization of these findings (Reprinted from Claassen et al, *Stroke* 2002;33:1225–1232, with permission).

Fluid and Electrolyte Disturbances

Hyponatremia and intravascular volume contraction frequently occur after SAH and reflect homeostatic derangements that favor excessive free-water retention and sodium loss. Hyponatremia occurs in to 5% to 30% of patients after SAH and is primarily related to inappropriate secretion of antidiuretic hormone (SIADH) and free-water retention. This process may be further exacerbated by excessive natriuresis that occurs after SAH (cerebral salt-wasting), related to elevations of atrial natriuretic factor and the glomerular filtration rate. Whereas hyponatremia after SAH is usually asymptomatic, sodium loss and intravascular volume contraction increase the risk of ischemia in the presence of severe vasospasm. To minimize the development of hypovolemia and hyponatremia after SAH, patients should be given large volumes of isotonic crystalloid guided by central venous or pulmonary artery pressure monitoring, with restriction of other potential sources of free water.

Neurogenic Cardiac and Pulmonary Disturbances

Severe SAH is typically associated with a surge in catecholamine levels and sympathetic tone, which in turn may lead to neurogenic cardiac dysfunction, neurogenic pulmonary edema, or both. Transient electrocardiographic abnormalities occur in at least 50% to 80% of SAH patients but usually do not produce symptoms. In some poor-grade patients, however, cardiac enzyme release and a reversible form of neurogenic "stunned myocardium" may occur. Hypotension and reduction of cardiac output may result, leading to impaired cerebral perfusion in the face of increased intracranial pressure or vasospasm. Neurogenic pulmonary edema, characterized by increased permeability of the pulmonary vasculature, may occur in isolation or in combination with neurogenic cardiac injury.

TREATMENT OF ANEURYSMAL SUBARACHNOID HEMORRHAGE

The initial goal of treatment is to prevent rebleeding by excluding the aneurysmal sac from the intracranial circulation, while preserving the parent artery and its branches. Once the aneurysm has been secured, the focus shifts toward monitoring and treating vasospasm and other secondary complications of SAH. This is best performed in an ICU.

Surgical Management

Craniotomy for surgical clip application has long been considered the definitive treatment for patients with aneurysms. In the 1980s, neurosurgeons began to abandon the traditional practice of delaying surgery until several weeks after aneurysmal rupture, in favor of early clip application, within the first 48 to 72 hours. This change in practice became feasible with the advances in safer microsurgical techniques. Although early clip application was initially reserved only for patients in good clinical condition (Hunt and Hess grade I to grade III), this approach has since been extended to all but the most moribund patients. Nonetheless, aneurysm clip application still remains hazardous, with a 5% to 10% risk of major morbidity or mortality when the aneurysm is acutely ruptured. In comparison, the risk of major morbidity or mortality from clip application of an unruptured aneurysm is 2% to 5%. The risks of surgery are highest when the aneurysm is large or when it is located on the basilar artery, and results are more favorable when the operation is performed by an experienced neurosurgeon in a high-volume center. If an intra- or postoperative angiogram demonstrates complete obliteration of the aneurysm after surgical clip application, the long-term risk of subsequent rebleeding is exceedingly small.

Endovascular Therapy

Since its introduction in the early 1990s, coil embolization has emerged as an important alternative to surgical clip application for the treatment of intracranial aneurysms (also discussed in chapter 17). Endovascular packing of aneurysms (Fig. 46.5) with soft, thrombogenic detachable platinum coils leads to short-term obliteration of small-necked aneurysms in 80% to 90% of cases, with a complication rate of approximately 9%. Aneurysms with wider necks are less amenable to this treatment because it is more difficult to attain complete obliteration and the coils or thrombus may migrate. A newer technique that may facilitate the treatment of wide-necked or complex aneurysms involves placing a flexible stent in the parent vessel that gives rise to the aneurysm, and then deploying coils through the stent into the aneurysm.

Endovascular coil insertion appears to be safer than surgical clip application, at least in the short term. In the International Subarachnoid Hemorrhage Aneurysm Trial, 2,134 patients (primarily with small [less than 10 mm] anterior circulation aneurysms) were randomly assigned to receive treatment with either clips or coils. At one year, 23.7% of the patients with coils were dead or dependent, compared to 30.6% of those treated with clip application. Although the exact reason for this discrepancy is unclear, the most likely explanation is a lower rate of intracranial complications, such as aneurysm rebleeding and brain retraction injury, with coil insertion.

The main disadvantage of endovascular treatment is the potential for rebleeding after several years, arising from coil compaction and aneurysm regrowth at the residual

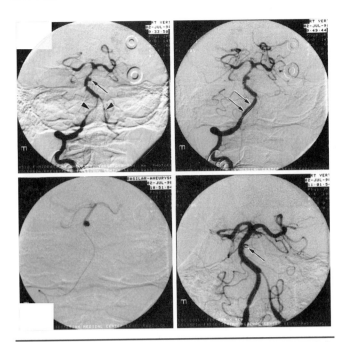

FIGURE 46-5. **A:** Cerebral angiogram demonstrates a left-pointing, 3-mm, midbasilar aneurysm *(closed arrow)* and vasospasm of both vertebral arteries *(open arrows)*, the distal basilar artery, and the proximal right posterior cerebral artery. **B:** Significant increase in luminal diameter of the right vertebral artery after balloon angioplasty *(arrows)*. **C:** Microcatheter positioned at the neck of the midbasilar aneurysm. **D:** Midbasilar aneurysm *(arrow)* with no residual filling after packing with a single platinum detachable coil. (Courtesy of Dr. Huang Duong.)

neck. Until long-term, follow-up studies define this risk more precisely, long-term serial angiography is recommended for patients with intracranial aneurysms treated with coils.

Intensive Care Management

A suggested algorithm for the postoperative management of SAH is outlined in Table 45.5.

All patients with SAH should be monitored in an ICU, where neurologic examinations may be performed frequently. Although the efficacy of blood pressure reduction in preventing early rebleeding has not been established, it seems prudent to maintain systolic pressure at 160 mmHg or less, until the aneurysm has been secured. Similarly, a loading dose of an intravenous anticonvulsant, such as fosphenytoin, is given to prevent early rebleeding related to seizures, although this risk is small. Anticonvulsants may be discontinued on the second postoperative day if the patient is stable and has not had a seizure.

Fluid resuscitation with isotonic crystalloid (approximately 1 mL/kg/hr, with or without additional colloids) should be given to counteract volume contraction resulting from natriuresis, which has been associated with an increased risk of infarction from vasospasm. A central-venous or pulmonary-artery catheter is used in high-risk patients to guide fluid administration on the basis of target cardiac-filling pressures. The calcium channel antagonist, nimodipine, reduced the frequency of delayed ischemic deterioration by about 30% in several clinical trials; this effect is presumably mediated by reduction of calcium entry into ischemic neurons or by improvement in microcollateral flow, since no effect was seen on angiographic spasm.

Use of dexamethasone in the treatment of acute SAH is controversial; it is often used in the perioperative period, for brain relaxation. There is no specific evidence to suggest that it is beneficial, although it may reduce the headache sometimes associated with vasospasm or SAH-induced sterile meningitis. Externalized ventricular drains are used to treat obstructive hydrocephalus in patients who are stuporous or comatose, but these devices carry a high risk of infection (15% overall) within the first 10 days. Serial lumbar puncture may be used to treat hydrocephalus in patients who are conscious and following commands.

Transcranial Doppler ultrasonography is widely used to diagnose vasospasm of the larger cerebral arteries after SAH. Accelerated blood-flow velocities, which occur as flow is maintained through narrowed arteries, have a sensitivity and specificity of 90% for angiographic vasospasm of the proximal middle cerebral artery, but they are less sensitive for detecting spasm of the anterior cerebral or basilar arteries.

Treatment of acute symptomatic vasospasm relies on increasing blood volume, blood pressure, and cardiac output in an attempt to improve cerebral blood flow through arteries in spasm that have lost the capacity to autoregulate. Crystalloid or colloid solutions are given to maintain pulmonary artery diastolic pressure (PADP) greater than 14 mmHg or central venous pressure (CVP) greater than 8 mmHg. Vasopressors, such as dopamine and phenylephrine, are used to elevate systolic blood pressure to levels as high as 180 mmHg to 220 mmHg. Hypertensive-hypervolemic hemodilution (triple-H therapy) of this type results in clinical improvement in about 70% of patients; cerebral angioplasty may lead to dramatic improvement in patients with severe deficits that are refractory to hemodynamic augmentation (Fig. 46.4).

Outcome After Subarachnoid Hemorrhage

In contrast to the severe physical handicaps that follow ischemic stroke, survivors of SAH are disabled primarily by cognitive impairment. Neuropsychologic testing reveals long-term problems in memory, concentration, psychomotor speed, visuospatial skills, or executive function in 60% to 80% of SAH patients. Depression

▶ **TABLE 46.5** Columbia University Medical Center Management Protocol for Acute SAH

Blood Pressure	■ Control elevated blood pressure during the preoperative phase (systolic BP <160 mmHg) with IV labetalol or nicardipine to prevent rebleeding.
IV Hydration	■ Preoperative: Normal (0.9%) saline at 80 mL/hr to 100 mL/hr. ■ Postoperative: Normal (0.9%) saline at 80 mL/hr to 100 mL/hr, and 250 mL 5% albumin every 2 hrs if the CVP is ≤ 5 mmHg.
Laboratory Testing	■ Periodically check CBC; transfuse for hematocrit <24% in stable patients, or <30% in patients with symptomatic vasospasm. ■ Periodically check electrolytes to detect hyponatremia. ■ Obtain serial ECGs and check admission cardiac troponin I (cTI) level to evaluate for cardiac injury; perform echocardiography in patients with abnormal ECG findings or cTI elevation.
Seizure Prophylaxis	■ Fosphenytoin or phenytoin IV load (20 mg/kg); discontinue on postoperative day 2 unless patient has seized or is unstable.
Vasospasm Prophylaxis Physiologic Homeostasis	■ Nimodipine 60 mg PO every 4 hrs for 21 days. ■ Cooling blankets to maintain T ≤ 37.5° C ■ Insulin drip to maintain glucose ≤ 120 mg/dL.
Ventricular Drainage Vasospasm diagnosis	■ Begin trials of clamping external ventricular drain and monitoring ICP on day 3 after placement ■ Transcranial Doppler sonography every 1 to 2 days until day 7 to 14 after SAH. ■ CT or MR perfusion on day 4 to day 8 after SAH, if high risk.
Therapy for Symptomatic Vasospasm	■ Place patient in Trendelenburg (head down) position. ■ Infuse 500 mL 5% albumin over 15 mins. ■ If the deficit persists, raise the systolic BP with phenylephrine or dopamine until the deficit resolves, up to a maximum of 200 mmHg to 220 mmHg. ■ 250 mL 5% albumin solution every 2 hrs if the CVP is ≤ 8 mmHg or the pulmonary artery diastolic pressure (PADP) is ≤ 14 mmHg. ■ If refractory, place pulmonary artery catheter and add dobutamine to maintain cardiac index ≥ 4.0 L/min/m². ■ Emergency angiogram for possible cerebral angioplasty unless the patient responds well to the above measures.

and anxiety are also common. These disturbances do not lead to the outward appearance of disability but may affect work capabilities, relationships, and quality of life; about 50% of SAH patients do not return to their previous level of employment. Cognitive and physical rehabilitation are essential to achieve maximal recovery in severely affected patients. Depression should be treated medically.

OTHER KINDS OF MACROSCOPIC ANEURYSMS

Fusiform or Dolichoectatic Aneurysms

These circumferential vessel dilations usually involve the carotid, basilar, or vertebral arteries. Atherosclerosis probably plays a role in their formation, but a develop-

mental defect of the wall may be present in some patients. Fusiform aneurysms seldom become occluded with thrombus and rarely rupture. If bleeding occurs, treatment often requires proximal vessel occlusion.

Mycotic Aneurysm

Mycotic aneurysms are caused by septic emboli, which are most often formed by bacterial endocarditis. They are usually only a few millimeters in size, and tend to occur on distal branches of pial vessels, especially those of the middle cerebral artery. Mycotic aneurysms have been reported in up to 10% of endocarditis patients, but arteriography is not routinely performed, and the incidence is probably underestimated. Pyogenic segmental arteritis from septic emboli, in the absence of frank aneurysm formation, may also lead to intracranial hemorrhage. As aneurysmal rupture is fatal in 80% of patients with mycotic aneurysms, cerebral arteriography should be performed when endocarditis is accompanied by suspicious headaches, stiff neck, seizure, focal neurologic symptoms, or CSF pleocytosis. Although mycotic aneurysms occasionally disappear radiographically, with antimicrobial therapy, the outcome may not be predicted and the aneurysm should be treated surgically as soon as possible.

Pseudoaneurysm

Dissection of an intracranial vessel, which usually results from trauma, may lead to extension of blood from the false lumen through the entire vessel wall. The extravasated blood is contained either by a thin layer of adventitia or by the surrounding tissues and does not have a true aneurysmal wall; hence the designation, *pseudoaneurysm*, is assigned. If a vessel traversing the subarachnoid space is affected, SAH may result. Treatment may require endovascular or surgical vessel occlusion or trapping, or angioplasty and stenting of the involved segment.

Vascular (Arteriovenous) Malformations (AVMs)

Vascular malformations account for less than 5% of all cases of SAH. Intracranial and spinal vascular malformations may be classified into five main types: (1) AVMs, which are high flow and most often symptomatic; (2) cavernous malformations; (3) capillary telangiectasias; (4) venous malformations; and (5) mixed malformations. More than 90% of vascular malformations are asymptomatic, throughout the life of the patient. Bleeding may occur in patients of any age but is most likely to occur in patients younger than 40 years. They are occasionally familial, and in 7% to 10% of cases, AVMs coexist with saccular aneurysms.

AVMs are a conglomerate of abnormal arteries and veins with intervening gliotic brain tissue; they resemble what could be called a bag of worms. When bleeding from an AVM occurs, reported initial mortality has ranged from 4% to 20%. Early rebleeding is far less likely than after aneurysm rupture, but recurrent hemorrhage occurs in 8% to 18% of patients, annually, over the next several years. For patients without hemorrhage, the risk of bleeding is 1% to 4% per year. Besides prior hemorrhage, reported risk factors for bleeding from an AVM include deep venous drainage, small size, a single draining vein, high feeding-artery pressure, male gender, and a diffuse nidus.

The diagnosis of AVM is made by MRI and arteriography. Small or thrombosed AVMs, especially in the brain stem, are occasionally missed by arteriography but may be detected by MRI, which better demonstrates the relationship of the malformation to surrounding brain and identifies its nidus. MRI is the preferred screening procedure for detecting vascular malformations; if surgery is contemplated, conventional angiography is required to delineate the vascular supply. Diagnosis of dural and spinal cord AVM should be kept in mind in patients with radiographically unexplained SAH.

Treatment depends on the location of the AVM and the age and condition of the patient. Direct surgical resection, endovascular glue embolization, and directed-beam radiation therapy with a linear accelerator or gamma-knife are the main treatment modalities. The long-term value of these treatments is unclear. Embolization is most useful for shrinking the malformation before surgery or radiation; it is occasionally curative as a single mode of therapy.

SUGGESTED READINGS

Aviv RI, Shad A, Tomlinson G, et al. Cervical dural arteriovenous fistulae manifesting as sub arachnoid hemorrhage: report of two cases and literature review. *AJNR Am J Neuroradiol* 2004;25(5):854–858.

Brust JCM, Dickinson PCT, Hughes JEO, et al. The diagnosis and treatment of cerebral mycotic aneurysms. *Ann Neurol* 1990;27:238–246.

Claassen J, Bernardini, GL, Kreiter K, et al. Effect of cisternal and ventricular blood on risk of delayed cerebral ischemia after subarachnoid hemorrhage: the Fisher scale revisited. *Stroke* 2001;32:2012–2020.

Feigin VL, Rinkel GJE, Algra A, et al. Calcium antagonists in patients with aneurysmal subarachnoid hemorrhage: a systematic review. *Neurology* 1998;50:876–883.

Fisher CM, Kistler JP, Davis JM. Relation of cerebral vasospasm to subarachnoid hemorrhage visualized by computerized tomographic scanning. *Neurosurgery* 1980;6:1–9.

Grosset DG, Straiton J, McDonald I, Cockburn M, Bullock R. Use of transcranial Doppler sonography to predict development of a delayed ischemic deficit after subarachnoid hemorrhage. *J Neurosurg* 1993;78:183–187.

Hop JW, Rinkel GJE, Algra A, van Gijn J. Case-fatality rates and functional outcome after subarachnoid hemorrhage: a systematic review. *Stroke* 1997;28:660–664.

Hunt WE, Hess RM. Surgical risk as related to time of intervention in the repair of intracranial aneurysms. *J Neurosurg* 1968;28:14–20.

International Subarachnoid Aneurysm Trial (ISAT) Collaborative Group, International Subarachnoid Aneurysm Trial (ISAT) of neurosurgical clip application versus endovascular coil insertion in 2143 patients with ruptured intracranial aneurysms: a randomised trial. *Lancet* 2002;360:1267–1274.

International Study of Unruptured Intracranial Aneurysms Investigators. Unruptured intracranial aneurysms: natural history, clinical outcome, and risks of surgical and endovascular treatment. *Lancet* 2003;362:103–110.

Kassell NF, Torner JC, Haley EC Jr, et al. The International Cooperative Study on the Timing of Aneurysm Surgery. 1. Overall management results. *J Neurosurg* 1990;73:18–36.

Kowalski RG, Claassen J, Kreiter KT, et al. Initial misdiagnosis and outcome after subarachnoid hemorrhage. *JAMA* 2004;291:866–869.

Longstreth WT Jr, Nelson LM, Koepsell TD, et al. Clinical course of spontaneous subarachnoid hemorrhage: a population-based study in King County, Washington. *Neurology* 1993;43:712–718.

Magnetic Resonance Angiography in Relatives of Patients with Subarachnoid Hemorrhage Study Group. Risks and benefits of screening for intracranial aneurysms in first-degree relatives of patients with sporadic subarachnoid hemorrhage. *N Engl J Med* 1999;341:1344–1350.

Manno EM. Subarachnoid hemmorhage. *Neurol Clin* 2004;22(2):347–366.

Mast H, Young WL, Koennecke HC, et al. Risk of spontaneous hemorrhage after diagnosis of cerebral arteriovenous malformation. *Lancet* 1997;350:1065–1068.

Mayberg MR, Batjer HH, Dacey R, et al. Guidelines for the management of subarachnoid hemorrhage: a statement for healthcare professionals from a special writing group of the Stroke Council, American Heart Association. *Circulation* 1994;90:2592–2605.

Mayer SA, Fink ME, Homma S, et al. Cardiac injury associated with neurogenic pulmonary edema following subarachnoid hemorrhage. *Neurology* 1994;44:815–820.

Murayama Y, Nien YL, Duckwiler G, et al. Guglielmi detachable coil embolization of cerebral aneurysms: 11 years' experience. *J Neurosurg* 2003;98:945–947.

Niskanen M, Koivisto T, Ron Kainen A, et al. Resource use after subarachnoid hemorrhage: comparison between endovascular and surgical treatment. *Neurosurgery* 2004;54(5):1081–1086.

Polin RS, Coenen VA, Hansen CA, et al. Efficacy of transluminal angioplasty for the management of symptomatic cerebral vasospasm following aneurysmal subarachnoid hemorrhage. *J Neurosurg* 2000;92:284–290.

Rhoney DH, Tipps LB, Murry KR, et al. Anticonvulsant prophylaxis and timing of seizures after aneurysmal subarachnoid hemorrhage. *Neurology* 2000;55:258–265.

Rinkel GJE, Djibuti M, Algra A, et al. Prevalence and risk of rupture of intracranial aneurysms: a systematic review. *Stroke* 1998;29:251–256.

Ronkainen A, Hernesniemi J, Puranen M, et al. Familial intracranial aneurysms. *Lancet* 1997;349:380–384.

Sahs AL, Nibbelink DW, Torner JC, eds. *Aneurysmal Subarachnoid Hemorrhage: Report of the Cooperative Study.* Baltimore: Urban & Schwartzenberg, 1981.

Schievink WI. Intracranial aneurysms. *N Engl J Med* 1997;336:28–40.

Teunissen LL, Rinkel GJ, Algra A. Risk factors for subarachnoid hemorrhage: a systematic review. *Stroke* 1996;27:544–549.

Topcuoglu MA, Ogilvy CS, Carter BS, et al. Subarachnoid hemorrhage without evident cause on initial angiography studies: diagnostic yield of subsequent angiography and other neuroimaging tests. *J Neurosurg* 2003;98:1235–1240.

Treggiari MM, Walder B, Suter PM, Romand JA. Systematic review of the prevention of delayed ischemic neurological deficits with hypertension, hypervolemia, and hemodilution therapy following subarachnoid hemorrhage. *J Neurosurg* 2003;98:978–984.

Tung P, Kopelnik A, Banki N, et al. Predictors of neurocardiogenic injury after subarachnoid hemorrhage. *Stroke* 2004;35(2):548–551.

Vinuela G, Duckwiler G, Mawad M. Guglielmi detachable coil embolization of acute intracranial aneurysm: perioperative anatomical and clinical outcome in 403 patients. *J Neurosurg* 1997;86:475–482.

Chapter 47

Cerebral Veins and Sinuses

Robert A. Fishman

Occlusion of the cerebral veins and sinuses occurs secondary to thrombus, thrombophlebitis, or tumors. Occlusion of the cortical and subcortical veins may cause focal neurologic symptoms and signs. The dural sinuses that are most frequently thrombosed are the lateral, cavernous, and superior sagittal sinuses. Less frequently affected are the straight sinus and the vein of Galen. Factors predis-

posing to thrombosis and associated disorders include the following:

Primary idiopathic thrombosis
Secondary thrombosis
    Pregnancy
    Postpartum
    Birth control pills
    Trauma—after open or closed head injury
    Tumors
        Meningioma
        Metastatic tumors
Malnutrition and dehydration (marantic thrombosis)
Infection—sinus thrombophlebitis, bacterial, fungal
Hematologic disorders
    Polycythemia
    Cryofibrinogenemia
    Sickle-cell anemia
    Leukemia
    Disseminated intravascular coagulation and other coagulopathies
Behçet syndrome

LATERAL SINUS THROMBOSIS

Thrombosis of the lateral sinus is usually secondary to otitis media and mastoiditis. Infants and children are most commonly affected. Thrombosis may be coincidental with the acute attack of otitis and mastoiditis, or it may occur in the chronic stage of infection.

Symptoms and Signs

Onset is usually heralded by fever and chills; however, fever may be absent. Septicemia most commonly occurs with hemolytic streptococci and is present in about 50% of patients. Petechiae in the skin and mucous membranes, and septic embolism of the lungs, joints, and muscles are infrequent complications of the septicemia.

The classic symptoms of lateral sinus thrombosis are fever, headache, nausea, and vomiting. The latter signs are effects of increased intracranial pressure (ICP) and are most apt to occur when the right sinus is occluded; in most individuals, the right sinus drains the greater portion of blood from the brain. Local signs of thrombosis of the sinus are usually absent, but occasionally there is swelling over the mastoid region with distention of the superficial veins and tenderness over the jugular vein in the neck.

Papilledema develops in about 50% of patients. It is usually bilateral but is occasionally unilateral, possibly the result of asymmetric extension of the process to the cavernous sinuses. ICP may cause separation of the sutures or bulging of the fontanels in infants.

Drowsiness and coma are common symptoms. Convulsive seizures may also occur. Jacksonian seizures, followed by hemiplegia, may reflect extension of the infection into the cerebral veins. However, these signs often indicate a brain abscess. Diplopia may result from injury to the sixth cranial nerve by increased ICP or from involvement of the nerve by extension of the infection in the petrous bone. The combination of sixth-nerve palsy (lateral rectus weakness) and pain in the face as the result of damage to the fifth nerve is the Gradenigo syndrome. There may be signs of damage to the ninth, tenth, and eleventh cranial nerves. These signs are attributed to pressure on these nerves by the distended jugular vein, as the nerves pass through the jugular foramen. In some cases these cranial nerve palsies are caused by extension of the infection into the bone (osteomyelitis) adjacent to these structures.

Laboratory Data

Leukocytosis is present in the blood, and the causative agent is recovered from the blood in 50% of septic cases. The CSF may show changes characteristic of an aseptic meningeal reaction. The pressure is increased. The fluid is usually slightly turbid or cloudy and contains several to many hundred leukocytes per cubic millimeter. The glucose content of the fluid is normal, and cultures are sterile, unless bacterial meningitis has developed.

Diagnosis

The diagnosis of lateral sinus thrombosis is usually made based on signs of increased ICP in a patient with an acute or chronic otitis and mastoiditis. The development of a hemiplegia, aphasia, or hemianopia favors the possibility of an intracerebral abscess or infarction, which should be excluded with imaging studies.

Course and Prognosis

The mortality rate is high in untreated lateral sinus thrombosis. Occasionally, the infected thrombus may heal by complete organization but more commonly, death results from septicemia, meningitis, extension of the infection to the cavernous or longitudinal sinus, or abscess of the brain. When patients recover, ICP may continue to be elevated for some months, especially if the jugular vein on the right side is ligated, as a result of pulmonary embolism.

Treatment

The occurrence of a thrombosis of the lateral sinus should be prevented by the prompt treatment of infections of the middle ear. Treatment of a thrombosis involves antibiotics and surgical drainage. Infected bone should be removed, the sinus should be exposed and drained, and the jugular vein should be ligated if necessary. Nonseptic patients may be candidates for thrombolytic therapy.

CAVERNOUS SINUS THROMBOSIS

Cavernous sinus thrombosis usually originates in suppurative processes of the orbit, nasal sinuses, or the upper one-half of the face. The infection commonly involves only one sinus at the onset but rapidly spreads to the opposite side. One or both sides may be secondarily involved, by extension of infection to the other dural sinuses. Nonseptic thrombosis of the cavernous sinus is rare. The sinus may be partially or totally occluded by tumor masses, trauma, or arteriovenous aneurysms.

Symptoms and Signs

The onset of symptoms of a septic thrombosis is usually sudden and dramatic. The patient appears acutely ill and there is a septic-related fever. There is pain in the eyes and the orbits are painful to applied pressure. The globes are proptosed by orbital edema and chemosis of the conjunctivae and eyelids. Diplopia follows involvement of the oculomotor nerves. Ptosis may be present and may be obscured by exophthalmos. The optic discs are usually swollen, and there are numerous small or large hemorrhages around the disc if the orbital veins are occluded. The corneas are cloudy and ulcers may develop. The pupils may be dilated or constricted. Pupillary reactions may be lost. Visual acuity may be normal or moderately impaired. The laboratory findings in patients with cavernous sinus thrombosis are similar to those in patients with lateral sinus thrombosis.

Diagnosis

Cavernous sinus thrombosis must be distinguished from other conditions that produce exophthalmos and congestion in the orbit. These include orbital tumors, meningiomas and other tumors in the region of the sphenoid, malignant exophthalmos, and arteriovenous fistulas. The evolution of symptoms is usually slow in the latter conditions, except with arteriovenous fistulas. These may be identified by the presence of pulsating exophthalmos and an orbital bruit, and recession of the exophthalmos when the carotid artery is occluded by digital pressure. CT, MRI, and MR venography (MRV) are valuable in establishing the diagnosis.

Treatment

Septic thrombosis of the cavernous sinus was once, almost invariably fatal because of the development of an acute meningitis. Cures now are possible, with appropriate antibiotics and anticoagulation therapy.

SUPERIOR SAGITTAL SINUS THROMBOSIS

The superior sagittal sinus is less commonly the site of an infective thrombosis than either the lateral or cavernous sinuses. Infections may reach the superior sagittal sinus from the nasal cavities or as secondary extensions from the lateral or cavernous sinuses. The superior sagittal sinus may also be occluded by extension of infection from osteomyelitis or from epidural or subdural infection.

The superior sagittal sinus is the most common site of nonseptic sinus thrombosis, and is associated with dehydration and marasmus in infancy. It may also be occluded by trauma or by tumors (meningiomas). Sagittal sinus thrombosis has also been associated with oral contraceptive use, pregnancy, hemolytic anemia, sickle-cell trait, thrombocytopenia, ulcerative colitis, diabetes mellitus, Behçet syndrome, and other diseases. Nonseptic thrombosis of the sinus occasionally occurs in adults without any known cause.

Symptoms and Signs

The general signs are prostration, fever, headache, and papilledema. Local signs include edema of the forehead and anterior part of the scalp and engorgement of the veins in the area of the anterior or posterior fontanels (in infants), with the formation of a caput medusae.

Focal neurologic signs and symptoms may be absent, entirely, in nonseptic thrombosis, with increased ICP as the only presenting sign. However, extension of the clot into the larger cerebral veins is commonly accompanied by the onset of dramatic signs caused by hemorrhage into the cerebrum. Extension into these veins is common in septic thrombosis and in a high percentage of the nonseptic type. Convulsive seizures (often unilateral), hemiplegia, aphasia, or hemianopia may occur. The diagnosis of nonseptic (marantic) thrombosis should be considered in all infants who show signs of increased ICP and cerebral symptoms, during the course of severe nutritional disturbances and cachexia.

The laboratory findings with septic thrombosis of the superior sagittal sinus are similar to those in patients with lateral sinus thrombosis. Occasionally, the CSF is bloody or xanthochromic as the result of cortical and meningeal hemorrhage.

Diagnosis

The diagnosis may be established by MRV. CT and MRV may show multiple, often bilateral lesions, some hemorrhagic and others ischemic (Figs. 47.1 and 47.2).

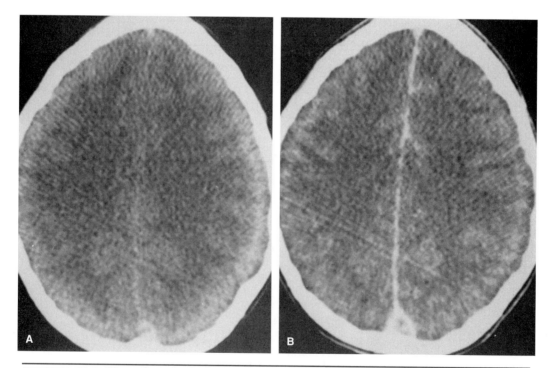

FIGURE 47-1. Sinus thrombosis, hemorrhagic venous infarction. A: Axial CT without contrast enhancement demonstrates density in the sagittal sinus posteriorly. **B:** At the same level, postcontrast, the empty delta sign is noted in the affected sinus. Thrombus density caused a central-filling defect within the sinus. Triangular enhancement at the periphery is related to collateral venous channels within the dura. (Courtesy of Drs. S.K. Hilal and J.A. Bello.)

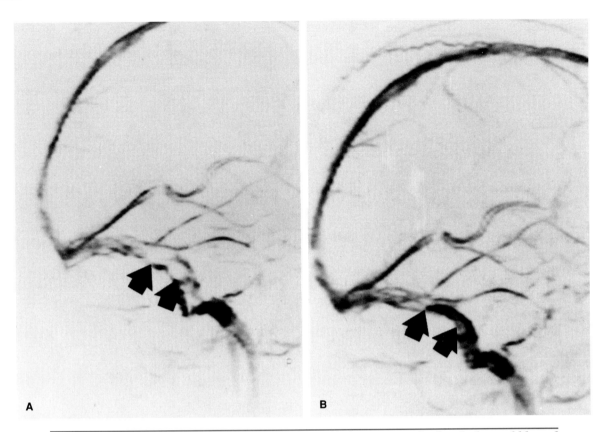

FIGURE 47-2. A 34-year-old man with bilateral papilledema, increasing headache, and blurred vision. Routine spin-echo MR image was normal. **A:** Two-dimensional (2D) time-of-flight (TOF) MRV at time of symptoms shows filling defects at the junction of right transverse and sigmoid sinuses *(arrows)*. **B:** 2D TOF MRV after local infusion of urokinase shows near-total resolution of filling defects *(arrows)*. The patient's symptoms were markedly improved. (Courtesy of Drs. Phillip Baum and David Norman.)

The *cord sign* is a linear area of increased density related to clots in veins or sinuses. The *empty delta sign* appears in the torcula after injection of contrast material, which outlines the periphery of the sinus where blood still flows, leaving the central area of the clot dark; there may also be enhancement of the gyri or tentorium. Ventricles may be large or small. Cerebral angiography is definitive, showing the venous block or collateral flow.

Prognosis

The prognosis is guarded in patients with septic thrombosis. Death may result from meningitis or hemorrhagic lesions in the brain. Survivors may have focal neurologic deficits and recurrent convulsive seizures. The prognosis is less grave in patients with nonseptic thrombosis. Symptoms may recede weeks or months after recanalization of the sinus or after development of collateral circulation.

Treatment

Antibiotics should be administered to patients with septic thrombosis. Craniotomy with evacuation of subdural or epidural abscess should be performed when these are present. Heparin or thrombolytic therapy (endovascular chemical thrombolysis) has been beneficial in some patients, despite the risks of hemorrhagic infarction. Acetazolamide reduces CSF secretion and may be useful in lowering ICP. The role of steroids has not been established.

THROMBOSIS OF OTHER DURAL SINUSES

Thrombosis of the inferior longitudinal sinus, the straight sinus, the petrosals, or the vein of Galen rarely occurs alone. These sites are usually involved by secondary extension of a septic or nonseptic thrombosis of the lateral, superior sagittal, or cavernous sinuses. Any signs or symptoms that may be produced by thrombosis of the inferior longitudinal, straight, or petrosal sinuses are usually masked by those resulting from involvement of the more important sinuses. Thrombosis of the great vein of Galen may cause hemorrhages in the central white matter of the hemispheres, or in the basal ganglia and lateral ventricles. Anticoagulation is indicated in most cases. Endovascular chemical thrombolysis with urokinase or tissue plasminogen activator (tPA) has proved effective in some patients. Mechanical clot thrombolysis is effective in opening occluded sinuses but may cause cerebral hemorrhage.

DURAL ARTERIOVENOUS MALFORMATIONS

Dural arteriovenous malformations (AVMs) are more common in women than men, and occur more often in the posterior fossa than above the tentorium. They may cause multiple cranial nerve involvement (most commonly, third, seventh, eighth, and twelfth) or central nervous system manifestations. The latter are attributed to intracranial venous hypertension, decreased CSF absorption, venous sinus thrombosis, or minimal subarachnoid bleeding. Seizures, motor weakness, and brain-stem and cerebellar syndromes have been observed, depending on the region involved. Some patients experience subarachnoid hemorrhaging or papilledema and headache only, as in idiopathic pseudotumor.

Diagnosis usually requires detailed cerebral angiography, including selective injection of the external carotid and both vertebral arteries. Therapy with selective embolization, using silicone or other agents, may be beneficial and may require direct surgical excision. Spontaneous thrombosis of a dural AVM with remission of symptoms is not unusual; many lesions have a benign prognosis. Dural AVMs also occur in the spinal cord, often presenting as an insidiously progressive paraparesis. The role of interventional neuroradiologists in the management of AVMs has become increasingly important.

SUGGESTED READINGS

Berroir S, Grabli D, Heran F, Bakouche P, Bousser MG. Cerebral sinus venous thrombosis in two patients with spontaneous intracranial hypotension. *Cerebrovasc Dis* 2004;17(1):9–12. Epub 2003 Oct 03.

Bousser MG, Russell RR. *Cerebral venous thrombosis*. Philadelphia: WB Saunders, 1997:175.

Crassard I, Bousser MG. Cerebral venous thrombosis. *J Neuroophthalmol* 2004 Jun;24(2)156–63.

Favrole P, Guichard JP, Crassard I, Bousser MG, Chabriat H. Diffusion-weighted imaging of intravascular clots in cerebral venous thrombosis. *Stroke* 2004 Jan;35(1):99–103.

Horowitz M, Purdy P, Unwin H, et al. Treatment of dural sinus thrombosis using selective catheterization and urokinase. *Ann Neurol* 1995;38:58–67.

Gee JH, Lee HK, Lark JK, et al. Cavernous sinus syndrome: clinical features and differential diagnosis with MR imaging. *Am J Roentgenol* 2003;181(2):583–590.

Masuhr F, Mehraein S, Einhaupl K. Cerebral venous and sinus thrombosis. *J Neurol* 2004 Jan;251(1):11–23.

Schreiber SJ, Diehl RR, Weber W, Henkes H, Nahser HC, Lehmann R, Doepp F, Valdueza JM. Doppler sonographic evaluation of shunts in patients with dural arteriovenous fistulas. *AJNR Am J Neuroradiol* 2004 May;25(5):775–80.

Smith TP, Higashida RT, Barnwell SL, et al. Treatment of dural sinus thrombosis by urokinase infusion. *ANJR* 1994;15:801–807.

Soleau SW, Schmidt R, Stevens S, et al. Extensive experience with dural sinus thrombosis. *Neurosurgery* 2003;52(3):534–544.

Southwick FS, Richardson EP, Swartz MN. Septic thrombosis of the dural venous sinuses. *Medicine* 1986;65:82–106.

Steinmetz MP, Chow MM, Krishnaney AA, et al. Andrews-Hinders D, Benzel EC, Masaryk TJ, Mayberg MR, Rasmussen PA. Outcome after the treatment of spinal dural arteriovenous fistulae: a contemporary single-institution series and meta-analysis. *Neurosurgery* 2004 Jul;55(1):77–87.

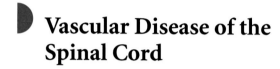

Chapter 48

Vascular Disease of the Spinal Cord

Leon A. Weisberg

Blood supply to the spinal cord and nerve roots originates in the vertebral, thyrocervical, costocervical, intercostal, and lumbar arteries, these give rise to radicular and medullary arteries. Segmental radicular arteries supply nerve roots, originating near the vertebral foramina. Six to nine large medullary arteries originate from the vertebral, subclavian, or iliac arteries and aorta (Fig. 48.1).

ANATOMY

Branches of medullary arteries form a single, anterior, median spinal artery and two posterior spinal arteries, which perfuse the spinal cord. The anterior median spinal artery arises from the vertebral artery, and runs along the entire length of the cord. The pial arteriolar plexus and posterior spinal arteries supply dorsal aspects of the cord.

In the cervical region, the anterior median artery has collateral vessels at several levels in unpaired medullary arteries derived from the vertebral and subclavian arteries; this blood supply is rich in collateral branches. In the thoracic region, the anterior median spinal artery is joined by only a few branches from the thoracic aorta, and blood supply is relatively sparse, especially in lower segments.

The midthoracic spinal cord is supplied by terminal vessels descending from the subclavian and vertebral arteries or ascending from the abdominal aorta; this watershed is particularly vulnerable to vascular insufficiency, and spinal-cord infarction is most likely to occur at levels T-4 to T-9. Owing to its relative hypovascularity, the midthoracic region is particularly vulnerable to effects of

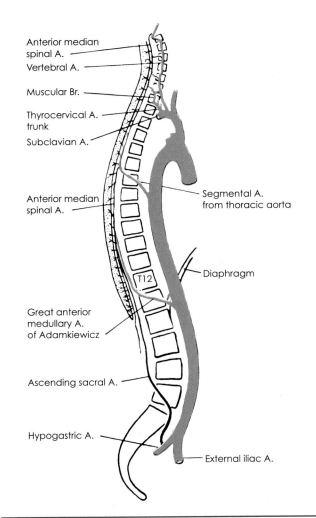

FIGURE 48-1. The anterior median spinal artery is joined at various levels by arteries arising from the vertebral and subclavian arteries, the aorta, and the iliac arteries.

hypotensive infarction. The midthoracic spinal syndrome (e.g., T-4 myelopathy) actually may be false localizing, and apparent clinical dysfunction at this level may actually be the result of impaired perfusion at higher or lower cord levels, or to global ischemia.

Lumbar and sacral spinal areas are supplied by the largest and most constant of medullary arteries, the great anterior radicular artery of Adamkiewicz. This is usually found at level L-1 or L-2 (occasionally as high as T-12 or as low as L-4). This artery, paired or single, travels through the vertebral foramen and anastomoses with the anterior medial spinal artery; the largest branch supplies the lumbosacral spinal cord and conus medullaris. Conus and cauda equina are also supplied by sacral branches ascending from the iliac arteries.

The central (sulcal) arteries originate in the anterior spinal artery to supply the anterior two-thirds and central area of the spinal cord. Penetrating branches from the pial arterial plexus supply the periphery and posterior

one-third of the cord. Within the spinal cord, these arterial feeders anastomose in their most distal parts, creating border zones similar to those in the brain. These vascular border zones may explain the development of incomplete or partial syndromes seen after some spinal-cord infarctions (Fig. 48.1). The plexiform venous system interconnects freely with the radicular arteries within subarachnoid space. The radicular veins empty into the epidural venous plexus, which in turn communicates with the inferior vena cava and azygos system, through the perivertebral plexus.

INFARCTION OF THE SPINAL CORD

Softening or infarction of the spinal cord (myelomalacia) results from occlusion of major vessels. Anterior spinal artery infarction is much more common than the posterior spinal artery syndrome because of the difference in collateral supply between these two regions.

Etiology

Spinal-cord infarction is most often caused by atheromas involving the aorta and is a potential complication of thoracoabdominal aneurysm repair. In one series, spinal infarction accounted for 1.2% of stroke admissions. Less common causes of spinal-cord infarction (i.e., acute spinal ischemic syndrome) include collagen vascular disease (e.g., systemic lupus and polyarteritis), syphilitic angiitis, dissecting aortic aneurysm, embolic infarction (e.g., bacterial endocarditis, nucleus pulposus), pregnancy, sickle-cell disease (SCD), neurotoxic effects of iodinated contrast material used in angiography, compression of spinal arteries by tumor, systemic arterial hypotension as a consequence of cardiac arrest, and decompression sickness. In 36% of cases, there is no obvious cause or identifiable vascular risk factor. Paraplegia may follow surgical repair of an aortic aneurysm if the cross-clamp time exceeds 25 minutes; neurologic injury consequences are made less likely by avoiding systemic arterial hypotension, by placing the shunt around the cross-clamp, and by using thiopental anesthesia. Spinal-cord ischemia may occur as an early complication of spinal arteriovenous malformation (AVM) repair (e.g., surgery, embolization).

Symptoms and Signs

The symptoms of spinal stroke usually appear within minutes or hours of the onset of ischemia. The first symptom may be radicular back pain, either lancinating or burning in quality. There may also be diffuse, deep, aching pain in both legs, or a burning, dysesthetic pain in the feet, rapidly ascending to the calves, thighs, and abdomen. These sensory symptoms are followed by the rapid onset of leg weakness. Occlusion of the cervical part of the anterior spinal artery causes tetraplegia, incontinence of urine and feces, and sensory impairment below the level of the lesion. In cervical lesions, breathing impairment may be caused by involvement of the voluntary and autonomic ventilatory pathways and lower motor neurons that innervate the diaphragm. Proprioception and vibratory sensation are spared because the posterior columns are supplied by the posterior arterial plexus. If proprioception and vibration sensation are impaired, the lesion is most likely not an anterior spinal artery infarction, but is rather a myelopathy of nonvascular origin. Spastic weakness in the legs results from lesions of the lateral corticospinal tract.

Sometimes, signs are restricted to those of either upper or lower motor neurons (or both) in a pattern similar to that of amyotrophic lateral sclerosis (ALS), but with major differences in the mode of onset and in its lack of progressive worsening in spinal stroke. If spinal ischemia involves only the gray matter supplied by sulcal arterial branches, there may be only lower motor neuron signs (i.e., amyotrophy). Sudden onset of the motor syndrome is consistent with vascular etiology; however, if symptoms appear more slowly and progressively, clinical differentiation from ALS or spinal-cord tumor may be difficult. The spinal level of abnormal signs in spinal ischemia may involve the high-cervical or low-sacral regions, with a mean level at T-8.

Most clinical spinal-cord strokes affect the midthoracic region, where levels are localized in paraplegia, urinary incontinence, loss of pain and temperature sensation, and sparing of proprioception and vibration. The weakness is flaccid at first but Babinski signs are seen, and spasticity and hyperreflexia usually appear in a few weeks. Arterial insufficiency of the lumbar region causes paraplegia, sphincter symptoms, and loss of cutaneous sensation with sacral sparing. The weakness is more likely to remain flaccid because the anterior horn cells are affected.

TIAs of the spinal cord and cauda equina may occur but there is no way to confirm this clinical impression. These attacks may precede spinal artery infarction, sometimes in association with lumbar spondylosis and stenosis. Symptoms may be precipitated by postural change in patients with lumbar stenosis. In cervical spondylosis, the role of arterial compression in the subsequent development of myelopathy is uncertain.

Diagnosis

MRI is the most sensitive imaging study; cord enlargement may be seen on T-1 and linear hyperintensity seen on T-2. MRI also is needed to rule out spinal-cord neoplasm or cervical spondylosis, which may simulate spinal-cord stroke, clinically. Lumbar puncture assay excludes hemorrhagic or infectious disorders. In spinal-cord infarction, the CSF may show a slight rise in protein content but the gamma globulin content is normal.

Two conditions that may simulate spinal infarction are multiple sclerosis (MS) and cord neoplasm. In MS or transverse myelitis, the CSF frequently shows an elevated gamma globulin content. Neoplasms are more likely to increase the CSF protein content to several hundred milligrams per deciliter. In spinal-cord infarction, edema may cause signs of an intramedullary mass and subarachnoid block; MRI is preferred to myelography to differentiate. Spinal angiography may cause cord infarction, and is contraindicated unless spinal vascular malformation is considered likely; angiography results are usually normal in spinal ischemia.

Treatment and Prognosis

The general principles of care for patients with quadriplegia or paraplegia should be followed. Naloxone and calcium channel antagonists have been used, experimentally, to treat spinal-cord ischemia, but no studies have been undertaken in humans. There is no evidence to support the use of antiplatelet or anticoagulant medication for prevention of spinal ischemia. The prognosis for recovery is uncertain. In one review, the mortality rate was 22%. At discharge from spinal-cord injury unit, 57% were in wheelchairs, 25% were ambulatory with technical aids, and 18% were fully ambulatory. Two-thirds required indwelling bladder catheters and one-third used intermittent catheterization.

The major predisposing factor for spinal ischemia is surgical reconstruction of thoracoabdominal aortic aneurysm. The potential for spinal ischemia and resulting neurologic deficit depends on aneurysm extension and whether or not dissection has occurred. Despite the use of hypothermia, intraoperative somatosensory monitoring, reanastomosis of intercostal arteries, short clamp time, distal aortic perfusion, and CSF drainage techniques, spinal ischemia is a possible risk of aortic aneurysm repair.

VENOUS DISEASE

Venous disorders of the spinal cord are even less common than arterial lesions. Venous infarction may occur in patients with sepsis, systemic malignancy, or spinal vascular malformation. Patients experience sudden back pain, and motor, sensory, and autonomic dysfunctions develop. Sensory impairment does not necessarily spare the posterior columns, as it may, characteristically, in anterior spinal artery ischemia. CSF examination is necessary to exclude infectious, inflammatory or neoplastic conditions in patients with spinal-cord ischemia. CT or MRI is necessary to exclude alternative lesions, including vascular malformations.

The Foix-Alajouanine syndrome (i.e., subacute or progressive necrotic myelopathy) is characterized by spinal-cord necrosis and evidence of enlarged, tortuous, thrombosed veins. Although this necrotic myelitis is attributed to venous thrombosis, there usually is no angiographic evidence of venous thrombosis or vascular spinal-cord malformation. Instead, the pathologic evidence points to vascular malformations, with spontaneous vascular thrombosis causing multiple, small infarcts and hemorrhagic spinal lesions. Pathologically for the most part, the necrosis involves the corticospinal tract, sparing anterior horn cells, and the lesion is most prominent in the thoracolumbar region.

Clinically, subacute and progressive worsening of symptoms continues for several weeks. The prodrome may include back or leg pain. Symptoms include leg weakness, incontinence, and sensory loss. Findings usually include spastic paraparesis, hyperreflexia, bilateral Babinski signs, and a sensory level below the lesion. CSF may show a markedly elevated protein content, leukocytic pleocytosis, and the presence of red blood cells. Treatment with anticoagulants or corticosteroids has not been effective. Some venous infarctions of the spinal cord are hemorrhagic, so anticoagulation is potentially dangerous in this condition.

SPINAL CORD HEMORRHAGE

Hemorrhage in the spinal cord is rare and may be epidural, subdural, subarachnoid, or intramedullary in location. Hematomyelia (i.e., hemorrhage into the substance of the spinal cord) usually follows a spinal injury immediately; however, it may be delayed for hours or days. Nontraumatic causes of spinal-cord hemorrhage include blood disorders (e.g., leukemia), anticoagulation therapy, AVM, venous spinal-cord infarction, and epidural anesthesia.

Pathology

In intramedullary spinal-cord hemorrhage, the spinal cord is swollen because of an intramedullary central blood clot. The blood dissects longitudinally, for several segments below and above the hemorrhage, most severely affecting the gray matter and contiguous white matter. The clot is usually surrounded by a rim of normal nerve tissue. With time, the blood is liquefied and removed by phagocytes. Glial replacement is usually incomplete, resulting in a syrinx-like cavity that extends over several cord segments.

Signs and Symptoms

In spinal-cord hemorrhage, localized back pain or radicular pain is sudden in onset. If hemorrhage is small, there may be only spastic weakness, associated with hyperreflexia in the legs, and bladder dysfunction. If the hemorrhage is large, signs of cord transection include: flaccid paralysis, complete sensory loss below the lesion, absent reflexes, Babinski signs, and loss of sphincter control. Autonomic disturbance and vasomotor instability may result in cardiovascular shock. If the patient survives, the hematoma is reabsorbed and symptoms may improve, but outcome is uncertain. Spinal subdural or epidural hemorrhage is usually caused by trauma (e.g., lumbar puncture) or coagulopathy. Initially, patients experience neck or back pain and radiculopathy, or myelopathy may subsequently develop.

Diagnosis

The CSF is bloody or xanthochromic, especially if there is an associated subarachnoid hemorrhage, and protein content is increased. CT may show the hyperdense hematoma more clearly than MRI. Spinal angiography may be indicated in nontraumatic cases if spinal vascular malformation is suspected.

Spinal epidural or subdural hemorrhage may cause mass effect that rapidly compresses the cord. This may follow spinal trauma, even without evidence of bone fracture; other causes include neoplasm, abscess anticoagulation, and blood dyscrasias, and there are cases without obvious etiology. This spinal hemorrhage is most common in cervical and thoracic region. Epidural hemorrhage may follow lumbar puncture in patients with a coagulation disorder, including those who are taking warfarin or other anticoagulant therapy. The symptoms of epidural and subdural spinal hematoma are similar.

Symptoms of epidural hemorrhage appear rapidly, with back pain, sensory loss, and sphincter impairment. The diagnosis is now established by MRI, which directly visualizes the hemorrhage. On sagittal sections, MRI shows biconvex mass located dorsally to the thecal sac, with tapering superior and inferior margins. The dura appears curvilinear and is separate from the cord. Spinal subarachnoid hemorrhage may arise from vascular malformation, spinal neoplasm (e.g., most commonly, ependymoma), blood dyscrasia, or periarteritis nodosa: it is characterized by sudden, severe back pain at the level of the lesion. Symptoms may be caused by blood in the subarachnoid space, or by blood dissecting into the spinal cord or along the nerve-root sheaths. The CSF is bloody and xanthochromic. MRI shows the hemorrhage.

Spinal angiography is necessary to establish the cause of the hemorrhage. Ruptured intracranial aneurysm occasionally causes severe back pain, with clinical findings indicative of spinal hemorrhage; in these cases, cerebral angiography may be necessary to determine the etiology, especially if the patient also reports headache and has nuchal rigidity.

Treatment

Treatment of spinal-cord hemorrhage depends on the cause and location of the hemorrhage. For subdural and epidural hemorrhage, surgery is necessary with laminectomy to remove the clot is necessary, but the prognosis is poor when paraplegia is present and if there is a delay in surgical intervention. In some cases, the clots may re-solve spontaneously. Patients with spinal-cord hematomas caused by anticoagulant therapy should receive fresh, whole blood and vitamin K. Spinal-cord decompression is carried out if effective hemostasis may be achieved, but should be avoided if bleeding impairment is not correctable.

SUGGESTED READINGS

Alexander RT, Cummings TJ. Pathologic quiz case: acute-onset paraplegia in a 60-year-old woman. Spinal cord infarction secondary to fibrocartilaginous (intervertebral disk) embolism. *Arch Pathol Lab Med* 2003;127(8):1047–1048.

Benavente O, Barnett HJM. Spinal cord ischemia in stroke. In: Barnett HJM, Mohr JP, Stein BM, Yatsu FM, eds. *Stroke* 3rd ed. New York: Churchill Livingstone, 1998:751–766.

Cheshire WP, Santos CC, Massey EW, Howard JF. Spinal cord infarction: etiology and outcome. *Neurology* 1996;47:321–330.

Crawford ES, Crawford JL, Safi HJ. Thoraco-abdominal aortic aneurysms: preoperative and intraoperative factors determining immediate and long-term results of operations in 605 patients. *J Vasc Surg* 1986;3:389–404.

Fukui M, Swarnkar A, Williams R. Acute spontaneous spinal epidural hematomas. *Am J Neuroradiol* 1999;20:1365–1372.

Garland H, Greenberg J, Harriman DGF. Infarction of the spinal cord. *Brain* 1966;89:645–662.

Hughes JT. Venous infarction of the spinal cord. *Neurology* 1971;21:794–800.

Kim RC, Smith HR, Henbest ML. Nonhemorrhagic venous infarction of the spinal cord. *Ann Neurol* 1984;15:379–385.

Kim SW, Kim RC, Choi BH, Gordon SK. Non-traumatic ischemic myelopathy: a review of 25 cases. *Paraplegia* 1988;26:262–272.

Loher TJ, Bassetti CL, Lovblad KO, et al. Diffusion-weighted MRI in acute spinal cord ischaemia. *Neuroradiology* 2003;45(8):557–561.

Mair WCP, Folkerts JF. Necrosis of spinal cord due to thrombophlebitis (subacute necrotic myelitis). *Brain* 1953;76:536–572.

Maroon JC, Abla AA, Wilberger JI, Bailes JE, Sternau LL. Central cord syndrome. *Clin Neurosurg* 1991;37:612–621.

Nedeltchev K, Loher TJ, Stepper F, et al. Long-term outcome of acute spinal cord ischemia syndrome. *Stroke* 2004;35(2):560–565.

Ross RT. Spinal cord infarction in disease and surgery of the aorta. *Can J Neurol Sci* 1985;12:289–295.

Russel NA, Benoit BG. Spinal subdural hematoma: a review. *Surg Neurol* 1983;20:133–137.

Salvador de la Barrera S, Barca-Buyo A. Spinal cord infarction: prognosis and recovery in a series of 36 patients. *Spinal Cord* 2001;39:520–525.

Sandson TA, Friedman JH. Spinal cord infarction: report of 8 cases and review of the literature. *Medicine* 1989;68:282–292.

Satran R. Spinal cord infarction. *Stroke* 1988;19:529–532.

Silver JR, Buxton PH. Spinal stroke. *Brain* 1974;97:539–550.

Sliwa JA, Maclean IC. Ischemic myelopathy: a review of spinal vasculature and related clinical syndromes. *Arch Phys Med Rehabil* 1992;73:365–372.

Zull D, Cydulka R. Acute paraplegia and aortic dissection. *Am J Med* 1988;84:765–770.

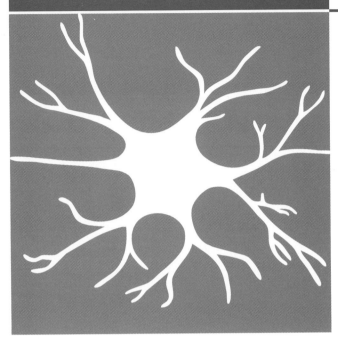

Disorders of Cerebrospinal and Brain Fluids

Chapter 49

▶ Hydrocephalus

Leon D. Prockop

Hydrocephalus is characterized by increased CSF volume and dilation of the cerebral ventricles. Although various classifications have evolved historically, the following types are recognized:

Obstructive hydrocephalus (intraventricular, or IVOH, and extraventricular, or EVOH)
    Congenital malformations
    Postinflammatory or posthemorrhagic
    Mass lesions
Communicating hydrocephalus
    Overproduction of CSF
    Defective absorption of CSF
    Venous drainage insufficiency
Normal pressure hydrocephalus
Hydrocephalus *ex vacuo*

When clinical signs or symptoms of intracranial hypertension are not apparent, hydrocephalus is labeled *occult*. It is *active* when the disease is progressive, and there is increased intracranial pressure (ICP). Hydrocephalus is considered *arrested* when ventricular enlargement has ceased. Dandy and Blackfan introduced the terms *communicating* and *noncommunicating hydrocephalus* to describe the flow of CSF. To make this determination, they injected a tracer dye into one lateral ventricle. If the dye appeared in lumbar CSF, the hydrocephalus was termed *communicating;* if the dye did not appear in the lumbar CSF, the hydrocephalus was termed *noncommunicating.* This functional classification was widely accepted because it proved useful in surgical-shunt placement; however, by this definition, noncommunicating hydrocephalus refers only to that caused by obstruction within the ventricular system. Currently, the term *obstructive hydrocephalus* is used to describe conditions after obstruction of either intraventricular or extraventricular pathways. In communicating hydrocephalus, no obstruction may be demonstrated by standard tests. *Normal pressure hydrocephalus* warrants separate classification and discussion. These forms of hydrocephalus are distinguished from *hydrocephalus ex vacuo* in which CSF volume increases without change in CSF pressure because of cerebral atrophy, as in Alzheimer disease (Fig. 49.1).

OBSTRUCTIVE HYDROCEPHALUS

Obstructive hydrocephalus is best characterized as the most common form of hydrocephalus. The term noncommunicating hydrocephalus is sometimes used. To facilitate clinical diagnosis and management, obstructive hydrocephalus is further classified as IVOH or EVOH. In IVOH, the obstruction site causes proximal dilatation of the ventricles with preservation of normal ventricular size distal to the blockage. Obstruction may occur at the Foramen of Monro, the third ventricle, the aqueduct of Sylvius, the fourth ventricle, or the outflow of the foramina of Luschka and Magendie.

In obstruction of extraventricular CSF pathways, absolute or relative reduction of flow may occur in the subarachnoid spaces at the base of the brain, at the tentorial level, or over the hemisphere convexities. The limitations of the clinical tests discussed later mean that the precise location of the obstruction or absorptive block may not always be determined. Obstructive hydrocephalus is caused by congenital malformations, developmental lesions, postinflammatory fibrosis, posthemorrhagic fibrosis, or mass lesion.

Congenital Malformations and Developmental Lesions

Congenital hydrocephalus occurs with an incidence of 0.5 to 1.8 per 1,000 births and may result from either genetic or nongenetic causes. Common nongenetic causes include intrauterine infection, intracranial hemorrhage secondary to birth trauma or prematurity, and meningitis. Genetically, an X-linked hydrocephalus has been described. In most of these cases, aqueductal stenosis has been documented

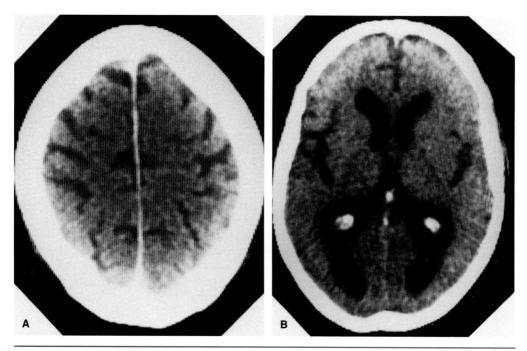

FIGURE 49.1. Brain CT. Marked ventricular dilatation **(A)** and widening of cortical sulci **(B)** are indicative of hydrocephalus *ex vacuo* in a 64-year-old woman with dementia.

by MRI or at postmortem examination. In some families, the occurrence of aqueductal stenosis, hydrocephalus of undetermined anatomic type, and the Dandy-Walker syndrome in siblings of both sexes suggests other modes of inheritance. In the Dandy-Walker syndrome, there is expansion of the fourth ventricle and the posterior fossa, with obstruction of the foramina of Luschka and Magendie (Fig. 49.2).

It is not clear whether or not aqueductal lesions (e.g., gliosis or fibrosis) occur developmentally or are the residue of prior viral inflammatory disease contracted *in utero* or in early life (Fig. 49.3). The Arnold-Chiari malformation may be associated with hydrocephalus at birth or it may develop later.

Postinflammatory or Posthemorrhagic Hydrocephalus

Posthemorrhagic hydrocephalus is a major complication of cerebral intraventricular hemorrhage (IVH) in low-birth-weight infants, with an incidence of 26% to 70%, depending on the severity of the hemorrhage. Hydrocephalus results when a clot within the ventricular system obstructs CSF flow by obliterative basilar arachnoiditis or by cortical arachnoiditis. After subarachnoid hemorrhage (SAH), the fact that the arachnoid villi are distended with packed red cells suggests an absorptive defect as a pathogenic mechanism for hydrocephalus. Consequently, fibrotic impairment of extraventricular CSF pathways after intracranial hemorrhage (ICH) may be complicated by dysfunc-

tion of arachnoid villi. In preterm infants, there is a predisposition to germinal matrix (GM) hemorrhage, leading to periventricular hemorrhagic infarction (PHI) and intraventricular hemorrhage (IVH) hydrocephalus. Such status as GM to IVH is graded by severity, as I through IV,

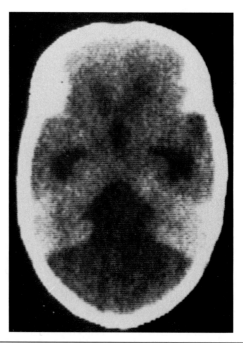

FIGURE 49.2. Brain CT. Hydrocephalus associated with Dandy-Walker malformation in a 4-month-old child with increasing head circumference and bulging fontanels.

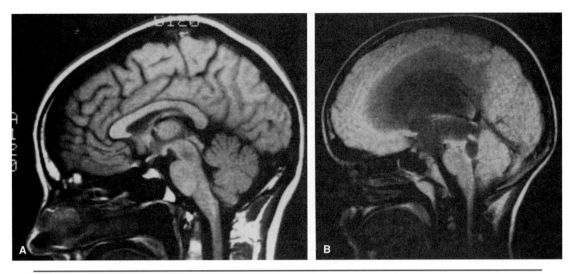

FIGURE 49.3. A: Normal midsagittal brain anatomy demonstrated by T1-weighted MRI. **B:** On a similar scan of a child, abnormal membranous structures within the fourth ventricle and aqueduct of Sylvius caused dilation of the upper fourth, third, and lateral ventricles. (Courtesy of Dr. Reed Murtagh.)

whereby grades III and IV usually develop progressive hydrocephalus which requires shunting.

Intramedullary or intraventricular hemorrhage in adults also causes hydrocephalus, especially if there are clots in the ventricles (Fig. 49.4A). Hydrocephalus also occurs in adults after subarachnoid bleeding caused by head trauma or ruptured aneurysm (Fig. 49.4B).

In some patients the obstruction of CSF flow is transient. As a result, ICP increases, and hydrocephalus appears but then disappears spontaneously. Other patients exhibit progressive hydrocephalus. This form of obstructive hydrocephalus is due to extraventricular obstruction to CSF flow and may be a form of, or may cause NPH (Fig. 49.5).

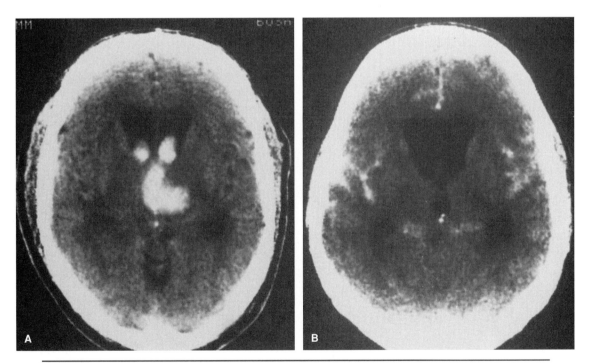

FIGURE 49.4. A: Brain CT in a 58-year-old individual several hours after the sudden development of coma and right hemiparesis. Blood in the left thalamus and within the third and lateral ventricles is associated with hydrocephalus. **B:** Similar scan of adult 24 hrs after the sudden onset of severe headache and meningism. Acute hydrocephalus with subarachnoid space blood is seen.

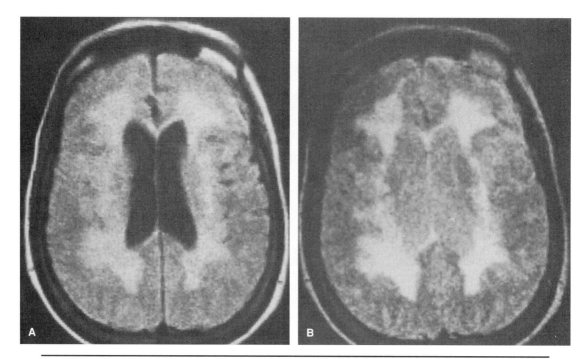

FIGURE 49.5. A: Axial T1-weighted MRI of the brain shows lateral ventricular dilatation in a 42-year-old woman with dementia, ataxia, and urinary incontinence 3 months after subarachnoid hemorrhage. **B:** Axial, more T2-weighted image in this woman demonstrates periventricular increased signal intensity consistent with transependymal migration of CSF. Her condition improved after CSF-shunt procedure was done.

Among infectious diseases, tuberculous and luetic meningitis may cause hydrocephalus secondary to basal arachnoiditis. CT and MRI have demonstrated that hydrocephalus may also follow other forms of meningitis (e.g., bacterial, fungal, viral, carcinomatous) (Fig. 49.6). Among parasitic infections, neurocysticercosis may produce both IVOH and EVOH.

Mass Lesions

Intracranial neoplasms may cause obstructive hydrocephalus (Fig. 49.7). Tumors clustered about the third or fourth ventricles or the aqueduct of Sylvius are commonly implicated in IVOH, including pineal tremors, colloid cysts, gliomas, ependymoma and metastases. Prognosis, after shunting, is largely related to the type of tissue in the tumor. Other mass lesions, such as intraparenchymal cerebral hemorrhage, cerebellar infarction or cerebellar hemorrhage, may lead to acute hydrocephalus. Basilar artery ectasia and other vascular abnormalities (e.g., vein of Galen malformation) have also been associated with hydrocephalus.

COMMUNICATING HYDROCEPHALUS

When impairment of neither intraventricular nor extraventricular CSF flow may be documented, three other mechanisms may cause hydrocephalus: oversecretion of CSF, venous insufficiency, or impaired absorption of CSF by arachnoid villi.

When CSF *oversecretion* occurs, the absorptive capacity of the subarachnoid space is about three times the normal CSF formation rate of 0.35 mL per minute; formation rates greater than 1.0 mL per minute may produce hydrocephalus. Clinically, *choroid plexus papilloma* is the only known cause of oversecretion hydrocephalus.

Otitic hydrocephalus occurs in children after chronic otitis media or mastoiditis with lateral sinus thrombosis; otherwise, impaired cerebral *venous drainage* (e.g., thrombosis of cortical veins or intracranial venous sinuses) rarely causes hydrocephalus. Hydrocephalus owing to impairment of extracranial venous drainage only rarely follows radical neck dissection or obstruction of the superior vena cava.

Communicating hydrocephalus has been attributed to *congenital agenesis of the arachnoid villi*, with consequent impairment of CSF absorption. Detailed pathologic study of the number of villi and their structural characteristics is difficult and rarely performed; as a result, this defect may be more common than statistics indicate. Likewise, dysfunction of arachnoid villi, without obstruction of basilar or transcortical CSF pathways, may not be assessed easily.

Hydrocephalus has also been described when lumbar CSF protein content exceeds 500 mg/dL, (e.g. in cases of polyneuritis or spinal-cord tumor). The protein may interfere with CSF absorption. Ependymoma, the most

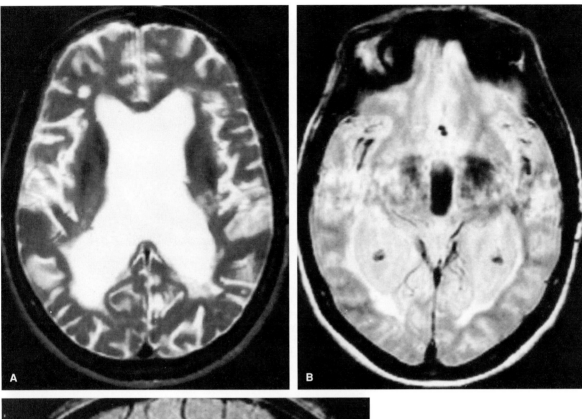

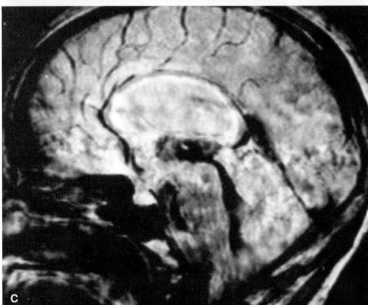

FIGURE 49.6. Normal pressure hydrocephalus (NPH). A: Axial T2-weighted MR image shows dilated lateral ventricles with no evidence of sulcal effacement. **B:** and **C:** Axial and sagittal proton-density MRI shows increased signal intensity around both lateral ventricles consistent with interstitial edema within the periventricular white matter. Pronounced flow void is seen within the third ventricle on the axial view; the sagittal view shows extension of the flow void down the aqueduct of Sylvius and into the fourth ventricle. This indicates abnormally increased CSF pulsations through these structures and may represent a prognostic marker for successful ventricular shunt placement for NPH. A ventricular shunt was placed, and this patient showed improvement in mental status and gait difficulty. (Courtesy of Dr. R. Murtagh.)

common spinal-cord tumor associated with hydrocephalus, may be due to tumor seeding of the arachnoid villi.

NORMAL PRESSURE HYDROCEPHALUS

As a potentially treatable cause of dementia, NPH has captured wide attention. The syndrome was first delineated in 1964, as an occult form of hydrocephalus. The absence of papilledema, with normal CSF pressure at lumbar puncture, led to the term *normal pressure hydrocephalus;* however, ICH probably occurs before diagnosis. Intermittent ICH has been noted during pressure monitoring of suspected cases. The syndrome may follow head trauma, SAH, or meningitis, or it may be associated with an occult mass lesion.

There is much speculation about the pathophysiology of NPH. Obliteration or insufficiency of the cortical subarachnoid space may occur alone, or with an impaired

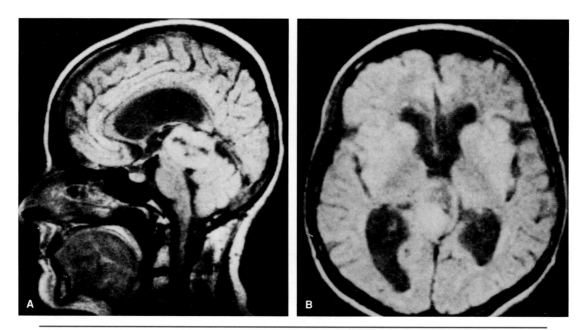

FIGURE 49.7. **A:** Midsagittal T1-weighted MRI in a 42-year-old woman demonstrates a pinealoma causing lateral ventricular dilation with a normal fourth ventricle. **B:** Axial T1-weighted imaging demonstrates the pineal region tumor and dilation of the proximal third and lateral ventricles.

absorption defect at the arachnoid villi, leading to reduced conductance to CSF outflow.

General Clinical Data

Signs and Symptoms

In children, before the cranial sutures fuse, hydrocephalus causes skull enlargement and widened fontanels. The face, although of normal size, appears small relative to the enlarged head. Exophthalmos and scleral prominence result from downward displacement of the orbits. Severe ICH produces sluggish pupillary reaction, absence of upward gaze, impaired lateral gaze, paralysis or spasm of conversion, nystagmus, retractions, and absence of visual fixation or response to visible threat.

Untreated hydrocephalic infants fail to thrive and show retardation of motor and intellectual development. Limb movements, particularly of the legs, show progressive weakness and spasticity, and seizures are common. Prominent skull veins are evident and percussion of the skull evokes a sound similar to that made by a cracked pot. In addition, wasting of trunk and limb muscles is apparent, with spasticity, overactive tendon reflexes, and Babinski signs. With progression, the child is unable to lift the enlarged head. Visual loss is followed by optic atrophy. Scalp necrosis in these children may lead to CSF leakage, infection, and death.

In otitic hydrocephalus, the child may be febrile and listless. Eardrum perforation and purulent otic discharge usually occur. Often, ipsilateral sixth nerve paralysis and papilledema are noted.

In adults, symptoms include headache, lethargy, malaise, incoordination, and weakness. Seizures are uncommon. Findings may include dementia, altered consciousness, ocular nerve palsies, papilledema, ataxia, or corticospinal tract signs. Ventricular enlargement is not usually a uniform process and frequently occurs at the expense of periventricular white matter with relative preservation of gray matter. Therefore, severe hydrocephalus may remain occult, and even though uncomplicated by brain tumor or other obvious causes, may be found by CT in adults with preserved mental state with signs limited to pyramidal tract or cerebellar dysfunction.

NPH is characterized by insidious onset and gradual development for weeks or months of the triad of dementia, ataxia of gait, and urinary incontinence. Headache and signs of increased ICP do not occur. Symptoms may begin weeks after head trauma or SAH. In advanced disease, there may be frontal release signs, with hyperactive tendon reflexes and Babinski signs.

Laboratory Data

In infants, hydrocephalus must be distinguished from other forms of macrocephaly, such as subdural hematoma. Skull transillumination should be performed. Plain-skull radiographs and skull measurements are useful, to follow the course of hydrocephalus in infants and children. Overall, CT and MRI are the best diagnostic aids for all forms of hydrocephalus.

Lumbar puncture is sometimes indicated to measure CSF pressure and to determine whether it contains blood, or signs of inflammatory or infectious disease. Continuous monitoring of intraventricular pressure (IVP) may differentiate arrested from progressive disease when lumbar-sac CSF pressure is normal, and may not accurately reflect the IVP. Likewise, CSF pulse-wave analysis may be more reliable than CSF pressure, alone, in diagnosis of hydrocephalus.

Ultrasonography is useful in evaluating subependymal and intraventricular hemorrhage in high-risk premature infants and in following the infants for possible later development of progressive hydrocephalus. Results correlate well with CT. As a bedside procedure, ultrasonography requires minimal manipulation of critically ill infants.

In adult-onset NPH, many clinicians believe that the best results from the CSF-shunt procedure are achieved in patients who have the full clinical triad, or who show improvement when a volume of 30 mL to 50 mL of CSF is removed by lumbar puncture. However, because NPH is a potentially reversible form of dementia, other diagnostic techniques are used to improve the selection of patients most likely to benefit from the CSF-shunt procedure.

The following tests are preferred by one or more groups, but none is universally accepted as reliably prognostic of a favorable outcome: CT or MRI evidence of transependymal diffusion of fluid; isotope cisternography, a measure of the direction of CSF flow, showing CSF reflux from the subarachnoid space to the lateral ventricles (reversing the normal flow), and delayed clearance or intraventricular transependymal penetration of the isotope; CSF compartment infusion or perfusion tests; ICP monitoring to assess high-pressure waves; measurement of CSF blood flow; and dynamic MRI cine and ventriculography studies to determine the direction and volume of CSF flow. Cerebral angiography is occasionally indicated in when diagnosing hydrocephalus is problematic, owing to intracranial mass lesions.

Prognosis and Treatment

In the rare choroid plexus papilloma, surgical removal may be associated with favorable outcome.

Hydrocephalus in children is not a specific disease but results from diverse conditions that affect the fetus, infant, or child and is not an all-or-nothing condition. Some children may be managed with observation, if hydrocephalus is mild. Adequate treatment did not exist before the valve-regulated shunt was developed in the early 1950s. The valves now used include: differential pressure regulators (static and programmable), flow regulators, siphon-resistive devices, and gravity-activated valves. All CSF-shunt systems contain a proximal ventricular catheter, a one-way valve, and a distal catheter terminating in the peritoneum or the venous system or, less commonly, the pleural space. Details of the technologies involved are beyond the scope of this chapter, and may be provided by selections from Suggested Readings.

If data from *in vivo* animal studies may be applied to humans, early intervention is indicated. For example, ventricular enlargement began immediately and was grossly evident within 3 hours of experimental obstruction of the fourth ventricle, in monkeys. After 3 weeks, brain damage was irreversible. Overall, results vary with the procedures used, operative technique, patient status, cause and duration of the hydrocephalus, and the incidence of complications such as infection, subdural hematoma, and seizures.

Shunt failure is also sometimes a problem, despite the sophistication of the shunt system. Prognosis is sometimes related to an underlying disease (e.g., cerebral neoplasm). In such cases, treatment of hydrocephalus may be only palliative. However, because management of eventually terminal conditions prolongs life with quality, relief of obstructive hydrocephalus by a shunting procedure is often indicated to prevent acute brain herniation and death. Likewise, in nonneoplastic but serious conditions, such as the Dandy-Walker syndrome or postbasal arachnoiditis, shunting is indicated but eventual outcome depends on the underlying disease. In still other cases, such as in benign infantile communicating hydrocephalus, shunting allows the condition to stabilize or arrest.

If untreated, progressive infantile hydrocephalus carries a mortality rate as high as 50% at age 1 year and 75% at age 10 years. Treatment greatly improves these figures. For example, with shunting the survival rate is at least 50% after age 15 years, but with a 15% incidence of mental retardation. If ICH leads to hydrocephalus in high-risk premature infants, the outcome is usually related to factors (e.g., asphyxia) other than shunt responsiveness.

In many adults with hydrocephalus (e.g., those with adult aquadental stenosis), shunting leads to an excellent long-term prognosis. In adult onset IVOH, endoscopic III ventriculostomy (ETV) is a well established treatment modality, with success rates of 60% to 85% in hydrocephalus caused by aqueductal stenosis. Success rates approach 80% in children with aqueduct stenosis and tectal plate gliomas. This procedure allows diversion of CSF from the third ventricle to the basal cisterns, obviating the need for a shunt. Its role in infantile posthemorrhagic and postinflammatory hydrocephalus is being debated.

Complications of shunting must be considered. For instance, shunt infection rates may be as high as 10%. Likewise, shunt failure rates, requiring revision, may be as high as 44%. Furthermore, ETV has a failure rate of 20% to 30% in various series. Problems arise in selecting patients with idiopathic NPH for shunting, as opposed to those who have had prior SAH or meningitis. Tests, such as phase-contrast MRI and temporary external-lumbar CSF drainage, are useful in diagnosis and in predicting shunt-procedure outcome. In the series of Viennese and colleagues (1992), 36% of patients with idiopathic NPH improved (Table 49.1), and 28% suffered complications of the procedure, with death or persistent disability in 7%.

▶ **TABLE 49.1 Results of CFS Shunting for NPH**

Cause of NP	Patients (n)	Grade of Improvement		
		None	Slight	Marked
Idiopathic	127	87	21	19 (15%)
Known cause				
Communicating	11	7	0	4 (36%)
Noncommunicating	14	3	2	9 (64%)
Total	152	97	23	32
Percent		64%	15%	21%

Modified from Vanneste et al., 1992.

Complications included cerebral infarction and hemorrhage, subdural hematoma or effusion, intracranial and extracranial infection, and seizures. In 166 patients, 32 had shunt revisions. More recently, Meier and colleagues (2004) found excellent results in 63% of 128 patients, satisfactory results in 16%, and unsatisfactory or negative outcome in 21%. The infection rate was 9%.

In all forms of hydrocephalus including NPH, pharmacologic therapy is of limited value; however, there have been favorable reports of acetazolamide, furosemide, and isosorbide use, with or without repeated lumbar punctures. With respect to shunt procedures in NPH, the success rate is best in those with recent-onset, progressive dementia and ataxia, without urinary incontinence, or with imaging evidence of chronic hydrocephalus, normal CSF on lumbar puncture, and no adverse risk factors. Under those circumstances, 60% of patients may show improvement. Gait impairment remains the cardinal symptom. Higher rates of improvement have been reported; however favorable results are more likely to be reported than adverse ones.

SUGGESTED READINGS

Arthur AS, Whitehead WE, Kestle JRW. Duration of antibiotic therapy for the treatment of shunt infection: a surgeon and patient survey. *Pediatr Neurosurg* 2002;36(5):256–259.

Boon AJ, Tans JT, Delwel EJ, et al. Dutch normal-pressure hydrocephalus study: prediction of outcome after shunting by resistance to outflow of cerebrospinal fluid. *J Neurosurg* 1997;87:687–693.

Bradley WG. Normal pressure hydrocephalus: new concepts on etiology and diagnosis. *Am J Neuroradiol* 2000;21(9):1586–1590.

Callen PW, Hashimoto BE, Newton TH. Sonographic evaluation of cerebral cortical mantle thickness in the fetus and neonate with hydrocephalus. *J Ultrasound Med* 1986;5:251–255.

Carrion E, Hertzog JH, Medlock MD, Hauser GJ, Dalton HJ. Use of acetazolamide to decrease cerebrospinal fluid production in chronically ventilated patients with ventribulopleural shunts. *Arch Dis Child* 2001;84:68–71.

Duinkerke A, Williams MA, Rigamonti D, Hillis AE. Cognitive recovery in idiopathic normal pressure hydrocephalus after shunt. *Cogn Behav Neurol* 2004 Sep;17(3):179–84.

Edwards RJ, Dombrowski SM, Luciano MG, Pople IK. Chronic hydrocephalus in adults. *Brain Pathol* 2004 Jul;14(3):325–36.

Ginsberg HJ. Physiology of cerebrospinal fluid shunt devices. In: Winn HR, ed. *Youmans Neurological Surgery*, 5th ed. Philadelphia: WB Saunders Co., 2004;3374–3385.

Gnanalingham KK, Lafuente J, Thompson D, Harkness W, Hayward R. The natural history of ventriculomegaly and tonsillar herniation in children with posterior fossa tumors—an MRI study. *Pediatr Neurosurg* 2003;39(5):246–253.

Goh D, Minns RA, Hendry GM, et al. Cerebrovascular resistive index assessed by duplex Doppler sonography and its relationship to intracranial pressure in infantile hydrocephalus. *Pediatr Radiol* 1992;22:246–250.

Gradin WC, Taylon C, Fruin AH. Choroid plexus papilloma of the third ventricle: case report and review of the literature. *Neurosurgery* 1983;12:217–220.

Greitz D. Radiological assessment of hydrocephalus: new theories and implications for therapy. *Neurosurg Rev* 2004 Jul;27(3):145–65; discussion 166–7. Epub 2004 May 26.

Hakim R, Black PM. Correlation between lumbo-ventricular perfusion and MRI-CSF flow studies in idiopathic normal pressure hydrocephalus. *Surg Neurol* 1998;49:14–19.

Hakim S, Adams RD. The special clinical problem of symptomatic hydrocephalus with normal cerebrospinal fluid pressure. *J Neurol Sci* 1965;2:307–327.

Johnston I, Teo C. Disorders of CSF Hydrodynamics. *Child's Nerv Syst* 2000;16:776–799.

Joseph VB, Rahuram L, Korah P, Chacko AG. MR ventriculography for the study of CSF flow. *AJNR Am J Neuroradiol* 2003;24(3):373–381.

Khoromi S, Prockop LD. Disturbances of cerebrospinal fluid circulation, including hydrocephalus and meningeal reactions. In: Greenburg JO, ed. *Neuroimaging*, 2nd ed. New York: McGraw-Hill, 1999;335–374.

Klinge P, Fischer J, Heissler HE, et al. PET and CBF studies of chronic hydrocephalus: a contribution to surgical indication and prognosis. *J Neuroimaging* 1998;8:205–209.

Krauss JK, Regel JP. The predictive value of ventricular CSF removal in normal pressure hydrocephalus. *Neurol Res* 1997;19:357–360.

Lan CC, Wong TT, Chen SJ, Liang ML, Tang RB. Early diagnosis of ventriculoperitoneal shunt infections and malfunctions in children with hydrocephalus. *J Microbiol Immunol Infect* 2003;36(1):47–50.

Lazareff JA, Peacock W, Holly L, et al. Multiple shunt failures: an analysis of relevant factors. *Childs Nerv Syst* 1998;14(6):271–275.

Luciano M, Pattisapu JV, Wickremesekera A. Infantile posthemorrhagic hydrocephalus. In: Winn HR, ed. *Youmans Neurological Surgery*, 5th ed. Philadelphia: WB Saunders Co., 2004;3405–3417.

Luetmer PH, Huston J, Friedman JA, et al. Measurement of cerebrospinal fluid flow at the cerebral aqueduct by use of phase-contrast magnetic resonance imaging: technique validation and utility in diagnosing idiopathic normal pressure hydrocephalus. *Neurosurgery* 2002;50(3):534–542.

Meier U, Bartels P. The importance of the intrathecal infusion test in the diagnostic of normal-pressure hydrocephalus. *J Clin Neurosci* 2002;9(3):260–267.

Meier U, Kiefer M, Sprung C. Evaluation of the Miethke dual-switch valve in patients with normal pressure hydrocephalus. *Surg Neurol* 2004;61:119–128.

Meier U, Konig A, Miethke C. Predictors of outcome in patients with normal-pressure hydrocephalus. *Eur Neurol* 2004;51(2):59–67. Epub 2003 Dec 04.

Miyati T, Mase M, Banno T, Kasuga T, et al. Frequency analyses of CSF flow on cine MRI in normal pressure hydrocephalus. *Eur Radiol* 2003;13(5):1019–1024.

Mohanty A, Vasudev MK, Sampath S, et al. Failed endoscopic third ventriculostomy in children: management options. *Pediatr Neurosurg* 2002;37(6):304–309.

Racette BA, Esper GJ, Antenor J, Black KJ, Burkey A, Moerlein SM, Videen TO, Kotagal V, Ojemann JG, Perlmutter JS. Pathophysiology of parkinsonism due to hydrocephalus. *J Neurol Neurosurg Psychiatry* 2004 Nov;75(11):1617–9.

Rekate HL. Hydrocephalus in children. In: Winn HR, ed. *Youmans Neurological Surgery*, 5th ed. Philadelphia: WB Saunders Co., 2004;3387–3404.

Sgouros S, John P, Walsh AR, Hockley AD. The value of colour Doppler imaging in assessing flow through ventriculo-peritoneal shunts. *Childs Nerv Syst* 1996;12:454–459.

Siomin V, Cinalli G, Grotenhuis A, et al. Endoscopic third ventriculostomy in patients with cerebrospinal fluid infection and/or hemorrhage. *J Neurosurg* 2002;97(3):519–524.

Vanneste JAL. Diagnosis and management of normal pressure hydrocephalus. *J Neurol* 2000;247:5–14.

Vanneste J, Augustijn P, Dirven C, et al. Shunting normal pressure hydrocephalus: do the benefits outweigh the risks? A multicenter study and literature review. *Neurology* 1992;43:54–59.

Volpe JJ. Brain injury in the premature infant: neuropathology, clinical aspects, pathogenesis, and prevention. *Clin Perinatol* 1997;24(3):567–587.

Walchenbach R, Geiger E, Thomeer R, Vanneste J. The value of temporary external lumbar CSF drainage in predicting the outcome of shunting on normal pressure hydrocephalus. *J Neurol Neurosurg Psychiatry* 2002;72(4):503–506.

Yasuda T, Tomita T, McLone DG, Donovan M. Measurement of cerebrospinal fluid output through external ventricular drainage in one hundred infants and children: correlation with cerebrospinal fluid production. *Pediatr Neurosurg* 2002;36(1):22–28.

Chapter 50

▶ # Brain Edema and Disorders of Intracranial Pressure

Robert A. Fishman

BRAIN EDEMA

Brain edema accompanies a wide variety of pathologic processes. It plays a major role in head injury, stroke, and brain tumor, as well as in cerebral infections, including brain abscess, encephalitis, and meningitis; lead encephalopathy; hypoxia; hypoosmolality; the dysequilibrium syndromes associated with dialysis and diabetic ketoacidosis; Reye syndrome; fulminant hepatic encephalopathy; and hydrocephalus. Brain edema occurs in several different forms; clearly it is not a single pathologic or clinical entity.

Brain edema is defined as an increase in brain volume caused by an increase in water and sodium content. Brain edema, when well localized or mild in degree, is associated with little or no clinical evidence of brain dysfunction; however, when severe, it causes focal or generalized signs of brain dysfunction, including various forms of brain herniation and medullary failure of respiration and circulation. The major forms of herniation are uncal, cerebellar tonsillar, upward cerebellar, cingulate, and transcalvarial herniation.

Brain edema and brain engorgement are different processes. *Brain engorgement* is an increase in the blood volume of the brain caused by obstruction of the cerebral veins and venous sinuses or by arterial vasodilatation, such as that caused by hypercapnia. Focal or generalized brain edema results in intracranial hypertension when it is severe enough to exceed the compensatory mechanisms modulating intracranial pressure.

Brain edema is classified into three major categories: vasogenic, cellular (cytotoxic), and interstitial (hydrocephalic). The features of the three forms of cerebral edema are summarized in Table 50.1 in terms of pathogenesis, location and composition of the edema fluid, and changes in capillary permeability.

Vasogenic Edema

Vasogenic edema is characterized by increased permeability of brain capillary endothelial cells to macromolecules, such as the plasma proteins whose entry is limited by the capillary endothelial cells. The increase in permeability is visualized when contrast enhancement is observed with CT. Increased CSF protein levels are also indicative of increased endothelial permeability. MRI is more sensitive than CT in demonstrating the increases in brain water and extracellular volume that characterize vasogenic edema.

Vasogenic edema is characteristic of clinical disorders in which contrast-enhanced CT is frequently positive or MRI shows increased signal intensity. These disorders include brain tumor, abscess, hemorrhage, infarction, and contusion. These radiologic changes are also seen with acute demyelinating lesions in multiple sclerosis. They also occur with lead encephalopathy or purulent meningitis. The functional manifestations of vasogenic edema include focal neurologic deficits, focal EEG slowing, disturbances of consciousness, and severe intracranial hypertension. In patients with brain tumor, whether primary or metastatic, the clinical signs are often caused more by the surrounding edema than by the tumor mass itself.

Cellular (Cytotoxic) Edema

Cellular edema is characterized by swelling of all the cellular elements of the brain (neurons, glia, and endothelial cells), with a concomitant reduction in the volume of the extracellular fluid space of the brain. Capillary permeability is not usually affected in the various cellular edemas; patients so affected have a normal CSF protein and isotopic brain scan. CT does not reveal contrast enhancement, and MRI is usually normal.

There are several causes of cellular edema: hypoxia, acute hypoosmolality of the plasma, and osmotic dysequilibrium syndromes. *Hypoxia* after cardiac arrest or asphyxia results in cerebral energy depletion. The cellular swelling is determined by the appearance of increased intracellular osmoles (especially sodium, lactate, and hydrogen ions) that induce the rapid entry of water into cells.

▶ **TABLE 50.1 Classification of Brain Edema**

	Vasogenic	*Cytotoxic*	*Interstitial (hydrocephalic)*
Pathogenesis	Increased capillary permeability	Cellular swelling (glial, neuronal, endothelial)	Increased brain fluid due to block of CSF absorption
Location of edema	Chiefly, white matter	Gray and white matter	Chiefly, periventricular white matter in hydrocephalus
Edema fluid composition	Plasma filtrate including plasma proteins	Increased intracellular water and sodium	CSF
Extracellular fluid volume	Increased	Decreased	Increased
Capillary permeability to large molecules (radioiodinated serum albumin, inulin)	Increased	Normal	Normal
Clinical disorders			
Syndromes	Brain tumor, abscess, infarction, trauma, hemorrhage, lead encephalopathy	Hypoxia, hypoosmolality (e.g., water intoxication); dysequilibrium syndromes	Obstructive hydrocephalus, pseudotumor (begin intracranial hypertension)
	Ischemia	Ischemia	–
	Purulent meningitis (granulocytic edema)	Purulent meningitis (granulocytic edema) fulminant hepatic encephalopathy	Purulent meningitis (granulocytic edema)
EEG changes	Focal slowing common	Generalized slowing	Often normal
Therapeutic effects			
Steroids	Beneficial in brain tumor, abscess	Not effective (? fulminant hepatic encephalopathy)	Uncertain effectiveness
Osmotherapy	Reduces volume of normal brain tissue only, *acutely*	Reduces brain volume *acutely*	Rarely useful

Modified from Fishman RA. Brain edema. In: *Cerebrospinal fluid in diseases of the nervous system.* Philadelphia: WB Saunders, 1992:116–137.

Acute hypoosmolality of the plasma and extracellular fluid is caused by acute dilutional hyponatremia, inappropriate secretion of antidiuretic hormone, or acute sodium depletion. *Osmotic dysequilibrium syndromes* occur with hemodialysis or diabetic ketoacidosis, in which excessive brain intracellular solutes result in excessive cellular hydration when the plasma osmolality is rapidly normalized with therapy. In uremia, the intracellular solutes presumably include a number of organic acids recovered in the dialysis bath. In diabetic ketoacidosis, the intracellular solutes include glucose and ketone bodies; however, there are also unidentified, osmotically active, intracellular solutes, termed *idiogenic osmoles,* that favor cellular swelling.

Major changes in cerebral function occur with the cellular edemas, including stupor, coma, EEG changes, asterixis, myoclonus, and focal or generalized seizures. The encephalopathy is often severe with acute hypoosmolality, but in more chronic states of hypoosmolality of the same severity, neurologic function may be spared. Acute hypoxia causes cellular edema that is followed by vasogenic edema as infarction develops. Vasogenic edema increases progressively for several days after an acute arterial occlusion. The delay in obtaining contrast enhancement with CT following an ischemic stroke illustrates that time is needed for defects in endothelial cell permeability to develop.

Ischemic Brain Edema

Most patients with arterial occlusion have a combination of cellular edema first and then vasogenic edema, together termed *ischemic brain edema.* The cellular phase takes place after acute ischemia over minutes to hours and may be reversible. The vasogenic phase takes place over hours to days and results in infarction, a largely irreversible process, although the increased endothelial cell permeability usually reverts to normal within weeks.

Fulminant Hepatic Encephalopathy

Acute hepatocellular failure occurs secondary to acute viral or toxic hepatitis and in Reye syndrome, a disorder affecting children. The resulting encephalopathy is characterized by progressive stupor and coma. Severe intracranial hypertension with cytotoxic brain edema is a major and often fatal complication. Imaging studies reveal a "tight" brain with normal vascular permeability to contrast material.

Interstitial (Hydrocephalic) Edema

Interstitial edema is the third type of edema, best characterized in obstructive hydrocephalus, in which the water and sodium content of the periventricular white matter is increased because of the movement of CSF across the ventricular ependymal surface. Obstruction of the CSF outflow results in the transependymal movement of CSF and thereby an absolute increase in the volume of the extracellular fluid of the brain. This is observed in obstructive hydrocephalus with CT and MRI. Low-density changes are observed at the angles of the lateral ventricles. The chemical changes are those of edema, with one exception: The volume of periventricular white matter is reduced rather than increased. After successful shunting of CSF, interstitial edema is reduced, and the thickness of the mantle is restored.

Functional manifestations of interstitial edema are usually relatively minor in chronic hydrocephalus, unless the changes are advanced, when dementia and gait disorder become prominent. The EEG is often normal in interstitial edema. This finding indicates that the accumulation of CSF in the periventricular extracellular fluid space is much better tolerated than is the presence of plasma in the extracellular fluid space, as seen with vasogenic edema, which is characterized by focal neurologic signs and EEG slowing.

Granulocytic Brain Edema

Severe brain edema occurs with brain abscess and purulent meningitis originating from collections of pus that are often sterile as a result of antibiotic treatment. Such edema, associated with membranous products of granulocytes (pus), has been termed *granulocytic brain edema*. The features of cellular and vasogenic edema occur concurrently in purulent meningitis, and in severe cases hydrocephalic edema also develops, so that granulocytic brain edema may include the features of all three types of brain edema.

Therapeutic Considerations

The therapy of brain edema depends on the cause. Appropriate and early treatment of intracranial infection is essential. Surgical therapy is directed toward alleviating the cause by excision or decompression of intracranial mass lesions as well as by a variety of shunting procedures. A patent airway, maintenance of an adequate blood pressure, and the avoidance of hypoxia are fundamental requirements in the care of these patients. The surgical technique of optic nerve decompression to treat severe papilledema has been largely abandoned.

The administration of appropriate parenteral fluids to meet the needs of patients is also essential. Administration of salt-free fluids to patients with cerebral edema should be avoided because serum hypoosmolality increases brain swelling. The pharmacologic treatment of brain edema is based on the use of glucocorticoids, osmotherapy, and drugs that reduce CSF formation. Hyperventilation, hypothermia, and barbiturate therapy have also been tested experimentally but in clinical practice they are little used.

Glucocorticoids

The rationale for the use of steroids is largely empiric. Glucocorticoids dramatically and rapidly (in hours) begin to reduce the focal and general signs of brain edema around tumors. The major mechanism explaining their usefulness in vasogenic brain edema is a direct normalizing effect on endothelial cell function and permeability.

The biochemical basis of the changes in membrane integrity that underlie vasogenic and cellular edema is now under study. Attention has focused on the role of free radicals (i.e., superoxide ions, hydroxyl radicals, singlet oxygen, and nitric oxide) and on the effects of polyunsaturated fatty acids, most notably arachidonic acid, in the peroxidation of membrane phospholipids. The ability of adrenal glucocorticoids to inhibit the release of arachidonic acid from cell membranes may explain their beneficial effects in vasogenic edema; however, steroids have not been shown to be therapeutically useful in the cellular brain edema of hypoxia or ischemia. Cellular necrosis is more important than brain edema in these conditions.

Long-acting, high-potency glucocorticoids are the most widely used. The usual dosage of dexamethasone is a starting dose of 10 mg followed by 4 mg administered four times a day thereafter—a dose equivalent in potency to 400 mg of cortisol daily. These large doses are about 20 times the normal rate of human endogenous cortisol production. Even larger dosages are sometimes used. Insufficient data are available to establish a formal dose–response curve for steroids in the treatment of brain edema; dosage schedules remain empiric.

Although any of the usual complications of steroid therapy are to be expected, gastric hemorrhage is usually the most troublesome. Fortunately, convulsive seizures apparently have not been increased in frequency by high dosages of the glucocorticoids. The risks of increased wound infection and impaired wound healing appear to be outweighed by the therapeutic effects in most patients receiving short-term therapy.

Although published data indicate that dexamethasone is valuable in the treatment of vasogenic edema associated with brain tumor and abscess, the literature recommending its use in stroke has, in general, been poorly documented and is controversial. Steroids may be useful in the treatment of intracerebral hematoma with extensive vasogenic edema that stems from the mass effect of the clot. In head injury, steroid therapy has frequently been used. Although some effectiveness following trauma has been documented, reductions in morbidity and mortality attributable to steroids are not great. The role of megadose steroids in the treatment of acute spinal cord injury is discussed elsewhere.

There are no convincing data, clinical or experimental, that glucocorticoids have beneficial effects in the cellular edema associated with hypoosmolality, asphyxia, or hypoxia in the absence of infarction with mass effects. There is little basis for recommending steroids in the treatment of the cerebral edema associated with cardiac arrest or asphyxia. The use of steroids in the management of fulminant hepatic encephalopathy is controversial. There are no controlled data regarding its effectiveness.

When intracranial hypertension and obstructive hydrocephalus occur because of inflammatory changes in the subarachnoid space or at the arachnoid villi, whether attributable to leukocytes or to blood, there is a reasonable rationale for the use of steroids. Despite the frequent use of steroids in purulent or tuberculous meningitis, however, few data are available to document the effectiveness of steroids against the acute disease. There are conflicting reports about the efficacy of steroids in acute bacterial meningitis or tuberculous meningitis. Use of steroids has not been shown to affect the subsequent incidence of chronic sequelae, such as obstructive hydrocephalus or seizures. Steroids do reduce the incidence of deafness in infants with bacterial meningitis. Steroids appear useful in the management of other conditions characterized by an inflammatory CSF, such as chemical meningitis following intrathecal injection of pharmaceuticals, meningeal sarcoidosis, or cerebral cysticercosis.

Osmotherapy

Intravenous hypertonic mannitol is the most widely used solute for the treatment of intracranial hypertension associated with brain edema. The effectiveness of osmotherapy depends on several factors. First, it is effective in reducing brain volume and elastance only as long as an osmotic gradient exists between blood and brain. Second, osmotic gradients obtained with hypertonic parenteral fluids are short-lived because the solute reaches an equilibrium concentration in the brain after a delay of only a few hours. Third, the parts of the brain most likely to "shrink" are normal areas; thus, with focal vasogenic edema, the normal regions of the hemisphere shrink, but edematous regions with increased capillary permeability do not. Fourth, a rebound in the severity of the edema may follow use of any hypertonic solution because the solute is not excluded from the edematous tissue; if tissue osmolality rises, the tissue water is increased. Finally, there is scant rationale for long-term use of hypertonic fluids, either orally or par-

enterally, because the brain adapts to sustained hyperosmolality with an increase, a therapeutically significant decrease in brain volume and intracranial pressure in brain intracellular osmolarity, as a result of the administrated solute and idiogenic osmoles.

There is some uncertainty about the size of an increase in plasma osmolality required to cause humans. Acute increases as small as 10 mOsm/L may be therapeutically effective. It should be emphasized that accurate dose–response relationships in different clinical situations have not been well-defined with mannitol.

Other Therapeutic Measures

Hyperventilation, hypothermia, and barbiturates have been used in the management of intracranial hypertension, but none is established, and the extensive literature is not reviewed here. Acetazolamide and furosemide reduce CSF formation in animals and have limited usefulness in the management of interstitial brain edema.

IDIOPATHIC INTRACRANIAL HYPERTENSION

Idiopathic intracranial hypertension (IIH) describes a heterogeneous group of disorders characterized by increased intracranial pressure when intracranial mass lesions, obstructive hydrocephalus, intracranial infection, and hypertensive encephalopathy have been excluded. IIH is also termed *pseudotumor cerebri*. In the past, it has also been referred to as "serous meningitis" and "otitic hydrocephalus." The term *benign* has also been used because spontaneous recovery is characteristic, but serious threats to vision make accurate diagnosis and therapeutic intervention a necessity.

Various pathologic conditions are associated with IIH, although in most cases the pathogenesis of the intracranial hypertension (ICH) is poorly understood. Conditions associated with IIH include the following:

Endocrine and Metabolic Disorders
    Obesity and menstrual irregularities
    Pregnancy and postpartum (without sinus thrombosis)
    Menarche
    Female sex hormones
    Addison disease
    Adrenal steroid withdrawal
    Hyperadrenalism
    Acromegaly
    Hypoparathyroidism
Intracranial Venous-Sinus Thrombosis
    Mastoiditis and lateral sinus thrombosis
    After head trauma
    Pregnancy and postpartum

Oral progestational drugs
"Marantic" sinus thrombosis
Cryofibrinogenemia
Primary (idiopathic) sinus thrombosis
Drugs and Toxins (*Rare, Isolated Case Reports)
    Vitamin A
    Retinoic acid
    Tetracycline
    Nalidixic acid
    Chlordecone*
    Danazol*
    Amiodarone hydrochloride*
    Lithium carbonate
    Nitrofurantoin*
Hematologic and Connective Tissue Disorders
    Iron deficiency anemia
    Infectious mononucleosis
    Lupus erythematosus
High CSF Protein Content
    Spinal cord tumors
    Polyneuritis
Miscellaneous
    "Meningism" with systemic bacterial or viral infections
    Empty-sella syndrome
    Sydenham chorea
    Familial syndromes
    Rapid growth in infancy
Idiopathic Conditions

Symptomatic ICH without localizing signs may simulate IIH. Such conditions include obstructive hydrocephalus, chronic meningitis (i.e., sarcoid, fungal, or neoplastic), hypertensive encephalopathy, pulmonary encephalopathy resulting from paralytic hypoventilation, obstructive pulmonary disease (OPD), or the pickwickian syndrome (morbid obesity). High-altitude cerebral edema is a manifestation of hypoxia.

Clinical Manifestations

Typically, the first symptoms are headache and impaired vision. The headache may be worse on awakening and aggravated by coughing and straining. It is often mild or may be entirely absent. The most common ocular complaint is visual blurring, a manifestation of papilledema. Some patients complain of brief, fleeting moments of dimming or complete loss of vision, occurring many times during the day (amaurosis fugax), at times accentuated or precipitated by coughing and straining. This ominous symptom indicates that vision is in jeopardy. Visual loss may be minimal despite severe chronic papilledema, including retinal hemorrhages; however, blindness occasionally develops rapidly (i.e., less than 24 hours). Visual fields characteristically show enlargement of the blind spots, and may show constriction of the peripheral fields, and cen-

tral or paracentral scotoma. Diplopia caused by unilateral or bilateral sixth-nerve palsy may develop as a result of increased ICP. The neurologic examination is otherwise normal. A major clinical point is that patients with IIH usually look well; their apparent well being belies the ominous appearance of the papilledema. Although the disorder most often lasts for months, it may persist for years without serious sequelae. Remissions may be followed by one or more recurrences in 5% to 10% of cases. In some patients, IIH may be responsible for development of the *empty-sella syndrome,* in which radiographic image showing enlargement of the sella turcica simulates the appearance of a pituitary tumor. CT reveals that the enlarged sella is filled with CSF flowing from a defect of its diaphragm.

Pathophysiology of IIH

Several mechanisms have been considered as possible explanations for the pathophysiology of IIH. These include an increased rate of CSF formation, a sustained increase in intracranial venous pressure, a decreased rate of CSF absorption by arachnoid villi apart from venous occlusive disease, and an increase in brain volume caused by an increase in blood volume or extravascular fluid volume, simulating a form of brain edema.

No data are available regarding the rate of CSF formation in IIH because the only reliable method for measurement (ventriculocisternal perfusion) is not applicable to these patients. The only condition in which increased CSF formation has been demonstrated is choroid plexus papilloma. Increased CSF production might explain the pathophysiology in some of the diverse conditions associated with IIH, but this mechanism remains unproven. A sustained increase in intracranial venous pressure associated with decreased CSF absorption readily explains the pathophysiology of IIH associated with venous-sinus thrombosis. Increased venous-sinus pressures are readily transmitted to the CSF and would also interfere with CSF absorption. Decreased CSF absorption (in the absence of venous occlusion) resulting from altered function of the arachnoid villi would explain the occurrence of IIH in some cases; this reasonable hypothesis is also unproven. The fact that IIH is associated with normal or smaller-than-normal ventricles rather than hydrocephalus is consonant with such a mechanism. Abnormal spinal infusion tests do not differentiate between impairment of CSF absorption and decreased intracranial compliance. The occurrence of IIH in patients with polyneuritis or spinal-cord tumors appears to support the hypothesis that defective CSF absorption may be the basis for the syndrome. This is not directly correlated with the degree of CSF protein elevation; it is presumed to depend on an alteration of the function of the arachnoid villi.

The hypothesis that IIH might be caused by an increase in brain volume (a special form of brain edema) secondary to an increase in blood or extracellular fluid volume is supported by the presence of small ventricles, although this is an uncommon finding. An increase in brain volume would be expected if the extracellular space of the brain were expanded; this might occur if there were an excessive amount of CSF in the brain owing to either increased formation or decreased absorption.

Any theory of the pathogenesis of IIH must be consonant with the rapid therapeutic response of IIH to shunting of CSF by an implanted lumbar peritoneal shunt. Impaired CSF absorption or increased CSF formation would explain the occurrence of IIH in most cases; however, the limited data available, currently, do not allow any firm conclusions.

Endocrine and Metabolic Disorders

IIH is most commonly seen in healthy women with a history of menstrual dysfunction. Frequently, the women are moderately or markedly overweight (without evidence of alveolar hypoventilation). Menstrual irregularity or amenorrhea is common. Galactorrhea is an unusual associated symptom. The histories often emphasize excessive premenstrual weight gain. Endocrine studies have not revealed specific abnormalities of urinary gonadotropins or estrogens, and the pathogenesis is unknown. IIH has a complex relationship to adrenal hormones. Rarely, IIH is a complication of Addison disease or Cushing disease. Improvement occurs after restoration of a normal adrenal state; the mechanism in either circumstance is unknown.

IIH has also occurred in patients treated with adrenal corticosteroids for prolonged periods. Many of the patients had allergic skin disorders or asthma during childhood; IIH generally occurred when the steroid dosage was reduced, but evidence of hyperadrenalism persisted. Hypoparathyroidism may also present with increased intracranial pressure; hypocalcemic seizures or cerebral calcifications may further complicate the clinical picture. IIH has been reported in women taking oral progestational drugs when angiography has excluded sinus thrombosis.

Intracranial Venous-Sinus Thrombosis

Intracranial hypertension occurs secondarily to occlusion of the intracranial venous sinuses, as a consequence of acute or chronic otitis media with extension of the infection into the petrous bone and lateral sinus. The sixth cranial nerve may also be involved, giving rise to diplopia on lateral gaze. Thrombosis of the superior longitudinal sinus may occur after mild closed-head injury, giving rise to IIH. Occlusion of this sinus, which normally drains both cerebral hemispheres, is more likely to result in hemorrhagic infarction of the cerebrum as the thrombosis extends into the cerebral veins, giving rise to bilateral signs. In such cases, the course is frequently fulminant and the prognosis guarded, although complete recovery may occur. Aseptic or primary thrombosis of the superior longitudinal sinus may also be responsible for a pseudotumor syndrome, especially as a complication of pregnancy; it has been reported in the first 2 to 3 weeks postpartum, as well as at the end of the first trimester of pregnancy. Sinus thrombosis has been reported with the use of oral progestational drugs. A coagulopathy is suggested as the basis for these events, although rarely has this been substantiated. Sinus thrombosis occurs as a complication of dehydration and cachexia (i.e., marantic thrombosis), particularly in infancy.

Drugs and Toxins

IIH has been reported in otherwise healthy adolescents who are taking huge doses of vitamin A for the treatment of acne. Oral doses as low as 25,000 IU, daily, may cause headache and papilledema, with rapid improvement after cessation of the therapy. The syndrome is said to have occurred in Arctic explorers who consumed polar-bear liver, a great source of vitamin A. Some cases of IIH that are manifested by bulging fontanel and papilledema, have been reported in children given tetracycline or nalidixic acid. The mechanisms involved are obscure. Spontaneous, rapid recovery occurs when the drugs are stopped. The insecticide chlordecone, as well as amiodarone and lithium carbonate, have also been reported to cause IIH.

Hematologic and Connective Tissue Disorders

Papilledema and increased ICP have been attributed to severe iron-deficiency anemia, with striking improvement after treatment of the anemia. Presumably, the mechanism partly reflects the marked increase in cerebral blood flow that accompanies profound anemia. IIH has been reported with infectious mononucleosis, but the mechanism is not known. It has also been observed as a manifestation of systemic lupus erythematosus (SLE).

Pulmonary Encephalopathy

IIH may be a major complication of chronic, hypoxic hypercapnia, caused by paralytic states such as muscular dystrophy and cervical myelopathy; it may also be a major complication of obstructive pulmonary disease and the pickwickian syndrome. There is a chronic increase of cerebral blood flow because of the anoxemia and carbon dioxide retention. Patients usually appear mentally dull and encephalopathic, and thus differ from most patients with IIH.

Spinal Cord Diseases

IIH rarely occurs with tumors of the spinal cord or cauda equina, or with polyneuritis. Papilledema and headache disappear with treatment of the spinal lesion or regression of the polyneuropathy. The mechanism may involve the effects of an elevated CSF protein on CSF absorption, at the arachnoid villi in both cranial and spinal subarachnoid spaces. Occurrence of this syndrome, however, does not correlate with the degree of protein elevation.

Meningism is an old term that is applied to patients with stiff neck, increased ICP (usually 200 mmHg to 300 mmHg), but an otherwise normal CSF. This syndrome occurs in patients with acute systemic viral infections such as influenza. The mechanism of the ICH is unknown.

One of the more common forms of IIH appears in otherwise healthy persons in the absence of any of the aforementioned etiologic factors. Both genders are affected, and the occurrence is most often in patients who are between the ages of 10 and 50 years.

Diagnosis

The patient with headache and papilledema without other neurologic signs must be considered to have symptomatic ICH due from intracranial infection, until proven otherwise. This is true in about 35% of cases. Although the diagnosis of IIH may be suspected by the appearance of well being and a history of some of the associated etiologic features listed previously, the diagnosis is essentially one of exclusion, and depends on ruling out the more common causes of increased ICP. Brain tumor, particularly when located in relatively "silent" areas such as the frontal lobes or right temporal lobe, or when obstructing the ventricular system, may be manifested only by headache and papilledema. Patients with chronic subdural hematoma, without a history of significant trauma, may have the same symptoms.

Diagnostic evaluation depends on CT or MRI, which have obviated conventional angiography in most cases. MR venography promises to be the procedure of choice to exclude venous occlusion. Lumbar puncture should be deferred until CT indicates that the ventricular system is normal in size and location. Diagnostic lumbar puncture is mandatory to establish the diagnosis of IIH. In obesity, the normal upper limit of CSF pressure is 250 mmHg. In IIH, the CSF pressure is elevated, usually between 250 mmHg and 600 mmHg, but the fluid is otherwise normal. The protein content is often in the lower range of normal, and lumbar CSF protein levels of 10 mg/dL to 20 mg/dL are common. A CSF protein content greater than 50 mg/dL, decreased CSF glucose, or increased cell count throws doubt on the diagnosis of IIH and suggests other disease conditions.

Pseudopapilledema may be a source of diagnostic confusion. In this developmental anomaly of the fundus, the ophthalmic appearance may be indistinguishable from true papilledema; there is elevation of the optic disc, although exudates and hemorrhages are absent. Visual acuity is normal, but visual fields may show enlargement of the blind spots. The unchanging appearance of the fundus in subsequent examinations favors the diagnosis of pseudopapilledema, as does the finding of normal CSF pressure on lumbar puncture. Optic neuritis is differentiated from IIH by visual loss and normal CSF pressure.

Treatment

The common form of IIH in patients with menstrual disorders and obesity requires individualized management. This syndrome is self limited in most cases, and after some weeks or months, spontaneous remissions occur, making evaluation of therapy outcomes difficult. Recurrent episodes have been noted in about 5% to 10% of patients, and the illness seldom lasts for years. In the extremely obese patient, weight reduction is recommended. Daily lumbar puncture was used in the past to lower CSF pressure to normal levels by removing sufficient fluid; 15 mL to 30 mL of fluid may be removed, but the value of this procedure is dubious. A CSF-shunt procedure, such as a lumboperitoneal shunt, is useful in patients with intractable headache and progressive visual impairment. It may dramatically relieve symptoms. Optic nerve decompression has its advocates as the procedure of choice to preserve vision.

Dexamethasone has been used empirically because it minimizes cerebral edema of diverse causes and seems effective in some patients. However, steroids should be avoided unless acetazolamide and furosemide fail, because hyperadrenocorticism may precipitate IIH. Acetazolamide has been used because this carbonic anhydrase inhibitor reduces CSF formation. Furosemide also reduces CSF formation in animals and is similarly useful in humans. Hypertonic intravenous solutions (25% mannitol) to lower ICP may be used in acute situations when there is rapidly failing vision and surgical intervention is awaited; however, prolonged dehydration therapy is deleterious. Use of oral glycerol has the disadvantage of high-caloric intake for obese patients. Subtemporal decompression was widely used in the past, but its efficacy has been questioned. Either lumboperitoneal shunts or optic-nerve decompression is used to treat progressive visual loss. Their comparative risks and benefits should be assessed on an individual basis.

In patients with lateral sinus thrombosis caused by chronic infection in the petrous bone, surgical decompression may be indicated. When the pseudotumor syndrome is a manifestation of hypoadrenalism or hypoparathyroidism, replacement therapy is indicated. Vitamin A intoxication disappears when administration of the vitamin is stopped. Anticoagulation therapy is recommended for some patients with dural-sinus thrombosis; however, even with extension of the clot into cerebral veins, and hemorrhagic infarction of tissue, anticoagulation is useful despite its hazards. Thrombolytic therapy has been used successfully in recent reports.

SPONTANEOUS INTRACRANIAL HYPOTENSION (SIH)

In 1938, Schaltenbrand described the occurrence of primary spontaneous intracranial hypotension, or *essential aliquorrhea*. The symptoms were self limited, resolving spontaneously within several weeks to several months. Decreased choroidal secretion and increased CSF reabsorption were suggested as possible mechanisms, but evidence for either was lacking. SIH may simulate an acquired-Chiari I malformation. Less commonly, multiple cranial nerve signs have been noted, including binasal field defects, diplopia, tinnitus, and hearing loss.

Spontaneous, cryptic CSF leaks via dural fistulas adjacent to the spinal roots have been identified on radionuclide cisternography and contrast myelography. Such defects commonly reflect rupture of arachnoid (Tarlov cysts) that occur without trauma. The rapid urinary excretion of radioisotope, following intrathecal injection of the tracer, reflects such spinal-dural deficits. This diagnosis has been established with an intraspinal, combined injection of technetium-albumin and myelographic contrast material.

In some cases, one agent alone may identify the leak, which explains the advantage of the double injection. Cervical subarachnoid injection (C-2 or C-3 level) is often preferred over lumbar injection because it is less likely to result in a postlumbar-puncture headache, and the cervical region is distant from the more common. . . MRI commonly reveals striking, diffuse dural enhancement with CSF hypotension and CSF hypovolemia that are the result of a CSF fistula associated with a *sagging brain* (i.e., sites of leakage in the thoracolumbar region).

Gadolinium-enhanced MRI commonly reveals flattening of the optic chiasm, displacement of the pons against the clivus, and the cerebellar tonsils below the foramen magnum, simulating a Chiari malformation). Engorgement of the dural venous sinuses is also observed. These changes resolve rapidly after closure of the CSF fistula. Figure 50.1. shows the characteristic MR findings in the sagging brain, together with their resolution 5 days after a successful, large-volume, epidural lumbar blood patch. The dural enhancement reflects the Monro-Kellie rule: Intracranial venous engorgement results from a reduced CSF volume.

SIH usually resolves spontaneously or with bedrest, analogous to postlumbar-puncture headache. For intractable cases, treatment with a large-volume lumbar epidural blood patch is usually preferred, with the head and spine then tilted downward (30° for 10 minutes) to facilitate the movement of blood, extradurally, to the thoracic and cervical regions. In persistent cases, surgical closure of the fistula may be necessary. This requires CT myelography to identify the precise location of the fistula.

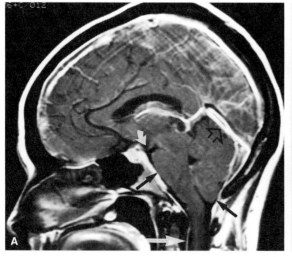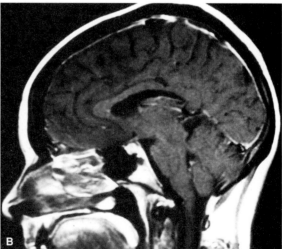

FIGURE 50.1. Sagging brain in spontaneous intracranial hypotension. A: Gadolinium-enhanced T1-weighted sagittal MR image prior to lumbar epidural blood patch demonstrates enhancement of the dura, venous engorgement, displacement of the pons and cerebellum below the level of the prepontal cistern *(arrow)*, and inferior displacement of the optic chiasm and third ventricle *(arrow)*. **B:** Gadolinium-enhanced T1-weighted images 5 days after large-volume (20 mL) lumbar epidural blood patch show resolution of dural enhancement and restoration of the cisterns, with elevation of the pons, tonsils, and optic chiasm. (From Fishman RA, Dillon WP. *Neurology* 1993;43:609–610. With permission.)

Although postural headaches in the erect position are typical of SIH, some patients are headache free, despite characteristic radiologic changes. The occurrence of somnolence and stupor caused by a sagging brain has been observed. Restoration of CSR volume and pressure to normal by the intrathecal injection of normal saline or preferably Elliott's B solution (a pH-adjusted buffered saline) dramatically and rapidly restores consciousness and a normal mental state.

SUGGESTED READINGS

Brain Edema

Fishman RA.Brain edema. In: *Cerebrospinal Fluid in Diseases of the Nervous System*, 2nd ed. Philadelphia: WB Saunders, 1992:116–137.

Levine BD, Yoshimuri K, Kobayashi T, et al. Dexamethasone for the treatment of acute mountain sickness. *N Engl J Med* 1989;32:1707–1713.

Idiopathic Intracranial Hypertension

Binder DK, Horton JC, Lawton, MT, McDermott MW. Idiopathic intracranial hypertension. *Neurosurgery* 2004;54:538–552.

Duncan FJ, Corbett JJ, Wall M. The incidence of pseudotumor cerebri. *Arch Neurol* 1988;45:875–877.

Fishman RA. Pseudotumor cerebri. In: *Cerebrospinal Fluid in Diseases of the Nervous System*, 2nd ed. Philadelphia: WB Saunders, 1992:138–151.

Higgins JN, Gillard H, Owler BK, Harkness K, Pickard JD. MR venography in idiopathic intracranial hypertension: unappreciated and misunderstood. *J Neurol Neurosurg Psychiatry* 2004;75(4):621–625.

Bastin, ME, Sinha, S, Farrall, AJ, et al. Diffuse brain edema in idiopathic intracranial hypertension: a quantitative magnetic resonance in an ongoing study. *J Neurol Neurosurg Psychiatry* 2003;74:1693–1696.

Ridsdale L, Moseley I. Thoracolumbar intraspinal tumors presenting features of raised intracranial pressure. *J Neurol Neurosurg Psychiatry* 1978;41:737–745.

Intracranial Hypotension

Atkinson JLD, Weinshenker BG, Miller GM, et al. Acquired Chiari I malformation secondary to spontaneous spinal cerebrospinal fluid leakage and chronic intracranial hypotension syndrome in seven cases. *J Neurosurg* 1998;88:237–242.

Fishman RA, Dillon WP. Dural enhancement and cerebral displacement secondary to intracranial hypotension. *Neurology* 1993;43:609–610.

Horton JC, Fishman RA. Neurovisual findings in the syndrome of spontaneous intracranial hypotension from dural cerebrospinal fluid leak. *Ophthalmology* 1994;101:244–251.

Mokri B, Piepgras DG, Miller GM. Syndrome of orthostatic headaches and diffuse pachymeningeal gadolinium enhancement. *Mayo Clin Proc* 1997;72:400–413.

Pleasure SJ, Abosch A, Friedman J, et al. Spontaneous intracranial hypotension resulting in stupor caused by diencephalic compression. *Neurology* 1998;50:1854–1857.

Rando TA, Fishman RA. Spontaneous intracranial hypotension: report of two cases and review of the literature. *Neurology* 1992;42:481–487.

Samadani, U, Huang, JH, Baranov, D, et al. Intracranial hypotension after intraoperative lumbar cerebrospinal fluid drainage. *Neurosurgery* 2003;52:148–152.

Schaltenbrand VG. Normal and pathological physiology of the cerebrospinal fluid circulation. *Lancet* 1953;1:805–808.

Schievink, WI, Gordon, OK, Tourje, J. Connective tissue disorders with spontaneous spinal cerebrospinal fluid leaks and intracranial hypotension: a prospective study. *Neurosurgery* 2004;54:65–71.

Tarlov IM. Spinal perineurial and meningeal cysts. *J Neurol Neurosurg Psychiatry* 1970;33:833–843.

C h a p t e r   5 1

Superficial Siderosis of the Central Nervous System

Robert A. Fishman

SIGNS AND SYMPTOMS

Superficial siderosis is the deposition of hemosiderin over the pial surfaces and superficial neuropil of the brain and spinal cord. It is usually characterized by sequential development of sensorineural deafness and cerebellar ataxia, followed by myelopathy, anosmia, and dementia. The condition usually evolves for many years as a consequence of chronic, intermittent, or persistent oozing of blood into the CSF. The bleeding may be cryptic, that is, asymptomatic and unassociated with headache, backache, or signs of meningeal irritation. A common error is the faulty clinical diagnosis of a neurodegenerative disorder, cerebellar degeneration with deafness.

DIAGNOSIS

In the past, the condition was recognized chiefly at autopsy, by its rust-colored appearance of the affected structures. CT and particularly MRI have shown that the incidence of the condition is far more frequent than previously suspected. MRI has greater sensitivity because the strong paramagnetic effect of iron-containing compounds allows better visualization of T2-weighted images, which show striking rims of hypointensity over the surfaces of the cerebrum, and particularly over the cerebellar vermis and adjacent cortical sulci. Hypointensities are observed rimming the brain stem and especially along the eighth cranial nerve, which is the most vulnerable cranial nerve because it is covered in the subarachnoid space by oligodendroglia, and not by the Schwann cells that cover the nerve roots and peripheral nerves. The first and second cranial nerves and spinal cord are similarly vulnerable. The Bergmann radial glia of the cerebellum are also susceptible to the deposition of iron pigments, perhaps because they can synthesize ferritin more readily than do other neural cells. The presence of xanthochromic CSF, often without a cellular reaction, should alert the clinician that a patient with insidiously progressive ataxia and deafness may have superficial siderosis. T2-weighted MRI is more likely to establish the diagnosis than CT, which is less sensitive (Fig. 51.1).

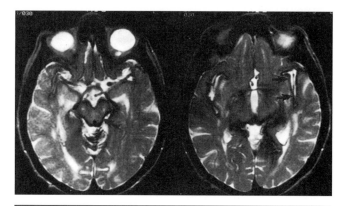

FIGURE 51.1. Patient with 10-year history of progressive cerebellar ataxia, deafness, cognitive impairment, spasticity, and xanthochromic CSF. T2-weighted MRI shows deposition of low-signal hemosiderin on the surfaces of the midbrain, cerebellar folia, and cerebral cortex adjacent to the sylvian cisterns *(arrows)*. (Courtesy of Dr. William P. Dillon.)

TREATMENT

The treatment of superficial siderosis requires identifying and treating the bleeding source, which is usually obvious in patients with aneurysms, vascular malformations, and tumors—especially ependymomas—of the brain or spinal cord. Fearnley and colleagues (1995) reported identifying the precise source of bleeding in only about 50% of patients with this diagnosis. Improvements in MRI should increase the success rate for identification. There have been several reports of siderosis developing in patients with a variety of spinal-dural defects, such as posttraumatic root avulsions, or with postoperative pseudomeningoceles following laminectomy. Closure of these dural defects arrests the progressive neurologic injury that results from chronic subarachnoid bleeding. Iron chelating agents have been ineffective in experimental animal models. Theoretically, antioxidants might be of some benefit but to date, this has not been established.

SUGGESTED READINGS

Anderson NE, Sheffield S, Hope JKA. Superficial siderosis of the central nervous system: a late complication of cerebellar tumors. *Neurology* 1999;52:163–169.

Fearnley JM, Stevens JM, Rudge P. Superficial siderosis of the central nervous system. *Brain* 1995;118:1051–1066.

Kale SU, Donaldson I, West RJ, Shehu A. Superficial siderosis of the meninges and its otolaryngologic connection: a series of five patients. *Otol Neurotol* 2003;24(1):90–5.

Fishman RA. Superficial siderosis. *Ann Neurol* 1993;34:635–636.

Koeppen AH, Dickson AC, Chu RC, Thach RE. The pathogenesis of superficial siderosis of the central nervous system. *Ann Neurol* 1993;34:646–653.

Leussink VI, Flachenecker P, Brechtelsbauer D, Bendszus M, Sliwka U, Gold R, Becker G. Superficial siderosis of the central nervous system: pathogenetic heterogeneity and therapeutic approaches. *Acta Neurol Scand.* 2003;107(1):54–61.

McCarron MO, Flynn PA, Owens C, Wallace I, Mirakhur M, Gibson JM, Patterson VH. Superficial siderosis of the central nervous system

many years after neurosurgical procedures. *J Neurol Neurosurg Psychiatry* 2003;74(9):1326–8.

Messori A, Di Bella P, Herber N, Logullo F, Ruggiero M, Salvolini U. The importance of suspecting superficial siderosis of the central nervous system in clinical practice. *J Neurol Neurosurg Psychiatry* 2004;75(2):188–90.

Tapscott SJ, Askridge J, Kliot M. Surgical management of superficial siderosis following cervical nerve root avulsion. *Ann Neurol* 1996;40:936–949.

Chapter 52

Hyperosmolar Hyperglycemic Nonketotic Syndrome

Stephan A. Mayer and Leon D. Prockop

The hyperosmolar hyperglycemic nonketotic syndrome (HHNS) is characterized by an abnormally high serum-glucose level, high osmolality, and a depressed level of consciousness in the absence of ketoacidosis. Modern awareness of the syndrome is ascribed to Sament and Schwartz; in 1957 they described diabetic stupor without ketosis. By 1968, the neurologic symptoms and signs of seizures and metabolic encephalopathy were well recognized. HHNS occurs in 10% to 20% of all patients with severe hyperglycemia; it is most common in elderly patients with mild adult-onset diabetes mellitus. Death ensues in 20% to 40%, usually related to medical comorbidity or neurologic complications.

HHNS is defined by serum osmolality greater than 350 mOsm/kg, plasma glucose content greater than 600 mg/dL, and no ketosis in a patient with depressed consciousness. Often, the patient is lethargic or stuporous; coma is unusual. The degree of lethargy correlates with the level of hyperosmolarity. Serum glucose levels are usually much higher than in diabetic ketoacidosis.

The average age of patients with HHNS is 60 years; men and women are affected equally. In many patients, the diabetes was not previously recognized. The majority of cases of HHNS are precipitated by an illness that precludes fluid intake and insulin or oral hypoglycemic therapy. One of the most common precipitants is stroke.

Other frequently associated illnesses include pneumonia or sepsis, gastrointestinal hemorrhage, myocardial infarction, pulmonary embolism, subdural hematoma, chronic renal insufficiency, pancreatitis, and burns. Medications implicated in HHNS include diuretic agents such as hydrochlorothiazide and furosemide, corticosteroids, phenytoin, propranolol, chlorpromazine hydrochloride (Thorazine), and immunosuppressive agents. Hyperalimentation, peritoneal dialysis or hemodialysis, and recent cardiac surgery have also been implicated.

Symptoms begin with several days or weeks of polyuria and polydipsia followed by dehydration and altered mental status. Depressed consciousness plays a key role in the development of the syndrome by preventing the patient from taking fluids in response to thirst. Confusion or unresponsiveness usually precipitates medical attention. Other neurologic findings include seizures (sometimes status epilepticus or epilepsia partialis continua), hemiparesis, aphasia, hemianopsia, visual loss, visual hallucinations, nystagmus, pupillary reflex abnormalities, asymmetric caloric responses, dysphagia, hyperreflexia, myoclonus, Babinski signs, and urinary retention. Systemic signs of dehydration include orthostatic hypotension, poor skin turgor, dry mucous membranes, and reduced sweating. The differential diagnosis includes diabetic ketoacidosis, alcoholic ketoacidosis, lactic acidosis, hepatic failure, uremia, hypoglycemia, drug ingestion, and stroke.

DIAGNOSIS

The diagnosis of HHNS is made in the laboratory. The serum glucose level ranges from 600 mg/dL to 2,700 mg/dL, and serum osmolality is in the range of 325 mOsm/kg to 425 mOsm/kg. The existence of a difference between the measured and calculated osmolality (calculated osmolality (mOsm/L) = $2 \times [Na^+] + [glucose]/18 + [BUN]/2.8$) indicates the presence of an unmeasured solute, such as mannitol or ethylene glycol. Although ketones are absent, mild acidosis with an elevated anion gap is present in 50% of patients (pH range, 6.8 to 7.4). In some patients, an element of lactic acidosis may result from hypotension and poor tissue perfusion, although this never completely accounts for the anion gap. Mixed acid–base disturbances may be present in patients with a metabolic alkalosis resulting from diuretic use.

Plasma sodium concentrations vary over a wide range (120 mEq/L to 180 mEq/L), although most patients are mildly hypernatremic. Elevated plasma-glucose levels tend to depress the plasma-sodium concentration (for every 100 mg/dL increment in glucose, sodium falls by 1.8 mEq/L). Therefore, a substantial free-water deficit may exist, even if the plasma sodium concentration is normal. Hypokalemia usually results from the sustained osmotic diuresis, and severe prerenal azotemia is the rule. In addition to laboratory studies, search for an underlying illness should include an electrocardiogram to rule out myocardial ischemia, blood and urine cultures, a chest xray to rule out infection, and brain CT or MRI if focal neurologic signs are present.

HHNS evolves when a physiologic stress and decreased insulin activity induce hyperglycemia. The hyperglycemia, in turn, induces an osmotic diuresis that continues until intravascular volume depletion reduces renal perfusion. The resulting free-water deficit and hyperosmolality cause cellular dehydration in both cerebral and extracerebral tissues, as water moves down the osmotic gradient from the intracellular to the extracellular compartment.

Sodium and potassium losses occur as the osmotic diuresis interferes with normal tubular reabsorption, but water is always lost out of proportion to sodium, resulting in further extracellular hypertonicity. Cerebral dehydration is thought to be the primary cause of the neurologic changes seen with HHNS.

TREATMENT

Treatment focuses on replacing volume deficits, correcting hyperosmolality, normalizing plasma glucose levels, and managing any underlying illnesses. Patients in shock need immediate resuscitation with normal saline. The average total fluid deficit is 9 L to 12 L. Central venous pressure monitoring (target 5 mmHg to 8 mmHg) may be useful in guiding therapy. Normal saline should be given until the blood pressure and urine output stabilize, at which point, half-normal saline may be used to replace any free-water deficits that still exist. It is recommended that one-half of the estimated fluid deficit be replaced in the first 12 to 24 hours, and the remainder replaced over the next few days.

Insulin is usually required to control hyperglycemia and limit ongoing osmotic diuresis in the initial management of HHNS. Serum glucose levels may drop by 25% with fluid replacement alone. A decrease in the plasma glucose concentration indicates response to therapy, especially to rehydration; the goal is for the plasma-glucose level to decline by at least 75 mg/dL to 100 mg/dL per hour. Insulin is mandatory if the patient is acidotic, hyperkalemic, or in renal failure. If insulin is used, an initial intravenous bolus of 0.1 IU/kg of regular insulin, followed by a continuous intravenous infusion of 0.1 IU/kg per hour may be given. To avoid overshooting the target serum glucose to levels of hypoglycemia, once glucose levels fall below 200 mg/dL, 5% dextrose should be added to the infusion.

Most patients have total-body potassium deficits. Hydration and insulin administration further depress the serum potassium level. Therefore, potassium should be administered early in treatment. Electrolytes such as calcium, phosphate, and magnesium may need to be replaced as well.

If seizures develop, intravenous benzodiazepines may be given as an alternative to phenytoin until the metabolic disturbance is corrected. Long-term anticonvulsant therapy after the acute phase of illness is usually unnecessary. Owing to the high mortality rate of patients with HHNS and the meticulous monitoring that their treatments require, these patients are best managed in an intensive care unit. A smooth transition to a long-term treatment regimen and a plan to prevent recurrence are also critical components of care.

SUGGESTED READINGS

Arieff AI, Ayus JC. Strategies for diagnosing and managing hypernatremic encephalopathy. *J Crit Illness* 1996;11:720–727.

Arieff A, Carroll HJ. Non-ketotic hyperosmolar coma with hyperglycemia: clinical features, pathophysiology, renal function, acid–base balance, plasma-cerebrospinal fluid equilibrium and the effects of therapy on 37 cases. *Medicine* 1972;51:73–96.

Chiasson JL, Aris-Jilwan N, Belanger R, et al. Diagnosis and treatment of diabetic ketoacidosis and the hyperglycemic hyperosmolar state. *Can Med Assoc J* 2003;168:859–866.

Daugirdas JT, Knonfol NO, Tzamaloukas AH, et al. Hyperosmolar coma: cellular dehydration and the sodium concentration. *Ann Intern Med* 1989;110:855–857.

Delaney MF, Zisman A, Kettyle WM. Diabetic ketoacidosis and hyperglycemic hyperosmolar nonketotic syndrome. *Endocrin Metab Clin N Am* 2000;29:683–705.

English P, Williams G. Hyperglycaemic crises and lactic acidosis in diabetes mellitus. *Postgrad Med J* 2004;80(943):253–261.

Gaglia JL, Wyckoff J, Abrahamson MJ. Acute hyperglycemic crises in the elderly. *Med Clin North Am* 2004;88(4):1063–1084.

Gullans SR, Verbalis JG. Control of brain volume during hyperosmolar and hyposmolar conditions. *Ann Rev Med* 1993;44:289–301.

Hennis A, Corbin D, Fraser H. Focal seizures and nonketotic hyperglycemia. *J Neurol Neurosurg Psychiatry* 1992;55:195–197.

Maccario M. Neurological dysfunction associated with nonketotic hyperglycemia. *Arch Neurol* 1968;19:525–534.

MacIsaac RJ, Lee LY, McNeil KJ, Tsalamandris C, Jerums G. Influence of age on the presentation and outcome of acidotic and hyperosmolar diabetic emergencies. *Int Med J* 2002;32:379–385.

Matz R. Management of the hyperosmolar hyperglycemic syndrome. *Am Fam Phys* 1999;60:1468–1476.

Prockop LD. Hyperglycemia, polyol accumulation and increased intracranial pressure. *Arch Neurol* 1971;25:126–140.

Singh BM, Strobos RJ. Epilepsia partialis continua associated with nonketotic hyperglycemia: clinical and biochemical profile of 21 patients. *Ann Neurol* 1980;8:155–160.

Umpierrez GE, Khajavi M, Kitabchi AE. Review: diabetic ketoacidosis and hyperosmolar nonketotic syndrome. *Am J Med Sci* 1996;311:225–233.

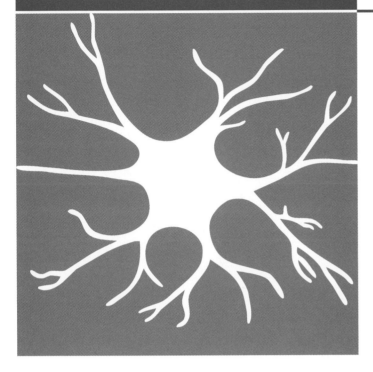

Tumors

Chapter 53

General Considerations

Lisa M. DeAngelis

CNS tumors are relatively uncommon but are among the most feared of cancers. Cancers of other organs may cause pain, disability and death but CNS tumors attack the patient's sense of self by causing paralysis, seizures, cognitive impairment and personality changes. CNS tumors are also among the most intractable of malignancies partly because their location in the brain restricts vigorous therapy.

Surgery is the most important treatment, but the wide margins so critical to successful surgical treatment of other cancers may not be achieved. New techniques have allowed more precise delivery of radiotherapy, but normal CNS tolerance limits the dose. Chemotherapy has been improving for some CNS tumors, but most are largely resistant to conventional agents. However, increased understanding of the biology of CNS tumors has led to trials of exciting new agents.

Long considered a set of orphan diseases, brain tumors are emerging as a major focus of research, as some recent success stories (e.g., oligodendrogliomas and primary CNS lymphoma) indicate that patients may be treated successfully and may recover neurologic function. This chapter addresses the general principles governing all CNS tumors, including the use of standard symptomatic treatments that apply to all tumor types. Each individual tumor type is discussed in detail in the following chapters. Comprehensive texts are available for the interested reader.

EPIDEMIOLOGY

Two large epidemiologic studies, one from the Mayo Clinic and the second from the Central Brain Tumor Registry of the United States (CBTRUS) give a remarkably similar incidence of symptomatic brain tumors with a rate of about 12 per 100,000 population per year. Given the current United States population, this comes to about 35,000 new patients with symptomatic brain tumors who are diagnosed each year. In the Mayo Clinic study, full population records were available from Olmstead County, Minnesota and the incidence of all primary intracranial tumors was 19.1 per 100,000 persons per year for the period 1950 through 1989. This includes a rate of 7.3 per 100,000 persons per year for asymptomatic tumors that were diagnosed at autopsy or by neuroimaging. Intracranial tumors may occur at any age but the incidence and histologic type varies by age. There is a small peak before age 10 years and a steady rise in the incidence from the age of 15 years on, with the highest incidence between ages 75 and 84 years (Fig. 53.1).

In children, brain tumors are the most common solid tumor of childhood and are second only to leukemia in their overall incidence of malignancies in the pediatric population. In children, low grade astrocytomas and medulloblastomas predominate. In adults, malignant astrocytoma and meningioma are the most common tumors. In general, most tumor subtypes predominate in men with the exception of the meningioma, which has a strong female predominance.

Several studies suggest that the incidence of brain tumors has been steadily rising in the US. Some of this may be an ascertainment bias, particularly in older people because the evaluation of neurologic symptoms is more easily accomplished with neuroimaging and because physicians and families are now more willing to investigate neurologic symptoms in older patients. However, ascertainment is not the only explanation for this seemingly higher incidence of tumors. There has also been a change in the type of tumors diagnosed. For instance, there the incidence of primary CNS lymphoma has certainly increased, particularly in the elderly. A similar increase in the incidence of oligodendrogliomas may have had more to do with the willingness of the neuropathologists to recognize oligodendroglial features within a glioma; this would not have been considered important previously, but is now recognized to have therapeutic implications. Data also show that the increased prevalence of elderly in the population may contribute to the increased incidence of brain tumors. As people survive longer and do not die at a younger age of more common diseases, such as cardiovascular

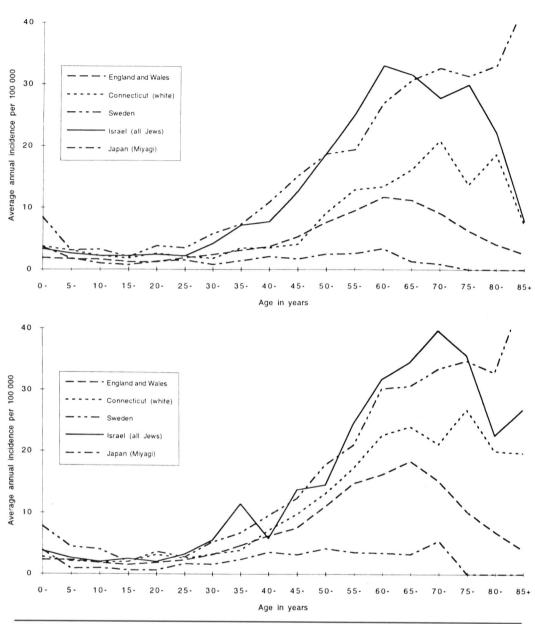

FIGURE 53.1. Female **(top)** and male **(bottom)** age-specific incidence rates for malignant CNS tumors, 1978–1982. (From Muir et al.; with permission.)

conditions, they live long enough to become vulnerable to rare diseases, such as brain tumors. It is doubtful that there is a single explanation for the apparent increased incidence, but rather all of these factors are contributing to a greater number of patients being diagnosed with brain tumors each year.

ETIOLOGY

No known life-style factors contribute to the risk of developing a brain tumor, but a few environmental risk factors do contribute. The first is high-dose irradiation, which increases the risk of gliomas, meningiomas, and nerve sheath tumors. Modern dental x-rays do not increase the risk of brain tumors.

Acquired immune suppression, such as HIV infection or chronic immunosuppressive therapy after organ transplant, increases the risk of primary CNS lymphoma. There may be a slight increased risk of gliomas in HIV infected individuals and there is a definite increased incidence of intracranial leiomyosarcomas in these patients.

Other environmental risk factors such as head trauma, dietary exposure to N-nitrosourea compounds, industrial exposure to polyvinyl chloride and other occupational exposures have not been convincingly demonstrated to increase the risk of brain tumors. Cell-phone use has been excluded as a cause of either gliomas or meningiomas.

Several genetic syndromes substantially increase the risk of intracranial neoplasms. The most common are neurofibromatosis type-1, which leads to gliomas, and neurofibromatosis type-2, which includes vestibular schwannomas and meningiomas. The Li-Fraumeni syndrome, which is associated with mutation in the *p53* gene, causes glioma and medulloblastoma. Tuberous sclerosis, an autosomal dominant trait, leads to subependymal giant cell astrocytomas and cortical tubers. In the Von Hippel-Lindau syndrome, also autosomal dominant, hemangioblastomas are seen in the brain, spinal cord and retina. Burkitt syndrome and hereditary nonpolyposis colorectal cancer syndrome may be either autosomal recessive or autosomal dominant, and include glioblastoma and medulloblastoma. These syndromes are important to recognize because advice includes genetic counseling and surveillance for other cancers, such as renal cell cancer in Von Hippel-Lindau disease.

BIOLOGY OF INTRACRANIAL NEOPLASMS

All tumors are genetic in the sense that tumor-cell development requires enhanced growth signals, disruption of normal cell-cycle controls, and inhibition of apoptosis; these changes are mediated through point mutation, deletion, or duplication. In brain tumors, multiple genetic disruptions are necessary to produce an intracranial neoplasm. These include an amplification of growth factor pathways, particularly those of the epidermal growth factor receptor and the platelet-derived growth factor and its receptor. Most of these changes occur in mutations of proto-oncogenes, which increase the signaling for growth. Most tumors also show loss of tumor suppressor genes, which function in controlling the internal machinery or the cell cycle and its regulatory factors. These include loss of the *PTEN* gene, which enhances signal transduction pathways leading to activation of the cell cycle. Lastly, most tumors have alterations in apoptotic mechanisms, such as p53 mutations, with impairment of normal apoptosis. In addition to the genetic changes that define the malignant phenotype, other mutations enable the tumor to support growth, such as the development of new blood vessels. Tumor cells may secrete angiogenic factors, such as vascular endothelial growth factor (VEGF), which stimulate the formation of new blood vessels for the growing tumor.

These complex genetic changes may be acquired through serial mutations as tumors progress from low- to high-grade malignancy or may lead to a high-grade tumor *de novo*. Although most tumors have alterations in these three basic mechanisms, the specific alteration may vary from one tumor to the next and not all changes are seen in every single tumor cell within a particular category. Consequently, this degree of heterogeneity makes targeted therapy challenging and suggests that it is not likely to find an effective therapy if it controls only intracellular pathways.

CLINICAL DIAGNOSIS

Neurologic symptoms and signs of brain tumors may be similar regardless of the specific histologic type of each neoplasm. Symptoms and signs may be due to brain invasion with destruction of underlying tissue; brain compression with expansion of an intracranial mass; CSF obstruction with increased intracranial pressure (ICP); or herniation. Specific symptoms and signs are due to tumor location and the development of symptoms depends largely on the rapidity of tumor growth. Rapidly growing tumors create symptoms over weeks (e.g., CNS lymphoma) whereas slowly growing tumors may remain asymptomatic for years, or until they reach a critical size that causes symptoms from brain compression (e.g., subfrontal meningioma).

Most brain tumors are accompanied by edema of the surrounding brain. This may be seen on CT or MRI and is responsible for many of the symptoms. Symptoms and signs arise from the aggregate mass of tumor plus edema, and are not due simply to the size of the tumor alone. In general, the more rapidly growing the tumor, the greater the surrounding edema.

SYMPTOMS AND SIGNS

Symptoms may be generalized or focal. Generalized symptoms are frequently due to increased ICP. Headache, the most common, generalized symptom, is the first symptom in 30% to 40% of patients with brain tumors. It may sometimes indicate the laterality of the tumor but most of the time, the headache is not specific and is not localizing. Classically, headaches are worse in the morning and improve over the course of the day. Nausea and vomiting are common indications of raised ICP, and projectile or explosive vomiting may occur without preceding nausea. This is seen more commonly in children than adults, particularly with tumors involving the posterior fossa where they may compress the emetic center of the brainstem. Vertigo and dizziness are also common, particularly with vestibular schwannomas, but they may occur with any kind of brain tumor. Mental and cognitive abnormalities are frequently nonspecific; patients may develop apathy, irritability or personality changes that are attributed to depression by family members or physicians. Specific cognitive abnormalities, such as aphasia or agnosia, localize the tumor to a particular region of the brain.

Episodic symptoms may arise from plateau waves that are caused by fluctuations of ICP. They are typically triggered by a change in body position and may be manifest as transient severe headache, nausea, vomiting, ataxia, visual loss, or bilateral leg weakness. They may last for only a few minutes and then may resolve completely. Episodic symptoms may occasionally be accompanied by loss of consciousness and are frequently confused with seizures. However, they are easily discriminated from seizures by eliciting the history that they are usually preceded by changes in body position, typically going from lying or sitting to standing.

Focal symptoms and signs occur in almost all patients with a brain tumor. Seizures are the most common, affecting about one-third of the patients. Although the seizures may appear to be generalized, all seizures from a brain tumor are focal in origin, whether the focal signature is clinically apparent or not. Other focal symptoms and signs include hemiparesis, visual field defect, and aphasia.

Tumors in different locations tend to create a typical constellation of symptoms. For example, tumors in the frontal lobe frequently cause seizures, behavioral changes, dementia, gait disorders, hemiparesis, and expressive aphasia from the dominant hemisphere. Occipital lobe tumors are associated with hemianopia and unformed visual disturbances. Temporal lobe tumors usually cause behavioral changes, including language disturbance from the dominant hemisphere, olfactory and partial-complex seizures, or visual field deficit. Tumors in the corpus callosum may cause dementia when the anterior callosum is involved, behavioral changes and severe memory loss with an amnestic syndrome when the splenium is involved, or no symptoms at all. Tumors in the cerebellopontine angle may cause ipsilateral deafness and facial numbness, weakness, and ataxia. Pineal tumors cause the Parinaud syndrome with impaired upgaze and pupillary abnormalities, as well as hydrocephalus. Cerebellar tumors cause headache, ataxia, nystagmus and occasionally neck pain.

Skull-base tumors affect the cranial nerves. Meningioma of the olfactory groove causes anosmia. Optic nerve meningioma causes unilateral visual loss. Pituitary tumors cause bitemporal hemianopia from chiasmal compression. Extraocular abnormalities occur with cavernous sinus or brainstem tumors. Hearing loss and, less commonly, facial weakness may be seen with acoustic neuroma. Multiple cranial nerve signs are seen with leptomeningeal metastasis.

False localizing signs may arise from increased ICP. The most common is a sixth nerve palsy produced by compression of the abducens nerve as it passes over the petrous ridge. The nerve is particularly vulnerable because of its long course. Ipsilateral hemiparesis may occur as a herniating uncus compresses the contralateral cerebral peduncle against the tentorium. Hydrocephalus may lead to personality changes, gait abnormalities, and urinary incontinence. Tinnitus is a common symptom of increased ICP from any cause. Cortical blindness or hemianopia may result from compression of the posterior cerebral arteries with occipital infarction from herniation though the tentorial notch.

NEUROOPHTHALMOLOGIC SIGNS

Oculomotor problems are common with tumors of the pineal area. The Parinaud syndrome consists of light-near dissociation, as well as paralysis of convergence and upgaze. It is common with pineal tumors that compress adjacent midbrain. Pineal tumors may also lead to other disorders of ocular motility, such as convergence-retraction nystagmus, ptosis, or lid retraction (i.e., Collier sign). In children, a setting-sun sign consisting of downward deviation of the eyes and lid retraction may occur, along with hydrocephalus.

Papilledema is a rare sign in patients with brain tumors because neuroimaging now leads to earlier evaluation of symptoms such as headache. Papilledema develops after sustained increased ICP elevations for weeks or months (Fig. 53.2) and is attributed to transmission of pressure along the optic nerve sheath and to blockade of axoplasmic transport and venous return.

Papilledema resulting from increased ICP affects both eyes. Unilateral papilledema is caused by asymmetric swelling of the optic nerve because of the location of the lesion or because of a congenital anomaly in which the optic nerve sheath does not fully envelop both nerves equally,

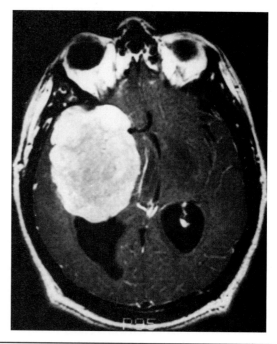

FIGURE 53.2. **Temporal meningioma (a large, slowly growing tumor affecting a "silent" area of the brain).** This 38-year-old man had mild papilledema on routine eye examination. Gadolinium-enhanced MRI shows a 7-cm right temporal lobe meningioma.

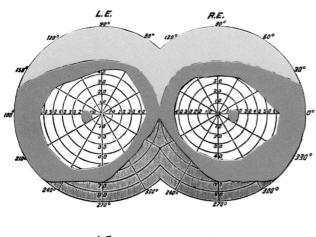

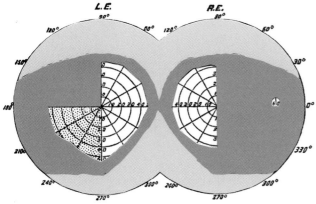

FIGURE 53.3. Visual-field defects in intracranial tumors. A: Enlargement of blind spots and constriction of peripheral fields with increased cranial pressure. **B:** Bitemporal hemianopia with pituitary adenoma. (From Merritt H, Mettler FA, Putnam TJ. *Fundamentals of Clinical Neurology.* New York: Blakiston Co, 1947; with permission.)

preventing symmetric transmission of increased ICP. On visual field testing, characteristic findings are enlargement of the blind spot and constriction of the visual fields (Fig. 53.3).

The Foster Kennedy syndrome, ipsilateral optic nerve atrophy and contralateral papilledema, is associated with orbital tumors that compress the ipsilateral optic nerve to cause optic atrophy but also lead to increased ICP, causing contralateral papilledema.

LABORATORY EXAMINATION

Imaging

MRI is the test of choice to evaluate suspected intracranial tumor. It is far superior to CT, which may miss lesions in the posterior fossa where bone creates substantial artifact. In addition, low-grade infiltrating lesions are often difficult to see on CT or may be confused with strokes. For patients who may not undergo MRI (e.g., patients with pacemakers), CT may exclude a majority of intracranial neoplasms

successfully, but it does not show the anatomic relationships as well as MRI.

CT and MRI must be performed without and with contrast material. Contrast highlights areas of blood-brain barrier disruption, which is characteristic of most high-grade brain tumors. It also highlights extra-axial tumors and may define their relationship to surrounding neural structures (e.g., vestibular schwannoma and meningioma). In general, parenchymal brain tumors or any lesion that enhances with contrast is usually a high-grade malignant tumor, whereas low-grade tumors such as astrocytomas or oligodendrogliomas tend to be nonenhancing. Although this general rule applies to the majority of patients, there are certainly nonenhancing tumors that turn out to be high-grade and there are specific low-grade tumors, such as the pilocytic astrocytoma, that brightly enhance with contrast.

Both CT and MRI may visualize hemorrhage within a tumor. Hemorrhage is bright on CT before administration of contrast agent, but the MRI appearance of hemorrhage depends on how long the hemorrhage has been present. Hyperacute hemorrhages may appear isointense on T1-weighted MRI, but may be discerned on gradient-echo MRI. With the passage of 1 to 2 days, hemorrhage may become hyperintense on precontrast T1 MRI.

There is no role for skull x-rays or angiography. Occasionally, the vascular anatomy needs to be elucidated to assist the surgeon in preoperative planning such as ascertaining the patency of a venous sinus prior to tumor resection (e.g., parasagittal meningioma). However, MRA or MRV usually suffices to delineate these structures. Formal angiography is reserved for patients who need preoperative embolization to reduce the vascularity of a lesion before resection (e.g., glomus jugulare tumor).

EEG is almost never helpful in the diagnosis of brain tumor. It may be useful if the patient is unresponsive and nonconvulsive status epilepticus is a consideration. CSF analysis is useful only for the neurologic staging required for some malignancies such as primary CNS lymphoma, intracranial germ-cell tumors, medulloblastoma or pineoblastoma. Occasionally the diagnosis may be established on a CSF evaluation for tumors such as lymphoma, but lumbar puncture is not necessary for most intracranial neoplasms.

Functional MRI is a useful preoperative test for noninvasive evaluation of the relationship between a tumor and surrounding eloquent cortex. It may determine whether speech or motor activity resides within the parenchyma occupied by a tumor, or is adjacent to it. This may enable the surgeon to ascertain the safety of a complete resection before taking the patient to the operating room. Cortical representation of function may be confirmed intraoperatively with cortical mapping, which guides the resection during the procedure.

Positron emission tomography (PET) using ^{18}F-fluorodeoxyglucose (FDG) is useful to measure tumor metabolism. Occasionally this is helpful in the diagnosis of patients with presumed low-grade gliomas who show nonenhancing lesions on CT or MRI. PET is performed to ascertain whether there is a focus of hypermetabolism within the lesion that may indicate an area of anaplasia to be included in any biopsy being performed for diagnosis. FDG-PET may also be useful in discriminating tumor recurrence from radiation necrosis. This is particularly important for patients who have received focal therapy, such as stereotactic radiosurgery, and who develop progressive enhancing lesions that could be either tumor recurrence or treatment-related cerebral injury. PET can usually discriminate between the two because tumor is characterized by hypermetabolism of FDG, whereas radionecrosis is characterized by hypometabolism. Amino acid imaging, particularly with ^{11}C-methionine, may be more sensitive and specific in the diagnosis of low-grade tumors, but it is not yet widely available.

SPECT involves the administration of radioactive tracers for functions similar to those of FDG-PET. It is widely available and less expensive than PET, but it is also less sensitive. MR spectroscopy (MRS) is being performed with increasing frequency as are MR perfusion scans. MRS identifies intracellular metabolites that are characteristic of high-grade tumors; for instance, increased choline, decreased N-acetylaspartic acid, and high lipid and lactate levels suggest a high-grade neoplasm. Perfusion MRI delineates the hypervascularity associated with high-grade malignancies and provides indirect evidence of a malignant brain tumor. These techniques are widely used, but it is not clear that they are sufficiently sensitive or specific to establish a diagnosis.

SYMPTOMATIC MANAGEMENT OF BRAIN TUMORS

Corticosteroids

Corticosteroids may relieve the symptoms of brain tumors rapidly and dramatically by reducing peritumoral edema and decreasing intracranial pressure (ICP). The standard drug used is dexamethasone, owing to its relatively low mineralocorticoid activity. Patients often experience symptomatic improvement within an hour of receiving a dose of dexamethasone, but full effect often takes 24 to 48 hours. The mechanisms of glucocorticoid activity are unclear, but they seem to reconstitute the disrupted blood-brain barrier characteristic of malignant brain tumors.

Corticosteroids are indicated in all symptomatic patients with brain tumors. In particular, they are essential in any symptomatic patient or patient with substantial peritumoral edema seen on neuroimaging if radiotherapy is to be used. The only exception is in a patient with suspected

▶ **TABLE 53.1** Side Effects of Corticosteroids

Common but mild
Insomnia
Increased appetite
Visual blurring
Acne
Urinary frequency
Oral candidiasis
Nonneurologic but serious
GI bleeding
Osteoporosis
Avascular necrosis
Hyperglycemia
Neurologic
Common
Myopathy
Depression
Agitation
Hiccoughs
Tremor
Uncommon
Psychosis

lymphoma, where corticosteroids may cause regression of the tumor, preventing an accurate histologic diagnosis from being established if given before the biopsy.

Although beneficial, long-term administration of corticosteroids may result in substantial clinical toxicity (Table 53.1). Patients expected to be on corticosteroids for more than 6 weeks should receive prophylactic antibiotics to prevent *Pneumocystis carinii* infection.

Once a patient's symptoms are controlled with corticosteroids and specific tumor therapy has been instituted, the dose of corticosteroids should be reduced. Most patients may discontinue steroids once treatment has been completed and those who require chronic corticosteroids should be maintained on the lowest dose that minimizes symptoms. The standard dose of dexamethasone is 16 mg per day, in divided doses, but lower doses are frequently sufficient, and doses as high as 100 mg per day are occasionally necessary to manage severe symptoms of increased ICP.

Anticonvulsants

Anticonvulsants are given to all patients who have had a seizure. However, most patients with brain tumors do not have a seizure as the first symptom. Randomized controlled trials have documented that prophylactic anticonvulsants in brain tumor patients do not protect these patients against future seizures and may have substantial toxicity. Therefore, brain tumor patients who have not had a seizure should never be given prophylactic anticonvulsants. For those who are given anticonvulsants, it is preferable to use agents that do not activate the hepatic microsomal system. These include valproic acid, lamotrigine, topiramate, gabapentin, and levetiracetam. Drugs such as phenytoin, phenobarbital and carbamazepine may cause rash or, rarely, the Stevens-Johnson syndrome. More important, they have drug interactions. Specifically, they may enhance the metabolism of chemotherapeutic agents, effectively reducing levels to sub-therapeutic values. Interactions with other agents such as corticosteroids may also affect the metabolism of the anticonvulsants themselves, making it difficult to maintain therapeutic blood levels.

COMPLICATIONS OF BRAIN TUMORS

Thromboembolism

Thromboembolism is a common complication of all brain tumors and their therapy. Deep vein thrombosis occurs in at least 25% of patients with gliomas and pulmonary embolism is common. Many factors contribute to thromboembolic disease in brain tumor patients, including immobility, surgery, hypercoagulability from chemotherapy or the presence of systemic cancer and the release of thromboplastins from the brain. Many episodes occur in the postoperative period so pneumatic compression boots should be used postoperatively in all patients. The addition of low-molecular-weight heparin, combined with use of the boots, affords even greater protection and is safe even after craniotomy.

When thromboembolism develops, there is frequently great concern that anticoagulation is not safe for use in patients with an intracranial neoplasm. However, numerous studies on patients with gliomas, as well as CNS metastases, have shown the safety of full-dose anticoagulation in this population. This is far preferable to the use of inferior vena cava filters that, in brain tumor patients, may lead to pulmonary embolism from the filter itself. These complications frequently result in full-dose anticoagulation of the patient even though a filter is in place. It is preferable to treat these patients with low-molecular-weight heparin and then convert them to warfarin, which is maintained for at least 3 to 6 months.

SUGGESTED READINGS

Ahsan H, Neugut AI, Bruce JN. Trends in incidence of primary malignant brain tumors in the USA, 1981–1990. *Int J Epidemiol* 1995;24:1078–1085.

Auguste KI, Quinones-Hinojosa A, Gadkary C, et al. Incidence of venous thromboembolism in patients undergoing craniotomy and motor mapping for glioma without intraoperative mechanical prophylaxis to the contralateral leg. *J Neurosurg* 2003;99:680–684.

Becherer A, Karanikas G, Szabo M, et al. Brain tumour imaging with PET: a comparison between [18F] fluorodopa and [11C] methionine. *Eur J Nucl Med Mol Imaging* 2003;30:1561–1567.

Bell D, Grant R, Collie D, et al. How well do radiologists diagnose intracerebral tumour histology on CT? Findings from a prospective multicentre study. *Br J Neurosurg* 2002;16:573–577.

Bohnen NI, Kurland LT. Brain tumor and exposure to pesticides in humans: a review of the epidemiologic data. *J Neurol Sci* 1995;132:110–121.

Carman TL, Kanner AA, Barnett Gh, Deitcher SR. Prevention of thromboembolism after neurosurgery for brain and spinal tumors. *South Med J* 2003;96:17–22.

CBTRUS. Statistical Report: Primary brain tumors in the United States. 1995–1999. Central Brain Tumor Registry of the United States, 2002.

Cersosimo RJ, Brophy MT. Hiccups with high dose dexamethasone administration. A case report. *Cancer* 1998;82:412–414.

Counsell CE, Grant R. Incidence studies of primary and secondary intracranial tumors: a systematic review of their methodology and results. *J Neurooncol* 1998;37:241–250.

DeAngelis LM. Brain tumors. *N Engl J Med* 2001;344(2):114–123.

DeAngelis LM, Gutin PH, Leibel SA, Posner JB. *Diagnosis and Treatment of Intracranial Tumors: The Memorial Sloan-Kettering Experience.*:Martin Dunitz, Ltd., 2001.

Forsyth P, Posner JB. Headaches in patients with brain tumors: a study of 111 patients. *Neurology* 1993;43:1678–1683.

Forsyth PA, Weaver S, Fulton D, et al. Prophylactic anticonvulsants in patients with brain tumour. *Can J Neurol Sci* 2003;30:106–112.

Gassel MM. False localizing signs: a review of the concept and analysis of the occurrence in 250 cases of intracranial meningioma. *Arch Neurol* 1961;4:526–554.

Giles GG. What do we know about risk factors for glioma? *Cancer Causes Control* 1997;8:3–4.

Girard N, Wang ZJ, Erbetta A, et al. Prognostic value of proton MR spectroscopy of cerebral hemisphere tumors in children. *Neuroradiology* 1998;40:121–125.

Glantz MJ, Cole BF, Forsyth PA, et al. Practice parameter. Anticonvulsant prophylaxis in patients with newly diagnosed brain tumors: report of the Quality Standards Subcommittee of the American Academy of Neurology. *Neurology* 2000;54:1886–1893.

Glantz MJ, Cole BF, Friedberg MH, et al. A randomized, blinded, placebo-controlled trial of divalproex sodium prophylaxis in adults with newly diagnosed brain tumors. *Neurology* 1996;46:985–991.

Goldhaber SZ, Dunn K, Gerhard-Herman M, et al. Low rate of venous thromboembolism after craniotomy for brain tumor using multimodality prophylaxis. *Chest* 2002;122:1933–1937.

Goldschmidt N, Linetsky E, Shalom E, et al. High incidence of thromboembolism in patients with central nervous system lymphoma. *Cancer* 2003;98:1239–1242.

Hartmann M, Heiland S, Harting I, et al. Distinguishing of primary cerebral lymphoma from high-grade glioma with perfusion-weighted magnetic resonance imaging. *Neurosci Lett* 2003;338:119–122.

Hirsch J, Ruge MI, Kim KH, et al. An integrated functional magnetic resonance imaging procedure for preoperative mapping of cortical areas associated with tactile, motor, language, and visual functions. *Neurosurgery* 2000;47:711–721.

Honing PJ, Charney EB. Children with brain tumor headaches: distinguishing features. *Am J Dis Child* 1982;136:121–124.

Hutter A, Schwetye KE, Bierhals AJ, McKinstry RC. Brain neoplasms: epidemiology, diagnosis, and prospects for cost-effective imaging. *Neuroimaging Clin N Am* 2003;23:237–250.

Karlsson P, Holmberg E, Lundell M, et al. Intracranial tumors after exposure to ionizing radiation during infancy: a pooled analysis of two Swedish cohorts of 28,008 infants with skin hemangioma. *Radiat Res* 1998;15:357–364.

Koehler PJ. Use of corticosteroids in neuro-oncology. *Anticancer Drugs* 1995;6:19–33.

Krabbe K, Gideon P, Wagn P, et al. MR diffusion imaging of human intracranial tumours. *Neuroradiology* 1997;39:483–489.

Kumar PP, Good RR, Skultety M, et al. Radiation-induced neoplasms of the brain. *Cancer* 1987;59:1274–1282.

Kuratsu J, Ushio Y. Epidemiological study of primary intracranial tumours in elderly people. *J Neurol Neurosurg Psychiatry* 1997;63:116–118.

Mahindra AK, Grossman SA. Pneumocystis carinii pneumonia in HIV negative patients with primary brain tumors. *J Neurooncol* 2003;63:263–270.

Mason WP. Anticonvulsant prophylaxis for patients with brain tumours: insights from clinical trials. *Can J Neurol Sci* 2003;30:89–90.

Nafe R, Herminghaus S, Raab P, et al. Correlation between preoperative magnetic resonance spectroscopic data on high grade gliomas and morphology of Ki 67-positive tumor cell nuclei. *Anal Quant Cytol Histol* 2003;25:131–138.

Non R, Modan B, Boice JDJ, et al. Tumors of the brain and nervous system after radiotherapy in childhood. *N Engl J Med* 1988;319:1033–1039.

Olivero WC, Dulebohn SC, Lister JR. The use of PET in evaluating patients with primary brain tumours: is it useful? *J Neurol Neurosurg Psychiatry* 1995;58:250–252.

Padma MV, Said S, Jacobs M, et al. Prediction of pathology and survival by PDG PET in gliomas. *J Neurooncol* 2003;64:227–237.

Preul MC, Leblanc R, Caramanos Z, et al. Magnetic resonance spectroscopy guided brain tumor resection: differentiation between recurrent glioma and radiation change in two diagnostically difficult cases. *Can J Neurol Sci* 1998;25:13–22.

Rutz HP. Effects of corticosteroid use on treatment of solid tumours. *Lancet* 2002;360:1969–1970.

Saag KG, Emkey R, Schnitzer TJ, et al. Alendronate for the prevention and treatment of glucocorticoid-induced osteoporosis. *N Engl J Med* 1998;339:292–299.

Sherwood PR, Stommel M, Murman DL, Given CW, Given BA. Primary malignant brain tumor incidence and medicaid enrollment. *Neurology* 2004;62(10):1788–1793.

Soffer D, Pittaluga S, Feiner M, et al. Intracranial meningiomas following low-dose irradiation to the head. *J Neurosurg* 1983;59:1048–1053.

Tabori U, Beni-Adani L, Dvir R, et al. Risk of venous thromboembolism in pediatric patients with brain tumors. *Pediatr Blood Cancer* 2004;43(6):633–636.

Walker AE, Robins M, Weinfeld FD. Epidemiology of brain tumors: the National Survey of Intracranial Neoplasms. *Neurology* 1985;35:219–226.

Wen PY, Marks PW. Medical management of patients with brain tumors. *Curr Opin Oncol* 2002;14:299–307.

Zingale A, Musumeci S, Nicoletti G, et al. Thallium-201-SPECT and 99Tc-HM-PAO SPECT imaging to study functionally cerebral supratentorial neoplasms: the biological basis of the functional imaging interpretation. *J Neurosurg Sci* 1995;39:227–235.

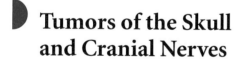

Chapter 54

Tumors of the Skull and Cranial Nerves

Lisa M. DeAngelis and Jeffrey N. Bruce

BENIGN TUMORS OF THE SKULL

Osteoma

An osteoma is a benign growth of mature, dense, cortical bone, arising from either the outer or inner table of the skull. The tumor often arises in a paranasal sinus but may occur in the cranial vault, mandible, or in a mastoid sinus. It has been associated with Gardner syndrome, an autosomal-dominant disorder that includes colonic polyps and soft-tissue fibromas.

In most cases, the tumor is asymptomatic because it is slow growing. In the paranasal sinuses, it may cause local pain, headache, or recurrent sinusitis. Proptosis may result from growth into the orbit, but dural erosion, CSF rhinorrhea or direct brain compression is rare (Fig. 54.1). Mucoceles may be associated with osteomas that obstruct the frontal sinuses. In the calvarium, tumors are hard but painless, localized masses without much intracranial extension.

Diagnosis is made on the characteristic radiographic appearance of a circumscribed homogeneous bone density best seen on CT, with bone windows. Symptomatic tumors are treated surgically, and reconstruction may be needed if the mass is extensive.

Chondroma

A chondroma is a rare, slowly growing, benign tumor arising from the cartilaginous portion of bones formed by enchondral ossification. The bones of the cranial vault are formed by membranous ossification, so chondromas are mainly limited to the skull base and paranasal sinuses. Lesions in the parasellar area or cerebellopontine angle often cause cranial nerve palsies. Radiographically, the tumors appear as lytic lesions, with sharp margins and erosion of surrounding bone. Stippled calcification within the lesion helps distinguish it from a metastasis or chordoma. Treatment of symptomatic lesions is radical resection, extending back to normal bone margins, to prevent recurrence. Progression to a malignant chondrosarcoma is rare.

Hemangioma

Hemangioma is a benign, vascular bone tumor comprising capillary or cavernous vascular channels. It occurs more commonly in the vertebral column than in the cranial vault. Skull hemangiomas vary from small, solitary lesions to huge lesions that receive blood from the scalp or meningeal vessels and that may cause headache by periosteal involvement. The cavernous sinus is a common location for intracranial hemangiomas, especially in middle-aged women. Radiographically, an hemangioma may show flow voids on MRI, suggesting a vascular lesion. Surgical resection is curative. Radiation therapy is sometimes recommended for incompletely resected or multiple tumors (particularly in the spine), but this treatment is of uncertain efficacy.

Dermoid and Epidermoid Tumors

Dermoid and epidermoid tumors occur in the cranial vault, paranasal sinuses, orbit, and petrous bone. They are among the most common benign skull lesions in

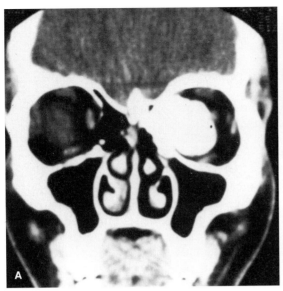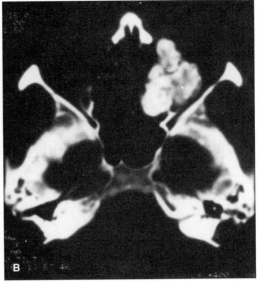

FIGURE 54.1. Orbital osteoma. Coronal **(A)** and axial **(B)** CT with bone windows show an osteoma involving the orbit. The tumor, which had caused proptosis, was successfully resected.

children. Radiographically, they produce rounded or ovoid lytic lesions with sharp, sclerotic margins that involve all three layers of bone. Treatment is rarely necessary.

Other Benign Tumors of the Skull

Aneurysmal bone cysts are lytic lesions composed of large vascular spaces separated by trabeculae of connective tissue and bone. They usually occur in the shaft of long bones, but occasionally involve the skull, causing painful local swelling. Ossifying and nonossifying fibromas, osteoid osteoma, and osteoblastoma are related tumors that contain varying degrees of fibrous tissue and mature bone. Giant-cell tumors are composed of giant cells interspersed with indistinct stromal cells. Some giant-cell tumors are benign but others are aggressive and malignant. As with most benign tumors of the skull, these are best viewed on CT with

bone windows, where they appear as well demarcated areas of bony erosion. MRI may help detail intracranial extension. Treatment is by surgical resection.

MALIGNANT TUMORS INVOLVING THE SKULL AND SKULL-BASE

Metastasis to the Skull-Base

As the cranial nerves exit through the bony foramina of the skull, they are vulnerable to entrapment and compression by osseous metastasis. Skull-base metastases most commonly arise from a prostate, breast, lung, head-and-neck cancer, or a lymphoma. Localized cranial or facial pain at the site of tumor invasion may be a symptom, but metastases to the skull-base are often painless. The cardinal sign is cranial neuropathy, which is typically sudden in onset (Table 54.1).

▶ **TABLE 54.1 Clinical Syndromes Associated with Metastases to the Base of the Skull**

Syndrome	Symptoms	Cranial Nerves Affected
Orbital	Proptosis, diplopia, facial numbness, pain	II, V_1
Parasellar	Unilateral frontal headache, diplopia, facial numbness	II, IV, VI, V_1
Petrous apex	Facial pain, diplopia	V, VI
Middle fossa or gasserian ganglion	Facial pain, facial numbness, diplopia	V_2, V_3, VI
Jugular foramen	Hoarseness, dysphagia, pain in pharynx	IX, X, XI
Occipital condyle or hypoglossal canal	Occipital pain, unilateral tongue weakness	XII

Diagnosis is usually easy with MRI, which may detect even small skull-base lesions. Occasionally a tumor may not be visualized, especially in the cavernous sinus. However, empiric treatment without radiographic documentation may be necessary if the clinical picture is clear, symptoms are progressive, and alternative diagnoses excluded. Biopsy is difficult and hazardous, even with stereotactic approaches.

The most important differential diagnosis is leptomeningeal metastasis, which may co-exist with skull-base metastases. Subarachnoid tumor often affects other sites as well as cranial nerves, especially those of spinal roots. Therefore, careful neurologic examination, enhanced MRI, and CSF examination are needed to exclude CNS disease.

Palliative radiotherapy is recommended with a total dose of at least 3,000 cGy given in 300 cGy fractions. Relief of symptoms is accomplished in almost all patients.

Extension of Malignant Tumors to the Skull-Base

Several malignant tumors involve the base of the skull by direct extension (Fig. 54.2). These include squamous cell carcinoma (nasal sinuses and temporal bone), adenoid cystic carcinoma (salivary glands), esthesioneuroblastoma (olfactory mucosa), and nasopharyngeal carcinoma.

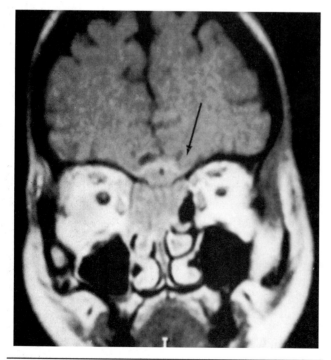

FIGURE 54.2. Esthesioneuroblastoma. Coronal MRI demonstrates an esthesioneuroblastoma in the ethmoid sinus with intradural extension *(arrow)*. This tumor arises from the olfactory mucosa.

These tumors cause pain and involve the cranial nerves. Erosion of the skull-base and the presence of a soft-tissue mass are seen on CT or MRI; and biopsy is diagnostic. Small tumors may sometimes be cured with wide surgical excision before they invade sensitive neural structures. However, most tumors are more extensive when detected, and despite treatment with radical excision and radiation therapy, the prognosis is often poor.

Primary Malignant Tumors of the Skull

Chondrosarcoma is a malignant cartilage tumor originating in the enchondral bones of the skull-base. It is most common in men during the fourth decade. It usually occurs in the parasellar areas, cerebellopontine angle, or paranasal sinuses. Chordoma is a tumor derived from primitive notochord tissue; it characteristically develops in the clivus or sacrum. Clival chordoma is locally invasive, and may extend into the middle fossa or brainstem. It recurs despite resection and radiotherapy, and may destroy surrounding tissues, but rarely metastasizes.

Osteogenic sarcoma (osteosarcoma) is the most commonly found malignant primary tumor of bone. It occurs most frequently in the second decade of life (Fig. 54.3) and may be associated with prior radiation, Paget disease, fibrous dysplasia, or chronic osteomyelitis.

Fibrous sarcoma is a soft-tissue tumor that arises from bone, periosteum, scalp, or dura. It is often accompanied by bony destruction, showing a regular but discrete lytic radiographic picture.

Treatment for all these malignant tumors is radical surgical resection with extensive margins, although complete excision is often impossible for lesions at the skull-base. Radiotherapy is usually given postoperatively. Charged-particle irradiation, such as proton beam or helium, is particularly effective for chordoma or chondrosarcoma of the skull-base and, if available, is the technique of choice. Despite aggressive therapy, recurrence is common.

Glomus Jugulare Tumors

Glomus jugulare tumors, or paragangliomas, arise from chromaffin cells in the region of the jugular bulb and invade the neighboring temporal or occipital bones. They are locally invasive, although metastasis is rare. They may extend into the middle ear and posterior fossa to cause tinnitus, audible bruit, deafness, and lower cranial neuropathies. Larger tumors may cause cerebellar and brainstem symptoms. Occasionally, they are discovered as small vascular masses protruding into the middle-ear cavity. The differential diagnosis includes neurinoma, cholesteatoma, chondrosarcoma, carcinoma, metastatic tumor, and meningioma. The tumors are visualized by MRI or CT with contrast, and MRA reveals their extensive vascularity.

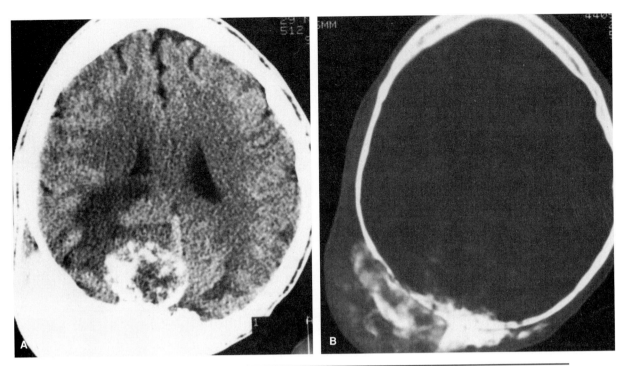

FIGURE 54.3. Osteosarcoma. A: Noncontrast axial CT shows a calcified mass within the medial right parietooccipital lobes with massive extracranial soft tissue swelling. **B:** Corresponding bone window shows thinning and erosive changes of calvarium with several large areas of calcification and ossification within extracranial soft tissues in the right parietooccipital region. These findings are classic for osteosarcoma.

Some paragangliomas secrete catecholamines, which may be ascertained by a 24-hour urinary assay. Catecholamine secretion must be blocked prior to surgery. Preoperative embolization is essential to decrease tumor vascularity and facilitate resection. Surgery offers the best chance of cure, or extended control, of the disease. Recurrence is common after partial resection, even if followed by radiotherapy. Radiosurgery may decrease tumor volume and provide local disease control.

NEOPLASTIC-LIKE LESIONS AFFECTING THE SKULL

Hyperostosis

Hyperostosis of nonneoplastic etiology may involve either the outer or inner table of the skull. Outer-table involvement is insignificant, except for disfigurement from extensive growth. Hyperostosis of the inner table is rarely large enough to compress intracranial contents. Hyperostosis of the inner table of the frontal bone (i.e., hyperostosis frontalis interna) is often asymptomatic and may be found coincidentally by CT or MRI; it is most common in middle-aged or elderly women. Attempts have been made to associate these changes in the skull with headache and other symptoms common at menopause, but this seems unlikely because hyperostosis rarely distorts intracranial structures and is so often asymptomatic.

Fibrous Dysplasia

Fibrous dysplasia is more common in men and rarely occurs after age 40 years (Fig. 54.4).

Localized involvement of the skull-base and sphenoid wing, particularly by the sclerotic variety, may become symptomatic by compressing nerves exiting the foramina at the skull-base. Nerve decompression is usually effective treatment because the process is rarely progressive. The etiology of fibrous dysplasia is unknown.

Paget Disease

Paget disease (osteitis deformans) is usually a multicentric disease that frequently involves the skull. Skull xrays show a characteristically diffuse, mottled, thickening of the cranial vault and often discrete lytic lesions. Symptoms result when bony lesions compromise the neural foramina of the skull-base. Pain, loss of vision, and hearing loss are the most common symptoms.

Mucocele

Obstruction of a nasal sinus ostium may result in an encapsulated, thick-fluid collection known as a mucocele (Fig. 54.5).

Mucoceles may erode through the base of the skull and result in intracranial compression. Surgery with reconstruction is the treatment of choice.

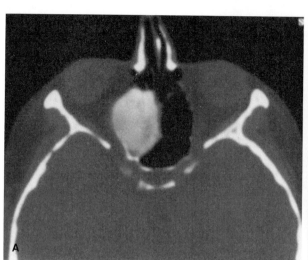

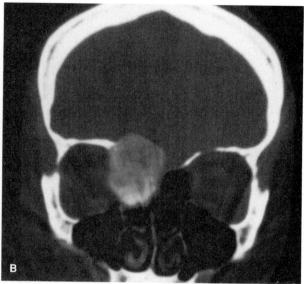

FIGURE 54.4. Fibrous dysplasia. Axial **(A)** and coronal **(B)** CT with bone windows demonstrates fibrous dysplasia of the orbit and ethmoid sinus. This lesion was cured by surgical resection.

Miscellaneous Diseases Involving the Skull

Systemic diseases may involve the skull. These include xanthomatosis (Hand-Schüller-Christian disease), multiple myeloma and plasmacytoma, and osteitis fibrosa cystica. The symptoms and signs of these conditions are considered in detail elsewhere.

Other disorders that simulate skull tumors include leptomeningeal cysts (e.g., growing skull fractures), sinus pericranii, metabolic diseases such as hyperparathyroidism, infections, sarcoidosis, and histiocytosis X. Neuroectodermal dysplasia commonly involves the cranial bones, as well.

NERVE-SHEATH TUMORS

There are four groups of nerve-sheath tumors: neurofibromas, schwannomas, malignant peripheral nerve-sheath tumors, and the rare benign perineurioma, not further discussed here. Nerve-sheath tumors may occur sporadically

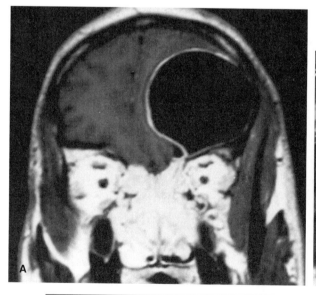

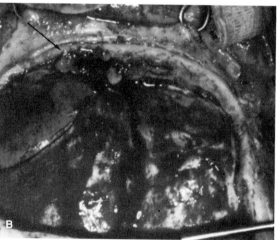

FIGURE 54.5. Frontal mucocele. A: Coronal MRI with contrast enhancement shows a large mucocele compressing the frontal lobe, with chronic inflammation of the nasal mucosa obstructing the nasal sinuses. **B:** Intraoperative photograph shows the mucocele before its resection and subsequent reconstruction of the cranial base defect. The frontal sinus contains inflammatory tissue *(arrow)*, which had caused obstruction of the sinus.

or as part of the genetic syndromes, neurofibromatosis-1 (NF-1) and neurofibromatosis-2 (NF-2). They are usually multiple when part of an hereditary syndrome and typically single in sporadic cases. They occur along any cranial or peripheral root or nerve. In the intracranial cavity the major nerve-sheath tumor is the vestibular schwannoma; occurring much less frequently is the trigeminal schwannoma. Neurofibromas and schwannomas are well encapsulated and usually may be completely resected, although the involved nerve is often sacrificed. The malignant, peripheral nerve-sheath tumor is highly aggressive and infiltrating, and may not be cured by excision.

Vestibular Schwannoma

Vestibular schwannoma (e.g., acoustic neuroma, acoustic neurofibroma) is a benign tumor arising from Schwann cells of the vestibular branch of the eighth cranial nerve, in more than 90% of cases; less than 10% arise from the cochlear branch of the eighth nerve. Vestibular schwannoma accounts for 5% to 10% of all intracranial tumors and is the most commonly occurring tumor of the cerebellopontine angle. The peak age of patients is between 40 and 60 years and the tumors occur twice as frequently in women as in men. Bilateral tumors occur in less than 5% of patients and are the defining characteristic of NF-2 (Fig. 54.6).

Vestibular schwannomas grow slowly, usually at a rate of less than 2 mm per year, but there is wide variability. They grow into the internal auditory meatus and the cerebellopontine angle, displacing adjacent cerebellum, pons, or the fifth and seventh cranial nerves. Because growth is slow, many tumors are large and even cystic before they become symptomatic. The growth rate may increase during pregnancy.

Macroscopically, the neuroma is usually yellowish, sometimes with areas of cystic degeneration. Microscopically, the tumors appear to be composed of mature Schwann cells with abundant cytoplasm. Mitoses and nuclear atypia do not indicate malignancy. Antoni-A areas show with densely packed tumor cells and Antoni-B areas have a looser pattern of stellate cells, with long irregular processes.

Increased clinical awareness and MRI have allowed earlier detection, so the clinical picture has changed in the last decade (Table 54.2). Progressive, unilateral hearing loss occurs in nearly all patients. Hearing loss is often preceded by difficulty with speech discrimination, especially when the patient is talking on the telephone. Tinnitus (70%) and unsteady gait (70%) are common. Patients sometimes note true vertigo, but typical Ménière syndrome is rare. Further growth may cause facial numbness (30%) or, less often, facial weakness, loss of taste, and otalgia. Trigeminal neuralgia is rare. Larger tumors grow into the cerebellopontine angle, causing headache, nausea, vomiting, diplopia, and ataxia, or symptoms of increased intracranial pres-

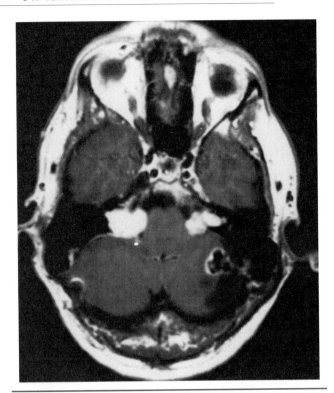

FIGURE 54.6. Bilateral vestibular schwannomas. T1-weighted axial MR scan after gadolinium administration shows enhancing masses within both cerebellopontine angles and internal auditory canals, most consistent with bilateral acoustic schwannomas. (Courtesy of Dr. S. Chan, Columbia University College of Physicians and Surgeons, New York, NY.)

sure and hydrocephalus. Other signs include nystagmus and cerebellar ataxia. This constellation of symptoms may occur with any mass in the cerebellopontine angle, including meningioma, cholesteatoma or trigeminal neuroma. However, only rarely do these other tumors begin with tinnitus or hearing dysfunction.

Gadolinium-enhanced MRI is the best technique to diagnose a vestibular schwannoma (Fig. 54.7). The tumor

▶ **TABLE 54.2 Symptoms and Signs in 76 Patients with Surgically Confirmed Acoustic Neuroma**

	%		%
Hearing loss	97	Decreased corneal reflex	37
Dysequilibrium	70	Nystagmus	34
Tinnitus	70	Facial hypesthesia	29
Headache	38	Abnormal eye movement	14
Facial numbness	33	Facial weakness	13
Nausea	13	Papilledema	12
Otalgia	11	Babinski sign	8
Diplopia	9		
Facial palsy	9		
Loss of taste	9		

From Harner SG, Laws ER Jr. Diagnosis of acoustic neuroma. *Neurosurgery* 1981;9:373–379; with permission.

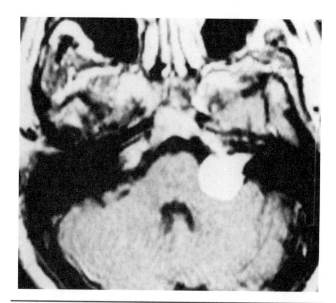

FIGURE 54.7. Vestibular schwannomas. T1-weighted axial MRI with gadolinium shows a vestibular schwannoma with flaring of the internal auditory canal.

image enhances vigorously and its origin in the internal auditory canal distinguishes a vestibular schwannoma from a meningioma (Fig. 54.8).

CT with contrast demonstrates nearly all tumors greater than 1.5 cm in diameter. Brainstem auditory-evoked poten-

tials, caloric stimulation with electronystagmography, and audiometry may all be used to evaluate hearing function, but none are as sensitive as MRI for this diagnosis.

The goals of treatment are to cure the tumor and preserve intact neurologic function. Surgery is highly effective, using current microsurgical techniques. Facial nerve function may be preserved in more than 95% of patients with small tumors (e.g., less than 2 cm) but in less than 50% of patients if the tumor is larger than 3 cm. If useful hearing was present preoperatively, it may be preserved in patients with tumors smaller than 2 cm in diameter, but is usually lost with resection of larger lesions. Complete resection cures these tumors, but because of the slow growth rate, subtotal resection or conservative treatment may be indicated in elderly patients with minimal symptoms. Radiosurgery is an excellent alternative to surgical resection of tumors of less than 3 cm in diameter. Local control is achieved in more than 90% of patients, and hearing has been preserved in a greater proportion of patients with this treatment than after standard surgery. However, delayed hearing loss, delayed facial weakness, and delayed trigeminal sensory loss have been reported in some patients as long as 2 to 3 years after radiosurgery. Radiosurgery avoids surgical morbidity, and for well selected patients, radiosurgery with an experienced surgeon at an experienced center is the treatment of choice.

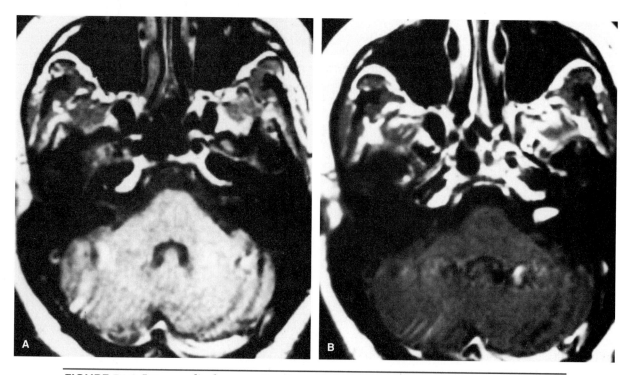

FIGURE 54.8. Intracanalicular acoustic schwannoma. A: T1-weighted axial MR image before contrast administration shows no definite mass within the internal auditory canals. **B:** With gadolinium, there is clear-cut contrast enhancement within the left internal auditory canal, most consistent with intracanalicular acoustic schwannoma. (Courtesy of Dr. S. Chan, Columbia University College of Physicians and Surgeons, New York, NY.)

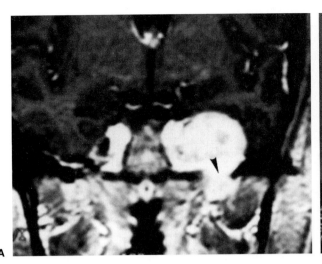
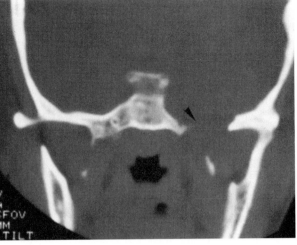

A
B

FIGURE 54.9. Trigeminal schwannoma. A: Coronal gadolinium-enhanced MRI shows a trigeminal schwannoma that has extended through the foramen ovale *(arrowhead).* **B:** Coronal CT with bone windows shows the widening of the foramen ovale by the tumor *(arrowhead).*

Trigeminal Schwannoma

Trigeminal schwannomas are rare and originate within the ganglion, nerve root, or one of the three divisions of the trigeminal nerve. Nearly all patients develop numbness and pain in the trigeminal distribution, and about 40% have some weakness in the muscles of mastication. True trigeminal neuralgia is exceptional. Extension of the tumor into the posterior fossa is associated with seventh and eighth nerve dysfunction and cerebellar and pyramidal tract signs. About 50% of these tumors are limited to the middle fossa, while 30% extend into the posterior fossa, and 20% are dumbbell-shaped and extend into both fossae. Diagnosis is established by MRI or CT with bone windows (Fig. 54.9).

The differential diagnosis includes meningioma, acoustic neuroma, epidermoid lesions, and primary bone tumors of the skull-base. Surgical resection is highly successful in providing cure or long-term control of the tumor. Radiosurgery may also afford disease control in some patients.

SUGGESTED READINGS

Al-Mefty O, Borba LAB. Skull base chordomas: a management challenge. *J Neurosurg* 1997;86:182–189.

Amaral L, Chiurciu M, Almeida JR, et al. MR imaging for evaluation of lesions of the cranial vault: a pictorial essay. *Arq Neuropsiquiatr* 2003;61:521–542.

Bederson JB, von Ammon K, Wichman WW, et al. Conservative treatment of patients with acoustic tumors. *Neurosurgery* 1991;28:646–651.

Bloch DC, Oghalai JS, Jackler RK, et al. The fate of the tumor remnant after less-than-complete acoustic neuroma resection. *Otolaryngol Head Neck Surg* 2004;130:104–112.

Capobianco DJ, Brazis PW, Rubino FA, Dalton JN. Occipital condyle syndrome. *Headache* 2002;42:142–146.

Casali PG, Messina A, Stacchiotti S, et al. Imatinib mesylate in chordoma. *Cancer* 2004 Nov 1;101(9):2086–2097.

Castro JR, Linstadt DE, Bahary JP, et al. Experience in charged particle irradiation of tumors of the skull base: 1977–1992. *Int J Radiat Oncol Biol Phys* 1994;29:647–655.

Chakrabarti I, Apuzzo ML, Giannota SL. Acoustic tumors: operation versus radiation—making sense of opposing viewpoints. Part I. Acoustic neuroma: decision making with all the tools. *Clin Neurosurg* 2003;50:293–312.

Crossley GH, Dismukes WE. Central nervous system epidermoid cyst: a probable etiology of Mollaret's meningitis. *Am J Med* 1990;89:805–806.

Day JD, Chen DA, Arriaga M. Translabyrinthine approach for acoustic neuroma. *Neurosurgery* 2004;54:391–395.

Glasscock ME, Hays JW, Minor LB, et al. Preservation of hearing in surgery for acoustic neuroma. *J Neurosurg* 1993;78:864–870.

Greenberg H, Deck MDF, Vikram B, et al. Metastases to the base of the skull: clinical findings in 43 cases. *Neurology* 1981;31:530–537.

Gwak HS, Hwang SK, Paek SH, et al. Long-term outcome of trigeminal neurinomas with modified classification focusing on petrous erosion. *Surg Neurol* 2003;60:39–48.

Igaki H, Tokuuye K, Okumura T, et al. Clinical results of proton beam therapy for skull base chordoma. *Int J Radiat Oncol Biol Phys* 2004 Nov 15;60(4):1120–1126.

Kondziolka D, Lunsford LD, Flickinger JC. Acoustic tumors: operation versus radiation—making sense of opposing viewpoints. Part II. Acoustic neuromas: sorting out management options. *Clin Neurosurg* 2003;50:313–328.

Kwan TL, Tang KW, Pak KK, Cheung JY. Screening for vestibular schwannoma by magnetic resonance imaging: analysis of 1821 patients. *Hong Kong Med J* 2004;10:38–43.

Landy HJ, Markoe AM, Wu X, et al. Safety and efficacy of tiered limited-Dose gamma knife stereotactic radiosurgery for unilateral acoustic neuroma. *Stereotact Funct Neurosurg* 2004 Oct 4;82(4):147–152.

Lim M, Gibbs IC, Adler JR Jr, et al. The efficacy of linear accelerator stereotactic radiosurgery in treating glomus jugulare tumors. *Technol Cancer Res Treat* 2003;2:261–265.

Loevner LA, Sonners AI. Imaging of neoplasms of the paranasal sinuses. *Magn Reson Imaging Clin N Am* 2002;10:467–493.

Maarouf M, Voges J, Landwehr P, et al. Stereotactic linear accelerator-based radiosurgery for the treatment of patients with glomus jugulare tumors. *Cancer* 2003;97:1093–1098.

McCormick PC, Bello JA, Post KD. Trigeminal schwannoma: surgical series of 14 cases with review of the literature. *J Neurosurg* 1988;69:850–860.

Naka T, Boltze C, Samii A, et al. Skull base and nonskull base chordomas: clinicopathologic and immunohistochemical study with special reference to nuclear pleomorphism and proliferative ability. *Cancer* 2003;98:1934–1941.

O'Connell JX, Renard LG, Liebsch NJ, et al. Base of skull chordoma: a correlative study of histological and clinical features of 62 cases. *Cancer* 1994;74:2261–2267.

Sanna M, Khrais T, Russo A, et al. Hearing preservation surgery in vestibular schwannoma: the hidden truth. *Ann Otol Rhinol Laryngol* 2004;113:156–163.

St Martin M, Levine SC. Chordomas of the skull base: manifestations and management. *Curr Opin Otolaryngol Head Neck Surg* 2003;11:324–327.

Storper IS, Glasscock ME 3rd, Jackson CG, et al. Management of nonacoustic cranial nerve neuroma. *Am J Otol* 1998;19:484–490.

Tos T, Caye-Thomasen P, Stangerup SE, et al. Long-term socio-economic impact of vestibular schwannoma for patients under observation and after surgery. *J Laryngol Otol* 2003;117:955–964.

Tos M, Stangerup SE, Caye-Thomasen P, et al. What is the real incidence of vestibular schwannoma? *Arch Otolaryngol Head Neck Surg* 2004;130:216–220.

Turowski B, Zanella FE. Interventional neuroradiology of the head and neck. *Neuroimaging Clin N Am* 2003;13:619–645.

Zhou LF, Mao Y, Chen L. Diagnosis and surgical treatment of cavernous sinus hemangiomas: an experience of 20 cases. *Surg Neurol* 2003;60:31–36.

Chapter 55

Tumors of the Meninges

Lisa M. DeAngelis and Jeffrey N. Bruce

MENINGIOMAS

Meningiomas originate from the arachnoid coverings of the brain, and they account for 20% of all intracranial tumors. When asymptomatic meningiomas are included, meningiomas may comprise 40% or more of intracranial neoplasms, 7% of all posterior fossa tumors, and 3% to 12% of cerebellopontine angle tumors. Most tumors are diagnosed in the sixth or seventh decades of life. Meningiomas are more common in women, and female:male ratios are 3:2 to 2:1; spinal meningiomas occur 10 times more often in women. Meningiomas are rare in children; childhood meningiomas are more common in boys, rarely have a dural attachment, are usually intraventricular or in the posterior fossa, and commonly show sarcomatous changes that render surgical resection difficult. In children, meningiomas are frequently associated with neurofibromatosis-2 (NF-2). Multiple meningiomas occur in 5% to 15% of patients, especially those with NF-2. More than 90% of tumors are intracranial and 10% are intra spinal.

Etiology

Radiotherapy is the only established risk factor for meningiomas. Low-dose radiation for tinea capitis and high-dose radiation for the treatment of other brain tumors (e.g. medulloblastoma) both increase the risk for a meningioma. Standard dental xrays are probably not a risk factor. High-dose radiotherapy is associated with a shorter latency (i.e., 5 to 10 years) to develop a meningioma, whereas low-dose irradiation may take several decades to cause a meningioma. Radiation-induced tumors tend to occur over the convexities, are more likely to be multiple and histologically malignant, and are more likely to recur. Head trauma has been suggested but not confirmed as a risk factor.

Endogenous and perhaps exogenous stimulation via hormones may play a role in etiology. Estrogen and progesterone have been implicated because of the higher rate of meningiomas in women, an apparent association with breast cancer, and the frequent increase in size of the tumor during pregnancy. Estrogen receptors are marginally present in meningiomas; binding occurs to a type-II receptor that does not have as much affinity for estrogen as the receptor found in breast carcinomas. In contrast, the progesterone receptor is expressed in about 80% of meningiomas occurring in women and 40% in men. Binding sites for progesterone are less common in aggressive meningiomas. The role for these receptors is unknown, but estrogen and progesterone inhibitors have been tried therapeutically, without success.

Viral infections, particularly SV-40, have been implicated in meningioma pathogenesis but the data are unconvincing. Meningiomas are thought to arise through a multistep process involving both oncogene activation and loss of tumor suppressor genes. Molecular genetic studies have shown several alterations, most commonly loss of 22q in 80% of all sporadic meningiomas. This results in deletion of the NF-2 tumor suppressor gene located at 22q11 and lack of the protein product, merlin. Almost all familial meningiomas occur with NF-2; likewise, patients with NF-2 are at increased risk for meningiomas as well as vestibular schwannomas, and both tumors are frequently multiple in these patients. Abnormalities have been observed in other chromosomes, suggesting that several oncogenes or tumor suppressor genes are involved in meningioma formation; chromosomal changes are more extensive in the atypical and anaplastic tumors.

Biology

With a paucity of animal models, most studies have used cell cultures. Several growth factor receptors, including those for epidermal growth factor, PDGF, insulin-like growth factors, transforming growth factor-β, and somato-statin, are overexpressed and may stimulate meningioma-cell proliferation. Meningiomas are highly vascular and they contain vascular endothelial growth factor (VEGF). PDGF and fibroblast growth factor are also angiogenic. The secretory and microcystic subtypes of meningioma contain particularly high levels of VEGF.

Pathology

Meningiomas are thought to arise from the mening-othelial-cap cells that are normally distributed through the arachnoid trabeculations. The highest concentration of meningothelial cells is found in the arachnoid villi at dural sinuses, cranial nerve foramina, middle cranial fossa, and the cribriform plate. Therefore, meningiomas are commonly found over the convexity, along the falx, and at the skull-base. On gross examination, the tumors are nodular and compress adjacent structures. Occasionally, they are distributed in sheath-like formations (e.g., meningioma *en plaque*), especially at the sphenoid ridge. The tumors are encapsulated and attach to the dura, which provides blood supply from the external-carotid circulation; there may be hyperostosis of the adjacent bone. Microscopically, meningiomas appear histologically benign. There is no characteristic cytologic marker, and diagnosis is based on the typical features: whorls of arachnoid cells surrounding a central hyaline material that eventually calcifies to form psammoma bodies. Cells are arranged in sheaths separated by connective tissue trabeculae.

A variety of meningioma subtypes includes meningotheliomatous (syncytial), fibrous, transitional, or psamommatous tumors, but this division has little prognostic value. There are only a few subtypes that have clinical meaning: clear-cell meningioma may behave more aggressively; the secretory meningioma secretes VEGF and is associated with extensive edema, and papillary or rhabdoid variants must be treated as malignant tumors. Grading meningiomas is important and the World Health Organization grading system classifies tumors as typical or benign, atypical, or malignant on the basis of cellularity, cytologic atypia, mitosis and necrosis. Malignant meningiomas are rare but aggressive; systemic metastases are seen in about half of these patients, and are usually found in bone, liver or lung. Benign meningiomas recur in about 7% to 20%, atypical tumors in 29% to 40%, and anaplastic tumors in 50% to 78%. Brain invasion may occur with all three histologic grades of meningioma. It connotes a greater likelihood of recurrence but does not upgrade the pathologic diagnosis to a malignant meningioma. However, a relatively high proliferation index (greater than 5%) predicts a poor outcome.

Clinical Manifestations

Meningiomas may be asymptomatic and found incidentally by MRI. When symptoms are present, they are determined by tumor location, and are usually caused by compression of underlying neural structures. Convexity and falx lesions may cause seizures, hemiparesis, or gait difficulties. Skull-base lesions cause diplopia, visual loss, or other cranial neuropathies. Tumor growth may be very slow, so that tumors may reach a large size, particularly in the subfrontal location, causing only subtle personality changes before coming to medical attention. Hydrocephalus may also result from intraventricular tumors or large lesions that cause secondary communicating hydrocephalus, likely from increased CSF protein.

Imaging

On CT, the tumor appears isointense or slightly hyperdense compared with brain tissue. The mass is smooth, sometimes lobulated, and may be calcified. Enhancement is strong and homogeneous. If calcification is dense, enhancement may not be evident. Margins are distinct, and the tumor is dural-based. Edema is variable. Hyperostosis is seen in 25% of patients.

On MRI, the tumor is isointense (65%) or hypointense (35%) compared with normal brain tissue on T1-weighted and T2-weighted imaging. Enhancement with gadolinium is intense and homogeneous (Fig. 55.1).

There may be a dural tail of attachment, which may also be seen in vestibular schwannomas or dural metastases. MRI clearly defines the relationship of the tumor to the surrounding neural structures and blood vessels.

Angiography typically shows a hypervascular mass. The venous phase may assess flow in the sinuses (e.g., compressed or thrombosed by tumor), internal jugular vein, and the vein of Labbé. Angiography is performed only if preoperative embolization is planned to reduce the risk of intraoperative bleeding. MR angiography and venography may outline the relationship of the tumor to critical vessels and has replaced standard angiography for preoperative definition of vascular structures.

Atypical radiographic features such as cysts, hemorrhage, and central necrosis, which may mimic gliomas, occur in about 15% of meningiomas. Malignant meningiomas commonly show bone destruction, necrosis, irregular enhancement, and extensive edema; brain invasion is occasionally seen radiographically on MRI. The differential diagnosis includes dural metastasis, other primary meningeal tumors (e.g., sarcoma), granuloma or aneurysm. Metastases are commonly associated with abundant surrounding edema and bone destruction; in contrast, hyperostosis and moderate edema suggest meningioma.

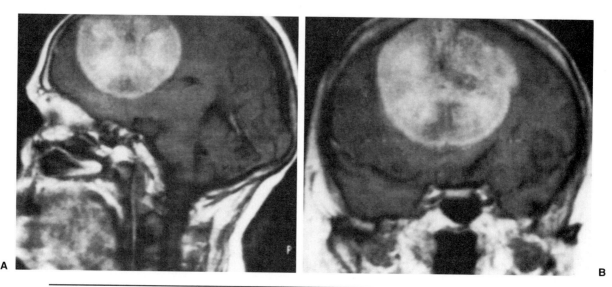

FIGURE 55.1. Parasagittal falx meningioma. Sagittal **(A)** and coronal **(B)** T1-weighted, contrast-enhanced MRIs show an enormous tumor arising from the falx.

Treatment

The diagnosis of a meningioma can usually be established by the patient's clinical presentation and imaging features. Once the diagnosis is clear, the most important decision is whether or not treatment is necessary. Many meningiomas are asymptomatic, present with seizures that are easily controlled, or involve structures that make resection impossible. Many of these tumors do not require immediate intervention and may be followed for years with no apparent growth. Among 41 patients with asymptomatic meningiomas who were followed, 66% had growth rates of less than 1 cm per year and tumor-doubling time ranged from 1.27 to 14.35 years. Therefore, many patients may be followed safely. If the patient has significant symptoms, such as a hemiparesis, or there is clear progression of a lesion being followed on serial images, then intervention is appropriate. The most important treatment is surgery.

Surgery

Complete excision may cure many meningiomas. Factors that influence surgery include tumor location, preoperative cranial-nerve deficits, vascularity, invasion of venous sinuses, and encasement of arteries. Partial resection is an option if total tumor removal will risk unacceptable loss of function.

New techniques include the use of computerized virtual reality, a three-dimensional reconstruction of the brain that assists the surgeon in planning the procedure; it is an invaluable technique in establishing the relationship of the tumor to brainstem, vessels, or cranial nerves. Intraoperative MRI shows real-time images during surgery.

Preoperative embolization is performed to decrease tumor vascularity, facilitate removal, and decrease blood loss. Embolization of the dural tail may decrease recurrence. The procedure is not done routinely because most surgical centers lack experienced embolization personnel or because small lesions may be removed without much blood loss.

In convexity meningiomas, the dura is resected to decrease the chances of recurrence. If venous sinuses are totally occluded or thrombosed, the involved segment may be resected without influencing flow. Meningiomas of the medial sphenoid wing, orbit, sagittal sinus, cerebral ventricles, cerebellopontine angle, optic nerve sheath, or clivus may be difficult to remove entirely. For cavernous sinus meningiomas, the risk of injury to cranial nerves or the internal carotid artery is a concern, and surgical cure is rarely feasible.

Surgery may reverse some neurologic signs, although cranial neuropathies are the most intractable to improvement. Operative morbidity ranges from 1% to 14%. The extent of resection is the most important factor in determining recurrence; age affects prognosis inversely. After complete resection, the recurrence rate for a low-grade meningioma is about 20% at 5 years and 25% at 10 years. If the tumor recurs, reresection should be considered. Overall, the 5-year survival rate for patients younger than 65 years is about 80% but is closer to 50% for those aged 65 years and older.

Radiation Therapy

Current indications for radiation include residual tumor after surgery in some patients, recurrent tumor, or atypical or malignant histology; some irradiate patients with

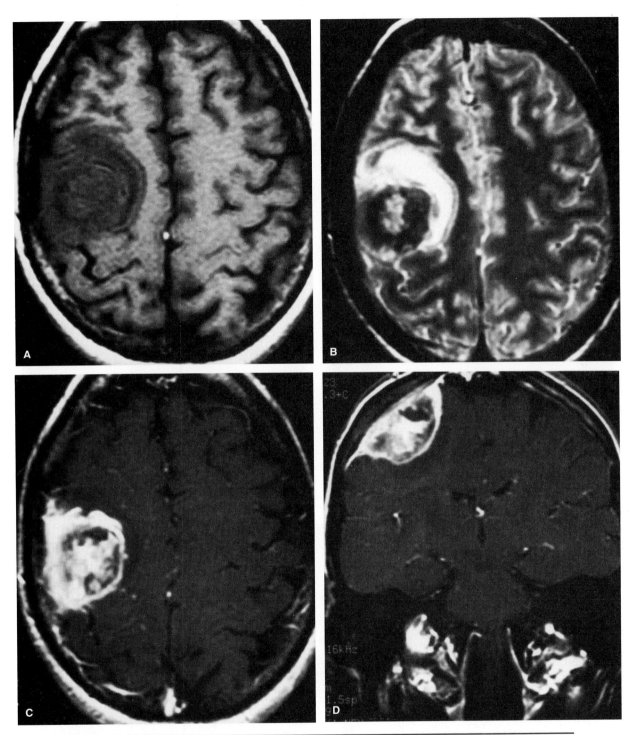

FIGURE 55.2. Convexity meningioma. T1-weighted **(A)** and proton-density **(B)** axial MRIs show a heterogeneous mass in the right parietal region. Surrounding edema is noted medial to the mass, and buckling of the cerebral white matter medially is also present. White matter buckling is considered a sign of extraaxial mass. T1-weighted axial **(C)** and coronal **(D)** MR images after gadolinium administration show marked enhancement within the lesion, with smaller nonenhancing areas correlating with known calcified portions. Coronal view shows dural enhancement and thickening both medially and laterally. The "dural tail" sign is most often seen with meningiomas but is occasionally seen with other tumors. (Courtesy of Dr. S. Chan, Columbia University College of Physicians and Surgeons, New York, NY.)

atypical meningiomas. Radiotherapy has been occasionally as primary therapy, if the tumor is inaccessible surgically, or there is a medical contraindication to surgery. Local control, defined as tumor regression or stability, is seen in 95% at 5 years and 92% at 10 and 15 years; it may be achieved with radiotherapy, with or without subtotal excision. The 10-year local control rate for combined, subtotal resection and radiation is 82%, compared to 18% for subtotal resection alone. Time to recurrence was 125 months for subtotal resection and irradiation, and 66 months for subtotal resection alone. For malignant meningiomas, overall 5-year survival after surgery and radiation is 28%. The recurrence rate for malignant meningiomas is 90% after subtotal resection and 41% after resection plus radiation. The long survival time of patients with benign meningiomas means radiation-induced secondary tumors are a concern in these patients.

The proton beam delivers heavy charged particles; it may be more effective for deep therapy and may minimize damage to normal tissue in brainstem meningiomas. Radiosurgery involves focused radiation given in one large dose, in an attempt to minimize damage to adjacent structures. Radiosurgery is done with a linear accelerator or gamma rays (i.e., gamma knife) as energy sources. It is limited to tumors of up to 3 cm in diameter, but is particularly useful in older or infirm patients who cannot undergo surgery. Excellent control may be achieved, 93.2% at 5 and 10 years, in patients treated with gamma-knife

radiosurgery alone. Another approach is stereotactic radiotherapy, in which radiation is given in multiple, small fractions for optic nerve tumors, cavernous sinus meningiomas, or tumors close to the brain stem, in an effort to avoid the ill effects of single large doses. With this method, 71% of patients survived for 5 years, and 72% of symptomatic patients showed neurologic improvement, particularly those with cavernous sinus meningiomas. If feasible, radiosurgery has become the preferred method for delivering radiotherapy to most patients with meningiomas.

Medical Treatment
Hormonal Treatment

Antiestrogen therapy has been ineffective. Mifepristone (RU-486), an anti-progesterone agent, has five times the affinity of progesterone, and crosses the blood–brain barrier. There are isolated reports of tumor control with this agent, but large clinical trials have been disappointing.

Chemotherapy

Chemotherapy is the last resort and may be indicated for patients with a recurrent meningioma who have had multiple resections and maximum irradiation. There are isolated patient reports of response to hydroxyurea, octreotide, and other agents, but clinical

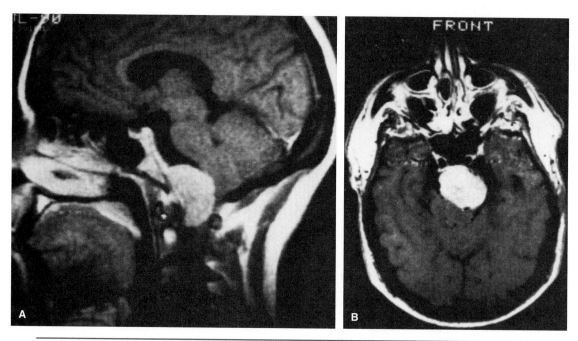

FIGURE 55.3. **Clivus meningioma.** Contrast-enhanced sagittal **(A)** and axial **(B)** T1-weighted MRI show a lower clivus–foramen magnum meningioma, with marked compression of the medulla.

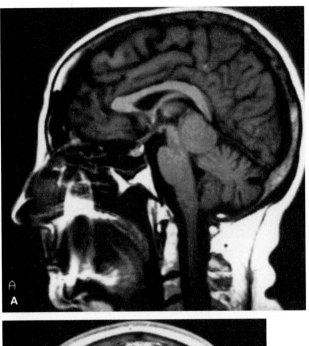

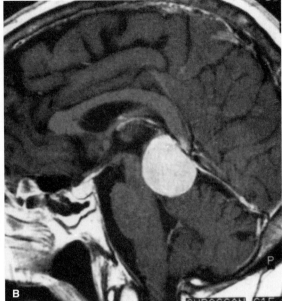

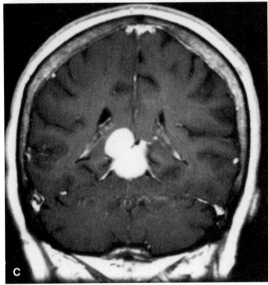

FIGURE 55.4. Tentorial meningioma. A: T1-weighted sagittal MRI shows a large infratentorial mass that is isointense to brain and causing anterior displacement of the midbrain and inferior displacement of the superior vermis. T1-weighted sagittal **(B)** and coronal **(C)** MRI after gadolinium administration demonstrate marked homogeneous enhancement of this mass, consistent with meningioma. The coronal view demonstrates the supratentorial component of the tumor. (Courtesy of Dr. S. Chan, Columbia University College of Physicians and Surgeons, New York, NY.)

trials of these drugs have been disappointing because meningioma is largely chemoresistant. Clinical trials in progress are evaluating growth factor and angiogenesis inhibitors.

Supportive Treatment

Corticosteroids are useful to manage peritumoral edema but should be tapered off as rapidly as possible because of side effects. As with other brain tumors, thromboembolism is a hazard, warranting the use of antiembolic stockings, subcutaneous heparin, and early postoperative mobilization. There is no role for prophylactic anticonvulsant drugs.

Specific Tumor Locations

Convexity meningiomas are the most amenable to surgical cure because wide dural margins may be achieved (Fig. 55.2). If the tumor invades an eloquent area of brain, complete resection may not be feasible.

Parasagittal meningiomas tend to involve the superior sagittal sinus (Fig. 55.1). If the sinus is patent, a subtotal resection may prevent occlusion and venous infarction. *Olfactory groove meningiomas* with invasion of the frontal sinuses usually require a bifrontal craniotomy. Piece-meal resection may preserve the optic nerves. *Tuberculum sellae meningiomas* usually cause visual loss, anosmia, headache, or hypopituitarism. Up to 42% of these patients have visual improvement after surgery, 30% do not change, and 28% become worse.

Meningiomas may occur within the sella region, originating from the diaphragma sellae. Radiographic evidence of sellar enlargement or calcification may help differentiate the tumor from a pituitary adenoma. *Optic-sheath meningiomas* are difficult to resect, and surgery is reserved for patients with visual loss. Radiation may slow the growth of tumors that do not yet affect vision, but there may be delayed radiation toxicity to the optic nerves or retina.

Cerebellopontine angle meningiomas cause hearing loss and facial pain or numbness. Meningiomas are the second most common tumor of the posterior fossa, after acoustic neuromas, and here they often have a characteristic *en plaque* shape. By the time eighth-nerve dysfunction is evident, the tumor is usually large; meningiomas in this location recur more often than vestibular schwannomas because they invade bone and cranial nerves. MRI usually differentiates a meningioma from a vestibular schwannoma because the latter begins within the internal auditory canal. Abnormalities on electronystagmogram, audiogram, and brainstem auditory evoked-potentials testing are less common than with vestibular schwannomas, but these tests are rarely needed with current imaging techniques. *Clivus meningiomas* grow from the dura anterior to the brainstem (Fig. 55.3). Lateral extension into the petrous bone may complicate surgery because cranial nerves are affected.

Tentorial meningiomas cause headache and cerebellar signs (Fig. 55.4). The major concern at surgery is the transverse sinus; if patent, it is not sacrificed.

Foramen magnum meningiomas cause pain, gait difficulties, and hand muscle wasting. They are intimately entwined with the cranial nerves, making a complete resection difficult to achieve.

Therapy for *cavernous sinus meningiomas* presents a challenge because resection may damage the cranial nerves. In young patients with no ocular muscle palsy, some recommend subtotal resection and radiotherapy. *Intraventricular meningiomas* arise from the arachnoid cells in the choroid plexus and account for 1% of all intracranial meningiomas. Surgical approaches include cortical or transcallosal incisions. The callosal approach is contraindicated in patients with a right homonymous hemianopsia because it may cause the syndrome of alexia without agraphia.

Sphenoid wing meningiomas include the *en plaque* meningiomas characterized by marked sphenoid hyperostosis, proptosis, visual loss, and third nerve palsy (Fig. 55.5). Surgery may include removal of the sphenoid wing itself. Some meningiomas here encase the middle cerebral artery.

Spinal meningiomas are most common in the thoracic region and account for 25% to 46% of primary spinal tu-

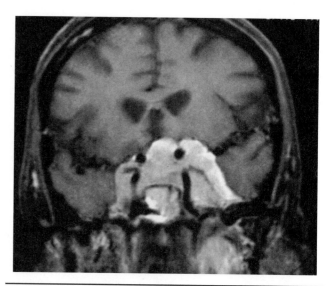

FIGURE 55.5. Sphenoid-ridge meningioma. Contrast-enhanced T1-weighted MR image shows an extensive sphenoid-ridge meningioma with bilateral cavernous sinus invasion and encasement of both carotid arteries.

mors. Clinical signs and symptoms include radicular pain (72%), paraparesis (76%), tendon reflex changes (77%), and sphincter dysfunction (37%). Symptoms usually antedate the diagnosis by months or years. Paraparesis or paraplegia is seen in 80% of patients with this diagnosis, but most patients (67%) are still walking. The most commonly seen pathology are the meningothelial and psammomatous tumors. Complete removal is possible for most patients, but tumors anterior to the spinal cord and those with calcification may be technically challenging to resect. After surgical resection, 82% of patients show improvement, 13% are stable, and 2% become worse. Postoperative mortality is low; pia-mater invasion or adhesion to the surface of the cord increases the risk.

HEMANGIOPERICYTOMAS

Hemangiopericytomas are meningeal tumors that are not derived from meningothelial cells but from the pericytes, smooth-muscle cells associated with small blood vessels. They were formerly considered angioblastic meningiomas, but ultrastructural studies revealed their distinct origin. They account for up to 7% of all meningeal tumors and are highly aggressive. Local recurrence develops in about 90% of patients after 15 years. Up to 65% of CNS hemangiopericytomas metastasize at 15 years, most often to bone, liver or lung. Surgical excision is the most common therapy, and postoperative irradiation to doses greater than 55 Gy have led to a significantly improved, relapse-free survival; however, recurrences are invariable despite irradiation, and survival is about 2 years after systemic metastases develop.

SUGGESTED READINGS

Bondy M, Ligon BL. Epidemiology and etiology of intracranial meningiomas: a review. *J Neurooncol* 1996;29:197–205.

Custer BS, Koepsell TD, Mueller BA. The association between breast carcinoma and meningioma in women. *Cancer* 2002;94:1626–1635.

Davis C. Surgical and non-surgical treatment of symptomatic intracranial meningiomas. *Br J Neurosurg* 1995;9:295–302.

De Monte F. Current management of meningiomas. *Oncology* 1995;9:83–91.

Flickinger JC, Kondziolka D, Maitz AH, Lunsford LD. Gamma knife radiosurgery of imaging-diagnosed intracranial meningioma. *Int J Radiat Oncol Biol Phys* 2003;56:801–806.

Ginsberg LE. Radiology of meningiomas. *J Neurooncol* 1996;29:229–238.

Hart MJ, Lillehei KO. Management of posterior cranial fossa meningiomas. *Ann Otol Rhinol Laryngol* 1995;104:105–116.

Hug EB, DeVries A, Thornton AF, et al. Management of atypical and malignant meningiomas: role of high-dose, 3D-conformal radiation therapy. *J Neurooncol* 2000;48:151–160.

Iwai Y, Yamanaka K, Morikawa T. Adjuvant gamma knife radiosurgery after meningioma resection. *J Clin Neurosci* 2004 Sep;11(7):715–718.

Jhawar BS, Fuchs CS, Colditz GA, Stampfer MJ. Sex steroid hormone exposures and risk for meningioma. *J Neurosurg* 2003;99:848–853.

Johannesen TB, Lien HH, Hole KH, Lote K. Radiological and clinical assessment of long-term brain tumour survivors after radiotherapy. *Radiother Oncol* 2003;69:169–176.

Kokubo M, Shibamoto Y, Takahashi JA, et al. Efficacy of conventional radiotherapy for recurrent meningioma. *J Neurooncol* 2000;48:51–55.

Kondziolka D, Nathoo N, Flickinger JC, et al. Long-term results after radiosurgery for benign intracranial tumors. *Neurosurgery* 2003;53:815–821.

Longstreth WT Jr, Phillips LE, Drangsholt M, et al. Dental X-rays and the risk of intracranial meningioma. *Cancer* 2004;100:1026–1034.

Lusis E, Gutmann DH. Meningioma: an update, *Curr Opin Neurol* 2004;17:687–692.

Maxwell M, Shih SD, Galanopoulos T, et al. Familial meningioma: analysis of expression of neurofibromatosis 2 protein Merlin. Report of two cases. *J Neurosurg* 1998;88:562–569.

McMullen KP, Stieber VW. Meningioma: current treatment options and future directions. *Curr Treat Options Oncol* 2004 Dec;5(6):499–509.

Mendenhall WM, Morris CG, Amdur RJ, et al. Radiotherapy alone or after subtotal resection for benign skull-base meningiomas. *Cancer* 2003;98:1473–1482.

Nakamura M, Roser F, Michel J, et al. The natural history of incidental meningiomas. *Neurosurgery* 2003;53:62–70.

Nappi O, Ritter JH, Pettinato G, Wick MR. Hemangiopericytoma: histopathological pattern or clinicopathologic entity? *Semin Diagn Pathol* 1995;12:221–232.

Nunes F, MacCollin M. Neurofibromatosis 2 in the pediatric population. *J Child Neurol* 2003;18:718–724.

Perry A, Chicoine MR, Filiput E, et al. Clinicopathologic assessment and grading of embolized meningiomas. *Cancer* 2001;92:701–711.

Rochat P, Johannesen HH, Gjerris F. Long-term follow-up of children with meningiomas in Denmark 1935 to 1984. *J Neurosurg* 2004;100:179–182.

Roux FX, Nataf FM, Borne G, et al. Intraspinal meningiomas: review of 54 cases with discussion of poor prognostic factors and modern therapeutic management. *Surg Neurol* 1996;46:458–463.

Sadetzki S, Flint-Richter P, Ben-Tal T, Nass D. Radiation-induced meningioma: a descriptive study of 253 cases. *J Neurosurg* 2002;97:1078–1082.

Takahashi JA, Ueba T, Hashimoto N, et al. The combination of mitotic and Ki-67 indices as a useful method for predicting short-term recurrence of meningiomas. *Surg Neurol* 2004;61:149–155.

Tucha O, Smely C, Preier M, et al. Preoperative and postoperative cognitive functioning in patients with frontal meningiomas. *J Neurosurg* 2003;98:21–31.

Chapter 56

Gliomas

Lisa M. DeAngelis

EPIDEMIOLOGY

Gliomas are the most commonly occurring primary brain tumors, accounting for about half of all symptomatic intracranial neoplasms. The incidence increases with advancing age, reaching a peak in the eighth and ninth decades. Several but not all studies have suggested that the incidence of gliomas is increasing, particularly among the elderly; however, improved ascertainment probably accounts for the apparent increase. More accurate diagnosis with the easy availability of noninvasive neuroimaging has created more willingness to evaluate neurologic symptoms in the elderly. In addition, better control of more common conditions such as heart disease allows patients to live long enough to develop less common illnesses, such as brain tumors. The male to female ratio is about 1:1.6 for all age groups, and the overall incidence of gliomas is higher in Caucasians than in African Americans.

There are no known environmental factors that lead to a brain tumor. There has been concern that cell phones may contribute to gliomagenesis, but well-designed epidemiologic studies failed to identify any increased risk associated with cell phone use. There are no behavioral or life-style choices, such as smoking, that influence the development of a glioma. Immunosuppression, such as HIV-1 infection, may slightly increase the risk of gliomas, but this is not well-established.

The only clear risk factor is ionizing radiation. Low-dose irradiation, such as was used to treat fungal infections of the scalp, or higher dose radiation, such as that used to treat a prior malignancy (e.g., medulloblastoma), may increase the risk of a glioma. The latency may be as long as 10 or more years. Radiation-induced gliomas are often malignant.

PATHOLOGY

Gliomas are believed to originate from glial cells or their stem-cell precursors and include astrocytoma, oligodendroglioma and ependymoma. All of these tumors exist along a spectrum of malignancy based on their histologic grade. The World Health Organization classification is universally accepted as the standard. It is based on the

▶ TABLE 56.1 WHO* Classification of Glial Tumors

Grade	WHO Designation	Criteria for Tumor Type	Criteria for Grade
I	Pilocytic astrocytoma	Bipolar and multipolar astrocytes, long processes, microcysts	Piloid cells, Rosenthal fibers, eosinophilic granular bodies, low cellularity
II	Astrocytoma	Well-differentiated fibrillary or neoplastic astrocytes	Nuclear atypia, increased cellularity
III	Anaplastic astrocytoma		Nuclear atypia and mitosis
IV	Glioblastoma multiforme		Nuclear atypia, mitoses plus endothelial proliferation and/or necrosis
II	Oligodendroglioma	Rounded tumor cells "fried egg" appearance, network of branching capillaries	Nuclear atypia, occasional mitosis
III	Anaplastic oligodendroglioma		Nuclear atypia, mitoses, microvascular proliferation, necrosis
II	Ependymoma	Perivascular pseudorosettes	Well-delineated, moderately cellular and ependymal rosettes
III	Anaplastic ependymoma		Mitoses, microvascular proliferation, pseudopalisading necrosis

*World Health Organization

presence or absence of increased cellularity, nuclear atypia, mitosis, endothelial proliferation and necrosis (Table 56.1).

Astrocytomas are assigned to one of four grades; each grade is associated with a clinically important prognosis. The pilocytic astrocytoma (Grade I) is a unique entity that occurs primarily in children or young adults, and carries an unusually excellent prognosis. It is a focal astrocytoma that may be associated with neurofibromatosis type 1 (NF-1). It will not be considered further here. The diffuse or fibrillary astrocytoma (Grade II) is considered a low-grade tumor ("benign"), but it typically transforms over time to a Grade III or even Grade IV astrocytoma, at which point it has the prognosis of these higher grade (malignant) neoplasms. The low-grade astrocytoma is not a benign neoplasm because of its latent potential for malignant transformation and the anatomic complexity that leads to the inability to fully excise it. The anaplastic astrocytoma (Grade III) is a malignant tumor, but it carries a modestly better prognosis than the most malignant astrocytoma, the glioblastoma multiforme (Grade IV). Although called malignant, glioma almost never metastasizes outside of the CNS.

Oligodendrogliomas and ependymomas are divided into only two grades, the low-grade and the anaplastic variant. Anaplastic oligodendrogliomas carry a worse prognosis than a lower grade tumor, but there is controversy regarding whether or not an anaplastic ependymoma confers a significantly worse prognosis than a low-grade ependymoma.

A substantial proportion of glial tumors elude easy histologic classification for several reasons: First, many tumors have features that are both astrocytic and oligodendroglial. These mixed gliomas are common, particularly among lower grade tumors. The neuropathologist frequently has difficulty assigning these tumors to one category or another and often makes the designation of a mixed glioma or an oligoastrocytoma. While ependymal features are occasionally seen in some astrocytic tumors, they are uncommon, and usually do not cause classification difficulties. Second, foci of high-grade glioma may occur within a low-grade neoplasm. A tumor is always classified according to the highest grade apparent on the specimen. However, if the high-grade component is not part of the sample sent to the neuropathologist, then the tumor will be undergraded, and the choice of treatment potentially incorrect. The challenges associated with classification and grading are amplified by the small specimens frequently received by the pathologist. When a complete excision of a glioma is performed, there is ample material for the pathologist to review and accurately classify the neoplasm. However, when a needle biopsy is performed and only a tiny portion of the tumor is sampled, different histologic features as well as the grade of malignancy may be missed.

The pathologist will occasionally use an index that labels the cells actively in the cell cycle, such as the Ki-67 antigen or MIB-1 index, to help classify the malignant potential of the tumor. In general, a labeling index that exceeds 5% is associated with a worse prognosis; however, the spectrum of labeling indices for either a low- or high-grade tumor is wide, and it is difficult to interpret this prognostically for an individual patient. It may be feasible to classify tumors by molecular analysis. For instance, about 40% of glioblastomas have a mutated version of the epidermal growth factor receptor (EGFR) vIII that, when present, defines the neoplasm as a glioblastoma. Loss of heterozygosity of chromosomes 1p and 19q is associated with oligodendroglial neoplasms, and identifies oligodendroglial tumors that show a better response to treatment and a better prognosis than more aggressive tumors. It seems likely that classification of primary brain tumors will be based on genetic abnormalities to distinguish less aggressive from more aggressive neoplasms.

One of the most striking features of gliomas (except the pilocytic astrocytoma) is their highly infiltrative nature. Although the mass may seem quite discrete on neuroimaging, it has long been established, pathologically, that infiltrating tumor cells may extend for many centimeters beyond the area of bulk disease. This capacity to infiltrate the brain widely is one of the features that make gliomas so difficult to treat. Metalloproteinases are overexpressed in gliomas and are thought to facilitate tumor-cell infiltration. In high-grade tumors the area of bulk disease has a distorted blood-brain barrier, but the infiltrating margin of tumor has tumor cells that penetrate normal brain tissue and reside behind an intact blood-brain barrier.

The disrupted biology that leads to a malignant glioma is an area of intense investigation. Investigators recognize two pathways that lead to histologically identical glioblastomas: the primary or *de novo* glioblastoma, and the secondary glioblastoma that arises from a preexisting low-grade tumor. The *de novo* glioblastoma usually develops in older people and has a short duration of symptoms. The secondary glioblastoma develops in younger people, who may have a 3- to 10-year history of a low-grade lesion. The genetic alterations that characterize the two different glioblastomas have been delineated; however, the histologic appearance of these lesions and their prognosis, once they become glioblastomas, is identical. The primary glioblastoma typically has overexpression, mutation or amplification of the epidermal growth factor receptor, deletion of p16 and loss of heterozygosity on 10q, or loss of the tumor suppressor gene, PTEN. The secondary glioblastoma is characterized by a sequential accumulation of genetic abnormalities: the low-grade astrocytoma has p53 mutations and overactivity of the platelet-derived growth factor (PDGF) pathway; acquisition of retinoblastoma gene alterations or loss of heterozygosity of 19q leads

to an anaplastic astrocytoma; and subsequent loss of PTEN and loss of another tumor-suppressor gene, DCC (deleted in colorectal cancer), lead to secondary glioblastoma multiforme formation. To date, recognition of these different pathways has not segregated the glioblastoma into two clinically different groups. However, it clearly indicates that different mutations may produce an identically appearing neoplasm. This strongly suggests that genetic characterization of individual tumors may be necessary before therapy directed to these genetic impairments is useful.

Many drugs are being developed that target the downstream effects of these genetic abnormalities, some of which are found in many types of cancer. Activation of EGFR, PDGFR and loss of PTEN all result in overactivity of the Ras pathway, and an increase in activity of the kinase, Akt, whose downstream effects control the cell cycle and apoptotic pathways. In addition, the vascular proliferation characteristic of glioblastomas is driven by increased expression of vascular endothelial growth factor (VEGF). VEGF may also contribute to the development of edema surrounding high-grade brain tumors. VEGF is a major target of antiangiogenic drugs.

FAMILIAL CONDITIONS

Most gliomas occur sporadically but about 5% are familial, not all belonging to recognized syndromes. The identifiable familial syndromes are characterized by germ-line loss of a tumor-suppressor gene, which predisposes to the development of brain tumors as well as other malignancies. The most common syndromes are detailed below.

Li Fraumeni Syndrome

The Li Fraumeni syndrome is defined by a germ-line mutation of *p53*, a gene that mediates cell repair and apoptosis. It is an autosomal-dominant disorder; about 10% of affected patients develop gliomas, often in young adulthood. Other cancers common in the Li Fraumeni syndrome are breast cancer, bone or soft tissue sarcomas, and leukemia. In addition to gliomas, medulloblastomas and primitive neuroectodermal tumors, choroid plexus tumors, ependymomas and schwannomas have all been reported. There is often a strong family history of similar malignancies in first-degree relatives.

Neurofibromatosis Type 1

Neurofibromatosis type 1 (NF-1) is an autosomal-dominant disorder caused by an abnormality of the NF-1 gene on chromosome 17q11.2. This is one of the most common genetic syndromes that predispose to cancer and 30% to 50% of patients represent new mutations, so a family history may be absent. The NF-1 gene encodes for neurofibromin, a Ras GTPase that converts the Ras protein from the active to the inactive form. Loss of neurofibromin results in unrestrained cell proliferation and tumor development. The most common tumors of NF-1 are neurofibromas and brain tumors such as pilocytic astrocytomas typically occurring in the optic nerve, hypothalamus or brainstem of children. There is also an increased frequency of diffuse astrocytomas and glioblastomas, but these are much less common.

Neurofibromatosis Type 2

Neurofibromatosis type 2 (NF-2) is an autosomal-dominant disorder characterized by bilateral vestibular schwannomas, meningiomas and gliomas. The incidence is much less than that of NF-1, but new mutations account for about half of all tumor patients. The NF-2 gene has been mapped to chromosome 22 q11 and the gene product is called merlin. Gliomas of all grades may be seen with increased incidence in patients with NF-2.

Turcot Syndrome

Turcot syndrome refers to several disorders that all include multiple colorectal tumors, other polyps or carcinomas, and CNS neuroepithelial tumors, including all grades of astrocytomas, medulloblastomas and ependymomas. Several genetic abnormalities have been identified. Patients with familial adenomatosis-polyposis syndrome have germ-line mutations in the APC gene located on chromosome 5q21. Other patients have mutations similar to those found in patients with hereditary nonpolyposis-colorectal cancer, in which there are mutations of genes that control DNA repair mechanisms. These include mutations of hMLH-1 or hPMS-2 genes. Both encode proteins responsible for DNA mismatch repair.

CLINICAL FEATURES

Symptoms and signs of intrinsic brain tumors are similar regardless of type or grade of the lesion. Generalized symptoms include headache, nausea, vomiting, lethargy and personality or behavioral changes. Focal symptoms and signs include seizures, hemiparesis, language difficulties, and ataxia, or cranial neuropathies for tumors in the posterior fossa. Many patients have what seem to be generalized seizures, but in patients with brain tumors, all seizures are focal, even if the focal onset is not appreciated clinically.

Although the spectrum of symptoms is similar in all grades of glial tumors, the frequency of different symptoms varies depending on whether the lesion is low- or high-grade. For example, low-grade gliomas start with seizures in more than 80% of patients and most of them have no other abnormality on neurologic examination; about 25% of patients with glioblastoma have seizures at onset but most also have prominent lateralizing sensory or motor symptoms.

IMAGING

Specific neuroimaging characteristics help define the type of glial tumor. Low grade gliomas, either astrocytic or oligodendroglial, are typically nonenhancing and are best appreciated on T2 or FLAIR MRI (Fig. 56.1). They are

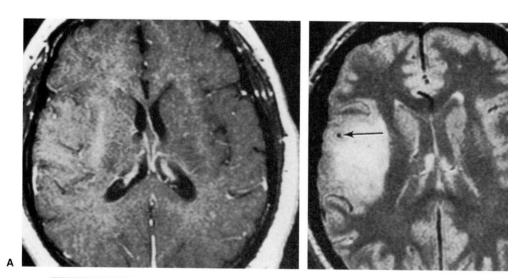

FIGURE 56.1. Low-grade infiltrative astrocytoma. Contrast-enhanced T1-weighted **(A)** and T2-weighted **(B)** MRIs show a right frontal low-grade infiltrative astrocytoma. There is faint contrast enhancement. The site of the stereotactic biopsy is visible *(arrow)*. The lesion is unchanged for 3 years without treatment.

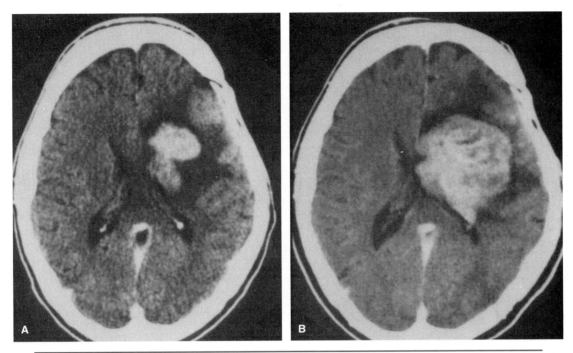

FIGURE 56.2. Glioblastoma. A: and B: Contrast-enhanced CT in a patient with an extremely rapidly recurring left frontotemporal glioblastoma shows a dramatic increase in tumor size in the intervening 8 weeks between the two scans.

often large, extensively infiltrative lesions, and typically involve the frontal or temporal lobes. Despite their large size on MRI, they are rarely associated with neurologic deficits and patients usually exhibit normal abilities and patterns. Malignant gliomas are typically characterized by large contrast enhancing lesions with surrounding edema (Fig. 56.2).

The development of the uptake of contrast enhancement in a previously nonenhancing low-grade lesion is often an indicator of malignant transformation. However, approximately 30% of nonenhancing lesions may harbor features of an anaplastic glioma, making accurate radiographic diagnosis difficult. Fluorodeoxyglucose PET imaging or ^{11}C-methionine PET may indicate foci of higher grade within a predominantly low-grade tumor. ^{11}C-methionine PET may also be able to differentiate astrocytic from oligodendroglial tumors. Magnetic resonance spectroscopy (MRS) is being explored as a potential means of identifying foci of high-grade disease.

THERAPY OF ANAPLASTIC ASTROCYTOMA AND GLIOBLASTOMA MULTIFORME

All three of the major modalities of cancer treatment, surgery, radiation therapy, and chemotherapy, are used for the treatment of malignant astrocytomas. The approach is identical for both the anaplastic astrocytoma and glioblas-

toma, but the prognosis differs. With identical treatment, the median survival time for patients with an anaplastic astrocytoma is about 3 years, with some patients surviving a decade or longer. However, overall survival is only about 1 year for patients with glioblastoma multiforme, and 3-year survivors are rare.

Treatment may affect function and outcome, but pretreatment prognostic factors give greater insight to projected outcome than most therapies. The importance of both patient-related and tumor-related prognostic factors has been confirmed in every large study of gliomas. Age is the most powerful prognostic factor. Young adults have significantly longer survival than older patients, even when they receive identical therapy. In particular, patients over the age of 65 years have a poor prognosis. Performance status also exerts a powerful effect. Patients in good clinical condition survive longer than those in poor condition. Patients with anaplastic astrocytomas fare better than those with glioblastoma multiforme. In addition, patients with oligodendroglial tumors have a better outcome than those with a comparably graded astrocytoma. Patients with long histories of symptoms, such as seizures, live longer than those with short histories of symptoms; this likely points to preexisting low-grade gliomas.

The fact that these prognostic factors that are immutable for a given patient are so powerful speaks to the poor efficacy of existing therapy. Surgery, radiotherapy and chemotherapy may help control disease for a time, but tumor recurs in almost every patient, typically at the original site. Thus, current treatment leaves residual viable tumor, even when none is visible on imaging studies. Therefore, there is an acute need for new and better treatments and this is an area of active research.

Surgery

Aggressive surgical resection with complete removal of all bulky disease is the surgical goal for the treatment of malignant gliomas. There has never been a randomized, prospective trial comparing biopsy with gross total excision, but there are substantial retrospective data that support the therapeutic and survival benefits of debulking surgical procedures. For most patients, gross total excision substantially improves neurologic function, reduces surrounding edema and with it, concomitant dependence on corticosteroids, and prolongs survival. Even when tumors involve eloquent areas of brain, presurgical evaluation with functional MRI (fMRI) and intraoperative mapping often enable a skilled neurosurgeon to perform a complete excision of these lesions. Gross total excision also provides the pathologist with extensive material to make an accurate diagnosis.

The extent of surgical resection should be measured by a postoperative MRI, obtained within 72 hours of surgery, because the intraoperative assessment of tumor removal is often inaccurate. For imaging performed within this time frame, any residual contrast enhancement seen at the surgical site represents residual disease, whereas such enhancement seen from a few days to even months after surgery may represent postoperative change. Tumors that are multifocal, bilateral, or involve critical structures, such as the thalamus, may not be removed surgically. In these patients, stereotactic biopsy is performed for tissue diagnosis.

Radiotherapy

Radiotherapy is the most important nonsurgical treatment for high-grade gliomas. Focal radiotherapy is administered to a total dose of about 60 Gy, delivered in 30 to 33 fractions over 6 to 7 weeks. The field is defined by the area of involvement seen on MRI, as well as a 1.5-cm to 2-cm margin to encompass the region most heavily infiltrated by microscopic disease. Modern techniques using 3D-conformal radiotherapy and more recently intensity modulated radiotherapy (IMRT) allow a focal port to be delivered to the exact configuration of the tumor, thus minimizing the amount of normal brain tissue included in the radiotherapy port.

Numerous efforts have been devoted to enhancing the beneficial effect of radiotherapy in patients with malignant gliomas. A series of radiosensitizers such as metronidazole, lonidamine, halogenated pyrimidine analogs, and most recently, motexafin gadolinium, have failed to enhance disease control. A recent study using RSR-13, an allosteric modifier of hemoglobin that improves oxygenation within anaerobic regions of tumor thus, enhancing the efficacy of radiotherapy, has shown promise in phase II studies as an effective radiation sensitizer. It is currently being evaluated in a phase III trial.

Despite high-dose focal radiotherapy, more than 80% of malignant gliomas recur at their original site, suggesting substantial local disease remains after effective therapy. Numerous efforts to increase the dose of radiotherapy only within the region of tumor to protect normal brain from radiation toxicity have been tried. These include brachytherapy with focal implantation of temporary radioactive seeds, stereotactic radiosurgery with the delivery of a focal boost of high-dose radiotherapy, hyperthermia to enhance radiotherapy, hyperfractionation to increase the dose to a total of 80 Gy, and accelerated fractionation to increase the daily fraction and shorten the course of radiotherapy. All have failed to prolong survival or improve disease control in patients with malignant astrocytomas. At this point, there is no role for any of these approaches in the standard treatment of patients with malignant gliomas unless the patients are enrolled in clinical trials.

Recent data have demonstrated that elderly patients with malignant gliomas, who have particularly poor prognoses, have a similar survival and outcome when shorter courses of radiotherapy are used (e.g., 300 cGy in ten fractions). Shorter courses of radiotherapy are advantageous in patients whose median survival is only about 6 months because they afford equivalent palliation with less treatment time. Studies also show that treatment with temozolomide, alone, offers an equivalent alternative to radiotherapy for elderly patients, and is very well tolerated. Either approach is a considerable advance for patients for whom 6 to 7 weeks of radiotherapy may represent half of their remaining lifespans.

Chemotherapy

Adjuvant chemotherapy with a nitrosourea has never been shown in a randomized prospective study to prolong median survival in patients with high-grade gliomas. However, in many phase III trials, there is a suggestion that 20% of such patients appear to have prolonged survival with the addition of chemotherapy. As only a small proportion of patients benefit, the median survival of the population as a whole is not affected. This small benefit of adjuvant chemotherapy reaches statistical significance when a meta-analysis of multiple phase III trials is performed. Two such analyses demonstrate that adjuvant chemotherapy significantly prolongs survival in patients with malignant gliomas.

The standard drug tested in all of these trials was a nitrosourea, usually carmustine. However, many physicians now use temozolomide instead of the nitrosoureas.

Temozolomide is an alkylating agent given orally. It has established efficacy in the treatment of patients with recurrent, malignant gliomas and has become the standard in that situation. As it is so easily administered, is well tolerated by patients, and has no organ toxicity other than mild myelosuppression, it is often used as an adjuvant drug even though it is not approved for this use by the FDA. In a phase II trial, temozolomide administered concurrently during radiotherapy, and followed by adjuvant temozolomide, appeared to prolong survival in patients with newly diagnosed glioblastomas. A large, randomized phase III study established the efficacy of temozolomide given during radiation and followed by adjuvant temozolomide. However, the control arm in that study consisted of patients treated with radiotherapy alone and no chemotherapy. Unfortunately, this study does not answer the question of whether the concurrent temozolomide during radiotherapy adds to the improved outcome over what is seen with adjuvant temozolomide alone.

Recurrent Malignant Astrocytoma

At recurrence, patients may be eligible for reresection and additional chemotherapy. If not used as part of therapy for the initial diagnosis, the first conventional drug option is temozolomide followed by the nitrosoureas. Other agents that have activity against malignant astrocytomas include etoposide, procarbazine, carboplatin, and thalidomide, but the proportion of responders is small. Optimally, these patients should be enrolled in clinical trials of new agents.

Prognosis

Despite recent advances, the median survival for patients with malignant gliomas has not changed significantly. Patients with glioblastomas have a median survival of 1 year and those with anaplastic astrocytomas survive 3 years. Recurrence is almost always local and patients rapidly become refractory to therapy. However, a subset of patients may do well. For example, young patients with completely resected anaplastic astrocytomas may survive for 10 years or longer, without recurrence.

THERAPY OF LOW-GRADE ASTROCYTOMA

The treatment of low-grade astrocytoma is both complicated and controversial. Treatment involves surgery and radiotherapy, but the main issue is the timing. Optimally, treatment of a low-grade glioma would: (1) ameliorate current symptoms, and (2) delay or prevent transformation to a high-grade neoplasm. To date, evidence for true benefit from immediate intervention is lacking. This is one of the most challenging aspects of managing patients with low-grade gliomas, who often find it difficult to accept a recommendation of watchful waiting even when it is the most appropriate course of action. This does seem to run counter to the understanding the general public has of the benefits of early detection of cancer and rapid treatment. However, at the present time current therapies are not sufficiently potent to prevent malignant transformation, and thereby to improve patient survival.

Surgery

There are no prospective, randomized studies that assess the efficacy of surgery in patients with low-grade gliomas. Retrospective studies are about equally divided. Some clearly show that gross total excision improves survival and outcome, whereas other studies fail to show this relationship. The difficulty with interpreting these retrospective data is the selection bias of those patients chosen to undergo extensive resection. In addition, the highly infiltrative nature of low-grade gliomas makes it even more difficult to effect a gross total excision in the majority of patients. Frequently, a lesion involves extensive regions of the frontal and temporal lobes and insular cortex, and cannot be removed. However, in the occasional patient who presents with a lesion radiographically confined to the frontal pole, particularly in the nondominant hemisphere, where a gross total excision may be safely performed, it is generally recommended. Furthermore, extensive tumor removal also helps provide more accurate pathologic examination. However, needle biopsy is more commonly the only diagnostic option in patients with low-grade tumors, as compared with that of patients with malignant lesions; preoperative PET or MRS may indicate a suspicious focus of high-grade disease that should be the target for a diagnostic stereotactic biopsy.

Radiotherapy

Focal radiotherapy has been the mainstay for treating astrocytomas. There have been a series of randomized, phase III trials that define the role of radiotherapy. Two studies have evaluated the effective dose of radiotherapy. A European Organization for Research and Treatment of Cancer (EORTC) study compared 45 Gy with 59.4 Gy and a second study compared 50.4 Gy with 64.8 Gy. Both of these phase III trials found that survival was not compromised by using the lower dose of radiotherapy. Furthermore, radiation-related toxicities such as fatigue, malaise, insomnia, and emotional functioning were significantly less frequent in patients receiving lower doses of radiotherapy. Even though the EORTC established the efficacy of 45 Gy, many radiotherapists continue to treat patients with 50 Gy to 54 Gy, which is a significantly lower dose than the 60 Gy used to treat high-grade gliomas.

The second critical issue is the timing of treatment. The EORTC conducted a second randomized clinical trial in which patients with the histologic diagnosis of low-grade glioma were randomly assigned to receive either immediate radiotherapy or delayed radiotherapy at the time of clinical or radiographic progression. The progression-free survival was significantly prolonged in patients who received immediate radiotherapy, but overall survival was unaffected. While the authors of this study interpreted the results as demonstrating the importance of administering radiotherapy immediately after diagnosis, many have also interpreted these data as showing that radiotherapy may be deferred safely until clinically indicated. Therefore, patients who present with seizures that may be well controlled on anticonvulsants, who have no other neurologic symptoms, and whose tumors are followed with serial imaging, may have their radiotherapy deferred. Patients with significant cognitive or lateralizing signs at presentation, or whose tumors have clearly progressed radiographically during follow-up imaging, require immediate radiotherapy.

The major reason to defer radiotherapy in this young population, with a likely prolonged survival, is the potential for them to develop significant neurotoxicity as a consequence of treatment, particularly if overall survival is not affected favorably by the institution of immediate therapy. The role of radiotherapy in causing cognitive dysfunction in such patients is also controversial. A series of studies has suggested that the disease itself may be more important in causing cognitive impairment than the treatment. A recent study has also shown that anticonvulsant use in this population is associated with significant cognitive dysfunction and may be more important than any radiation-related neurotoxicity. However, there remains substantial concern that radiation to large regions of the brain may result in cognitive impairment, particularly in loss of executive function that may adversely affect a patient's ability to perform at high-level, job-related tasks.

Lastly, while investigators agree that a growing astrocytoma requires treatment with radiotherapy, it is not always easy to ascertain when growth is occurring. Frequently, one must compare a neuroimaging study with not only the immediate-past prior scan, but with images obtained 2, 3, or more years previously, in order to detect accurately changes that are difficult to appreciate when only a few months separate scans. Recent work has shown that even when the lesion appears radiographically stable, all low-grade astrocytomas grow inexorably, at a rate of about 4 mm per year, until they reach a critical size in which the change in growth is easily appreciated on MRI, or when it results in new symptoms. Therefore, when a decision is made to defer treatment, these patients must be followed very closely in order to determine, accurately, when therapy should be instituted.

Prognosis

Patients with low-grade astrocytomas survive a median of 5 years. The range of survival is broad, with some patients succumbing within a year and others surviving a decade or more. Most die from tumor that has transformed to a higher grade.

THERAPY OF OLIGODENDROGLIAL TUMORS

Oligodendrogliomas are highly infiltrative neoplasms that often involve critical areas of cortex or large regions of brain. Unlike the astrocytic tumors where 70% to 80% are high-grade malignant neoplasms, the majority of oligodendroglial tumors are low-grade lesions. The low-grade oligodendroglioma has the potential to transform, over time, to an anaplastic oligodendroglioma, but these tumors may also acquire astrocytic features and may even develop into typical-appearing glioblastoma multiforme. The treatment is determined by the histologic grade of the tumor and the clinical condition of the patient.

Anaplastic Oligodendroglioma

Surgery

Complete surgical resection should be performed for any patient with an anaplastic oligodendroglioma, if feasible. Extirpation affords accurate pathologic diagnosis, usually improves the patient's neurologic function, and affords a more rapid taper off corticosteroid therapy by decompressing the mass effect.

Radiotherapy

Radiotherapy has been the standard treatment for patients with anaplastic oligodendrogliomas. It prolongs disease control and survival. A total dose of about 60 Gy in 30 to 33 fractions is given to a focal region.

Chemotherapy

The choice and timing of chemotherapy in the treatment of patients with anaplastic oligodendrogliomas is the most controversial aspect of its therapy. The unique chemosensitivity of oligodendroglial neoplasms was first noticed in patients with recurrent anaplastic tumors. Marked responses were observed to the triple-drug regimen of procarbazine, CCNU and vincristine (PCV). As many as 75% of patients had either complete or partial response of their recurrent tumor to this regimen (Fig. 56.3).

Furthermore, survival and disease control were directly related to the degree of response observed on MRI. This marked tumor response was subsequently correlated with

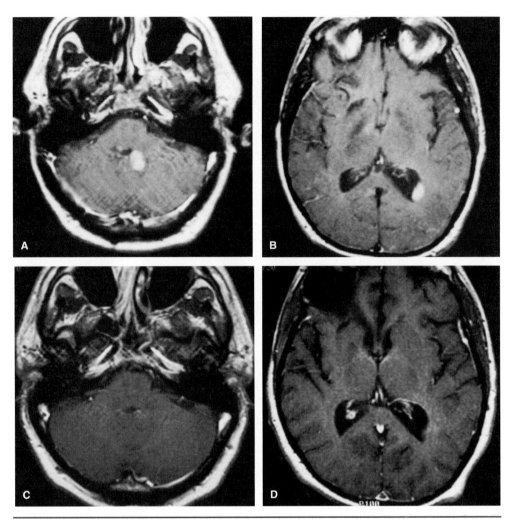

FIGURE 56.3. Disseminated oligodendroglioma. Contrast-enhanced MRI in a patient with recurrent anaplastic oligodendroglioma shows ependymal seeding of the left lateral **(A)** and fourth **(B)** ventricles. **C: and D:** In the same patient 4 months later, there is complete response of both intraventricular lesions after two cycles of PCV chemotherapy.

the loss of heterozygosity of chromosomes 1p and 19q. While some oligodendroglial neoplasms with intact 1p and 19q may also respond to treatment, their overall outcome is not as favorable as those tumors that have 1p/19q LOH.

The chemosensitivity of the oligodendroglial tumors has introduced some degree of controversy regarding the use of chemotherapy as part of the initial treatment. A recent study was completed by the Radiation Therapy Oncology Group (RTOG) in which patients with newly diagnosed, anaplastic oligodendroglial tumors were randomized to receive radiotherapy alone, versus three cycles of intensive PCV followed by radiotherapy. Patients who received chemotherapy had significantly longer times to disease progression (2.6 years for PCV and RT and 1.9 years for RT alone) but overall survival between the groups was identical (4.8 years for PCV and RT, and 4.5 years for RT alone). This was largely related to the fact that patients who received radiation alone received PCV at recurrence.

Alternatively, some investigators have used chemotherapy as the initial treatment for patients with newly diagnosed anaplastic oligodendrogliomas. If the patient has a significant response, they may defer radiotherapy until the time of recurrence. This approach is based on the rationale that patients will be spared the long-term side effects of radiotherapy until absolutely necessary. Although this has been an approach used by neuro-oncologists, it has not been validated in any clinical trial. However, the principle of deferring radiotherapy by using intensive chemotherapy has been shown effective in a recent report. A multicenter, phase II trial, using high-dose chemotherapy with autologous stem-cell rescue in patients with newly diagnosed anaplastic oligodendrogliomas, reported a median progression-free survival of 5.8 years, and the median overall survival was not reached. These patients were treated with chemotherapy alone and no radiotherapy was administered, but radiotherapy was usually used at recurrence.

The survival of this selected population is favorable compared to that of patients treated with standard radiotherapy and chemotherapy. This study establishes the feasibility, safety and efficacy of this chemotherapy-only approach. A second study of high-dose chemotherapy with autologous stem-cell rescue is underway, but this treatment should be confined to a clinical trial. Therefore, patients with newly diagnosed anaplastic oligodendrogliomas could be treated in a conventional fashion, with radiotherapy and adjuvant chemotherapy. Most neuro-oncologists use chemotherapy initially, and defer radiotherapy until there is clinical or radiographic progression. However, all such patients require immediate treatment.

Prognosis

Patients with an anaplastic oligodendrogliomas survive a median of 5 years, almost as long as those with low-grade astrocytomas. Some may survive considerably longer and they almost always have tumors that are 1p/19q deleted.

Low-Grade Oligodendroglioma

Like patients with low-grade astrocytomas, many of these patients may be followed clinically and radiographically, until clinical symptoms or radiographic progression dictate treatment. If possible, all low-grade tumors should be resected, although this is rarely feasible. For those patients who require immediate treatment because of significant neurologic deficits, such as hemiparesis or cognitive problems, or for those who have tumor progression, there are several options. A standard approach would be focal radiotherapy to a dose of about 54 Gy. Alternatively, many patients are treated with chemotherapy, initially, as the sole modality. Most published studies describe responses to PCV; however, increasingly for low-grade and anaplastic oligodendrogliomas, temozolomide is used as a first-line agent. The efficacy of temozolomide has been established at recurrence, but there have been no substantial studies evaluating its role in initial treatment. However, because it is an alkylating agent (like CCNU and procarbazine), has excellent penetration behind the blood-brain barrier, has documented efficacy and much less toxicity than PCV, it is the agent of choice. Patients are usually treated with standard 5-day regimens, at doses of 150 mg/m^2 to 200 mg/m^2 per day. Patients tolerate this extremely well and many have no interruptions in their normal lives during this therapy.

Recurrence

At recurrence, radiotherapy should be used, if not already administered. Likewise, chemotherapy, such as temozolomide or PCV, if not used as part of the initial regimen, would be an option. Other agents that have been re-

ported to be efficacious include melphalan, the platins, and etoposide. If there is malignant transformation at recurrence, the patient should be treated accordingly. High-dose chemotherapy with autologous stem-cell rescue has been established as being too toxic and ineffective for use as treatment at relapse.

Prognosis

The median survival of patients with low-grade oligodendrogliomas ranges from 8 to 16 years in different reports, with some patients surviving decades without recurrence. Tumors that have 1p/19q LOH clearly have the best prognosis. Most patients die from malignant transformation of their tumors.

Oligoastrocytomas

Tumors that contain significant elements of both oligodendroglial and astrocytic components may account for as many as 10% of all gliomas. In general, these tumors have prognoses that are intermediate, and fall between the prognoses of the pure astrocytic and pure oligodendroglial varieties. This is the area where pathologists disagree most frequently, and determination of a mixed glioma is very subjective. However, if 1p/19q LOH can be demonstrated in a histologically mixed glioma, it is treated as an oligodendroglial neoplasm. Mixed tumors tend to have better responses to chemotherapy and radiotherapy than pure astrocytic tumors, but have higher recurrence rates and shorter times to progression than pure oligodendroglial neoplasms.

GLIOMATOSIS CEREBRI

Gliomatosis cerebri is characterized by diffuse infiltration of neoplastic glial cells throughout a hemisphere or even the entire brain. This variant of a glioma may occur in adults of all ages. Patients often present with personality or cognitive changes, and MRI typically reveals diffuse, nonenhancing abnormalities seen in the white matter of the hemispheres (Fig. 56.4). The brain may have a swollen appearance, with loss of the normal sulci and small ventricles. Occasionally, tiny focal areas of contrast enhancement may be seen, but the predominant disease is nonenhancing. A biopsy typically reveals a diffuse astrocytoma. Occasionally, oligodendroglial-type tumors may present in this fashion. Frequently, foci of anaplasia can exist within this predominantly low-grade tumor. The clinical course may be quite variable. Some patients progress rapidly, whereas others may be followed for years without the need for immediate treatment. Radiotherapy is the predominant treatment for gliomatosis cerebri, but frequently, the whole brain must be included within the radiotherapy port.

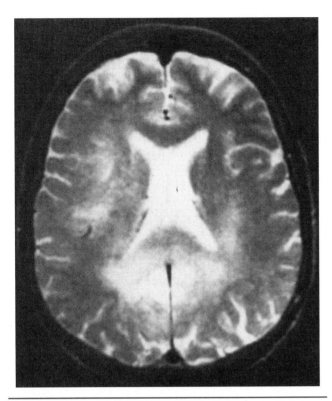

FIGURE 56.4. Gliomatosis cerebri. T2-weighted MRI shows widespread areas of increased signal in both cerebral hemispheres. Stereotactic biopsy revealed anaplastic astrocytoma.

EPENDYMOMAS

Ependymomas arise from the ependymal cells that line the ventricular system and the central canal of the spinal cord. They are more common in childhood, accounting for about 10% of pediatric intracranial tumors, but only 5% of adult intracranial neoplasms. Ependymomas of the spinal cord are discussed in detail in Chapter 63.

Intracranial ependymomas may arise anywhere ependymal cells are present, but the most common intracranial site is the fourth ventricle. Supratentorial ependymomas may grow into or abut the lateral ventricles, or may grow in the brain parenchyma without obvious attachment to the ventricular system.

Histologically, ependymomas are characterized by perivascular pseudorosettes and ependymal or Homer-Wright rosettes. Pseudorosettes are identified when tumor cells arrange themselves radially around blood vessels, whereas ependymal rosettes occur when tumor cells arrange themselves around a central lumen. There are a series of histologic subtypes of intracranial ependymoma, including clear cell, cellular, and papillary, but these subtypes have no prognostic significance. In general, ependymomas are divided into low-grade or anaplastic neoplasms. Initial data failed to demonstrate that histologic features of anaplasia conferred worse prognoses in patients harboring such lesions. However, recent studies have all conclusively indicated that anaplastic features carry worse prognoses. Ependymomas have been associated with loss of chromosome 22, particularly 22q, but a specific gene has not yet been identified in this area.

Clinical features depend upon the site of the tumor. Fourth ventricle tumors typically cause symptoms by obstructing the egress of CSF from the fourth ventricle. Patients commonly present with headaches, nausea, vomiting, ataxia, and vertigo. Patients with supratentorial lesions present with focal neurologic symptoms and signs appropriate to their tumor locations.

MRI demonstrates a heterogeneous, well-delineated lesion that usually contrast enhances prominently. Hemorrhage and calcification are occasionally seen. The most important treatment for ependymomas is gross total excision. Patients with anaplastic tumors should be followed with focal postoperative radiotherapy. There is controversy about whether craniospinal irradiation is necessary for infratentorial lesions. However, in the absence of demonstrable CSF seeding by the tumor, focal radiotherapy usually suffices. There is no role for craniospinal irradiation in supratentorial ependymomas. The need to follow surgery with radiotherapy in patients who have had completely resected, low-grade ependymomas is less clear. Data in the literature are conflicting, with some studies suggesting that focal radiotherapy improves disease-free time and overall survival, whereas other studies suggest that it may be withheld until recurrence, without a negative impact on outcome.

Prognosis

The overall 5-year survival rate ranges from 40% to 80% and 10-year survival ranges from 47% to 68% in some series. Outcome is largely determined by young age, infratentorial location, gross total excision and low-grade histology, all of which point to a better prognosis.

NEURONAL AND NEURONAL GLIAL TUMORS

Central Neurocytomas

Central neurocytomas represent less than 1% of intracranial neoplasms and have a peak incidence at between 20 and 40 years of age; they affect both genders equally. Central neurocytomas arise from the subependymal matrix cells close to the lateral ventricles, and usually present as an intraventricular mass spanning the frontal horns of both lateral ventricles. Histologically they may mimic oligodendrogliomas, including the presence of calcifications and occasionally of hemorrhage. The tumors consist of round cells with a round or oval nucleus and a prominent nucleolus. The correct diagnosis may be established by synaptophysin immunohistochemistry, which demonstrates the tumors to be of neuronal origin. Mitoses and necrosis are rarely seen.

The tumor usually causes obstruction of the ventricular system with blockage of the foramen of Monro leading to headache, nausea, vomiting and diplopia. Pressure on the optic chiasm with bitemporal hemianopia may occur. Some patients develop pituitary insufficiency and other hormonal dysfunctions, such as inappropriate secretion of antidiuretic hormone (SIADH). Focal neurologic deficits including seizures and hemiparesis may occur when tumors invade the parenchyma.

MRI of neurocytomas demonstrates characteristic intraventricular masses with intense contrast enhancement. The lesion is well-circumscribed and has numerous microcystic regions that may give it a honeycombed appearance (Fig. 56.5). Calcifications or hemorrhage may also be evident on MRI.

Surgery is the treatment of choice. Gross total excision may lead to a 5-year local control rate of 100%. Owing to their locations, complete removal of these tumors is not always possible. However, partial resections may also be associated with prolonged survival. Recurrence may be treated with additional surgery, followed by radiotherapy, or by radiotherapy alone. Radiosurgery is also an option. Despite the benign behavior of central neurocytomas, they may occasionally seed the leptomeninges, which would ne-

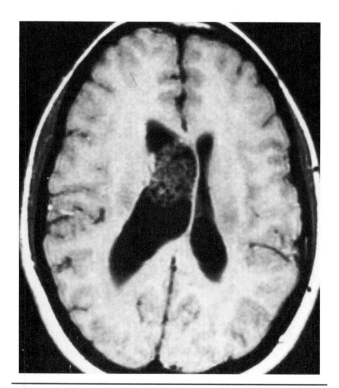

FIGURE 56.5. Intraventricular neurocytoma. Gadolinium-enhanced MRI of a 24 year old woman with a one year history of headache due to a right lateral ventricular neurocytoma obstructing the foramen of Monro. The tumor was completely resected.

cessitate treatment with radiotherapy if not already administered, and chemotherapy.

Ganglioglioma and Gangliocytomas

These low-grade tumors are composed of neoplastic neurons (i.e., gangliocytomas) or a combination of neoplastic neurons and glial cells (i.e., gangliogliomas). These tumors are almost always low-grade but the glial components may become anaplastic and behave aggressively, even disseminating throughout the subarachnoid space. These tumors represent about 1% of primary intracranial tumors but up to 4% of pediatric brain tumors. They may occur anywhere in the brain but the majority are found in the temporal lobes and many are associated with resistant focal epilepsy.

Pathologically, gangliocytomas have large pleomorphic neurons embedded in a network of collagen fibers. Lymphocytic infiltrates might be focal and prominent. In gangliogliomas, the neural elements may be prominent or sparse. The tumors frequently contain microcysts and calcifications. The mixed population is identified when the glial cells stain positively for GFAP and the neuronal component is positive for synaptophysin. Pleomorphism is occasionally seen and a few mitotic figures might be present, but these features do not delineate an anaplastic tumor. The MIB-1 labeling indices are typically less than 3%.

The symptoms and signs of these tumors depend upon their location in the brain, but overall the majority of patients present with seizures, particularly of the partial-complex variety. On MRI, the tumors usually contrast enhance but occasionally no enhancement is seen. At least one-half of these tumors have large cystic components, and edema surrounding the tumors is uncommon. Hemorrhage and necrosis are rare.

The treatment is surgical; complete resection may be achieved in most patients and may be curative. The seizures may improve even if partial resection is accomplished. Patients should be followed closely and if there is evidence of progression, second resections, followed by focal radiotherapy, should be performed. Even gangliogliomas with anaplastic glial elements may be treated with resection alone and then followed. Immediate radiotherapy is not necessary and may be reserved for use at progression. Chemotherapy is used only at recurrence. Nitrosoureas, retinoic acid, and cisplatin have all been reported to be effective in some patients.

Dysembryoplastic Neuroepithelial Tumor (DNT)

This is a low-grade, cortical-based tumor of mixed glial and neuronal origin that occurs predominantly in the temporal cortex. DNTs are encountered relatively frequently in patients undergoing epilepsy surgery. The MRI may be characteristic. Typically, the tumor expands the cortex and appears as multiple firm nodules; some tumors are poorly demarcated whereas about half are sharply delineated. Some are cystic and there may be local mass effect; edema is rare. Calcification and occasionally hemorrhage may occur. Contrast enhancement is seen in about half of these tumors but is absent in the other half.

Clinically, the symptoms in almost all patients start with seizures. The epilepsy is usually longstanding, drug resistant, and frequently begins in childhood. Treatment is surgical and gross total excision is curative. Partial resection may improve seizure control and should be performed even if complete removal is not possible. No additional therapy is required.

SUGGESTED READINGS

General Considerations in Glioma

Barnholtz-Sloan JS, Sloan AE, Schwartz AG. Racial differences in survival after diagnosis with primary malignant brain tumor. *Cancer* 2003;98:603–609.

DeAngelis LM, Gutin PH, Leibel SA, Posner JB. Glial tumors. In: *Intracranial Tumors: Diagnosis and Treatment.* London: Martin Dunitz, 2002:149–188.

DeAngelis LM. Brain tumors. *N Engl J Med* 2001;344:114–123.

De Roos AJ, Stewart PA, Linet MS, et al. Occupation and the risk of adult glioma in the United States. *Cancer Causes Control* 2003;14:139–150.

Inskip PD, Tarone RE, Hatch EE, et al. Cellular-telephone use and brain tumors. *N Engl J Med* 2001;344:79–86.

Kleihues P, Cavenee WK, eds. *World Health Organization Classification of Tumours. Pathology & Genetics. Tumors of the Nervous System.* Cedex, France: International Agency for Research on Cancer Press, 2000.

Muscat JE, Malkin MG, Thompson S, et al. Handheld cellular telephone use and the risk of brain cancer. *JAMA* 284;3001–3007.

Wang LE, Bondy ML, Shen H, et al. Polymorphisms of DNA repair genes and risk of glioma. *Cancer Res* 2004 Aug 15;64(16):5560–5563.

Astrocytic Gliomas

Bampoe J, Bernstein M. The role of surgery in low-grade gliomas. *J Neurooncol* 1999;42:259–269.

Barnholtz-Sloan JS, Sloan AE, Schwartz AG. Relative survival rates and patterns of diagnosis analyzed by time period for individuals with primary malignant brain tumor, 1973–1997. *J Neurosurg* 2003;99:458–466.

Bauman G, Lote K, Larson D, et al. Pretreatment factors predict overall survival for patients with low-grade glioma: a recursive partitioning analysis. *Int J Radiat Oncol Biol Phys* 1999;45:923–929.

Brown PS, Bruckner JC, O'Fallon JR. Effects of radiotherapy on cognitive function in patients with low-grade glioma measured by the Folstein mini-mental state examination. *J Clin Oncol* 2003;21:2519–2524.

Chinot OL, Barrie M, Frauger E, et al. Phase II study of temozolomide without radiotherapy in newly diagnosed glioblastoma multiforme in an elderly population. *Cancer* 2004;100:2208–2214.

Chung JK, Kim YK, Kim SK, et al. Usefulness of 11C-methionine PET in the evaluation of brain lesions that are hypo-or isometabolic on 18F-FDG PET. *Eur J Nucl Med Mol Imaging* 2002;29:176–182.

Collins VP. Brain tumors: classification and genes. *J Neurol Neurosurg Psychiatry* 2004;75:2–11.

Fisher BJ, Naumova E, Leighton CC, et al. Ki-67: a prognostic factor for low-grade glioma? *Int J Radiat Oncol Biol Phys* 2002;52:996–1001.

Hirsch J, Ruge MI, Kim KH, et al. An integrated functional magnetic resonance imaging procedure for preoperative mapping of cortical areas associated with tactile, motor, language, and visual functions. *Neurosurgery* 2000;47:711–721.

Johannesen TB, Langmark F, Lote K. Progress in long-term survival in adult patients with supratentorial low-grade gliomas: a population-based study of 993 patients in whom tumors were diagnosed between 1970 and 1993. *J Neurosurg* 2003;99:854–862.

Karim AB, Afra D, Cornu P, et al. Randomized trial on the efficacy of radiotherapy for cerebral low-grade glioma in the adult: European Organization for Research and Treatment of Cancer Study 22845 with the Medical Research Council study BRO4: an interim analysis. *Int J Radiat Oncol Biol Phys* 2002;52:316–324.

Kiebert GM, Curran D, Aaronson NK, et al. Quality of life after radiation therapy of cerebral low-grade gliomas of the adult: results of a randomized phase III trial on dose response (EORTC trial 22844). EORTC Radiotherapy Cooperative Group. *Eur J Cancer* 1998;34:1902–1909.

Klein M, Heimans JJ, Aaronson NK, et al. Effect of radiotherapy and other treatment-related factors on mid-term to long-term cognitive sequelae in low-grade gliomas: comparative study. *Lancet* 2002;360:1361–1368.

Lo SS, Cho KH, Hall WA, et al. Does the extent of surgery have an impact on the survival of patients who receive postoperative radiation therapy for supratentorial low-grade gliomas? *Int J Cancer* 2001;96:71–78.

Marquez A, Wu R, Zhao J, et al. Evaluation of epidermal growth factor receptor (EGFR) by chromogenic in situ hybridization (CISH) and immunohistochemistry (IHC) in archival gliomas using bright-field microscopy. *Diagn Mol Pathol* 2004;113 :1–8.

Pignatti F, van de Bent M, Curran D, et al. Prognostic factors for survival in adult patients with cerebral low-grade glioma. *J Clin Oncol* 2002;20:2076–2084.

Ribom D, Eriksson A, Hartman M, et al. Positron emission tomography 11C-methionine and survival in patients with low-grade gliomas. *Cancer* 2001;92:1541–1549.

Rich JN, Bigner DD. Development of novel targeted therapies in the treatment of malignant glioma. *Nat Rev Drug Discov* 2004 May;3(5):430–446.

Roa W, Brasher PM, Bauman G, et al. Abbreviated course of radiation therapy in older patients with glioblastoma multiforme: a prospective randomized clinical trial. *J Clin Oncol* 2004;22:1583–1588.

Schiffer D, Cavil P, Chio A, et al. Proliferative activity and prognosis of low-grade astrocytomas. *J Neurooncol* 1997;34:31–35.

Selker RG, Shapiro WR, Burger P, et al. The Brain Tumor Cooperative Group NIH Trial 87-01: a randomized comparison of surgery, external radiotherapy, and carmustine versus surgery, interstitial radiotherapy boost, external radiation therapy, and carmustine. *Neurosurgery* 2002;51:343–355.

Shaw E, Arusell R, Scheithauer B, et al. Prospective randomized trial of low- versus high-dose radiation therapy in adults with supratentorial low-grade glioma: initial report of a North Central Cancer Treatment Group/Radiation Therapy Oncology Group/Eastern Cooperative Oncology Group study. *J Clin Oncol* 2002;20:2267–2276.

Stupp R, Mason WP, van den Bent MJ, et al. Concomitant and adjuvant temozolomide (TMZ) and radiotherapy (RT) for newly diagnosed glioblastoma multiforme (GBM). Conclusive results of a randomized phase III trial by the EORTC Brain & RT Groups and NCIC Clinical Trials Group.

Surma-aho O, Niemela M, Vilkki J, et al. Adverse long-term effects of brain radiotherapy in adult low-grade glioma patients. *Neurology* 2001;56:1285–1290.

Van Veelen ML, Avezaat CJ, Kros JM, et al. Supratentorial low grade astrocytoma: prognostic factors, dedifferentiation, and the issue of early versus late surgery. *J Neurol Neurosurg Psychiatry* 1998;64:581–587.

Whittle IR. The dilemma of low grade glioma. *J Neurol Neurosurg Psychiatry* 2004 Jun; 75 Suppl 2:ii31–36. 3:

Oligodendroglial Tumors

Abrey LE, Childs BH, Paleologos N, et al. High-dose chemotherapy with stem cell rescue as initial therapy for anaplastic oligodendroglioma. *J Neurooncol* 2003;65:127–134.

Brandes AA, Basso U, Vastola F, et al. Carboplatin and teniposide as third-line chemotherapy in patients with recurrent oligodendroglioma or oligoastrocytoma: a phase II study. *Ann Oncol* 2003;12:1727–1731.

Cairncross G, Seiferheld W, Shaw E, et al. An intergroup randomized controlled clinical trial (RCT) of chemotherapy plus radiation (RT) versus RT alone for pure and mixed anaplastic oligodendrogliomas: *Proc. Amer Soc Clin Oncol* 23:107,2004, New Orleans, LA initial report of RTOG 94-02.

Felsberg J, Erkwoh A, Sabel MC, et al. Oligodendroglial tumors: refinement of candidate regions on chromosome arm 1p and correlation of 1p/19q status with survival. *Brain Pathol* 2004;14:121–130.

Huang H, Okamoto Y, Yokoo H, et al. Gene expression profiling and subgroup identification of oligodendrogliomas. *Oncogene* 2004;23(35):6012–6022.

Jeremic B, Milicic B, Grujicic D, et al. Combined treatment modality for anaplastic oligodendroglioma and oligoastrocytoma: a 10-year update of a phase II study. *Int J Radiat Oncol Biol Phys* 2004;59:509–514.

Kaleita TA, Wellisch DK, Cloughesy TF, et al. Prediction of neurocognitive outcome in adult brain tumor patients. *J Neurooncol* 2004;67:245–253.

Lebrun C, Fontaine D, Ramaioli A, et al. Long-term outcome of oligodendrogliomas. *Neurology* 2004;62:1783–1787.

Mandonnet E, Delattre JY, Tanguy ML, et al. Continuous growth of mean tumor diameter in a subset of grade II gliomas. *Ann Neurol* 2003;53:524–528.

Olson JD, Riedel E, DeAngelis LM. Long-term outcome of low-grade oligodendroglioma and mixed glioma. *Neurology* 2000;54:1442–1448.

Puduvalli VK, Hashmi M, McAllister LD, et al. Anaplastic oligodendrogliomas: prognostic factors for tumor recurrence and survival. *Oncology* 2003;65:259–266.

Van den bent MJ, Taphoorn MJ, Brandes AA, et al. Phase II study of first-line chemotherapy with temozolomide in recurrent oligodendroglial tumors: the European Organization for Research and Treatment of Cancer Brain Tumor Group Study 26971. *J Clin Oncol* 2003;21:2525–2528.

Van den Bent M, Chinot OL, Cairncross JG. Recent developments in the molecular characterization and treatment of oligodendroglial tumors. *Neurooncol* 2003;5:128–138.

Ependymoma

Gornet MK, Buckner JC, Marks RS, et al. Chemotherapy for advanced CNS ependymoma. *J Neurooncol* 1999;45:61–67.

Guyotat J, Signorelli F, Desme S, et al. Intracranial ependymomas in adult patients: analyses of prognostic factors. *J Neurooncol* 2002;60:225–268.

Huang B, Starostik P, Kuhl J, et al. Loss of heterozygosity on chromosome 22 in human ependymomas. *Acta Neuropathol* 2002;103:415–420.

Korshunov A, Golanov A, Sycheva R, Timirgaz V. The histologic grade is a main prognostic factor for patients with intracranial ependymomas treated in the microneurosurgical era: an analysis of 258 patients. *Cancer* 2004;100:1230–1237.

Mansur DB, Drzymala RE, Rich KM, Klein EE, Simpson JR. The efficacy of stereotactic radiosurgery in the management of intracranial ependymoma. *J Neurooncol* 2004 Jan;66(1–2):187–190.

Massimino M, Gandola L, Giangaspero F, et al. Hyperfractionated radiotherapy and chemotherapy for childhood ependymoma: final results of the first prospective AIEOP (Associazione Italiana di Ematologia-Oncologia Pediatrics) study. *Int J Radiat Oncol Biol Phys* 2004;58:1336–1345.

Oya N, Shibamoto Y, Nagata Y, et al. Postoperative radiotherapy for intracranial ependymoma: analysis of prognostic factors and patterns of failure. *J Neurooncol* 2002;56:87–94.

Reni M, Brandes AA, Vavassori V, et al. A multicenter study of the prognosis and treatment of adult brain ependymal tumors. *Cancer* 2004;100:1221–1229.

Taylor RE. Review of radiotherapy dose and volume for intracranial ependymoma. *Pediatr Blood Cancer* 2004;42:457–460.

Neuronal and Neuronal Glial Neoplasms

Blumcke I, Wiestler OD. Gangliogliomas: an intriguing tumor entity associated with focal epilepsies. *J Neuropathol Exp Neurol* 2002;61:575–584.

Choi JY, Chang JW, Park YG, et al. A retrospective study of the clinical outcomes and significant variables in the surgical treatment of temporal lobe tumor associated with intractable seizures. *Stereotact Funct Neurosurg* 2004;82:35–42.

Hukin J, Siffert J, Velasquez L, Zagzag D, Allen J. Leptomeningeal dissemination in children with progressive low-grade neuroepithelial tumors. *Neurooncol* 2002;4:253–260.

Luyken C, Blumcke I, Fimmers R, et al. The spectrum of long-term epilepsy–associated tumors: long-term seizure and tumor outcome and neurosurgical aspects. *Epilepsia* 2003;44:822–830.

McLendon RE, Provenzale J. Glioneuronal tumors of the central nervous system. *Brain Tumor Pathol* 2002;19:51–58.

Park JY, Suh YL, Han J. Dysembryoplastic neuroepithelial tumor. Features distinguishing it from oligodendroglioma on cytologic squash preparations. *Acta Cytol* 2003;47:624–629.

Schmidt MH, Gottfried ON, von Koch CS, et al. Central neurocytoma: a review. *J Neurooncol* 2004;66:377–384.

C h a p t e r   5 7

Lymphomas

Lisa M. DeAngelis and Casilda M. BalmaCeda

LYMPHOMA METASTATIC TO THE NERVOUS SYSTEM

Systemic lymphoma may metastasize to the CNS at any time throughout the course of the illness. Nervous system involvement may be present at diagnosis or may appear during treatment, but it is usually seen at advanced stages of disease associated with systemic metastases. It occurs almost exclusively with non-Hodgkin lymphoma (NHL), and typically the intermediate and high-grade subtypes. NHL most commonly involves the leptomeninges (10%), the epidural space (3% to 5%) and rarely the brain (less than 1%). This pattern of involvement is different from primary central nervous system lymphoma (PCNSL) where parenchymal brain disease occurs in more than 90% of patients. CNS involvement is much less common in Hodgkin disease. Epidural cord compression may occur, but leptomeningeal and brain involvement are rare. Epidural spinal cord compression is considered here because the first symptoms may indicate a myelopathy, but the tumor does not involve the CNS directly; the disease is outside the dura.

Factors that predispose to CNS involvement include older age, bone marrow or retroperitoneal involvement, high serum lactic dehydrogenase (LDH) and involvement of specific sites, such as nasal sinus disease. Some authors recommend CNS prophylaxis with intrathecal chemotherapy for high-risk groups, including Burkitt lymphoma.

Leptomeningeal lymphoma is seen in 4% to 11% of all NHL patients, and higher frequency is seen in some histologic subtypes. Symptoms include visual disturbances, headache, limb weakness, drowsiness or confusion, nausea and vomiting, numbness, or back pain. On examination, cranial nerve palsies, spinal nerve or root signs, and behavioral changes are common. The oculomotor, abducens, and facial nerves are the most commonly affected cranial nerves. The diagnosis is established by finding leptomeningeal tumor on MRI of the head or spine, or identification of lymphoma cells in CSF. Sometimes multiple lumbar punctures are necessary, although the diagnosis may remain elusive in 10% of patients, even after three spinal taps. The tumor marker β_2 microglobulin may be particularly useful when measured in the CSF of patients with NHL. Other techniques that may secure the identification of lymphoma cells in the CSF include flow cytometry, immunohistochemistry for B- and T-cell markers, and molecular biologic tests for monoclonality. Treatment often requires focal radiotherapy to a symptomatic site and intrathecal chemotherapy. Median survival is about 4 months, but some patients live for years and may be cured with treatment.

Epidural spinal cord compression occurs in about 5% of NHL patients. Noncontrast MRI of the spine is the only test necessary to diagnose epidural disease; the entire spine should be imaged to identify the 5% to 10% of patients with multifocal epidural tumor. Most patients have direct involvement from vertebral body metastases that encroach on epidural spaces. However, some have disease that directly infiltrates through the neural foramina, leaving bone structure intact. Predilection for the thoracic cord is well-known with this disease. Patients usually have back pain and signs of spinal cord or nerve root compression. Treatment is focal radiotherapy.

Brain metastasis is rare. It causes headache, seizures or lateralizing signs. MRI reveals a diffusely enhancing mass that may be multifocal. Occasionally, biopsy is necessary to establish the diagnosis, particularly if the patient is otherwise thought to be in remission. Treatment may involve radiotherapy; patients with good performance status may benefit from a chemotherapy program identical to regimens designed for PCNSL.

PRIMARY CNS LYMPHOMA IN THE IMMUNOCOMPETENT PATIENT

Epidemiology

PCNSL currently accounts for about 3% of all intracranial neoplasms and 7% of all malignant lymphomas. Its incidence was steadily rising in both the immunocompromised and immunocompetent populations after 1970, and continues to rise in patients over the age of 60 years. The incidence has plateaued in younger patients and decreased in immunocompromised patients, specifically in people with AIDS. The peak incidence occurs in the fifth to seventh decade, with a male to female ratio of 3:2 in immunocompetent patients.

Clinical Manifestations

The most common symptoms are behavioral changes and lateralizing symptoms, such as hemiparesis, aphasia, or visual field deficits. Seizures, ataxia, and cranial nerve palsies occur occasionally. The eye is involved in about 20% of patients with PCNSL and may be the sole site of disease in some patients. Typical ocular symptoms include blurred vision, floaters, and visual loss resulting from retinal detachment.

Pathology

The tumor was first described in the early 1900s and was called perivascular sarcoma or reticulum cell sarcoma. Later the tumor was called a microglioma, to reflect the presumed cell of origin; it was not until the 1970s that the lymphocytic nature of this tumor was recognized. Theories on pathogenesis include migration of malignant lymphocytes to the CNS or transformation of lymphocytes within the CNS, but there are no clear data to support either hypothesis.

PCNSL is manifest as a brain tumor with single or multiple parenchymal lesions in more than 90% of patients. However, PCNSL may develop exclusively in the leptomeninges, as in primary leptomeningeal lymphoma. Uveal or vitreous lesions may be the first site of disease, resulting in primary ocular lymphoma. The rarest manifestation is primary intramedullary lymphoma of the spinal cord. However, ocular, leptomeningeal, or spinal cord involvement frequently coexists with brain disease, necessitating treatment of all these compartments.

Almost all PCNSLs (98%) are B-cell tumors, and most are of the diffuse large-cell subtype, although other types are seen occasionally. About 2% of PCNSLs are T-cell tumors, but reactive T-lymphocytes may infiltrate malignant B-cell neoplasms as host responses to the tumors. This may make diagnosis difficult, particularly if a small sample has been obtained, and a mixed-lymphocyte population identified. Evidence of immunoglobulin gene rearrangement may help determine monoclonality.

Grossly, the tumors have a fleshy appearance with ill-defined borders. Hemorrhage and necrosis are rare in immunocompetent patients. Histologically, the cells are closely packed and have a characteristic perivascular concentration. They infiltrate the brain widely and tumor has been identified remote from the main lesion and in areas that are completely normal radiographically.

Imaging

The lesions may be single or multiple, and are often periventricular. The most common location is supratentorial, particularly in the frontal lobes; however, PCNSL may occur anywhere in the brain. Lesions are usually iso- or hyperdense on precontrast CT (Fig. 57.1A). On MRI the lesions are usually hypointense on T1 images relative to gray matter.

On both CT and MRI, contrast enhancement is dense and homogeneous in immunocompetent patients (Figs. 57.1, and 57.2). The borders are not well demarcated. MRI may show diffuse ependymal spread that is not appreciated on CT (Fig. 57.3).

Ring enhancement, calcification, and hemorrhage are rare in immunocompetent patients, but common in immunodeficient patients. The differential diagnosis includes high-grade gliomas, metastasis, abscess, sarcoid, tuberculosis, or active areas of demyelination. Edema on MRI is moderate to severe in abscess or metastasis, and mild to moderate in PCNSL, a difference that may aid in diagnosis.

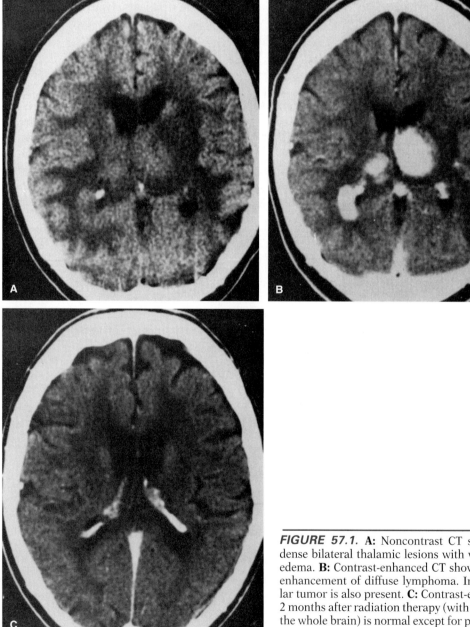

FIGURE 57.1. A: Noncontrast CT showing iso-dense bilateral thalamic lesions with white matter edema. **B:** Contrast-enhanced CT showing marked enhancement of diffuse lymphoma. Intraventricular tumor is also present. **C:** Contrast-enhanced CT 2 months after radiation therapy (with 5,000 cGy to the whole brain) is normal except for persistence of white matter lucency.

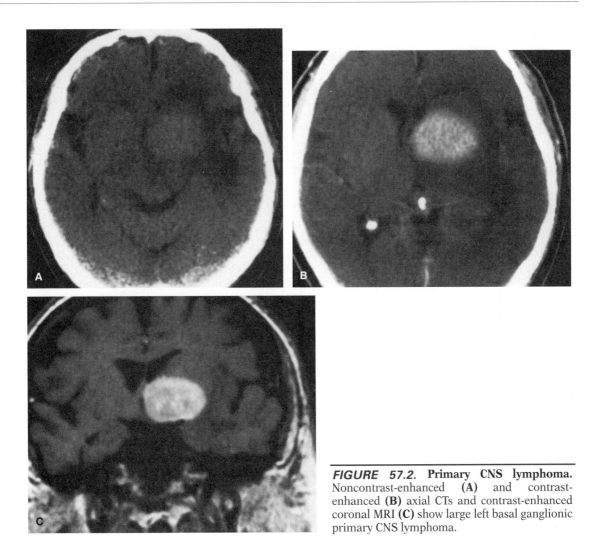

FIGURE 57.2. Primary CNS lymphoma. Noncontrast-enhanced **(A)** and contrast-enhanced **(B)** axial CTs and contrast-enhanced coronal MRI **(C)** show large left basal ganglionic primary CNS lymphoma.

Diagnosis

Diagnosis requires histologic confirmation, usually from brain tissue, but CSF or vitreous humor may also establish the diagnosis. Leptomeningeal disease may be documented in about 40% of patients and CSF establishes the diagnosis in about 15%. A comprehensive neurologic extent of disease evaluation must be done for every patient (Table 57.1) including lumbar puncture and slit-lamp examination.

Body imaging reveals systemic disease in no more than 3% of patients, so bone marrow and chest, abdomen, and pelvic CT scans are not required for routine treatment of every patient unless required by a protocol. Each patient should have a test for HIV antibodies.

Treatment

Corticosteroids

Response is usually dramatic, with a decrease in edema and a cytotoxic effect on lymphoma cells. Rarely, steroids alone may induce tumor regression lasting months after steroids have been discontinued. Corticosteroids should be withheld until biopsy and staging have been completed, to avoid false-negative results, unless a mass is rapidly expanding and herniation is imminent. Response to steroids is not pathognomonic for PCNSL because demyelinating conditions or sarcoidosis may behave similarly.

Surgery

Because the tumors are infiltrative and sometimes bilateral, surgical resection is not helpful, therapeutically. The goal of surgery is to provide tissue diagnosis, and stereotactic biopsy is often the procedure of choice. Complete resection of even a single lesion does not contribute to survival.

Radiation

PCNSL is highly responsive to radiotherapy. Patients are given whole-brain radiotherapy (WBRT) because of the widespread disease present, even if only a single lesion

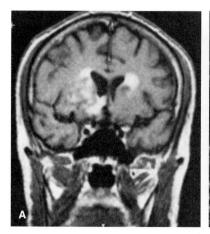
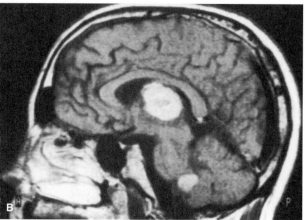

FIGURE 57.3. Primary CNS lymphoma (PCNSL): ependymal spread. A: Contrast-enhanced coronal MRI of a patient with progressive cognitive impairment and diabetes insipidus shows bilateral periventricular and hypothalamic lesions that enhance markedly after contrast administration. **B:** Sagittal contrast-enhanced MRI of a different patient with gait ataxia caused by fourth ventricular spread of a thalamic PCNSL.

is seen on imaging. Patients receive a total dose of 45 Gy. There is no benefit from higher doses, or a boost to the involved area. For ocular involvement, 36 Gy is given to both eyes. The median survival after WBRT, alone, is 10 to 18 months, and only 3% to 4% live 5 years. Age less than 60 years and good performance status predict better outcome.

Chemotherapy

PCNSL is a chemosensitive tumor and the most effective drug therapy is high-dose methotrexate, which penetrates the blood-brain barrier and reaches all areas of disease, including the CSF or eyes. Other active agents include high-dose cytarabine, procarbazine, temozolomide, and nitrosoureas. High-dose methotrexate and high-dose cytarabine may also treat ocular and leptomeningeal disease. Standard NHL regimens are ineffective in part because they incorporate agents unable to pen-

etrate the blood-brain barrier, and therefore should not be used.

When methotrexate is used as a single agent or in combination with other drugs, the response rate exceeds 90% and most patients enjoy a complete response. When high-dose methotrexate-based regimens are combined with WBRT, median survival may reach 60 months. However, this combination may cause permanent, severe, long-term neurotoxicity, particularly in patients over the age of 60 years. Therefore, approaches using chemotherapy alone are being studied, and preliminary data suggest that results comparable to those seen with chemotherapy plus WBRT may be achieved, but without neurotoxicity. All patients, regardless of age, should be considered for chemotherapy as the initial treatment of PCNSL.

Prognosis

Outcome has markedly improved with the introduction of chemotherapy as the initial treatment of PCNSL. The median survival for patients treated with combined modality regimens is 30 to 60 months, whereas it is 12 to 18 months for those treated with irradiation alone. Patients treated with chemotherapy alone may have a median survival time of about 36 months, but many studies have not yet achieved adequate follow-up to reach a median. Fifty percent of patients relapse, usually within 2 years of diagnosis. Recurrence is mostly in the brain, but may also involve the CSF or eyes. Extraneural relapse is seen in less than 10% of patients and usually involves other extranodal sites, such as breast or kidney. Salvage treatment may include chemotherapy or radiotherapy if not already administered. Second remission

▶ **TABLE 57.1 Patient Evaluation at Diagnosis of PCNSL**

1. Ophthalmologic examination including slit-lamp
2. CSF examination
   cytology
   tumor markers
3. Spine MRI with gadolinium if appropriate
4. HIV-1 serology
5. Chest, abdomen and pelvic CT scan
6. Bone marrow biopsy

may be achieved in more than 60% of patients and many have prolonged survival, so vigorous treatment may be beneficial.

PCNSL IN THE IMMUNOCOMPROMISED PATIENT

Epidemiology

The most common immunocompromised state associated with PCNSL is AIDS. Other conditions associated with an increased incidence of PCNSL include renal transplantation, Wiskott-Aldrich syndrome, ataxia, telangiectasia, IgA deficiency, and rheumatoid arthritis. PCNSL is the most common brain tumor in AIDS patients and is the second most common cause of an intracranial mass in this population, after toxoplasmosis. When PCNSL develops, most AIDS patients have profound immunosuppression and marked T4-cell depletion (median CD4 counts are less than $50/mm^3$). In immunosuppressed subjects, PCNSL occurs in the third or fourth decade, with demographic features comparable to those of HIV-1 infection. PCNSL formerly developed in about 6% of HIV-infected patients, but the incidence has fallen dramatically since the introduction of highly active antiretroviral therapy (HAART).

Pathology and Pathogenesis

The gross and microscopic pathology of PSNCL is identical in immunocompetent and immunodeficient individuals, except for the increased preponderance of the immunoblastic subtype in immunocompromised patients. In immunocompromised patients, PCNSL is associated with the Epstein-Barr virus (EBV). After acute EBV infection, usually in childhood, a small population of latently infected B-cells are immortalized and persist for the life of the individual. With cellular immunodeficiency, these B-cells grow and transform into a malignant clone, leading to lymphoma. Such lymphomas may occur anywhere in the body, but they have a predilection for the brain because of the relatively immunoprivileged environment of the CNS. These issues account, in part, for the marked incidental increase in PCNSL in immunodeficient individuals.

Clinical Manifestations

Manifestations are identical in immunocompetent and immunodeficient patients. Symptoms are typical of a space-occupying lesion and include headache, lateralizing signs, and personality changes.

Imaging

Unlike PCNSL in immunocompetent hosts, in immunosuppressed patients the tumors usually show ring enhancement (corresponding to necrosis), and may be impossible to distinguish from infection or other tumors. The lesions are almost always multiple and do not have typical periventricular locations. SPECT or PET may discriminate PCNSL from toxoplasmosis. SPECT and positron emission tomography (PET) typically reveal hypermetabolic lesions for PCNSL, in contradistinction to the hypometabolism associated with focal infections such as toxoplasmosis.

Diagnosis

The diagnosis may be established by brain biopsy, but the risk of cerebral hemorrhage after stereotactic biopsy is much greater in AIDS patients than in immunocompetent individuals. Therefore, a noninvasive approach is preferable if a definite diagnosis may be made. CSF may be evaluated by PCR for the presence of EBV DNA. This is associated with a high likelihood that an intracranial lesion is PCNSL. If a patient has a hypermetabolic lesion on PET or SPECT, and EBV DNA in CSF, the diagnosis of PCNSL may be established with 100% accuracy. If both are negative, then the patient does not have PCNSL. If only one of the two tests is positive, a biopsy must be performed to confirm the diagnosis.

Treatment

The standard antitumor treatment is WBRT to a total dose of 45 Gy. For patients in poor condition where rapid palliation is the goal, 3 Gy in 10 fractions for a total of 30 Gy is a reasonable alternative. Most patients have clinical responses to radiotherapy. High-dose methotrexate is effective in AIDS-related PCNSL and may be tolerated well in selected patients. Some patients enjoy prolonged survival when treated with both high-dose methotrexate and radiation, or methotrexate alone. The best candidates for chemotherapy are those patients with good performance status, no coexisting medical conditions, and CD4 counts greater than $200/mm^3$. However, most AIDS patients with PCNSL do not have such high CD4 counts. Nevertheless, some with counts of less than $50/mm^3$ may still benefit from chemotherapy. Institution of HAART may have a dramatic effect on AIDS-related PCNSL. Tumor regression has been reported with HAART alone. Others have combined it with antiviral agents, such as ganciclovir, that target EBV. Attempts to reconstitute the immune system, if possible, should be a feature of PCNSL therapy for all immunosuppressed patients.

Prognosis

The median survival is about 4 months with radiotherapy. Patients selected to receive high-dose methotrexate regimens may survive years. Survival correlates closely with performance status at diagnosis and the presence of coexistent opportunistic infections. Patients who have effective therapy commonly die of opportunistic infections, whereas patients who do not usually die of PCNSL.

INTRAVASCULAR LYMPHOMA

Intravascular lymphoma is a rare condition first described in 1959 by Pfleger and Tappeiner; it has also been known as *neoplastic angioendotheliomatosis* or *angiotropic lymphoma*. It is a B-cell NHL that grows within the lumen of blood vessels and has a predilection for the skin and CNS. There are three main forms: a mild cutaneous form, a progressive form with both skin and visceral organ involvement, and an aggressive form with multiorgan involvement.

Clinically, the symptoms usually develop over weeks or months. A stroke-like syndrome may occur as a result of occlusion of cerebral vessels, but progressive encephalopathy is the most common manifestation. Seizures are common. Focal signs include hemiparesis, myelopathy, and aphasia. A patient may have multifocal signs that wax and wane; progressive dementia and lethargy are common. Unexplained fever is seen in 25% of patients. The median age at onset is 60 years (range, 12 to 87 years). Systemic signs other than skin lesions are rare; the common skin lesions include telangiectasias, hemorrhagic nodules, and leg lymphedema.

Diagnosis usually requires a brain biopsy. Pathologically, neoplastic cells are seen within and may occlude the lumen of capillaries, venules, arterioles, and small arteries. Only rarely do neoplastic cells extend beyond the vessel wall. Blood vessels in the subarachnoid space, cortex, white matter, and deep gray matter are involved. Immunohistochemical staining is positive for B-cell markers. Rearrangement of immunoglobulin heavy chain genes may be detected by PCR and is useful to confirm the presence of a monoclonal B-cell population in specimens where the diagnosis is uncertain on histologic examination. The mechanism of intravascular lymphoma is unknown; the cells may have surface properties that favor attachment to the blood vessels of skin, CNS, and peripheral nerves. Owing to the nonspecific clinical features and imaging characteristics, the disease is often difficult to diagnose and frequently is found only at autopsy.

Laboratory results are mostly nonspecific. Anemia is seen in up to 73% of patients, elevated ESR in 83%, and elevated LDH in 89%. CSF protein content is increased in 90% of patients and a mild pleocytosis in more than half of patients; oligoclonal bands are present in 77%. Neoplastic cells in the CSF are seen in only 3%.

Imaging usually reveals multifocal abnormalities reflecting diffuse brain involvement. The most common lesion is a mass with increased signal on T2-weighted images, which correlates with areas of gliosis and edema, pathologically. The white matter is most commonly affected, but lesions may also be seen in the gray matter. Typical strokes may be seen with gyriform enhancement. There may be subependymal and leptomeningeal enhancement. Angiography may show multifocal vessel stenosis or occlusion, as in vasculitis. Other conditions that may mimic this disease include multiinfarct dementia, vasculitis, Creutzfeldt-Jakob disease, progressive multifocal leucoencephalopathy, or gliomatosis cerebri.

Treatment includes corticosteroids, a combination of chemotherapy and radiation, plasmapheresis, and intrathecal chemotherapy. Although complete responses have been observed, median survival is only 6 months.

LYMPHOMATOID GRANULOMATOSIS

This is an angiocentric and angiodestructive, EBV-associated, B-cell lymphoproliferative process that preferentially involves the lungs. It was first described in 1972 by Liebow. Pathologically, there is a lymphoid infiltrate (i.e., plasma cells, histiocytes, and lymphoreticular cells), with vascular proliferation, and necrosis. The malignant B-cells are accompanied by an exuberant reaction, mediated in part by high doses of cytokines that result in vascular damage and granuloma formation. The perivascular spaces are infiltrated with neoplastic cells, differing from angiotropic lymphoma where the neoplastic cells are within the vessel lumen. Extrathoracic manifestations include the skin (37%) and the CNS (30%). Neurologic symptoms include headache, altered consciousness, cranial nerve palsies or a multiinfarct dementia. Peripheral neuropathy affects 25% of patients.

On cranial MRI, lesions are seen in the gray and white matter, accompanied by edema. Multiple, punctate foci of enhancement and hemorrhage may be seen; the brainstem and cerebellum are frequently involved. Treatment with corticosteroids, cyclophosphamide, and radiotherapy has been tried. Prognosis is poor; median survival is about 2 years.

SUGGESTED READINGS

Systemic Lymphoma

Batchelor T, ed. *Lymphoma of the Nervous System*. New York: Butterworth-Heinemann, 2004.

Bekkenk MW, Postma TJ, Meijer CJ, et al. Frequency of central nervous system involvement in primary cutaneous B-cell lymphoma. *Cancer* 2000;89:913–919.

Chahal S, Lagera JE, Ryder J, et al. Hematological neoplasms with first presentation as spinal cord compression syndromes: a 10-year retrospective series and review of the literature. *Clin Neuropathol* 2003;22:282–290.

Fonseca R, Habermann TM, Colgan JP, et al. Testicular lymphoma is associated with a high incidence of extranodal recurrence. *Cancer* 2000;88:154–161.

Gray JR, Wallner KE. Reversal of cranial nerve dysfunction with radiation therapy in adults with lymphoma and leukemia. *Int J Radiat Oncol Biol Phys* 1990;19:439–444.

Mackintosh FR, Colby TV, Podolsky WJ, et al. Central nervous system involvement in non-Hodgkin's lymphoma: an analysis of 105 cases. *Cancer* 1982;49:586–595.

Recht L, Straus DJ, Cirrincione C, et al. Central nervous system metastases from non-Hodgkin's lymphoma: treatment and prophylaxis. *Am J Med* 1988;84:425–435.

Primary Central Nervous System Lymphoma

Abrey LE, DeAngelis L, Yahalom J. Long-term survival in primary CNS lymphoma. *J Clin Oncol* 1998;16:859–863.

Abrey LE, Moskowitz CH, Mason WP, et al. Intensive methotrexate and cytarabine followed by high-dose chemotherapy with autologous stem-cell rescue in patients with newly diagnosed primary CNS lymphoma: an intent-to-treat analysis. *J Clin Oncol* 2003;21:4151–4156.

Balmaceda CM, Gaynor JJ, Sun M, et al. Leptomeningeal involvement in primary central nervous system lymphoma: recognition, significance and implications. *Ann Neurol* 1995;38:202–209.

Batchelor T, Carson K, O'Neill A, et al. Treatment of primary CNS lymphoma with methotrexate and deferred radiotherapy: a report of NABTT 96-07. *J Clin Oncol* 2003;21:1044–1049.

Carlson CL, Hartman R, Ly JQ, et al. Primary leptomeningeal lymphoma of the lumbar spine. *Clin Imaging* 2003;27:389–393.

Castellano-Sanchez AA, Li S, Qian J, et al. Primary central nervous system posttransplant lymphoproliferative disorders. *Am J Clin Pathol* 2004;121:246–253.

Corn BW, Trock BJ, Curran WJ. Management of primary central nervous system lymphoma for the patient with acquired immunodeficiency syndrome. Confronting a clinical catch 22. *Cancer* 1995;76:163–166.

Correa DD, DeAngelis LM, Shi W, et al. Cognitive functions in survivors of primary central nervous system lymphoma. *Neurology* 2004;62:548–555.

DeAngelis LM, Hormigo A. Treatment of primary central nervous system lymphoma. *Semin Oncol* 2004 Oct;31(5):684–692.

DeAngelis LM, Seiferheld W, Schold SC, et al. Combination chemotherapy and radiotherapy for primary central nervous system lymphoma: Radiation Therapy Oncology Group 93-10. *J Clin Oncol* 2002;20:4615–4617.

DeAngelis LM, Yahalom J, Thaler HT, et al. Combined modality therapy for primary CNS lymphoma. *J Clin Oncol* 1992;10:635–643.

DeAngelis LM. Current management of primary central nervous system lymphoma. *Oncology* 1995;9:63–71.

Dubuisson A, Kaschten B, Lenelle J, et al. Primary central nervous system lymphoma; Report of 32 cases and review of the literature. *Clin Neurol Neurosurg* 2004 Dec;107(1):55–63.

Ferreri AJ, Abrey LE, Blay JY, et al. Summary statement of primary central nervous system lymphoma from the Eighth International Conference on Malignant Lymphoma: Lugano, Switzerland, 2002. *J Clin Oncol* 2003;21:2407–2414.

Ferreri AJ, Guerra E, Regazzi M, et al. Area under the curve of methotrexate and creatinine clearance are outcome-determining factors in primary CNS lymphomas. *Br J Cancer* 2004;90:353–358.

Forsyth P, Yahalom J, DeAngelis LM. Combined modality therapy in the treatment of primary central nervous system lymphoma in AIDS. *Neurology* 1994;44:1473–1479.

Hoang-Xuan K, Taillandier L, Chinot O, et al. Chemotherapy alone as initial treatment for primary CNS lymphoma in patients older than 60 years: a multicenter phase II study (26952) of the European Organization for Research and Treatment of Cancer Brain Tumor Group. *J Clin Oncol* 2003;21:2726–2731.

Hormigo A, DeAngelis LM. Primary intraocular lymphoma: clinical features, diagnosis and treatment. *Clin Lymphoma* 2003;4:22–29.

Khalfallah S, Stamatoullas A, Fruchart C, et al. Durable remission of a relapsing primary central nervous system lymphoma after autologous bone marrow transplantation. *Bone Marrow Transplant* 1998;18:1021–1023.

Lai R, Rosenbaum MK, DeAngelis LM. Primary CNS lymphoma: a whole-brain disease? *Neurology* 2002;59:1557–1562.

Newell ME, Hoy JF, Cooper SG, DeGraaff B, Grulich AE, Bryant M, Millar JL, Brew BJ, Quinn DI. Human immunodeficiency virus-related primary central nervous system lymphoma: factors influencing survival in 111 patients. *Cancer* 2004 Jan 15;100(12):2627–2636.

O'Neill BP, O'Fallon JR, Earle JD, et al. Primary central nervous system non-Hodgkin's lymphoma: survival advantages with combined initial therapy? *Int J Radiat Oncol Biol Phys* 1995;33:663–673.

Pels H, Schmidt-Wolf IG, Glasmacher A, et al. Primary central nervous system lymphoma: results of a pilot and phase II study of systemic and intraventricular chemotherapy with deferred radiotherapy. *J Clin Oncol* 2003;21:4489–4495.

Poortmans PM, Kluin-Nelemans HC, Haaxma-Reiche H, et al. High-dose methotrexate-based chemotherapy followed by consolidating radiotherapy in non-AIDS-related primary central nervous system lymphoma: European Organization for Research and Treatment of Cancer Lymphoma Group Phase II Trial 20962. *J Clin Oncol* 2003;21:4483–4488.

Raval S, Yahalom J, DeAngelis LM. Management of central nervous system lymphoma. In: Mauch P, Armitage JO, Harris NL, et al., eds *Non-Hodgkins Lymphoma.* Philadelphia: Lippincott, Williams & Wilkins, 2003:643–655.

Sandor V, Stark Vancs V, Pearson D, et al. Phase II trial of chemotherapy alone for primary CNS and intraocular lymphoma. *J Clin Oncol* 1998;16:3000–3006.

Schiff D, Suman VJ, Yang P, et al. Risk factors for primary central nervous system lymphoma: a case-control study. *Cancer* 1998;82:975–982.

Schultz C, Scott C, Sherman W, et al. Preirradiation chemotherapy with cyclophosphamide, doxorubicin, vincristine, and dexamethasone for primary CNS lymphomas: initial report of Radiation Therapy Oncology Group protocol 88-06. *J Clin Oncol* 1996;14:556–564.

Skiest DJ, Crosby C. Survival is prolonged by highly active antiretroviral therapy in AIDS patients with primary central nervous system lymphoma. *AIDS* 2003;17:1787–1793.

Intravascular Lymphoma

Anghel G, Petrinato G, Severino A, et al. Intravascular B-cell lymphoma: report of two cases with different clinical presentation but rapid central nervous system involvement. *Leuk Lymphoma* 2003;44:1353–1359.

Baehring JM, Longtine J, Hochberg FH. A new approach to the diagnosis and treatment of intravascular lymphoma. *J Neurooncol* 2003;61:237–248.

Beristain X, Azzarelli B. The neurological masquerade of intravascular lymphomatosis. *Arch Neurol* 2002;59:439–443.

Davis TS. Intravascular lymphoma presenting with cauda equina syndrome: treated with CHOP and rituxan. *Leuk Lymphoma* 2003;44:887–888.

Imai H, Kajimoto K, Taniwaki M, et al. Intravascular large B-cell lymphoma presenting with mass lesions in the central nervous system: a report of five cases. *Pathol Int* 2004;54:231–236.

Liu PC, Wong GK, Poon WS, et al. Intravascular lymphomatosis. *J Clin Pathol* 2003;56:468–470.

Martin-Duverneuil N, Mokhtari K, Behin A, et al. Intravascular malignant lymphomatosis. *Neuroradiology* 2002;44:749–754.

Wick MR, Mills SE. Intravascular lymphomatosis: clinicopathologic features and differential diagnosis. *Semin Diagn Pathol* 1991;8:91–101.

Williams RL, Meltzer CC, Smirniotopoulos JG, et al. Cerebral MR imaging in intravascular lymphomatosis. *Am J Neuroradiol* 1998;19:427–431.

Lymphomatoid Granulomatosis

Beaty MW, Toro J, Sorbara L, et al. Cutaneous lymphomatoid granulomatosis: correlation of clinical and biologic features. *Am J Surg Pathol* 2001;25:1111–1120.

Jaffe ES, Wilson WH. Lymphomatoid granulomatosis: pathogenesis, pathology and clinical implications. *Cancer Surv* 1997;30:233–248.

Miura H, Shimamura H, Tsuchiya K, et al. Magnetic resonance imaging of lymphomatoid granulomatosis: punctate and linear enhancement preceding hemorrhage. *Eur Radiol* 2003;13:2192–2195.

Mizuno T, Takanashi Y, Onodera H, et al. A case of lymphomatoid granulomatosis/angiocentric immunoproliferative lesion with long clinical course and diffuse brain involvement. *J Neurol Sci* 2003;15:67–76.

Petrella TM, Walker IR, Jones GW, et al. Radiotherapy to control CNS lymphomatoid granulomatosis: a case report and review of the literature. *Am J Hematol* 1999;62:239–241.

Tateishi U, Terae S, Ogata A, et al. MR imaging of the brain in lymphomatoid granulomatosis. *Am J Neuroradiol* 2001;22:1283–1290.

Chapter 58

Pineal Region Tumors

Lisa M. DeAngelis and Jeffrey N. Bruce

The pineal gland is composed of glandular tissue, glia, endothelial cells, and sympathetic nerve terminals. The numerous cell types that make up the normal gland and surrounding periventricular region may lead to a diverse group of tumors (Table 58.1), all of which may have a similar clinical presentation.

Pineocytomas and pineoblastomas arise from pineal glandular elements, astrocytomas and oligodendrogliomas from glial cells, hemangioblastomas from endothelial cells, and chemodectomas from sympathetic nerve cells. Arachnoid cells in the reflections of the tela choroidea, adjacent to the pineal gland, give rise to meningiomas. Ependymomas arise from ependymal cells that line the third ventricle. Germ-cell tumors (GCTs) derive from primitive germ-cell rests that are retained in the pineal and other midline structures after embryologic migration.

Pineal tumors account for about 1% of all intracranial tumors in the United States. In Asia, where GCTs are common, pineal-cell tumors constitute 4% to 7% of all intracranial tumors.

GERM-CELL TUMORS

GCTs account for approximately one-third of all pineal tumors and are histologically identical to gonadal GCTs. They predominate in men and usually occur in children and adolescents. Pineal GCTs occur almost exclusively in boys, but suprasellar tumors occur equally in boys and girls. GCTs fall into 2 major categories: germinomas and nongerminomatous (NGGCT) that include choriocarcinomas, embryonal-cell carcinomas, teratocarcinomas, and endodermal sinus tumors. Benign, mature teratomas may also be seen.

Germinomas arise in the midline, usually in the pineal area and suprasellar cistern, and occasionally in both areas simultaneously. Rarely do they develop in the cerebral hemispheres. Germinomas account for about half of all intracranial GCTs. They are histologically identical to the testicular seminoma and ovarian dysgerminoma.

Germinomas are highly malignant; pathologically they are frequently infiltrated by lymphocytes, which may occasionally confuse the diagnosis. Germinomas label with placental alkaline phosphatase; some contain syncytiotrophoblastic elements that produce beta human chorionic gonadotropin (β-hCG), which confers a slightly worse prognosis in some studies (Table 58.2).

Germinomas may occasionally seed the CSF. NGGCTs are highly malignant and more aggressive than germinomas; they metastasize to the CSF more frequently than germinomas. Choriocarcinoma contains cyto- and syncytiotrophoblastic cells that produce β-hCG. Endodermal sinus tumors contain yolk sac elements that produce alpha-fetoprotein (AFP). High levels of β-hCG or AFP in the CSF or serum indicate the presence of malignant germ-cell elements. All patients with GCTs should have serum and CSF tested for markers, a complete-spine MRI with

▶ **TABLE 58.1** **Summary of Pathologically Verified Pineal Tumors at the New York Neurological Institute (1978–1998)**

Type	Benign	Malignant	Male: Female	Average Age (yr)
Germ cell	13	51	58/6	20.2
Pineal cell	9	41	25/25	36.2
Glial cell	19	34	27/26	25.6
Meningioma	10	0	6/4	50.8
Pineal cyst	10	0	3/7	33.8
Miscellaneous	3	5	4/4	50.6
Total	64	131	123/72	29.3

TABLE 58.2 Biologic Markers in Germ Cell Tumors

Tumors	βhCG	AFP
Immature teratoma	?	+/−
Germinoma	−	−
Germinoma with syncytiotrophoblastic cells	+	−
Embryonal cell carcinoma	+/−	+/−
Choriocarcinoma	++	−
Endodermal sinus tumor	−	++

β-hCG: beta human chorionic gonadatropin; AFP, alpha-fetoprotein.

gadolinium, and CSF for cytologic examination to complete staging prior to treatment.

Treatment first involves surgical resection to establish the diagnosis and debulk the tumor; if possible, gross total excision is the surgical goal. Patients with pure germinomas should be treated with radiotherapy, usually to 50.4 Gy; the port must include the whole ventricular system, and some radiotherapists treat the whole brain. If the tumor is disseminated in the CSF, craniospinal radiation is required. Chemotherapy may be useful at recurrence but is not recommended at diagnosis because most germinoma patients are cured with radiotherapy alone. NGGCTs require craniospinal radiotherapy and adjuvant chemotherapy in all cases after maximal resection. Benign GCTs such as teratomas, dermoids, and epidermoids are generally curable with surgery alone.

PINEAL CELL TUMORS

Primary pineal-cell tumors are classified as low-grade pineocytomas, intermediate-grade or the highly malignant pineoblastoma. The higher grade tumors tend to occur in children and young adults, whereas pineocytomas usually occur in adults. Pineal tumors of all histologic grades may seed the leptomeninges, but pineocytomas do so only rarely. Complete resection of a pineocytoma does not require additional therapy but incomplete resection should be followed by radiation. Intermediate-grade pineocytomas require radiotherapy and pineoblastomas require neuraxis radiation and chemotherapy.

GLIOMAS

Gliomas account for one-third of pineal tumors. Most are invasive and have a prognosis comparable to astrocytomas of the upper brainstem. Some gliomas are low-grade, cystic, and may be surgically curable. Anaplastic astrocytomas and glioblastomas are less common. Oligodendrogliomas and ependymomas may also occur. Treatment of these tumors is identical to the treatment of gliomas in other areas of the CNS.

MENINGIOMAS

Meningiomas may arise from the velum interpositum or from the tentorial edge. They occur predominantly in middle age patients and in the elderly. They are amenable to surgical resection.

METASTASIS AND OTHER MISCELLANEOUS TUMORS

The pineal gland does not have a blood–brain barrier and, like the pituitary gland, may be underrecognized as a site of CNS metastasis from systemic tumors. Miscellaneous

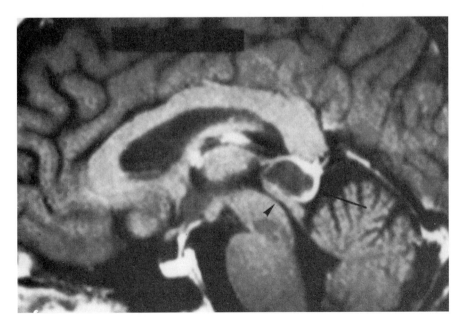

FIGURE 58.1. Sagittal T1-weighted gadolinium enhanced MRI of a pineal cyst. These cysts may have rim enhancement (*arrow*) and may be up to 3 cm in diameter. They rarely cause compression of the Sylvian aqueduct (*arrowhead* on patent aqueduct) and are rarely symptomatic. Histologically, they are normal variants of the pineal gland and require no treatment; they must be distinguished from cystic tumors. Growth of the cyst on serial MRIs or the development of hydrocephalus is sufficient cause to doubt the diagnosis, and surgical resection should be considered.

tumors include sarcoma, hemangioblastoma, choroid plexus papilloma, lymphoma, and chemodectoma.

PINEAL CYSTS

Benign cysts of the pineal gland are often found incidentally on imaging studies, and it is important to distinguish them from cystic tumors. They are normal variants of the pineal gland and consist of a cystic structure surrounded by normal pineal parenchymal tissue (Fig. 58.1).

Radiographically, they are up to 2 cm in diameter and often have some degree of peripheral enhancement as a result of the compressed normal pineal gland. Pineal cysts may be found in 4% of all MRI scans. These cysts are static, anatomic variants and need no treatment unless they become symptomatic. The most common symptoms are headaches, followed by visual symptoms. The cysts may be sufficiently large to cause obstructive hydrocephalus. Decompression can occasionally be accomplished by third-ventricular endoscopic resection of the cyst.

General Considerations for Pineal Region Tumors

Symptoms

Pineal region tumors may become symptomatic from one of three mechanisms: increased intracranial pressure from hydrocephalus, direct compression of brainstem and cerebellum, or endocrine dysfunction. Headache, associated with hydrocephalus, is the most common symptom at onset, and is caused by obstruction of third-ventricular outflow at the aqueduct of Sylvius (Table 58.3).

More advanced hydrocephalus may result in papilledema, gait disorder, nausea, vomiting, lethargy, and memory disturbance. Direct midbrain compression may cause disorders of ocular movements, such as Parinaud syndrome (paralysis of upgaze, convergence or retraction nystagmus, and light-near pupillary dissociation) or the Sylvian aqueduct syndrome (paralysis of downgaze or horizontal gaze superimposed upon a Parinaud syndrome). Either lid retraction (Collier sign) or ptosis may follow dorsal midbrain compression or infiltration. Fourth nerve palsy with diplopia and head tilt may be seen. Ataxia and dysmetria may result from direct cerebellar compression.

Endocrine dysfunction is rare, usually arising from secondary effects of hydrocephalus or tumor spread to the hypothalamic region (Fig. 58.2). The symptoms may occur early, before any radiographic documentation of hypothalamic seeding.

Although precocious puberty has been linked with pineal masses, documented cases are rare. Precocious puberty is actually precocious pseudopuberty because the hypothalamic-gonadal axis is not mature. It occurs in boys with choriocarcinomas or germinomas with syncytiotro-

▶ **TABLE 58.3**   Presenting Symptoms and Signs in 100 Consecutive Patients with Pineal Region Tumors at the New York Neurological Institute

Symptoms	Number	Signs	Number
Headache	87	Parinaud syndrome	75
Nausea/vomiting	32	Ataxia	39
Gait unsteadiness	32	Papilledema	36
Diplopia	31	Normal exam	12
Blurred vision	19	4th nerve palsy	5
Memory impairment	16	Obtundation	4
Lethargy	11	6th nerve palsy	3
Altered consciousness	9	Spasticity	3
Personality change	9	Visual field deficit	1
Visual obscurations	4	Psychomotor retardation	1
Syncope	3		
Polyuria/polydipsia	3		
Seizures	3		
Tremor	3		
Neck stiffness	2		
Numbness	2		
Developmental delay	2		
Incontinence	2		
Precocious puberty	1		
Rigidity	1		
Amenorrhea	1		
Subarachnoid hemorrhage	1		

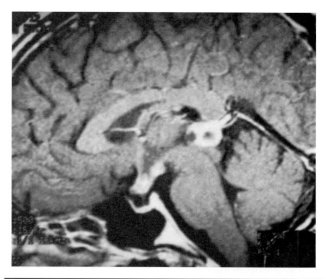

FIGURE 58.2. Sagittal MRI with gadolinium showing multicentric germinoma involving the pineal region and infiltrating the mammillary bodies, optic chiasm, and pituitary stalk. This patient presented with diminished visual fields and diabetes insipidus.

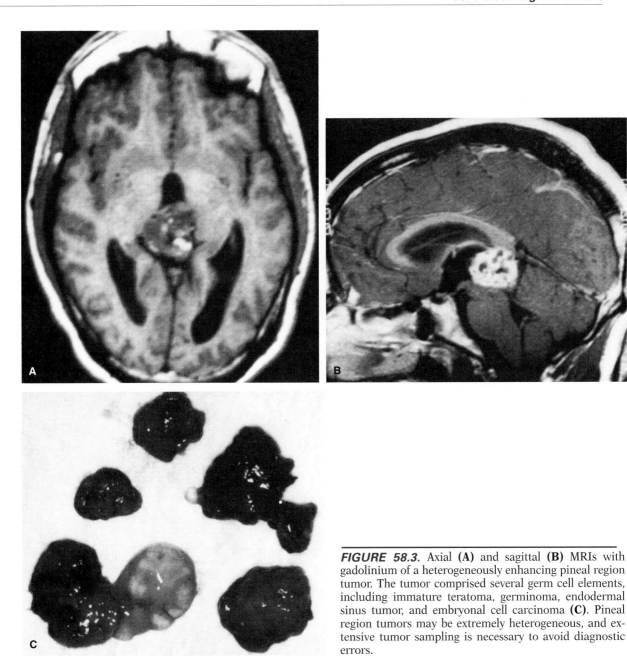

FIGURE 58.3. Axial **(A)** and sagittal **(B)** MRIs with gadolinium of a heterogeneously enhancing pineal region tumor. The tumor comprised several germ cell elements, including immature teratoma, germinoma, endodermal sinus tumor, and embryonal cell carcinoma **(C)**. Pineal region tumors may be extremely heterogeneous, and extensive tumor sampling is necessary to avoid diagnostic errors.

phoblastic cells and ectopic secretion of β-hCG. In boys, the luteinizing hormone-like effects of β-hCG may stimulate Leydig cells to produce androgens that induce development of secondary sexual characteristics and pseudopuberty. This phenomenon does not occur in girls with pineal region tumors because GCTs are rare in females, and both luteinizing hormone and follicle-stimulating hormone are necessary to trigger ovarian estrogen production.

Diagnosis

MRI with gadolinium is mandatory for all pineal tumors to determine the presence of hydrocephalus, and to eval-

uate tumor size, vascularity, and homogeneity. In particular, sagittal MRI reveals the relationship of the tumor to surrounding structures, and also evaluates possible ventricular seeding. Angiography is not performed unless a vascular anomaly is suspected. Measurement of AFP and β-hCG in serum and CSF is required in the preoperative workup. If β-hCG or AFP levels are elevated, malignant germ-cell elements are present even if histologic examination fails to reveal NGGCT elements because a small island of these cells within a large tumor may be overlooked. Despite improved imaging and CSF markers, a definite histologic diagnosis requires pathologic examination of tumor tissue and all patients should undergo surgery.

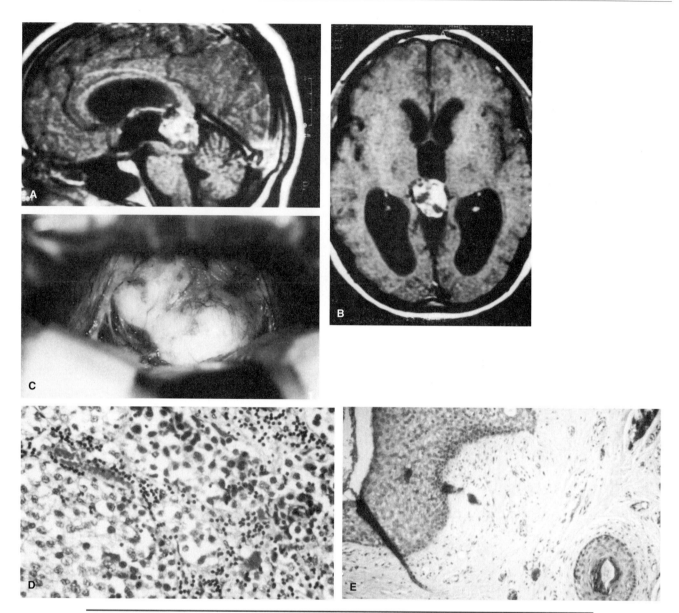

FIGURE 58.4. Sagittal (**A**) and axial (**B**) MRIs with gadolinium of a mixed dermoid/germinoma causing hydrocephalus. **C:** Intraoperative photograph shows the tumor, which was completely resected through a supracerebellar-infratentorial approach without neurologic deficits (cerebellum is at the bottom of the photograph covered by a retractor). **D:** and **E:** Histologic analysis revealed a mixed dermoid/germinoma.

Surgery

Owing to the wide variety of pineal region tumor subtypes, a histologic diagnosis is mandatory for optimal patient management (Fig. 58.3). The pineal region may be reached surgically from one of several approaches, above or below the tentorium, depending upon tumor size and coexistent hydrocephalus (Fig. 58.4).

Complete excision is the goal for any pineal tumor. Nearly one-third of pineal tumors are benign and curable with complete resection alone. With malignant tumors, aggressive tumor resection provides the best opportunity for accurate histologic diagnosis and may

increase the effectiveness of adjuvant radiotherapy or chemotherapy. The overall operative mortality is about 4%, with an additional 3% permanent major morbidity. The most serious complication of surgery is hemorrhage into a partially resected malignant tumor. The most common postoperative complications are ocular palsies, altered mental status, and ataxia, which are usually transient. For patients with obviously disseminated tumor or those with medical problems that pose excessive surgical risks, stereotactic biopsy is a reasonable alternative for obtaining diagnostic tissue. Although gaining in popularity, stereotactic biopsy is not performed routinely because of possible sampling error through insufficient

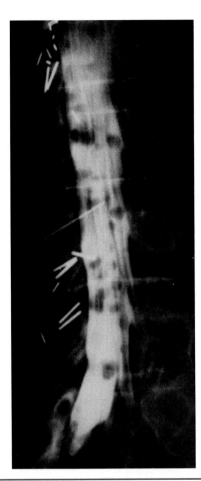

FIGURE 58.5. Intradural seeding from a pineal tumor. Lumbar myelography, oblique view, demonstrates intradural filling defects studding the lumbar nerve roots. These represent "drop" metastases. (Courtesy of Drs. J. A. Bello and S. K. Hilal.)

tissue analysis, increased risk of hemorrhage from the adjacent deep venous system and highly vascular pineal tumors, and a better prognosis that follows aggressive resection.

Postoperative Staging

All patients with pineal-cell tumors and GCTs are evaluated for CSF seeding (Fig. 58.5). High-resolution gadolinium enhanced MRI of the complete spine should be performed. Even if the spine MRI is negative, CSF analysis for cytology and markers is still required in all patients.

Radiotherapy

All patients with pineoblastomas, NGGCT, and disseminated germinomas require neuraxis radiotherapy, usually to a total dose of about 36 Gy with a boost to the primary site to achieve a dose of at least 54 Gy. Ger-

minomas and pineal-parenchymal tumors of intermediate differentiation require local radiation to a dose of 50 Gy to 60 Gy. Gliomas are treated according to histologic subtype.

Experience with stereotactic radiosurgery is limited because pineal tumors are rare. It has been used with some success for tumors less than 3 cm in diameter at recurrence, provided there is no evidence of CSF dissemination. There are reports of disease control using radiosurgery as the sole treatment for pineocytoma, but it rarely produces complete tumor regression and is probably not optimal initial therapy.

Chemotherapy

Chemotherapy has been of most benefit with NGGCTs and pineoblastomas. The most commonly used regimens are combinations of cisplatin, vinblastine, and bleomycin or cisplatin and VP-16 (e.g., etoposide). Chemotherapy is usually given after completion of neuraxis radiation, except in young children in whom radiotherapy is avoided because of the risk of severe, long-term effects on growth and cognition. Young children are treated with chemotherapy alone and radiotherapy is deferred until they are at least 3 years of age or older. Initial attempts to avoid radiation in all patients by using aggressive chemotherapy resulted in an unacceptably high incidence (50%) of recurrence at 2 years, including patients with germinoma, which is curable with radiation alone. Therefore, chemotherapy is not used as part of the initial treatment of localized germinomas.

Long-Term Outcome

Generally, benign pineal tumors and pineal cysts are curable with surgery alone. Among malignant tumors, the prognosis depends on tumor histology (Table 58.1). Germinomas have an 80% to 90% 5-year survival rate following surgery and radiotherapy. Patients with NGGCT usually relapse within 2 years, but some may be salvaged with additional chemotherapy. About 80% of patients with pineocytomas survive 5 years, but the 5-year survival rate is only 50% for pineoblastomas.

SUGGESTED READINGS

Balmaceda C, Heller G, Rosenblum M, et al. Chemotherapy without irradiation-a novel approach for newly diagnosed CNS germ cell tumors: results of an international cooperative trial. *J Clin Oncol* 1996;14:2908–2915.

Balmaceda C, Finlay J. Current advances in the diagnosis and management of intracranial germ cell tumors. *Curr Neurol Neurosci Rep* 2004;May;4(3):253–262.

Bruce JN, Stein BM, Connolly ES. Pineal and germ cell tumors. In: Kaye AH, Laws ER, eds. *Brain Tumors: An Encyclopedic Approach*, 2nd ed. London: Churchill Livingstone, 2001:771–800.

Choi JU, Kim DS, Chung SS, Kim TS. Treatment of germ cell tumors in the pineal region. *Childs Nerv Syst* 1998;14:41–48.

Dattoli MJ, Newall J. Radiation therapy for intracranial germinoma: the case for limited volume treatment. *Int J Radiat Oncol Biol Phys* 1990;19:429–433.

Engel U, Gottschalk S, Niehaus L, et al. Cystic lesions of the pineal region—MRI and pathology. *Neuroradiology* 2000;42:399–402.

Fetell MR, Bruce JN, Burke AM, et al. Nonneoplastic pineal cysts. *Neurology* 1991;41:1034–1040.

Gururangan S, McLaughlin C, Quinn J, et al. High-dose chemotherapy with autologous stem-cell rescue in children and adults with newly diagnosed pineoblastomas. *J Clin Oncol* 2003;21:2187–2191.

Hasegawa T, Kondziolka D, Hadjipanayis CG, Flickinger JC, Lunsford LD. Stereotactic radiosurgery for CNS nongerminomatous germ cell tumors. Report of four cases. *Pediatr Neurosurg* 2003;38:329–333.

Herrmann HD, Westphal M, Winkler K, Laas RW, Schulte FJ. Treatment of nongerminomatous germ cell tumors of the pineal region. *Neurosurgery* 1994;34:524–529.

Hirato J, Nakazato Y. Pathology of pineal region tumors. *J Neurooncol* 2001;54:239–249.

Kakita A, Kobayashi K, Aoki N, et al. Lung carcinoma metastasis presenting as a pineal region tumor. *Neuropathology* 2003;23:57–60.

Kellie SJ, Boyce H, Dunkel IJ, et al. Primary chemotherapy for intracranial nongerminomatous germ cell tumors: results of the second international CNS germ cell study group protocol. *J Clin Oncol* 2004;22:846–853.

Knierim DS, Yamada S. Pineal tumors and associated lesions: the effect of ethnicity on tumor type and treatment. *Pediatr Neurosurg* 2003;38:307–323.

Kobayashi T, Yoshida J, Ishiyama J, et al. Combination chemotherapy with cisplatin and etoposide for malignant intracranial germ cell tumors. *J Neurosurg* 1989;70:676–681.

Kochi M, Itoyama Y, Shiraishi S, et al. Successful treatment of intracranial nongerminomatous malignant germ cell tumors by administering neoadjuvant chemotherapy and radiotherapy before excision of residual tumors. *J Neurosurg* 2003;99:106–114.

Kondziolka D, Hadjipanayis CG, Flickinger JC, Lunsford LD. The role of radiosurgery for the treatment of pineal parenchymal tumors. *Neurosurgery* 2002;51:880–889.

Korogi Y, Takahashi M, Ushio Y. MRI of pineal region tumors. *J Neurooncol* 2001;54:251–261.

Lutterbach J, Fauchon F, Schild SE, et al. Malignant pineal parenchymal tumors in adult patients: patterns of care and prognostic factors. *Neurosurgery* 2002;51:44–55.

Mandera M, Marcol W, Bierzynska-Macyszyn G, Kluczewska E. Pineal cysts in childhood. *Childs Nerv Syst* 2003;19:750–755.

Matsutani M, Sano K, Takakura K, et al. Primary intracranial germ cell tumors: a clinical analysis of 153 histologically verified cases. *J Neurosurg* 1997;86:446–455.

Matsutani M. Clinical management of primary central nervous system germ cell tumors. *Semin Oncol* 2004;Oct;31(5):676–683.

Michielsen G, Benoit Y, Baert E, et al. Symptomatic pineal cysts: clinical manifestations and management. *Acta Neurochir* 2002;144:233–242.

Nogueira K, Liberman B, Pimentel-Filho FR, et al. hCG-secreting pineal teratoma causing precocious puberty: report of two patients and review of the literature. *J Pediatr Endocrinol Metab* 2002;15:1195–1201.

Ogawa K, Toita T, Nakamura K, et al. Treatment and prognosis of patients with intracranial nongerminomatous malignant germ cell tumors. *Cancer* 2003;98:369–376.

Packer RJ, Cohen BH, Coney K. Intracranial germ cell tumors. *Oncologist* 2000;5:312–320.

Patel SR, Buckner JC, Smithson WA, et al. Cisplatin-based chemotherapy in primary central nervous system germ cell tumors. *J Neurooncol* 1992;12:47–52.

Plowman PN, Pizer B, Kingston JE. Pineal parenchymal tumors: II. On the aggressive behaviour of pineoblastoma in patients with an inherited mutation of the RBI gene. *Clin Oncol (R Coll Radiol)* 2004; Jun;16(4):244–247.

Regis J, Bouillot P, Rouby-Volot F, et al. Pineal region tumors and the role of stereotactic biopsy: review of the mortality, morbidity, and diagnostic rates in 370 cases. *Neurosurgery* 1996;39:907–914.

Sawamura Y, de Tribolet N, Ishii N, Abe H. Management of primary intracranial germinomas: diagnostic surgery or radical resection? *J Neurosurg* 1997;87:262–266.

Smith AA, Weng E, Handler M, Foreman NK. Intracranial germ cell tumors: a single institution experience and review of the literature. *J Neurooncol* 2004; Jun;68(2):153–159.

Spunt SL, Walsh MF, Krasin MJ, Helton KJ, Billups CA, Cain AM, Pappo AS. Brain metastases of malignant germ cell tumors in children and adolescents. *Cancer* 2004; Aug 1;101(3):620–626.

Timmermann B, Kortmann RD, Kuhl J, et al. Role of radiotherapy in the treatment of supratentorial primitive neuroectodermal tumors in childhood: results of the prospective German brain tumor trials HIT 88/89 and 91. *J Clin Oncol* 2002;20:842–849.

Wolden SL, Wara WM, Larson DA, et al. Radiation therapy for primary intracranial germ cell tumors. *Int J Radiat Oncol Biol Phys* 1995;32:943–949.

Yoshida J, Sugita K, Kobayashi T, et al. Prognosis of intracranial germ cell tumours: effectiveness of chemotherapy with cisplatin and etoposide (CDDP and VP-16). *Acta Neurochir* 1993;120:111–117.

C h a p t e r   5 9

Tumors of the Pituitary Gland

Lisa M. DeAngelis, Pamela U. Freda, and Jeffrey N. Bruce

The true incidence of pituitary adenomas is difficult to ascertain because they are often asymptomatic; autopsy estimates of incidence range from 1.7% to 24%. There is no sexual predilection, but the tumors are most common in adults, peaking in the third and fourth decades; children and adolescents account for about 10% of cases. These tumors are not hereditary except for rare families with multiple endocrine neoplasia I (MEN-I), an autosomal-dominant condition manifested by a high incidence of pituitary adenomas and tumors of other endocrine glands.

PATHOLOGY

Pituitary tumors are classified in four ways: (1) size (e.g., microadenomas are less than 1 cm in diameter and macroadenomas are larger than 1 cm); microadenomas cause symptoms by excess hormone secretion whereas macroadenomas usually cause symptoms by compressing normal glandular or neural structures; (2) endocrine function: this is based on the particular hormones being oversecreted; (3) clinical findings; and (4) histology. Almost all pituitary tumors are histologically benign; pituitary carcinomas are rare.

Functional classification is based on endocrinologic activity, dividing tumors into secreting and nonsecreting types. Secreting tumors are less common and produce one or more anterior pituitary hormones, including prolactin (the prolactinoma is the most common endocrinologically active tumor), growth hormone, adrenocorticotropic hormone (ACTH) causing Cushing disease, follicle-stimulating hormone (FSH), or luteinizing hormone. Mixed secretory tumors account for 10% of adenomas; interestingly, even multihormone adenomas have a monoclonal origin. Secretion of more than one hormone has implications for medical therapy because all excess hormone secretion must be treated. *Null cell* or nonsecreting adenomas demonstrate no clinical or immunohistochemical evidence of hormone secretion.

Macroadenomas may invade the dura or bone, and may infiltrate surrounding structures such as the cavernous sinus, cranial nerves, blood vessels, sphenoid bone, and sinus or brain. Locally invasive pituitary adenomas are nearly always histologically benign. In some studies, but not all, the proliferation index correlates with growth velocity and recurrence. However, their invasive character may be independent of the growth rate.

In general, older patients have adenomas that grow more slowly than the lesions in younger patients do. *Pituitary carcinomas* are highly invasive, rapidly growing, and anaplastic, but unequivocal diagnosis relies on the presence of distant metastases. Pleomorphism and mitotic figures are insufficient histologic features to justify the diagnosis of carcinoma because they may be seen in benign adenomas.

The posterior pituitary, which contains the terminal processes of hypothalamic neurons and supporting glial cells, is a rare site of neoplasia. *Infundibulomas* are rare tumors of the neurohypophysis; they are variants of pilocytic astrocytomas. *Granular-cell tumors* (e.g., *myoblastomas* or *choristomas*), also rare tumors of the neurohypophysis, are of uncertain origin.

CLINICAL FEATURES

Clinical manifestations stem either from endocrine dysfunction or mass effect with invasion or compression of surrounding neural and vascular structures. The manifestations and management of hormonally active tumors are discussed in Chapter 146. Here, we limit discussion to nonsecretory tumors, most of which are macroadenomas when they come to clinical attention. Macroadenomas may present with panhypopituitarism when the normal pituitary gland is destroyed. Headaches result from stretching of the diaphragma sellae and adjacent dural structures that transmit sensation through the first branch of the trigeminal nerve. Visual field abnormalities are caused by compression of the crossing fibers in the optic chiasm, first affecting the superior temporal quadrants and then the inferior temporal quadrants, leading to a bitemporal hemianopia. Further expansion compromises the noncrossing fibers and affects the lower nasal quadrants and finally the upper nasal quadrants (Fig. 59.1).

Visual loss may be accompanied by optic disc pallor and loss of central visual acuity, but papilledema is rare. Patients usually complain of blurring or dimming of vision or they may be unaware of loss of their peripheral vision. Formal visual field testing is important because some tumors affect only the macular fibers, causing central hemianopic scotomas that may be missed on routine screening. Bitemporal hemianopia is most common, but any pattern

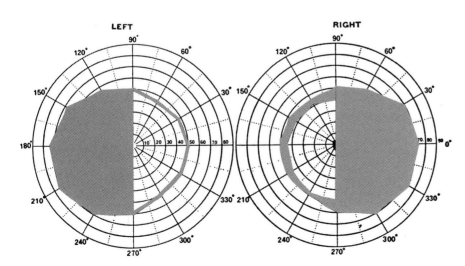

FIGURE 59.1. Pituitary macroadenoma. Bitemporal hemianopia; visual acuity O.D. 15/200, O.S. 15/30. The blind half-fields are black. (Courtesy of Dr. Max Chamlin.)

of visual loss is possible, including unilateral or homonymous hemianopia.

Lateral extension of the tumor with compression or invasion of the cavernous sinus may compromise third, fourth, or sixth cranial nerve functions, manifesting as diplopia. The third cranial nerve is most commonly affected. There may be numbness in the V1 or V2 distribution. Overall, however, cranial nerve dysfunction is not a common feature of adenomas and may be more suggestive of other neoplasms of the cavernous sinus.

Adenomas may become very large before causing symptoms. Suprasellar extension may compress the foramen of Monro, to cause hydrocephalus and symptoms of increased intracranial pressure (ICP). Hypothalamic dysfunction may lead to diabetes insipidus; however, diabetes insipidus is relatively rare with adenomas and, if present, is more suggestive of conditions associated with inflammation, or possible tumor invasion of the pituitary stalk. Extensive subfrontal extension with compression of both frontal lobes may cause personality changes or dementia. There may be seizures or motor and sensory dysfunction. Erosion of the skull base may cause CSF rhinorrhea.

Complete endocrine evaluation is necessary for all patients with pituitary tumors, not only to establish the diagnosis of a secreting adenoma but also to determine the presence of hypopituitarism (Table 59.1), which may result from compression of the normal pituitary gland.

Serum hormone levels should be obtained in all patients, and adequate hormone replacement, usually for thyroid, sex and adrenal hormones, is required. Long-term follow-up monitoring is essential because hypopituitarism may develop years after diagnosis and treatment. Nonse-creting tumors cause slight elevations of serum prolactin levels to about 100 ng/mL, which is attributed to compression of the pituitary stalk, interrupting dopaminergic fibers that inhibit prolactin release. Mild elevations are common and must be distinguished from prolactin-secreting tumors that typically produce prolactin levels of more than 200 ng/mL. This distinction is important therapeutically because nonsecreting tumors do not respond to dopamine agonists (e.g., cabergoline or bromocriptine).

In about 5% of pituitary tumors, the first symptoms are those of pituitary apoplexy caused by hemorrhage or infarction of the adenoma. Symptoms include sudden onset of severe headache, oculomotor palsies, nausea, vomiting, altered mental state, diplopia, and rapidly progressive visual loss. Apoplexy is diagnosed by CT or MRI and occasionally is an indication for emergency surgery (Fig. 59.2).

Histologically, the adenoma shows massive necrosis and hemorrhage. Apoplexy is almost always caused by a pituitary tumor, but it has been reported in other conditions, such as lymphocytic hypophysitis. Pituitary adenomas may enlarge during pregnancy, causing acute symptoms or even apoplexy.

RADIOGRAPHIC FEATURES

MRI is the best way to evaluate pituitary pathology, because soft tissue is seen clearly without interference from the bony surroundings of the sella. MRI also produces images in any plane, which helps define the relationship of the tumor to the surrounding structures. Vascular structures such as the adjacent carotid artery are easily visualized by signal void. Normally, the anterior lobe of the pituitary gland has the same signal as white matter on T1-weighted imaging. With gadolinium, the normal gland enhances homogeneously. Small punctate areas of heterogeneity may be the result of local variations in vascularity, microcyst formation, or granularity within the gland. The posterior lobe shows increased signal on T1-weighted images, probably representing neurosecretory granules in the antidiuretic hormone (ADH)–containing axons.

Microadenomas are sometimes difficult to see directly on MRI but may be inferred by glandular asymmetry, focal sellar erosion, asymmetric convexity of the upper margin of the gland, or displacement of the infundibulum (Fig. 59.3).

The normal gland usually shows more enhancement than the microadenoma (Fig. 59.4). In the presence of a macroadenoma, the normal gland may not be visualized and the bright signal of the posterior lobe may be absent. Areas of increased signal on the T1-weighted image may stem from hemorrhage; areas of low signal may represent cystic degeneration. MRI alone is usually

▶ **TABLE 59.1 Symptoms of Pituitary Failure**

1. Gonadotroph Failure
   Loss of libido
   Impotence
2. Thyrotroph Failure
   Fatigue
   Malaise
   Apathy
   Constipation
   Weight gain
3. Somatotroph Failure
   Weight gain
   Depression
   Premature atherosclerosis
   Muscle weakness
4. Corticotroph Failure
   Fatigue
   Weight gain
   Hypoglycemia

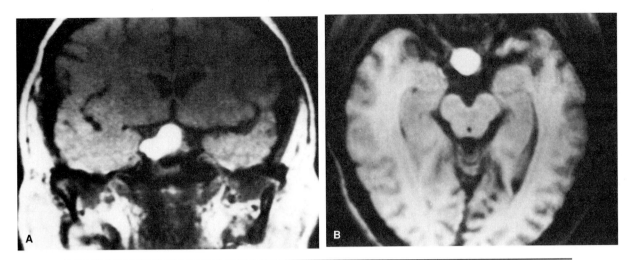

FIGURE 59.2. Coronal (**A**) and axial (**B**) MRIs demonstrating a high signal pituitary mass that turned out to be a hemorrhage in a patient with apoplexy. This patient had a successful tumor resection through a standard transsphenoidal approach.

sufficient, but CT may show the bony anatomy in better detail. MRI usually excludes an aneurysm, but MRA or an angiogram is indicated if aneurysm is a serious diagnostic concern.

ACTH-secreting tumors may be too small to visualize on MRI. Diagnosis is suggested by the clinical fea-

tures of Cushing disease, elevated 24-hour urinary free-cortisol levels, loss of ACTH suppression by glucocorticoids, and elevated ACTH levels. However, the specific diagnosis of an ACTH-secreting pituitary tumor may require measurement of ACTH in each inferior petrosal sinus, which drains the pituitary gland.

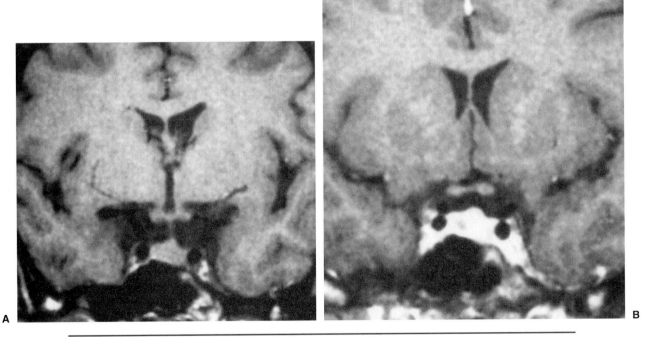

FIGURE 59.3. Pituitary microadenoma. A: T1-weighted coronal MRI shows slight tilting of the pituitary stalk to the left, with questionable fullness of the right pituitary gland. These are secondary signs of pituitary microadenoma but are not sufficient to establish the diagnosis radiographically. **B:** T1-weighted coronal scan after gadolinium enhancement demonstrates a tiny focus of relative hypointensity within the right pituitary gland. This is consistent with right pituitary microadenoma. (Courtesy of Dr. S. Chan.)

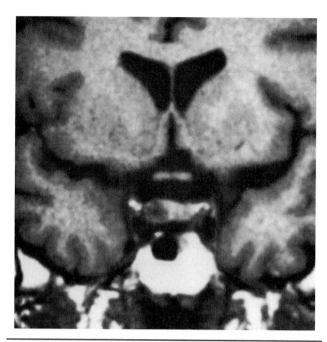

FIGURE 59.4. Pituitary adenoma. T1-weighted coronal MRI after gadolinium enhancement demonstrates a discrete focus of hypointensity in the right pituitary gland, most consistent with pituitary adenoma. (Courtesy of Dr. S. Chan.)

DIFFERENTIAL DIAGNOSIS

Most lesions in the differential diagnosis have characteristic radiographic or clinical syndromes that distinguish them from pituitary adenomas. Craniopharyngiomas have a predilection for children, are calcified, and usually include cystic areas that contain highly proteinaceous fluid with cholesterol crystals. Rathke cleft cysts are similar to craniopharyngiomas but have a cystic appearance, without any solid component. Meningiomas are commonly found in the diaphragma sellae, planum sphenoidale, and tuberculum sellae, and may be difficult to distinguish from a macroadenoma.

Distinguishing characteristics of meningiomas include enhancement, visualization of a cleavage plane between the mass and the sellar contents, normally sized sella, and the presence of a dural tail of enhancement. Optic glioma, hypothalamic glioma, germinoma, dermoid tumor, metastasis, and nasopharyngeal carcinoma are less commonly seen entities that should be considered. Chordomas characteristically show extensive bony destruction of the clivus. Mucoceles of the sphenoid sinus may simulate pituitary adenoma. Visual symptoms and sellar enlargement may also result from chronic, increased ICP of any origin. Characteristic signal voids on MRI usually distinguish an aneurysm. The differential diagnosis also includes sarcoidosis, lymphoma, lymphocytic hypophysitis, and other granulomatous diseases.

Herniation of the subarachnoid space into the sella through an incompetent diaphragma sellae may produce the empty sella syndrome, with enlargement of the sella and flattening of the pituitary gland on its floor (Fig. 59.5). This syndrome may be associated with pseudotumor cerebri or CSF rhinorrhea. Although most are not symptomatic, an empty sella may be associated with headaches and occasionally with mild hypopituitarism, but the visual fields are usually normal. The condition is readily seen on MRI and may be a complication of previous transphenoidal surgery.

TREATMENT

Pituitary tumors are histologically benign tumors, but they are associated with a significant decrease in a patient's quality of life and functional capacity. Early intervention may minimize disability and must address both endocrinologic and neurologic function.

Treatment of pituitary adenomas begins with replacement of pituitary hormones if deficient; replacement of thyroid and adrenal hormones is most important. Steroid replacement must be adequate for stressful situations, including for surgery on the pituitary lesion. Data from a randomized, controlled trial demonstrated that a low-dose protocol for steroid replacement reduced the incidence of postoperative diabetes insipidus more effectively than a higher dose conventional protocol; also, patients with small tumors and normal preoperative cortisol levels did not require perioperative hydrocortisone.

The goals of treatment differ according to the functional activity of the tumor. For endocrinologically active tumors, an aggressive approach toward reversing hypersecretion is essential while preserving normal pituitary function. This may often be achieved by surgical excision, although prolactinomas are better controlled by giving dopamine agonists, such as cabergoline, that achieve tumor shrinkage and normalization of prolactin levels in almost all microadenomas and in about 60% of macroadenomas (Fig. 59.6).

Candidates for surgical treatment include patients with prolactinomas who fail to respond medically or those who do not tolerate the side effects of medication. The treatment strategies for secretory adenomas are covered in detail in Chapter 146.

Nonsecreting tumors are best treated by surgical reduction of the mass, while maintaining pituitary function. Resection also offers the advantage of establishing the correct diagnosis. Incidentally discovered, asymptomatic adenomas require no intervention but should be followed with periodic visual field examination and MRI. Onset of symptoms or MRI documentation of growth are indications for treatment.

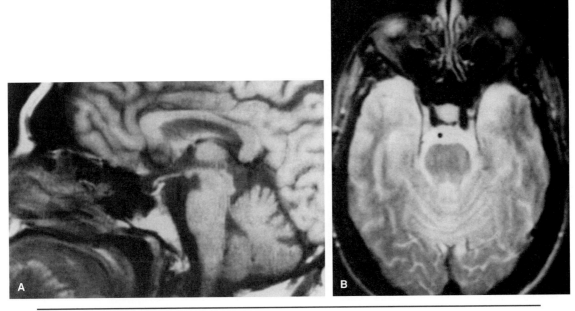

FIGURE 59.5. Empty sella. A: Sagittal T1-weighted MRI demonstrates low-intensity intrasellar signal representing CSF compare with signal within the fourth ventricle). **B:** Axial T2-weighted MRI on a different patient shows increased signal within the sella representing CSF on this pulse sequence (compare with signal from incidentally noted anterior temporal arachnoid cysts). (Courtesy of Drs. J. A. Bello and S. K. Hilal.)

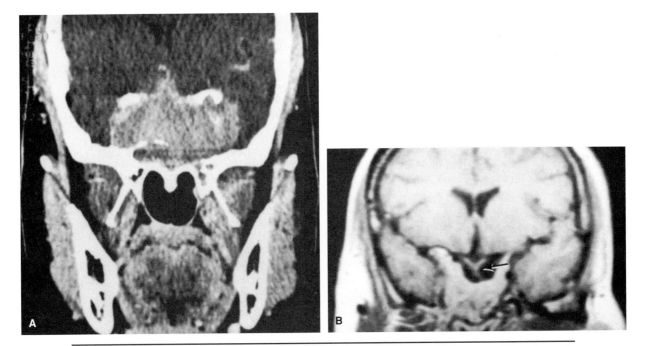

FIGURE 59.6. A: Coronal CT with contrast from a 40-year-old man with bitemporal hemianopsia and a markedly elevated serum prolactin level. A large pituitary adenoma with suprasellar and parasellar extension may be easily seen. **B:** Coronal MRI with contrast after bromocriptine therapy shows marked decrease in the tumor size such that the infundibulum and optic chiasm are decompressed (*arrow*).

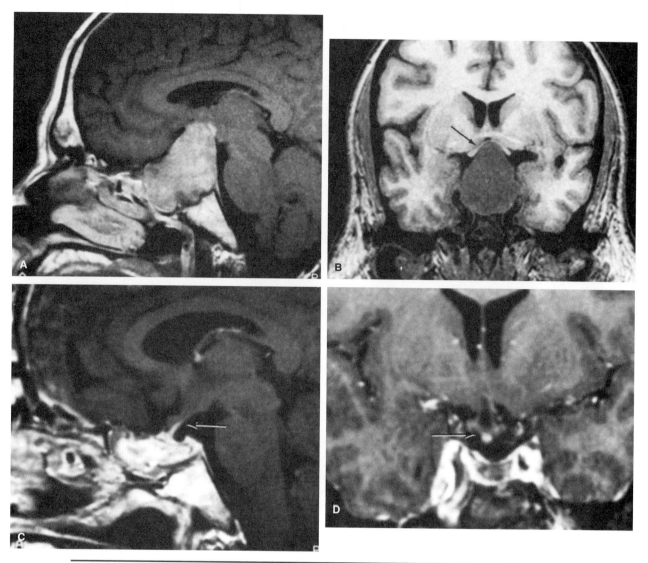

FIGURE 59.7. A: Sagittal MRI showing a large pituitary adenoma filling the sphenoid sinus and extending into the floor of the third ventricle. **B:** On the coronal view, the suprasellar component may be seen compressing the optic chiasm (*arrow*). A large tumor such as this often requires a craniotomy to decompress the optic structures adequately. **C:** Sagittal MRI after a gross total resection of the pituitary adenoma through an extended frontal craniotomy. There are postoperative changes in the sella and sphenoid sinus, and the infundibulum is well decompressed (*arrow*). **D:** On the coronal view, there is no residual tumor, and the optic chiasm and a portion of the infundibulum may be seen clearly (*arrow*).

Surgery

The efficacy and safety of the transsphenoidal approach make it the procedure of choice for the removal of adenomas. Most tumors are soft and friable; transsphenoidal access, although limited, permits complete removal even if there is suprasellar extension or the sella is not enlarged. Transsphenoidal surgery was originally developed by Cushing, but refinements in microsurgery and the availability of steroid replacement and antibiotics have dramatically improved the results. Mortality rates are less than 1%. Major morbidity is less than 3.5%, including stroke,

visual loss, meningitis, CSF leak or cranial nerve palsy. Diabetes insipidus may also develop but is usually transient, requiring temporary hormonal replacement.

A transcranial approach may be preferred for resection of tumors extending into the middle fossa, or if there is suprasellar growth through an intact diaphragm a sellae, with a waistband constriction of the tumor (Fig. 59.7).

A transcranial approach may be necessary to decompress the optic structures before radiation, when a transsphenoidal approach fails to adequately debulk the tumor, or there is persistent major visual loss.

Radiation Therapy

Radiation therapy is complementary to surgery in preventing progression or recurrence. Standard radiation now uses conformal treatment planning to avoid unnecessary dosage to the temporal lobes. Doses of 4,500 cGy to 5,000 cGy, delivered in 180 cGy fractions, are recommended. Radiation may be the only treatment for patients who are poor operative risks, but histologic confirmation is generally desired. Radiation therapy is usually not the initial treatment for hormonally active tumors because it rarely lowers hormone levels to normal and then only after a delay of months or years.

Radiation therapy is indicated for patients with recurrent, medically refractory, hypersecreting tumors or administered postoperatively to patients with invasive or large, incompletely removed adenomas. It is not routinely administered after gross total resection; these patients are followed with serial MRI and visual field examination, and radiation is reserved for documented tumor regrowth.

Early complications of radiation therapy are transient and involve minor inconveniences such as epilation, dry mouth, and altered taste or smell. The most common and important delayed complication is hypopituitarism, which may occur any time from 6 months to 10 years after treatment. Some degree of hypopituitarism occurs in 30% to 50% of patients. Annual endocrine evaluation is necessary to treat this appropriately. Other rare complications include visual loss, radiation necrosis of the temporal lobes, and radiation-induced tumors. To minimize risk of visual loss, optic structures should be decompressed before radiation therapy.

New techniques, such as radiosurgery using proton beam, gamma knife, or the linear accelerator, are being investigated. In these methods, a single high-dose fraction is directed to a limited volume, giving a high biologic effect. These methods may produce more rapid clinical and hormonal responses, potentially with less toxicity. However, there is concern about damage to the optic chiasm or cranial nerves. Radiosurgery is not used for large tumors or those of less than 3 mm distance from the optic apparatus; this therapy may also be associated with a higher incidence of hypopituitarism.

Recurrent Tumors

Patients with recurrent tumors are difficult to manage and treatment must be individualized. If the patient has not had prior radiation, then radiation would be the treatment of choice. Otherwise, repeat transsphenoidal surgery is usually indicated. Other treatment options include stereotactic radiosurgery, which may be effective and safe even in the patient who has had standard external beam radiotherapy.

SUGGESTED READINGS

Bills DC, Meyer FB, Laws ER Jr, et al. A retrospective analysis of pituitary apoplexy. *Neurosurgery* 1993;33:602–609.

Black PM, Hsu DW, Klibanski A, et al. Hormone production in clinically nonfunctioning pituitary adenomas. *J Neurosurg* 1987;66:244–250.

Bradley KM, Adams CBT, Potter CPS, et al. An audit of selected patients with nonfunctioning pituitary adenoma treated by transsphenoidal surgery without irradiation. *Clin Endocrinol* 1994;41:655–659.

Breen P, Flickinger JC, Kondziolka D, Martinez AJ. Radiotherapy for nonfunctional pituitary adenoma: analysis of long-term tumor control. *J Neurosurg* 1998;89:933–938.

Ebersold MJ, Laws ER, Scheithauer BW, Randall RV. Pituitary apoplexy treated by transsphenoidal surgery. A clinicopathological and immunocytochemical study. *J Neurosurg* 1983;58:315–320.

Gertner ME, Kebebew E. Multiple endocrine neoplasia type 2. *Curr Treat Options Oncol* 2004;5(4):315–325.

Goel A, Nadkarni T, Muzumdar D, et al. Giant pituitary tumors: a study based on surgical treatment of 118 cases. *Surg Neurol* 2004;61(5):436–445.

Hall WA, Luciano MG, Doppman JL, et al. Pituitary magnetic resonance imaging in normal human volunteers: occult adenomas in the general population. *Ann Intern Med* 1994;120:817–820.

Honegger J, Prettin C, Feuerhake F, et al. Expression of Ki-67 antigen in nonfunctioning pituitary adenomas: correlation with growth velocity and invasiveness. *J Neurosurg* 2003;99:674–679.

Ibrahim AE, Pickering RM, Gawne-Cain ML, et al. Indices of apoptosis and proliferation as potential prognostic markers in non-functioning pituitary adenomas. *Clin Neuropathol* 2004;23:8–15.

Johnson MD, Woodburn CJ, Vance ML. Quality of life in patients with a pituitary adenoma. *Pituitary* 2003;6:81–87.

Komninos J, Vlassopoulou V, Protopapa D, et al. Tumors metastatic to the pituitary gland: case report and literature review. *J Clin Endocrinol Metab* 2004;89(2):574–580.

Kreutzer J, Fahlbusch R. Diagnosis and treatment of pituitary tumors. *Curr Opin Neurol* 2004;17(6):693–703.

Lee MS, Pless M. Apoplectic lymphocytic hypophysitis. *J Neurosurg* 2003;98:183–185.

Ma W, Ikeda H, Yoshimoto T. Clinicopathologic study of 123 cases of prolactin-secreting pituitary adenomas with special reference to multihormone production and clonality of the adenomas. *Cancer* 2002;95:258–266.

Mejico LS, Miller NR, Dong LM. Clinical features associated with lesions other than pituitary adenoma in patients with an optic chiasmal syndrome. *Am & Ophthalmol* 2004;137(5):908–913.

Nishizawa S, Ohta S, Yokoyama T, Uemura K. Therapeutic strategy for incidentally found pituitary tumors ("pituitary incidentalomas"). *Neurosurgery* 1998;43:1344–1350.

Pollock BE, Carpenter PC. Stereotactic radiosurgery as an alternative to fractionated radiotherapy for patients with recurrent or residual nonfunctioning pituitary adenomas. *Neurosurgery* 2003;53:1086–1091.

Rajaratnam S, Seshadri MS, Chandy MJ, Rajshekhar V. Hydrocortisone dose and postoperative diabetes insipidus in patients undergoing transsphenoidal pituitary surgery: a prospective randomized controlled study. *Br J Neurosurg* 2003;17:437–442.

Scheithauer BW, Kovacs KT, Laws EWJ, et al. Pathology of invasive pituitary tumors with special reference to functional classification. *J Neurosurg* 1986;65:733–744.

Steiner E, Imhof H, Knosp E. Gd-DTPA-enhanced high resolution MR imaging of pituitary adenomas. *Radiographics* 1989;9:587–598.

Swords FM, Allan CA, Plowman PN, et al. Stereotactic radiosurgery XVI: a treatment for previously irradiated pituitary adenomas. *J Clin Endocrinol Metab* 2003;88:5334–5340.

Tanaka Y, Hongo K, Tada T, et al. Growth pattern and rate in residual nonfunctioning pituitary adenomas: correlations among tumor volume doubling time, patient age, and MIB-1 index. *J Neurosurg* 2003;98:359–365.

Tsang RW, Brierley JD, Panzarella T, et al. Radiation therapy for pituitary adenoma: treatment outcome and prognostic factors. *Int J Radiat Oncol Biol Phys* 1994;30:557–565.

Chapter 60

Congenital and Childhood Central Nervous System Tumors

James H. Garvin, Jr., Neil A. Feldstein, and Saadi Ghatan

Childhood brain tumors range from benign congenital lesions to aggressive, infiltrative cancers. Cure rates for malignant brain tumors are less than those of most other common childhood cancers, but research advances and refinement of treatment techniques give a sense of cautious optimism. Research focuses on identifying molecular targets for novel therapies.

EPIDEMIOLOGY

Malignant and benign tumors of the CNS may arise at any time in infancy and childhood. Astrocytomas are the largest group, mostly of low-grade histology, and pilocytic astrocytomas account for 24% of all childhood brain tumors. Next are medulloblastomas, the most frequent malignant tumor (16%). After these are congenital and acquired lesions, a diverse group that includes high-grade astrocytomas (14%), ependymomas (10%), craniopharyngiomas (5.6%), germ-cell tumors (2.5%), and choroid plexus tumors (0.9%). Apart from high-grade astrocytomas, the usual tumors of adults (glioblastoma multiforme, meningioma, oligodendroglioma, pituitary adenoma) are rarely seen. Moreover, tumorigenesis of high-grade astrocytomas in children differs from that in adults, as deduced from comparative genomic hybridization studies. CNS metastases from solid tumors are also uncommon in children. Cerebral metastases are reported in germ-cell tumors (13.5% incidence), osteosarcoma (6.5%), neuroblastoma (4.4%), melanoma (3.6%), Ewing sarcoma (3.3%), rhabdomyosarcoma (1.9%), and Wilms tumor (1.3%).

Primary CNS tumors account for 20% of all childhood cancers, second only to leukemia. Approximately 2,200 cases are diagnosed annually in the United States in children under age 15 years, an incidence of 2.8 per 100,000 population. The reported annual incidence of childhood brain tumors in the United States increased by 35% between 1973 and 1994, led mainly by supratentorial low-grade gliomas and brainstem tumors diagnosed by MRI.

The causes of congenital and childhood CNS tumors remain unknown. A meta-analysis of 10,582 childhood brain tumors from 16 international surveys revealed a male: female ratio of 1.29. Most CNS tumors are sporadic, but some are seen in inherited disorders, especially neurocutaneous syndromes. As described in chapter 100, those with *neurofibromatosis type 1 (NF-1)* have a 10% chance of developing an intracranial tumor, including optic pathway gliomas and astrocytomas elsewhere in the brain and spinal cord. The NF-1 gene maps to chromosome 17q11.2, and loss of one NF-1 allele is evident in nearly all NF1-associated pilocytic astrocytomas, but only rarely in sporadic pilocytic astrocytomas, suggesting different mechanisms of tumor formation. In the less common *neurofibromatosis type 2 (NF-2)*, there is a predisposition to bilateral vestibular schwannomas, with chromosome 22q deletions and NF-2 gene mutations in at least half of cases. NF-2 also predisposes to ependymomas, which commonly show a chromosome 22q deletion, but analysis of the NF-2 gene in ependymomas has revealed only a single mutation in a tumor that had lost the remaining wild-type allele.

Children with *tuberous sclerosis* may have a subependymal giant cell astrocytoma or ependymoma. Tuberous sclerosis genes map to chromosomes 9q and 16p, and allelic loss at these loci has been found in some subependymal giant-cell astrocytomas, suggesting a tumor-suppressor function. Hemangioblastomas of the cerebellum, medulla, and spinal cord are associated with *von Hippel-Lindau disease,* and choroid plexus tumors have occasionally been reported. Loss of chromosome 3p sequences has been described in one choroid plexus tumor, suggesting involvement of the VHL gene. There is an increased risk of brain tumors in the Li-Fraumeni syndrome, involving mutations in p53 on chromosome 17.

Combined cytogenetic and molecular studies of the common sporadic childhood brain tumors have identified genomic alterations that may lead to the identification of genes contributing to tumorigenesis. Isochromosome 17q is found in half of all medulloblastomas (primitive neuroectodermal tumors, or PNETs), implicating a tumor suppressor gene. Clinical outcome is now predictable by gene expression profiles. For example, overexpression of p53 in malignant gliomas of childhood is associated with adverse outcome. In medulloblastoma, low MYC oncogene mRNA expression and high TrkC neurotrophin receptor mRNA expression identify a good outcome; the desmoplastic subtype of medulloblastoma is specifically associated with the basal-cell nevus syndrome (BCNS) (e.g., Gorlin syndrome), in which the molecular defect is thought to be a mutation in the human homologue of the Drosophila patched gene. Identification of a novel polymorphism in this gene allows direct detection of allelic loss in BCNS. Desmoplastic medulloblastoma in infants from affected families is reported to have a good prognosis. Conversely, the large-cell, anaplastic variant of medulloblastoma and the atypical teratoid/rhabdoid tumor (ATRT) have an unfavorable prognosis. Diagnosis of these variants is based on light microscopic and immunohistochemical findings, and ATRT is further distinguished by chromosome 22q11 deletion with inactivation of the hSNF5/INI1 gene.

Environmental risk factors for CNS tumors include ionizing radiation, even for benign conditions such as tinea capitis. In children treated for acute lymphoblastic leukemia, there is a 1.39% cumulative incidence of secondary brain tumors (i.e., gliomas and meningiomas) at 20 years, and cranial irradiation is a dose-dependent predisposing factor. PNETs may also follow cranial irradiation. There is no conclusive evidence of risk from electromagnetic fields (by use of electric blankets or other residential exposure). Studies have shown an association between farm and animal exposures and childhood brain tumors, but dietary exposure to N-nitroso compounds, implicated in experimental brain tumors in animals, is not a risk factor in children. Maternal intake of folic acid in pregnancy may protect against PNETs and in England, the incidence of medulloblastoma declined after 1984 when multivitamin supplementation in pregnancy became widespread, following reports that folate reduced the risk of neural-tube defects.

DEVELOPMENTAL BIOLOGY

Current research on CNS tumorigenesis is based on the molecular genetics of tumor-associated syndromes, rodent models of pediatric brain tumors, and technologic advances in efforts to identify genes that regulate normal and neoplastic cells in the developing CNS.

Sonic Hedgehog (Shh), Wnt Signaling, Cerebellar Development and Medulloblastoma

In the 19th century, Obersteiner described the cells of the external granular layer (EGL) in the developing cerebellum. Based on morphologic similarity, granule cell precursors (GCPs) there were considered the cells of origin in medulloblastoma. Now, gene chip analysis and mouse models have linked medulloblastoma to molecular markers of GCPs. Only medulloblastomas carry these molecular markers of developing cells, and other PNETs do not.

The cerebellum matures through a complex interplay of genes of general CNS development and specifically cerebellar genes. For instance, sonic hedgehog (Shh) is a glycoprotein involved in the development of the CNS. In cerebellar development, Purkinje cells secrete Shh to activate genes in GCPs and stimulate proliferation of these cells. Activating mutations of the Shh pathway account for desmoplastic medulloblastoma in the nevoid basal-cell carcinoma syndrome (Gorlin syndrome), 10% to 20% of sporadic medul-

loblastomas, and histologically similar tumors in mice that are heterozygous for the equivalent genes.

Wnt proteins also play a role in CNS development and have been linked to medulloblastoma. Patients with Turcot syndrome, which involves defects in the APC (*Adenomatous Polyposis Complex*) gene, are susceptible to colorectal and brain tumors, notably medulloblastoma. APC is an element of the Wnt signaling pathway, and up to 30% of spontaneous medulloblastomas show mutations in APC and other components of this neurodevelopmental signaling cascade.

Wnt proteins bind to receptors and modulate C-myc, a transcription factor that promotes cell-cycle progression. Activation of C-myc and N-myc leads to proliferation, cell growth, and maintenance of an undifferentiated cellular phenotype; these genes are amplified in some medulloblastomas, and are associated with a poor clinical outcome. The same genes are amplified by the Shh pathway.

Wnt1 is required for mesencephalon/metencephalon patterning early in development. Cerebellar primordia fail to develop in mice lacking Wnt1, and mutations in other Wnt pathway components have been implicated not only in medulloblastoma, but also in colon cancer, hepatocellular carcinoma, and prostate and ovarian cancers.

A tumor-suppressor gene on *chromosome 17p* has yet to be identified but deletions or rearrangements of 17p are seen in 30% to 50% of medulloblastoma, and are also seen in leukemias, lymphomas, stomach, colon, and cervical cancers. Inactivation of the tumor suppressor p53, also a resident of chromosome 17, may contribute to the growth of tumors resembling medulloblastoma in mice, but there is neither an increased incidence of medulloblastoma in humans lacking p53 nor a change in p53 within the medulloblastoma cells.

The gene Bmi1, which induces leukemia through repression of tumor suppressors, is overexpressed in many medulloblastomas, and promotes cerebellar granule cell precursor proliferation.

ASTROCYTOMAS: GROWTH FACTORS, TUMOR SUPPRESSORS, AND ASTROCYTE DEVELOPMENT

Like the delayed maturation of the cerebellum discussed above, astrocytes develop later than neurons and continue to do so long after neurogenesis stops. Astrocytes retain the capacity for division throughout life and are more susceptible to transformation. Control over astrocyte proliferation and differentiation may be divided into two main categories: cell signaling and cell-cycle arrest pathways.

During glial development, precursor cells respond to growth factors such as epidermal growth factor (EGF) or platelet derived growth factor (PDGF). Their receptors (EGFR and PDGFR) are activated to stimulate tyrosine kinase activity and intracellular pathways that control proliferation and differentiation, programmed-cell death, migration, cellular shape, and metabolism.

Amplification and mutation of EGFR are among the most common genetic abnormalities found in glioblastomas. These tumors contain ligands that may activate the receptor, stimulating a pathway that results in tumor progression. In addition, the receptor may be mutated to a constitutively activated form, unable to bind ligand but generating unregulated tyrosine kinase activity. Mice lacking EGFR have fewer glial fibrillary acidic protein (GFAP)-positive cells, and massive neuronal degeneration is attributed to a lack of trophic support from the missing glial cells. Attempts to block glioma progression through disruption of the EGFR pathway have led to development of drugs targeting EGFR or PDGFR.

Ras is a downstream effector of several growth factor receptors, signaling through both mitogenic and antiapoptotic pathways. It is under control of the NF-1 gene neurofibromin, and mutations in that gene cause neurofibromatosis type-1, which includes optic-nerve glioma, astrocytoma, and glioblastoma. While ras mutations have not been detected in spontaneous malignant gliomas, they are used in generating mouse models of glial tumors.

The tumor suppressor, phosphatase with homology to tensin (PTEN) is mutated or lost in most high-grade astrocytomas. PTEN is expressed throughout the embryo and is critical in CNS development. PTEN mutations are thought to cause Lhermitte-Duclos disease, characterized by enlarged cerebellar foliae, distorted cerebellar cortex, abnormally myelinated axon bundles, and dysplastic neurons. Conditional inactivation of the gene in the cerebellum of developing mice has generated a mammalian model of that disease.

Loss of PTEN promotes astrocytic growth and survival, because it would otherwise act as a repressor of antiapoptotic signaling pathways. PTEN is also thought to regulate astrocyte migration and invasion by effects on cell shape and movement. When PTEN is overexpressed it inhibits tumor-cell movement; conversely, reduction of PTEN activity promotes cell movement, invasiveness, and perhaps metastasis.

The tumor suppressors *Retinoblastoma (Rb) protein* and *p53* are also regulators of cell survival and programmed-cell death, and are intimately involved with astrocytoma. Rb mutations in children lead to tumors in the retina, while mice null for Rb do not survive because of lethally abnormal patterns of neuronal development, with pronounced CNS programmed-cell death. Rb encodes a phosphoprotein important in cell-cycle regulation, blocking transcription factors that promote proliferation. In the developing CNS, Rb is found in the ventricular zone where neuroblasts proliferate.

Rb is also involved in the regulation of apoptosis through interactions with the tumor suppressor *p53*, a transcription factor upregulated in response to cellular stress to facilitate arrest of the cell cycle for either DNA repair or cell death. Humans with the Li-Fraumeni syndrome lack p53 and show marked susceptibility to gliomas. p53 mutant mice develop tumors early in life.

Under conditions of Rb inactivation, many cells enter the cell cycle inappropriately, and subsequently undergo apoptosis. However, Rb loss may synergize with the loss of apoptotic regulators, such as p53 to promote tumor formation. With the loss of Rb, transcription factors go unchecked, which then promotes cell proliferation. Loss of Rb might normally lead to apoptosis, but if p53 is also missing, apoptosis is impaired and tumorigenesis is enhanced. In fact, approximately 75% of glioblastomas show impaired apoptotic mechanisms and p53-pathway defects.

Symptoms

Children with brain tumors most often present with symptoms and signs of increased ICP because obstruction of normal CSF pathways leads to ventriculomegaly, and also because of the mass effects of the tumors. Characteristic signs are headache, vomiting, and diplopia, but the onset may be gradual and nonfocal. Fatigue, personality change, or worsening school performance may be described. Symptoms in infants are nonspecific and include irritability, anorexia, persistent vomiting, and developmental delay or regression, with macrocephaly, and seemingly forced-downward deviation of the eyes ("sunset sign"). The median duration of symptoms before diagnosis was 2 months in one series; only one-third of the patients were diagnosed in the first month after onset of symptoms. Persistent vomiting, recurrent headache (awakening the child from sleep), neurologic findings (ataxia, head tilt, vision loss, papilledema), endocrine disturbance (growth deceleration, diabetes insipidus), and stigmata of neurofibromatosis should all prompt immediate evaluation for the presence of a CNS tumor.

Symptoms and signs reflect tumor location, and in children (unlike adults), CNS tumors are divided about equally between supratentorial and infratentorial sites (Table 60.1).

In a meta-analysis, the ratio of supra- to infratentorial tumors was 0.92, and infratentorial location was more common between the ages of 3 and 11 years. *Supratentorial tumors*, which predominate in infants and toddlers and also occur in older children, cause headache, limb weakness, sensory loss, and occasionally seizures, deteriorating school performance, or personality change. Frontal-lobe tumors affect personality and movement. Temporal-lobe tumors may cause partial-complex seizures or fluent aphasias. The incidence of underlying neoplasm in children with intractable epilepsy approaches 20%, and the increased risk of having a brain tumor is noted even 10 or more years after a diagnosis of epilepsy.

Parietal-lobe tumors affect reading ability and awareness of contralateral extremities (hemineglect).

▶ **TABLE 60.1** Location of Central Nervous Systems Tumors in Infants, Children, and Adolescents

Location	Infants	Children	Adolescents
Supratentorial	Teratoma Cerebral astrocytoma Choroid plexus tumor PNET (primitive neuroectodermal tumor) Craniopharyngioma Optic glioma Dermoid	Cerebral astrocytoma Optic pathway or diencephalic glioma Craniopharyngioma Suprasellar germ cell tumor Ependymoma Ganglioglioma	Cerebral astrocytoma Glioblastoma multiforme Pineal germ cell tumor Craniopharyngioma Oligodendroglioma Meningioma Lymphoma Colloid cyst
Infratentorial	Medulloblastoma Ependymoma Astrocytoma	Medulloblastoma Brainstem glioma Ependymoma Cerebellar astrocytoma	Medulloblastoma Cerebellar astrocytoma Ependymoma Epidermoid

Occipital-lobe tumors cause visual-field disturbance and occasionally, hallucinations. Suprasellar lesions may cause both visual-field defects and endocrine dysfunction. The Parinaud syndrome (upgaze paresis and mild pupil dilatation with better reaction to accommodation than light, retraction or convergence nystagmus, and lid retraction) is found in pineal-region tumors.

Infratentorial tumors, which predominate from ages 4 to 11 years, typically cause headache, vomiting, diplopia, and imbalance. Bilateral sixth cranial-nerve palsy is a frequent sign of increased ICP. Brainstem tumors cause facial and extraocular muscle palsies, ataxia, and hemiparesis. Leptomeningeal spread occurs at diagnosis or recurrence in up to 15% of children with CNS tumors (more often in medulloblastoma/PNET) and may be asymptomatic, or may cause pain, irritability, weakness, or bowel and bladder dysfunction.

Diagnosis and Management

MRI is cost effective for children with headache of less then 6 months' duration and abnormal signs on neurologic examination or other clinical predictors of brain tumor. Compared with CT, MRI is more sensitive, especially for nonenhancing, infiltrative tumors and leptomeningeal involvement, may generate images in any plane (e.g., axial, coronal, sagittal), and is not compromised in the posterior fossa by bone artifact. Nonetheless, it may be difficult to distinguish tumor from surrounding edema or residual tumor from postoperative changes; for these reasons, postoperative studies should be obtained within 48 hours of surgery.

MRI of the spine has replaced myelography as the standard procedure for evaluation of spinal cord lesions (e.g., drop metastases) and leptomeningeal disease, in cases of medulloblastoma, ependymoma, choroid-plexus carcinoma, and pineal-region tumors, and should be obtained preoperatively if one of these diagnoses is suspected.

Lumbar puncture for CSF cytology and tumor markers should be done in children with these diagnoses. Recommended baseline and surveillance studies, based on tumor aggressiveness and patterns of recurrence, are shown in Table 60.2.

Treatment responses are determined by change in tumor size on MRI. Surveillance imaging may detect asymptomatic relapses. PET characterizes metabolic abnormalities that distinguish residual or recurrent tumor from cerebral necrosis. *Thallium-201* SPECT is sensitive for recurrent tumors; MRS offers similar capability and is more widely available.

The mainstay of therapy is *surgery,* which may be curative by itself in congenital and benign tumors. Gross total resection is also attempted, generally, in malignant tumors, and contributes to the cure rates of high-grade astrocytoma, medulloblastoma, or ependymoma. Resection is generally not attempted for lesions deep in the thalamus, or for diffuse, intrinsic brain-stem tumors. The introduction of the operating microscope and ultrasonic aspirator has improved both the safety and effectiveness of surgery. Stereotactic (e.g., CT- or MRI-guided) techniques are used for biopsy or subtotal resection in difficult-to-reach areas such as the basal ganglia. However, even a 99% resection of a lesion that is 10 cm^3 in size will leave 10^8 tumor cells behind, and additional postoperative treatment will be necessary to prevent the lesion from regrowing. Surgery is important for establishing a tissue diagnosis and relieving obstructive hydrocephalus. With placement of an external drain or endoscopic third ventriculostomy, followed by tumor resection, it may be possible to avoid the need for a permanent ventriculoperitoneal shunt, in most patients.

Operative mortality is generally not more than 1%, but morbidity varies according to the site and extent of surgery and the condition of the child. Complications of posterior-fossa surgery include occasional mutism, which is generally transient but may be accompanied by other

▶ **TABLE 60.2 Staging and Surveillance of Children with CNS Tumors (21 Months from End of Treatment)**

Tumor Category	Baseline Evaluation	Survelliance (mo)
Medulloblastoma/PNET High-grade astrocytoma Posterior fossa ependymoma Germ cell tumor/pineocytoma	Head/spine MR w/Gd CSF exam including cytology	Head 3, 6, 9, 12, 16, 20, 24, 30, 36, 48, 60, 84, 120 Spine 12, 24*, 36, 48* (* if residual or dissemination)
Brainstem glioma Supratentorial ependymona Oligodendroglioma	Head/spine MR w/Gd CSF exam for ependymoma	Head 4, 8, 12, 16, 20, 24, 30*, 36, 48, 60, 84, 120 Spine 18*, 48* (* if residual or dissemination)
Cerebellar astrocytoma Supratentorial astrocytoma Hypothalamic/chiasmatic glioma Craniopharyngioma Choroid plexus papilloma	Head MR w/GD CSF exam optional	Head 6, 12, 18*, 24, 36*, 48*, 60, 84, 120 (* if residual, and all craniopharyngioma)

PNET, primitive neuroectodermal tumor; MR, magnetic resonance; Gd, gadolinium.
From Kramer ED, Vezine LG, Packer RJ, et al. Staging and survellance of children with central nervous system
  neoplasms; recommendations of the Neurology and Tumor Imaging Committees of the Children's Cancer Group.
  Pediatr Neurosurg 1994;20:254-263

neurologic deficits. A cerebellar cognitive-affective syndrome has been described following surgical treatment alone. Surgery may be facilitated by intraoperative monitoring of sensory and other evoked potentials. Adjunctive measures include the use of corticosteroids, which counteract tumor edema, and are often used in the perioperative period, but should be tapered within 1 to 2 weeks, if possible. Patients undergoing surgery for supratentorial tumors are placed on anticonvulsants if they have had seizures or if the surgical approach is likely to cause seizures. Prophylactic anticonvulsants are generally continued for 1 week to 12 months.

Pathologic diagnosis is based on the revised World Health Organization (WHO) classification published in 2000. This classification distinguishes astrocytic tumors, oligodendroglial tumors and mixed gliomas, ependymal tumors, choroid plexus tumors, and neuronal and mixed neuronal-glial tumors. Among entities newly incorporated in the revised classification are atypical teratoid/rhabdoid tumor (AT/RT) and large-cell medulloblastoma. Some childhood brain tumors, such as supratentorial astrocytomas, are difficult to characterize in the WHO classification. A proposed pediatric classification divides tumors into glial, mixed glial-neuronal, neural, embryonal, and pineal categories. Glial tumors include astrocytoma, ependymoma, oligodendroglioma, and choroid-plexus tumor. Mixed glial-neuronal tumors include ganglioglioma and subependymal giant-cell tumor. Neural tumors include gangliocytoma. Embryonal tumors are primitive neuroectodermal tumor (PNET), atypical teratoid/rhabdoid tumor (ATRT), and medulloepithelioma. Pineal tumors are represented by pineocytoma.

Pathologic diagnosis is greatly facilitated by immunostaining for specific markers such as glial fibrillary acidic protein (GFAP) in glial tumors and neurofilament or synaptophysin in PNETs and gangliogliomas. Other markers have been developed for different tumors. An important trend in tumor pathology is the application of cytogenetic and DNA approaches. Examples are isochromosome 17q in medulloblastoma, chromosome 1p and 19q deletions in oligodendroglioma, and monosomy or deletion of chromosome 22 (hSNF/INI-1 locus) in ATRT.

Radiation therapy is used for nearly all malignant CNS tumors and for some benign lesions. Standard doses used to achieve local control range from 45 Gy to 55 Gy, in divided fractions of 150 cGy to 200 cGy, to the tumor as localized on MR plus 1- to 2-cm margin. Higher doses may be given, often in smaller twice-daily doses (e.g., hyperfractionated technique), but with high total doses there is increased risk of injuring normal brain tissue. The volume irradiated depends on tumor histology, and may include an involved field, or whole brain and spine. Presymptomatic craniospinal irradiation is almost always given for medulloblastoma, because of its propensity to disseminate throughout the neuraxis. Doses of 36 Gy have been used conventionally, but lower doses (23.4 Gy) are adequate in standard-risk patients if supplemented with adjuvant chemotherapy.

Newer radiotherapy techniques may increase the effective tumor dose and limit toxicity to the surrounding brain. Stereotactic irradiation techniques, in conjunction with rigid head fixation systems include single high-dose delivery (e.g., radiosurgery), fractionated-convergence therapy, and 3D-conformal therapy. Interstitial radioactive implants (e.g., brachytherapy) may be appropriate in some cases. Neutron-beam protons are of advantageous use in skull-base tumors such as chordomas. Use of radiation sensitizers, including chemotherapy agents and gadolinium compounds, is currently under study. Acute side effects of radiation therapy include headache, nausea, alopecia, skin hyperpigmentation and desquamation, and a transient "somnolence syndrome," occurring 4 to 8 weeks after treatment.

Chemotherapy is used as an adjunct to radiotherapy, as primary postsurgical treatment in infants, and in recurrent tumors. Chemotherapy may increase survival for children with medulloblastoma and high-grade astrocytoma, and may be effective in delaying the need for radiotherapy in children with malignant CNS tumors. Effective agents include the nitrosoureas (e.g., carmustine, lomustine), vincristine, cisplatin, carboplatin, etoposide, and cyclophosphamide. Temozolomide appears promising. Chemotherapy is generally given systemically, and in combination, because of complementary mechanisms of action of different agents and to subvert potential tumor resistance. Regional delivery of drugs (e.g., intraarterial, intrathecal, intratumor), has not yet been shown to improve survival in childhood CNS tumors, but responses to intraarterial carboplatin- or methotrexate-based chemotherapy with osmotic blood-brain barrier disruption are reported for germ-cell tumors or primary CNS lymphoma. The dose intensity of conventional, systemic chemotherapy may be increased with the use of hematopoietic growth factors, which shorten the period of myelosuppression and permit the use of higher doses or shorter intervals between treatments. A related approach is the use of extremely high doses of chemotherapy, supported by autologous hematopoietic stem-cell rescue for recurrent tumors, or as an intensive consolidation therapy for infants.

Biological agents in clinical trials include differentiation agents (e.g., retinoic acid), agents targeting tumor growth factor receptors (e.g., gefitinib, imatinib), farnesyltransferase inhibitors (e.g., tipifarnib), agents interfering with

angiogenesis (e.g., bevicizumab); and immunologic therapies, such as interferon.

CONGENITAL TUMORS

Craniopharyngiomas originate from rests of embryonic tissue located in the Rathke pouch, which later form the anterior pituitary gland. They may appear clinically at any age, even later adulthood, and constitute 6% to 10% of intracranial tumors in children. They vary from small, well-circumscribed, solid nodules to huge, multilocular cysts invading the sella turcica. The cysts are filled with turbid fluid that may contain cholesterin crystals. Craniopharyngiomas are histologically benign and may be categorized as mucoid-epithelial cysts, squamous epitheliomas, or adamantinomas. Total surgical removal may be difficult because the tumor may invade the hypothalamus or third ventricle and adhere to optic nerves or blood vessels. Manifestations include short stature, hypothyroidism, and diabetes insipidus, with vision loss, and signs of increased ICP. Although CT is useful for demonstrating calcification and bony expansion of the sella, MRI is preferred for better definition of the relationship of the tumor to neighboring vessels, optic chiasm and nerves, and the hypothalamus (Fig. 60.1).

A conservative approach is to drain the cyst and resect nonadherent tumor, and then administer radiation therapy to the involved area. Alternatively, gross total resection may be attempted, avoiding irradiation. Recurrence rates are similar (20% to 40%), and radical surgery is likely to be accompanied by panhypopituitarism, necessitating life-long hormonal replacement therapy, whereas irradiation has lesser hormonal sequelae but causes cognitive deficits, especially in younger children. Focused treatment

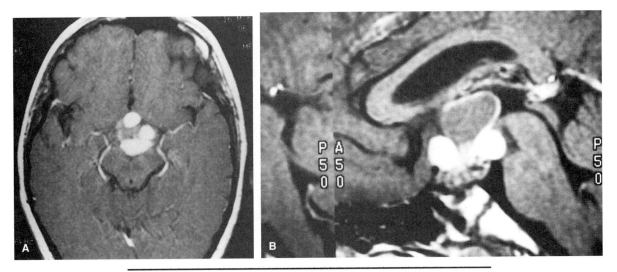

FIGURE 60.1. Axial (**A**) and sagittal (**B**) MRIs of a craniopharyngioma.

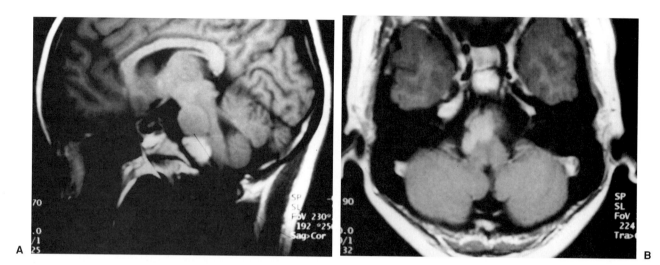

FIGURE 60.2. Sagittal **(A)** and axial **(B)** MR images of a pontomedullary epidermoid.

by stereotactic radiosurgery (e.g., gamma knife) may be advantageous in this regard. Interferon alpha-2a has been used in recurrent craniopharyngiomas.

Epidermoids (*cholesteatomas*) are the most common, embryonal CNS tumors and account for about 2% of all intracranial tumors. They arise within skull tables or adjacent to the dura, usually in the suprasellar region, skull base, brain-stem or cerebellopontine angle, or within a ventricle. They are encapsulated, have a pearly appearance, and may contain cyst fluid with cholesterol crystals. Clinical onset is usually in young adulthood, with variable rate of progression depending on location. MRI demonstrates a lesion with low T1- and high T2-weighted signal intensity (Fig. 60.2).

Diffusion imaging may be helpful. Treatment is surgical resection, with radical removal of the tumor capsule. *Dermoid tumors* are also cystic, and sebaceous gland secretions impart a dark yellow color to the cyst fluid. Intracranial dermoids are associated with Goldenhar syndrome (i.e., oculo-auriculo-vertebral dysplasia). Treatment is surgical resection.

Teratomas occur in infants and young children. Prenatal diagnosis of an intracranial teratoma has been reported. Mature teratomas are generally lobulated and cystic, often containing differentiated tissues such as bone, cartilage, teeth, hair, or intestine. Immature and malignant teratomas are less common. Teratomas tend to occur in the pineal region, presenting with Parinaud syndrome and hydrocephalus. They comprise about 4% of childhood intracranial tumors and also occur in the spine. Treatment is surgical resection.

Chordomas develop from remnants of the embryonic notochord. Half are in the sacrococcygeal region, one-third at the sphenoid-occipital junction, and the remainder elsewhere along the spinal column. They are rare, accounting for less than 1% of CNS tumors, and usually remain asymp-

tomatic until adulthood. These tumors are locally invasive and cause vision loss or cranial-nerve dysfunction. They may invade the nasopharynx or intracranial sinuses and may extend into the neck, causing torticollis.

Chordomas have a smooth, nodular surface that resembles cartilage; the characteristic histologic feature is the presence of large masses of physaliferous cells, round or polygonal cells arranged in cords and having large cytoplasmic vacuoles containing mucin. Chordomas grow slowly but may recur after excision. A chondroid variant contains prominent cartilage. A malignant variant is distinguished by mitotic spindle cells and may metastasize to the lung. Chordoma should be suspected in a patient presenting with multiple cranial-nerve palsies or erosion of the skull base. Treatment is surgical resection, although gross total resection is rarely achieved, occasionally with postoperative irradiation. Radiation therapy may be used postoperatively or at recurrence. Proton radiotherapy is advocated because it may confer effective local control and possibly better cosmetic outcome than with conventional irradiation.

Choroid-plexus tumors are rare congenital tumors found in, or near, a lateral ventricle. They may cause symptoms shortly after birth, and most are diagnosed before age 2 years. About two-thirds are benign papillomas, and the remainder are carcinomas. The first manifestation is likely to be macrocephaly resulting from hydrocephalus, with bulging fontanelle and split sutures noted in infants. Excess CSF production arising from the tumor may approach 2,000 mL per day. Papillomas usually grow into the ventricle and tend not to be invasive. Carcinomas typically invade the parenchyma and cause hydrocephalus (Fig. 60.3).

Surgical resection stops the excessive production of CSF. Carcinomas are invasive and nearly half of them disseminate in the leptomeninges. Total excision of localized

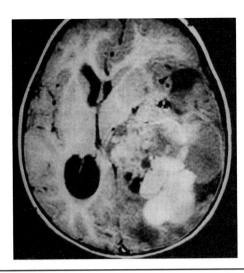

FIGURE 60.3. MRI of a choroid-plexus carcinoma of the lateral ventricle, with parenchymal invasion.

lesions may be curative, but malignant transformation of incompletely resected papillomas has been reported; adjuvant chemotherapy or irradiation has been advocated for carcinomas, even following gross total resection, owing to their guarded prognosis (median survival 6 months in one series). For patients undergoing subtotal resection of carcinomas, both chemotherapy and craniospinal irradiation are recommended.

Colloid cysts of the third ventricle presumably arise from the anlage of the paraphysis. These lesions grow in the anterior, superior portion of the third ventricle as small, white cysts filled with homogeneous, gelatinous material. They do not usually cause symptoms until adulthood, when there may be intermittent hydrocephalus. Disturbance of the limbic system may cause emotional and behavioral changes, in some instances. Treatment is surgical excision. Endoscopic procedures are gaining acceptance as an alternative to microsurgical resection.

Gangliogliomas are rare, glioneural tumors that account for 2.5% of pediatric brain tumors. The peak age incidence is 10 to 20 years. They arise mainly in the temporal lobe, but also in other lobes or spinal cord. The usual syndrome is a long history of refractory epilepsy. Imaging reveals a solid-to-cystic lesion, with calcification on CT and hypometabolic activity on PET. Histologically, there is a mixture of neoplastic astrocytes and abnormal ganglion cells, which together with perivascular lymphoplasmacytic infiltrates, distinguishes these tumors from pilocytic astrocytoma.

Total surgical resection is recommended. Malignant transformation to glioblastoma may follow incomplete resection. Radiation therapy and chemotherapy are of uncertain benefit, and are reserved for malignant variants, unresectable tumors, or disease progression. *Desmoplastic infantile ganglioglioma (DIG)* is a rare cerebral glioneural

tumor of early childhood. DIGs are large hemispheric tumors that are generally benign, but deep lesions may be aggressive. Treatment is resection. Radiation therapy and chemotherapy after incomplete resection are of uncertain benefit. Related glioneural tumors include *desmoplastic astrocytoma of infancy (DACI)* and *pleomorphic xanthoastrocytoma (PXA)*, which usually cause seizures and headache. *Dysembryoplastic neuroepithelial tumor (DNT)* is a rare, low-grade mixed neuronal and glial tumor often associated with intractable seizures. These tumors may appear malignant histologically and PXA may invade meninges, but surgical excision is generally curative.

ASTROCYTOMAS

Cerebellar astrocytomas constitute approximately 12% of childhood brain tumors and 30% to 40% of posterior-fossa tumors. The peak incidence is early in the second decade. These tumors arise most often in the lateral, cerebellar hemispheres rather than in the vermis. Symptoms of clumsiness and unsteadiness may be present for months and eventually, are accompanied by intermittent morning headache and vomiting. Midline lesions have a shorter symptom interval. Truncal ataxia, dysmetria, and papilledema are usually present at diagnosis. Head tilt may be present, but other cranial-nerve palsies or long-tract signs are infrequent and suggest brain-stem invasion. Cerebellar astrocytomas may be primarily cystic or solid, and cystic lesions may have a nodule (Fig. 60.4).

Most are histologically benign. The typical juvenile pilocytic astrocytoma contains areas of compact fibrillated cells with microcysts and eosinophilic structures called Rosenthal fibers. These lesions have greater than 90%

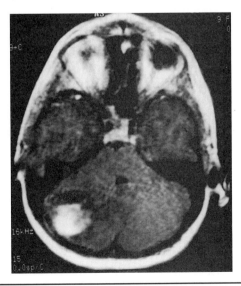

FIGURE 60.4. MRI showing lateral location of a partly cystic, partly solid cerebellar astrocytoma.

survival with surgery, alone. The tumor and associated cyst should be removed completely. If there is residual tumor, reresection should be considered; focal radiotherapy may be offered if there is disease progression. Some patients have infiltrating tumors with hypercellularity or frank anaplasia; these have been considered diffuse or anaplastic astrocytomas, are harder to resect because of brainstem invasion, and have approximately 30% recurrence-free survival. Local radiotherapy does not appear to improve survival, and the value of craniospinal irradiation or chemotherapy is unclear.

Brain-stem gliomas are heterogeneous. The diffuse, intrinsic pontine lesions carry the worst prognosis of any childhood brain tumor. In contrast, small, intrinsic, tectal gliomas are indolent and may be managed conservatively. Brain-stem tumors constitute 10% to 20% of posterior fossa tumors, with a peak incidence at ages 5 to 8 years. Most arise in the pons, and there may be contiguous spread to the medulla or midbrain. Despite the clinical aggressiveness of these tumors, the histologic appearance at initial diagnosis is quite variable, but at autopsy a substantial portion shows anaplastic features. This may reflect sampling error at initial biopsy or subsequent malignant transformation. These tumors infiltrate the brain stem and compress normal structures, while extending superiorly and inferiorly to produce diffuse enlargement of the brain stem. Diffuse, intrinsic, pontine lesions are nearly uniformly fatal, within 18 to 24 months. Some tumors extend ventrally, laterally, or posteriorly, and the primarily exophytic tumors tend to be more accessible to surgical resection and carry a better prognosis, as do focal midbrain lesions.

The course is insidious, with slowly progressive cranial neuropathy, motor symptoms, and disturbance of gait, swallowing, and speech. Vomiting and headache indicate the presence of hydrocephalus, which is generally a late finding. Children with dorsal exophytic lesions may have more unsteadiness and less evidence of cranial-nerve dysfunction. CT shows a low-density lesion in the brain stem, with compression and obliteration of surrounding cisterns, but little if any contrast enhancement. Uncommonly, brain-stem tumors may be isodense or hyperdense, with cystic areas. MRI is preferred because of the detail appreciated on sagittal images, typically revealing more extensive disease than appreciated on CT. The MR appearance is of decreased signal intensity on T1-weighted images (Fig. 60.5A) and increased T2-weighted signal. MRI may also demonstrate infiltration of the medulla (Fig. 60.5B) or thalamus.

Given the accuracy of MR diagnosis, the morbidity of surgery, and the variable prognostic impact of biopsy, it has been accepted that surgery is not warranted for the 70% of patients with diffuse intrinsic pontine lesions, in whom major resection when attempted has not improved survival. Patients with exophytic, cervico-medullary tumors are more likely to benefit from surgery, as are patients with atypical clinical courses or MR findings (e.g., symptom duration exceeding 6 months, absence of cranial-nerve findings, primarily exophytic or focal ring-enhancing lesions). Standard treatment is field-radiation therapy, except for completely resected focal lesions. Most children with brain-stem gliomas benefit at least transiently from radiation therapy to a dose of 54 Gy to 56 Gy. Hyperfractionated irradiation to a dose of 72 Gy to 78 Gy, in smaller twice-daily fractions did not alter survival for patients with diffuse pontine lesions, nor did accelerated radiotherapy in standard fractions, given twice daily. Although leptomeningeal dissemination may occur, the main risk is for local recurrence. Chemotherapy and immunotherapy have been unsuccessful in this condition, although new agents

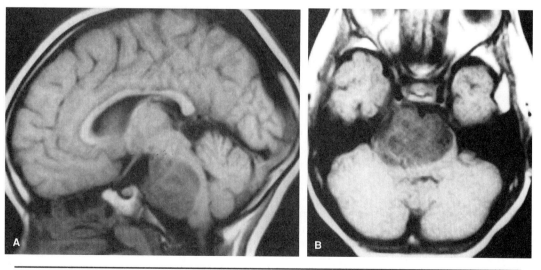

FIGURE 60.5. A: Sagittal MRI of a diffuse brainstem glioma. **B:** Axial image showing infiltration of the medulla.

continue to be studied. Children with brain-stem tumors should be monitored for signs of hydrocephalus, because CSF diversion by shunting or third ventriculostomy may improve quality of life.

Diencephalic and optic pathway gliomas constitute up to 5% of childhood CNS tumors. Unilateral optic nerve tumors are generally diagnosed in the first decade of life, and optic-chiasm tumors tend to present either in infancy or the second decade. An association with NF-1 is present in 50% to 70% of patients with isolated optic-nerve tumors and 10% to 20% of patients with optic-chiasm tumors. Adolescents are more likely to complain of slowly progressive vision loss. Infants are more likely to be evaluated because of strabismus, nystagmus, or developmental delay. Patients with contiguous optic-nerve involvement, usually present with proptosis, and optic pallor or atrophy. Intraorbital lesions usually cause decrease in central vision, whereas chiasmatic tumors produce bitemporal hemianopic field cuts. Nystagmus may be present in the more involved eye, and amblyopia is common. With routine MRI of NF-1 patients, lesions may be detected before onset of symptoms. There may be endocrine disturbances, such as growth deceleration, precocious puberty, and diencephalic emaciation. Thalamic lesions may cause acute hemiparesis or hemisensory loss, signs of increased ICP, seizures, or involuntary movements. Infants tend to have macrocephaly, psychomotor delay, and vision deficits. Hypothalamic tumors have insidious onset and may be associated with altered mental status, endocrine dysfunction, and focal neurologic deficits.

On CT or MRI, diencephalic gliomas are hypo- or isodense lesions with variable contrast enhancement. Larger lesions may be cystic (Fig. 60.6, A and B).

Visual-pathway tumors may be confined to the optic chiasm (Fig. 60.7, A and B) or may show abnormal enhancement along the optic tracts and radiations.

This streaking phenomenon is best appreciated on MRI, particularly with FLAIR sequence. Most diencephalic tumors are low-grade fibrillary or pilocytic astrocytomas. The natural history of these lesions is unpredictable. Spontaneous regression has been noted. An increased MIB-1 labeling index identifies more aggressive pilocytic astrocytomas. Visual-pathway tumors have a particular tendency to spread to contiguous structures. The role of surgery is unclear.

In patients with diffusely infiltrating lesions, especially with NF-1, diagnosis may be confirmed with near certainty on neuroimaging alone, and surgery may be deemed of little benefit. In patients with unilateral blindness, surgery may be recommended for treatment of a severely proptotic eye. However, if some vision persists, local radiotherapy may be recommended. Radiotherapy at doses of 45 Gy to 55 Gy generally reverses tumor progression in nearly all patients, and stabilizes or improves vision in most. There may be apparent tumor enlargement at 6 to 12 weeks, as a transient effect of the radiation. Patients with very large lesions may benefit from preliminary surgical debulking.

The major disadvantages of radiotherapy are adverse endocrine and neurocognitive effects, especially in younger children. Chemotherapy (vincristine and carboplatin) has been beneficial as initial treatment in children under 5 years of age who have progressive optic-pathway and hypothalamic/chiasmatic gliomas, delaying the need for radiotherapy by a median of 4 years; most eventually relapse, however, except for NF-1 patients who tend to have indolent disease. The same chemotherapy

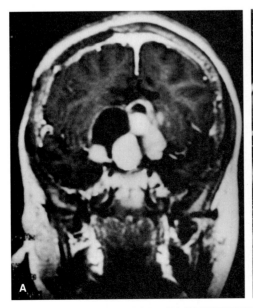
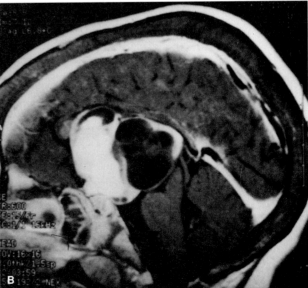

FIGURE 60.6. Coronal **(A)** and sagittal **(B)** MRIs of a large hypothalamic glioma.

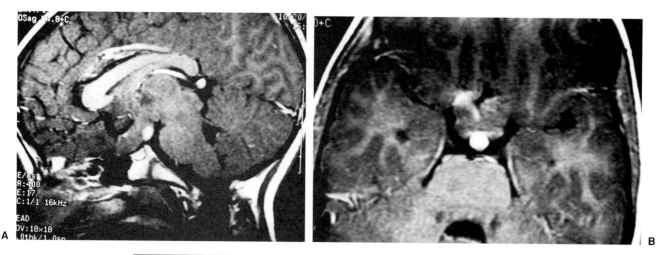

FIGURE 60.7. Sagittal (**A**) and coronal (**B**) MRIs of an optic pathway tumor.

regimen has been advocated as initial treatment for infants with tumor-associated diencephalic syndrome of emaciation.

Cerebral-hemisphere low-grade gliomas have a peak incidence between ages 2 and 4 years and again in early adolescence. In toddlers, there may be symptoms of increased ICP, developmental delay, and growth retardation, and specific signs such as weakness, sensory loss, or vision deficit. These slow-growing pediatric tumors are far less likely than adult gliomas to undergo malignant degeneration. They are infiltrating, however, and may cause seizures, either generalized or focal, the latter particularly suggestive of an occult brain tumor such as a ganglioglioma.

CT often reveals a relatively homogeneous, low-density, variably enhancing lesion with indistinct margins. MRI is more sensitive, showing decreased T1- and increased T2-weighted signal and providing better resolution of tumor and edema. Gross total resection often affords long-term disease control but may not be curative. Five-year survival rates are 75% to 85%. Radiation therapy at doses of 50 Gy to 55 Gy may be given postoperatively, following incomplete resection, or at progression, at least in older children but reoperation should also be considered. If radiation therapy is used, stereotactically guided conformal techniques are recommended because there is the potential for reduction in late toxicity. For younger children with residual or recurrent tumor, chemotherapy (e.g., vincristine and carboplatin) has been used in an attempt to defer radiotherapy, and prospective trials evaluating this approach are in progress.

Cerebral-hemisphere high-grade astrocytomas account for about 11% of childhood brain tumors. High-grade astrocytomas may be classified according to cytologic appearance (e.g., fibrillary, pilocytic, gemistocytic, xanthomatous, or protoplasmic) and by degree of anaplasia. Kernohan classification grades astrocytomas on a scale of 1 to 4, with grade 3 (i.e., *anaplastic astrocytoma*) and grade 4 (i.e., *glioblastoma multiforme*) representing high-grade lesions.

The WHO classification emphasizes degree of cellularity, nuclear and cellular pleomorphism, mitosis, endothelial proliferation, and necrosis, and identifies three gradations: astrocytomas, anaplastic astrocytomas, and glioblastoma multiforme. In general, *anaplastic astrocytomas* are composed of astrocytes with increased cellularity, pleomorphism, and numbers of mitoses. There may be focal necrosis, but it may not be so extensive as to form pseudopalisades. In contrast to low-grade pilocytic tumors, anaplastic astrocytomas have an unstable vasculature, with a predominance of immature vessels distinguished by negative immunostaining for alpha smooth-muscle actin.

Vascular endothelial growth factor and anti-*flt-1/VEGF receptor-1* immunoreactivity was detected in anaplastic astrocytomas, but not pilocytic astrocytomas. *Glioblastoma multiforme* has prominent vascular proliferation and a pseudopalisading pattern of necrosis. Cytogenetic analyses developed mainly of tumors from adults has shown consistent, chromosomal abnormalities in all tumor grades; however, one aberration—the loss of part or all of chromosome 10—has been specifically associated with glioblastoma multiforme, and amplification and rearrangement of the epidermal growth factor receptor (EGFR) gene have also been associated with malignant histology. Gene profiling shows overexpression of hypoxia-inducible transcription factor (HIF)-2 alpha and FK506-binding protein (FKBP) 12-associated genes, including EGFR and insulin-like growth factor-binding protein 2.

Common symptoms include headache, vomiting, seizures, motor weakness, and behavioral abnormalities. Symptom duration is generally less than 3 months. Diagnosis is made by CT or MRI. Surgery is important for diagnosis and for removing tumor; major resection improves survival. However, these infiltrative tumors may disseminate in the CSF and will almost certainly recur without further therapy. Postoperative involved-field irradiation (59 Gy to 60 Gy) and adjuvant chemotherapy both increase survival. Adjuvant vincristine plus lomustine was effective in one trial but survival rates remain below 35%. Survival is influenced by extent of tumor resection, and by histology (e.g., anaplastic astrocytoma vs. glioblastoma multiforme). In a major study, there was a significant association between the MIB-1 proliferation index and progression-free survival. Tumors with labeling indices above 36% had nearly uniform poor outcome, regardless of histology. These highly proliferative cancers may be susceptible to intensive chemotherapy, augmented by hematopoietic stem-cell rescue.

Spinal cord astrocytomas account for about 4% of childhood CNS neoplasms. Other primary spinal-cord tumors in children include gangliogliomas and ependymomas. Spinal high-grade astrocytomas and PNETs are uncommon. Astrocytomas may occur in any part of the cord, but are seen most often in the cervical region, with the solid component extending an average of five spinal segments. Most have benign histologic appearance and grow slowly. Symptoms and signs may include pain (i.e., localized or radicular), weakness or spasticity, gait disturbance, and bowel or bladder dysfunction. Gadolinium-enhanced MRI is preferred for demonstrating the location of the solid tumor, associated cysts, and edema. Treatment may be attempted gross-total or near-total resection or partial resection with decompression of cysts with postoperative radiotherapy.

The degree of neurologic recovery depends on the preoperative condition of the patient. A potential complication is spinal deformity, resulting from laminectomy, radiotherapy, or both. About one-third of patients require a spine-stabilization procedure. For children with low-grade tumors, survival rates of 55% at 10 years have been reported after partial resection and radiotherapy. Chemotherapy has been substituted for radiotherapy in very young children. The prognosis for children with high-grade tumors is worse, although 5-year progression-free survival of 46% was reported in a study using combined radiation therapy and chemotherapy.

EMBRYONAL TUMORS: MEDULLOBLASTOMAS, SUPRATENTORIAL PRIMITIVE NEUROECTODERMAL TUMORS, AND ATYPICAL TERATOID/RHABDOID TUMORS

Medulloblastoma and supratentorial PNETs, collectively, are the most common malignant CNS tumors of childhood. Most PNETs arise in the posterior fossa and are specifically called medulloblastomas. Posterior fossa and supratentorial PNETs are histologically identical and have similar epidemiologic profiles. The incidence of medulloblastoma/PNET before age 20 years rose 23% from 1973–77 to 1993–98.

As described above, the presumed cell of origin of medulloblastoma/PNET is derived from fetal external-granular cells of the cerebellum or rests in the posterior medullary velum. These tumors account for about 30% of infratentorial tumors in children but are uncommon in adults. Medulloblastomas typically involve the cerebellar vermis, grow to fill the fourth ventricle, and may infiltrate the floor of the ventricle and adjacent structures. The tumor may arise more laterally, especially in older patients. Supratentorial PNETs generally arise in the cerebral cortex or pineal region.

The histologic appearance is of a small, round, cell tumor with glial or other types of differentiation, in some cases. There may be positive staining for both neurofilament protein and glial fibrillary acidic protein but also for synaptophysin, which is more specific for PNET. Desmoplastic medulloblastoma has a unique nodular histology and better outcome, while large cell medulloblastoma is an anaplastic variant with worse outcome. Most medulloblastomas fall between these histologic extremes, but one-quarter exhibit at least moderate anaplasia and an associated, aggressive clinical behavior. In infants, medulloblastoma must be distinguished from the ATRT, which has a small-cell component resembling medulloblastoma but also cords of cells in a mucinous background that resemble chordoma, with a rhabdoid appearance of the cytoplasm of the larger cells.

A specific chromosome abnormality, isochromosome 17q (i.e., duplication of the long arm or deletion of the short arm of chromosome 17), is seen in one-third of cases of medulloblastoma. This could result in inactivation of a tumor-suppressor gene located on chromosome 17 but is apparently distinct from p53. It is unclear whether chromosome 17p deletions impart poor prognosis, but diploid tumors have worse outcome than aneuploid or hyperdiploid tumors. Relatively less is known about the cytogenetic and molecular features of supratentorial PNETs, but gene expression analysis shows distinct patterns of gene activation that differ from those of medulloblastoma. ATRTs have monosomy or deletion of chromosome 22, and inactivating mutations of the hSNF5/INI-1 gene at 22q11.2 are considered fundamental to pathogenesis. Loss of chromosome 19 has been reported in ATRT.

Children with medulloblastoma typically have symptoms of increased ICP (e.g., vomiting, lethargy, morning headache), unsteadiness, and diplopia. The median age is 5 years. Symptom duration is generally of less than 3 months. There may be recent onset of head tilt resulting from ophthalmoparesis or incipient cerebellar herniation. Laterally situated lesions present slightly differently, with symptoms of cerebellopontine angle disturbance or limb

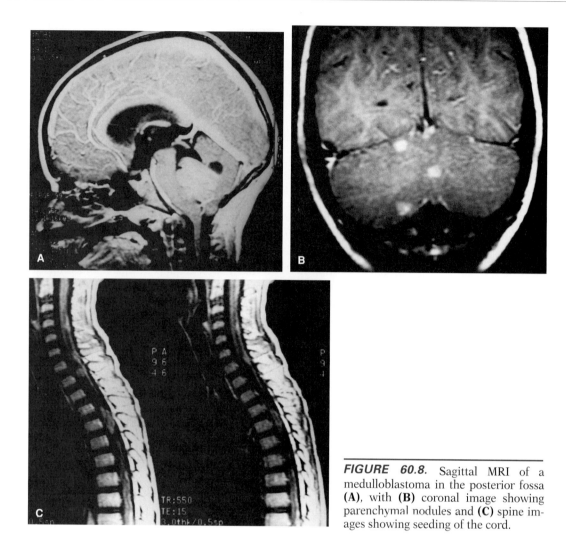

FIGURE 60.8. Sagittal MRI of a medulloblastoma in the posterior fossa **(A)**, with **(B)** coronal image showing parenchymal nodules and **(C)** spine images showing seeding of the cord.

ataxia. These tumors appear isodense or hyperdense on CT and usually enhance homogeneously. Hydrocephalus is seen in more than 80% of patients. Other CT features include small cysts, calcification, and hemorrhage.

MRI may give better indication of tumor extent (Fig. 60.8A) and possible leptomeningeal dissemination (Fig. 60.8, B and C).

MRI is also preferred to facilitate evaluation of disseminated spinal tumor, which is found in up to one-third of patients with medulloblastomas. Surgery achieves complete or near-complete resection of medulloblastomas in most cases, limited mainly by tumor infiltration of the fourth ventricle, the brain stem, or one of the cerebellar peduncles. Morbidity may include the posterior-fossa syndrome of aseptic meningitis or less commonly, of mutism, pharyngeal dysfunction, and ataxia. Preoperative ventriculoperitoneal shunting is not done routinely owing to the risk of upward herniation and because hydrocephalus will be relieved by tumor removal in most patients. About 30% to 40% of patients require permanent shunting.

Postoperative CT or MRI is indicated to confirm the extent of resection, and this study should be done within 48 hours, when there is less edema than later. Patients may be stratified clinically as average risk (i.e., localized posterior fossa medulloblastoma with no more than 1.5 cm² postoperative residual tumor), and high risk (i.e., more than 1.5 cm² residual, or dissemination outside the posterior fossa, including positive CSF cytology). The overall 5-year disease-free survival rate is approximately 55%. Children with completely resected, localized tumors have up to 70% disease-free survival rates. Infants below age 3 years have inferior outcome and are considered high-risk patients.

Radiation therapy is the standard postoperative treatment for medulloblastoma, and craniospinal irradiation is given because the entire neuraxis is at risk for tumor recurrence. Conventional doses are 36 Gy to the brain and spine, with an 18-Gy to 20-Gy boost to the local tumor site. Reduction of the neuraxis dose to 23.4 Gy in average risk patients with nondisseminated tumors resulted in an inferior 5-year survival rate (52% vs 67%). Adjuvant (postirradiation) chemotherapy with vincristine and lomustine improved survival in advanced stages of medulloblastoma, and the addition of cisplatin afforded a remarkable

5-year progression-free survival rate of 85% in one series.

Preirradiation chemotherapy did not improve survival. Reduced neuraxis irradiation, followed by vincristine, lomustine, and cisplatin chemotherapy, in average-risk children aged 3 to 10 years with nondisseminated medulloblastoma, resulted in a 5-year progression-free survival rate of 79%. Chemotherapy has also been used as primary postoperative treatment in infants, to avoid radiotherapy. Current protocols for infants up to age 3 years use this approach, with increasingly intensive regimens to enhance the response rate to chemotherapy, and to improve the control of leptomeningeal disease. Because early tumor progression on chemotherapy remains a major problem, some protocols for older infants combine local tumor irradiation (i.e., using confocal techniques) and chemotherapy. Finally, chemotherapy with hematopoietic stem-cell rescue is used for selected patients with recurrent medulloblastoma, and in some infant protocols.

Supratentorial PNETs are histologically equivalent to medulloblastoma and are treated with the same approach of resection, craniospinal irradiation, and chemotherapy. Prognosis is worse for these patients, however, with only a 37% 5-year survival rate. As with medulloblastoma, preirradiation chemotherapy seems to compromise survival. Pineal-region PNETs (i.e., pineoblastomas) have a better outcome. These tumors must be distinguished from pineal germ-cell tumors (see below) and pineocytomas (i.e., benign pineal parenchymal tumors treated by surgery alone or with radiotherapy). Pineal tumors are also discussed in Chapter 58.

Atypical teratoid/rhabdoid tumors generally affect infants and toddlers, and may account for up to one-quarter of primitive CNS tumors in this age group. ATRTs usually arise in the cerebellum or cerebellar-pontine angle, but may also occur in supratentorial and pineal locations, and are occasionally multifocal. Diagnosis is based on distinctive-light microscopy and molecular-genetic analysis. Treatment includes surgery, radiation therapy, and chemotherapy but outcome is almost uniformly poor, except occasionally in older patients. Mean survival rate is less than 1 year, and both local and disseminated tumor-recurrence patterns are seen.

EPENDYMOMAS

Ependymomas usually arise within or adjacent to the ependymal lining of the ventricular system, with 60% to 75% of all tumors found in the posterior fossa. They constitute 5% to 10% of all primary childhood brain tumors. Ependymomas are glial neoplasms, derived from ependymal cells, and most appear to be histologically mature. Variants include anaplastic ependymoma, which carries

a worse outcome in some series, and subependymoma, a lower grade lesion in which the fibrillary subependymal astrocyte predominates.

Ependymoblastoma, a primitive tumor, is better categorized as a type of PNET. Simian virus 40-related DNA sequences have been demonstrated in ependymomas and choroid-plexus carcinomas, suggesting a viral etiology. Cytogenetic and molecular studies of childhood ependymomas have revealed isochrome 1q as an early genetic event, as well as rearrangements or deletions of chromosomes 6, 17, and 22.

Clinical symptoms depend on tumor location. Children with ependymomas filling or compressing the fourth ventricle have obstructive hydrocephalus with nausea, vomiting, and morning headaches. Tumors arising low in the fourth ventricle and extending into the lower medulla may cause neck pain, whereas cranial-nerve palsies may result from brain-stem invasion or compression of cranial nerves. In patients with supratentorial lesions, seizures and focal deficits are seen. Features on CT include calcification and variable enhancement. MRI may better demonstrate the invasion by posterior-fossa lesions into the brainstem (Fig. 60.9) or upper cervical spinal cord.

The most important predictor of outcome in these cases is the extent of surgical resection as confirmed by postoperative imaging. In posterior-fossa lesions, resectability may be limited by infiltration of the brain stem, extension into the cerebellar pontine angle, or involvement of cranial-nerve nuclei. Supratentorial lesions may also be quite infiltrative and difficult to remove. Total resection of ependymomas affords up to a 75% survival rate at 10 years, whereas local recurrence is the rule following subtotal resection, where survival rates drop to 15%. Patients with

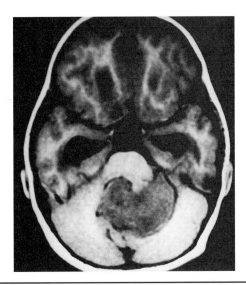

FIGURE 60.9. MR appearance of an ependymoma, showing tumor extension through the foramen of Luschka and invasion of the brainstem.

tumor dissemination at diagnosis (i.e., usually fewer than 10% of cases) also do poorly.

Postoperative radiation therapy increases survival rates for patients with localized ependymoma, and treatment to an involved field (at a dose of 55 Gy) is generally considered sufficient because relapses are overwhelmingly local. The need for larger volumes of radiation therapy to anaplastic lesions or for presymptomatic irradiation to the neuraxis with posterior fossa lesions has not been established definitely. Adjuvant chemotherapy may improve outcome, based on the responses of recurrent ependymomas to cisplatin and other agents; preirradiation chemotherapy is being evaluated in patients with postoperative residual tumor. Recurrent ependymomas are managed by reresection and chemotherapy or by stereotactic radiosurgery.

GERM-CELL TUMORS

Germ-cell tumors tend to arise in the pineal and suprasellar regions. They account for about half of all pineal tumors and 5% to 10% of parasellar lesions. Pineal germ-cell tumors have a male preponderance and usually present in adolescence, whereas suprasellar germ-cell tumors predominate in younger females. About 50% to 65% of germ-cell tumors are germinomas, histologically primitive lesions resembling gonadal germ-cell tumors, and presumably derived from embryonic migration of totipotent germ cells. Teratomas and mixed germ-cell tumors are variously comprised of mature, immature, and malignant elements. Choriocarcinomas are rare but highly malignant.

Symptoms and signs of pineal-region germ-cell tumors most often include headaches and Parinaud syndrome of upgaze paresis. With extension to the overlying thalamus there may be hemiparesis, incoordination, vision disturbances, or movement disorders. Suprasellar germ-cell tumors produce pituitary and hypothalamic dysfunctions but usually not vision loss. CT appearance is of an irregular lesion of mixed density, occasionally with calcification, and with variable enhancement.

MRI is more sensitive for purposes of follow-up evaluation. MRI may reveal a pineal cyst in otherwise healthy children being evaluated for headache; lack of hydrocephalus and Parinaud syndrome should lead one away from the diagnosis of a pineal tumor. Diagnosis may be aided by measurement of alpha-fetoprotein and beta-subunit of human chorionic gonadotropin, which are secreted by germ-cell tumors, but not pineal parenchymal-cell tumors or cysts, and are detectable in serum and CSF. Alpha-fetoprotein is elevated in endodermal-sinus tumors and some immature teratomas; human chorionic gonadotropin is elevated in choriocarcinoma and embryonal carcinomas. Elevations associated with both indicate the presence of mixed malignant elements. Even with tumor-marker elevation, however, histologic confirmation is recommended.

Surgery for pineal-region tumors is technically difficult, but major resections may be achieved with acceptable morbidity rates by the use of supratentorial suboccipital or infratentorial supracerebellar approaches. Most patients require CSF shunting. There may be transient visual migraines caused by occipital-lobe contusions. Teratomas may be encapsulated and are therefore easier to remove. Germ-cell tumors may disseminate throughout the neuraxis, in up to 10% of cases. Radiotherapy is the standard treatment for pure germinomas, given typically as 35 Gy to 45 Gy to the brain and spine, with a 10-Gy to 15-Gy boost to the area of the tumor, affording a 90% survival rate at 5 years. Chemotherapy may allow reductions in the extent of irradiation, lessening the considerable endocrine, neuro-ophthalmologic, and neuropsychologic sequelae of treatment.

Survival rates for mixed malignant germ-cell tumors are considerably lower, rates of less than 30% with radiotherapy alone, but have improved with the addition of chemotherapy. Current protocols are based on cisplatin-containing regimens active in gonadal germ-cell tumors; patients achieving a complete response to intensive chemotherapy may receive no further treatment, while those with incomplete response undergo second-look surgery or irradiation. Five-year overall survival rates are about 75% and the event-free survival rate is 36%.

LYMPHOMAS

Primary CNS lymphomas are rare, constituting fewer than 1% of intracranial tumors and are discussed in Chapter 57. They may occur at any age and are generally of B-lymphocyte origin, including Burkitt type, often seen with congenital or acquired immunodeficiency. The tumor location most commonly seen is the cerebral cortex. CNS lymphomas appear isodense or hyperdense on CT, with enhancement. MRI shows an iso- to hypointense lesion on T1-weighted images and iso-, hypo-, or slightly hyperintense lesion on T2-weighted images, with variable enhancement. Whole-brain irradiation has produced survival rates of 20% to 30%. A prospective trial in immunocompetent adults with primary CNS lymphoma showed that preirradiation, high-dose methotrexate chemotherapy improved survival rates over whole-brain irradiation alone. In addition, there was a 94% objective-response rate to preirradiation chemotherapy, but there was also a 15% incidence of life-threatening, delayed neurologic toxicity. For these reasons, methotrexate-based chemotherapy without irradiation is now the preferred treatment.

MENINGIOMAS

Meningiomas are rare in childhood, accounting for 2.5% of pediatric brain tumors. There is an association with neurofibromatosis type 2, and this diagnosis should be sought

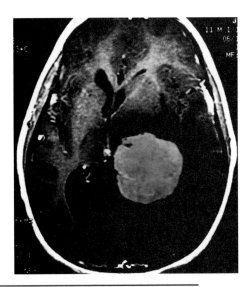

FIGURE 60.10. Axial MRI of a meningioma.

in any child with meningioma. These tumors usually arise on the meningeal surface but (in contrast to adults) may grow as parenchymal lesions, presumably from meningeal cell rests. CT and MRI show an isointense or hyperintense lesion enhancing with contrast (Fig. 60.10).

Most lesions are clinically benign, although 10% of pediatric or NF-2 associated tumors show anaplasia and 50% have atypical features. High mitotic index, MIB-1 labeling index, and variant histology (e.g., papillary, clear cell) are associated with invasiveness and adverse outcome. Deletions of NF2, DAL-1, and chromosome 1p and 14q are common. Surgery is the primary treatment. Radiotherapy is of uncertain value but has been used for recurrent tumors, especially after unsuccessful reresection. Meningiomas may occasionally involve the leptomeninges, primarily, and these tumors (i.e., meningeal sarcomas), tend to behave aggressively. Treatment has been combined radiation and chemotherapy.

LATE EFFECTS OF TREATMENT AND QUALITY OF LIFE

The health of children surviving brain tumors is generally worse than that of survivors of other childhood cancers. Children with supratentorial astrocytomas or craniopharyngioma have a lower health-status index than children with other types of brain tumors. A survey of health-related quality of life in childhood brain tumor survivors found cognitive impairment in two-thirds of the children and pain in almost one-third. Global health status was lowest in children given radiation therapy before age 5 years, and in those with residual disease.

Another survey of residual physical handicap in survivors found motor impairment in 56% of patients, cognitive impairment (i.e., IQ score less than 80) in 30%, visual impairment in 24%, and epilepsy in 21%.

A study of psychologic outcomes in long-term survivors found that the prevalence of psychologic distress (11%) exceeded that in siblings (5%) and was not a direct result of cancer treatment but rather was associated with diminished social-functioning and vocational skills. Another report found increased risk of hospital admission was the focus for psychiatric disorders among patients with brain tumors who had survived at least 3 years from diagnosis, compared to other childhood cancer survivors, in whom there was no increased risk.

Radiation effects include a transient somnolence syndrome of sleepiness, irritability, anorexia, and headaches, lasting about a week. Radiation necrosis develops in 0.1% to 5.0% of patients after conventional treatment at 50 Gy to 60 Gy, in daily fractions of 180 cGy to 200 cGy. The onset may be within 3 months and is usually seen by 3 years, although occasionally not until much later; the symptoms and signs are those of a recurrent intracranial mass, with possible seizures and progressive neuropsychologic impairment. Surgical resection should be attempted; unresectable lesions may be treated with corticosteroids, but it may be difficult to reduce the dose later. Children younger than 2 to 3 years of age are particularly susceptible to radiation injury because of incomplete development of the CNS. Large-vessel thrombosis is a rare complication of radiation therapy, occurring between 2 and 30 years after cranial irradiation. Treatment is symptomatic.

Endocrine dysfunction may follow irradiation to the hypothalamus and pituitary. Doses as low as 18 Gy may produce growth-hormone deficiency, and doses above 36 Gy may cause hypothyroidism and gonadal dysfunction in more than half of patients Nearly 40% of brain-cancer survivors in the Childhood Cancer Survivor Study were below the 10th percentile for height. Risk factors included age below 5 years at diagnosis, and radiation therapy to the hypothalamic-pituitary axis. Growth-hormone deficiency in the absence of other anterior-pituitary hormone deficiencies in children receiving cranial irradiation for posterior-fossa tumors suggests growth hormone is the hormone most sensitive to radiation injury. Hypothalamic obesity, a syndrome of intractable weight gain, is an uncommon but serious complication of hypothalamic irradiation at doses exceeding 50 Gy.

Brain tumor survivors are at risk for hypothyroidism as a collateral effect of cranial or craniospinal irradiation. The incidence of hypothyroidism appears to be considerably lower in children receiving hyperfractionated irradiation, compared to those receiving conventional once-daily dosing. Precocious puberty has been noted in nearly one-quarter of girls treated with irradiation. Frank adrenal insufficiency is uncommon, but subtle abnormalities in adrenal function may be present. There is also an increased incidence of osteoporosis.

Children should be followed for measurement of linear growth, periodic thyroid-function studies, and additional endocrine evaluation if there is precocious or delayed-onset puberty. Growth-hormone treatment improves final height in children with growth-hormone deficiency after brain-tumor therapy. Growth-hormone response depends on adequate thyroid function, and thyroid supplementation may be required. In the subset of patients in whom growth was further limited by early puberty, the combination of gonadotrophin-releasing hormone analogs and growth hormone is reported to improve prospects for attainment of target height. A survey of growth-hormone replacement therapy in patients with medulloblastoma suggests a trend toward underutilization, despite ample evidence that there is no increased risk of brain-tumor recurrence associated with growth-hormone therapy.

Cardiovascular late effects in children treated for brain tumors include increased risk of stroke, blood clots, and angina-like symptoms. Late effects are common in those treated with surgery and radiation, and higher still in those treated with surgery, radiation, and chemotherapy. Cardiovascular problems may be compounded by restrictive-lung disease and cardiotoxicity in recipients of craniospinal irradiation or intensive chemotherapy. Among survivors of childhood brain cancer, whose mean age was 26 years and mean posttreatment interval was 16 years, systolic blood pressures and waist:hip ratios were higher than controls, as were blood-lipid abnormalities. These findings identify dyslipidemia, central obesity, and hypertension as controllable risk factors for cardiovascular disease.

Neurologic and neurosensory sequelae in adult survivors of childhood brain tumors include hearing loss, blindness, cataracts, and diplopia. Nearly half of the survivors have coordination problems, and one-quarter have motor-control problems after radiation doses of 50 Gy to frontal-brain regions. Seizures are reported in one-quarter of patients, especially after radiation doses of 30 Gy or more. Atonic seizures in particular are difficult to control, and are associated with pervasive cognitive impairments. Patients treated with surgery alone generally have no more than minor neurologic impairment that does not interfere with activities of daily living, but one-third have severe ataxia, spastic paresis, visual impairment, or epilepsy.

Radiation therapy is a principal cause of *neurocognitive disorders* in children with CNS tumors. Other factors include acute or chronic increased ICP, tumor-mass effect, poorly controlled seizure disorders, and complications of surgery and chemotherapy. Radiologic evaluation of patients treated for medulloblastoma with craniospinal irradiation, with or without chemotherapy, showed reduced volumes of normal white matter, which correlated with full-scale IQ. Neurocognitive problems are more likely in children treated at a young age or with high doses of radiation, especially when applied to cerebral-cortical areas associated with higher functions. The effects may be progressive for years and may include attention deficit, impaired memory, and lowering IQ. In one series, mean observed full-scale IQ was 97.1 for nonirradiated patients and 78.8

for irradiated patients. These children generally require psychologic intervention and special education programs.

Chronic neurotoxicity of chemotherapy used in treating CNS tumors includes hearing loss (e.g., especially after cisplatin therapy) and peripheral neuropathy (e.g., with vincristine or occasionally cisplatin and etoposide). Osteopenia is found in half of the children surviving brain tumors, and bone pain may limit physical activity. Chemotherapy may potentiate the deleterious effect of craniospinal irradiation on growth. There is an increased risk (3% to 5%) of second tumors, including meningiomas and sarcomas arising 10 to 20 years after cranial irradiation treatment. Secondary leukemia has been reported after chemotherapy with alkylating agents and etoposide.

SUGGESTED READINGS

Epidemiology

Amlashi SF, Riffaud L, Brassier G, et al. Nevoid basal cell carcinoma syndrome: Relation with desmoplastic medulloblastoma in infancy. A population-based study and review of the literature. *Cancer* 2003;98:618–624.

Bergsagel DJ, Finegold MJ, Butel JS, et al. DNA sequences similar to those of simian virus 40 in ependymomas and choroid plexus tumors of childhood. *N Engl J Med* 1992;326:988–993.

Biegel JA. Genetics of pediatric central nervous system tumors. *J Pediatr Hematol Oncol* 1997;19:492–501.

Blamires TL, Maher ER. Choroid plexus papilloma. A new presentation of von Hippel-Lindau (VHL) disease. *Eye* 1992;6:90–92.

Bunin G. What causes childhood brain tumors? Limited knowledge, many clues. *Pediatr Neurosurg* 2000;32:321–326.

Bunin GR, Buckley JD, Boesel CP, et al. Risk factors for astrocytic glioma and primitive neuroectodermal tumor of the brain in young children: a report from the Children's Cancer Group. *Cancer Epidemiol Biomarkers Prev* 1994;3:197–204.

Bunin GR, Kuijten RR, Buckley JD, et al. Relation between maternal diet and subsequent primitive neuroectodermal brain tumors in young children. *N Engl J Med* 1993;329:536–541.

Curless RG, Toledano SR, Ragheb J, et al. Hematogenous brain metastasis in children. *Pediatr Neurol* 2002;26:219–221.

Gold DR, Cohen BH. Brain tumors in neurofibromatosis. *Curr Treat Options Neurol* 2003;5:199–206.

Green AJ, Smith M, Yates JR. Loss of heterozygosity on chromosome 16p13.3 in hamartomas from tuberous sclerosis patients. *Nat Genet* 1994;6:193–196.

Gurney JG, Mueller BA, Preston-Martin S, et al. A study of pediatric brain tumors and their association with epilepsy and anticonvulsant use. *Neuroepidemiology* 1997;16:248–255.

Gurney JG, Severson RK, Davis S, et al. Incidence of cancer in children in the United States. Sex-, race-, and 1-year age-specific rates by histologic type. *Cancer* 1995;75:2186–2195.

Hader WJ, Drovini-Zis K, Maguire JA. Primitive neuroectodermal tumors in the central nervous system following cranial irradiation: A report of four cases. *Cancer* 2003;97:1072–1076.

Holly EA, Bracci PM, Mueller BA, et al. Farm and animal exposures and pediatric brain tumors: results from the United States West Coast Childhood Brain Tumor Study. *Cancer Epidemiol Biomark Prev* 1998;7:797–802.

Kheifets LI, Sussman SS, Preston-Martin S. Childhood brain tumors and residential electromagnetic fields (EMF). *Rev Environ Contam Toxicol* 1999;159:111–129

Kluwe L, Hagel C, Tatagiba M, et al. Loss of NF1 alleles distinguish sporadic from NF1-associated pilocytic astrocytomas. *J Neuropathol Exp Neurol* 2001;60:917–920.

Louis DN, Ramesh V, Gusella JF. Neuropathology and molecular genetics of neurofibromatosis 2 and related tumors. *Brain Pathol* 1995;5:163–172.

Nabbout R, Santos M, Rolland Y, et al. Early diagnosis of subependymal giant cell astrocytoma in children with tuberous sclerosis. *J Neurol Neurosurg Psychiatry* 1999;66:370–375.

Rickert CH, Paulus W. Epidemiology of central nervous system tumors in childhood and adolescence based on the new WHO classification. *Childs Nerv Syst* 2001;17:503–511.

Rickert CH, Sträter R, Kaatsch P, et al. Pediatric high-grade astrocytomas show chromosomal imbalances distinct from adult cases. *Am J Pathol* 2001;158:1525–1532.

Rubio MP, Correa KM, Ramesh V, et al. Analysis of the neurofibromatosis 2 gene in human ependymomas and astrocytomas. *Cancer Res* 1994;54:45–47.

Shore RE, Moseson M, Harley N, et al. Tumors and other diseases following childhood x-ray treatment for ringworm of the scalp (Tinea capitis). *Health Phys* 2003;85:404–408.

Smith MA, Freidlin B, Ries LA, et al. Trends in reported incidence of primary malignant brain tumors in children in the United States. *J Natl Cancer Inst* 1998;90:1269–1277.

Van Wijngaarden E, Stewart PA, Olshan AF, et al. Parental occupational exposure to pesticides and childhood brain cancer. *Am J Epidemiol* 2003;157:989–997.

Walter AW, Hancock ML, Pui CH, et al. Secondary brain tumors in children treated for acute lymphoblastic leukemia at St Jude Children's Research Hospital. *J Clin Oncol* 1998;16:3761–3767.

Developmental Biology

Biegel JA, Tan L, Zhang F, et al. Alterations of the hSNF5/INI1 gene in central nervous system atypical teratoid/rhabdoid tumors and renal and extrarenal rhabdoid tumors. *Clin Cancer Res* 2002;8:3461–3467.

Ding H, Roncari L, Shannon P, et al. Astrocyte-specific expression of activated p21-RAS results in malignant astrocytoma formation in a transgenic mouse model of human gliomas. *Cancer Res* 2001;61:3826–3836.

Hesselager G, Holland EC. Using mice to decipher the molecular genetics of brain tumors. *Neurosurgery* 2003;53:685–694.

Holland EC, Celestino J, Dai C, et al. Combined activation of RAS and AKT in neural progenitors induces glioblastoma formation in mice. *Nat Genet* 2000;25:55–57.

Judkins AR, Mauger J, Rorke LB, Biegel JA. Immunohistochemical analysis of hSNF5/INI1 in pediatric CNS neoplasms. *Am J Surg Pathol* 2004;28:644–650.

Leung C, Lingbeek M, Shakhova O, et al. Bmi1 is essential for cerebellar development and is overexpressed in human medulloblastomas. *Nature* 2004;428:337–341.

Li J, Yen C, Liaw D, et al. PTEN, a putative protein tyrosine phosphatase gene mutated in human brain, breast, and prostate cancer. *Science* 1997;275:1943–1947.

Merlo A. Genes and pathways driving glioblastomas in humans and murine disease models. *Neurosurg Rev* 2003;26:145–158.

Pomeroy SL, Tamayo P, Gaasenbeek M, et al. Prediction of central nervous system embryonal tumour outcome based on gene expression. *Nature* 2002;415:436–442.

Rubin JB, Rowitch DH. Medulloblastoma: a problem of developmental biology. *Cancer Cell* 2002;2:7–8.

Wang VY, Zoghbi HY. Genetic regulation of cerebellar development. *Nat Rev Neurosci* 2001;2:484–491.

Wechsler-Reya R, Scott MP. The developmental biology of brain tumors. *Ann Rev Neurosci* 2001;24:385–428.

Wechsler-Reya RJ. Analysis of gene expression in the normal and malignant cerebellum. *Recent Prog Horm Res* 2003;58:227–248.

Zedan W, Robinson PA, High AS. A novel polymorphism in the PTC gene allows easy identification of allelic loss in basal cell nevus syndrome lesions. *Diagn Mol Pathol* 2001;10:41–45.

Symptoms, Diagnosis, and Management

Cochrane DD, Gustavsson B, Poskitt KP, et al. The surgical and natural morbidity of aggressive resection for posterior fossa tumors in childhood. *Pediatr Neurosurg* 1994;20:19–29.

Dahlborg SA, Petrillo A, Crossen JR, et al. The potential for complete and durable response in nonglial primary brain tumors in children and young adults with enhanced chemotherapy delivery. *Cancer J Sci Am* 1998;4:110–124.

Dobrovoljac M, Hengartner H, Boltshauser E, et al. Delay in the diagnosis of paediatric brain tumours. *Eur J Pediatr* 2002;161:663–667.

Duffner PK, Horowitz ME, Krischer JP, et al. Postoperative chemotherapy and delayed radiation in children less than three years of age with malignant brain tumors. *N Engl J Med* 1993;328:1725–1731.

Duffner PK, Horowitz ME, Krischer JP, et al. The treatment of malignant brain tumors in infants and very young children: An update of the Pediatric Oncology Group experience. *Neuro-oncol* 1999;1:152–161.

Finlay JF, Goldman S, Wong MC, et al. Pilot study of high-dose thiotepa and etoposide with autologous bone marrow rescue in children and young adults with recurrent CNS tumors. *J Clin Oncol* 1996;14:2495–2503.

Gilles FH, Brown WD, Leviton A, et al. Limitations of the World Health Organization classification of childhood supratentorial astrocytic tumors. Childhood Brain Tumor Consortium. *Cancer* 2000;88:1477–1483.

Gilles FH, Leviton A, Tavare CJ, et al. Clinical and survival covariates of eight classes of childhood supratentorial neuroglial tumors. *Cancer* 2002;95:1302–1310.

Habrand JL, De Crevoisier R. Radiation therapy in the management of childhood brain tumors. *Childs Nerv Syst* 2001;17:121–133.

Hug EB, Sweeney RA, Nurre PM, et al. Proton radiotherapy in management of pediatric base of skull tumors. *Int J Radiat Oncol Biol* 2002;52:1017–1024.

Kalifa C, Valtreau D, Pizer B, et al. High-dose chemotherapy in childhood brain tumours. *Childs Nerv Syst* 1999;15:498–505.

Kellie SJ. Chemotherapy of central nervous system tumours in infants. *Childs Nerv Syst* 1999;15:592–612.

Kestle JR. Pediatric hydrocephalus: Current management. *Neurol Clin* 2003;21:883–895.

Kleihues P, Burger PC, Scheithauer BW. The new WHO classification of brain tumours. *Brain Pathol* 1993;3:255–268.

Kleihues P, Louis DN, Scheithauer BW, et al. The WHO classification of tumors of the central nervous system. *J Neuropathol Exp Neurol* 2002;61:215–225.

Kortmann RD, Timmermann B, Becker G, et al. Advances in treatment techniques and time/dose schedules in external radiation therapy of brain tumors in childhood. *Klin Pediatr* 1998;210:220–226.

Kramer ED, Vezine LG, Packer RJ, et al. Staging and surveillance of children with central nervous system neoplasms: recommendations of the Neurology and Tumor Imaging Committees of the Children's Cancer Group. *Pediatr Neurosurg* 1994;20:254–263.

Lashford LS, Campbell RH, Gattamaneni HR, et al. An intensive multiagent chemotherapy regimen for brain tumours occurring in very young children. *Arch Dis Child* 1996;74:219–223.

Levisohn L, Cronin-Golomb A, Schmahmann JD. Neuropsychological consequences of cerebellar tumour resection in children: Cerebellar cognitive affective syndrome in a paediatric population. *Brain* 2000;123(Pt 5):1041–1050.

Maria BL, Drane WE, Mastin ST, et al. Comparative value of thallium and glucose SPECT imaging in childhood brain tumors. *Pediatr Neurol* 1998;19:351–357.

Mason WP, Grovas A, Halpern S, et al. Intensive chemotherapy and bone marrow rescue for young children with newly diagnosed malignant brain tumors. *J Clin Oncol* 1998;16:210–221.

Medina LS, Kuntz KM, Pomeroy S. Children with headache suspected of having a brain tumor: A cost-effectiveness analysis of diagnostic strategies. *Pediatrics* 2001;108:255–263.

Minn AY, Pollock BH, Garzarella L, et al. Surveillance neuroimaging to detect relapse in childhood brain tumors: a Pediatric Oncology Group study. *J Clin Oncol* 2001;19:4135–4140.

Noel G, Habrand JL, Helfre S, et al. Proton beam therapy in the management of central nervous system tumors in childhood: The preliminary experience of the Centre de Protontherapie d'Orsay. *Med Pediatr Oncol* 2003;40:309–315.

Steinbok P, Cochrane DD, Perrin R, et al. Mutism after posterior fossa tumour resection in children: Incomplete recovery on long-term follow-up. *Pediatr Neurosurg* 2003;39:179–183.

Taylor JS, Langston JW, Reddick WE, et al. Clinical value of proton magnetic resonance spectroscopy for differentiating recurrent or residual brain tumor from delayed cerebral necrosis. *Int J Radiat Oncol Biol Phys* 1996;36:1251–1261.

Tzika AA, Vajapeyam S, Barnes PD. Multivoxel proton MR spectroscopy and hemodynamic MR imaging of childhood brain tumors: preliminary observations. *Am J Neuroradiol* 1997;18:203–218.

Utriainen M, Metsahonkala L, Salmi TT, et al. Metabolic characterization of childhood brain tumors: Comparison of 18F-fluorodeoxyglucose and ^{11}C-methionine positron emission tomography. *Cancer* 2002;95:1376–1386.

Warren KE, Frank JA, Black JL, et al. Proton magnetic resonance spectroscopic imaging in children with recurrent primary brain tumors. *J Clin Oncol* 2000;18:1020–1026.

Warren KE, Patronas N, Aikin AA, et al. Comparison of one-, two-, and three-dimensional measurements of childhood brain tumors. *J Natl Cancer Inst* 2001;93:1401–1405.

Congenital Tumors

Adamek D, Korzeniowska A, Morga R, et al. Dysembryoplastic neuroepithelial tumor (DNT). Is the mechanism of seizures related to glutamate? An immunohistochemical study. *Folia Neuropathol* 2001;39:111–117.

Allen J, Wissof J, Helson L, et al. Choroid plexus carcinoma: responses to chemotherapy alone in newly diagnosed young children. *J Neurooncol* 1992;12:69–74.

Bachli H, Avoledo P, Gratzl O, et al. Therapeutic strategies and management of desmoplastic infantile ganglioglioma: two case reports and literature review. *Childs Nerv Syst* 2003;19:359–366.

Chow E, Reardon DA, Shah AB, et al. Pediatric choroid plexus neoplasma. *Int J Radiat Oncol Biol Phys* 1999;44:249–254.

Dash RC, Provenzale JM, McComb RD, et al. Malignant supratentorial ganglioglioma (ganglion cell–giant cell glioblastoma): a case report and review of the literature. *Arch Pathol Lab Med* 1999;123:342–345.

Ferreira J, Eviatar L, Schneider S, et al. Prenatal diagnosis of intracranial teratoma. Prolonged survival after resection of a malignant teratoma diagnosed prenatally by ultrasound: a case report and literature review. *Pediatr Neurosurg* 1993;19:84–88.

Fischer EG, Welch K, Shillito J Jr, et al. Craniopharyngiomas in children. Long-term effects of conservative surgical procedures combined with radiation therapy. *J Neurosurg* 1990;73:534–540.

Fisher PG, Jenab J, Gopldthwaite PT, et al. Outcomes and failure patterns in childhood craniopharyngiomas. *Childs Nerv Syst* 1998;14:558–563.

Fornari M, Solero C, Lasio G, et al. Surgical treatment of intracranial dermoid and epidermoid cysts in children. *Childs Nerv Syst* 1990;6:66–70.

Fouladi M, Jenkins J, Burger P, et al. Pleomorphic xanthoastrocytoma: Favorable outcome after complete surgical resection. *Neuro-oncol* 2001;3:184–192.

Hayward R. The present and future management of childhood craniopharyngioma. *Childs Nerv Syst* 1999;15:764–769.

Hellwig D, Bauer BL, Schulte M, et al. Neuroendoscopic treatment for colloid cysts of the third ventricle: The experience of a decade. *Neurosurgery* 2003;52:525–533.

Hoffman HJ, DeSilva M, Humphreys RP, et al. Aggressive surgical management of craniopharyngiomas in children. *J Neurosurg* 1992;76:47–52.

Im SH, Chung CK, Cho BK, et al. Intracranial ganglioglioma: Preoperative characteristics and oncologic outcome after surgery. *J Neurooncol* 2002;59:173–183.

Jakacki RI, Cohen BH, Jamison C, et al. Phase II evaluation of interferon-alpha-2a for progressive or recurrent craniopharyngiomas. *J Neurosurg* 2000;92:255–260.

Lunardi P, Missori P. Supratentorial dermoid cysts. *J Neurosurg* 1991;75:262–266.

Mallucci C, Lellouch-Tubiana A, Salazar C, et al. The management of desmoplastic neuroepithelial tumours in childhood. *Childs Nerv Syst* 2000;16:8–14.

McEvoy AW, Harding BN, Phipps KP, et al. Management of choroid plexus tumours in children: 20 years experience at a single neurosurgical center. *Pediatr Neurosurg* 2000;32:192–199.

Sarkar C, Sharma MC, Gaikwad S, et al. Choroid plexus papilloma: a clinicopathological study of 23 cases. *Surg Neurol* 1999;52:37–39.

Souveidane MM, Johnson JH Jr, Lis E. Volumetric reduction of a choroid plexus carcinoma using preoperative chemotherapy. *J Neurooncol* 1999;43:167–171.

Stripp DC, Maity A, Janss AJ, et al. Surgery with or without radiation therapy in the management of craniopharyngiomas in children and young adults. *Int J Radiat Oncol Biol Phys* 2004;58:714–720.

Zentner J, Wolf HK, Ostertun B, et al. Gangliogliomas: clinical, radiological, and histopathological findings in 51 patients. *J Neurol Neurosurg Psychiatry* 1994;57:1497–1502.

Astrocytomas

Albright AL, Packer RJ, Zimmerman R, et al. Magnetic resonance scans should replace biopsies for the diagnosis of diffuse brain stem gliomas: A report from the Children's Cancer Group. *Neurosurgery* 1993;33:1026–1029.

Allen JC, Aviner S, Yates AJ, et al. Treatment of high-grade spinal cord astrocytoma of childhood with "8-in-1" chemotherapy and radiotherapy: a pilot study of CCG-945. Children's Cancer Group. *J Neurosurg* 1998;88:215–220.

Amano T, Inamura T, Nakamizo A, et al. Case management of hydrocephalus associated with the progression of childhood brain stem gliomas. *Childs Nerv Syst* 2002;18:599–604.

Bowers DC, Gargan L, Kapur P, et al. Study of the MIB-1 labeling index as a predictor of tumor progression in pilocytic astrocytomas in children and adolescents. *J Clin Oncol* 2003;21:2968–2973.

Bowers DC, Krause TP, Aronson LJ, et al. Second surgery for recurrent pilocytic astrocytoma in children. *Pediatr Neurosurg* 2001;34:229–234.

Bredel M, Pollack IF, Hamilton RL, et al. Epidermal growth factor receptor expression and gene amplification in high-grade non-brainstem gliomas of childhood. *Clin Cancer Res* 1999;5:1786–1792.

Daglioglu E, Cataltepe O, Akalan N. Tectal gliomas in children: the implications for natural history and management strategy. *Pediatr Neurosurg* 2003;38:223–231.

Finlay JL, August C, Packer R, et al. High-dose multi-agent chemotherapy followed by bone marrow "rescue" for malignant astrocytomas of childhood and adolescence. *J Neurooncol* 1990;9:239–248.

Finlay JL, Boyett JM, Yates AJ, et al. Randomized phase III trial in childhood high-grade astrocytoma comparing vincristine, lomustine, and prednisone with the eight-drugs-in-1-day regimen. *J Clin Oncol* 1995;13:112–123.

Gajjar A, Heideman RL, Kovnar EH, et al. Response of pediatric low-grade gliomas to chemotherapy. *Pediatr Neurosurg* 1993;19:113–120.

Gesundheit B, Klement G, Senger C, et al. Differences in vasculature between pilocytic and anaplastic astrocytomas of childhood. *Med Pediatr Oncol* 2003;41:516–526.

Gropman AL, Packer RJ, Nicholson HS, et al. Treatment of diencephalic syndrome with chemotherapy: growth, tumor response, and long term control. *Cancer* 1998;83:166–172.

Heidemen RL, Kuttesch J Jr, Gajjar AJ, et al. Supratentorial malignant gliomas in childhood. A single institution perspective. *Cancer* 1997;80:497–504.

Jallo GI, Biser-Rohrbaugh A, Freed D. Brainstem gliomas. *Childs Nerv Syst* 2004;20:143–153.

Jallo GI, Freed D, Epstein F. Intramedullary spinal cord tumors in children. *Childs Nerv Syst* 2003;19:641–649.

Janss AJ, Grundy R, Cnaan A, et al. Optic pathway and hypothalamic/chiasmatic gliomas in children younger than age 5 years with a 6-year follow-up. *Cancer* 1995;75:1051–1059.

Khatua S, Peterson KM, Brown KM, et al. Overexpression of the EGFR/FKBP12/HIF-2alpha pathway identified in childhood astrocytomas by angiogenesis gene profiling. *Cancer Res* 2003;63:1865–1870.

Lashford LS, Thiesse P, Jouvet A, et al. Temozolomide in malignant gliomas of childhood: a United Kingdom Children's Cancer Study Group and French Society for Pediatric Oncology Intergroup Study. *J Clin Oncol* 2002;20:4684–4691.

Lewis J, Lucraft H, Gholkar A. UKCCSG study of accelerated radiotherapy for pediatric brain stem gliomas. United Kingdom Childhood Cancer Study Group. *Int J Radiat Oncol Biol Phys* 1997;38:925–929.

Listernick R, Louis DN, Packer RJ, et al. Optic pathway gliomas in children with neurofibromatosis 1: consensus statement from the NF1 Optic Pathway Glioma Task Force. *Ann Neuro* 1997;41:143–149.

Lowis SP, Pizer BL, Coakham H, et al. Chemotherapy for spinal cord astrocytoma: can natural history be modified? *Childs Nerv Syst* 1998;14:317–321.

Martinez-Lage JF, Perez-Espejo MA, Esteban JA, et al. Thalamic tumors: clinical presentation. *Childs Nerv Syst* 2002;18:405–411.

Packer RJ, Boyett JM, Zimmerman RA, et al. Hyperfractionated radiation therapy (72 Gy) for children with brain stem gliomas: a Children's Cancer Group phase I/II trial. *Cancer* 1993;72:1414–1421.

Packer RJ, Prados M, Phillips P, et al. Treatment of children with newly diagnosed brain stem gliomas with intravenous recombinant beta-interferon and hyperfractionated radiation therapy: a Children's Cancer Group phase I/II study. *Cancer* 1996;77:2150–2152.

Pencalat P, Maixner W, Sainte-Rose C, et al. Benign cerebellar astrocytomas in children. *J Neurosurg* 1999;90:265–273.

Pollack IF. The role of surgery in pediatric gliomas. *J Neurooncol* 1999;42:271–288.

Pollack IF, Boyett JM, Finlay JL. Chemotherapy for high-grade gliomas of childhood. *Childs Nerv Syst* 1999;15:529–544.

Pollack IF, Finkelstein SD, Woods J, et al. Expression of p53 and prognosis in children with malignant gliomas. *N Engl J Med* 2002;346:420–427.

Pollack IF, Hamilton RL, Burnham J, et al. Impact of proliferation index on outcome in childhood malignant gliomas: Results in a multi-institutional cohort. *Neurosurgery* 2002;50:1238–1244.

Sanghavi SN, Needle MN, Krailo MD, et al.. A phase I study of topotecan as a radiosensitizer for brainstem glioma of childhood: first report of the Children's Cancer Group-0952. *Neuro-oncol* 2003;5:8–13.

Saran FH, Baumert BG, Khoo VS, et al. Stereotactically guided conformal radiotherapy for progressive low-grade gliomas of childhood. *Int J Radiat Oncol Biol Phys* 2002;53:43–51.

Schmandt SM, Packer RJ, Vezina LG, et al. Spontaneous regression of low-grade astrocytomas in childhood. *Pediatr Neurosurg* 2000;32:132–136.

Sposto R, Ertel IH, Jenkin RD, et al. The effectiveness of chemotherapy for treatment of high grade astrocytoma in children: results of a randomized trial. A report from the Children's Cancer Study Group. *J Neurooncol* 1989;7:165–177.

Tao ML, Barnes PD, Billett AL, et al. Childhood optic chiasm gliomas: radiographic response following radiotherapy and long-term clinical outcome. *Int J Radiat Oncol Biol Phys* 1997;39:579–587.

Wisoff JH, Boyett JM, Berger MS, et al. Current neurosurgical management and the impact of the extent of resection in the treatment of malignant gliomas of childhood: a report of the Children's Cancer Group Trial No. CCG-945. *J Neurosurg* 1998;89:52–59.

Embryonal Tumors: Medulloblastomas, Primitive Neuroectodermal Tumors, and Atypical Teratoid/Rhabdoid Tumors

Aldosari N, Bigner SH, Burger PC, et al. MYCC and MYCN oncogene amplification in medulloblastoma. A fluorescence in situ hybridization study on paraffin sections from the Children's Oncology Group. *Arch Pathol Lab Med* 2002;126:540–544.

Biegel JA, Janss AJ, Raffel C, et al. Prognostic significance of chromosome 17p deletions in childhood primitive neuroectodermal tumors (medulloblastomas) of the central nervous system. *Clin Cancer Res* 1997;3:473–478.

Biegel JA, Kalpana G, Knudsen ES, et al. The role of INI1 and the SWI/SNF complex in the development of rhabdoid tumors: meeting summary from the workshop on childhood atypical teratoid/rhabdoid tumors. *Cancer Res* 2002;62:323–328.

Burger PC, Yu IT, Tihan T, et al. Atypical teratoid/rhabdoid tumor of the central nervous system: a highly malignant tumor of infancy and childhood frequently mistaken for medulloblastoma. A Pediatric Oncology Group study. *Am J Surg Pathol* 1998;22:1083–1092.

Cogen PH, Daneshvar L, Metzger AK, Edwards MS et al. Deletion mapping of the medulloblastoma locus on chromosome 17p. *Genomics* 1990;8:279–285.

Cohen BH, Zeltzer PM, Boyett JM, et al. Prognostic factors and treatment results for supratentorial primitive neuroectodermal tumors in children using radiation and chemotherapy: A Children's Cancer Group randomized trial. *J Clin Oncol* 1995;13:1687–1696.

Dunkel IJ, Boyett JM, Yates A, et al. High-dose carboplatin, thiotepa, and etoposide with autologous stem-cell rescue for patients with recurrent medulloblastoma. *J Clin Oncol* 1998;16:222–228.

Eberhart CG, Kepner JL, Goldthwaite PT, et al. Histopathologic grading of medulloblastomas: a Pediatric Oncology Group study. *Cancer* 2002;94:552–560.

Evans AE, Jenkin RDT, Sposto R, et al. The treatment of medulloblastoma. Results of a prospective randomized trial of radiation therapy with and without CCNU, vincristine, and prednisone. *J Neurosurg* 1990;72:572–582.

Gajjar AJ, Heideman RL, Douglass EC, et al. Relation of tumor-cell ploidy to survival in children with medulloblastoma. *J Clin Oncol* 1993;11:2211–2217.

Gajjar A, Hernan R, Kocak M, et al. Clinical, histopathologic, and molecular markers of prognosis: Toward a new disease risk stratification system for medulloblastoma. *J Clin Oncol* 2004;22:984–993.

Goldwein JW, Radcliffe J, Packer RJ, et al. Results of a pilot study of low-dose craniospinal radiation therapy plus chemotherapy for children younger than 5 years with primitive neuroectodermal tumors. *Cancer* 1993;71:2647–2652.

Grotzer MA, Hogarty MD, Janss AJ, et al. MYC messenger RNA expression predicts survival outcome in childhood primitive neuroectodermal tumor/medulloblastoma. *Clin Cancer Res* 2001;7:2425–2433.

Grotzer MA, Janss AJ, Phillips PC, et al. Neurotrophin receptor Trk C predicts good clinical outcome in medulloblastoma and other primitive neuroectodermal brain tumors. *Klin Padiatr* 2000;212:196–199.

Jakacki RI, Zeltzer PM, Boyett JM, et al. Survival and prognostic factors following radiation and/or chemotherapy for primitive neuroectodermal tumors of the pineal region in infants and children: a report of the Children's Cancer Group. *J Clin Oncol* 1995;13:1377–1383.

Kortmann RD, Kuhl J, Timmermann B, et al. Postoperative neoadjuvant chemotherapy before radiotherapy as compared to immediate radiotherapy followed by maintenance chemotherapy in the treatment of medulloblastoma in childhood: results of the German prospective randomized trial HIT 91. *Int J Radiat Oncol Biol Phys* 2000;46:269–279.

Kun LE, Constine LS. Medulloblastoma: caution regarding new treatment approaches. *Int J Radiat Oncol Biol Phys* 1991;20:897–899.

Lusher ME, Lindsey JC, Latif F, et al. Biallelic epigenetic inactivation of the RASSF1A tumor suppressor gene in medulloblastoma development. *Cancer Res* 2002;62:5906–5911.

McNeil DE, Cote TR, Clegg L, et al. Incidence trends in pediatric malignancies medulloblastoma/primitive neuroectodermal tumor: a SEER update. Surveillance Epidemiology and End Results. *Med Pediatr Oncol* 2002;39:190–194.

Michaels EM, Weiss MM, Hoovers JM, et al. Genetic alterations in childhood medulloblastoma analyzed by comparative genomic hybridization. *J Pediatr Hematol Oncol* 2002;24:205–210.

Packer RJ, Biegel JA, Blaney S, et al. Atypical teratoid/rhabdoid tumor of the central nervous system: Report on workshop. *J Pediatr Hematol Oncol* 2002;24:337–342.

Packer RJ, Goldwein J, Nicholson HS, et al. Treatment of children with medulloblastomas with reduced-dose craniospinal radiation therapy and adjuvant chemotherapy: a Children's Cancer Group Study. *J Clin Oncol* 1999;17:2127–2136.

Packer RJ, Sutton LN, Elterman R, et al. Outcome for children with medulloblastoma treated with radiation and cisplatin, CCNU, and vincristine chemotherapy. *J Neurosurg* 1994;81:690–698.

Pigott TJ, Punt JA, Lowe JS, et al. The clinical, radiological and histopathological features of cerebral primitive neuroectodermal tumours. *Br J Neurosurg* 1990;4:287–297.

Pomeroy SL, Tamayo P, Gaasenbeek M, et al. Prediction of central nervous system embryonal tumour outcome based on gene expression. *Nature* 2002;415:436–442.

Reddy AT, Janss AJ, Phillips PC, et al. Outcome for children with supratentorial primitive neuroectodermal tumors treated with surgery, radiation, and chemotherapy. *Cancer* 2000;88:2189–2193.

Rickert CH, Paulus W. Chromosomal imbalances detected by comparative genomic hybridization in atypical teratoid/rhabdoid tumours. *Childs Nerv Syst* 2004;20:221–224.

Schabet M, Martos J, Buchholz R, et al. Animal model of human medulloblastoma: clinical, magnetic resonance imaging, and histopathological findings after intra-cisternal injection of MHH-MED-1 cells into nude rats. *Med Pediatr Oncol* 1997;29:92–97.

Tait DM, Thornton-Jones H, Bloom HJ, et al. Adjuvant chemotherapy for medulloblastoma: the first multi-centre control trial of the International Society of Pediatric Oncology (SIOP I). *Eur J Cancer* 1990;26:464–469.

Thomas PR, Deutsch M, Kepner JL, et al. Low-stage medulloblastoma: final analysis of trial comparing standard-dose with reduced-dose neuraxis irradiation. *J Clin Oncol* 2000;18:3004–3011.

Timmermann B, Kortmann RD, Kuhl J, et al. Role of radiotherapy in the treatment of supratentorial primitive neuroectodermal tumors in childhood: results of the prospective German brain tumor trials HIT 88/89 and 91. *J Clin Oncol* 2002;20:842–849.

Weil MD, Lamborn K, Edwards MS, et al. Influence of a child's sex on medulloblastoma outcome. *JAMA* 1998;279:1474–1476.

Weiner HL, Bakst R, Hurlbert MS, et al. Induction of medulloblastomas in mice by sonic hedgehog, independent of Gli1. *Cancer Res* 2002;62:6385–6389.

Ependymomas

Goldwein JW, Leahy JM, Packer RJ, et al. Intracranial ependymomas in children. *Int J Radiat Oncol Biol Phys* 1990;99:1497–1502.

Good CD, Wade AM, Hayward RD, et al. Surveillance neuroimaging in childhood intracranial ependymomas: How effective, how often, and for how long? *J Neurosurg* 2001;94:27–32.

Granzow M, Popp S, Weber S, et al. Isochromosome 1q as an early genetic event in a child with intracranial ependymoma characterized by molecular cytogenetics. *Cancer Genet Cytogenet* 2001;130:79–83.

Korshunov A, Golanov A, Sycheva R, et al. The histologic grade is a main prognostic factor for patients with intracranial ependymomas treated in the microneurosurgical era: an analysis of 258 patients. *Cancer* 2004;100:1230–1237.

Kramer DL, Parmiter AH, Rorke LB, et al. Molecular cytogenetic studies of pediatric ependymomas. *J Neurooncol* 1998;37:25–33.

Needle MN, Goldwein JW, Grass J, et al. Adjuvant chemotherapy for the treatment of intracranial ependymoma of childhood. *Cancer* 1997;80:341–347.

Sutton LN, Goldwein J, Perilongo G, et al. Prognostic factors in childhood ependymomas. *Pediatr Neurosurg* 1990;16:57–65.

Timmermann B, Kortmann RD, Kuhl J, et al. Combined postoperative irradiation and chemotherapy for anaplastic ependymomas in childhood: results of the German prospective trials HIT 88/89 and HIT 91. *Int J Radiat Oncol Biol Phys* 2000;46:287–295.

Van Veelen-Vincent ML, Pierre-Kahn A, Kalifa C, et al. Ependymoma in childhood: prognostic factors, extent of surgery, and adjuvant therapy. *J Neurosurg* 2002;97:827–835.

Germ-Cell Tumors

Benesch M, Lackner H, Schagerl S, et al. Tumor- and treatment-related side effects after multimodal therapy of childhood intracranial germ cell tumors. *Acta Paediatr* 2001;90:264–270.

Drummond KJ, Rosenfeld JV. Pineal region tumours in childhood. A 30-year experience. *Childs Nerv Syst* 1999;15:119–126.

Kellie SJ, Boyce H, Dunkel IJ, et al. Primary chemotherapy for intracranial nongerminomatous germ cell tumors: Results of the second international CNS germ cell study group protocol. *J Clin Oncol* 2004;22:846–853.

Lymphomas

Cheng AL, Yeh KH, Uen WC, et al. Systemic chemotherapy alone for patients with non-acquired immunodeficiency syndrome-related central nervous system lymphoma. A pilot study of the BOMES protocol. *Cancer* 1998;82:1946–1951.

DeAngelis LM. Primary central nervous system lymphomas. *Curr Treat Options Oncol* 2001;2:309–318.

DeAngelis LM, Seiferheld W, Schold SC, et al. Combination chemotherapy and radiotherapy for primary central nervous system lymphoma: Radiation Therapy Oncology Group Study 93-10. *J Clin Oncol* 2002;20:4643–4648.

DeAngelis LM, Yahalom J, Thaler HT, et al. Combined modality therapy for primary CNS lymphoma. *J Clin Oncol* 1992;10:635–643.

Silfen ME, Garvin JH Jr, Hays AP, et al. Primary central nervous system lymphoma in childhood presenting as progressive panhypopituitarism. *J Pediatr Hematol Oncol* 2001;23:130–133.

Meningiomas

Amirjamshidi A, Mehrazin M, Abbassioun K. Meningiomas of the central nervous system occurring below the age of 17: report of 24 cases not associated with neurofibromatosis and review of the literature. *Childs Nerv Syst* 2000;16:406–416.

Erdincler P, Lena G, Sarioglu AC, et al. Intracranial meningiomas in children: review of 29 cases. *Surg Neurol* 1998;49:136–140.

Greenberg SB, Schneck MJ, Faerber EN, et al. Malignant meningioma in a child: CT and MR findings. *Am J Radiol* 1993;160:1111–1112.

Perry A, Giannini C, Raghavan R, et al. Aggressive phenotypic and genotypic features in pediatric and NF2-associated meningiomas: a clinicopathologic study of 53 cases. *J Neuropathol Exp Neurol* 2001;60:994–1003.

Late Effects of Treatment and Quality of Life

Andersen PB, Krabbe K, Leffers AM, et al. Cerebral glucose metabolism in long-term survivors of childhood primary brain tumors treated with surgery and radiotherapy. *J Neurooncol* 2003;62:305–313.

Barr RD, Simpson T, Webber CE, et al. Osteopenia in children surviving brain tumors. *Eur J Cancer* 1998;34:873–877.

Barr RD, Simpson T, Whitton A, et al. Health-related quality of life in survivors of tumours of the central nervous system in childhood—A preference-based approach to measurement in a cross-sectional study. *Eur J Cancer* 1999;35:248–255.

Carlson-Green B, Morris RD, Krawiecki N. Family and illness predictors of outcome in pediatric brain tumors. *J Pediatr Psychol* 1995;20:769–784.

Constine LS, Woolf PD, Cann D, et al. Hypothalamic-pituitary dysfunction after radiation for brain tumors. *N Engl J Med* 1993;328:87–94.

Foreman NK, Faestel PM, Pearson J, et al. Health status in 52 long-term survivors of pediatric brain tumors. *J Neurooncol* 1999;41:47–53.

Gleeson HK, Stoeter R, Ogilvy-Stuart AL, et al. Improvements in final height over 25 years in growth hormone (GH)-deficient childhood survivors of brain tumors receiving GH replacement. *J Clin Endocrinol Metab* 2003;88:3682–3689.

Gurney JG, Kadan-Lottick NS, Packer RJ, et al. Endocrine and cardiovascular late effects among adult survivors of childhood brain tumors: Childhood Cancer Survivor Study. *Cancer* 2003;97:663–673.

Gurney JG, Ness KK, Stovall M, et al. Final height and body mass index among adult survivors of childhood brain cancer: Childhood cancer survivor study. *J Clin Endocrinol Metab* 2003;88:4731–4739.

Heikens J, Ubbink MC, van der Pal HP, et al. Long term survivors of childhood brain cancer have an increased risk for cardiovascular disease. *Cancer* 2000;88:2116–2121.

Jakacki RI, Goldwein JW, Larsen RL, et al. Cardiac dysfunction following spinal irradiation during childhood. *J Clin Oncol* 1993;11:1033–1038.

Jakacki RI, Schramm CM, Donahue BR, et al. Restrictive lung disease following treatment for malignant brain tumors: a potential late effect of craniospinal irradiation. *J Clin Oncol* 1995;13:1478–1485.

Khan RB, Marshman KC, Mulhern RK. Atonic seizures in survivors of childhood cancer. *J Child Neurol* 2003;18:397–400.

Lustig RH, Post SR, Srivannaboon K, et al. Risk factors for the development of obesity in children surviving brain tumors. *J Clin Endocrinol Metab* 2003;88:611–616.

Macedoni-Luksic M, Jereb B, Todorovski L. Long-term sequelae in children treated for brain tumors: Impairments, disability, and handicap. *Pediatr Hematol Oncol* 2003;20:89–101.

Mulhern RK, Reddick WE, Palmer SL, et al.. Neurocognitive deficits in medulloblastoma survivors and white matter loss. *Ann Neurol* 1999;46:834–841.

Oberfield SE, Chin D, Uli N, et al. Endocrine late effects of childhood cancers. *J Pediatr* 1997;131(Pt 2):S37–S41.

Olshan JS, Gubernick J, Packer RJ, et al. The effects of adjuvant chemotherapy on growth in children with medulloblastoma. *Cancer* 1992;70:2013–2017.

Packer RJ, Boyett JM, Janss AJ, et al. Growth hormone replacement therapy in children with medulloblastomas: use and effect on tumor control *J Clin Oncol* 2001;19:480–487.

Packer RJ, Gurney JG, Punyko JA, et al. Long-term neurologic and neurosensory sequelae in adult survivors of a childhood brain tumor: Childhood cancer survivor study. *J Clin Oncol* 2003;21:3255–3261.

Reimers TS, Ehrenfels S, Mortensen EL, et al. Cognitive deficits in long-term survivors of childhood brain tumors: Identification of predictive factors. *Med Pediatr Oncol* 2003;40:26–34.

Ross L, Johansen C, Dalton SO, et al. Psychiatric hospitalizations among survivors of cancer in childhood or adolescence. *N Engl J Med* 2003;349:650–657.

Silber JH, Radcliffe J, Peckham V, et al. Whole-brain irradiation and decline in intelligence: the influence of dose and age on IQ score. *J Clin Oncol* 1992;10:1390–1396.

Sklar CA, Mertens AC, Mitby P, et al. Risk of disease recurrence and second neoplasms in survivors of childhood cancer treated with growth hormone: a report from the Childhood Cancer Survivor Study. *J Clin Endocrinol Metab* 2002;87:3136–3141.

Sonderkaer S, Schmiegelow M, Carstensen H, et al. Long-term neurological outcome of childhood brain tumors treated by surgery only. *J Clin Oncol* 2003;21:1347–1351.

Spoudreas HA, Charmandari E, Brook CG. Hypothalamo-pituitary-adrenal axis integrity after cranial irradiation for childhood posterior fossa tumours. *Med Pediatr Oncol* 2003;40:224–229.

Swerdlow AJ, Reddingius RE, Higgins CD, et al. Growth hormone treatment of children with brain tumors and risk of tumor recurrence. *J Clin Endocrinol Metab* 2000;85:4444–4449.

Zebrack BJ, Gurney JG, Oeffinger K, et al. Psychological outcomes in long-term survivors of childhood brain cancer: A report from the childhood cancer survivor study. *J Clin Oncol* 2004;22:999–1006.

Chapter 61

Vascular Tumors and Malformations

J. P. Mohr and John Pile-Spellman

This chapter includes reviews of a heterogeneous group of vascular lesions, some of which are true vascular malformations, some acquired fistulas, a few that belong to a category of neoplasms, and a few that are difficult to classify, as follows:

Vascular Malformations
Arteriovenous malformations
Venous malformations
Cavernous malformations
Telangiectases
Sturge-Weber disorder
Sinus pericranii

Vascular Tumors
Angioblastic meningiomas
Hemangiopericytomas
Hemangioblastomas

VASCULAR MALFORMATIONS

Vascular lesions regarded as malformations (i.e., arteriovenous malformation [AVM]) of the brain have been confused with vascular neoplasms because the clinical course may be progressive and the angiographic picture is sometimes indistinguishable from a neoplasm of blood vessels. However, although they may enlarge in size, and in some instances proliferate in complexity, none are true neoplasms if, by definition, that means having a capacity for metastasis. Further, despite repeated search, none of them have shown any mitotic features on histologic study. Although the term malformation suggests a congenital lesion, some arteriovenous fistulae are acquired from trauma and some from arterial or venous occlusions.

Arteriovenous Malformations

Whether congenital or acquired, AVMs are limited to the brain, dura, or both. Those confined to the brain are the more commonly seen. At the main site of linkage between the arteries and veins, histologic study finds no capillaries; the nidus is a tangle of abnormal arteries and veins with

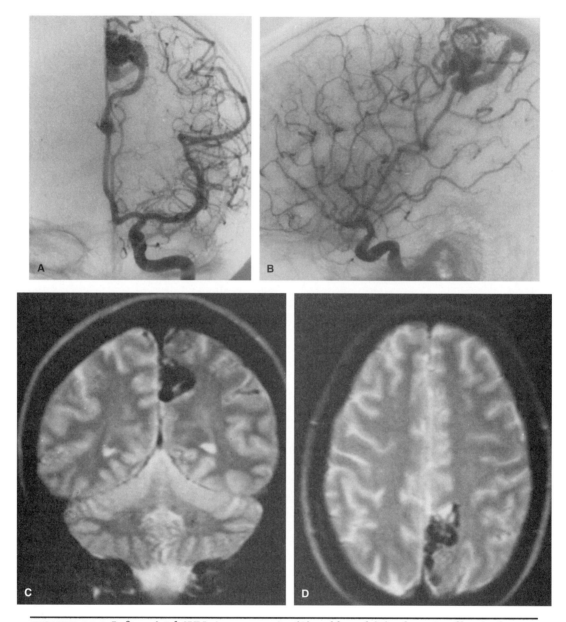

FIGURE 61.1. Left parietal AVM. Anteroposterior **(A)** and lateral **(B)** subtraction films in the arterial phase of a left internal-carotid injection show the anterior cerebral artery (ACA) supply and early superficial-venous drainage of a left-parietal AVM. Coronal **(C)** and axial **(D)** T2-weighted MRIs of the same patient show a serpiginous pattern of signal void, representing flow in vascular structures. (Courtesy of Drs. J. A. Bello and S. K. Hilal.)

interposed sinuses of irregularly sized vascular channels, lacks a media, and neither arteries nor veins are clearly delineated. Only rarely is an AVM found in newborns or infants, suggesting a congenital origin is so well hidden that only growth over decades brings the lesion to clinical attention, through hemorrhage or mass effect from displacement of adjacent brain tissue. AVM location varies widely; some are limited to the surface of one cerebral hemisphere. Others have their major focus in the subsurface white matter; a few are confined to the deep structures (e.g., basal

ganglia, thalamus), and a small number are found in the cerebellum or the brain stem, even in arteries leading to the choroid plexus, alone. Those on the brain surface in the border zone between the major cerebral arteries typically draw supply from more than one of the adjacent cerebral-arterial branches. Collaterals may come from the adjacent dura. Those that penetrate to the ventricular wall often draw collaterals from the deep vasculature supplying the basal ganglia. Venous drainage may be by superficial means or the deep venous systems.

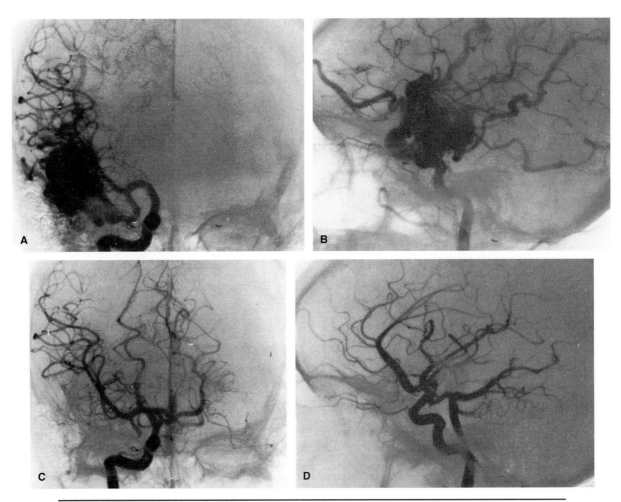

FIGURE 61.2. **Right temporal AVM. A:** Anteroposterior view from arterial phase of right internal-carotid arteriogram shows a large, enhancing vascular lesion in right temporal region, supplied by enlarged branches of the right middle cerebral artery. **B:** Lateral view demonstrates prominent early draining of cortical veins emanating from AVM. Postembolization antero-posterior (**C**) and lateral (**D**) views of right internal-carotid arteriogram show interval disappearance of right-temporal AVM with multiple metallic coils seen within right middle-cerebral arterial feeders. Note the normal filling of both anterior cerebral arteries and both posterior cerebral arteries, thereby confirming increase in blood flow to normal brain structures. Patient did well after embolization with no complications. Follow-up definitive surgery found no evidence of flow within AVM, and the nidus was removed to prevent recurrence. (Courtesy of Drs. S. Chan and S. K. Hilal, Columbia University College of Physicians and Surgeons, New York, NY.)

Risks

Based on current population studies, incident discovery is 1.5 per 100 000 population; hemorrhage leads to discovery in approximately half of the cases. The threat to health is hemorrhage. Although the annual risk of bleeding has been considered comparable to that of cerebral aneurysms, the morbidity differs; although usually far less serious clinically, some AVMs are barely symptomatic, but a few are devastating. The risk for hemorrhage is well correlated with the presence of deep-venous drainage and a deep location of the lesion; risks are far lower when the lesion is on the brain surface and drains to surface veins. The hemorrhage usually arises from the nidus, displacing adjacent healthy brain, with varying degrees of resulting damage. For those with ready venous access to the ventricular system, the main effect of bleeding may be ventricular, mainly causing a hemocephalus or hydrocephalus. Uncommonly, the hemorrhage arises on or near the brain surface, spreading into the subarachnoid space. Arteries feeding the AVM nidus may develop flow-related aneurysms, and these may bleed separately, causing typical subarachnoid-hemorrhage syndromes. Hemorrhage occurs most commonly in the middle decades of life.

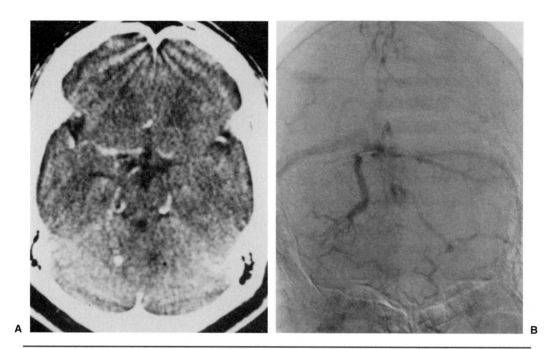

A   **B**

FIGURE 61.3. **Venous angioma. A:** Postcontrast CT demonstrates a round, enhancing structure in the right-cerebellar hemisphere, seen on contiguous axial sections as well, and therefore consistent with a single prominent vessel, as seen end on. This is the typical CT appearance of a venous angioma. **B:** An anteroposterior subtraction film in the venous phase of a vertebral angiogram shows medullary veins in the right-cerebellar hemisphere, converging toward a single vertically oriented draining vein that corresponds to the vessel seen in cross section on CT. The arterial phase was typically normal. (Courtesy of Drs. J. A. Bello and S. K. Hilal.)

Clinical Presentation and Diagnosis

AVMs are less often associated with seizures or headaches. No distinctive features separate either the seizures or the types of headaches (including migraines) from non-AVM causes (Figs. 61.1 through 61.3).

CT or MRI detects acute hemorrhage; MRI and MRA document the AVM, any prior major hemorrhage, intranidal aneurysms, and the main sources of vascular supply. In cases intended for treatment, the vascular anatomy is best defined by angiography, the use of which should be reserved for such times (Figs. 61.4 and 61.5).

Treatment

Once the first hemorrhage has occurred, recurrence is common enough to require that a treatment plan be made. The annual hemorrhage risk for those patients with AVMs who are increasingly being discovered prior to hemorrhage is far less clear, and plans for intervention should be based on the feasibility of eradication with a minimum of neurologic disturbance. For those undergoing treatment, intravascular occlusive therapy using quick-acting glues and other agents may obliterate some AVMs feeders or, rarely, even the whole AVM. More commonly, the

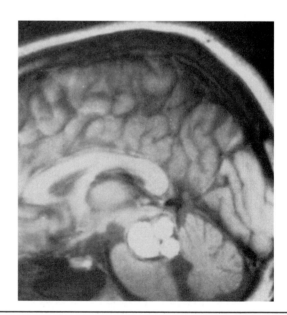

FIGURE 61.4. **Cavernous malformation, brainstem.** Sagittal T1-weighted MRI demonstrates a loculated-appearing midbrain lesion of increased signal intensity, surrounded by ring of decreased signal intensity, which is characteristic of a subacute hemorrhage surrounded by a ring of hemosiderin. Cavernous vascular malformations typically show evidence of previous hemorrhage. (Courtesy of Drs. J. A. Bello and S. K. Hilal.)

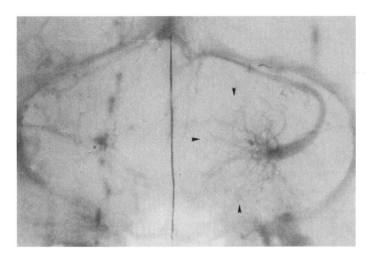

FIGURE 61.5. Subtraction posterior-fossa angiogram, venous phase. In this anteroposterior view, the characteristic venous malformation is demonstrated (*arrows*).

reduction of flow by embolization in the pathways creates a more favorable setting for operation. Surgery remains the most effective means of eliminating AVMs. For the smaller (less than 2.5 cm) deeply lying lesions not suitable for embolization or surgery, focused-beam radiotherapy (i.e., radiosurgery) is an alternative therapy. Despite eradication as documented by postoperative MRA, still a small number of lesions recur. The vein of Galen malformation is a special AVM associated with the deep-venous system, often with marked aneurysmal dilatation of the vein of Galen region. The arterial supply may be complex and difficult to occlude by intravascular or surgical techniques. These lesions are symptomatic in neonates or young children; severe vascular shunting leads to cardiac failure and compression of the midbrain, which subsequently causes hydrocephalus. The currently accepted treatment

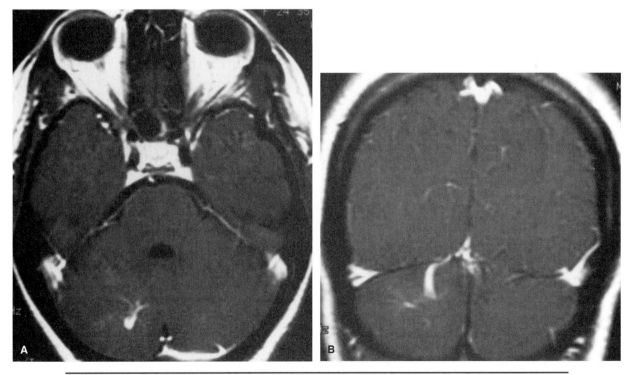

FIGURE 61.6. Venous angioma. T1-weighted gadolinium-enhanced axial **(A)** and coronal **(B)** MR scans demonstrate prominent vascular enhancement within the right-cerebellar hemisphere, with prominent venous radicles draining into an enlarged draining vein. This configuration is characteristic of venous angioma. (Courtesy of Dr. S. Chan, Columbia University College of Physicians and Surgeons, New York, NY.)

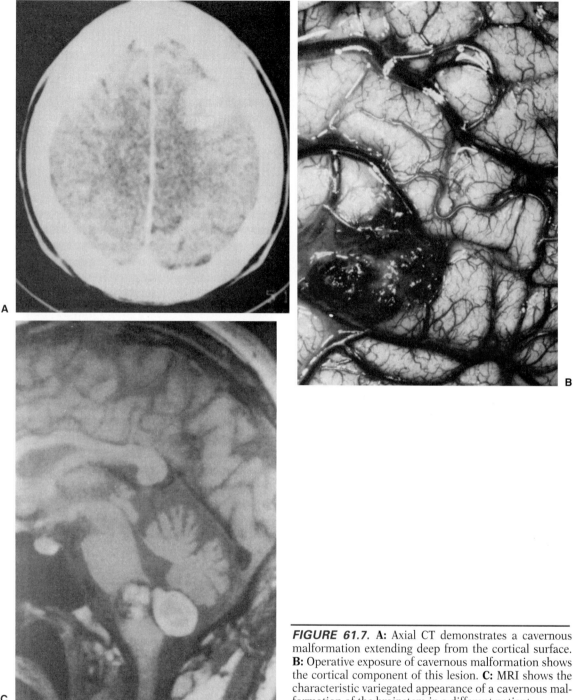

A

B

C

FIGURE 61.7. A: Axial CT demonstrates a cavernous malformation extending deep from the cortical surface. **B:** Operative exposure of cavernous malformation shows the cortical component of this lesion. **C:** MRI shows the characteristic variegated appearance of a cavernous malformation of the brainstem in a different patient.

of these lesions is embolization, occasionally followed by surgery.

Venous Malformations

Venous malformations (e.g., deep-venous anomalies) are characterized by no apparent arterial supply. They may cause headaches, seizures, and rarely, hemorrhage (Fig. 61.6).

They are easily recognized using CT because of their characteristic contrast enhancement. They generally lie in the deep white matter, portions of the brain stem, and cerebellum, and are often spider-like (e.g., caput medusa), diffuse, ill-defined, are not amenable to obliteration by occlusion of the arterial supply (the lesion is entirely venous), and are thus not suitable candidates for safe surgical resection. These lesions generally follow a benign course. The symptoms produced by the lesion are treated individually.

Only under extenuating circumstances is surgical resection considered.

Cavernous Malformation

Cavernous malformations are highly focal anomalies, varying in size; most are less than 1 cm in diameter. Histologically, they show a distinct cluster of tiny vessels of uniform size, hence the basis of the name cavernous. The vessels are too small to be seen on angiogram and are rarely documented by CT. They may cause a limited local hemorrhage, and it may recur, but bleeding sufficient to cause major disability is uncommon. Multiple lesions have been documented in families. They may occur anywhere in the brain. Owing to hemosiderin residua from inferred, prior, asymptomatic hemorrhage, the lesion may be visible on CT or MRI. Some may be mistaken for a vascular tumor, however, even without displacement of the surrounding structures. MRI is characterized by a target appearance (Fig. 61.7). Seizures, headaches, or vague neurologic symptoms may occur. If hemorrhage has occurred and the lesion is readily accessible, surgery is usually recommended.

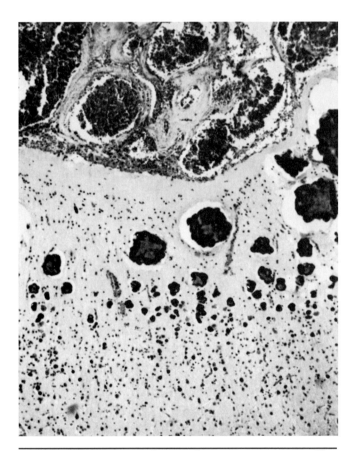

FIGURE 61.8. Sturge-Weber syndrome. Angiomatous malformation in meninges and calcification in cortex. Hematoxylin and eosin stain. (Courtesy of Dr. P. Duffy.)

Telangiectasias

Telangiectasias are collections of engorged capillaries or cavernous spaces separated by relatively normal brain tissue. Telangiectasias are usually small and poorly circumscribed, and may be found in any portion of the CNS but have a propensity for the white matter. In the *Rendu-Osler-Weber syndrome* (the exact order of authors sometimes varying, according to the country using the term), brain telangiectasias are associated with telangiectasia of the skin (i.e., mucous membranes, respiratory, gastrointestinal, and genitourinary tracts). The presence of the tiny fistula, however difficult it may be to demonstrate as a pulmonary shunt, may nonetheless provide a path for septic material instigating brain-abscess formation. Major hemorrhage is rare. For the most part, these are neurologic curiosities; they may not be identified on angiography or CT and have no surgical significance. They are usually recognized only at autopsy. However, rare cases of large, map-like brain-surface lesions have been described. Interest in genetic mapping for the remarkable variety of telangiectasias has increased greatly, and may well lead to a total reclassification of these lesions that is separate from the classic, clinical description. For the present, a clinical description is still popular. Future editions of this book may no longer give prominent place to the disorders mentioned below.

Sturge-Weber Disease (Krabbe-Weber-Dimitri Disease)

Whether to consider this disease as an example of AVM or as a member of the telangiectasia group is open to argument, but genetic mapping has been achieved. The two cardinal features are (1) a localized atrophy and calcification of the cerebral cortex associated with capillary malformation (CM), and (2) an ipsilateral port wine-colored facial nevus, usually in the distribution of the first division of the trigeminal nerve. Angiomatous malformation in the meninges, ipsilateral exophthalmos, glaucoma, buphthalmos, angiomas of the retina, optic atrophy, and dilated vessels in the sclera may also be present. Any portion of the cerebral cortex may be affected by the atrophic process, but the occipital and parietal regions are most commonly involved. In the atrophic cortical areas, there is loss of nerve cells and axons and proliferations of the fibrous glia. The small vessels are thickened and calcified, particularly in the second- and third-cortical layers. Small calcium deposits are also present in the cerebral substance (Fig. 61.8); rarely are there large, calcified nodules.

When an angioma is present, it is limited to the meninges overlying the area of shrunken cortex. It is now generally agreed that the atrophy and calcification of the cortex are not secondary to the angiomatous malformations of the leptomeninges.

Clinical Presentation and Diagnosis

It is possible for the combination of a port-wine facial nevus and localized cortical atrophy to exist without clinical symptoms but in most patients, convulsive seizures are present from infancy. Mental retardation, glaucoma, contralateral hemiplegia (Fig. 61.9), and hemianopia are also present in most cases. Sturge-Weber disease may be diagnosed without difficulty from the clinical syndrome. The presence of the cortical lesion may be demonstrated in most cases by the appearance of characteristic shadows in the radiographs (Fig. 61.10).

The calcified area in the cortex appears as a sinuous shadow with a double contour, showing both the gyri and sulci of the affected cerebral convolutions. The lesions in the occipital or parietal lobes are usually more definitely calcified than are those that occur in the frontal lobe.

Treatment

The treatment of Sturge-Weber disease is essentially symptomatic. Anticonvulsive drugs are given for the seizures. Radiation therapy has been recommended, but there is no evidence that it is of any benefit. Hemispherectomy may control the convulsive seizures but is avoided because of its high rate of complications.

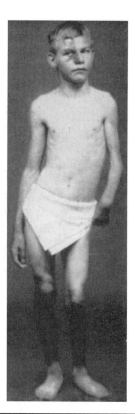

FIGURE 61.9. Sturge-Weber disease. Right facial nevus in a patient with convulsions and left hemiparesis. (Courtesy of Dr. P. I. Yakovlev.)

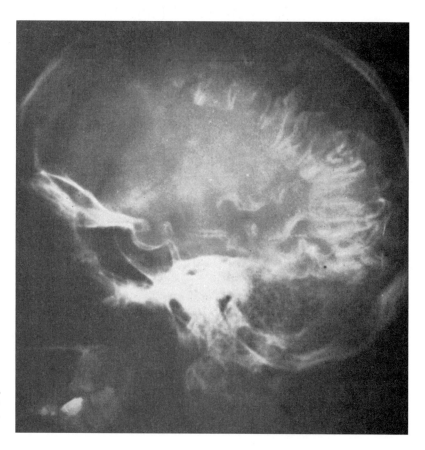

FIGURE 61.10. Radiograph shows the intracerebral calcification in Sturge-Weber disease. (Courtesy of Dr. P. I. Yakovlev.)

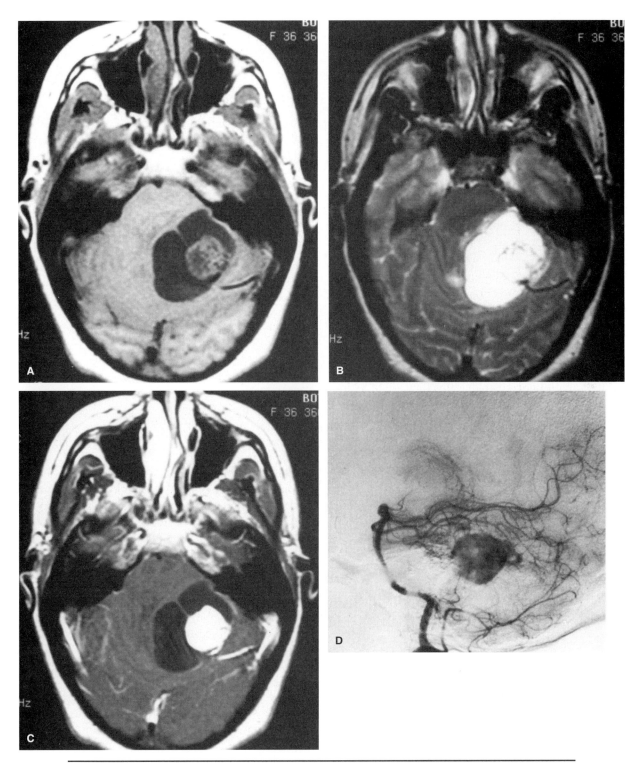

FIGURE 61.11. Cerebellar hemangioblastoma. T1-weighted **(A)** and T2-weighted **(B)** axial MR scans demonstrate a large, fluid-filled cyst in the left-cerebellar hemisphere that appears dark on T1 scan and bright on T2 scan. A mass of heterogeneous signal intensity present within the left-posterior aspect of the cyst appears attached to the wall of the cyst. Note prominent blood vessel projecting to the left from the posterior aspect of this mural nodule, probably representing draining vein. **C:** T1-weighted axial MR scan with gadolinium enhancement shows marked enhancement of mural nodule and no enhancement of the cyst. Note prominent enhancement of enlarged draining vein. **D:** Lateral view from late-arterial phase of conventional vertebral arteriogram shows densely enhancing mass in posterior fossa with posterior draining vein. (Courtesy of Drs. S. Chan and A. G. Khandji, Columbia University College of Physicians and Surgeons, New York, NY.)

Sinus Pericranii

Sinus pericranii is composed of thin-walled vascular spaces interconnected by numerous anastomoses that protrude from the skull and communicate with the superior longitudinal sinus. The malformation appears early in life and is soft and compressible; it increases in size when the venous pressure in the head is raised by coughing, straining, or lowering the head. It may enlarge slowly over a period of years. The external protuberance may be seen at any portion of the midline of the skull, including the occiput, but is most often found in the mid-portion of the forehead. Except for the external swelling, there are usually no symptoms. Occasionally, there may be pulsating tinnitus, increased intracranial pressure (ICP), or a variety of cerebral symptoms. Radiographs show a defect of the underlying bone, through which the lesion communicates with the longitudinal sinus.

VASCULAR TUMORS

The three forms of the neoplastic lesions may be variations of the same tumor. Histologically, they are indistinguishable. The hemangioblastoma is confined to the posterior fossa and has no dural attachment. The angioblastic meningioma is, grossly, identical to other meningiomas but has a significant dural attachment and is located either above or below the tentorium. The hemangiopericytoma originates in other areas of the body, presumably from blood vessel elements.

Angioblastic Meningiomas

These tumors are included here because they are histologically similar to the other tumors reviewed in this section.

Hemangiopericytomas

The hemangiopericytoma arises from the endothelial elements of blood vessels and is recognized elsewhere in the body. It is histologically similar to the angioblastic meningioma and the hemangioblastoma, especially when the vascular spaces are separated more widely and the stroma cells are collected about the vascular spaces. It may be that the pial and endothelial cells are interconvertible.

Hemangioblastomas

Hemangioblastomas are composed of primitive vascular elements and are rare, accounting for only 1% to 2% of all intracranial neoplasms. They occur at all ages, but young and middle-aged adults are more frequently afflicted. In children, they occur almost as commonly in the posterior fossa as do meningiomas (Fig. 61.11).

Clinical Manifestations and Diagnosis

Symptoms are generally present for approximately a year before the diagnosis is made. Male incidence predominates. *Von Hippel-Lindau disease* is defined by the coexistence of hemangioblastoma and multiple angiomatoses of the retina, cysts of the kidney and pancreas, and occasionally, of renal cell carcinomas and capillary nevi of the skin. There is a familial incidence in 20% of cases. Only 10% to 20% of the hemangioblastomas, however, are associated with the systemic signs known as the Lindau syndrome. All gradations of clinical expression between the full syndrome and incomplete manifestations may be seen in the same family. Pheochromocytoma and syringomyelia may occur, especially when the hemangioblastoma site is in the spinal cord. Polycythemia disappears after resection of the neoplasm, but returns with tumor recurrence; an erythropoietic substance from the cystic fluid has been identified.

These tumors are seen predominantly in the cerebellum, are often associated with large cysts surrounded by a glial wall and contain yellow, proteinaceous fluid, which may be the result of secretion and hemorrhage from the tumor. It resembles the cyst and mural nodule of the cystic-cerebellar astrocytoma but shows a distinctive vascular appearance on angiogram. The tumors may be multiple, in which case it may be difficult to achieve cure or total removal of the lesion. They have no dural attachment and only rarely occur in the supratentorial area, where they may be mistaken for angioblastic meningiomas. The most common site of the hemangioblastoma is in the paramedian cerebellar hemispheric area; the second most common site is the spinal cord. Hemangioblastomas also occur in the medulla, in the area postrema. Clinical features of the hemangioblastoma of the cerebellum are symptoms typical of any cerebellar mass, such as headaches, papilledemas, and ataxia. When the tumor is multiple, lesions may involve the brain stem and upper cervical cord as well. Hemangioblastoma of the cerebellum may be diagnosed without difficulty from the CT and posterior-fossa angiogram. The diagnosis is even more certain when the tumor is associated with angiomas of the retina and polycythemia.

Treatment

Treatment is surgical, with evacuation of the cyst and removal of the mural nodule; 85% of all patients who undergo this treatment are alive and well 5 to 20 years after surgery. There is a high incidence of recurrence, however, if the tumor is only partially removed or the patient has multiple tumors.

SUGGESTED READINGS

Brancati F, Valente EM, Tadini G, et al. Autosomal dominant hereditary benign telangiectasia maps to the CMC1 locus for capillary malformation on chromosome 5q14. *J Med Genet* 2003;40:849–853.

Comi AM. Pathophysiology of Sturge-Weber syndrome. *Child Neurol* 2003;18:509–16.

Cushing H, Bailey P. *Tumors Arising from the Blood Vessels of the Brain.* Springfield, IL: Charles C Thomas, 1928.

Eerola I, Boon LM, Mulliken JB, et al. Capillary malformation-arteriovenous malformation, a new clinical and genetic disorder caused by RASA1 mutations. *Am J Hum Genet* 2003;73:1240–9.

Gold AP, Ransohoff J, Carter S. Vein of Galen malformation. *Acta Neurol Scand* 1964;40(suppl 11):1–31.

Guttmacher AE, Marchuk DA, White RI. Hereditary hemorrhagic telangiectasia. *N Engl J Med* 1995;333:918–924.

Kruse F Jr. Hemangiopericytomas of the meninges (angioblastic meningioma of Cushing and Eisenhardt). Clinicopathologic aspects and follow-up studies in 8 cases. *Neurology* 1961;11:771–777.

Lasjaunias P. *Vascular Diseases in Neonates, Infants and Children. Interventional Neuroradiology Management.* Berlin, Germany: Springer-Verlag, 1997.

Mast H, Young WL, Koennecke HC, et al. Risk of spontaneous hemorrhage after diagnosis of cerebral arteriovenous malformations. *Lancet* 1997;350:1065–1068.

McLaughlin MR, Kondziolka D, Flickinger JC, Lunsford S, Lunsford LD. The prospective natural history of cerebral venous malformations. *Neurosurgery* 1998;43:195–200.

Mohr JP, Stein BM, Pile Spellman J. Arteriovenous malformations. In: Barnett JM, Mohr JP, Stein BM, Yatsu FM, eds. *Stroke. Pathophysiology, Diagnosis and Management.* Philadelphia, PA: Churchill Livingstone, 1998:725–750.

Naff NJ, Wemmer J, Hoenig-Rigamonti K, Rigamonti DR. A longitudinal study of venous malformations: documentation of a negligible risk and benign natural history. *Neurology* 1998;50:1709–1714.

Neumann HP, Lips CJ, Hsia YE, Zbar B. Von Hippel-Lindau syndrome. *Brain Pathol* 1995;5:181–193.

Retta SF, Avolio M, Francalanci F, et al. Identification of Krit1B: a novel alternative splicing isoform of cerebral cavernous malformation gene-1. *Gene* 2004;325:63–78.

Richard S, Graff J, Lindau J, Resche F. Von Hippel-Lindau disease. *Lancet* 2004;363(9416):1231–1234.

Romanowski CW, Cavallin LI. Tuberous sclerosis, von Hippel-Lindau disease, Sturge-Weber syndrome. *Hosp Med* 1998;59:226–231.

Schaller C, Pavlidis C, Schramm J. Differential therapy of cerebral arteriovenous malformations. An analysis with reference to personal microsurgery experience. *Nervenarzt* 1996;67:860–869.

Sheu M, Fauteux G, Chang H, et al. Sinus pericranii: dermatologic considerations and literature review. *J Am Acad Dermatol* 2002;46(6): 934–941.

Stapf C, Mast H, Sciacca RR, et al. The New York Islands AVM Study: design, study progress, and initial results. *Stroke* 2003;34:e29–e33.

Slater A, Moore NR, Huson SM. The natural history of cerebellar hemangioblastomas in von Hippel-Lindau disease. *Am J Neuroradiol* 2003;24:1570–1574.

Sung DI, Thang CH, Harisiadis L. Cerebellar hemangioblastomas. *Cancer* 1982;49:553–555.

Tang SC, Jeng JS, Liu HM, Yip PK. Diffuse capillary telangiectasia of the brain manifested as a slowly progressive course. *Cerebrovasc Dis* 2003;15:140–142.

Thomas-Sohl KA, Vaslow DF, Maria BL. Sturge-Weber syndrome: a review. *Pediatr Neurol* 2004;30(5):303-10303–310.

Chapter 62

Metastatic Tumors

Lisa M. DeAngelis

EPIDEMIOLOGY

At autopsy, 25% of all patients with systemic cancer have intracranial metastases: 15% have metastases to the brain, 5% to the leptomeninges and 5% to the dura. The incidence of CNS metastases may be increasing as improved therapies prolong survival from systemic disease. This may permit microscopic tumor in sanctuary sites such as the CNS to grow and become symptomatic. Brain metastases are about eight times more common than primary brain tumors; 12,000 people die annually, in the United States, with primary brain tumors but 93,000 die with symptomatic brain metastases each year.

BRAIN METASTASIS

Brain metastases are usually found with disseminated systemic disease. However, in some patients the symptoms and signs of intracranial disease appear before the systemic cancer is found. Evaluation of the neurologic symptoms reveals the CNS metastases, and after systemic evaluation, the underlying malignancy. In some patients, the systemic source is never found. At other times, the CNS disease appears after the systemic disease has been eradicated and the brain is an isolated site of relapse. These different clinical scenarios may affect the choice of treatment. Therapy is also determined by the number of metastatic lesions seen at diagnosis. Approximately half of all patients with brain metastases have single lesions and an additional 20% have only two lesions. Thus, 70% of patients are potentially eligible for focal therapy.

Non-small cell lung cancer is the most common primary lesion leading to a brain metastasis, but melanoma and small-cell lung cancer have the greatest propensity to metastasize to the brain. Other primary cancers that commonly spread to the brain include breast, renal, and GI cancers. Almost every malignancy has been reported to metastasize to brain, but tumors that rarely do include prostate, pancreas and uterine cancers.

Clinical Findings

Symptoms are similar to those of any space-occupying lesion. There is frequently more edema surrounding a small brain metastasis than a primary brain tumor and this may cause increased intracranial pressure (ICP). Symptoms include headaches (25%), hemiparesis (25%), cognitive or behavioral changes (15%) and seizures (15%). Multiple, small brain metastases in a miliary pattern may produce a clinical picture identical to that of diffuse encephalopathy but without lateralizing signs (Fig. 62.1).

Most patients have subacute courses, with progressive dysfunction over 1 or 2 weeks. Occasionally, the onset is acute and stroke-like, especially when there has been an intratumoral hemorrhage. The most common cause of hemorrhagic metastasis is lung cancer because it is the most common primary, but melanoma, thyroid, renal and choriocarcinoma all have a greater propensity to bleed.

Imaging

MRI with administration of gadolinium is the only important diagnostic test for brain metastases (Fig. 62.2). The lesions are contrast enhancing, usually diffusely so when small, and ring-enhancing when larger. They are typically spherical and often occur at the junction between gray and white matter. If a patient cannot undergo MRI (e.g., owing to presence of pacemaker), then contrast-enhanced CT may identify most brain metastases, but some lesions are missed on CT that would be visualized on MRI, particularly subcentimeter lesions and those in the posterior fossa.

Clinical Evaluation

In the patient without a known primary tumor and with suspected brain metastases on MRI, systemic evaluation is appropriate. Physical examination should address possible breast, testicular, prostate, or rectal lesions. Stool should be examined for occult blood. The standard imaging approach has been chest, abdomen and pelvic CT, with bone scan and mammogram. This may be replaced by performing a total body PET with fluorodeoxyglucose, the most sensitive approach to identifying a systemic source of metastasis.

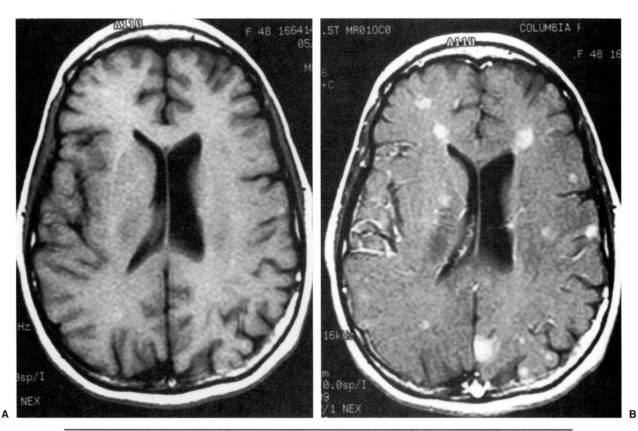

FIGURE 62.1. Miliary brain metastases. Noncontrast-enhanced **(A)** and contrast-enhanced **(B)** MRIs of a patient with breast cancer. Note that the nonenhanced scan appears almost normal. The contrast-enhanced scan shows greater than 20 separate, metastatic lesions with no significant surrounding edema. This patient was neurologically normal at the time of this scan, which was performed after a cervical spine MRI showed a cerebellar metastasis.

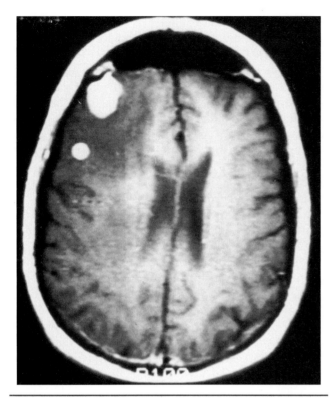

FIGURE 62.2. Melanoma brain metastases. Noncontrast-enhanced, T1-weighted MRI of a patient with recurrent melanoma. The metastases are high signal because of either the presence of melanin within the tumor, or hemorrhage. Note the extensive surrounding edema.

Differential Diagnosis

When a patient with cancer develops neurologic symptoms and has intracranial lesions on MRI, the first consideration is metastatic disease; however, the MRI may not differentiate metastases from other processes. The diagnosis may be suspect when the location of the lesion is atypical for a metastasis, such as within the corpus callosum. Rarely, a biopsy may be necessary to establish the diagnosis with certainty.

Other intracranial processes may occur in cancer patients—such as infection, primary brain tumors, and demyelination—that can mimic brain metastases. In one study of patients with a single brain metastasis, all of whom had resection or biopsy, 11% had some other diagnosis once the pathology was reviewed. In patients who have been immunosuppressed by chemotherapy, pulmonary infection may lead to septic emboli and brain abscess. Multiple, small, contrast-enhancing lesions may be seen in tuberculosis or fungal abscesses. On MRI, abscesses have thin-walled rings of contrast enhancement, different from the thicker, nodular enhancement usually seen with metastatic lesions. Multifocal gliomas may mimic brain metastases.

Demyelinating disease can occasionally appear on CT or MRI as a large contrast-enhancing lesion with mass ef-fect. The clinical disorder may be acute and monophasic rather than the typical relapsing and remitting pattern of multiple sclerosis. Histologically, large, reactive astrocytes seen in active demyelinating lesions may be misinterpreted as neoplastic. Multifocal demyelination can occur in cancer patients after treatment with 5-fluorouracil and levamisole. These lesions have often been confused with brain metastases.

Delayed radiation necrosis can cause a contrast-enhancing mass that may enlarge on subsequent scans and may occur in patients treated with whole-brain radiotherapy, or more often radiosurgery, for their metastatic lesions. Stroke may mimic metastasis clinically and radiographically, with discrete lesions and contrast enhancement. With time, the infarct improves radiographically.

Pathophysiology

In 1889, Paget proposed the soil-seed hypothesis, according to which tumors (the "seed") metastasize preferentially to organs (the "soil") that provide a favorable environment. In 1928, Ewing speculated that the distribution of metastases is directly related to the vascular supply of the target organ. Data support both theories.

Spread to the brain occurs when the primary tumor sheds tumor cells into the circulation. The pulmonary capillary bed effectively filters larger tumor emboli, which may lead to development of a lung metastasis if the patient does not have a pulmonary primary; lung metastasis is present in more than 70% of patients with nonpulmonary cancers when brain metastases are diagnosed. Alternatively, circulating tumor cells may bypass the lungs via a patent foramen ovale. Regardless of how tumor cells enter the arterial circulation, they are carried to the brain by the 20% of cardiac output that supplies the CNS. Generally, the distribution of brain metastases follows the proportion of blood flow to the supra- and infratentorial compartments. About 85% occur in the cerebral hemispheres, 5% in the brainstem and about 10% in the cerebellum. This suggests that tumor cells are carried in the bloodstream by bulk flow. However, metastases are not uniformly distributed in the cerebral hemispheres. The watershed areas of the brain are overrepresented as sites for brain metastases, likely because small tumor emboli lodge in terminal arterioles, with slower flow in these regions. There are other factors that influence the development of brain metastases. For example, not all primaries have an identical distribution in the brain; pelvic and gastrointestinal (GI) primaries preferentially metastasize to the posterior fossa, whereas lung cancer and melanoma tend to spread to the cerebral hemispheres, suggesting there are preferential areas for growth of specific tumor types.

Once tumor cells are delivered to the brain via the circulation, they must be capable of adhering to the endothelial wall, extravasating into the interstitial space, and growing in the CNS microenvironment. The new tumor must develop a vasculature (e.g., angiogenesis) to sustain any growth beyond 1 mm in diameter. Only by forming its own vessels can a metastasis grow sufficiently large to produce symptoms. At any point along this complicated process, a tumor cell may fail to have the necessary machinery to sustain spread and growth in its host organ. It is estimated that less than 0.01% of all tumor cells that reach the circulation are ever able to form a metastatic focus. Nevertheless, there are clearly sufficient numbers of them, making brain metastases a major clinical problem.

Treatment

Radiotherapy

Radiotherapy has been the standard of care for patients with brain metastases for decades. Whole-brain radiotherapy (WBRT) is delivered to treat the disease visible on MRI as well as micrometastases that may be present. The intention is that WBRT would prevent these unseen lesions from growing into clinically important metastases. WBRT is usually delivered in 10 fractions of 300 cGy each, for a total of 3000 cGy. Other fractionation schedules are equivalent but take longer to administer, or are associated with greater neurologic side effects if the daily fraction size exceeds 300 cGy. WBRT is effective palliation, relieving neurologic symptoms in about 80% of patients, but median survival is only 4 to 6 months. All patients should have received at least 48 hours of dexamethasone (e.g., usually 16 mg/d) before WBRT is delivered, to minimize any acute radiation toxicity symptoms such as headaches and nausea and vomiting caused by enhanced disruption of the blood-brain barrier by the WBRT, subsequently exacerbating edema and increasing ICP. WBRT for brain metastases is never an emergency, so this brief delay for cortisone therapy is acceptable and makes treatment safer. Despite a good initial response, most patients progress, with about half of the patients dying of progressive CNS tumor and half from their systemic disease. Rare patients have prolonged survival and those are at risk for late complications of WBRT, such as leukoencephalopathy.

Stereotactic Radiosurgery

Stereotactic radiosurgery delivers a single, high dose of radiotherapy to a confined region of brain, using a gamma knife or linear accelerator. The spherical nature and defined borders of brain metastases make these patients ideal candidates for radiosurgery. Radiosurgery should be used only for brain metastases that are up to 3 cm in diameter and it should be used for no more than three lesions. The local control rate with radiosurgery, defined as tumor regression or stability, is about 90%. Melanoma and renal-cell carcinoma, traditionally resistant to WBRT, may respond favorably to radiosurgery (Fig. 62.3).

Radiosurgery may be used at recurrence after WBRT, but increasingly is used as initial treatment. There is controversy regarding whether or not radiosurgery should be combined with WBRT. The addition of WBRT may reduce relapse in the brain, but at the cost of increased neurotoxicity. Given that the median survival after radiosurgery for brain metastasis is about 1 year, neurotoxicity is a valid concern. Therefore, radiosurgery is often used as sole treatment, especially in elderly patients. In addition, it is useful therapy for single metastases that may not be surgically excised, such as tumors in the brainstem, or in patients whose condition makes them unable to undergo resection. Radiosurgery may produce focal radionecrosis, usually months after treatment. Radiographically, this is indistinguishable from recurrent tumor, with increased enhancement and edema. In most patients, the diagnosis may be determined by PET or MR spectroscopy. However, resection is occasionally necessary to establish the diagnosis, so appropriate treatment may be instituted if recurrent tumor is present. Furthermore, resection is the treatment of choice for radionecrosis and may be helpful for tumor recurrence as well.

Surgery

Two randomized, controlled trials established that resection followed by WBRT is superior to WBRT alone, for patients with single brain metastases. A third trial failed to show a difference, but some factors may explain this discrepancy. Survival may not have been different in this study because many patients in the WBRT arm had surgery at recurrence; in addition, many patients were in poor medical condition at entry into the trial and may not have been good surgical candidates initially, dying quickly of their systemic disease. At this time, it is generally accepted that surgical resection of single brain metastases in patients with controlled systemic disease significantly prolongs survival (median 40 to 50 weeks), improves neurologic function, and helps patients retain independence for a longer period of time.

No prospective studies have evaluated surgery for more than one lesion, but retrospective data suggest that patients who have had excision of two or three lesions may fare as well as those with single metastases and therefore may be candidates for tumor resection. This may be preferred to stereotactic radiosurgery when the metastases have extensive surrounding edema that might be exacerbated by radiosurgical treatment.

A controlled trial demonstrated that postoperative WBRT after resection of a single metastasis reduced the frequency of CNS relapse at the surgical site and elsewhere

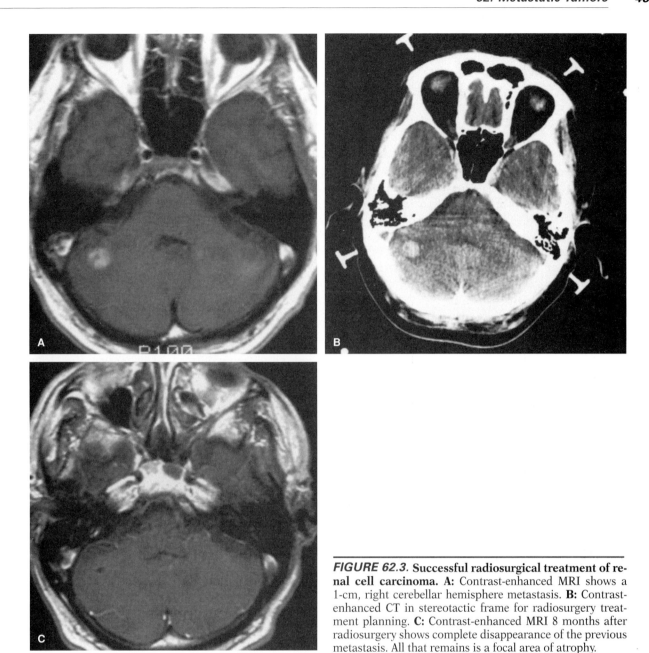

FIGURE 62.3. Successful radiosurgical treatment of renal cell carcinoma. A: Contrast-enhanced MRI shows a 1-cm, right cerebellar hemisphere metastasis. **B:** Contrast-enhanced CT in stereotactic frame for radiosurgery treatment planning. **C:** Contrast-enhanced MRI 8 months after radiosurgery shows complete disappearance of the previous metastasis. All that remains is a focal area of atrophy.

in the brain, and also reduced the number of neurologic deaths. However, overall survival was unaffected because patients died of systemic tumor. Therefore, the use of postoperative WBRT has become controversial. Some withhold it until recurrence, especially in older patients or in those likely to live years, or who are at increased risk for neurotoxicity; others administer it to all patients because it helps control neurologic disease.

When choosing focal therapy, no clear data have prospectively compared surgery and radiosurgery. From most retrospective analyses, they appear to have a comparable outcome. Surgery is superior for large lesions and those with marked surrounding edema. Radiosurgery may be the preferred choice for poor surgical candidates, for patients with multiple lesions, and for patients whose tumors are in surgically inaccessible sites.

Chemotherapy

Chemotherapy has a limited role in treating brain metastases and is used only at recurrence and after surgical and radiotherapeutic options have been exhausted. The main problem is chemoresistance of the metastasis; however, some patients with brain metastases from relatively chemosensitive primaries may respond to drugs appropriate to the underlying malignancy. This is best seen in patients with breast cancer, small-cell lung cancer, or chorio-carcinoma. Brain metastases from lung cancer may respond to temozolomide.

DURAL METASTASIS

Dural metastasis is seen primarily in patients with breast or prostate cancer. Occasionally chloromas (i.e., focal sites of acute myelogenous leukemia) may also occur in the dura. Dural lesions usually arise from direct extension of a calvarial metastasis (Fig. 62.4). They may become very extensive and may grow to invade the subarachnoid space and underlying brain. They may be accompanied by subdural hematoma or effusion, and in some patients the hematomas predominate and the thin layers of tumor cells adherent to the dura are missed.

Patients may present with painless, growing skull lesions. Common neurologic symptoms include seizures, headaches, and hemiparesis. MRI establishes the diagnosis. However, the tumors may appear identical to meningiomas, the main diagnostic consideration. When the lesion is close to the vertex, involvement and occlusion of the superior sagittal sinus is a concern; patency of the sinus may be determined by MR venography. The treatment is focal radiotherapy.

LEPTOMENINGEAL METASTASIS

Leptomeningeal metastasis develops in about 8% of all patients with cancer. The most common cancers associated with leptomeningeal metastases are the hematologic malignancies, especially acute lymphocytic leukemia. Of the solid tumors, the most frequent sources are breast, lung, melanoma, and gastrointestinal cancers. Most patients have active systemic disease when their leptomeningeal metastases are diagnosed, although patients with lymphomas or leukemias, and rarely breast cancer, may have isolated leptomeningeal metastases.

Pathogenesis

Metastatic cells reach the leptomeninges by various routes: hematogenous dissemination, and spread from bone metastases via the venous sinuses and brain metastases that abut the CSF. Surgical resection of a brain metastasis may seed the subarachnoid space; leptomeningeal metastases develop in 40% of patients following resection of cerebellar lesions, but only in 3% of those who undergo surgery on supratentorial lesions. Cells in the subarachnoid space spread along the leptomeninges and enter the Virchow-Robin spaces, where they can penetrate the pia to infiltrate the brain, cranial nerves or spinal roots. Hy-

drocephalus may develop if tumors obstruct the ventricles, basal cisterns, or arachnoid granulations.

Diagnosis

The clinical hallmark of leptomeningeal metastasis is multilevel symptoms and signs that affect three main areas: (1) cranial nerves, (2) spinal roots and cord, and (3) cerebrum. Often the examining physician finds more signs than symptoms. At presentation, cerebral symptoms and signs include headaches (40%), mental status changes (50%), difficulty walking (45%), nausea and vomiting (12%), and seizures (15%). Cranial nerve symptoms include diplopia (30%), facial weakness (25%), hearing loss (20%), optic neuropathy (2%), and trigeminal neuropathy (12%). Spinal findings comprise reflex asymmetry (60%), limb weakness (78%), paresthesias (10%), radicular pain (25%), and sphincter dysfunction (2%). The diagnosis requires demonstration of tumor cells in the CSF or definitive findings on neuroimaging (Fig. 62.5). CSF abnormalities include elevated pressure (50%), pleocytosis (60%), elevated protein (80%), and low glucose (25%). Tumor cells are identified in only 50% of patients on the first lumbar puncture, and repeated puncture assays are often needed. Positive cytology is found in 90% of patients following the third lumbar puncture, but 10% of patients still have false-negative results even at that point. Occasionally, sampling CSF from cisternal taps may yield the diagnosis, particularly in patients who have cerebral or cranial nerve symptoms. Evaluating tumor markers in the CSF may help provide circumstantial evidence for leptomeningeal metastasis. The best markers are those specific for the primary (e.g., cancer antigen 15-3 for breast cancer) but nonspecific markers such as lactate dehydrogenase isoenzymes may also be useful.

MRI may establish the diagnosis of leptomeningeal metastasis when clear evidence of subarachnoid tumor is visualized. Definite findings include tumor nodules on the cauda equina, enhancing cranial nerves, enhancing tumor in the cortical sulci, and subependymal enhancement (Fig. 62.6).

Complete neuraxis imaging should be performed in all patients (Fig. 62.7). If definite leptomeningeal metastasis tumor is identified on MRI, there is no need to perform a lumbar puncture for cytologic examination. However, negative imaging does not exclude the diagnosis and such patients should have CSF analysis repeatedly, if necessary, to confirm the diagnosis. Patients with symptoms of increased ICP should also have a lumbar puncture to measure the opening pressure, even if imaging has established the diagnosis of subarachnoid tumor. Elevated ICP may need specific treatment, especially if intrathecal chemotherapy is planned. Instillation of drug into the CSF is contraindicated in the presence of uncontrolled, high ICP.

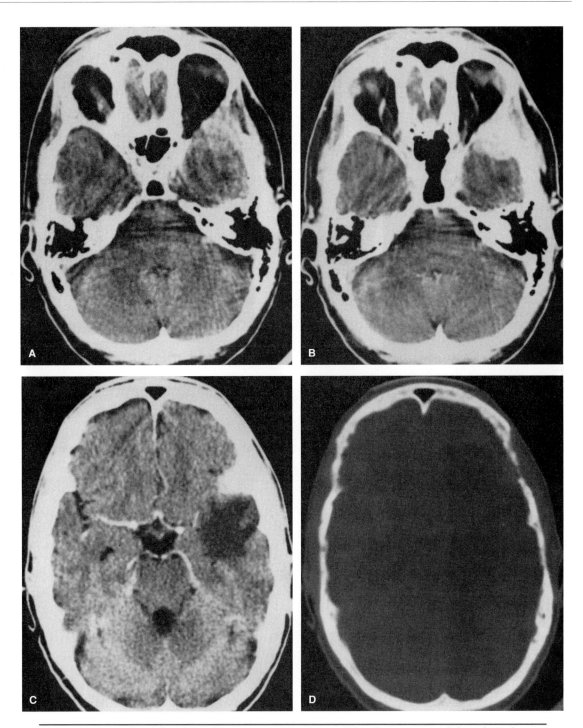

FIGURE 62.4. Calvarial and dural metastases. Precontrast **(A)** and postcontrast **(B)** axial CTs demonstrate that the anterior wall of the middle cranial fossa is missing; it is replaced by an enhancing metastasis from breast carcinoma, with an dural component anterior to the left temporal lobe. The patient had left V1 sensory loss. Higher postcontrast cut **(C)** and bone window **(D)** at the same level demonstrate extension of the epidural metastasis. Transdural involvement is suggested by the prominent white matter edema in the underlying temporal lobe, with effacement of the left Sylvian fissure resulting from mass effect. Note the extensive calvarial involvement in **D.** Malignant cells were recovered from CSF, thus indicating coexistent meningeal carcinomatosis. (Courtesy of Drs. J. A. Bello and S. K. Hilal.)

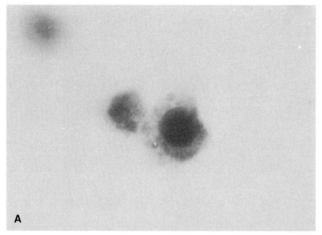

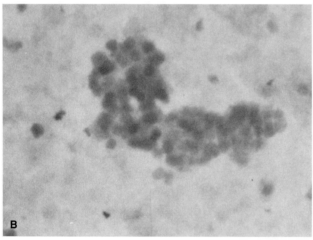

FIGURE 62.5. Malignant cells in spinal fluid. Formalin-fixed millipore filtrates of lumbar CSF in two patients with meningeal spread of neoplasms. **A:** Isolated large cells with increased nuclear-to-cytoplasm ratio and fine clumps of cytoplasmic pigment in a patient with meningeal carcinomatosis caused by malignant melanoma (hematoxylin stain, ×450). **B:** A clump of cohesive cells in a patient with a primitive neuroectodermal tumor and extensive meningeal seeding (hematoxylin stain, ×180).

Other imaging findings suggestive of leptomeningeal metastasis include communicating hydrocephalus, multiple brain metastases on the surface of the brain or in the cortical sulci, and intraventricular nodules. These findings deserve evaluation of the CSF, even if the patient does not have specific symptoms of leptomeningeal metastasis. Radionuclide CSF-flow studies with ^{111}In-DTPA, injected into either the ventricles or lumbar CSF compartment, are abnormal in 40% of patients. Any patient with large, bulky, subarachnoid nodules seen on MRI may be presumed to have altered CSF dynamics because of partial or complete obstruction of CSF flow. However, patients without obvious structural disease in the subarachnoid space may also have poor CSF circulation. The importance of determining if there is altered CSF flow is that it impairs homogeneous distribution of intrathecal chemotherapy.

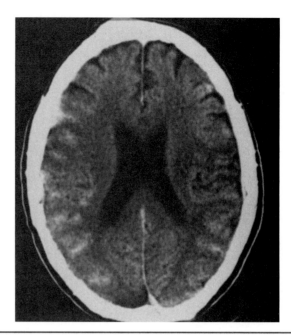

FIGURE 62.6. Meningeal carcinomatosis. An axial, contrast-enhanced CT demonstrates abnormal sulcal enhancement causing sulcal effacement in a patient with metastatic breast carcinoma.

Treatment

Leptomeningeal metastasis affects the entire neuraxis, and treatment must encompass the whole CSF compartment. Treatment is palliative. Radiotherapy is given to symptomatic sites (e.g., the brain for cranial neuropathies), and may be given to sites of bulky disease seen on neuroimaging. Craniospinal radiotherapy is not given because of myelosuppression and it does not improve disease control.

Chemotherapy is usually administered directly into CSF, where it circulates via bulk flow to reach all areas of the subarachnoid space. It is usually delivered via an Ommaya reservoir, which is connected to the ventricular system via catheter. Intrathecal chemotherapy is limited to three agents (methotrexate, cytarabine or liposomal cytarabine, and thiotepa). The ventricular route achieves more uniform drug distribution than lumbar injections, is easier to achieve, and is more reliable. Efficacy of intrathecal drug administration is limited by altered CSF flow dynamics and poor drug distribution, but more importantly, by intrinsic or acquired drug resistance to the limited number of agents deemed safe to be instilled into the CSF. Most complications of intraventricular treatment are transient, and are characterized by aseptic meningitis. Patients may experience myelosuppression, particularly if they are receiving concurrent systemic therapy. Chemotherapy-related leukoencephalopathy may develop in long-term survivors, especially if they received WBRT as well as intrathecal drug.

Systemic chemotherapy is not routine for leptomeningeal metastasis, owing to the poor CSF penetration

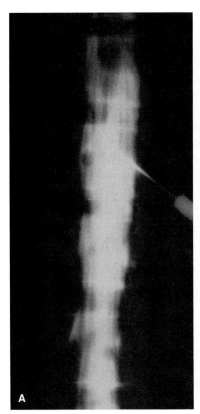

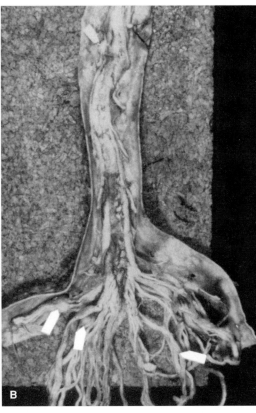

FIGURE 62.7. Meningeal carcinomatosis. Myelogram and autopsy specimen of spinal cord from same patient with meningeal carcinomatosis. Note the intradural filling defects in the myelogram **(A)** that correspond to tumor nodules (*arrows*) seen on multiple nerve roots and thoracic spinal cord in pathologic specimen **(B)**.

of most agents. However, recent data suggest that some drugs (e.g., high-dose methotrexate, capecitabine or others) may be useful. Median survival of patients with leptomeningeal metastasis is 4 to 6 months, but treatment may prevent neurologic deterioration. Prognosis is worse with widespread systemic disease, CSF block, and coexistent bulky CNS metastases. However, good outcome with prolonged survival, and even cure, may be seen in some patients with hematologic cancers and occasionally in patients with breast cancer.

EPIDURAL SPINAL CORD METASTASIS

Epidural spinal cord compression occurs in 5% of patients with cancer, usually in those with known bone metastases; however, spinal cord compression may be the first sign of a malignancy or the development of metastatic disease. The most common cancers leading to epidural tumors include breast, lung, and prostate. The level of compression is at the thoracic cord in 70%; lumbar in 20% and cervical in 10%. Multiple sites of epidural tumor may be found in 5% to 15% of patients.

Pathogenesis

The vertebral column is the most common site of skeletal metastases. First, it represents a large proportion of the skeleton. Second, bone marrow has a high concentra-

tion of growth factors that may stimulate tumor growth. Third, the vertebral venous plexus of Batson is the site of drainage for pelvic, abdominal, and thoracic organs, so tumors in these sites have direct access to the spine. Fourth, the lymphatic system, which anastomoses with the vertebral plexus, may also provide a conduit to the spine for tumor cells from the major visceral sites in the chest and abdomen. In the majority of patients, epidural cord compression results from direct extension of tumors from the vertebral column into the anterior epidural spaces. Some tumors, such as lymphomas, may grow in the paravertebral spaces and grow through the neural foramina without affecting the bone. The mechanism of cord injury includes direct compression and impairment of venous drainage, with resultant cord edema and ischemia.

Clinical Presentation

Pain is the first symptom in 97% of patients with epidural tumors. Pain may be local or radicular, and may be aggravated by movement. Pain from epidural metastases may arise at any spinal level, but it usually arises from thoracic involvement and may be band-like across the chest or abdomen, whereas degenerative arthritic pain is usually lumbar or cervical. Lying supine usually alleviates arthritic pain but aggravates metastatic pain. Limb weakness (76%), autonomic disturbance (57%), and sensory dysfunction (51%) develop as compression progresses. Urinary incontinence is a late symptom.

Diagnostic Evaluation

Noncontrast MRI is the only test necessary to diagnose epidural tumor, and should be obtained in any patient suspected of the diagnosis. Gadolinium is not necessary to evaluate the epidural space, but is essential if leptomeningeal metastasis is being considered. However, epidural tumor is a neurologic emergency and a complete noncontrast spine MRI is sufficient to establish or exclude the diagnosis; the patient can always return for a contrast-enhanced study, if necessary. This is one of the few neurooncologic situations in which it is appropriate to eliminate contrast on the first image because complete-spine MRI, with and without gadolinium, takes at least 1.5 hours to perform, and patients with epidural tumors are often too uncomfortable to complete the entire study at once. Therefore, getting the noncontrast film first enables the entire spine to be imaged, and the most serious diagnostic consideration to be eliminated immediately. Complete-spine MRI should be obtained in all patients to exclude multifocal disease. Patients unable to undergo MRI should have CT myelogram.

Therapy

The most important aspects of management of these patients are preservation of neurologic function and alleviation of pain. Immediate treatment is essential because patients may deteriorate abruptly, probably from venous infarction leading to paraplegia. Early recognition and treatment are crucial. Corticosteroids are given immediately and may alleviate pain rapidly. Data suggest that high doses of corticosteroids may relieve pain more rapidly and effectively, starting with an intravenous bolus of 100 mg of dexamethasone, followed by 24 mg given four times a day. The steroids should be tapered rapidly once definitive therapy (e.g., radiotherapy) is started.

Radiotherapy is the standard treatment, usually for a total dose of 3000 cGy in 10 fractions. Radiation usually includes two vertebral bodies above and two below the lesion site. Highly focused, intensity-modulated radiotherapy is being explored as a potential technique to deliver a second course of radiotherapy safely, if recompression occurs at a previously irradiated site. As an alternative to radiotherapy, surgery is playing an increasing role in the management of spinal cord compression. Posterior tumors are best approached by laminectomy; however, most patients with epidural cord compression have anterior lesions that require thoracotomy, vertebral body resection, and spinal stabilization. Surgery is considered in the following circumstances: cord compression and unknown primary tumor, progressive epidural tumor in a previously irradiated site, spinal instability, and radioresistant tumors. Surgery may be preceded by embolization of the tumor to decrease vascularity, particularly from highly vascular primaries such as renal or thyroid cancer. A randomized trial comparing surgery to radiotherapy in newly diagnosed patients with epidural metastases showed that neurologic function and survival were superior in patients who had resections, compared to those who had radiotherapy alone. Therefore, all appropriate surgical candidates should be considered for resection if an experienced surgeon is available. Most patients who undergo surgical excision receive postoperative radiotherapy, if it was not administered previously.

The most important prognostic factor for outcome is neurologic status at the time of treatment. Up to 80% of ambulatory patients remained ambulatory, whereas only 50% of those with leg weakness and 10% of those with paralysis walked after radiotherapy. Complete resection may afford a greater opportunity for paraplegic patients to regain leg strength. Pain may be relieved in 96% of patients treated with corticosteroids and radiation. Patients with compression fractures are less likely to have favorable responses to external radiotherapy, and early surgery should be considered. Survival depends mostly on control of the underlying malignancy.

SUGGESTED READINGS

Brain Metastasis

Abrey LE, Olson JD, Raizer JJ, et al. A phase II trial of temozolomide for patients with recurrent or progressive brain metastases. *J Neurooncol* 2001;53:259–265.

Akeson P, Larsson EM, Kristoffersen DT, et al. Brain metastases—comparison of gadodiamide injection-enhanced MR imaging at standard and high dose, contrast-enhanced CT and non-contrast-enhanced MR imaging. *Acta Radiol* 1995;36:300–306.

Barker FG II. Craniotomy for the resection of metastatic brain tumors in the U.S., 1988–2000: decreasing mortality and the effect of provider caseload. *Cancer* 2004;100:999–1007.

Bartelt S, Lutterbach J. Brain metastases in patients with cancer of unknown primary. *J Neurooncol.* 2003;64:249–253.

Bindal AK, Bindal RK, Hess KR, et al. Surgery versus radiosurgery in the treatment of brain metastasis. *J Neurosurg* 1996;84:748–754.

Chang EL, Hassenbusch SJ III, Shiu AS, et al. The role of tumor size in the radiosurgical management of patients with ambiguous brain metastases. *Neurosurgery* 2003;2:272–280.

Cormio G, Gabriele A, Maneo A, et al. Complete remission of brain metastases from ovarian carcinoma with carboplatin. *Eur J Obstet Gynecol Reprod Biol* 1998;78:91–93.

Das A, Hochberg FH. Clinical presentation of intracranial metastases. *Neurosurg Clin N Am* 1996;7:377–391.

Fan G, Sun B, Wu Z, et al. In vivo single-voxel proton MR spectroscopy in the differentiation of high-grade gliomas and solitary metastases. *Clin Radiol* 2004;59:77–85.

Flannery TW, Suntharalingam M, Kwok Y, et al. Gamma knife stereotactic versus metachronous solitary brain metastases from non-small cell lung cancer. *Lung Cancer* 2003;42:327–333.

Flickinger JC, Kondziolka D. Radiosurgery instead of resection for solitary brain metastasis: the gold standard redefined. *Int J Radiat Oncol Biol Phys* 1996;35:185–186.

Hiraki A, Tabata M, Ueoka H, et al. Direct intracerebral invasion from skull metastasis of large cell lung cancer. *Intern Med* 1997;36:720–723.

Hwang TL, Close TP, Grego JM, et al. Predilection of brain metastasis in gray and white matter junction and vascular border zones. *Cancer* 1996;77:1551–1555.

Johnson JD, Young B. Demographics of brain metastasis. *Neurosurg Clin N Am* 1996;7:337–344.

Kimura T, Sako K, Tohyama Y, et al. Diagnosis and treatment of progressive space-occupying radiation necrosis following sterotactic radiosurgery for brain metastasis: value of proton magnetic resonance spectroscopy. *Acta Neurochir (Wein)* 2003;145:557–564.

Lassman AB, DeAngelis LM. Brain metastases. *Neurol Clin N Am* 2003;21:1–23.

Lee JS, Pisters KM, Komaki R, et al. Paclitaxel/carboplatin chemotherapy as primary treatment of brain metastases in non-small cell lung cancer: a preliminary report. *Semin Oncol* 1997;24:S12–S55.

Lesser GJ. Chemotherapy of cerebral metastases from solid tumors. *Neurosurg Clin N Am* 1996;7:527–536.

McWilliams RR, Brown PD, Buckner JC, et al. Treatment of brain metastasis from melanoma. *Mayo Clin Proc* 2003;78:1529–1536.

Mintz AH, Kestle J, Rathbone MP, et al. A randomized trial to assess the efficacy of surgery in addition to radiotherapy in patients with a single cerebral metastasis. *Cancer* 1996;78:1470–1476.

Nieder C, Berberich W, Schnabel K. Tumor-related prognostic factors for remission of brain metastases after radiotherapy. *Int J Radiat Oncol Biol Phys* 1997;39:25–30.

Noel G, Valery CA, Boisserie G, et al. LINAC radiosurgery for brain metastasis of renal cell carcinoma. *Urol Oncol* 2004;22:25–31.

Orhan B, Yalcin S, Evrensel T, et al. Successful treatment of cranial metastases of extrapulmonary small cell carcinoma with chemotherapy alone. *Med Oncol* 1998;15:66–69.

Patchell RA. The management of brain metastases. *Cancer Treat Rev* 2003;29:533–540.

Patchell RA, Tibbs PA, Walsh JW, et al. A randomized trial of surgery in the treatment of single metastases to the brain. *N Engl J Med* 1990;322:494–500.

Pollack BE, Brown PD, Foote RL, et al. Properly selected patients with multiple brain metastases may benefit from aggressive treatment of the intracranial disease. *J Neurooncol* 2003;61:73–80.

Roberts WS, Sell JJ, Orrison WW Jr. Multiple ischemic infarcts versus metastatic disease. *Acad Radiol* 1994;1:75–77.

Schouten LJ, Rutten J, Huveneers HAM, et al. Incidence of brain metastases in a cohort of patients with carcinoma of the breast, colon, kidney, lung and melanoma. *Cancer* 2002;94:2698–2705.

Shirato H, Takamura A, Tomita M, et al. Stereotactic irradiation without whole-brain irradiation for single brain metastasis. *Int J Radiat Oncol Biol Phys* 1997;37:385–391.

Dural Metastasis

Johnson MD, Powell SZ, Boyer PJ, et al. Dural lesions mimicking meningiomas. *Hum Pathol* 2002;33:1211–1226.

Raizer JJ, DeAngelis LM. Cerebral sinus thrombosis diagnosed by MRI and MR venography in cancer patients. *Neurology* 2000;54:1222–1226.

Richiello A, Sparano L, Del Basso De Caro ML, Russo G. Dural metastasis mimicking falx meningioma. Case report. *J Neurosurg Sci* 2003;47:167–171.

Tseng SH, Liao CC, Lin SM, et al. Dural metastasis in patients with malignant neoplasm and chronic subdural hematoma. *Acta Neurol Scand* 2003;108:43–46.

Leptomeningeal Metastasis

Abrey LE. Leptomeningeal neoplasms. *Curr Treat Options Neurol* 2002;4(2):147–156.

Berg SL, Chamberlain MC. Systemic chemotherapy, intrathecal chemotherapy, and symptom management in the treatment of leptomeningeal metastasis. *Curr Oncol Rep* 2003;5:29–40.

Bokstein F, Lossos A, Siegal T. Leptomeningeal metastases from solid tumors: a comparison of two prospective series treated with and without intra-cerebrospinal chemotherapy. *Cancer* 1998;82:1756–1763.

Collie DA, Brush JP, Lammie GA, et al. Imaging features of leptomeningeal metastases. *Clin Radiol* 1999;54:765–771.

Demopoulos A, DeAngelis LM. Neurologic complications of leukemia. *Curr Opin Neurol* 2002;15:691–699.

Freilich RJ, Krol D, DeAngelis LM. Neuroimaging and cerebrospinal fluid cytology in the diagnosis of leptomeningeal metastasis. *Ann Neurol* 1995;38:51–57.

Kesari S, Batchelor T. Leptomeningeal metastases. *Neurol Clin N Am* 2003;21:25–66.

Mason WP, Yeh SDJ, DeAngelis LM. Indium-diethylenetriamine pentaacetic acid cerebrospinal fluid flow studies predict distribution of intrathecally administered chemotherapy and outcome in patients with leptomeningeal metastases. *Neurology* 1998;50:438–444.

Moots PL, Harrison MB, Vandenberg SR. Prolonged survival in carcinomatous meningitis associated with breast cancer. *South Med J* 1995;88:357–362.

Norris LK, Grossman SA, Olivi A. Neoplastic meningitis following surgical resection of isolated cerebellar metastasis: a potentially preventable complication. *J Neurooncol* 1997;32:215–223.

Rogers LR, Remer SE, Tejwani S. Durable response of breast cancer leptomeningeal metastasis to capecitabine monotherapy. *Neuro-oncol* 2004;6:63–64.

Sandberg DI, Bilsky MH, Souweidane MM, et al. Ommaya reservoirs for the treatment of leptomeningeal metastases. *Neurosurgery* 2000;47:49–54.

Siegal T. Leptomeningeal metastases: rationale for systemic chemotherapy or what is the role of intra-CSF-chemotherapy? *J Neurooncol* 1998;38:151–157.

Tetef ML, Margolin KA, Doroshow, et al. Pharmacokinetics and toxicity of high-dose intravenous methotrexate in the treatment of leptomeningeal carcinomatosis. *Cancer Chemother Pharmacol* 2000;46:19–26.

Wasserstrom W, Glass J, Posner J. Diagnosis and treatment of leptomeningeal metastases from solid tumors: experience with 90 patients. *Cancer* 1982;49:759–772.

Epidural Spinal Cord Compression

Cook AM, Lau TN, Tomlinson MJ, et al. Magnetic resonance imaging of the whole spine in suspected malignant spinal cord compression: impact on management. *Clin Oncol R Coll Radiol* 1998;10:39–43.

Faul CM, Flickinger JC. The use of radiation in the management of spinal metastases. *J Neurooncol* 1995;23:149–161.

Harris JK, Sutcliffe JC, Robinson NE. The role of emergency surgery in malignant spinal extradural compression: assessment of functional outcome. *Br J Neurosurg* 1996;10:27–33.

Helweg-Larsen S, Johnsen A, Boesen J, Sorensen PS. Radiologic features compared to clinical findings in a prospective study of 153 patients with metastatic spinal cord compression treated by radiotherapy. *Acta Neurochir (Wien)* 1997;139:105–111.

Loblaw DA, Laperriere NJ. Emergency treatment of malignant extradural spinal cord compression: an evidence-based guideline. *J Clin Oncol* 1998;16:1613–1614.

Prabhu VC, Bilsky MH, Jambhekar K, et al. Results of preoperative embolization for metastatic spinal neoplasms. *J Neurosurg* 2003;98:156–164.

Schiff D, O'Neill BP. Intramedullary spinal cord metastases: clinical features and treatment outcome. *Neurology* 1996;47:906–912.

Yenice KM, Lovelock DM, Hunt MA, et al. CT image-guided intensity-modulated therapy for paraspinal tumors using stereotactic immobilization. *Int J Radiat Oncol Biol Phys* 2003;55:583–593.

Chapter 63

Spinal Tumors

Paul C. McCormick and Lewis P. Rowland

Tumors of the spinal cord or nerve roots are similar to intracranial tumors in cellular type. They may arise from the parenchyma of the cord, nerve roots, meninges, intraspinal blood vessels, sympathetic nerves, or vertebrae. Metastases may arise from remote tumors.

Spinal tumors are divided by location into three groups: intramedullary, intradural, or extradural. Occasionally, an extradural tumor extends through an intervertebral foramen to be partially within and partially outside the spinal canal (e.g., dumbbell or hourglass tumors).

PATHOLOGY

The histologic characteristics (Table 63.1) of primary and secondary tumors are similar to those of intracranial tumors. Intramedullary tumors are rare, accounting for about 10% of all spinal tumors. In contrast, benign, encapsulated tumors (Figs. 63.1 and 63.2), meningiomas, and neurofibromas comprise about 65% of all primary spinal tumors. Intramedullary tumors are more common in children, and extramedullary tumors are more common in adults.

The most common primary sites of metastatic tumors to the spine in order of frequency are lung, breast, and prostate. Other origins include tumors of the gastrointestinal tract, lymphomas, melanomas, kidney, sarcomas, thyroid, and myelomas.

▶ TABLE 63.1 Relative Frequency of Different Types of Spinal Tumors

Type	Percent
Neurofibromas	29
Meningiomas	26
Ependymomas	13
Miscellaneous	12
Astrocytomas	7
Metastatic and other	13
Total	100

FREQUENCY

Spinal cord tumors are much less prevalent than intracranial tumors, in a ratio of 1:4, but this varies by histology. The intracranial-to-spinal ratio of astrocytoma is 10:1, and the ratio for ependymomas varies from 3:1 to 20:1. Men and women are affected equally often, except that meningiomas are more common in women and ependymomas are more common in men. Spinal tumors occur predominantly in young or middle-aged adults and are less common in childhood or after age 60 years (Table 63.2).

Spinal tumors appear most often in the thoracic region, but if the relative lengths of the divisions of the spinal cord are considered, the distribution is comparatively equal. Ependymomas may be either intramedullary or extramedullary; at the conus, an ependymoma may be wholly or partially extramedullary.

SYMPTOMS

Extramedullary tumors cause symptoms by compressing nerve roots or spinal cord or by occluding the spinal blood vessels. The symptoms of intramedullary tumors result from direct interference with the intrinsic structures of the spinal cord from mass effect, edema, or development of syringomyelia. Descriptions of special syndromes follow.

EXTRAMEDULLARY TUMORS

These tumors may be either intradural or extradural. They usually involve a few cord segments and cause focal signs by compressing nerve roots, especially the dorsal roots. Extramedullary tumors may ultimately affect the spinal cord, with complete loss of function below the level of the lesion. The first symptoms are focal pain and paresthesias, arising from pressure on the dorsal nerve roots; neurofibromas originate from these structures. This symptom pattern is soon followed by sensory loss, weakness, and muscular wasting in the distribution of the affected roots. Compression of the spinal cord first interrupts the functions of the pathways that lie at the periphery of the spinal cord. The early signs of cord compression include spastic weakness below the lesion; impairment of cutaneous and proprioceptive sensation below the lesion; impaired control of the bladder and, less often, the rectum; and increased tendon reflexes, Babinski signs, and loss of superficial abdominal reflexes. If untreated, this syndrome may lead to signs and symptoms of complete transection of spinal cord, with wasting and atrophy of muscles at the level of the root lesion and, below the lesion, paraplegia or quadriplegia in flexion.

The severity and distribution of weakness and sensory loss varies, depending in part on the location of the tumor

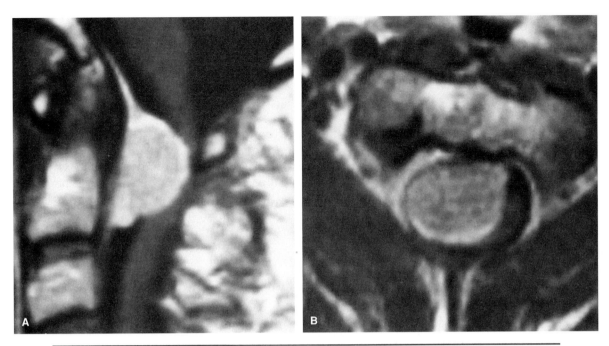

FIGURE 63.1. Cervical meningioma. A: T-1 weighted contrast-enhanced sagittal MRI demonstrates a large intradural mass at C1-2. **B:** Axial MRI demonstrates the large size of this lesion, probably a meningioma. Despite marked spinal cord compression, the patient had no abnormality on neurologic examination.

in relation to the anterior, lateral, or posterior portion of the spinal cord. Eccentrically placed tumors may cause a typical Brown-Séquard syndrome, namely, ipsilateral signs of posterior column and pyramidal tract dysfunction, with contralateral loss of pain and temperature due to involvement of the lateral spinothalamic tract. Usually, however, the Brown-Séquard features are incomplete.

Spinal vessels may be occluded by extradural tumors, particularly metastatic carcinoma, lymphoma, or abscess.

When the arteries destined for the spinal cord are occluded, the resulting myelomalacia causes signs and symptoms similar to those of severe intradural compression and necrosis of the spinal cord. Occlusion of major components of the anterior spinal artery, however, results in segmental lower motor-neuron signs at the appropriate level, bilateral loss of pain and temperature sensation, and upper motor-neuron signs below the lesion. The posterior columns are generally spared.

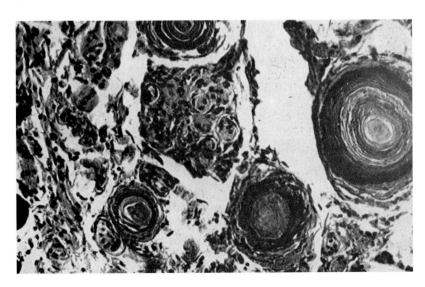

FIGURE 63.2. Meningioma of the spinal cord with whorls.

▶ **TABLE 63.2** **Age Incidence of Spinal Tumors of All Types**[a]

Age (yrs)	No. of Cases	Percent
0–9	19	2
10–19	98	10
20–29	156	16
30–39	177	18
40–49	238	25
50–59	186	19
Over 60	101	10
Total	975	100

[a]Data compiled from the literature.

SPINAL METASTASES

Epidural Spinal Cord Compression

Epidural-spinal metastases may be considered a disorder of the vertebral column; the neurologic consequences result from extension of tumor into the spinal canal. Patients with primary malignant tumors now survive longer, and the incidence of epidural spinal cord compression has increased to about 5% to 10% of all cancer patients. Treatment of cord compression does not prolong survival but may relieve pain and may prevent neurologic disability.

Signs and symptoms of epidural spinal cord compression are easily overlooked in a patient with cancer who is often wracked by asthenia and diffuse pain. The physician, however, must respond to neck or back pain that is relentless and persists when the patient lies in bed, even if the pain is relieved by analgesics. Limb weakness, paresthesias in the distribution of a nerve root, and bowel or bladder dysfunction create a neurooncologic emergency that commands prompt evaluation and treatment. Rarely, the only manifestation of cord compression is a gait disorder, often due to sensory ataxia, without overt evidence of weakness or cutaneous sensory loss. It may even be difficult to demonstrate impaired proprioception. The ataxia may be caused by compression of spinocerebellar pathways. The tumor in more than 50% of cases of epidural cord compression arises from lung or breast; more than 80% of cases arise from primary tumors in lung, breast, gastrointestinal system, prostate, melanoma, or lymphoma.

These tumors spread to the epidural space by direct, centripetal invasion from a paravertebral focus through a nerve root foramen, hematogenous metastasis to the vertebrae with extension from bone into the epidural space, or retrograde spread along the venous plexus of Batson. Hematogenous spread is the most common, and CT shows lytic or blastic changes in 85% of patients. Osteoblastic changes are common with myeloma, prostate carcinoma, and Hodgkin disease and are occasionally seen with breast cancer. CT and MRI are sensitive techniques for the detection of spinal osseous metastases (Figs. 63.3 and 63.4).

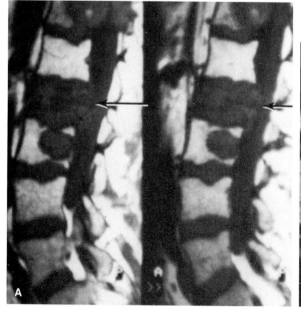 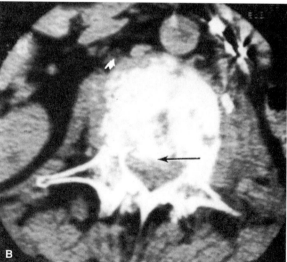

FIGURE 63.3. **A:** Epidural spinal metastases. T1-weighted sagittal MRI demonstrates multiple levels of spinal involvement from metastatic renal carcinoma. The L2 vertebra (*arrow*) is collapsed, and there is epidural extension of tumor and bone at this level. **B:** Axial computed tomography demonstrates the degree of bone destruction at the L2 level. Note the retropulsion of bone fragments into the epidural space (*arrow*).

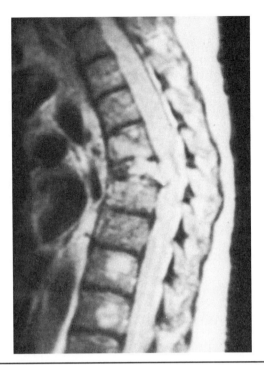

FIGURE 63.4. Epidural spinal metastases. T1-weighted sagittal MRI demonstrates destruction and collapse of the T6 vertebra in a patient with multiple myeloma. In addition to spinal cord compression from epidural extension of the neoplasm, there is a kyphotic deformity of the spine, indicating instability. Note the hyperintense marrow signal in the bodies of T9 and T10, indicating additional metastatic deposits.

Treatment of Epidural Metastatic Disease

Treatment of epidural metastasis is palliative in nearly all patients. Patient management must be individually tailored to consider age, clinical state, extent of systemic disease, life expectancy, tumor pathology if known, and extent of spinal lesions. The keys to successful management are timely diagnosis and prompt treatment. Persistent back or neck pain in a patient with known cancer is presumed to indicate metastatic spinal disease until proved otherwise. Emergency treatment of the patient with rapidly progressive paraparesis rarely reverses the neurologic signs. Loss of bowel or bladder function is an ominous prognostic sign and is usually irreversible. Among patients diagnosed and treated early (e.g., while they may still walk), 94% remain ambulatory until they die.

Radiation is the treatment of choice for most patients with spinal metastases, with therapy comprising 3,000 cGy in 10 fractions of 300 cGy each. It is tolerated well even by patients who are seriously ill, and in most cases, palliation is achieved with relief of pain, local tumor control, and prevention or reversal of neurologic impairment. Indications for surgery include tumors such as melanoma and other radioresistant tumors, recurrent tumor at a site of prior radiation therapy, spinal instability, unknown tissue diagnosis,

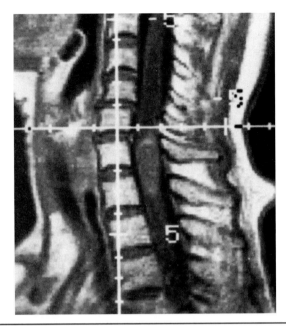

FIGURE 63.5. Intramedullary metastasis. Sagittal T1-weighted contrast-enhanced MRI shows a faintly contrast-enhancing tumor at C6-7 expanding the cervical cord in a patient with widely metastatic small cell lung cancer. Biopsy was not performed, and the tumor receded with radiation therapy.

or rapid progression of neurologic disorder. Patients with advanced systemic disease are poor surgical candidates. The choice of operative approach is debated; some surgeons advocate an anterior approach over radiation therapy or posterior laminectomy. The attendant surgical risks of anterior decompression have to be considered.

INTRAMEDULLARY METASTASES

The most common tumors that cause intramedullary metastases are lung cancer or breast cancer (Fig. 63.5). Intramedullary metastases occur with advanced metastatic disease, and at autopsy, 61% of patients with intramedullary metastases are found to have had multiple sites of cerebral or spinal lesions. MRI is the preferred diagnostic method for detection of intramedullary metastases. Reversal or stabilization of neurologic signs depends on early diagnosis, but survival is poor; 80% of patients in one series died within 3 months of diagnosis.

PRIMARY INTRAMEDULLARY TUMORS

Primary intramedullary tumors usually extend over many segments, sometimes involving the whole length of the spinal cord. For this reason, the signs and symptoms of intramedullary tumors are more variable than those of extramedullary tumors (Fig. 63.6).

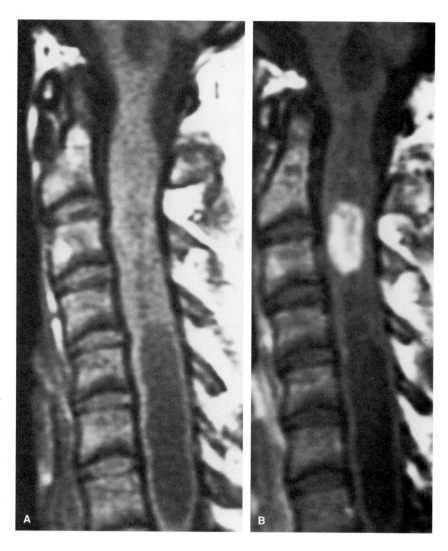

FIGURE 63.6. Intramedullary astrocytoma. A: T1-weighted sagittal MRI demonstrates a large cyst in the lower cervical spinal cord and a smaller cyst extending up into the medulla. The intervening spinal cord is slightly enlarged but demonstrates no signal abnormality. **B:** T1-weighted MRI shows a contrast-enhancing intramedullary tumor at the C2-3 level. At operation, a well-circumscribed pilocytic astrocytoma was removed.

If the tumor is restricted to one or two segments, the syndrome is similar to that of an extramedullary tumor. Commonly, however, the tumor involves several segments. Pain may be an early manifestation if the dorsal-root entry zone is affected. Compression of the crossing pain fibers in the central cord may cause loss of pain and temperature only in the affected segments. As the tumor spreads peripherally, the spinothalamic tracts may be affected; in the thoracic and cervical areas, pain and temperature fibers from the sacral area lie near the external surface of the cord and may be spared (e.g., sacral sparing). Involvement of the central gray matter destroys the anterior horn cells, with local weakness and atrophy resulting. However, pyramidal fibers may be spared. The clinical picture may be identical to that of syringomyelia.

INTRADURAL TUMORS

Neurofibromas, schwannomas, and *meningiomas* are the most commonly occurring primary intradural tumors of the spinal cord. On MRI after the administration of gadolinium, the lesions enhance brightly (Fig. 63.7). Meningiomas may be identified by the presence of a dural tail, where the tumor attaches to the dura. *Leptomeningeal metastasis* and *drop metastases* of intracranial tumors also involve the intradural space but typically, they appear as small nodules attached to the surface of the cord or cauda-equina nerve roots (Fig. 63.8).

REGIONAL SYNDROMES

Foramen Magnum Tumors

Tumors in the region of the foramen magnum may extend up into the posterior fossa or down into the cervical region. The syndrome is typified by signs and symptoms of dysfunction of the lower cranial nerves, primarily those pertaining to the eleventh, twelfth, and rarely, the ninth and tenth. The most characteristic foramen magnum tumor, the ventrolateral meningioma, compresses the spinal cord at the cervicomedullary junction to cause posterior column signs: loss of position, vibratory, and light touch

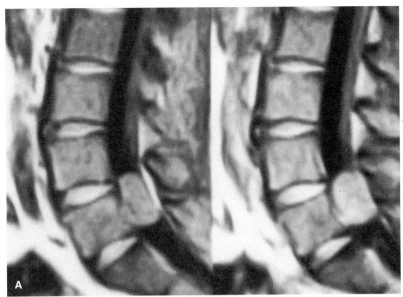

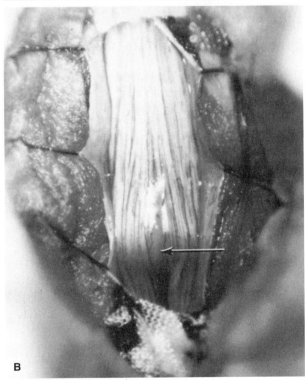

FIGURE 63.7. Schwannoma. A: Gadolinium-enhanced T1-weighted sagittal MRI demonstrates large intradural tumor at the L5 level. Differential diagnosis includes nerve sheath tumor, meningioma, filum terminale ependymoma, and intradural ("drop") metastases. **B:** Intraoperative photograph demonstrates a large intradural schwannoma (*arrow*) that displaces the cauda equina dorsally.

perception, and more prominent in the arms than in the legs. Upper motor-neuron signs are seen in all four limbs. There may be cutaneous sensory loss in distribution of C2 or the occiput, with posterior cranial headaches and high cervical pain. Progression of sensory and motor symptoms may involve the limbs asymmetrically.

Cervical Tumors

Tumors of the upper cervical segments cause pain or paresthesias in the occipital or cervical region, with stiff neck, weakness, and wasting of neck muscles. Below the lesion,

there may be a spastic tetraplegia or hemiplegia. Cutaneous sensation may be affected below the lesion, and the descending trigeminal nucleus may be involved. Characteristic findings make it possible to localize the upper level of spinal tumors in the middle and lower cervical segments or T1 as follows:

C4: Paralysis of the diaphragm.
C5: Atrophy and paralysis of the deltoid, biceps, supinator longus, rhomboid, and spinati muscles. The upper arms hang limp at the side. The sensory level extends to the outer surface of the arm. The biceps and supinator reflexes are lost.

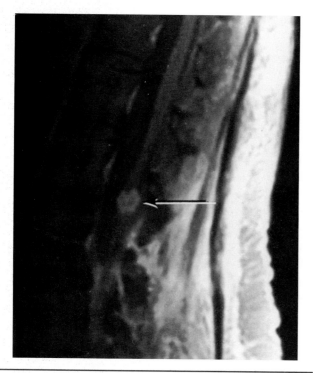

FIGURE 63.8. Drop metastases. Sagittal T1-weighted contrast-enhanced MRI shows an intradural module (*arrow*) of a fourth ventricular choroid plexus papilloma that has seeded the cauda equina.

C6: Paralysis of triceps and wrist extensors. The forearm is held semiflexed and there is a partial wrist-drop. The triceps reflex is lost. Sensory impairment extends to a line running down the middle of the arm slightly to the radial side.

C7: Paralysis of the flexors of the wrist and of the flexors and extensors of the fingers. Efforts to close the hands result in extension of the wrist and slight flexion of the fingers (e.g., preacher's hand). The sensory level is similar to that of the sixth cervical segment but slightly more to the ulnar side of the arm.

C8: Atrophy and paralysis of the small muscles of the hand with resulting clawhand (main-en-griffe). *Horner syndrome*, unilateral or bilateral, results from lesions at this level and is characterized by the triad of ptosis, small pupil (i.e., miosis), and loss of sweating on the face. Sensory loss extends to the inner aspect of the arm and involves the fourth and fifth fingers and the ulnar aspect of the middle finger.

T1: Lesions rarely cause motor symptoms because the T1 nerve root normally provides little functional innervation of the small hand muscles.

Other signs of cervical tumors include nystagmus, which is attributed to involvement of the descending portion of the median longitudinal fasciculus. A Horner syndrome may be found with intramedullary lesions in any portion of the cervical cord if the descending sympathetic pathways are affected.

Thoracic Tumors

Clinical localization of tumors in the thoracic region of the cord is best made by the sensory level. It is not possible to determine the location of a lesion in the upper half of the thoracic cord by testing the strength of intercostal muscles. Lesions that affect the abdominal muscles below T10 but spare the upper ones may be localized by the Beevor sign (i.e., the umbilicus moves upward when the patient, lying in the supine position, attempts to flex the neck against resistance). Abdominal skin reflexes are absent below the lesion.

Lumbar Tumors

Lesions in the lumbar region may be localized by the level of the sensory loss and motor weakness. Tumors that compress only the L1 and L2 segments cause loss of the cremasteric reflexes. The abdominal reflexes are preserved, as are the knee and ankle jerks.

If the tumor affects the L3 and L4 segments and does not involve the cauda equina, the signs are weakness of the quadriceps, loss of the patellar reflexes, and hyperactive Achilles reflexes. More commonly, lesions at this level also involve the cauda equina to cause flaccid paralysis of the legs with loss of knee and ankle reflexes. If both the spinal cord and cauda equina are affected, there may be spastic paralysis of one leg with an overactive ankle reflex on that side and flaccid paralysis with loss of reflexes on the other side.

Tumors of the Conus and Cauda Equina

The first symptom of a tumor that involves the conus or cauda equina is pain in the back, rectal area, or both lower legs, often leading to the preliminary diagnosis of sciatica. Loss of bladder function and impotence are seen early. As the tumor grows, there may be flaccid paralysis of the legs, with atrophy of leg muscles, and foot drop. Fasciculation may be evident. Sensory loss may affect the perianal or saddle area, and the remaining sacral and lumbar dermatomes. This loss may be slight or may be so severe that a trophic ulcer develops over the lumbosacral region, buttocks, hips, or heels.

Signs of raised ICP may be seen with ependymomas of this region if the CSF protein content is over 100 mg/dL.

DIAGNOSIS OF SPINAL TUMORS

Tumors compressing the spinal cord or the cauda equina cause radicular pain, and the slow evolution of signs of an incomplete transverse lesion of the cord, or signs of compression of the cauda equina. Extradural tumors that do not compress the spinal cord may obstruct the blood supply to the cord; if this occurs, the symptoms are often of sudden onset, and the tumor is either metastatic or a granuloma of the Hodgkin type. In a patient with von Recklinghausen disease, the skin lesions may suggest the presence of a neurofibroma, glioma, or ependymoma.

The diagnosis of an intraspinal tumor may be established before operation, with absolute certainty, by CT, MRI, or myelography. Vascular malformations or vascular tumors may be visualized by spinal angiography. Examination of the CSF may also be helpful.

Radiography

CT and MRI have largely replaced standard radiographic films but are these more sensitive scans not available everywhere. In about 15% of spinal neoplasms, one or more of the following abnormalities are seen in standard radiographs:

1. Localized destruction of the vertebrae is manifested by scalloping of the posterior margin of the vertebral body or lucency of a portion of the vertebra or pedicle.
2. Changes occur in the contour or separation of the pedicles (e.g., the interpediculate distance may be measured and compared with normal values). Localized enlargement of foramina is seen in the dumbbell neurofibroma. Localized enlargement of the spinal canal is usually diagnostic of an intraspinal tumor, but enlargement of many segments may be a developmental anomaly.
3. Paraspinal tissues are distorted by tumors, frequently neurofibromas that extend through the intervertebral foramen or by tumors that originate in the paraspinal structures.
4. Proliferation of bone, which is rare except in osteomas and sarcomas, is also occasionally seen in hemangiomas of bone and meninges.
5. Calcium deposits are occasionally present in meningiomas or congenital tumors.

Diagnostic Imaging

MRI has largely supplanted myelography. In patients with partial spinal block, myelography may alter CSF pressure relationships, causing complete spinal block and neurologic deterioration. MRI is the most useful test for evaluating spinal tumors. The vertebral bodies, spinal canal, and spinal cord, itself, are clearly delineated. Injection of gadolinium assists because most spinal neoplasms display contrast enhancement. When a metastatic tumor is demonstrated, it is advisable to image the entire cord because more than one lesion may be present.

CT is more limited than MRI. Without the intrathecal instillation of a contrast agent, CT may not be relied on to demonstrate the soft-tissue changes of intraspinal tumors. However, the extraspinal aspects, such as metastatic cancer, may be identified. With intrathecal injection of contrast agents, intraspinal tumors are usually seen. The contrast material may leach into the cavity to establish the diagnosis of syringomyelia or cystic tumor.

Cerebrospinal Fluid

When there is a complete subarachnoid block, the CSF is xanthochromic as a result of the high protein content. It may be only slightly yellow, or colorless, if the subarachnoid block is incomplete. The cell count is usually normal, but a slight pleocytosis is found in about 30% of patients. Cell counts of between 25/mm^3 and 100/mm^3 are found in about 15% of the patients. The protein content is increased in more than 95%. Values of over 100 mg/dL are present in 60% of the patients and values of over 1,000 mg/dL are present in 5% and may, in rare cases, lead to communicating hydrocephalus. The glucose content is normal unless there is meningeal spread. Cytologic evaluation of the CSF is useful when malignant tumors are suspected.

Differential Diagnosis

Spinal tumors must be differentiated from other disorders of the spinal cord, including transverse myelitis, multiple sclerosis, syringomyelia, combined system disease, syphilis, amyotrophic lateral sclerosis, anomalies of the cervical spine and base of the skull, spondylosis, adhesive arachnoiditis, radiculitis of the cauda equina, hypertrophic arthritis, ruptured intervertebral discs, and vascular anomalies. *Epidural lipomatosis* is a complication of prolonged steroid therapy but sometimes occurs without apparent cause; the fat accumulations act as an intraspinal mass lesion, causing low back pain and compression of the spinal cord or cauda equina.

Multiple sclerosis, with a complete or incomplete transverse lesion of the cord, may usually be differentiated from spinal-cord tumors by the remitting course, signs and symptoms of more than one lesion, evoked-potential studies, cranial MRI, and the presence of CSF oligoclonal bands. Acute transverse myelitis may occasionally enlarge the cord to simulate an intramedullary tumor.

Determining the differential diagnosis between syringomyelia and intramedullary tumors is complicated because intramedullary cysts are commonly associated with these tumors. Extramedullary tumors in the cervical region may give rise to localized pains and muscular atrophy in conjunction with a Brown-Séquard syndrome, producing a clinical picture similar to that of syringomyelia. The diagnosis of syringomyelia is likely when trophic disturbances are present. The differential diagnosis may often be made by contrast-enhanced MRI that reveals a tumor nodule (Fig. 63.6).

The combination of atrophy of hand muscles and spastic weakness in the legs in amyotrophic lateral sclerosis may suggest the diagnosis of a cervical cord tumor. Tumor is excluded by the lack of paresthesias, and normal sensation on examination, and by the presence of fasciculation or atrophy in leg muscles.

Cervical spondylosis, with or without rupture of the intervertebral disks, may cause symptoms and signs of root irritation and compression of the spinal cord. The osteoarthritis may be diagnosed by findings in plain radiographs, but this is so common in asymptomatic people that MRI may be necessary to determine whether there is spondylotic myelopathy or an extramedullary tumor. Even MRI may show spondylosis in asymptomatic people.

Anomalies in the cervical region or at the base of the skull, such as *platybasia* or *Klippel-Feil syndrome*, are diagnosed by CT or MRI. Occasionally, arachnoiditis may interfere with the circulation in the cord, causing signs and symptoms of a transverse lesion. The CSF protein content is elevated. Diagnosis is made by complete or partial arrest of the contrast column on myelography, or by fragmentation of the material at the site of the lesion. Separation of the adhesions and removal of the thickened arachnoid

by surgery have been of little benefit; steroid therapy is no better.

COURSE AND PROGNOSIS

Benign tumors of the spinal cord are characterized by slow progression for years. If a neurofibroma arises from a dorsal root, there may be years of radicular pain before the tumor is evident from other manifestations of growth. Intramedullary tumors are generally benign and slow growing; they may attain enormous size (over the course of 6 to 8 years) before they are discovered.

Conversely, the sudden onset of a severe neurologic disorder, with or without pain, is usually indicative of a malignant extradural tumor, such as metastatic carcinoma or lymphoma.

TREATMENT OF PRIMARY SPINAL TUMORS

Once the diagnosis of an intraspinal tumor has been made, the treatment is surgical removal of the tumor whenever possible. When the neurologic disorder is severe or rapidly progressing, emergency surgery is indicated. With

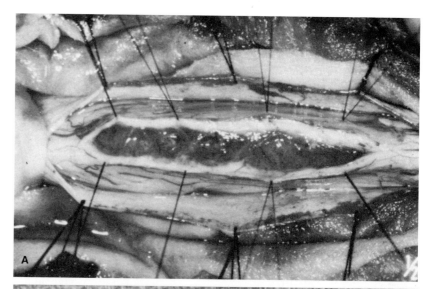

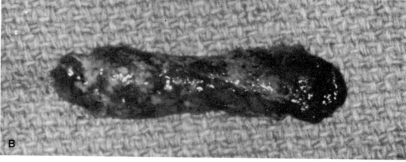

FIGURE 63.9. Intramedullary ependymoma. A: Operative photograph. Myelotomy exposes the dorsal surface of the tumor. Note the clear demarcation of the tumor from the surrounding spinal cord. **B:** Operative photograph of the tumor specimen that has been completely removed.

microneurosurgery, the best results are obtained when the signs and symptoms are due solely to compression of the spinal cord by a meningioma, neurofibroma, or other benign encapsulated tumor. Some of these tumors, especially meningiomas, may lie anterior to the spinal cord and require the most delicate expertise of the neurosurgeon.

Function may be completely restored even when severe spastic weakness has been present for years. The postoperative results, however, are often predicated on the severity of preoperative neurologic disability, which is a strong point in favor of early diagnosis and surgery for these tumors. Radiotherapy is not indicated for most intradural extramedullary tumors, even when removal has been incomplete, because these tumors are usually benign.

The most common intramedullary tumors are ependymomas and astrocytomas. In almost all ependymomas, the tumor may be resected by myelotomy and microsurgery (Fig. 63.9). Radiotherapy is not indicated after total removal of the tumor and is rarely indicated after partial removal; the patient should be observed for recurrence. Additional operative procedures should be considered if they are indicated. Perhaps half of all intramedullary astrocytomas are resectable by microsurgery; again, postoperative radiotherapy is not indicated. When radiotherapy is given after incomplete removal of an astrocytoma, the results are discouraging. In the uncommon presence of other intramedullary tumors, such as hemangioblastomas, teratomas, or dermoids, complete removal without adjuvant radiotherapy is the rule.

After radical and extensive surgery for these tumors, spinal deformities that may have been present preoperatively may appear or increase, requiring fixation. If allowed to progress, these deformities may in turn create neurologic syndromes resulting from spinal cord compression. This condition is especially pertinent in children. Some surgeons have advocated replacement of the lamina after definitive surgery, rather than the standard laminectomy. The additional use of radiotherapy for intraspinal tumors in children may affect the growth of the spine, leading to or increasing preexisting deformities of the spine.

SUGGESTED READINGS

Cook AM, Lau TN, Tomlinson MJ, et al. MRI of the whole spine in suspected malignant spinal cord compression: impact on management. *Clin Oncol R Coll Radiol* 1998;10:39–43.

Aryan HE, Farin A, Nakaji P, Imbesi SG, Abshire BB. Intramedullary spinal cord metastasis of lung adenocarcinoma presenting as Brown-Sequard syndrome. *Surg Neurol* 2004;61(1):72–76.

Elsberg CA. *Surgical Diseases of the Spinal Cord, Membranes and Nerve Roots.* New York: Paul B Hoeber, 1941.

George B, Lot G, Boissonnet H. Meningioma of the foramen magnum: a series of 40 cases. *Surg Neurol* 1997;47:371–379.

Goel A, Bhatjiwale M, Desai K. Basilar invagination: a study based on 190 surgically treated patients. *J Neurosurg* 1998;88:962–968.

Goh KY, Velasquez L, Epstein FJ. Pediatric intramedullary spinal cord tumors: is surgery alone enough? *Pediatr Neurosurg* 1997;27:334–339.

Greenberg HS, Kim JH, Posner JB. Epidural spinal cord compression from metastatic tumor: results with a new treatment protocol. *Ann Neurol* 1980;8:361–366.

Grem JL, Burgess J, Trump DL. Clinical features and natural history of intramedullary spinal cord metastasis. *Cancer* 1985;56:2305–2314.

Hainline B, Tuszynski MH, Posner JB. Ataxia in epidural spinal cord compression. *Neurology* 1992;42:2193–2195.

Hanbali F, Fourney DR, Marmor E, et al. Spinal cord ependymoma: radical surgical resection and outcome. *Neurosurgery* 2002;51(5):1162–1174.

Harrison SK, Ditchfield MR, Waters K. Correlation of MRI and CSF cytology in the diagnosis of medulloblastoma spinal metastases. *Pediatr Radiol* 1998;28:571–574.

Hirano A. Neuropathology of tumors of the spinal cord: the Montefiore experience. *Brain Tumor Pathol* 1997;14:1–4.

Jallo GI, Danish S, Velasquez L, Epstein F. Intramedullary low-grade astrocytomas: long-term outcome following radical surgery. *J Neurooncol* 2001;53(1):61–66.

Jallo GI, Freed D, Epstein F. Intramedullary spinal cord tumors in children. *Childs Nervous System* 2003;19(9):641–649.

Jenis LG, Dunn EJ, An HS. Metastatic disease of the cervical spine. A review. *Clin Orthop* 1999;359:89–103.

Katzman H, Waugh T, Berdon W. Skeletal changes following irradiation of childhood tumors. *J Bone Joint Surg* 1969;51A:825–843.

King AT, Sharr MM, Gullan RW, Bartlett JR. Spinal meningiomas: a 20 year review. *Br J Neurosurg* 1998;12:521–526.

Lee M, Epstein FJ, Rezai AR, Zagzag D. Nonneoplastic intramedullary spinal cord lesions mimicking tumors. *Neurosurgery* 1998;43:788–794.

Lee TT, Gromelski EB, Green BA. Surgical treatment of spinal ependymoma and postoperative radiotherapy. *Acta Neurochir* 1998;140:309–313.

Lefton DR, Pinto RS, Martin SW. MRI features of intracranial and spinal ependymomas. *Pediatr Neurosurg* 1998;28:97–105.

Lonser RR, Weil RJ, Wanebo JE, DeVroom HL, Oldfield EH. Surgical management of spinal cord hemangioblastomas in patients with von Hippel-Lindau disease. *J Neurosurg* 2003;98(1):106–116.

Maranzano E, Trippa F, Chirico L, Basagni ML, Rossi R. Management of metastatic spinal cord compression. *Tumori* 2003;89(5):469–475.

Mathew P, Todd NV. Intradural conus and cauda equina tumours: a retrospective review of presentation, diagnosis and early outcome. *J Neurol Neurosurg Psychiatry* 1993;56:69–74.

Matson DD. *Neurosurgery of Infancy and Childhood*, 2nd ed. Springfield, IL: Charles C Thomas, 1969.

McCormick PC, Stein BM. Intramedullary tumors in adults. *Neurosurg Clin North Am* 1990;1:609–630.

McCormick PC, Torres R, Post K, et al. Intramedullary ependymoma of the spinal cord. *J Neurosurg* 1990;72:523–532.

McLain RF, Bell GR. Newer management options in patients with spinal metastasis. *Cleve Clin J Med* 1998;65:359–366.

Nadkami TD, Rekate HL. Pediatric intramedullary spinal cord tumors. Critical review of the literature. *Childs Nerv Syst* 1999;15:17–28.

O'Toole JE, McCormick PC. Midline ventral intradural schwannoma of the cervical spinal cord resected via anterior corpectomy with reconstruction: technical case report and review of the literature. *Neurosurgery* 2003;52(6):1482–1485.

Pollono D, Tomarchia S, Drut R, Ibanez O, Ferreyra M, Cedola J. Spinal cord compression: a review of 70 pediatric patients. *Pediat Hematol Oncol* 2003;20(6):457–466.

Robertson SC, Traynelis VC, Follett KA, Meunezes AH. Idiopathic spinal epidural lipomatosis. *Neurosurgery* 1997;41:68–74.

Santi M, Mena H, Wong K, Koeller K, Olsen C, Rushing EJ. Malignant astrocytomas. Clinicopathologic features in 36 cases. *Cancer* 2003;98(3):554–561.

Schiffer D, Gordana MT. Prognosis of ependymoma. *Childs Nerv Syst* 1998;14:357–361.

Schild SE, Nisi K, Scheithauer BW, et al. The results of radiotherapy for ependymomas: the Mayo Clinic experience. *Int J Radiat Oncol* 1998;42:953–958.

Stein BM, Leeds NE, Taveras JM, et al. Meningiomas of the foramen magnum. *J Neurosurg* 1963;20:740–751.

Sun B, Wang C, Wang J, Liu A. MRI features of intramedullary spinal cord ependymomas. *J Neuroimag* 2003;13:346–351.

Takacs I, Hamilton AJ. Extracranial stereotactic radiosurgery: applications for the spine and beyond. *Neurosurg Clin North Am* 1999;10:257–270.

Turner S, Marosszeky B, Timms I, et al. Malignant spinal cord compression: a prospective evaluation. *Int J Radiat Oncol Biol Phys* 1993;26:141–146.

Vindlacheeruvu RR, McEvoy AW, Kitchen ND. Intramedullary thoracic cord metastasis managed effectively without surgery. *Clin Oncol R Coll Radiol* 1997;9:343–345.

Williams AL, Haughton VM, Pojunas KW, et al. Differentiation of intramedullary neoplasms and cysts by MR. *Am J Radiol* 1987;149:159–164.

Winkleman MD, Adelstein DJ, Karlins NL. Intramedullary spinal cord metastasis. Diagnostic and therapeutic considerations. *Arch Neurol* 1987;44:526–531.

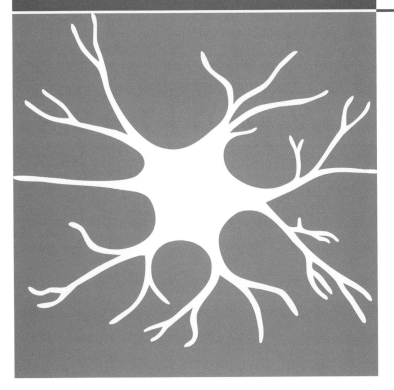

Trauma

Chapter 64

Head Injury

Stephan A. Mayer

EPIDEMIOLOGY

Traumatic brain injury (TBI) is a modern scourge of industrialized society. It is a major cause of death, especially in young adults, and a major cause of disability. The costs in human misery and dollars are exceeded by few other conditions.

More than 2 million patients with head injuries are seen annually, in U.S. emergency rooms, and 25% of these patients are admitted to a hospital. Almost 10% of all deaths in the United States are caused by injury, and about half of traumatic deaths involve the brain. In the United States, a head injury occurs every 7 seconds and a death every 5 minutes. About 200,000 people are killed or permanently disabled annually as a result.

Brain injuries occur at all ages, but the peak is in young adults between the ages of 15 and 24. Head injury is the leading cause of death among people under the age of 24 years. Men are affected three or four times as often as women. The major causes of brain injury differ in different parts of the United States; in all areas, motor vehicle accidents are prominent, and in metropolitan areas, personal violence is prevalent.

PATHOLOGY AND PATHOPHYSIOLOGY OF CRANIOCEREBRAL TRAUMA

Skull Fractures

Skull fractures may be divided into linear, depressed, or comminuted types. If the scalp is lacerated over the fracture, it is considered an open or *compound fracture*. Skull fractures are important markers of potentially serious in-

jury but rarely cause problems by themselves; prognosis depends more on the nature and severity of injury to the brain than on the severity of injury to the skull.

About 80% of fractures are linear. They occur most commonly in the temporoparietal region, where the skull is thinnest. Detection of a linear fracture often raises the suspicion of serious brain injury, but CT in most patients is otherwise normal. Nondisplaced, linear skull fractures generally do not require surgical intervention and may be managed conservatively.

In *depressed fracture* of the skull, one or more fragments of bone are displaced inward, compressing the underlying brain. In comminuted fracture there are multiple, shattered-bone fragments, which may or may not be displaced. In 85% of cases, depressed fractures are open (or compound) and liable to become infected, or leak CSF. Even when closed, most depressed or comminuted fractures require surgical exploration for debridement, elevation of bone fragments, and repair of dural lacerations. The underlying brain is injured in many cases. In some patients, depressed skull fractures are associated with tearing, compression, or thrombosis of underlying venous dural sinuses.

Basilar skull fractures may be linear, depressed, or comminuted. They are frequently missed by standard skull x-rays and are best identified by CT with bone windows. There may be associated cranial-nerve injury or a dural tear, adjacent to the fracture site, which may lead to delayed meningitis if bacteria enter the subarachnoid space. Signs that lead the physician to suspect a fracture of the petrous portion of the temporal bone include hemotympanum or tympanic perforation, hearing loss, CSF otorrhea, peripheral facial-nerve weakness, or ecchymosis of the scalp overlying the mastoid process (Battle sign). Anosmia, bilateral periorbital ecchymosis, and CSF rhinorrhea suggest possible fracture of the sphenoid, frontal, or ethmoid bones.

Cerebral Concussion and Axonal Shearing Injury

Loss of consciousness at the moment of impact is caused by acceleration-deceleration movements of the head, which result in the stretching and shearing of axons. When the alteration of consciousness is brief (e.g., less than

6 hours), the term *concussion* is used. These patients may be completely unconscious or remain awake but appear dazed; most recover within seconds to minutes, rather than hours, and may have retrograde and anterograde amnesia surrounding the event.

The mechanism by which concussion leads to loss of consciousness is believed to be transient functional disruption of the reticular-activating system, caused by rotational forces on the upper brainstem. Experimentally, violent head rotation may produce concussion without impact to the head. Most patients with concussion have normal CT or MRI findings, because concussion results from physiologic, rather than structural injury to the brain. Only 5% of patients who have sustained a concussion and are otherwise intact have an intracranial hemorrhage (ICH) on CT.

The term *diffuse axonal injury* (DAI) is applied to traumatic coma lasting more than 6 hours. In these cases, when no other cause of coma is identified by CT or MRI, it is presumed that widespread microscopic and macroscopic axonal-shearing injury has occurred. Coma of 6 to 24 hours in duration is deemed mild DAI; coma lasting more than 24 hours is referred to as moderate or severe DAI, depending on the absence or presence of brain-stem signs, such as decorticate or decerebrate posturing (Table 64.1).

Autonomic dysfunction (e.g., hypertension, hyperhidrosis, hyperpyrexia) is common in patients with acute severe DAI and may reflect brain-stem or hypothalamic injury. Patients may remain unconscious for days, months, or years and those who recover may be left with severe cognitive and motor impairment, including spasticity and ataxia. DAI is considered the single most important cause of persistent disability after traumatic brain damage.

Axonal-shearing injury tends to be most severe in specific brain regions that are anatomically predisposed to maximal stress from rotational forces. At the time of injury, microscopic damage occurs diffusely, as manifest by axonal-retraction bulbs throughout the white matter of the cerebral hemispheres. Macroscopic tissue tears, best visualized by MRI, tend to occur in midline structures, including the dorsolateral midbrain and pons, posterior corpus callosum, parasagittal white matter, periventricular regions, and internal capsule. Prolonged loss of consciousness from DAI tends to be associated with bilateral, asymmetric, focal lesions of the midbrain tegmentum, a region densely populated with reticular-activating system neurons. Small hemorrhages, known as gliding contusions, are sometimes associated with focal-shearing lesions (Fig. 64.1).

Axonal shearing is thought to initiate a dynamic sequence of pathologic events that evolve over days to weeks. Initially, injury causes physical transection of some neurons and internal axonal damage to many others. In both cases, the process of axoplasmic transport continues, and materials flow from the cell body to the site of damage. These materials accumulate and may lead to secondary axonal transection, with formation of a "retraction ball" from 12 hours to several days after the injury. Membrane channels may open to admit toxic levels of calcium. If the patient survives, there may be later evidence of Wallerian degeneration and gliosis.

Brain Swelling and Cerebral Edema

Brain swelling after head injury is a poorly understood phenomenon that may result from several different mechanisms. Posttraumatic brain swelling may result from *cerebral edema* (e.g., an increase in the content of extravascular brain water), an increase in cerebral blood volume (CBV) resulting from abnormal vasodilatation, or both.

▶ **TABLE 64.1 Clinical Characteristics and Outcome of Diffuse Brain Injuries**

	Mild Concussion	Cerebral Contusion	Diffuse Axonal Injury		
			Mild	**Moderate**	**Severe**
Loss of consciousness	None	Immediate	Immediate	Immediate	Immediate
Length of unconsciousness	None	<6 hr	6–24	>24 hr	Days–weeks
Decerebrate posturing	None	None	Rare	Occasionally	Present
Posttraumatic amnesia	Minutes	Minutes-hours	Hours	Days	Weeks
Memory deficit	None	Mild	Mild-mod	Mild-mod	Severe
Motor deficits	None	None	None	Mild	Severe
Outcome at 3 months (%)					
Good recovery	100	95	63	38	15
Moderate deficit	0	5	15	21	13
Severe deficit	0	0	6	12	14
Vegetative	0	0	1	5	7
Death	0	0	15	24	51

Adapted from Gennarelli TA. Cerebral concussion and diffuse brain injuries. In: Cooper PR, ed. *head injury*, 3rd ed. Baltimore: Williams & Wilkins, 1993:140.

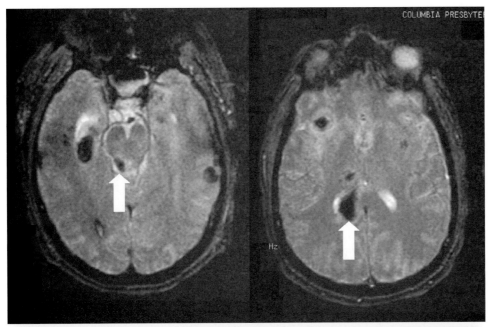

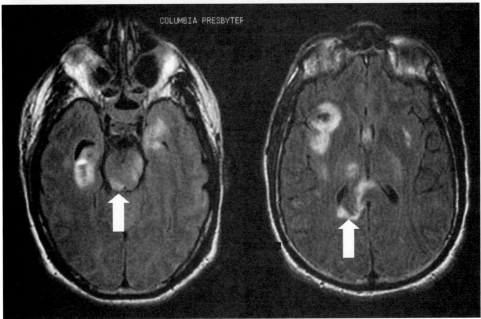

FIGURE 64.1. Focal MRI findings characteristic of diffuse axonal shearing injury after neurotrauma. Top: Gradient echo (T2*) images demonstrating hemorrhagic lesions (gliding contusions) of the right dorsolateral midbrain and splenium of the corpus callosum. Bottom: Fluid-attenuated inversion recovery (FLAIR) images showing edema in these regions.

Cerebral edema may be further classified as cytotoxic, vasogenic, or interstitial (see Chapter 50). The swelling may be diffuse or focal, adjacent to a parenchymal or extradural hemorrhage.

Brain swelling may follow any type of head injury. Curiously, the magnitude of swelling does not always correlate well with the severity of injury. In some cases, particularly in young people, severe diffuse brain swelling that may be fatal occurs minutes to hours after a minor concussion. Abnormal dilation of the cerebral blood vessels is thought to lead to increased CBV, hyperperfusion, and increased vascular permeability, resulting in secondary leakage of plasma and vasogenic cerebral edema.

Cerebral blood flow studies indicate that some degree of hyperemia occurs in nearly all patients 1 to 3 days after severe head injury. Severe brain swelling may be related to this phenomenon or may result from damage to cerebral vasomotor regulatory centers in the brain stem.

Parenchymal Contusion and Hemorrhage

Cerebral *contusions* are focal parenchymal hemorrhages that result from scraping and bruising of the brain as it moves across the inner surface of the skull. The inferior

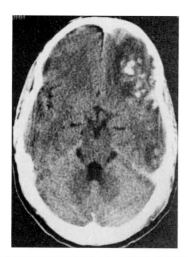

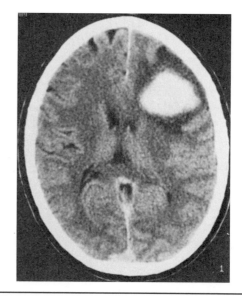

FIGURE 64.2. **Traumatic contusions**. Axial noncontrast view demonstrates areas of contusion with small focal hemorrhages involving the lower poles of the left frontal and temporal lobes adjacent to the rough cranial vault. (Courtesy of Drs. S. K. Hilal, J. A. Bello, and T. L. Chi.)

FIGURE 64.3. **Traumatic intracerebral hemorrhage, frontal lobe.** Axial noncontrast computed tomography demonstrates left frontal lobe density (hemorrhage), surrounding lucency (edema), and mass effect (sulcal and ventricular effacement). (Courtesy of Drs. S. K. Hilal and J. A. Bello.)

frontal and temporal lobes, where brain tissue comes in contact with irregular protuberances at the base of the skull, are the most common sites of traumatic contusion (Fig. 64.2). Tearing of the meninges or cerebral tissue, usually a result of cuts from the sharp edges of depressed skull fragments, are called *lacerations*.

Contusions may occur at the site of a skull fracture, but more often occur without a fracture and with the overlying pia and arachnoid left intact. In most patients, contusions are small and multiple. With lateral forces, contusions may occur at the site of the blow to the head (coup lesions) or at the opposite pole as the brain impacts on the inner table of the skull (contrecoup lesions). Contusions frequently enlarge over 12 to 24 hours, especially in the setting of coagulopathy. In some cases, contusions appear in delayed fashion 1 or more days after injury.

When rotational forces lead to tearing of a small- or medium-sized vessels within the parenchyma, a intracerebral *hematoma* may occur (Fig. 64.3). Hematomas are focal collections of blood clots that displace the brain, in contrast to contusions, which resemble bruised and bloodied brain tissue (Fig. 64.4). Most parenchymal hematomas are located in the deep white matter, in contrast to contusions, which tend to be cortical.

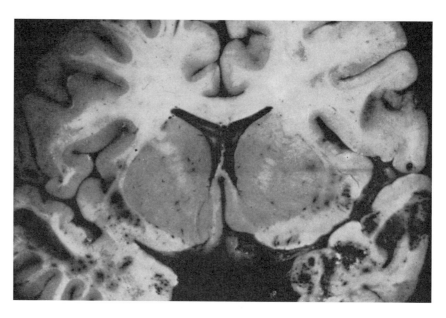

FIGURE 64.4. Pathologic specimen demonstrating traumatic contusions in the temporal lobes.

If there is no DAI, brain swelling, or secondary hemorrhage, recovery from one or more small contusions may be excellent. Healed contusions are often found at autopsy of people with no clinical evidence of permanent brain damage. Large, parenchymal hematomas with mass effect may require surgical evacuation.

Contusions are often managed conservatively unless they lead to significant symptomatic mass effect, because they often consist of hemorrhagic or ecchymotic (but potentially viable) brain tissue.

Subdural Hematoma

Subdural hematomas usually arise from a venous source, with blood filling the potential space between the dural and arachnoid membranes. In most cases, the bleeding is caused by movements of the brain within the skull that may lead to stretching and tearing of veins that drain from the surface of the brain to the dural sinuses. Less often, the source of the hematoma is the result of a ruptured, small pial artery.

Most subdural hematomas are located over the lateral cerebral convexities, but subdural blood may also collect along the medial surface of the hemisphere, between the tentorium and occipital lobe, between the temporal lobe and the base of the skull, or in the posterior fossa. CT usually reveals a high-density, crescentic collection across the entire hemispheric convexity (Fig. 64.5).

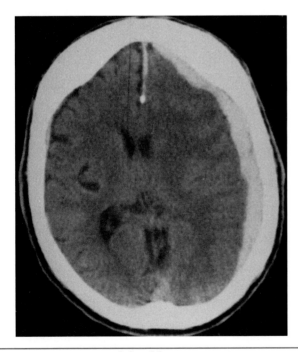

FIGURE 64.5. Acute subdural hematoma. Noncontrast axial CT demonstrates a hyperdense, crescent-shaped, extra-axial collection showing mass effect (sulcal and ventricular effacement) and midline shift from left to right. (Courtesy of Drs. J. A. Bello and S. K. Hilal.)

Elderly or alcoholic patients with cerebral atrophy are particularly prone to subdural bleeding; in these patients, large hematomas may result from trivial impact or even from pure acceleration-deceleration injuries, such as whiplash.

Acute subdural hematomas, by definition, are symptomatic within 72 hours of injury, but most patients have neurologic symptoms from the moment of impact. They may occur after any type of head injury but seem to be less common after vehicular trauma and relatively more common after falls or assaults. Half of all patients with an acute subdural hematoma lose consciousness at the time of injury; 25% are in coma when they arrive at the hospital, and half of those who awaken, lose consciousness for a second time after a "lucid interval" of minutes to hours, as the subdural hematoma grows in size. Hemiparesis and pupillary abnormalities are the most common focal neurologic signs; each occur in one-half to two-thirds of patients. The usual picture is ipsilateral pupillary dilation and contralateral hemiparesis. However, so-called false localizing signs are common with acute subdural hematoma because uncal herniation may lead to compression of the contralateral cerebral peduncle or third cranial nerve, against the tentorial edge (*Kernohan notch*).

Chronic subdural hematomas become symptomatic after 21 days or later. They are more likely to occur in patients after age 50 years. In 25% to 50% of cases, there are no recognized head traumas. Almost half of the patients have histories of alcoholism or epilepsy and the trauma may have been forgotten. Other risk factors for chronic subdural hematomas include overdrainage of ventriculoperitoneal shunts and bleeding disorders, including conditions relevant to anticoagulant medication.

In most cases of chronic subdural hematoma, the bleeding results from trivial trauma with little or no brain compression, owing to coexisting cerebral atrophy. After 1 week, fibroblasts on the inner surface of the dura form a thick outer membrane; after 2 weeks a thin inner membrane develops, resulting in encapsulation of the clot, which begins to liquefy. Enlargement of the hematoma may then result from recurrent bleeding (e.g., acute-on-chronic subdural hematoma) or because of osmotic effects related to a high-protein content of the fluid. Symptoms may be restricted to altered mental status, a syndrome sometimes mistaken for dementia. CT typically shows an isodense or hypodense, crescent-shaped mass that deforms the surface of the brain, and the membranes may enhance with intravenous contrast (Fig. 64.6). Longstanding, chronic subdural hematomas eventually liquefy, forming *hygromas,* and in some cases the membranes may calcify.

Acute and chronic subdural hematomas with significant mass effect should be evacuated. The main indication for surgery is the presence of symptomatic mass effect in the form of focal neurologic deficits, or seizures.

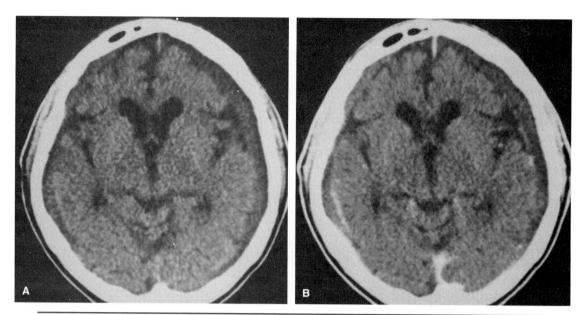

FIGURE 64.6. Bilateral chronic subdural hematoma. A: Noncontrast axial CT shows bilateral iso-dense extra-axial collections, larger on the left. **B:** These are better demonstrated on the post-contrast scan, in which enhancing membranes, typical of the subacute phase, may be seen. (Courtesy of Drs. J. A. Bello and S. K. Hilal.)

Surgical evacuation of the thick, clotted blood that constitutes an acute subdural hematoma usually requires a large-window craniotomy. Outcome after surgical evacuation depends primarily on the severity of the initial deficit, and the interval from injury to surgery. Liquefied chronic subdural hematomas may often be evacuated with drainage of the collections via a series of burr holes. Reoperations for acute and chronic subdural hematomas are required in about 15% of cases. Glucocorticoids have no role in the conservative management of smaller, minimally symptomatic, subdural hematomas.

Epidural Hematoma

Epidural hematoma is a rare complication of head injury. It occurs in less than 1% of all cases but is found in 5% to 15% of autopsy series, attesting to the potential seriousness of this complication.

Bleeding into the epidural space is generally caused by a tear in the wall of one of the meningeal arteries, usually the middle meningeal artery, but in 15% of patients the bleeding is from one of the dural sinuses. Seventy-five percent are associated with a skull fracture. The dura is separated from the skull by the extravasated blood, and the size of the clot increases until the ruptured vessel is compressed or occluded by the hematoma.

Most epidural hematomas are located over the convexity of the hemisphere in the middle cranial fossa, but occasionally hemorrhages may be confined to the anterior fossa, possibly as a result of tearing of anterior meningeal arteries. Extradural hemorrhage in the posterior fossa may occur when the torcula Herophili is torn. In most cases, the hematoma is ipsilateral to the site of impact.

Epidural hematoma is primarily a problem of young adults; it is rarely seen in the elderly because the dura becomes increasingly adherent to the skull with advanced age. The clinical course, in one-third of patients, proceeds from an immediate loss of consciousness caused by concussion, to a lucid interval, and then to a relapse into coma, with hemiplegia as the epidural hematoma expands. The ipsilateral pupil becomes fixed and dilated because the third cranial nerve is compressed by the hippocampal gyrus as it herniates over the free edge of the tentorium; the pupillary change signals impending brain-stem compression (Fig. 64.7).

As with acute subdural hematomas, false localizing signs may occur. The presence of cerebellar signs, nuchal rigidity, and drowsiness, together with a fracture of the occipital bone, should prompt suspicion of a clot in the posterior fossa.

Epidural blood takes on a bulging convex pattern on CT (Fig. 64.8) because the collection is limited by firm attachments from the dura to the cranial sutures.

Progression to herniation and death may occur rapidly because the bleeding is arterial. The mortality rate approaches 100% in untreated patients and ranges from 5% to 30% in treated patients. As the interval between injury and surgical intervention decreases, survival improves. If there is little coexisting brain damage, functional recovery may be excellent.

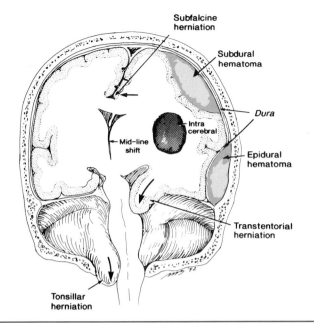

FIGURE 64.7. Patterns of traumatic intracranial hemorrhage and brain herniation. (From White RJ, Likavei MJ, 1992.)

Subarachnoid Hemorrhage

Some extravasation of blood into the subarachnoid spaces is to be expected in any patient with head injury. In most cases, subarachnoid blood is detected only by CSF examination, and is of little clinical importance. With more serious injuries, when larger vessels traversing the sub-arachnoid space are torn, focal or diffuse *subarachnoid hemorrhage* may be detected by CT. In these cases, blood is often distributed over the convexities; in contrast, aneurysmal bleeding results in collections of blood that are restricted to the basal cisterns. Although the presence of a large amount of subarachnoid blood is a poor prognostic sign, delayed complications of aneurysmal subarachnoid hemorrhage, such as hydrocephalus and ischemia from vasospasm, are unusual after traumatic subarachnoid hemorrhage.

INITIAL ASSESSMENT AND STABILIZATION

On admission to the emergency room, resuscitation measures, history taking, and examination should begin simultaneously. The immediate goals of management are to assess and stabilize the airway, respiration, and circulation; to classify the severity of the head injury as low, moderate, or high risk; to rule out a fracture of the cervical spine; and to identify any extracranial injuries. All moderate- and high-risk patients require a CT to rule out fractures or intracranial bleeding.

Hypoxia and *hypotension* may have devastating effects in head-injured patients. If the patient is hypoxic or in respiratory distress, endotracheal intubation is performed, ensuring that the spine remains immobilized during the procedure. Hypotension should be corrected with intravenous boluses of isotonic fluids such as normal saline or

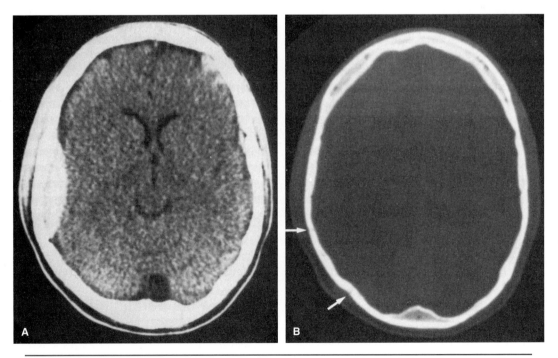

FIGURE 64.8. **A:** Epidural hematoma is evident on CT. **B:** CT with bone windows shows two adjacent fractures (*arrows*); the anterior fracture is at the site of the groove for the middle meningeal artery.

lactated Ringer solution, blood transfusions, or vasopressors. Systolic blood pressure during the stabilization phase should be maintained above 90 mmHg to ensure adequate cerebral blood flow. If the patient is hypotensive, exclude bleeding into the abdomen, thorax, retroperitoneal space, or tissues surrounding a long bone fracture. Hypotension may also reflect *spinal shock* related to a coexisting spinal cord injury (see Chapter 65). Hypertension associated with wide pulse pressure and bradycardia (Cushing reflex) may reflect increased intracranial pressure (ICP) or focal brainstem injury.

A baseline neurologic evaluation should be performed immediately, while airway, respiration, and circulation are assessed. Injuries may be ranked as low, moderate, or high risk, according to risk factors and a rapid initial neurologic assessment (Table 64.2). The Glasgow Coma Scale (Table 64.3) is based on eye opening and the patient's best verbal and motor responses. It is widely used as a semiquantitative, clinical measure of the severity of brain injury; it also provides a guide to prognosis (Table 64.4).

Except for asymptomatic patients in the low-risk group, all patients with suspected trauma should have head

▶ **TABLE 64.3 Glasgow Coma Scale**

Activity/Response	Score[a]
Eye opening	
Spontaneous	4
To voice	3
To pain	2
None	1
Best motor response	
Obeys commands	6
Localizes to pain	5
Withdraws to pain	4
Flexor posturing	3
Extensor posturing	2
None	1
Best verbal response	
Conversant and oriented	5
Conversant and disoriented	4
Inappropriate words	3
Incomprehensible sounds	2
None	1

[a] Total score = sum of the score for each of the three components.
From Teasdale G, Jennett B, 1974.

▶ **TABLE 64.2 Risk Stratification of Patients with Head Injury**

Risk Category	Characteristics
Mild	Normal neurologic examination
	No concussion
	No drug or alcohol intoxication
	May complain of headache and dizziness
	May have scalp abrasion, laceration, or hematoma
	Absence of moderate or severe injury criteria
Moderate	Glasgow coma score of 9–14 (confused, lethargic, stuporous)
	Concussion
	Posttraumatic amnesia
	Vomiting
	Seizure
	Signs of possible basilar or depressed skull fracture of serious facial injury
	Alcohol or drug intoxication
	Unreliable or no history of injury
	Age <2 years, >65 years
Severe	Glasgow coma score of 3–8 (comatose)
	Progressive decline in level of consciousness ("talked and deteriorated")
	Focal neurologic signs
	Penetrating skull injury or palpable depressed skull fracture

Adapted from Masters SJ, McClean PM, Arcanese MS, et al. 1987.

CT. Even before CT is performed, patients who are comatose (Glasgow Coma Scale Score ≤8), or who show clinical signs of herniation, require emergency measures to reduce ICP, including those of head elevation, hyperventilation, and the administration of mannitol (Table 64.5).

Before a cervical collar may be removed, the cervical spine must be cleared completely from C1 to C7. In most patients, lateral cervical spine xrays may be performed to rule out unstable fractures. A cervical-spine CT may be obtained as an alternative, and is more sensitive for fractures of the upper three cervical vertebrae than standard radiographic assay. In addition, unstable ligamentous injuries should be ruled out with the use of flexion-extension cervical xrays in awake patients, or MRI in comatose patients.

DIAGNOSIS

History

The circumstances of the accident and the clinical condition of the patient before admission to the emergency room should be ascertained from emergency medical services records, the patient (if possible), and eyewitnesses. The force and location of head impact should be determined as precisely as possible. Specific inquiry should be made regarding concussion; because patients are amnestic during concussion, only an eyewitness may accurately gauge the duration of loss of consciousness.

▶ **TABLE 64.4 Estimated Mortality Based on Various Features of Head Injury**

	Mortality (%)
Glasgow Coma Scale score	
15	<1
11–14	3
8–10	15
6–7	20
4–5	50
3	80
Age, among comatose patients	
16–35	30
36–45	40
46–55	50
≥56	80
CT abnormalities, among comatose patients	
None	10
Intracranial pathology without diffuse swelling or midline shift	15
Intracranial pathology with diffuse swelling (cisterns compressed or absent)	35
Intracranial pathology with midline shift (>5 mm)	55
Intracranial pressure, among comatose patients	
<20 mm Hg	15
>20 mm Hg, reducible	45
>20 mm Hg, not reducible	90
Pathologic entity	
Epidural hematoma	5–15
Gunshot wound	55
Acute subdural hematoma	
Simple	20–25
Complicated	40–75
Bilateral	75–100

Percentages are adapted from several sources and have been rounded.
From Greenberg J, Brawanaki A. Cranial trauma. In: Hacke W, *Neurocritical care.* New York: Springer-Verlag; 1994:705; Vollmer DG, Torner JC, Jane LA, et al. *J Neurosurg* 1991;75 (Suppl 1):S37–S49; Marshall LF, Gautille T, Klauber MR, et al. *J Neurosurg* 1991;75 (Suppl 1):S28–S36; Miller JD, Becker DP, Ward JD, et al. *J Neurosurg* 1977;47:503–516.

▶ **TABLE 64.5 Emergency Measures for ICP Reduction in an Unmonitored Patient with Clinical Signs of Herniation**

1. Elevate head of bed 15–30 degrees
2. Normal saline (0.9%) at 80–100 mL/hr (avoid hypotonic fluids)
3. Intubate and hyperventilate (target $Pco_2 = 28$–32 mm Hg)
4. Mannitol 20% 1–1.5 g/kg via rapid i.v. infusion
5. Foley catheter
6. Neurosurgical consulation

ICP, intracranial pressure.
From Mayer SA, Dennis L, 1998.

Patients who have "talked and deteriorated" should be assumed to have an expanding intracranial hematoma until proven otherwise. Reports of headache, nausea, vomiting, confusion, or seizure activity must be noted. A medical history, including medications, and drug and alcohol use, should be obtained. Recent drug and alcohol use occurs in a large percentage of trauma patients, and intoxication status may confound assessments of mental status.

Examination

After the initial neurologic assessment, a more detailed physical and neurologic examination should be performed. The skull should be palpated for fractures, hematomas, and lacerations. A step-off or palpable bony shelf, is presumed to represent a depressed skull fracture. The patient should be thoroughly examined for external signs of trauma to the neck, chest, back, abdomen, and limbs. A bloody discharge from the nose or ear may indicate leakage of CSF; bloody CSF may be differentiated from blood by a positive halo test (i.e., a halo of CSF forms around the blood when dropped on a white cloth sheet). If there is no admixture of blood, CSF may be distinguished from nasal secretions because the CSF glucose concentration is 30 mg/dL or more, whereas lacrimal secretions and nasal mucus usually contain less than 5 mg/dL glucose.

After determining the patient's level of consciousness (e.g., alert, lethargic, stuporous, or comatose), a focused mental-status examination should be performed if the patient is conversant. Particular attention should be paid to attention capabilities, concentration (e.g., counting backward from 20 to 1, or reciting the months in reverse), orientation, and memory, including assessment for retrograde and anterograde amnesia.

Eye movements, pupillary size and shape, and reactivity to light should be noted. A sluggishly reactive or dilated pupil suggests transtentorial herniation with compression of the third cranial nerve. A midposition, poorly reactive, irregular pupil may result from injury to the oculomotor nucleus in the midbrain tegmentum. Nystagmus often follows a concussion. In comatose patients, the oculocephalic and oculovestibular reflexes should be tested (see Chapter 4).

Motor examination should focus on identifying asymmetric weakness or posturing. Spontaneous movements should be assessed for preferential use of the limbs on one side. If the patient is not fully cooperative, lateralized weakness may be detected by assessment of an asymmetry in tone or tendon reflexes, or by the presence of an arm drift, preferential localizing response to sternal rub, or extensor plantar reflex. Noxious stimuli, such as pinching the medial arm or applying nailbed pressure, may reveal subtle motor posturing in a limb that otherwise moves purposefully. *Decorticate posturing* (i.e., flexion of arms, extension of legs) results from injury to the corticospinal pathways at the level of the diencephalon or upper midbrain. *Decerebrate posturing* (i.e., extension of legs and arms) implies injury to the motor pathways at the level of the lower midbrain, pons, or medulla.

Gait is particularly important to check in low-risk patients who are treated and scheduled for release without CT scanning. Balance and equilibrium, tested by tandem heel-to-toe walking, are frequently impaired after a concussion.

Radiography and Imaging

CT is the emergency imaging method of choice for head injury. CT is more informative than standard skull radiographic films for detecting skull fractures, and provides unsurpassed sensitivity for detecting intracranial blood. In general, all patients with head injuries should have CT, except for those who are classified as low risk (e.g., without concussion, with no neurologic abnormalities on examination, and with no evidence or suspicion of a skull fracture, alcohol or drug intoxication, or other moderate-risk criteria) (Table 64.2). The likelihood of detecting ICH by CT in these patients is only 1 in 10,000. MRI is better for detecting subtle injury to the brain, particularly for focal lesions related to DAI, but is generally not used for emergency evaluations unless it is rapidly and readily available.

CT images should be assessed for evidence of the presence of epidural or subdural hematoma, subarachnoid or intraventricular blood, parenchymal contusions and hemorrhages, cerebral edema, and gliding contusions related to DAI. With bone-window settings, fractures, sinus opacification, and pneumocephalus may be identified. CT evidence of mass effect and brain-tissue displacement—compression or obliteration of the mesencephalic cisterns or midline shift—correlates with increased ICP and a decreased chance of survival.

MANAGEMENT

Admission to the Hospital

Low-Risk Group

Low-risk patients who meet all criteria described in Table 64.2, generally may be discharged from the emergency room without CT, so long as a responsible person is available to observe the patient for the next 24 hours. In general, these are patients who did not sustain a concussion and have normal findings on neurologic examination. Patients are given a checklist of symptoms (e.g., headache, vomiting, confusion) and instructed to return immediately to the emergency room if any occur.

▶ **TABLE 64.6   Criteria for Hospital Admission After Head Injury**

- Intracranial blood or fracture identified on head CT
- Confusion, agitation, or depressed level of consciousness
- Focal neurologic signs or symptoms
- Posttraumatic seizure
- Alcohol or drug intoxication
- Significant comorbid medical illness
- Lack of a reliable home environment for observation

Moderate-Risk Group

Among patients who have experienced a concussion, a normal Glasgow Coma Scale score of 15 (e.g., alert, fully oriented, and following commands) and normal CT eliminate the need for hospital admission. These patients may be discharged to home for observation with a warning card, even in the presence of headache, nausea, vomiting, dizziness, or retrograde amnesia, because the risk of a significant intracranial lesion developing thereafter is minimal. Criteria for hospital admission for patients with head injury are listed in Table 64.6.

Patients with mild-to-moderate neurologic deficits (generally corresponding to Glasgow Coma Scale scores of 9 to 14) and CT findings that do not require neurosurgical intervention should be admitted to an intermediate or intensive care unit (ICU) for observation. A follow-up CT at 24 hours is often helpful to check for progression of bleeding.

High-Risk Group

All patients with a serious head injury are admitted to the hospital. An early neurosurgical consultation is crucial, because once the patient has been stabilized, assessed, and imaged, the immediate consideration is whether emergency surgery is indicated. If the decision is made to operate, surgery should proceed immediately because delays only increase the likelihood of further brain damage during the waiting period. Medical management of severe-injury patients should take place in an ICU. Although little may be done about the brain damage that occurs on impact, ICU care may play a major role in reducing secondary brain injury that develops over hours or days.

Surgical Intervention

Simple wounds of the scalp should be thoroughly cleaned and sutured. Compound fractures of the skull should be completely debrided. Operative treatment of compound fractures should be performed as soon as possible but may be delayed for 24 hours until the patient is transported to a hospital equipped for this purpose or until the patient is hemodynamically stable. Elevation of small, depressed fractures need not be performed immediately, but the depressed fragments should be elevated before the patient is discharged from the hospital, particularly if the inner table of the skull is involved.

The treatment of massive acute subdural, epidural, or parenchymal hematomas with mass effect is *craniotomy* and surgical removal of the clot. The bleeding point should be identified and either ligated or clipped. The operative results depend to a great extent on the degree of associated brain damage. In the absence of coexisting brain injury, remarkable improvement may occur after evacuation of a subdural or epidural hematoma, with disappearance of the hemiplegia or other focal neurologic signs.

Burr-hole or *twist-drill* evacuation is insufficient for acute, large, subdural and epidural hematomas but for liquefied, chronic, subdural hematomas it is associated with better outcomes than craniotomy. A plastic catheter (e.g., Jackson-Pratt drain) is usually placed in the subdural space for several days until the drainage subsides.

Intracranial Pressure Management

As a general rule, an ICP monitor should be placed in all head-injured patients who are comatose (i.e., Glasgow Coma Scale score 8) after resuscitation, unless the prognosis is sufficiently dismal that aggressive care is unwarranted. Intracranial hypertension occurs in over 50% of comatose patients with CT evidence of mass effect from ICH or cerebral edema and in 10% to 15% of patients with normal scans. A ventricular catheter or fiberoptic parenchymal monitor may be used. Ventriculostomy has the advantage of allowing CSF drainage to reduce ICP but has a high risk of infection (approximately 15%). The risk of infection or hemorrhage is substantially lower with parenchymal ICP monitors (approximately 1% to 2%).

Normal ICP is less than 15 mmHg, or 20 cm H_2O. Cerebral perfusion pressure (CPP) is routinely monitored in conjunction with ICP because it is an important determinant of cerebral blood flow; CPP is defined as mean arterial blood pressure minus ICP. The goal of ICP management after head injury is to maintain ICP less than 20 mmHg and CPP greater than 60 mmHg. The magnitude and duration of derangements beyond these targets is highly correlated with poor outcome after severe TBI.

Treatment of elevated ICP is most successful when a preestablished protocol is used. The Columbia University Medical Center step-wise management protocol for treating ICP elevations in monitored ICU patients is shown in Table 64.7.

An acute, severe increase in ICP always prompts a repeat CT to assess the need for a definitive neurosurgical procedure. If the patient is agitated or appears to be

TABLE 64.7 Stepwise Treatment Protocol for Elevated ICP (>20 mm Hg for More Than 10 min) in A Monitored Patient

1. Consider repeat CT and surgical removal of an intracranial mass lesion or ventricular drainage.
2. i.v. sedation to attain a motionless quiet state.
3. Pressor infusion if CPP <70 mm Hg, or reduction of blood pressure if CPP remains >120 mm Hg.
4. Mannitol 0.25–1 g/kg i.v. every 2–6 h as needed.
5. Hyperventilation to Pco$_2$ levels of 28–32 mm Hg.
6. High-dose pentobarbital therapy (load with 5–20 mg/kg, maintain with 1–4 mg/k/h).
7. Systemic hypothermia. (T = 33%)

See text for details.
CPP, cerebral perfusion pressure.
From Mayer SA, Dennis L, 1998.

fighting the ventilator, a short-acting intravenous sedative agent, such as propofol, fentanyl, or sodium thiopental, should be given to attain a quiet, motionless state. Thereafter, if CPP is less than 60 mmHg, vasopressors such as dopamine or phenylephrine may lead to reduction of ICP by decreasing cerebral vasodilation that occurs in response to inadequate perfusion. Alternately, if CPP exceeds 120 mmHg, blood pressure reduction with intravenous labetalol or nicardipine may sometimes lead to a parallel decrease of ICP. The relationship between extremes of CPP and ICP in states of reduced intracranial compliance is shown in Figure 64.9.

Mannitol and hyperventilation are used only after sedation and CPP management fail to normalize ICP. Mannitol, an osmotic diuretic, lowers ICP via its cerebral dehydrating effects. The initial dose of mannitol 20% solution is 1.0 g/kg to 1.5 g/kg, followed by doses of 0.25 g/kg to 1.0 g/kg as needed. Further doses should be given individually, on the basis of ICP measurements, rather than on a standing basis. Mannitol boluses may also be used to reverse acute herniation syndromes (i.e., a blown pupil) resulting from compartmental mass effect and intracranial ICP gradients. The effect of mannitol is maximal when given rapidly; ICP reduction occurs within 10 to 20 minutes and may last for 2 to 6 hours. Serum osmolality should be monitored closely, with a secondary goal of attaining levels of 300 mOsm/kg to 320 mOsm/kg. Urinary losses should be compensated for with intravenous normal saline, to avoid secondary hypovolemia. Central venous pressure (CVP) monitoring is generally recommended.

More recently, 23.4% hypertonic saline solution (0.5 mL/kg to 2.0 ml/kg) has been used as an alternative to mannitol bolus therapy for the acute treatment of ICP elevations and herniation syndromes. Studies evaluating equi-osmolar doses of mannitol and hypertonic saline indicate that in most cases mannitol is at least equivalent, if not superior, for lowering ICP, although one trial failed to show that hypertonic saline was superior to normal saline

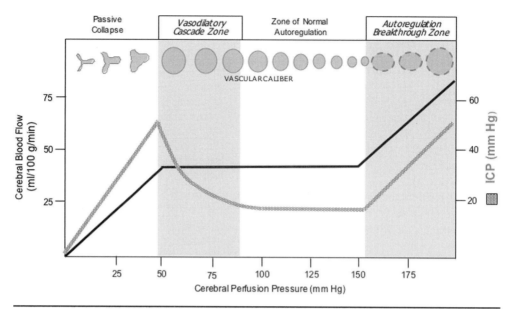

FIGURE 64.9. Relationship between extremes of CPP and ICP in states of reduced intracranial compliance. In the vasodilatory cascade zone, CPP insufficiency and intact pressure autoregulation leads to reflex cerebral vasodilation and increased ICP; the treatment is to raise CPP. In the autoregulation breakthrough zone, pressure and volume overload which overwhelms the brains capacity to autoregulate leads to increased CBV and ICP; the treatment is to lower CPP. Reproduced with permission from Rose JA, Mayer SA. *Neurocritical Care* 2004 (in press).

as the initial treatment for acute fluid resuscitation in severe TBI. As a general rule, hypertonic saline is generally preferred in patients who are hypotensive or hypovolemic, whereas mannitol is preferable for patients who are, relatively, volume overloaded.

Hyperventilation lowers ICP by inducing cerebral alkalosis and reflex vasoconstriction, with a concomitant reduction of CBV. Hyperventilation to PCO_2 levels of 28 mmHg to 32 mmHg may lower ICP within minutes, although the effect gradually diminishes over as little as 1 to 3 hours, as acid-base buffering mechanisms correct the alkalosis within the CNS. Overly aggressive hyperventilation to PCO_2 levels less than 26 mmHg may potentially exacerbate cerebral ischemia, and in general should be avoided unless jugular venous oxygen saturation or brain tissue oxygen monitoring is available to ensure that cerebral hypoxia does not occur.

High-dose barbiturate therapy with pentobarbital, given in doses equivalent to those used for general anesthesia (10 mg/kg to 20 mg/kg as a loading dose, followed by 1 mg/kg/hr to 4 mg/kg/hr) effectively lowers ICP in most patients who are refractory to the steps outlined above. The effect of pentobarbital is multifactorial but most likely stems from a coupled reduction in cerebral metabolism, blood flow, and blood volume. Pentobarbital may cause profound hypotension and usually requires the use of vasopressors to maintain CPP of at least 60 mmHg.

Mild-to-moderate systemic hypothermia (33°C) has been shown to reduce ICP in patients with intracranial hy-

pertension refractory to pentobarbital. The application of hypothermia is complex, and requires a management protocol that emphasizes the use of agents such as meperidine, fentanyl, or dexmedetomidine, and neuromuscular blocking agents if necessary, to prevent shivering that increases cerebral and metabolic stress and fights the cooling process. The routine application of mild-to-moderate hypothermia within 8 hours of TBI, as a form of neuroprotection, was tested in a large clinical trial and was shown not to be of benefit. For this reason, its use should be limited to the management of refractory intracranial hypertension.

Intensive Care Unit Management of Severe Head Injury

Patients with severe head injuries are best treated in an ICU. In some hospitals, patients with head injuries are treated in a special neurologic or neurosurgical ICU. A time-coded flow sheet is helpful to allow for meticulous, continuous updating of the patient's clinical, neurologic, and physiologic status.

Serial Neurologic Evaluation

The patient should be examined repeatedly to evaluate level of consciousness and the presence or absence of signs of injury to the brain or cranial nerves. Variations in level of consciousness, reflected by changes in the Glasgow Coma

Scale score, or the appearance of hemiplegia or other focal neurologic signs should prompt repeat CT.

Airway and Ventilation

In general, patients who are unable to protect their airways because of depressed levels of consciousness should be intubated with an endotracheal tube. Routine hyperventilation is not recommended; in the absence of increased ICP, ventilatory parameters should be set to maintain PCO_2 at 35 mmHg to 40 mmHg and PO_2 at 90 mmHg to 100 mmHg.

Blood Pressure Management

If the patient shows signs of hemodynamic instability, a radial-artery catheter should be placed to monitor blood pressure. Because cerebral blood flow autoregulation is frequently impaired in acute head injury, mean blood pressure (or CPP if ICP is being monitored) must be carefully regulated to avoid hypotensionthat may lead to cerebral ischemia, or hypertension that may exacerbate cerebral edema. Continuous-infusion, short-acting vasopressors (e.g., phenylephrine and norepinephrine) and antihypertensive agents (e.g., labetalol and nicardipine) are preferable because of their abilities to stabilize blood pressure within a narrow therapeutic range. Sodium nitroprusside should be avoided because it may dilate cerebral vessels and raise ICP.

Fluid Management

Only *isotonic fluids*, such as 0.9% (i.e., normal) saline or lactated-Ringer solution, should be administered to head-injured patients because the extra free water in half-normal saline or D5W may exacerbate cerebral edema. Hypertonic saline (i.e., 3% sodium chloride/acetate solution) with a target osmolality of 300 mOsms/L to 320 mOsms/L may be used as an alternative in patients with significant brain edema, and has been shown to reduce the number of ICP elevations. CVP monitoring is helpful to guide fluid management in hypotensive or hypovolemic patients. Negative fluid balance is associated with poor outcome after TBI, and should be avoided.

Nutrition

Severe head injury leads to a generalized hypermetabolic and catabolic response, with caloric requirements that are 50% to 100% higher than normal. Enteral feedings via a nasogastric or nasoduodenal tube should be instituted as soon as possible (e.g., usually after 24 to 48 hours). Early enteral feeding on day 1 after injury is generally well tolerated, and has been shown to improve outcome, compared to delayed feeding. Parenteral nutrition carries significant risks, primarily those of infection and electrolyte derangements, and should be used only if enteral feeding may not be tolerated.

Sedation

Patients may be agitated or delirious, which may lead to self injury, forcible removal of monitoring devices, systemic and cerebral hypermetabolism, and increased ICP. Intubated patients may be sedated using a continuous intravenous infusion of a rapid-acting sedative agent, such as propofol or fentanyl, that may be turned off periodically to allow neurologic assessments. Nonintubated patients with delirium may be treated with haloperidol 2 mg to 10 mg, intramuscularly, every 4 hours as needed.

Temperature Management

Fever (i.e., greater than 38.3°C) is common after TBI, and may be the result of infection or of central fever. Even small temperature elevations may exacerbate traumatic and ischemic brain injury and should be aggressively treated. Newer cooling devices utilizing adhesive cooling pads or intravascular heat-exchange catheters have been shown to be superior to standard water-circulating cooling blankets for maintaining normothermia in comatose brain-injured patients.

Anticonvulsants

Phenytoin or fosphenytoin (15 mg/kg to 20 mg/kg loading dose, then 300 mg/day) reduced the frequency of early (i.e., first week) posttraumatic seizures from 14% to 4% in a clinical trial of patients with intracranial hemorrhage but did not prevent later seizures. Intravenous valproic acid is an acceptable alternative for patients with phenytoin allergy. If the patient has not had a seizure, prophylactic anticonvulsants should be discontinued after 7 days. Anticonvulsant serum levels of head-injured patients should be monitored closely, because subtherapeutic levels frequently result from drug hypermetabolism, particularly in younger men. Nonconvulsive seizures and status epilepticus, which is diagnosable only with continuous EEG monitoring, occur in over 10% of comatose TBI patients, are associated with poor outcome, and generally warrant aggressive treatment with continuous infusion midazolam or similar agents.

Nimodipine for Subarachnoid Hemorrhage

In a clinical trial, nimodipine 60 mg orally every 6 hours was credited with improved outcome in head-injury patients with evidence of subarachnoid hemorrhage on admission CT. Nimodipine may increase neuronal is-chemic tolerance at the cellular level or may improve collateral blood flow. Hypotension was the most common adverse event.

Intensive Insulin Therapy

Continuous insulin infusion therapy to control blood glucose to between 90 mg/dL and 110 mg/dL in hyperglycemic patients has been shown to reduce mortality in critically-ill surgical patients, and is increasingly being adopted as a practice option in the ICU management of severe TBI.

Steroids

Glucocorticoids have been used to treat cerebral edema for years, but have not been shown to favorably alter outcomes or lower ICP in head-injured patients and may, in fact, increase the risk of infection, hyperglycemia, or other complications. For these reasons, dexamethasone and other steroids are not recommended for use in patients with head injury.

Deep-Vein Thrombosis Prophylaxis

Patients with head injury who are immobilized are at high risk for deep vein thrombosis in the legs and pulmonary thromboembolism. Pneumatic compression boots should be used routinely to protect against this risk, and also given subcutaneous heparin 5,000 U or enoxaparin 30 mg, every 12 hours, which may be safely added 48 hours after injury, even in the presence of intracranial hemorrhage.

Gastric Stress Ulcer Prophylaxis

Patients on mechanical ventilation or with coagulopathy are at increased risk of gastric stress ulceration and should receive pantoprazole 40 mg daily, intravenously, famotidine 20 mg intravenously, every 12 hours, or sucralfate 1 g, orally, every 6 hours.

Antibiotics

The routine use of prophylactic antibiotics in patients with open skull injuries is controversial, and opinions are sharply divided. Prophylactic antibiotics with gram-positive activity, such as oxacillin, are often used to reduce the risk of meningitis in patients with CSF otorrhea, rhinorrhea, or intracranial air; however, these agents may increase the risk of infection with more virulent or resistant organisms.

ACUTE COMPLICATIONS OF HEAD INJURY

Cerebrospinal Fluid Fistula

CSF fistulas result from tearing of the dura and arachnoid membranes. They occur in 3% of patients with closed head injury and in 5% to 10% of those with basilar skull fractures. They are usually associated with fractures of the ethmoid, sphenoid, or orbital plate of the frontal bone.

CSF leakage ceases after head elevation, alone, for a few days in 85% of cases. If it persists, the insertion of a lumbar drain may lower CSF pressure, reduce flow through the fistula, and hasten spontaneous closure of the dural tear. Patients with dural leaks are at increased risk for meningitis, and although the use of prophylactic antibiotics is controversial, most physicians use them. Persistent CSF otorrhea or rhinorrhea for more than 2 weeks calls for surgical repair, as does recurrent meningitis. If there is a leak and the site of the fracture is not evident, a metrizamide CT study is the diagnostic method of choice.

Pneumocephalus

Pneumocephalus is a collection of air in the intracranial cavity, usually in the subarachnoid space. It usually occurs with a fracture of a frontal sinus. The air may not appear for several days after injury, and then only after patients sneeze or blow their noses. The presence of intracranial air has the same implications as a CSF fistula. Most pneumoceles are asymptomatic, but headaches or mental symptoms may result from intracranial hypotension. The diagnosis is made by CT, and the site of the dural defect may be identified by CT-metrizamide studies. If spontaneous resorption of the air does not occur, the opening in the frontal sinus should be surgically repaired through a transfrontal craniotomy.

Carotid-Cavernous Fistula

Carotid-cavernous fistulae are characterized by the clinical triad of pulsating exophthalmos, ocular chemosis, and orbital bruit. They result from traumatic laceration of the internal carotid artery as it passes through the cavernous sinus; approximately 20% of cases are nontraumatic, and most of these are related to spontaneous rupture of an intracavernous, internal carotid-artery aneurysm. Other symptoms may include distended orbital and periorbital veins and paralysis of the cranial nerves (e.g., III, IV, V, and VI) that pass through or within the wall of the cavernous sinus.

Traumatic carotid-cavernous fistulae may develop immediately, or within days after injury. Angiography is required to confirm the diagnosis (Fig. 64.8). Endovascular treatment, with a balloon placed through the defect in the arterial wall into the venous side of the fistula, is the most effective means of repair and may prevent permanent visual loss caused by venous retinal infarction, if performed as soon as possible after injury.

Vascular Injury and Thrombosis

Traumatic injuries may be associated with dissections of the extracranial or intracranial internal carotid or vertebral arteries, which may lead to thrombosis at the site of the intimal flap and stroke resulting from distal thromboembolism. The diagnosis is established by conventional MR or MRA; anticoagulation should be used to prevent thrombosis and infarction, although this may be contraindicated if there is coexisting intracranial hemorrhage.

Basilar skull fractures are sometimes associated with thrombosis of adjacent dural sinuses. In most cases, *dural sinus thrombosis* takes several days to develop; the sphenoid and transverse sinuses are most commonly involved. Symptoms are related to increased ICP or associated venous infarction and may include headache, vomiting, seizures, depressed level of consciousness, or hemiparesis. The diagnosis is established by angiography or MR venography, and anticoagulation is the treatment of choice (see Chapter 47).

In patients with large epidural or subdural hematomas and subfalcine herniation, secondary cerebral infarction may sometimes result from compression of the ipsilateral anterior cerebral artery against the falx, or contralateral posterior-cerebral artery against the tentorium.

Cranial Nerve Injury

Injury to the cranial nerves is a frequent complication of fracture at the base of the skull (see Chapter 69). The facial nerve is the most commonly injured nerve in these cases, complicating 0.3% to 5% of all head injuries. Occasionally, the paralysis may not develop until several days after the injury. Partial or complete recovery of function is the rule with traumatic injuries to the cranial nerves, with the exception of injury to the first or second cranial nerve.

Infections

Infections within the intracranial cavity after injury to the head may be extradural (e.g., osteomyelitis), subdural (e.g., empyema), subarachnoid (e.g., meningitis), or intracerebral (e.g., abscess). For more information, refer to Chapter 22.

Extradural infections are usually accompanied by, and are secondary to, infection of the external wound or osteomyelitis of the skull. *Subdural empyema* is a closed-space infection between the dura and arachnoid. *Intracerebral abscess* may follow compound fractures of the skull or penetrating injuries to the brain. All these infections usu-ally develop in the first few weeks after injury but may be delayed. Diagnosis is suggested by CT and MRI, and confirmed by culture of the infected tissue. Treatment includes surgical debridement and administration of antibiotics.

Meningitis may follow any type of open fracture associated with tearing of the dura, including compound skull fractures, penetrating missiles, or linear fractures that extend into the nasal sinuses or the middle ear. Within the past decade, there have been reports of meningitis in as few as 2% and as many as 22% of patients with basilar skull fractures. Meningitis commonly develops 2 to 8 days after injury but may be delayed for several months, particularly in patients with fractures penetrating through the mastoid or nasal sinuses. Cases of meningitis that develop within a few days after injury are almost always caused by pneumococcus or other gram-positive bacteria, but any pathogenic organism may be the cause. Diagnosis depends on the CSF findings after lumbar puncture. The principles of treatment are those recommended for meningitis in general. The presence of a persistent CSF fistula with rhinorrhea or otorrhea favors the recurrence of meningitis; as many as seven or eight attacks have been reported. Treatment in such cases must include surgical closure of the fistula.

OUTCOMES

The outcomes that may be expected after head injury are often matters of great concern, particularly in those with serious injuries. *Depth of coma, CT findings,* and *age* are the medical and demographic variables most predictive of late outcome. Other factors of prognostic importance include pupillary responses, hypotension or hypoxemia on admission, persistently elevated ICP, and critically-reduced (less than 10 mmHg) brain-tissue oxygen levels. In the Traumatic Coma Data Bank, an observational study of 746 patients, 33% died, 14% became vegetative, 28% remained dependent with severe disability, 19% regained independence with moderate disability, and only 7% made a full or near-complete recovery.

Severity of coma may be quantified using the admission Glasgow Coma Scale score (Table 63.3), which has substantial prognostic value. Patients scoring 3 or 4 (deep coma) have an 85% chance of dying or remaining vegetative, whereas these outcomes occur in only 5% to 10% of patients scoring 12 or more. In general, elderly patients do very poorly. In one series of comatose patients older than 65 years, only 10% survived, and only 4% regained functional independence. Death may result from the direct effect of the injury or from the complications that ensue. Attempts to make a firm prognosis in severe head injuries, especially in the early stages, are hazardous because the outcome depends on so many variables. Some indices, however, are valuable as prognostic indicators (Table 64.4).

Persistent vegetative state is a much feared potential outcome of traumatic coma. In general, the prospects of recovery from trauma-induced coma is better than recovery from coma of other causes. Fifty percent of adults and 60% of children who experience trauma-induced coma for 30 days will recover consciousness within 1 year, compared with 15% of patients in coma from nontraumatic causes. Recovery of consciousness is operationally defined as the ability to follow commands convincingly and consistently.

Almost every patient with severe brain injury shows mental changes after recovery of consciousness from prolonged coma; disorientation and agitation are particularly common. With time, there is usually considerable improvement in the signs and symptoms of brain damage, but permanent sequelae are common. In addition to cognitive and motor deficits, headache, dizziness, or vertigo may be present in the immediate posttraumatic period. These symptoms usually disappear in a few weeks but persist and prolong for months.

Disabling cognitive problems include: impaired memory, attention, and concentration; slowing of psychomotor speed and mental processing; and changes in personality. There may be loss of memory for the events that occurred in the immediate period after recovery of consciousness (i.e., *posttraumatic amnesia*) and a similar amnesia for the events immediately preceding the injury (i.e., *pretraumatic amnesia*). These periods of amnesia may encompass days, weeks, or years. Depression occurs in up to 40% of TBI survivors during the first year of recovery, and is highly amenable to medical therapy.

Early cognitive, physical, and occupational therapy is an important part of optimizing recovery after TBI. Physical therapy, including range-of-motion exercises to prevent limb contractures, may begin even while patients are still in the ICU. Once the patient is stabilized, they should be transferred to an acute or subacute rehabilitation facility. Whether cognitive rehabilitative measures truly improve neuropsychologic outcome remains to be established.

In a study of patients with moderate or severe injuries, only 46% returned to work 2 years later, and most of those who did return to work did not go back to their preinjury occupations. Only 18% were financially independent, inducing considerable stress on the family. Vocational training may play a key role in helping patients reintegrate into the workplace.

Postconcussion Syndrome

Approximately 40% of patients who have sustained minor or severe injuries to the head complain of headache, dizziness, fatigue, insomnia, irritability, restlessness, and inability to concentrate. Often, there is overlap with symptoms of anxiety and depression. This group of symptoms, which may be present for only a few weeks or may persist for years, is known as *postconcussion syndrome*.

Postconcussion syndrome is somewhat misleadingly named, because affected individuals need not have suffered loss of consciousness. There are no criteria to define the role of either physiologic or psychologic factors in the etiology of postconcussion syndrome. Patients may be severely disabled, yet have normal findings on neurologic examination and no MR evidence of brain injury. The correlation between the severity of the original injury and the severity and duration of later symptoms is poor. For instance, the incidence of postconcussion syndrome is not related to the duration of retrograde amnesia, coma, or the posttraumatic amnesia. In some patients, the symptoms may be related to the brain damage; in others, they seem to be entirely psychogenic. In practice, it is often difficult to sort out the complicated origins of this disorder.

Posttraumatic symptoms may develop in patients who had previously shown normal adjustment but are more likely to occur in patients who had psychiatric symptoms before the injury. Factors such as domestic or financial difficulties, unrewarding occupations, and the desire to obtain compensation, financial or otherwise, tend to produce and may prolong the symptoms once they have developed.

The prognosis of the postconcussion syndrome is uncertain. In general, progressive improvement may be expected. The duration of symptoms is not related to the severity of the injury. In some patients with only mild injuries, symptoms continue for long periods, whereas patients with severe injuries may have only mild or transient symptoms. By and large, however, it is a matter of 2 to 6 months before the headache and dizziness, and the more definite mental changes, show much improvement. Treatment for postconcussion syndrome is based on psychotherapy, cognitive and occupational therapy, vocational rehabilitation, and treatment with antidepressant or antianxiety agents.

Seizures and Posttraumatic Epilepsy

Posttraumatic seizures may be immediate (i.e., within 24 hours), early (i.e., within the first week), or late (i.e., occurring after the first week).

The exact incidence of seizures after head injury is unknown, but figures in the literature vary from 2.5% to 40%. As a rule, the more severe the injury, the greater the likelihood that seizures will develop. The overall incidence of seizures is about 25% in those with brain contusion or hematoma, and as high as 50% in those with penetrating head injury.

Immediate seizures are infrequent; they are risk factors for further early seizures but not for late seizures. Early seizures occur in 3% to 14% of patients with head injury who are admitted to the hospital. Risk factors include depressed skull fracture, penetrating head injury, intracranial hemorrhage (i.e., epidural, subdural, or intraparenchymal), prolonged unconsciousness (i.e., more than 24 hours), coma, and immediate seizures; the risk of early seizures in patients with any of these risk factors is 20% to 30%. Children are more likely to develop early posttraumatic seizures than are adults. Patients who experience early seizures remain at risk for late seizures and should be maintained on anticonvulsants after discharge from the hospital.

The overall incidence of late seizures (e.g., posttraumatic epilepsy) after closed-head injury is 5%, but the risk is as high as 30% among patients with intracranial hemorrhage or a depressed skull fracture, and 50% among patients who have experienced early seizures. About 60% of patients experience their initial seizures during the first year, but the risk of seizures remains increased for up to 15 years after a severe head injury. Because 25% of patients have only a single late seizure, many practitioners begin anticonvulsants only after a second seizure occurs. Therapy of posttraumatic epilepsy is discussed further in Chapter 141.

Posttraumatic Movement Disorders

Movement disorders are rare sequelae of head injury. Action tremor is most common, although its pathogenesis remains obscure. Cerebellar ataxia, rubral tremor, and palatal myoclonus have been described in patients with focal shearing injuries of the superior cerebellar peduncle, midbrain, and dentato-rubro-olivary triangle, respectively. Parkinsonism and other basal ganglia syndromes have been reported after a single episode of head trauma.

PEDIATRIC TRAUMA

Injuries are the leading cause of death in children, and brain injury is the most common cause of pediatric traumatic death. Motor vehicle accidents account for the largest number of severe injuries in children, but children are also prone to unique forms of injury, such as birth injury and child abuse. Children are more likely than adults to experience brain swelling and seizures after head injury, and in general make better recoveries than do adults.

Birth Injuries

The most common neurosurgical lesions of neonates are skull fractures, subarachnoid hemorrhage; and epidural, subdural, and intracerebral hematomas. Extracranial, subgaleal, and subperiosteal hematomas resulting from trauma at the time of delivery are fairly common and rarely need treatment. Acute subdural hematoma was once considered the most common intracranial birth injury, but this syndrome seems to be disappearing with improved obstetric care. Diagnosis by subdural puncture has been supplanted by the use of CT. Surgical evacuation is accomplished through craniotomy, rather than through a burr hole.

Leptomeningeal Cysts

A rare complication of head injury is the formation of a leptomeningeal cyst in the space between the pia mater and the arachnoid membrane. This complication is most common in infants and children of less than 2 years of age; the clinical hallmark is a palpable, nontender swelling that is getting larger, in the area of a previous fracture. Also known as a growing fracture, leptomeningeal cysts may develop when a linear fracture of the skull is associated with laceration of the dura; pulsation of the brain forces CSF into a cyst formed between the edges of the fracture, producing erosion of the skull. The diagnosis is made from radiographic evidence of a circular or oval area of erosion of the skull in a patient who has had a previous fracture of the skull. Treatment consists of excision of the cyst and repair of the dural defect.

Child Abuse

Child abuse is an important causal consideration in the care of children who present with head trauma. Certain characteristics may enable the physician to identify an abused child. There is often a delay in seeking medical care, and there may be a history of multiple previous injuries. Details of the history may be sketchy or may be inconsistent with the severity or nature of the child's injury. Examination may reveal bruises or injuries that do not normally result from the day-to-day activities of a child, including injuries between the shoulder blades, circumferentially around the arm, or behind the legs. A skeletal survey may reveal multiple healed fractures.

The shaken-baby syndrome should be suspected in children with significant neurologic injury but with little evidence of external trauma. Retinal hemorrhages occur frequently and may be pathognomonic for this syndrome, and subdural hematoma is also common. MRI may play a pivotal role in the diagnosis by identifying intracranial lesions of varying ages. Established protocols should be followed once there is suspicion of child abuse, to ensure that the child will not be subjected to further injury.

NEUROLOGY OF PROFESSIONAL BOXING

The term punch drunk is ascribed to a 1928 paper by Martland; another term is dementia pugilistica. The current nonperjorative, three-word term used to describe the condition is *chronic traumatic encephalopathy*. Whatever the name, there seems to be little doubt that professional boxers are especially at risk for a syndrome that is dominated by parkinsonism and other extrapyramidal features of tremor, ataxia, cerebellar signs, and in some cases, dementia. The disorder is attributed to the cumulative effects of repetitive, subconcussive blows to the head. Pathology studies show hypothalamic abnormalities, degeneration of substantia nigra, widespread neurofibrillary changes, and scarring of cerebellar folia.

Although the syndrome is well known, few prospective studies have been done to determine precise risk factors, to define whether or not signs may be seen early enough to prevent the severe late syndrome, whether or not the syndrome could be prevented by offering protective guidelines for boxing matches (e.g., neurologic examination, including CT and MRI, better head protection, different gloves), and whether not it is a progressive disorder after the boxer has ceased to fight. According to the early study of Critchley (1957), manifestations begin from 6 to 40 years after starting a boxing career, with an average elapsed time of 16 years.

Other sports involve the risk of serious injury, but only boxing includes the goal of deliberately injuring the opponent's brain. Knockout is the prized achievement. Many neurologists have therefore urged the abolition of boxing, but this has not yet been achieved, and it may never be; many powerful social forces promote the sport in the United States and elsewhere. If boxing is not to be banned, physicians and other health-care workers must take every opportunity to regulate the profession. Physicians must stop matches when there is evidence of brain injury. Better protection for boxers must be available during training and in the ring. Once the symptoms of chronic, traumatic encephalopathy have become evident, no therapy is effective, and a degenerative course over years may occur.

SUGGESTED READINGS

Head Injury, General Considerations

Adams JH, Graham DI, Gennarelli TA, et al. Diffuse axonal injury in non-missile head injury. *J Neurol Neurosurg Psychiatry* 1991;54:481–483.

Bullock MR, Chestnut RM, Clifton G, et al. Guidelines for the management of severe head injury. *J Neurotrauma* 1996;13:639–734.

Clifton GL, Miller ER, Choi SC, et al. Lack of effect of induction of hypothermia after acute brain injury. *N Engl J Med* 2001;344:556–563.

Clifton GL, Miller ER, Choi SC, Levin HS. Fluid thresholds and outcome from severe brain injury. *Crit Care Med.* 2002;30:739–475.

Cruz J, Minoja G, Okuchi K, Facco E. Successful use of the new high-dose mannitol treatment in patients with Glasgow Coma Scale scores of 3 and bilateral abnormal pupillary widening: a randomized trial. *J Neurosurg* 2004;100:376–383.

Eisenberg HM, Frankowski RF, Contant CF, et al. High-dose barbiturate control of elevated intracranial pressure in patients with severe head injury. *J Neurosurg* 1988;69:15–23.

Ghajar J. Traumatic brain injury. *Lancet* 2000;356:923–929.

Gruen P, Liu C. Current trends in the management of head injury. *Emerg Med Clin North Am* 1998;16:63–83.

Harders A, Kakarieka A, Braakman R, et al. Traumatic subarachnoid hemorrhage and its treatment with nimodipine. *J Neurosurg* 1996;85:82–89.

Ibanez J, Arikan F, Pedraza S, et al. Reliability of clinical guidelines in the detection of patients at risk following mild head injury: results of a prospective study. *J Neurosurg* 2004;100(5):825–834.

Jane JA, Anderson DK, Torner JC, Young W. *Central Nervous System Trauma Status Report—1991.* New York: Mary Ann Liebert, 1992.

Marshall LF, Marshall SB, Klauber MR, et al. A new classification of head injury based on computerized tomography. *J Neurosurg* 1991;75(suppl 1):S14–S20.

Martin NA, Patwardhan RV, Alexander MJ, et al. Characterization of cerebral hemodynamic phases following severe head trauma: hypoperfusion, hyperemia, and vasospasm. *J Neurosurg* 1997;87:9–19.

Mayer SA, Chong J: Critical care management of increased intracranial pressure. *J Intensive Care Med* 2002;17:55–67.

Merritt HH. Head injury. *War Med* 1943;4:61–82.

Muizelaar JP, Marmarou A, Ward JD, et al. Adverse effects of prolonged hyperventilation in patients with head injury: a randomized clinical trial. *J Neurosurg* 1991;75:731–739.

Oertel M, Kelly DF, McArthur D, et al. Progressive hemorrhage after head trauma: predictors and consequences of the evolving injury. *J Neurosurg* 2002;96:109–116.

Pearl GS. Traumatic neuropathology. *Clin Lab Med* 1998;18:39–64.

Rosner MJ, Rosner SD, Johnson AH. Cerebral perfusion pressure: management protocol and clinical results. *J Neurosurg* 1995;83:949–962.

Stiell IG, Wells GA, Vandemheen K, et al. The Canadian CT Head Rule for patients with minor head injury. *Lancet* 2001;357:1391–1396.

Symonds C. Concussion and its sequelae. *Lancet* 1962;1:1–5.

Taylor SJ, Fettes SB, Jewkes C, Nelson RJ. Prospective, randomized, controlled trial to determine the effect of early enhanced enteral nutrition on clinical outcome in mechanically ventilated patients suffering head injury. *Crit Care Med* 1999;27:2525–2531.

Teasdale G, Jennett B. Assessment of coma and impaired consciousness. A practical scale. *Lancet* 1974;2:81–83.

Teasdale GM, Murray G, Anderson E, et al. Risks of acute traumatic intracranial hematoma in children and adults: implications for management of head injuries. *BMJ* 1990;300:363–367.

Temkin NR, Dikman SS, Wilensky AJ, et al. A randomized, double-blind study of phenytoin for the prevention of posttraumatic seizures. *N Engl J Med* 1990;323:497–502.

Temkin NR, Haglund MM, Winn HR. Causes, prevention and treatment of post-traumatic epilepsy. *New Horizons* 1995;3:518–522.

Vespa PM, Nuwer MR, Nenov V, et al. Increased incidence and impact of nonconvulsive and convulsive seizures after traumatic brain injury as detected by continuous electroencephalographic monitoring. *J Neurosurg* 1999;91:750–760.

Vialet R, Albanese J, Thomachot L, et al. Isovolume hypertonic solutes (sodium chloride or mannitol) in the treatment of refractory posttraumatic intracranial hypertension: 2 mL/kg 7.5% saline is more effective than 2 mL/kg 20% mannitol. *Crit Care Med* 2003;31:1683–1687.

Imaging

Bigler ED. Neuroimaging in pediatric traumatic head injury: diagnostic considerations and relationships to neurobehavioral outcome. *J Head Trauma Rehab* 1999;14:406–423.

Brisman MH. Camins MB. Radiologic evaluation in patients with head injury. *Mt Sinai J Medicine* 1997;64(3):226–232.

Glauser J. Head injury: which patients need imaging? Which test is best? *Cleveland Clinic J Med* 2004;71(4):353–357.

Jeret JS, Mandell M, Anziska B, et al. Clinical predictors of abnormality disclosed by computed tomography after mild head trauma. *Neurosurgery* 1993;32:9–16.

Schaefer PW, Huisman TA, Sorensen AG, et al. Diffusion-weighted MR imaging in closed head injury: High correlation with initial Glasgow coma scale score and score on modified Rankin scale at discharge. *Radiology* 2004;233(1):58–66.

Schenarts PJ, Diaz J, Kaiser C, et al. Prospective comparison of admission computed tomographic scan and plain films of the upper cervical spine in trauma patients with altered mental status. *J Trauma Inj Infection Crit Care* 2001;51:663–668.

Zee CS, Go JL. CT of head trauma. *Neuroimag Clin North Am* 1998;8:525–539.

Epidural Hematoma

Borzone M, Rivano C, Altomonte M, Baldini M. Acute traumatic posterior fossa haematomas. *Acta Neurochir* 1995;135:32–37.

Bricolo AP, Pasut LM. Extradural hematoma: toward zero mortality. *Neurosurgery* 1984;14:8–12.

Bullock R, Smith RM, van Dellen JR. Nonoperative management of extradural hematoma. *Neurosurgery* 1985;16:602–606.

Dhellemmes P, Lejeune JP, Christiaens JL, et al. Traumatic extradural hematomas in infancy and childhood. *J Neurosurg* 1985;62:861–865.

Huda MF, Mohanty S, Sharma V, et al. Double extradural hematoma: An analysis of 46 cases. *Neurol India* 2004;52(4):450–452.

Subdural Hematoma

Bender MB. Recovery from subdural hematoma without surgery. *Mt Sinai J Med* 1960;26:52–58.

Lee KS. The pathogenesis and clinical significance of traumatic subdural hygroma. *Brain Injury* 1998;12:595–603.

Lee JY, Ebel H, Ernestus RI, et al. Various surgical treatments of chronic subdural hematoma and outcome in 172 patients: Is membranectomy necessary? *Surg Neurol* 2004;61(6):523–527.

Munro D, Merritt HH. Surgical pathology of subdural hematoma. *Arch Neurol Psychiatry* 1936;35:64–78.

Munro PT, Smith RD, Parke TR. Effect of patients' age on management of acute intracranial haematoma: prospective national study. *BMJ* 2002;325:1001.

Rohde V, Graf G, Hassler W. Complications of burr-hole craniostomy and closed-system drainage for chronic subdural hematomas: a retrospective analysis of 376 patients. *Neurosurg Rev* 2002;25:89–94.

Weigel R, Schmiedek P, Krauss JK. Outcome of contemporary surgery for chronic subdural haematoma: evidence based review. *J Neurol Neurosurg Psychiatry* 2003;74:937–943.

Complications of Head Injury

Bell RB, Dierks EJ, Homer L, Potter BE. Management of cerebrospinal fluid leak associated with craniomaxillofacial trauma. *J Oral Maxillofacial Surg* 2004;62(6):676–684.

Davis JM, Zimmerman RA. Injury to the carotid and vertebral arteries. *Neuroradiology* 1983;25:55–70.

Dott NM. Carotid-cavernous arteriovenous fistula. *Clin Neurosurg* 1969;16:17–21.

Friedman AP, Merritt HH. Damage to cranial nerves resulting from head injury. *Bull Los Angel Neurol Soc* 1944;9:135–139.

Hemphill JC III, Gress DR, Halbach VV. Endovascular therapy of traumatic injuries of the intracranial cerebral arteries. *Crit Care Clin* 1999;15:811–829.

Klisch J, Huppertz HJ, Spetzger U, et al. Transvenous treatment of carotid cavernous and dural arteriovenous fistulae: results for 31 patients and review of the literature. *Neurosurgery* 2003;3(4):836–856.

Luo CB, Teng MM, Yen DH, et al. Endovascular embolization of recurrent traumatic carotid-cavernous fistulas managed previously with detachable balloons. *J Trauma* 2004;56(6):1214–1220.

Morgan MK, Besser M, Johnston I, et al. Intracranial carotid artery injury in closed head trauma. *J Neurosurg* 1987;66:192–197.

Scott BL, Jancovic J. Delayed-onset progressive movement disorders after static brain lesions. *Neurology* 1996;46:68–74.

Pediatric Trauma

Adelson PD, Kochanek PM. Head injury in children. *J Child Neurol* 1998;13:2–15.

Carbaugh SF. Understanding shaken baby syndrome. *Adv Neonatal Care* 2004;4(2):105–114.

Duhaime AC, Christian CW, Rorke LB, Zimmerman RA. Nonaccidental head injury in infants—the "shaken baby syndrome." *N Engl J Med* 1998;338:1822–1829.

Hylton C, Goldberg MF. Images in clinical medicine. Circumpapillary retinal ridge in the shaken-baby syndrome. *N Engl J Med* 2004;8;351:170.

Schutzman SA, Barnes P, Duhaime AC, et al. Evaluation and management of children younger than two years old with apparently minor head trauma: proposed guidelines. *Pediatrics* 2001;107:983–993.

Ward JD. Pediatric issues in head trauma. *New Horizons* 1995;3:539–545.

Outcome

Anderson VA, Morse SA, Catroppa C, Haritou F, Rosenfeld JV. Thirty month outcome from early childhood head injury: A prospective analysis of neurobehavioural recovery. *Brain* 2004 Dec;127(Pt 12):2608–2620. Epub 2004 Dec.

Annegers JF, Grabow JD, Groover RV, et al. Seizures after head trauma: a population study. *Neurology* 1980;30:683–689.

Brooke OG. Delayed effects of head injuries in children. *BMJ* 1988;296:948.

Cifu DX, Kreutzer JS, Marwitz JH, et al. Functional outcomes of older adults with traumatic brain injury: a prospective, multicenter analysis. *Arch Phys Med Rehab* 1996;77:883–888.

Dennis M, Levin HS. New perspectives on congnitive and behavioral outcome after childhood closed head injury. *Dev Neuropsychol* 2004;25(1–2):1–3.

Dikman S, Machamer J, Temkin N. Psychosocial outcome in patients with moderate to severe head injury: 2-year follow-up. *Brain Injury* 1993;7:113–124.

Englander J, Bushnik T, Duong TT, et al. Analyzing risk factors for late posttraumatic seizures: a prospective, multicenter investigation. *Arch Phys Med Rehab* 2003;84:365–373.

Gordon E, von Holst H, Rudehill A. Outcome of head injury in 2298 patients treated in a single clinic during a 21-year period. *J Neurosurg Anesth* 1995;7:235–247.

Klonoff H, Clark C, Klonoff PS. Long-term outcome of head injuries: 23-year follow-up of children. *J Neurol Neurosurg Psychiatry* 1993;56:410–415.

Levin HS, Amparo E, Eisenberg HM, et al. MRI and CT in relation to the neurobehavioral sequelae of mild and moderate head injuries. *J Neurosurg* 1987;66:706–713.

Levin HS, Gary HS Jr, Eisenberg MM, et al. Neurobehavioral outcome one year after severe head injury: experience of the Traumatic Coma Data Bank. *J Neurosurg* 1990;73:699–709.

Lishman WA. Physiogenesis and psychogenesis in the "postconcussional" syndrome. *Br J Psychiatry* 1988;153:460.

Macciocchi SN, Barth JT, Littlefield LM. Outcome after mild head injury. *Clin Sports Med* 1998;17:27–36.

Pohlmann-Eden B, Bruckmeir J. Predictors and dynamics of posttraumatic epilepsy. *Acta Neuro Scand* 1997;95:257–262.

Rovlias A, Kotsou S. Classification and regression tree for prediction of outcome after severe head injury using simple clinical and laboratory variables. *J Neurotrauma* 2004 Jul;21(7):886–893.

Sakas DE, Bullock MR, Teasdale GM. One-year outcome following craniotomy for traumatic hematoma in patients with fixed dilated pupils. *J Neurosurg* 1995;82:961–965.

Temkin NR, Holubkov R, Machamer JE, et al. Classification and regression trees (CART) for prediction of function 1 year following head trauma. *J Neurosurg* 1995;82:764–771.

Neurology of Boxing

Critchley M. Medical aspects of boxing, particularly from a neurological standpoint. *Br Med J* 1957;1:351–357.

Jordan BD. Neurologic aspects of boxing. *Arch Neurol* 1987;44:453–459.

Jordan BD, Lahre C, Hauser WA, et al. CT of 338 professional boxers. *Radiology* 1992;185:509–512.

Martland HS. Punch drunk. *JAMA* 1928;91:1103–1107.

Moriarity J, Collie A, Olson D, Buchanan J, Leary P, McStephen M, McCrory P. A prospective controlled study of cognitive function during an amateur boxing tournament. *Neurology* 2004 May 11;62(9):1497–1502.

Ross RJ, Cole M, Thompson JS, et al. Boxers—computed tomography, EEG, and neurological examination. *JAMA* 1983;249:211–213.

Spriggs M. Compulsory brain scans and genetic tests for boxers–or should boxing be banned? *J Med Ethics* 2004 Oct;30(5):515–516.

Zazryn TR, Finch CF, McCrory P. A 16-year study of injuries to professional boxers in the state of Victoria, Australia. *Br J Sports Med* 2003;37:321–324.

Chapter 65

Spinal Injury

Christopher Commichou, Joseph T. Marrotta, and Nazli Janjua

Traumatic spinal cord injury (TSCI, SCI) is often acute and unexpected, causing irreversible damage and dramatically changing the course of an individual's life. The social and economic consequences to patient, family, and society may be catastrophic.

The annual incidence of SCI, worldwide, is estimated at 15 to 50 cases per 1,000,000 persons, with about 12,000 new cases per year in the U.S. These numbers may be underestimates because many patients succumb to the injuries prior to hospitalization. Mortality at the scene is probably in excess of 50%. Of those who survive to hospitalization, mortality at one year is 13%. Acute, traumatic, spinal cord injuries account for 2.5% of admissions to trauma centers. The prevalence is 900 cases per 1,000,000 admissions, affecting up to 250,000 patients in the United States. The median age of this group is a sobering 27 years. Sixty-five percent of those with SCI are younger than 35 years of age. The greatest incidence occurs between ages 20 to 24 years. The male-to-female ratio is nearly 4:1. The incidence of injury is highest during the summer months and on weekends.

The most common level of injury is cervical, specifically C-5 followed by C-4 and C-6. The most common lower level is T-12 followed by L-1 and T-10.

ETIOLOGY

Vehicular accidents are the most common cause of traumatic paraplegia and tetraplegia. Patients in this group (i.e., those involved in single and multiple motor vehicle accidents, motorcycle accidents, and injuries to pedestrians), account for approximately 48% of all new cases of SCI. Other causes include falls (21%), sports and recreational injuries (13%), industrial accidents (12%), and acts of violence (16%). In the elderly, falls are an increasingly common cause of SCI. There are regional differences in causation (i.e., in large cities, gunshot wounds and stabbings are seen more frequently) and the relative frequency of these causes differs in different societies (Table 65.1). Birth injuries, particularly in breech deliveries, may result in a stretched or compressed spinal cord

TABLE 65.1 Causes of Spinal Cord Injury: New Admissions to Duke of Cornwall Spinal Treatment Center 1989–1991

Causes	%
Motor vehicle accidents	51.5
Car, truck	27
Motorcycle	21
Bicycle	3
Pedestrian	1
Domestic and industrial accidents	27
Domestic	
Falls in house; stairs, ladders, trees	16
Industrial	
Falls from scaffolds, ladders; crush injuries	11
Athletic injuries	16
Diving in shallow water	7
Rugby	3
Horse riding	1
Gymnastics, skiing, others	5.5
Personal injury	5
Self-harm	4.5
Criminal assault	0.5
Major catastrophe	
Air crash	0.5

Modified from Grundy D, Swain A, eds. *ABC of spinal cord injury*, 2nd ed. London: BMJ Publishing Group, 1993.

caused by traction and hyperextension of the cervical spine.

MECHANISM OF INJURY

The most frequent mechanism of SCI is indirect translational force, such as that generated by sudden flexion, hyperextension, vertebral compression, or rotation of the vertebral column. This may result in dislocation of facet joints, fracture of vertebral bodies, misalignment of the vertebral canal, herniation of disc material, and bone splintering. The spinal cord may consequently be contused, stretched, lacerated, or crushed. When there is preexisting cervical spondylosis or spinal stenosis, a trivial injury may cause major neurologic damage, even without fracture or dislocation. MRI has been instrumental in defining mechanistic processes of injury, especially in determining the frequency of disc herniation.

Direct injury to the spinal cord results from high velocity missiles, foreign bodies and bony fragments, and from sharp objects that are able to bypass or destroy the bony protection of the spinal column. Direct injuries, like indirect injuries, may be partial or complete in their destruction of the cord.

Appreciation of the mechanism of injury provides insight into the potential instability of spinal injury. Sudden, violent flexion, particularly in the cervical and thoracic regions, may cause anterior compression fractures of vertebral bodies and unilateral or bilateral facet joint dislocation. Rupture of longitudinal or interspinous ligaments may occur. As a result of severe compression injuries, a vertebral body may burst, so that bone splinters and disc material are pushed into the spinal canal. Rotational injuries may result in unilateral fracture–dislocation with variable trauma to the cord. Hyperextension injuries may result in fracture of the posterior elements of the vertebral bodies. Any combination of forces may occur in a single case. It is important to recognize the mechanism of injury, as it permits assessment not only of the nature, level, and extent of underlying cord injury, but also of the stability of the spinal column at the site of injury.

Secondary injury has been recognized increasingly as a source of ongoing SCI. Much focus has been placed on unraveling these mechanisms in order to intervene and halt these processes. They are generally considered a cascade of events triggered by the initial insult that continue to cause damage to neural tissue on the cellular level. These include vascular changes, effects of excitatory amino acids and cell membrane destabilization, free radical production, inflammatory mediators production, and apoptosis. These events are described in detail by Sekhon (2001).

PATHOLOGY

The type and severity of spinal column injury help determine the nature and extent of the underlying cord damage. There may be contusion and compression of the cord, partial or complete laceration, and discrete or gross destruction of spinal tissue. There is often a combination of injury type. There may also be significant SCI without any evident bony or structural abnormality. This is often the case in younger patients with ligamentous injury.

Traumatic SCI results from a direct mechanical blow causing cord dysfunction of varying degree. This is acute and immediate. Macroscopic examination in acute SCI reveals a swollen, reddish, soft, and friable cord. Contusion, extradural hemorrhages of modest size, subdural hemorrhages, and subarachnoid hemorrhage may be seen. Complete transection is rare.

Hyperemia is obvious within 12 to 24 hours. The vascular changes are likely caused by the presence of vasoactive agents, triggered by prostaglandins and catecholamines. Cross sections of the swollen cord reveal centrally placed hemorrhages, softening, or necrosis. Microscopic investigation reveals fragmented myelin sheaths, splayed myelin lamellae, broken axons, and eosinophilic neurons. The exudate consists of red cells, polymorphonuclear leukocytes, lymphocytes, and plasma cells. These changes extend several segments above and below the level of injury. The edema and acute reaction usually subside within several weeks; hemorrhages are absorbed, and the acute exudate is replaced by macrophages, with the most prominent cell being a lipid phagocyte. This reparative stage may persist for 2 years, resulting in cavitation, gliosis, and fibrosis. In 5 years or more post injury, the damaged area shrinks, and the cord is replaced by fibrous tissue. There is progressive proliferation of acellular connective tissue, resulting in dense and chronic adhesive arachnoiditis. The chronic results of SCI may include traumatic neuroma from injured nerve roots, posttraumatic syringomyelia, or spinal stenosis secondary to disc protrusion and associated osteophyte formation.

In traumatic hematomyelia, hemorrhage occurs within the central gray matter. It is limited in extent and is eventually absorbed, leaving a centrally placed, smooth-walled cyst. This differs from the much more common hemorrhagic softening and necrosis that occur as described above.

In some patients, after several years of neurologic stability, residual intramedullary cysts may become distended, leading to progressive neurologic deterioration. There is no clear understanding of this delayed myelopathy, which is called traumatic syringomyelia. Similarly, delayed myelomalacia may appear on MRI as atrophic spinal cord, often with cystic components, with or without symptoms.

NEUROLOGIC ASSESSMENT AND CLASSIFICATION

A comprehensive, thorough neurologic assessment is pivotal in determining the level, type, and severity of cord injury. The American Spinal Injury Association (ASIA) and the International Medical Society of Paraplegia (IMSOP) jointly published the *International Standards for Neurological and Functional Classification of Spinal Cord Injury* (Maynard et al., 1997). This is an excellent guide for evaluation and clinical neurologic assessment, allowing comparison of findings from center to center and investigator to investigator (Fig. 65.1).

The ASIA/IMSOP have also published an impairment scale that consists of the following categories:

Complete: No motor or sensory function preserved in the sacral segments S-4 and S-5.
Incomplete: Sensory but not motor function is preserved below the neurologic level and extends through to the sacral segments S-4 and S-5.

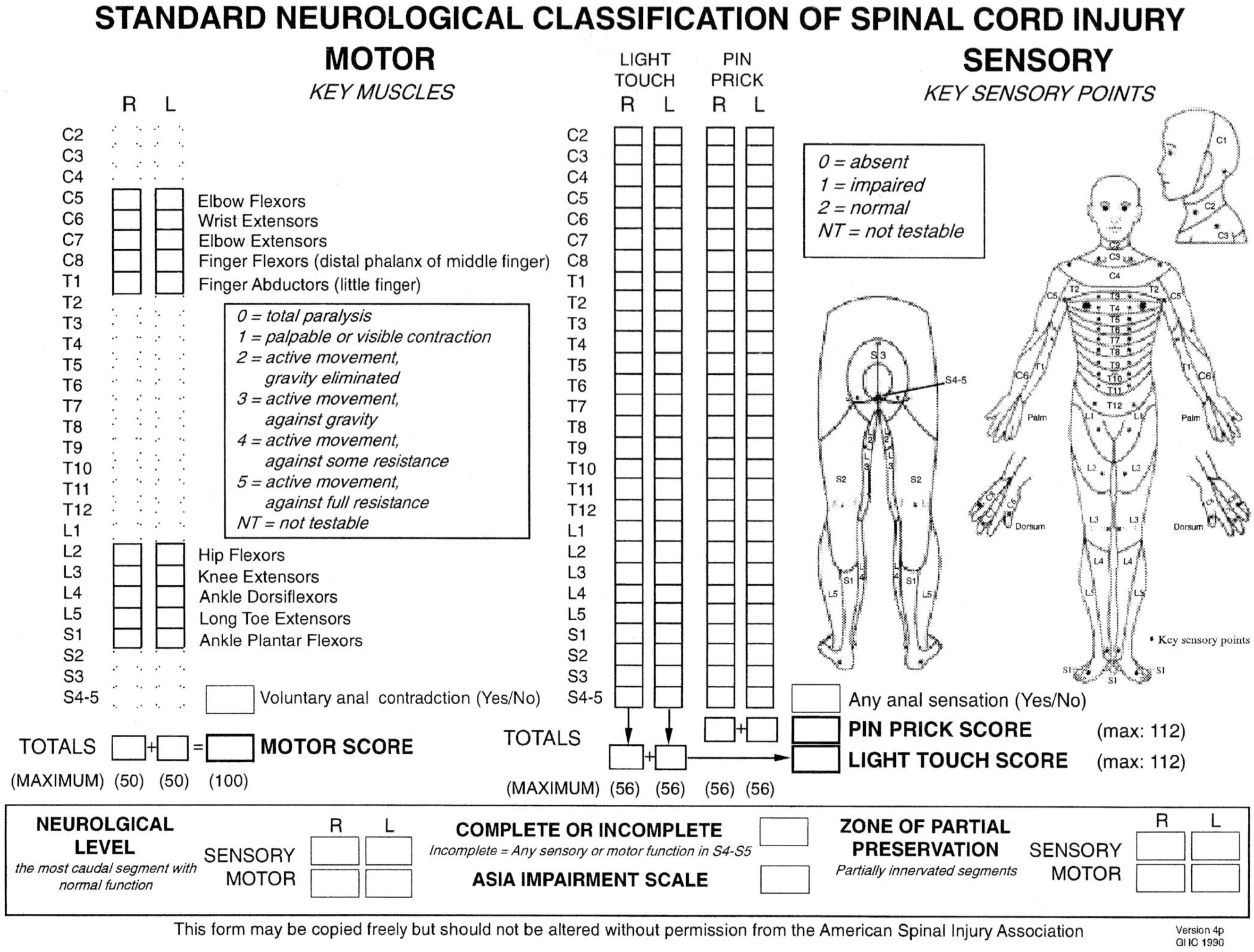

STANDARD NEUROLOGICAL CLASSIFICATION OF SPINAL CORD INJURY

MOTOR
KEY MUSCLES

R L

C2
C3
C4
C5 — Elbow Flexors
C6 — Wrist Extensors
C7 — Elbow Extensors
C8 — Finger Flexors (distal phalanx of middle finger)
T1 — Finger Abductors (little finger)
T2
T3
T4
T5
T6
T7
T8
T9
T10
T11
T12
L1

| 0 = total paralysis |
| 1 = palpable or visible contraction |
| 2 = active movement, gravity eliminated |
| 3 = active movement, against gravity |
| 4 = active movement, against some resistance |
| 5 = active movement, against full resistance |
| NT = not testable |

L2 — Hip Flexors
L3 — Knee Extensors
L4 — Ankle Dorsiflexors
L5 — Long Toe Extensors
S1 — Ankle Plantar Flexors
S2
S3
S4-5 — Voluntary anal contradction (Yes/No)

TOTALS ☐ + ☐ = ☐ **MOTOR SCORE**

(MAXIMUM) (50) (50) (100)

SENSORY
KEY SENSORY POINTS

LIGHT TOUCH   PIN PRICK
R L   R L

C2
C3
C4
C5
C6
C7
C8
T1
T2
T3
T4
T5
T6
T7
T8
T9
T10
T11
T12
L1
L2
L3
L4
L5
S1
S2
S3
S4-5

| 0 = absent |
| 1 = impaired |
| 2 = normal |
| NT = not testable |

TOTALS

(MAXIMUM) (56) (56)   (56) (56)

☐ + ☐ **PIN PRICK SCORE** (max: 112)
☐ **LIGHT TOUCH SCORE** (max: 112)

☐ Any anal sensation (Yes/No)

* Key sensory points

NEUROLGICAL LEVEL *the most caudal segment with normal function*		R	L	**COMPLETE OR INCOMPLETE** *Incomplete = Any sensory or motor function in S4-S5* **ASIA IMPAIRMENT SCALE**	☐	**ZONE OF PARTIAL PRESERVATION** *Partially innervated segments*		R	L
	SENSORY						SENSORY		
	MOTOR				☐		MOTOR		

This form may be copied freely but should not be altered without permission from the American Spinal Injury Association

Version 4p
GI IC 1990

FIGURE 65.1. ASIA neurologic examination form for spinal cord injury.

Incomplete: Motor function is preserved below the neurologic level, and the majority of key muscles below the neurologic level have a muscle grade of less than 3.

Incomplete: Motor function is preserved below the neurologic level, and the majority of key muscles have a muscle grade of 3 or greater.

Normal: Motor and sensory function is normal.

The following definitions are noted:

Incomplete SCI: if partial preservation of sensory or motor functions is found below the neurologic level, and includes the lowest sacral segment, the injury is defined as incomplete. Sacral sensation also includes deep anal sensation. Voluntary contraction of the anal sphincter muscle is used to demonstrate preserved muscle function.

Complete SCI: this term is used when there is no sensory or motor function in the lowest sacral segment. The neurologic level is given as the lowest level where there is still some evidence of muscle function or sensation but no preservation in the sacral area.

Zone of Partial Preservation: this refers to dermatomes and myotomes below the neurologic level that remain partially innervated. When some impaired sensory or motor function is found below the lowest normal segment, the exact number of segments so affected constitutes the zone of partial preservation. This term is used only with incomplete injuries.

Several clinical patterns seen in spinal injury deserve attention:

Cauda equina lesions
Conus medullaris lesions
Mixed cauda–conus lesions
Brown-Séquard syndrome
    Complete cord transection
    Incomplete cord transection
Central-cord syndrome
Anterior-cord syndrome

Posterior-cord syndrome
Spinal cord injuries
    Spinal-cord concussion
    Spinal shock

Damage to the cauda equina causes flaccid, areflexic paralysis, and sensory loss in the area supplied by the affected roots, with paralysis of bladder and rectum. The findings may be symmetric or asymmetric. The cauda equina syndrome tends to have a better prognosis, possibly because of the higher threshold to injury of the roots. If the conus is damaged, symptoms include urinary and fecal incontinence, failure of erection and ejaculation in men, paralysis of the pelvic floor muscles, and sensory impairment, frequently with sacral sparing. In a pure conus lesion, tendon reflexes are frequently preserved, but occasionally the ankle jerks are lost. A mixture of anatomically appropriate clinical signs is commonly seen because conus and cauda injuries often occur together.

The *Brown-Séquard syndrome* refers to hemisection of the spinal cord and may result from blunt trauma as well as from direct, penetrating injuries. The following signs are found: ipsilateral paresis, ipsilateral corticospinal signs, contralateral loss of pain and temperature sensation, and ipsilateral impairment of vibration and joint-position sense. There is usually little loss of tactile sensation. There may be ipsilateral segmental loss of sensation or weakness appropriate to the level of the lesion. Complete transection of the cord results in permanent motor, sensory, and autonomic paralysis below the level of the lesion. Incomplete transverse section results in different clinical pictures, depending on the pathways involved.

The *central-cord syndrome* is characterized by weakness that is more marked in the arms than the legs, with urinary retention and sensory loss below the level of the lesion. The arms or hands may be paralyzed or moderately weak; in the legs there may be severe paresis or only minimal weakness, overactive tendon reflexes, and Babinski signs. Micturition may be normal. Complete-cord transection may be diagnosed at first because there seems to be no cord function below the level of the lesion. Careful testing, however, may reveal sacral sparing and therefore an incomplete lesion. If so, the potential for recovery without operative intervention is better and depends on the degree of central hemorrhage.

In the *anterior-cord syndrome*, immediate complete paralysis is associated with mild-to-moderate impairment of pinprick response and light touch, below the injury, with preservation of position and vibration sense. This syndrome may be caused by an acutely ruptured disc, with or without fracture or fracture, dislocation in the cervical region impinging on the anterior spinal artery and compromising blood flow to the anterior cervical spine. Recovery from this syndrome is often poor.

The *posterior-cord syndrome* is characterized by pain and paresthesia in the neck, upper arms, and trunk. Paresthesia is usually symmetric and has a burning quality. The sensory manifestations may be combined with mild paresis of the arms and hands, but the long tracts are only slightly affected.

Spinal-cord concussion is the term for transient, neurologic symptoms with recovery in minutes or hours. Symptoms develop below the level of the blow. *Spinal shock* occurs after an abrupt injury of the spinal cord, whether complete or incomplete. There is immediate complete paralysis and anesthesia below the lesion, with hypotonia, areflexia, and potentially life-threatening autonomic disturbances, such as bradycardia or hypotension. Spinal shock is seen in its most severe form in cervical injuries, and stems from the disruption of sympathetic transmission. The plantar responses may be absent, extensor, or equivocal. The areflexic, hypotonic state is gradually replaced by pyramidal signs, usually within 3 or 4 weeks. Stabilization from this state may be delayed by urinary tract and pulmonary infections, skin breakdown, anemia, or malnutrition, or combinations of these conditions.

Clear demarcation between incomplete and complete spinal cord syndromes may be clinically difficult to ascertain at the time of injury. An accurate neurologic examination may not be feasible for hours to days after the injury if the course is complicated by severe shock. The accuracy of acute assessment must take into account the effects of alcohol, drugs, or multiple trauma.

DIAGNOSIS

After clinical neurologic assessment and stabilization, it is essential to obtain accurate and complete imaging of the spinal column soon after the time of injury. This is done to enhance diagnostic accuracy and to rule out unsuspected pathology, a possibility especially in the comatose, incoherent, or uncooperative patient.

Anteroposterior (AP) and lateral plain-film x-rays must be taken at the appropriate level as directed by the clinical evaluation. Lateral xrays of the cervical spine, encompassing the lower cervical region, are mandatory. Open-mouth, odontoid radiographic views should form part of the initial examination. In thoracic and lumbar injuries, AP, lateral, oblique, and extension views may be required.

CT is the best procedure for evaluating uncertain findings seen on plain xrays, as well as for detecting bone pathology. High-resolution CT with sagittal reconstruction enhances radiologic diagnosis to 95% accuracy.

In general, MRI is the best technique for soft-tissue imaging and CT is best for detecting bone pathology. Multiplanar, high-resolution MRI, with T1-weighted and gradient-echo or T2-weighted imaging, is the most specific and sensitive technique for assessing soft-tissue paraspinal lesions, disc herniation, spinal-cord hemorrhage, spinal-cord edema, and intra- or extradural hemorrhage. Monitoring of severely injured patients during MRI procedures, although improved, is still inadequate in many institutions. The ability to monitor the critically injured must be a priority when MRI is considered. If MRI is not available, intrathecally enhanced CT is the current best alternative.

Neurophysiologic assessment of spinal cord function is feasible with the use of sensory- and motor-evoked responses. Mixed nerve-evoked potentials may be useful in determining the integrity of particular spinal-cord pathways, such as the dorsal columns. These procedures are used at times in ICUs, or intraoperatively, for monitoring spinal cord function and identifying spinal-conduction blockade.

COURSE AND PROGNOSIS

Long-term survival depends on the level and extent of the lesion, patient age, and the availability of special treatment units that include multidisciplinary personnel. Co-existing injuries, notably head injuries, increase mortality rates and leave survivors with more disability than SCI, alone. Patients with high cervical injuries are more likely to succumb to their injuries than those injured at lower levels. As might be expected, the mortality rate escalates with higher cervical lesions.

Of those who survive their injuries and acute hospital periods, the leading causes of death are pneumonia, cardiac dysfunction, septicemia, pulmonary emboli, suicide, and accidents. Renal failure was long believed to be a leading cause of death in this group, but that notion has not been borne out by recent data. In younger patients, suicide and accidents become more prevalent.

De Vivo and colleagues (1987) studied the 7-year survival period following SCI. Patients with complete lesions, predictably, did less well than those with incomplete lesions. The cumulative, 7-year survival rate among neurologically complete quadriplegics, who were at least 50 years old when injured, was only 22.7%. The cumulative 7-year survival rate for all groups was 86.7%.

Neurologic recovery is assessed by changes in the ASIA impairment-scale grade and by changes in spinal cord level damage. Knowledge of the site and severity of the injury, and the degree of neurologic dysfunction, are critical in predicting the recovery of function. It is important to differentiate between neurologic recovery and functional recovery.

The role and timing of surgery continue to be controversial issues. Currently, immediate surgery is recommended for release of cord compression and many also be advocated for early intervention of unstable spine injury. Beyond that obvious cord compression, the optimal timing for surgery is not clear. Advocates of early surgery believe that any incomplete cord injury deserves surgical evaluation prior to the onset of cord edema and subsequent worsening. Recovery rates related to operative or nonoperative care indicate no significant differences in neurologic outcome between the two groups. Early surgery seems to be safe, and in specific situations, may lead to earlier rehabilitation. Opponents of early surgery would cite the need for medical stabilization and resolution of edema, prior to any operative procedure.

In summary, neurologic assessment within the first 24 to 48 hours after SCI offers the best method of predicting the eventual outcome. The initial assessment must be done in an alert, cooperative patient, without the presence of alcohol intoxication, drug toxicities, or refractory shock interfering with the assessment. In both complete and incomplete lesions, predictors for return of neurologic function are inconsistent. A sign of serious injury is failure of return of any function within 48 hours of the accident.

TREATMENT

Treatment of the spinal cord-injured patient encompasses five phases: (1) emergency treatment with attention to circulation, respiration, patent airway, appropriate immobilization of the spine, and transfer to a specialized center; (2) treatment of general medical problems (e.g., hypotension, hypoxia, poikilothermy, ileus); (3) spinal alignment; (4) surgical decompression of the spinal cord, if indicated; and (5) a well structured rehabilitation program.

Prehospital management is critical in preventing further complications. Treatment at the site may not change the primary SCI, but it does have a significant effect on preventing secondary damage. Secondary injury of the spinal cord may result from hypotension, hypoxia, lack of immobilization of the spine, poor methods of extrication, inexact monitoring of the patient in transit to hospital, inability to communicate with the physicians at the accepting trauma center during transfer, and failure to recognize severity and mechanism of injury.

Extrication of the patient from an automobile after a crash must be attempted only after the patient's head and back have been immobilized in a neutral position on a firm base. There must be similar concern for head and neck stability in victims of diving accidents. Rapid evacuation to a hospital is essential. It is estimated that 10% of patients suffer progressive cord or nerve-root damage between the time of diagnosis at the site of the accident, and the beginning of appropriate treatment by trained personnel in the hospital.

At the trauma center, the ABCs are reviewed: airway, breathing, and circulation. In addition, D and E have been added, representing "disability" and "exposure." Disability refers to the assessment of neurologic status; exposure refers to the necessity for removal of all clothing to conduct a complete examination.

Clinical signs of shock require the insertion of an arterial infusion line and often, a Swan-Ganz catheter. Meticulous attention must be paid to cardiac output and mean blood pressure to prevent the cardiopulmonary complications that frequently accompany cord injuries.

As cord injury may result in loss of sympathetic tone, with peripheral vasodilation, bradycardia, and hypotension, secondary ischemic damage may aggravate the primary SCI. Treatment of this potential hazard includes judicious administration of intravenous fluids, blood pressure augmentation with vasopressors if hypotension is refractory to fluid administration, and occasionally, intravenous atropine sulfate to counter unopposed parasympathetic activity. Vasomotor paralysis may also cause loss of thermal control and lead to poikilothermy, which usually may be treated by the appropriate use of warming blankets.

In the acute phase (within 8 hours of injury) methylprednisolone therapy is indicated. The National Acute Spinal Cord Injury Study (NASCIS) 2 demonstrated the benefit of high-dose methylprednisolone in reducing the severity of neurologic damage (Bracken and Holford, 1993). Patients are given a bolus of 30 mg/kg over 15 minutes, which is followed by a 5.4-mg/kg infusion over 23 hours. NASCIS 3 further demonstrated that patients who were treated in the period between 3 and 8 hours post injury benefitted from continuing the infusion for 48 hours. The effectiveness of methylprednisolone was confirmed in a Cochrane analysis but there is still some doubt about the benefits of steroid therapy. Methylprednisolone is thought to improve spinal cord function by inhibiting lipid peroxidase.

Other pharmacologic agents being tested include antioxidants and gangliosides (e.g., acidic glycosphingolipids). Preliminary results are promising with the gangliosides. These agents are thought to become part of the lipid bilayer of the plasma membrane and simulate formation of endogenous gangliosides. Benefit was found for both complete and incomplete spinal-cord lesions. Medical complications and mortality rates for these patients were unchanged, however. This treatment must be started within 8 hours of injury.

In the acute phase, intermittent bladder catheterization must be instituted to prevent permanent bladder atony that may result from urinary retention. A nasogastric tube may control abdominal distention, reducing the risks of aspiration and pneumonitis.

With control of systemic functions, attention is directed toward correcting malalignment or instability of the vertebral column. In cervical fracture-dislocation, this is usually done by external skeletal traction (e.g., with Crutchfield tongs, Gardner-Wells tongs, or halo fixation). Cervical traction must be delayed until adequate radiologic studies may be done.

Thoracolumbar injuries do not lend themselves to external traction, and accordingly, surgical stabilization is attempted with devices such as Harrington rods or Weiss springs.

Surgery has little effect on the neurologic outcome of the primary injury. When cord compression is evident, or the neurologic disorder progresses, benefit may follow immediate decompression (i.e., 1 to 2 hours after injury). There are no set rules for determining appropriate selection of early or late surgical intervention. Clinical judgment and physician experience continue to direct the surgical timing in each case.

Patients with SCI need the facilities of a special spinal care unit with staff well versed in neurologic nursing. After the acute treatment phase, specialized and continuing therapy is required. Frequent turning of patients and the use of pillows or pads prevent pressure sores. Antiembolic stockings reduce the incidence of venous thrombosis, and administration of low-dose heparin or other heparinoids reduces the risks of pulmonary embolus. Intermittent catheterization of the bladder has replaced the use of an indwelling catheter and suprapubic cystostomy. Bladder regimens are designed to reduce the stress of detrussor hyperreflexia. An appropriate bowel regimen should be instituted early on, with stool softeners and motility agents if needed. Rehabilitation therapy should be started as soon as possible. Psychosocial support needs to be available to patients and their families from the beginning.

COMPLICATIONS

Dysautonomia

Autonomic dysreflexia is a serious and frequent complication in patients incurring cord injury at the midthoracic level or higher. Dysautonomia may continue for days and weeks after the injury, but usually peaks on the fourth day. Loss of inhibition of higher sympathetic outflow, and abnormal reorganization of preafferent neurons and interneurons, lead to precipitous changes in blood pressure, heart rate, and temperature. Sudden tachycardia and hypertension may be triggered by pain, fecal impaction, and abdominal distension and voiding. Attention to bowel and bladder functions are instrumental in promoting recovery.

Pulmonary Function

Pulmonary complications are a leading cause of morbidity and mortality in patients with SCI, especially in those with cervical lesions. Pulmonary function (i.e., vital capacity and negative inspiratory force) should be monitored closely and often, for several days after injury. For those requiring intubation, early tracheostomy should be considered, regardless of eventual weaning potential. Prevention of atelectasis, aspiration, deep vein thrombosis (DVT), and pulmonary embolism (PE) are paramount. Assessment of adequate ventilation should take place immediately in the field, and continue through the patient's hospitalization. The prevention of DVT and PE begins on admission. Pneumatic compression devices and elastic stockings should be standard orders. Lacking any definite contraindication, enoxaparin or low-dose heparin should also be used. In patients with complete injuries and no hope of recovery, some experts advocate a prophylactic inferior vena-cava filter.

Bladder Function

Restoration of a balanced bladder implies achieving a balance between storage and evacuation of urine. A balanced bladder shows no outlet obstruction, a sterile urine, low residual volume (i.e., less than 100 mL), and low voiding pressures. Failure to attain this requires further urodynamic studies to determine whether the problem is an obstruction (i.e., bladder neck hypertrophy, prostatism, sphincter-detrusor dyssynergia) or a disturbance of storage (i.e., uninhibited bladder contractions, outflow incontinence, decreased outlet resistance). Intermittent catheterization (no-touch technique) is superior to the use of indwelling catheters in reducing complications and developing bladder training. In cases of detrussor hyperreflexia, antispasmodic agents may be used.

Urinary-tract complications are the result of high residual-urine volume and infection. Cystitis and pyelitis respond to antibiotics. Complications occurring months or years after injury include renal and bladder stones, hydronephrosis, pyonephrosis, bladder diverticula, and ureteral reflux. The incidence of these complications has been markedly reduced in the past few decades.

Bowel Training

For several weeks after acute spinal injury, laxatives and digital removal of feces are necessary. Glycerin suppositories are useful at this time. Stretching of the anus (i.e., vagal response) must be avoided. Subsequent training for regular defecation includes the use of laxatives on alternate days, and the judicious use of glycerin suppositories that are inserted approximately 20 minutes before the desired time of evacuation. The goal is to achieve a consistent schedule of bowel evacuation. Safety testing of a novel, selective serotonin-4 receptor agonist with enterokinetic properties is underway.

Pressure Sores

Decubitus ulcers develop in almost all patients with complete cord transection unless preventive measures are vigorously pursued. These ulcers develop wherever bony prominences are covered by skin; the sacrum, trochanters, heels, ischium, knees, and anterosuperior iliac spine are the most common sites. Preventive measures include eliminating pressure points by padding, frequent changing of patient position, and keeping the bed scrupulously clean. Sheepskin, alternating (air) pressure mattresses, gel pads, and waterbeds are also commonly used for prevention. Mechanical aids (e.g., Foster or Stryker frame, or CircOlectric beds) are rarely necessary in well organized and well staffed nursing units.

Once pressure sores have developed, repeated changes of dressings, topical agents, and systemic antibiotics may be used, but these are not always successful. The most effective treatment is repositioning the patient so that pressure is continuously removed and the surface is kept as dry as possible. Conservative therapy may be beneficial, but surgical debridement and early closure are usually required.

Nutritional Deficiency

Attention to general nutrition is paramount in the treatment of patients with SCI. Early weight loss occurs in many patients because of anorexia. In addition, protein may be lost through serous drainage from bedsores. A diet high in protein, calories, and vitamins is advised. If the patient can not eat sufficient quantities by mouth, parenteral hyperalimentation is recommended. Anemia may be treated with iron, and when severe, by blood transfusion.

Muscle Spasms

Flexor or extensor spasms require treatment when they are painful, interfere with rehabilitation, or delay healing of bedsores. The aims are reduction in the number of painful and disabling flexor spasms and a decrease in muscle tone when it interferes with function, nursing care, or rehabilitation. The most useful drugs are dantrolene sodium, diazepam, and baclofen. Intrathecal administration of baclofen has become increasingly popular. It is most effective in relieving flexor spasms, may relieve other adverse effects of spasticity and hypertonia, and may be given safely with appropriate precautions. Neurosurgical implantation of an intrathecal baclofen pump is an option in severe cases. Physical therapy, including stretching and passive range-of-movement should be instituted early. Botox injection may be helpful, especially if contractures develop. For refractory cases, surgical options must be explored, including percutaneous radiofrequency rhizotomy of the lower lumbar and upper sacral roots.

Sexual Function

Several forms of treatment are available for neurogenic erectile dysfunction. These include a vacuum device that fits over the penis and is kept in place by a constricting ring around the base of the penis; injection of vasoactive agents such as phentolamine mesylate, papaverine, or prostaglandin E_1 into the corpora cavernosa; and use of an implantable prosthesis. Sildenafil has been reported to be useful in erectile dysfunction secondary to traumatic spinal-cord disease. Sexual function among women after TSCI has been little investigated. About 50% of patients fail to achieve orgasms or may note decreased libido. Sildenafil, ephedrine, phentolamine, arginine, and apomorphine are potential therapeutic options for women yet to be investigated.

Pain

Pain may affect anesthetic areas after complete lesions. There may be sharp shooting pains in the distribution of one or more roots; burning pain may be poorly localized; or deep pain may be localized in the viscera. Pain should be treated effectively to avoid reflex dysautonomia. Treatment includes repositioning, nonsteroidal analgesia, and occasionally narcotics. Gabapentin is increasingly used in these patients. All analgesics, but particularly narcotics, should be used cautiously. Spinal anesthesia, posterior rhizotomy, sympathectomy, cordotomy, and posterior-column tractotomy have all been performed. None has been uniformly successful. Transcutaneous electrical neurostimulation (TENS) is reported to be effective.

Rehabilitation

The ultimate aim for all patients with SCI is recovery of maximal independence or ambulation. This has increasingly become an achievable goal and may be accomplished in many patients who have injuries below the cervical area. It is best done in a rehabilitation center with trained personnel and adequate equipment. Such facilities are studying the use of functional electrical stimulation to augment partial weight-bearing, supported-treadmill training in patients with incomplete SCI, with promising initial results. When the arms are paralyzed, the therapeutic goal is more limited, but devices controlled by intact muscles and appropriate surgery may permit useful motion of paralyzed arms. Implantation of diaphragmatic stimulators has permitted survival of high-cervical cord injured patients.

The development of spinal-cord care units specializing in the care of tetraplegia and paraplegia is important. An increase in life expectancy, reduction in the frequency of complications, and development of new techniques that allow greater patient autonomy and improve quality of life are areas of focus.

New hope has been stimulated by stem-cell research and SCI is a major focus. Although it is still embroiled in political controversy, the potential for recovery and repair of damaged neural tissue leading to functional improvement of these devastating injuries may not be denied. Current research is still mainly in the laboratory, but in the era of molecular biology, clinical trials may not be so remote an eventuality.

Finally, the best treatment must be prevention. Nationwide educational programs should be concerned with causes of SCI: motor vehicle safety, water and occupational safety, eliminating drunk driving, adhering to speed limits, and mandatory use of seatbelts and other protective gear.

SUGGESTED READINGS

Baskin DS. Spinal cord injury. In: Evans RW, ed. *Neurology and Trauma.* Philadelphia: WB Saunders, 1996:276–299.

Blackmer J. Rehabilitation medicine: 1. Autonomic dysreflexia. *CMAJ* 2003;169(9):931–935.

Bracken MB. Steroids for acute spinal cord injury. *Cochrane Database of Systematic Reviews* 2002(3):CD001046.

Bracken MB, Holford TR. Effects of timing of methylprednisolone or naloxone administration on recovery of segmental and long-tract neurological function in NASCIS 2. *J Neurosurg* 1993;79:500–507.

Bracken MB, Shepard MJ, Holford TR, et al. Administration of methylprednisolone for 24 or 48 hours or tirilazad mesylate for 48 hours in the treatment of acute spinal cord injury: results of the Third National Acute Spinal Cord Injury Randomized Controlled Trial. National Acute Spinal Cord Injury Study. *JAMA* 1997;277:1597–1604.

Burney RE, Maio RF, Maynard F, Karunas R. Incidence, characteristics, and outcome of spinal cord injury at trauma centers in North America. *Arch Surg* 1993;128:596–599.

Derry F. Sildenafil (Viagra): a double-blind, placebo controlled, single-dose, two-way crossover study in men with erectile dysfunction caused by traumatic spinal cord injury. *J Urol* 1997;157(suppl): 181(abstr 702).

De Vivo MJ, Kartus PL, Stover SL, Rutt RD, Fine PR. Seven-year survival following spinal cord injury. *Arch Neurol* 1987;44:872–875.

Donovan WH. Rehabilitation treatment of complications of spinal cord injury. In: Evans RW, ed. *Neurology and Trauma.* Philadelphia: 1996: 300–322.

Duh MS, Shephard MJ, Wilberger JE, Bracken MB. The effectiveness of surgery on the treatment of acute spinal cord injury and its relation to pharmacological treatment. *Neurosurgery* 1994;35:240–248; discussion 248–249.

Formal CS, Ditunno JF Jr. Rehabilitation of patients with traumatic spinal cord injury. In: Frymoyer JW, Ducker TB, Hadler NM, et al., eds. *The Adult Spine: Principles and Practice,* 2nd ed. Philadelphia: Lippincott–Raven Publishers, 1997;1:931–947.

Geisler FH, Coleman WP, Grieco G, et al. The Sygen multicenter acute spinal cord injury study. *Spine* 2001;26(suppl):S87–S98.

George ER, Scholten DJ, Buechler CM, et al. Failure of methylprednisolone to improve outcome of spinal cord injuries. *Am Surg* 1995;61: 659–663; discussion 663–664.

Guest J, Eleraky MA, Apostolides PJ, Dickman CA, Sonntag VK. Traumatic central cord syndrome: results of surgical management. *J Neurosurg* 2002;97(1):25–32.

Kakulas BA, Taylor JR. Pathology of injuries of vertebral column and spinal cord. *Spinal Cord Trauma. Handbook of Clinical Neurology, vol 61.* Amsterdam: Elsevier, 1992:21–51.

Korenkov AI, Niendorf WR, Darwish N, Glaeser E, Gaab MR. Continuous intrathecal infusion of baclofen in patients with spasticity caused by spinal cord injuries. *Neurosurg Rev* 2002;25:228–230.

Krough K, Jensen MB, Gandrup P, et al. Efficacy and tolerability of prucalopride in patients with constipation due to spinal cord injury. *Scand J Gastroenterol* 2002;37:431–436.

Lee TT, Arias JM, Andrus HL, et al. Progressive post-traumatic myelomalacic myelopathy: treatment with untethering and expansive duraplasty. *J Neurosurg* 1997;86:624–628.

Levendoglu F, Ogun CO, Ozerbil O, Ogun TC, Ugurlu H. Gabapentin is a first line drug for the treatment of neuropathic pain in spinal cord injury. *Spine* 2004;29:743–751.

Lewis KS, Mueller WM. Intrathecal baclofen for severe spasticity secondary to spinal cord injury. *Ann Pharmacother* 1993;27:767–774.

Madersbacher HG. Neurogenic bladder dysfunction. *Curr Opin Urol* 1999;9:303–307.

Maynard FM Jr, Bracken MB, Creasey G, et al. International standards for neurological and functional classification of spinal cord injury. American Spinal Injury Association. *Spinal Cord* 1997;35:266–274.

McDonald JW, Becker D, Holekamp TF, et al. Repair of the injured spinal cord and the potential of embryonic stem cell transplantation. *J Neurotrauma* 2004;21(4):383–393.

Postans NJ, Hasler JP, Granat MH, Maxwell DJ. Functional electric stimulation to augment partial weight-bearing supported treadmill training for patients with incomplete spinal cord injury: a pilot study. *Arch Phys Med Rehabil* 2004;85:604–610.

Profyius C, Cheema SS, Zang D, et al. Degenerative and regenerative mechanisms governing spinal cord injury. *Neurobiol Dis* 2004;15:415–436.

Sekhon LHS, Fehings MG. Epidemiology, demographics, and pathophysiology of acute spinal cord injury. *Spine* 2001;26(24):2–12.

Sipski ML. Central nervous system based neurogenic female sexual dysfunction: current status and future trends. *Arch Sex Behav* 2002;31:421–424.

Smith EM, Bodner DR. Sexual dysfunction after spinal cord injury. *Urol Clin North Am* 1993;20:535–542.

Sonntag VKH, Francis PM. *Patient Selection and Timing of Surgery in Contemporary Management of Spinal Cord Injury.* Park Ridge, IL: AANS Publication Committee, 1995:97–107.

Spinalith Cord Injury Thromboprophylaxis Investigators. Prevention of venous thromboembolism in the rehabilitation phase after spinal cord injury: prophylaxis with low-dose heparin or enoxaparin. *J Trauma* 2003;54(6):1111–1115.

Stringer WA, Andersen BJ. Imaging after spine trauma. In: Evans RW, ed. *Neurology and trauma.* Philadelphia: WB Saunders, 1996;251–275.

Winslow C., Rozovsky J. Effect of spinal cord injury on the respiratory system. *Am J Phys Med & Rehab* 2003;82(10):803–814.

Chapter 66

Intervertebral Discs and Radiculopathy

Paul C. McCormick

Rupture of an intervertebral disc into the body of a vertebra was first described by Schmorl in 1927. Earlier, in a 1909 text on neurologic surgery, Krause described operating on an iceman who had been diagnosed by Oppenheimer as suffering from a lesion localized to L-4. Krause found an extradural mass that was described, pathologically, as a chondroma; the operation apparently effected a cure. There were other reports of chondromas removed at explorations of the intervertebral area. It remained for Mixter and Barr in 1934 to point out that these lesions were actually fragments of intervertebral discs and that they were responsible for sciatica.

PATHOGENESIS

Displaced disc material may create signs and symptoms by bulging or protruding beneath an attenuated annulus fibrosus, or the material may extrude through a tear in the annulus and project directly into the spinal canal. In either case, the encroaching disc material may irritate or compress nerve roots that are coursing to foramina of exit. In the cervical or thoracic regions, the problem is more complex, neurologically, because the spinal cord itself, as well as the adjacent nerve roots, may be involved. There, signs and symptoms are either caused by cord compression or a combination of cord and root compression. In the lumbar region, signs and symptoms relate to an individual root lesion (i.e., compressed laterally) or to compression of the cauda equina if the disc is large enough to crowd the entire spinal canal.

In the cervical region, the levels most commonly affected are in the C-5 to C-7 segments (Table 66.1). In the lumbar area, most disc protrusions occur at L4-5 and L5-S1. This pattern suggests that the dynamics of pathologic change are partly related to the trauma of motion, wear, and tear. Thoracic disc protrusion, except at the lower thoracic levels, differs from cervical and lumbar disorders in genesis and histopathology. Motion plays no role there because the thoracic vertebrae are designed for stability rather than motion, and the heavy rib cage contributes to the rigidity of this structure. One must therefore look elsewhere for the cause of thoracic disc rupture. On gross and microscopic examination: the lesion is unique, markedly degenerated, and characterized by gritty calcified deposits; it almost never has the consistency of cervical and lumbar ruptured discs; and thoracic disc protrusion is more granular and yellowish.

Although trauma has been accepted as the prime cause of disc herniation, it is not the only cause. There seems to be a genetic predisposition, too. Trauma may aggravate this susceptibility and ultimately cause rupture. In the most florid, preordained syndrome, there may be multiple levels of severe disc degeneration throughout the spine, with progressive clinical involvement in different areas. That syndrome may explain why fusion often fails to prevent recurrent symptoms.

Spinal stenosis, which is an abnormally narrow spinal canal, is an example of an inherited anomaly, as are the spinal abnormalities of achondroplastic dwarfism. These abnormal spinal configurations, along with spondylosis, are major contributors to compression syndromes of the spinal cord and cauda equina. When disc protrusion occurs in a patient with spinal stenosis, it further compromises an already limited canal, as do changes

▶ **TABLE 66.1 Common Root Syndromes of Intervertebral Disc Disease**

Disc space	L3-4	L4-5	L5-S1	C4-5	C5-6	C6-7	C7-T1
Root affected	L-4	L-5	S-1	C-5	C-6	C-7	C-8
Muscles affected	Quadriceps	Peroneals, anterior tibial, extensor hallucis longus	Gluteus maximus, gastrocnemius, plantar flexors of toes	Deltoid, biceps		Triceps, wrist extensors	Intrinsic hand muscles
Area of pain and sensory loss	Anterior thigh, medial shin	Great toe, dorsum of foot	Lateral foot, small toe	Shoulder, anterior arm, radial forearm		Thumb, middle fingers	Index, fourth fifth finger
Reflex affected	Knee jerk	Posterior tibial	Ankle jerk	Biceps		Triceps	Triceps
Straight leg raising	Many not increase pain	Aggravates root pain	Aggravates root pain	—	—	—	

caused by arthritic proliferation or ligamentous degeneration.

The signs and symptoms of herniated discs relate not only to the size and strategic location of the disc fragments, but also to the size and configuration of the canal. The anteroposterior and lateral dimensions of the canal, particularly the foramina, play key roles. Spinal stenosis and osteoarthritic changes may compress roots, even with small protrusions. In a canal of normal dimensions, the severity of compression depends more on the site of rupture and the volume of the extruded material. There may be single-root compression or cauda equina compression. A laterally placed lesion in the cervical region may involve a single root, but if it is large enough, it may compress the cord. This is also true in the thoracic region. Although single-root syndromes in the lumbar region are usual, truly ventral or large lesions may lead to less easily recognized clinical pictures. For instance, scoliosis may be the major feature, with severe back pain and muscle splinting, but without signs of mechanical root compression in the straight leg-raising test.

INCIDENCE

Rupture of an intervertebral disc is common, especially in the fourth to sixth decades of life. It is rare before age 25 years and uncommon after age 60 years. About 80% of patients are men. Many patients have had earlier trauma.

LUMBAR INTERVERTEBRAL DISC RUPTURE

Signs and Symptoms

Root syndromes of intervertebral disc disease are often episodic, so remissions are characteristic. Pain may be aggravated by Valsalva maneuvers (e.g., coughing, sneezing, or straining at defecation). The pain may be restricted to the back or follow a radicular distribution in one or both legs. Lumbar pain may increase after heavy lifting or twisting of the spine. No matter how severe the pain is when the patient is erect, characteristically it is promptly relieved when the patient lies down. Some patients, however, are more comfortable sitting, and some may find no comfortable position. Relief of pain on bedrest is useful in diagnosing disc disease from intraspinal tumor, in which pain is often not relieved or may be worsened.

Examination reveals loss of lumbar lordosis or flattening of the lumbar spine, with splinting and asymmetric prominence of the long erector muscles. A list or tilt may be present, with one iliac crest elevated. This asymmetry is responsible for the commonly diagnosed longer-leg-on-one-side and the erroneous assignment of the back pain to asymmetry of leg length. This asymmetry often causes a patient to raise the heel on the shoe of what appears to be the short leg, to level the pelvis.

Range of motion of the lumbar spine is reduced by the protective splinting of paraspinal muscles, and attempted movement in some planes induces severe back pain. There may be tenderness of the adjacent vertebrae. When the patient is erect, one gluteal fold may hang down and show added skin creases because the gluteus is wasted, evidence of involvement of the S-1 root. Passive straight leg raising is reduced in range and increases back and leg pain. Muscle atrophy and weakness or sciatic tenderness and discomfort may occur on direct pressure at some point along the nerve from the sciatic notch to the calf. This is particularly true in older patients. Paresthesia in the realm of the involved root is common; fasciculation is rare.

The typical syndromes of root compression at lumbar levels are given in Table 66.2, although the signs may not be as distinct in actual practice as the table implies. More than 80% of syndromes affect L-5 or S-1 (Figs. 66.1 and 66.2). When the lesion affects L-4 or higher roots, straight-leg raising does not stretch the roots above L-5. The affected roots may be tensed, however, by extension of the limb with the knee flexed when the patient is prone, thus reproducing the typical radicular spread of pain.

▶ **TABLE 66.2   Signs of Lumbar Disc Herniation in 97 Patients**

Disc Space	L2-3	L3-4	L4-5	L5-S1
Patients (n)	1	9	45	42
Weak muscles				
Anterior tibial, extensor hallucis	0	3	13	3
Gastrocnemius, plantar responses of foot	0	0	2	3
Quadriceps	0	3	0	0
Reflex affected				
Knee jerk	1	6	4	0
Ankle jerk	0	1	12	23

Data from Hardy RW Jr, Plank NM. Clinical diagnosis of herniated lumbar disc. In: Hardy RW, ed. *Lumbar disc disease*. New York: Raven Press, 1982.

Diagnosis

About 10% of lumbar disc herniations occur lateral to the spinal canal and root sleeve. Myelography is unrevealing in these cases. These far lateral disc herniations compress the rostral lumbar nerve root at the affected level. A far lateral L3-4 lumbar disc herniation, for example, may compress the L-3 nerve root either within the foramen or more distally as the root passes over the disc space (Fig. 66.3).

These herniations often affect higher lumbar (e.g., L3-4) levels and are likely to cause objective neurologic deficit. A far lateral disc herniation should be suspected with acute onset of an isolated upper lumbar radiculopathy, one that affects L-2, L-3, or L-4. Diagnosis of far lateral lumbar disc herniation is made by CT or MRI.

THORACIC INTERVERTEBRAL DISC RUPTURE

Because the thoracic spine is designed for rigidity rather than excursion, wear and tear from motion and stress may not cause thoracic disc protrusion, and clinical disorders are rare. Thoracic disc disease may result from chronic vertebral changes incident to Scheuermann disease or juvenile osteochondritis with later trauma. The radiographic changes of Scheuermann disease, when seen with thoracic cord compression, should raise the possibility of disc protrusion (Fig. 66.4). Calcific changes in the intervertebral disc and the typical vertebral changes of that disease are diagnostic markers.

The small capacity of the thoracic canal makes clinical syndromes of cord compression more critical than at other levels. By the same token, decompressive operations are more precarious and require meticulous care to avoid damaging the spinal cord. The lower thoracic levels, however, are more capacious, and although the conus medullaris or cauda equina may be damaged by disc pro-

trusions, surgical approaches are less hazardous than at higher levels.

CERVICAL DISC DISEASE

Cervical disc herniation may involve both the root and the spinal cord, depending on the volume of the canal and the size of the lesion. Cord compression is uncommon, except with spinal stenosis or massive rupture of a disc. The sites of the most frequent disc herniations are C5-6 (Fig. 66.5) and C6-7; C4-5 and C7-T1 are less frequently affected, and other levels are rarely involved (Table 66.3).

Because movement of the cervical spine is normally incremental, any process contributing to focal stress at individual levels adds to local wear and tear, to progressive pathologic changes in the disc, and to deficits in joint mechanics. Development of a new fulcrum of motion above a fusion or congenital block vertebrae increases susceptibility to these changes.

Signs and Symptoms

The signs and symptoms of cervical disc disease usually begin with stiff neck, reactive splinting of the erector capital muscles, and discomfort at the medial order of the scapula. Radicular paresthesia and pain supervene when the root is more severely compromised. These symptoms are worsened by movements of the head and neck and often, also by stretching of the dependent arm. For relief, the patient often adopts a position with the arm elevated and flexed behind the head, unlike the patient with shoulder disease who maintains the arm in a dependent position, avoiding elevation or abduction at the shoulder joint.

As compression proceeds, discrete root syndromes appear (Tables 66.1 and 66.2). C-5 lesions cause pain in the shoulder and dermatomic sensory diminution with weakness and atrophy of the deltoid. C-6 lesions cause paresthesia of the thumb and depression of the biceps reflex with weakness and atrophy of that muscle. In C-7 lesions, paresthesia may involve the index and middle fingers, and even the thumb, with atrophy and weakness in the triceps muscles, wrist extensors, and pectoral muscles, as well as a parallel reflex depression. C-8 subserves important intrinsic muscle functions in the hand and sensation in the fourth and fifth fingers. Because these are important in discriminatory and fine-finger maneuvers, C-8 damage may be disabling. Large disc protrusions, particularly with spinal stenosis, may cause clinical syndromes of cord compression.

Diagnosis

Lesions such as supraspinatus tendinitis, arthritic changes in the acromioclavicular joint, and rotator cuff tears may be difficult to differentiate from cervical root compression,

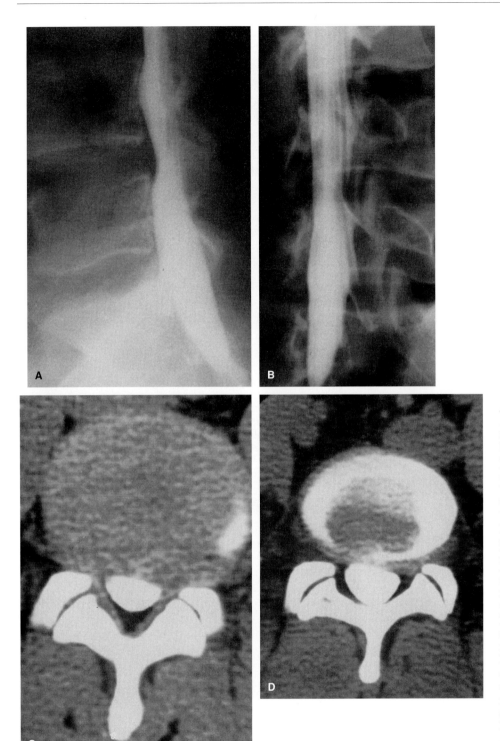

FIGURE 66.1. Lumbar disc herniation. A: Lateral film from a lumbar myelogram demonstrates a large ventral defect at L4-5. The L5-S1 level is unremarkable. **B:** Left posterior oblique projection demonstrates swelling and amputation of the left L-5 root and possible compression of the left S-1 root with subtle thinning of the contrast. **C:** Post myelogram axial CT at the L4-5 level confirms a large herniated nucleus pulposus obliterating the neural foramina bilaterally with eccentric deformity of the sac on the left. **D:** At the L5-S1 level, CT is more sensitive than myelography in diagnosing lateral disc herniation into the left foramen. Compare its appearance with that of the preserved lucent fat in the right foramen. Minimal deformity of the sac ventrally accounts for the unimpressive myelogram at this level. (Courtesy of Dr. J. A. Bello, Dr. T. L. Chi, and Dr. S. K. Hilal.)

especially because prolonged pain and lack of range of motion lead to atrophy and frozen shoulder in these syndromes. C-8 and T1 lesions commonly cause a partial Horner syndrome. A diagnostic workup for syndromes of these levels must include apical lordotic views of the chest, and special care must be taken to rule out sulcus neoplasms or abnormal cervical ribs.

OTHER DIAGNOSTIC FEATURES

Because many disc syndromes are genetic, abnormal skeletal features throughout the spine should be sought on radiographs. These include spinal stenosis, spondylolisthesis, widespread disc disease, or Marfan syndrome. Acquired disorders, such as osteochondritis juvenilis, and

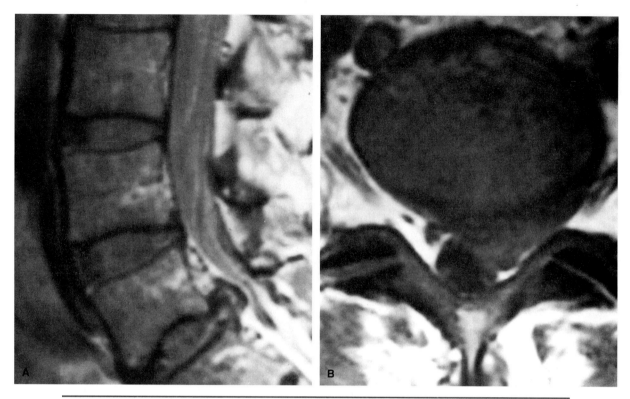

FIGURE 66.2. Lumbosacral disc herniation. Sagittal proton-density **(A)** and axial T1-weighted **(B)** MRI demonstrate a large L5-S1 disc herniation on the left side. Clinically, this patient had an S-1 radiculopathy that did not respond to conservative therapy. Complete relief of symptoms followed lumbar discectomy.

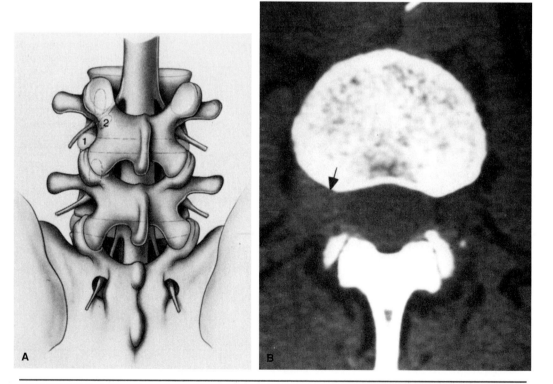

FIGURE 66.3. A: Two sites of possible upper nerve root compression from a far lateral disc herniation. Root compression may occur at the level of the disc space (1) or from a rostrally migrated fragment into the foramen of the upper nerve root (2). **B:** CT demonstrates a large far lateral disc herniation (arrow).

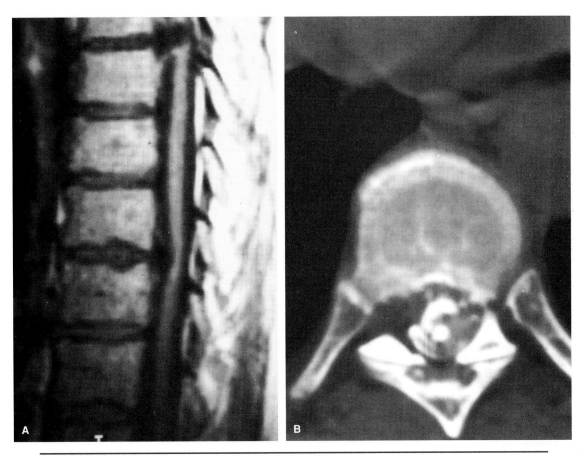

FIGURE 66.4. **A:** Sagittal T1-weighted MRI demonstrates two large thoracic discs in a patient with a subacute myelopathy. **B:** Post myelographic CT in the same patient demonstrates a large calcified thoracic disc at T-6 compressing the spinal cord.

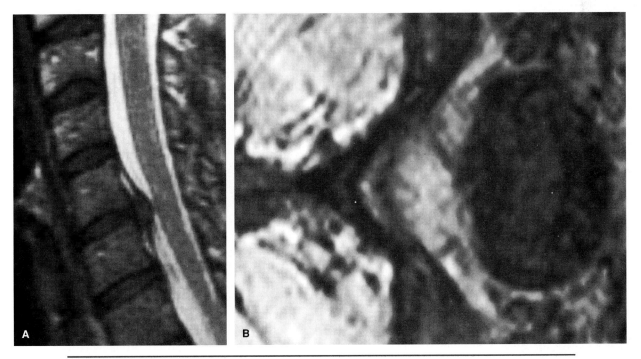

FIGURE 66.5. **A:** Sagittal T2-weighted MRI shows C5-6 disc herniation. **B:** Axial MRI demonstrates foraminal disc herniation in a patient with radiculopathy.

▶ **TABLE 66.3** **Frequency of Compression of the Cervical Roots by Ruptured Intervertebral Disc**

Root	%
C-5	2
C-6	19
C-7	69
C-8	10

Modified from Yoss et al., 1957.

metabolic states such as osteoporosis, may contribute to pathologic changes in the disc and adjacent joints, as do several forms of arthritis.

Imaging

MRI is the imaging procedure of choice for disc disorders. MRI identifies spinal cord or root compression and also shows the degree of degenerative change within the disc. It clearly delineates both intra- and extradural structures and is the ideal screening procedure for the differential diagnosis of structural disorders affecting the spinal cord and nerve roots.

Myelography has largely been replaced by MRI in the evaluation of disc disease. However, myelography does allow scrutiny of the entire spinal canal and may identify dynamic changes of spinal-canal size that may occur with standing and flexion or extension of the spine. Post-myelography CT is useful as an adjunct to MRI if equivocal or multilevel disc disease is present; it is particularly useful in evaluating foraminal-nerve root compression.

Electromyography and evoked-potentials studies may be helpful in localizing root involvement but are not essential. The CSF level is only rarely higher than 100 mg/dL; higher values are more characteristic of tumors.

Disc syndromes may be duplicated by tumors (e.g., primary or metastatic), infections (e.g., epidural abscess), and arachnoiditis. Epidural lipomatosis, a rare cause of low-back syndromes, is a complication of steroid therapy.

TREATMENT

Most acute attacks of back pain improve in days or weeks. In one meta-analysis, 82% of patients with acute low-back pain returned to work within a month of onset. Many patients may have difficulty standing because attempts to do so increase the pain; for them, bed rest comes naturally and conservative treatment continues so long as the patient improves, with analgesics and bedrest for lumbar-

disc disorders, and immobilization of the neck by a collar for cervical-disc disorders. Surgery for a lumbar-disc disorder is indicated when there is no improvement over a reasonable period of strict bedrest or when a severe neurologic disorder is found on examination. Some clinicians use epidural steroid injections, which presumably decrease edematous swelling and thereby relieve pressure on the affected nerve root.

Discectomy of a herniated lumbar-disc fragment almost always results in long-term, satisfactory relief of symptoms. Lumbar fusion is rarely required for treatment of radiculopathy from a herniated lumbar disc. Microsurgery has shortened recovery time and is as effective as open surgery, according to randomized trials.

Excessively prolonged physiotherapy and bedrest may cause emotional exhaustion, muscle loss, or drug dependence. Chemonucleosis, or injections of chymopapain or collagenase to digest the disc material, has been controversial.

Cord compression requires consideration of decompressive measures as soon as it is recognized. Root syndromes of the cervical spine may be separated into those that require careful supervision and early operation, and those that tolerate and may respond to conservative care. The muscles served by C-5 may rapidly atrophy, leaving abduction paresis, poor prognosis for restoration of function, and a painful frozen shoulder. C-8 is also vulnerable, and unrelieved compression may lead to irreversible atrophy with complex shoulder-arm-hand disorders that include circulatory and sweating abnormalities.

C-6 and C-7 subserve large muscles and tolerate pressure more benignly, even for long periods, and may have good functional return. Cervical-root syndromes are less likely to recur than lumbar disorders, and conservative therapy is worthwhile within the outlines described.

Removal of a cervical herniated disc may be performed either through a posterior laminotomy or an anterior approach. Excellent results may be anticipated in appropriately selected patients. Success in disc surgery also includes adequate evaluation of psychologic patterns and motivation.

CHRONIC LOW-BACK PAIN

In the United States back pain is the most common reason for limiting physical activity in people younger than age 45 years; it is the second-most frequent cause of visits to a physician, the fifth cause of hospital admissions, and the third leading cause of surgery. In many countries it is the most common cause of absenteeism from work, accounting for more than 12% of sick days. The economic costs in the Netherlands were probably typical, coming to 1.7% of the gross national product.

According to Andersson,

"chronic low back pain has become a diagnosis of convenience for many people who are actually disabled for socioeconomic, work-related, or psychological reasons."

The complexity of the problem is measured in a huge literature and a long list of approaches to therapy. Medications and other therapies include: nonsteroidal antiinflammatory drugs, opiates, and antidepressants; extradural injection of steroids; decompressive surgery; physical therapy, including massage and exercise; chiropractic treatment; and acupuncture. In Finland, a third of the direct costs were spent on complementary therapies. Multidisciplinary spine centers and pain centers may be sources of the most effective approach to management.

SUGGESTED READINGS

Andersson GBJ. Epidemiological features of chronic low back pain. *Lancet* 1999;354:581–585.

Atlas SJ, Nardin RA. Evaluation and treatment of low back pain: an evidence-based approach to clinical care. *Muscle & Nerve* 2003;27(3):265–284.

Awwad EE, Martin DS, Smith KR Jr, Baker BK. Asymptomatic versus symptomatic herniated thoracic discs: frequency and characteristics as detected by computed tomography after myelography. *Neurosurgery* 1991;28:180–186.

Borre DG, Borre GE, Aude F, Palmieri GN. Lumbosacral epidural lipomatosis: MRI grading. *Europ Radiology* 2003;13(7):1709–1721.

Butterman GR. Treatment of lumbar disc herniation: epidural steroid injection compared with diskectomy. A prospective, randomized study. *J Bone Joint Surg* 2004;86A(4):670–679.

Charlesworth CH, Savy LE, Stevens J, et al. MRI demonstration of arachnoiditis in cauda equina syndrome of ankylosing spondylitis. *Neuroradiology* 1996;38:462–465.

Conforti R, Scuotto A, Muras I, et al. Herniated disk in adolescents. *J Neuroradiol* 1993;20:60–69.

Deyo RA. Low back pain. *N Engl J Med* 2001;344:363–370.

Deyo RA, Cherkin DC, Loeser JD, et al. Morbidity and mortality in association with operations on the lumbar spine. *J Bone Joint Surg Am* 1992;74:536–543.

Deyo RA, Nachemson A, Kirza SK. Spinal-fusion surgery–the case for restraint. *N Engl J Med* 2004;350:722–726.

Esses SI, Morley TP. Spinal arachnoiditis. *Can J Neurol Sci* 1983;10:2–10.

Fessler RG, Johnson DL, Brown FD, et al. Epidural lipomatosis in steroid-treated patients. *Spine* 1992;17:183–188.

Fiirgaard B, Marsden FH. Spinal epidural lipomatosis: case report and review of the literature. *Scand J Med Sci Sports* 1997;7:354–357.

Frost H, Lamb SE, Doll HA, Carver PT, Stewart-Brown S. Randomised controlled trial of physiotherapy compared with adivce for low back pain. *BMJ* 2004 Sep; 25;329 (7468):708. Epub 2004 Sep 17.

Haggman S, Maher CG, Refshauge KM. Screening for symptoms of depression by physical therapists managing low back pain. *Phys Ther* 2004; Dec;84(12):1157–1166.

Hansen FR, Bendix T, Skov P, et al. Intensive, dynamic back muscle exercises, conventional physiotherapy, or placebo-control treatment of low back pain: a randomized, observer-blind trial. *Spine* 1993;18:98–108.

Hemmila HM. Quality of life and cost of care of back pain patients in Finnish general practice. *Spine* 2002;27(6):647–653.

Hutubessy RC, Van Tulder MW, Vondeling H, Bouter LM. Indirect costs of back pain in the Netherlands; a comparison of the human capital method with the friction cost method. *Pain* 1999;80 (1–2):201–207.

Koenigsberg RA, Klahr J, Zito JL, et al. Magnetic resonance imaging of cauda equina syndrome in ankylosing spondylitis: a case report. *J Neuroimaging* 1995;5:46–48.

Maroon JC, Kupitnik TA, Schulhuf LA. Diagnosis and microsurgical approach to far lateral disc herniations in the lumbar spine. *J Neurosurg* 1990;72:378–382.

Martin DS, Awwad EE, Pittman T, et al. Current imaging concepts of thoracic intervertebral disks. *Crit Rev Diagn Imaging* 1992;33:109–181.

Mixter WJ, Barr JS. Rupture of the intervertebral disc with involvement of the spinal canal. *N Engl J Med* 1934;211:210.

Mohanty S, Sutter B, Mokry M, Ascher PW. Herniation of calcified cervical intervertebral disk in children. *Surg Neurol* 1992;38:407–410.

Noel P, Pepersack T, Vanbinst A, Alle JL. Spinal epidural lipomatosis in Cushing's syndrome secondary to an adrenal tumor. *Neurology* 1992;42:1250–1251.

Onel D, Sari H, Donmez C. Lumbar spinal stenosis: clinical/radiologic therapeutic evaluation in 145 patients: conservative treatment or surgical intervention? *Spine* 1993;18:291–298.

Pengel LHM, Herbert RD, Maher CG, Refshauge KM. Acute low back pain: systematic review of its prognosis. *BMJ* 2003;327:323–328.

Pyeritz RE, Sack GH Jr, Udvarhelyi GB. Thoracolumbosacral laminectomy in achondroplasia: long-term results in 22 patients. *Am J Med Genet* 1987;28:433–444.

Robertson SC, Traynelis VC, Follett KA, et al. Idiopathic spinal epidural lipomatosis. *Neurosurgery* 1997;41:68–74.

Shapiro S. Cauda equina syndrome secondary to lumbar disc herniation. *Neurosurgery* 1993;332:743–747.

Shaw MDM, Russell JA, Grossart KW. Changing pattern of spinal arachnoiditis. *J Neurol Neurosurg Psychiatry* 1978;41:97–107.

Turner JA, Ersek M, Hernon L, et al. Patient outcomes after lumbar spinal fusions. *JAMA* 1992;268:907–911.

Yoss RE, Corbin KB, MacCarty CS, Love JG. Significance of symptoms and signs in localization of involved root in cervical disc protrusion. *Neurology* 1957;7:673–683.

Chapter 67

Cervical Spondylotic Myelopathy

Lewis P. Rowland and Paul C. McCormick

Cervical spondylosis is a condition in which progressive degeneration of the intervertebral discs leads to proliferative changes in surrounding structures, especially in the bones, meninges, and supporting tissues of the spine. Damage to the spinal cord may be demonstrated at autopsy.

The myelopathy is attributed to one or more of three possible mechanisms: (1) direct compression of the spinal cord by bony or fibrocalcific tissues, (2) ischemia caused by compromise of the vascular supply to the cord, and (3) repeated trauma in the course of normal flexion and extension of the neck. It is difficult, however, to be precise in identifying this type of myelopathy in living patients. The very concept may be one of the persistent myths of clinical neurology, and the situation begs for critical review.

INCIDENCE

Radiographic evidence of cervical spondylosis increases with each decade of life. It is seen in 5% to 10% of people between 20 and 30 years of age, increases to more than 50% by age 45 years, and to more than 90% after age 60 years. Signs of cervical myelopathy of unknown cause appear in only a few patients. Those with myelopathy do not usually have a history of repeated single-root syndromes; that is, radiculopathy caused by cervical disc herniation and myelopathy seem to be distinct syndromes affecting different populations.

PATHOLOGY

The water content of the intervertebral disc and annulus fibrosus declines progressively with advancing age. Concomitantly, there are degenerative changes in the disc. The intervertebral space narrows and may be obliterated, and the annulus fibrosus protrudes into the spinal canal. Osteophytes form at the margins of the vertebral body, converge on the protruded annulus, and may convert it into a bony ridge or bar. The bar may extend laterally into the intervertebral foramen; there is also fibrosis of the dural sleeves of the nerve roots. All these changes narrow the canal, a process that may be aggravated by fibrosis and hypertrophy of the ligamenta flava. The likelihood of cord compression or vascular compromise increases in direct relation to the decrease in the original diameter of the spinal canal.

Spondylotic bars may leave deep indentations (e.g., visible at autopsy) on the ventral surface of the spinal cord. At what may be several levels of lesions, there is degeneration of the gray matter, sometimes with necrosis and cavitation. Above the compression, there is degeneration of the posterior columns; below the compression, corticospinal tracts are demyelinated.

Dense ossification of the posterior longitudinal ligament is a variant of cervical spondylosis that may also cause progressive myelopathy. The condition may be fo-

cal or diffuse and seems to be most common in people of Asian heritage.

One theory of pathogenesis holds that the cord is damaged by tensile stresses transmitted from the dura, via the dentate ligaments. The spondylotic bar increases dentate tension by displacing the cord dorsally, while the ligaments are anchored.

SYMPTOMS AND SIGNS

Neck pain may be prominent. Root pain is uncommon, but paresthesias may indicate the most affected root. The most common symptom is spastic gait disorder (Table 67.1). Weakness and wasting of the hands may be seen. Fasciculations may also be noted. Urinary sphincter symptoms occur in a minority of patients. Overt sensory loss is uncommon, but the diagnosis is facilitated if there is a sensory level, or if there is sensory loss that occurs in the distribution of a cervical dermatome. The course of the disorder is slowly progressive, but the natural history is not well delineated. Study of patients who were not treated surgically indicates that the condition may become arrested or even improve spontaneously. In one report, 39 of 45 patients were unchanged or

▶ **TABLE 67.1 Clinical Manifestations of Cervical Spondylotic Myelopathy**

Symptom or Sign	% of Patients
Reflexes	
Hyperreflexia	87
Babinski sign	51
Hoffmann sign	13
Spastic gait disorder	49
Bladder symptoms	49
Sensation	
Vague sensory level	41
Proprioceptive sensory loss	39
Cervical dermatome sensory loss	33
Motor functions	
Arm weakness	31
Paraparesis	21
Hemiparesis	18
Quadriparesis	10
Brown-Sequard syndrome	18
Hand atrophy	13
Fasciculation	13
Pain	
Radicular arm	41
Radicular leg	13
Neck	8

Data from Lunsford et al., 1980.

fared better without surgery, many years after the original diagnosis.

LABORATORY DATA

Formerly, the most important diagnostic tests were plain radiographs of the cervical spine and myelography. Plain radiographs show narrowing of the disc spaces and the presence of osteophytes, especially at C5–C6 and C6–C7. Posterior osteophytes tend to be smaller than anterior projections and may not be seen without CT. The disc bodies may be normal or may show sclerosis. Changes in the zygapophyseal joints account for the designation of osteoarthritis and may encroach on the intervertebral foramen; the changes may cause subluxation of the articular surfaces or compression of vertebral arteries.

MRI is the imaging procedure of choice; it is noninvasive and provides exquisite resolution of spinal cord structures (Figs. 67.1 and 67.2). MRI allows evaluation of spondylosis and the alternative possibilities: Chiari malformation, arteriovenous malformation, extramedullary tumor, syringomyelia, or multiple sclerosis (MS). In time, technical advances in MRI may make myelography obsolete.

Somatosensory evoked responses have been used to aid in diagnosis but are not crucial. The CSF is usually normal or has a protein concentration of 50 mg/dL to 100 mg/dL. Higher protein levels or CSF pleocytosis should

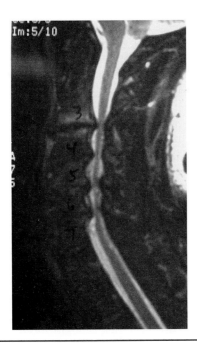

FIGURE 67.1. Sagittal proton-density MRI demonstrates extensive spinal-cord compression caused by a combination of ventral bone spurs and preexisting (i.e., congenital) canal stenosis.

raise the question of MS or tumor, including meningeal carcinomatosis. The role of transcranial magnetic stimulation in diagnosis remains to be ascertained but motor-evoked potentials may be more contributory than sensory potentials.

DIFFERENTIAL DIAGNOSIS

There are two types of problems in the differential diagnosis. In one group, there is compression of the cervical spinal cord, but not by spondylosis, or at least not by spondylosis alone. Cervical spinal tumors are the best example of this kind of problem. These lesions are revealed by MRI. In other compressive lesions, the primary bony changes are congenital (e.g., anomalies of the craniocervical junction) or acquired (e.g., rheumatoid arthritis or basilar impression) and may be further complicated by spondylosis. These disorders are recognized by CT or MRI. Arteriovenous malformations (AVMs) may also be found.

Another group of myelopathies presents more of a diagnostic problem. Cervical spondylosis is so common in the general population that it may be present by chance, and may be harmless in a person with another disease of the spinal cord. The ultimate test of the pathogenic significance of spondylosis would be complete relief of symptoms after decompressive surgery, but this is rarely seen. Among the other diseases that may cause clinical syndromes similar to those attributed to spondylosis are MS, amyotrophic lateral sclerosis (ALS), neurosyphilis, and possibly subacute combined-system disease. In 12% of patients diagnosed with spondylotic myelopathy, some other diagnosis was ultimately made.

MS is probably the most common cause of spastic paraplegia in middle life and is probably the actual cause of the disorder in some people who have had cervical laminectomies. Therefore, before laminectomy it is imperative to test for MS by use of visual, somatosensory, and brainstem-evoked responses; examine CSF for gamma globulin and oligoclonal bands; and do MRI examination of the cerebral white matter, foramen magnum, brainstem, and cervical spinal cord. Proper use and interpretation of the test results often remove diagnostic uncertainty.

ALS must be considered whenever wasting and fasciculations are seen in arm and hand muscles, and especially when there are fasciculations in the legs. The presence of overt fasciculation makes it unlikely that spondylotic myelopathy is the cause of symptoms; when fasciculation is visible, caution is warranted when laminectomy is being considered. There is no diagnostic test for ALS, however, and the distinction may be difficult.

Rare causes of spastic paraplegia in middle life are the myelopathy caused by human T-cell lymphotropic-virus

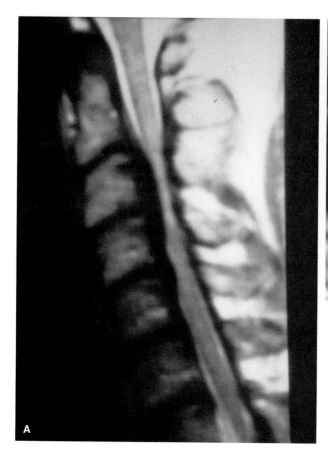

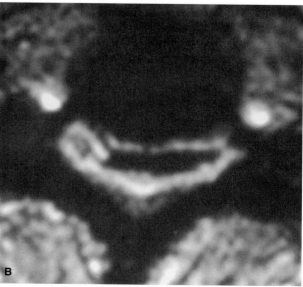

FIGURE 67.2. A: Sagittal T1-weighted MRI shows focal spinal cord compression from a single osteophyte at the C3-4 level. This dense calcification is typical of segmental ossification of the posterior longitudinal ligament. **B:** Axial CT in same patient.

type I or adult-onset adrenoleukodystrophy. The diagnosis of exclusion, when no other cause is identified, is primary lateral sclerosis, which is almost as common a cause of spastic paraparesis as MS.

In northern England, a prospective survey of 585 patients with nontraumatic spastic paraparesis gave the following order of frequency of diagnosis: cervical spondylotic myelopathy, 24%; tumor, 16%; MS, 18%; diagnosis uncertain, 19%; and ALS, 4%. The absence of primary lateral sclerosis from this list suggests regional differences in making a diagnosis. Of course, the real problem is ascertaining the diagnosis of spondylotic myelopathy.

An old adage: Be wary of the diagnosis of cervical spondylotic myelopathy if there is no sensory loss.

TREATMENT

The natural history of cervical spondylotic myelopathy varies greatly and is unpredictable in individual patients. The Cochrane Library lists a single, controlled trial for spondylotic myelopathy, that of Bednarik et al, who found an early benefit for surgery over conservative therapy but did not find differences after one year. However, they studied only 49 patients. Therefore, there have been no adequately controlled trials of surgical therapy. Additionally,

several different operations have been advocated (e.g., with or without fusion, and with or without different kinds of stabilizing hardware). Therefore, uniform recommendations for treatment have been difficult to establish. Decompressive operations include posterior laminectomy, anterior discectomy, or vertebrectomy; these procedures are widely used but are associated with a high failure rate. Although contemporary surgical series report a 70% to 80% rate of improvement, only about 50% of patients show satisfactory functional improvement or complete reversal of symptoms that is maintained for a long time. The efficacy of surgical decompression seems to have been established in these improved patients. The others show little or no improvement, and their conditions may even become worse as a result of surgery. Sometimes, symptoms return and progress, even immediately after postoperative improvement.

Sooner or later, an attempt will be made to standardize data collection to evaluate the outcome of these operations, and there might even be a therapeutic trial. Surgeons still contend that a controlled trial is neither feasible nor necessary. However, one randomized trial of corpectomy for single-level disc disease found that fusion added nothing to decompression alone. Commenting on the trial, orthopedist Jeremy Fairbank noted all the problems to be faced but nevertheless reaffirmed the need to document the advantages of surgery over nonsurgical management. Others have questioned the need for spinal fusion.

In the absence of clear guidelines, management is tailored to the specific circumstances of individual patients and to the experiences of the treating physicians and surgeons. Conservative treatment with physical therapy for gait training and with neck immobilization with a firm collar is appropriate for patients with mild myelopathy. Surgery should be considered if the myelopathy progresses despite conservative treatment.

SUGGESTED READINGS

Adams CBT, Logue V. Movement and contour of spine in relation to neural complications of cervical spondylosis. *Brain* 1971;94:569–586.

Adams CBT, Logue V. Some functional effects of operations for cervical spondylotic myelopathy. *Brain* 1971;94:587–594.

Barnes MP, Saunders M. The effect of cervical mobility on the natural history of cervical spondylotic myelopathy. *J Neurol Neurosurg Psychiatry* 1984;47:17–20.

Bednarik J, Kadanka Z, Vohanka S, et al. The value of somatosensory- and motor-evoked potentials in predicting and monitoring the effect of therapy in spondylotic cervical myelopathy. Prospective randomized study. *Spine* 1999;24(15):1593–1598.

Braakman R. Management of cervical spondylotic myelopathy and radiculopathy. *J Neurol Neurosurg Psychiatry* 1994;57:257–263.

Caruso PA, Patel MR, Joseph J, Rachlin J. Primary intramedullary lymphoma of the spinal cord mimicking cervical spondylotic myelopathy. *AJR* 1998;171:526–527.

Crockard HA, Heilman AE, Stevens JM. Progressive myelopathy secondary to odontoid fractures: clinical, radiological and surgical features. *J Neurosurg* 1993;78:579–586.

Deyo RA, Nachemson A, Kirza SK. Spinal-fusion surgery–the case for restraint. *N Engl J Med* 2004;350:722–726.

Ebara S, Yonenobu K, Fujiwara K, et al. Myelopathy hand characterized by muscle wasting: a different type of myelopathy hand in patients with cervical spondylosis. *Spine* 1988;13:785–791.

Emery SE, Bohlman HH, Bolesta MJ, Jones PK. Anterior cervical decompression and arthrodesis for the treatment of cervical spondylotic myelopathy. Two- to seventeen-year follow-up. *J Bone Joint Surg Am* 1998;80:941–951.

Fessler RG, Steck JC, Giovanni MA. Anterior cervical corpectomy for cervical spondylotic myelopathy. *Neurosurgery* 1998;43:257–265.

Fouyas IP, Statham PFX, Sandercock PAG, Lynch C. Surgery for cervical radiculomyelopathy (Cochrane Review). In: *The Cochrane Library*, Issue 2. Chichester, UK: John Wiley & Sons, Ltd., 2004.

Hirose G, Kadoya S. Cervical spondylotic radiculo-myelopathy in patients with athetoid-dystonic cerebral palsy: clinical evaluation and surgical treatment. *J Neurol Neurosurg Psychiatry* 1984;47:775–780.

Kardon D. Cervical spondylotic myelopathy with reversible fasciculations in the lower extremities. *Arch Neurol* 1977;34:774–776.

Lees F, Turner JWA. Natural history and prognosis of cervical spondylosis. *BMJ* 1963;2:1607–1610.

Lunsford LD, Bissonette DJ, Zorub DS. Anterior surgery for cervical disc disease. Part 2: treatment of cervical spondylotic myelopathy in 32 cases. *J Neurosurg* 1980;53:12–19.

Lyu RK, Tang LM, Chen CJ, et al. The use of evoked potentials for clinical correlation and surgical outcome in cervical spondylotic myelopathy with intramedullary high signal intensity on MRI. *J Neurol Neurosurg Psychiatry* 2004;75:256–261.

Moore AP, Blumhardt LD. A prospective survey of the causes of nontraumatic spastic paraparesis and tetraparesis in 585 patients. *Spinal Cord* 1997;5:361–367.

Nakamura K, Kurokawa T, Hoshino Y, et al. Conservative treatment for cervical spondylotic myelopathy: achievement and sustainability of a level of "no disability." *J Spinal Disord* 1998;11:175–179.

Nurick S. The pathogenesis of the spinal cord disorder associated with cervical spondylosis. *Brain* 1972;95:87–100.

Nurick S. The natural history and results of surgical treatment of the spinal cord disorder associated with cervical spondylosis. *Brain* 1972;95:101–108.

Olive PM, Whitecloud TS 3rd, Bennett JT. Lower cervical spondylosis and myelopathy in adults with Down's syndrome. *Spine* 1988;13:781–784.

Persson LCG, Carlsson C-A, Carlsson JY. Long-lasting cervical radicular pain managed with surgery, physiotherapy, or a cervical collar. A prospective, randomized study. *Spine* 1997;22(7):751–758.

Restuccia D, DiLazzaro V, Valeriani M, et al. Segmental dysfunction of the cervical cord revealed by abnormalities of the spinal N13 potential in cervical spondylotic myelopathy. *Neurology* 1992;42:1054–1063.

Rowland LP. Surgical treatment of cervical spondylotic myelopathy: time for a controlled trial. *Neurology* 1992;42:5–13.

Saunders RL, Bernini PM, Shirreffs TG, Reeves AG. Central corpectomy for cervical spondylotic myelopathy: a consecutive series with long-term follow-up evaluation. *J Neurosurg* 1991;74:163–170.

Sampath P, Bendebba M, Davis JD. Outcome of patients treated for cervical myelopathy. A prospective multicenter study with independent clinical review. *Spine* 2000;25:670–676.

Szpalski M, Gunzburg R, eds. *The Degenerative Cervical Spine.* Baltimore: Lippincott Williams & Wilkins, 2001.

Tavy DLJ, Wagner GL, Keunen RWM, et al. Transcranial magnetic stimulation in patients with cervical spondylotic myelopathy: clinical and radiological correlations. *Muscle Nerve* 1994;17:235–241.

Wang MY, Shah S, Green BA. Clinical outcomes following cervical laminoplasty for 204 patients with cervical spondylotic myelopathy. *Surg Neurol* 2004 Dec;62(6):487–492.

Wilkinson M, ed. *Cervical Spondylosis: Its Early Diagnosis and Treatment.* Philadelphia: WB Saunders, 1971.

Chapter 68

Lumbar Spondylosis

Lewis P. Rowland and Paul C. McCormick

The same pathologic changes that define cervical spondylosis may affect the lower spine. Here, however, the roots of the cauda equina are affected rather than the spinal cord. The spinal cord becomes narrow because of age-related degenerative changes that affect the vertebral column articulations, including disc bulging and spur formation, facet-joint enlargement, and hypertrophy of the ligamenta flava and facet capsule. Encroachment is usually maximal at the disc spaces. *Spinal stenosis* is the term for this narrowing. Congenital stenosis makes a person more vulnerable to these changes.

The stenosis caused by spondylosis may be diffuse, but it is usually confined to one or two lumbar levels. Isolated

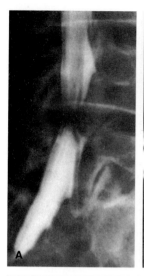 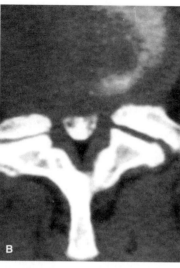

FIGURE 68.1. A: Lumbar myelogram demonstrates focal high-grade stenosis at L4-5. **B:** Post myelographic CT at the L4-5 interspace demonstrates circumferential stenosis caused by disc bulging, enlarged facets, and hypertrophy of the ligamenta flava.

L4-L5 disorder, with unilateral or bilateral L-5 radiculopathy, is the most common syndrome (Fig. 68.1). The L3-L4 segment is less often affected either alone or in combination with L4-L5 stenosis. Disorders at other levels are rare.

The resulting syndrome differs from acute herniation in many respects. Most patients are older than age 40 years, and many are older than age 60 years. Progression of symptoms is likely to be gradual rather than acute. Twisting of the back, lifting, or falling are precipitating factors in fewer than one-third of cases, and back pain is not the dominant symptom, but may be reported by more than 50% of patients. Leg pain, when present, is as often bilateral as unilateral. Weakness of the legs and urinary incontinence are symptoms in a minority of patients, but many show weakness of isolated muscles and loss of reflexes on examination. Straight-leg raising is limited in a few patients.

SYMPTOMS AND SIGNS

The characteristic symptom is *pseudoclaudication,* seen in almost all patients, and is defined as unilateral or bilateral discomfort in buttock, thigh, or leg on standing or walking that is relieved by rest. Patients use the words pain, numbness, or weakness to describe the discomfort, but there is often no objective sensory loss or focal muscle weakness. The discomfort is relieved by lying down, sitting, or flexing at the waist. Sometimes, pain persists in recumbency until the spine is flexed. Unlike vascular claudication, the pain persists if the patient stops walking without flexing the spine, and sometimes the discomfort is brought on by prolonged standing without walking.

PATHOLOGY

The pathogenesis of pseudoclaudication is uncertain. Sometimes, myelography shows that hyperextension of the spine increases the protrusion of intervertebral discs, with relief of nerve root compression in flexed postures. In addition, blood flow to the lumbar spinal cord may increase when leg muscles are exercised. As a result, vessels on nerve roots dilate, but are then confined by the bony changes and thus compress the nerve roots. This is relieved by cessation of activity.

DIAGNOSIS

The diagnosis is made from the characteristic history, clinical findings, and radiography. Formerly, the syndrome was defined by changes in plain spine radiographs and by evidence of partial or complete subarachnoid block, found by contrast myelography. Diagnosis was facilitated by the advent of CT, with or without contrast enhancement (Fig. 68.1). Now, however, MRI alone usually suffices to show the specific patterns and extent of compression. Electromyography may reveal that denervation is restricted to muscles innervated by lumbosacral roots. The CSF protein level may be normal if the puncture is performed above the level of the block, but values greater than 100 mg/dL may be found if there are multiple blocks.

The differential diagnosis includes intermittent claudication caused by peripheral-arterial occlusive disease, which is recognized by the loss of pulses and characteristic trophic changes in the skin of the feet. Aortoiliac occlusive disease may spare peripheral pulses, but the femoral pulse is usually affected; it may cause claudication and wasting of leg muscles but does not cause postural claudication. The pain of aortoiliac disease is localized to exercising muscles. The radicular pattern of spinal claudication is not seen. The pain of aortoiliac disease persists as long as exercise is continued, regardless of body position. Vascular sonography may be a necessity.

Osteoarthritis of the hip joint may also cause activity-induced leg pain that is relieved by rest. The pain originates in the hip and usually radiates into the groin or anterior thigh, but does not extend below the knee. Pain and limitation of hip rotation are the usual findings. The diagnosis is confirmed radiographically.

TREATMENT

The treatment of lumbar stenosis varies according to the severity of the symptoms. Mild symptoms often respond to nonsteroidal antiinflammatory drugs (NSAIDs) and physical therapy. The symptoms of lumbar stenosis may be episodic; even severe pain should be treated conservatively because a prolonged remission may ensue.

Surgical treatment consists of decompressive laminectomy, with medial facetectomy and resection of the ligamenta flava at the stenosed levels. One meta-analysis found improvement after surgery in 64% of the patients. The Cochrane Library found trials comparing different methods of fusion but not one adequately controlled trial comparing surgery to natural history. Epidural injection of steroids does not relieve the pain of spinal claudication. The outcome of surgery may be less favorable in people over age 70 years who have diabetes mellitus.

Surgery is reserved for patients who have pain and claudication severe enough to affect the quality of life and who do not respond to conservative therapy. Surgery is usually well tolerated and is highly effective; about two-thirds of the patients report considerable improvement that is sustained for years after surgery. In one study, the following features indicated a favorable prognosis for patients with weak legs: disc herniation, stenosis at one level, duration of leg weakness of less than 6 weeks, and age younger than 65 years. In another study, the radiographic severity of stenosis was the best predictor of long-term outcome, regardless of therapy, surgical or nonsurgical. There have been no controlled trials of surgical treatment.

SUGGESTED READINGS

Arinzon Z, Adunsky A, Fidelman Z, Gepstein R. Outcomes of decompression surgery for lumbar spinal stenosis in elderly diabetic patients. *Eur Spine J* 2004;13:32–37.

Bischoff RJ, Rodriguez RP, Gupta K, et al. Comparison of CT, MRI and myelography in the diagnosis of herniated nucleus pulposus and spinal stenosis. *J Spinal Disord* 1993;6:289–295.

Caputy AJ, Lessenhup AJ. Long-term evaluation of decompressive surgery for degenerative lumbar stenosis. *J Neurosurg* 1992;77:669–678.

DeVilliers JC. Combined neurogenic and vascular claudication. *S Afr Med J* 1980;57:650–654.

Epstein NE, Maldonado VC, Cusick JF. Symptomatic lumbar spinal stenosis. *Surg Neurol* 1998;50:3–10.

Fukusaki M, Kobayashi I, Hara T, Sumikawa K. Symptoms of spinal stenosis do not improve after epidural steroid injection. *Clin J Pain* 1998;14:148–151.

Gibson JNA, Waddell G, Grant IC. Surgery for degenerative lumbar spondylosis (Cochrane Review). In: *The Cochrane Library,* Issue 2. Chichester UK, John Wiley & Sons, Ltd., 2004.

Giugui P, Benoist M, Delecourt C, Delhoume J, Deburge A. Motor deficit in lumbar spinal stenosis: a retrospective study of a series of 50 patients. *J Spinal Disorder* 1998;11:283–288.

Goh KJ, Khlifa W, Anslow P, Cadoux-Hudson T, Donaghy M. The clinical syndrome associated with lumbar spinal stenosis. *Eur Neurol* 2004 Dec 1;52(4):242–249.

Hall S, Bartelson JD, Onofrio BM, et al. Lumbar spinal stenosis: clinical features, diagnostic procedures, and results of surgical treatment in 68 patients. *Ann Intern Med* 1985;103:271–275.

Hurri H, Slatis P, Soini J, et al. Lumbar spinal stenosis: assessment of long-term outcome 12 years after operative and conservative treatment. *J Spinal Disord* 1998;11:110–115.

Javid MJ, Hadar EJ. Long-term follow-up review of patients who underwent laminectomy for lumbar stenosis. *J Neurosurg* 1998;89:1–7.

Lange M, Hamburger C, Waldhauser E, Beck OJ. Surgical treatment and results in patients with lumbar spinal stenosis. *Neurosurg Rev* 1993;16:27–33.

Onel D, Sari H, Donmez C. Lumbar spinal stenosis: clinical-radiologic therapeutic evaluation in 145 patients: conservative treatment or surgery? *Spine* 1993;18:291–298.

Sanderson PL, Wood PL. Surgery for lumbar spinal stenosis in old people. *J Bone Joint Surg Br* 1993;75:393–397.

Silvers HR, Lewis PJ, Asch HL. Decompressive lumbar laminectomy for spinal stenosis. *J Neurosurg* 1993;78:695–701.

Spivak JM. Degenerative lumbar spinal stenosis. *J Bone Joint Surg Am* 1998;80:1053–1066.

Chapter 69

Cranial and Peripheral Nerve Lesions

Clifton L. Gooch, Dale J. Lange, and Werner Trojaborg

GENERAL PRINCIPLES OF NERVE INJURY

Trauma, infections, tumors, toxins, and vascular or metabolic disorders may injure the peripheral and cranial nerves. Trauma is the most common cause of localized injury to a single nerve (mononeuropathy), while inflammatory, metabolic, toxic and other disorders often affect the peripheral nervous system diffusely or attack multiple individual nerves over a short period (symmetric polyneuropathy or mononeuropathy multiplex). This section focuses on the mechanisms, clinical features, and treatment of focal nerve injury, while more generalized polyneuropathies are covered in Chapters 104, 105, and 106.

PATHOPHYSIOLOGY

The type and severity of nerve injury determines the degree of pathologic change, the capacity for regeneration, and the prognosis for recovery. Seddon's classification of mechanical nerve injury includes three major categories: nerve transection (*neurotmesis*); axonal interruption with distal degeneration but preservation of the endoneurium (*axonotmesis*); and mild ischemic or compressive injury resulting in conduction block at the site of the lesion but without axonal or endoneurial disruption, without degeneration of distal axons (*neurapraxia*).

Within the first 24 hours, focal swelling appears adjacent to the site of injury, with fragmentation of the endoplasmic reticulum, neurotubules, and neurofilaments. The axolemma becomes discontinuous, with axonal swelling at some sites and narrowing at others, resulting in a beaded appearance. This process begins between the nodes of Ranvier and appears first in smaller fibers. Changes in myelin sheaths lag behind those in axons but progress in a similar way along the entire distal stump, again affecting the small fibers first. The myelin surrounding the fragmented axons breaks up to form rows of elliptoids. Finally, Schwann cells and macrophages degrade the axon and myelin debris. In addition to these distal nerve changes, a *retrograde axon reaction* or *chromatolysis* is seen with retraction of axons proximal to the lesion and cell body swelling, disruption of the Nissl substance, migration of the nucleus and increases in the size of the nucleoli. Presynaptic terminals gradually withdraw and synaptic transmission is reduced until dorsal root stimulation fails to excite the motor neuron.

The pathologic distal changes of degeneration and retrograde axon reaction are similar in crush injury or complete nerve transection, but axonal outgrowth may repair some of the injury by reestablishing connection with the severed portion. However, if the distance between the proximal stump, which is still attached to the cell body, and the severed distal stump is too great, regeneration is not possible unless the ends are apposed, which may require microsurgery in some cases. If the distance is small, the fine processes of the axon penetrate the fibrin and connective tissue in the scar and enter the distal end of the nerve. Some of these may be deflected from the proper path by the scar and become entangled to form a *neuroma*.

CLINICAL MANIFESTATIONS

The symptoms and signs of nerve injury depend on the type of nerve affected. If the nerve is predominately motor, flaccid paralysis ensues with wasting of the muscles innervated by the nerve. If the nerve contains sensory fibers, the result is loss of sensation in an area that is usually smaller than the anatomic distribution of the nerve. Vasomotor disorders and trophic disturbances are more common when a sensory or mixed-type of nerve is injured than when a motor nerve is damaged. Partial injury or incomplete division of a nerve may be accompanied by pain that may be described as stabbing, pricking (pins-and-needles) or burning, sometimes resulting in the clinical syndrome of *causalgia*. Complete or incomplete interruption of a nerve may be followed by trophic changes in the skin, mucous membranes, bones, and nails.

DIAGNOSIS

The diagnosis of injury to one or more peripheral nerves may usually be made clinically by assessment of the distribution of the motor and sensory abnormalities. The dif-

ferentiation between lesions of the spinal roots and one or more peripheral nerves may be made by determining whether muscular weakness and sensory loss are segmental, rather than in the pattern of a peripheral nerve. EMG may be used to better define the extent and pattern of denervation and more chronically, of reinnervation; nerve conduction studies may ascertain the site and the nature of the injury. The differential diagnosis of polyneuropathy and other causes of generalized weakness is reviewed in Chapters 104 and 105.

PROGNOSIS

The prognosis after injury of peripheral nerves is related to the degree of axonal injury and to some extent, to the site of the injury. As a rule, the nearer the injury is to the CNS, the lower the probability will be that a completely severed nerve will regenerate (e.g., the cranial nerves). When injury to a peripheral nerve involves little or no axonal loss, recovery is complete within a few days or weeks. If axonal loss is severe, recovery is slow because axonal regeneration is required for recovery of function. If the nerve is severed or the damage is so great that axons may not grow along the appropriate tubules, recovery may fail or be incomplete, with permanent neuronal dysfunction.

TREATMENT

When a peripheral nerve is severed by trauma, the ends should be surgically anastomosed. There is no agreement about the best time to explore and repair lesions of peripheral nerves, if it may not be determined whether or not there has been anatomic or physiologic interruption of the nerve. Most clinicians believe that surgery should be performed as soon as possible if there is any doubt about the state of the nerve. After surgical therapy, or in patients who do not need operative therapy, rehabilitation measures should commence immediately, with passive range-of-motion exercises for paralyzed muscles and restorative exercises for weak muscles. Electrical stimulation is of unproven value in preventing permanent weakness. Splints, braces, and other corrective devices should be used when the lesion produces a deformity, but should be removable to allow physiotherapy.

CRANIAL NERVE INJURY

The Olfactory Nerve (Cranial Nerve I)

The ability to smell is a special quality relegated to the olfactory cells in the nasal mucosa. The molecular biology of smell is uncertain, but transcription-activating factors, such as Olf-1, found exclusively in neurons with olfactory receptors, probably direct cellular differentiation. Smell may be impaired after injury of the nasal mucosa, the olfactory bulb or its filaments, or CNS connections. Lesions of the nerve cause diminution or loss of the sense of smell. Occasionally, olfactory hallucinations of a transient and paroxysmal nature may occur with lesions in the temporal lobe. The most common, chief complaint of patients afflicted with olfactory nerve injury, however, is not loss of smell but diminished taste, as olfaction plays a key role in taste perception because of the volatile substances in many food and beverages. The sense of smell is most commonly impaired, transiently, because of allergic nasal congestion or the common cold. The most common traumatic injury of the olfactory nerve occurs in head injury, usually of the acceleration-deceleration variety, as in motor vehicle accidents. The delicate filaments of the olfactory nerve are sheared where they pass through the perforations of the cribiform plate. The olfactory bulb may also be contused or lacerated in head injuries. Leigh and Zee (1991) reported altered olfactory sense in 7.2% of patients with head injuries at a military hospital, with complete loss in 4.1% and partial loss in 3.1%. Recovery of smell occurred in only 6 of 72 patients. In a study of head injuries in civilians, Friedman and Merritt (1944) found that the olfactory nerve was damaged in 11 (2.6%) of 430 patients. In all patients, anosmia was bilateral. In three, the loss was transient and disappeared within 2 weeks of injury.

Inflammatory or neuritic lesions of the bulb or tract are uncommon, but these structures are sometimes affected in meningitis or in mononeuritis multiplex. Rarely, patients with diabetes mellitus may have an impaired sensation of smell, sometimes stemming from vascular infarction of the olfactory nerve. Hyposmia or anosmia is also common early in Refsum disease. The olfactory bulb or tract may be compressed by meningiomas, metastatic tumors, or aneurysms in the anterior fossa or by infiltrating tumors of the frontal lobe. *Parosmia* (i.e., perversion of sense of smell) was present in 12 patients.

Parosmia is not accompanied by impairment of olfactory acuity and is most commonly caused by lesions of the temporal lobe, although it has been reported with injury to the olfactory bulb or tract. Olfactory hallucinations may occur in psychosis or as an aura in patients with seizures that involve the hippocampal or uncinate gyrus, and are described as strange, unpleasant and ill-defined odors. Increased sensitivity to olfactory stimuli is generally rare, though it may occur in migraneurs and in patients with reactive-airways disease, perhaps because of prior sensitization to olfactory triggers. Cases in which the sense of smell is so acute that it is a source of continuous discomfort, however, may be psychogenic.

The Optic Nerve (Cranial Nerve II)

Retina, optic nerve, and optic tract injuries have many etiologies and cause loss of vision, impairment of pupillary light reflexes, and abnormalities in pupillary size and reactivity (Table 69.1). Disorders of the visual pathway are discussed in more detail in Chapter 7.

Injury to the retina or optic nerve may result from direct trauma, inflammation (e.g., optic neuritis, multiple sclerosis), systemic diseases (e.g., diabetes mellitus, chronic renal failure, leukemia, anemia, polycythemia, nutritional deficiencies, syphilis, tuberculosis, the lipodystrophies,

▶ **TABLE 69.1** Effects of Lesions of the Optic, Oculomotor, and Sympathetic Pathways on the Pupils

Site of Lesion on Right Side	Size of Pupil		Reaction of Homolateral Pupil to Stimulation by Light Directed into		Consensual Reaction of Contralateral Pupil to Stimulation by Light Directed Into		Accommodation–Convergence Reaction
	Right	Left	Right	Left	Right	Left	
Retina	Normal	Normal	Impaired	Normal	Impaired	Normal	Normal
Optic nerve	Normal	Normal	Lost	Normal	Lost	Normal	Normal
Optic chiasm	Normal	Normal	Normal[a]	Normal[a]	Normal[a]	Normal[a]	Normal
Optic tract	Normal	Normal	Normal[a]	Normal[a]	Normal[a]	Normal[a]	Normal
Optic radiation	Normal	Normal	Normal	Normal	Normal	Normal	Normal
Periaqueductal region[b]	Contracted	Normal	Lost	Normal	Normal	Lost	Normal
Oculonuclear complex or nerve	Dilated	Normal	Lost	Normal	Normal	Lost	Lost on right
Sympathetic pathways	Contracted	Normal	Normal	Normal	Normal	Normal	Normal

[a]No reaction of the pupils if the beam of light is focused sharply on the amblyopic portions of the retina.
[b]Argyll-Robertson pupil.

giant cell arteritis, or generalized arteriosclerosis), toxins (e.g., methyl alcohol, ethyl alcohol, tobacco, quinine, pentavalent arsenicals, thallium, lead, or mercury), hereditary disorders, intraocular disease (e.g., chorioretinitis, glaucoma, tumors, congenital anomalies, or thrombosis or embolism of the veins or arteries of the retina, etc.), infiltration or compression of the nerve (e.g., glioma, meningioma, pituitary tumor, craniopharyngioma, metastatic tumor, or aneurysm), and increased intracranial pressure (e.g., papilledema).

Optic Neuritis

Optic neuritis is a term used loosely to describe lesions of the optic nerve. Patients present with decreased visual acuity and predominate central visual-field loss. It is caused by inflammatory, degenerative, demyelinating, or toxic disorders (Fig. 69.1).

On ophthalmoscopic examination, the disc may appear normal initially, with rapid swelling and congestion of the nerve appearing shortly after injury. Later, the disc becomes pale and smaller than normal. Optic neuritis most commonly occurs either as a spontaneous, likely autoimmune, self-limited phenomenon, or as a part of multiple sclerosis for which it may be the presenting symptom.

Alcohol-Tobacco Amblyopia

Alcohol-tobacco amblyopia describes the optic nerve injury resulting from the long and continued use of both tobacco and ethyl alcohol. The lesion may be an interstitial neuritis with destruction of the papillomacular bundle, or may result from injury to the ganglion cells in the macula. It is most common in middle-aged men who smoke and drink alcohol in large quantities and usually affects both eyes. At onset, a partial central or paracentral scotoma appears, with diminished color perception, eventually progressing to a complete central scotoma. Peripheral vision remains normal. Alcohol-tobacco amblyopia is associated with pernicious anemia and many authorities believe the condition is primarily a nutritional disorder, and in alcoholics is related to poor nutrition. Absolute withdrawal of all forms of alcohol and tobacco may improve vision if the retinal cells of the optic nerve have not completely atrophied.

The Oculomotor, Trochlear, and Abducens Nerves (Cranial Nerves III, IV, and VI)

Injury to the nerves or nuclei that innervate the ocular muscles causes diplopia, deviation of the eye, and impairment of ocular movement. Complete lesions of the *oculomotor (third cranial) nerve* produces paralysis of the extraocular muscles it supplies (i.e., medial rectus, superior rectus, inferior rectus, inferior oblique, and levator palpebrae superior), as well as the papillary constrictor and levator palpebrae muscles. Clinically, a full oculomotor-nerve lesion manifests with unilateral ptosis, progressing to inability to open the eye, lateral and slightly inferior deviation of the eye, dilation of the pupil, and loss of direct reaction to light but preservation of the consensual papillary response. Partial lesions of the third nerve produce differing combinations of these symptoms, according to the extent of involvement of the nerve fibers or neurons. A full discussion of the pathways for papillary function and accommodation appears in Chapter 7.

Lesions of the *trochlear (fourth cranial) nerve* cause paralysis of the superior oblique muscle, with impairment of the ability to move the eye inferiorly and medially. Deviation at rest is slight, and diplopia is corrected by inclination of the head forward and toward the side of the unaffected (i.e., contralateral) eye. Injury to the *abducens (sixth*

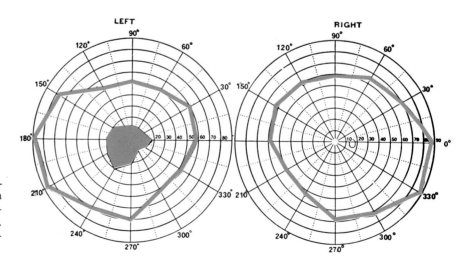

FIGURE 69.1. Chart of visual fields in a patient with retrobulbar optic neuritis indicates large central scotoma in left eye. Visual acuity: OD 15/15, OS 1/400. (Courtesy of Dr. M. Chamlin.)

cranial) nerve causes paralysis of the lateral rectus muscle. The eye is deviated medially, and diplopia is present in almost all directions of gaze, though not when gaze is directed to the side opposite the lesion (i.e., contralaterally). Lesions in the brain stem that involve the sixth-nerve nucleus are also accompanied by paralysis of lateral gaze. If both the sixth nerve and its medial longitudinal fasciculus are injured within the brain stem, neither eye will move past midline during attempted gaze towards the side of the lesion. Both accommodation and convergence are spared, and no ptosis or papillary abnormalities are present under these circumstances, supporting the integrity of the oculomotor (third cranial) nerve. Paralysis of the ocular muscles may result from injury to the corresponding motor nerves or cells of origin by many conditions, including: trauma, neurosyphilis, multiple sclerosis (MS) and other demyelinating diseases, tumors or aneurysms at the base of the skull, acute or subacute meningitis, thrombosis of intracranial venous sinuses, encephalitis, acute anterior poliomyelitis, diphtheria, diabetes mellitus, syringobulbia, vascular accidents in the brainstem, lead poisoning, botulism, alcoholic polioencephalitis (Wernicke encephalitis), osteomyelitis of the skull, and following spinal anesthesia, or simple lumbar puncture. Intraorbital lesions may cause ophthalmoplegia, proptosis, and local pain; retroorbital lesions may cause similar symptoms.

Inflammation of the cavernous sinus may cause a painful ophthalmoplegia known as the *Tolosa-Hunt syndrome*, but the precise pathology has been documented in only a few cases. Most of these would also be considered examples of *orbital myositis* or *orbital pseudotumor*, in which swelling of the muscles within the orbit may be demonstrated by CT. Ocular palsies are also frequently seen in myasthenia gravis, ocular myopathy, and rarely polyneuropathy, among many others. Increased intracranial pressure (ICP) is a particularly important cause of these symptoms, which often serve as the sentinel signs of serious CNS disease. The sixth nerve has a long course from its point of exit from the brain stem to the lateral rectus muscle. Although it lies in a fluid-cushioned channel for a portion of its course, it is especially prone to compression against the floor of the skull with increased ICP, causing unilateral or bilateral paralysis of the lateral rectus muscles, and acting as a false localizing sign.

Although commonly compressed by aneurysm, the third cranial nerve is less commonly injured by chronic increased ICP, alone. However, signs of third-nerve injury, typically including a dilated pupil unresponsive to light (i.e., a "blown" pupil) appearing suddenly in a patient with altered consciousness, must be considered supratentorial herniation of the uncinate gyrus through the tentorial notch until proven otherwise.

Massive intracerebral hemorrhage, extradural and subdural hematomas, are common causes of acute uncal herniation. As these patients are often comatose, oculovestibular testing by the doll's-eyes maneuver or caloric testing is usually necessary to determine the integrity of the vestibular and oculomotor systems.

The Trigeminal Nerve (Cranial Nerve V)

Injury to the fifth cranial nerve causes loss of soft-tactile, thermal, and pain sensation in the face, loss of the corneal and sneezing (i.e., sternutatory) reflexes and paralysis of the muscles of mastication. The dorsal root ganglia for the sensory fibers of the trigeminal nerve reside in the trigeminal (i.e., gasserian) ganglion in the middle cranial fossa, from which afferent sensory fibers pass into the mid-pons. Fibers subserving light touch ascend to terminate in the chief sensory nucleus of the fifth cranial nerve. Fibers subserving pain and temperature sense descend to terminate in the nucleus of the spinal tract of the fifth cranial nerve, while fibers subserving proprioception for jaw muscles course to the mesencephalic nucleus.

Lesions of the trigeminal pathways in the pons usually affect the motor and chief sensory nuclei, causing paralysis of the muscles of mastication and loss of sensation of light touch in the face, while lesions in the medulla affect only the descending tract and cause loss of the sensation of light touch in the face. MRI of the head with contrast is often a useful diagnostic test to search for mass lesions, ischemia, and inflammation, while electrophysiologic testing (e.g., blink-reflex testing) may help quantitate both the afferent (i.e., trigeminal nerve) and efferent (i.e., facial nerve) components of the corneal reflex. The fifth nerve may be injured by trauma, neoplasm, aneurysm, or meningeal infection. Rarely, it may be involved in poliomyelitis and polyneuropathy. Infarcts and other vascular lesions, as well as intramedullary tumors, may damage the sensory and motor nuclei in the pons and medulla. Isolated lesions of the descending tract may occur in syringobulbia or in multiple sclerosis. Common causes of trigeminal-nerve injury with facial numbness include dental trauma, herpes zoster, cranial trauma, head and neck tumors, intracranial tumors, and idiopathic trigeminal neuropathy. Less common causes include multiple sclerosis, systemic sclerosis, mixed connective-tissue diseases, amyloidosis, and sarcoidosis. Isolated facial numbness may also occur without a clearly identifiable cause (i.e., *idiopathic trigeminal neuropathy*), but these patients must be carefully evaluated to ensure an occult process is not overlooked. Although restricted loss of sensation over the chin (i.e., the *numb-chin syndrome*) usually is caused by dental trauma, dental or surgical procedures, or even poorly fitting dentures, this syndrome may also be the presenting feature of a systemic malignancy such as lymphoma, metastatic breast carcinoma, melanoma, or prostate cancer. MRI of the mandible may help identify these disorders. Painful facial numbness, particularly, may herald nasopharyngeal or metastatic carcinoma.

Trigeminal Neuralgia

Trigeminal neuralgia (i.e., tic douloureux) is a syndrome of extremely severe facial pain in the absence of numbness or other objective findings caused by fifth-nerve dysfunction. This disorder of the trigeminal nerve is characterized by recurrent paroxysms of sharp, stabbing pains in the distribution of one or more branches of the nerve. The cause is unknown. In most cases, no organic disease of the fifth nerve or the CNS may be identified. Degenerative or fibrotic changes in the gasserian ganglion have been described, but are too variable to be considered causal. Some investigators believe that most patients with idiopathic trigeminal neuralgia experience nerve compression related to an anomalous blood vessel, usually in the vicinity of the ganglion. Painful symptoms typical of trigeminal neuralgia occasionally occur with demyelinating lesions of the brain stem and may be caused by multiple sclerosis, as well as vascular ischemia affecting the descending root of the fifth nerve. Although trigeminal neuralgia usually follows other symptoms of multiple sclerosis rather than preceding them, up to 10% of patients may have facial pain as part of their initial presentation. The paroxysmal attacks of facial pain in trigeminal neuralgia may be related to excessive discharge within the descending nucleus of the nerve, triggered by an influx of impulses. Relief of symptoms by section of the greater auricular or occipital nerves in some patients suggests a role for peripheral excitation, and interruption of an episode by intravenous phenytoin, as well as a general therapeutic response to antiepileptic agents, suggests aberrant neuronal discharge may also play an important part in the pathophysiology of this disorder. Trigeminal neuralgia is the most common of all neuralgias.

Onset is usually in middle or late life but may occur at any age. Typical trigeminal neuralgia occasionally affects children but rarely occurs before age 35 years. The incidence is slightly greater in women than in men. The pain is extremely severe, is described by many patients as among the worst pain imaginable, and in severe and refractory cases, the risk of suicide for these patients is increased. The pain appears in paroxysms. Between episodes, the patient is free of symptoms, except for fear of an impending attack. The pain is searing or burning, coming in lightning-like jabs. A paroxysm may last 15 minutes or more. The frequency of attacks varies from many times a day to a few times a month. The patient ceases to talk when the pain strikes and may rub or pinch the face; movements of the face and jaw may accompany the pain. Sometimes, ipsilateral lacrimation is prominent. No objective loss of cutaneous sensation is found during or after the paroxysms, but the patient may complain of facial hyperesthesia.

A characteristic feature in the presentation is the *trigger zone*, stimulation of which sets off a typical paroxysm of pain. This zone is a small area on the cheek, lip, or nose that may be stimulated by facial movement, chewing, or touch. The patient may avoid making facial expressions during conversation, may go without eating for days, or may avoid the slightest breeze to prevent an attack. The pain is limited strictly to one or more branches of the fifth nerve and does not spread beyond the distribution of that nerve. The second division is involved more frequently than the third. The first division is primarily affected in less than 5% of patients. Pain may spread to one or both of the other divisions. In cases of long duration, all three divisions are affected in 15% of patients. The pain is occasionally bilateral (5%) for some, but rarely occurs at the same time. Bilateral trigeminal neuralgia is encountered most often in patients with MS.

Diagnosis

The diagnosis of trigeminal neuralgia is usually made from the history. Neurologic examination in patients with trigeminal neuralgia is usually normal, though some patients may also have concurrent hemifacial spasm, and patients whose attacks are provoked by eating may appear thin or cachectic. The results of serum studies and other diagnostic evaluations are also normal. Characteristically, patients avoid touching the area of origin when asked to point it out, instead holding the tip of the index finger a short distance from the face.

Trigeminal neuralgia must be differentiated from other types of pain that occur in the face or head, especially that of infections of the teeth and nasal sinuses. These pains are usually steady instead of episodic, are often throbbing and persist for many hours. However, it is not uncommon for patients with trigeminal neuralgia to undergo surgical treatment of the sinuses and/or tooth extractions before the diagnosis is established. Conversely, patients with diseased teeth may be referred to neurology with a diagnosis of trigeminal neuralgia, though careful dental examination usually identifies primary dental pathology in these patients.

Temporomandibular joint disease may also mimic trigeminal neuralgia, but the pain is not paroxysmal and, although exacerbated by eating, no trigger point may be identified and symptoms are usually less severe between meals. Cluster headaches are also in the differential but occur in protracted clusters rather than as brief events and are accompanied by ipsilateral nasal congestion, ipsilateral conjuctival injection and lacrimation, and an ipsilateral Horner syndrome. Atypical facial pain may have a trigeminal distribution but the individual paroxysms always last longer than a few seconds (usually minutes or hours). The pain itself is dull, aching, crushing, or burning. Surgical treatment is not effective in atypical facial pain and its etiology remains obscure, though it may be associated with depression.

Trigeminal neuralgia is most effectively treated with carbamazepine at 800 mg/d to 1200 mg/d, in four divided doses. However, dosing should be titrated to effect, and doses producing serum levels above the therapeutic range for seizure control may be needed, so long as dose-limiting side effects do not appear. Overdosage is manifested by drowsiness, dizziness, ataxia, unsteady gait, and nausea. Hepatotoxicity may occur, but is usually reversible with discontinuation. Another more rare but serious complication is aplastic anemia, and both periodic liver function testing and monitoring of the blood count are needed. In some patients, tolerance may develop over time. Baclofen is also effective in many cases, while phenytoin is less effective but may be used as adjunctive therapy. Some of the newer antiepileptic agents may also provide some relief. Surgical procedures used to treat this condition include microvascular decompression, radiofrequency ablation, and chemical gangliolysis and rhizotomy. Of these methods, radiofrequency ablation has met with the greatest success in initial treatment, though recurrence rates have not been studied carefully. As compression of the trigeminal nerve by arterial loops may play a role in some cases, posterior fossa exploration with decompression has sometimes been used for refractory cases. Other chronic masses, such as arteriovenous malformation, aneurysm, and cholesteatoma, may also cause compression of the ganglion and may be more amenable to surgical correction.

The Facial Nerve (Cranial Nerve VII)

On exiting the brain stem ventrally, near the pontomedullary junction, the facial nerve forms two divisions: the nervus intermedius and the motor root. The nervus intermedius relays afferent taste sensation from the anterior two-thirds of the tongue and also sends autonomic fibers to the submaxillary and sphenopalatine ganglia, which then innervate the salivary and lacrimal glands. The seventh cranial nerve may also relay proprioceptive impulses from the facial muscles and cutaneous sensation from the posteromedial surface of the pinna and the external auditory canal.

Lesions near the origin of the nerve, or in the vicinity of the geniculate ganglion, are accompanied by loss of motor, gustatory, and autonomic functions. Lesions between the geniculate ganglion and the origin of the chorda tympani, typically spare lacrimation, whereas lesions near the stylomastoid foramen spare taste and lacrimation, causing only ipsilateral facial paralysis of the upper and lower face. Lesions of the facial nerve nucleus in the brain stem also cause ipsilateral paralysis of all facial muscles, both upper and lower.

The pattern of peripheral or nuclear injury (the peripheral seventh-nerve lesion) must be distinguished from that associated with central motor pathway lesions above the level of the nucleus, which cause weakness and paralysis in the lower half of the face while sparing forehead wrinkling, because of the redundancy of the central pathways subserving the muscles of the upper face (the central seventh-nerve lesion, a supranuclear palsy). In supranuclear lesions, voluntary contractions of the face differ, being more or less intense, from those occurring during spontaneous emotional expression, particularly when accompanied by laughing or crying. Depending upon the precise site and extent of associated injury within the CNS, other neurologic signs may also appear.

Owing to this anatomic organization, the signs of peripheral facial nerve injury are somewhat variable. More severe injury produces obvious facial paralysis at rest, with sagging of the muscles of the lower ipsilateral face. The normal folds and lines around the lips, nose, and forehead are attenuated, the palpebral fissure is wider than normal, and voluntary movement of the facial and platysmal muscles is completely absent. Attempted smile contrasts normal activation of the unaffected orbicularis oris with the droop of the affected side. Although weakness of both the upper and lower halves of the face is seen, occasionally the lower muscles may be weaker than the upper, or more rarely, the upper muscles may be weaker than the lower, with partial nerve injury. Saliva may seep from the paralyzed side of the mouth at rest, and food or fluids may leak out when eating. Closure of the eyelid is incomplete, and the upward and inward deviation of the eye may be seen during examination when eye closure is attempted (Bell phenomenon). This common complication assumes great importance, as early patching and lubrication of the affected eye after seventh-nerve injury is critical to prevent corneal desiccation with permanent scarring. Actual tear production is diminished only if the lesion is proximal to the geniculate ganglion. With lesions peripheral to the ganglion, lacrimation is spared but tears may still be sequestered in the conjunctival sac because incomplete eyelid closure no longer moves them effectively through the lacrimal duct. The corneal reflex is also impaired by paralysis of the upper lid, though preservation of corneal sensation and the afferent portion of the reflex is confirmed by consensual blinking of the contralateral eyelid, during corneal-reflex testing. Decreased salivation and loss of taste in the anterior two-thirds of the tongue are present when the chorda tympani is affected. Loss of somatic sensation to the external auditory canal, however, is less common. The seventh nerve also supplies the stapedius muscle and patients may develop increased sensitivity to loud sounds (i.e., hyperacusis) when it is paralyzed and its dampening effect on the tympanic membrane is lost. Recovery from facial paralysis depends on the severity of the lesion and also on its specific cause. If the nerve is completely crushed or severed, the chances of even partial recovery are remote because even the intraneural scaffolding necessary to guide axonal regeneration properly is lost. In contrast, with purely demyelinative lesions without axonal injury, excellent and often complete recovery is the rule. When the facial nerve attempts to regenerate through proximal axonal growth across an injured segment, axonal extension sometimes results in aberrant reinnervation. This faulty circuit results in the movement of previously unrelated facial muscles when the patient attempts isolated activation of a separate muscle, a process known as *synkinesis*. In such patients, for example, a slight twitch of the labial muscles may occur with each blink of the eyes. Aberrant reinnervation may also cause excessive lacrimation during activation of the facial muscles, or when the salivary glands are activated during eating (e.g., producing "crocodile tears"). In addition, some patients develop paroxysmal clonic contractions of the hemi-facial muscles (i.e., hemifacial spasm; see below) that may simulate focal seizures

Bell Palsy

Bell palsy is a clinical syndrome of uncertain etiology in which acute, unilateral paresis, or paralysis of muscles innervated by the facial nerve appears spontaneously, over hours to days, and is the most common cause of facial-nerve injury. It occurs at all ages but is slightly more common in the third to fifth decades, and is equally likely to affect the right or left sides. Recurrence, either on the same or on the opposite side, is rare and raises the question of a more generalized disorder. Familial Bell palsy has been reported, but is also extremely unusual. Risk factors have not been well defined, though many patients report exposure of the affected side to a steady breeze or fan for several hours just prior to onset. Pain is not typical except in the Ramsay Hunt syndrome, which is caused by herpes zoster and is usually accompanied by vesicular eruption in the sensory distribution of the seventh nerve in the ear ipsilateral to the facial paralysis. The prognosis of facial nerve injury after Bell palsy has also been the focus of much discussion. Nerve conduction studies (NCS) of the extracranial portion of the facial nerve may be performed, along with needle recordings from its myotomes (e.g., facial-muscle EMG) to help determine the nature and degree of injury. Injury to the intracranial portion sometimes also may be detected by electrical blink-reflex testing, as well as with the use of long-latency late responses, in which an impulse is sent retrograde up the motor nerve and rebounds in the anterior horn-cell pool to cause a small, but recordable response in the muscle. In general, preservation of motor amplitudes on NCS after 7 to 10 days supports axonal continuity (i.e., consistent with a principally demyelinating lesion) and suggests a good prognosis for recovery. In contrast, rapid loss of motor amplitudes following acute injury suggests more axonal involvement and poorer odds for functional improvement. Needle EMG examina-

tion may also aid in detecting denervation change supporting axonal injury. Though permanent deficits may occur in severe cases, the vast majority of patients with Bell palsy experience full, functional recovery, with minimal to no residual signs. Inflammation, herpes simplex virus infection, and swelling with compression may be involved in the pathogenesis of Bell palsy, so steroids, antiviral medication (acyclovir) and surgical decompression have been advocated as acute therapy. A practice parameter on therapy of Bell palsy, prepared by the Quality Standards Subcommittee of the American Academy of Neurology, reviewed the literature supporting each of these interventions, rating steroids probably effective and acyclovir possibly effective, but the quality of the studies assessing surgical treatment was insufficient to draw any conclusions regarding its effectiveness. Most practitioners now administer brief courses of both steroids and acyclovir to patients in the acute phase, as the risks of such therapy are very low.

Other Causes of Facial Nerve Injury

Many other processes may significantly damage the facial nerve. Intracranially, it may be injured by tumors, aneurysms, meningeal infections, leukemia, osteomyelitis, herpes zoster, Paget disease, sarcomas, and bony tumors, among others. It may also be damaged by leprous polyneuritis, Guillain-Barré syndrome, and diphtheritic polyneuropathy. Diabetic seventh-nerve lesions may also occur, but are less common than other cranial mononeuropathies in that disorder. The peripheral segment of the nerve may be compressed by tumors of the parotid gland, sarcoidosis, and more rarely, mumps. Bilateral facial palsy also may be caused by many of the same conditions producing unilateral paralysis, but is most often seen in sarcoidosis, Guillain-Barré syndrome, leprosy, leukemia, and meningococcal meningitis. The facial nucleus, itself, may be damaged by vascular lesions, MS, intraparenchymal tumors, inflammatory lesions, and acute poliomyelitis, among others. The relatively superficial peripheral branches of the seventh nerve are vulnerable to stab and gunshot wounds, cuts, and in neonates, birth trauma. Occasionally, the nerve is also injured in surgeries involving the mastoid and parotid glands, acoustic neuroma resection, and trigeminal ganglion decompression, as well as in fractures of the temporal bone.

Cases of facial nerve injury with a specific, identifiable cause may require aggressive intervention. Microsurgical anastomosis may be performed in some cases of transection of the extracranial nerve or its branches. However, when the nerve is damaged proximal to the stylomastoid foramen, such anastamosis becomes more difficult. Surgery may still be indicated, however, if a mass lesion is found before excessive damage is done. In cases of partial or inaccessible intracranial facial-nerve injury, compensatory surgical reinnervation may be provided by suturing the distal portion of the seventh nerve to the central portion of either the eleventh nerve or the twelfth nerve. With rehabilitative training, these patients may learn to reroute impulses formerly destined for the sternocleidomastiod muscle, or half of the tongue, to the newly rewired facial musculature. However, use of the eleventh nerve for this procedure causes permanent paralysis of the sternocleidomastoid and upper fibers of the trapezius muscle, while use of the twelfth nerve causes atrophy and paralysis of one-half of the tongue. Anastomosis of the facial nerve with either the eleventh or the twelfth nerve should be performed as soon as possible following acute injury, such as with surgical misadventure by surgery of the mastoid or removal of an acoustic neuroma, for instance. In other situations, surgery may need to be delayed for up to 6 months or more to determine whether spontaneous regeneration occurs.

Hemifacial Spasm

Hemifacial spasm is characterized by clonic spasms of the facial muscles, usually starting around the eye and often spreading to other muscles of one side of the face. It increases in intensity during stress and may occur during sleep. EMG needle recordings of the facial muscles reveal regular or irregular bursts of muscle activation, occurring at 5 Hz to 20 Hz.

Unlike facial myokymia, hemifacial spasm is not typically associated with a more severe underlying disease, but the cosmetic effects may be distressing. It often occurs spontaneously, but may follow facial-nerve trauma or Bell palsy and its pathophysiology remains obscure. Ephaptic transmission from aberrant reinnervation may play a role, and may occur at several locations along the course of the nerve, including the pontocerebellar angle, inside the petrous bone, and extracranially. Treatment with antiepileptic drugs, such as carbamazepine, may help control these symptoms. Botulinum toxin is also effective and widely available. Surgical therapy may be needed in severe, refractory cases and involves chemical neurolysis of the facial nerve through injection, or partial section, when the spasms are localized. These operations occasionally give permanent relief but in most cases, the spasms recur when the nerve regenerates. Permanent relief usually results with section of the seventh nerve and reanastomosis of with the eleventh or twelfth cranial nerve; occasionally hemifacial spasm may arise as a complication of such reanastamoses when they are performed to alleviate permanent facial weakness after Bell palsy.

The Acoustic Nerve (Cranial Nerve VIII)

Eighth nerve disorders are described in Chapter 6.

The Glossopharyngeal Nerve (Cranial Nerve IX)

The ninth cranial nerve contains both motor and sensory fibers. The motor fibers supply the stylopharyngeus muscle and the constrictors of the pharynx, while other efferent fibers innervate secretory glands in the pharyngeal mucosa. The sensory fibers carry general sensation from the upper part of the pharynx, and the special sensation of taste from the posterior one-third of the tongue. Isolated lesions of the nerve, or its nuclei, are rare and are not accompanied by perceptible disability. Taste is lost on the posterior one-third of the tongue, and the gag reflex is absent on the side of the lesion. Injuries of the ninth nerve by infections or tumors are rarely isolated, and are usually accompanied by signs of injury to nearby cranial nerves. As the ninth, tenth and eleventh nerves exit the jugular foramen together, tumors at that point produce multiple cranial-nerve palsies (i.e., *jugular foramen syndrome*). Within the brain stem, the tractus solitarius receives taste fibers from both the seventh and the ninth nerves and is commonly injured by vascular or neoplastic lesions in the brain stem.

Glossopharyngeal Neuralgia

Glossopharyngeal neuralgia (i.e., tic douloureux of the ninth nerve) is characterized by paroxysms of excruciating pain in the region of the tonsils, posterior pharynx, back of the tongue, and middle ear. The cause of glossopharyngeal neuralgia is unknown, and no significant pathologic changes occur in most cases. Pain in the distribution of the nerve occasionally follows injury of the nerve in the neck, by tumors. Glossopharyngeal neuralgia is rare, with a frequency of approximately 5% that of trigeminal neuralgia. The paroxysms consist of burning or stabbing pain and may occur spontaneously, but are often precipitated by swallowing, talking, or touching the tonsils or posterior pharynx. The attacks usually last only a few seconds but sometimes may last several minutes, and they may occur many times daily, or once every few weeks. Patients may become emaciated because of the fear that chewing each morsel of food will precipitate a pain paroxysm; general quality of life may be seriously affected, especially in severe cases.

The diagnosis of glossopharyngeal neuralgia may often be made by history, and may be confirmed by provocative testing (e.g., precipitation by stimulation of the tonsils, posterior pharynx, or base of the tongue) or by transient relief of pain following the application of topical anesthetic to the ninth-nerve dermatome. Following this procedure, the pain may no longer be precipitated by stimulation, and the patient may swallow food, and talk without discomfort, until the anesthetic wears off. The differential diagnosis is highly limited, but includes neuralgia of the mandibular branch of the fifth nerve. There may be long remissions, during which pain may no longer be triggered. The pains usually recur, however, unless prevented by medical therapy or surgical resection of the nerve. Carbamazepine, alone or in combination with phenytoin, may provide effective control and induce a pharmacologic remission. The newer antiepileptic drugs such as neurontin, topiramate, and lamotrigine might also be effective.

If medical therapy is unsuccessful, intracranial transection of the nerve may provide relief. Following this procedure, the mucous membrane supplied by the ninth nerve is permanently anesthetized, with ipsilateral loss of the gag reflex and ipsilateral loss of taste on the posterior one-third of the tongue. Motor symptoms, such as dysphagia or dysarthria, are not typical unless the tenth nerve is injured during surgery.

The Vagus Nerve (Cranial Nerve X)

Efferent fibers of the vagus nerve arise from both the nucleus ambiguous and the dorsal-motor nucleus. Fibers from the nucleus ambiguous ultimately innervate the somatic muscles of the pharynx and larynx, while those from the dorsal motor nucleus supply autonomic innervation to the heart, lungs, esophagus, and stomach. The vagus nerve also relays sensory fibers, from the mucosa in the oropharynx and upper part of the gastrointestinal tract to the spinal nucleus of the trigeminal nucleus, and relays sensory fibers from the thoracic and abdominal organs to the tractus solitarius. Central lesions of the above nuclei in the brain stem cause a number of symptoms. Unilateral lesions of the nucleus ambiguus result in dysarthria and dysphagia, though rarely is the condition severe. However, because the nucleus has a considerable longitudinal extent in the medulla, such lesions may produce dysarthria without dysphagia, or vice versa (i.e., caudal nuclear lesions cause dysphagia, whereas rostral lesions produce dysarthria). Hoarseness may also occur, but speech is usually intelligible. Dysphagia is usually slight, although occasionally a more severe transient aphagia necessitates the use of a feeding tube for days to weeks. On examination, contraction of the palatal muscles is absent on the affected side, during gag-reflex testing. The palate on the affected side is lax at rest, and the uvula deviates to the opposite side on phonation, drawn away from the paralyzed muscles by normal, contralateral, palatal contraction (i.e., contralateral uvular deviation).

In contrast to the mild deficits typically seen with unilateral lesions, bilateral lesions of the nucleus ambiguous cause complete aphonia and aphagia. Focused bilateral injury of this type is rare, but may be seen in advanced ALS. Selective destruction of portions of the nucleus ambiguus may been produced by syringobulbia, intramedullary tumors, or ischemia, and may cause a clinical syndrome of vocal-cord paralysis during adduction. The patient may talk and swallow without difficulty, but inspiratory stridor and dyspnea may appear and progress sufficiently to re-

quire tracheotomy. Unilateral lesions of the dorsal-motor nucleus are not accompanied by any significant symptoms, but bilateral lesions may produce life-threatening autonomic instability. The dorsal nucleus may be damaged by infection (e.g., acute poliomyelitis), intramedullary tumor, ischemia, and polyneuropathy, especially that associated with diphtheria and Guillain-Barré syndrome. Injury to the pharyngeal branches of the vagus nerve causes dysphagia, while lesions of the superior laryngeal nerve produce anesthesia of the upper part of the larynx and paralysis of the cricothyroid muscle. In these cases, the voice is weak and easily fatigueable. Injury to a single, recurrent laryngeal nerve (i.e., frequently seen with aneurysms of the aorta and occasionally after operations in the neck) causes unilateral paralysis of the vocal cords, with hoarseness and dysphonia; bilateral injury causes complete vocal-cord paralysis, with aphonia and inspiratory stridor. Partial bilateral paralysis may produce a paralysis of both abductors, with severe dyspnea and inspiratory stridor, but does not usually cause any alteration in the voice.

The Spinal Accessory Nerve (Cranial Nerve XI)

The spinal portion of the accessory nerve innervates the sternocleidomastoid and part or all of the trapezius muscles. Its fibers originate in the upper-cervical spinal cord (C2, C3, and C4), enter the skull via the foramen magnum, and travel through the jugular foramen along the carotid artery, to innervate the sternocleidomastoid (SCM) muscle. Another branch emerges in the mid-SCM at its posterior border, and crosses the posterior triangle of the neck to innervate the upper trapezius.

Lesions of the spinal portion of the eleventh nerve produce weakness and atrophy of the trapezius muscle, impairing rotary movements of the neck and chin to the opposite side, and weakness of shrugging movements of the shoulder. Weakness of the upper portion of the trapezius results in winging of the scapula, which must be differentiated from that produced by weakness of the serratus anterior. Scapular winging from weakness of the trapezius is present at rest (e.g., arms at side) and becomes worse on abduction of the shoulder. Scapular winging from weakness of the serratus anterior is negligible at rest and worsens during flexion of the shoulder. The accessory, or cranial portion of the nerve originates in the nucleus ambiguous and passes through the jugular foramen with the tenth nerve, traveling with the spinal fibers (see above), eventually innervating the larynx, and functionally, is considered by some to be a part of the vagus-nerve complex.

The nucleus of the eleventh nerve may be destroyed by infections and degenerative disorders in the medulla, such as syringobulbia or amyotrophic lateral sclerosis. The nerve itself may be injured by polyneuropathy, meningeal infection, extramedullary tumor (e.g., meningioma and neurinoma) or by destructive processes in the occipital bone. It is particularly vulnerable to damage during lymph-node biopsy, cannulation of the internal jugular vein, or carotid endarterectomy along its course, in the posterior triangle of the neck.

The Hypoglossal Nerve (Cranial Nerve XII)

The hypoglossal nerve emerges from the medulla between the ventrolateral sulcus, between the olive and the pyramids, as a number of rootlets that converge into the hypoglossal nerve. The nerve then exits the cranium through the hypoglossal foramen in the posterior cranial fossa, traveling close to cranial nerves IX, X, and XI and passing downward, near the inferior ganglion of the vagus, to lie between the internal carotid artery and internal jugular vein. It then crosses laterally to the bifurcation of the common carotid artery, and loops above the hyoid bone, before moving ventrally to supply the genioglossus and other muscles of the tongue. The twelfth nerve and its nucleus may be injured by most of the same processes that damage the tenth and eleventh nuclei. Occlusions of the short branches of the basilar artery supplying the paramedian medulla cause paralysis of the tongue on one side, and paralysis of the arm and leg on the opposite side (i.e., alternating hemiplegia). Unilateral injury to the nucleus results in atrophy and paralysis of the muscles of one-half of the tongue, causing deviation toward the paralyzed side, with protrusion.

Fibrillation of the muscles is seen with chronic injury to the hypoglossal nerve or its nucleus in syringobulbia or ALS, and may be observed as miniscule twitching of the surface of the tongue, on visual inspection. Bilateral paralysis of the nucleus or nerve produces atrophy of both sides of the tongue, and paralysis of all movements, with severe dysarthria and difficulty manipulating food while eating. The tongue is only rarely affected by supranuclear lesions within the CNS; unilateral weakness may accompany severe hemiplegia, with slight deviation of the tongue to the paralyzed side, when protruded. Moderate weakness of the tongue may accompany pseudobulbar palsy, but is never as severe as that caused by destruction of both medullary nuclei.

PERIPHERAL NERVE INJURY

Individual peripheral nerves may be injured by anatomic compression, trauma (e.g., lacerations, perforating injury, fractures of nearby bones, stretch, etc.), and ischemia, among other causes. They may also be involved in syndromes of multiple mononeuropathy, such as those seen in vasculitis and diabetes mellitus. Diffuse injury of the peripheral nerves, or polyneuropathy, also may sometimes include disproportionate injury to a specific nerve. The hereditary and acquired polyneuropathies are discussed in detail in Chapters 104, 105, and 106. Among the peripheral nerves, the median, ulnar, and radial nerves of the arm, and the common peroneal nerve in the leg, are prone to compressive injury, either from external pressure or anatomic compression. The axillary nerve may be damaged by shoulder dislocation. The sciatic and femoral nerves are less commonly affected by external compression, but may be damaged in association with pelvic and hip trauma, and the direct injection of drugs.

UPPER EXTREMITY NERVE INJURY

The Spinal Roots and Brachial Plexus

At each cervical spinal level, numerous rootlets containing both motor and sensory fibers join after leaving the spinal cord, to form the spinal roots that exit the spinal canal through the intervertebral foramen of the spinal column, immediately branching into anterior and posterior rami. The nerve roots are commonly injured by degenerative-joint disease and disc herniation at the cervical and lumbosacral levels. Importantly, the dorsal-root ganglia (i.e., the cell bodies of the sensory nerves) are located outside the foramen and are spared in foraminal compression, meaning the remainder of the sensory nerve will remain viable and will appear normal on nerve conduction studies, even though it is disconnected from the CNS, and the patient reports numbness and pain. Before going on to form the brachial plexus, the C5 nerve root gives off a proximal branch, the *dorsal scapular nerve* (to the rhomboid muscles), while the C5, C6, and C7 roots give proximal branches that join to form the *long thoracic nerve*, supplying the serratus anterior muscle. The C5 and C6 roots then join to form the *upper trunk* of the brachial plexus, while the C7 root forms the *middle trunk*, and the C8 and T1 roots form the *lower trunk*. The upper trunk gives off a small branch, the *suprascapular* nerve, which supplies the supra- and infraspinatus muscles. All trunks pass through the supraclavicular fossa, under the cervical and scalene muscles. Each trunk then forms two branches and these branches regroup to form new divisions, the cords, as they course through the *thoracic outlet*, between the first rib and the clavicle, along with the subclavian artery. The lateral branches of the upper and middle trunks contribute to the *lateral cord* (i.e., C5, C6, C7), while the medial branches join with the lateral branch of the lower trunk, and move dorsally to form the *posterior cord* (i.e., C5, C6, C7, C8). Finally, the lower trunk gives rise to the *medial cord* (i.e., C8, T1). The *lateral and medial pectoral nerves* branch off near the juncture of the trunks and the lateral and medial cords, respectively, supplying the pectoralis major muscle.

The *thoracodorsal nerve* that supplies the latissimus dorsi, and the *subscapular* nerve that supplies the teres major, each branch medially off the posterior cord. The posterior cord persists distally, becoming the *radial nerve*,

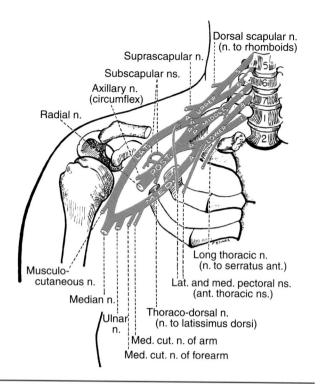

FIGURE 69.2. The brachial plexus. (From Haymaker W., Woodhall B. *Peripheral Nerve Injuries.* Philadelphia: WB Saunders, 1945; with permission.)

after giving off a smaller lateral branch, the *axillary nerve,* which supplies the deltoid. The lateral and medial cords then each contribute a branch to form the *median nerve,* composed of the medial branch of the lateral cord and the lateral branch of the medial cord, joined in the middle of the plexus. The lateral branch of the lateral cord persists distally, becoming the *musculocutaneous nerve,* while the medial branch of the medial cord becomes the *ulnar nerve* (Fig. 69.2; Table 69.2; Table 69.3)

The brachial plexus may be injured by traumatic, neoplastic, infectious and other processes. Careful history and neurologic examination, in concert with a detailed understanding of plexus anatomy, is the first step in recognizing plexus injury and differentiating it from injury to the nerve roots or peripheral nerves. Electrophysiologic assessment with electromyography and nerve conductions is often critical in confirming the diagnosis, and imaging studies may also be indicated. Mixed syndromes of radicular-plexus and peripheral nerve injury may also occur, making localization even more challenging. However, in these cases it is highly important to recognize the full spectrum of nerve injury contributing to the patient's symptoms, to ensure appropriate diagnosis and treatment. The roots or trunks of the brachial plexus may be damaged by lacerations, gunshot wounds or direct trauma. They may be compressed by tumors or aneurysms, or stretched and torn by violent movements of the shoulder

▶ **TABLE 69.2** **Innervation of the Muscles of the Shoulder Girdle**

Muscle	*Nerve*	*Spinal Nerve Roots*
Sternocleidomastoid	Accessory	X-1, C-2, C-3
Trapezius	Accessory	C-3, C-4
Serratus anterior	Long thoracic	C-5, C-7
Levator scapulae	Dorsal scapular	C-5, C-6
Rhomboideus major	Dorsal scapular	C-5, C-6
Rhomboideus minor	Dorsal scapular	C-5, C-6
Subclavius	Subclavian	C-5, C-6
Supraspinatus	Suprascapular	C-5, C-6
Infraspinatus	Suprascapular	C-5, C-6
Pectoralis major	Medial and lateral pectoralis	C-5, C-6
Pectoralis minor	Medial pectoralis	C-5, C-6
Teres major	Subscapular	C-5, C-6
Latissimus dorsi	Thoracodorsal	C-6, C-7
Subscapularis	Subscapular	C-5, C-6
Deltoid	Axillaris	C-5, C-6
Teres minor	Axillaris	C-5, C-6

in falls, dislocation of the shoulder, carrying heavy loads on or over the shoulder, and by traction during birth. The syndromes of the roots and trunks cause deficits principally in the distribution of the affected nerve roots. Partial paralysis and incomplete sensory loss are common because many muscles of the arm receive innervation from two or more roots. Compression at the level of the thoracic

▶ **TABLE 69.3** **Innervation of Muscles of the Arm and Forearm**

Muscle	*Nerve*	*Root*
Biceps brachii / Brachialis	Musculocutaneous	C-5, C-6
Triceps	Radialis	C-7, C-8
Anconeus	Radialis	C-7, C-8
Brachioradialis	Radialis	C-5, C-6
Extensor carpi radialis	Radialis	C-6, C-7
Pronator teres	Medianus	C-6, C-7
Flexor carpi radialis	Medianus	C-7, C-8
Palmaris longus	Medianus	C-7, C-8
Flexor digitorum sublimis	Medianus	C-7, C-8
Flexor digitorum profundus	Medianus, ulnaris	C-7, C-8
Flexor carpi ulnaris	Ulnaris	C-7, C-8
Supinator	Radialis	C-7, C-8
Extensor digitorum communis	Radialis	C-7, C-8
Extensor digiti minimi	Radialis	C-7, C-8
Extensor carpi ulnaris	Radialis	C-7, C-8
Abductor pollicis longus and brevis	Radialis	C-7, C-8
Extensor indicis proprius	Radialis	C-7, C-8

outlet (*thoracic outlet syndrome*) is addressed separately in Chapter 70.

Trunk and Root Injury

Upper Radicular Syndrome

Upper radicular syndrome (Erb or Erb-Duchenne palsy) results from damage to the upper roots (C4, C5 or C6) or the upper trunk. Such lesions are most commonly the result of stretch injuries during difficult deliveries, especially when forceps are used, and cause paralysis of the deltoid, biceps, brachioradialis, pectoralis major, supraspinatus, infraspinatus, subscapularis, and teres major muscles in varying combinations. If the lesion is near the roots, the serratus, rhomboids, and levator scapulae are also paralyzed. Clinically, this causes weakness of flexion at the elbow and of abduction and internal and external rotation of the arm. There is also weakness or paralysis of apposition of the scapula and backward-inward movements of the arm. Sensory loss is incomplete and consists of hypesthesia on the outer surface of the arm and forearm. The biceps reflex is absent. Unless treated by passive range-of-motion exercise, these patients may develop chronic contractures with the arm extended at the side, fully adducted, and pronated, with the hand flexed and facing rearward (e.g., the waiter's tip position).

Middle Radicular Syndrome

Middle radicular syndrome results from damage to the seventh cervical root (C7) or the middle trunk. Such lesions cause paralysis primarily of the muscles supplied by the radial nerve except the brachioradialis, which is entirely spared. Clinical weakness parallels that of injury to the radial nerve below the level of its branch to the brachioradialis. Sensory loss is variable and when present, is limited to hypesthesia over the dorsal surface of the forearm and the external part of the dorsal surface of the hand.

Lower Radicular Syndrome (Klumpke Palsy)

Lower radicular syndrome (Klumpke palsy) results from injury to the lower trunk or lower roots (C7-T1), which causes paralysis of the flexor carpi ulnaris, the flexor digitorum, the interossei, and the thenar and hypothenar muscles. This pattern mimics a combined lesion of the median and ulnar nerves. Clinically, a flattened or simian hand is seen, with loss of all intrinsic hand musculature, and with loss of sensation on the inner side of the arm and forearm and on the ulnar side of the hand. The triceps reflex is abolished. If the communicating branch to the inferior cervical ganglion is injured, there is paralysis of the sympathetic nerves, causing the Horner syndrome.

Cord Injury

Lesions of the cords cause motor and sensory loss resembling that seen after injury to two or more peripheral nerves. *Lateral cord* injury causes weakness in the distribution of the musculocutaneous nerve and the lateral head of the median nerve, including weakness in the pronator teres, almost complete paralysis of the flexor carpi radialis, and weakness of the flexor pollicis and opponens. *Posterior cord* injury causes weakness paralleling that resulting from combined damage to the radial and axillary nerves, while *medial cord* injury mimics combined damage to the ulnar nerve and the medial head of the median nerve (finger-flexion weakness).

Diffuse Plexus Injury

Generalized injury to the brachial plexus is usually unilateral, but occasionally appears bilaterally. Such injury result from a more diffuse polyneuropathy, such as chronic inflammatory demyelinating neuropathy, or from multifocal motor neuropathy. A variety of insults may produce injury selectively affecting the brachial plexus, but tumor infiltration, radiation plexitis, and idiopathic plexitis are among the most important. Almost any neoplasm with a propensity for the chest may affect the plexus, but those cancers originating locally, such as lung and breast cancer, are most likely to cause injury. Such tumors may cause extrinsic compression of the plexus as they grow, or may directly infiltrate the nervous tissue. Other neoplasms, such as lymphoma, may infiltrate the plexus and cause progressive deficits, without any apparent mass effect or enlargement of the plexus itself in the initial stages. MRI with contrast is the best way to confirm these lesions.

Idiopathic brachial plexitis (also known as the *Parsonage-Turner syndrome* or *neuralgic amyotrophy*) usually begins with a sudden, sharp pain affecting one shoulder, often with radiation down the ipsilateral arm, followed by arm or shoulder weakness. The pain persists for hours or a few days with gradual improvement, and usually resolves completely within days to weeks, leaving some sensory and motor dysfunction. Localization is often difficult, because plexus involvement ranges from diffuse to multifocal, and often includes patchy injury to the nerve branches off the plexus (e.g., the axillary nerve).

Electrodiagnostic studies, if performed at least 14 to 21 days after onset, usually may localize the injury to the plexus, but may demonstrate multifocal-plexus injury. Patterns of both axonal and demyelenative injury have been reported, and percutaneous electrical stimulation of the cervical roots and brachial plexus may reveal proximal conduction block not otherwise detectable. Although most patients recover well over 6 to 12 months, some are left with permanent disability. Although presumed autoimmune, no specific cause has been identified, and there is no evidence that immunosuppressive therapy alters the course of the disease. However, short courses of tapering oral steroids are often prescribed if the patient presents shortly after symptom onset. Variants of this syndrome have also been described, including one with isolated, pure sensory injury affecting the lateral, antebrachial, cutaneous nerves and the median nerves.

Ischemic paralysis of the arm may follow injury to the large arteries of the arm or chest. Ischemic paralysis may follow ligation of the major vessels, or prolonged constriction of the arm by plaster casts or tourniquets. In the initial stages, the distal part of the limb becomes cyanotic and edematous. Active movements of the finger and wrist muscles are possible but are of a limited range. Diminished cutaneous sensibility follows; all stimuli are poorly localized and have a painful quality. With chronic ischemia, cyanosis and edema disappear, the skin becomes atrophic (e.g., smooth and shiny), the muscles undergo fibrotic changes, and anesthesia extends in a glove-like distribution to the wrist or middle of the forearm. The hand is held extended, and the fingers are slightly flexed, except when there are associated nerve lesions. Ischemic paralysis may be differentiated from paralysis caused by lesions of the nerves by signs of vascular lesions on examination (e.g., absence of the radial pulse), the glove-like distribution of sensory loss, and the fibrous consistency of the tissues. Ischemic paralysis is often permanent, and treatment depends upon correction of the vascular insufficiency. If blood flow may not be restored primarily, symptomatic improvement may be seen in some patients by the use of hot baths, massage, passive range-of-motion exercises, and electrical stimulation.

The Proximal Nerves
The Axillary Nerve

The axillary nerve is the last branch of the posterior cord of the brachial plexus before it becomes the radial nerve. It arises from C5 and C6, supplies the deltoid muscle and transmits cutaneous sensation from a small area on the lateral surface of the shoulder. Lesions of the axillary nerve may be caused by trauma, fracture, or dislocation of the head of the humerus, and by brachial plexitis, and usually also include injury to other portions of the plexus. Lesions of the axillary nerve are characterized, primarily, by weakness of abduction of the arm at the shoulder after the first 15° to 30° of movement of the hand away from the hip. Outward, backward, and forward movements of the arm are also weakened, though less dramatically. Sensory loss is highly restricted, and usually appears only in the upper lateral arm just over the body of the mid-portion of the deltoid.

The Long Thoracic Nerve

The long thoracic nerve arises from C5, C6, and C7, and supplies the serratus anterior muscle. This nerve is most commonly injured in isolation by forceful, downward pressure on the shoulder, which stretches and compresses it. Typically, such pressure is caused by carrying excessively heavy loads on the shoulder (e.g., furniture, carpets, heavy sacks, backpacks slung over one shoulder, etc.), though it may also appear after acute impact, such as that occurring while playing football. A more archaic term, though one still in use, is hod-carrier's palsy, in reference to the hod or container bricklayers formerly placed on their shoulder to carry bricks up to roof tops when constructing chimneys. Injury of this nerve destabilizes the scapula, causing winging, and prevents the rotation of the scapula needed to enable the last few degrees of abduction of the arm from 90° to 180° over the head. Injury following acute or chronic trauma is characterized by weakness in elevation of the arm above the horizontal plane. Winging of the scapula is most prominent when the arm is fully abducted or elevated anteriorly (Fig. 69.3). Winging is often not readily apparent with the arm resting at the side.

The Brachial Cutaneous and Antebrachial Cutaneous Nerves

The brachial and antebrachial cutaneous nerves branch from the C8–T1 plexus and provide sensation to the medial arm and upper two-thirds of the forearm. These nerves are usually injured in conjunction with the medial cord of the brachial plexus, and are rarely injured in isolation. When they are damaged, sensation is lost in the above distributions.

The Suprascapular Nerve

The suprascapular nerve fibers arise in C5 and C6, ultimately branching from the upper trunk of the brachial plexus. It is primarily motor and innervates the supraspinatus and infraspinatus muscles. Clinically, patients with lesions of this nerve have difficulty moving the arm from the side through the first 15° to 30° of abduction and with external rotation of the shoulder. It is most commonly damaged in association with shoulder trauma or more diffuse injury of the brachial plexus, and isolated injury of this nerve is rare.

The Peripheral Nerves
The Radial Nerve

The radial nerve is a continuation of the posterior cord and contains elements of the C5, C6, C7, C8, and T1 nerve roots. It is predominantly a motor nerve, and innervates the chief extensors of the forearm, wrist, and fingers. It

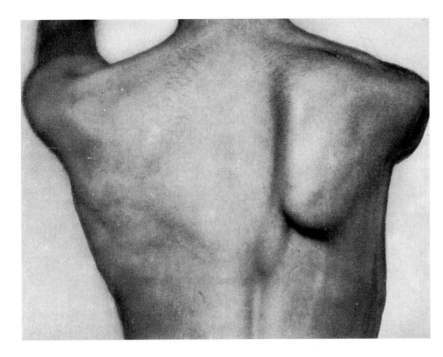

FIGURE 69.3. Paralysis of the serratus anterior muscle with winging of the scapula.

descends through the axilla to supply the triceps, giving off three minor sensory branches to the upper arm, then winds posteriorly around the humerus in the spiral groove. It exits the spiral groove and innervates the brachioradialis and extensor carpi radialis muscles, then moves laterally to enter the forearm between the brachialis and brachioradialis muscles. There, it branches into a primary sensory component, the *superficial radial nerve*, that supplies sensation to the dorso-radial aspect of the distal forearm and the dorsal surface of the hand, and a motor component, the *posterior interosseous nerve*, which supplies all the remaining forearm extensor muscles and often the supinator as well. (Table 69.4).

The clinical findings after radial nerve injury depend on the level of the lesion. Injury in the axilla, classically caused by improperly fitting crutches that are too long, causes triceps weakness as well as weakness of the remaining radial myotome and in the radial dermatomes. Injury in the spiral groove, caused by both humeral fracture and extrinsic compression (e.g., a head resting on the inner arm during sleep or honeymooners' palsy) causes weakness of the radial myotome below the elbow, with prominent wrist drop,

weakness of finger extension, and sensory loss in the distribution of the superficial radial nerve, but preserved elbow extension. Mild elbow flexor weakness may be present as a result of involvement of the brachioradialis, which should be easy to distinguish on physical examination. The posterior interosseous branch may also be injured by entrapment as it passes through the supinator muscle in the tight space of the arcade of Frohse.

In contrast to injury of the radial nerve at the spiral groove, injury of the posterior interosseous nerve spares the brachioradialis and the long end of the extensor carpi radialus, as well as the superficial radial nerve, causing radial deviation of the wrist with attempted wrist extension, but without any sensory loss (i.e., posterior interosseous nerve syndrome). Damage to the superficial radial branch may occur at the wrist, as a result of tight-fitting jewelry or handcuffs, causing pure sensory loss over the dorsum of the hand without weakness. Evaluation of radial nerve injury often includes electrodiagnostic studies and may include imaging studies, depending upon the site of the lesion. Treatment focuses on relieving the cause of compressive injury, if possible. Posterior interosseous nerve syndrome is sometimes treated with surgical release.

The Median Nerve

The median nerve derives from the C6 through T1 nerve roots, passing through the lateral and medial cords of the brachial plexus, which each contribute a segment to the nerve. The median nerve passes down the arm and through the two heads of the pronator teres, at the level of the forearm, ultimately supplying the pronator teres as well as the flexor carpi radialis, palmaris longus, and flexor digitorum

▶ **TABLE 69.4 Muscles Innervated By the Radial Nerve**

Triceps	Extensor digiti minimi
Anconeus	Extensor carpi ulnaris
Brachioradialis	Abductor pollicis longus
Extensor carpi radialis longus and brevis	Extensor pollicis longus and brevis
Supinator	Extensor indicis proprius
Extensor digitorum communis	

▶ TABLE 69.5 **Muscles Innervated by the Median Nerve**

Pronator teres	Abductor pollicis brevis
Flexor carpi radialis	Opponens pollicis
Palmaris longus	Flexor pollicis brevis
Flexor digitorum sublimis	Lumbricales (digits one and two)
Flexor digitorum profundus	
Flexor pollicis longus	
Pronator quadratus	

superficialis muscles. It then branches into the pure motor *anterior interosseous nerve*, which supplies the flexor pollicis longus, pronator quadratus, and flexor digitorum profundus I and II, and into a main branch, which passes through the carpal tunnel, further branching into the *recurrent thenar nerve*, supplying the abductor and the lateral flexor pollicis brevi and the opponens pollicis before terminating in the palm, where it supplies lumbricals I and II. Pronation is mediated by the pronator quadratus and pronator teres, wrist flexion by the flexor carpi radialis and palmaris longus, flexion of the thumb and the index and middle fingers by the superficial and deep flexors, and opposition of the thumb by the opponens pollicis (Table 69.5).

The median nerve supplies sensation to the radial side of the palm, the ventral thumb, index and middle fingers, the radial half of the ring finger, as well as the dorsal surfaces of the distal phalanx of the thumb, and the middle and terminal phalanges of the index and middle fingers. Isolated lesions of the median nerve cause weakness and sensory loss in the above distributions, but only a few movements are absolutely paralyzed because of the synergistic contributions of muscles innervated by other nerves to these movements. However, there is absence of flexion in the index finger and near complete paralysis of the opponens pollicis. The median nerve may be injured by trauma, ischemia and other processes, but most commonly is damaged by anatomic compression. It may be entrapped between the heads of the pronator teres muscle, causing weakness and sensory loss in the above distributions, with sparing of the pronator teres itself, which is innervated more proximally (i.e., the pronator teres syndrome).

Entrapment of the anterior interosseous nerve (i.e., the anterior interosseous syndrome) often presents with pain, but does not produce sensory deficits, as it is a pure motor branch. Symptoms include weakness of the flexor pollicis longus, flexor digitorum profundus I and II, and the pronator quadratus. Attempts to make the "OK" sign with the thumb and index finger produces a triangle rather than a circle (e.g., the pinch sign). The most common of all the nerve entrapment syndromes is the *carpal tunnel syndrome*. This syndrome results from entrapment of the median nerve as it passes through the tunnel defined by the carpal bones and the transverse ligament, resulting in pain and sensory loss in a median distribution, and wasting and

weakness of the median myotomes of the hand, particularly the thenar eminence. It is associated with repetitive-stress injury involving flexion/extension movements of the wrist and hand, such as typing on a keyboard or knitting, or prolonged wrist flexion. Although the diagnosis is a clinical one, electrophysiologic studies may confirm the lesion and special studies may localize the compression within one centimeter (e.g., segmental nerve conductions, or "inching"). Conservative treatment with application of a neutral position wrist splint is often effective. More severe or refractory cases, particularly those in which motor deficits appear, may be treated by surgical release of the carpal tunnel.

The Ulnar Nerve

The ulnar nerve arises from C8 and T1 roots and the medial cord of the brachial plexus. It passes between the biceps and triceps, moving posteriorly to pass behind the medial epicondyle in the ulnar groove. It enters the forearm through the cubital tunnel, supplying the flexor carpi ulnaris and the flexor digitorum profundus II and IV, then moves medially to enter the hand through Guyan's canal, where it divides into a superficial sensory branch and a deep motor branch, which supplies the abductor, opponens and flexor digiti minimi medially. It then moves laterally to the adductor pollicis and the medial half of the flexor pollicis brevis (Table 69.6).

It supplies sensation to the palmar and dorsal surfaces of the little finger, the medial half of the ring finger, and both the palmar and dorsal sides of the ulnar portion of the hand. Complete lesions of the proximal ulnar nerve are characterized by weakness of flexion and adduction of the wrist and of flexion of the ring and the little fingers, paralysis of abduction and opposition of the little finger, paralysis of adduction of the thumb, and paralysis of adduction and abduction of the fingers, along with atrophy of the hypothenar muscles and the interossei. Atrophy of the first dorsal interosseous is especially obvious on the dorsum of the hand, between the thumb and the index finger. Sensory loss is greatest in the little finger and is present to a lesser extent on the inner side of the ring finger. Chronic lesions result in clawing of the hand. The ulnar nerve may also be injured by trauma, ischemia, and other causes but like the median nerve, it is most commonly injured by anatomic

▶ TABLE 69.6 **Muscles Innervated by the Ulnar Nerve**

Flexor carpi ulnaris	All interossei
Flexor digitorum profundus (digits four and five)	Lumbricales (digits three and four)
Palmaris brevis	Flexor pollicis brevis
Abductor digiti minimi	
Opponens digiti minimi	
Flexor digiti minimi	

compression. It may become entrapped in three primary locations. The most common site of entrapment is at the elbow, in or just proximal to the ulnar groove. Moving just distally to the elbow, the nerve may become entrapped in the cubital tunnel, the tunnel formed by the aponeuroisis connecting the two heads of the flexor carpi ulnaris. Proximal nerve injury causes weakness in the ulnar myotomes of the hand, and may include the flexor carpi ulnaris (FCU) and flexor digitorum profundus (FDP) III and IV, depending on the precise site of the compression. Guyon canal stenosis, most commonly associated with a ganglion cyst, causes weakness and atrophy of the hand intrinsic muscles. Sensory symptoms may be minimal, though nerve-conduction studies to the digits are abnormal. However, the FCU and FDP III and IV are spared, along with the dorsal surface of the ulnar hand, which is innervated by the dorsal ulnar cutaneous nerve that has a more proximal origin and is normal, if tested electrophysiologically. The innervation of the muscles of the hand is summarized in Table 69.7.

The Musculocutaneous Nerve

The musculocutaneous nerve originates from the C5 and C6 nerve roots and the main branch of the upper trunk of the brachial plexus. It provides innervation to the coracobrachialis, biceps brachii, and brachialis muscles, and provides sensation to the ventrolateral forearm, as well as to a small area on the dorsolateral outer surface of the forearm. Isolated injuries of the nerve are rare and it is not typically prone to compression, though it may be involved in traumatic lesions of the brachial plexus. Lesions of the

▶ **TABLE 69.7 Innervation of Muscles of the Arm and Forearm**

Muscle	Nerve	Root
Biceps brachii } Brachialis }	Musculocutaneous	C-5, C-6
Triceps	Radialis	C-7, C-8
Anconeus	Radialis	C-7, C-8
Brachioradialis	Radialis	C-5, C-6
Extensor carpi radialis	Radialis	C-6, C-7
Pronator teres	Medianus	C-6, C-7
Flexor carpi radialis	Medianus	C-7, C-8
Palmaris longus	Medianus	C-7, C-8
Flexor digitorum sublimis	Medianus	C-7, C-8
Flexor digitorum profundus	Medianus, ulnaris	C-7, C-8
Flexor carpi ulnaris	Ulnaris	C-7, C-8
Supinator	Radialis	C-7, C-8
Extensor digitorum communis	Radialis	C-7, C-8
Extensor digiti minimi	Radialis	C-7, C-8
Extensor carpi ulnaris	Radialis	C-7, C-8
Abductor pollicis longus and brevis	Radialis	C-7, C-8
Extensor indicis proprius	Radialis	C-7, C-8

musculocutaneous nerve produce weakness of flexion and supination of the forearm, sensory loss in the musculocutaneous myotomes, and loss of the biceps reflex. Forearm flexion may still be performed by the brachioradialis muscle, innervated by the radial nerve. However, because the bicep is the chief supinator of the forearm, this movement is paralyzed.

LOWER EXTREMITY NERVE INJURY

The Spinal Roots and Lumbar and Sacral Plexi

The Lumbar Plexus

The spinal roots at L2, L3, and L4 join to form the *lumbar plexus* in the psoas major muscle. This plexus gives off a number of principally sensory nerves, including the iliohypogastric, the ilioinguinal, the genitofemoral, and the lateral femoral cutaneous. The *femoral nerve* is derived from the L2, L3, and L4 roots, passing to the anterior leg along the lateral aspect of the psoas muscle (which it supplies), exiting the pelvis, and passing under the inguinal ligament to supply the pectineus, sartorius, rectus femoris, vastus lateralis, vastus intermedius, and vastus medialis muscles. It also contributes to another pure sensory branch to the saphenous nerve.

The *obturator nerve* arises from anterior branches of the L2, L3, and L4 roots, forming in the psoas muscle and entering the pelvis anteriorly to the sacroiliac joint. It passes through the obturator canal, branching anteriorly to supply the adductor longus and brevis, and the gracilis, as well as posteriorly to supply the obturator externus, and half of the adductor magnus. It carries sensation from a small area on the inner surface of the middle side of the hip, thigh, and knee joint. A sensory anastomosis also contributes to the saphenous nerve.

The Sacral Plexus

The sacral plexus is formed from the L5, S1, and S2 roots, with variable contributions from L4. The *superior gluteal nerve* arises from the L4, L5, and S1 roots, and supplies the gluteus medius and minimus, and tensor fascia lata, while the *inferior gluteal nerve* arises from the L5 and S1 roots and supplies the gluteus maximus.

The *sciatic nerve* is formed from the posterior fusion of the L4, L5, and S1 roots, exiting the pelvis via the greater sciatic foramen. It is functionally divided into a lateral peroneal portion, which supplies the short head of the biceps femoris, and a medial tibial portion, which supplies the long head of the biceps femoris, the semitendinosus, and the semimembranosus. The sciatic enters the thigh, passing inferiorly where these segments physically divide into the common peroneal and tibial nerves.

The *common peroneal nerve* branches laterally from the sciatic trunk in the popliteal fossa, then moves superficially to wind around the head of the fibula. It then divides into the *superficial peroneal nerve* to supply the peroneus longus and peroneus brevis, and the *deep peroneal nerve*, which supplies the tibialis anterior, extensor hallucis longus, peroneus tertius and extensor digitorum brevis. The *tibial nerve* supplies the medial and lateral gastrocnemius and soleus, tibialis posterior, flexor digitorum longus, and flexor hallucis longus. It descends through the lower leg between the medial malleolus and the flexor retinaculum, dividing into the *medial plantar nerve* to supply the abductor hallucis, flexor digitorum brevis and flexor hallucis brevis, and the *lateral plantar nerve* to supply the abductor digiti minimi, flexor digiti minimi, abductor hallucis and interosseous muscles. Both the tibial and peroneal nerves supply sensory branches, which join to form the *sural nerve* below the popliteal space.

THE NERVES OF THE LEG

The Obturator Nerve

Lesions of the obturator nerve are uncommon and may be caused by pelvic tumors, obturator hernias, and by passage of the head of the fetus during difficult labor. Injuries to the obturator nerve result in severe weakness of adduction and to a lesser extent, internal and external rotation of the thigh. Pain in the knee joint is sometimes caused by pelvic involvement of the geniculate branch of the obturator.

The Iliohypogastric Nerve

The iliohypogastric nerve is a predominately sensory nerve that originates from the uppermost part of the lumbar plexus. It provides sensation to the outer and upper parts of the buttocks and the lower part of the abdomen, and supplies partial innervation to the internal oblique and transversalis muscles. Lesions of the iliohypogastric nerve are rare. It may be divided by incisions in kidney operations or together with the ilioinguinal nerve in operations in the inguinal region. Lesions of these nerves produce no significant motor loss, and only a small area of cutaneous anesthesia.

The Ilioinguinal Nerve

The ilioinguinal nerve is also a branch of the upper lumbar plexus. It provides sensation to the upper inner portion of the thigh, the pubic region, and the external genitalia, and supplies the transversalis, internal oblique, and external oblique muscles. The ilioinguinal nerve is usually injured in concert with the iliohypogastric nerve, and is only rarely injured in isolation.

The Genitofemoral Nerve

This predominately sensory nerve originates from the second lumbar root, and provides sensation to the scrotum and the contiguous area of the inner surface of the thigh. Lesions of the genitofemoral nerve are rare. Irritative lesions of the nerve in the abdominal wall are accompanied by painful hyperesthesia at the root of the thigh and the scrotum.

The Lateral Femoral Cutaneous Nerve of the Thigh

This nerve is formed by fibers from the second- and third-lumbar roots. It crosses beneath the fascia iliaca to emerge at the anterosuperior iliac spine, descends in the thigh beneath the fascia lata, and divides into two branches. The posterior branch passes obliquely backward through the fascia lata and provides sensation to the superior external buttock. The anterior branch, which is more important clinically, pierces the fascia lata through a small fibrous canal located about 10 cm below the ligament, and provides sensation to the outer surface of the thigh.

Lesions to this nerve principally affect the anterior branch, causing the clinical syndrome of *meralgia paresthetica*, and includes dysesthesias and sensory loss along the lateral thigh. The use of tight, heavy, utility belts or corsets, obesity, and pregnancy have been implicated as possible contributors to compression. Pains in the lateral thigh may also be caused by spinal lesions or pelvic tumors, which must be excluded as sources by appropriate diagnostic studies. The course of meralgia paresthetica is variable. Occasionally, symptoms disappear spontaneously, after a few weeks. In most patients, removal of contributors aids resolution of symptoms (e.g., weight loss, cessation of utility belt use).

The Femoral Nerve

The femoral nerve arises from the second-, third-, and fourth-lumbar nerves. It innervates the iliacus, psoas magnus, pectineus, sartorius, and quadriceps femoris muscles, and provides sensation to the anterior surface of the thigh, and by its internal saphenous branch, to the entire inner surface of the leg and the anteriomedial surface of the knee. The femoral nerve may be compressed by tumors and other lesions in the pelvis, or it may be injured by fractures of the pubic ramus or femur, as well as by ischemia in diabetic neuropathy and other conditions.

Injury to the nerve produces paralysis of extension of the leg and weakness of flexion of the thigh. Walking on level ground is possible so long as the leg may be kept extended, but if the slightest flexion occurs, the patient's knee may collapse. Climbing stairs or walking uphill is difficult or impossible. The quadriceps reflex is lost on the affected side. In severe cases, orthopedic appliances that fix the knee joint in extension, or tendon transposition may be considered.

The Sciatic Nerve

The main trunk of the sciatic nerve is derived from the lower lumbosacral nerve roots, and retains a strict segregation of peroneal and tibial fibers, ultimately terminating into the common peroneal and tibial nerves. The sciatic nerve innervates the semitendinosus, the long- and short-heads of the biceps, the adductor magnus, and the semimembranosus muscles. Total paralysis of muscles innervated by the sciatic nerve is rare. Even with a lesion in the thigh, the common peroneal division is often more severely damaged than the tibial.

The sciatic nerve is frequently injured by gunshot, shrapnel, or stab wounds to the leg or pelvis, and may be injured by fractures of the pelvis or femur, dislocations of the hip, pressure of the fetal head on the plexus in the mother's pelvis, or pelvic tumors. The nerve is sometimes inadvertently injured by intramuscular injection of drugs, especially in infants. *Sciatica* is a term used to describe pain in the low back and in the leg along the course of the nerve, but the vast majority of these patients have nerve root injury at the L5–S1 level, often caused by intervertebral disc herniation. The clinical features of cervical and lumbar disc herniation are considered in Chapters 67 and 68.

Complete injury of the sciatic nerve causes paralysis of all the movements of the ankle and toes, as well as weakness or paralysis of knee flexion. Gait is marked by foot drop and the ankle jerk is lost, along with sensation on the outer surface of the leg, on the instep and sole of the foot, and over the toes.

The Common Peroneal Nerve

The common peroneal branch of the sciatic nerve is a mixed nerve, innervating the extensor muscles of the ankle and toes, and the foot evertors. It provides sensation from the outer side of the leg, the front of its lower one-third, the instep, and the dorsal surface of the four inner toes over their proximal phalanges. The common peroneal nerve is highly subject to trauma. It may be damaged by wounds near the knee or in the trunk of the sciatic nerve, in the thigh. Owing to its superficial position in close relationship to the head and neck of the fibula, it is readily compressed by sitting with the legs crossed, squatting, or resting the edge of the leg against a hard surface while a patient is asleep, intoxicated, or under anesthesia. The nerve may also be injured by ganglion cysts, which usually may be palpated at the head of the fibula. Paralysis of the common peroneal nerve results in foot drop and inversion of the foot. The patient may not dorsiflex the ankle, straighten or extend the toes, or evert the foot, and there is sensory loss in the distribution of the nerve. Recovery is dependent upon the extent of injury, which usually correlates with the degree and duration of extrinsic compression. Control of foot drop during ambulation may be greatly aided by the use of ankle-foot orthoses.

The Tibial Nerve

The tibial branch of the sciatic nerve innervates the calf muscles and the plantar muscles of the foot, and provides sensation to the entire sole of the foot, the back and lower middle third of the leg, the outer dorsal surface of the foot, and the terminal phalanges of the toes. Lesions of the tibial nerve are uncommon. It may be injured by gunshot wounds or fractures of the legs. A complete lesion of the nerve is characterized by paralysis of plantar flexion and inversion of the foot, flexion and separation of the toes, and sensory loss in the distribution of the nerve. The ankle jerk and plantar reflex are lost. Rarely, compression of the posterior tibial branch of the nerve at the medial malleolus produces pain and paresthesia in the soles of the feet in a manner similar to compression of the median nerve at the wrist (*tarsal tunnel syndrome*). In severe cases, surgical decompression may be curative.

SUGGESTED READINGS
General

Aminoff MJ. *Electromyography in Clinical Practice,* 3rd ed. New York: Churchill Livingstone, 1997.
Carlson N, Logigian E. The radial nerve. *Neurolog Clin North Amer.* 1999:17;499–523.
Dyck PJ, Thomas PK, Griffin JW, Low PA, Poduslo JF, eds. *Peripheral Neuropathy,* 3rd ed. Philadelphia: WB Saunders, 1993.
Haymaker W, Woodhall B. *Peripheral Nerve Injuries,* 2nd ed. Philadelphia: WB Saunders, 1953.
Kimura J. *Electrodiagnosis in Diseases of Nerve and Muscle: Principles and Practice,* 3rd ed. Philadelphia: FA Davis Co, 2001.
Liguori R, Krarup C, Trojaborg W. Determination of the segmental sensory and motor innervation of the lumbosacral spinal nerves. *Brain* 1992;115:915–934.
Parry GJ. Electrodiagnostic studies in the evaluation of peripheral nerve and brachial plexus injuries. *Neurol Clin* 1992;10:921–934.
Petrera J, Trojaborg W. Conduction studies of the long thoracic nerve in serratus anterior palsy of different etiology. *Neurology* 1984;34:1033–1037.
Stuart JD. *Focal Peripheral Neuropathies,* 3rd ed. New York: Raven Press, 2000.
Sunderland S. *Nerves and Nerve Injuries,* 2nd ed. Edinburgh: Churchill Livingstone, 1979.
Tinel J. *Nerve Wounds: Symptomatology of Peripheral Nerve Lesions Caused by War Wounds.* London: Balliere, Tindall and Cox, 1917.

Cranial Nerves

Ashkan K, Marsh H. Microvascular decompression for trigeminal neuralgia in the elderly: a review of the safety and efficacy. *Neurosurgery* 2004 Oct;55(4):840–848.
Auger RG, Pipegras DG, Laws ER Jr. Hemifacial spasm: results of microvascular decompression of the facial nerve in 54 patients. *Mayo Clin Proc* 1986;61:640–644.
Axelsson S, Lindberg S, Stjernquist-Desatnik A. Outcome of treatment with valacyclovir and prednisone in patients with Bell's palsy. *Ann Otol Rhinol Laryngol* 2003;112(3):197–201.
Boghen DR, Glaser JS. Ischemic optic neuropathy: the clinical profile and natural history. *Brain* 1975;98:689–708.

Brin MF, Blitzer A, Stewart C, Fahn S. Treatment of spasmodic dysphonia (laryngeal dystonia) with local injections of botulinum toxin: review and technical aspects. In: Blitzer A, Brin MF, Sasaki CT, Fahn S, Harris KS, eds. *Neurological Disorders of the Larynx.* New York: Thieme Medical Publishers, 1992.

Brisman R. Trigeminal neuralgia and multiple sclerosis. *Arch Neurol* 1987;44:379–381.

Brisman R. Repeat gamma knife radiosurgery for trigeminal neuralgia. *Stereotact Funct Neurosurg* 2003;81(1-4):43–49.

Ceylan S, Karakus A, Duru S, Koca O. Glossopharyngeal neuralgia: a study of 6 cases. *Neurosurg Rev* 1997;20:196–200.

Cheuk AV, Chin LS, Petit JH, Herman JM, Fang HB, Regine WF. Gamma knife surgery for trigeminal neuralgia: outcome, imaging, and brainstem correlates. *Int J Radiat Oncol Biol Phys* 2004 Oct1;60(2):537–541.

De Diego JI, Prim MP, De Sarria MJ, et al. Idiopathic facial paralysis: a randomized, prospective, and controlled study using single-dose prednisone versus acyclovir three times daily. *Laryngoscope* 1998;108:573–575.

Dunphy EB. Alcohol-tobacco amblyopia: a historical survey. *Am J Ophthalmol* 1969;68:569–578.

Eldridge PR, Sinha AK, Javadpour M, Littlechild P, Varma TR. Microvascular decompression for trigeminal neuralgia in patients with multiple sclerosis. *Stereotact Funct Neurosurg* 2003;81(1-4):57–64.

Evidente VG, Adler CH. Hemifacial spasm and other craniofacial movement disorders. *Mayo Clin Proc* 1998;73:67–71.

Ford FR, Woodhall B. Phenomena due to misdirection of regenerating fibers of cranial, spinal and autonomic nerves: clinical observations. *Arch Surg* 1938;36:480–496.

Friedman AP, Merritt HH. Damage to cranial nerves resulting from head injury. *Bull Los Angeles Neurol Soc* 1944;9:135–139.

Fukuda H, Ishikawa M, Okumura R Demonstration of neurovascular compression in trigeminal neuralgia and hemifacial spasm with magnetic resonance imaging: comparison with surgical findings in 60 consecutive cases. *Surg Neurol* 2003;59(2):93–99.

Furuta Y, Fukuda S, Chida E, et al. Reactivation of herpes simplex virus type 1 in patients with Bell's palsy. *J Med Virol* 1998;54:162–166.

Glocker FX, Krauss JK, Deuschl G, et al. Hemifacial spasm due to posterior fossa tumors: the impact of tumor location on electrophysiological findings. *Clin Neurol Neurosurg* 1998;100:104–111.

Gouda JJ, Brown JA. Atypical facial pain and other pain syndromes: differential diagnosis and treatment. *Neurosurg Clin N Am* 1997;8:87–100.

Jankovic J, Ford J. Blepharospasm and orofacial-cervical dystonia: clinical and pharmacological findings in 100 patients. *Ann Neurol* 1983;13:402–411.

Jannetta P. Observations on the etiology of trigeminal neuralgia, hemifacial spasm, acoustic nerve dysfunction and glossopharyngeal neuralgia: definitive microsurgical treatment and results in 11 patients. *Neurochirurgie* 1977;20:145–154.

Jitpimolmard S, Tiamkao S, Laopaiboon M. Long-term results of botulinum toxin type A (Dysport) in the treatment of hemifacial spasm: a report of 175 cases. *J Neurol Neurosurg Psychiatry* 1998;64:751–757.

Juncos JL, Beal MF. Idiopathic cranial polyneuropathy: a 5-year experience. *Brain* 1987;110:197–212.

Kalovidouris A, Mancuso AA, Dillon W. A CT-clinical approach to patients with symptoms related to the V, VII, IX–XII cranial nerves and cervical sympathetics. *Radiology* 1984;151:671–676.

Kemp LW, Reich SG. Hemifacial Spasm. *Curr Treat Options Neurol* 2004 May;6(3):175–179.

Kondziolka D, Perez B, Flickinger JC, et al. Gamma knife radiosurgery for trigeminal neuralgia: results and expectations. *Arch Neurol* 1998;55:1524–1529.

Lecky BRF, Hughes RAC, Murray NMF. Trigeminal sensory neuropathy. *Brain* 1987;110:1463–1486.

Leigh RJ, Zee DS. *The Neurology of Eye Movements,* 2nd ed. Philadelphia: FA Davis Co, 1991.

Lopez BC, Hamlyn PJ, Zakrzewska JM. Stereotactic radiosurgery for primary trigeminal neuralgia: state of the evidence and recommendations for future reports. *J Neurol Neurosurg Psychiatry* 2004 Jul;75(7):1019–1024.

Lossos A, Siegal T. Numb chin syndrome in cancer patients: etiology, response to treatment, and prognostic significance. *Neurology* 1992;42:1181–1184.

Ludlow CL, Naunton RF, Fujita M, et al. Effects of botulinum toxin injections on speech in adductor spasmodic dysphonia. *Neurology* 1988;38:1220–1225.

Majoie CB, Hulsmans FJ, Castelijns JA, et al. Symptoms and signs related to the trigeminal nerve: diagnostic yield of MR imaging. *Radiology* 1998;209:557–562.

Murakami S, Nakashiro Y, Mizobuchi M, et al. Varicella-zoster virus distribution in Ramsay Hunt syndrome revealed by polymerase chain reaction. *Acta Otolaryngol* 1998;118:145–149.

Nadeau SE, Trobe JD. Pupil sparing in oculomotor palsy: a brief review. *Ann Neurol* 1983;13:143–148.

Nielsen VK. Electrophysiology of the facial nerve in hemifacial spasm: ectopic/ephaptic excitation. *Muscle Nerve* 1985;8:545–555.

Pearce JM. Melkersson's syndrome. *J Neurol Neurosurg Psychiatry* 1995;58:340.

Pollock BE, Gorman DA, Schomberg PJ, Kline RW. The Mayo Clinic gamma knife experience: indications and initial results. *Mayo Clin Proc* 1999;74:5–13.

Portenoy RK, Duma C, Foley KM. Acute herpetic and postherpetic neuralgia: clinical review and current management. *Ann Neurol* 1986;20:651–664.

Rozen TD. Trigeminal neuralgia and glossopharyngeal neuralgia. *Neurol Clin* 2004 Feb;22(1):185–206.

Rush JA, Younge BR. Paralysis of cranial nerves III, IV and VI: cause and prognosis in 1,000 cases. *Arch Ophthalmol* 1981;99:76–79.

Ryu H, Yamamoto S, Sugiyama K, et al. Hemifacial spasm caused by vascular compression of the distal portion of the facial nerve: report of seven cases. *J Neurosurg* 1998;88:605–609.

Searles RP, Mladinich K, Messner RP. Isolated trigeminal sensory neuropathy: early manifestations of mixed connective tissue disease. *Neurology* 1978;28:1286–1289.

Shaya M, Jawahar A, Caldito G, et al. Gamma knife radiosurgery for trigeminal neuralgia: a study of predictors of success, efficacy, safety, and outcome at LSUHSC. *Surg Neurol* 2004;61(6):529–534.

Spillane JD, Wells CEC. Isolated trigeminal neuropathy. *Brain* 1959;82:391–416.

Stevens H. Melkersson's syndrome. *Neurology* 1965;15:263–266.

Tan EK, Chan LL. Clinico-radiologic correlation in unilateral and bilateral hemifacial spasm. *J Neurol Sci* 2004 Jul 15;222(1–2):59–64.

Tankere F, Maisonobe T, Lamas G, et al. Electrophysiological determination of the site involved in generating abnormal muscle responses in hemifacial spasm. *Muscle Nerve* 1998;21:1013–1018.

Taylor FH. Idiopathic Bell's facial palsy: natural history defies steroid and surgical treatment. *Laryngoscope* 1985;95:406–409.

Tenser RB. Trigeminal neuralgia: mechanisms of treatment. *Neurology* 1998;51:17–19.

Troost BT, Daroff RB. The ocular motor defects in progressive supranuclear palsy. *Ann Neurol* 1977;2:397–403.

Van Zandycke M, Martin JJ, Vande Gaer L, Van den Heyning P. Facial myokymia in the Guillain-Barré syndrome: a clinicopathologic study. *Neurology* 1982;32:744–748.

Victor M, Dreyfus PM. Tobacco-alcohol amblyopia: further comments on its pathology. *Arch Ophthalmol* 1965;74:649–657.

Wang A, Jankovic J. Hemifacial spasm: clinical findings and treatment. *Muscle Nerve* 1998;21:1740–1747.

Wartenberg R. *Hemifacial Spasm: a Clinical and Pathological Study.* London: Oxford University Press, 1952.

Willoughby EW, Anderson NE. Lower cranial nerve motor function in unilateral vascular lesions of the cerebral hemisphere. *BMJ* 1984;289:791–794.

Yoshino N. Akimoto H. Yamada I, et al. Trigeminal neuralgia: evaluation of neuralgic manifestation and site of neurovascular compression with 3D CISS MR imaging and MR angiography. *Radiology* 2003;228(2):539–545.

Peripheral Nerves

Bowsher D. The management of postherpetic neuralgia. *Postgrad Med J* 1997;73:623–629.

Buchthal F, Rosenfalck A, Trojaborg W. Electrophysiological findings in entrapment of the median nerve at the wrist and elbow. *J Neurol Neurosurg Psychiatry* 1974;37:340–360.

Choi PD, Novak CB, Mackinnon SE, Kline DG. Quality of life and functional outcome following brachial plexus injury. *J Hand Surg [Am]* 1997;22:605–612.

D'Amour ML, Lebrun LH, Rabbat A, et al. Peripheral neurological complications of aortoiliac vascular disease. *Can J Neurol Sci* 1987;14:127–130.

Dawson DM. Entrapment neuropathies of the upper extremities. *N Engl J Med* 1993;329:2013–2018.

Dubinsky RM, Kabbani H, El-Chemi Z, Boutwell C, Ali H; Quality Standards Subcommittee of the American Academy of Neurology. Practice parameter: Treatment of postherpetic neuralgia: an evidence-based report of the Quality Standards Subcommittee of the American Academy of Neurology *Neurology* 2004 Sep 28;63(6):959–965.

Dubuisson A, Kline DG. Indications for peripheral nerve and brachial plexus surgery. *Neurol Clin* 1992;10:935–951.

Friedman AH, Nashold BS Jr, Ovelmen-Levitt J. Dorsal root entry zone lesions for the treatment of postherpetic neuralgia. *J Neurosurg* 1984;60:1258–1262.

Gilliatt RW. Acute compression block. In: Sumner AJ, ed. *The Physiology of Peripheral Nerve Disease.* Philadelphia: WB Saunders, 1980.

Gilliatt RW, Willison RG, Dietz V, et al. Peripheral nerve conduction in patients with a cervical rib and band. *Ann Neurol* 1978;4:124–129.

Gossett JG, Chance PF. Is there a familial carpal tunnel syndrome? An evaluation and literature review. *Muscle Nerve* 1998;21:1533–1536.

Jung BF, Johnson RW, Griffin DR, Dworkin RH. Risk factors for postherpetic neuralgia in patients with herpes zoster. *Neurology* 2004 May 11;62(9):1545–1551.

Kline DG, Kim D, Midha R, et al. Management and results of sciatic nerve injuries: a 24-year experience. *J Neurosurg* 1998;89:13–23.

Kori SH, Foley KM, Posner JB. Brachial plexus lesions in patients with cancer: 100 cases. *Neurology* 1981;31:45–50.

Liguori R, Krarup C, Trojaborg W. Determination of the segmental sensory and motor innervation of the lumbosacral spinal nerves. *Brain* 1992;115:915–934.

Mastroianni PP, Roberts MP. Femoral neuropathy and retroperitoneal hemorrhage. *Neurosurgery* 1983;13:44–47.

Miller RG. Injury to peripheral nerves. *Muscle Nerve* 1987;10:698–710.

Morris HH, Peters PH. Pronator syndrome: clinical and electrophysiological features in seven cases. *J Neurol Neurosurg Psychiatry* 1976;39:461–464.

Nakano KK, Lundergan C, Okharo MM. Anterior interosseous syndromes: diagnostic methods and alternative treatments. *Arch Neurol* 1977;34:477–480.

Oberle J, Kahamba J, Richter HP. Peripheral nerve schwannomas: an analysis of 16 patients. *Acta Neurochir (Wien)* 1997;139:949–953.

Petrera J, Trojaborg W. Conduction studies of the long thoracic nerve in serratus anterior palsy of different etiology. *Neurology* 1984;34:1033–1037.

Rempel D, Evanoff B, Amadio PC, et al. Consensus criteria for the classification of carpal tunnel syndrome in epidemiologic studies. *Am J Public Health* 1998;88:1447–1451.

Rowbotham M, Harden N, Stacey B, et al. Gabapentin for the treatment of postherpetic neuralgia: a randomized, controlled trial. *JAMA* 1998;280:1837–1842.

Seddon HJ. *Peripheral Nerve Injuries: Medical Research Council Special Report, Series No. 282.* London: Her Majesty's Stationery Office, 1954.

Thomas JE, Pipegras DG, Scheithauer B, et al. Neurogenic tumors of the sciatic nerve: a clinicopathologic study of 35 cases. *Mayo Clin Proc* 1983;58:640–647.

Trojaborg W. Rate of recovery in motor and sensory fibres of the radial nerve. *J Neurol Neurosurg Psychiatry* 1970;33:625–638.

Trojaborg W. Early electrophysiological changes in conduction block. *Muscle Nerve* 1978;1:400–403.

Watson CP, Babul N. Efficacy of oxycodone in neuropathic pain: a randomized trial in postherpetic neuralgia. *Neurology* 1998;50:1837–1841.

Watson CP, Vernich L, Chipman M, et al. Nortriptyline versus amitriptyline in postherpetic neuralgia: a randomized trial. *Neurology* 1998;51:1166–1171.

Wiles CM, Whitehead S, Ward AB, Fletcher CDM. Not tarsal tunnel syndrome: a malignant "triton" tumour of the tibial nerve. *J Neurol Neurosurg Psychiatry* 1987;50:479–482.

Wulff CH, Hansen K, Strange P, Trojaborg W. Multiple mononeuritis and radiculitis with erythema, pain, elevated CSF protein and pleocytosis (Bannwarth's syndrome). *J Neurol Neurosurg Psychiatry* 1983;46:485–490.

Brachial Plexus and Lumbosacral Plexus

Cruz-Martinez A, Barrio M, Arpa J. Neuralgic amyotrophy: variable expression in 40 patients. *J Periph Nerv Syst* 2002;7(3):198–204.

Evans BA, Stevens JC, Dyck PJ. Lumbosacral plexus neuropathy. *Neurology* 1981;31:1327–1331.

Hunermund G, Schirmacher A, Ringelstein B, et al. Genomic organization and mutation analysis of three candidate genes for hereditary neuralgic amyotrophy. *Muscle Nerve* 2004;29(4):601–604.

Lo Y-L, Mills KR: Motor root conduction in neuralgic amyotrophy: evidence of proximal conduction block. *J Neurol Neurosurgery Psychiatry* 1999;66:586–590.

Parry GJ. Electrodiagnosis studies in the evaluation of peripheral nerve and brachial plexus injuries. *Neurol Clin* 1992;10:921–934.

Seror P. Isolated sensory manifestations in neuralgic amyotrophy: Report of eight cases. *Muscle Nerve* 2004;29:134–138.

Shinder N, Polson A, Pringle E, O'Donnell DE. Neuralgic amyotrophy: a rare cause of bilateral diaphragmatic paralysis. *Can Respir J* 1998;5:139–142.

Swash M. Diagnosis of brachial root and plexus lesions. *J Neurol* 1986;233:131–135.

Thyagarajan D, Cascino T, Harms G. Magnetic resonance imaging in brachial plexopathy of cancer. *Neurology* 1995;45:421–427.

Trojaborg W. Electrophysiological finding in pressure palsy of the brachial plexus. *J Neurol Neurosurg Psychiatry* 1977;40:1160–1167.

Tsairis P, Dyck P, Mulder D. Natural history of brachial plexus neuropathy. *Arch Neurol* 1972;27:109–117.

Wouter van Es H, Engelen AM, Witkamp TD, et al. Radiation-induced brachial plexopathy: MR imaging. *Skeletal Radiol* 1997;26:284–288.

Chapter 70

▶ Thoracic Outlet Syndrome

*Lewis P. Rowland and
Louis H. Weimer*

The term *thoracic outlet syndrome* (TOS) encompasses different syndromes that arise from compression of the nerves in the brachial plexus or blood vessels (i.e., subclavian or axillary arteries, or veins in the same area). The putative compression sources are also diverse.

How often these lesions are actually responsible for symptoms and how the symptoms should be treated are matters of intense debate. Studies done mainly by orthopedists, vascular surgeons, and neurosurgeons have included reports on several hundred patients who were treated surgically for this syndrome. When neurologists write about the neurogenic form of TOS, however, the tone is always skeptical, and the syndrome is described as exceedingly rare, with an annual incidence of about 1 per 1 million persons.

PATHOLOGY

The T1 and C8 nerve roots and the lower trunk of the brachial plexus are exposed to compression and angulation by anatomic anomalies that include cervical ribs and fibrous bands of uncertain origin. Other nearby structures, such as scalene muscles, are dubious sources of compression. Cervical ribs are commonly found in asymptomatic people, and it is therefore difficult to assume that the presence of a cervical rib necessarily explains local symptoms. In addition to the neural syndromes, the same anomalies may compress local blood vessels and cause vascular syndromes, usually separated into arterial and venous entities. These conditions are also rare and may cause neurogenic symptoms by distal nerve ischemia but not pressure on the brachial plexus. Some cases follow local trauma.

SYMPTOMS AND SIGNS

Patients have pain in their shoulders, arms, and hands, or sometimes in all three locations. The hand pain is often most severe in the fourth and fifth fingers. The pain is aggravated by use of the arm and arm "fatigue" may be prominent. There may or may not be hypesthesia in the affected area.

Critics have divided cases into two groups: the *true* neurogenic thoracic outlet syndrome and the *disputed* syndrome. In the *true* syndrome, there are definite clinical and electrodiagnostic abnormalities. This disorder is rare and is almost always caused by a taut fibrous band extending from a cervical rib or abnormally elongated C7 transverse process; the band stretches the distal C8 and T1 roots or lower brachial plexus trunk. There is unequivocal wasting and weakness of hand muscles innervated by these segments. Changes are unilateral in almost all cases.

EMG and nerve conduction studies demonstrate a pattern of low-amplitude median motor, ulnar sensory, and medial antebrachial cutaneous-evoked responses. Ulnar-motor responses to hypothenar muscles may be involved to a lesser degree. EMG signs of active and chronic denervation are limited to involved muscles, most severely in the abductor pollicis brevis, and are attributed to a major contribution from T1.

In the *disputed* form, there are no objective motor or sensory signs or consistent laboratory abnormalities. Attempts to reproduce the syndrome by passive abduction of the arm (i.e., the Adson test) or other maneuvers have been cited, but the same abnormalities may be found in normal people and have no specific diagnostic value. The

diagnosis is usually made by the treating surgeon; symptoms are frequently bilateral, and complicated by legal or other nonmedical issues.

Similarly, studies of the application of electrodiagnostic techniques have not been blinded or controlled, so less specific abnormalities have been noted; the findings include isolated abnormalities of ulnar sensory-nerve amplitude, conduction velocity after stimulation of the Erb point, ulnar F-waves, and ulnar somatosensory-evoked potentials. MRI may show deviation or distortion of nerves or blood vessels, bands extending from the C7 transverse process, or other local anomalies. MRI quantitative estimates of the size of the thoracic outlet may show smaller than average dimensions, as were the cases in blinded reviews of series that compared vascular and neurogenic patients together with controls, but do not prove that the differences are causative. MRA and Doppler ultrasonography may help assess possible vascular compression.

DIAGNOSIS AND MANAGEMENT

In cases of *true* thoracic outlet syndrome, diagnosis must exclude entrapment syndromes in the arm and compressive lesions in the cervical spine. Rarely, arteriography may be indicated if there is any suggestion of a subclavian-artery aneurysm. Surgery is indicated when the diagnosis is unequivocal. Surgical methods and approaches also vary between surgeons.

In the *disputed* form, when no objective findings are noted on neurologic examination, there are problems. Each case must be evaluated separately, but caution is reasonable when symptoms are not accompanied by objective changes. Conservative therapy should be given an adequate trial; postural adjustments, passive exercise to increase mobility of shoulder muscles, and an exercise program have all been advocated. The results of surgery are difficult to evaluate without objective signs or diagnostic laboratory abnormalities to track; placebo effects are rarely considered in the evaluation of surgery. Success rates of 90% for a particular operation may be followed by equally enthusiastic reports for reoperation after the failed procedure. Symptomatic improvement also appears to be unrelated to the surgical procedure or the particular structure that has been excised or resected. Surgery is not without hazard; complications may include causalgia, injury of the long thoracic nerve, infection, and laceration of the subclavian artery.

SUGGESTED READINGS

Bhattacharya V, Hansrani M, Wyatt MG, Lambert D, Jones NA. Outcome following surgery for thoracic outlet syndrome. *Eur J Vasc Endovasc Surg* 2003;26:170–175.
Cherington M, Cherington C. Thoracic outlet syndrome: reimbursement patterns and patient profiles. *Neurology* 1992;42:943–945.

Demondion X, Bacqueville E, Paul C, et al. Thoracic outlet: assessment with MR imaging in asymptomatic and symptomatic populations. *Radiology* 2003;227:461–468.

Gilliatt RW, Le Quesne PL, Logue V, Sumner AJ. Wasting of the hand associated with a cervical rib or band. *J Neurol Neurosurg Psychiatry* 1977;33:615–624.

Gregoudis R, Barnes RW. Thoracic outlet arterial compression: prevalence in normal persons. *Angiology* 1980;31:538–541.

Kenny RA, Traynor GB, Withington D, Keegan DJ. Thoracic outlet syndrome: a useful exercise treatment option. *Am J Surg* 1993;165:282–284.

Kothari MJ, Macintosh K, Heistand M, Logigian EL. Medial antebrachial cutaneous sensory studies in the evaluation of neurogenic thoracic outlet syndrome. *Muscle Nerve* 1998;21:647–649.

LeForestier N, Moulonguet A, Maisonobe T, et al. True neurogenic thoracic outlet syndrome: electrophysiological diagnosis in six cases. *Muscle Nerve* 1998;21:1129–1134.

Levin KH, Wilbourn AJ, Maggiano HJ. Cervical rib and median sternotomy-related brachial plexopathies: a reassessment. *Neurology* 1998;50:1407–1413.

Maxey TS, Reece TB, Ellman PI, et al. Safety and efficacy of the supraclavicular approach to thoracic outlet decompression. *Ann Thorac Surg* 2003;76:396–399.

Panegyres PK, Moore N, Gibson R, Rushworth G, Donaghy M. Thoracic outlet syndromes and magnetic resonance imaging. *Brain* 1993;116:823–841.

Roos DB. Thoracic outlet syndrome is underdiagnosed. *Muscle Nerve* 1999;22:126–129.

Smith T, Trojaborg W. Diagnosis of thoracic outlet syndrome. *Arch Neurol* 1987;44:1161–1166.

Stalberg E, Incesu L, Basoglu A. Bilateral neurogenic thoracic outlet syndrome. *MuscleNerve* 2004;29(1):147–150.

Tilki HE, Stalberg E, Incesu L, Basoglu A. Bilateral neurogenic thoracic outlet syndrome. *Muscle Nerve* 2004;29:147–150.

Veilleux M, Stevens JC, Campbell JK. Somatosensory evoked potentials: lack of value for diagnosis of thoracic outlet syndrome. *Muscle Nerve* 1988;11:571–575.

Wilbourn AJ. Thoracic outlet syndrome is overdiagnosed. *Muscle Nerve* 1999;22:130–136.

Chapter 71

▶ Neuropathic Pain

Clifton L. Gooch

At once, neuropathic pain is a bane for its victims, clinically counterintuitive and scientifically fascinating. Damage to any level of the sensory pathway, from the small nerve fibers to the sensory cortex, may produce pain, in addition to numbness, and this large category includes some of the most agonizing of human afflictions. In this chapter we will review the normal neurologic processing of pain, the mechanisms underlying neurogenic pain, its clinical features, and the broad range of its pharmacologic therapies, with a particular emphasis on painful polyneuropathy.

DEFINITIONS

Pain is an unpleasant sensory and emotional experience associated with actual or potential tissue damage or described in terms of such damage. Acute pain clearly serves a protective function and is frequently the decisive factor prompting a patient to seek medical care. However, when it persists after recovery from injury, it may become the primary problem. Chronic pain is defined as long-term pain that invades patients' lives and affects their behaviors, work, daily tasks, emotional states, and social interactions. Chronic pain may follow lesions at virtually any level of the neuraxis, including peripheral nerves, dorsal roots, spinal cord, brain stem, subcortex, and cortex.

Neurogenic pain is defined as pain resulting from noninflammatory dysfunction of the peripheral nervous system or CNS, without peripheral nociceptor stimulation or trauma. It must be distinguished from primary nociceptive pain, which arises when the process injuring tissue stimulates pain receptors. *Deafferentation pain* follows interruption of the primary afferent nociceptive pathways at any point, though this term most often refers to syndromes following CNS injury.

Neuropathic pain, in contrast, usually refers to pain associated with peripheral nervous system injury. This general term is often used, synonymously, with *painful polyneuropathy*, although it also encompasses pain syndromes that follow focal peripheral-nerve injury. *Neuralgia* refers more specifically to pain in the distribution of a single peripheral nerve.

Other clinical syndromes with neurogenic pain include the *complex regional pain syndromes* (CPRS). CPRS I was formerly known as *reflex sympathetic dystrophy*, and CPRS II was formerly *causalgia*. Some neurogenic pain syndromes are so unique that they have individual designations, including thalamic pain syndrome, trigeminal neuralgia, and post-herpetic neuralgia.

THE NORMAL PROCESSING OF PAIN

Peripheral Nociception

Following noxious chemical, mechanical, or thermal stimulation, transduction occurs at the peripheral sensory-nerve terminal through a poorly understood process, causing depolarization of the distal nerve fibers and transmission of nociceptive impulses up the sensory axons to the dorsal-root ganglion and dorsal-nerve roots. Axons carrying nociceptive information are divided into three primary groups: (1) the heavily myelinated, rapidly conducting, intermediate diameter beta fibers; (2) the finely myelinated, slower conducting, small diameter A-delta fibers; and (3) the unmyelinated, very slowly conducting, very small diameter C fibers. Local factors at the site of injury may sensitize nociceptors and cause hyperalgesia, including potassium leaked from damaged cells, histamine, and bradykinin, while prostaglandin and leukotriene formation concurrently cause vasodilation, local edema, and erythema.

A normally propagated nociceptive-action potential may also rebound antidromically through other axonal branches at a site of injury, resulting in the release of substance P from the distal sensory-nerve terminal. Substance P activates other C fibers and also contributes to the release of histamine, further promoting nociception, vasodilation, and enlarging the region of hypersensitivity. Substance P also acts as a nociceptive neurotransmitter in the dorsal horn of the spinal cord, exciting the relay neurons that modulate pain transmission.

Central Nociception

Sensory axons carrying nociceptive impulses project to the spinal cord via the dorsal root ganglion and terminate in the dorsal horn. There, Rexed's laminae I, II, and V play a role in modulating nociceptive transmission. Layer I, the marginal zone, caps the top of the dorsal horn and the A-delta nociceptors largely terminate here. Most lamina I cells are nociceptive specific, responding only to noxious stimuli, and ultimately project to the contralateral midbrain and thalamus. The majority of C-fiber nociceptors terminate in lamina II (i.e., substantia gelatinosa). Very few laminae-II neurons project to sites rostral to the spinal cord, instead forming interneuronal connections that modify input from the primary sensory neurons. Lamina V receives some direct input from the A-delta neurons, but the receptive fields of the neurons in this lamina are larger than those in the lamina I, suggesting more neuronal convergence at this level, and some dendrites from laminae V extend dorsally into lamina I and II. Cells in the deeper layers of the spinal-cord gray matter have extremely complex receptive fields and wide areas of cutaneous input, with some input from deeper tissues.

Many nociceptive impulses ultimately pass contralaterally, across the spinal cord through the anterior commissure, to the spinothalamic tract, before ascending to brain-stem targets, including the reticular formation in the rostral medulla and the periaqueductal gray matter in the dorsal midbrain. Most of the spinothalamic neurons ultimately ascend to the ventroposterolateral (VPL) nucleus of the thalamus, though they may branch to provide input to these brain-stem targets. However, some axons terminate solely in these bulbar regions, which then send projections to thalamic nuclei.

The periaqueductal gray matter, the reticular formation, and the raphe magnus nucleus also harbor neurons containing endorphins or having endorphin receptors. *Endorphins* are endogenous chemical transmitters whose receptors may also be activated by morphine and other exogenous narcotics; this collection of neurons is known as the *enkephalinergic system*. After synapsing in the thalamus, a final group of neurons convey primary nociceptive information through the posterior limb of the internal capsule to the postcentral gyrus. Many nociceptive axons also project to a much wider area, the full range of which has not been fully defined.

The sensation and the subjective experience of pain are produced by a complex series of interactions. Transmission of nociception in spinal neurons depends not only on input from peripheral nociceptive neurons but also on input from non-nociceptive primary afferents, as well as modulation at several levels. Enkephalinergic neurons play a critical role in the modulation of nociceptive input, extending from the cortex and hypothalamus through the periaqueductal gray matter of the midbrain and the rostral medulla, to the dorsal horn of the spinal cord. Nociceptive, cortical, and other inputs activate neurons in the reticular formation and the raphe magnus, which then descend to the substantia gelatinosa (Rexed lamina II) in the dorsal horn of the spinal cord, to inhibit nociceptive input from peripheral neurons, thereby diminishing pain.

The affective component of pain has also been studied extensively. Unlike the discriminative somatosensory experience, it varies considerably between individuals and may help explain the substantial differences in pain tolerance in the general population. Central pathways proposed as mediators of the affective experience of pain include the reticular formation and its projections to the thalamus, as well as the medial thalamic nuclei and their projections to the frontal lobes. The discharge of neurons within the reticular formation correlates with escape behavior in animals, and frontal lobe lesions (e.g., frontal lobotomy) as well as bilateral medial thalamic lesions, produce subjective indifference to pain in humans, despite normal somatosensory discrimination. Psychologic factors, including the anxiety level, unpleasant memories of physically painful experiences, the anticipation of imminent physical injury or possible death, and others may also bear on our perception of pain. Both psychologic factors and the physiologic modulation of the nociceptive impulse are influenced by changes in serotonergic activity.

THE PATHOPHYSIOLOGY OF NEUROPATHIC PAIN

Peripheral Mechanisms

Transection of a peripheral nerve induces retrograde shrinkage of both myelinated and unmyelinated axons and reduced conduction velocities. Axonal sprouting from the proximal nerve stump is a normal reaction to such injury, and these sprouts grow towards the distal-nerve stump in an attempt to restore axonal continuity. Within 1 to 2 days, multiple unmyelinated sprouts appear and grow from transected axons. If these sprouts fail to enter a Schwann-cell tube in the distal-nerve segment, they curl to form a mass containing fibrous tissue, blood vessels, clusters of unmyelinated axons, and Schwann cells, known as a *neuroma*. Division of an entire nerve trunk with prevention of regeneration (e.g., amputation) yields a nerve-end neuroma, whereas total division with partial regeneration (e.g., surgical nerve repair) may create a neuroma-in-continuity at the site of the anastomosis. Trauma over the length of a nerve, even without transection (e.g., stretch injury), may damage small-axon fascicles or individual axons at multiple levels, creating disseminated microneuromas. Neuromas may also appear following crush injury. Unfortunately, neuroma formation favors nociceptive afferents.

Neuromas are a source of both spontaneous and evoked electrical discharges, as indicated by recording from dorsal-root filaments with the injured nerve at rest. These discharges increase with mechanical stimulation at the site of the neuroma, and are more likely to affect sensory rather than motor or autonomic fibers. Chronic discharges, particularly, appear to originate primarily in the C-fibers. Ectopic neuropacemakers remain near thresholds for repetitive firing and often generate repetitive afterdischarges following a single depolarization. This activity may be due to the high density of sodium channels, originally destined for the transected distal axon, that accumulate in the stump neuroma, enhancing sodium influx and chronically lowering the membrane potential towards the depolarization threshold. Close contact between the disorganized axonal sprouts within the neuroma may also cause current to be passed laterally from one axon to another, a short circuit called *ephaptic transmission*. Recurrent after discharges and other sustained activity may also result from the cyclic passage of current back and forth in a loop between two ephapses (i.e., *circus propagation,* as seen in some cardiac arrhythmias).

Faulty axonal regeneration and ephapse formation and may also appear in nerves chronically injured by demyelination or axonal degeneration, in the absence of external trauma. Spontaneous discharges may be induced not only by mechanical stimulation, but also by heat, cold, ischemia, chemical irritation, and metabolic stimuli. Mechanical stimulation may induce a burst of discharges and afterdischarges, and heating and cooling modulate discharge rates and patterns. Peptides and other neuroactive substances, especially alpha-adrenergic agonists, increase activity in experimental neuromas.

Ectopic pacemaker activity has been recorded in the phantom-limb syndrome, and may explain the hypersensitivity to heat and cold in that syndrome. Many of the core features of painful neuropathy and neuralgia, such as spontaneous electric, burning, and aching dysesthesias and hyperesthesia, could also be related to ectopic discharges. Sensitivity to mechanical stimulation in neuralgia or compressive mononeuropathy, which may provoke pain long outlasting the inciting stimulus, may result from the repetitive discharges and afterdischarges provoked by neuroma compression.

Central Mechanisms

Although the above peripheral mechanisms undoubtedly play a role in neuropathic pain, central mechanisms are also important and may predominate in chronic peripheral-nerve injury. The failure of measures designed to interrupt peripheral input from the painful region to fully relieve the pain of phantom limb syndrome including pharmacologic blockade of the damaged nerve proximal to the site of injury, dorsal rhizotomy, and even spinal and other CNS block, illustrates the confounding influence of central mechanisms. After peripheral-nerve injury, the aberrant rerouting of impulses within the brain and spinal cord may result in the diversion of impulses from non-nociceptive pathways to nociceptive pathways. This has been demonstrated experimentally in mapping studies of the spinal cord and brain, done before and after transection of a single peripheral nerve in one limb. Initially, the central-pain pathways serving the denervated area fall silent, but electrical activity gradually resumes within a few days. Some of this activity may be induced by non-nociceptive stimulation of areas supplied by an uninjured nerve that is remote from the dermatomes supplied by the injured nerve, suggesting spread of non-nociceptive impulses from normal routes into nociceptive pathways that were previously supplied by the injured nerve.

This phenomenon, known as *somatotopic reorganization,* could result from limited axonal sprouting over short distances within the spinal cord, and the formation of new synapses, prompted when primary sensory input is interrupted. However, the distance over which central spinal axons can sprout is highly limited and this hypothesis does not explain the degree of somatotopic reorganization documented experimentally. A more likely explanation is that the loss of primary afferent input to a central-spinal pathway following peripheral-nerve injury may unmask previously quiescent synapses. These synapses, supplied by nearby spinal axons serving sensation in other regions, enable surreptitious stimulation of the denervated pathway and produce phantom sensations, including pain.

Mapping CNS pathways during selective stimulation of cutaneous fields demonstrates wide-ranging synaptic inputs that reach well beyond their normal functional boundaries within the spinal cord. Similar phenomena have also been demonstrated at more rostral levels of the nervous system, including the thalamic nuclei. These phenomena could explain the phantom limb syndrome, in which a patient has the sensation that an amputated limb is still present. They may also play a role in some of the features of neuropathic pain, including the perception of one type of stimulus as another (i.e., *allesthesia*), when touch is perceived as heat, or when a non-nociceptive stimulus is perceived as painful (i.e., *allodynia*).

THE CLINICAL FEATURES OF NEUROPATHIC PAIN

Neuropathic pain is estimated to affect up to 1% of the population, and is even more prevalent in the elderly. It affects 10% of people with diabetic neuropathy and is often the complication having the greatest impact on the quality of life for the patient with diabetes. Fortunately, the repertoire of agents effective for the control of this potentially debilitating symptom has expanded considerably in the last decade.

Trauma to the peripheral nervous system can take a variety of forms; it may be predominantly axonal or predominantly demyelinating and may disproportionately affect the sensory or motor nerves, or the small or large nerve fibers. It may begin acutely or chronically, depending upon the cause. Small-fiber dysfunction classically produces loss of temperature and pain sensation, with subjective feelings of numbness, most often starting in a distal, symmetric pattern in the feet, with gradual ascension. However, pure small-fiber injury often presents with paresthesias (e.g., tingling, cold, or burning sensations) and neuropathic pain (e.g., electric, lancinating, stabbing or aching quality). Patients classically also complain of allodynia, and are particularly bothered by contact of their feet and bed sheets. Unlike large-fiber, sensory-nerve injury, tendon reflexes may be preserved in these patients. The most common cause is diabetes mellitus, but many other causes have also been identified (e.g., Sjögren syndrome, alcohol or drug toxicity, AIDS, hyperlipidemia, amyloidosis, Tangier disease, and Fabry disease). The unusual syndrome of *diabetic neuropathic cachexia* also includes subacute small-fiber neuropathy and mimics malignancy, as discussed in Chapter 106.

Large-fiber, sensory-nerve injury typically causes loss of vibration and position sense, with subjective numbness. Also, it usually begins in a distal symmetric pattern, affecting the feet and gradually ascending. With sufficient progression, it causes lower-limb incoordination and unsteadiness of gait. Tendon reflexes are diminished or absent, and motor-nerve involvement may produce weakness. Neuropathic pain may follow injury to the large sensory fibers, though concurrent small-fiber injury is also present in most of these cases. Patients with symptoms suggesting painful polyneuropathy must undergo a thorough neurologic evaluation, including: detailed history, physical examination, electrophysiologic studies, imaging, and serum studies. Other, non-neurogenic causes of pain must be excluded. Patients with pure small-fiber neuropathy, however, may have normal electrophysiologic studies, leading to quantitative sensory testing and skin biopsy for counts of small sensory fibers. Treatment of these patients focuses on the cause of nerve injury, if reversible.

THE TREATMENT OF NEUROPATHIC PAIN

General Principles

Patients with neuropathic pain vary more in response to treatments than patients with other disorders, and the course of neuropathic pain may be difficult to predict, with unexpected exacerbations and spontaneous remissions. The therapeutic goal of treatment is to return the patient to normal functioning, with reduction of pain to tolerable levels. The patient should understand and accept this goal at the outset, and not expect complete elimination of pain. Furthermore, the patient should also understand that numbness, weakness, and other neuropathic symptoms will not be improved by these medications. Patients often benefit from physical therapy, regular exercise, and constructive activity. Refractory symptoms may lead to treatment by a multidisciplinary team, in a reputable pain clinic. This team should include not only a physician specialist, but also a psychiatrist or psychologist trained in pain management, who may assist with analysis of the affective component of the patient's symptoms and issues such as secondary gain, as well as with conditioning and psychotherapy. Some patients may also benefit from adjunctive (i.e., complementary) biofeedback and meditation methods.

Surgical Therapy

Surgical therapy does not have a role in generalized neuropathic pain. Although a variety of surgical therapies directed at interruption of the nociceptive pathways have been attempted, over the years, for the treatment of focal neuropathic pain syndromes, such measures often provide only transient relief of symptoms and usually worsen somatosensory deficits. Techniques have included dorsal rhizotomy and thalamotomy. Sympathectomy has been attempted for the complex regional-pain syndromes, but remains controversial.

Pharmacologic Therapy

A summary of the major drugs evaluated for the treatment of neuropathic pain, along with their efficacy, is presented in Table 71.1.

▶ **TABLE 71.1 Drug Therapy for Painful Neuropathy**

Drug	Efficacy	Evidence
Tricyclic antide-pressants	Effective	Double blind, controlled trial
Tramadol hydrochloride	Effective	Double blind, controlled trial
Gabapentin	Effective	Double blind, controlled trial
Carbamazepine	Effective	Small, randomized trial
Capsaicin cream	Effective	Blinded controlled trials
Lidocaine patch	Effective	Blinded, controlled trial
Citalopram	Effective	Double blind, controlled trial
Isosorbide dinitrate spray	Effective	Double blind, controlled trial
Paroxetine	Effective	Controlled trial
Zonisamide	Effective	Open label pilot trial
Venlafaxine	Effective	Randomized comparative trial
Lamotrigine	Variably effective	Multiple trial designs
Narcotic analgesics	Possibly effective	Multiple trial designs
Phenytoin	Conflicting trial data	Mutliple trial designs
Fluoxetine	Not effective	Double blind, controlled trial

Antinociceptive Agents

Unlike primary nociceptive pain, neuropathic pain is often resistant to traditional analgesic therapy, including that of nonsteroidal antiinflammatory agents such as ibuprofen and aspirin. Acetaminophen is generally minimally effective. Narcotic analgesics are also less likely to provide chronic relief than in other pain states, although they may be useful as part of a multimodal regimen in refractory patients. Physicians regularly employing narcotics for the treatment of neuropathic pain should be trained in chronic use, and must be vigilant in monitoring patients' patterns of drug consumption and response to avoid addictive patterns. Refer patients taking narcotic therapy to a reputable pain clinic for appropriate long-term monitoring and evaluation of tolerance, dependence, and drug abuse, when appropriate.

Tramadol Hydrochloride

Tramadol hydrochloride, unlike most other analgesics, has been proved effective for the treatment of painful neuropathy in a placebo-controlled, double-blind, randomized trial. It is a weak inhibitor of norepinephrine and serotonin reuptake, and has low affinity for the μ-opioid receptors (i.e., approximately one-tenth the strength of codeine). Its beneficial effects in neuropathic pain are at-tributed to serotonergic modulation of pain transmission within the brain and spinal cord. It is well tolerated, but may cause mild constipation, headache, or sedation. Therapy is usually initiated at 50 mg per day, gradually increasing on a weekly schedule to 150 mg daily to 200 mg daily, or the maximal effective dose, whichever is lower. Some relief may appear almost immediately, but maximal benefit may not be seen for 1 to 2 weeks after initiation or dosage change. The opioid effects are weak and tolerance does not develop, simplifying its use as chronic therapy.

Anticonvulsants

The antiexcitatory properties of the antiepileptic drugs (AEDs) make them attractive agents for the suppression of the spontaneous neuronal discharges underlying neuropathic pain. Early trials of phenytoin gave conflicting results, but carbamazepine was effective in two placebo-controlled and one comparative study (vs. tricyclic antidepressants) at doses of 300 mg daily to 1000 mg daily. Common adverse effects of carbamazepine include somnolence, dizziness, and gait disturbances, and rarely, leukopenia, hepatotoxicity, and inappropriate secretion of antidiuretic hormone. Oxcarbazepine may also be effective, with fewer side effects.

Gabapentin appears to be the most effective AED for suppressing neuropathic pain thus far, proven in placebo-controlled trials for painful diabetic neuropathy, postherpetic neuralgia, and other neuropathic pain syndromes. Side effects are generally mild, although sedation is often a limiting factor in the elderly. Initial doses of 300 mg per day to 600 mg per day, in three divided doses, are gradually increased to efficacy over several weeks; the slow increase may prevent excessive sedation. Daily doses of 1000 mg daily to 2000 mg daily are given for adequate pain control in most patients, but some take up to 3600 mg daily. One to 2 weeks of continuous therapy, after initiation or dosage increase, is needed before maximal effect appears.

Lamotrigine, a voltage-dependent sodium-channel blocker, proved effective in treating the pain of HIV neuropathy and in trigeminal neuralgia, but was negative in a large neuropathic pain trial. In those studies demonstrating efficacy, doses of 50 mg per day to 400 mg per day were used. Lamotrigine has a less favorable side-effect profile than gabapentin, causing dizziness, ataxia, constipation, nausea, and somnolence, and these effects may be dose limiting. Zonisamide, a sodium- and T-type calcium-channel blocker and enhancer of GABA release, may have a role in the treatment of neuropathic pain. Other agents, such as tiagabine and topiramate, are under study and may also ultimately have a role in the therapy of painful neuropathy.

Tricyclic Antidepressants

Amitriptyline was one of the first agents proven effective for the treatment of painful neuropathy. The tricyclic antidepressants (TCAs) block serotonin and noradrenalin reuptake, and modulate pain transmission within the CNS. They may also inhibit sodium-channel function, and the pain relief they provide is independent of any effect on mood. Amitriptyline has been effective in numerous double-blind, placebo-controlled trials and proved equivalent to gabapentin in head-to-head comparative studies. Other TCAs, such as desipramine and nortriptyline may also be effective and may sometimes work when amitriptyline does not. Although less potent, side effects are also generally milder Unfortunately, the TCAs have anticholinergic effects including sedation, orthostatic hypotension, and urinary retention that often limit their use in diabetic and elderly subjects. Sedation during initial therapy may improve over 1 or 2 weeks. Typical starting doses are 10 mg to 25 mg at bedtime, gradually increasing every 2 weeks to effect or maximally tolerated dose (i.e., not more than 150 mg per day). If no benefit appears after 4 to 6 weeks at maximally tolerated doses, another agent should be tried. The TCAs are often especially helpful for severe nocturnal pain and insomnia, as they relieve pain while restoring sleep quality, but once steady-state blood levels are achieved, they also provide relief throughout the day.

Selective Serotonin Reuptake Inhibitors

The selective serotonin reuptake inhibitors (SSRIs) have not been studied so extensively as the TCAs in the treatment of neuropathic pain. However, paroxetine and citalopram were more effective than placebo but less effective than the TCAs, in treating neuropathic pain, while fluoxetine has not been effective in the limited studies performed thus far.

Other Drugs

Venlafaxine is a serotonin and weak noradrenalin reuptake inhibitorthat demonstrated efficacy equivalent to imipramine in a randomized trial. Both intravenous lidocaine and its oral conjoiner, mexiletine, have great potential, theoretically, for the suppression of aberrant neuronal excitation, but results have been inconsistent. The lidocaine patch delivers topical agent to an affected area, decreasing spontaneous discharge in cutaneous nerves. It may reduce regional pain in severely affected areas, such as the soles of the feet. However, this drug transiently worsens numbness and may increase the likelihood of insensate-skin injury, especially in patients with diabetes. Capsaicin cream, which depletes substance P from the cutaneous-sensory nerves with chronic topical use, is effective. However, patients find this drug inconvenient, because topical application is required three times per day. It is caustic and irritates any mucous membranes it may contact (e.g., eye and mouth, after accidental transfer from the hand during application). It also actually increases neuropathic pain during the initial 1 to 2 weeks of therapy (i.e., the early depletion phase), before producing relief. Isosorbide dinitrate (ISDN), a nitric-oxide donor and a local vasodilator, was effective in one study.

SUGGESTED READINGS

Neuropathic Pain

Dworkin RH, Backonja M, Rowbotham MC, et al. Advances in neuropathic pain. *Arch Neurol* 2003;60:1524–1534.

Lacomis D. Small-fiber neuropathy. *Muscle Nerve* 2002;26:173–188.

Mendell JR, Sahenk Z. Painful sensory neuropathy. *N Engl J Med* 2003;27;348:1243–1255.

Podwall D, Gooch C. Diabetic neuropathy: clinical features, etiology, and therapy. *Curr Neurol Neurosci Rep* 2004;4:55–56.

Rho RH, Brewer RP, Lamer TJ, Wilson PR. Complex regional pain syndrome. *Mayo Clin Proc* 2002;77:174–180.

Wolfe GI, Trivedi JR. Painful peripheral neuropathy and its nonsurgical treatment. *Muscle Nerve* 2004;30(1):3–19.

Woolf CJ. Dissecting out mechanisms responsible for peripheral neuropathic pain: implications for diagnosis and therapy. *Life Sci* 2004;74:2605–2610.

Treatment of Neuropathic Pain

Backonja M, Beydoun A, Edwards KR, et al. Gabapentin for the symptomatic treatment of painful neuropathy in patients with diabetes mellitus: a randomized controlled trial. *JAMA* 1998;280:1831–1836.

Backonja M, Glanzman RL. Gabapentin dosing for neuropathic pain: evidence from randomized, placebo-controlled clinical trials. *Clin Ther* 2003;25(1).81–104.

Backonja MM. Use of anticonvulsants for treatment of neuropathic pain. *Neurology* 2002;59(5)(suppl 2):S14–S17.

The Capsaicin Study Group. Treatment of painful diabetic neuropathy with topical capsaicin: a multicenter, double-blind, vehicle-controlled study. *Arch Intern Med* 1991;151:2225–2229.

Dejgård A, Petersen P, Kastrup J. Mexiletine for treatment of chronic painful diabetic neuropathy. *Lancet* 1988;1:9–11.

Gomez-Perez FJ, Choza R, Rios JM, et al. Nortriptyline-fluphenazine vs. carbamazepine in the symptomatic treatment of diabetic neuropathy. *Arch Med Res* 1996;27:525–529.

Harati Y, Gooch CL, Swenson M, et al. A double-blind, randomized trial of tramadol for treatment of the pain of diabetic neuropathy. *Neurology* 1998;50:1842–1846.

Harati Y, Gooch CL, Swenson M, et al. Maintenance of the long-term effectiveness of tramadol in treatment of the pain of diabetic neuropathy. *J Diabetes Complications* 2000;14:65–70.

Heit HA. Addiction, physical dependence, and tolerance: precise definitions to help clinicians evaluate and treat chronic pain patients. *J Pain Palliat Care Pharmacother* 2003;17:15–29.

Kastrup J, Petersen P, Dejgård A et al. Intravenous lidocaine infusion—a new treatment of chronic painful diabetic neuropathy? *Pain* 1987;28:69–75.

Max MB, Culnane M, Schafer SC, et al. Amitriptyline relieves diabetic neuropathy pain in patients with normal or depressed mood. *Neurology* 1987;37(4):589–596.

Max MB, Lynch SA, Muir J, et al. Effects of desipramine, amitriptyline, and fluoxetine on pain in diabetic neuropathy. *N Engl J Med* 1992;326:1250–1256.

McCleane G. 200 mg daily of lamotrigine has no analgesic effect in neuropathic pain: a randomised, double-blind placebo controlled trial. *Pain* 1999;83:105–107.

Oskarsson P, Ljunggren JG, Lins PE. Efficacy and safety of mexiletine in the treatment of painful diabetic neuropathy. *Diabetes Care* 1997;20:1594–1597.

Polydefkis M, Hauer P, Griffin JW, McArthur JC. Skin biopsy as a tool to assess distal small fiber innervation in diabetic neuropathy. *Diabetes Technol Therapeut* 2001;3:23–28.

Rull JA, Quibrera R, Gonzalez-Millan H, Lozano Castaneda O. Symptomatic treatment of peripheral diabetic neuropathy with carbamazepine: double-blind crossover study. *Diabetologia* 1969;5:215–220.

Saudek DC, Werns S, Reidenberg MM. Phenytoin in the treatment of diabetic symmetrical polyneuropathy. *Clin Pharmacol Therapeut* 1977;22(2):196–199.

Scheffler NM, Sheitel PL, Lipton MN. Treatment of painful diabetic neuropathy with capsaicin 0.075%. *J Am Podiatr Med Assoc* 1991;81:288–293.

Simpson DM, Onley R, McArthur JC, et al. A placebo-controlled trial of lamotrigine for painful HIV-associated neuropathy. *Neurology* 2000;54:2115–2119.

Sindrup SH, Gram LF, Brcsen K, et al. The selective serotonin reuptake inhibitor paroxetine is effective in the treatment of diabetic neuropathy symptoms. *Pain* 1990;42:135–144.

Sindrup SH, Bjerre U, Dejgaard A, et al. The selective serotonin reuptake inhibitor citalopram relieves the symptoms of diabetic neuropathy. *Clin Pharmacol Therapeut* 1992;52:547–552.

Sindrup SH, Bach FW, Madsen C, et al. Venlafaxine versus imipramine in painful polyneuropathy. *Neurology* 2003;60:1284–1289.

Stracke H, Meyer UE, Schumacher HE, Federlin K. Mexiletine in the treatment of diabetic neuropathy. *Diabetes Care* 1992;15:1550–1555.

Tandan R, Lewis GA, Krusinski PB, et al. Topical capsaicin in painful diabetic neuropathy: controlled study with long-term follow-up. *Diabetes Care* 1992;15:8–14.

Wolfe GI, Trivedi JR. Painful peripheral neuropathy and its nonsurgical treatment. *Muscle Nerve* 2004;30:3–19.

Wright JM, Oki JC, Graves L III. Mexiletine in the symptomatic treatment of diabetic peripheral neuropathy. *Ann Pharmacother* 1997;31:29–34.

Yuen K, Baker N, Rayman G. Treatment of chronic painful diabetic neuropathy with isosorbide dinitrate spray. *Diabetes Care* 2002;25:1699–1703.

Zakrzewska JM, Chaudhry Z, Nurmikko TJ, et al. Lamotrigine (Lamictal) in refractory trigeminal neuralgia: results from a double-blind placebo-controlled crossover trial. *Pain* 1997;73:223–230.

Chapter 72

▶ Radiation Injury

Steven R. Isaacson, Casilda Balmaceda, and Michael D. Daras

Since the first description of radionecrosis in 1930, injury to the brain or spinal cord is a feared complication of radiation therapy, even though this treatment is essential for many CNS malignancies. Healthy tissue may be exposed when the target of radiation is nearby in the brain or spinal cord, or even after non-neural structures have been irradiated, if the peripheral or cranial nerves are within the field. Neurologic injury may follow scalp irradiation for tinea capitis, prophylactic whole-brain radiotherapy for small-cell carcinoma of the lung or acute lymphocytic leukemia, or radiotherapy to the neck for systemic malignancy. Three major categories are identified: acute reactions (i.e., 1 to 6 weeks after radiotherapy), early-delayed reactions (i.e., within 6 months afterward), and late-delayed reactions (i.e., months or years afterward).

EARLY (ACUTE) EFFECTS

Radiotherapy is usually tolerated well during the treatment period. The only acute CNS injury is edema, days or weeks after starting therapy. Headache, nausea, and vomiting may occur with high daily-dose fractions. Fractions of 750 cGy generate a complication rate of 49%, but daily doses of 200 cGy or less are seldom toxic. The acute lesions appear on MRI as localized swelling, without enhancement. Steroids may reduce symptoms and are commonly given during radiotherapy to reduce the likelihood of this complication.

Tissues that have the fastest turnover rate are most often affected after CNS irradiation, causing alopecia and skin erythema. Otitis media or externa, and pharyngitis, may follow radiotherapy to the posterior fossa or brain stem because of eustachian-tube obstruction by swelling. Temporary hearing loss may occur, but deafness is rare. Bone-marrow depression after craniospinal radiotherapy is particularly frequent, especially with concomitant chemotherapy, and may lead to infection or hemorrhage.

EARLY-DELAYED SYNDROMES

Reactions occurring 1 month to several years after radiotherapy are divided into early and late categories, but there are no clearly defined boundaries. Two main clinical syndromes are seen. Somnolence and headache may occur in children given prophylactic whole-brain radiotherapy for acute lymphocytic leukemia or tinea capitis. The syndrome appears 24 to 66 days after radiotherapy, and recovery is spontaneous. Focal signs are uncommon but may simulate tumor progression.

Rhombencephalitis with ataxia, dysarthria, and nystagmus may follow irradiation to the middle ear area for glomus jugulare tumors. Severe leukoencephalopathy may occur within the first 6 months. Early-delayed radiation myelopathy may present with the Lhermitte symptom, a sensation of electrical current radiating down the back or limbs, induced by flexing the neck. It may be present in up to 15% of patients receiving mantle irradiation for

Hodgkin lymphoma. This symptom may be distinguished from delayed-radiation myelopathy because it is transient and appears within 6 months of the completion of treatment. The Lhermitte symptom is also seen in multiple sclerosis, vitamin B_{12} deficiency, and after cisplatin chemotherapy, as well as epidural-cord compression by tumor, when it is usually painful.

The latent period for early-delayed effects is thought to correspond to the turnover time of myelin, and these syndromes are attributed to transient demyelination. Pathologic data are scarce because the syndrome is rarely lethal, but the few autopsies have shown areas of demyelination.

LATE-DELAYED SYNDROMES

Radiation Necrosis

It is not known how adverse effects relate to total dose of radiotherapy, fraction size, treatment time, volume of tissue irradiated, and host factors such as age. To standardize the biologic effects of different treatment regimens, Sheline and colleagues developed the concept of *neuroret,* to specifically address brain tolerance to irradiation. The value is derived from a graph representing fractions (i.e., abscissa) and total dose (i.e., ordinate), to determine the threshold for necrosis. It occurs at doses greater than 1,000 neurorets to 1,100 neurorets (i.e., equivalent to 6,000 cGy, given in 30 fractions for 6 weeks, a treatment commonly used for primary brain tumors).

Necrosis develops in about 5% of patients given total doses greater than 5,000 cGy, with daily fraction sizes greater than 200 cGy. It may also follow irradiation of extracranial malignancies, such as squamous-cell carcinoma, or stereotactic radiosurgery, proton-beam irradiation, or brachytherapy (i.e., implantation of radioactive sources into the tumor bed). The median time for onset of symptoms is 14 months after radiotherapy, but symptoms may occur as early as 6 months afterward. In 75% of the patients, symptoms appear within 3 years of the treatment but may be seen as late as 7.5 years post therapy. The clinical manifestations may simulate those of the original tumor, with lateralizing signs, headache, or increased intracranial pressure (ICP). Patients irradiated for nasopharyngeal carcinoma may have lesions in the temporal lobe with or without hypothalamic dysfunction.

Radiation necrosis shows a predilection for the *white matter.* The underlying mechanisms are thought to be either loss of oligodendrocytes, with demyelination and necrosis (i.e., *glial hypothesis*), or a *vasculopathy,* with ischemia and infarction leading to necrosis. Current views point to a vascular-mediated response resulting in delayed white-matter necrosis. Glial cells, particularly oligodendrocytes, and the vascular endothelium are the major targets, not the neurons. Histologic changes include white-matter necrosis, cystic cavitation with gliosis, and patchy demyelination. Vascular changes include endothelial proliferation, fibrinoid degeneration, perivascular lymphocytic infiltration, capillary occlusion, and intraluminal thrombosis of medium- and small-sized arteries.

Vasogenic edema follows endothelial-cell damage. The *immunologic hypothesis* speculates that irradiated glial cells release antigens that induce an autoimmune reaction. A *mineralizing microangiopathy* is seen at autopsy in up to 17% of patients who received cranial irradiation and were usually asymptomatic. Radiographically, calcification may be seen at the gray–white matter junction, basal ganglia, or pons.

Neuroradiologic abnormalities are of two types. The first is a *mass lesion,* located at the original tumor site or within the path of radiation. Ring-like or heterogeneous enhancement is usually seen mimicking the original neoplasm. Angiography shows that the lesion is avascular. CT or MRI demonstrate that that the lesion may resolve with time. Neuroimaging may often differentiate between early, transient and more progressive, and later injury. Imaging may differentiate mild edema from noxious edema and frank necrosis. Early changes are confined to white matter, but after 6 months to 1 or 2 years, gray matter lesions may be evident.

The second abnormality consists of diffuse *white-matter changes,* appearing as areas of hypodensity on CT, or increased signal intensity on MRI (Fig. 72.1).

The imaging abnormalities vary from mild to severe and are usually irreversible. Mild changes (i.e., grade 1) lie adjacent to the frontal and occipital horns of the lateral ventricles. Grade 2 (i.e., intermediate) change affects the centrum semiovale, and grades 3 to 4 show diffuse white-matter lesions with a characteristic scalloped configuration. Mass effect is rare. Accompanying changes include cortical atrophy or ventricular dilation. MRI is more sensitive than CT in detecting these white-matter abnormalities. Imaging abnormalities correlate poorly with symptoms; many patients with severe white-matter changes are asymptomatic.

Distinguishing tumor recurrence from radiation necrosis may be difficult. Provided that steroid dosage is not increasing, radiation effect is suggested by clinical improvement, accompanied by a decrease of mass effect on CT or MRI. Although PET may show hypometabolic areas of radiation necrosis, a tissue biopsy is usually needed to establish the diagnosis. Single-photon emission CT (SPECT) and PET are complementary. *MR spectroscopy* may document metabolic changes in brain *N*-acetylaspartate, choline, creatine, and lactate that appear after radiation and later return to normal. A reduction in choline levels, with radiation, indicates the transformation of tumor to necrotic tissue, while an increase in choline levels is associated with tumor recurrence. Steroid therapy may lead to clinical stabilization, but when there is

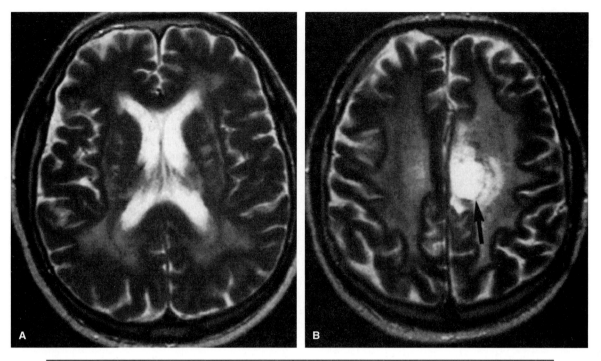

FIGURE 72.1. Radiation leukoencephalopathy. A: Axial T2-weighted MR scan shows diffuse increased signal intensity involving the periventricular white matter of both frontal lobes and parietal lobes, as well as the corona radiata and external capsules bilaterally. **B:** Axial T2-weighted MR scan at the level of the centrum semiovale demonstrates similar changes within the hemispheric white matter bilaterally. The known malignant glioma is identified in the posteromedial left frontal lobe *(arrow)*, for which the patient had received cranial radiation therapy. (Courtesy of Dr. S. Chan, Columbia University College of Physicians and Surgeons, New York, NY.)

marked mass effect, surgical resection may improve neurologic function and may be life saving. Radiation necrosis may be progressive and fatal.

Radiation Myelopathy

Delayed injury to the spinal cord, *radiation myelopathy*, develops 1 to 3 years after radiotherapy, with one peak at 12 to 14 months and another at 24 to 28 months. The average latent period is 12 months, and in 75% of the patients, radiation myelopathy occurs within 30 months. In patients with shorter intervals, the total dose of radiation and the average dose per fraction were higher. The incidence is about 5% when doses between 57 Gy and 61 Gy are given to the spinal cord. Latency periods are shorter in children, after a second course of radiation, or for lumbar lesions. The latency bimodality is attributed to dual mechanisms of injury. Higher doses cause white-matter necrosis and early myelopathy; lower doses preferentially cause vascular damage and delayed manifestations. Syrinx formation after radiation to the spinal cord has been described in a patient with a cervical astrocytoma.

The true incidence of radiation myelopathy is not known. Wara and associates (1975) suggested a 5% risk in patients who received 4,500 cGy, at fraction doses of 180 cGy, but the specifics of cord tolerance remain elusive. Symptoms are associated with increased fraction size, shorter treatment time, higher total dose, and cord exposure greater than 10 cm in length. Additional risk factors (e.g., diabetes mellitus, hypertension) may contribute to its development.

The clinical syndrome includes painless, subacute numbness, and paresthesia, followed by progression of spastic gait, sphincter symptoms, and limb weakness. MRI may be normal or show cord swelling, atrophy, or complete subarachnoid block. Low-signal intensity on T1-weighted imaging, high-signal on T2-weighted imaging, and focal enhancement may be seen as early as 1 month after the clinical manifestations. Diagnosis must exclude extra- or intramedullary tumors, leptomeningeal metastases, or vertebral-body abnormalities causing cord compression.

As early as 10 months after the onset of symptoms, one may see cord atrophy or resolution of contrast enhancement. There is no effective treatment, although steroids may transiently improve symptoms. Pathologically, spinal-cord infarction is associated with necrosis, hemorrhage, and demyelination. After experimental radiation, asymptomatic animals showed spongy vacuolation of the spinal-cord white matter only, whereas those with paralysis had large areas of tissue destruction and vascular changes, particularly in the posterior and lateral columns. Other rare syndromes attributed to radiation-induced cord damage include acute paraplegia that progresses for hours to days (possibly induced by vascular damage to the cord with infarction), anterior horn-cell damage, and a delayed clinical syndrome that simulates motor-neuron disease, but is arrested spontaneously after 1 to 2 years.

Radiation-Induced Vasculopathy

Both intra- and extracranial circulation may be affected. Most patients have had neck irradiation for head-and-neck cancer or for optic-nerve or suprasellar tumors. The latent period may be up to 23 years. Angiography reveals localized stenosis, an irregular contour of the vessel involved, or even complete occlusion of the portion of the artery in the radiation portal. Extracranially, internal- and common-carotid artery occlusion may be seen, with premature atherosclerosis and endothelial proliferation compromising vessel patency, and leading to thrombosis and infarction. Intracranially, the supraclinoid carotid is most commonly affected, and a moyamoya pattern may develop. Autopsy studies reveal myointimal proliferation, hyalinization, and occlusion. Clinically, radiation-induced vasculopathy causes transient ischemic attacks or ischemic stroke. Cerebrovascular malformations have also been observed in the irradiated field. Aneurysm formation is rare. Stenting is a promising treatment for large-artery stenotic lesions.

Radiation-Induced Plexopathy

Either brachial- or lumbar plexus may be affected; most commonly the arm is affected after radiotherapy for breast carcinoma. Three different syndromes are observed. *Transient plexus injury* occurs in 1.4% of the patients treated with doses of 5,000 cGy to the area, with paresthesia, or less commonly, pain or weakness. Median onset is 4.5 months after radiotherapy. *Acute ischemic brachial neuropathy* follows subclavian artery occlusion, owing to prior irradiation. The lesion is acute, nonprogressive, and painless. *Radiation fibrosis* appears about 4 years after radiotherapy, with paresthesia or swelling of the arm; the signs are sensorimotor, most commonly affecting the upper plexus. Pathologically, local fibrosis or scarring entraps the plexus or nerves. *Brachial plexopathy* was reported in the treatment of breast cancer when the fraction size was greater than 2 Gy. Patients may have symptoms of paresthesia, hypesthesia, and weak hands. *Lumbosacral plexopathy* is a rare occurrence in patients treated for cervical or endometrial carcinoma, even when total doses approach 70 Gy to 80 Gy, by a combination of brachytherapy and external-beam radiation.

Clinically, the major difficulty lies in trying to differentiate radiation-induced plexopathy from tumor. Lymphedema, painless paresis and sensory loss, and upper-plexus involvement suggest radiation plexopathy. Pain, lack of edema, and lower-plexus involvement suggest recurrent tumor. *Myokymia*, when present on electromyography, strongly favors the diagnosis of radiation fibrosis. Typically, radiation fibrosis of the plexus appears on CT as diffuse involvement without a discrete mass. MRI may reveal radiation changes in the soft tissue or bone. Gadolinium enhancement of the irradiated area may occur and persist, even two decades after irradiation. Although the presence of enhancement is usually suggestive of recurrent tumor, the radiographic stability is more consistent with necrosis. When ancillary studies are ambiguous, surgical exploration of the plexus may be considered. Once the diagnosis of radiation plexopathy is established, attention should be given to preventing shoulder subluxation, treating lymphedema, and relieving pain. The plexopathy is usually irreversible.

Endocrine Dysfunction

Irradiation of the brain or neighboring sites may cause neuroendocrine disorders. These are primarily to the result of radiation effects on the hypothalamic–pituitary axis when this structure is included in the radiation field for treatment of primary brain tumors or head-and-neck cancer. For unknown reasons, the posterior pituitary is remarkably resistant to the effects of radiation. Several clinical syndromes may be evident. *Growth-hormone function* is the most vulnerable. *Growth arrest* may occur in children treated with spinal radiotherapy because radiation impairs vertebral development and is exaggerated by endocrine deficiency. It is most visible in growing children; the rate of growth slows and stature is short for age.

Adults may exhibit a decrease in muscle mass and an increase in adipose tissue. These effects may become evident in children with doses of fractionated radiation as low as 18 Gy, or single fractions of 9 Gy to 10 Gy. Adults have a higher threshold. Among children treated for acute lymphoblastic leukemia, who received moderate doses of prophylactic cranial radiation (2,000 cGy to 3,000 cGy), 65% have impaired growth-hormone responses. Treatment includes growth-hormone replacement. Modern treatment for chemosensitive tumors therefore emphasizes chemotherapy to reduce or avoid radiation.

Gonadotropin deficiency (i.e., luteinizing hormone [LH] and follicle-stimulating hormone [FSH]) may develop, with failure to enter puberty, and amenorrhea. Adults may demonstrate infertility, sexual dysfunction, and decreased libido. The tolerance dose appears to be between 40 Gy and 50 Gy. *Thyrotropin deficiency* may be manifested as weight gain and lethargy. *Adrenocorticotropic-hormone deficiency* is rarely seen, but shows lethargy, decreased stamina, fasting, hypoglycemia, and dilutional hyponatremia. *Hyperprolactinemia* may cause delay in puberty, galactorrhea, or amenorrhea. Men may experience decreased libido and impotence. These findings may be found in 20% to 50% of patients receiving greater than 50 Gy of radiation.

Neuropsychologic Sequelae

Cognitive impairment is a delayed complication of radiation, especially in long-term survivors who have been cured of the original disease. There usually has been concomitant use of intrathecal chemotherapy, but radiation, itself, may be the culprit. Children younger than 5 years of age are particularly susceptible to cognitive sequelae. In the treatment of *childhood* brain tumors, survivors demonstrate a 40% to 100% incidence of cognitive dysfunction on formal neuropsychologic testing. Cranial irradiation in children may be associated with mild-delayed IQ decline, learning disability, and academic failure.

In spite of the considerable pediatric literature, cognitive outcome in adults has not been adequately studied. In most studies there were lacks of controls, or the most appropriate neuropsychologic tests were not used. A syndrome of ataxia, cognitive disturbance, and urinary incontinence, sometimes ameliorated by ventriculoperitoneal shunting, has been described in adults treated with irradiation for brain tumors. Memory seems to be sensitive to radiotherapy. Local-field irradiation to the posterior fossa may also be accompanied by significant cognitive impairment. There have been few studies of the *quality of life* of patients surviving irradiation.

Other Complications of Radiation

Peripheral Nerves

Peripheral nerves are seldom damaged with fractionated doses of less than 6,000 cGy. Fraction size appears to play a significant role as a causative factor. There may be two phases of injury to nerves following radiation. First, direct effects may cause changes in electrophysiology and histochemistry. Fibrosis may occur later and surround the nerve. Vascular injury to nutrient vessels may also occur.

Radiation-Induced Tumors

As the survival of cancer patients increases, secondary tumors become an important treatment complication. Radiation has been implicated in the development of secondary tumors. The association between radiation and CNS tumors is especially strong for *meningiomas*, which may follow irradiation for brain or spinal-cord tumors, or doses of less than 850 cGy to the scalp for tinea capitis. The mean latency is 37 years if low-dose irradiation was given, and 18 months for doses greater than 2,000 cGy. Compared with spontaneously arising tumors, radiation-induced meningiomas are more likely to undergo malignant transformation, and recur after surgical excision. Radiation-

induced *sarcomas* are seen in the third, fourth, or fifth decades after radiation for pituitary adenomas or gliomas. The latency period is 8 to 11 years, with doses greater than 5,000 cGy.

The possible role of cranial irradiation in the pathogenesis of CNS *gliomas* is controversial. The main diagnostic problem is differentiation of radiation-induced malignancy from recurrence of the original tumor. *Peripheral-nerve tumors*, benign or malignant, arising within the radiation port may occur in up to 9% of patients, particularly those treated for breast cancer or lymphoma. Tumors are most frequently located in the brachial plexus, followed by those of spinal roots or nerve. Clinically, they present as an enlarging, painful mass that causes progressive motor and sensory signs of plexopathy. The mean interval between irradiation and diagnosis of these tumors is 16 years. Patients with neurofibromatosis are particularly prone to radiation-induced peripheral-nerve tumors. Treatment is surgical resection, but the prognosis for malignant tumors is poor.

Radiation Optic Neuropathy

Radiation-induced optic neuropathy follows treatment directed to the orbit, sinuses, pituitary, or intracranial tumors. There is painless visual loss, usually monocular, but both eyes may be affected. Symptoms develop within 3 years. Findings include decreased visual acuity, abnormal visual fields (especially altitudinal defects), papilledema followed by optic atrophy, and hemorrhagic exudates. About 50% of the patients experience improvement of the condition, but some become blind. Steroids are ineffective. Measures to shield the optic nerve from the radiation portals may reduce the incidence of this rare but devastating complication.

SUGGESTED READINGS
Radiation: CNS Effects

Al-Mefty O, Kersh JE, Routh A, et al. The long-term side effects of radiation therapy for benign brain tumors in adults. *J Neurosurg* 1990;73:502–512.

Archibald Y, Lunn D, Ruttan L, et al. Cognitive functioning in long-term survivors of high-grade gliomas. *J Neurosurg* 1994;80:247–253.

Ball WS, Prenger EC, Ballard ET. Neurotoxicity of radio/chemotherapy in children: pathologic and MR correlation. *AJNR* 1992;13:761–776.

Curnes J, Laster D, et al. MRI of radiation injury to the brain. *Am J Roentgenol* 1986;147:119–124.

DeAngelis LM, Delattre JY, Posner JB. Radiation-induced dementia in patients cured of brain metastases. *Neurology* 1989;39:789–796.

Donahue B. Short- and long-term complications of radiation therapy for pediatric brain tumors. *Pediatr Neurosurg* 1992;18:207–217.

Giglio P. Gilbert MR. Cerebral radiation necrosis. *Neurologist* 2003;9(4):180–188.

Glass JP, Hwang TL, Leavens ME, et al. Cerebral radiation necrosis following treatment of extracranial malignancies. *Cancer* 1984;54:1966–1972.

Grattan-Smith PJ, Morris JG, Langlands AO. Delayed radiation necrosis of the central nervous system in patients irradiated for pituitary tumours. *J Neurol Neurosurg Psychiatry* 1992;55:949–955.

Kaufman M, Swartz BE, Mandelkern M, et al. Diagnosis of delayed cerebral radiation necrosis following proton beam therapy. *Arch Neurol* 1990;47:474–476.

McIver JI, Pollock BE. Radiation-induced tumor after stereotactic radiosurgery and whole brain radiotherapy: case report and literature review. *J Neurooncol* 2004 Feb;66(3):301–305.

Meadows A, Massari D, Ferguson J, et al. Declines in IQ scores and cognitive dysfunctions in children with acute lymphocytic leukemia treated with cranial irradiation. *Lancet* 1981;2:1015–1018.

Mitomo M, Kawai R, Miura T, et al. Radiation necrosis of the brain and radiation-induced vasculopathy. *Acta Radiol* 1986;369(suppl):227–230.

Monje ML, Palmer T. Radiation injury and neurogenesis. *Curr Opin Neurol* 2003;16(2):129–134.

Mostow EN, Byrne J, Connelly RR, et al. Quality of life in long-term survivors of CNS tumors of childhood and adolescence. *J Clin Oncol* 1991;9:592–599.

Norris AM, Carrington BM. Late radiation change in the CNS: MR imaging following gadolinium enhancement. *Clin Radiol* 1997;52:356–362.

Plowman PN. Haematologic toxicity during craniospinal irradiation—the impact of prior chemotherapy. *Med Pediatr Oncol* 1997;28:238–239.

Pomeranz HD, Henson JW, Lessell S. Radiation-associated cerebral blindness. *Am J Ophthalmol* 1998;126:609–611.

Rock JP, Hearshen D, Scarpace L. et al. Correlations between magnetic resonance spectroscopy and image-guided histopathology, with special attention to radiation necrosis. *Neurosurgery* 2002;51(4):912–919.

Schlemmer HP, Bachert P, Henze M, et al. Differentiation of radiation necrosis from tumor progression using proton magnetic resonance spectroscopy. *Neuroradiology* 2002;44(3):216–222.

Schultheiss TE, Kun LE, Ang KK, Stephens LC. Radiation response of the central nervous system. *Int J Radiat Oncol Biol Phys* 1995;31:1093–1112.

Sheline GE, Wara WM, Smith V. Therapeutic irradiation and brain therapy. *Int J Radiat Oncol Biol Phys* 1980;6:1215–1228.

Sonoda Y, Kumabe T, Takahashi T, et al. Clinical usefulness of ^{11}C-MET PET and ^{201}Tl SPECT for differentiation of recurrent glioma from radiation necrosis. *Neurol Med Chir (Tokyo)* 1998;38:342–347.

Tada E, Matsumoto K, Nakagawa M, Tamiya T, Furuta T, Ohmoto T. Serial magnetic resonance imaging of delayed radiation necrosis treated with dexamethasone: case illustration. *Neurosurgery* 1997;86:1067.

Twijnstra A, Boon PJ, Lormans ACM, et al. Neurotoxicity of prophylactic cranial irradiation in patients with small cell carcinoma of the lung. *Eur J Cancer Clin Oncol* 1987;23:983–986.

Valk PE, Budinger TF, Levin VA, et al. PET of malignant cerebral tumors after interstitial brachytherapy. *J Neurosurg* 1988;69:830–838.

Wald LL, Nelson SJ, Day MR, et al. Serial proton magnetic resonance spectroscopy imaging of glioblastoma multiforme after brachytherapy. *J Neurosurg* 1997;87:525–534.

Radiation Myelopathy

Alfonso ED, De Gregorio MA, Mateo P, et al. Radiation myelopathy in over-irradiated patients: MR imaging findings. *Eur Radiol* 1997;7:400–404.

Grunewald R, Panayiotopoulos C, Enevoldson T. Late onset radiation-induced motor neuron syndrome. *J Neurol Neurosurg Psychiatry* 1992;55:741–742.

Hopewell JW. Radiation injury to the central nervous system. *Med Pediatr Oncol* 1998;(suppl 1):1–9.

Jeremic B, Djuric L. Mijatovic L. Incidence of radiation myelitis of the cervical spinal cord at doses of 5,500 cGy or greater. *Cancer* 1991;68:2138–2141.

Koehler PJ, Verbiest H, Jager J, Vecht CJ. Delayed radiation myelopathy: serial MR imaging and pathology. *Clin Neurol Neurosurg* 1996;98:197–201.

Komachi H, Tsuchiya K, Ikeda M, et al. Radiation myelopathy: a clinicopathological study with special reference to correlation between MRI findings and neuropathology. *J Neurol Sci* 1995;132:228–232.

Lengyel Z, Reko G, Majtenyi K, et al. Autopsy verifies demyelination and lack of vascular damage in partially reversible radiation myelopathy. *Spinal Cord* 2003;41(10):577–585.

Melki PS, Halimi P, Wibault P, et al. MRI in chronic progressive radiation myelopathy. *J Comput Assist Tomogr* 1994;18:1–6.

Mut M, Cataltepe O, Soylemezoglu F, Akalan N, Ozgen T. Radiation-induced malignant triton tumor associated with severe spinal cord compression. Case report and review of the literature. *J Neurosurg Spine* 2004 Mar;100(3):298–302.

Phuphanich S, Jacobs M, Murtagh FR, Gonzalvo A. MRI of spinal cord recognition necrosis stimulating recurrent cervical cord astrocytoma and syringomyelia. *Surg Neurol* 1996;45:362–365.

Tashima T, Morioka T, Nishio S, et al. Delayed cerebral radionecrosis with a high uptake of ^{11}C-methionine on positron emission tomography and ^{201}Tl-chloride on single-photon emission computed tomography. *Neuroradiology* 1998;40:435–438.

Thorton AF, Zimberg SH, Greenberg HS, et al. Protracted Lhermitte's sign following head and neck irradiation. *Arch Otolaryngol Head Neck Surg* 1991;117:1300–1303.

Wang PY, Shen WC, Jan JS. Serial MRI changes in radiation myelopathy. *Neuroradiology* 1995;37:374–377.

Radiation: Vascular Complications

Benson PJ, Sung JH. Cerebral aneurysms following radiotherapy for medulloblastoma. *J Neurosurg* 1989;70:545–550.

Chang SD, Vanefsky MA, Havton LA, et al. Bilateral cavernous malformations resulting from cranial irradiation of a choroid plexus papilloma. *Neurol Res* 1998;20:529–532.

Houdart E, Mounayer C, Chapot R, et al. Carotid stenting for radiation-induced stenosis. *Stroke* 2001;32:118–121.

McGuirt WF, Feehs RS, Strickland JL, et al. Irradiation-induced atherosclerosis: a factor in therapeutic planning. *Ann Otol Rhinol Laryngol* 1992;101:222–228.

Murros KE, Toole JF. The effect of radiation of carotid arteries: a review article. *Arch Neurol* 1989;46:449–455.

Pozzati E, Giangaspero F, Marliani F, Acciarri N. Occult cerebrovascular malformations after irradiation. *Neurosurgery* 1996;39:677–682.

Steele SR, Martin MJ, Mullenix PS, Crawford JV, Cuadrado DS, Andersen CA. Focused high-risk population screening for carotid arterial stenosis after radiation therapy for head and neck cancer. *Am J Surg* 2004 May;187(5):594–598.

Radiation-Induced Plexopathy

Bowen BC, Verma A, Brandon AH, Fiedler JA. Radiation-induced brachial plexopathy: MR and clinical findings. *AJNR* 1996;17:1932–1936.

Georgion A, Grigsby PW, Perez CA. Radiation-induced lumbosacral plexopathy in gynecologic tumors: clinical findings and dosimetric analysis. *Int J Radiat Oncol Biol Phys* 1993;26:479–482.

Jaeckle KA, Young DF, Foley KM. The natural history of lumbosacral plexopathy in cancer. *Neurology* 1985;35:8–15.

Kori SH, Foley KM, Posner JB. Brachial plexus lesions in patients with cancer: 100 cases. *Neurology* 1981;31:45–50.

Olsen NK, Pfeiffer P, Johannsen L. Radiation-induced brachial plexopathy: neurological follow-up in 161 recurrence-free breast cancer patients. *Int J Radiat Oncol Biology Phys* 1993;26:43–49.

Thomas JE, Cascino TL, Earle JD. Differential diagnosis between radiation and tumor plexopathy of the pelvis. *Neurology* 1985;35:1–7.

Thyagarajan D, Cascino T, Harms G. Magnetic resonance imaging in brachial plexopathy of cancer. *Neurology* 1995;45(3)(Pt 1):421–427.

Wouter van Es H, Engelen AM, Witkamp TD, et al. Radiation-induced brachial plexopathy: MR imaging. *Skeletal Radiol* 1997;26:284–288.

Endocrine Dysfunction

Burstein S. Poor growth after cranial irradiation. *Pediatr Rev* 1997;18:442–444.

Constine LS, Woolf PD, Cann D, et al. Hypothalamic-pituitary dysfunction after radiation for brain tumors. *N Engl J Med* 1993;328:87–94.

Duffner PK, Cohen ME, Voorhess ML, et al. Long-term effects of cranial irradiation on endocrine function in children with brain tumors: a prospective study. *Cancer* 1985;56:2189–2193.

Mechanik JI, Hochberg FH, LaRocque A. Hypothalamic dysfunction following whole-brain irradiation. *J Neurosurg* 1986;65:490–494.

Rappaport R, Brauner R. Growth and endocrine disorders secondary to cranial irradiation. *Pediatr Res* 1989;25:561–567.

Shalet SM. Radiation and pituitary dysfunction. *N Engl J Med* 1993; 238:131–133.

Woo E, Lam K, Yu YL, Ma J, Wang C, Yeung RT. Temporal lobe and hypothalamic-pituitary dysfunctions after radiotherapy for nasopharyngeal carcinoma: a distinct clinical syndrome. *J Neurol Neurosurg Psychiatry* 1988;51:1302–1307.

Radiation: Neuropsychologic Effects

Anderson V, Godber T, Smibert E, Ekert H. Neurobehavioural sequelae following cranial irradiation and chemotherapy in children: an analysis of risk factors. *Pediatr Rehabil* 1997;1:63–76.

Armstrong C, Ruffer J, Corn B, De Vries K, Mollman J. Biphasic patterns of memory deficits following moderate-dose partial-brain irradiation: neuropsychologic outcome and proposed mechanisms. *J Clin Oncol* 1995;13:2263–2271.

Crossen JR, Garwood D, Glatstein E, et al. Neurobehavioral sequelae of cranial irradiation in adults: a review of radiation-induced encephalopathy. *J Clin Oncol* 1994;12:627–642.

Duffey P, Chari G, Cartlidge NEF, et al. Progressive deterioration of intellect and motor function occurring several decades after cranial irradiation. *Arch Neurol* 1996;53:814–818.

Iuvone L, Mariotti P, Colosimo C, et al. Long-term cognitive outcome, brain computed tomography scan, and magnetic resonance imaging in children cured for acute lymphoblastic leukemia. *Cancer* 2002;95(12):2562–2570.

Roman DD, Sperduto PW. Neuropsychological effects of cranial radiation: current knowledge and future directions. *Int J Radiat Oncol Biol Phys* 1998;31:983–998.

Sklar CA, Copstine LS. Chronic neuropsychological sequela of radiation therapy. *Int J Radiat Oncol Biol Phys* 1995;31:1113–1121.

Radiation Damage to Peripheral Nerves

Giese WL, Kinsella TJ. Radiation injury to peripheral and cranial nerves. In: Gutin PH, Leibel SA, Sheline GE, eds. *Radiation Injury to the Nervous System*. New York: Raven Press, 1991:383–403.

Gillette EL, Mahler PA, Powers BE, Gillette SM, Vujaskovic Z. Late radiation injury to muscle and peripheral nerves. *Int J Radiat Oncol Biol Phys* 1995;31:1309–1318.

Radiation-Induced Tumors

Dweik A, Maheut-Lourmiere J, Lioret E, Jan M. Radiation-induced meningioma. *Childs Nerv Syst* 1995;11:661–663.

Foley KM. Radiation-induced malignant and atypical peripheral nerve sheath tumors. *Ann Neurol* 1980;7:311–318.

Harrison MJ, Wolfe DE, Lau TS, et al. Radiation-induced meningiomas: experience at the Mount Sinai Hospital and review of the literature. *J Neurosurg* 1991;75:564–574.

Nadeem SQ, Feun LG, Bruce-Gregorios JH, et al. Post-radiation sarcoma (malignant fibrous histiocytoma) of the cervical spine following ependymoma: a case report. *J Neurooncol* 1991;11:263–268.

Ron E, Modan B, Boice JD Jr, et al. Tumors of the brain and nervous system after radiotherapy in childhood. *N Engl J Med* 1988;319:1033–1039.

Salvati M, Frati A, Russo N, et al. Radiation-induced gliomas: report of 10 cases and review of the literature. *Surg Neurol* 2003;60(1):60–67.

Radiation Optic Neuropathy

Piquemal R, Cottier JP, Arsene S, et al. Radiation-induced optic neuropathy 4 years after radiation: report of a case followed up with MRI. *Neuroradiology* 1998;40:439–441.

McClellan RL, el Gammal T, Kline LB. Early bilateral radiation-induced optic neuropathy with follow-up MRI. *Neuroradiology* 1995;37:131–133.

Macdonald D, Rottenberg D, Schutz J, et al. Radiation-induced optic neuropathy. In: Rottenberg D, ed. *Neurological Complications of Cancer Treatment*. Boston: Butterworth-Heinemann, 1991:37–61.

Chapter 73

Electrical and Lightning Injury

Lewis P. Rowland

PATHOLOGY

High-voltage electric shock or lightning stroke may damage the CNS, motor neurons, or peripheral nerves. James Parkinson, himself, was one of the early observers of the syndrome. The lesions may involve either the brain or the spinal cord. In the spinal cord, myelomalacia may result without change in blood vessels, inflammation, or gliosis. Similarly, nonspecific lesions are found in the brain, and gray matter may be affected. In death from acute injury, cerebral lesions seem to be dominated by the effects of cardiac arrest and anoxia, with edema, perivascular hemorrhage, and neuronal loss.

PATHOGENESIS

The mechanism of injury is not clear. Investigators have stated that resistance to the flow of electric current is lower in neural tissue than in other organs and that the consequent syndromes result from the direct effects of high-voltage electricity on neural cells. Cerebellar injury has been attributed to heat injury as part of the insult. Demyelination does not seem to be the result of vascular injury, and it is not clear why symptoms are immediate in most patients, but delayed in many. Nor is it clear why different parts of the nervous system are affected in different victims.

EPIDEMIOLOGY

In earlier times, electrocution was the result of accidents at work or in the home. With technologic advances, these causes have become less common but still account for about 1,000 deaths per year in the United States; lightning strikes account for about 100 deaths per year. Lightning strikes may be occupational hazards (e.g., farming, ranching, roofing) or recreational (e.g., water sports, hiking, camping, or other outdoor activities) hazards. Men outnumber women by 4.5:1, as victims.

SYMPTOMS AND SIGNS

Among survivors, the first signs occur immediately after the shock and may be transient. Unconsciousness and amnesia are common, and there may be transient limb paralysis or paresthesia. Cerebral infarction may result from cardiac arrhythmia and embolization. Posthypoxic encephalopathy or cerebral hemorrhage may occur. Days or weeks later, progressive disorders begin, and resemble one or another of several syndromes, such as parkinsonism, cerebellar disorders, myelopathy, spinal-muscular atrophy, or sensorimotor peripheral neuropathy. Because there are so few cases, it is not possible to determine whether all reported cases are consequences of the electric shock or are a coincidental occurrence of two conditions.

TREATMENT

Acutely, attention is directed to the cardiac disorder. The delayed-onset syndromes may only be managed symptomatically because no specific treatment exists.

SUGGESTED READINGS

Cherington M. Neurologic manifestations of lightning strikes. *Neurology* 2003;60:182–185.

Cherington M, Parkinson J. Links to Charcot, Lichtenberg, and lightning. *Arch Neurol* 2004;61:977.

Cherington M, Yarnell P, Hallmark D. MRI in lightning encephalopathy. *Neurology* 1993;43:1437–1438.

Cherington M, Yarnell P, Lammereste D. Lightning strikes: nature of neurological damage in patients evaluated in hospital emergency departments. *Ann Emerg Med* 1992;21:575–578.

Critchley M. Neurological effects of lightning and electricity. *Lancet* 1934;1:68–72.

Davidson GS, Deck JH. Delayed myelopathy following lightning strike: a demyelinating process. *Acta Neuropathol* 1988;77:104–108.

Gallagher JP, Talbert OR. Motor neuron syndrome after electric shock. *Acta Neurol Scand* 1991;83:79–82.

Fahmy FS, Brinsden MD, Smith J, Frame JD. Lightning: the multisystem group injuries. *J Trauma* 1999;46:937–940.

Hawke CH, Thorpe JW. Acute polyneuropathy due to lightning injury. *J Neurol Neurosurg Psychiatry* 1992;55:388–390.

Kleinschmidt-DeMasters DK. Neuropathology of lightning-strike injuries. *Semin Neurol* 1995;15:323–328.

Panse F. Electrical trauma. In: Vinken PJ, Bruyn GW, Braakman R, eds. *Injuries of the Brain and Skull. Handbook of Clinical Neurology,* Vols 23-24. Amsterdam: North-Holland Publishing, 1975:683–729.

Sirdofsky MD, Hawley RJ, Manz H. Progressive motor neuron disease associated with electrical injury. *Muscle Nerve* 1991;14:977–980.

Stanley LD, Suss RA. Intracerebral hematoma secondary to lightning stroke: case report and review of the literature. *Neurosurgery* 1985;16:686–688.

Chapter 74

Decompression Sickness

Leon D. Prockop

In scuba diving, caisson work, flying, and simulated altitude ascents, rapid reduction in ambient pressure may allow the formation of bubbles from inert gases, especially nitrogen, that are normally dissolved in body tissues. Barotrauma encompasses disorders related to over- expansion of gas-filled cavities, such as the lung or inner ear.

Arterial gas embolism (AGE) describes penetration of gas bubbles into the systemic circulation as a result of pulmonary barotrauma, transpulmonary passage after massive bubble formation (i.e., chokes), or cardiac shunting. Decompression sickness (DCS) is caused by the growth of gas nuclei in predominately fatty tissues. The resulting lesions involve the limbs, cardiopulmonary system, and CNS. In divers, DCS affects the spinal cord, primarily. Aviators may develop typical musculoskeletal or neurological DCS symptoms while at altitude, with resolution of symptoms frequently occurring on return to sea level. AGE is frequently related to a rapid ascent, and is far more common in diving than altitude exposure.

INCIDENCE

The incidence of decompression sickness in divers is between 1% and 30%. Although the spinal cord is the most common site of neurologic lesions, encephalopathy is also well described. Electrophysiologic studies, experimental models, and isolated postmortem examinations of patients show predominant involvement of the posterolateral and posterior columns in the watershed areas of the thoracic, upper lumbar, and lower cervical cord. Ischemic perivascular lesions are usually confined to the white matter, but subsequent petechial hemorrhage may occur and extend into the gray matter. Lesions result from bubbles occluding vessels or directly disrupting tissue. Coincident intraarterial embolism may cause cerebral damage.

SIGNS AND SYMPTOMS

With cord damage, radicular symptoms are followed by leg paresthesia, paresis, and bladder and bowel dysfunction. When the brain is affected, neurologic signs and symptoms include visual impairment, vertigo, hemiparesis, loss of consciousness, and seizures. Unless recompression is achieved promptly, the signs, including paralysis, may become permanent.

TREATMENT

Manifestations of decompression sickness, including any neurologic symptoms and signs, are a medical emergency. Current therapy consists of recompression in a hyperbaric chamber and the concurrent administration of 100% oxygen. Results of treatment vary, but the sooner recompression is begun, the better the outcome. Although the use of drugs to improve outcomes is being investigated, no particular adjunctive pharmacotherapy has been proved effective. Some advise the use of steroids or lidocaine. Intravenous fluids are important. MRI can document the extent of brain and spinal cord damage. Although the issue is controversial, patent foramen ovale (PFO) may be a cause of unexplained DCS or AGE in sports divers. For chamber locations and emergency information, physicians should contact The Divers Alert Network, at 919-681-4326, a 24-hour hotline.

SUGGESTED READINGS

Aharon-Peretz J, Adir Y, Gordon CR, et al. Spinal cord decompression sickness in sport diving. *Arch Neurol* 1993;50:753–756.

Balldin UI, Pilmanis AA, Webb JT. Central nervous system decompression sickness and venous gas emboli in hypobaric conditions. *Aviat Space Environ Med* 2004 Nov;75(11):969–972.

Bond JP, Kirschner DA. Spinal cord myelin is vulnerable to decompression. *Mol Chem Neuropathol* 1997;30:273–288.

Doolett DJ, Mitchell SS. The physiological kinetics of nitrogen and the prevention of decompression sickness. *Clin Pharmacokinet* 2001;40(1):1–14.

Dutka AJ. Long term effects on the central nervous system, In: Brubakk AO, Neuman TS, eds. *Bennett and Elliott's Physiology and Medicine of Diving*, 6th ed. New York: WB Saunders, 2003.

Dutka AJ, Francis TF. Pathophysiology of decompression sickness, In: Bove AA, ed. *Bove and Davis' Diving Medicine*, 3rd ed. Philadelphia: WB Saunders, 1997.

Green RD, Leitch DR. Twenty years of treating decompression sickness. *Aviat Space Environ Med* 1987;58:362–366.

Haymaker W, Johnston AD. Pathology of decompression sickness: comparison of lesions in airmen with those in caisson workers and divers. *Mil Med* 1955;117:285–306.

Lambersten CJ. Concepts for advances in the therapy of bends in undersea and aerospace activity. *Aerospace Med* 1968;39:1086–1093.

Mitchell SJ. Lidocaine in the treatment of decompression sickness: a review of the literature. *Undersea Hyperb Med* 2001;28(3):165–174.

Moon RE, Gorman DF. Treatment of decompression disorders, In: Brubakk AO, Neuman TS, eds. *Bennett and Elliott's Physiology and Medicine of Diving*, 5th ed. New York: WB Saunders, 2003.

Reuter M, Tetzlaff K, Hutzelmann A, et al. MR imaging of the central nervous system in diving-related decompression illness. *Acta Radiol* 1997;38(6):940–994.

Schwerzmann M, Seiler C. Recreational scuba diving, patent foramen ovale, and their associated risks. *Swiss Med Wkly* 2001;131(25-26):365–374.

U.S. Navy Diving Manual, 4 Change A, 20 Jan 1999; Naval Sea Systems Command.

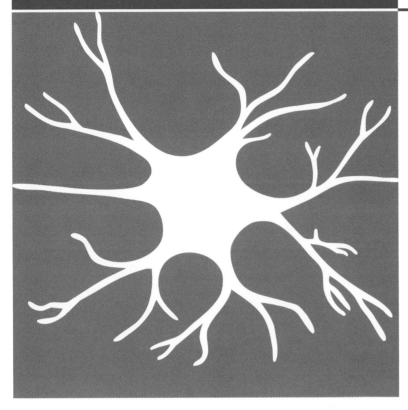

Birth Injuries and Developmental Abnormalities

Chapter 75

▶ # Neonatal Neurology

M. Richard Koenigsberger,
Ram Kairam,
Douglas R. Nordli, Jr., and
Timothy A. Pedley

Many children come to pediatric neurology clinics with static brain injuries that originate in the perinatal period and cause mental retardation, cerebral palsy or seizures. Intracranial hemorrhage, periventricular leukomalacia, neonatal encephalopathy, neonatal seizures and neonatal infection account for many of these problems as described in this chapter. Metabolic and congenital disorders, many inherited, are discussed in Sections VIII and IX.

INTRACRANIAL HEMORRHAGE

Gestational age and mode of delivery are the best statistical indicators of the probable site of intracranial hemorrhage (ICH). *Supratentorial subdural hemorrhage* has become rare and occurs almost exclusively in full-term or large infants after difficult deliveries. *Parenchymal cerebral hemorrhage* originating in the periventricular area with or without secondary subarachnoid bleeding is common in infants of 32 weeks' gestation or less. *Primary subarachnoid supratentorial hemorrhage* of venous origin occurs in full-term newborns who may have focal seizures and a benign clinical course. *Subarachnoid hemorrhage* may be found at autopsy in premature infants, but there is no recognized clinical syndrome. *Posterior fossa hemorrhages* are now more readily recognized in newborns, some needing only careful clinical observation, while others require urgent surgical intervention.

PERIVENTRICULAR INTRAVENTRICULAR HEMORRHAGE

Incidence

With the advent of cranial ultrasonography, the incidence of parenchymal hemorrhage—more precisely, periventricular intraventricular hemorrhage (IVH) was about 40% among newborns weighing less than 1,500 g in 1980. In the past two decades, the incidence has declined to 10% to 20%. The incidence is most frequent in infants weighing less than 900 gm. Prenatal corticosteroid therapy and the use of a surfactant after birth have contributed to the decline of IVH.

Pathology and Pathophysiology

In most patients, the hemorrhage arises in the vascular germinal plate located in the region of the caudate near the foramen of Monro (Fig. 75.1). Bleeding may be confined to this friable matrix area (grade I), but more than 50% of such hemorrhages rupture into the lateral ventricles (grade II), and these sometimes progressively enlarge (grade III). Grade IV, formerly attributed to parenchymal extension of grade III hemorrhage, is now thought to originate in the brain parenchyma itself; its location and size are main contributors to neonatal mortality and neurologic morbidity.

It is not known whether IVH of grades I through III originates from an arterial source, the recurrent artery of Heubner, or from the thalamostriate veins. Proponents of the arterial theory cite hypotension followed by hypertension in a hypoxic brain that has lost autoregulation. The venous hypothesis suggests that increased venous pressure leads to stasis, thrombosis, and rupture of thin-walled vessels of the germinal plate. This mechanism of increased venous pressure is thought to produce a concurrent white matter parenchymal infarct, which may become bloody (grade IV).

Signs and Symptoms

Grade I hemorrhage is usually asymptomatic. In grade II, there is nonspecific irritability or lethargy. Some grade III hemorrhages are clinically silent in spite of ventriculomegaly, whereas others produce hydrocephalic

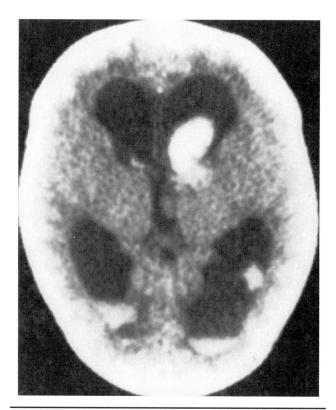

FIGURE 75.1. Germinal matrix hemorrhage. Noncontrast axial CT shows small, focal hemorrhage in the region of the left caudate head near the left thalamus with extension into the frontal horn of the left lateral ventricle. There is spread of hemorrhage into both occipital horns. This represents grade III germinal matrix hemorrhage. (Courtesy of Dr. S. Chan, Columbia University College of Physicians and Surgeons, New York, NY.)

symptoms of varying severity. When observed in combination with grade IV hemorrhage, deterioration may ensue soon after onset, with at least a 50% chance of mortality; signs include severe apnea, bradycardia, extensor posturing and opisthotonus, ocular conversion or diversion, and pupillary fixation, usually in mid position. Many neonates become flaccid and unresponsive and die within minutes or hours. Clonic limb movements may occur concurrently. The posturing and movements have been called "seizures," but there is little, if any, EEG correlation. Less dramatic deterioration may occur over a few days.

Diagnosis

Gestation of less than 32 weeks places an infant at risk for periventricular IVH. A 20% or greater fall in the hematocrit suggests IVH. The CSF contains many red blood cells and has a protein content of 250 mg/dL to 1,200 mg/dL. Days later, the CSF becomes xanthochromic with white and red blood cells and low glucose content; meningitis is ruled out by cultures.

Sonography is the cornerstone of diagnosis. This portable cribside technique delineates the site of blood in the parenchyma and ventricles, ventricular size, and shifts of major structures. Cystic periventricular leukomalacia can also be identified.

Prognosis and Therapy

In grades I and II IVH, prognosis is good, with an 80% to 90% survival rate without obvious neurologic abnormality. Many of these children, however, may show later disorders of learning and behavior. Morbidity is attributed to coexisting hypoxic damage (see PVL that follows). Grade III hemorrhage may develop into a static or reversible ventriculomegaly with normal pressure or may be followed by progressive hydrocephalus with at least a 40% incidence of cerebral palsy and mental retardation. Along with the dramatic decrease in the incidence of IVH, there has been a corresponding decrease in post-hemorrhagic hydrocephalus. Grade IV hemorrhage has a high mortality, particularly when large lesions occur. Morbidity can be predicted by the size of hemorrhage. Those with large, echodense parenchymal lesions have a universally poor outcome.

No treatment is needed for grades I and II hemorrhages. In grade III, serial lumbar punctures are most effective when large volumes can be drained (e.g., 10 mL) or when sonography after lumbar puncture shows diminished ventricular size. If sonographic evidence of ventricular enlargement and signs of intracranial pressure persist one option is to place a temporary ventriculo-subgaleal shunt. If that fails, external ventriculostomy is used for periods not exceeding 5 days (because of the danger of infection). These therapies usually serve only to postpone an inevitable ventriculoperitoneal shunt. This procedure has a high complication rate in small infants. Every attempt should be made to delay shunting until the infant attains as much somatic growth as possible. Although treatment with acetazolamide (Diamox) to decrease production of CSF is only sometimes efficacious, it may postpone placement of a shunt.

Prevention

Many treatments for the prevention of germinal hemorrhage have been attempted. Of pharmacologic agents administered to small preterm infants, indomethacin seems to be most effective in lowering the incidence of IVH. Antenatal corticosteroids are used primarily to induce maturation of the fetal lung, but reduce neonatal mortality, as well as the overall incidence and severity of IVH. The best prevention of ICH remains, when possible, the avoidance of premature birth.

PERIVENTRICULAR LEUKOMALACIA

Periventricular leukomalacia (PVL) may not cause overt symptoms during a newborn's hospital stay or even in the neonatal period. At the same time, imaging has shown PVL in 10% of surviving very-low birth-weight (VLBW) babies (birth weight less than 1500 g), and 50% in extremely-low birth-weight (ELBW) infants (birth weight 500 g to 1000 g). Consequently, when premature infants as young as 24 weeks gestational age are seen in follow-up examination, PVL becomes the leading cause of subsequent cerebral palsy, in the form of spastic diplegia. Therefore, a working knowledge of the condition, its pathology, presumptive pathophysiology, therapy and prevention are useful to the clinician.

Pathology

First described at autopsy as punctate bleeding and cystic necrosis in the periventricular white matter of premature infants, the definition of PVL has expanded to encompass not only these focal lesions, but also more extensive, diffuse, white-matter pathology. Cystic PVL may be diagnosed in the newborn by ultrasound examination, accomplished through the anterior fontanelle. Cysts are found in the periventricular region and are characterized by focal necrosis of axons, oligodendrocytes, and astrocytes. The more common entity of diffuse white-matter hypomyelination in the centrum semiovale is characterized, histologically, by astrocytosis, loss of oligodendrial cells, and by impaired myelinogenesis. Lesions are evident at 40 weeks postconception age in as many as 50% of these same VLBW survivors, appearing as diffuse areas of high-signal density in the centrum semiovale on T2 MRI. PVL of this variety is usually not evident on ultrasound.

Pathophysiology

Current thinking about the genesis of PVL suggests two triggers that initiate the process. In the immature infant, the blood vessels supplying the white matter are arrayed radially, to create end zones. These vessels lack autoregulation and are therefore susceptible to changes in cerebral blood pressure. In this setting, systemic hypotension leads to brain tissue hypoxia, followed by glutamate toxicity, and free radical damage to preoligodendrocytes, the predominant cell in the white matter at this early gestational age. The preoligodendrocytes are then destroyed or so altered that they do not mature into normal, myelin-producing cells. Hypomyelination is seen in descending fibers, from the frontal lobes to neurons of leg muscles, as they proceed in the posterior limb of the internal capsule, the corpus callosum, pes pedunculi, and the corticospinal tract. This result is spastic diplegia of varying degrees, usually evident clinically in the first or second year of life as increased tone and hyperreflexia in the legs. In the newborn period, hypotonia may precede spasticity.

If the visual radiations in the posterior white matter are affected, visual abnormality occurs in surviving ELBW infants. With white-matter dropout, an ex vacuo ventriculomegaly may ensue, sometimes accompanied by decreased gray-matter volume with underdeveloped gyration; this may explain the subnormal IQ scores and behavioral aberrations observed in many of these infants.

Maternal or fetal infection, as well as hypoxia, may contribute to the development of PVL in the VLBW newborn. Maternal infection begets premature labor and birth, so more VLBW newborn become candidates for PVL. Also, maternal infections, such as amnionitis, not only cause umbilical-cord funisitis, but also produce proinflammatory cytokines in the amniotic fluid, as well as in the blood and CSF of the fetus. The cytokines TNF α and IL-6 set off a cascade release of free radicals that could cause PVL by activating microglia, which in turn secrete products toxic to preoligodendrocytes. Finally, low birth weight (LBW) neonates who survive sepsis demonstrate a higher incidence of PVL and cerebral palsy at follow-up examination than do controls, possible induced by either the hypotensive/anoxic or the humoral/cytokine pathways.

Thus, it may be anticipated that a reduction in the incidence of spastic diplegia will be linked to the prevention of prematurity and maternal infection, as well as to the ability to maintain adequate perfusion of the brains of VLBW infants.

HYPOXIC-ISCHEMIC ENCEPHALOPATHY

Incidence

The incidence of acute encephalopathy at birth, or shortly after, in infants of 36 weeks gestational age is 2 to 4 infants per 1000 live births. Perinatal anoxia or hypoxia was believed to be the main cause. However, it has become evident that other events are important; maternal infection or amnionitis, inborn metabolic errors, congenital CNS malformations, as well as undetermined causes, may also present with neonatal depression, seizures with cerebral palsy, and even death, as a result. Hypoxic-ischemic encephalopathy (HIE), however, still accounts for many clinical neonatal encephalopathies, often occurring precipitously, despite optimal obstetric management.

Pathology and Pathophysiology

The most common events associated with HIE are severe maternal hypotension, rupture of the uterus, abruptio placenta, and placental or umbilical-cord dysfunction.

Concomitant hypoxic cardiopulmonary, hepatic, and renal dysfunction may add to the cerebral insult. The resultant brain pathology depends on the maturity of the brain at the time of insult, as well as the duration and location of the insult. PVL prevails in infants of low gestation, (e.g., less than 32 weeks). After 36 weeks gestation, hypoxic-anoxic lesions involve the cerebral gray matter, the basal ganglia and thalamus, brain stem, and cerebellar Purkinje cells. Acute neuronal loss, in a laminar distribution in the depths of the cerebral sulci of the cortex, is often accompanied by edema and infarction. The chronic picture reveals neuronal loss and astrocytosis, along with atrophy, cystic change and ulegyria of the cortex, status marmoratus of the basal ganglia, and cerebellar atrophy (see Chapter 77).

Severe, brief, total HIE results in diffuse deep and superficial lesions that may be incompatible with life. Experimentally, similar lesions may be produced, in monkeys, by instituting complete intrauterine asphyxia for 13 minutes. In humans, these lesions may be caused by abruptio placenta, uterine rupture, or umbilical-cord occlusion. Near-total asphyxia by the same mechanisms results in injury to the putamen, thalamus, and peri-Rolandic cerebral cortex. Sometimes the brain stem is involved.

Partial HIE for minutes or hours, results in predominantly supratentorial lesions, which may show a parasagittal-watershed distribution. This subacute variant is often recognized in the neonatal period and may be due to impaired placental exchange. Less severe episodes of hypoxia-ischemia of undetermined frequency, duration, and timing, may diffusely involve neurons or preferentially affect the hippocampal area.

At the cellular level, magnetic resonance spectroscopy (MRS), MRI, PET, and in particular, experimental animal studies, continue to add to knowledge of the pathophysiology of HIE. The data suggest that not all brain cells undergo immediate necrotic death following anoxic energy failure. After the anoxic insult, many cells go through reoxygenation and reperfusion. During this time, glutamate accumulates in hypoxic glial cells. The excess of glutamate contributes to further cellular damage in at least two ways. First, it stimulates neurons with NMDA and AMPA receptors, leading to cytosolic accumulation of calcium ions in neurons, and then a cascade of events resulting in secondary-cell death. The glutamate excitotoxicity leads to the release of nitric oxide, which combines with free radicals to induce apoptotic cell death. Second, the same NMDA receptors also release calpains that activate caspase-3, which leads to apoptosis and further neural degeneration. Moreover, mitochondrial failure contributes in causing brain-cell injury and death. Increased lactic acid is detectable in the brain, by MRS, and in the CSF of affected newborns, confirming mitochondrial breakdown.

The problems of ischemia-reperfusion seem to start 5 to 6 hours after the first ischemic event and may last for hours or even days. There may be time enough for therapeutic interventions that could limit the injurious cascade by preventing glutamate toxicity or mitochondrial injury. In animal studies, damage has been reduced by pretreatment with MK 801, an NMDA-uptake inhibitor that blocks the glutamate. Also, L-carnitine reduces the accumulation of acyl-CoA in the mitochondrial matrix, and hypothermia is protective in animals.

Signs and Symptoms

A strict definition of HIE would include a sentinel obstetric event occurring immediately before, or during labor, abnormal fetal heart-rate pattern in this same period, metabolic acidosis as measured by a pH of less than 7.0 in fetal umbilical blood, Apgar scores of 0 to 3 for 5 minutes or longer, and imaging evidence of acute, nonfocal, cerebral damage. Clinically, the low Apgar scores translate into reduced heart rate, depressed or absent respiration, diminished responsivity, and decreased muscle tone and tendon reflexes. This picture evolves into one of three clinical patterns: an awake, even hyperalert baby, with mild-to-moderate lethargy and hypotonia, those symptoms plus seizures, or an apathetic infant with severe hypotonia and severe depression or coma, almost invariably with accompanying seizures.

Newborns in the first two categories gradually improve in alertness, tone, and ability to feed. Those with seizures recover a little more gradually, partly retarded by drug therapy for seizures. Infants with severe encephalopathy become more stuporous in the first 24 hours and develop frequent seizures, respiratory depression, brain-stem abnormalities, and intermittent signs of decerebration. They lose Moro and sucking reflexes, and become unresponsive. Even with vigorous anticonvulsant and supportive therapy, 20% to 30% of these infants die. If an infant survives the first 48 to 72 hours, the seizures usually stop. The infant remains in stupor for a variable period, depending on the severity of brain injury and the blood level of anticonvulsants; it then shows variable recovery, often appearing almost normal, but then developing slowly, and exhibiting spastic quadriparesis or choreoathetosis, mental retardation, and often, seizures.

Laboratory Data

During labor, nonreassuring fetal-heart patterns indicating placental insufficiency or fetal distress may herald HIE. Although providing a warning for appropriate action, such as emergency cesarean section, abnormal fetal-heart tones do not necessarily correlate with the degree of subsequent brain damage.

After birth, umbilical arterial blood gasses with a low PO_2, a pH of less than 7.0, or a base excess of greater than 12, are significant. Reduced or absent renal flow, abnormal liver function, depressed serum glucose or sodium levels, and elevated creatine kinase B-B or CSF lactate levels, also are indicators of an hypoxemic event. EEG may reveal seizure activity that is inapparent, clinically. In the interictal period, a relatively inactive background and burst suppression patterns on EEG imply poor outcome, as do impaired VER and persistently abnormal BAER. CT evidence of extensive areas of hypodensity of both gray and white matter suggest a guarded outlook. MRI with diffusion-weighted imaging (DWI) on day 1 or 2 demonstrates early, bright signaling in the basal ganglia and other deep structures. Subsequent laminar necrosis and infarction are also evident in the gray matter on DWI, before they appear on T1 or FLAIR sequences. Cystic parenchymal changes, as well as atrophy, may be evident by 2 weeks of life. Assessing the severity of these changes is helpful in establishing a prognosis. A lactate peak may be seen on MRS, which is helpful in both diagnosis and prognosis of HIE.

Treatment and Prognosis

Because the hypoxic-ischemic insult involves several body systems in addition to the brain, measures include respiratory support, maintenance of normal blood pressure and renal output, and adequate supply of energy to the brain in the form of 10% D/W intravenous fluid replacement therapy. The treatment of seizures is discussed later. Steroids and osmotic agents have been used to treat brain edema but with little success. In addition, given the limitations of the therapeutic window described above, treatments effective in animals with NMDA-receptor antagonists or antioxidative substances have not been successful in humans. A 48- to 72-hour period of brain cooling, beginning less than 6 hours after birth, has been effective in animal studies, and may have success in infants with mild or moderate disease, but not severe encephalopathy.

The prognosis is always guarded. The more rapid the recovery from the initial depression, the better the outlook appears, in the absence of MRI abnormalities. Of infants with a benign neonatal course 20% to 30% may still have neurologic sequelae ranging from spastic quadriparesis or choreoathetotic cerebral palsy, to intellectual impairment and seizures. At least 50% of those with neonatal seizures have serious morbidity. Prevention by rapid delivery (i.e., cesarean section) when there is evidence of intrauterine distress is still the best method of avoiding sequelae.

NEONATAL INFECTIONS

Bacterial infections are commonly acquired perinatally. Viral or protozoan infections may be acquired in utero from the first trimester until delivery. Infections constituting the TORCH syndrome (toxoplasmosis, other agents, rubella, cytomegalovirus, herpes simplex) are discussed in Section III, Infections of the Nervous System. Only some features of perinatally-acquired herpes simplex virus (HSV) infection are dealt with here.

Neonatal Herpes Encephalitis

Estimates of the incidence of active neonatal HSV infection are 1 to 3 per 10,000 live births. HSV infection may be acquired *in utero* or during passage through the birth canal. Most neonatal HSV infections are caused by HSV type 2, rather than HSV type 1. Some infants have only skin-eye-mouth disease, but 70% have either systemic or CNS disease. Infants with CNS involvement usually have symptoms in the second or third weeks of life; those with HSV septicemia may have respiratory disease, jaundice, fever, and CNS symptoms, without skin or mucous membrane vesicles, much like those with only CNS involvement, who have fever, irritability, and seizures.

Laboratory investigation reveals lymphocytosis and increased protein in the CSF. Viral amplification with the polymerase-chain reaction in the CSF has made diagnosis of HSV encephalitis quicker and more reliable. Neuroimaging results may be normal, but two-thirds of the children show diffuse, or occasionally, focal abnormalities.

Infants with suspected HSV infection should be treated with acyclovir, 60 mg/kg, intravenously, for 21 days. The mortality rate is about 15% when there is only CNS disease, but increases to 45% with disseminated infection. Only 30% of infants with CNS disease develop normally, and severe sequelae are invariably present when multicystic encephalomalacia is seen on imaging.

Neonatal Meningitis

Neonatal bacterial meningitis shows two clinical patterns. Early-onset sepsis with meningitis is a fulminant, systemic disease, occurring during the first 4 to 5 days of life. It is associated with complications of labor and delivery, including premature birth, premature or prolonged rupture of membranes, maternal colonization with group B-streptococcal infection, and maternal chorioamnionitis. The incidence of sepsis neonatorum varies from 1 to 8 per 1000 births. The meninges are infected in one of four cases. At present, despite a lower incidence of maternal disease owing to intrapartum treatment, *group B-streptococcus*, is still the predominant causative organism, followed by gram-negative organisms *Escherichia coli, Proteus vulgaris*, and *Pseudomonas aeruginosa*. *Listeria monocytogenes* and other organisms are also encountered. Pathologic changes in the newborn are similar to those in older children.

The clinical manifestations of meningitis in the newborn are subtle. Meningeal signs are rarely elicited; lassitude and poor feeding may be the only abnormalities. Hypothermia is as likely as fever. Seizures may be the first sign. Only when the course is advanced, does the fontanel bulge and the infant assume a position of opisthotonus. CSF changes are similar to those in older children, but CSF protein levels up to 100 mg/dL may be normal in term newborns. The blood-to-CSF ratio is less valid, because newborns normally have blood glucose levels as low as 40 mg/dL. Cultures of the CSF may remain positive for 3 or 4 days, even after initiation of proper therapy.

As the disease may be advanced when it is clinically manifest, both mortality and morbidity remain high. Appropriate intravenous antibiotic therapy should be given for 3 weeks. Intrathecal and intraventricular therapy have not been effective. Gram-negative organisms, particularly *Citrobacter*, are most frequently implicated in neonatal abscess, which is rare.

NEONATAL SEIZURES

Seizures are the most common symptoms of neonatal brain dysfunction, and they frequently indicate major injury to the developing brain. Seizures occur in 0.5% to 1% of all newborns and in many babies seen in a neonatal intensive care unit, it becomes an urgent clinical problem that requires prompt diagnosis and treatment.

Classification

The clinical and EEG features of neonatal seizures differ from those of older children. Classification schemes for older patients are not appropriate for newborns. Instead, neonatal seizures are most often classified by dominant clinical features, although there is disagreement about which patterns are epileptic, in the sense that the term is used in older children. Simultaneous video and EEG recordings have revealed that not all paroxysmal behaviors are accompanied by changes in the EEG (Table 75.1). Focal clonic, focal tonic, and some myoclonic seizures do exhibit ictal EEG discharges. Generalized tonic postures, motor automatisms (mouthing, pedaling, and rotatory-arm movements) have unreliable or inconsistent EEG equivalents. Classifying these as *subtle seizures* may lead to unnecessary anticonvulsant drug treatment. Such abnormal movements, often seen with HIE, imply a guarded prognosis, and likely reflect basal-ganglia dysfunction or release phenomena involving frontal or brain-stem structures. Apnea is only rarely the sole manifestation of an ictal event. Generalized tonic-clonic seizures do not occur in newborns because of brain immaturity.

EEG Patterns

Neonatal EEG seizure patterns also differ from those seen in older children. For example, it is common to see rhyth-

▶ **TABLE 75.1 Classification of Neonatal Seizures**

Clinical Seizures	Electrographic Seizure	
	Common	Uncommon
Autonomic phenomena		+
Oral-buccal lingual movements		+
Motor automatisms		+
Clonic		
Focal	+	
Multifocal	+	
Tonic		
Focal	+	
Generalized		+
Myoclonic		
Focal, multifocal		+
Generalized	+	

Modified from Volpe JJ. *Pediatrics* 1989;84:422–428.

mic runs of delta waves, alpha-frequency discharges, recurrent sharp waves or mixed sharp and slow waves (Fig. 75.2). EEG discharges are mostly located in the temporal regions, but any brain area may be involved and multifocal discharges are common, particularly with diffuse encephalopathies. Ictal patterns are not etiologically specific.

Not all EEG discharges produce clinical changes. In fact, many treated infants have EEG seizure patterns without clinical signs. Neither gestational age, nor severity of EEG background activity correlates with the appearance of subclinical seizures. Interictal-EEG patterns are useful in determining the prognosis of seizures (see below).

Etiology

Although the incidence of neonatal seizures has remained relatively constant for several decades, the frequency with which different etiologies are encountered has changed considerably. Causes of seizures, such as hypocalcemia and obstetrical injury, once common in the newborn, are rare today. Now, neonatal encephalopathy (e.g., often HIE) in term infants and IVH in premature babies account for about one-third of seizures in newborns. Other important causes include intracerebral hemorrhage, infarction, intrauterine or postnatal infection, cerebral malformations, and metabolic disorders, including hypoglycemia, hypocalcemia, hypomagnesemia, and inborn errors of metabolism (e.g., nonketotic hyperglycinemia, urea-cycle defects, phenylketonuria, maple-sugar urine disease, lactic and organic acidurias). In many babies, multiple factors coexist. Some refractory neonatal seizures are responsive to vitamin treatment, including B-6, pyridoxal phosphate, and folinic acid. Withdrawal seizures may occur

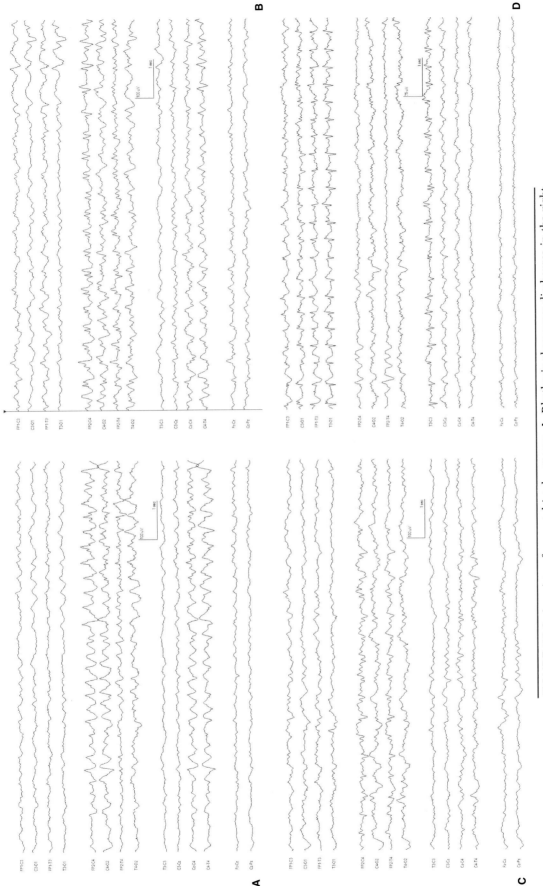

FIGURE 75.2. A variety of neonatal ictal patterns. **A.** Rhythmic slow wave discharges in the right central region. **B.** Rhythmic spikes in the right anterior region. **C.** Bursts of fast activity. **D.** Rhythmic positive sharp waves in the left temporal region.

▶ **TABLE 75.2 Relationship of Neurologic Disease to Prognosis in Neonatal Seizures**

Disease	Children Who Survive and Become Normal (%)	Comment
Perinatal asphyxia	50	Most common cause of neonatal encephalopathy
Subarachnoid Hemorrhage	90	Seen in difficult deliveries
Intraventricular Hemorrhage	10	Seizures rare in premature
Hypoglycemia	50	Outcome may be related to early onset therapy
Late hypocalcemia	90	Presents days 5 to 10
Early hypocalcemia	50	Presents days 1 to 3 with other encephalopathies
Hypomagnesemia	75	Often seen with resistant hypocalcemia
Inborn metabolic errors	10	Some with phenylketonuria or pyridoxine dependency do well
Bacterial meningitis	30	Mortality higher in "early onset" type
Congenital anomalies	0	Includes lissencephaly, polymicrogyria, pachygria, and others
Drug withdrawal	?	Good follow-up unavailable; drugs include heroin, methadone
Cause unknown Includes BFNC	67	10% to 20% of neonatal seizures

secondary to maternal drug use. No cause may be found in at least 25% of cases.

Epilepsy Syndromes

Neonatal seizures are only rarely due to epilepsy. Four neonatal epilepsy syndromes have been widely recognized: benign neonatal convulsions, benign familial neonatal convulsion (BFNC), early infantile epileptogenic encephalopathy (EIEE, or Ohtahara syndrome), and early myoclonic epilepsy (EME, as described by Aicardi). The first two are benign, occurring in neonates who are otherwise well, and both carry a good prognosis. BFNC is an autosomal-dominant disorder linked to 20Q13.2-q13.3 (EBN1) in some families, and 8q24 (EBN2) in others. It is caused by defects in either the KCNQ2 or KCNQ3 genes. Both encode voltage-gated potassium channels, similar to those found in prolonged-QT syndrome. Seizures are focal, but they may begin with tonic postures. Interictal EEGs are normal but during the seizures the EEG may show diffuse flattening. Seizures remit spontaneously by 40 days of life, in the majority of cases.

EIEE and EME, in contrast, are symptomatic types of epilepsy with invariably poor outcomes. These syndromes are characterized by encephalopathy, burst-suppression pattern on EEG, and frequent prominent seizures. The seizures described in the Ohtahara syndrome are mostly tonic, and a burst-suppression EEG pattern is invariably present. Seizures in EME are myoclonic and tend to occur erratically. The burst-suppression EEG and may be present only during sleep. Structural brain lesions are commonly found in EIEE, while inborn errors of metabolism, especially those of nonketotic hyperglycinemia, are frequent in EME.

Evaluation

As in older patients with seizures, the history—including family history and details of the infant's gestation and delivery—is central to the evaluation. Particularly useful is information on specific features on the general physical examination, including head circumference, identification of any congenital anomalies, evidence of a neurocutaneous disorder, or organomegaly. Neurologic examination should note the quality of spontaneous movements as well as any abnormal postures or movements that may be elicited by stimulation or positioning.

Laboratory tests should first focus on the common metabolic and infectious disorders that require treatment. High priorities are the exclusion of hypoglycemia with a dip-stick test, and evaluating possible meningitis or hemorrhage with lumbar puncture. Blood should be taken for measurement of glucose, calcium, magnesium, sodium and acid-base levels, as well as a blood culture. An EEG should be obtained promptly if abnormal movements are present or if there are unexplained fluctuations in behavior. Bedside ultrasound may identify hemorrhage and hydrocephalus. CT also shows hemorrhage and hydrocephalus and in addition, demonstrates parenchymal calcifications and major cerebral malformations. MRI is usually necessary to detect more subtle developmental abnormalities, such as partial lissencephaly, polymicrogyria, or cortical dysplasia. Properly timed, particularly in cases of HIE, high-resolution MRI will demonstrate brain abnormalities in two-thirds of newborns with seizures.

The timing of the first seizure helps to prioritize diagnostic possibilities. Seizures due to severe brain malformations, intracerebral hemorrhage, and hypoxic-ischemic injury occur within 24 to 48 hours. Seizures caused by infection and inborn errors of metabolism typically begin later in the first week of life. Seizures related to passive drug withdrawal usually occur within the first 3 days (e.g., alcohol or short-acting barbiturates) but may not appear for 2 to 3 weeks (e.g., methadone). Seizures resulting from sepsis occur at any time.

Seizures must be distinguished from other paroxysmal phenomena that occur in newborns, including jitteriness, which can be triggered or stopped by manipulation of a limb, benign sleep myoclonus, dyskinesias (i.e., common with severe bronchopulmonary dysplasia), and the movements that occur during rapid-eye-movement (REM) sleep. Brief, generalized, tonic postures that occur with poor cerebral perfusion or with resolving encephalopathies are usually not epileptic seizures. They are not accompanied by ictal changes in the EEG and are likely the result of different pathophysiologic mechanisms. They respond poorly or not at all to antiepileptic drugs. Deep sedation, however, may eliminate these clinical phenomena.

Are Seizures Harmful?

Immature experimental animals are more resistant than older animals to the effects of prolonged or repeated seizures. However, absence of cell death does not mean absence of long-term consequences. Immature animals have lower thresholds for inducing seizures later in life, and they also exhibit developmental effects (defects). The resistance to cell death is an area of active research. Some investigators have proposed that mitochondrial-uncoupling protein-2 protects the immature brain from neuronal death, and that this protein is upregulated by diets high in fat.

Treatment

Painter and colleagues found that either phenobarbital or phenytoin is effective in only 45% of cases. Still, most authorities recommend beginning with one drug, and if ineffective, to proceed to the next. In most nurseries, phenobarbital is the first medication administered, followed by fosphenytoin, for babies with persistent clinical seizures. However, serial video-EEG studies have shown that while antiepileptic-drug treatment often suppresses clinical manifestations, electrical-seizure activity frequently persists. It is still not clear to what extent continuing electrical discharges, by themselves cause neuronal injury and in the absence of hypoxia and ischemia, lead to permanent neurologic sequelae. From a practical standpoint, it is useful to administer antiepileptic drugs to the point that clinical seizures are eliminated or high-therapeutic blood levels are achieved without compromising respiratory or circulatory function. The authors attempt to suppress EEG ictal activity that continues after clinical seizures end, but will not push medications to the point of semicoma, respiratory failure, or cardiac depression.

Phenobarbital is the antiepileptic drug most frequently used in newborns. Typical starting doses of 20 mg/kg should be given intravenously, over 5 minutes. If seizures persist, additional 5-mg/kg increments of phenobarbital may be administered every 20 minutes, up to a total loading dose of 40 mg/kg. The maintenance dose for phenobarbital is 3 mg/kg to 6 mg/kg per day. Therapeutic levels are 15 μg/mL to 35 μg/mL; levels higher than 40 μg/mL produce lethargy.

Fosphenytoin is an alternative drug when phenobarbital fails. A loading dose of 20 mg/kg of phenytoin equivalents (PE) is given intravenously, over a period of about 20 minutes. Some clinicians advise dividing the loading dose into two 10-mg/kg increments, to minimize cardiac toxicity. Maintenance doses are 4 mg/kg to 7 mg/kg, per day. Fosphenytoin is the water-soluble phosphorylated form of phenytoin and has been administered safely to small groups of neonates as young as 26 weeks conceptional age. Midazolam, 0.1 mg/kg to 0.4 mg/kg, per hour, administered by continuous intravenous infusion, may be useful in suppressing seizures refractory to phenobarbital and fosphenytoin.

Hypoglycemia should be treated using a 10%-glucose solution, infused in a dosage of 2 mL/kg. Hypocalcemia should be treated intravenously, with concomitant EKG monitoring when levels fall below 7 mg/dL. Failure of response may be due to hypomagnesemia; treatment may be administered intramuscularly, as magnesium sulfate. Some neonates with refractory seizures respond to vitamin therapy. If these are not included in the protocol for refractory neonatal seizures, they will almost certainly be missed, and irreversible damage may occur. Small-group case studies have been reported of neonates responding to vitamin B-6 (50 mg to 100 mg, intravenously), pyridoxal phosphate 30 mg/kg per day for 3 days, or folinic acid 1 mg/kg per day, for 3 days.

When to stop antiepileptic drugs is a matter of judgment. If the infant is normal and the EEG is normal or near normal, the authors generally discontinue antiepileptic drug therapy before the child is discharged from the hospital. In other cases, we wait 1 to 3 months after the last seizure.

Prognosis

About 15% of infants with seizures die, and 35% to 40% have permanent neurologic sequelae. Seizures are associated with high rates of morbidity and mortality, because many of the etiologies that cause seizures in newborns lead to permanent damage. HIE, severe IVH, and cerebral malformations are particularly associated with poor outcomes. The presence of suppression-burst activity, an unreactive low-voltage background, and continuous multifocal discharges reliably predict disabling brain damage more than 90% of the time. In contrast, a normal EEG at the time of the first seizure is usually associated with a good outcome. EEG findings are less useful in predicting which infants will continue to have seizures beyond the neonatal period, or which will develop epilepsy later in life. About 15% to 30% of infants with neonatal seizures develop epilepsy.

SUGGESTED READINGS

Intracranial Hemorrhage

Bergman I, Bauer RE, Barmada MH. Intracerebral hemorrhage in the full-term neonatal infant. *Pediatrics* 1985;75:488–496.

Fulmer BB, Grabb PA, Oakes WJ, Mapstone TB. Neonatal ventriculosubgaleal shunts. *Neurosurgery* 2000;47:80–84.

Horbar JD. Antenatal corticosteroid treatment and neonatal outcomes for infants 501 to 1500 gm in the Vermont-Oxford Trials Network. *Am J Obstet Gynecol* 1995;173:275–281.

Ment LR, Oh W, Ehrenkranz RA, et al. Low-dose indomethacin and prevention of intraventricular hemorrhage: a multicenter randomized trial. *Pediatrics* 1994;93:543–550.

O'Shea TM, Doyle LW. Perinatal glucocorticoid therapy and neurodevelopmental outcome: an epidemiological perspective. *Sem Neonatol* 2002;6:293–297.

Osborn DA, Evans N, Kluckow M. Hemodynamics and antecedent risk factors of early and late periventricular/intraventricular hemorrhage in premature infants. *Pediatrics* 2003;112:33–39.

Pape KE, Wigglesworth JS. Hemorrhage, ischemia and the perinatal brain. Philadelphia: JB Lippincott Co, 1979.

Perrin RG, Rutha JT, Drake JM, et al. Management and outcome of posterior fossa subdural hematomas in neonates. *Neurosurgery* 1997;40:1190–1199.

Roland EH, Hill A. Intraventricular hemorrhage and posthemorrhagic hydrocephalus: current and potential future interventions. *Clin Perinatol* 1997;24:589–605.

Roland EH, Hill A. Germinal matrix-intraventricular hemorrhage in the premature newborn: management and outcome. *Neurol Clin* 2003;21:833–851.

van de Bor M, den Ouden L. School performance in adolescents with and without periventricular-intraventricular hemorrhage in the neonatal period. *Semin Perinatol* 2004 Aug;28(4):295–303.

Vergani P, Locatelli A, Doria V, Assi F, Paterlini G, Pezzullo JC, Ghidini A. Intraventricular hemorrhage and periventricular leukomalacia in preterm infants. *Obstet Gynecol* 2004 Aug;104(2):225–231.

Vohr BR, Allan WC, Westerfeld M, et al. School age outcomes of very low birth weight infants in the indomethacin intraventricular prevention trial. *Pediatrics* 2003;111:340–346.

Volpe JJ. *Neurology of the Newborn*, 4th ed. Philadelphia: WB Saunders, 2001.

Welch K, Strand R. Traumatic parturitional intracranial hemorrhage. *Dev Med Child Neurol* 1986;28:156–164.

Whitelaw A. Intraventricular hemorrhage and posthemorrhagic hydrocephalus: pathogenesis, prevention and future interventions. *Sem Neonatol* 2001;6:135–146.

Periventricular Leukomalacia

Banker BA, Larroche JC. Periventricular leukomalacia of infancy. *Arch Neurol* 1962;7:386–410.

Bracewell M, Marlow N. Patterns of motor disability in very preterm children. *Ment Retard Devel Disabil Res Rev* 2002;8:241–248.

Counsell SJ, Allsop JM, Harrison MC, et al. Diffusion-weighted imaging of the brain in preterm infants with focal and diffuse white matter abnormality. *Pediatrics* 2003;112:1–7.

Hagberg H, Peebles D, Mallard C. Models of white matter injury: comparison of infectious, hypoxic-ischemic and excitotoxic insults. *Ment Retard Devel Disabil Res Rev* 2002;8:30–38.

Hamrick SE, Miller SP, Leonard C, Glidden DV, Goldstein R, Ramaswamy V, Piecuch R, Ferriero DM. Trends in severe brain injury and neurodevelopmental outcome in premature newborn infants: the role of cystic periventricular leukomalacia. *J Pediatr* 2004 Nov;145(5):593–599.

Inder TE, Anderson NJ, Spencer C, et al. White matter injury in the premature infant; a comparison between serial cranial sonographic MR findings at term. *AJNR* 2003;5:805–809.

Inder TE, Huppi RS, Warfield S, et al. Periventricular white matter injury in the premature infant is associated with a reduction in cerebral gray matter volume at term. *Ann Neurol* 1999;46:755–760.

Murata Y, Itakura A, Matsuzawa K, Okumura A, Wakai K, Mizutani S. Possible antenatal and perinatal related factors in development of cystic periventricular leukomalacia. *Brain Dev* 2005 Jan;27(1):17–21.

Nosarti C, Al-Asady MH, Frangaou S, et al. Adolescents who were born very preterm have decreased brain volumes. *Brain* 2002:125;1616–1623.

Tsuji M, Saul P, du Plessis A, et al. Cerebral intravascular oxygenation correlates with mean arterial pressure in critically ill premature infants. *Pediatrics* 2000;106;625–632.

Volpe JJ. Cerebral white matter injury of the premature infant—more common than you think. *Pediatrics* 2003;112:176–180.

Hypoxic-Ischemic Encephalopathy

Badawi N, Kurinczuk JJ, Keogh JM, et al. Intrapartum risk factors for newborn encephalopathy: the Western Australian case-control study. *BMJ* 1998;317:1554–1548.

Barkovich AJ, Baranski K, Vigneron D. Proton MR spectroscopy for the evaluation of brain injury in asphyxiated term neonates. *AJNR* 1999;20:1399–1405.

Biagioni E, Mercuri E, Rutherford M, et al. Combined use of electroencephalogram and magnetic resonance imaging in full-term infants with acute encephalopathy. *Pediatrics* 2001;107:461–468.

Cowan F, Rutherford M, Groenendaal F. Origin and timing of brain lesions in term infants with neonatal encephalopathy. *Lancet* 2003; 361:736–742.

Inder TE, Hunt RW, Morley CJ, et al. Randomized trial of systemic hypothermia selectively protects the cortex on MRI in hypoxic-ischemic encephalopathy. *J Pediatr* 2004;145:835–837.

Jacobs S, Hunt R, Tarnow-Mordi W. Cooling for newborns with hypoxic-ischemic encephalopathy. *Cochrane Database Syst Rev* 2003;(4): CD003311.

Johnston MV, Nakajima W, Hagberg H. Mechanisms of hypoxic neurodegeneration in the developing brain. *Neuroscientist* 2002;8:212–220.

Nelson KB, Leviton A. How much of neonatal encephalopathy is due to birth asphyxia? *Am J Dis Child* 1991;145:325–1331.

Painter MJ. Fetal heart rate patterns, perinatal asphyxia, and brain injury. *Pediatr Neurol* 1989;5:137–144.

Pasternak JF, Gorey MT. The syndrome of acute near-total intrauterine asphyxia in the term infant. *Pediatr Neurol* 1998;18:391–398.

Rivkin MJ. Hypoxic-ischemic brain injury in the term newborn: neuropathology, clinical aspects, and neuroimaging. *Clin Perinatol* 1997;24:607–626.

Roth SC, Edwards AD, Cady EB, et al. Relation of deranged neonatal cerebral oxidative metabolism asphyxia, with neurodevelopmental outcome and head circumference at 4 years. *Dev Med Child Neurol* 1997;39:758–773.

Takeoka M, Sosman TB, Yoshii A, et al. Diffusion-weighted images in neonatal cerebral hypoxic-ischemic injury. *Pediatr Neurol* 2002;26:274–281.

Vannucci SJ, Hagberg H. Hypoxia-ischemia in the immature brain. *J Exp Biol* 2004;207:3149–3154.

Volpe JJ. Perinatal brain injury: from pathogenesis to neuroprotection. *Ment Retard Devel Disabil Res Rev* 2001;7:56–54.

Wainwright MS, Mannix MK, Brown J, Stumpf DA. Carnitine reduces brain injury after hypoxia-ischemia in newborn rats. *Ped Res* 2003;54:688–695.

Infections

Bale JF Jr, Murph JR. Infections of the central nervous system in the newborn. *Clin Perinatol* 1997;24:787–806.

Edwards MS, Rench MA, Haffer AA, et al. Long-term sequelae of group B streptococcal meningitis in infants. *J Pediatr* 1985;106:717–722.

Kimberlin DW, Chin-Yu L, Jacobs RF, et al. Natural history of neonatal herpes simplex viral infection in the Acyclovir era. *Pediatrics* 2000;108:230–238.

Kline M. Citrobacter meningitis and brain abscess in infancy: epidemiology, pathogenesis and treatment. *J Pediatr* 1988;113:430–434.

Klinger G, Choy-Nyok C, Beyene J, Perlman M. Predicting the outcome of neonatal bacterial meningitis. *Pediatrics* 2000;106:447–482.

Polin RA, Harris MC. Neonatal bacterial meningitis. *Semin Neonatol* 2001;6:157–172.

Seizures

Bye AM, Cunningham CA, Chee KY, Flanagan D. Outcome of neonates with electrographically identified seizures, or at risk of seizures. *Pediatr Neurol* 1997;16:225–231.

Clancy RR, Legido A, Lewis D. Occult neonatal seizures. *Epilepsia* 1988;29:256–261.

Holmes GL, Ben-Ari Y. The neurobiology and consequences of epilepsy in the developing brain. *Pediatr Res* 2001;49:320–325.

Leth H, Toft PB, Herning M, et al. Neonatal seizures associated with cerebral lesions shown by magnetic resonance imaging. *Arch Dis Child Fetal Neonat Med* 1997;77:F105–F110.

Lynch BJ, Rust RS. Natural history of neonatal hypocalcemic and hypomagnesemic seizures. *Pediatr Neurol* 1994;11:23–27.

Mizrahi EM, Kellaway P. Characterization and classification of neonatal seizures. *Neurology* 1987;37:1837–1844.

Ortibus EL, Sum JM, Hahn JS. Predictive value of EEG for outcome and epilepsy following neonatal seizures. *Electroencephalogr Clin Neurophysiol* 1996;98:175–185.

Painter MJ, Scher MS, Stein AD, et al. Phenobarbital compared with phenytoin for the treatment of neonatal seizures. *N Engl J Med* 1999;341:485–489.

Patrizi S, Holmes GL, Orzalesi M, Allemand F. Neonatal seizures: characteristics of EEG ictal activity in preterm and full term infants. *Brain Devel* 2003;25:427–437.

Ronen GM, Penney S, Andrews W. The epidemiology of clinical neonatal seizures in Newfoundland: a population-based study. *J Pediatr* 1999;134:71–75.

Ronen, GM, Rosales TO, Connolly M, Anderson VE, Leppert M. Seizure characteristics in chromosome 20 benign familial neonatal convulsions. *Neurology* 1993;43:1355–1360.

Scher MS. Seizures in the newborn infant. Diagnosis, treatment, and outcome. *Clin Perinatol* 1997;24:735–772.

Scher MS. Neonatal seizures and brain damage. *Pediat Neurol* 2003; 29:391–390.

Sheth RD, Buckley DJ, Gutierrez AR, et al. Midazolam in the treatment of refractory neonatal seizures. *Clin Neuropharmacol* 1996;19:156–170.

Strober JB, Bienkowski RS, Maytal J. The incidence of acute and remote seizures in children with intraventricular hemorrhage. *Clin Pediatr* 1997;36:643–647.

Sullivan PG, Dubé C, Dorenbos K, Steward O, Baram TZ. Mitochondrial uncoupling protein-2 protects the immature brain from excitotoxic neuronal death. *Ann Neurol* 2003;53:711–717.

Tharp BR. Neonatal seizures and syndromes. *Epilepsia* 2002;43(suppl 3): 2–10.

Volpe JJ. Neonatal seizures: current concepts and revised classification. *Pediatrics* 1989;84:422–428.

Chapter 76

Floppy Infant Syndrome

Juan M. Pascual and Darryl C. De Vivo

When a normal infant is suspended in the prone position, the arms and legs move out, and the head is held in line with the body. In many different disorders, a child does not respond in this fashion. Rather, the limbs and head all hang limply, like a rag doll. That is why the *floppy infant syndrome* has caught on as a popular term. In addition to children with these abnormal postures, some clinicians have extended the use of the term to include those whose limbs have diminished resistance to passive movement.

The number of conditions that cause these manifestations seems endless, including disorders of the brain, spinal cord, peripheral nerves, neuromuscular junction, muscles and ligaments, as well as some disorders of unknown origin. There are almost always clues of some kind, however, that narrow the list of possible causes to a few choices. An essential division separates conditions found in the newborn infant from those occurring later (Table 76.1).

A second division separates patients with conditions characterized by true weakness of skeletal muscle (often with total loss of tendon reflexes) from those without true limb weakness but who have evidence on examination of brain injury or encephalopathy. Among the latter, there are likely to be skeletal anomalies of dysmorphism, which may be a manifestation of chromosomal abnormality, or an abnormal mental state as a result of metabolic encephalopathy.

A third diagnostic consideration concerns illness in the mother, and the perinatal history. If the mother is known to have myotonic muscular dystrophy, myasthenia gravis, or ulcerative colitis, depressed movement in the infant is immediately recognized. The correct diagnosis in the child may be the first clue to explain previously unrecognized manifestations of illness in the mother. Similarly, maternal narcotic drug abuse, alcoholism, or use of anticonvulsant medications may affect the infant. Adverse perinatal events may lead to suspicion of asphyxia or cerebral hemorrhage.

A fourth consideration is the distribution of the abnormality. Are all four limbs involved, or are only the legs or one arm affected? Is sucking, swallowing, or ventilation impaired? The answers have different diagnostic implications.

▶ **TABLE 76.1 Floppy Infant Syndromes**

	Neuromuscular Disorders (weakness prominent)	Central Disorders with Abnormal Neurologic Signs or Peripheral Disorders (little or no weakness)
Neonate	Infantile spinal muscular atrophy Congenital myotonic dystrophy Neonatal myasthenia gravis Congenital myopathies[a,b] Metabolic myopathies[c] Congenital muscular dystrophies	Perinatal asphyxia Cerebral hemorrhage Sepsis Intoxication Spinal cord injury or malformation Failure-to-thrive syndromes Congenital hypothyroidism Neurotransmitter disorders Down syndrome Prader-Willi syndrome Other dysgenetic syndromes
Age 1 to 6 months (or later)	Infantile spinal muscular atrophy Infantile Guillain-Barré syndrome or other neuropathies Congenital myasthenic syndromes[d] Botulism	Metabolic cerebral degenerations[e] Tissue disorders[f] Metabolic and endocrine diseases[g] Hypotonic cerebral palsy Benign congenital hypotonia
Failure to reach developmental stages but not really floppy	Congenital myopathies[b] Duchenne muscular dystrophy	

[a]Spinal muscular atrophy and congenital myopathies are more likely to become symptomatic *after* the neonatal period.
[b]Congenital myopathies include those characterized by specific histochemical abnormality (e.g., nemaline, central cores, myotubules, and other structures).
[c]Metabolic myopathies include infantile acid-maltase deficiency (i.e., Pompe disease), mitochondrial DNA-depletion syndrome, and benign and fatal infantile cytochrome-C-oxidase deficiency.
[d]Congenital myasthenic syndromes do not usually cause infantile symptoms other than ophthalmoplegia.
[e]Leukodystrophies, lipid-storage diseases, peroxisomal diseases, mucopolysaccharidosis, aminoacidurias, Leigh syndrome.
[f]Congenital laxity of ligaments, Ehler-Danlos syndrome, Marfan syndrome.
[g]Organic acidemia, hypocalcemia, hypercalcemia, hypothyroidism, renal tubular acidosis.

ETIOLOGY

The most common causes of hypotonia are perinatal hypoxia-ischemia of the brain or spinal cord, spinal-muscular atrophy, and dysgenetic syndromes. About 75% of cases fall into these categories. Spinal-muscular atrophy, however, is only rarely evident immediately after birth. The neonatologist first considers common perinatal insults, such as birth asphyxia, intracranial hemorrhage, bacterial or viral infections, metabolic disturbances, and extreme prematurity as principal causes of hypotonia in the newborn. Congenital hypoglycemia or hypothyroidism may be suggested by hypothermia in the infant. Spinal-cord injuries usually follow intrauterine malpositioning or traumatic birth, and may occur without encephalopathy. Severe asphyxia may also affect the lower motor neurons of the spinal cord. Autopsy studies of fatally asphyxiated neonates with flaccidity and areflexia demonstrate prominent, ischemic necrosis of anterior spinal-cord gray matter in a radially oriented, watershed distribution that is consistent with hypoperfusion between the anterior spinal artery and the paired dorsal-spinal arteries.

In these conditions, the perinatal history is informative, and the hypotonic infant has associated behavioral alterations, including decreased responsiveness (e.g., sometimes manifest as a reduction of vigil time) or seizures. Dysmorphic features are absent, and tendon reflexes are present.

FOCAL NEONATAL HYPOTONIA

This disorder may be caused by trauma or developmental abnormality. A flaccid arm usually implies brachial plexus injury. Signs of injury to the upper brachial plexus (i.e., Klumpke palsy) may be associated with ipsilateral paralysis of the diaphragm; lower brachial plexus lesions (i.e., Erb palsy) may be accompanied by an ipsilateral Horner syndrome. Electromyography and spinal-evoked potentials help define the severity of the nerve-root injury. Spinal cord imaging may document nerve-root avulsion.

Hypotonia and weakness of the legs indicate spinal-cord pathology. Spinal dysraphism and the caudal-regression syndrome are obvious, on inspection and palpation of the back. An arthrogrypotic-leg deformity or gross maldevelopment of the legs is associated with sacral agenesis.

Fifteen percent of patients with sacral agenesis are infants of diabetic mothers.

DYSGENETIC SYNDROMES

These syndromes are often associated with distinctive, dysmorphic physical features. The neurologic disorder may not be recognized until the infant fails to reach certain developmental stages. Common syndromes associated with hypotonia are Down syndrome, Prader-Willi syndrome, Lowe syndrome, Zellweger syndrome, Smith-Lemli-Opitz syndrome, molybdenum cofactor (i.e., sulfite oxidase) deficiency syndrome, and the Riley-Day (i.e., familial dysautonomia) syndrome. Environmental toxins may also produce hypotonia and dysmorphism. Common examples include fetal exposure to heroin, phenytoin, trimethadione, or alcohol intoxication. Strength is normal in these syndromes, but the tendon reflexes may vary from absent to brisk.

Neurotransmitter Disorders

Disorders of central neurotransmission may cause neonatal hypotonia. In the recessively inherited disorders of tetrahydrobiopterin synthesis, tyrosine hydroxylase, and aromatic L-amino acid decarboxylase, symptoms appear within the first few months of life. Symptoms may also include ptosis, severe irritability, oculogyric crises, temperature instability, and tremor, with or without other parkinsonian features. The investigation of infants and children with suspected neurotransmitter diseases of serotonin and catecholamine (i.e., dopamine and norepinephrine) metabolism is complicated because the measurement of metabolites in peripheral fluids is generally uninformative. Disorders that affect catecholamine and serotonin neurotransmission, and that do not present with hyperphenylalaninemia, require a lumbar puncture and measurement of specific metabolites in CSF.

NEUROMUSCULAR DISORDERS

Neuromuscular disorders that cause infantile hypotonia do not impair alertness but are characterized by decreased limb movement owing to weakness, and decreased tendon reflexes. Dysmorphic features accompany many congenital myopathies. After the immediate neonatal period, *spinal muscular atrophy* is the most common cause of infantile hypotonia. This autosomal-recessive disorder (Werdnig-Hoffmann disease), with a carrier frequency of 1 in 40 in the normal population, may sometimes be evident at birth. The characteristic findings include limb weakness, areflexia, and fasciculations of the tongue. Although most affected infants die before age 2 years, some may survive for decades.

Poliomyelitis is a rare cause of limb weakness. The neurologic findings are asymmetric, and are accompanied by signs of meningeal irritation, with CSF pleocytosis and elevated protein content.

Infantile peripheral neuropathies are uncommon causes of weakness, areflexia, and hypotonia. Examples include metachromatic leukodystrophy, globoid-cell leukodystrophy, infantile-neuroaxonal dystrophy, giant-axonal neuropathy, neonatal adrenoleukodystrophy, hypertrophic interstitial polyneuropathy, and peroneal-muscular atrophy. Important clues may include a family history, palpably enlarged peripheral nerves, upper motor-neuron signs, elevated CSF protein concentration, and slowed nerve-conduction velocities. Guillain-Barré syndrome occasionally affects infants. Diphtheria, caused by *Corynebacterium diphtheriae*, produces a generalized, demyelinating polyneuropathy that is clinically similar to Guillain-Barré syndrome. A protein exotoxin secreted by the organism inhibits myelin synthesis, and may also activate cytotoxic mechanisms.

Tick paralysis has a rapid onset, producing a hypotonic picture also similar to Guillain-Barré syndrome, and usually occurs in the spring and summer months. The paralysis is caused by a tick that is continuously attached, and secreting toxin-laden saliva; removal of the tick is rapidly curative.

Disorders of the neuromuscular junction may cause limb, bulbar, or diaphragmatic weakness. Fluctuating signs intensified by vigorous crying, or limb activity, are important observations. *Congenital myasthenic syndromes* often affect siblings, and are inherited as an autosomal-recessive disorder. These conditions are caused by mutations in the genes for proteins of the junctional apparatus. Clinically, the infant may display external ophthalmoplegia and generalized weakness; sudden respiratory failure may also occur later in life. Autoimmune forms of myasthenia gravis in infancy include the transient *neonatal form* in infants of myasthenic mothers. The *juvenile form* ordinarily does not cause symptoms before age 2 years. Circulating acetylcholine-receptor antibodies, and responsiveness to immunotherapy distinguish these myasthenic syndromes from heritable, nonimmunologic forms, as discussed in Chapter 121 (myasthenia gravis).

Another condition affecting neuromuscular transmission is *infantile botulism*, which results from ingestion of *Clostridium botulinum* spores that germinate in the intestinal tract. Manifestations include ileus, constipation, hypotonia, weakness, pupillary dilation and paralysis, and apneic spells. The clinical picture is distinctive, and diagnosis may be confirmed by the recovery of the bacterium and the exotoxin, in the feces. A facilitating response to repetitive stimulation, such as that of the Eaton-Lambert syndrome, may usually be demonstrated and may be an important diagnostic clue. Attention should be paid to avoiding any medications that might exacerbate the neuromuscular-transmission deficit, in particular aminoglycoside antibiotics that are sometimes initiated empirically, at presentation, for possible sepsis. Complete recovery follows appropriate supportive care.

Myopathies that cause infantile limb weakness include the *congenital myopathies* with specific structural abnormalities, myotonic muscular dystrophy, and metabolic myopathies. Although the term *muscular dystrophy* usually implies progressive disease, the term has been applied to apparently static, congenital disorders in which the changes in muscle biopsy are myopathic, but that have no specific features. In Japan, the Fukuyama type of *congenital muscular dystrophy* is characterized by severe mental retardation in all cases, and seizures in about 50% of the cases. Symptoms may start soon after birth, with difficulty nursing and impoverished movement. The children never walk but may live for decades. The cerebral pathology is distinctive, with polymicrogyria of the occipital lobes in a pattern that may be recognized by MRI. Similar cases have been seen in the United States and Europe. Walker-Warburg syndrome and muscle-eye-brain disease are related clinically, although they are genetically distinct entities.

The *histochemically defined myopathies* may be inherited as autosomal-dominant or autosomal-recessive traits, or as a sex-linked recessive trait. These disorders share many phenotypic features that overlap with other syndromes. Examples include: central core disease, multicore disease, nemaline myopathy, myotubular (centronuclear) myopathy, congenital fiber-type disproportion, sarcotubular myopathy, fingerprint-body myopathy, and reducing-body myopathy. Limb weakness, decreased tendon reflexes, dysmorphic physical features, a predisposition to congenital hip dislocation, and later development of scoliosis characterize most of the histochemically defined myopathies. The similarities often outweigh the differences.

Infantile acid-maltase deficiency (i.e., *Pompe disease*) is the classic example of a combined, metabolic myopathy and motor-neuron disease that causes infantile hypotonia. The infant is mentally alert but limb movements are feeble and limited, and the child is weak. The tongue and heart are enlarged, limb muscles may feel and appear robust, and congestive heart failure (CHF) is the cause of death before age 6 months.

Other *metabolic myopathies* that may cause infantile hypotonia and weakness include cytochrome-*c*-oxidase deficiency (e.g., benign reversible, and fatal forms), the mitochondrial DNA-depletion syndrome, glycogenosis type IV (debrancher-enzyme deficiency), and glycogenosis type V (myophosphorylase deficiency). Cytochrome-*c*-oxidase deficiency and mitochondrial DNA-depletion syndrome are associated with lactic acidosis.

A few hypotonic infants eventually develop normally, after several years. The term *essential* or *benign-congenital*

hypotonia should be reserved to describe an otherwise healthy infant with unexplained hypotonia, and normal strength, tendon reflexes, and general physical features.

SUGGESTED READINGS

Bamford NS, Trojaborg W, Sherbany AA, De Vivo DC. Congenital Guillain-Barré syndrome associated with maternal inflammatory bowel disease is responsive to intravenous immunoglobulin. *Eur J Paediatr Neurol.* 2002;6:115–119.

Brooke MH, Carroll JE, Ringel SP. Congenital hypotonia revisited. *Muscle Nerve* 1979;2:84–100.

Dubowitz V. *The Floppy Infant.* Cambridge UK: Cambridge University Press, 1993.

Dubowitz V. *Muscle Disorders in Childhood, 2nd ed.* Philadelphia: WB Saunders, 1995.

Engel AG, Gilman S, eds. *Myasthenia Gravis and Myasthenic Syndromes.* Philadelphia: FA Davis, 1998.

Engel AG, Ohno K, Sine SM. Sleuthing molecular targets for neurological diseases at the neuromuscular junction. *Nat Rev Neurosci.* 2003;4:339–352.

Hagberg B, Sanner G, Steen M. The dysequilibrium syndrome in cerebral palsy: clinical aspects and treatment. *Acta Paediatr Scand Suppl* 1972;226:1–63.

Hirano M, DiMauro S. Metabolic myopathies. *Adv Neurol* 2002;88:217–234.

Hyland K. The lumbar puncture for diagnosis of pediatric neurotransmitter diseases. *Ann Neurol* 2003;54(suppl):S13–S17.

Jones HR, De Vivo DC, Darras BT, eds. *Neuromuscular Diseases of Infancy, Childhood, and Adolescence.* Philadelphia: Butterworth-Heinemann, 2003.

Pickett J, Berg B, Chaplin E, Brunstetter-Shaffer MA. Syndrome of botulism in infancy: clinical and electrophysiological study. *N Engl J Med* 1976;295:770–772.

Schaumburg HH, Kaplan JG. Toxic peripheral neuropathies. In: Asbury AK, Thomas PK, eds. *Peripheral Nerve Disorders 2.* Oxford: Butterworth-Heinemann, 1995:238–261.

Chapter 77

Static Disorders of Brain Development

Isabelle Rapin

The immature brain can be adversely affected at any time, from fertilization (conception) to maturity, because genetic or acquired disorders may disrupt developmental programs or inflict physical damage. Among the causes are genetic-nongenetic cerebral malformations or dysgeneses, intrauterine or extrauterine infections or strokes, and perinatal trauma or ischemic-anoxic insults that may, or may not, lead to gross-motor impairments (e.g., cerebral palsy) or learning disorders. Genetic factors play a major etiologic role in developmental disabilities, such as learning disabilities not associated with detectable lesions or overt sensorimotor abnormalities.

DEVELOPMENTAL DISORDERS OF MOTOR FUNCTION

Minor Motor Disability

This term refers to subtle impairments of motor coordination, such as clumsiness, maladroitness, or developmental dyspraxia. Some, such as reflex asymmetry or hyperactivity and minor dysmetria, are mild or pastel classic neurologic signs; others may be due to delayed acquisition of independent coordination of the two hands, and maintenance of posture without adventitious movements. The neurologic basis of these soft signs is rarely known. They may occur in isolation but are often seen in children with other specific learning disabilities or mild mental deficiency.

Cerebral Palsy

This term has no etiologic specificity and refers to any nonprogressive motor disorder of cerebral or cerebellar origin. The term cerebral palsy (CP) does not apply to disorders of the spinal cord, peripheral nerves, or muscles. The signs are present from early life and are evident on a standard neurologic examination. The cause of cerebral palsy is often, although not invariably, an acquired lesion that is evident on neuroimaging (Table 77.1). The type of cerebral palsy depends on the location of the lesion.

Spastic Hemiparesis

Spastic hemiparesis (*hemiplegia*) arises from a lesion of the corticospinal system of one cerebral hemisphere. A common cause is an intrauterine stroke that results in congenital porencephaly, in the territory of the trunk or a branch of the middle cerebral artery. Strokes can also occur during the birth process and in infancy (i.e., acute infantile hemiplegia). Another common cause of hemiplegic CP is intraventricular hemorrhage, complicated by intraparenchymal hemorrhage, which occurs in small, premature infants and starts as a germinal-matrix hemorrhage. In late childhood, neuroimaging may reveal smallness of the entire hemisphere and an old infarct; the skull is thicker on that side, the sphenoid wing and petrous bone are elevated, and the frontal sinuses and mastoid air cells are larger. These changes are called the *Davidoff-Dyke-Masson syndrome*.

Typically the hemiparesis affects the arm and hand, more than the leg. All children with hemiplegic CP walk, albeit often later and on the toes of the affected foot because of a tight heel cord that may necessitate surgical lengthening. Growth arrest of the arm and leg is frequent in lesions that also involve the parietal lobe; the arm and leg are shorter and thinner, and there may be a compensatory scoliosis. In mild cases, decreased associated movements of the arm may be seen only in running or walking on the heels. Comparing fingernails on the two sides may demonstrate minor growth arrest.

A purely motor hemiparesis may be the result of a frontal lesion, or one that affects the head of the caudate nucleus and adjacent internal capsule. Larger lesions are associated with a cortical sensory loss, involving position sense, stereognosis, neglect, and lack of use of the affected hand except as a prop. The tone in the hand may be decreased rather than increased, and there may be severe laxity of hand and finger ligaments, sometimes with joint deformities. Prognosis for habilitation of the hand is poor. Posterior lesions are associated with a contralateral hemianopsia or spatial neglect.

Hemiparesis may not be evident until the child starts to grab for objects and shows precocious handedness or failure of hand use; this delay does not imply that the lesion was acquired postnatally. Spasticity tends to increase in the first and second years and is more evident when the child is erect than supine.

Seizures are frequent when the lesion affects the cortex. Children with large, unilateral lesions, intractable seizures, and severe behavior disorders may be candidates for hemispherectomy or other excisional surgery. Speech may be delayed but competent in children with hemiplegic CP, and may stem from a strictly unilateral lesion in either hemisphere. Intelligence may be spared despite subtle neuropsychologic differences between right and left lesions; children with right lesions tend to pay more attention to details of a visual display than to the overall pattern, whereas those with left lesions attend to the overall pattern but overlook details. Drawings done by young children with right-sided lesions are more disorganized than those of children with left-sided lesions. As infants, children with right-sided lesions tend to be more irritable, and cry more than those with left-sided lesions.

▶ **TABLE 77.1 Clinical Variants of Cerebral Palsy (CP)**

Spastic hemiparesis (hemiplegia)
Spastic diparesis (diplegia), Little disease
Spastic quadriparesis (quadriplegia)
Hypotonic CP
Dyskinetic CP (athetosis, choreoathetosis)
Ataxic CP
Mixed CP

Spastic Diplegia or Diparesis

In *spastic diplegia* or *diparesis* or *Little disease*, spasticity predominates in the legs, less severely affecting the hands and face. Tendon reflexes are hyperactive and the toes upgoing. The most common causes are prematurity with bilateral germinal-matrix hemorrhage—with or without intraventricular hemorrhage and hydrocephalus—and perinatal ischemia in the watershed-parasagittal zone between the territories of the anterior and posterior cerebral arteries. Adductor spasm is responsible for scissoring of the legs, and marked spasticity may preclude ambulation, if attempted without a walker and long-leg braces. Intelligence and language are often unimpaired, but there may be variable clumsiness of the hands.

Spastic Quadriplegia

Spastic quadriplegia is the most severe variant of CP, often associated with moderate-to-severe mental deficiency. It denotes diffuse damage or malformation in the brain, such as multicystic leukomalacia following severe ischemia, or lissencephaly. In some cases, bilateral porencephalies cause a double hemiplegia, with the hands more severely affected than the legs. Severe limb spasticity may be associated with axial- and neck hypotonia. Children with quadriparesis are rarely able to walk; most are totally dependent and require wheelchairs with neck and trunk supports. Pseudobulbar manifestations often preclude speech and severe dysphagia may require a feeding gastrostomy. Seizures are frequent and difficult to control.

Poor hand use almost always prevents the acquisition of signing, making the assessment of cognition very difficult. Every effort must be made to provide an alternate means of expression, such as pointing. A child who understands that pointing means "I want" may learn to use a communication board, and potentially, a computer with voice. Even such a rudimentary means for communication greatly enhances the quality of life for these children and their caretakers.

To relieve spasticity, dantrolene produces weakness, diazepam drowsiness, and oral baclofen has a modest effect. Baclofen is more effective in spastic quadriplegia when administered by continuous intrathecal infusion. Injection of botulinum toxin into spastic muscles decreases spasticity for a number of months, but requires reinjection. Selective dorsal rhizotomy relieves spasticity without causing weakness, and may enhance function. In most cases, ongoing physical therapy, orthoses, and orthopedic procedures are still needed.

Other Forms of CP

Children with *hypotonic CP* are floppy but most have hyperactive tendon reflexes, contrary to those with lower motor-neuron or primary-muscle diseases. The pathophysiology of this syndrome is not understood, but there is usually severe mental deficiency, with evidence of diffuse brain involvement, for example, a major malformation.

In children with *dyskinetic CP*, basal ganglia lesions lead to abnormal involuntary movements, including athetosis, choreoathetosis, or dystonia. Most dyskinetic CP follows neonatal hyperbilirubinemia (i.e., kernicterus) or severe anoxia. The main cause of hyperbilirubinemia is neonatal blood group incompatibility, a preventable cause of CP that has become rare in the United States.

Unconjugated bilirubin damages the basal ganglia, central auditory and vestibular pathways, and the deep cerebellar nuclei, selectively sparing the cortex. As a result, these children, who may be unable to speak because of facial dyskinesia and hearing loss, and have little or no hand use, may be normally intelligent. In contrast, children with dyskinetic CP following anoxia are likely to have both cortical and subcortical damage (e.g., status marmoratus of the basal ganglia), with intellectual as well as motor handicaps. Rare metabolic disorders, such as glutaric aciduria Type I, must be ruled out. It is crucial to test the hearing of all children with dyskinetic CP. The hearing loss of kernicterus is typically a high-tone loss; the children are not deaf but cannot discriminate the consonants that convey most of the meaning of speech. Assessment of cognitive skills is difficult because of the motor handicap and hearing loss but is crucial; it may have to rely on interest in the environment, development of nonverbal communication, and the views of parents.

Athetosis is not present at birth; the movements emerge usually after age 1 year. In early infancy, the children are hypotonic, with poor head and trunk control and little or no use of the hands. The first sign of athetosis may be tongue thrusting that makes spoon feeding difficult. Severely affected children are helpless and unable to walk. Some gain sufficient control of a fist or a foot, or of the head, to manipulate a wand and communicate with a computer or a communication board. Some children walk but assume grotesque postures and have stigmatizing facial grimaces, dysarthria, and dysphagia.

Many drugs have been tried in athetosis, but none is adequately effective. High doses of trihexyphenidyl pushed to tolerance may have a modest effect on dystonia; carbidopa is sometimes effective; chlorpromazine is sedative and may have long-term side effects. Chronic stimulation of the globus pallidus pars interna may be a treatment option for severe medication-resistant cases but experience with this treatment is limited.

Ataxic CP is rare and usually denotes maldevelopment of the cerebellum or its pathways, for example Joubert syndrome. If severe, cerebellar dysgenesis may be associated with significant cognitive impairment. The differential diagnosis includes benign familial tremor, which may be seen in the preschool years, as well as a slowly progressive genetic-metabolic disease, rather than a static condition. Truncal and gait ataxia are more striking than limb ataxia, but some children take a long time to learn to feed themselves and have severe difficulty writing. The children eventually learn to walk but fall frequently. Nystagmus is uncommon. Speech may be slow and scanning. Ataxic CP does not respond well to physical therapy, nor to any drug, but may improve with age.

Mixed CP refers to the combination of dyskinetic and spastic CP, or ataxia and athetosis. It is also used to describe children who do not meet strict criteria for one of the major forms.

Management of Cerebral Palsy

Children with CP should be referred to a specialized assessment center as soon as they are identified. Children with significant CP should undergo neuroimaging to determine the basis of the motor disorder and to be sure that there is no remediable condition, such as hydrocephalus. Hearing must be tested early, using brain-stem evoked responses or cochlear emissions in children who cannot cooperate for behavioral audiometry. Vision must be assessed, as many children with CP have strabismus or a refractive error; myopia is particularly frequent in children born prematurely. Early evaluations of communication and cognitive skills, although essential, are descriptive and not necessarily predictive; response to intervention is a more reliable gauge of abilities than is a one-shot test.

Early intervention programs typically provide all required therapies in one center. Physical therapy is essential to train ambulation, stretch spastic muscles, and prevent deformities; however, it may not avoid the need for surgical procedures, such as botulinum toxin injections, tendon releases, or transplants, and for those described earlier. Occupational therapy focuses on self-help skills, and language therapy emphasizes interpersonal communication. These centers teach parents to foster independence, and help them get needed appliances and services, provide support groups for parents, and are often a source for babysitting and respite care. In severely affected children with CP and cognitive impairment, the thrust is to foster feeding, toileting, and dressing; most end up in a nursing home when their parents can no longer care for them.

Less affected school-age children need an education tailored to their intellectual abilities. Sooner or later, they require counseling for adapting to the fact that they will always remain different from other people. Educated adults with CP provide excellent role models, who can spur the CP child to fight for independence and achievement.

DEVELOPMENTAL DISORDERS OF HIGHER CEREBRAL FUNCTIONS

All of these disorders are defined behaviorally. Their severity varies greatly. Comorbidity (e.g., more than one developmental disorder in a given child, for example, dyslexia and Tourette syndrome) is frequent and may result from lack of selectivity of the underlying pathology, genetic linkage, or fuzzy boundaries because diagnostic criteria are quantitative rather than dichotomous.

If general intelligence (i.e., cognition) is affected (e.g., *mental deficiency or retardation*, now officially referred to as *global developmental delay*), there is generally a diffuse disorder of neocortical or cortical-subcortical development and function, or of multiple widespread lesions. Disorders that affect certain cognitive abilities selectively are considered *specific developmental disorders* and are generally classified according to their main functional consequence (Table 77.2).

Progress in functional brain imaging and electrophysiology, methods that are rapidly identifying brain regions activated selectively by particular cognitive tasks, indicate that the responsible circuits are both modular and distributed. A particularly striking discovery is the unanticipated participation of the cerebellum and basal ganglia in many cognitive tasks.

Etiology

The label *minimal brain damage* (MBD), later replaced by *minimal brain dysfunction* (also MBD), was applied to clumsy, hyperkinetic, inattentive children with school problems when MBD was viewed as a global disorder with perinatal traumatic or ischemic-anoxic insult as its most common etiology. The Collaborative Perinatal Study of

▶ **TABLE 77.2 Developmental Disorders of Higher Cerebral Function**

Disorder	*Function Affected*	*Location of Brain Dysfunction*
Mental deficiency (mental retardation)	Cognition	Diffuse or multifocal (nonspecific?)
Developmental language disorders (dysphasias)	Oral language	Language systems
Dyslexias (reading disability)	Written language	Language systems (usually), especially phonology
Dyscalculias (several variants)	Mathematics	Specific systems?
Attention deficit disorder with/without hyperactivity	Focused attention	Cingulate gyrus, fronto-striate network, others?
Autistic spectrum disorders (pervasive developmental disorder)	Sociability, language, range of activities and interests	Undefined cortical/subcortical systems

the 1960s and 1970s showed that, in contrast to severe prematurity, isolated perinatal insults account for fewer than 10% of the cases of CP and severe mental deficiency, and play a minor role in milder cognitive impairments like learning disabilities. Mild mental subnormality is, to a large degree, attributable to environmental factors such as poverty, social deprivation, inadequate nutrition, or substance abuse during gestation, and low level of maternal education.

Genetics rather than exogenous factors plays a major causal role in the developmental disorders. Some, like autism, are polygenic, with several genes required to produce the full phenotype. Polygenic causation provides an explanation for overlapping and borderline phenotypes. Some families with many dyslexic members have linkages to different chromosomes, which suggests that dyslexia is not linked to a single-gene defect. The effects of genes responsible for developmental disorders on brain development are unknown. Perhaps some exert their effect by enhancing susceptibility to generally well tolerated environmental exposures.

Mental Deficiency

This term is preferred instead of the term mental retardation or global developmental delay, because it implies that it is unrealistic to expect catch-up skills and the achievement of normalcy. The best definition of mental deficiency is not a low score on an intelligence test but the inability to function independently, arising from general incompetence. Before assuming general incompetence, it is necessary to exclude specific impairments in sensorimotor, visual, auditory, language, and other specific cognitive and social skills that might account for failure to perform at a level commensurate with chronologic age and cultural opportunity; these impairments may make valid assessment difficult because there are few standardized intelligence tests for children with CP, deafness, blindness, or autism.

Measurement of Intelligence and Neuropsychologic Skills

A modular view of brain function negates the concept of a single construct, intelligence; it posits that intelligence or cognitive competence depends on the functional integrity of many discrete brain circuits, whose coordinated activity underlies adaptive responses to unpredictable endogenous and exogenous conditions. Intelligence-test batteries are used to predict likely success in school or in a particular vocation. These tests are generally well standardized for normal people of a particular culture, and sample a range of verbal and nonverbal abilities, but the scores must be applied cautiously whenever they are used in other cultures, or with handicapped persons. Brief screening tests,

such as the Peabody Picture Vocabulary Test or the non-verbal Raven Progressive Matrices, may be adequate for some limited purposes.

For the practical purpose of assessing and predicting ability to function in real life, the Revised Vineland Adaptive Behavior Scales provide measures of communication, sociability, motor skills, and adaptive function. The data are derived from an interview with the parents or caretaker, do not require participation of the person being assessed, and are less culturally biased than test data.

The Revised Wechsler scales (e.g., Wechsler Preschool and Primary Scale of Intelligence–WPPSI, Wechsler Intelligence Scale for Children–WISC, and Wechsler Adult Intelligence Scale–WAIS) and the Stanford-Binet, 4th edition, provide verbal and nonverbal summary scores as well as an overall IQ score, and extend from preschool children to adults. The most commonly used test-based criterion for mental deficiency is departure from the mean score of 100 (standard deviation 15) in the general population. Likely functional outcomes as a function of IQ score are listed in Table 77.3.

IQ scores must be used cautiously: Tests in preschool and young school-age children may provide valid comparisons with peers, and have satisfactory predictive validity when applied to groups, but they are not necessarily valid for long-term prediction in the individual child, especially in the face of a handicap, or at very early ages.

In addition to associated handicaps, what determines the functional level of a mentally deficient person with a particular IQ level are motivation, the efficacy of habilitation, and a supportive environment. Adequate self-help and social skills, rather than academic skills, may determine outcome. Severe behavior disorders that worsen functional outcome increase with the severity of the mental deficiency.

A quite different use of psychologic test data from the measure of intelligence is the identification of specific cognitive impairments. Neuropsychologic batteries incorporate tests to detect inadequacies in language; memory and learning; attention; visual, auditory, and somatosensory perception and processing; intersensory integration; fine motor abilities; planning; and even affect recognition, mood, and social cognition. Neuropsychologic tests generate a useful profile of strengths and weaknesses for planning remediation. Appropriately designed neuropsychologic measures are required to identify the neurologic basis of cognitively demanding tasks, using functional brain imaging and electrophysiology.

Developmental Language Disorders (or Dysphasias)

There is considerable variation in the manner and age at which normal children acquire various aspects of language. This makes the definition of *developmental*

▶ **TABLE 77.3 Functional Ability and Level of Cognitive Competence***

		Abilities			
IQ	Mental	Language	Education	Work	Daily Living
>115	Superior				
85–115	Average				
70–85	Borderline	Usually normal	Remediation needed	Employable	Independent ADL, may need some living help
55–70	Mild mental deficiency	Normal or impaired	Limited ability	Employable at selected tasks	Need variable amount of living help
40–55	Moderate mental deficiency	Normal or impaired	Very limited	May be capable of simple tasks	Dependent for living, may need ADL help
25–40	Severe mental deficiency	Limited or absent	Minimal functional	None or minimal	Need ADL help
<25	Profound mental deficiency	Absent			Usually totally dependent, often nonambulatory, incontinent

*The American Association on Mental Retardation recommends a new classification of persons with IQs below 70 to 75,
  based on limitations in two or more adaptive skills and on the kinds and intensities of needed supports.
ADL: Activities of daily living.

language disorders (DLD) controversial because it depends on departure from some expected language age, or on a discrepancy between verbal and nonverbal cognitive skills. The term *developmental language delay* is widely used because most children with DLD learn to speak before school age; the term is inappropriate for the many children who later have trouble learning to read or express themselves coherently orally, or in writing.

Neurologic Basis of the Dysphasias

Focal brain lesions are rare, in part because unilateral focal lesions acquired in early life do not preclude the acquisition of language, reflecting greater potential for reorganization in the immature than in the mature brain. Most people, regardless of handedness, are genetically destined to develop language in the left hemisphere. Yet language may develop and be sustained in either hemisphere, as shown by adequate development of language in young children with large hemispheric lesions, or following hemispherectomy; albeit, there are subtle but demonstrable differences in language and nonverbal skills in those with right and left pathology. Dysphasic children are therefore thought to have bilateral dysfunction in circuits critical to language development.

Subtypes of Developmental Language Disorders

There is no fully accepted classification of the dysphasias. Despite some similarities, models based on the acquired aphasias of adults do not fully apply to disorders of language acquisition, yet focal brain lesions in adults have provided crucial information on the circuits required for particular aspects of language.

Some dysphasias, like Broca aphasia in adults, are predominantly expressive and affect phonology (i.e., the production of the sounds of speech) and syntax (i.e., the grammar of language), whereas semantics (i.e., the meaning of language) and pragmatics (i.e., the communicative use of language) are spared.

Receptive dysphasias preclude or severely jeopardize the processing of phonology and syntax, and as a consequence, semantics and the acquisition of expressive language; they are therefore always mixed (e.g., receptive and expressive), in contrast to Wernicke aphasia of adults, in which automatic speech continues unabated, albeit with abnormal content. The closest analogy between adult aphasia and childhood dysphasia is word deafness (i.e., *verbal auditory agnosia* [*VAA*]), the most severe variant of receptive DLD, with the difference that adults with bilateral temporal lesions may speak normally and can read and write, whereas children with VAA are nonverbal because profound impairment of comprehension precludes all language skills, with the possible exception of nonverbal pragmatics (i.e., communicative gestures). VAA is especially frequent in children with acquired epileptic aphasia (i.e., *Landau-Kleffner syndrome*), which consists of chronic loss of speech, or failure to develop speech in the case of developmental VAA, associated with a seizure disorder or a frankly paroxysmal EEG without clinical seizures. Children with developmental or very early VAA are often autistic, with no sparing of pragmatics.

A third type of DLD largely spares the development of receptive and expressive phonology and syntax but impairs semantic processing; these children have difficulty understanding complex sentences, answering open-ended questions, retrieving vocabulary, and formulating coherent discourse. They may speak clearly but when younger, often produced a fluent, incomprehensible jargon, with word approximations. Some have an excellent rote verbal memory and impaired pragmatic skills; they are likely to be chatterboxes who rely on overlearned scripts. They often perseverate and speak to themselves aloud without a conversational partner. This semantic-pragmatic syndrome is particularly frequent in verbal autistic children.

Etiology and Pathophysiology

DLD clearly does not have a single cause. Genetics plays a major but not an exclusive role. A few known syndromes are associated with particular subtypes of dysphasia, e.g., hydrocephalus and Williams syndrome with the semantic-pragmatic syndrome. Dysphasia is significantly more frequent in boys than girls. Disorders of the acquisition of phonology may be linked to a more general impairment of rapid-auditory processing that jeopardizes the detection of the brief acoustic stimuli that differentiate one consonant from another. VAA is linked to dysfunction in temporal-auditory cortices. The pathophysiology of other dysphasic syndromes is not understood.

Reading Disability (Dyslexia)

Learning to read is learning to decode written (e.g., visually coded) language. It may be difficult to distinguish true dyslexia from poor reading attributable to impoverished language stimulation, poor teaching, lack of motivation, or borderline intellectual competence. As in the case of dysphasia, there are subtypes of dyslexia.

Visual-perceptual problems play a minor pathophysiologic role in dyslexia, which is almost always the consequence of a language problem. The most prevalent subtype involves inadequate phonologic processing, such as difficulty segmenting speech into component phonemes (e.g., speech sounds), sequencing them, learning the relationship between graphemes (e.g., letters) and phonemes, sounding out strings of letters (e.g., nonwords), and spelling. Some children have more difficulty learning to read whole words than analyzing them phonologically. Others have visual problems in association with phonologic deficits, making learning to read arduous, or nearly impossible. Poor readers may be more generally learning disabled. Some are clumsy and have poor handwriting, difficulty with mathematics, or an attention deficit, with or without hyperactivity.

Specific reading disability is virtually never the consequence of a detectable, structural brain lesion, although brain imaging may show statistic linkage to atypical hemispheric asymmetry. Galaburda describes minor migration-cell defects and tiny scars located selectively in the perisylvian areas of the left hemisphere in dyslexics. Functional MRI shows that training in phonologic skills may mitigate dyslexia, and reverse previously inadequate activation of left posterior-cortical regions during reading.

Genetics, including linkage to chromosomes 6 or 15 in some families, plays a major but not exclusive etiologic role. Outcome depends in part on the general intellectual level and adequacy of intervention. Most intelligent dyslexics eventually learn to read more or less efficiently, but they tend to be poor spellers, have difficulty reading nonwords, and may not read for pleasure.

Other Learning Disabilities

There are at least two clearly differentiable reasons for difficulty in writing (i.e., *dysgraphia*): dysorthographia—the consequence of dyslexia, and poor handwriting—caused by a minor motor or visuomotor disability. There are also several variants of *dyscalculia*: a lack of understanding of the rules for calculation, spatial problems resulting in place errors while setting up written calculations, and difficulty with geometry, higher-order language deficits interfering with the solving of word problems, and inadequate attention impairing short-term memory essential for mental arithmetic.

Children with *nonverbal learning disabilities* have lower performance than verbal abilities and dyscalculia. Many have social deficits that place them on the autistic spectrum. *Memory disorders* for specific types of materials and tasks resemble those of adults. *Executive* and *planning disorders* have a profound impact on organizational and reasoning abilities, which as in adults, depend on the integrity of prefrontal-striatal circuits.

Disorders of Attention

Attention deficit disorder (ADD) is reportedly more frequent in boys, because ADD is genuinely more frequent in boys, because boys are more likely to have ADD with hyperactivity (ADHD) than girls, or because boys are generally more active and aggressive than girls and ADD is therefore more conspicuous and difficult to tolerate in boys. ADD may be evident in infancy by reduced need for sleep, later by difficulty falling asleep, waking too early in the morning, or by multiple awakenings during the night. Children with ADD are restless, have a short attention span, go from one toy to another without getting engaged, and in school get up from their seats or wander in the classroom. They are impulsive, disorganized, and forgetful, and may have a labile affect. Other features, such as clumsiness and learning disability, are associated rather than intrinsic manifestations. Marked distractibility may interfere with the acquisition of reading and arithmetic, but most ADHD children of normal intelligence are not learning disabled. ADD persists in adult life, although motor hyperactivity usually abates in adolescence. Prognosis varies; ADHD tends to abate with maturation, but distractibility, impulsivity, a disorganized lifestyle, accident-proneness, and a short temper may be lifelong liabilities. The high level of energy and curtailed need for sleep may be assets in otherwise well functioning adults.

The most widely used criteria for diagnosing ADD and gauging the efficacy of medication are found in Conner's questionnaire, administered to parents or teachers. Assessment of ADHD may include written or computerized tests of attention, or direct recording of amount of movement.

Management of ADD and ADHD

Management combines parental counseling, environmental manipulations, such as removing distractions, providing the opportunity for frequent breaks, and opportunities to move about, and often, medication. ADHD is disruptive because it affects family, peers, and teachers alike. Medication alone is rarely sufficient, and in severe cases, counseling of the family, adjustments of school routines, and in older children, teaching strategies to minimize the consequences of ADD, are necessary.

Methylphenidate is the safest and most frequently prescribed drug. Its short half-life is advantageous for gauging efficacy but requires divided doses. There are now slow-release preparations and most recently a nonstimulating analog. In a young child, one starts with a small dose given in the morning and at midday, progressively increasing until the desired effect is achieved, or until the appearance of sleeplessness, oversedation, increased hyperkinesia, or tics. Drug holidays in the summer are reasonable to gauge whether the child can do without, but if the drug is truly effective, giving it only on school days risks committing the child to an emotional roller-coaster.

Dextroamphetamine, especially its timed-release capsules, may also be tried, in doses half those of methylphenidate. Pemoline has a long half-life and is quite effective, but it is rarely used because of the risk of fatal liver damage. Sedatives should be avoided because some, notably phenobarbital, may precipitate ADHD. There is no evidence that avoidance of sugar, foods with red dye, or those rich in salicylates, and megadoses of vitamins help either ADD or the learning disabilities. The prescription of drugs such as thioridazine, chlorpromazine, and haloperidol, and even risperidone is contraindicated because they are sedating and have potential long-term, irreversible side effects.

Autism Spectrum Disorders: Pervasive Developmental Disorders

The term pervasive developmental disorder (PDD) is used in the *Diagnostic and Statistical Manual of the American Psychiatric Association* as an umbrella term for persons with classically autistic symptomatology, referred to as autistic disorder, as well as for others with similar but fewer, less severe symptoms. Using PDD to avoid mentioning autism, considered stigmatizing because of the discredited theory that poor parenting was responsible, and because it was erroneously thought to be hopeless, is confusing.

Etiology

Autism is one of the developmental disorders of brain function; as do the others, it has several causes. Judging from twin and family studies, polygenic inheritance accounts for most cases with an unknown cause. In some cases there may be an inherited susceptibility to some environmentally determined stress or insult. A minority of individuals with autism have tuberous sclerosis, fragile X, Rett or Angelman syndromes, phenylketonuria, congenital rubella, neonatal herpes simplex, hydrocephalus, a brain malformation, or other static encephalopathy. Perinatal brain injury and measles-mumps-rubella and other vaccines are not credible causes of autism without other evidence of brain damage.

Symptoms

There is great variability in severity and range of symptoms. The core problems involve sociability and lack of insight into other people's thinking, inadequate verbal and nonverbal communication and imagination, and a limited range of interests and activities. Intelligence is not a defining feature but strongly influences prognosis. There may be profound mental deficiency or superior ability, often with areas of major impairment coupled to normal or even prodigious rote memory, calculation, or music ability (i.e., *savant syndrome*).

Problems in sociability range from almost total lack of interest in others, inability to engage another person in play or conversation, and gaze aversion, to inappropriate intrusiveness, failure to maintain appropriate interpersonal distance, and lack of empathy. Impaired ability to read facial expression, body language, and tone of voice may contribute to these deficits and to heightened anxiety. Children with autism may be affectionate, but very selectively so.

The second core problem, communicative incompetence, regularly presents as failure to learn to speak, and limited comprehension of language. Nonverbal communication is affected as young autistic children may not point to request or draw attention, or shake the head "yes" or "no." The most severely affected preschoolers may understand little or nothing; they may remain nonverbal into adulthood, even when comprehension has improved. Others learn to speak after age 3 or 4 years, but with inadequate syntax and phonology. Still others, once they start to speak, progress rapidly to full, clearly articulated sentences. Echolalia, use of verbatim scripts, stilted or wooden prosody (melody of language), and a high-pitched or sing-song voice, are frequent. A large and inappropriately sophisticated vocabulary may mask impaired comprehension of discourse, and especially of questions. Some preschool autistic children are fascinated with letters and numbers and may learn to read without instruction, albeit often with limited comprehension (i.e., *hyperlexia*).

The third core characteristic of autism is a narrow range of interests, unusual preoccupations and choices of activities, inadequate play, perseveration, resistance to change, and tolerance for monotony. Young children may look at the same video or book for hours, play with a string or spin wheels of a car, and prefer to line up or classify toys rather than play with them. Imaginative play is absent or minimal in early childhood. Older autistic children may become engrossed in studying time-tables or collecting bottle caps or sports statistics.

Frequent motor problems in autistic children include toe-walking, hypotonia, stereotypies, and apraxia (failure to imitate gestures and inadequate mastery of complex motor tasks). Stereotypies may be tic-like; they are most prevalent in low-functioning autistic persons but may persist in miniature even in high-functioning adults and be associated with obsessive preoccupations. Stereotypies may consist of flapping the hands when excited, wringing or licking the hands, fiddling with clothing or a lock of hair, or twisting the fingers or gazing at them. There are few facts about the neurologic basis for self-injury, head-banging, or self-biting; failure to respond to sound but intolerance of certain sounds; withdrawal from tactile contact but enjoyment of tickling; excessive sniffing and licking; a narrow range of food choices; and enjoyment of staring at rotating objects, running around in circles, and antigravity play. Sleep disorders, over-focused attention or distractibility, labile mood, destructiveness, self-injury, and seemingly unprovoked temper tantrums and aggression are frequent and troublesome complaints.

Children with autism may have epileptic seizures of any type. The probability of epilepsy is highest in autistic children with mental deficiency, or with frank motor abnormality. It is high in infancy and early childhood, and increases to a second peak in adolescence. Autism may follow infantile spasms or the Lennox-Gastaut syndrome.

Course and Prognosis

In retrospect, signs of autism may already have been present in infancy. In almost half the cases, signs of autism appear in the toddler or early preschool years, either in a perfectly normal or less severely developmentally affected child. Inadequate language is usually the presenting complaint. A third of parents report language regression at a mean age of 21 months, together with regression of sociability and play, but without regression of motor skills. Regression may be insidious or may follow an acute illness or environmental stress. Development resumes after a plateau lasting weeks or months, although complete recovery is exceptional. In some children, regression is associated with a paroxysmal EEG, with or without clinical seizures, and falls within the definition of acquired epileptic aphasia (Landau-Kleffner syndrome).

Disintegrative disorder refers to autistic regression after age 2 years in completely normal, fully verbal children. The neurologic basis of autistic regression, including the potential role of subclinical epilepsy, is not known because autistic regression is often overlooked, precluding early investigation. No reliably effective medical treatment for autistic regression is known; anecdotal reports of the effectiveness of spike-suppressant anticonvulsant drugs, steroids, or intravenous immunoglobulins still lack empiric support.

Like other developmental disorders, autism is a lifelong condition, although sociability and language tend to improve. Unless an early history is available, autistic adults are likely to be diagnosed as mentally retarded, obsessive-compulsive, schizophrenic, manic-depressive, or as having an antisocial or inadequate personality. Some intelligent, verbal persons with autism lead independent lives. In general, they remain single and are likely to be underemployed but remarkably faithful workers. The brightest may function in suitable professions like mathematics or taxonomy. Less intelligent and multiply handicapped autistic persons need supervision throughout life, and the most severely affected require institutionalization.

Pathology and Pathophysiology

Information is scanty. Except in cases with a known cause, there is no evidence for gross malformation or destructive or inflammatory pathology. There may be developmental cellular anomalies in the limbic system, parts of the cerebellar and cerebral cortex, and the inferior olive. Even high-resolution MRI is usually normal; therefore MRI is not indicated clinically, unless the neurologic examination mandates it, even if the patient's head circumference is larger than average. Standard EEG and evoked-potential studies are generally normal unless there are seizures, although recent loss of language mandates a prolonged-sleep EEG to detect subclinical epilepsy. Research MRI morphometry reveals subtle differences in the size of various structures such as vermal lobules VI and VII of the cerebellum, or the size of focal areas of the cerebral white matter, in some groups of individuals with autism. Event-related potentials and functional imaging with appropriate ligands during the performance of cognitive and language tasks are starting to provide insights into the pathophysiology of autism and abnormalities of neurotransmitter metabolism, notably serotonin, but a fully coherent hypothesis regarding the neurologic basis of autism has yet to emerge.

Management

Early, individualized education, based in part on operant principles that address both the behavioral and the communication needs of children with autistic spectrum disorders is the backbone of management. Parents need instruction in behavior management. Neurologists should discourage the squandering of resources on the many well meaning but unproven behavioral and dietary treatments offered to desperate parents.

No drug cures autism, but psychotropic drugs may be targeted to specific behavioral problems, although empiric studies are largely lacking. Risperidone has been shown to decrease irritability and perseveration, and perhaps, enhance some functional skills. Specific serotonin-reuptake inhibitors are widely prescribed clinically, as is clonidine, a central alpha 2-adrenergic agonist. Aggressive outbursts may respond to large doses of propranolol, given in progressive increments to tolerance, and in a crisis, to parenteral haloperidol or phenothiazines which must be avoided long-term because of their potentially irreversible side effects. The use of naltrexone to mitigate self-injury has been disappointing. Anxiolytic drugs and tricyclic antidepressants have their places and methylphenidate may help ADHD, although stimulants are generally contraindicated in autism. Anticonvulsants may be tried in children with frankly paroxysmal EEGs without clinical seizures, and may also have mood stabilizing efficacy.

SUGGESTED READINGS

Developmental Disorders of Motor Function–Cerebral Palsy

Crothers B, Paine RS. *The Natural History of Cerebral Palsy.* Cambridge UK: Harvard University Press, 1959.

Ferriero DM. Neonatal brain injury. *N Engl J Med* 2004 Nov 4; 351(19):1985–1995.

Filloux FM. Neuropathophysiology of movement disorder in cerebral palsy. *J Child Neurol* 1996;11(suppl 1):S5–S12.

Hoon AH Jr, Reinhardt EM, Kelley RI, et al. Brain magnetic imaging in suspected extrapyramidal cerebral palsy: observations in distinguishing genetic-metabolic from acquired causes. *J Pediatr* 1997;131:240–245.

Jacobs JM. Management options for the child with spastic cerebral palsy. *Orthop Nurs* 2001;20:53–59.

Johnston MV. Hypoxic and ischemic disorders of infants and children. *Brain Devel* 1997;19:235–239.

Krauss JK, Loher TJ, Weigel R, et al. Chronic stimulation of the globus pallidus internus for treatment of non-dYT1 generalized dystonia and choreoathetosis: 2-year follow up. *J Neurosurg* 2003;98:785–792.

Little WJ. On the influence of abnormal parturition, difficult labor, premature birth, and asphyxia neonatorum on the mental and physical conditions of the child, especially in relation to deformities. *Clin Orthop* 1966;46:7–22.

Morota N, Kameyama S, Masuda M, et al. Functional posterior rhizotomy for severely disabled children with mixed type cerebral palsy. *Acta Neurochir Suppl* 2003;87:99–102.

Murphy NA, Irwin MC, Hoff C. Intrathecal baclofen therapy in children with cerebral palsy: efficacy and complications. *Arch Phys Med Rehabil* 2002;83:1721–1725.

Nelson KB. Can we prevent cerebral palsy? *N Engl J Med* 2003;349:1765–1769.

Okumura A, Kato T, Kuno K, Hayakawa F, Watanabe K. MRI findings in patients with spastic cerebral palsy. II: Correlation with type of cerebral palsy. *Dev Med Child Neurol* 1997;39(6):369–372.

Ramaswamy V, Miller SP, Barkovich AJ, Partridge JC, Ferriero DM. Perinatal stroke in term infants with neonatal encephalopathy. *Neurology* 2004;62:2088–2091.

Stevenson DK, Sunshine P, eds. *Fetal and Neonatal Brain Injury: Mechanisms, Management, and Risks.* New York: Oxford University Press, 1997.

Tilton AH. Injectable neuromuscular blockade in the treatment of spasticity and movement disorders. 2003;18(suppl 1):S50–S66.

Developmental Disorders of Higher Cerebral Functions

American Association on Mental Retardation. *Mental Retardation: Definition, Classification, and Systems of Supports,* 9th ed. Washington, DC: American Association on Mental Retardation, 1992.

Barkley RA. Issues in the diagnosis of attention-deficit/hyperactivity disorder in children. *Brain Devel* 2003;25:77–83.

Bates E, Thal D, Finlay B, Clancy B. Early language development and its neural correlates. In: Segalowitz SJ, Rapin I, eds. *Handbook of Neuropsychology,* 2nd ed. Vol 8: *Child Neuropsychology* Part II. Amsterdam: Elsevier, 2003.

Broman S, Nichols PL, Shaughnessy P, et al. *Retardation in Young Children.* Hillsdale, NJ: L Erlbaum Associates, 1987.

Colvin M, McGuire W, Fowlie PW. Neurodevelopmental outcomes after preterm birth. *BMJ* 2004 Dec 11;329(7479):1390–1393.

Deuel RK. Motor soft signs and development. In: Segalowitz SJ, Rapin I, eds. *Handbook of Neuropsychology,* 2nd ed. Vol 8: *Child Neuropsychology* Part I. Amsterdam: Elsevier Science, 2002.

Eden GF, Jones KM, Cappell K, Gareau L, Wood FB, Zeffiro TA, Dietz NA, Agnew JA, Flowers DL. Neural changes following remediation in adult developmental dyslexia. *Neuron* 2004 Oct 28;44(3):411–422.

Fisher SE, Lai CS, Monaco AP. Deciphering the genetic basis of speech and language disorders. *Annu Rev Neurosci* 2003;26:57–80. Epub 2003 Jan 08.

Garcia O'Shea A, et al. The neuropsychological assessment of the preschool child. In: Segalowitz SJ, Rapin I, eds. *Handbook of Neuropsychology,* 2nd ed. Vol 8: *Child Neuropsychology* Part I. Amsterdam: Elsevier Science, 2002.

Gillberg C, Coleman M. *The Biology of the Autistic Syndromes,* 3rd ed. Oxford: Mac Keith Press, 2000.

Juranek J, Filipek PA. Neuroimaging in developmental disorders. In: Segalowitz SJ, Rapin I, eds. *Handbook of Neuropsychology,* 2nd ed. Vol 8: *Child Neuropsychology* Part I. Amsterdam: Elsevier Science, 2002.

Marlow N, Wolke D, Bracewell MA, Samara M; EPICure Study Group. Neurologic and developmental disability at six years of age after extremely preterm birth. *N Engl J Med* 2005 Jan 6;352(1):9–19.

Mattis S, Luck DZ. Neuropsychological assessment of school-aged children. In: Segalowitz SJ, Rapin I, eds. *Handbook of Neuropsychology,* 2nd ed. Vol 8: *Child Neuropsychology,* Part I. Amsterdam: Elsevier Science, 2002.

Muhle R, Trentacoste SV, Rapin I. The genetics of autism. *Pediatrics* 2004;113:e472–e486.

Nordentoft M, Lou HC, Hansen D, et al. Intrauterine growth retardation and premature delivery: the influence of maternal smoking and psychosocial factors. *Am J Publ Health* 1996;86:347–354.

Rapin I. Developmental language disorders: a clinical update. *J Child Psychol Psychiat* 1996;37:643–655.

Rapin I. Autism. *New Engl J Med* 1997;337:97–104.

Schmahmann JD, ed. *The Cerebellum and Cognition.* San Diego: Academic Press, 1997.

Shaywitz SE, Shaywitz BA, Fulbright RK, et al. Neural systems for compensation and persistence: young adult outcome of childhood reading disability. *Biol Psychiatry* 2003;54:25–33.

Steinschneider M, Dunn M. Electrophysiology in developmental neuropsychology. In: Segalowitz SJ, Rapin I eds. *Handbook of Neuropsychology,* 2nd ed. Vol 8: *Child Neuropsychology* Part I. Amsterdam: Elsevier Science, 2002.

Shalev RS. Developmental dyscalculia. In: Segalowitz SJ, Rapin I, eds. *Handbook of Neuropsychology,* 2nd ed. Vol 8: *Child Neuropsychology* Part II. Amsterdam: Elsevier Science, 2003.

Tuchman RF, Rapin I. Epilepsy in autism. *Lancet Neurology* 2002;1:352–358.

Weiss G, Trockenberg-Hechtman L. *Hyperactive Children Grown Up.* New York: Guilford Press, 1986.

Chapter 78

Laurence-Moon-Biedl Syndrome

Melvin Greer

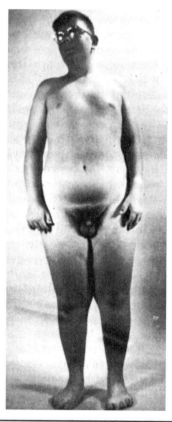

FIGURE 78.1. Laurence-Moon-Biedl syndrome. A 19-year-old patient with obesity, hypogenitalism, polydactyly (toes), retinitis pigmentosa, and mental retardation.

A variable group of clinical features manifested primarily by obesity and hypogonadism was described in 1866 by Laurence and Moon. Subsequent redefinition of the syndrome by Bardet and Biedl may have established a new entity, but the clustering of manifestations was similar. The features include obesity (85% to 95%); mental retardation (70% to 85%); retinal dystrophy and coloboma (92% to 95%); hypogenitalism and hypogonadism (74% to 86% of males, 45% to 53% of females); and polydactyly, syndactyly, or both (75% to 80%). Added to this were renal dysfunction and hypertension, and with lesser frequency, cardiac and hepatic defects. Isolated case reports include cranial-nerve palsy, diabetes mellitus, diabetes insipidus, spinocerebellar degeneration, spastic quadriparesis with severe cervical stenosis, hydrocephalus, and facial dysostosis.

The salient early characteristic is obesity (Fig. 78.1). During the first decade of life, impaired night vision is the hallmark of retinitis pigmentosa, which progresses, and by age 20, 73% of the patients are blind. McKusick-Kaufman syndrome is another variant, which may be diagnosed in infancy. Vaginal atresia and postaxial polydactyly exist. Later, obesity and retinal dystrophy become evident.

Testicular atrophy, a decrease in the number of germinal cells, and spermatogenic arrest have been described, but no identifiable endocrine cause explains the gonadal dysfunction. Indeed, in adolescence, some patients improve spontaneously. Testosterone therapy is ineffective in treating hypogonadism or hypogenitalism.

The mode of inheritance is autosomal recessive. Although the condition is compatible with a normal lifespan, longevity may be shortened by renal or cardiac defects. No specific neuropathologic changes have been described. Several hereditary syndromes associated with pigmentary retinopathy include manifestations that loosely fit the Laurence-Moon-Biedl syndrome. For instance, the Alström-Hallgren syndrome, transmitted as an autosomal-recessive disorder, includes obesity, hypogonadism, nerve deafness, diabetes mellitus, and retinitis pigmentosa. The Biemond syndrome is characterized by hypogonadotropic hypogonadism, obesity, postaxial polydactyly, mental retardation, and coloboma of the iris rather than retinitis pigmentosa. The Prader-Willi syndrome is also manifested by obesity, hypogonadism, and mental retardation, but there are no visual problems. DNA samples from 29 families with these disorders have identified loci in chromosome regions 11q13, 15q22.3-q23, 16q21, 3p13-p12, 2q31, and 20p12. Genetic interactions are thought to modulate phenotypes, as well.

SUGGESTED READINGS

Biedl A. Aduber das Laurence-Biedlsche Syndrome. *Med Klin* 1933; 29:839–840.

Beales PL, Badano JL, Ross AJ, et al. Genetic interaction of BBS1 mutations with alleles at other BBS loci can result in non-Mendelian Bardet-Biedl syndrome. *Am J Hum Genet* 2003;72:1187–1199.

Buford EA, Riise R, Teague PW, et al. Linkage mapping in 29 Bardet-Biedl syndrome families confirms loci in chromosomal regions 11q13, 15q22.3-q23 and 16q21. *Genomics* 1997;41:93–99.

Badano JL, Kim JC, Hoskins BE, et al. Heterozygous mutations in BBS1, BBS2 and BBS6 have a potential epistatic effect on Bardet-Biedl patients with two mutations at a second BBS locus. *Hum Mol Genet* 2003;15:1651–1659.

Cantani A, Bellioni P, Bamonte G, et al. Seven hereditary syndromes with pigmentary retinopathy. *Clin Pediatr* 1985;24:578–583.

David A, Bitoun P, Lacombe D, et al. Hydrometrocolpos and polydactyly: a common neonatal presentation of Bardet-Biedl and McKusick-Kaufman syndromes. *J Med Genet* 1999;36:599–603.

Kim JC, Badano JL, Sibold S, et al. The Bardet-Biedl protein BBS4 targets cargo to the pericentriolar region and is required for microtubule anchoring and cell cycle progression. *Nat Genet* 2004;36(5):462–470. Epub 2004 Apr 25.

Koepp P. Laurence-Moon-Biedl syndrome associated with diabetes insipidus neurohormonalis. *Eur J Pediatr* 1975;121:59–62.

Mehrotra N, Taub S, Covert RF. Hydrometrocolpos as a neonatal manifestation of the Bardet-Biedl syndrome. *Am J Med Genet* 1997;69:220.

Moore SJ, Green JS, Fan Y, et al. Clinical and genetic epidemiology of Bardet-Biedl syndrome in Newfoundland: A 22-year prospective, population-based, cohort study. *Am J Med Genet A* 2005 Jan 6; [Epub ahead of print]

Pagon RA, Haas JE, Bunt AH, et al. Hepatic involvement in the Bardet-Biedl syndrome. *Am J Med Genet* 1982;13:373–381.

Soliman AT, Rajab A, Al Salmi I, et al. Empty sellae, impaired testosterone secretion, and defective hypothalamic-pituitary growth and gonadal axes in children with Bardet-Biedl syndrome. *Metabolism* 1996;45:1230–1234.

Verloes A, Temple IK, Bonnet S, Bottani A. Coloboma, mental retardation, hypogonadism, and obesity: critical review of the so-called Biemond syndrome type 2, updated nosology, and delineation of three "new" syndromes. *Am J Med Genet* 1997;69:370–379.

Chapter 79

Structural Malformations

Melvin Greer

MALFORMATIONS OF CEREBRAL HEMISPHERES AND AGENESIS OF CORPUS CALLOSUM

Before day 23 of human gestation, failure of cleavage of the telencephalon and diencephalon results in a single-lobed structure with an undivided ventricle. This is *alobar holoprosencephaly* or *arhinencephaly*. It is commonly associated with defects and anomalies of the skull base, dura, face, eyes, and olfactory apparatus. Semilobar and lobar holoprosencephaly are variations wherein the hemispheres are partly or completely separated and are invariably associated with multiple deformities of cerebral architecture, ranging from absence or primitive appearance of gyri (*lissencephaly*) to heterotopias and migration defects.

Cerebellar cortical dysplasias may be seen as incidental findings on MR studies or as another component of a disturbance of cortical layering attributed to genetic factors or prenatal insults. Perisylvian polymicrogyria may be familial and in some families, mothers and daughters have band heterotropia and their sons have lissencephaly. Linkage to xq21.3-24 has been reported. Multiple genetic defects have been identified, including these that encode inductive signals, allowing the prenatal amniocentesis diagnosis.

Lissencephaly with malformations of muscle and eye have been identified in Fukuyama congenital muscular dystrophy and the Walker-Warburg syndrome. Common clinical manifestations noted early are facial dysmorphism, apneic episodes, seizures, and delayed psychomotor development. Causal mechanisms include chromosomal abnormalities and intrauterine acquired factors, such as maternal diabetes, toxoplasmosis, rubella, syphilis, or the fetal-alcohol syndrome.

Endocrine disorders include pituitary, thyroid, and adrenal hypoplasia. Septooptic dysplasia, another midline-developmental defect, includes hypoplasia of the optic nerve, lateral geniculate, hypothalamic, or posterior pituitary, in addition to cerebral and cerebellar dysplasia.

Complete or partial agenesis of the corpus callosum is commonly noted in association with the holoprosencephalic brain. Callosal agenesis, unassociated with the major holoprosencephalic anomalies, is more common. This may be present in an otherwise clinically normal person, and is attributed to impairment in development between gestation weeks 11 through 20. It may be partial or complete, familial or sporadic, and has been described as an autosomal-dominant, autosomal-recessive, or sex-limited recessive trait.

CT or MRI shows that the lateral ventricles are widely separated and angular (Fig. 79.1).

The medial ventricular wall is convex, and the cavity is small. The septum pellucidum is superiorly displaced. When the agenesis is partial, the body and splenium are missing; the genu is present as a poorly formed, anterior-callosal rudiment. The third ventricle is wide and higher than normal.

Both microcephaly and macrocephaly, in association with other cerebral malformations including hydrocephalus, may be noted with agenesis of the corpus callosum. Seizures and mental retardation are seen in more than 50% of patients; other anomalies seen with lesser frequency include defects of the skeleton, heart, craniofacial structures, gastrointestinal system, and genitourinary system. In some metabolic degenerative disorders, corpus callosum shrinkage may be postnatal in origin. This has been seen in the nonketotic hyperglycinemia, Menkes syndrome, Zellweger syndrome, adrenoleukodystrophy, pyruvate-dehydrogenase deficiency, adenyl-succinate deficiency, and glutaric aciduria type II.

Structural changes within the affected corpus callosum may include a lipoma, or more rarely, a midline meningioma, dermoid cyst, or hamartoma. Chromosome defects, including trisomy 8, 9, 13, and 18, may be seen with agenesis of the corpus callosum. Syndrome complexes that include agenesis of the corpus callosum are listed in Table 79.1.

The acallosal but clinically normal person has alternative pathways of information transfer, probably via intercollicular connections and posterior commissure.

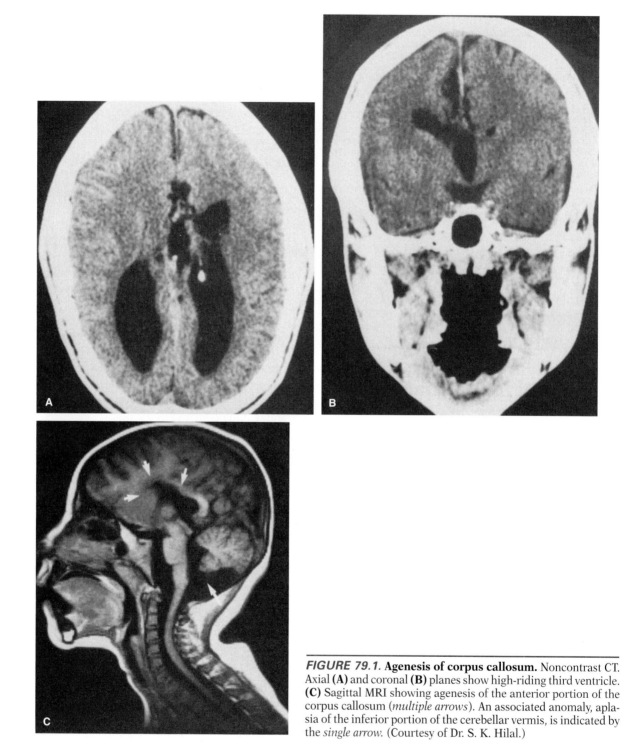

FIGURE 79.1. Agenesis of corpus callosum. Noncontrast CT. Axial **(A)** and coronal **(B)** planes show high-riding third ventricle. **(C)** Sagittal MRI showing agenesis of the anterior portion of the corpus callosum (*multiple arrows*). An associated anomaly, aplasia of the inferior portion of the cerebellar vermis, is indicated by the *single arrow.* (Courtesy of Dr. S. K. Hilal.)

Myelination of the corpus callosum is accomplished, in large measure, by age 6 years but may not be complete before age 10 years. Callosotomy, as a treatment of refractory seizures in children, did not result in the same psychologic changes identified as the disconnection syndrome in the adult callosotomy patient. This difference implies plasticity of neuronal pathways.

MACROCEPHALY AND MEGALENCEPHALY

Head-size enlargement greater than 2 standard deviations above the mean, for age, is *macrocephaly*. Progressive hydrocephalus and mass lesions are common causes of an enlarged head size in the infant and young child. Closure

▶ **TABLE 79.1** Syndromes Associated with Agenesis of the Corpus Callosum

Syndrome	Characteristics
Apert	Megalencephaly; anomalies of the skull base, hands, and feet; cerebral malformations including limbic system changes and polygyria
Aicardi	Females affected, mental retardation and seizures (infantile spasms), vertebral abnormalities, chorioretinopathy
Oral-facial digital	Mental retardation, midline oral and facial defects, hand and finger abnormalities, renal microcysts, cerebral migration defects
Miller-Dieker	Profound clinical cerebral dysfunction with death in first decade; chromosome 17 abnormality in most; anteverted nostrils, micrognathia, lissencephaly and other cerebral migration defects, cardiac anomalies
Neu-Laxova	Autosomal recessive; death in weeks; ocular abnormalities, everted lips, short neck, ichthyosis, edema, limb deformities, lissencephaly and cerebral, cerebellar, and brainstem atrophy
Fanconi anemia	Autosomal recessive, pancytopenia, skeletal anomalies including radial aplasia
Sensorimotor neuropathy and agenesis of corpus callosum	Autosomal recessive; sensorimotor agenesis of corpus callosum neuropathy, dysmorphism
Shapiro	Genitourinary and cardiac defects, mental retardation, hydrocephalus, holoprosencephaly, episodic hyperhidrosis, and hypothermia or hyperthermia
Osteochondrodysplasia	Nonlethal rhizomelic osteochondrodysplasia, hypertension, thrombocytopenia, hydrocephalus
XK syndrome	Aprosencephaly, congenital heart disease, preaxial limb malformation, abnormal genitalia, adrenohypoplasia, 13q32 deletions.

of the suture in the pubertal child prevents skull enlargement in the presence of these pressure-inducing disorders. Benign states of macrocephaly may be familial. Not infrequently, imaging studies reveal mildly dilated lateral ventricles and an increase in subarachnoid fluid. Children who exhibit such features on CT or MRI have been identified as having *hydrocephalus ex vacuo*, but CSF shunts should be reserved for conditions in which there is progressive enlargement of the CSF spaces, and additionally, evidence of neurologic dysfunction.

Megalencephaly is an enlarged brain. Brain weight 2.5 standard deviations above the mean, for sex and age, or brain weight greater than 1,600 g, qualifies for the diagnosis. Primarily, megalencephaly may be an isolated finding. It has been described in families as an autosomal-recessive trait and attributed to a disturbance of developmental-cell proliferation.

A broad spectrum of mutations have been identified in the MLC1 gene associated with megalencephalic leucoencephalopathy and subcortical-cyst syndrome.

Progressive enlargement of the brain with deterioration of neurologic function is seen in children with neurocutaneous syndromes, neuronal storage, or degenerative diseases such as mucopolysaccharidoses or leukodystrophies. Pathologic changes include new growths, such as the tubers of tuberous sclerosis, that may occlude ventricular-fluid flow to cause hydrocephalus. The degenerative diseases are associated with a myriad of pathologic changes associated with megalencephaly, including cystic changes and extensive gliosis. Developmental brain defects causing macrocephaly, and megalencephaly may be associated

with other organ-system defects and are often noted at birth (Table 79.2).

Unilateral megalencephaly is associated with unilateral-hemisphere defects, such as an altered gyral pattern, including pachygyria and polymicrogyria, thickened cortex, and disorganization of gray matter. Such features are similar to the Lhermitte-Duclos syndrome, in which cerebellar granular-cell hypertrophy and other cerebellar hamartomatous growths create a mass effect.

Children with hemimegalencephaly commonly have seizures, hemiparesis, and mental retardation. MRI depicts the structural changes and may also identify the asymptomatic hemi-megalencephalic child with white-matter low-attenuation features, early in life, that may later disappear.

MALFORMATIONS OF OCCIPITAL BONE AND CERVICAL SPINE

The defects in the development of the cervical spine and base of the skull may be divided into the following groups:

1. Basilar impression;
2. Malformation of the atlas and axis; and
3. Malformation or fusion of other cervical vertebrae (i.e., Klippel-Feil anomaly) (Table 79.3).

Any of these malformations may occur singly or together; they also may be associated with developmental

▶ **TABLE 79.2 Macrocephaly and Megalencephaly**

Developmental Defects	Characteristics
Cerebral gigantism (Sotos syndrome)	Macrocephaly with mildly dilated ventricles; precocious increased size including enlarged hands and feet, dolichocephaly, hypertelorism, macroglossia, prognathism; often associated mental retardation, seizures, and clumsiness; frequent early respiratory and feeding problems; may be autosomal dominant
Trisomy 9p syndrome	Macrocephaly with somatic and genital growth delay; facial, hand, and feet deformities, periscapular muscle hypoplasia, delayed bone maturation; severe mental retardation
Robinow syndrome	Macrocephaly with macroglossia and other facial deformities; hemivertebrae and limb defects; genital hypoplasia; seizures may be present, variable degree of mental deficiency
FG syndrome	Megalencephaly with facial dysmorphism, imperforate anus, joint and hand deformities; occasional hydrocephalus, agenesis of corpus callosum, intestinal abnormalities, sensorineural deafness, cardiac and genitourinary defects
Achondroplasia	Macrocephaly with associated cranial defects; short cranial base, early sphenooccipital stenosis, depressed nasal bridge and facial hypoplasia. Skeletal deformities. May have hydrocephalus; spinal cord and foraminal narrowing with compression in about 46%, normal intelligence. Short stature. Frequency 1:26,000, autosomal dominant transmission
Greig cephalopolysyndactyly	Macrocephaly, frontal bossing and hypertelorism, broad thumbs and other hand deformities; autosomal dominant
Osteopetrosis	Macrocephaly with progressive compression of cranial foramina; multiple skeletal defects; increased alkaline phosphatase; autosomal recessive
Osteopathia striata with cranial sclerosis	Macrocephaly, linear striations of long bones, hypertelorism, palate anomalies, hearing deficits, mental retardation
Storage diseases/metabolic	
Tay-Sachs disease–infantile (GM$_2$ ganliosidosis)	Megalencephaly secondary to neuronal swelling and astrocytic hyperplasia; myoclonic seizures and rapidly progressive dementia, quadriparesis, hyperacusis with onset in first months of life; cherry-red spot in fundus; blindness; autosomal recessive
Hurler (mucopolysaccharidosis IH)	Macrocephaly with occasional hydrocephalus secondary to arachnoid mucopolysaccharide accumulation; growth retardation, mental retardation, coarse facial features, corneal and retinal changes, macroglossia, kyphosis and other skeletal deformities, deafness, hepatosplenomegaly, cardiac defects; autosomal recessive
Hurler-Scheie (mucopolysaccharidosis IH/S)	Macrocephaly with facial dysmorphism, corneal clouding; mild mental deficiency to normal; dysostosis multiplex, mild joint contractures, deafness, hepatosplenomegaly, cardiac defects
Maroteaux-Larny Mucopolysaccharidosis (mucopolysaccharidosis VI)	Occasional macrocephaly with coarse facial features, growth delay, joint and skeletal changes, hepatosplenomegaly, deafness; autosomal recessive
Mucopolysaccharidosis VII (Sly syndrome; glucuronidase deficiency)	Macrocephaly with mental deficiency; joint and skeletal deformities, hepatosplenomegaly, corneal clouding; autosomal recessive
Fucosidosis	Megalencephaly with progressive psychomotor retardation; hepatosplenomegaly, dysostosis multiplex
Mitochondrial respiratory chain	
Mitochondrial respiratory chain in complex I deficency	Fatal progressive macrocephaly and hypertrophic cardiomyopathy. Cerebral small vessel proliferation and gliosis
Leukodystrophies	
Spongy degeneration (Canavan)	Megalencephaly with progressive psychomotor retardation, seizures; vacuolation and Alzheimer type II astrocytes prominent
Alexander disease	Megalencephaly with progressive psychomotor retardation, seizures; Rosenthal fibers deep to internal and external brain surfaces
Neurocutaneous disorders	
Tuberous sclerosis	Megalencephic brain with cortical tubers, subependymal nodules, heterotopias; mental retardation, seizures, hypomelanotic macules, facial angiofibromas; ocular, cardiac, and renal defects; autosomal dominant
Klippel-Trenaunay-Weber	Macrocephaly with limb hypertrophy; hemangiomata, hyperpigmented nevi, and other skin lesions, ocular abnormalities, visceromegaly; may be mentally deficient; seizures
Ruvalcaba-Myhre syndrome	Macrocephaly and tan spots on penis; mental deficiency, intestinal hamartomas; macrosomia at birth; lipid storage myopathy
Proteus syndrome	Macrocephaly associated with hemihypertrophy, thickened skin, hyperpigmented areas, hemangiomata and lipomata, bony defects, macrodactyly, mental deficiency
Cowden disease	Megalencephaly associated with Lhermitte-Duclos cerebellar dysplasia; facial, oral, and acral papules, tumors of breast and ovary; may see mental deficiency, seizures, tremor

▶ TABLE 79.3 Uncommon Syndromes Associated with Cervicomedullary and Cervical Spine Malformations

Syndromes	Characteristics
Craniometaphyseal dysplasia	Hyperostosis and skull sclerosis, long bone metaphyseal widening, cranial nerve compression, foramen magnum narrowing causing hydrocephalus, cord and brainstem compression. Calcitrol treatment
MURCS (Müllerian duct aplasia, renal aplasia, cervicothoracic somite dysplasia)	Klippel-Feil anomaly with absence of vagina and uterus, absence or hypoplasia, renal agenesis or ectopy: other bony defects; hearing and gastrointestinal defects
Goldenhar	Cervical hemivertebrae or hypoplasia with associated facial bone, ear, and oral hypoplasias; deafness; occasional defects of heart, kidney, other bones; may be unilateral; mental deficiency in some
Escobar	Cervical vertebral fusion and other bony defects, ptosis, hypertelorism, pterygia of neck, axillae, and other joints; genital anomalies; small stature; autosomal recessive

defects in the skull, spine, CNS, or other organs. These deformities may be present without clinical symptoms, but symptoms may appear because of mechanical compression of the neuraxis or as the result of an associated malformation of the nervous system.

Basilar Impression

Platybasia, basilar impression, and basilar invagination are names frequently used interchangeably for the skeletal malformation in which the base of the skull is flattened on the cervical spine. *Platybasia* (i.e., flat-base skull) is present if the angle formed by a line connecting the nasion, tuberculum sella, and anterior margin of the foramen magnum is greater than 143° (Fig. 79.2).

Basilar invagination refers to an upward indentation of the base of the skull, which may be present in Paget disease, osteomalacia, or other forms of bone disease associated with softening of the bones of the skull. An upward displacement of the occipital bone and cervical spine, with protrusion of the odontoid process into the foramen magnum, constitutes *basilar impression*. Compression of the

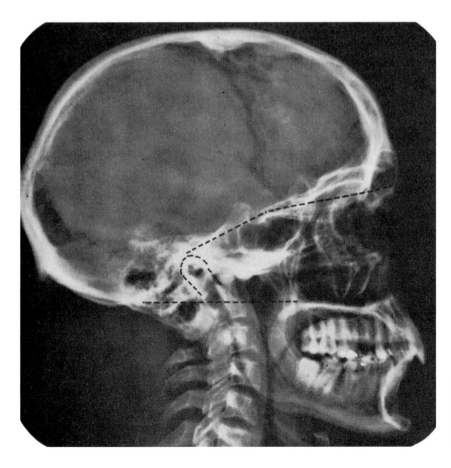

FIGURE 79.2. Basilar impression with platybasia. The odontoid process is entirely above Chamberlain's line (hard palate to base of skull). Basal angle is flat. (Courtesy of Dr. Juan Taveras.)

pons, medulla, cerebellum, and cervical cord, and stretching of the cranial nerves, may result from the upward ascent of the occipital bone and cervical spine, and from narrowing of the foramen magnum.

Pathology and Pathogenesis

Minor degrees of platybasia and basilar invagination may not produce symptoms. In most symptomatic cases, the deformity is caused by a congenital maldevelopment or hypoplasia of the basiocciput, which causes basilar impression, platybasia, partial- or complete-atlantooccipital fusion, atlantoaxial dislocation, and a narrowed foramen magnum. The pons, medulla, and cerebellum may be distorted and the cranial nerves stretched. Vertebral artery obstruction may be significant in the production of brainstem symptoms (e.g., vertigo and drop attacks with head turning) in basilar impression.

Symptoms and Signs

Basilar impression is rare. Neurologic symptoms, when present, usually develop in childhood or early adult life. The head may appear to be elongated and its vertical diameter reduced. The neck appears shortened, and its movements may be limited by anomalies of the upper cervical vertebrae. Neurologic symptoms include spastic paraparesis, unsteady gait, cerebellar ataxia, nystagmus, and paralyses of the lower cranial nerves. Papilledema and signs of increased pressure may occur if the deformity interferes with the circulation of the CSF. Partial- or complete-subarachnoid block is present at lumbar puncture, in most cases. CSF protein levels are increased in 50% of patients.

Diagnosis

The diagnosis of basilar impression is usually obvious from the general appearance of the patient. It may be established, with certainty, by the characteristic radiographic or CT appearance of the base of the skull. The clinical syndromes produced by the anomaly may simulate those of multiple sclerosis, syringomyelia, the Arnold-Chiari malformation, and posterior-fossa tumors. These diagnoses are readily excluded on CT and MRI.

Treatment

The treatment is surgical decompression of the posterior fossa and the upper cervical cord.

Malformations of the Atlas and Axis

Maldevelopments of the atlas and axis may be found with basilar impression or may occur independently. Congenital defects resulting in weakness, or absence of the structures maintaining stability of the atlantoaxial joints, predispose to subluxation and dislocation. These include dens aplasia, a condition in which part of the odontoid process remains on the body of the second cervical vertebra, thereby reducing the stability of the joint.

Neurologic symptoms may be produced by anterior dislocation of the atlas and compression of the cord, between the protruding odontoid process and the posterior rim of the foramen magnum. There may be mild or severe spastic quadriparesis, with or without evidence of damage to the lower cranial nerves. Head movement causes pain. Sensory loss may be mild. Transitory signs or symptoms of a progressive myelopathy may occur, often after exaggerated movements of the neck. Respiratory embarrassment is prominent when the thoracic muscles are affected.

The diagnosis is made by finding anterior dislocation of the atlas in CT. When the bony changes are slight, and especially when there is little or no posterior dislocation of the odontoid process, the symptoms may be caused by other congenital defects, such as syringomyelia or Arnold-Chiari malformation.

Fusion of the Cervical Vertebrae

Fusion of the upper thoracic vertebrae and the entire cervical spine into a single, bony mass was reported by Klippel and Feil in 1912. Since that time, numerous cases have been reported with variations of this deformity. In most, the abnormality consists of the fusion of the cervical vertebrae into one or more separate masses (Fig. 79.3). This vertebral fusion is the result of maldevelopment *in utero*, and there is evidence of both autosomal-dominant and autosomal-recessive transmission. This anomaly is associated with a short neck, low hairline, and limitation of neck movement, especially in the lateral direction. Fusion of the vertebrae is not, in itself, of any great clinical importance except for the resulting deformity in the appearance of the neck.

Clinical symptoms are usually caused by the presence of syringomyelia or other developmental defects of the spinal cord, brain stem, or cerebellum. Congenital cardiovascular defects have been reported in 4% of cases and genitourinary anomalies in 2% of patients. Congenital deafness arising from faulty development of the osseous inner ear was estimated to occur in up to 30% of patients. More frequently, there may be fusion of only two adjacent cervical vertebrae causing only accentuation of symptoms in the presence of cervical osteoarthritis.

PREMATURE CLOSURE OF CRANIAL SUTURES

Craniosynostosis or premature closure of cranial sutures occurs in childhood if cerebral growth is impaired. This is commonly manifested by a uniform closure of all

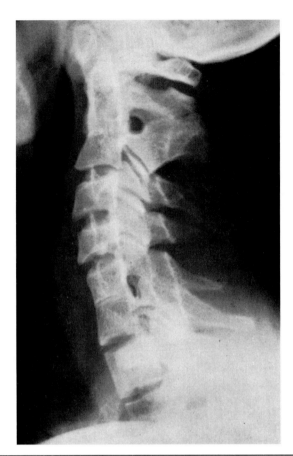

FIGURE 79.3. Fusion of cervical vertebrae (Klippel-Feil syndrome).

sutures and microcephaly. True microcephaly is defined by a head circumference less than 3 standard deviations below the mean for age and sex. Rarely, early closure of the sutures may occur as a consequence of metabolic diseases, including rickets and hyperthyroidism.

Craniosynostosis is usually a primary congenital disturbance of skull growth with no neurologic disorder. The frequency is about 1 in 1,900 births. In 10% to 20%, there is a mendelian inheritance. Sixty-four mutations of six genes have been described in craniosynostosis syndromes commonly associated with limb malformations. Accompanying facial and other tissue deformities also may be seen in recognized syndromes (Table 79.4).

In essence, the skull deformity in primary craniosynostosis reflects the inhibition of growth perpendicular to the closed suture, with compensatory overgrowth in directions perpendicular to the unaffected sutures. Closure of a single suture is most common. Sagittal suture closure alone, seen in 55% of all patients with craniosynostosis, is clinically identified by a child with an oblong-shaped skull (*dolichocephalic* or *scaphocephalic*), often with visible ridging of the closed suture (Fig. 79.4).

Unilateral closure of the coronal suture is seen in about 24% of all patients, appearing as a misshapen and unilat-

erally flattened head (plagiocephaly). Metopic suture closure occurs in about 5% of all craniosynostosis patients, with a prominent midforehead brow appearance (*trigonocephaly*).

Single suture closure does not lead to compression of intracranial tissues. Multiple suture closure occurs commonly with other skull and facial defects and may lead to increased intracranial pressure because of interference with intracranial CSF flow. The optic and acoustic nerves may be compressed, especially in infants with bilateral coronal suture closure (about 9% of all patients with craniosynostosis). These infants have a broad biparietal diameter skull (*brachycephaly*). Rarer forms of multiple suture disorder include some infants with closure of all sutures, resulting in a tower-shaped skull (oxycephaly) or a grossly distorted skull with an asymmetric, often bizarre cloverleaf shape (*Kleeblattschädel*).

Early diagnosis of primary craniosynostosis is essential because the best cosmetic results from surgery are accomplished before the infant is 3 months old. The longer the delay, the greater the compensatory deformity in other areas of the skull and the more complex the surgery. Three-dimensional CT identifies the overall craniofacial contours and guides the surgical procedures needed for the complicated deformities of infants with more than one closed suture. In these infants, the cosmetic benefits are less important than prevention of intracranial hypertension and cranial nerve compression.

Craniectomy to open up closed sutures is of no value in infants with craniostenosis and microcephaly in whom the injured brain has not grown adequately.

SPINA BIFIDA AND CRANIUM BIFIDUM

Both environmental factors and genetics may produce structural malformations of the developing nervous system. Moreover, the damaged fetal brain may be more vulnerable to hypoxic perinatal insults. Teratogenetic factors including certain anticonvulsants probably cause malformations in 1 of every 400 births; genetic factors account for about a third of the malformations, and the cause is unknown in more than 50%.

Pathogenesis and Diagnosis

The neural tube begins to fuse on about day 27 and closes about day 28 of gestation. The primordium of the vertebrae forms from the mesoderm that, similar to the adjacent developing ectoderm, separates from the neural tube. Failure of closure of the neural tube and associated primitive mesodermal and ectodermal elements accounts for the appearance of congenital midline defects, termed dysraphism (Table 79.5).

▶ TABLE 79.4 Syndromes Associated with Craniosynostosis

Syndromes	Characteristics
Apert (acrocephalosyndactyly) (Fig. 79.4)	Coronal suture closure, shallow orbits, hypertelorism, small nose, maxillary hypoplasia, narrow and occasional cleft palate; syndactyly and other skeletal deformities; occasional cardiac, gastrointestinal, and genitourinary malformations; autosomal dominant; mental deficiency often seen
Carpenter	Synostosis of coronal and often sagittal and lambdoid sutures, shallow supraorbital ridges, laterally displaced inner canthi; brachydactyly and other skeletal deformities; hypogenitalism, obesity; occasional cardiac and renal malformations; neurosensory and conductive hearing loss; probably autosomal recessive; may be mentally deficient
Crouzon (craniofacial dysostosis)	Coronal, lambdoid, and sagittal suture closure of variable degree, ocular proptosis and shallow orbits, hypertelorism, conductive hearing loss; autosomal dominant; may be mentally deficient and have agenesis of corpus callosum, optic atrophy, and seizures
Saethre-Chotzen	Coronal suture closure, maxillary hypoplasia, shallow orbits, hypertelorism, ptosis, small ears; cutaneous syndactyly and other skeletal deformities; short stature; may have renal and cardiac abnormalities; autosomal dominant; mental deficiency may be seen
Pfeiffer	Coronal and perhaps sagittal suture closure with hypertelorism, narrow maxilla. Broad distal phalanges, thumb, and hallux; other skeletal deformities including Arnold-Chiari malformation. Autosomal dominant
Autley-Bixler	Multiple suture closure, brachycephaly with midfacial hypoplasia, proptosis choanal stenosis, dysplastic ears; arachnodactyly, joint contractures, and other skeletal deformities; may have genitourinary anomalies, multiple hemangiomas; probable autosomal recessive
Baller-Gerold	One or more suture synostosis (usually metopic), radial hypoplasia, and other preaxial limb anomalies; other skeletal, genitourinary, and cardiac deformities; anal malformation; autosomal recessive; mental deficiency
Chromosome (9p monosomy)	Metopic suture closure, midfacial hypoplasia, poorly formed ears; long mid-phalanges of fingers with extra flexion creases, short distal phalanges with short nails; other skeletal anomalies, cardiac and genitourinary defects; deletion of distal portion of short arm chromosome 9

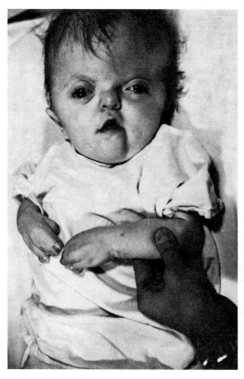 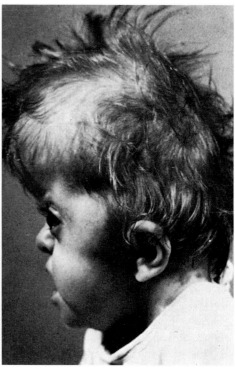

FIGURE 79.4. **Acrocephalosyndactyly (Apert syndrome).** Head is shortened in anteroposterior dimension, forehead is prominent, and occiput flat. Typical facies showing shallow orbits and proptosis of eyes, downward slanting palpebral fissures, small nose, and low-set ears. Osseous and cutaneous syndactyly of hands and feet.

▶ TABLE 79.5 Neural Tube Closure Malformations

Malformation	Characteristics
Anencephaly	Absence of brain with associated defects in skull, meninges, and scalp; minimal hind brain structures may present. Frequency 1:1,000 deliveries
Iniencephaly	Retroflexed head with defects of cervical spine; often combined with anencephaly or encephaloceles
Craniorachischisis	Brain and spinal cord necrosis secondary to exposure to amniotic fluid
Cephalocele	Partial brain protrusion through skull defect (cranium bifidum) with variable covering of meninges and skin; common in occipital region but may be parietal or anterior skull
Meningocele	Skull or spine defect associated with meningeal protrusion
Dermal sinus tract	Incomplete separation of neural and epithelial ectoderm; may be associated with dermoid; marked external skin and hair changes; point of entry for bacteria with subsequent meningitis
Spina bifida	Varying degree of vertebral abnormality
Spina bifida occulta	Vertebral arch defect only. Up to 24% of population
Spina bifida cystica	Dura and arachnoid herniation through vertebral defect
Myelomeningocele	Herniation of spinal cord and meninges through defect

Severe malformations may be detected *in utero* by ultrasonography and by finding elevated maternal serum levels of alpha-fetoprotein (AFP). AFP is the major circulating protein of early fetal life, synthesized in the fetal liver and yolk sac. Peak levels are found about 16 weeks after the last menstrual period, making that the optimum time for testing. The exposed fetal membranes and blood vessel surfaces increase the AFP levels in both maternal serum and amniotic fluid if there is an open neural tube.

If results are ambiguous or in circumstances in which there is increased risk of a defect because of genetic factors, measurement of AFP and acetylcholinesterase by amniocentesis is warranted. Measurement of amniotic acetylcholinesterase activity helps to detect an open dysraphic state *in utero* because amniotic AFP levels may be high in gastroschisis, omphalocele, and nephrosis. Increased levels of amniotic AFP and acetylcholinesterase detect at least 90% of open spina bifida fetuses and almost all of the anencephalics, whereas maternal serum AFP levels detect 60% to 80% of open spina bifida fetuses and 90% of the anencephalics.

The use of folic acid or vitamin supplements containing folic acid during the periconceptional period significantly decreases the risk of neural tube closure defects in the offspring. The risk of another child born with a neural tube defect in a family with two unaffected parents is 3% to 5%. Although familial clustering of neural tube defects has been identified, the pattern best fits a polygenic model of inheritance.

The simplest defect, *spina bifida occulta*, is characterized by a lack of vertebral arch closure without any other associated defect. It is usually localized to L5-S1 and does not seem to have an increased risk of neural tube closure malformations in that individual's progeny. This is in contrast to anencephaly and other forms of spina bifida in which there is a close genetic relationship and in which the recurrence risk is equally distributed.

Many severely affected fetuses are spontaneously aborted. Associated anomalies of other organ systems include congenital heart disorders, diaphragmatic defects, and esophageal atresia. Other central nervous system anomalies are common but may not be clinically apparent in the newborn infant with neural tube closure defect. Abnormalities of the basal ganglia, hippocampi, commissural pathways, brainstem, and cerebellum may be seen in infants born with occipital encephaloceles. Ventricular wall deformities, corpus callosum defects, and hydrocephalus may be noted with parietal encephaloceles. Basal ganglia and commissural anomalies may be seen with anterior encephaloceles that are most common in the frontoethmoidal junction.

Spina bifida deformities commonly include other nervous system abnormalities: tethering of the cord (Fig. 79.5), diastematomyelia, hydromyelia, and hydrocephalus usually associated with Arnold-Chiari type II malformation.

Occult spinal dysraphic states reflect other defects of ectodermal and mesodermal origin, including pelvic meningoceles, hamartomas, lipomas, and dermoid tumors, and may be suspected if there are skin markers: skin tags, hair tufts, abnormal dimpling, or aplasia cutis congenita.

The congenital syndromes associated with defects of neural tube closure include the *Meckel-Gruber syndrome* (posterior encephalocele, microcephaly, cerebral and cerebellar hypoplasia, and associated defects of face, neck, limbs, kidney, liver, and genitalia) and the *Walker-Warburg syndrome* (occipital encephalocele, Dandy-Walker cyst, hydrocephalus, cerebellar hypoplasia, and eye defects).

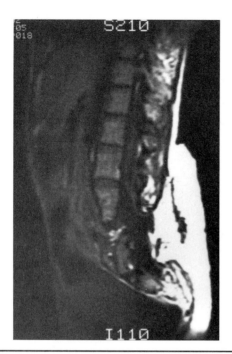

FIGURE 79.5. Lumbosacral myelomeningocele. Sagittal MRI shows spinal dysraphism and tethered cord.

Treatment

MRI of the brain and spine has enhanced an understanding of the extent of the primary defect and the associated anomalies. MRI also guides treatment. Neurologic evaluation defines the level of function by evaluating anal reaction and sensory, reflex, and motor functions.

Surgical excision of the meningocele and the encephalocele must include meticulous protection of the neural elements underlying and sometimes adherent to the tissue to be excised. Post-excision assessment is vital to detect complications or the emergence of secondary or associated abnormalities (e.g., hydrocephalus after closure of a spinal meningocele or tethering of the spinal cord). Orthopedic and urologic approaches are essential for maximizing functional ability and preventing skin, bone, and renal problems. Concomitant or resultant bone and joint changes include the Klippel-Feil syndrome, foot deformities, scoliosis, and hip dysplasia, which may point to an associated disorder, such as cord tethering, hydromyelia, adhesive arachnoiditis, or a lipoma.

In a series of 286 patients who had surgical closure of a spinal defect within 48 hours of birth, 42% had a thoracic defect and 58% had a lumbar or sacral defect. With an average age at follow-up of 61.4 months, 11% had lost quadriceps function between birth and the most recent examination. This was attributed to the development of a tethered cord. Only 24% of the thoracic-level patients could walk, whereas 92% of the lumbosacral-level patients did

so. Prevalence of quadriceps function was critical. Ninety-three percent of all patients had shunts placed for the treatment of clinically overt hydrocephalus; 74% had more than one shunt.

Psychologic development depends on the extent of cerebral pathology stemming from associated congenital defects or the sequelae of an open spina bifida such as neonatal meningitis, hydrocephalus, and shunting plus the emotional impact of the multiplicity of treatment regimens.

ARNOLD-CHIARI MALFORMATION

A congenital anomaly of the hindbrain characterized by a downward elongation of the brainstem and cerebellum into the cervical portion of the spinal cord was originally described by Arnold in 1894 and Chiari in 1895.

Pathology

Because of its common association with spina bifida occulta or the presence of a meningocele or meningomyelocele in the lumbosacral region, the downward displacement of the brainstem and cerebellum was attributed to fixation of the cord at the site of the spinal defect early in fetal life. This hypothesis is not applicable to the many cases in which there is no defect in the lower spine, and the theory fails to account for the other anomalies commonly associated with the hindbrain malformation (e.g., absence of the septum pellucidum, fusion of the thalami, hypoplasia of the falx cerebri, fusion of the corporea quadrigemina and microgyri). Some type of developmental arrest and overgrowth of the neural tube in embryonic life is a more plausible explanation of the anomaly.

The gross description of the abnormality has been remarkably similar in all the reported cases. The inferior poles of the cerebellar hemispheres extend downward through the foramen magnum in two tonguelike processes and are often adherent to the adjacent medulla; more than half is usually below the level of the foramen magnum (Fig. 79.6). The medulla is elongated and flattened anteroposteriorly, and the lower cranial nerves are stretched.

Chiari I malformation identifies the intracranial anomaly whereas Chiari II includes the spinal changes as well. The posterior fossa is smaller than normal, adhesions may be prominent with accompanying crowding of normal structures.

Incidence

The Arnold-Chiari malformation is not as rare as would be expected from the small number of reported cases. Ingraham and Swan found 20 instances of this

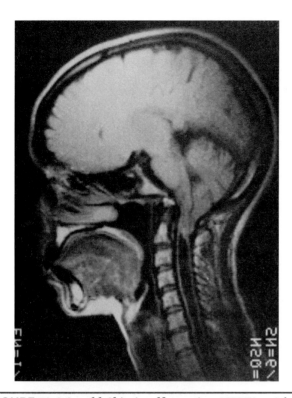

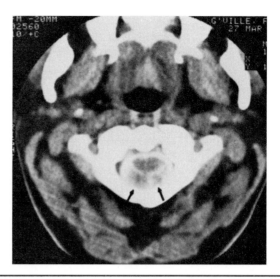

FIGURE 79.7. Arnold-Chiari malformation. Postmyelography CT. At level of odontoid in high cervical region, spinal cord is flattened by cerebellar tonsils (*arrows*). (Courtesy of Drs. S. K. Hilal and M. Mawad.)

FIGURE 79.6. Arnold-Chiari malformation. MRI T1-weighted image of midsagittal section of brain and cervical cord. Note small and elongated fourth ventricle, low position of obex of fourth ventricle below plane of foramen magnum, cerebellar-tonsillar ectopia, short clivus, wide foramen magnum, kinked cervical-medullary junction, and prominent superior vermis. Large hydromyelia in cervical cord.

abnormality among 290 patients with myelomeningoceles. The defect is almost always, but not invariably, associated with a meningomyelocele or spina bifida occulta in the lumbosacral region. Hydrocephalus is present in most cases. Other associated defects of development include rounded defects in the bones of the skull (craniolacunia, Lückenschädel), defects in the spinal cord (hydromyelia, syringomyelia, double cord), and defects in the spinal column (basilar impression).

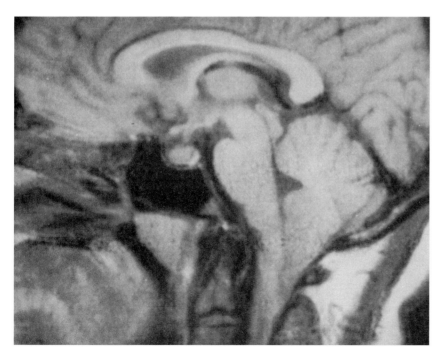

FIGURE 79.8. Type I Arnold-Chiari malformation. Sagittal T1-weighted scan shows tonsillar herniation through foramen magnum. Fourth ventricle is of normal size and position, as are aqueduct and brain stem. There is no hydrocephalus. (Courtesy of Drs. J. A. Bello and S. K. Hilal.)

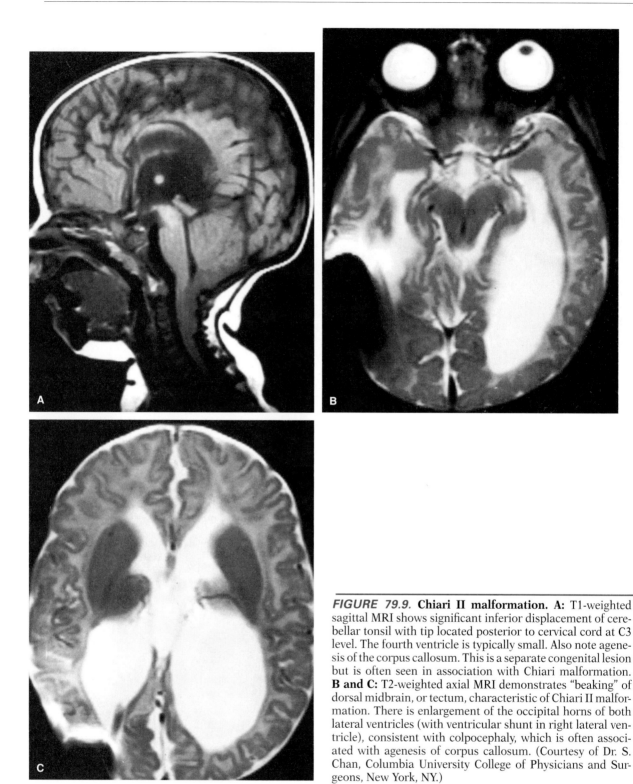

FIGURE 79.9. Chiari II malformation. A: T1-weighted sagittal MRI shows significant inferior displacement of cerebellar tonsil with tip located posterior to cervical cord at C3 level. The fourth ventricle is typically small. Also note agenesis of the corpus callosum. This is a separate congenital lesion but is often seen in association with Chiari malformation. **B and C:** T2-weighted axial MRI demonstrates "beaking" of dorsal midbrain, or tectum, characteristic of Chiari II malformation. There is enlargement of the occipital horns of both lateral ventricles (with ventricular shunt in right lateral ventricle), consistent with colpocephaly, which is often associated with agenesis of corpus callosum. (Courtesy of Dr. S. Chan, Columbia University College of Physicians and Surgeons, New York, NY.)

Symptoms and Signs

The neurologic signs and symptoms of the Arnold-Chiari malformation that appear in the first few months of life are usually prompted by hydrocephalus and other developmental defects in the nervous system. The prognosis is poor in these cases. The onset of symptoms may be delayed until adult life. There may be signs and symptoms of injury to the cerebellum, medulla, and the lower cranial nerves, with or without evidence

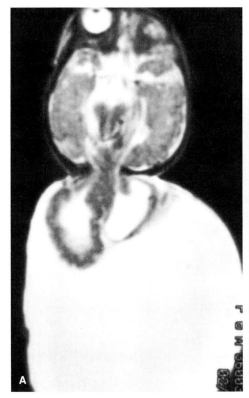
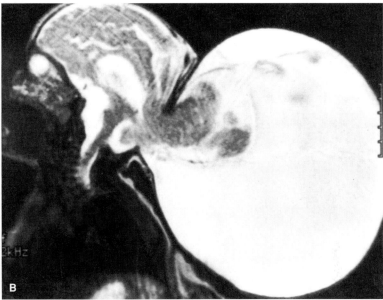

FIGURE 79.10. Encephalocele with Chiari III malformation. A and B: T2-weighted sagittal and axial MRIs demonstrate a huge fluid-filled sac external to the skull posteriorly, with patent communication to intracranial structures. There is herniation of both cerebellar hemispheres into the extruded cerebrospinal fluid-filled sac, most consistent with occipital encephalocele. Distortion of the brain stem and absence of the corpus callosum are also apparent. (Courtesy of Dr. S. Chan, Columbia University College of Physicians and Surgeons, New York, NY.)

of increased intracranial pressure. Progressive ataxia, leg weakness, and visual complaints are characteristic. Oscillopsia at rest and visual blurring of fixated targets are described. Downbeat nystagmus and seesaw nystagmus may be noted in lesions of the cervicomedullary region. About one-third of patients with descent of cerebellar tonsils noted on cranial MRI are asymptomatic.

Diagnosis

The presence of an Arnold-Chiari malformation is probable when there is a coincidence of meningomyelocele, hydrocephalus, and craniolacunia in infancy. The diagnosis in adults should be considered whenever there are signs and symptoms of damage to the cerebellum, medulla, and lower cranial nerves. The signs and symptoms of the Arnold-Chiari malformation in adults may simulate the syndromes produced by tumors of the posterior fossa, multiple sclerosis, syringomyelia, or basilar impression. The diagnosis may be established by CT (Fig. 79.7) and MRI (Figs. 79.8, 79.9, and 79.10).

Treatment

Treatment of the malformation, in infants, includes excision of the sac in the spinal region and a ventriculoperitoneal shunt to relieve the hydrocephalus. Early hind-brain decompression is needed in symptomatic neonates with vocal-cord paralysis. In adults, the posterior fossa should be decompressed. The best results are obtained when there are few neurologic symptoms caused by the spinal defect or other congenital anomalies.

SUGGESTED READINGS

Agenesis of the Corpus Callosum

Barkovich AJ, Kuzniecky RI, Jackson GD, et al. Classification system for malformations of cortical development. *Neurology* 2001;57:2168–2178.

Berg MJ, Sohifitto G, Powers JM, et al. X-linked female band heterotropia-male lissencephaly syndrome. *Neurology* 1998;50:1143–1146.

Bertoni JM, von Loh S, Allen RJ. The Aicardi syndrome: report of 4 cases and review of the literature. *Ann Neurol* 1979;5:475–482.

Dobyns WB. Agenesis of the corpus callosum and gyral malformations are frequent manifestations of nonketotic hyperglycinemia. *Neurology* 1989;39:817–820.

Dobyns WB, Truwit CL. Lissencephaly and other malformations of cortical development. *Neuropediatrics* 1995;26:132–147.

Faye-Peterson OM, Ward K, Carey JC, Kinsley AS. Osteochondrodysplasia with rhizomelia, platyspondyly, callosal agenesis, thrombocytopenia, hydrocephalus and hypertension. *Am J Med Genet* 1991;40:183–187.

Guala A, Dellavecchia C, Mannarino S. Ring chromosome 13 with loss of the region D13S317-D13S285: phenotypic overlap with XK syndrome. *Am J Med Genet* 1997;72:319–323.

Haltia M, Leivo I, Samer H, et al. Muscle-eye-brain disease: a neuropathological study. *Ann Neurol* 1997;41:173–180.

Harding BN. Malformation of the nervous system. In: Adams JH, Duchen LW, eds. *Greenfield's Neuropathology*, 5th ed. New York: Oxford University Press, 1992.

Jeret JS, Serur D, Wisniewski KE, et al. Clinicopathological findings associated with agenesis of the corpus callosum. *Brain Dev* 1987;9:255–264.

Jones KL. *Smith's Recognizable Patterns of Human Malformation*, 4th ed. Philadelphia: WB Saunders, 1988.

Koening R, Bach A, Woelki U, et al. Spectrum of the acrocallosal syndrome. *Am J Med Genet* 2002;108(1):7–11.

Loeser JD, Alvord EC. Agenesis of the corpus callosum. *Brain* 1968;91:553–570.

Pavlakis, SG, Frissora, CL, Giampietro PF, et al. Fanconi anemia, a model for genetic causes of abnormal brain development. *Dev Med Child Neurol* 1992;34:1081–1084.

Richards LJ, Plachez C, Ren T. Mechanisms regulating the development of the corpus callosum and its agenesis in mouse and human. *Clin Genet* 2004 Oct;66(4):276–289.

Rosser, T. Aicardi Syndrome. *Arch Neurol* 2003;60:1471–1473.

Saito Y, Kobayashi M, Itoh M, et al. Aberrant neuronal migration in the brainstem of Fukuyama-Type congenital Muscular Dystrophy, *J Neuropath Experimental Neuro* 2003;62:497–508.

Sarnat H. Molecular genetic classification of central nervous system malformations. *J Child Neurol* 2000;15:675–687.

Sicca F, Kelemen A, Genton P, et al. Mosaic mutations of the LIS1 gene cause subcortical band heterotopia. *Neurology* 2003;61:1042–1046.

Soto-Ares G, Devisme L, Jorriot S, et al. Neuropathologic and MR imaging correlation in a neonatal case of cerebellar cortical dysplasia. *Am J Neuroradiol* 2002;23:1101–1104.

Uyanik G, Aigner L, Martin P, et al. ARX mutations in X-linked lissencephaly with abnormal genitalia. *Neurology* 2003;61:232–235.

Verlinsky Y, Rechitsky S, Verlinsky O, et al. Preimplantation diagnosis for sonic hedgehog mutation causing familial holoprosencephaly. *N Engl J Med* 2003;348:1449–1454.

Macrocephaly and Megalencephaly

DeMeyer W. Megalencephaly: types, clinical syndromes, and management. *Pediatr Neurol* 1986;2:321–328.

Dionisi-Vici C, Ruitenbeek W, Fariello G, et al. New familial mitochondrial encephalopathy with macrocephaly, cardiomyopathy, and complex I deficiency. *Ann Neurol* 1997;42:661–665.

Elson E, Perveen R, Donnai, et al. De novo GL13 mutation in acrocallosal syndrome: broadening the phenotypic spectrum of GL13 defects and overlap with murine models. *J Med Genet* 2002;39:804–806.

Fusco L, Ferracuti S, Fariello G, et al. Hemimegalencephaly and normal intellectual development. *J Neurol Neurosurg Psychiatry* 1992;55:720–722.

Gontieres F, Boulloche J, Bourgeois M, Aicardi J. Leucoencephalopathy, megalencephaly, and mild clinical course. A recently individualized familial leucodystrophy. *J Child Neurol* 1996;11:439–444.

Harding BN. Malformation of the nervous system. In: Adams JH, Duchen LW, eds. *Greenfield's Neuropathology*, 5th ed. New York: Oxford University Press, 1992.

Lapunzina P, Gairi A, Delicado A, Mori MA, Torres ML, Goma A, Navia M, Pajares IL. Macrocephaly-cutis marmorata telangiectatica congenita: report of six new patients and a review. *Am J Med Genet A* 2004 Sep 15;130(1):45–51. Review

Laubscher B, Deonna T, Uske A, et al. Primitive megalencephaly in children: natural history, medium term prognosis with special reference to external hydrocephalus. *Eur J Pediatr* 1990;149:502–507.

Padberg GW, Schot JD, Vielvoye GJ, et al. L'hermitte-Duclos disease and Cowden disease: a single phakomatosis. *Ann Neurol* 1991;29:517–523.

Patrono C, Di Giacinto G, Eymard-Pierre E, et al. Genetic heterogeneity of megalencephalic leukoencephalopathy and subcortical cysts. *Neurology* 2003;61:534–537.

Saijo H, Nakayama H, Ezoe T, et al. A case of megalencephalic leukoencephalopathy with subcortical cysts (van der Knaap disease): molecular genetic study. *Brain Dev* 2003;25:362–366.

Suara RO, Trouth AJ, Collins M. Benign subarachnoid space enlargement of infancy. *J Natl Med Assoc* 2001;93:70–73.

Malformations of Occipital Bone and Cervical Spine

DeBarros MC, Farias W, Ataide L, et al. Basilar impression and Arnold-Chiari malformation. *J Neurol Neurosurg Psychiatry* 1968;31:596–605.

Dehaene I, Pattyn G, Calliauw L. Megadolicho-basilar anomaly, basilar impression and occipitovertebral anastomosis. *Clin Neurol Neurosurg* 1975;78:131–138.

Dunsker SB, Brown O, Thomson N. Craniovertebral anomalies. *Clin Neurosurg* 1980;27:430–439.

Gunderson CH, Greenspan RH, Glaser GH. The Klippel-Feil syndrome: genetic and clinical reevaluation of cervical fusion. *Medicine (Baltimore)* 1967;46:491–512.

Janeway R, Toole JF, Leinbach LB, et al. Vertebral artery obstruction with basilar impression. *Arch Neurol* 1966;15:211–214.

Jones KL. *Smith's Recognizable Patterns of Human Malformations*, 4th ed. Philadelphia: WB Saunders, 1988.

Kaplan JG, Rosenberg RS, DeSouza T, et al. Atlantoaxial subluxation in psoriatic arthropathy. *Ann Neurol* 1988;23:522–524.

Norot JC, Stauffer ES. Sequelae of atlanto-axial stabilization in two patients with Down's syndrome. *Spine* 1981;6:437–440.

Sakai M, Shinkawa A, Miyake H, et al. Klippel-Feil syndrome with conductive deafness: histological findings of removed stapes. *Ann Otol Rhinol Laryngol* 1983;92:202–206.

Stevens JM, Chong WK, Barber C, Kendall BE, Cockard HA. A new appraisal of abnormalities of the odontoid process associated with atlanto-axial subluxation and neurological disability. *Brain* 1994;117:133–148.

Vangilder JC, Menezes AH, Dlan KD. *The Craniovertebral Junction and Its Abnormalities.* Mt. Kisco, NY: Futura Publishing Co, 1987.

Premature Closure of Cranial Sutures

Carmel PW, Luken MG III, Ascherl GF. Craniosynostosis: computed tomographic evaluation of skull base and calvarial deformities and associated intracranial changes. *Neurosurgery* 1981;9:366–372.

Cohen MM. Merging the old skeletal biology with the new. II. Molecular aspects of bone formation and bone growth. *J Craniofac Genet Develop Biol* 2000;20:94–106.

Cohen MM. Craniosynostosis and syndromes with craniosynostosis: incidence, genetics, penetrance, variability, and new syndrome updating. *Birth Defects* 1979;15:13–63.

Crouzon Q. Dysostose cranio-faciale hereditaire. *Bull Mem Soc Med Hop Paris* 1912;33:545.

Gorlin RJ, Cohen MM Jr, Levin LS. *Syndromes of the Head and Neck*, 3rd ed. New York: Oxford University Press, 1990.

Gripp KW, McDonald-McGinn DM, Gaudenz K, et al. Identification of a genetic cause for isolated unilateral coronal synostosis: a unique mutation in the fibroblast growth factor receptor 3. *J Pediatr* 1998;132:714–716.

Hoffman HS, Epstein F. *Disorders of the Developing Nervous System: Diagnosis and Treatment.* Boston: Blackwell Scientific Publications, 1986.

Jones KL. *Smith's Recognizable Patterns of Human Malformation*, 4th ed. Philadelphia: WB Saunders, 1988.

Pellegrino JE, McDonald-McGinn DM, Schneider A. Further clinical delineation and increased morbidity in males with osteopathia striata with cranial sclerosis: an x-linked disorder? *Am J Med Genet* 1997;70:159–165.

Shillito J Jr. A plea for early operation for craniostenosis. *Surg Neurol* 1992;37:182–188.

Wilkie AOM. Craniosynostosis: genes and mechanisms. *Hum Mol Genet* 1997;6:1647–1656.

Zhang XL, Kuroda S, Carpenter D, et al. Craniosynostosis in transgenic mice over expressing Nell-1. *J Clin Invest* 2003;110:861–870.

Spina Bifida and Cranium Bifidum

Czeizel AE, Duda I. Prevention of the first occurrence of neural tube defects by periconceptional vitamin supplementation. *N Engl J Med* 1992;327:1832–1835.

Gorlin RJ, Cohen MM Jr, Levin LS. *Syndromes of the head and neck,* 3rd ed. New York: Oxford University Press, 1990.

Harding BN. Malformation of the nervous system. In: Adams JH, Duchen LW, eds. *Greenfield's Neuropathology,* 5th ed. New York: Oxford University Press, 1992.

Harper PS. *Practical Genetic Counseling,* 3rd ed. London: Wright, 1988.

Hoffman HS, Epstein F. *Disorders of the Developing Nervous System: Diagnosis and Treatment.* Boston: Blackwell Scientific Publications, 1986.

Kawamura T, Morioka T, Nishio S, et al. Cerebral abnormalities in lumbosacral neural tube closure defect: MR imaging evaluation. *Childs Nerv Syst* 2001;17:405–410.

Mitchell LE, Adzick NS, Melchionne J, Pasquariello PS, Sutton LN, Whitehead AS. Spina bifida. *Lancet* 2004 Nov 20;364(9448):1885–1895.

Patterson RS, Egelhoff JC, Crone KR, et al. Atretic parietal cephaloceles revisited: an enlarging clinical and imaging spectrum. *Am J Neuroradiol* 1998;19:791–795.

Robert E, Guiband P. Maternal valproic acid and congenital neural tube defects. *Lancet* 1982;2:934.

Salonen R. The Meckel syndrome: clinicopathological findings in 67 patients. *Am J Med Genet* 1984;18:671–689.

Schijman E. Split spinal cord malformations: report of 22 cases and review of the literature. *Childs Nerv Syst* 2003;19:104–105.

Arnold-Chiari Malformation

Arnett B. Arnold Chiari Malformation. *Arch Neurol* 2003;60:898–900.

Arnold J. Myelocyste. Transposition von Gewebskeimen und Sympodie. *Beitr Pathol Anat* 1894;16:1–28.

Balagura S, Kuo DC. Spontaneous retraction of cerebellar tonsils after surgery for Arnold-Chiari malformation and posterior fossa cyst. *Surg Neurol* 1988;29:137–140.

Banerji NK, Millar JHD. Chiari malformation presenting in adult life. Its relationship to syringomyelia. *Brain* 1974;97:157–168.

Brill CB, Gutierrez J, Mishkin MM. Chiari I malformation: association with seizures and developmental disabilities. *J Child Neurol* 1997;12:101–106.

Caviness VS Jr. The Chiari malformations of the posterior fossa and their relation to hydrocephalus. *Dev Med Child Neurol* 1976;18:103–116.

Chiari H. Adüber Vererungen des Kleinhirns, des Pons und der Medulla oblongata in Folge von congenitaler Hydrocephalie des Grosshirns. *Denkschr Akad Wiss Wien* 1896;63:71–116.

DeBarros MC, Farias W, Ataide L, et al. Basilar impression and Arnold-Chiari malformation. *J Neurol Neurosurg Psychiatry* 1968;31:596–605.

Dehaene I, Pattyn G, Calliauw L. Megadolicho-basilar anomaly, basilar impression and occipito-vertebral anastomosis. *Clin Neurol Neurosurg* 1975;78:131–138.

el Gammal T, Mark EK, Brooks BS. MR imaging of Chiari II malformation. *AJR* 1988;150:163–170.

Elster AD, Chen MY. Chiari I malformations: clinical and radiologic reappraisal. *Radiology* 1992;183:347–353.

Gilbert JN, Jones KL, Rorke LB, et al. Central nervous system anomalies associated with meningomyelocele hydrocephalus and the Arnold-Chiari malformation. *Neurosurgery* 1986;18:559–564.

Hershberger ML, Chidekel A. Arnold Chiari malformation type I and sleep-disordered breathing: an uncommon manifestation of an important pediatric problem. *J Pediatr Health Care* 2003;17:190–197.

Kumar A, Patni AH, Charbel F. The Chiari I malformation and the neurotologist. *Otol Neurotol* 2002;23:727–735.

Levy WJ, Mason L, Hahn JF. Chiari malformation presenting in adults: a surgical experience in 127 cases. *Neurosurgery* 1983;12:377–390.

Pollach IF, Dachling P, Albright AL, et al. Outcome following hindbrain decompression of symptomatic Chiari malformations in children previously treated with myelomeningocele closure and shunts. *J Neurosurg* 1992;77:881–888.

Salam MZ, Adams RD. The Arnold-Chiari malformation. In: Vinken P, Bruyn G, eds. *Handbook of Clinical Neurology.* Vol. 32. New York: American Elsevier-North Holland, 1978;99–110.

C h a p t e r 8 0

Marcus Gunn and Möbius Syndromes

Lewis P. Rowland and Marc C. Patterson

MARCUS GUNN SYNDROME

Among the more bizarre and unexplained neurologic phenomena is *jaw winking*. The phenomenon was described by Marcus Gunn in 1863, and there have been many descriptions since then. The patient has congenital and unilateral ptosis. When the mouth is opened, the lid rises and there may even be retraction of the lid. Conversely, when the jaw closes, the lid comes down in a wink. Lateral movements of the jaw may substitute for opening. The patient may raise the lid voluntarily and on upward gaze, but the movements are exaggerated in response to movements of the jaw. There is also an inverted or reversed Marcus Gunn phenomenon. The eye closes when the jaw opens. One case of congenital, inverse Marcus Gunn syndrome with apparent autosomal-dominant transmission has been reported.

How the Marcus Gunn syndrome arises is still not known; it is presumably a congenital error of neuronal wiring in the brain stem. In that respect, it is similar to the Duane retraction syndrome (i.e., retraction of the globe and narrowing of the palpebral fissure on attempted adduction). Another syndrome sometimes seen with the

Marcus Gunn phenomenon and also attributed to neuronal miswiring is *synergistic divergence,* in which there is simultaneous abduction of both eyes on attempted gaze into the field of action of a paretic medial rectus; both eyes abduct on attempted lateral gaze. It is sometimes associated with other congenital anomalies that suggest an anomaly of tissues derived from the neural crest, or there may be restriction of all ocular movements in a pattern suggesting congenital fibrosis of ocular muscles.

The Marcus Gunn syndrome is sometimes an autosomal-dominant familial trait. The risk is increased in infants after a pregnant woman has used misoprostol as an abortifacient. Abnormal brain-stem auditory-evoked responses suggest that the problem is in the brain stem, but the levator muscle of the eyelid may show neurogenic changes, suggesting that the oculomotor nerve is affected. There have not been enough anatomic, imaging, or physiologic studies, however, to come to any conclusion.

The syndrome accounts for about 5% of all cases of congenital ptosis and may be so mild that it is of no functional consequence. The cosmetic distortion, however, has sometimes been sufficient to lead to surgical therapy in the form of operations on the levator or facial muscles.

The Marcus Gunn syndrome should not be confused with the Marcus Gunn pupil, for he also described what is now known as the *afferent-pupillary defect.* Jaw winking is an abnormal *synkinesis,* simultaneous movements effected by muscles innervated by different nerves. Formally, this is a trigeminal-oculomotor synkinesis.

MÖBIUS SYNDROME

The usual definition of this syndrome is the combination of *congenital facial diplegia* and bilateral abducens palsies. Other cranial nerves, however, may be affected, with hearing loss, dysarthria, and dysphagia. Associated conditions include congenital anomalies of limbs or heart, Kallmann syndrome (hypogonadism and anosmia), or mental retardation. A syndrome of brain-stem dysgenesis has been described in Native Americans of Athabascan descent; it is distinguished from the Möbius syndrome by the presence of sensorineural hearing loss, horizontal-gaze palsy, and central hypoventilation. Another syndrome of brain-stem dysgenesis, as yet lacking acronym or eponym, features severe congenital hypotonia, facial diplegia, jaw ankylosis, velo-pharyngeal incoordination, pyramidal-tract signs, and oculomotor apraxia.

Möbius syndrome is often evident in the neonatal period because the children have difficulty sucking, and they lack facial expression when they cry. Vertical gaze and convergence are preserved; there is usually a convergent squint. If facial paralysis is incomplete, as in almost one-half the cases, the syndrome may not be recognized until later in childhood. Then, in contrast to other supranu-

clear or lower motor-neuron causes of facial paralysis, the weakness is more severe in the upper face than below; there is more of a problem with eye closure than in moving the lips. There may be complete ophthalmoplegia, ptosis, lingual hemiatrophy, and in a few cases, mental retardation.

There is probably more than one mechanism in the pathogenesis of the facial paralysis. For instance, physiologic studies have shown cocontraction of the horizontal recti, but other cases have shown evidence of aplasia of ocular muscles or agenesis of motor neurons. In one autopsy, the facial muscles were absent but ocular muscles, nerves, and motor-nerve cells were normal; there were, however, developmental anomalies of the brain stem, which may be evident on CT or MRI. In other autopsies, there was hypoplasia or degeneration of motor nuclei, but in some, no abnormality was seen in the CNS. Loci linked to Möbius syndrome include 13q12.2-q13, 3q21-q22, and 10q21.3-q22, in various inheritance patterns, in different kindreds. Exposure to misoprostol during pregnancy was linked to Möbius syndrome and central hypoventilation in case reports, an association supported by a subsequent case-control study, but not by an underpowered prospective study. Some cases later prove to be caused by facioscapulohumeral muscular dystrophy. Congenital, myotonic muscular dystrophy is another cause of facial diplegia.

Treatment of the syndrome is generally symptomatic and unsatisfactory, but bilateral gracilis-muscle implantation with masseter-nerve innervation has improved speech intelligibility, facial mobility and self esteem in one series of children with Möbius syndrome.

SUGGESTED READINGS

Marcus Gunn Syndrome

Bowyer JD, Sullivan TJ. Management of Marcus Gunn jaw winking synkinesis. *Ophthal Plast Reconstr Surg* 2004 Mar;20(2):92–98.

Brodsky MC, Pollock SC, Buckley EG. Neural misdirection in congenital ocular fibrosis syndrome; implications and pathogenesis. *J Pediatr Ophthalmol Strabis* 1989;26:159–161.

Clausen N, Andersson P, Tommerup N. Familial occurrence of neuroblastoma, von Recklinghausen neurofibromatosis, Hirschsprung's aganglioss and jaw-winking syndrome. *Acta Paediatr Scand* 1989;78:736–741.

Creel DJ, Kivlin JD, Wolfley DE. Auditory brain stem responses in Marcus Gunn ptosis. *Electroencephalogr Clin Neurophysiol* 1984;59:341–344.

Falls HF, Kruse WT, Cotterman CW. Three cases of Marcus Gunn phenomenon in two generations. *Am J Ophthalmol* 1949;32:53–59.

Grant FC. The Marcus Gunn phenomenon. *Arch Neurol Psychiatry* 1936;35:487–500.

Hamed LM, Dennehy PJ, Lingua RW. Synergistic divergence and jaw-winking phenomenon. *J Pediatr Ophthalmol Strabis* 1990;27:88–90.

Lewy FH, Groff RA, Grant FC. Autonomic innervation of the eyelids and the Marcus Gunn phenomenon. *Arch Neurol Psychiatry* 1937;37:1289–1297.

Lyness RW, Collin JR, Alexander RA, Garner A. Histologic appearances of the levator palpebral superioris muscle in the Marcus Gunn phenomenon. *Br J Ophthalmol* 1988;72:104–109.

Meirez F, Standaert L, Delaey JJ, Zeng LH. Waardenberg syndrome, Hirschprung megacolon, and Marcus Gunn ptosis. *Am J Med Genet* 1987;27:683–686.

Oh JY, Kim JE, Kim YJ, Park KD, Choi KG. A case of familial inverse Marcus Gunn phenomenon. *J Neurol Neurosurg Psychiatry.* 2003; 74:278.

Pratt SG, Beyer CK, Johnson CC. The Marcus Gunn phenomenon. A review of 71 cases. *Ophthalmology* 1984;91:27–30.

Möbius Syndrome

Abid F, Hall R, Hudgson P, Weiser R. Möbius syndrome, peripheral neuropathy and hypogonadotrophic hypogonadism. *J Neurol Sci* 1978;35:309–315.

Bavinck JN, Weaver DD. Subclavian artery supply description sequence: hypothesis of a vascular etiology for Poland, Klippel-Feil, and Möbius anomalies. *Am J Med Genet* 1986;23:903–918.

Brackett LE, Demers LM, Mamourian AC, et al. Möbius syndrome in association with hypogonadotropic hypogonadism. *J Endocrinol Invest* 1991;14:599–607.

Goldberg C, DeLorie R, Zuker RM, Manktelow RT. The effects of gracilis muscle transplantation on speech in children with Moebius syndrome. *J Craniofac Surg* 2003;14:687–690.

Hanson PA, Rowland LP. Möbius syndrome and facioscapulohumeral muscular dystrophy. *Arch Neurol* 1971;24:31–39.

Henderson JL. The congenital facial diplegia syndrome. *Brain* 1939;62: 381–403.

Holve S, Friedman B, Hoyme HE, et al. Athabascan brainstem dysgenesis syndrome. *Am J Med Genet* 2003;120A(2):169–173.

Hopper KD, Haas DK, Rice MM, et al. Poland-Möbius syndrome: evaluation by computerized tomography. *South Med J* 1985;78:523–527.

Jennings JE, Costigan C, Reardon W. Moebius sequence and hypogonadotrophic hypogonadism. *Am J Med Genet* 2003;123A(1):107–110.

Kumar D. Möbius syndrome. *J Med Genet* 1990;27:122–126.

Lorenz B. Genetics of isolated and syndromic strabismus: facts and perspectives. *Strabismus* 2002;10:147–156.

Nunes ML, Friedrich MA, Loch LF. Association of misoprostol, Moebius syndrome and congenital central alveolar hypoventilation. Case report. *Arq Neuropsiquiatr* 1999;57:88–91.

Olson WH, Bardin CW, Walsh GO, Engel WK. Möbius syndrome, lower motor neuron involvement and hypogonadotropic hypogonadism. *Neurology* 1970;20:1002–1008.

Pastuszak AL, Schuler L, Speck-Martins CE, et al. Use of misoprostol during pregnancy and Möbius syndrome in infants. *N Engl J Med* 1998;359:1553–1554.

Pitner SE, Edwards JE, McCormick WF. Observations on the pathology of the Möbius syndrome. *J Neurol Neurosurg Psychiatry* 1965;28:362–374.

Roig M, Gratacos M, Vazquez E, et al. Brainstem dysgenesis: report of five patients with congenital hypotonia, multiple cranial nerve involvement, and ocular motor apraxia. *Dev Med Child Neurol* 2003;45:489–493.

Rojas-Martinez A, Garcia-Cruz D, Rodriguez-Garcia A, et al. Poland-Möbius syndrome in a boy and Poland syndrome in his mother. *Clin Genet* 1991;40:225–228.

Rubenstein AE, Lovelace RE, Behrens MM, Weisberg LA. Moebius syndrome in Kallmann syndrome. *Arch Neurol* 1975;32:480–482.

Schuler L, Pastuszak A, Sanseverino TV, et al. Pregnancy outcome after exposure to misoprostol in Brazil: a prospective, controlled study. *Reprod Toxicol* 1999;13:147–151.

Slee JJ, Smart RD, Viljoen DL. Deletion of chromosome 13 in Möbius syndrome. *J Med Genet* 1991;28:413–414.

Towfighi J, Marks K, Palmer E, Vanucci R. Möbius syndrome. Neuropathologic observations. *Acta Neuropathol (Berl)* 1979;48:11–17.

Vargas FR, Schuler-Faccini L, Brunoni D, et al. Prenatal exposure to misoprostol and vascular disruption defects: a case-control study. *Am J Med Genet* 2000;95(4):302–306.

Verloes A, Bitoun P, Heuskin A, et al. Mobius sequence, Robin complex, and hypotonia: severe expression of brainstem disruption spectrum versus Carey-Fineman-Ziter syndrome. *Am J Med Genet* 2004 Jun 15;127A(3):277–287.

Ziter FA, Wiser WC, Robinson A. Three generation pedigree of a Möbius syndrome variant with chromosome translocation. *Arch Neurol* 1977;34:437–442.

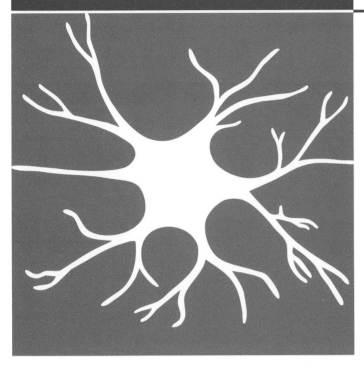

Genetic Diseases of the Central Nervous System

Chapter 81

Chromosomal Diseases

Ching H. Wang and
Marc C. Patterson

Human chromosomal anomalies are manifest as change in the total number of chromosomes, or as structural rearrangements. Examples of abnormal chromosome number (i.e., aneuploidy) are sex-chromosomal aneuploidy, such as 45,X (Turner syndrome) and autosomal aneuploidy, such as 47,XX +21 (trisomy 21, Down syndrome). Structural abnormalities include regional deletions or insertions, segmental translocations (i.e., reciprocal or robertsonian) or inversions (i.e., pericentric or paracentric), duplications, and ring chromosomes. The chromosomal syndromes are many, but they result primarily from these numeric or segmental anomalies, producing a functional change of gene dosage. The most common manifestation of chromosomal anomalies is mental retardation. Congenital malformations are seen with variable frequency and differences in severity. In the sex-chromosome disorders, infertility is the most common feature. In this section, as examples, we discuss four chromosomal syndromes: trisomy 21, Prader-Willi, and Angelman syndromes; and a common idiopathic mental retardation syndrome caused by subtelomeric anomalies of chromosomes.

TRISOMY 21 (DOWN SYNDROME)

Down syndrome was named after the English physician, John Langdon Down, who described the clinical features in 1866. The chromosomal abnormality, the first described in humans, was identified only 3 years after the normal human chromosome number was established in 1956. Down syndrome is also named *trisomy 21* because there is usually an extra copy of chromosome 21. The syndrome is encountered in about 1 in 800 live births, with a male-to-female ratio about 3:2. The risk of occurrence increases sharply with increased maternal age: 1 in 350 at maternal age 35 years and 1 in 110 at maternal age 40 years. A 45-year-old woman is 60 times more likely to have an affected child than is a 20-year-old woman.

Clinical Features

The typical facial features include a round face and a short nose with flat nasal bridge. The eyes show upward slanting of the lateral palpebral fissures, with epicanthal folds. Brushfield spots are often seen arranged in a circular ring around the outer third of the iris. The mouth is small and kept open by a large protruding tongue. The palate is high-arched or cleft. Structural anomalies of the middle and inner ear lead to frequent bouts of otitis. Conductive-hearing loss and visual problems (e.g., cataracts, strabismus, and refractive errors) require periodic assessment. Skeletal anomalies include short stature, stubby fingers and toes, an increased space between the first and second toes, and clinodactyly (inward curvature) of the fifth finger. The pelvis is small with diminished iliac and acetabular angles. Atlantoaxial or atlanto-occipital instability is found in 15% to 20% of patients. Unique dermatoglyphic features include the simian crease in the palm and unusual hand- and footprints.

An increased incidence of congenital heart diseases includes septal and endocardial-cushion defects. The genitalia are poorly developed in males, resulting in infertility. In women, ovarian defects and irregular menstruation commonly occur. Intestinal atresia, imperforate anus, and Hirschsprung disease are common. Hematologic abnormalities include an increased risk of leukemia. Thyroid-hormone abnormalities and depression occur in adolescent and adult patients. Infantile hypotonia and later, mental retardation, are the major neurologic signs. The IQ scores vary from 20 to 70, depending on the genetic background and environmental factors. Starting at ages 35 to 40 years, a further decline of cognitive function is attributed to dementia. Seizures occur more frequently in persons with Down syndrome, usually infantile spasms and tonic-clonic seizures, with myoclonus in early life and partial-simple or partial-complex seizures in the later years.

Neuropathology

The brain is spherical and small, with fewer secondary sulci than normal. The superior temporal lobes are hypoplastic, and the sylvian fissure is prominent. Microscopically, there is a reduction of neuronal density in diverse cortical areas. The pyramidal cells show a reduced number of apical dendrites and synapses. The cerebellum is small and includes an accumulation of undifferentiated fetal cells. There are striking microscopic similarities in the brains of those with Down syndrome and those with Alzheimer disease (AD), including degeneration of the cells in the nucleus basalis of Meynert, with decreased choline acetyltransferase; pigmentary degeneration of neurons, and accumulation of senile plaques and neurofibrillary tangles; and calcium deposits in the hippocampus, basal ganglia, and cerebellar folia. Almost all Down syndrome adults over age 30 years have plaques and tangles, but owing to the life-long mental retardation, it is difficult to discern whether these neuropathologic findings contribute to clinical dementia.

Cytogenetics and Molecular Genetics

In 90% to 95% of cases, karyotype analysis showed trisomy 21, with a complete, extra chromosome 21. In a few cases, trisomy is to the result of a translocation. Most free trisomy 21 results from meiotic nondisjunction in meiosis II, which correlates with advancing maternal age. Traditional cytogenetic techniques show maternal nondisjunction in about 80% and paternal in 20% of cases. With DNA analysis of polymorphisms, using highly informative markers and the polymerase-chain reaction, the origin is paternal in only about 5% of cases. All of chromosome 21 need not be triplicated to produce the syndrome. In a few cases, the only extra chromosomal 21 material is the distal half of the long arm, specifically, a region within bands q21.2 and q22.3 around a microsatellite marker D21S55. Many candidate genes have been isolated from this region. It is likely that multiple genes are responsible for the phenotypic variations in Down syndrome. The mosaic pattern (46/47, +21) occurs in 2% to 3%. The clinical features of these individuals range from virtually normal physical and intellectual characteristics, to that of typical trisomy 21.

Down Syndrome and Familial Alzheimer Disease

In addition to the neuropathologic similarities of Down syndrome and AD, linkage studies indicate that one of the early-onset familial AD genes is linked to chromosome 21. In these families, a single-base mutation in the amyloid-precursor protein (APP) gene in 21q21.3 segregates with the disease. Mutations in the APP gene prevent the normal proteolytic breakdown of Ab core (a portion of APP) and result in accumulation of amyloid protein in the senile plaques. In one study, three copies of the amyloid gene were seen in three patients with AD and also in two patients with nontrisomy Down syndrome. This finding suggested a common genetic and pathophysiologic basis for the two diseases. In Down syndrome, a triplicated region that includes the APP gene on chromosome 21 may be responsible for the increased APP production and the similar histopathology as seen in AD.

Management

There is no specific therapy for the neurologic or the cognitive impairment of Down syndrome. Several therapeutic trials using neurochemical (e.g., 5-hydroxytryptophan) or vitamin supplements have been unsuccessful. Management is addressed to the treatment of the medical and surgical conditions that accompany the syndrome. CT screening for atlantoaxial instability is indicated before a child participates in contact sports.

PRADER-WILLI AND ANGELMAN SYNDROMES

These clinically distinct syndromes are both associated with a DNA deletion within chromosome 15q11-13. The clinical differences are attributed to the derangements of the genes preferentially expressed on either the maternally or paternally derived chromosome, a process that is called genomic imprinting.

Prader-Willi Syndrome (PWS)

First described by Prader in 1956, this syndrome occurs in about 1 in 25,000 live births. It is usually sporadic, with an empiric risk of recurrence in siblings of less than 1:1,000. The clinical features may be divided into two stages. The first stage is characterized by neonatal hypotonia. A poor sucking reflex causes feeding difficulty that may lead to failure to thrive, and requires tube feeding. The external genitalia are small. The hypotonia improves at ages 8 to 11 months. Electromyography, motor nerve-conduction velocity, serum creatine kinase, and muscle biopsy are usually normal. The second stage, usually observed between ages 1 and 2 years, is characterized by delayed psychomotor development and childhood obesity. As the hypotonia improves, the infant becomes more alert. Increased appetite causes excessive weight gain. Speech delay and cognitive dysfunction are mild or moderately severe. Other typical features include short stature, small hands and feet, almond-shaped eyes, strabismus, and poor dentition.

The syndrome is attributed to defective hypothalamic function. Thermoinstability, hyperphagia, hypogonadism, and growth-hormone deficiency with short stature are clinical manifestations of hypothalamic dysfunction. However, no specific lesion of the hypothalamus has been identified at autopsy. Hyperphagia is correlated with abnormally high levels of serum ghrelin in patients with PWS. Early death is occasionally caused by morbid obesity or cardiopulmonary complications.

Angelman Syndrome

In 1965, Angelman described three children with "flat heads, jerky movements, protruding tongues, and bouts of laughter, giving them a superficial resemblance to puppets." The prevalence was estimated at 1 in 12,000. Most Angelman syndrome (AS) cases occur sporadically, but some are familial. There is no association with advanced maternal or paternal age. The infants are usually normal at birth. Feeding difficulty is noted at ages 1 to 2 months, with a period of failure to thrive. Head circumference stays at less than the fifth percentile. The children may not sit alone until age 1 year and may only learn to walk at ages 3 to 5 years. There is little or no development of speech. The child is usually happy and smiling. There is a large mouth with a protruding tongue. The skin and hair colors are usually lighter than the other family members. Hyperactivity is common. The gait is wide-based and ataxic, with tremulous movements. EEG abnormalities and seizures of various severities occur frequently in early infancy. The child is usually unable to perform activities of daily living. Pubertal development is delayed, and the adult height is less than the third percentile.

Molecular Basis

More than 50% of the PWS patients studied with high-resolution banding techniques showed some chromosome 15 anomalies. More than 90% of the abnormalities involve a deletion in band 15q11-13, and an equal proportion of AS patients have a similar deletion at 15q11-13. Using both cytogenetic techniques and DNA polymorphisms, it is possible to identify the parental origin of the deleted chromosome; all PWS patients inherit a deleted chromosome 15 from the father, and all AS patients inherit a similar chromosome 15 deletion from the mother. In PWS, maternal heterodisomy (i.e., two different chromosome 15 derived from the mother) is found in some of those without a cytogenetic deletion. Therefore, loss of the expressed paternal allele, as a result of interstitial deletion or uniparental disomy, may be responsible for the specific PWS phenotype.

Six paternally expressed genes (SNRPN, IPW, ZNF127, PAR-1, PAR-5, and NDN) have been isolated from the PWS critical region. However, no mutation or deletion of any single gene may produce the full, clinical phenotype of PWS. These findings suggest that PWS may be a contiguous-gene syndrome. In AS, recent progress in the molecular genetics has led to the identification of a strong AS-candidate gene, UBE3A, located closely to but distal from the PWS critical region within chromosome 15q12. Mutations of UBE3A gene alone were sufficient to produce a full, clinical AS phenotype. Using a mouse model, the UBE3A gene is maternally expressed in the hippocampal and Purkinje neurons. The other molecular causes of AS include *de novo* maternal deletions at 15q11-13 (about 70%), paternal uniparental disomy of chromosome 15 (about 2%), and mutations in the imprinting center (about 2% to 3%).

Genomic Imprinting

This epigenetic phenomenon illustrates an interesting non-Mendelian mode of inheritance in the mammalian genome. Several autosomal genes are inherited, in a silent state, on one parental allele, and in an active state on the other parental allele. This parent-of-origin–specific gene expression is called *genomic imprinting*. The diseases that arise from these genes are mostly caused by mutation of the active allele, duplication of the nonactive allele, or imprinting errors resulting in silencing of the active allele. Over 20 imprinted genes have now been identified in the mouse genome; many of them have human homologs. For example, the insulin-like growth-factor type 2 (IGF-2) gene is paternally active, and only when the gene defect is inherited from the father do the offspring express the dwarfing phenotype. In PWS and AS, deletions in the PWS critical region on the paternal chromosome, or maternal uniparental disomy result in silencing the paternally active allele and the PWS phenotype, whereas deletion of the AS critical region on the maternal chromosome, or paternal uniparental disomy results in the silencing of the maternal allele and the AS phenotype.

The PWS and AS critical regions are physically close to each other on chromosome 15q12. Evidence of other human genomic imprinting includes the following. First, in germline tumors such as hydatidiform moles, there are only paternally derived haploid sets of chromosomes. The lack of maternal chromosomes results in the tumor formation. Ovarian teratomas have two sets of maternal chromosomes. In fetal triploids, diandric triploids (i.e., two paternal chromosomes) are found in large cystic placentas. Conversely, in the digynic fetus (i.e., two maternal chromosomes), fetal development is severely retarded, and the placentas are small and usually nonmolar. Second, in somatic-cell tumors such as retinoblastoma and Wilms tumor, inactivation of one allele by imprinting, and a second step of chromosomal loss or mutation, result in loss of heterozygosity and tumorigenesis.

The molecular mechanism of genomic imprinting is largely unknown. The isolation of a cis-acting imprinting center, located upstream to the promotor region of the SNRPN gene, has helped us understand the molecular basis of genomic imprinting. Deletions or mutations in this imprinting center have been shown to associate with PWS or AS, depending on the origin of parental germlines. It is postulated that the imprinting center confers a male or female imprint by use of an imprinting switch during gametogenesis. In the female germline, the imprinting switch is needed to reset the male chromosome from the maternal grandfather, to confer the characteristics of a female chromosome. In the male germline, the same process is needed to reset the female chromosome from the paternal grandmother, to confer the characteristics of a male chromosome. This epigenetic mark is thought to be achieved by DNA methylation. In the case of PWS, the inactive allele on the maternal chromosome is hypermethylated, which suppresses gene transcription. The hypermethylated cytosine residues on the DNA sequences may repel the transcription factors needed for the activation of gene transcription. In other imprinted genes such as the IGF-2 receptor, DNA methylation is associated with the active allele on the maternal chromosome. Therefore, other factors in addition to DNA methylation may be involved in genomic imprinting.

SUBTELOMERIC CHROMOSOMAL ANOMALIES

A new class of chromosomal disease, the subtelomeric-chromosomal anomalies, has gained importance in the field of clinical genetics. Current fluorescent *in situ* hybridization (FISH) techniques, using a set of newly isolated subtelomeric probes, provide diagnostic insights for many human diseases, including idiopathic mental retardation and cancers. The telomere structure and its role in chromosomal disease warrant a discussion in this section.

Telomeres and Chromosomal Stability

Telomeres are the chromosome ends that contain complex DNA-protein structures. The DNA sequence is a repetitive-hexanucleotide motif, TTAGGG, ranging from 2 kb to 15 kb in length. This repetitive sequence and its specific DNA-binding proteins form a cap structure at the chromosome ends. This cap structure enables cells to distinguish chromosome ends, prevents fusion or degradation of chromosomes, and facilitates chromosomal segregations during cellular divisions. A reverse transcriptase named telomerase recognizes this terminal repetitive-DNA sequence and works to maintain the chromosomal integrity by adding telomeric DNA onto chromosome ends, when a lagging strand is created during replication. Anomalies of these DNA-protein structures change the chromosomal length. Shortening of telomeric length is seen in normal aging of somatic cells, while unchecked telomerase activation results in chromosomal fusion, as is often seen in cancer cells.

Mental Retardation Associated with Subtelomeric Chromosomal Anomalies

Mental retardation is a common, human-developmental disorder. The etiology of about 30% to 40% of moderate-to-severe mental retardation (IQ of less than 50) remains unknown, despite extensive diagnostic testing. Normal karyotype is observed in these patients using routine- or high-resolution chromosomal-banding techniques. Since early 1990s, researchers have developed DNA probes to detect subtle subtelomeric-chromosomal anomalies in humans. At least 6% of children with idiopathic mental retardation were found to harbor subtelomeric-chromosomal rearrangements, using a set of subtelomeric probes for FISH studies. These rearrangements include subtelomeric deletions, duplications, or derivative chromosomes resulting in partial monosomy-trisomy states. Positive detection rate increased to 25% when screening criteria included severe mental retardation, positive family history of mental retardation, and at least one physical dysmorphism. These results suggest that subtelomeric FISH study is a useful tool for identifying the etiology of the disorders of patients with idiopathic mental retardation.

22q11 Deletion Syndrome

Eponyms and acronyms have been applied to children with varying combinations of cardiac malformations, facial clefts, other cranial and brachial arch anomalies, dysmorphism, and learning problems, and psychiatric disorders. The terms include syndromes labelled DiGeorge, Opitz, conotruncal anomaly face, and velocardiofacial (VCFS) syndromes, as well as CATCH 22 or Pierre-Robin. All are associated with deletion of genes on the long arm of chromosome 22, leading to the term "22q11 deletion syndrome" (22q11DS), with an incidence of 1:4,000 births.

People with 22q11 have a markedly increased frequency of cognitive impairment including mental retardation (mean IQ is in the mid seventies) and psychiatric morbidity, including schizophrenia, obsessive-compulsive disorder, PDD and attention deficit hyperactivity disorder. In one study, even experienced observers had little better than a random chance of correctly identifying 22q11 deletions in patients and controls, emphasizing the importance of cytogenetic and molecular testing in patients with mild and fragmentary phenotypes.

SUGGESTED READINGS

Down Syndrome

Antonarakis SE, Down syndrome collaborative group. Parental origin of the extra chromosome in trisomy 21 as indicated by analysis of DNA polymorphisms. *N Engl J Med* 1991;324:872–876.

Antonarakis SE, Lyle R, Dermitzakis ET, Reymond A, Deutsch S. Chromosome 21 and down syndrome: from genomics to pathophysiology. *Nat Rev Genet* 2004 Oct;5(10):725–738.

Capone GT. Down syndrome: advances in molecular and biology and the neurosciences. *Devel Behav Pediat* 2001;22:40–59.

Epstein CJ. Down syndrome. In: Rosenberg RN, Prusiner SB, DiMauro S, et al., eds. *The Molecular and Genetic Basis of Neurologic and Psychiatric Disease.* Boston: Butterworth-Heinemann, 2003:125–134.

Head E, Lott IT. Down syndrome and beta-amyloid deposition. *Curr Opin Neurol* 2004 Apr;17(2):95–100.

Prader-Willi and Angelman Syndromes

Albrecht U, Sutcliffe JS, Cattanach BM, et al. Imprinted expression of the murine Angelman syndrome gene, Ube3a, in hippocampal and Purkinje neurons. *Nat Genet* 1997;17:75–78.

Clayton-Smith J, Laan L. Angelman syndrome: a review of the clinical and genetic aspects. *J Med Genet* 2003;40:87–95.

DelParigi, Tschop M, Heiman ML, et al. High circulating ghrelin: a potential cause for hyperphagia and obesity in Prader-Willi syndrome. *J Clin Endocrin Metab* 2002;87:5461–5464.

Runte M, Kroisel PM, Gillessen-Kaesbach G, et al. SNURF-SNRPN and UBE3A transcript levels in patients with Angelman syndrome. *Hum Genet* 2004;114:553–561.

Whittington J, Holland A, Webb T, et al. Relationship between clinical and genetic diagnosis of Prader-Willi syndrome. *J Med Genet* 2002;39:926–932.

Genomic Imprinting

Bartolomei MS, Tilghman SM. Genomic imprinting in mammals. *Annu Rev Genet* 1997;31:493–525.

Buiting K, Saitoh S, Gross S, et al. Inherited microdeletions in the Angelman and Prader-Willi syndromes define an imprinting centre on human chromosome 15. *Nat Genet* 1995;9:395–400.

Egger G, Liang G, Aparicio A, et al. Epigenetics in human disease and prospects for epigenetic therapy. *Nature* 2004;429:457–463.

Goto Y, Feil R. Genomic imprinting and its effects on genes and chromosomes in mammals. *Methods in Mol Biol* 2004;240:53–75.

Okamato I, Otte AP, Allis C, et al. Epigenetic dynamics of imprinted X inactivation during early mouse development. *Science* 2004;303:644–649.

Subtelomeric Chromosomal Anomalies

Baker E, Hinton L, Callen DF, et al. Study of 250 children with idiopathic mental retardation reveals nine cryptic diverse subtelomeric chromosome anomalies. *Am J Med Genet* 2001;107:285–293.

Chan SR, Blackburn EH. Telomeres and telomerase. *Philosophical Transaction of the Royal Society of London–Series B: Biol Sci* 2004;359 (1441):109–121.

de Vries BBA, Winter R, Schinzel A, et al. Telomeres: a diagnosis at the end of the chromosomes. *J Med Genet* 2003;40:385–398.

Knight SJL, Flint J. Perfect endings: a review of subtelomeric probes and their use in clinical diagnosis. *J Med Genet* 2000;37:401–409.

Meeker AK, De Marzo AM. Recent advances in telomere biology: implications for human cancer. *Curr Opin Oncol* 2003;16:32–38.

22q11 Deletion Syndrome

Bearden CE, Jawad AF, Lynch DR, Sokol S, Kanes SJ, McDonald-McGinn DM, Saitta SC, Harris SE, Moss E, Wang PP, Zackai E, Emanuel BS, Simon TJ. Effects of a functional COMT polymorphism on prefrontal cognitive function in patients with 22q11.2 deletion syndrome. *Am J Psychiatry* 2004 Sep;161(9):1700–1702.

Becker DB, Pilgram T, Marty-Grames L, Govier DP, Marsh JL, Kane AA. Accuracy in identification of patients with 22q11.2 deletion by likely care providers using facial photographs. *Plast Reconstr Surg* 2004 Nov;114(6):1367–1372.

D'Antoni S, Mattina T, Di Mare P, Federico C, Motta S, Saccone S. Altered replication timing of the HIRA/Tuple1 locus in the DiGeorge and Velocardiofacial syndromes. *Gene* 2004 May 26;333:111–119.

Gothelf D, Presburger G, Zohar AH, Burg M, Nahmani A, Frydman M, Shohat M, Inbar D, Aviram-Goldring A, Yeshaya J, Steinberg T,

Finkelstein Y, Frisch A, Weizman A, Apter A. Obsessive-compulsive disorder in patients with velocardiofacial (22q11 deletion) syndrome. *Am J Med Genet B Neuropsychiatr Genet* 2004 Apr 1;126(1):99–105.

Maynard TM, Haskell GT, Peters AZ, Sikich L, Lieberman JA, LaMantia AS. A comprehensive analysis of 22q11 gene expression in the developing and adult brain. *Proc Natl Acad Sci USA* 2003 Nov 25;100(24):14433–14438.

Mehendale FV, Birch MJ, Birkett L, Sell D, Sommerlad BC. Surgical management of velopharyngeal incompetence in velocardiofacial syndrome. *Cleft Palate Craniofac J* 2004 Mar;41(2):124–135.

Roubertie A, Semprino M, Chaze AM, Rivier F, Humbertclaude V, Cheminal R, Lefort G, Echenne B. Neurological presentation of three patients with 22q11 deletion (CATCH 22 syndrome). *Brain Dev* 2001 Dec;23(8):810–814.

van Amelsvoort T, Daly E, Henry J, Robertson D, Ng V, Owen M, Murphy KC, Murphy DG. Brain anatomy in adults with velocardiofacial syndrome with and without schizophrenia: preliminary results of a structural magnetic resonance imaging study. *Arch Gen Psychiatry* 2004 Nov;61(11):1085–1096.

Vogels A, Fryns JP. The velocardiofacial syndrome: a review. *Genet Couns* 2002;13(2):105–113.

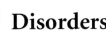

Chapter 82

Disorders of Amino Acid Metabolism

John H. Menkes

There has been an exponential growth in our understanding of the multiplicity of genetic defects that cause the diverse disorders of amino acid metabolism. Rather than elaborate on the molecular biology of these conditions, this chapter focuses on the neurologic aspects, diagnosis, and management. For more details, the interested reader is referred to chapters dealing with the disorders of amino acid metabolism in the volumes edited by Scriver et al.

Mass screening for disorders of amino acid metabolism has resulted in early biochemical diagnosis of phenylketonuria (PKU) and other aminoacidopathies. In one screening program, the incidence of PKU was 1:10,000 in New South Wales, Australia, the incidence of defects of amino acid transport was about 2:10,000, and the combined incidence of all other aminoacidopathies was less than 8:100,000. Although these conditions are rare, they are important because neurologic damage is frequently preventable with early treatment and because neurologic damage is frequently preventable with early treatment and because they provide information about the development and functions of the brain.

PHENYLKETONURIA (MIM 261600)

Phenylalanine hydroxylase deficiency (PKU) is an inborn error of metabolism transmitted as an autosomal-recessive trait and manifested by impairment in the hepatic hydroxylation of phenylalanine to tyrosine. Untreated, the disorder causes a clinical picture highlighted by mental retardation, seizures, and imperfect hair pigmentation. Inasmuch as PKU is the epitome of a metabolic disorder, demonstrating the interrelation between genetic alterations in intermediary metabolism and neurologic dysfunction, it deserves more space than its frequency in the panoply of neurologic disorders would otherwise warrant.

The disease has been found in all parts of the world. The frequency in the general population of the United States, as determined by screening programs, is about 1:11,700.

Pathogenesis and Pathology

The hydroxylation of phenylalanine to tyrosine is an irreversible and complex reaction that requires phenylalanine hydroxylase and five other enzymes, in addition to several nonprotein components. Phenylalanine hydroxylase is normally found in liver, kidney, and pancreas but not in brain or skin fibroblasts.

In classic PKU, as a result of multiple and distinct mutations in the gene for phenylalanine hydroxylase, enzyme activity is completely or nearly completely abolished. Cloning of a full-length, complementary DNA has enabled characterization of the normal and mutant genes. Some 500 mutations in the phenylalanine hydroxylase gene, the majority of which result in deficient-enzyme activity and cause hyperphenylalaninemia, have been found in all 13 exons of the gene and flanking sequence. Some cause phenylketonuria; others cause non-PKU hyperphenylalaninemia, while still others are silent polymorphisms present on both normal and mutant chromosomes. Missense mutations predominate, although every other type of mutation has also been found. A high proportion of patients are compound heterozygotes rather than homozygotes.

In some 1% to 3% of subjects, hyperphenylalaninemia results from a deficiency of tetrahydrobiopterin (BH$_4$). The BH$_4$-deficient hyperphenylalaninemias comprise a genetically heterogeneous group of disorders caused by mutations in the genes encoding enzymes involved in the synthesis or regeneration of the coenzyme BH$_4$. Three genetic defects in the synthesis of BH$_4$ have been described. These involve GTP cyclohydrolase I (OMIM 233910), 6-pyruvoyl-tetrahydropterin synthase (OMIM 261640), and sepiapterin reductase (OMIM 181125). In addition there are two disorders in the regeneration of the aromatic amino acid-hydroxylating system: dihydropteridine reductase (OMIM 261630), and pterin-4a-carbinolamine

dehydratase. All these conditions lead to hyperphenylalaninemia, which in most instances is accompanied by a syndrome of progressive neurologic deterioration, accompanied by a variety of dyskinesias.

Children suffering from classic PKU are born with only slightly elevated phenylalanine blood levels, but because of the defect in phenylalanine hydroxylase, the amino acid derived from food proteins accumulates in serum and cerebrospinal fluid, and is excreted in large quantities. In lieu of the normal degradative pathway, phenylalanine is converted to phenylpyruvic acid, phenylacetic acid, and phenylacetylglutamine.

The transamination of phenylalanine to phenylpyruvic acid is sometimes deficient for the first few days of life, and the age when phenylpyruvic acid may be first detected ranges from 2 to 34 days.

Alterations within the brain are nonspecific and diffuse, and involve both gray and white matter. There are three types of alterations within the brain:

1. Interference with normal maturation of the brain. Brain growth is reduced; there is microscopic evidence of impaired cortical layering, delayed outward migration of neuroblasts, and heterotopic gray matter. These changes suggest a period of abnormal brain development during the last trimester of gestation.
2. Defective myelination. This may be generalized or limited to areas in which postnatal deposition of myelin is normal. Except in some older patients, products of myelin degeneration are not seen. Generally, there is relative pallor of myelin, sometimes with mild gliosis and irregular areas of vacuolation (i.e., status spongiosus). The vacuoles are usually seen in central white matter of the cerebral hemispheres and in the cerebellum.
3. Diminished or absent pigmentation of the substantia nigra and locus ceruleus.

Symptoms and Signs

Patients suffering from PKU exhibit a wide range of clinical and biochemical severity. In the classic form, caused by a virtual absence of phenylalanine hydroxylase activity, untreated infants appear normal at birth. During the first 2 months, there is vomiting (i.e., sometimes projectile) and irritability. Delayed intellectual development is apparent by 4 to 9 months; mental retardation may be severe, precluding speech or toilet training. Seizures, common in more severely retarded infants, usually start before age 18 months and may cease spontaneously. In infants, seizures may appear as infantile spasms, later changing to grand mal attacks.

The typical affected, untreated child is blond and blue-eyed, with normal and often pleasant features. The skin is rough and dry, sometimes with eczema. A peculiar musty odor, attributable to phenylacetic acid, may suggest the diagnosis. Significant focal neurologic abnormalities are rare. Microcephaly may be present, and there may be a mild increase in muscle tone, particularly in the legs. A fine, irregular tremor of the hands is seen in about 35% of subjects. The plantar response is often variable or extensor. EEG abnormalities include hypsarrhythmia, recorded even in the absence of seizures, and single or multiple foci of spike and polyspike discharges.

MRI is almost invariably abnormal, even in early treated patients. On T2-weighted images, high signal areas are seen in white matter. These are mainly located in the posterior temporal- and occipital-periventricular regions, notably in the watershed between the posterior- and middle-cerebral arteries. They are probably caused by abnormalities of myelin formation and maintenance.

Diagnosis

Most PKU patients are identified through a newborn screening program. Although most infants whose blood phenylalanine levels are above the threshold value of 2 mg/dL to 4 mg/dL (120 μM/L to 240 μM/L) do not have PKU, such patients will require prompt reevaluation by an appropriate laboratory to determine whether hyperphenylalaninemia is persistent, and whether it is caused by phenylalanine hydroxylase deficiency. As the urine of most phenylketoneuric newborns does not contain appreciable amounts of phenylpyruvic acid, the ferric chloride and 2,4- dinitrophenylhydrazine tests are inadequate during the neonatal period. If the diagnosis of a case of classic PKU is missed, the most likely reason is laboratory error, rather than insufficient protein intake, or too early testing of the infant.

A combination of haplotype and mutation analysis has facilitated carrier detection and the prenatal diagnosis of PKU, in families with at least one previously affected child. The widespread screening programs that detect newborns with blood-phenylalanine concentrations higher than normal have also uncovered other conditions in which blood phenylalanine levels are increased in the neonatal period. Patients with moderate and mild PKU, and mild hyperphenylalaninemia, as these entities are termed, have phenylalanine levels that tend to be lower than those seen in classic PKU. As Scriver (2002) has pointed out, the correlation between genotype and phenotype in even this well understood, monogenic disorder is complex and at this point unpredictable.

Treatment

On referral of an infant with a positive screening test, the first step is quantitative determination of serum phenylalanine and tyrosine levels. All infants whose blood-phenylalanine concentration is greater than 10 mg/dL (600 μM/L) and whose tyrosine concentration is low or normal (i.e., 1 mg/dL to 4 mg/dL) should be started on a low-phenylalanine diet immediately. Infants whose blood phenylalanine concentrations remain in the range of 6.6 mg/dL to 10.0 mg/dL (400 μM/L to 600 μM/L) on an unrestricted diet are generally not treated, and on follow-up evaluations this group of children have normal intelligence and a normal MRI.

The generally accepted therapy for classic PKU is restriction of the dietary intake of phenylalanine by placing the infant on one of several low-phenylalanine formulas. To avoid symptoms of phenylalanine deficiency, milk is added to the diet in amounts sufficient to maintain blood levels of the amino acid between 2 mg/dL and 6 mg/dL (120 μM/L to 360 μM/L). Generally, patients tolerate this diet quite well, and within 1 to 2 weeks, the serum concentration of phenylalanine becomes normal.

Weekly serum-phenylalanine determinations are essential, to ensure adequate regulation of diet. Strict dietary control should be maintained for as long as possible, and most centers strive to keep levels below 6.0 mg/dL (360 μM/L), even in patients with moderate and mild PKU. Dietary lapses are frequently accompanied by progressive white-matter abnormalities, on MRI. Some workers have suggested supplementation of the low-phenylalanine diet with tyrosine, but there is no statistical evidence that this regimen results in a better intellectual outcome. Vectors for efficient gene transfer have yet to be developed.

Treatment of phenylalaninemia caused by BH$_4$ deficiency involves control of blood phenylalanine, administration of BH$_4$ or a synthetic pterin, and replacement therapy with neurotransmitter precursors (L-dopa/carbidopa and 5-hydroxytryptophan), because synthesis of these substances is also impaired.

Early detection and dietary control of PKU has increased the number of homozygous PKU women who are of childbearing age. The harmful effects of maternal hyperphenylalaninemia on the heterozygous offspring include mental retardation, microcephaly, seizures, and congenital heart defects. Women who conceive while their blood phenylalanine levels are 15 mg/dL or above (i.e., greater than 900 μM/L) are at high risk for these malformations and should be offered termination of pregnancy. In mothers whose blood phenylalanine levels are maintained below 10 mg/dL (600 μM/L) prior to conception, intelligence in offspring is normal. Otherwise, the 7-year Wechsler Intelligence Scales for Children (WISC) score of offspring depends on the gestational age at which maternal blood-phenylalanine was brought down below 10 mg/dL (600 μM/L). There is, however, no linear regression of offspring IQ versus average maternal-phenylalanine levels. During pregnancy, phenylalanine levels should be monitored as closely as during infancy, because the fetus is exposed to even higher phenylalanine concentrations than the mother.

Prognosis

When a child with classic PKU is maintained on a low-phenylalanine diet, seizures disappear and the EEG tends to revert to normal. Abnormally blond hair regains natural color, and any microcephaly tends to revert to normal.

The effects on mental ability are less clearcut. In most studies, some deficit in intellectual development has been found, even in infants who had been diagnosed and treated as neonates, and there appears to be no threshold below which phenylalanine has no effect on cognition. When the measured IQ is normal, children may exhibit impaired perceptual functions, and progress in school is poorer than expected from the IQ score. Neurologic deterioration during adult life has been seen in some patients. This is generally the consequence of dietary lapses.

Failure to prevent mild mental retardation or cognitive deficits, even with optimal control, may be a consequence of prenatal brain damage induced by high phenylalanine levels in the fetus.

MAPLE SYRUP URINE DISEASE (MIM 248600)

Maple syrup urine disease (MSUD) is a familial, cerebral degenerative disease caused by a defect in branched-chain amino acid metabolism, and marked by the passage of urine with a sweet maple syrup–like odor. Its incidence is 1:220,000 to 1:400,000 newborns. In the Mennonite population of Pennsylvania, the incidence of the classic form of the disease is 1:176 births. The disorder is characterized by accumulation of three branched-chain ketoacids: α-keto-isocaproic acid, α-keto-isovaleric acid, and α-keto-β-methylvaleric acid, which are the respective derivatives of leucine, valine, and isoleucine. Accumulation of these substances results from an autosomal-recessively inherited deficiency in the mitochondrial branched-chain α-ketoacid dehydrogenase. This is a multienzyme complex comprising six proteins: $E_{1\alpha}$ and $E_{1\beta}$, which form the decarboxylase; E_2 and E_3; and a branched-chain specific kinase and phosphatase. Mutations in the genes for $E_{1\alpha}$, $E_{1\beta}$, E_2, and E_3 have been described. These induce a continuum of disease severity that ranges from the severe, classic form of MSUD, to mild and intermittent forms. Patients with the severe, classic phenotype may be compound heterozygote or homozygotes for defects in the genes for $E_{1\alpha}$ or $E_{1\beta}$.

Plasma levels of the corresponding amino acids are also elevated because the ketoacids are transaminated. In some cases, the branched-chain α-hydroxyacids, most prominently α-hydroxyisovaleric acid, are also excreted; a sotolone derivative of α-ketobutyric acid, whose decarboxylation is impaired by accumulation of α-keto-β-methylvaleric acid, is responsible for the characteristic odor of the urine and sweat. Sotolone, a furanone derivative, is also found in maple syrup and fenugreek.

Structural alterations in the brain are similar to, but more severe than, those in PKU. The cytoarchitecture of the cortex is generally immature, with fewer cortical layers, persistence of ectopic foci of neuroblasts, and abnormal dendritic development.

Manifestations of the untreated classic form of the condition include opisthotonos, intermittent increase of muscle tone, seizures, and rapid deterioration of all cerebral functions. Some patients have presented with pseudotumor cerebri, or with fluctuating ophthalmoplegia. About half the infants develop hypoglycemia. In the acute stage of the disease, MRI demonstrates both diffuse edema, and a severe edema characteristically localized to the cerebellar deep white matter, the posterior part of the brain stem, the cerebral peduncles, the posterior limb of the internal capsule, and the posterior part of the centrum semiovale. The condition is suggested by the characteristic odor of the patient's urine and perspiration. It is confirmed by quantitation of plasma amino acids.

Treatment

Treatment is based on a commercially available diet that contains restricted amounts of leucine, isoleucine, and valine. For optimal results, dietary management must be initiated during the first few days of life. The regimen is complex and requires frequent quantitative measurement of serum amino acids. Children with the classic form of the disease, who have been maintained on this regimen, have achieved near-normal intellectual development, although a residual picture resembling mild spastic diplegia may be seen.

A subset of MSUD patients exhibits intermittent periods of ataxia, drowsiness, behavior disturbances, and seizures that appear between 6 and 9 months of age. In some of these subjects, there is a defect in the gene coding for the E_2 subunit. In other children, there is only mild or moderate mental retardation. In yet another group of MSUD patients, the biochemical abnormality may be corrected by the administration of thiamin.

DEFECTS IN THE METABOLISM OF SULFUR AMINO ACIDS

Of the several defects in the metabolism of sulfur-containing amino acids, the most common is homocystinuria (MIM 236200) (Table 82.1).

This inborn error of methionine metabolism is manifested by multiple thromboembolic episodes, ectopia lentis, and mental retardation. It is transmitted by an autosomal-recessive gene. The condition occurs in 1:45,000 newborns; it is second in frequency only to PKU, among metabolic errors responsible for brain damage.

In the most common form of homocystinuria, the metabolic defect affects cystathionine β-synthase, the

▶ **TABLE 82.1** **Disorders of Sulfur Amino Acids**

Disorder	Enzyme Deficiency	Neurological Picture
Homocystinuria	Cystathionine-β-synthase	Multiple thromboembolic episodes starting in first year of life, mental retardation, ectopia lentis
Homocystinuria and mild homocysteinemia	$N^{5,10}$-methylenetetrahydrofolate reductase	Seizures, microcephaly, spastic paraparesis, ataxia
Cystathioninuria	γ-Cystathionase	Asymptomatic
Homocystinuria with megaloblastic anemia		
Cbl E	Methionine synthase reductase	Severe developmental delay, lethargy, staring spells, hypotonia
Cbl G	Methionine synthase	Failure to thrive, mental retardation, cerebral atrophy
Cbl C	Synthesis of methyl and adenosyl cobalamin	Marfanoid habitus, mental retardation, acute psychosis, subacute spinal cord degeneration
Cbl D	Synthesis of methyl and adenosyl cobalamin	Acute psychosis, mental retardation, subacute spinal cord degeneration, Marfanoid habitus.
Cbl F	Cobalamin lysosomal release	Developmental delay, sudden death in infancy
Sulfite oxidase deficiency	Sulfite oxidase	Seizures starting in neonatal period, profound mental retardation, subluxation of lens
Molybdenum cofactor deficiency	Molybdenum cofactor deficiency	See Chapter 89

enzyme that catalyzes the formation of cystathionine from homocysteine and serine. In most homocystinuric subjects, activity of this enzyme is completely absent, but there is residual enzyme activity in members of a significant proportion of affected families. In the latter group, about 25% to 50% of patients with homocystinuria, the addition of pyridoxine stimulates enzyme activity and partially, or completely, abolishes the excretion of homocystine, the oxidized derivative of homocysteine. Such patients tend to have a milder phenotype of the disease. As a result of the enzymatic block, increased amounts of homocystine and its precursor, methionine, are found in urine and plasma.

Primary structural alterations are noted in blood vessels of all calibers. In most vessels, there is intimal thickening and fibrosis; in the aorta and its major branches, fraying of elastic fibers may be found. Both arterial and venous thromboses are common in different organs. In the brain, there are usually multiple infarcts of varying age. Dural-sinus thrombosis has been recorded. The relationships between the metabolic defect and the predisposition to vascular thrombosis are multiple. Homocysteine is toxic to vascular endothelium, inhibiting intracellular protein transport; it potentiates the autooxidation of low-density lipoprotein cholesterol and promotes thrombosis by inhibiting the activation of anticoagulant protein C.

Homocystinuric infants appear normal at birth, and early development is unremarkable until seizures, developmental slowing, or strokes occur between 5 and 9 months of age. Ectopia lentis has been recognized by age 18 months and is invariable in older children. The typical older homocystinuric child's hair is sparse, blond, and brittle. There are multiple erythematous blotches over the skin, particularly across the maxillary areas and cheeks.

The gait is shuffling, the limbs and digits are long, and genu valgum is usually present.

In about half of the cases, major thromboembolic episodes occur once, or more. These include fatal thrombosis of the pulmonary artery or vein. Multiple major strokes may result in hemiplegia, and ultimately, in pseudobulbar palsy. Minor and unrecognized cerebral thrombi may be the direct cause of the mental retardation that occurs in more than 50% of homocystinuric patients. The observation that homocysteine acts as an agonist at the glutamate-binding site of the *N*-methyl-D-aspartate

▶ **TABLE 82.2** **Aminoacidurias Detected by Newborn-Infant Urine Screening**

Condition	Cases/100,000 6-Week-Old Infants
Disorders of amino-acid metabolism	
Phenylketonuria	10
Histidinemia	5.2
Hyperprolinemia	1.0
Cystathioninuria	0.33
Tyrosinemia	0.33
Argininosuccinic aciduria	0.25
Hyperlysinemia	0.1
Nonketotic hyperglycinemia	0.1
Homocystinuria	0.1
α-Ketoadipic aciduria	0.1
Others	0
Disorders of amino-acid transport	
Iminoglycinuria	10
Cystinuria	5.8
Hartnup disease	4.0
Cystinosis	0.33

▶ **TABLE 82.3 Some Uncommon Errors of Amino Acid Metabolism**

Disease[a]	Enzymatic Defect	Clinical Features	Diagnosis
Argininosuccinic aciduria (207900)	Argininosuccinase	Recurrent generalized convulsions, poorly pigmented hair, ataxia, hepatomegaly, mental retardation	CSF shows large amounts of argininosuccinic acid, elevated blood ammonia
Citrullinemia (215700)	Argininosuccinic acid synthetase	Mental retardation, vomiting, irritability, seizures	Serum and urine citrulline elevated blood ammonia
Hyperammonemia	Ornithine transcarbamylase (311250)	Seizures, recurrent changes in consciousness, hepatomegaly, males succumb early. Ataxia in older children	Elevated blood ammonia, assay liver enzymes
	Carbamyl phosphate synthetase (237300)	Episodic vomiting, lethargy	Elevated blood ammonia, assay liver enzymes
Hyperlysinemia (238700)	Lysine-α-ketoglutarate reductase	Probably asymptomatic	Elevated plasma lysine, elevated urine lysine, also seen in heterozygotes for cystinuria
Saccharopinuria (268700)	Aminoadipic semialdehydeglutamate reductase	Mental retardation, progressive spastic diplegia	Elevated urine, serum lysine, saccharopine in urine and serum
Aspartylglucosaminuria (208400)	Aspartylglucosaminidase	Mental retardation, hepatosplenomegaly, vacuolated lymphocytes in 75%, coarse facial features	Elevated urine aspartylglucosaminuria
Carnosinemia (212200)	Carnosinase	Mental retardation, mixed major and minor motor seizures	Elevated serum, urine carnosine elevated CSF homocarnosine
Argininemia (207800)	Arginase	Spastic diplegia, seizures	Elevated plasma and CSF argininemia; elevated blood ammonia
Valinemia (277100)	Valine transaminase	Vomiting, failure to thrive, nystagmus, mental retardation	Increase blood and urine valine, no increase in ketoacid excretion
Sarcosinemia (folic acid dependent) (268900)	Impaired sarcosine-glycine conversion	Emotional disturbance in some; normal intelligence in most others	Increased blood and urine sarcosine, ethanolamine
Hyper-beta-alaninemia (237400)	β-Alanine-α-ketoglutarate transaminase	Seizures commencing at birth, somnolence	Plasma, urine β-alanine and β-aminoisobutyric acid elevated urinary γ-amino butyric acid elevated
β-Methylcrotonylglycinuria (210200)	β-Methylcrotonyl-CoA carboxylase	Similar to infantile spinal muscular atrophy, persistent vomiting, mental retardation, urine smells like that of cat	Increased urine β-hydroxyisovaleric acid, β-methylcrotonylglycine; some patients are biotin-responsive
α-Methylacetoacetic aciduria (203750)	3-Ketothiolase	Recurrent severe metabolic acidosis	α-Methyl acetoacetate and α-methyl-β-hydroxy-butyric acid in urine
Cytosol tyrosine aminotransferase deficiency (276600)	Soluble tyrosine amino transferase	Herpetiform corneal ulcers, palmoplantar keratoses, mental retardation	ρ-Hydroxyphenylpyruvic and p-Hydroxyphenyl lactic acid excretion increased
Tryptophanuria with dwarfism (276100)	Tryptophan pyrrolase	Ataxia, spasticity, mental retardation, pellagra-like skin rash	Elevated serum tryptophan, diminished kynurenine
Glutathione synthetase deficiency (231900)	γ-Glutamylcysteine synthetase	Hemolytic anemia, spinocerebellar degeneration, peripheral neuropathy	Reduced erythrocyte glutathione generalized aminoaciduria
Pyroglutamic aciduria (266130)	Glutathione synthetase	Mental retardation, metabolic acidosis	Elevated urinary 5-oxoproline

[a]The numbers in parentheses refer to McKusick's *Mandelian Inheritance in Man* (MIM), as explained in the preface.

receptor suggests that overstimulation of this receptor contributes to the pathogenesis of neurologic symptoms.

The diagnosis of homocystinuria is suggested by the appearance of the patient and may be confirmed by a positive urinary cyanide-nitroprusside reaction, by the increased urinary excretion of homocystine, and by elevated levels of plasma homocystine and methionine. The diagnosis is further established by assays of cystathionine β-synthase in skin fibroblasts or liver.

Administration of a commercially available, low-methionine diet supplemented with cysteine, lowers plasma-methionine content and eliminates the abnormally high homocystine excretion. In some centers, the diet is further supplemented with betaine, to use alternative pathways for removal of homocysteine. Pyridoxine (i.e., 50 mg to 500 mg per day, combined with folic acid) reduces the homocystine excretion of pyridoxine-responsive patients. Although the biochemical picture may be improved by these means, the variable clinical picture, particularly the thromboembolic episodes and mental retardation, has up to now rendered useless any evidence for clinical benefit.

Heterozygotes for homocystinuria have an increased propensity to peripheral-vascular disease and premature cerebrovascular accidents, and one-third of all patients with premature arterial-thrombotic disease have elevated blood levels of homocysteine. The incidence of myocardial infarcts in this population, however, is no higher than normal.

Several other genetic entities manifest themselves by increased excretion of homocystine (Table 82.1). In some, the conversion of homocysteine to methionine is impaired. The most important of these entities is $N^{5,10}$-methylenetetrahydrofolate-reductase deficiency. Children with this disorder may present with ataxia, spastic paraparesis, and mental retardation. Several conditions result from a deficiency of methyl cobalamine, the active cofactor for the conversion of homocysteine to methionine. These entities are summarized in Table 82.1. The characteristic biochemical feature of these diseases is that the excretion of homocystinuria is accompanied by methylmalonic aciduria.

OTHER DEFECTS OF AMINO ACID METABOLISM

There have been numerous reports of a neurologic disorder apparently associated with some abnormality in the amino-acid pattern of serum or urine. The frequency in the general population may be gauged by routine, mass, newborn screening, such as the one by Wilcken et al. (Table 82.2). Other screening programs have found similar incidences.

Neurologic complications are also common in disorders of the urea cycle. These are discussed in Chapter 88. The neurologic deficits reported in some of the other more common conditions (e.g., histidinemia, sarcosinemia, hyperprolinemia, and cystathioninuria) are considered to be unrelated to the metabolic defect, but are the result of screening a selected population, namely mentally retarded individuals. Some of the less uncommon disorders are summarized in Table 82.3.

▶ **TABLE 82.4 Defects in Amino-acid Transport**

Transport System	Condition	Biochemical Features	Clinical Features
Basic amino acids	Cystinuria (three types) (220100)[a]	Impaired renal clearance, defective intestinal transport of lysine, arginine, ornithine, and cystine	Renal stones, no neurologic disease
	Lowe syndrome (309000)	Impaired intestinal transport of lysine and arginine, impaired tubular transport of lysine	Severe mental retardation, congenital glaucoma, cataracts, myopathy
Acidic amino acids	Dicarboxylic aminoaciduria (222730)	Increased excretion of glutamic, aspartic acids	Severe mental retardation glaucoma, cataracts, myopathy, sex-linked transmission
Neutral amino acids	Hartnup disease (234500)	Defective intestinal and renal tubular transport of tryptophan and other neutral amino acids	Intermittent cerebellar ataxia, photosensitive rash
Proline, hydroxyproline, glycine	Iminoglycinuria (242600)	Impaired tubular transport of proline, hydroxyproline, and glycine	Harmless variant
β-Amino acids	None known	Excretion of β-aminoisobutyric acid and taurine in β-alaninemia is increased due to competition at the tubular level	Harmless variant

[a]Numbers are taken from *Mendelian Inheritance in Man*, as explained in the Preface.

DISORDERS OF AMINO ACID TRANSPORT

Renal amino-acid transport is handled by five specific systems that have nonoverlapping substrate preferences. The disorders that result from genetic defects in each of these systems are listed in Table 82.4.

Lowe Syndrome (MIM 309000)

Lowe syndrome (*oculocerebrorenal syndrome*) is a sex-linked, recessive disorder characterized clinically by severe mental retardation, delayed physical development, myopathy, congenital glaucoma or cataract, and renal Fanconi syndrome. The condition results from mutations in the OCRL1 gene, which has been mapped to the long arm of the X chromosome. The gene encodes a phosphatidylinositol 4,5 biphosphate-5-phosphatase located in the trans-Golgi network. The fundamental biochemical defect is believed to be a defect in the actin cytoskeleton, with impaired polymerization and consequent defects in the formation and maintenance of tight junctions that are involved in the function of renal proximal tubules, and the differentiation of the lens. Biochemically, there is generalized aminoaciduria, with renal tubular acidosis, and rickets. There are no consistent neuropathologic findings. MRI shows different degrees of white matter involvement. Urinary levels of lysine are more elevated than those of the other amino acids, and defective uptake of lysine and arginine by the intestinal mucosa has been demonstrated in some patients.

Hartnup Disease (MIM 236200)

This rare familial condition is characterized by photosensitive dermatitis, intermittent cerebellar ataxia, mental disturbances, and renal aminoaciduria. The name is that of the family in which the disorder was first detected.

Symptoms are caused by an extensive disturbance in the transport of neutral amino acids. There are four main biochemical abnormalities: renal aminoaciduria, increased excretion of indican, increased excretion of nonhydroxylated indole metabolites, and increased fecal amino acids.

Symptoms usually occur in mildly malnourished children. When present, they are intermittent and variable, tending to improve with age. They include a red scaly rash on the exposed areas of the body (resembling the dermatitis of pellagra), intermittent personality disorders, migraine-like headaches, photophobia, and bouts of cerebellar ataxia. Neuroimaging studies are nonspecific; MRI shows delayed myelination. There are no consistent neuropathologic findings.

The similarity of Hartnup disease to pellagra has prompted treatment with nicotinic acid. The tendency, however, for symptoms to remit spontaneously and for general improvement to occur with improved dietary intake and advancing age, makes such therapy difficult to evaluate.

SUGGESTED READINGS

General

Wilcox WR, Cedarbaum SD. Amino acid metabolism. In: Rimoin DL, Connor JM, Pyeritz RE, Korf BR, eds. *Principles and Practice of Medical Genetics,* 4th ed. New York: Churchill Livingstone, 2002:2405–2440.

Menkes JH, Wilcox WR. Inherited metabolic diseases of the nervous system. In: Menkes JH, ed. *Textbook of Child Neurology,* 7th ed. Baltimore: Lippincott Williams & Wilkins, 2005.

Scriver CR, Beaudet AL, Sly WS, et al., eds. *The Metabolic Bases of Inherited Disease,* 8th ed. New York: McGraw-Hill, 2001.

Phenylketonuria

Anderson PJ, Wood SJ, Francis DE, et al. Neuropsychological functioning in children with early-treated phenylketonuria: impact of white matter abnormalities. *Develop Med Child Neurol* 2004;46(4):230–238.

Baumeister AA, Baumeister AA. Dietary treatment of destructive behavior associated with hyperphenylalaninemia. *Clin Neuropharmacol* 1998;21:18–27.

Cederbaum S. Phenylketonuria: an update. *Curr Opin Pediatr* 2002; 14:702–708.

Green A. Neonatal screening: current trends and quality control in the United Kingdom. *Jpn J Clin Pathol* 1998;46:211–216.

Guldberg P, Rey F, Zschocke J, et al. A European multicenter study of phenylalanine hydroxylase deficiency: classification of 105 mutations and a general system for genotype-based prediction of metabolic phenotype. *Am J Hum Genet* 1998;63:71–79.

Hanley WB. Adult phenylketonuria. *Am J Med* 2004 Oct 15;117(8):590–595.

Holtzman NA, Kronmal RA, van Doorninck W, et al. Effect of age at loss of dietary control of intellectual performance and behavior of children with phenylketonuria. *N Engl J Med* 1986;314:593–598.

Kalsner LR, Rohr FJ, Strauss KA, et al. Tyrosine supplementation in phenylketonuria: Diurnal blood tyrosine levels and presumptive brain influx of tyrosine and other large neutral amino acids. *J Pediatr* 2001;139:421–427.

Kaufman S, Kapatos G, Rizzo WB, et al. Tetrahydropterin therapy for hyperphenylalaninemia caused by defective synthesis of tetrahydrobiopterin. *Ann Neurol* 1983;14:308–315.

Koch R, Hanley W, Levy H, et al. The maternal phenylketonuria international study: 1984–2002. *Pediatrics* 2003;112:1523–1529.

Lou HC, Toft PB, Andresen J, et al. An occipito-temporal syndrome in adolescents with optimally controlled hyperphenylalaninemia. *J Inher Metab Dis* 1992;15:687–695.

Malamud N. Neuropathology of phenylketonuria. *J Neuropathol Exp Neurol* 1966;25:254–268.

MRC Working Party on Phenylketonuria. Recommendations on the dietary management of phenylketonuria. *Arch Dis Child* 1993;68:426–427.

MRC Working Party on Phenylketonuria. Phenylketonuria due to phenylalanine hydroxylase deficiency: an unfolding story. *BMJ* 1993; 306:115–119.

Schneider AJ. Newborn phenylalanine tyrosine metabolism. Implications for screening for phenylketonuria. *Am J Dis Child* 1983;137:427–432.

Scriver CR. Why mutation analysis does not always predict clinical consequences: Explanations in the era of genomics. *J Pediatr* 2002;140:502–506.

Smith I, Leeming RJ, Cavanagh NPC, et al. Neurologic aspects of biopterin metabolism. *Arch Dis Child* 1986;61:130–137.

Smith ML, Hanley WB, Clarke JT, et al. Randomized controlled trial of tyrosine supplementation on neuropsychological performance in phenylketonuria. *Arch Dis Child* 1998;78:116–121.

Thompson AJ, Smith I, Brenton D, et al. Neurological deterioration in young adults with phenylketonuria. *Lancet* 1990;336:602–605.

Weglage J, Pietsch M, Feldmann R, et al. Normal clinical outcome in untreated subjects with mild hyperphenylalaninemia. *Pediatr Res* 2001;49:532–536.

Welsh MC, Pennington BF, Ozonoff S, et al. Neuropsychology of early-treated phenylketonuria: specific executive function deficits. *Child Dev* 1990;61:1697–1713.

Maple Syrup Urine Disease

Brismar J, Aqeel A, Brismar G, et al. Maple syrup urine disease: findings on CT and MR scans of the brain in 10 infants. *Am J Neuroradiol* 1990;11:1219–1228.

Chuang DT. Maple syrup urine disease: it has come a long way. *J Pediatr* 1998;132:S17–S23.

Di Rocco M, Biancheri R, Rossi A, Allegri AE, Vecchi V, Tortori-Donati P. MRI in acute intermittent maple syrup urine disease. *Neurology* 2004 Sep 8;63(6):1078.

Kamei A, Takashima S, Chan F, et al. Abnormal dendritic development in maple syrup urine disease. *Pediatr Neurol* 1992;8:145–147.

Mantovani JF, Naidich TP, Prensky AL, et al. MSUD: presentation with pseudotumor cerebri and CT abnormalities. *J Pediatr* 1980;96:279–281.

Menkes JH. Maple syrup disease: isolation and identification of organic acids in the urine. *Pediatrics* 1959;23:348–353.

Menkes JH, Hurst PL, Craig JM. A new syndrome: progressive familial infantile cerebral dysfunction associated with unusual urinary substance. *Pediatrics* 1954;14:462–466.

Morton DH, Strauss KA, Robinson DL, et al. Diagnosis and treatment of maple syrup disease: a study of 36 patients. *Pediatrics* 2002;109:999–1008.

Parmar H, Sitoh YY, Ho L. Maple syrup urine disease: diffusion-weighted and diffusion-tensor magnetic resonance imaging findings. *J Comput Assist Tomogr* 2004;28(1):93–97.

Podebrad F, Heil M, Reichart S, et al. 4,5-dimethyl-3-hydroxy-2[5H]-furanone (sotolone)—the odor of maple syrup urine disease. *J Inherit Metab Dis* 1999;22:107–114.

Schadewaldt P, Wendel U. Metabolism of branched-chain amino acids in maple syrup urine disease. *Eur J Pediatr* 1997;156[Suppl 1]:S62–S66.

Schonberger S, Schweiger B, Schwahn B, Schwarz M, Wendel U. Dysmyelination in the brain of adolescents and young adults with maple syrup urine disease. *Mol Genet Metab* 2004 May;82(1):69–75.

Tsuruta M, Mitsubuchi H, Mardy S, et al. Molecular basis of intermitted maple syrup urine disease: novel mutations in the E2 gene of the branched-chain alpha-keto acid dehydrogenase complex. *J Hum Genet* 1998;43:91–100.

Wynn RM, Davie JR, Chuang JL, et al. Impaired assembly of E1 decarboxylase of the branched-chain alpha-ketoacid dehydrogenase complex in type IA maple syrup urine disease. *J Biol Chem* 1998;273:13110–13118.

Defects in the Metabolism of Sulfur Amino Acids

Dixon MA, Leonard JV. Intercurrent illness in inborn errors of intermediary metabolism. *Arch Dis Child* 1992;67:1387–1391.

Kelly PJ, Furie KL, Kistler JP, et al. Stroke in young patients with hyperhomocysteinemia due to cystathionine beta-synthase deficiency. *Neurology* 2003;60:275–279.

Lentz SR, Sadler JE. Homocysteine inhibits von Willebrand factor processing and secretion by preventing transport from the endoplasmic reticulum. *Blood* 1993;81:683–689.

Lipton SA, Kim WK, Choi YB, et al. Neurotoxicity associated with dual actions of homocysteine at the *N*-methyl-D-aspartate receptor. *Proc Natl Acad Sci USA* 1997;94:5923–5928.

Mitchell GA, Watkins D, Melancon SB, et al. Clinical heterogeneity in cobalamin C variant of combined homocystinuria and methylmalonic aciduria. *J Pediatr* 1986;108:410–415.

Schimke RN, McKusick VA, Huang T. Homocystinuria: studies of 20 families with 38 affected members. *JAMA* 1965;193:711–719.

Singh RH, Kruger WD, Wang L, Pasquali M, Elsas LJ 2nd. Cystathionine beta-synthase deficiency: effects of betaine supplementation after methionine restriction in B6-nonresponsive homocystinuria. *Genet Med* 2004 Mar–Apr;6(2):90–95.

Walter JH, Wraith JE, White FJ, et al. Strategies for the treatment of cystathionine beta-synthase deficiency: the experience of the Willink Biochemical Genetics Unit over the past 30 years. *Eur J Pediatr* 1998;157(suppl 2):S71–S76.

Disorders of Amino Acid Transport

Lowe Syndrome

Charnas L, Bernar J, Pezeshkpour GH, et al. MRI findings and peripheral neuropathy in Lowe's syndrome. *Neuropediatrics* 1988;19:7–9.

Charnas LR, Gahl WA. The oculocerebrorenal syndrome of Lowe. *Adv Pediatr* 1991;38:75–107.

Demmer LA, Wippold FJ II, Dowton SB. Periventricular white matter cystic lesions in Lowe (oculocerebrorenal) syndrome. A new MR finding. *Pediatr Radiol* 1992;22:76–77.

Lin T, Orrison BM, Leahey AM, et al. Spectrum of mutations in the OCR1 gene in the Lowe oculocerebrorenal syndrome. *Am J Hum Genet* 1997;60:1384–1388.

Lowe CU, Terrey M, MacLachlan EA. Organic aciduria, decreased renal ammonia production, hydrophthalmos, and mental retardation. *Am J Dis Child* 1952;83:164–184.

Martin MA, Sylvester PE. Clinico-pathological studies of oculo-cerebral-renal syndrome of Lowe, Terrey and MacLachlan. *J Ment Defic Res* 1980;24:1–16.

Sener RN. Lowe syndrome: proton MR spectroscopy, and diffusion MRI. *J Neuroradiol* 2004 Jun;31(3):238–240.

Suchy SF, Nussbaum RL. The deficiency of PIP2 5-phosphatase in Lowe syndrome affects actin polymerization. *Am J Hum Genet* 2002;71:1420–1427.

Hartnup Disease

Baron DN. Hereditary pellagra-like skin rash with temporary cerebellar ataxia, constant renal aminoaciduria, and other bizarre chemical features. *Lancet* 1956;2:421–428.

Erly W, Castillo M, Foosaner D, et al. Hartnup disease: MR findings. *AJNR* 1991;12:1026–1027.

Jepson JB. Hartnup disease. In: Stanbury JB, Wyngaarden JB, Fredrickson DS, eds. *The Metabolic Basis of Inherited Disease,* 4th ed. New York: McGraw-Hill, 1978:1563–1577.

Wilcken B, Yu JS, Brown DA. Natural history of Hartnup disease. *Arch Dis Child* 1977;52:38–40.

Chapter 83

Disorders of Purine and Pyrimidine Metabolism

Marc C. Patterson and Lewis P. Rowland

Purines and pyrimidines are heterocyclic compounds that play a number of roles in intermediary metabolism, including nucleotide synthesis, generation of energy compounds (i.e., ADP and ATP), and in signaling pathways (i.e., cyclic AMP). Several disorders of purine and pyrimidine metabolism have been recognized. Findings include anemia, immunodeficiency, hypo- or hyperuricemia (i.e., with nephrolithiasis and renal failure in severe cases), and a variety of neurologic phenotypes. The latter range through sensorineural hearing loss, developmental delays, mental retardation, autism, seizures and movement disorders. The archetype, and most frequently recognized of these disorders is the Lesch-Nyhan syndrome, described in more detail below. The other disorders are summarized in Table 83.1.

LESCH-NYHAN SYNDROME (MIM 308000)

In 1964, Lesch and Nyhan described two brothers with hyperuricemia, mental retardation, choreoathetosis, and self-destructive biting of the lips and fingers. Most cases recorded since that time have affected boys, but at least one symptomatic female with skewed X-inactivation has been described. The trait is inherited as an X-linked recessive trait, and the gene has been localized to the long arm of the X chromosome. The basic defect is the lack of hypoxanthine-guanine phosphoribosyltransferase (HPRT) in all body fluids. The gene was one of the first human genes to be cloned. Owing to the enzyme deficiency, the rate of purine biosynthesis is increased, and the content of the end product of purine metabolism, uric acid, reaches high values in blood, urine, and CSF. Deposits of urate are found in the kidneys and joints, and may result in debilitating nephropathy and gout.

The neurologic manifestations include severe mental retardation, spasticity, and choreoathetosis that each start in the first year of life. The characteristic self-mutilating behavior appears in the second year. Death is usually caused by renal failure and may occur in the second or third decade of life. The pathogenesis of the cerebral symptoms is not known. Although low levels of dopamine metabolites have been found in postmortem samples of tissue from the basal ganglia, it is not known how these abnormalities lead to the symptoms, or how they relate to the enzyme disorder.

Diagnosis depends on recognition of the clinical manifestations and may be made, precisely, by biochemical assay of the enzyme in erythrocyte hemolysates or cultured fibroblasts. Hair-root analysis of HPRT has become a convenient way to analyze activity. Prenatal enzymatic diagnosis is possible in the first trimester with chorionic villus sampling. DNA analysis may be used for prenatal diagnosis and carrier detection, but is not yet adequate to diagnose all individual cases. The gene, however, has been mapped to Xq26.1, and numerous point mutations have been found.

Treatment

Treatment is not satisfactory. Gout may be treated with allopurinol, but the neurologic disorder is daunting. Restraints may be needed to prevent the child from damaging himself or others; sometimes teeth must be removed. In one subject, bilateral stimulation of the globus pallidus was intended to control the movement disorder, but also abolished self mutilation.. Enzyme-replacement therapy, with long-term erythrocyte transfusions, in three patients gave only modest improvement of the neurologic symptoms, and drug therapy to modify dopamine metabolism has not yet been effective. Gene therapy is being evaluated in animals because the human gene has been introduced into transgenic mice, and enzyme activity is expressed in the brain of the recipient animals.

There is evidence of both clinical and biochemical heterogeneity. Hyperuricemia and cerebellar ataxia have been noted in individuals with normal HPRT activity. Patients with partial enzyme deficiency may have gout without neurologic symptoms, or there may be various degrees of severity of mental retardation, movement disorders, spastic tetraplegia, or seizures. The self-mutilating behavior may be restricted to the classic form, which lacks all enzyme activity.

OTHER PURINE DISORDERS

Neurologic abnormalities are also seen in patients who are without other enzymes of purine-nucleoside metabolism. Adenosine-deaminase deficiency (MIM 102700) causes severe, combined immunodeficiency in infants; some patients have extrapyramidal or pyramidal signs and psychomotor development, and may be retarded. Partial exchange transfusion may be clinically beneficial. Also, a few patients lacking purine nucleoside phosphorylase (MIM 164050), with impaired cellular immunity, have shown a form of spastic paraparesis in childhood. 5'-nucleotidase

▶ **TABLE 83.1** Disorders of Purine and Pyrimidine Metabolism

Enzyme	Anemia	ID	Uric Acid	MR	SNHL	Seizures	Ataxia	MD	Other
NT	+	+	−	+		+	+	+	Symptoms improve with uridine
Purine pathway									
PRPS	−	−	+	+	+	−	+	−	Autism
ADSL	−	−	0	+	−	+	−	−	Autism
AMPD1	−	−	0	−	−	−	−	−	Muscle cramps, increased creatine kinase (CK)
ADA	−	+	0	+	−	−	−	+	Spasticity
NP	+	+	−	+	−	−	−	+	Spasticity
XDH	−	−	−	−	−	−	−	−	Myopathy, arthropathy
HPRT	−	−	+	+	−	+	−	+	Self mutilation, spasticity, 6-thioguanine resistance
APRT	−	−	+	−	−	−	−	−	
Pyrimidine pathway									
UMPS	+	−	0	+	−	−	−	−	
UMPH	+	−	0	−	−	−	−	−	
DPYD	−	−	0	+	−	+	−	−	Microcephaly, 5-fluorouracil sensitivity, autism
DPYS	−	−	0	+	−	+	−	−	
UP	−	−	0	+	−	+	−	+	

Key: NT–cytosolic 5′-nucleotidase superactivity [nucleotide depletion syndrome]; PRPS–Phosphoribosyl pyrophosphate synthetase superactivity; ADSL–Adenylosuccinate lyase deficiency; Muscle adenosine monophosphate deaminase deficiency; ADA–Adenosine deaminase deficiency; NP–nucleoside phosphorylase deficiency; XDH–xanthine dehydrogenase (= xanthine oxidase) deficiency [xanthinuria; secondary impairment in molybdenum cofactor deficiency]; HPRT–hypoxanthine-guanine phosphoribosyl transferase deficiency [Lesch-Nyhan syndrome]; APRT–adenine phosphoribosyltransferase deficiency [hereditary orotic aciduria]; UMPS–uridine monophosphate synthase deficiency [hereditary orotic aciduria]; UMPH–uridine monophosphate hydrolase (= pyrimidine 5′-nucleotidase) deficiency; DPYD–dihydropyrimidine dehydrogenase deficiency; DPYS–dihydropyrimidinase deficiency; UP–ureidopropionase deficiency; ID–immunodeficiency; MR–developmental delay, mental retardation; SNHL–sensorineural hearing loss; MD–movement disorder; + = present (or increased for uric acid); − = absent (or decreased for uric acid); 0 = unchanged.

superactivity produces a complex phenotype with all of the features of purine and pyrimidine disorders that responds to oral uridine therapy. These patients may have autistic features that may also be prominent in PRPS, ADSL and DPYD (Table 83.1).

SUGGESTED READINGS

Coleman MS, Danton MJ, Philips A. Adenosine deaminase and immune dysfunction. *Ann N Y Acad Sci* 1985;451:54–65.

DeGregorio L, Nyhan WL, Serafin E, Chamoles NA. An unexpected affected female patient in a classical Lesch-Nyhan family. *Molec Genet Metab* 2000;69:263–268.

Edwards NL. Immunodeficiencies associated with errors in purine metabolism. *Med Clin North Am* 1985;69:505–518.

Edwards NL, Jeryc W, Fox IH. Enzyme replacement in the Lesch-Nyhan syndrome with long-term erythrocyte transfusions. *Adv Exp Med Biol* 1984;165:23–26.

Graham GW, Aitken DA, Connor JM. Prenatal diagnosis by enzyme analysis in 15 pregnancies at risk for the Lesch-Nyhan syndrome. *Prenatal Diag* 1996;16:647–651.

Harris JC, Lee BR, Jinah HA, et al. Craniocerebral magnetic resonance imaging measurement and findings in Lesch-Nyhan syndrome. *Arch Neurol* 1998;55:547–553.

Hirschhorn R. Complete and partial adenosine deaminase deficiency. *Ann N Y Acad Sci* 1985;451:20–25.

Hirschhorn R, Ellenbogen A. Genetic heterogeneity in adenosine deaminase (ADA) deficiency: five different mutations in five new patients with partial ADA deficiency. *Am J Hum Genet* 1986;38:13–25.

Jankovic J, Caskey TC, Stout JT, Butler IJ. Lesch-Nyhan syndrome: motor behavior and CSF neurotransmitters. *Ann Neurol* 1988;23:466–468.

Kuehn MR, Bradley A, Robertson EJ, Evans MJ. A potential animal model for Lesch-Nyhan syndrome through introduction of HPRT mutations into mice. *Nature* 1987;326:295–298.

Marcus S, Stern AM, Andersson B, et al. Mutation analysis and prenatal diagnosis in Lesch-Nyhan syndrome showing non-random C-inactivation interferes with carrier detection tests. *Hum Genet* 1992;89:395–400.

Markert ML. Purine nucleoside deficiency. *Immunodefic Rev* 1991;3:45–81.

McCarthy G. Medical diagnosis, management and treatment of Lesch Nyhan disease. *Nucleosides Nucleotides Nucleic Acids* 2004 Oct;23:1147–1152.

Nyhan WL, Vuong LC, Broock R. Prenatal diagnosis of Lesch-Nyhan disease. *Prenat Diagn* 2003;23:807–809.

Nyhan WL. The recognition of Lesch-Nyhan syndrome as an inborn error of purine metabolism. *J Inherit Metabol Dis* 1997;20:171–178.

Nyhan WL, Parkman R, Page T, et al. Bone marrow transplantation in Lesch-Nyhan disease. *Adv Exp Med Biol* 1986;195:167–170.

Page T. Metabolic approaches to the treatment of autism spectrum disorders. *J Autism Dev Disord* 2000;30:463–469.

Page T, Yu A, Fontanesi J, Nyhan WL. Developmental disorder associated with increased cellular nucleotidase activity. *Proc Natl Acad Sci U S A* 1997;94(21):11601–11606.

Rijksen G, Kuis W, Wadman SK, et al. A new case of purine nucleoside phosphorylase deficiency with neurologic disorder. *Pediatr Res* 1987;21:137–141.

Rossiter BJF, Edwards A, Casket CT. HPRT mutations in Lesch-Nyhan syndrome. In: Brosis J, Frenau B, eds. *Molecular Genetic Approach to Neuropsychiatric Diseases.* New York: Academic Press, 1991.

Scully DG, Dawson PA, Emerson BT, Gordon RS. Review of the molecular basis of HPRT deficiency. *Hum Genet* 1992;90:195–207.

Shapira J, Ziberman Y, Becker A. Lesch-Nyhan syndrome: a nonextracting approach to prevent mutilation. *Spec Care Dentist* 1985;5:210–212.

Silverstein FS, Johnson MV, Hutchinson RJ, Edwards NL. Lesch-Nyhan syndrome: CSF neurotransmitter abnormalities. *Neurology* 1985;35:907–911.

Stout JT, Chen HY, Brennand J, et al. Expression of human HPRT in the central nervous system of transgenic mice. *Nature* 1985;317:250–251.

Taira T, Kobayashi T, Hori T. Disappearance of self-mutilating behavior in a patient with Lesch-Nyhan syndrome after bilateral chronic stimulation of the globus pallidus internus. Case report. *J Neurosurg.* 2003;98(2):414–416.

Watson AR, Simmonds HA, Webster DR, et al. Purine nucleoside phosphorylase (PNP) deficiency: a therapeutic challenge. *Adv Exp Med Biol* 1984;165:53–59.

Watts RWE, Spellacy E, Gibbs DA, et al. Clinical, postmortem, biochemical and therapeutic observations on the Lesch-Nyhan syndrome with particular reference to the neurological manifestations. *Q J Med* 1982;201:43–78.

Wilson JM, Stout JT, Palella TD, et al. A molecular survey of hypoxanthine-guanine phosphoribosyltransferase deficiency in man. *J Clin Invest* 1986;77:188–195.

Wu CL, Melton DW. Production of model for Lesch-Nyhan syndrome in hypoxanthine phosphoribosyl transferase-deficient mice. *Nat Genet* 1993;3:235–239.

Chapter 84

Lysosomal and Other Storage Diseases

Marc C. Patterson and William G. Johnson

In the lysosomal diseases, storage material accumulates within lysosomes because of genetically determined deficiency of a catabolic enzyme. The stored materials comprise complex lipids, saccharides, or proteins and the CNS is usually affected. Both autosomal and X-linked inheritance occur. Carrier detection and prenatal diagnosis are available for most of these disorders, but there is as yet no specific treatment, except for enzyme-replacement therapy for MPS 1, Gaucher, and Fabry disease. Hemopoietic-cell transplantation has been studied in several lysosomal-storage diseases with varying evidence of benefit.

LIPIDOSES

Lipid-storage diseases involve all three major lipid classes: neutral lipids (i.e., cholesterol ester, fatty acid, and triglycerides), polar lipids (i.e., glycolipids and phospholipids),

and very polar lipids (i.e., gangliosides). The largest group of stored lipids is the sphingolipids, based on sphingosine (Fig. 84.1A).

When a long-chain fatty acid is attached to the 2-amino group of sphingosine, the resulting compounds are called ceramides. Further hydrophilic residues are attached at the 1-hydroxyl group to give the sphingolipids (Fig. 84.1, B to E).

GM2-Gangliosidoses

Hexosaminidase-deficiency diseases result from a genetically determined deficiency of the enzyme hexosaminidase (reaction 3, Figs. 84.1, B and C, 84.2, and 84.3), which causes accumulation in cells (especially in neurons) of GM2-ganglioside, certain other glycosphingolipids, and other compounds containing a terminal β-linked, *N*-acetylgalactosaminide or *N*-acetylglucosaminide moiety.

For full activity, hexosaminidase requires two different subunits: the α-subunit, coded for by the HEXA locus on chromosome 15, and the β-subunit, coded for by the HEXB locus on chromosome 5. Three isozymes of hexosaminidase have a defined, subunit structure: hexosaminidase A ($\alpha\beta$), hexosaminidase B ($\beta\beta$), and hexosaminidase S ($\alpha\alpha$). Hexosaminidase A is required for cleavage of GM2-ganglioside, but the true substrate is the ganglioside bound to a protein activator whose deficiency also causes a GM2-gangliosidosis (the so-called AB variant). The GM2-gangliosidoses are classified according to the phenotype, the genetic locus, and the allele involved.

Progressive infantile encephalopathy was the most common clinical pattern in the past. The success of carrier screening, among couples of Ashkenazi Jewish background, dramatically reduced the incidence, and later onset variants are now seen more commonly. Hexosaminidase deficiencies show diverse phenotypes from infancy to adulthood. This diagnosis can be suspected with nearly any degenerative, neurologic disorder, except demyelinating neuropathy or myopathy. Sensory dysfunction, ocular palsies, neurogenic bladder, and extraneural involvement are not prominent features.

The diagnosis is made by measuring the amount of hexosaminidase in blood serum and leukocytes. Rectal biopsy for electron microscopy of neurons is useful to confirm the diagnosis in variant phenotypes. DNA-based diagnosis is useful to specify the mutation involved.

Infantile Encephalopathy with Cherry-red Spots

Three disorders in this group are well known: classic infantile Tay-Sachs disease (α locus), infantile Sandhoff disease (β locus), and the so-called AB variant (activator locus). Heterozygosity for α-locus mutations occurs in 1 in

30 Ashkenazi Jews (compared with 1 in 300 for the general population), accounting for the ethnic concentration of classic Tay-Sachs disease and genetic compounds containing α-locus mutations.

In all three conditions, the infants appear normal until 4 to 6 months of age. They learn to smile and reach for objects but do not sit or crawl. A myoclonic-jerk reaction to sound (i.e., hyperacusis) and the macular cherry-red spot (Fig. 84.4) are constant findings. The infants become floppy and weak but have hyperactive reflexes, clonus, and extensor plantar responses. Visual deterioration, apathy, and loss of developmental milestones lead to a vegetative state by the second year. Seizures and myoclonus are prominent for the first 2 years. The infants eventually become decorticate. They need tube feeding, have difficulty with secretions, and are blind. Head circumference enlarges progressively to about the 90th percentile, from ages 1 to 3 years, and then stabilizes. Death is due to intercurrent infection, usually pneumonia. The disease is confined to the nervous system, apart from variable hepatosplenomegaly in Sandhoff disease.

By light microscopy, grossly ballooned neurons (Fig. 84.5) are found throughout the brain, cerebellum, and spinal cord.

The cytoplasm is filled with pale, homogeneous-appearing material that pushes the nucleus and Nissl substrate to a corner of the cell. By electron microscopy, membranous cytoplasmic bodies (i.e., distended lysosomes) are seen with regularly spaced, concentric, dark and pale lamellae.

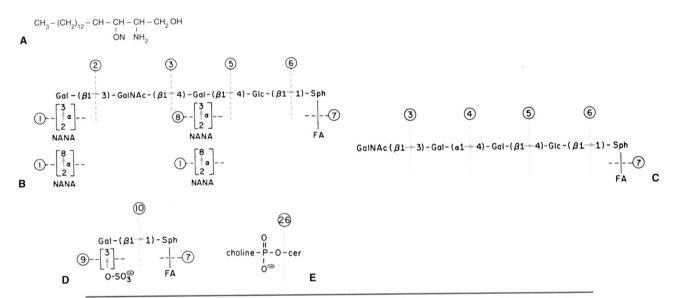

FIGURE 84.1. A: Sphingosine. Addition of fatty acid in amide linkage gives ceramide (Cer). **B:** Structure of a ganglioside (here, a tetrasialoganglioside, GQ1a) containing sphingosine (Sph), fatty acid (FA), neutral hexoses (glucose, Glc; galactose, Gal), hexosamine (GalNAc, *N*-acetylgalactosamine), and sialic acid (NANA, *N*-acetylneuraminic acid). **C:** Structure of a glycolipid, globoside (GL4), containing sphingosine, fatty acid, neutral hexoses, and hexosamine. **D:** Structure of sulfatide (a major glycolipid of myelin) containing sphingosine, fatty acid, and galactose, which is sulfated on the 3-hydroxyl group. **E:** Structure of sphingomyelin or ceramide phosphorylcholine. Reactions 1–26 are illustrated in Figs. 84.1–84.3. *1*, Sialidase (sialidoses). *2*, Beta-galactosidase (GM1-gangliosidoses, Morquio syndrome type B, secondarily deficient in galactosialidosis). *3*, Hexosaminidase (GM2-gangliosidoses). *4*, Alpha-galactosidase (Fabry disease). *5*, Ceramide lactosidase. *6*, β-Glucosidase (Gaucher disease). *7*, Ceramidase (Farber disease). *8*, Ganglioside sialidase. *9*, Sulfatase A (metachromatic leukodystrophy, mucosulfatidosis, MSD). *10*, Galactocerebrosidase (Krabbe disease). *11*, α-L-Iduronidase (Hurler syndrome, Scheie syndrome, Hurler-Scheie compound). *12*, Iduronate-2-sulfate sulfatase (Hunter syndrome, MSD). *13*, Sulfamidase (Sanfilippo A, MSD). *14*, α-*N*-acetylglucosaminidase (Sanfilippo B). *15*, *N*-acetyl transferase (Sanfilippo D, MSD). *16*, Galactose-6-sulfate sulfatase or *N*-acetylgalactosamine-6-sulfate sulfatase (Morquio syndrome type A, MSD). *17*, *N*-acetylgalactosamine-4-sulfate sulfatase or sulfatase B (Maroteaux-Lamy syndrome, MSD). *18*, β-Glucuronidase (Sly syndrome). *19*, Acetylglucosamine-6-sulfate sulfatase (Sanfilippo D, MSD). *20*, Dermatan sulfate *N*-acetylgalactosamine-6-sulfate sulfatase. *21*, α-L-Fucosidase (fucosidosis). *22*, α-Mannosidase (α-mannosidosis). *23*, Mannosidase (β-mannosidosis). *24*, Endoglucosaminidase. *25*, Aspartylglucosaminidase (aspartylglucosaminuria). *26*, Sphingomyelinase (Niemann-Pick disease, types A, B, and F).

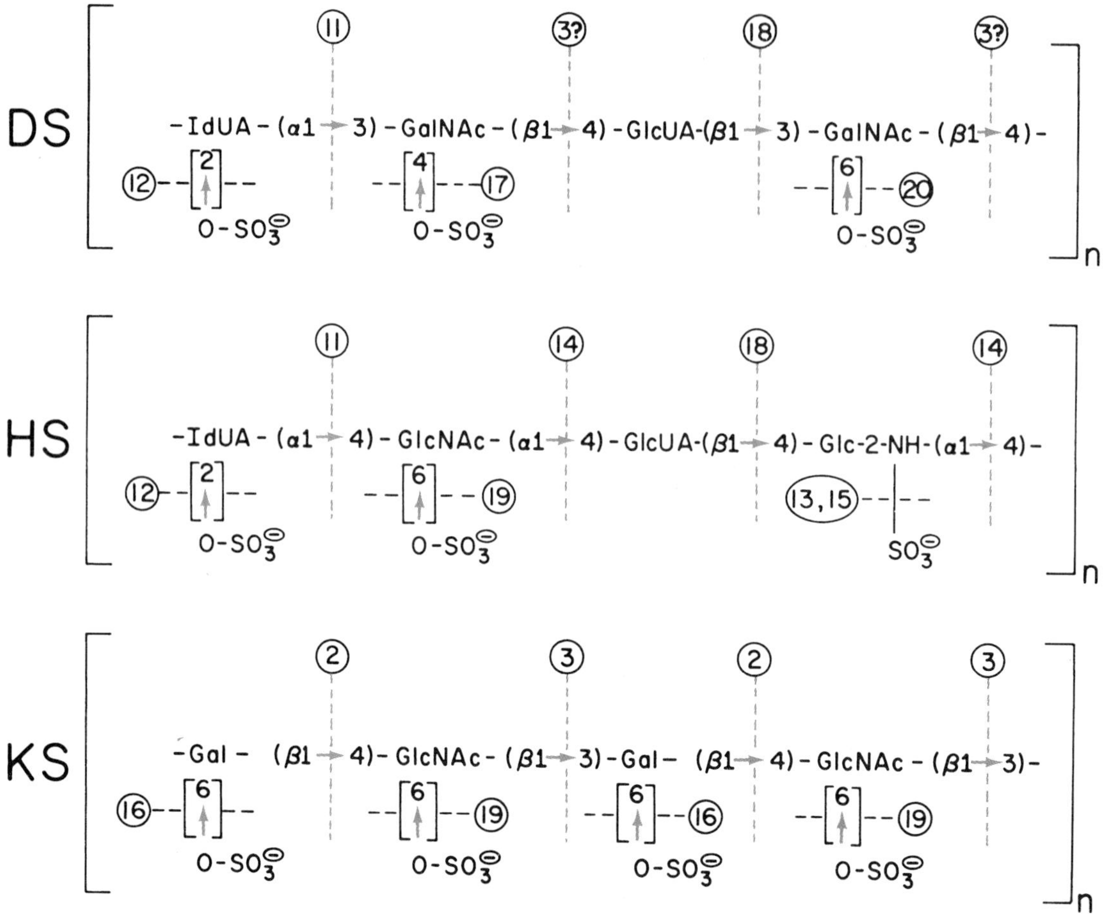

DS

⑪   ③?   ⑱   ③?

$-\text{IdUA}-(\alpha 1 \rightarrow 3)-\text{GalNAc}-(\beta 1 \rightarrow 4)-\text{GlcUA}-(\beta 1 \rightarrow 3)-\text{GalNAc}-(\beta 1 \rightarrow 4)-$

⑫$--\begin{bmatrix}2\\\uparrow\end{bmatrix}--$ $--\begin{bmatrix}4\\\uparrow\end{bmatrix}--$⑰ $--\begin{bmatrix}6\\\uparrow\end{bmatrix}--$⑳

$\text{O-SO}_3^{\ominus}$ $\text{O-SO}_3^{\ominus}$ $\text{O-SO}_3^{\ominus}$ $\rfloor_n$

HS

⑪   ⑭   ⑱   ⑭

$-\text{IdUA}-(\alpha 1 \rightarrow 4)-\text{GlcNAc}-(\alpha 1 \rightarrow 4)-\text{GlcUA}-(\beta 1 \rightarrow 4)-\text{Glc-2-NH}-(\alpha 1 \rightarrow 4)-$

⑫$--\begin{bmatrix}2\\\uparrow\end{bmatrix}--$ $--\begin{bmatrix}6\\\uparrow\end{bmatrix}--$⑲   (13,15)$--|--$

$\text{O-SO}_3^{\ominus}$ $\text{O-SO}_3^{\ominus}$ $\text{SO}_3^{\ominus}$ $\rfloor_n$

KS

②   ③   ②   ③

$-\text{Gal}-(\beta 1 \rightarrow 4)-\text{GlcNAc}-(\beta 1 \rightarrow 3)-\text{Gal}-(\beta 1 \rightarrow 4)-\text{GlcNAc}-(\beta 1 \rightarrow 3)-$

⑯$--\begin{bmatrix}6\\\uparrow\end{bmatrix}--$ $--\begin{bmatrix}6\\\uparrow\end{bmatrix}--$⑲ $--\begin{bmatrix}6\\\uparrow\end{bmatrix}--$⑯ $--\begin{bmatrix}6\\\uparrow\end{bmatrix}--$⑲

$\text{O-SO}_3^{\ominus}$ $\text{O-SO}_3^{\ominus}$ $\text{O-SO}_3^{\ominus}$ $\text{O-SO}_3^{\ominus}$ $\rfloor_n$

FIGURE 84.2. Structure of three clinically important mucopolysaccharides: dermatan sulfate (DS), heparan sulfate (HS), and keratan sulfate (KS). Each consists of repeating dimers of uronic acid (IdUA, iduronic acid; GlcUA, glucuronic acid), hexosamine (GlcNAc, N-acetylglucosamine; GalNAc, N-acetylgalactosamine), and sulfate (OSO3). In DS, the hexosamine is GalNAc. In HS, the hexosamine is α-linked glucosamine, sometimes N-acetylated, sometimes N-sulfated. In KS, uronic acid is replaced by galactose (Gal). The glycan portion is bound to protein (not shown).

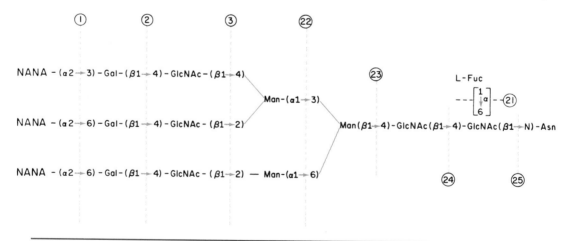

FIGURE 84.3. Structure of an asparagine-linked glycoprotein consisting of asparagine (Asn), neutral sugars (Man, mannose; Gal, galactose; L-Fuc, L-fucose), hexosamine (GlcNAc, N-acetylglucosamine), and sialic acid (NANA, N-acetylneuraminic acid). The mannose-6-phosphate recognition marker is formed by transfer of GlcNAc1P to the 6-hydroxyl groups of the α-linked mannose residues and subsequent removal of the phosphate-linked GlcNAc residues.

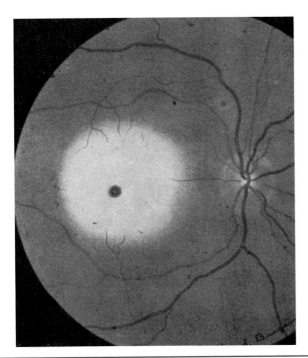

FIGURE 84.4. Macular cherry-red spot in Tay-Sachs disease. (Courtesy of Dr. Arnold Gold.)

GM2-ganglioside (Fig. 84.1B) content is markedly increased in the brain, and to a much lesser degree, in the viscera. Other glycosphingolipids with a terminal β-linked *N*-acetylgalactosamine moiety, such as asialo-GM2 (Fig. 84.1B) and globoside (Fig. 84.1C), accumulate to a lesser degree.

The storage results from the deficiency of hexosaminidase (reaction 3). In classic Tay-Sachs disease, hexosaminidase A is absent, and hexosaminidase B increased.

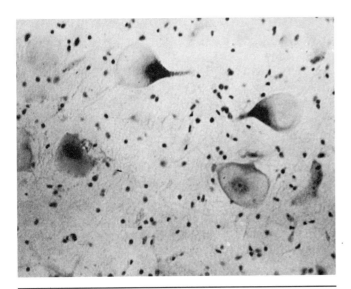

FIGURE 84.5. Ballooned spinal cord ventral horn cells in Tay-Sachs disease. (Courtesy of Dr. Abner Wolf.)

Heterozygous carriers have a partial decrease of hexosaminidase A.

In infantile Sandhoff disease, hexosaminidase A and B are deficient. Carriers have partially decreased hexosaminidase A and B. In one form of the AB variant, a hexosaminidase A-activating protein is missing. Although levels of hexosaminidase A and B are increased, GM2-ganglioside cannot be cleaved. Diagnosis requires the use of the radio-labeled natural substrate, M2-ganglioside, or direct testing for the activator or activator mutations. In a second form of the AB variant, the residual hexosaminidase A cleaves artificial but not sulfated-artificial or natural substrate. Although this is detected as an AB variant, it is an α-locus disorder.

Late Infantile, Juvenile, and Adult GM2-Gangliosidoses

These present with dementia and ataxia, with or without macular cherry-red spots. Spasticity, muscle wasting stemming from anterior horn-cell disease, and seizures are frequently seen. Hexosaminidase A deficiency or hexosaminidase A and B deficiency are found on biochemical study of serum, leukocytes, and cultured skin fibroblasts.

Other late-onset forms of GM2-gangliosidosis present as cerebellar ataxia or spinocerebellar ataxia. Hexosaminidase A or hexosaminidase A and B deficiency are found on biochemical study.

Motor-neuron disease may be the first evidence of late-onset GM2-gangliosidoses. Lower motor-neuron disease may resemble the Kugelberg-Welander or Aran-Duchenne syndrome. Upper motor-neuron disease may be present, giving an amyotrophic lateral sclerosis (ALS)-like phenotype.

Many, perhaps most, of these late-onset cases are genetic compounds. Rectal biopsy for electron microscopy of autonomic neurons, natural substrate hexosaminidase assays, and DNA-based diagnosis are important diagnostic tests for late-onset GM2-gangliosidosis.

GM1-Gangliosidosis

This group of disorders is characterized by the deficiency of GM1-ganglioside β-galactosidase (reaction 2, Figs. 84.1B, 84.2, and 84.3) and storage of compounds that contain a terminal β-linked galactose moiety. These include GM1-ganglioside, asialo-M1, keratan sulfate-like oligosaccharides, and glycoproteins. Other β-galactosidases, such as those that cleave galactosylceramide (reaction 10, Fig. 84.1D) and lactosylceramide (reaction 5, Fig. 84.1B and C) are not deficient, and those compounds do not accumulate. There are at least three forms of deficiency of this enzyme: primary deficiency of β-galactosidase, causing infantile and late-infantile GM1-gangliosidosis and an adult form; combined neuraminidase and β-galactosidase deficiency, galactosialidosis; and combined deficiency of β-galactosidase and several other lysosomal enzymes in I-cell disease, mucolipidosis II. The latter two types are discussed under mucolipidoses.

Infantile GM1-Gangliosidosis

Infantile GM1-gangliosidosis is earlier in onset, more severe, and more rapidly progressive than infantile Tay-Sachs disease. Soon after birth, these infants become hypotonic, with poor sucking ability, and slow weight gain. They have frontal bossing, coarsened features, large low-set ears, and an elongated philtrum. Gum hypertrophy, macroglossia, peripheral edema, and often faint corneal haze are noted. Strabismus and nystagmus may be seen. About half the patients develop macular cherry-red spots (Fig. 84.4). Development is slow, and they do not sit or crawl. By age 6 months, liver and spleen are enlarged; joint stiffness and claw-hand deformities may be seen, and the skin is coarse and thickened. Seizures may develop. The infants enter a vegetative state and die before age 2 years, of pneumonia or cardiac arrhythmias.

Bone radiographs after 6 to 12 months show changes similar to those of Hurler syndrome, with anterior beaking of vertebral bodies and J-shaped sella turcica. Peripheral-blood smears show vacuolated lymphocytes, and foamy histiocytes are found in the bone marrow.

Diagnosis is suggested by the characteristic oligosaccharide pattern in urine, and confirmed by assay of GM1-ganglioside β-galactosidase (reaction 2, Figs. 84.1B and 84.2) in blood leukocytes or cultured skin fibroblasts. Parents are obligate heterozygotes and have partially decreased enzyme levels. It is important to exclude sialidosis, and to be prepared for prenatal diagnosis. Specific mutations may be detected by DNA-based diagnosis.

Late Infantile GM1-Gangliosidosis

Symptoms begin between ages 1 and 3 years, with gait ataxia, hypotonia, hyperreflexia, dysarthria, and speech regression. Seizures, dementia, and spastic quadriplegia lead to death, usually by pneumonia. Optic atrophy and evidence of anterior horn-cell disease may be found. Corneas are clear, organomegaly is absent, and bone changes are scanty. Diagnosis is made in the same manner as for the infantile form.

Fabry Disease

Angiokeratoma corporis diffusum is an X-linked disorder in which the skin, kidney, peripheral- and autonomic-nervous systems, and blood vessels store trihexosylceramide (galactosyl galactosylglucosylceramide), a breakdown product of globoside (Fig. 84.1C). Trihexosylceramide accumulates because of a deficiency of trihexosylceramide β-galactosidase (reaction 4, Fig. 84.1C), also known as β-galactosidase A. Fabry disease is the only X-linked sphingolipidosis. It is incompletely recessive; that is, some female heterozygotes are clinically affected.

Symptoms usually commence in childhood or adolescence, with lancinating pains in the limbs, especially the feet and hands often brought on by temperature changes, and accompanied by paresthesia or abdominal crises. Anhydrosis and unexplained fever are common.

The characteristic skin lesions, which become more numerous with age, are purple, macular and maculopapular, hyperkeratotic, 1 to 3 mm in size, and with a predilection for the groin, buttocks, scrotum, and umbilicus. Glycolipid storage in the renal glomeruli and tubules begins with asymptomatic proteinuria in children; it progresses to renal failure and hypertension in the third or fourth decade. Glycolipid storage in blood-vessel walls may cause stroke. Edema of the limbs, whorled-corneal clouding (cornea verticillata) visible by slit lamp, and myocardial involvement may occur. Enzyme-replacement therapy has been demonstrated to reverse lipid storage in the kidney, heart, and blood vessels, and to produce corresponding improvement or reversal of renal impairment, pain, cardiac function, and cerebral blood flow. In some cases, renal transplant may still be required when renal failure supervenes. The lancinating pains may respond to phenytoin, carbamazepine, or gabapentin.

Heterozygous girls may also be affected, but manifestations are less marked. Skin lesions are few or absent. Corneal opacity is more common. If renal or cardiac involvement occurs, they are later in onset, and less severe. Fabry disease is diagnosed by finding decreased β-galactosidase activity in plasma and leukocytes, and a mutation in the β-galactosidase gene.

Gaucher Disease

Gaucher disease is an autosomal-recessive sphingolipidosis, in which glucocerebroside (Fig. 84.1B and C) is stored as a result of deficiency of glucocerebroside β-glucosidase (or glucocerebrosidase; reaction 6, Fig. 84.1, B and C). At least four forms have been described (Table 84.1): the infantile neuronopathic form, the juvenile neuronopathic form, the adult neuronopathic form, and the adult non-neuronopathic form.

These distinctions seem to be artificial, with overlapping manifestations occurring across a broad spectrum of phenotypes. The adult (nonneuropathic) form (Type I) is more common in Ashkenazi Jews than in the general population. Diagnosis of all forms is made by demonstrating reduced glucocerebroside β-glucosidase activity in cultured skin fibroblasts or blood leukocytes, and further refined by demonstrating mutations in the β-glucosidase gene.

▶ **TABLE 84.1** Lipidoses

Disorder	Defective Enzyme (Reaction Number)	Stored Material	Clinical Features
GM2-gangliosidoses	Hexosaminidase (3)	GM2, GA2, GL-4 globoside, OLS, ?GP, ?MPS	Infantile- to adult-onset phenotypes ranging from infantile encephalopathy with macular cherry-red spots to adult-onset spinal muscular atrophy
GM1-gangliosidoses	β-Galactosidase (2)	GM1, GA1, OLS, KS-like material	
Infantile form			Infantile encephalopathy, organomegaly, skeletal involvement, macular cherry-red spot (50%), corneal haze (occasionally)
Late-infantile form			Onset at age 1–3 yr of dementia, seizures, ataxia, dysarthria, spastic quadriplegia
Fabry disease	α-Galactosidase (4)	Ceramide trihexoside, ? blood group substance type B	Purple skin lesions, painful hands and feet, renal disease, leg edema, stroke
Gaucher disease	β-Glucosidase (6)	Glucocerebroside	
Infantile neuronopathic form			Onset at age 3 mo of dementia, organomegaly, poor suck and swallowing, opisthotonus, spasticity, seizures
Juvenile neuronopathic form			Variable onset of mental defect, splenomegaly, incoordination, seizures
Adult neuronopathic form			Splenomegaly (sometimes in infancy) and bony involvement; Ashkenazi Jewish predilection
Adult neuronopathic form			Splenomegaly, bony involvement, seizures, dementia
Niemann-Pick disease			
Infantile neuronopathic form, type A	Sphingomyelinase (26)	Sphingomyelin, cholesterol	Infantile encephalopathy, organomegaly, macular cherry-red spot (30%), lung infiltrates; Ashkenazi Jewish predilection
Juvenile nonneuronopathic form, type B	Sphingomyelinase (26)	Sphingomyelin, cholesterol	Hepatosplenomegaly
Juvenile neuronopathic form, type C	Endosomal trafficking defect (NPC1 or NPC2 gene)	Sphingomyelin, cholesterol	Onset at age 1–3 yr of dementia, seizures, spasticity, ataxia; hepatosplenomegaly less prominent
Nova Scotia variant, type D	Endosomal trafficking defect	Cholesterol, cholesterol ester, sphingomyelin, bis (monoacylglyceryl) phosphate	Infantile hepatosplenomegaly, onset age 2–5 yr of dementia, seizures, ataxia, spasticity
Adult nonneuronopathic from, type E	?	Sphingomyelin	Adult hepatosplenomegaly
Juvenile nonneuronopathic from, type F	Sphingomyelinase (26)	Sphingomyelin	Resembles type B, juvenile hepatosplenomegaly, sea-blue histiocytes, heat-labile sphingomyelinase
Farber disease	Acid ceramidase	Ceramide	Early infantile painful swollen joints, subcutaneous nodules, organomegaly, enlarged heart, dysphagia, vomiting, normal or impaired mentation
Wolman disease	Acid lipase	Cholesterol ester, triglyceride	Early infantile organomegaly, vomiting, diarrhea, jaundice, variable nervous system involvement
Refsum disease	Phytanic acid α-hydroxylase	Phytanic acid	Night blindness, retinitis pigmentosa, ataxia, demyelinating neuropathy, ichthyosis
Cerebrotendinous xanthomatosis	Mitochondrial enzyme 27-sterol hydroxylase (CYP 27)	Cholestanol, cholesterol	Static encephalopathy in first decade, adolescent or adult-onset cataracts, tendon xanthomas, ataxia, spasticity

(*continued*)

▶ **TABLE 84.1** Lipidoses (Continued)

Disorder	Defective Enzyme (Reaction Number)	Stored Material	Clinical Features
Neuronal lipofuscinoses (Batten disease)	CLN1, CLN2, CLN3, CLN4, CLN5 gene products	Retinoic acid derivatives, dolichol derivatives (whether this storage is primary or secondary is unclear)	
Infantile (Finnish) form (Santavuori disease)	Palmitoyl-protein thioesterase enzyme (CNL1 gene)		Infantile onset of progressive visual loss, retinal degeneration, myoclonic jerks, microcephaly
Late-infantile form (Jansky-Bielschowsky)	(CLN2 gene) Tripeptidyl peptidase 1		Onset at age 1–4 yr of seizures, ataxia, dementia, then visual deterioration and retinal degeneration
Juvenile form (Spielmeyer-Sjögren)	CLN3 gene product		Onset at age 5–10 yr of progressive visual loss and pigmentary retinal degeneration, then seizures and dementia
Adult form (Kufs)			Adult onset of dementia, ataxia, seizures, and myoclonus

GM2, GM2-ganglioside; GA2, asialo-GM2-ganglioside; OLS, oligosaccharide; GP, glycoprotein; MPS, mucopolysaccharide; GM1, GM1-ganglioside; GA1, asialo-GM1-ganglioside; KS, keratan sulfate; DS, dermatan sulfate; HS, heparan sulfate; GM3, GM3-ganglioside; GD3, GD3-ganglioside.

Type II (Infantile Neuronopathic) Gaucher Disease

This disease occurs in the first year of life, often in the first 3 months. The course is rapid, with developmental regression and death before age 2 years. Affected infants lose weight, reflecting the mechanical compression of the gut and the hypercatabolic state associated with pronounced hepatosplenomegaly. They have stridor, difficulty in sucking and swallowing, strabismus, retrocollis, spasticity, and hyperreflexia. Bilateral esotropia is typical. Later, they enter a vegetative state, becoming flaccid and weak. Seizures may occur. Macular cherry-red spots and optic atrophy do not occur.

Type III (Juvenile Neuronopathic) Gaucher Disease

The manifestations range from a severe form, presenting in infancy as pulmonary infiltrates, splenomegaly, and cardiorespiratory failure, to a progressive myoclonic dementia in adolescents or adults (i.e., the Norrbottnian form, common in the northern provinces of Sweden). Horizontal supranuclear-gaze palsy, with characteristic looping movements, is an important clue to the diagnosis

Type I (Adult) Gaucher Disease

These patients have visceral (e.g., liver, lymph nodes, lung) and skeletal manifestations, without primary neurologic disease. Multiple myeloma may be a late complication. It is most common in Ashkenazi Jews. Type 1 Gaucher disease presents at any age, from infancy to the seventh decade. Splenectomy should be avoided unless enzyme-replacement therapy is not possible, or the mechanical and

hematologic manifestations are not otherwise controlled. Lesions of long bones, pelvis, or vertebral bodies may be painful. Severe cases may require surgical intervention, including joint replacement. Enzyme-replacement therapy, with purified modified β-glucosidase, (i.e., alglucerase), or recombinant β-glucosidase, (i.e., imiglucerase), reverses all of the manifestations of Type 1 Gaucher disease, provided that treatment begins before severe tissue damage has occurred.

Adult Neuronopathic Gaucher Disease

Parkinsonism has been reported to be more frequent in some studies of adults with Gaucher disease. The subject is currently under investigation.

Niemann-Pick Disease

This group of disorders includes several diseases that were grouped together in 1958 by Crocker and Farber, on the basis of the overlapping pathology (i.e., visceral foam cells) and biochemistry (i.e., lysosomal storage of the glycosphingolipid sphingomyelin, ceramide phosphorylcholine) (Fig. 84.1E). Crocker subsequently proposed four groups. It is now recognized that his groups A and B are primary sphingomyelinase deficiencies, whereas groups C and D are allelic disorders, whose primary defect is not deficiency of a lysosomal hydrolase, but is in intracellular lipid trafficking. Patients with types A and B Niemann-Pick disease have deficient activity of the sphingomyelin-cleaving enzyme acid, sphingomyelinase (reaction 26, Fig. 84.1E). The diagnosis should be suspected in patients with progressive hepatosplenomegaly, with or without cerebral symptoms. The bone marrow contains characteristic mulberry storage cells (i.e., distinct from Gaucher cells). Decreased sphingomyelinase activity may be shown in cultured skin fibroblasts, leukocytes, or tissue.

Infantile Niemann-Pick Disease, Type A

This is the most common and most severe form of Niemann-Pick disease and occurs more commonly in Ashkenazi Jews. Transient neonatal jaundice is followed by progressive hepatosplenomegaly; developmental regression and weight loss lead to dementia, hypotonia, and death by age 2 years. About one-third of patients develop macular cherry-red spots (Fig. 84.4). Seizures are uncommon. Bone involvement is mild. Skin often has a brownish-yellow tinge. Most patients have diffuse haziness or patchy infiltrates in the lungs.

Diagnosis is made by the characteristic clinical picture, by finding foam cells in the bone marrow, and by demonstration of nearly total deficiency of sphingomyelinase (reaction 26, Fig. 84.1E) in leukocytes and cultured skin fibroblasts.

Juvenile Non-neuronopathic, Type B

This form presents with asymptomatic splenomegaly or hepatosplenomegaly, without neurologic disorder, in infants, children, or adults. Foam cells appear in the bone marrow, and sphingomyelinase (reaction 26, Fig. 84.1E) is reduced in cultured skin fibroblasts and leukocytes. These patients have more residual sphingomyelinase (i.e., 15% to 20% of normal) than those with type A (i.e., up to 10%).

Niemann-Pick Disease Type C

Niemann-Pick disease, type C (NPC), may arise at any age, from fetal life (i.e., with ascites) to the fifth or sixth decades. Early-onset disease is dominated by hepatic and pulmonary failure, which are usually lethal in infancy. Classic childhood-onset disease more often presents insidiously, with school failure and clumsiness that evolve into a progressive syndrome of ataxia, dystonia, and dementia. Vertical supranuclear-gaze palsy is characteristic and almost invariably presents early, although often unrecognized. About 50% of patients have seizures, and 20% experience gelastic cataplexy. Hepatosplenomegaly is variable, and its absence does not rule out NPC. Genetic isolates have been described in Nova Scotia (i.e., formerly Niemann-Pick disease, type D) and in Hispanics in Colorado and New Mexico.

Most patients with NPC are compound heterozygotes for mutations in NPC1; the gene product is a large transmembrane protein, localized to the late endosomal-lysosomal pathway. Dysfunction of this protein is associated with impaired trafficking of large molecules in this pathway, with accumulation of glycolipids, sphin-

gomyelin, and cholesterol in lysosomes. The diagnosis rests on demonstration of this defect. Direct DNA analysis is not practical as a first line diagnostic test, owing to the size of the gene and the large number of mutations (i.e., more than 150 recognized to date). The current diagnostic test requires demonstration of impaired esterification of radio-labeled, exogenous cholesterol in cultured fibroblasts, and its subsequent accumulation in lysosomes, identified by filipin staining. It should be borne in mind that this is an indirect index of the functional defect, with a significant number of variant cases with results that may be difficult to distinguish from heterozygotes.

A small number of cases of NPC are associated with mutations in a second gene, NPC2, and the gene product is a soluble, lysosomal protein of uncertain functional relationship to the NPC protein.

Farber Lipogranulomatosis

Infants with this disease present with painful swollen joints, hoarseness, vomiting, respiratory difficulty, or limb edema, in the first few months of life, sometimes as early as 2 weeks of age.

Subcutaneous nodules arise near joints and tendon sheaths, especially on the hands, arms, and at pressure points such as the occiput or lumbosacral spine. Other findings include cardiac enlargement and murmurs, lymphadenopathy, hepatomegaly, splenomegaly, enlarged tongue, difficulty in swallowing, and pulmonary granulomas. Tendon reflexes may be hyperactive or hypoactive. Mental development may be normal or impaired. Seizures do not occur. CSF protein may be elevated.

Ceramide (Fig. 84.1, B to E) and some related compounds accumulate in foam cells in affected tissues because of acid-ceramidase deficiency (reaction 7, Fig. 84.1, B to E). This enzyme catabolizes ceramide to sphingosine and fatty acid. Neutral ceramidase is not decreased. Diagnosis is made by demonstrating deficiency of acid-ceramidase activity in cultured skin fibroblasts or leukocytes. Prenatal diagnosis and carrier testing are possible. Most patients die of pulmonary disease before age 2 years, but some survive into adolescence.

Wolman Disease

Infants affected by Wolman disease are normal at birth but in the first few weeks of life have severe vomiting, abdominal distention, diarrhea, poor weight gain, jaundice, and unexplained fever. Hepatosplenomegaly may be massive, and there may be a papulo-vesiculo-pustular rash on face, neck, shoulders, and chest. The extent of neurologic disorder is not clear because the infants are so sick and die so early. Initially, they are active and alert, but activity decreases. Corticospinal tract signs have been found in some.

Laboratory findings include anemia and foam cells in bone marrow. Calcification of the adrenals on plain xrays is characteristic. The course is usually rapidly progressive. Death usually occurs within 3 to 6 months, but some patients survive into the second year. The lipid storage consists primarily of cholesterol ester and smaller amounts of triglyceride, because there is severe deficiency of a lysosomal fatty-acid ester acid-hydrolase (i.e., acid lipase, acid esterase, or acid cholesteryl ester hydrolase), which cleaves cholesterol ester, triglycerides, and artificial substrates. Nearly total deficiency of this acid lipase is found in tissues, leukocytes, and cultured fibroblasts from patients; carriers have been detected, and prenatal diagnosis is possible. The enzyme is coded for a gene on the long arm of chromosome 10 (10q23.2).

A milder allelic form of Wolman disease with deficiency of the same enzyme is called cholesterol-ester storage disease. These patients have hepatomegaly, with or without splenomegaly, hypercholesterolemia, and foam cells in the bone marrow.

Cerebrotendinous Xanthomatosis (Cholestanol Storage Disease)

Although patients with cholestanol storage disease often have mental defects of early onset, the diagnosis is difficult to make in the first decade because cataracts, tendon xanthomas, and progressive spasticity, usually associated with ataxia, commonly do not begin before adolescence or young adulthood. The spasticity and ataxia are severe and progressive. Speech is affected. Neuropathy may appear with distal-muscle wasting. Sensory deficits and Babinski signs are seen. Pseudobulbar palsy develops terminally. Death from neurologic disease or myocardial infarction usually occurs in the fourth to sixth decade. Some patients have apparently normal mental function.

Tendon xanthomas are almost always seen on the Achilles tendon and may occur elsewhere. The cerebellar hemispheres contain large (i.e., up to 1.5 cm), granulomatous, xanthomas with extensive demyelination. Microscopically, cystic areas of necrosis and clear needle-shaped clefts contain birefringent material surrounded by macrophages, with foamy vacuolated cytoplasm and multinucleated giant cells. The brain stem and spinal cord may be involved.

Cholestanol is increased in bile, plasma, brain, and tendon xanthomas. Cholesterol is increased in tendon xanthomas but is usually normal in plasma. Chenodeoxycholic acid, a major component of normal bile, is virtually absent.

Diagnosis is based on biochemical findings and demonstration of mutations in the sterol 27-hydroxylase gene (CYP27). Treatment with bile acids may be beneficial.

Neuronal Ceroid Lipofuscinoses

The neuronal ceroid lipofuscinoses (NCL) were previously defined by histologic and ultrastructural features, and a plethora of confusing and inconsistently applied eponyms, but are now classified according to genotypes or genetic linkage. The common pathologic features include neurons engorged with periodic acid-Schiff–positive and autofluorescent material on light microscopy, and abnormal lipopigments resembling ceroid and lipofuscin within distinctive abnormal cytosomes, such as curvilinear and fingerprint bodies, on electron microscopy. Although the signs and symptoms are confined to the nervous system, the abnormal cytosomes are widely distributed in skin, muscle, peripheral nerves, leukocytes, urine sediment, and viscera. Dolichol is elevated in tissue and urine sediment.

Genes for infantile- (CLN1), late infantile- (CLN2) and juvenile- (CLN3) neuronal ceroid lipofuscinoses have been cloned. CLN1 codes for the palmityl protein thioesterase enzyme; mutations in this gene also cause a juvenile form of neuronal-ceroid lipofuscinosis, with granular osmiophilic deposits. CLN2 also codes for a lysosomal enzyme, but the function of the CLN3 protein is not yet known. CLN5 codes for a putative, transmembrane protein.

Goebel and Wisniewski found that approximately 20% of a series of 520 patients with NCL could not be classified as CLN1, 2, 3 or 4. Turkish, Finnish, and Gypsy-Indian variants of LINCL (CLN2) have been identified as separate genotypes, as has a Northern epilepsy variant also characterized as progressive epilepsy with mental retardation. These new groups have been designated CLN 5 through 8.

The diagnosis of NCL1 and NCL2 may be made by enzyme assay and confirmed by mutational analysis. Diagnosis of NCL3 is confirmed by mutational analysis without a specific functional test. Linkage tests allow specific classification of several other subtypes. A database listing NCL mutations is available online at *http://www.ucl.ac.uk/ncl.*

Supporting investigations include an abnormal electroretinogram in the infantile, late-infantile, and juvenile forms, and electron microscopic examination of tissue (i.e., skin, nerve, muscle, or rectal biopsy for autonomic neurons). Abnormal autofluorescence is seen on examination of frozen section of biopsied muscle, enabling rapid diagnosis. The neuronal-ceroid lipofuscinoses are autosomal-recessive diseases.

NCL1: Infantile (Finnish) Variant (INCL, Haltia-Santavuori Disease)

Infantile (Finnish) Variant (INCL, Haltia-Santavuori Disease) is a variant of neuronal ceroid lipofuscinosis that begins at about 8 months of age, with progressive visual loss, loss of developmental milestones, myoclonic jerks, and microcephaly. There is optic atrophy, macular and retinal degeneration, and a flat electroretinogram. Progression is rapid, but some infants survive for several years.

NCL 2: Late-infantile Variant (LINCL, Jansky-Bielschowsky Disease)

This begins between 1.5 and 4 years of age, with seizures and ataxia. Seizures respond poorly to anticonvulsants. There is progressive visual deterioration, with abolished electroretinogram and retinal deterioration. Progression is usually rapid, leading to a vegetative state, but some affected children survive several years.

NCL3: Juvenile Variant (JNCL, Spielmeyer-Sjögren Disease)

This variant of neuronal ceroid lipofuscinosis begins with progressive visual loss occurring between the ages of 5 and 10 years, with pigmentary degeneration of the retina. Seizures, dementia, and motor abnormalities occur later, and progress to death by the end of the second decade. The storage material contains large amounts of the ATP-synthase subunit-C protein.

NCL4: Adult Variant (ANCL, Kufs Disease)

About half of these cases present before 10 years of age, and the remainder, as late as the third or fourth decade of life, with progressive dementia, seizures, myoclonus, and ataxia. Blindness and retinal degeneration are not features of the adult form.

LEUKODYSTROPHIES

The leukodystrophies are progressive, genetic metabolic disorders causing dysmyelination (Table 84.2).

Krabbe leukodystrophy (i.e., globoid-cell leukodystrophy) was initially defined by the presence of globoid cells in demyelinated portions of the brain. Metachromatic leukodystrophy (MLD) was set apart by abnormal tissue metachromasia. Adrenoleukodystrophy was set apart by involvement of adrenal glands and by X-linked inheritance (see Chapter 87 for a discussion of adrenoleukodystrophy). Classic Pelizaeus-Merzbacher disease was set apart by X-linked inheritance, early onset, a long course, and islands of preserved myelin in the demyelinated areas. Advanced imaging techniques and molecular biology have led to the identification of childhood ataxia with central hypomyelination, or CACH (also known as vanishing white-matter disease) and megencephalic leucoencephalopathy with subcortical cysts (MLC) in a at least two genetic variants. This leaves a heterogeneous, but shrinking group of unclassified leukodystrophies, sometimes called orthochromatic or sudanophilic leukodystrophies.

Metachromatic Leukodystrophy

MLD is a group of disorders with degeneration of central (Fig. 84.6) and peripheral myelin, striking metachromasia of the stored substances, primarily sulfatides, and deficiency of the sulfatide-cleaving enzyme, sulfatase A (reaction 9, Fig. 84.1D), also called arylsulfatase A. At least four forms are known, the late-infantile form being the most common. All have autosomal-recessive inheritance.

Alleles causing sulfatase A deficiency and MLD have either absent or low residual-enzyme activity. Patients with two alleles giving absent-enzyme activity have the severe, late-infantile MLD. Patients with two alleles giving low residual-enzyme activity have the mildest, adult-type MLD. Compound heterozygotes with one allele of each type have the intermediate, juvenile form of MLD.

The diagnosis of MLD is complicated by the existence of sulfatase A pseudodeficiency, an autosomal-recessive condition in which sulfatase A activity is greatly diminished by the usual enzyme assays, but there is no neurologic disease. An additional complication is the requirement of sulfatase A for the sulfatide-activator protein. Patients with genetic deficiency of sulfatide-activator protein may have MLD, but the commonly used enzyme assays may fail to diagnose this. Consequently, a high index of suspicion is required even if screening tests are apparently normal.

Late-Infantile Metachromatic Leukodystrophy

Affected infants have onset of difficulty in walking after the first year of life, usually between ages 12 and 30 months. Flaccid paresis and diminished, or absent, tendon reflexes are typical, but occasionally spastic paresis develops. Genu recurvatum may be noted. Progressive dementia and dysarthria follow.

Peripheral neuropathy leads to loss of tendon reflexes, and may be accompanied by limb pain. Later, patients become bedridden and quadriplegic, with feeding difficulties, bulbar and pseudobulbar palsies, and optic atrophy. Children so affected usually die in the first decade of life, blind and in a vegetative state. Investigations show increased CSF protein content, impaired gallbladder function, metachromatic lipids on sural nerve biopsy, and increased urinary-sulfatide excretion.

Sulfatide accumulates in brain, peripheral nerves, and some extraneural tissues (e.g., kidney). Sulfatide causes brown metachromasia, with acetic acid-cresyl violet staining in glial cells, Schwann cells, myelin lamellae, and neurons. Characteristic "tuffstone" bodies are seen by electron microscopy.

▶ **TABLE 84.2** Leukodystrophies

Clinical Disorder	Defective Enzyme (Reaction Number)	Stored Material	Clinical Features
Krabbe leukodystrophy (GLD)			
Infantile form	Galactocerebrosidase (10)	Psychosine Galacto-cerebroside	Onset at age 3–6 mo of irritability, spasticity, seizures, fevers. Progressive mental and motor loss to blind decerebrate vegetative state, with optic atrophy, decreased tendon reflexes, decreased nerve conduction velocities, increased CSF protein
Juvenile form	Galactocerebrosidase (10)	Galactocerebroside Psychosine	Juvenile onset of dementia, optic atrophy, pyramidal tract disorder
Adult form	Galactocerebrosidase (10)	Galactocerebroside Psychosine	Adult onset of slowly progressive dementia, optic atrophy, and pyramidal signs
Metachromatic leukodystrophy (MLD)			
Late-infantile form	Sulfatase A (9)	Sulfatide	Onset at age 1–2.5 yr of walking difficulty with weakness, ataxia or spasticity; progressive dementia, optic atrophy, loss of deep tendon reflexes; slow nerve conduction velocities, increased CSF protein
Juvenile form	Sulfatase A (9)	Sulfatide	Onset at age 3–10 yr of dementia, gait difficulty, neuropathy, elevated CSF protein; more slowly progressive
Adult form	Sulfatase A (9)	Sulfatide	Adult-onset dementia, often with ataxia and pyramidal findings; slowly progressive
MLD without sulfatase A deficiency	Sulfatase A (9) activator	Sulfatide	Same as late-infantile or juvenile form
Asymptomatic or presymptomatic adults with sulfatase A deficiency	Sulfatase A (9)	Sulfatide	Normal
Multiple sulfatase deficiency (mucosulfatidosis, MSD)	Sulfatase A (9) Sulfatase B (17) Sulfatase C Cholesterol sulfate sulfatase Dehydroepiandrosterone sulfate sulfatase Iduronate-2-sulfate sulfatase (12) Sulfamidase (13) N-acetylgalactosamine-6-sulfate sulfatase (16) N-acetylglucosamine-6-sulfate sulfatase (19) Basic defect presumed to be an enzyme affecting posttranslational modification of all sulfatases	Sulfatide MPS	Slowed early development. Onset at age 1–2 yr of mental and motor deterioration and seizures; mildly coarsened facial features, ichthyosis, organomegaly, skeletal changes

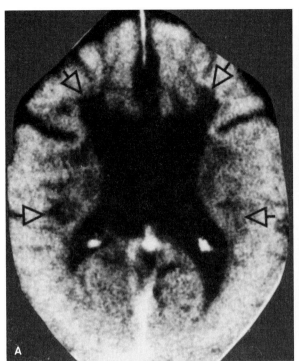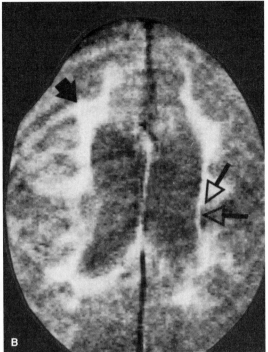

FIGURE 84.6. **A:** Standard CT projection through the center cerebrum. Open arrows indicate symmetrical lesions of markedly decreased absorption in white matter. Adult MLD, age 36. **B:** A more T₂-weighted MRI scan of the same patient. Black arrow shows the confluent hyperintense signal in diseased white matter. So shrunken is this white matter that gyri now extend down next to the ventricle (open arrows).

Sulfatide consists primarily of galactosylsulfatide (Fig. 84.1D), although a smaller amount of lactosylsulfatide is found. The diagnosis is based primarily on enzyme analysis, supported when necessary by demonstration of histologic and ultrastructural abnormalities in myelinated fibers of biopsied sural nerve or conjunctiva.

Juvenile Metachromatic Leukodystrophy

These patients have the clinical features of juvenile MLD, which are similar to those of late-infantile MLD, but for the later onset of symptoms (i.e., usually ages 3 to 10 years) and slower progression of the disease. Patients with juvenile MLD present more frequently with emotional disturbance or dementia, although gait disorder may be the initial symptom. Nystagmus and tremor may be noted. Nerve conduction velocities are slowed and CSF protein concentrations are elevated.

Adult Metachromatic Leukodystrophy

MLD commonly starts in adults in the third or fourth decade, as a psychiatric disorder or progressive dementia. Other findings may include truncal ataxia, hyperactive reflexes, and seizures. CSF protein concentration is usually not elevated. The illness runs a protracted course, averaging 15 years.

Multiple Sulfatase Deficiency

This rare disorder, also known as sulfatidosis, Austin-type, or mucosulfatidosis, has clinical features of MLD and mucopolysaccharidosis, with excretion of both sulfatide and mucopolysaccharide in urine, and deficiencies in at least nine sulfatases. Onset is usually earlier than with late-infantile MLD. Early development is slow. Patients do not achieve normal gait or speech, although they may walk and speak single words.

The disease resembles late-infantile MLD, with additional features including mildly coarsened facial features, ichthyosis, and sometimes hepatosplenomegaly and dysotosis multiplex. The histologic changes in brain and peripheral nerve resemble those of late-infantile MLD. Metachromatic material is found in liver, spleen, and kidney. The diagnosis is based on the characteristic clinical picture and the findings of deficiencies of sulfatase A and other sulfatases in cultured skin fibroblasts.

The biochemical basis for multiple-sulfatase deficiency rests on the requirement of posttranslational modification to activate sulfatases. This modification conversion of a cysteine residue, to 2-amino-3-oxopropionic acid, is believed to be defective in multiple-sulfatase deficiency.

Krabbe (Globoid-Cell) Leukodystrophy

Patients are normal at birth. Symptoms begin at ages 3 to 6 months, with irritability, inexplicable crying, fevers, rigidity, seizures, feeding difficulty, vomiting, and slowing of mental and motor development. Later, psychomotor regression occurs, accompanied by increasing tone and extensor posturing. Reflexes may be increased before being lost. Optic atrophy is frequent. Patients may develop flaccidity or flexor postures before death, at about 2 years of age.

Important diagnostic features are increased CSF protein content and decreased nerve-conduction velocities. On electron microscopy, sural-nerve biopsy specimens show needle-like inclusions in histiocytes and Schwann cells, also seen in globoid cells in demyelinated brain regions (Fig. 84.7).

Galactocerebrosidase (reaction 10, Fig. 84.1D) is deficient, as seen in serum, leukocytes, and cultured skin fibroblasts. Both galactosylcerebroside and galactosylsphingosine (i.e., psychosine) are substrates for that enzyme. Psychosine is increased at least 200-fold over levels in the normal brain, where it is barely detectable. Psychosine toxicity is probably the cause of the disease, based on studies showing its ability to produce characteristic lesions in animal models.

A few patients with juvenile-onset and slower progression of dementia, optic atrophy, and pyramidal tract signs, without neuropathy, have had galactocerebrosidase deficiency. An adult-onset disorder with a similar but more slowly progressive course has been described.

MUCOPOLYSACCHARIDOSES

The mucopolysaccharidoses (MPS) are defined by a characteristic phenotype and by the tissue storage and urinary excretion of acid mucopolysaccharide (Table 84.3). They were originally considered a single disease, but eight clinical types, and numerous subtypes, are now known. Each is caused by deficiency of a lysosomal hydrolase required for degradation of one or more of three sulfated mucopolysaccharides: dermatan sulfate, heparan sulfate, and keratan sulfate (Fig. 84.2).

Diagnosis is suspected based on the clinical picture, presence of excessive amounts of one or more acid mucopolysaccharides in urine, and is confirmed by demonstrating a specific-enzyme defect. Urine screening tests for excess mucopolysaccharides are useful but are subject to false-positive and false-negative results. Positive screening tests require confirmation by quantitative and qualitative determination of urinary mucopolysaccharides, radiographic and histologic evidence of tissue storage, and demonstration of the enzyme defect. False negatives are relatively frequent in Sanfilippo and Morquio syndromes. If clinical suspicion for a mucopolysaccharidosis is high, diagnostic evaluation should be pursued, despite a negative urine screening test. Prenatal diagnosis of these disorders is available.

Hurler Syndrome

This is the most severe of the mucopolysaccharidoses, characterized by onset in infancy, progressive disability, and death usually occurring before 10 years of age. Nearly all the features found in other types are present in Hurler syndrome. Corneal clouding and lumbar gibbus occur in the first year of life, followed by stiff joints with periarticular swelling, short, stubby hands and feet, claw hands, lumbar lordosis, chest deformity, and dwarfing by 2 or 3 years of age. The facial features become coarsened, with thickened eyelids and lips, frontal bossing, bushy eyebrows, a depressed nasal bridge, ocular hypertelorism, enlarged tongue, noisy breathing, rhinorrhea, and widely spaced, peg-like teeth. Psychomotor slowing is followed by dementia, but seizures are not typical. Deafness is frequent, and few patients develop speech. Leptomeningeal thickening, arachnoid cysts, and hydrocephalus may occur. Cardiac murmurs resulting from valvular heart disease, coronary

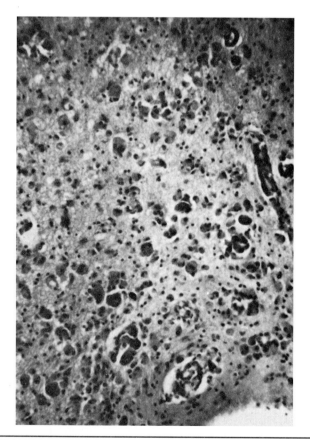

FIGURE 84.7. Globoid cells in white matter, Krabbe leukodystrophy (H&E stain).

▶ TABLE 84.3 Mucopolysaccharidoses

Syndrome Number	Syndrome Name	Stored Material	Deficient Enzyme	Reaction Number[a]	Mental Defect	Cloudy Corneas	Hearing Loss	Coarse Facial Features	Dwarfing	Dysostosis Multiplex	Heart Disease	Organomegaly	Other Features
MPS IH	Hurler	DS,HS	α-L-Iduronidase	11	3+	3+	2+	3+	3+	3+	3+	3+	Cord compression / Pigmentary retinopathy
MPS IH/S	Hurler-Scheie compound	DS,HS	α-L-Iduronidase	11	±	3+		2+	1+	2+	1+	2+	Severe arachnoid cysts / Pigmentary retinopathy
MPS IS	Scheie	DS	α-L-Iduronidase	11	0	3+	±	±	0	1+	1+	±	Carpal tunnel syndrome
MPS II A	Hunter (severe)	DS,HS	Iduronate-2-sulfate sulfatase	12	+	0	3+	2+	2+	2+	±	1+	Nodular skin lesions / Pigmentary retinopathy
MPS II B	Hunter (mild)	DS,HS	Iduronate-2-sulfate sulfatase	12	0	0	2+	1+	1+	1+	±	±	Carpal tunnel syndrome / Nodular skin lesions
MPS III A	Sanfilippo A	HS	Sulfamidase	13	3+	0	2+	1+	0	1+	1+	1+	Retinal degeneration / May have seizures
MPS III B	Sanfilippo B	HS	α-N-acetylglucosaminidase	14	3+	0	2+	1+	0	1+	1+	1+	Retinal degeneration
MPS III C	Sanfilippo C	HS	N-acetyltransferase	15	3+	0	2+	1+	0	1+	1+	1+	
MPS III D	Sanfilippo D	HS, KS	N-acetylglucosamine-6-sulfate sulfatase	19	2+	0	1+	0	1+	1+	0	1+	Odontoid hypoplasia
MPS IV A	Morquio A	KS	Galactose-6-sulfate sulfatase	16	0	2+	2+	1+	3+	3+	2+	±	Cord compression / Odontoid hypoplasia
MPS IV B	Morquio B	KS, OLS	β-Galactosidase	2	0	1+	0	0	0	2+	0	0	
MPS V	Category vacant	—	—										
MPS VI A	Maroteaux-Lamy (severe)	DS	Sulfatase B	17	0	2+	2+	2+	2+	2+	2+	±	Cord compression / Carpal tunnel syndrome / Hydrocephalus
MPS VI B	Maroteaux-Lamy (intermediate)	DS	Sulfatase B	17	0	2+		±	1+	2+	2+	0	Carpal tunnel syndrome
MPS VI C	Maroteaux-Lamy (mild)	DS	Sulfatase B	17	0	1+		±	1+	1+	1+	0	Cord compression / Carpal tunnel syndrome
MPS VII	Sly	DS,HS	β-Glucuronidase	18	2+	±		1+	2+	2+	1+	1+	Hydrocephalus

[a] See Figs 83.1 through 83.3. OLS, oligosaccharide; MPS, mucopolysaccharide; KS, keratan sulfate; DS, dermatan sulfate; HS, heparan sulfate.

occlusion, and cardiac enlargement may occur and cause death. Abdominal distention is common, with inguinal and umbilical hernias, and hepatomegaly. Corneal clouding progresses, and with retinal degeneration, impairs vision. Cervical-cord compression with quadriplegia may occur.

Radiographic changes support the diagnosis of mucopolysaccharidosis but do not, reliably, distinguish the various types. Findings include ovoid or beaked lumbar vertebrae, peg-shaped metacarpals, a J-shaped sella turcica, and spatulate ribs. Peripheral leukocytes and bone-marrow cells contain metachromatic granules. Clear vacuoles are seen in hepatocytes and other cells. Zebra bodies containing lipids occur in the brain. Both dermatan sulfate and heparan sulfate (Fig. 84.2) are stored. α-L-iduronidase (reaction 11, Fig. 84.2), required for degradation of both, is deficient. The diagnosis is made by demonstrating severe deficiency of α-L-iduronidase in cultured skin fibroblasts and leukocytes. The α-L-iduronidase gene is located on the short arm of chromosome 4.

Scheie syndrome (MPS IS), a milder allelic variant of Hurler syndrome, is characterized by juvenile onset of joint stiffness, with the development of claw hands and deformed feet. Corneal clouding causes visual impairment; corneal grafts may also become opacified. Other features are pigmentary degeneration of the retina, glaucoma, coarse facial features, genu valgus, carpal-tunnel syndrome, and involvement of the aortic valve. Deafness may occur. Stature and intelligence are normal. Psychologic disturbances have been reported. Lifespan is normal unless cardiac involvement is severe. A phenotype intermediate between that of the Hurler and Scheie syndromes is referred to as the Hurler-Scheie compound (MPS I HS). Distinction from other α-L-iduronidase deficiency disorders is solely clinical.

Hunter Syndrome (MPS II)

Hunter syndrome includes mild and severe forms. Both are X-linked recessive and show iduronate-2-sulfatase deficiency (reaction 12, Fig. 84.2). A Hunter-like phenocopy in girls with iduronate-2-sulfatase deficiency occurs in the context of total sulfatase deficiency (MLD, Austin-type).

Boys with the severe form experience juvenile-onset joint stiffness, coarse facial features, dysostosis multiplex, hepatosplenomegaly, diarrhea, dwarfing, and mental deterioration. Progressive deafness is prominent. Pigmentary retinal deterioration, papilledema, and hydrocephalus may be seen. Nodular or pebbled-skin change over the scapulae, and absence of corneal clouding are important features distinguishing Hunter from Hurler syndrome. Patients usually die by age 15 years.

Patients with the mild form of Hunter syndrome may be asymptomatic. They have short stature, joint stiffness and limitation of motion, coarse features, and hepatosplenomegaly. They may have hernias and carpal-tunnel syndrome. Intelligence is normal, but papilledema

and neurologic deterioration may occur late in the course. Lifespan may be normal.

Patients excrete excess urinary dermatan sulfate and heparan sulfate (Fig. 84.2). Diagnosis requires the demonstration of iduronate-2-sulfatase deficiency (reaction 12, Fig. 84.2) in serum or in cultured skin fibroblasts.

Sanfilippo Syndrome (MPS III)

Patients with this syndrome have progressive cognitive impairment, mild somatic involvement, and urinary excretion of heparan sulfate, alone. Four biochemically distinct forms reflect four metabolic steps required for the degradation of heparan sulfate, but not dermatan sulfate or keratan sulfate. Sanfilippo patients have juvenile-onset dementia, with delay or deterioration of speech or school performance. Children presenting with psychiatric disorder, mental retardation, or dementia should be carefully examined for mild coarsening of facial features, hepatosplenomegaly, hirsutism, joint stiffness, and radiographic changes of dysostosis multiplex. These patients deteriorate neurologically, with progressive dementia, spastic quadriparesis, tetraballism, athetosis, incontinence, and seizures. Cardiac involvement may occur. Corneal clouding is absent. Bone changes, dwarfing, and organ enlargement are slight. Patients may die in adolescence or survive into the third decade of life.

The diagnosis is made by the characteristic clinical picture, excess heparan sulfaturia, and demonstration of the enzyme defect. Screening tests for mucopolysacchariduria may be negative in Sanfilippo syndrome.

In Sanfilippo syndrome type A, the enzyme heparan sulfate N-sulfatase (i.e., sulfamidase; reaction 13, Fig. 84.2) is deficient. In type B, α-N-acetylglucosaminidase (reaction 14, Fig. 84.2) is lacking. In type C, an N-acetyltransferase is deficient (reaction 15, Fig. 84.2); this enzyme acetylates the amino group from which sulfamidase removes the sulfate (reaction 13, Fig. 84.2), thus allowing the N-acetylglucosaminidase (reaction 14, Fig. 84.2) to act. In type D, an N-acetylglucosamine-6-sulfatase is deficient (reaction 19, Fig. 84.2); this enzyme removes the 6-sulfate from N-acetylglucosamine in heparan sulfate and keratan sulfate. Type A is, by far, the most common phenotype.

Morquio Syndrome (MPS IV)

This mucopolysaccharidosis is characterized by a severe skeletal disorder, little neurologic abnormality, and the urinary excretion of keratan sulfate (Fig. 84.2). Two biochemically distinct forms are known, reflecting the two metabolic steps specifically required to degrade keratan sulfate.

Skeletal manifestations appear in the first year, as in Hurler syndrome, but corneal clouding is not prominent (i.e., corneas usually become mildly cloudy). Patients develop severe dwarfing, pectus carinatum, joint laxity, knock knees, short neck, sensorineural deafness, abnormal facies, and hepatosplenomegaly. Intelligence is normal. Owing to odontoid process hypoplasia and joint laxity, atlantoaxial subluxation may cause cervical-cord compression, even in young children; this may be prevented by posterior spinal fusion. Cardiac or respiratory disease may cause death in the third or fourth decade of life.

The diagnosis of type A is made by finding excess urinary keratan sulfate, and that of type B by finding excess urinary oligosaccharides, as well. Patients with type A Morquio syndrome lack an enzyme that cleaves 60 sulfate groups from galactose-6-sulfate (reaction 16, Fig. 84.2) and *N*-acetylgalactosamine-6-sulfate, causing the storage of keratan sulfate (i.e., which contains galactose-6-sulfate) and chondroitin-6-sulfate (i.e., which contains acetylgalactosamine-6-sulfate). The milder type-B form of Morquio syndrome is caused by deficiency of β-galactosidase (reaction 2, Fig. 84.2), the same enzyme that is deficient in GM1-gangliosidosis. Presumably, the Morquio mutation severely affects enzyme ability to cleave the β-galactoside linkage in keratan sulfate, but leaves sufficient activity against that linkage in GM1-ganglioside to prevent brain disease.

Maroteaux-Lamy Syndrome (MPS VI)

This syndrome resembles MPS type-I syndrome because of the prominent skeletal disease, but intelligence is normal, and the predominant urinary mucopolysaccharide is dermatan sulfate. It is distinguished from Scheie syndrome by the affected patient's short stature.

At least three forms of Maroteaux-Lamy syndrome are known, all with deficiency of *N*-acetylgalactosamine-4-sulfate sulfatase or arylsulfatase B (reaction 17, Fig. 84.2). In the severe form, growth retardation is apparent by ages 2 or 3 years. Coarse facial features, marked corneal clouding, and severe skeletal disease develop. Valvular disease and heart failure are common. Intelligence is normal, but neurologic complications include hydrocephalus and cervical-cord compression, resulting from instability of the craniocervical junction associated with hypoplasia of the odontoid process. Patients may survive into the second or third decade of life. In milder forms, cervical-cord compression and carpal-tunnel syndrome may occur.

MUCOLIPIDOSES

The mucolipidoses (Table 84.4) resemble the Hurler phenotype but lack excess urinary mucopolysaccharide, having instead, excess urinary oligosaccharides or glycopeptides, most of which are fragments of more complex structures (Fig. 84.3). Urinary thin-layer chromatography for oligosaccharides is a useful screening test.

Sialidosis

Patients with sialidoses have deficiency of α-L-neuraminidase, also known as sialidase (reaction 1, Figs. 84.1B and 84.3). In most forms, sialic acid-containing glycoproteins, oligosaccharides, and glycolipids accumulate in tissue, and sialyloligosaccharides are excreted in urine.

The diagnosis is based on clinical findings; the presence of abnormal sialyloligosaccharides in the urine; and deficiency of the appropriate sialidase in cultured skin fibroblasts, tissue, or leukocytes. There are at least two distinct lysosomal sialidases, one that cleaves the ($\alpha2,3$)-linked sialic acid in monosialoganglioside (reaction 8, Fig. 84.1B) and the other that cleaves ($\alpha2,3$)-linked and ($\alpha2,6$)-linked sialic acid in polysialogangliosides, oligosaccharides, and glycoproteins (reaction 1, Figs. 84.1B and 84.3). The latter enzyme is deficient in the other sialidoses.

In addition to the isolated sialidase deficiencies, two other groups of mucolipidoses have sialidase deficiency. In one, galactosialidosis and both sialidase and β-galactosidase are deficient because a stabilizing protein they share is defective. In the second group, mucolipidosis II and III, sialidase, and several other lysosomal hydrolases are deficient.

Sialidoses with isolated sialidase deficiency have a highly variable clinical picture. Neonates with congenital sialidoses have hydrops fetalis, hepatosplenomegaly, and short survival times. They resemble infants with congenital lipidosis of Norman and Wood. Infants with nephrosialidosis resemble the Hurler phenotype, and develop macular cherry-red spots and renal disease. Children with mucolipidosis I (i.e., lipomucopolysaccharidosis), a milder disorder, are similarly affected but develop ataxia, myoclonic jerks, and seizures. The mildest form is the cherry-red spot myoclonus disorder, in which adolescents who are usually mentally normal, develop macular cherry-red spots, myoclonus, and myoclonic seizures. There is a predilection for individuals of Italian descent.

Galactosialidosis

Sialidosis with combined sialidase and β-galactosidase deficiency (i.e., galactosialidosis) includes two forms: an infantile disorder with the clinical phenotype of GM1-gangliosidosis, and the Goldberg syndrome. The first disorder should be considered in any patient who is suspected of having GM1-gangliosidosis or is found to have β-galactosidase deficiency. Goldberg syndrome resembles mucolipidosis I, but is milder, with a predilection for those of Japanese origin; there is an adult form as well.

Free Sialic Acid Storage Diseases

Onset of Salla disease is between ages 4 and 12 months, with hypotonia, developmental delay, or both. Ataxia of trunk and limbs follows, and by age 2 years there is mental

▶ **TABLE 84.4 Mucolipidoses**

Clinical Disorder	Defective Enzyme (Reaction Number)[a]	Stored Material	Clinical Features
Sialidoses		GP, OLS, ? ganglioside	
Sialidoses with isolated sialidase deficiency			
Congenital sialidosis	Oligosaccharide sialidase (1)		Premature birth, congenital hydrops fetalis, organomegaly, severe mental and motor defect, death 0–5 mo
Severe infantile sialidosis	Oligosaccharide sialidase (1)		Similar to congenital sialidosis, but with renal disease and survival until age 2
Nephrosialidosis	Oligosaccharide sialidase (1)		Onset age 4–6 mo of organomegaly, facial dysmorphism and psychomotor retardation; progressive renal disease, macular cherry-red spot, and fine corneal opacities develop
Mucolipidosis I	Oligosaccharide sialidase (1)		Onset at age 6 mo of mild Hurler-like facial and skeletal changes, corneal clouding, macular cherry-red spot, mental defect, myoclonic jerks, cerebellar syndrome, seizures, neuropathy
Macular cherry-red spot myoclonus syndrome	Oligosaccharide sialidase (1)		Onset around age 10 yr of myoclonus, decreasing visual activity, and macular cherry-red spot; predilection for Italians
Sialidoses with additional β-galactosidase deficiency (galactosialidosis)			
Infantile sialidosis (GM$_1$-gangliosidosis phenotype)	Stabilizing protein for Oligosaccharide sialidase (1) and β-Galactosidase (2)		Same as GM$_1$-gangliosidosis
Goldberg syndrome	Stabilizing protein for Oligosaccharide sialidase (1) and β-galactosidase (2)		Similar to mucolipidosis I but juvenile or adolescent onset and slow progression, most common among Japanese
Salla disease	Sialic acid egress from lysosomes	Free sialic acid	Infantile onset of hypotonia, developmental delay; juvenile ataxia, mental and motor retardation, spasticity, athetosis, dysarthria, and sometimes convulsions; short stature
Fucosidosis	α-L-Fucosidase (21)	GP, OLS, fucolipids	Some resemble Hurler phenotype; some have coarse features and neurologic disorder resembling leukodystrophy
α-Mannosidosis	α-Mannosidase (22)	GP, OLS	Mild or severe disorder with mental defect, mild organomegaly, coarse features, and skeletal involvement; may have gingival hyperplasia, lenticular opacities, and survival into third decade
β-Mannosidosis	β-Mannosidase (23)	GP, OLS	Juvenile onset of mental retardation, speech delay, ± coarsened facial features, ± mild bony changes, ± angiokeratoma
Aspartylglycosaminuria	Aspartylglucosaminidase (25)	Aspartylglucosamine, OLS	Predilection for those of Finnish descent; characteristic facies, thickened skull, scoliosis, diarrhea, frequent respiratory infections, dementia, psychosis, and seizures
Mucolipidosis II (I-cell disease)	UDP-N-acetylgalactosamine-1-phosphate: glycoprotein N-acetylgalactosaminylphosphotransferase.	GP, OLS, MPS, ganglioside	Infantile onset of Hurler-like disorder, but corneas are usually clear
Mucolipidosis III (pseudopolydystrophy)	Same as mucolipidosis II	GP, OLS, MPS, ganglioside	Onset at age 2–4 of coarse facies, dwarfism, short neck, claw hands, shoulder stiffness; clear corneas, carpal tunnel syndrome, mental defect, and long survival
Mucolipidosis IV	Mucolipin (MCOLN 1 gene)	GM3, GD3	Early infantile corneal clouding; juvenile mental and motor defect; Ashkenazi Jewish predilection

[a]See Figs. 82.1 through 82.3.
OLS, oligosaccharide; GP, glycoprotein; MPS, mucopolysaccharide; GM3, GM3-ganglioside, GD3, GD3-ganglioside.

and motor retardation. Patients are, invariably, severely mentally retarded and may never speak or walk. Usually, they develop spasticity, athetosis, dysarthria, and sometimes convulsions. They are short, often with strabismus, and with thickened calvaria. Ultrastructural analysis of blood lymphocytes, skin, and liver reveals abnormal lysosomal morphology. Free sialic acid is markedly increased in urine; defective sialic-acid egress has been noted from isolated fibroblast lysosomes. Salla disease is largely restricted to the Finnish population.

Fucosidosis

Some patients with fucosidosis have severe neurologic disease that resembles a leukodystrophy; others show a Hurler phenotype. Some have survived into the second or third decade of life. Fucose residues form part of the structure of oligosaccharides, glycoproteins, and glycolipids, including fucogangliosides. Patients with fucosidosis excrete excessive-abnormal urinary oligosaccharides (Fig. 84.3). The diagnosis is made by demonstrating severely decreased α-L-fucosidase activity (reaction 21, Fig. 84.3) in serum, leukocytes, and cultured skin fibroblasts.

Mannosidoses

α-Mannosidosis shows a spectrum of phenotypes. In severely affected patients, the diagnosis has been confused with mucolipidosis I. Other patients have slower progression of the disorder with greater dysmorphism, cataracts, and longer survival. Still others have presented primarily with marked mental defect, striking gingival hyperplasia, and survival into the third decade of life, or longer. Facial dysmorphism, skeletal involvement, and organ enlargement are slight in these patients.

Screening shows excessive-abnormal urinary oligosaccharides. The diagnosis requires demonstration of decreased α-mannosidase activity (reaction 22, Fig. 84.3) in leukocytes and cultured skin fibroblasts.

β-Mannosidosis, originally described in goats, was subsequently recognized in humans. One patient presented at age 16 months with slowing of speech development, and at age 46 months had facial coarsening, mild bone changes, speech delay, and mental retardation. Two brothers, aged 44 and 19 years, had angiokeratomas on the penis and scrotum; mental retardation from age 5 years or earlier; and no coarsening, organomegaly, or bone changes. Investigation showed α-mannosidase deficiency in plasma, leukocytes, and fibroblasts, and a mannose-containing disaccharide in urine. The first patient had absent sulfamidase, low sulfamidase in one parent, and urinary mucopolysaccharide excretion, identical to that in Sanfilippo syndrome type A, a clinically similar disorder.

Aspartylglycosaminuria

Aspartylglycosaminuria occurs almost solely in Finland. Patients have juvenile-onset somatic and mental changes. Somatic changes include coarse facial features, anteverted nostrils, short neck, and scoliosis. Intellectual deterioration leads to severe mental defect in the adult. Episodic hyperactivity, psychotic behavior, and seizures may occur.

Patients excrete large amounts of aspartylglycosamine in their urine because of deficiency of N-aspartyl-β-glucosaminidase (reaction 25, Fig. 84.3). Diagnostic findings are aspartylglycosamine in the urine and deficiency of N-aspartyl-β-glucosaminidase (reaction 25, Fig. 84.3) in cultured skin fibroblasts.

Mucolipidoses II and III

Mucolipidosis II (ML II or I-cell disease) and mucolipidosis III (ML III or pseudo-Hurler polydystrophy) are allelic disorders associated with deficiency of the enzyme, UDP-N-acetylglucosamine (i.e., glycoprotein N-acetylglucosaminylphosphotransferase). This enzyme attaches the N-acetylglucosamine-1-phosphate of UDPGlc-NAc1P to the 6-position of α-linked mannose residues of glycoproteins. The N-acetylglucosamine is subsequently removed to leave a mannose-6-phosphate residue, an important recognition marker for uptake of certain glycoproteins, including many lysosomal hydrolase enzymes, into the cell.

ML II is a severe disorder that resembles Hurler syndrome without corneal clouding. Cultured fibroblasts contain coarse inclusions (I-cells). Diagnosis is made by finding excess sialo-oligosaccharides in the urine, and deficiencies of multiple lysosomal enzymes in cultured skin fibroblasts, with elevated levels of these enzymes in plasma. In brain and viscera, only β-galactosidase is consistently deficient.

MLIII is a milder clinical disorder than mucolipidosis II that may present with joint stiffness, carpal-tunnel syndrome, or mild intellectual impairment.

Mucolipidosis IV

Patients with mucolipidosis IV present with corneal clouding, as early as 6 weeks of age. Mild retardation progresses to severe mental and motor defect. The disease occurs almost exclusively in Ashkenazi Jews. Achlorhydria is universal, and measurement of elevated serum-gastrin levels is a convenient and reliable screening test for ML IV. Diagnosis may now be made by mutation analysis, supported by the clinical picture, light-microscopic findings (i.e., lipid-laden marrow histiocytes), and electron-microscopic findings (i.e., vacuoles and membranous bodies in skin, conjunctiva, and cultured fibroblasts).

Gangliosides GM3 and GD3 (Fig. 84.1B) accumulate in fibroblasts. Soluble ganglioside sialidase (reaction 8, Fig. 84.1B) is reportedly deficient, but the gene is not mutated. The primary defect is in the MCOLN 1 gene, which codes for mucolipin, a protein that may function in cation channels.

Therapy of Lysosomal Diseases

Several approaches are possible for therapy of lysosomal diseases, beyond symptomatic therapy. Enzyme-replacement therapy has been the most successful approach to date. FDA-approved recombinant-enzyme therapy is available for some disorders. For others, therapeutic trials are underway or trials of experimental drugs are planned.

FDA-approved enzyme-replacement therapy is available for Gaucher disease type I, Fabry disease, and MPS type I. Gaucher disease is successfully treated with imiglucerase, Fabry disease with alpha-galactosidase, and MPS-I with alpha-iduronidase. Trials of recombinant-enzyme therapy are underway for Pompe disease, MPS-II, and MPS-VI. A trial of recombinant-acid sphingomyelinase is planned for Niemann-Pick disease type B.

A second approach that has been successful is substrate-reduction therapy. The compound, N-butyldeoxynojirimycin (i.e., miglustat), an inhibitor of glucosylceramide synthase, has been used successfully for Gaucher disease type I, and has received FDA approval for this indication. Trials of miglustat are under way for late-onset Tay-Sachs disease and Niemann-Pick type C, and a trial is planned for GM1-gangliosidosis. This approach may be applicable to other lysosomal disorders that involve accumulation of glycosphingolipids.

Other approaches that have been tried or contemplated involve cellular replacement, especially with sources of stem cells (e.g., bone marrow transplantation, cord-blood transplantation, or mesenchymal stem cells).

Gene therapy is currently being studied in animal models of the lysosomal diseases, but human trials are not in immediate prospect.

SUGGESTED READINGS

Pastores GM. Expert opinion & therapeutic patents. Enzyme therapy for the lysosomal storage disorders: principles, patents, practice & prospects. *Expert Opin Ther Patents* 2003;13:1157–1172.

Cox TM, Aerts JM, Andria G, Beck M et al; Advisory Council to the European Working Group on Gaucher Disease. The role of the iminosugar N-butyldeoxynojirimycin (miglustat) in the management of type I (non-neuronopathic) Gaucher disease: a position statement. *J Inherit Metab Dis* 2003;26(6):513–526.

Desnick RJ, Brady RO. Fabry disease in childhood. *J Pediatr* 2004 May;144(5 Suppl):S20–S26.

Goker-Alpan O, Schiffmann R, LaMarca ME, Nussbaum RL, McInerney-Leo A, Sidransky E. Parkinsonism among Gaucher disease carriers. *J Med Genet* 2004 Dec;41(12):937–940.

Heitner R, Elstein D, Aerts J, Weely S, Zimran A. Low-dose N-butyldeoxynojirimycin (OGT 918) for type I Gaucher disease. *Blood Cells Mol Dis* 2002;28(2):127–133.

Pastores GM, Barnett NL. Expert Opinion in Investigational Drugs, Substrate reduction therapy: Miglustat as a remedy for symptomatic patients with Gaucher Disease Type I. *Expert Opin Investig Drugs* 2003;12:273–281.

Sidransky E. Gaucher disease: complexity in a "simple" disorder. *Mol Genet Metab* 2004 Sep–Oct;83(1–2):6–15.

Lysosomal Diseases

Gieselmann V. Lysosomal storage diseases [Review]. *Biochim Biophys Acta* 1995;1270:103–136.

Lipidoses and Leukodystrophies

Berger J, Loschl B, Bernheimer H, et al. Occurrence, distribution, and phenotype of arylsulfatase A mutations in patients with metachromatic leukodystrophy. *Am J Med Genet* 1997;69:335–340.

Beutler E. Enzyme replacement therapy for Gaucher's disease [Review]. *Baillieres Clin Haematol* 1997;10:751–763.

Beutler E. Gaucher disease [Review]. *Curr Opin Hematol* 1997;4:19–23.

Brady RO. Gaucher's disease: past, present and future. *Baillieres Clin Haematol* 1997;10:621–634.

Chen W, Kubota S, Teramoto T, et al. Genetic analysis enables definite and rapid diagnosis of cerebrotendinous xanthomatosis. *Neurology* 1998;51:865–867.

Crutchfield KE, Patronas NJ, Dambrosia JM, et al. Quantitative analysis of cerebral vasculopathy in patients with Fabry disease. *Neurology* 1998;50:1746–1749.

Eng CM, Ashley GA, Burgert TS, et al. Fabry disease: thirty five mutations in the alpha-galactosidase A gene in patients with classic and variant phenotypes. *Mol Med* 1997;3:174–182.

Goebel HH, Wisniewski KE. Current state of clinical and morphological features in human NCL. *Brain Pathol* 2004;14(1):61–69.

Grabowski GA, Horowitz M. Gaucher's disease: molecular, genetic and enzymological aspects [Review]. *Baillieres Clin Haematol* 1997;10:635–656.

Guimaraes J, Amaral O, Sa Miranda MC. Adult-onset neuronopathic form of Gaucher's disease: a case report. *Parkinsonism Relat Disord* 2003;9(5):261–264.

Jan MM, Camfield PR. Nova Scotia Niemann-Pick disease (type D): clinical study of 20 cases. *J Child Neurol* 1998;13:758.

Kaye EM, Shalish C, Livermore J, et al. Beta-galactosidase gene mutations in patients with slowly progressive GM1 gangliosidosis [Review]. *J Child Neurol* 1997;12:24–27.

Koch J, Gartner S, Li CM, et al. Molecular cloning and characterization of a full-length complementary DNA encoding human acid ceramidase (Farber disease). *J Biol Chem* 1996;271:33110–33115.

Lwin A, Orvisky E, Goker-Alpan O, LaMarca ME, Sidransky E. Glucocerebrosidase mutations in subjects with parkinsonism. *Mol Genet Metab* 2004;81(1):70–73.

Mehta A, Ricci R, Widmer U, et al. Fabry disease defined: baseline clinical manifestations of 366 patients in the Fabry Outcome Survey. *Eur J Clin Invest* 2004;34(3):236–242.

Mitchison HM, Hofmann SL, Becerra CH, et al. Mutations in the palmityl-protein thioesterase gene (PPT; CLN1) causing juvenile neuronal ceroid lipofuscinosis with granular osmiophilic deposits. *Hum Mol Genet* 1998;7:291–297.

Moore DF, Altarescu G, Ling GS, et al. Elevated cerebral blood flow velocities in Fabry disease with reversal after enzyme replacement. *Stroke* 2002;33(2):525–531.

Myerowitz R. Tay-Sachs disease-causing mutations and neutral polymorphisms in the Hex A gene [Review]. *Hum Mutat* 1997;9:195–208.

Nowaczyk MJ, Feigenbaum A, Silver MM, et al. Bone marrow involvement and obstructive jaundice in Farber lipogranulomatosis: clinical and autopsy report of a new case. *J Inherit Metab Dis* 1996;19:655–660.

Pagani F, Pariyarath R, Garcia R, et al. New lysosomal acid lipase gene mutants explain the phenotype of Wolman disease and cholesteryl ester storage disease. *J Lipid Res* 1998;39:1382–1388.

Schmidt B, Selmer T, Ingendoh A, et al. A novel amino acid modification in sulfatases that is defective in multiple sulfatase deficiency. *Cell* 1995;82:271–278.

Tylki-Szymanska AT, Czartoryska B, Lugowska A. Practical suggestions in diagnosing etachromatic leukodystrophy in probands and in testing family members. *Eur Neurol* 1998;40:67–70.

van Heijst AF, Verrips A, Wevers RA, et al. Treatment and follow-up of children with cerebrotendinous xanthomatosis. *Eur J Pediatr* 1998;157:31–36.

Wenger DA, Rafi MA, Luzi P. Molecular genetics of Krabbe disease (globoid cell leukodystrophy): diagnostic and clinical implications [Review]. *Hum Mutat* 1997;10:268–279.

Mucopolysaccharidoses and Mucolipidoses

Alkhayat AH, Kraemer SA, Leipprandt JR, et al. Human beta-mannosidase cDNA characterization and first identification of a mutation associated with human beta-mannosidosis. *Hum Mol Genet* 1998;7:75–83.

Altarescu G, Sun M, Moore DF, et al. The neurogenetics of mucolipidosis type IV. *Neurology* 2002;59(3):306–313.

Beck M, Barone R, Hoffmann R, et al. Inter and intrafamilial variability in mucolipidosis II (I-cell disease). *Clin Genet* 1995;47:191–199.

Chen CS, Bach G, Pagano RE. Abnormal transport along the lysosomal pathway in mucolipidosis, type IV disease. *Proc Natl Acad Sci USA* 1998;95:637–638.

Leppanen P, Isosomppi J, Schleutker J, et al. A physical map of the 6q14q15 region harboring the locus for the lysosomal membrane sialic acid transport defect (Salla disease and infantile free sialic acid storage disease). *Genomics* 1996;37:62–67.

Nilssen O, Berg T, Riise HM, et al. Alpha-mannosidosis: functional cloning of the lysosomal alpha-mannosidase cDNA and identification of a mutation in two affected siblings. *Hum Mol Genet* 1997;6:717–726.

Peltola M, Tikkanen R, Peltonen L, et al. Ser72Pro active-site disease mutation in human lysosomal aspartylglucosaminidase: abnormal intracellular processing and evidence for extracellular activation. *Hum Mol Genet* 1996;5:737–743.

Pshezhetsky AV, Richard C, Michaud L, et al. Cloning, expression and chromosomal mapping of human lysosomal sialidase and characterization of mutations in sialidosis. *Nat Genet* 1997;15:316–320.

Raychowdhury MK, Gonzalez-Perrett S, Montalbetti N, et al. Molecular pathophysiology of mucolipidosis type IV: pH dysregulation of the mucolipin-1 cation channel. *Hum Mol Genet* 2004;13(6):617–627.

Richard C, Tranchemontagne J, Elsliger MA, et al. Molecular pathology of galactosialidosis in a patient affected with two new frameshift mutations in the cathepsin A/protective protein gene. *Hum Mutat* 1998;11:461–469.

Umehara F, Matsumoto W, Kuriyama M, et al. Mucolipidosis III (pseudo-Hurler polydystrophy); clinical studies in aged patients in one family. *J Neurol Sci* 1997;146:167–172.

Wraith JE. The mucopolysaccharidoses: a clinical review and guide to management [Review]. *Arch Dis Child* 1995;72:26–37.

Therapy

Brady RO. Gaucher and Fabry diseases: from understanding pathophysiology to rational therapies. *Acta Paediatr Suppl* 2003;92:19–24.

Brady RO, Schiffmann R. Enzyme-replacement therapy for metabolic storage disorders. *Lancet Neurol* 2004 Dec;3(12):752–756.

Futerman AH, Sussman JL, Horowitz M, Silman I, Zimran A. New directions in the treatment of Gaucher disease. *Trends Pharmacol Sci* 2004;25(3):147–151.

Haltia M. The neuronal ceroid-lipofuscinoses. *J Neuropathol Exp Neurol* 2003;62(1):1–13.

Chapter 85

▶ Disorders of Carbohydrate Metabolism

Salvatore DiMauro

GLYCOGEN STORAGE DISEASES

Abnormal metabolism of glycogen and glucose may occur in a series of genetically determined disorders, each representing a specific enzyme deficiency (Table 85.1). The signs and symptoms of each disease are largely determined by the tissues in which the enzyme defect is expressed. Virtually all enzymes of glycogen metabolism, including tissue-specific isoforms or subunits, have been assigned to chromosomal loci and the corresponding genes have been cloned and sequenced. Numerous mutations have been identified and a genotype:phenotype correlation is taking shape. The disorders affecting the neuromuscular system primarily are discussed in Part XVIII, Myopathies.

Severe fasting hypoglycemia may result in periodic episodes of lethargy, coma, convulsions, and anoxic brain damage in *glucose-6-phosphatase deficiency* (*glycogenosis type I*) or in *glycogen synthetase deficiency*. The liver is enlarged in both diseases. Clinical manifestations tend to become milder in patients who survive the first few years of life.

The CNS is directly affected by the enzyme defect in generalized glycogen storage diseases, even though neurological symptoms are lacking in some disorders and in others may be ascribed to liver rather than to brain dysfunction. The following enzyme defects seem to be generalized: acid maltase (type II), debrancher (type III), brancher (type IV), and phosphoglycerate kinase (type IX).

In the infantile form of acid maltase deficiency (Pompe disease), pathologic involvement of the CNS has been documented, with accumulation of both free and intralysosomal glycogen in all cells, especially spinal motor neurons and neurons of the brain stem nuclei. Peripheral nerve biopsy specimens show accumulation of glycogen in Schwann cells. The profound generalized weakness of infants with Pompe disease is probably due to combined effects of glycogen storage in muscle, anterior horn cells, and peripheral nerves. In four patients with the childhood form of acid maltase deficiency, increased glycogen deposition in neurons of the brainstem was related to fatal intractable hyperpyrexia. No morphologic changes were seen in the CNS of a patient with adult-onset acid maltase deficiency despite marked decrease of enzyme activity.

▶ **TABLE 85.1 Classification of Glycogen Storage Disease**

Type	Affected Tissues	Clinical Presentation	Glycogen Structure	Enzyme Defect	Mode of Transmission
I	Liver and kidney	Severe hypoglycemia; hepatomegaly	Normal	Glucose-6-phosphatase	AR
II					
Infancy	Generalized	Cardiomegaly; weakness; hypotonia; death < age 1 yr	Normal		
Childhood	Generalized	Myopathy simulating Duchenne dystrophy; respiratory insufficiency	Normal	Acid maltase	AR
Adult	Generalized	Myopathy simulating limb-girdle dystrophy or polymyositis; respiratory insufficiency	Normal		
III	Generalized	Hepatomegaly; fasting hypoglycemia; progressive weakness	PLD	Debrancher	AR
IV	Generalized	Hepatosplenomegaly; cirrhosis of liver; hepatic failure	Polyglucosan	Brancher	AR
V	Skeletal muscle	Intolerance to intense exercise; cramps; myoglobinuria	Normal	Muscle phosphorylase	AR
VI	Liver; RBC	Mild hypoglycemia; hepatomegaly	Normal	Liver phosphorylase	AR
VII	Skeletal muscle; RBC	Intolerance to intense exercise; cramps; myoglobinuria	Normal (± polyglucosan)	Muscle phosphofructokinase (PFK-M)	AR
VIII	Liver	Asymptomatic hepatomegaly	Normal	Phosphorylase kinase	XR
	Liver and skeletal muscle	Hepatomegaly; growth retardation; hypotonia	Normal	Phosphorylase kinase	AR
	Skeletal muscle	Exercise intolerance; myoglobinuria	Normal	Phosphorylase kinase	AR
	Heart	Fatal infantile cardiomyopathy	Normal	Phosphorylase kinase	AR
IX	Generalized	Hemolytic anemia; seizures; mental retardation	Normal (?)	Phosphoglycerate kinase (PKG)	XR
		Intolerance to intense exercise; myoglobinuria			
X	Skeletal muscle	Intolerance to intense exercise; myoglobinuria	Normal (?)	Muscle phosphoglycerate mutase (PGAM-M)	AR
XI	Skeletal muscle	Intolerance to intense exercise; myoglobinuria	Normal (?)	Muscle lactate dehydrogenase (LDH-M)	AR
XII	Skeletal muscle RBC	Exercise intolerance	Normal (?)	Aldolase A	AR
XIII	Skeletal muscle	Exercise intolerance	Normal (?)	β-enolase	AR
	Generalized	Myoclonus epilepsy (Lafora Disease)	Polyglucosan	Laforin	AR
	Liver	Severe hypoglycemia; hepatomegaly		Glycogen synthetase	AR (?)

AR, autosomal recessive; XR, X-linked recessive; PLD, phosphorylase-limit dextrin; RBC, red blood cells.

Patients with debrancher deficiency (glycogenosis type III) have hepatomegaly, fasting hypoglycemia, and seizures in infancy and childhood, which usually remit around puberty. Although overt signs of peripheral neuropathy are rare, abnormal deposits of glycogen have been documented both in axons and in Schwann cells and may explain, in part at least, the distal wasting and mixed EMG pattern observed in adult patients with neuromuscular involvement.

In branching enzyme deficiency (glycogenosis type IV), the clinical picture is typically dominated by liver disease, with progressive cirrhosis and chronic hepatic failure causing death in childhood. Deposits of a basophilic, intensely PAS-positive material that is partially resistant to β-amylase digestion have been found in all tissues; in the CNS, spheroids composed of branched filaments were present in astrocytic processes, particularly in the spinal cord and medulla. Ultrastructurally the storage material was composed of aggregates of branched osmiophilic filaments, 6 nm in diameter often surrounded by normal glycogen particles.

In PGK deficiency (glycogenosis type IX), the type and severity of clinical manifestations vary in different genetic variants of the disease and are probably related to the severity of the enzyme defect in different tissues. In several families, the clinical picture was characterized by the association of severe hemolytic anemia, with mental retardation and seizures.

LAFORA DISEASE AND OTHER POLYGLUCOSAN STORAGE DISEASES

Myoclonus epilepsy with Lafora bodies (Lafora disease) is an autosomal recessive disease that is characterized by the triad of epilepsy, myoclonus, and dementia. Inconstant other neurologic manifestations include ataxia, dysarthria, spasticity, and rigidity. Onset is in adolescence, and the course progresses rapidly to death, which in 90% of patients occurs between 17 and 24 years of age. Negative criteria or manifestations that imply some other disease include onset before 6 or after age 20, optic atrophy, macular degeneration, prolonged course, or normal intelligence. Epilepsy, with predominantly occipital seizures, is the first manifestation in most patients; status epilepticus is common in terminal stages. Myoclonus usually appears 2 or 3 years after the onset of epilepsy, may affect any area of the body, is sensitive to startle, and is absent during sleep. Intellectual deterioration generally follows the appearance of seizures by 2 or 3 years and progresses rapidly to severe dementia. Therapy is symptomatic and is designed to suppress seizures and reduce the severity of myoclonus; some control of myoclonus is achieved with benzodiazepines.

Laboratory findings are normal except for EEG changes; bilaterally synchronous discharges of wave-and-spike formations are commonly seen in association with myoclonic jerks. EEG abnormalities may be found in asymptomatic relatives. The pathologic hallmark of the disease is the presence in the CNS of the bodies first described by Lafora in 1911: round, basophilic, strongly PAS-positive intracellular inclusions that vary in size from dustlike bodies less than 3 nm in diameter to large bodies up to 30 nm in diameter. The medium and large bodies often show a dense core and a lighter periphery. Lafora bodies are seen only in neuronal perikarya and processes and are most numerous in cerebral cortex, substantia nigra, thalamus, globus pallidus, and dentate nucleus.

Ultrastructurally, Lafora bodies are not membrane bound. They consist of two components in various proportions: amorphous, electron-dense granules and irregular filaments. The filaments, which are about 6 nm in diameter, are often branched and frequently continuous with the granular material.

Irregular accumulations of a material similar to that of the Lafora bodies are found in liver, heart, skeletal muscle, skin, and retina, suggesting that Lafora disease is a generalized storage disease. Both histochemical and biochemical criteria indicate that the storage material is a branched polysaccharide composed of glucose (polyglucosan) similar to the amylopectinlike polysaccharide that accumulates in branching enzyme deficiency. The activity of branching enzyme, however, was normal in several tissues, including brain, of patients with Lafora disease. Linkage analysis in nine families localized one gene responsible for Lafora disease (*EPM2A*) to chromosome 6q24. The gene product, named laforin, contains a carbohydrate-binding module in the N-terminus and a dual-specificity phosphatase domain in the C-terminus, whose substrate remains unknown. Two isoforms, A and B, are generated by alternative splicing: isoform A is cytoplasmic and is mutated in Lafora disease; isoform B is nuclear and is not involved in Lafora disease. About 30 mutations have been identified in the *EPM2A* gene in patients with Lafora disease. Genetic heterogeneity was expected because linkage to chromosome 6q24 was excluded in about 20% of families with Lafora disease. A genomewide linkage scan in French–Canadian families has revealed a second locus, *EPM2B*, at chromosome locus 6p22. Candidate affected proteins include kinesins and microtubular motor proteins, but pathogenic mutations remain to be documented.

A clinically distinct form of polyglucosan body disease (*adult polyglucosan body disease* or *APBD*) occurs in patients with a complex but stereotyped chronic neurologic disorder characterized by progressive upper and lower motor neuron involvement, sensory loss, sphincter problems, neurogenic bladder, and in about half of the cases, dementia; there is no myoclonus or epilepsy. Onset is in the fifth or sixth decade of life, and the course ranges from 3 to 20 years. Electrophysiologic studies show axonal neuropathy. In some cases the clinical picture simulates amyotrophic lateral sclerosis. Throughout the CNS, polyglucosan bodies are present in processes of neurons and astrocytes but not in perikarya. There are also polyglucosan accumulations in peripheral nerve and in other tissues, including liver, heart, and skeletal and smooth muscle. As in debranching enzyme deficiency and Lafora disease, the abnormal polysaccharide in APBD seems to have longer peripheral chains than normal glycogen. Branching enzyme activity was significantly decreased in leukocytes from Israeli patients, and this finding was confirmed in both leukocytes and peripheral nerve specimens from American Ashkenazi Jewish patients, whereas the activity was normal in tissues from three non-Jewish white patients and from one African American patient, suggesting genetic heterogeneity. A mutation in the gene encoding the branching enzyme (*GBE*) has been found in five Ashkenazi Jewish families with APBD, confirming that APBD is a clinical variant of branching deficiency, at least in Ashkenazi Jewish patients. Decreased branching enzyme activity was also reported in two non-Jewish patients: One was a compound heterozygote for two missense mutations in the *GBE* gene, whereas the other had no mutations in the *GBE* coding sequence.

Another form of polyglucosan is in *corpora amylacea*, which accumulate progressively and nonspecifically with age. They are more commonly seen within astrocytic processes in the hippocampus and in subpial and subependymal regions; however, they also occur in intramuscular nerves in patients older than 40 years.

SUGGESTED READINGS

Bruno C, Servidei S, Shanske S, et al. Glycogen branching enzyme deficiency in adult polyglucosan body disease. *Ann Neurol* 1993;33:88–93.

Bruno C, van Diggelen OP, Cassandrini D, et al. Clinical and genetic heterogeneity of branching enzyme deficiency (glycogenosis type IV). *Neurology* 2004 Sep 28;63(6):1053–1058.

Chan EM, Bulman DE, Paterson AD, et al. Genetic mapping of a new Lafora progressive myoclonus epilepsy locus (EPM2B) on 6p22. *J Med Genet* 2003;40:671–675.

Coleman DL, Gambetti PL, DiMauro S. Muscle in Lafora disease. *Arch Neurol* 1974;31:396–406.

DiMauro S, Lamperti C. Muscle glycogenoses. *Muscle and Nerve* 2001;24:984–999.

DiMauro S, Stern LZ, Mehler M, et al. Adult-onset acid maltase deficiency: a postmortem study. *Muscle and Nerve* 1978;1:27–36.

Gambetti PL, DiMauro S. Nervous system in Pompe's disease. *J Neuropath Exp Neurol* 1971;30:412–430.

Ianzano L, Young EJ, Zhao EC, et al. Loss of function of the cytoplasmic isoform of the protein laforin (EPM2A) causes Lafora progressive myoclonus epilepsy. *Hum Mutat* 2004;23:170–176.

Klein CJ, Boes CJ, Chapin JE, et al. Adult polyglucosan body disease: case description of an expanding genetic and clinical syndrome. *Muscle and Nerve* 2004;29:323–328.

Lafora GR. über das Vorkommen amyloider Körperchen in Innern der Ganglienzellen. *Virchows Arch Pathol Anat* 1911;205:295–303.

Lossos A, Barash V, Soffer D, et al. Hereditary branching enzyme dysfunction in adult polyglucosan body disease: a possible cause in two patients. *Ann Neurol* 1991;30:655–662.

Lossos A, Meiner Z, Barash V, et al. Adult polyglucosan body disease caused by the Tyr329Ser mutation in the glycogen branching enzyme gene in Ashkenazi Jews. *Arch Neurol* 1998;42:987.

McDonald ID, Faust PL, Bruno C, et al. Polyglucosan body disease simulating amyotrophic lateral sclerosis. *Neurology* 1993;43:785–790.

McMaster KR, Powers JM, Hennigar GR, et al. Nervous system involvement in type IV glycogenosis. *Arch Pathol Lab Med* 1979;103:105–111.

Minassian BA, Lee JR, Herbrick J-A, et al. Mutations in a gene encoding a novel protein tyrosine phosphatase cause progressive myoclonus epilepsy. *Nature Genet* 1998;20:171–174.

Minassian BA. Lafora's disease: towards a clinical, pathologic, and molecular synthesis. *Pediatr Neurol* 2001;25:21–29.

Page RA, Davie CA, MacManus D, Miszkiel KA, Walshe JM, Miller DH, Lees AJ, Schapira AH. Clinical correlation of brain MRI and MRS abnormalities in patients with Wilson disease. *Neurology* 2004 Aug 24;63(4):638–643.

Robitaille Y, Carpenter S, Karpati G, DiMauro S. A distinct form of adult polyglucosan body disease with massive involvement of central and peripheral neuronal processes and astrocytes. *Brain* 1980;103:315–336.

Serratosa JM, Delgado-Escueta AV, Posada I, et al. The gene for progressive myoclonus epilepsy of the Lafora type maps to chromosome 6q. *Hum Mol Genet* 1995;4:1657–1663.

Spencer-Peet J, Norman ME, Lake BD, et al. Hepatic glycogen storage disease. *Q J Med* 1971;40:95–114.

Ugawa Y, Inoue K, Takemura T, et al. Accumulation of glycogen in sural nerve axons in adult-onset type III glycogenosis. *Ann Neurol* 1986;19:294–297.

Chapter 86

Glucose Transporter Type 1 Deficiency Syndrome

Darryl C. De Vivo, Juan M. Pascual, and Dong Wang

CLINICAL SYNDROME

In 1991, De Vivo et al. described two children with infantile seizures, delayed motor and behavioral development, acquired microcephaly, and ataxia. Lumbar puncture revealed low cerebrospinal fluid glucose concentrations (hypoglycorrhachia) and low-normal to low cerebrospinal fluid lactate concentrations (Table 86.1). Since 1991, about 100 patients have been identified. The dominant clinical features are shown in Table 86.2.

Seizures begin in early infancy, and the seizure types vary with the age of the patient. In infancy, the dominant seizure types include behavioral arrest, pallor and cyanosis, eye deviation simulating opsoclonus, and apnea. The EEG at this stage may be normal or show focal spikes. In childhood, the seizures change in character and typically include astatic seizures, atypical absence seizures, and generalized tonic-clonic seizures. The EEG now shows a generalized spike-wave pattern. The seizures are refractory to antiepileptic drugs but respond promptly and dramatically to a ketogenic diet. Other phenotypes include isolated mental retardation or choreoathetosis.

LABORATORY DATA

Diagnosis requires awareness of the clinical manifestations and documentation of hypoglycorrhachia. A low or low-normal cerebrospinal fluid lactate concentration strengthens the presumptive diagnosis. Glucose uptake rates in vitro by intact washed erythrocytes are decreased in most patients by approximately 50%.

MOLECULAR GENETICS AND PATHOGENESIS

D-glucose is the obligate fuel for brain metabolism under virtually all circumstances. With acute or chronic fasting, the brain adapts metabolically to use ketone bodies (β-hydroxybutyrate and acetoacetate) in partial lieu of glucose. However, glucose is necessary as a permissive

▶ **TABLE 86.1** CSF Glucose and Lactate Values in GLUT1 Deficiency Syndrome

	n	Glucose (mg/dl)		Lactate (mM)
		CSF	CSF/blood	CSF
Disease controls	318	62 ± 1	0.65	1.3 ± 0.07
GLUT1 deficiency syndrome	69	32 ± 1	0.34	0.97 ± 0.03

Values are expressed as mean ± SEM.

substrate for brain ketone body use under these extreme physiologic conditions. The transport of D-glucose across the blood-brain barrier and into brain cells is selectively mediated by a facilitative carrier mechanism. The protein that facilitates glucose transport across these tissue barriers is glucose transporter 1 (GLUT1), a member of a multigene family of protein transporters that facilitate the diffusion of sugar molecules across tissue barriers. GLUT1 is encoded in chromosome 1p34.1 and is present in high abundance in brain capillaries, astroglial cells, and erythrocyte membranes.

The molecular basis of the syndrome is haploinsufficiency of the GLUT1 protein, which was found in 48 patients by Wang and De Vivo. Three patients were hemizygous as determined by a fluorescence in situ hybridization study, indicating a large-scale chromosomal deletion. The other 45 patients were heterozygous for nonsense mutations, missense mutations, frameshift mutations, or splice site mutations. The mutations were distributed throughout the gene, and several mutations were more common than others.

The GLUT1 cDNA is highly conserved, with 97% homology among men, rats, mice, and rabbits. The highly conserved nature of the gene increases the likelihood that pathogenicity is related to small-scale rearrangements.

The GLUT1 protein is responsible for the transport of glucose across both luminal and abluminal sides of the brain capillary endothelial cell and across the astroglial plasma membrane. GLUT1 haploinsufficiency may cause a severe decrease in the concentration of glucose in the interstitial space of the brain and in astroglial cells. This syndrome is the first genetically determined abnormality of the blood–brain barrier; it may be familial and transmitted as an autosomal dominant trait.

▶ **TABLE 86.2** Features of GLUT1 Deficiency Syndrome

Findings	Frequency (%)
Infantile seizures	97
Dysarthria	97
Motor delay	80
Microcephaly	75
Hypotonia	50
Ataxia	50
Spasticity	25
Hypoglycorrhachia	100

DIAGNOSIS

The differential diagnosis includes cerebral palsy, Rett syndrome, Angelman syndrome, neuroblastoma (with opsoclonus), hypoglycemia, infantile ataxia, and mitochondrial diseases. Seizures have been present in most but not all cases, but this observation could be an ascertainment bias. Lumbar puncture for measurement of glucose and lactate is a critical test in establishing the diagnosis. Confirmatory evidence is provided by decreased red cell glucose uptake, and supportive evidence by a characteristic pattern of cerebral FDG–PET abnormalities localized to cortex and thalami with otherwise relatively preserved basal ganglia uptake. DNA studies are diagnostic in over 95% of cases.

TREATMENT

Treatment is the ketogenic diet, which effectively controls the seizures but is less effective in improving cognition and behavior. Antiepileptic drugs have been uniformly ineffective. Thioctic acid may facilitate glucose transport and has been recommended as adjunctive therapy.

SUGGESTED READINGS

Brockmann K, Wang D, Korenke CG, et al. Autosomal dominant glut-1 deficiency syndrome and familial epilepsy. *Ann Neurol* 2001;50:476–485.

De Vivo DC, Garcia-Alvarez M, Roonen G, et al. Glucose transport protein deficiency. An emerging syndrome with therapeutic implications. *Int Pediatr* 1995;10:51–56.

De Vivo DC, Trifiletti RR, Jacobson RI, et al. Defective glucose transport across the blood-brain barrier as a cause of persistent hypoglycorrhachia, seizures, and developmental delay. *N Engl J Med* 1991;325:703–709.

Hirsch LJ. Absence epilepsy with onset before age three years: could this be Glut-1 deficiency syndrome (De Vivo syndrome)? *Epilepsia* 2004;45(Jan):92–93.

Overweg-Plandsoen WC, Groener JE, Wang D, et al. GLUT-1 deficiency without epilepsy—an exceptional case. *J Inherit Metab Dis* 2003;26:559–563.

Pardridge WM, Boado RJ, Farrell CR. Brain-type glucose transporter (Glut-1) is selectively localized to the blood-brain barrier. *J Biol Chem* 1990;265:18035–18040.

Pascual JM, Van Heertum RL, Wang D, et al. Imaging the metabolic footprint of Glut1 deficiency on the brain. *Ann Neurol* 2002;52:458–464.

Pascual JM, Van Heertum RL, Wang D, et al. (Updated 9 August 2002). Glucose transporter type 1 deficiency syndrome. In: *GeneReviews at GeneTests: Medical Genetics Information Resource* (database online). Copyright, University of Washington, Seattle. 1997–2004. Available at http://www.genetests.org. Accessed April 8, 2004.

Pascual JM, Wang D, Lecumberri B, Yang H, Mao X, Yang R, De Vivo

DC. GLUT1 deficiency and other glucose transporter diseases. *Eur J Endocrinol* 2004;150(5):627–633.

Seidner G, Garcia-Alvarez M, Jeh J-I, et al. GLUT-1 deficiency syndrome caused by haploinsufficiency of the blood-brain barrier hexose carrier. *Nat Genet* 1998;18:188–191.

Wang D, Kranz-Eble P, De Vivo DC. Mutational analysis of GLUT1 (SLC2A1) in Glut-1 deficiency syndrome. *Hum Mutat* 2000;16:224–231.

Chapter 87

Disorders of Deoxyribonucleic Acid (DNA) Maintenance, Transcription, and Translation

Marc C. Patterson

Except for components of the respiratory chain encoded by mitochondrial DNA, the DNA of the nucleus is responsible for the production of the molecules essential to the cellular economy. Disorders that impair the maintenance of the integrity of DNA, or its timely and accurate transcription and translation, frequently lead to neurodegeneration, impaired growth, premature aging, and a propensity to develop malignancies.

This chapter provides an introduction to the processes involved and the diseases resulting from derangement of these controls. Some conditions are treated in more detail elsewhere in the book. It is likely that the number of these disorders will continue to grow in parallel with the relevant basic science. Neurologists in the twenty-first century must have a firm grasp of the essential principles to diagnose and manage people with these diseases.

DNA MAINTENANCE AND TRANSCRIPTION

DNA is subject to errors in its duplication during cell division and during the process of repair following exposure to a variety of mutagens (environmental, toxic, and therapeutic). The elaborate machinery includes helicases that unwind the strands of DNA in preparation for transcrip-

tion into RNA; RNA polymerase, which directs the formation of messenger RNA (mRNA) on the DNA template; and DNA polymerase, which catalyses the duplication of DNA. The process is fine-tuned by a large and growing family of transcription factors.

When single bases are incorrectly inserted into the new DNA molecules, they are removed by the process of base excision repair, mediated by specific DNA glycolyases and endonucleases and DNA polymerases and ligases. Longer segments of 25 to 32 bases are frequently damaged by exposure to ultraviolet radiation and are removed by nucleotide excision repair, which requires its own family of proteins. Double-stranded DNA breaks activate a mechanism that requires the participation of DNA protein kinase and recombination proteins. The processes are even more complex than is implied by this brief overview, because many of the proteins involved play multiple, mutually modifying roles in repair and transcription.

Precursor-messenger RNA (pre-mRNA) is transcribed from the genomic DNA template and includes the sequences of both expressed sequences (exons) and intervening sequences (introns). Introns are removed from pre-mRNA by RNA splicing to produce the mRNA used in translation of the message into protein. This process requires the participation of five additional RNA molecules (small nuclear RNAs or snRNAs) and 50 proteins. The snRNAs are added to multiprotein complexes known as spliceosomes. The steps involved in pre-mRNA processing into mRNA occur in the nucleus and conclude with export of the mRNA to the cytoplasm by the nuclear pore complex.

DNA TRANSLATION AND MODIFICATION

Translation of mRNA requires intact ribosomal function, factors to control the initiation and duration of translation, and machinery to modify the nascent polypeptide chains by the addition of smaller molecules, particularly oligosaccharides. This modification amplifies the ability of the organism to respond to changing needs at different stages of development (such as differing proportions of enzyme or structural protein isoforms) or in response to external stimuli (as in the modification of T-cell receptor populations and other elements of the immune system to target invading micro-organisms). The most important such processes are N-linked and O-linked glycosylation.

CELL CYCLE CONTROL

The activity of the systems responsible for DNA transcription, maintenance, and translation is related to the phase of the cell cycle, which is regulated by a highly conserved family of protein kinases known as cyclin-dependent kinases (Cdks). Cdks are themselves regulated by inhibitory

▶ **TABLE 87.1** Selected Disorders of DNA Synthesis, Maintenance, Transcription, and Translation

Disorder	Inheritance	Gene and Protein	Mechanism (Known or Putative)	Specific Features
DNA maintenance and transcription				
Cockayne syndrome, Type 1 (CSA) MIM 216400	AR	*CSA (ERCC8)* Excision repair cross-complementing rodent repair deficiency 8 protein	CSA/ERCC8 interacts with p44, CSB, and TFIIH. Mutations thus lead to impaired RNA pol II dysfunction and impaired nucleotide excision repair.	Mental retardation. accelerated aging, pigmentary retinal degeneration, optic atrophy, deafness, marble epiphyses, photosensitivity, and basal ganglia/cerebellar calcification.
COFS MIM 214150	AR	*CSB (ERCC6)* Excision repair cross complementing rodent repair deficiency 6 protein	Abnormal nucleotide excision repair resulting from disturbed RNA polymerase I/TFIIH interaction within the CSBIP/150 complex, of which CSB/ERCC6 is a component	Microcephaly, microphthalmia, cataracts, dysmorphism, failure to thrive, recurrent pneumonias, axial hypotonia, appendicular hypertonia, hyperreflexia, and progressive contractures. Calcifications in the periventricular frontal white matter and basal ganglia.
Progeria MIM# 176670	AR	*LMNA* Lamin A	Lamin are structural components of the nuclear membrane. Mutations in LMNA are associated with both defective nuclear mechanics and impaired transcriptional activation	Postnatal onset of short stature, failure to thrive and accelerated aging, manifest as loss of scalp hair, subcutaneous fat, joint stiffness and early atherosclerosis leading to strokes and myocardial infarcts, and premature death. Cognition is spared.
Xeroderma pigmentosum (XP) (de Sanctis Cacchione syndrome-most commonly complementation group D-XPD) MIM 278730	AR	ERCC2 Excision repair cross-complementing rodent repair deficiency 2 protein	Abnormal nucleotide excision repair: XPD (ERCC2) interacts with the p44 subunit of TFIIH stimulating 5-prime-to-3-prime helicase activity. Mutations in the XPD prevent the interaction with p44, leading to decreased XPD helicase activity.	Mental retardation, short stature, facial freckling, spasticity, hypogonadism and olivopontocerebellar atrophy.
Trichothiodystrophy (TTD 1) MIM 601675	AR	ERCC2 Excision repair cross-complementing rodent repair deficiency 2 protein	As for XP	Mental retardation, hair shaft abnormalities, ichthyosis, immature sexual development, short stature, and facial dysmorphism

(*continued*)

▶ TABLE 87.1   Selected Disorders of DNA Synthesis, Maintenance, Transcription, and Translation (Continued)

Disorder	Inheritance	Gene and Protein	Mechanism (Known or Putative)	Specific Features
Rett syndrome MIM 312750	X linked	*MECP2* Methyl cGp binding protein 2	Regulation of gene expression, chromatin composition, and chromosomal architecture through binding to methylated DNA. MeCP2 is expressed ubiquitously by neurons; levels of MeCP2 expression increase during neuronal differentiation and remain at high levels in the adult brain.	Classic phenotype restricted to females. Normal development for first six months, followed by acquired microcephaly, loss of hand skills and replacement by stereotypies, regression of skills, seizures, spasticity, and scoliosis
Spinal muscular atrophy 1, 2, and 3 MIM 253300, 253550, 253400	AR	*SMN1* Survival motor neuron protein	SMN1 is a key component of the spliceosome complex; selective vulnerability of anterior horn cells is not yet understood	Loss of anterior horn cells (and neurons of brainstem and thalami in severe cases)
DNA translation and translational modification				
CACH, Cree leucoencephalopathy, ovarioleukodystrophy MIM 603896	AR	*e IF 2B* Eukaryotic translation initiation factor 2B	Translation initiation factor 2B catalyzes exchange of ADP for ATP, an essential stage in recycling of translation initiation factor 2 (eIF2). Mutations in any of the five genes coding for subunits of eIF2B are thought to cause loss of normal downregulation of protein translation under stress, resulting in protein denaturation and accumulation of aggregates producing cellular toxicity.	Slowly progressive ataxia with diffuse loss of white matter. Episodes of coma with fever and minor trauma
Congenital disorder of glycosylation 1a (CDG 1a) MIM 212065	AR	*PMM2* Phosphomannomutase 2	PMM2 is one of a family of enzymes catalyzing the assembly of the lipid-linked oligosaccharide precursor (LLO) that is attached to the nascent polypeptide chain during cotranslational modification by N-linked glycosylation	Mental retardation, short stature, progressive ataxia, peripheral neuropathy, stroke-like episodes, seizures, immune dysfunction, intermittent hepatic failure, coagulopathies

(*continued*)

▶ **TABLE 87.1** Selected Disorders of DNA Synthesis, Maintenance, Transcription, and Translation (Continued)

Disorder	Inheritance	Gene and Protein	Mechanism (Known or Putative)	Specific Features
Cell cycle regulation				
Angelman syndrome MIM 105830	Multiple mechanisms, including: maternal deletion of 15q11-13, paternal uniparental disomy, imprinting defects, and point mutations or small *UBE3A* intragenic deletions. Some patients have *MECP2* mutations.	*UBE3A* Ubiquitin-protein ligase E3A	The Ube3a gene encodes sense and antisense RNA transcripts in the brain with neuron-specific imprinting of Ube3a in primary brain cell cultures. The neuron-specific imprinting mechanism may be related to the lineage determination of neural stem cells.	Psychomotor retardation, ataxia, hypotonia, epilepsy, absence of speech, large mandible and tongue thrusting. Optic atrophy and albinism in some.
Ataxia telangiectasia MIM 208900	AR	*ATM* ATM (ataxia telangiectasia mutated) protein	The ATM protein is a phosphatidylinositol-3 kinase that phosphorylates key substrates involved in DNA repair and/or cell cycle control	Progressive ataxia, choreoathetosis, anterior horn cell loss, immune deficiency, scleral telangiectasia.
Seckel syndrome 1 MIM 210600	AR	*ATR* Ataxia telangiectasia and RAD 3 related protein	ATR is a PIK (phosphatidylinositol kinase) involved in cell cycle progression, DNA recombination, and the detection of DNA damage	Short stature, dysmorphism ("bird-headed dwarf"), congenital microcephaly, mental retardation. No immune deficiency or cancers

phosphorylation (Wee 1), dephosphorylation (Cdc25), the binding of inhibitor proteins (CKIs), and through cyclical proteolysis (ubiquitin ligases and activators—SCF, APC, Cdc20, Hct 1) and gene regulatory proteins (E2F, p53).

SPECIFIC DISORDERS

Table 87.1 summarizes the DNA disorders. The categorization of specific disorders in one category is an arbitrary oversimplification, because the gene products have multiple actions in many cases.

SUGGESTED READINGS

Akbarian S. The neurobiology of Rett syndrome. *Neuroscientist* 2003;9: 57–63.

Alberts B, Johnson A, Lewis J, et al. *Molecular Biology of the Cell*, 4th ed. New York: Garland Science, 2002.

Chen L, Lee L, Kudlow BA, et al. LMNA mutations in atypical Werner's syndrome. *Lancet* 2003;362:440–445.

Clayton-Smith J, Laan L. Angelman syndrome: a review of the clinical and genetic aspects. *J Med Genet* 2003;40:87–95.

Hou JW. Hallermann-Streiff syndrome associated with small cerebellum, endocrinopathy and increased chromosomal breakage. *Acta Paediatr* 2003;92:869–871.

Krokan HE, Kavli B, Slupphaug G. Novel aspects of macromolecular repair and relationship to human disease. *J Mol Med* 2004; 82:280–297.

Kruman II, Wersto RP, Cardozo-Pelaez F, et al. Cell cycle activation linked to neuronal cell death initiated by DNA damage. *Neuron* 2004;4:549–561.

Lammerding J, Schulze PC, Takahashi T, et al. Lamin A/C deficiency causes defective nuclear mechanics and mechanotransduction. *J Clin Invest* 2004;113:370–378.

Lee JH, Paull TT. Direct activation of the ATM protein kinase by the Mre11/Rad50/Nbs1 complex. *Science* 2004;304:93–96.

Lehmann AR. DNA repair-deficient diseases, xeroderma pigmentosum, Cockayne syndrome and trichothiodystrophy. *Biochimie* 2003;85: 1101–1111.

Perlman S, Becker-Catania S, Gatti RA. Ataxia-telangiectasia: diagnosis and treatment. *Semin Pediatr Neurol* 2003;10:173–182.

Robbins JH, Kraemer KH, Merchant SN, et al. Adult-onset xeroderma pigmentosum neurological disease—observations in an autopsy case. *Clin Neuropathol* 2002;21:18–23.

Runte M, Kroisel PM, Gillessen-Kaesbach G, et al. SNURF-SNRPN and UBE3A transcript levels in patients with Angelman syndrome. *Hum Genet* 2004;114:553–561.

Samaco RC, Nagarajan RP, Braunschweig D, et al. Multiple pathways regulate MeCP2 expression in normal brain development and exhibit defects in autism-spectrum disorders. *Hum Mol Genet* 2004;13:629–639.

Tuteja N, Tuteja R. Unraveling DNA repair in human: molecular mechanisms and consequences of repair defect. *Crit Rev Biochem Mol Biol* 2001;36:261–290.

Woods CG. Human microcephaly. *Curr Opin Neurobiol* 2004;14:112–117.

Worman HJ, Courvalin J-C. How do mutations in lamins A and C cause disease? *J Clin Invest* 2004;113:349–351

Yamasaki K, Joh K, Ohta T, et al. Neurons but not glial cells show reciprocal imprinting of sense and antisense transcripts of Ube3a. *Hum Mol Genet* 2003;12:837–847.

Chapter 88

Hyperammonemia

Marc C. Patterson

Hyperammonemia has many genetic and acquired causes (Table 88.1). The hepatic urea cycle is the major mammalian system for the detoxification of ammonia (Fig. 88.1), and defects have been described in all six urea cycle enzymes. An additional pathway from arginine to citrulline generates the putative second messenger and neurotransmitter, nitric oxide, catalyzed by nitric oxide synthetase. The enzyme is found in many tissues, including brain. The significance of this pathway is not yet clear, but it may be perturbed in urea cycle disorders. The differential diagnosis of hyperammonemia varies considerably with age (Table 88.1).

HYPERAMMONEMIA IN THE NEONATAL PERIOD

Transient hyperammonemia of the newborn is occasionally seen in otherwise well premature infants and is attributed to metabolic immaturity, analogous to physiologic hyperbilirubinemia of the newborn. Transient hyperammonemia is mild and reversible and rarely requires treatment. Hyperammonemia also reflects liver damage associated with birth asphyxia or congenital hepatic disease; the birth history may help to establish the diagnosis.

The ill neonate with hyperammonemia (especially marked hyperammonemia) without other explanation often has an inborn error of metabolism that, directly or indirectly, affects the urea cycle. Marked hyperammonemia,

▶ **TABLE 88.1 Major Causes of Hyperammonemia**

Newborn period
  Asymptomatic infant
    Transient hyperammonemia of the newborn
  Asymptomatic at birth; symptomatic after 24–72 h protein feeding
    Organic acidurias
      Methylmalonic acidemia
      Propionic acidemia
      Isovaleric acidemia
      Multiple carboxylase (biotinidase) deficiency
      Others
    Urea cycle enzymopathies other than arginase deficiency (see Fig. 86.1)
  Symptomatic at birth or within first day of life
      Asphyxia
      Congenital hepatic disease
      Congenital lactic acidosis
        Pyruvate dehydrogenase deficiency
        Pyruvate carboxylase deficiency (type B)
      Glutaric aciduria, type II
      Short-chain acyl Co-A dehydrogenase deficiency
Older child and adult
  Primary metabolic disease
    Urea cycle defects
      Incomplete blocks (i.e., ornithine carbamyl transferase deficiency heterozygotes)
      Arginase deficiency
    Dibasic aminoacidurias
      Lysinuric protein intolerance
      Hyperornithinemic states
        Partial defect of ornithine decarboxylase (hyperammonemia-hyperornithinemia-homocitrullinemia [HHH syndrome])
        Deficiency of ornithine-ketoacid aminotransferase
        Partial
        Severe—associated with gyrate atrophy of the retina
      Primary carnitine deficiency
  Drugs
    Valproic acid
    Salicylates
    Others

whatever the cause, produces a constellation of symptoms, including progressive lethargy, vomiting, poor feeding, apneic episodes, and seizures. These nonspecific symptoms occur in many disorders, such as sepsis, that can also precipitate hyperammonemia. The age at onset of these symptoms is a useful differential diagnostic point. Infants with hyperammonemia owing to urea cycle enzymopathies or organic acidurias typically are well until they have received 1 to 3 days of protein feeding. In contrast, infants with hyperammonemia secondary to impaired pyruvate metabolism are symptomatic within the first 24 hours. Pyruvate dehydrogenase and (type B) pyruvate carboxylase deficiencies feature lactic acidosis, and these diagnoses can be confirmed by an assay of enzyme activities in fibroblasts.

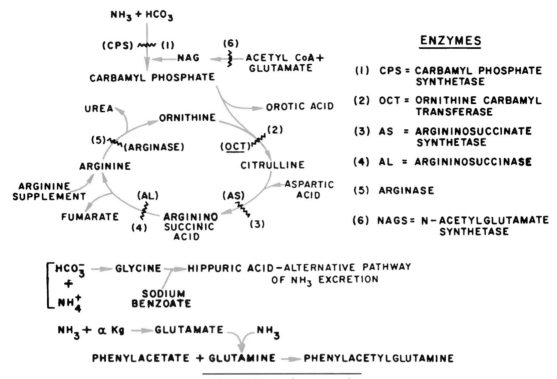

FIGURE 88.1. The urea cycle.

Organic acidurias lead to ketoacidosis (but maple syrup urine disease does not), which distinguishes them from urea cycle enzymopathies. Specific diagnosis of organic acidurias requires urine organic acid analysis, now performed by tandem mass spectrometry. Severe deficiency of the urea cycle enzymes listed in Fig. 88.1, other than arginase, causes similar clinical syndromes. The affected child is well for the first 24 hours of life, but signs of hyperammonemia appear as protein feedings continue. Respiratory alkalosis with hyperventilation is a classic finding, but is not always present, and infants with sepsis or vomiting may have metabolic acidosis or alkalosis. Quantitation of plasma citrulline and urinary orotic acid levels aids rapid determination of the site of block (Table 88.2). Confirmatory enzyme assays may then be performed; ornithine carbamyl transferase and carbamyl phosphate synthase activities can be measured only in liver, but other enzymes can be assayed in fibroblasts. All these enzymopathies are autosomal recessive diseases except for ornithine carbamyl transferase deficiency, which is X linked. Prenatal screening is available for some of these disorders.

Management of Neonatal Hyperammonemia

It is not known how elevated ammonia levels damage the brain, but the outcome is worst with long exposure to high levels. For this reason, acute hyperammonemic coma in the newborn is a medical emergency, and rapid reduction in ammonia levels is necessary. Peritoneal dialysis

▶ **TABLE 88.2 Plasma Amino Acid and Urinary Orotic Acid Findings in Urea Cycle Defects**

Enzymatic Deficiency	Citrulline	Argininosuccinic Acid	Orotic Acid	Arginine
Carbamyl phosphate synthetase (CPS deficiency)	0 to trace	0	↓	↓
Ornithine carbamyl transferase (OTC deficiencies)	0 to trace	0	↑ ↑	↓
Argininosuccinate synthetase (citrullinuria)	↑ ↑	0	↑	↓
Argininosuccinase (argininosuccinic aciduria)	↑	↑ ↑	nl	↓
Arginase	nl	0	↑	↑ ↑
Transient hyperammonemia of newborn	nl or sl ↑	0	nl	nl

nl, normal in plasma and urine; ↑, increased in plasma and urine; ↓, decreased.
Modified from Batshaw ML, Brusilow SW, Waber L, et al. *N Engl J Med* 1982;306:1387–1392.

is more effective than exchange transfusion; hemodialysis may also be effective. Useful adjuncts include intravenous administration of sodium benzoate (250 mg/kg body weight), followed by a constant infusion of 250 to 500 mg/kg body weight every 24 hours. The rationale for benzoate therapy is outlined in Fig. 88.1. An important metabolic consequence of a block in the urea cycle (other than at arginase) is that arginine is rendered an essential amino acid. Therefore, patients with hyperammonemia due to urea cycle enzymopathies should be given supplemental arginine. A loading dose of 0.8 mg/kg body weight of arginine hydrochloride is administered as a loading dose, followed by 0.2 mg/kg per day [N-acetyl-glutamate synthetase, carbamyl phosphate synthetase, or ornithine transcarbamoylase (OTC) deficiencies] or 0.8 mg/kg per day (argininosuccinate synthetase or argininosuccinate lyase deficiencies). Protein catabolism should be minimized by temporarily eliminating protein from the diet and by ensuring adequate caloric intake, principally as glucose. Long-term management depends on the specific enzyme defect.

OLDER CHILDREN AND ADULTS

As compared with the newborn, primary metabolic disease is much less likely a cause of hyperammonemia in an older child or adult. Incomplete urea cycle defects (as seen in female OTC-deficiency heterozygotes) may cause episodic hyperammonemia during periods of metabolic stress and should be considered, especially if there are affected relatives. A study of women heterozygous for OTC deficiency found evidence of a specific neuropsychological and metabolic phenotype, with worse performance in symptomatic compared to asymptomatic individuals. These findings emphasized the importance of impeccable metabolic control in preserving neurologic function. Dibasic amino acidurias and primary systemic carnitine deficiency (Table 88.1) are rare. More likely, the older child or adult with hyperammonemia has severe liver disease or drug-induced hyperammonemia.

Valproate-associated Hyperammonemia

Valproate therapy is one of the most common causes of hyperammonemia in clinical neurologic practice. Malnourished patients with carnitine deficiency and those with unrecognized urea cycle and fatty acid oxidation defects appear to be at higher risk of this complication. This silent dose-related laboratory finding may occur without hepatic dysfunction or clinical symptoms. The pathogenesis is obscure but may involve increased renal production of ammonia and decreased function of carbamyl phosphate synthetase. Inhibition of this enzyme may be a direct effect of the drug or may be related to reduced amounts of N-acetylglutamate because valproate depresses fatty acid metabolism. It is unclear whether patients sometimes become symptomatic from the increased ammonia under these circumstances. Lethargy may be associated with elevated ammonia values, but the encephalopathy may be owing to other substances, including known toxic metabolites of valproate or other organic acids. A patient with valproate encephalopathy showed symmetric T2 MRI signal hyperintensity in the globus pallidus and deep cerebellar white matter. MR spectroscopy showed depletion of myoinositol, choline, and n-acetylaspartate and increased glutamine, as seen in hepatic encephalopathy of other etiologies.

Laboratory studies suggest that L-carnitine supplementation can prevent the development of hyperammonemia in animals receiving valproate and in cultured rat hepatocytes. Supplementation with carnitine also reduces the elevated levels of ammonia in patients treated with valproate. The clinical significance of this reduction is unclear. Some authorities routinely measure serum carnitine levels in patients with marked hyperammonemia. If there is evidence of carnitine deficiency, the patient is given supplementary L-carnitine. In severe acute valproate hepatotoxicity with hyperammonemia, a disorder with high mortality, intravenous L-carnitine has been shown to improve survival compared to oral therapy with the same agent.

SUGGESTED READINGS

Bachmann C, Braissant O, Villard AM, et al. Ammonia toxicity to the brain and creatine. *Mol Genet Metab* 2004;81[Suppl 1]:S52–57.

Bohan TP, Helton E, McDonald I, et al. Effect of L-carnitine treatment for valproate-induced hepatotoxicity. *Neurology* 2001;56:1405–1409.

Brusilow SB, Horwich AL. Urea cycle enzymes. In: Scriver CR, Beaudet AL, Sly WS, et al., eds. *The Metabolic and Molecular Bases of Inherited Disease*, 8th ed. New York: McGraw-Hill, 2001:1909–1963.

Dawson TD, Dawson VL, Snyder SH. A novel neuronal messenger molecule in the brain: the free radical, nitric oxide. *Ann Neurol* 1992;32:297–311.

De Vivo DC, Bohan TP, Coulter DL, et al. L-carnitine supplementation in childhood epilepsy: current perspectives. *Epilepsia* 1998;39:1216–1225.

Gropman AL, Batshaw ML. Cognitive outcome in urea cycle disorders. *Mol Genet Metab* 2004;81(Suppl 1):S58–62.

Gyato K, Wray J, Huang ZJ, et al. Metabolic and neuropsychological phenotype in women heterozygous for ornithine transcarbamylase deficiency. *Ann Neurol* 2004;55:80–86.

Stanley CA, Lieu YK, Hsu BY, et al. Hyperinsulinism and hyperammonemia in infants with regulatory mutations of the glutamate dehydrogenase gene. *N Engl J Med* 1998;338:1352–1357.

Tein I. Role of carnitine and fatty acid oxidation and its defects in infantile epilepsy. *J Child Neurol* 2002;17(Suppl 3):3S57–82

Verrotti A, Trotta D, Morgese G, et al. Valproate-induced hyperammonemic encephalopathy. *Metab Brain Dis* 2002;17(Dec):367–373.

Ziyeh S, Thiel T, Spreer J, et al. Valproate-induced encephalopathy: assessment with MR imaging and 1H MR spectroscopy. *Epilepsia* 2002;43:1101–1105.

Peroxisomal Diseases: Adrenoleukodystrophy, Zellweger Syndrome, and Refsum Disease

Marc C. Patterson and Darryl C. De Vivo

▶ **TABLE 89.1 Human Genetic Diseases due to Peroxisomal Dysfunction**

Peroxisomal Biogenesis Disorders	Single Peroxisomal Enzyme Disorders
Zellweger syndrome	X-linked adrenoleukodystrophy
Neonatal adrenoleukodystrophy	Oxidase deficiency (Pseudoneonatal adrenoleukodystrophy)
Infantile Refsum disease	
Hyperpipecolic acidemia	
Rhizomelic chondrodysplasia punctata	Bifunctional enzyme deficiency
	Thiolase deficiency (pseudo-Zellweger)
	DHAP acyl transferase deficiency
	Alky1 DHAP synthase deficiency
	Glutaric aciduria type III (1 case only)
	Refsum disease
	Hyperoxaluria type 1
	Acatalasia

DHAP, dihydroxyacetone phosphate.

Peroxisomes are ubiquitous cellular organelles that participate in a variety of essential biochemical functions. Peroxisomes are enclosed by a single membrane and contain no DNA, implying that all peroxisomal-associated proteins are encoded by nuclear genes. A complex shuttle system transports peroxisomal enzymes and structural proteins from the cytosolic polyribosomes where they are made to the peroxisome. This system involves at least two recognition sequences (peroxisomal targeting sequences) that are embedded in the protein products themselves and several receptors or transporters; the system is ATP dependent.

Peroxisomes participate in both anabolic and catabolic cellular functions, especially in the metabolism of lipids. For example, peroxisomes contain a complete series of enzymes for the beta oxidation of fatty acids. These enzymes are distinct from the mitochondrial enzymes of beta oxidation in both genetic coding and substrate specificity. Because mitochondrial enzymes of beta oxidation cannot metabolize carbon chain lengths greater than 24, the peroxisomal system is required for the degradation of endogenous and exogenous very-long-chain fatty acids (VLCFA). The peroxisome is also the site of the initial and rate-limiting steps of the synthesis of plasmalogens, ether-linked lipids that constitute the major portion of the myelin sheath. Other key functions include cholesterol and bile acid biosynthesis, degradation of pipecolic and phytanic acids, and transamination of glyoxalate.

Human diseases caused by disruption of peroxisome function are divided into two broad categories (Table 89.1). The first is characterized by abnormalities in more than one metabolic pathway, often accompanied by morphologic changes of the peroxisome. The prototype of this class is Zellweger syndrome discussed below, although patients with milder phenotypes have been described under various names such as neonatal adrenoleukodystrophy, infantile Refsum disease, and hyperpipecolic acidemia. This overlapping range of phenotypes is referred to as the Zellweger spectrum. A second phenotype, distinct from the Zellweger spectrum and termed rhizomelic chondrodysplasia punctata (RCDP), is associated with severe growth failure, profound developmental delay, cataracts, rhizomelia, epiphyseal calcifications, and ichthyosis. Patients with RCDP have decreased plasmalogens and elevated phytanic acid, but unlike the Zellweger spectrum patients, the beta oxidation pathway and VLCFA levels are normal. In recognition of the similar cellular pathophysiology in these phenotypes, *peroxisome biogenesis disorder* (PBD) is now the preferred term for all Zellweger spectrum and RCDP conditions.

The second class of human peroxisomal diseases shows the genetic and biochemical features of single enzyme defects. In addition to X-linked adrenoleukodystrophy (ALD) and Refsum disease discussed below, this category includes defects in the beta oxidation pathway of VLCFA, which cause a Zellweger-like phenotype, and defects in plasmalogen synthesis, which result in an RCDP-like phenotype.

ZELLWEGER SYNDROME

The Zellweger syndrome (*cerebrohepatorenal syndrome*) is an autosomal recessive disease with no ethnic or racial predilection. Affected newborns are strikingly floppy and inactive; they lack the Moro, stepping, and placing reflexes. The characteristic facial appearance includes a high narrow forehead, round cheeks, flat root of the nose, wide-set eyes with shallow orbits, puffy eyelids, pursed lips, narrow high-arched palate, and small chin. The head circumference is normal, but the fontanels and sutures are widely open. Ophthalmologic findings include pigmentary retinopathy, retinal arteriolar attenuation, and optic atrophy. The pinnas may be abnormal and posteriorly rotated. Affected infants suck and swallow poorly and often require tube feeding. Some have congenital heart disease, notably patent ductus arteriosus or septal defects. The liver is cirrhotic and either enlarged or shrunken; some children are jaundiced, and some develop splenomegaly and a bleeding diathesis. Cystic dysplasia of the kidneys may be palpable and may cause mild renal failure. Genital anomalies include an enlarged clitoris, hypospadias, and cryptorchidism. Minor skeletal anomalies include contractures of large and small joints, polydactyly, low-set rotated thumbs, and clubfeet; there are also stippled calcifications of the patella and epiphyseal cartilage. The children are apathetic, poorly responsive to environmental stimuli, and limp. Tendon reflexes are absent or hypoactive. Many children have seizures and fail to thrive or develop; most succumb within the first few months of life.

The pathogenesis of the neurologic phenotype is uncertain. Studies in the Zellweger mouse have identified the diazepam binding inhibitor/acyl-CoA binding protein (DBI) as a candidate mediator of these effects, because it has a dual role as a neuropeptide antagonist of GABA(A) receptor signaling in the brain and as a regulator of lipid metabolism. Increased GABAergic signaling could account for the hypotonia and seizures, and for the structural abnormalities, which resemble those found in benzodiazepine fetopathy.

Typical but nonspecific laboratory findings include elevated bilirubin levels, abnormal liver function tests, elevated serum iron, saturated iron binding capacity, and transferrin. The CSF protein content may be elevated. The electroencephalogram is abnormal, and MRI shows poor myelination, brain atrophy, pachygyria, polymicrogyria, and neuronal heterotopias. Diffusion-weighted and tensor-diffusion MRI identify regions of injury in patients with PBD that are not apparent with conventional MRI.

The hallmark of Zellweger syndrome is dysfunction in multiple enzymatic pathways, including the following:

1. Levels of VLCFA—those with 24 or more carbons—are increased in plasma, fibroblasts, and chorionic villus;
2. In plasma and urine, increased content of intermediates of bile acid metabolism includes trihydroxycholestanoic acid and dihydroxycholestanoic acid;
3. Levels of pipecolic and phytanic acids increase;
4. Plasmalogen levels decrease.

In addition, levels of cholesterol and the fat-soluble vitamins may be low. Acylcarnitine screening of plasma and neonatal blood spots from PBD patients disclosed increased levels of hexadecanedioyl- and octadecanedioyl-carnitine, with a high dicarboxylycarnitine/monocarboxylylcarnitine ratio. This finding, if confirmed, could lead to a simpler and more sensitive screening test for PBDs, which might include neonatal screening.

PBD patients, including those with Zellweger syndrome, can be divided into at least 13 complementation groups, based on the ability of their cells to reconstitute peroxisomal structure and function in fusion experiments. These groups do not correspond to the clinical phenotypes, but rather to the underlying molecular defect (Table 89.2).

Pathologically, the absence of functional peroxisomes in hepatocytes is a pathognomonic feature of Zellweger syndrome and one that helps distinguish it from other PBDs and from single enzyme disorders such as pseudo-Zellweger disease. Membrane proteins may assemble with membrane lipids to form rudimentary "ghosts" of peroxisomes that seem unable to import enzymes. For reasons not well understood, secondary abnormalities are seen in mitochondria that show an abnormally dense matrix and distorted cristae. Lipid leaflets resembling those in adrenoleukodystrophy are found in several tissues, including the adrenal gland. The brain is dysgenic, with signs of disordered cell migration resulting in areas of pachygyria or micropolygyria and neuronal ectopias. The inferior olive is grossly disorganized. Myelination is severely affected. Neutral fat accumulates in fibrous astrocytes, hepatocytes, renal tubules and glomeruli, and muscle. Studies in the murine model of Zellweger syndrome show both developmental and degenerative abnormalities in the cerebellum, emphasizing the role of intact peroxisomal function in supporting normal development and survival of neurons.

Therapy for Zellweger syndrome is primarily supportive and limited because of the multisystem impairment already present at birth. Therapeutic trials of the polyunsaturated fatty acid docosahexaenate have shown some success in improving the visual function of mildly affected patients. Other potential therapies, including the peroxisomal proliferator clofibrate and bile acids, are of less clear benefit. Reliable prenatal diagnosis is available by enzymatic assays in chorionic villus or amniotic fluid cells.

ADRENOLEUKODYSTROPHY (ALD) (MIM 300100)

ALD is an X-linked incompletely recessive disorder with variable expressivity; it is well defined genetically, clinically, and pathologically. The most common phenotype is the childhood cerebral form, which appears in boys who have normal early development. Behavioral change

▶ TABLE 89.2 Molecular Basis of Peroxisomal Biogenesis Disorders (PBD)

Complementation Group	Percentage of Patients[a]	Gene Responsible	Function Gene Product
1	45	PEX1	ATPase of the AAA protein family
2	1	PEX5	PTS1 receptor
3	2	PEX12	48-kDa peroxisomal membrane protein
4	7	PEX6	Cytoplasmic ATPase
6–9	11	—	—
10	1	PEX2	35-kDa peroxisomal membrane protein
11	32	PEX7	PTS2 receptor

[a]Approximated from Moser et al. (1995) who found that 20% of patients initially thought to have a PBD actually had a single enzyme defect of the beta oxidation or plasmalogen synthesis pathway. Complementation groups 1–10 cause Zellweger spectrum phenotypes; all RCDP-type patients are in complementation group 11. PTS, peroxisomal transport signal.

is the most common initial feature, with abnormal withdrawal, aggression, poor memory, or difficulties in school. Ultimately, progressive dementia is evident. Visual loss with optic atrophy is a consistent feature owing to demyelination along the entire visual pathway. The outer retina is notably spared. Progressive gait disturbance with pyramidal tract signs is an important feature. Dysphagia and deafness may occur. Seizures are common late in the disease, but are occasionally the first manifestation. Some patients have overt signs of adrenal failure, including fatigue, vomiting, salt craving, and hyperpigmentation that is most prominent in skin folds. The course is relentlessly progressive. Patients enter a vegetative state and die from adrenal crisis or other causes 1 to 10 years after onset.

Several other clinical phenotypes have been described (Table 89.3). Adrenomyeloneuropathy (AMN) is the most common of the variant phenotypes. Typical features are spastic paraparesis, peripheral neuropathy, and adrenal insufficiency, beginning in the second decade. Hypogonadism, impotence, and sphincter disturbance are also seen. Cerebellar dysfunction and dementia have been reported. A similar syndrome is found in about 15% of women who are heterozygous for mutation at the *ALD* gene. MRI frequently reveals cortical demyelinating lesions in AMN patients, even in those without signs or symptoms of cortical involvement. Pathologic findings in AMN include demyelination and dying-back changes in the cord and lamellar cytoplasmic inclusions in brain, adrenal, and testis; the findings are similar to those of ALD.

A cerebral form of ALD is occasionally seen that is similar to the childhood form, but starts in adolescence. In adults, X-linked ALD may show symptoms of dementia, schizophrenia, or focal cerebral syndromes such as

▶ TABLE 89.3 Phenotypes Associated with Mutation at the *ALD* Locus

Form	Percentage of Patients	Age at Onset (yr)	Major Manifestations[a]
Childhood cerebral	50	5–9	Behavioral abnormalities, blindness, deafness, spasticity
Adolescent cerebral	5	10–21	Behavioral abnormalities, blindness, deafness, spasticity
Adrenomyeloneuropathy	25	18–36	Spastic paraparesis
Adrenal insufficiency only	10	1–14	Addison disease
Asymptomatic	10	—	Elevated VLCFA
Expressing carriers	(60% of obligate carriers)	20–50	Spastic paraparesis

[a]In all forms of ALD, radiographic abnormalities precede clinical findings.

aphasia, Klüver-Bucy syndrome, or hemianopia; usually there is also adrenal insufficiency. Adult ALD includes spastic paraparesis, cerebellar dysfunction, or olivopontocerebellar atrophy. Female heterozygotes may be symptomatic with adult ALD. Adrenal insufficiency can be seen without neurologic disorder; ALD should be considered in any boy with unexplained Addison disease. Finally, children and adults with the biochemical defect may be asymptomatic or presymptomatic. Phenotypic heterogeneity is the rule within families with multiple affected individuals; the disparate manifestations are probably the result of modifying genetic loci or environmental factors.

Laboratory evaluation of the patient with ALD reveals several abnormalities. The CSF protein content is often elevated. CT shows characteristic hyperdense and hypodense bandlike regions in parietooccipital white matter; if found, these are virtually diagnostic of ALD. MRI abnormalities are more diffuse and always predate clinical findings. Adrenal function tests, especially the corticotropin stimulation test, usually show adrenal insufficiency even in the absence of clinical signs. In the zona fasciculata and reticularis, adrenal biopsy shows many ballooned cortical cells and striated cytoplasm and microvacuoles, findings specific for ALD. Characteristic inclusions, accumulations of lamellar lipid profiles, may also be seen in the brain, sural nerve biopsy, or testis. The primary finding in the brain is extensive diffuse demyelination, sparing U-fibers in the centrum semiovale and elsewhere. In involved areas of white matter, perivascular infiltration of lymphocytes and plasma cells is prominent.

Diagnosis is suggested by the characteristic clinical findings of neurologic deterioration, demonstration of adrenal hypofunction, and MRI abnormalities. Definite diagnosis is made by finding elevated VLCFA levels in plasma and cultured skin fibroblasts without disruption of other peroxisomal functions. To date, elevated VLCFA levels in both tissues have been found only in patients with ALD, PBDs, and single enzyme defects involving the VLCFA oxidation pathway.

Studies in ALD mice did not confirm impaired peroxisomal VLCFA oxidation in association with elevated plasma levels. The presence of mitochondrial structural abnormalities in murine adrenal cortex supported the hypothesis that ALD protein functions to facilitate peroxisomal-mitochondrial interactions, rather than determining the rate of VLCFA beta oxidation. Markers of oxidative stress are elevated in the plasma of patients with X-ALD, suggesting that free radical injury contributes to the pathogenesis.

Unlike ALD patients, patients on the ketogenic diet may show elevated VLCFA levels in plasma but not cultured skin fibroblasts. Prenatal diagnosis of ALD is made by assay of VLCFA oxidation in amniotic fluid cells or chorionic villus sampling. Eighty-five percent of female carriers of ALD have elevated VLCFA levels in plasma and cultured skin fibroblasts.

The *ALD* gene has been cloned and encodes a member of the ATP binding cassette transporter class of proteins. Mutations at this locus have proven to be mostly private, limiting the usefulness of molecular analysis for diagnosis.

Several approaches have been taken to the rational treatment of ALD. Steroid replacement therapy is given during stressful periods, such as intercurrent illness, or if there is evidence of adrenal insufficiency. Dietary avoidance of VLCFA alone does not lead to biochemical change because of endogenous synthesis. Efforts to lower endogenous synthesis using glycerol trierucate oil and glycerol trioleate oil (Lorenzo oil) in conjunction with dietary restriction do produce a fall in VLCFA levels in both affected individuals and female carriers. Unfortunately, this striking biochemical change does not have an equally striking clinical correlate; its use is most likely limited to presymptomatic boys. Bone marrow transplantation cures the biochemical defect in ALD, but the morbidity and mortality are high, and neither neurologic defects nor radiologic abnormalities revert. In all cases, radiologic abnormalities and progression almost invariably precede neurologic progression; it is therefore imperative that every child whose family might consider bone marrow transplantation is closely followed radiographically. Immunotherapy has been considered in X-ALD because of the inflammatory component of the central lesions, but beta interferon and thalidomide have not been effective. Finally, the cloning and characterization of the *ALD* locus may lead to a gene or protein product replacement therapy.

REFSUM DISEASE (MIM 266510)

This autosomal recessive disease (also known as heredopathia atactica polyneuritiformis) is unique among the lipidoses because the stored lipid (phytanic acid) is not synthesized in the body but is exclusively dietary in origin. This has enabled successful therapy by dietary management. Symptoms begin in early childhood in some patients, but may be delayed until the fifth decade in others. Progressive night blindness usually appears in the first or second decade, followed by limb weakness and gait ataxia. Symptoms are progressive, but abrupt exacerbations and gradual remissions may occur with intercurrent illness or pregnancy. There are no seizures, but some patients have psychiatric symptoms. Peripheral neuropathy is manifest by loss of tendon reflexes, weakness and wasting, and distal sensory loss. Ataxia may be seen. A granular pigmentary retinopathy is universally present. Other findings include ichthyosis, nerve deafness (often severe), cataracts, miosis and pupillary asymmetry, pes cavus, and bone deformities with shortening of the metatarsal bones, epiphyseal dysplasia, and, in some, kyphoscoliosis. CSF protein content is elevated. Nerve conduction velocities are slowed. Electrocardiographic changes include conduction abnormalities. Peripheral nerves may feel thickened and, on histologic study, may show hypertrophic interstitial changes and onion-bulb formation. The course is generally progressive with exacerbations and remissions. Peripheral visual fields may ultimately be lost, with resulting telescopic vision. Sudden death may result from cardiac arrhythmia.

The biochemical defect in Refsum disease has been identified as phytanoyl-coenzyme A hydroxylase (PHYH) deficiency; the responsible gene in most cases is (*PAHX*). Several kindreds with typical Refsum disease have lacked *PAHX* mutations or linkage to chromosome 10; they proved to be heterozygous for mutations in *PEX 7*. That gene encodes the receptor for the type 2 peroxisomal targeting signal (PTS2), whose normal function is essential for PHYH import to peroxisomes. Diagnosis is made by the characteristic clinical picture and elevation of phytanic acid levels in the plasma. Studies in rat brain suggest that phytanic acid exerts direct neurotoxic effects by binding to the inner mitochondrial membrane, impairing mitochondrial ATP supply and membrane permeability.

Therapy limits dietary phytanic acid and its precursor, phytol, a branched chain fatty alcohol, which is abundantly present in nature as part of the chlorophyll molecule. When dairy products, ruminant fat, and chlorophyll-containing foods are eliminated, plasma phytanic acid levels are reduced and tissue stores are mobilized, with improvement of symptoms. Paradoxically, symptoms may worsen and plasma phytanic acid levels may rise shortly after institution of dietary therapy, especially if patients reduce caloric intake and lose weight. Increased plasma phytanic acid causes anorexia, increased weight loss, and still more severe symptoms. Adequate caloric intake helps prevent weight loss and abrupt fat mobilization. Plasmapheresis helps to prevent or treat exacerbations.

SUGGESTED READINGS

Peroxisomal Biogenesis and Biochemistry

Wanders RJ. Metabolic and molecular basis of peroxisomal disorders: a review. *Am J Med Genet* 2004;126A(May 1):355–375.

Peroxisomal Biogenesis Disorders

Braverman N, Dodt G, Gould S, et al. Disorders of peroxisome biogenesis. *Human Mol Genet* 1996;4:1791–1798.

Breitling R. Pathogenesis of peroxisomal deficiency disorders (Zellweger syndrome) may be mediated by misregulation of the GABAergic system via the diazepam binding inhibitor. *BMC Pediatr* 2004;4:5.

Faust PL. Abnormal cerebellar histogenesis in PEX2 Zellweger mice reflects multiple neuronal defects induced by peroxisome deficiency. *J Comp Neurol* 2003;461:394–413.

Martinez M, Vazquez E. MRI evidence that docosahexaenoic acid ethyl ester improves myelination in generalized peroxisomal disorders. *Neurology* 1998;51:26–32.

Martinez M, Vazquez E, Garcia-Silva MT, et al. Therapeutic effects of docosahexaenoic acid ethyl ester in patients with generalized peroxisomal disorders. *Am J Clin Nutr* 2000(Suppl)71:376S–385S.

Moser A, Rasmussen M, Naidu S, et al. Phenotype of patients with peroxisomal disorders subdivided into sixteen complementation groups. *J Pediatr* 1995;127:13–22.

Reuber B, Germain-Lee E, Collins C, et al. Mutations in PEX1 are the most common cause of peroxisome biogenesis disorders. *Nat Genet* 1997;17:445–452.

Rizzo C, Boenzi S, Wanders RJ, et al. Characteristic acylcarnitine profiles in inherited defects of peroxisome biogenesis: a novel tool for screening diagnosis using tandem mass spectrometry. *Pediatr Res* 2003;53:1013–1018

Santos MJ, Imanaka T, Shio H, et al. Peroxisomal membrane ghosts in Zellweger syndrome-aberrant organelle assembly. *Science* 1988;239:1536–1538.

Setchell K, Bragetti P, Zimmer-Nechemias L, et al. Oral bile acid treatment and the patient with Zellweger syndrome. *Hepatology* 1992;15:198–207.

Shimozawa N, Tsukamoto T, Nagase T, et al. Identification of a new complementation group of the peroxisome biogenesis disorders and PEX14 as the mutated gene. *Hum Mutat* 2004;23:552–558.

Ter Rahe BS, Majoie CB, Akkerman EM, et al. Peroxisomal biogenesis disorder: comparison of conventional MR imaging with diffusion-weighted and diffusion-tensor imaging findings. *Am J Neuroradiol* 2004;25:1022–1027.

Volpe JJ, Adams RD. Cerebro-hepato-renal syndrome of Zellweger: an inherited disorder of neuronal migration. *Acta Neuropathol (Berl)* 1972;20:175–198.

Adrenoleukodystrophy

Aubourg P, Adamsbaum C, Lavallard-Rousseau MC, et al. A two-year trial of oleic and erucic acids ("Lorenzo's oil") as treatment for adreno-myeloneuropathy. *N Engl J Med* 1993;329:745–752.

Aubourg P, Blanche S, Jambaque I, et al. Reversal of early neurologic and neuroradiologic manifestations of X-linked adrenoleukodystrophy by bone marrow transplantation. *N Engl J Med* 1990;322:1860–1866.

Bezman L, Moser H. Incidence of X-linked adrenoleukodystrophy and the relative frequency of its phenotypes. *Am J Med Genet* 1998;76:415–419.

McGuinness MC, Lu JF, Zhang HP, et al. Role of ALDP (ABCD1) and mitochondria in X-linked adrenoleukodystrophy. *Mol Cell Biol* 2003;23:744–753.

Moser H, Dubey P, Fatemi A. Progress in x-linked adrenoleukodystrophy. *Curr Opin Neurol* 2004 Jun;17(3):263–269.

Mosser J, Douar A, Sarde C, et al. Putative X-linked adrenoleukodystrophy gene shares unexpected homology with ABC transporters. *Nature* 1993;361:726–730.

Panegyres P, Goldswain P, Kakulas B. Adult-onset adrenoleukodystrophy manifesting as dementia. *Am J Med* 1989;87:481–482.

Sadeghi-Nejad A, Senior B. Adrenomyeloneuropathy presenting as Addison's disease in childhood. *N Engl J Med* 1990;322:13–16.

Shapiro E, Aubourg P, Lockman L, et al. Bone marrow transplant for adrenoleukodystrophy: 5 year follow-up of 12 engrafted cases. *Ann Neurol* 1997;42:498.

Shaw-Smith CJ, Lewis SJ, Reid E. X-linked adrenoleukodystrophy presenting as autosomal dominant pure hereditary spastic paraparesis. *J Neurol Neurosurg Psychiatry* 2004 May;75(5):686–688.

Vargas CR, Wajner M, Sirtori LR, et al. Evidence that oxidative stress is increased in patients with X-linked adrenoleukodystrophy. *Biochim Biophys Acta* 2004;1688:26–32.

Refsum Disease

Djupesland G, Flottorp G, Refsum S. Phytanic acid storage disease; hearing maintained after 15 years of dietary treatment. *Neurology* 1983;33:237–239.

Jansen GA, Waterham HR, Wanders RJ. Molecular basis of Refsum disease: sequence variations in phytanoyl-CoA hydroxylase (PHYH) and the PTS2 receptor (PEX7). *Hum Mutat* 2004;23:209–218.

Masters-Thomas A, Bailes J, Billimoria J, et al. Heredopathia atactica polyneuritiformis (Refsum's disease). *1. Clinical features and dietary management. J Hum Nutr* 1980;34:245–250.

Mihalik S, Morrell J, Kim D, et al. Identification of PAHX, a Refsum disease gene. *Nat Genet* 1997;17:185–189.

Refsum S. Heredopathia atactica polyneuritiformis. *Acta Psychiatr Scand* 1946(Suppl);38:9–303.

Schonfeld P, Kahlert S, Reiser G. In brain mitochondria the branched chain fatty acid phytanic acid impairs energy transduction and sensitizes for permeability transition. *Biochem J* 2004;383(Pt 1 Oct 1):121–128.

Other Single Enzyme Defects

Schram AW, Goldfischer S, van Roermund CWT, et al. Human peroxisomal 3-oxoacyl-coenzyme A thiolase deficiency. *Proc Natl Acad Sci USA* 1987;84:2494–2496.

Wanders R, Schumacher H, Heikoop H, et al. Human dihydroxyacetonephosphate acyltransferase deficiency: a new peroxisomal disorder. *J Inherit Metab Dis* 1992;15:389–391.

Watkins P, McGuinness M, Raymond G, et al. Distinction between peroxisomal bifunctional enzyme and acyl-CoA oxidase deficiencies. *Ann Neurol* 1995;38:472–477.

Chapter 90

Organic Acidurias

Stefano DiDonato and Graziella Uziel

DEFINITION

The organic acidurias are inborn errors of metabolism characterized by abnormal accumulation of one or more organic acids in plasma, urine, and CSF. Although individually rare, these diseases comprise more than 50 specific disorders and collectively are the most frequent cause of acute encephalopathy in early infancy. They may appear later in life with more complex features of chronic brain disorder, including dystonia, seizures, or myopathy, sometimes with liver and heart pathology.

The acute and frequently life-threatening manifestations in the newborn or young infant demand rapid differential diagnosis from the many acute encephalopathies of infancy such as cerebral infection, hypoxia, space-occupying lesions, and ingestion of drugs or toxins. The issue is urgent because some organic acidurias can be effectively cured, including multiple carboxylase deficiency responsive to biotin, methylmalonic aciduria responsive to vitamin B_{12}, and glutaric aciduria type II responsive to riboflavin. Early diagnosis is important because treatment may prevent acute metabolic attacks and subsequent mental retardation, epilepsy, severe brain damage, or death.

The most common inherited organic acidurias involve enzymes of two principal biochemical pathways. One is the stepwise degradation of amino acids, including methionine and threonine; the branched chain amino acids valine, leucine, and isoleucine; tryptophan and the basic aminoacid lysine. The other is the β-oxidation of straight chain fatty acids. Some of the final degradative pathways are the same in both amino acid and fatty acid catabolism; one example is the funneling of flavin-adenine-dinucleotide–linked reducing equivalents to the respiratory chain through the electron-transferring flavoproteins.

Lactic acidemia also results in an organic aciduria. Pyruvate dehydrogenase deficiency and respiratory chain defects, however, are the major causes of genetic lactic acidosis of infancy, so lactic acidemia is discussed in Chapter 98. In fact, most organic acidurias are mitochondrial disorders, caused by genetic deficiencies of enzymes that catalyze the oxidative degradation of some amino acids and the β−oxidation of straight chain fatty acids.

The organic acidurias that cause acute encephalopathy include multiple carboxylase deficiency, maple syrup urine disease, methylmalonic aciduria, propionic aciduria, isovaleric aciduria, fumaric aciduria, glutaric aciduria type I and type II, methylcrotonic aciduria, 3-hydroxy-3-methylglutaric aciduria, dicarboxylic acidurias, and 3-hydroxydicarboxylic aciduria (Table 90.1).

CLINICAL MANIFESTATIONS AND DIAGNOSIS

The signs and symptoms of organic acidurias in the newborn or infant are usually nonspecific. Acute episodes of nausea and vomiting, hypotonia, drowsiness, and coma do not discriminate acquired from inherited conditions. The presence of hypoglycemia, however, with glucose blood concentrations <2.5 mmol/liter, or metabolic acidosis with blood pH <7.30, and, in some instances, such as in propionic and methylmalonic acidurias, hyperammonemia with plasma ammonia values of more than 100 mmol/liter suggest organic acidurias. Acute hypoglycemia, particularly with acidosis, may be fatal. Some infants with these diseases die abruptly without any evident prodromal or accompanying symptoms. Similar features are also part of two relatively common but pathogenically ill-defined disorders of infancy: Reye disease or hepatic encephalopathy and the sudden infant death (SID) syndrome. Both syndromes, currently viewed as nongenetic, have much in common with inherited disorders of fatty acid metabolism

▶ **TABLE 90.1 Organic Acidurias**

Disease	Enzyme	OMIM
Amino acid metabolism		
Maple syrup urine disease	Branched-chain acyl-CoA dehydrogenase	248600
Propionic acidemia	Propionyl-CoA carboxylase	232050
Methylmalonic acidemia	Methylmalonyl-CoA mutase	251000
Isovaleric acidemia	Isovalery-CoA dehydrogenase	607036
Glutaric aciduria type I	Glutaryl-CoA dehydrogenase	231670
3-Methylcrotonic aciduria	3-Methylcrotonyl-CoA carboxylase	210200
2-Methylglutaconic acidemia	2-Methylglutaconyl-CoA hydratase	250950
3-Hydroxy-3-methylglutaric aciduria[a]	3-Hydroxy-3-methyl-glutaryl-CoA lyase (HMG-CoA lyase)	246450
Multiple carboxylase deficiency[b]	Holocarboxylase synthetase or biotinidase	253270 253260
4-Hydroxybutyric aciduria	Succinic semialdeide dehydrogenase	271980
Encephalopathy ethylmalonic	Not defined	608451
L-2 Hydroxyglutaric aciduria	Not defined	236792
Ethylmalonic aciduria	Not defined	602673
Krebs cycle		
Fumaric aciduria	Fumarase deficiency	606812
Fatty acid metabolism		
Dicarboxylic aciduria (VLCAD deficiency)	Very long-chain fatty acyl-CoA dehydrogenase	201475
Dicarboxylic aciduria (MCAD deficiency)	Medium-chain acyl-CoA dehydrogenase	201450
Ethylmalonic aciduria (SCAD deficiency)	Short-chain acyl-CoA dehydrogenase	201470
3-Hydroxydicarboxylic aciduria	Trifunctional protein or 3-hydroxy-acyl-CoA dehydrogenase	143450 600890
Glutaric aciduria type II[c]	Electron transfer flavoprotein (ETF) or ETF-coenzyme-Q reductase (ETF-QR)	231680 231675

[a]HMG-CoA lyase deficiency also affects fatty acid (ketone bodies) metabolism.
[b]Holocarboxylase synthetase and biotinidase deficiencies also affect fatty acid (synthesis) and glucose metabolism (gluconeogenesis).
[c]ETF and ETF-QR deficiencies also affect amino acid metabolism (valine, leucine, isoleucine, and lysine).

because dicarboxylic aciduria has been reported in the Reye syndrome, and SID has been observed in patients with β-oxidation defects such as medium-chain acyl-CoA dehydrogenase deficiency.

The only way to reach a definite diagnosis is laboratory examination, including the analysis of body fluids for accumulating metabolites and study of the patients' cells for the specific enzymes listed in Table 90.1. Molecular analysis of mutations of the corresponding genes usually follows biochemical diagnosis and is of less importance for early diagnosis. Analysis of amniotic fluid and enzyme assay in chorionic villi and amniocytes also are possible. However, DNA analysis is useful for prenatal diagnosis. Molecular diagnosis can be a first-choice diagnostic tool in case of prevalent mutations such as the A985G transition in medium-chain acyl-CoA dehydrogenase deficiency. Because most of these acids are effectively cleared from the blood by the kidneys, detection of abundant organic acids in urine is facilitated by gas chromatography–mass spectrometry of a 24-hour urine specimen, which generally reveals the pattern of urinary metabolites characteristic of one disease.

Some infants with organic aciduria survive the acute metabolic attack but show poor growth, macrocephaly, and impaired psychomotor development. Dystonia, spastic tetraplegia, and intractable seizures may also mark the devastating effects of acidosis, acute energy shortage, and the accumulation of toxic metabolites on the developing brain. A few organic acidurias may not damage the human brain acutely, but result in chronic neurological disorder. In general, early-onset forms are devastatingly lethal, whereas late-onset forms are less severe. Different amounts of residual enzyme activity may account for the clinical heterogeneity.

Therefore, in addition to acute acidosis, chronic neurological disorders of infancy or early childhood without evident cause should lead to a search for metabolic disease. Mental retardation, ataxia, and behavioral changes suggest maple syrup urine disease (MSUD), but are also seen in 4-hydroxybutyric aciduria. Spasticity, ataxia, mental retardation, and seizures are present in L-2-hydroxyglutaric aciduria. Severe hypotonia, epilepsy, spastic tetraparesis, and early death are features of fumaric aciduria. Dystonia and spasticity, often with normal intellectual development, may underlie glutaric aciduria type I. Choreoathetosis and dystonic posture are signs of 3-hydroxy-3-methylglutaric aciduria. Seizures and ataxia are classically seen with alopecia and skin rash, in late-onset multiple carboxylase deficiency. Ataxia, optic atrophy, and retinitis pigmentosa may be associated with 3-methylglutaconic aciduria. Some patients with late-onset 3-hydroxydicarboxylic aciduria associated with mitochondrial trifunctional protein deficiency in addition to retinitis pigmentosa show peripheral neuropathy. Infantile spinal muscular atrophy with mental retardation can suggest 3-methylcrotonic aciduria. Ethylmalonic encephalopathy is a devastating disease of infancy with developmental delay, orthostatic acrogenesis, and early death. Lipid storage myopathy and cardiomyopathy develop in patients with the rare late-onset β-oxidation defects associated with dicarboxylic aciduria, such as carnitine translocase deficiency, mitochondrial trifunctional protein deficiency, very long-chain acyl-CoA dehydrogenase deficiency, and the riboflavin-responsive form of glutaric aciduria type II.

NEUROIMAGING

Brain MRI and CT help in the diagnosis of organic acidurias, although they often lack specificity. Glutaric aciduria type I is characterized by abnormal signal intensity in the caudate and putamen, whereas MSUD and methylmalonic aciduria involve the pallidum. Leucoencephalopathy mainly involving the subcortical regions is seen in L-2-hydroxyglutaric aciduria.

THERAPY

Management of organic acidurias caused by defects in aminoacid metabolism is based on accurate early dietary treatment with protein modified diets that restrict the appropriate amino acids: leucine, valine, and isoleucine in MSUD; leucine in 3-hydroxy-methylglutaric aciduria; isoleucine, valine, threonine, and methionine in propionic and methylmalonic aciduria; lysine and tryptophan in glutaric aciduria type I. Patients with methylmalonic aciduria and propionic acidemia may also benefit from oral carnitine supplementation, which increases urinary excretion of propionyl carnitine. Carnitine and medium-chain triglycerides have been also used to treat β-oxidation disorders such as VLCAD deficiency and trifunctional protein deficiency. The use of carnitine in these disorders has been questioned because of possible cardiotoxicity of long-chain acylcarnitines.

SUGGESTED READINGS

Barth PG, Hoffmann GF, Jaeken J, et al. L-2-hydroxyglutaric acidemia: a novel inherited neurometabolic disease. *Ann Neurol* 1992;32:66–71.

Burri BJ, Sweetman L, Nyhan, WL. Mutant holocarboxylase synthetase: evidence for the enzyme defect in early infantile biotin-responsive multiple carboxylase deficiency. *J Clin Invest* 1981;68:1491–1495.

Frerman FE, Goodman SI. Defects of electron transfer flavoprotein and electron transfer flavoprotein-ubiquinone oxidoreductase: glutaric aciduria type II. In: Scriver CR, Beaudet AL, Sly WS, et al., eds. *The Metabolic and Molecular Bases of Inherited Disease.* New York: McGraw-Hill, 2001:2357–2365.

Gibson KM, Sherwood WG, Hoffmann GF, et al. Phenotypic heterogeneity in the syndromes of 3-methylglutaconic aciduria. *J Pediat* 1991;118:885–890.

Hoffmann GF, von Kries R, Klose D, et al. Frequencies of inherited organic acidurias and disorders of mitochondrial fatty acid transport and oxidation in Germany. *Eur J Pediatr* 2004 Feb;163(2):76–80.

Kuhara T. Diagnosis and monitoring of inborn errors of metabolism using urease-pretreatment of urine, isotope dilution, and gas chromatography-mass spectrometry. *J Chromatogr B Analyt Technol Biomed Life Sci* 2002;781(Dec 5):497–517.

Pearl PL, Gibson KM, Acosta MT, et al. Clinical spectrum of succinic semialdehyde dehydrogenase deficiency. *Neurology* 2003;60:1413–1417.

Strauss KA, Puffenberger EG, Robinson DL, et al. Type I glutaric aciduria, part 1: natural history of 77 patients. *Am J Med Genet* 2003;121C: 38–52.

Tiranti V, D'Adamo P, Briem E, et al. Ethylmalonic encephalopathy is caused by mutations in ETHE1, a gene encoding a mitochondrial matrix protein. *Am J Hum Genet* 2004;74:239–252.

Chapter 91

Disorders of Metal Metabolism

John H. Menkes

HEPATOLENTICULAR DEGENERATION (WILSON DISEASE; MIM 277900)

Wilson disease is an inborn error of copper metabolism that is associated with cirrhosis of the liver and degenerative changes in the basal ganglia. During the second half of the nineteenth century, a condition termed "pseudosclerosis" was distinguished from multiple sclerosis by the lack of nystagmus and visual loss. In 1902, Kayser observed green corneal pigmentation in one such patient; Fleischer commented on the association of the corneal rings with pseudosclerosis in 1903 and fully required it in 1912. In 1912, Wilson gave the classic description of the disease and its pathologic anatomy. The worldwide prevalence of the disease is about 30 in 1 million, with a gene frequency of 1:180.

Pathogenesis and Pathology

Wilson disease is an autosomal recessive disorder with the gene being located on the long arm of chromosome 13. The gene has been cloned. It encodes a copper-transporting P-type ATPase (ATP7b) that is expressed in liver and kidney. The protein is found in two forms: One is localized to the cellular trans-Golgi network and the other, probably representing a cleavage product, to mitochondria. Over 200 mutations have been characterized. Of these, about half are missense mutations, and most individuals are compound heterozygotes. There is little correlation between the type of mutation and the age when the disease makes its appearance or its severity. It is therefore likely that additional genetic and environmental factors influence the ultimate phenotype.

The mutation induces extensive changes in copper homeostasis. Normally, after hepatocyte uptake copper is bound to metallochaperones, which are a family of proteins that deliver copper to different pathways. The copper chaperone Atox1 delivers copper to the secretory pathway for incorporation into apoceruloplasmin and for excretion into bile by direct interaction with ATP7b. Normally the amount of copper in the body is kept constant through excretion of copper from the liver into bile. In Wilson disease, the two fundamental defects are reduced biliary transport of copper and an impaired formation of plasma ceruloplasmin. Ceruloplasmin is a plasma ferroxidase. It mediates oxidation of ferrous iron to ferric iron for insertion into apotransferritin.

In addition to these abnormalities, levels of nonceruloplasmin or free copper in serum are increased and plasma iron-binding globulin is low to low normal. These abnormalities occur in asymptomatic carriers and suggest that Wilson disease may also encompass a disorder of iron metabolism. This may result from the deficiency of ceruloplasmin that is directly involved in the transfer of iron from tissue cells to plasma transferrin.

Another metabolic feature is a persistent aminoaciduria. This is most marked during the later stages but may be noted in some asymptomatic patients. The presence of other tubular defects (e.g., impaired phosphate resorption in patients without aminoaciduria) suggests that a toxic action of the metal on renal tubules causes the aminoaciduria.

A defect in the gene encoding a different copper transporting P-type ATPase is responsible for Menkes disease.

▶ **TABLE 91.1** Molecular Biology of Menkes Disease and Wilson Disease

	Menkes	*Wilson*
Gene locus	Xq 13.3	13q 14.3
Gene product	Copper-binding p-type ATPase	Copper-binding P-type ATPase, 60% identity with Menkes
Expression	All tissues except liver	Liver, kidney, placenta
Mutations	16% deletions	Point mutations, small deletions
Clinical		
Age of onset	Birth	Late childhood, adolescence
Symptomatic organs	Brain, hair, skin	Liver, CNS, Kayser-Fleischer rings
Duration	<3y	Decades
Laboratory		
Serum copper	Decreased	Decreased
Ceruloplasmin	Decreased	Decreased
Renal copper	Increased	Increased
Urinary copper	—	Increased
Liver copper	Decreased	Increased
Cultured cells	Copper accumulation	Normal
	Decreased copper release	
Defect	Intestinal copper absorption	Biliary copper excretion
		Incorporation of copper into ceruloplasmin
	Deficiency copper-dependent enzymes	
Treatment	None effective	Penicillamine, zinc

a Modified from Chelly J, Monaco AP, *Nat Genet* 1993;5:317–318.

Although the gene for Menkes disease is located on the X chromosome, there is more than 60% identity between the two proteins. The similarities and differences between the two diseases are listed in Table 91.1.

The abnormalities in copper metabolism that occur in Wilson disease lead to accumulation of the metal in liver and consequently to progressive copper-mediated oxidative hepatocellular damage. Anatomically, the liver shows focal necrosis that leads to a coarsely nodular postnecrotic cirrhosis; the nodules vary in size and are separated by bands of fibrous tissue of different width. Some hepatic cells are enlarged and contain fat droplets, intranuclear glycogen, and clumped pigment granules; other cells are necrotic, and there are regenerative changes in the surrounding parenchyma.

Electron microscopic studies have shown that copper is sequestered by lysosomes that become more than normally sensitive to rupture and therefore lack normal

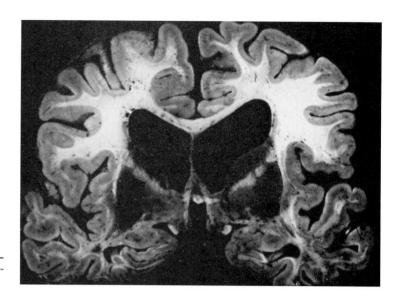

FIGURE 91.1. Wilson disease. Ventricular dilation, atrophy of caudate nucleus. Cyst in lower half of putamen.

alkaline phosphatase activity. Copper probably initiates and catalyzes oxidation of the lysosomal membrane lipids, resulting in lipofuscin accumulation. Subsequent overflow of copper from the liver produces accumulation in other organs, mainly brain, kidney, and cornea. Within the kidneys, the tubular epithelial cells may degenerate and the cytoplasm may contain copper deposits.

In brain, the basal ganglia show the most striking alterations (Fig. 91.1). They have a brick-red pigmentation; spongy degeneration of the putamen frequently leads to the formation of small cavities. Microscopic studies reveal a loss of neurons, axonal degeneration, and many protoplasmic astrocytes, including giant forms known as *Alzheimer cells*. The cortex of the frontal lobe may also show spongy degeneration and astrocytosis. Copper is deposited in the pericapillary area and within astrocytes, where it is located in the subcellular soluble fraction and bound not only to cerebrocuprein but also to other cerebral proteins. Copper is uniformly absent from neurons and ground substance. Lesser degenerative changes are seen in the brainstem, the dentate nucleus, the substantia nigra, and the convolutional white matter. Copper is also found throughout the cornea, particularly the substantia propria.

In the cornea, the metal is deposited in the periphery where it appears in granular clumps close to the endothelial surface of the Descemet membrane. The deposits in this area are responsible for the appearance of the Kayser-Fleischer ring. The color of this ring varies from yellow to green to brown. Copper is deposited in two or more layers, with particle size and distance between layers influencing the ultimate appearance of the ring.

Symptoms and Signs

Wilson disease is a progressive condition with a tendency toward temporary clinical improvement and arrest. The condition occurs in all races, with a particularly high incidence among Eastern European Jews, Italians from southern Italy and Sicily, and people from some of the smaller islands of Japan—groups in which there is a high rate of inbreeding.

In most patients, symptoms begin between the ages of 11 and 25 years. Onset as early as age 3 and as late as the fifth decade has been recorded.

The signs and symptoms of hepatolenticular degeneration are generally those of damage to the liver and brain. Signs of liver damage, ascites, or jaundice may occur at any stage of the disease. They have been observed in some cases several or many years before the onset of neurologic symptoms.

The neurologic manifestations are so varied that it is impossible to describe a clinical picture that is characteristic. In the past, texts have distinguished between pseudosclerotic and dystonic forms of the disease: the former dominated by tremor, the latter by rigidity and contractures. In actuality, most patients, if untreated, ultimately develop both types of symptoms. In essence, Wilson disease is a disorder of motor function; despite often widespread cerebral atrophy, there are no sensory symptoms or reflex alterations. Symptoms at onset are shown in Table 91.2. Symptoms of basal ganglia damage usually predominate, but cerebellar symptoms may occasionally be in the foreground. Tremors and rigidity are the most common early signs. The tremor may be of the intention type or it may be the alternating tremor of Parkinson disease. More commonly, however, it is a bizarre tremor, localized to the arms and best described by the term "wing beating" (Fig. 91.2). This tremor is usually absent when the arms are at rest; it develops after a short latent period when the arms are extended. The beating movements may be confined to the muscles of the wrist, but it is more common for the arm to be thrown up and down in a wide arc. The movements

TABLE 91.2 Clinical Manifestations at Onset of Wilson Disease

Symptoms	Percentage
Hepatic or hematologic abnormalities	35
Behavioral abnormalities	25
Neurologic symptoms	40
Pseudosclerotic form—one or more of the following:	40
Tremor at rest or purposive	
Dysarthria or scanning speech	
Diminished dexterity or mild clumsiness	
Unsteady gait	
Tremor, alone	33
Dysarthria, alone	5
Dystonic form—one or more of the following:	60
Hypophonic speech or mutism	
Drooling	
Rigid mouth, arms, or legs	
Seizures	1
Chorea or small-amplitude twitches	<1

Prepared with Drs. JH. Scheinberg and I. Sternlieb, Department of Medicine, Albert Einstein College of Medicine, Bronx, New York.

increase in severity and may become so violent that the patient is thrown off balance. A change in the posture of the outstretched arms may alter the severity of the tremor. The tremor may affect both arms but is usually more severe in one. The tremor may occasionally be present even when the arm is at rest. Many patients have a fixed open-mouth smile.

Rigidity and spasms of the muscles are often present. In some cases, typical parkinsonian rigidity may involve all muscles. Torticollis, tortipelvis, and other dystonic movements are not uncommon. Spasticity of the laryngeal and pharyngeal muscles may lead to dysarthria and dysphagia. Drooping of the lower jaw and excess salivation are common. Other symptoms include convulsions, transient periods of coma, and mental changes. Mental symptoms may dominate the clinical course for varying periods and simulate an affective disorder or a psychosis.

Tendon reflexes are increased, but extensor plantar responses are exceptional. Somatosensory evoked potentials are abnormal in most patients with neurologic symptoms. The prevalence of epileptic seizures is 10 times higher in patients with Wilson disease than in the general population. Seizures can occur at any stage of the disease, but most begin after the initiation of treatment.

Behavioral or personality disorders were noted in the original description of the disease by Wilson. In the experience of Akil and Brewer, the first symptoms of one third of patients are psychiatric abnormalities. These include impaired school performance, depression, labile moods, and frank psychosis. In those patients who show primarily neurologic symptoms, about two thirds have had psychiatric problems before the diagnosis was made. Symptoms in about one half of patients were sufficiently severe to require treatment by a psychiatrist or a hospital admission.

The intracorneal ring-shaped pigmentation first noted by Kayser (1902) and Fleischer (1912) may be evident to the naked eye or may be seen only by slit lamp examination. The ring may be complete or incomplete and is

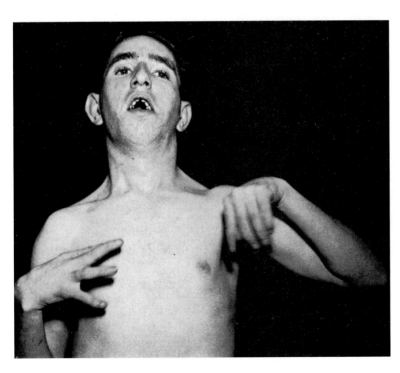

FIGURE 91.2. Wilson disease. Open mouth, athetoid posture of arms, and wing-beating movements of left hand.

present in 75% of patients who present with hepatic symptoms and in all patients with cerebral symptoms alone or both cerebral and hepatic symptoms. The Kayser-Fleischer ring may antedate overt symptoms and has been detected even with normal liver functions. In the larger clinical series of Arima and colleagues, it was never present before age 7 years.

MRI usually reveals ventricular dilatation and diffuse atrophy of the cortex, cerebellum, and brainstem. The basal ganglia are usually abnormal with the putamen, thalamus, the head of the caudate, and the globus pallidus the most likely areas to be involved in patients presenting with neurologic symptoms (Fig. 91.3). Most patients with hepatic symptoms have increased signal in the basal ganglia on T1-weighted images. Abnormalities are also seen in the tegmentum of the midbrain, the substantia nigra, and pons. In a few subjects there are focal white matter lesions. On CT, increased density owing to copper deposition is not observed. As a rule, MRI correlates better with the clinical symptoms than CT.

Diagnosis

The clinical picture of Wilson disease is fairly clear-cut when the disease is advanced. The Kayser-Fleischer ring is the most important diagnostic feature; absence of corneal pigmentation in untreated patients with neurologic symptoms rules out the diagnosis. The ring is not seen in most presymptomatic patients or in some children with hepatic symptoms. A low serum ceruloplasmin and elevated urinary copper support the diagnosis.

Although 96% of patients with Wilson disease have low or absent serum ceruloplasmin, some cases have been reported with normal ceruloplasmin levels. In affected families, the differential diagnosis between heterozygotes and presymptomatic homozygotes is of utmost importance because homozygotes should be treated preventively. Low ceruloplasmin levels in an asymptomatic patient suggest the presymptomatic stage of the disease. Because 6% of heterozygotes also have low ceruloplasmin levels, further studies are indicated. An elevation of urinary copper is diagnostic of a presymptomatic patient if the patient is 15 years or older. In children, urinary copper is not always elevated, and in such cases a liver biopsy to measure hepatic copper content is indicated to confirm the diagnosis. A screening test using penicillamine to stimulate urinary excretion of copper has not been standardized and is therefore of little value.

When a liver biopsy has been decided on, both histologic studies with stains for copper and copper-associated proteins and chemical quantitation for copper are performed. In all confirmed cases of Wilson disease, hepatic copper is >3.9 μmol/g dry weight (237.6 μg/g) compared with a normal range of 0.2 to 0.6 μmol/g. Because of the

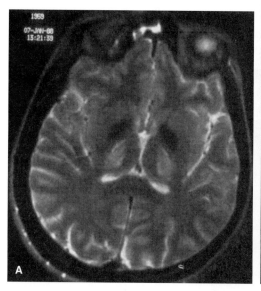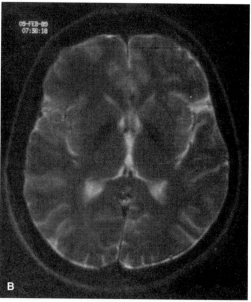

FIGURE 91.3. Wilson disease. Coronal T2-weighted magnetic resonance images of a 22-year-old woman with Wilson disease. **A.** Three months after the disease has been diagnosed and at start of penicillamine therapy, there is bilateral hyperintense thalamic lesions that were hypointense on T1-weighted images. **B.** The same patient after 13 months of penicillamine therapy shows a significant regression of the thalamic lesions. Spin-echo sequences TR 2.5 ms, TE 90 ms, using Siemens Magneton 63 operating at 1.5 T. (Reprinted with permission of Prayer I., Zentral Institut fur Radiodiagnose und Ludwig Boltzmann Institut, University of Vienna, Austria; and Rosenberg RN, Prusiner SB, DiMauro S, et al. Molecular and genetic basis of neurological disease. Boston: Butterworth-Heinemann, 1997.)

many mutations causing the disease, a combination of mutation and linkage analysis is required for prenatal diagnosis and as a rule is not useful in the diagnosis of an individual patient.

A variant of Wilson disease begins in adolescence and is marked by progressive tremor, dysarthria, disturbed eye movements, and dementia. Biochemically, it is characterized by low serum levels of copper and ceruloplasmin. Kayser-Fleischer rings are absent, and liver copper concentrations are low. Metabolic studies using labeled copper suggest a failure in copper absorption from the lower gut.

Treatment

All patients with Wilson disease, whether symptomatic or asymptomatic, require treatment. The aims of treatment are initially to remove the toxic amounts of copper and secondarily to prevent tissue reaccumulation of the metal.

Treatment can be divided into two phases: the initial phase, when toxic copper levels are brought under control, and maintenance therapy. There is no currently agreed on regimen for the treatment of the new patient with neurologic or psychiatric symptoms. In the past, most centers recommended starting patients on penicillamine (600 mg to 3,000 mg/day). Although this drug is effective in promoting urinary excretion of copper, adverse reactions during both the initial and maintenance phases of treatment are seen in about 25% of patients. These include worsening of neurologic symptoms during the initial phases of treatment, seen in up to 50% of patients and frequently irreversible. Skin rashes, gastrointestinal discomfort, and hair loss are also encountered. During maintenance therapy, one may see polyneuropathy, polymyositis, and nephropathy. Some of these adverse effects can be prevented by giving pyridoxine (25 mg/day).

Because of these side effects, many institutions now advocate initial therapy with ammonium tetrathiomolybdate (60 to 300 mg/day, administered in six divided doses, three with meals and three between meals). Tetrathiomolybdate forms a complex with protein and copper and when given with food blocks the absorption of copper. The major drawback to using this drug is that it still has not been approved for general use in this country.

Triethylene tetramine dihydrochloride (trientine; 250 mg four times a day, given at least 1 hour before or 2 hours after meals) is also a chelator that increases urinary excretion of copper. Its effectiveness is less than that of penicillamine, but the incidence of toxicity and hypersensitivity reactions is lower.

Zinc acetate (50 mg of elemental zinc acetate three times a day) acts by inducing intestinal metallothionein, which has a high affinity for copper and prevents its entrance into blood. Zinc is far less toxic than penicillamine but is much slower acting. Diet does not play an impor-

tant role in the management of Wilson disease, although Brewer recommended restriction of liver and shellfish during the first year of treatment.

Zinc is the optimum drug for maintenance therapy and for the treatment of the presymptomatic patient. Trientine in combination with zinc acetate has been suggested for patients who present in hepatic failure. Liver transplantation can be helpful in the patient who presents in end-stage liver disease. The procedure appears to correct the metabolic defect and can reverse neurologic symptoms.

Improvement of neurologic symptoms and signs and fading of the Kayser-Fleischer rings can be expected from therapy. As a rule, patients with the predominantly pseudosclerotic form of the disease fare better than those with dystonia as the main manifestation. Improvement of neurologic symptoms starts 5 to 6 months after therapy has begun and is generally complete in 24 months. Serial neuroimaging studies demonstrate progressive reduction of the abnormal areas in the basal ganglia (Fig. 91.3). Survival of patients who have completed the first few years of treatment is within the range of normal.

MENKES DISEASE (KINKY HAIR DISEASE; MIM 309400)

Menkes disease (kinky hair disease [KHD]) is a focal degenerative disorder of gray matter that is transmitted by a gene mapped to the long arm of the X chromosome. The gene codes for a copper-transporting ATPase (ATP7A) that has been localized to the trans-Golgi network. This transporter is required to translocate cytosolic copper across intracellular membranes. In response to exogenous copper, ATP7A moves from the trans-Golgi network to the plasma membrane and returns under low copper conditions. Numerous mutations have been documented. Complete and partial gene deletions are seen in some 15% to 20% of patients. About half of the mutations lead to splicing abnormalities. Other mutations that have been encountered include small duplications, nonsense mutations, and missense mutations. To date, all mutations detected have been unique for each given family, and almost all have been associated with a decreased level of the mRNA for the copper-transporting ATPase.

The result of this gene defect is maldistribution of body copper. The metal accumulates to abnormal levels in a location that makes it inaccessible for the synthesis of various copper enzymes. These include cytochrome c oxidase, lysyl oxidase, superoxide dismutase, and tyrosinase. Cytochrome c oxidase (complex IV) is a copper-containing enzyme located in the mitochondrial inner membrane. It is the terminal oxidase of the respiratory chain. In KHD there is a marked reduction in the enzyme in all portions of the central nervous system. Lysyl oxidase normally deaminates lysine and hydoxylysine as the first step in collagen cross-link formation. Several groups of workers have found that lysyl oxidase activity is markedly reduced in children with KHD. Tyrosinase, an enzyme involved in melanin biosynthesis, is thought to be responsible for reduced pigmentation in hair and skin.

Copper levels are low in liver and all areas of the brain but are elevated in some other tissues, notably intestinal mucosa and kidney. Patients absorb little or no orally administered copper, but when the metal is given intravenously, there is a prompt rise in serum copper and ceruloplasmin. In fibroblasts, the copper content is markedly elevated as is metallothionein; synthesis of metallothionein is increased as a consequence of abnormally high intracellular copper levels.

As a consequence of tissue copper deficiency, many pathologic changes are set into motion. Cerebral and systemic arteries are tortuous with irregular lumens and frayed and split intimal linings. In brain, there is extensive focal degeneration of cortical gray matter with neuronal loss and gliosis. MRI can show bilateral ischemic lesions in deep gray matter. Cellular loss is prominent in the cerebellum, where many Purkinje cells are lost; others show grotesque proliferation of the dendritic network. In the thalamus, there is primary cellular degeneration that spares the smaller inhibitory neurons.

The incidence of KHD is thought to be as high as 2 in 100,000 male live births. Symptoms appear in the neonatal period. Most commonly, hypothermia, poor feeding, and impaired weight gain are observed. Seizures soon become apparent with progressive deterioration of all neurologic functions. The most striking finding is the appearance of the hair, which is colorless and friable. On microscopic examination, a variety of abnormalities is evident, most often pili torti (twisted hair) and trichorrhexis nodosa (fractures of the hair shaft at regular intervals).

Radiographs of long bones reveal metaphyseal spurring and a diaphyseal periosteal reaction. On arteriography, the cerebral vessels are markedly elongated and tortuous. Similar changes are seen in systemic blood vessels. CT or MRI may reveal areas of cortical atrophy or tortuous and enlarged intracranial vessels. Subdural effusions are not unusual (Fig. 91.4).

The clinical history and appearance of the infant suggest the diagnosis. Because of an immature biliary secretion in utero, copper is unavailable to the hepatocyte secretory pathway, and the newborn liver predominantly secretes apoceruloplasmin. As a result, serum ceruloplasmin and copper levels are normally low in the neonatal period and do not reach adult levels until age 1 month. Thus, these determinations must be performed serially to demonstrate that the expected rise does not occur. The increased copper content of fibroblasts permits intrauterine diagnosis. Even though copper infusions raise serum copper and ceruloplasmin, neurologic symptoms

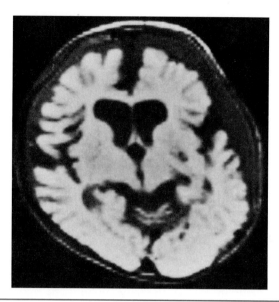

FIGURE 91.4. Axial T1-weighted magnetic resonance image in patient with Menkes disease. Patient was a 2-year-old girl with psychomotor retardation, seizures, and characteristic hair. No family history of neurologic disease. Chromosomal analysis revealed X/2 translocation. There is considerable periventricular and cortical atrophy. Fluid collection over left cortical margin represents an old subdural hematoma.

are neither alleviated nor prevented. In the experience of Christodoulou et al., early treatment with copper-histidine allowed normal or near-normal intellectual development but did not prevent some of the many somatic complications. Several variants of Menkes syndrome have been recognized based on the low serum copper concentrations. Symptoms include ataxia, mild mental retardation, and extrapyramidal movement disorders. In occipital horn syndrome, a condition allelic with KHD, the characteristic picture includes a hyperelastic and bruisable skin, hyperextensible joints, hernias, bladder diverticula or rupture, and multiple skeletal abnormalities, including Wormian bones in the skull.

ACERULOPLASMINEMIA (MIM 604290)

Aceruloplasminemia is an autosomal recessive disorder marked by the complete absence of ceruloplasmin. The condition is caused by a mutation in the gene encoding ceruloplasmin, localized to 3q23-24.

As a consequence of the absence of ceruloplasmin, ferroxidase activity is completely lacking and iron efflux from cells with mobilizable iron stores is impaired. There is iron accumulation and neuronal degeneration in the basal ganglia and dentate nucleus; astrocytes are more affected than neurons. Lesser degrees of iron storage are seen in the cerebral cortex. Abundant iron is also present in liver, spleen, and pancreas.

The disease manifests itself during adult life. It is seen with diabetes mellitus, dementia, various extrapyramidal movement disorders, ataxia, and retinal degeneration. The clinical diagnosis rests on the absence of serum ceruloplasmin, increased serum ferritin concentrations, and evidence of iron deposition within the brain on MRI. The distribution of abnormalities as seen on neuroimaging distinguishes this condition from Wilson disease.

Early treatment with the iron chelator desferrioxamine can prevent progression of the disease.

MOLYBDENUM COFACTOR DEFICIENCY (MIM 252150)

Three genetically distinct autosomal recessive conditions result in a deficiency of the molybdenum-containing cofactor that is essential to the function of three enzymes: sulfite oxidase, xanthine dehydrogenase, and aldehyde oxidase. More than 30 disease-causing mutations have been found at either of the two steps in the formation of the cofactor, as well as in the gene coding for gephyrin, a membrane-associated protein that catalyses the insertion of molybdenum into molybdopterin.

The clinical picture is marked by seizures commencing in infancy or during the neonatal period, feeding difficulties, craniofacial dysmorphic features, abnormal muscle tone, and frequently dislocation of the lens. The diagnosis rests on finding a low blood uric acid, or less reliably, increased urinary sulfites, particularly S-sulfo-L-cysteine. Neuroimaging studies demonstrate an encephalomalacia reminiscent of hypoxic ischemic encephalopathy.

No specific treatment is available. Diets supplemented with cysteine or molybdenum and restricted in methionine have been suggested.

SUGGESTED READINGS

Aisen AM, Martel W, Gabrielsen TO, et al. Wilson disease of the brain: MR imaging. *Radiology* 1985;157:137–141.

Akil M, Brewer GJ. Psychiatric and behavioral abnormalities in Wilson's disease. *Adv Neurol* 1995;65:171–178.

Arima M, Takeshita K, Yoshino K, et al. Prognosis of Wilson's disease in childhood. *Eur J Pediatr* 1977;126:147–154.

Brewer GJ. Practical recommendations and new therapies for Wilson's disease. *Drugs* 1995;50:240–249.

Brewer GJ, Hill GM, Prasad AS, et al. Oral zinc for Wilson's disease. *Ann Intern Med* 1983;99:314–320.

Brewer GJ, Yuzbasian-Gurkan V. Wilson disease. *Medicine (Baltimore)* 1992;71:139–164.

Chelly J, Monaco AP. Cloning the Wilson disease gene. *Nat Genet* 1993;5:317–318.

Christodoulou J, Danks DM, Sarkar B, et al. Early treatment of Menkes disease with parenteral copper-histidine: long-term follow-up of four treated patients. *Am J Med Genet* 1998;76:154–164.

Danks DM, Campbell PE, Stevens BJ, et al. Menkes' kinky hair syndrome: An inherited defect in copper absorption with widespread effects. *Pediatrics* 1972;50:188–201.

Davis W, Chowrimootoo GF, Seymour CA. Defective biliary copper excretion in Wilson's disease: the role of caeruloplasmin. *Eur J Clin Invest* 1996;26:893–901.

Ferenci P. Pathophysiology and clinical features of Wilson disease. *Metab Brain Dis* 2004 Dec;19(3–4):229–239.

Fleischer, B. Über einer der "Pseudosklerose" nahestehende bisher unbekannte Krankheit (gekennzeichnet durch Tremor, psychische Störungen, bräunliche Pigmentierung bestimmter Gewebe, insbesondere auch der Hornhautperipherie, Lebercirrhose). *Deutsch Z Nervenheilk* 1912;44:179–201.

Francis MJ, Jones EE, Levy ER, et al. A Golgi localization signal identified in the Menkes recombinant protein. *Hum Mol Genet* 1998;7:1245–1252.

Gitlin J. Aceruloplasminemia. *Pediatr Res* 1998;44:271–276.

Gitlin J. Wilson disease. *Gastroenterology* 2003;125:1868–1877.

Glass JD, Reich SG, Delong MR. Wilson's disease. Development of neurologic disease after beginning penicillamine therapy. *Arch Neurol* 1990;47:595–596.

Graf WD, Noetzel MJ, Radical reactions from missing ceruloplasmin. The importance of a ferroxidase as an endogenous antioxidant. *Neurology* 1999;53:446–447.

Grover WD, Johnson WC, Henkin RI. Clinical and biochemical aspects of trichopoliodystrophy. *Ann Neurol* 1979;5:65–71.

Heckmann J, Saffer D. Abnormal copper metabolism: another "non-Wilson's" case. *Neurology* 1988;38:1493–1496.

Hefter H, Rautenberg W, Kreuzpaintner G, et al. Does orthoptic liver transplantation heal Wilson's disease? Clinical follow-up of two liver-transplanted patients. *Acta Neurol Scand* 1991;84:192–196.

His G, Cox DW. A comparison of the mutation spectra of Menkes disease and Wilson disease. *Hum Genet* 2004;114:165–172.

Kayser, B. Ueber einen Fall von angeborener grünlicher Verfärbung der Cornea. *Klin Monatsbl Augenheilkd* 1902;40:22–25.

Lutsenko S, Petris MJ. Function and regulation of the mammalian copper-transporting ATPases: insights from biochemical and cell biological approaches. *J Membr Biol* 2003;191:1–12.

Menkes JH, Alter M, Steigleder GK, et al. A sex-linked recessive disorder with growth retardation, peculiar hair, and focal cerebral and cerebellar degeneration. *Pediatrics* 1962;29:764–779.

Miyajima H. Aceruloplasminemia, an iron metabolic disorder. *Neuropathology* 2003;23:345–350.

Nittis T, Gitlin JD. The copper-iron connection: hereditary aceruloplasminemia. *Semin Hematol* 2002;39:282–289.

Reiss J, Johnson JL. Mutations in the molybdenum cofactor biosynthetic genes MOCS1, MOCS2, and GEPH. *Hum Mutat* 2003;21:569–576.

Riordon SM, Williams R. The Wilson's disease gene and phenotypic diversity. *J Hepatol* 2001;34:165–171.

Roberts EA, Schilsky ML. A practice guideline on Wilson disease. *Hepatology* 2003;37:1475–1492.

Shah AB, Chernov I, Zhang HT, et al. Identification and analysis of mutation in the Wilson disease gene ATP7B. *Am J Hum Genet* 1997;61:317–339.

Starosta-Rubenstein S, Young AB, Kluin K, et al. Clinical assessment of 31 patients with Wilson's disease. *Arch Neurol* 1987;44:365–370.

Tanzi RE, Petrukhin K, Chernov I, et al. The Wilson disease gene is a copper-transporting ATPase with homology to the Menkes disease gene. *Nat Genet* 1993;5:344–350.

Vulpe C, Levinson B, Whitney S, et al. Isolation of a candidate gene for Menkes disease and evidence that it encodes a copper-transporting ATPase. *Nat Genet* 1993;3:7–13.

Wilson SAK. Progressive lenticular degeneration: a familial nervous disease associated with cirrhosis of the liver. *Brain* 1912;34:295–509.

Chapter 92

Acute Intermittent Porphyria

Lewis P. Rowland

Excessive excretion of porphyrins makes the urine appear bright red. The change is so dramatic that one form of genetic porphyria was among the first inborn errors of metabolism when that class of disease was identified by Garrod. We now recognize both acquired and heritable forms; the genetic categories are further divided into hepatic and erythropoietic types, depending on the site of the enzymatic disorder. Neurologic manifestations are encountered in two classes of porphyria. *Acute intermittent porphyria* (AIP; MIM 176000) occurs worldwide; *variegate porphyria* (MIM 176200) occurs in Sweden and South Africa. These two forms differ primarily in that a rash occurs in the variegate form but not in AIP. Both are inherited as autosomal dominant traits, with low penetrance.

PATHOGENESIS

There are eight steps in the biosynthesis of heme. The crucial steps in understanding porphyria are as follows: delta *aminolevulinic acid* (ALA) is formed from succinyl CoA and glycine under the influence of ALA synthetase; two molecules of ALA are joined by ALA-dehydratase to form a monopyrrole, *porphobilinogen* (PBG); four molecules of PBG are linked to form a *porphyrin* by *uroporphyrinogen-1 synthase*—rearrangements of the side chains of this tetrapyrrole follow under the action of a series of other enzymes, including *protoporphyrinogen oxidase*; and the process culminates in the formation of heme by the addition of an iron molecule.

In AIP, there is excessive urinary excretion of ALA, PBG, and several porphyrins. Suggestions of a block in an alternate pathway of ALA metabolism have not been confirmed. It is still not certain how this pattern of metabolite excretion arises. The dominant theory is of a block in the activity of PBG deaminase in AIP and of protoporphyrinogen oxidase in the variegate form; this causes decreased amounts of heme to be formed downstream, and the lack of normal inhibitory feedback from heme on ALA synthetase releases that enzyme, accounting for the overproduction of ALA and PBG. However, there is no deficiency of heme compounds in blood or tissues, and the activity of PBG

deaminase is about 50% of normal. This is the usual level of enzyme activity in asymptomatic heterozygote carriers of autosomal recessive diseases; it is not clear why the same level of activity should be linked to symptoms in AIP but not in so many other conditions. Moreover, the decreased activity of PBG deaminase has been demonstrated in liver biopsy specimens, cultured skin fibroblasts, amniotic cells, and erythrocytes. Inexplicably, the enzyme activity is normal in some unequivocally affected individuals.

Neurologic symptoms do not appear in other genetic disorders of porphyrin synthesis. It has not been possible to attribute the characteristic neuropathy of AIP to the increased amounts of circulating ALA or PBG. Clinical symptoms of porphyria are similar to those of lead poisoning, in which ALA excretion also increases, but PBG excretion is normal in lead intoxication.

Whatever the abnormality, clinical symptoms seem to be caused by the interaction of genetic and environmental factors. Porphyric crises result most often from ingestion or administration of drugs that adversely affect porphyrin metabolism, especially barbiturates taken for sedation or for general anesthesia. Attacks are also attributed to menses, starvation, emotional stress, intercurrent infections, or other drugs.

MOLECULAR GENETICS

Genetic heterogeneity was evident even before DNA analysis was possible. For instance, using antibodies to PBG deaminase, 74% to 85% of families show cross-reacting immunologic material, whereas others do not. In most families, the enzyme in red blood cells has about half of normal activity; in others, the erythrocyte enzyme is normal.

The enzyme has been mapped to 11q24.1-q24.2. DNA studies have revealed 14 different mutations in the gene. In Sweden, about half of all families had the same point mutation. In Switzerland, 60% of families have the same mutation. In France, however, only 5% of patients had that mutation, differences likely arising from founder effects. There have been a few patients who were homozygous for a mutation and had more severe symptoms; one child was a "compound" of two different mutations at the same locus on the two chromosomes. DNA analysis is important in family studies, identifying people at risk more reliably than assays of erythrocyte PBG deaminase activity, which, in one study, missed 28% of those who carried the mutation and therefore might be susceptible to symptoms if exposed to responsible drugs. Similarly, a study in Finland showed that measurement of urinary PBG was accurate in identifying symptomatic patients but missed 15% of asymptomatic people who had been identified by mutation analysis.

PATHOLOGY

The functional disorder is not due to structural change. Even in fatal cases, it may be difficult to demonstrate any histologic lesions. Demyelinating lesions of central and peripheral nerves have been observed, but modern electrophysiologic studies show normal or nearly normal conduction velocities with signs of denervation in muscle, the pattern of an axonal neuropathy. This view has been supported by morphometric studies of peripheral nerves and nerve roots, with evidence also of a dying-back process. Large and small fibers are affected in peripheral nerves, and autonomic fibers are also attacked.

INCIDENCE

In South Africa, Dean and Barnes traced most current cases to a single colonist who arrived there in 1688. In Sweden, the prevalence varies from 1:1,000 in the north to 1:100,000 population in other parts. Prevalence figures for other countries are also about 1:100,000. In one psychiatric hospital, the prevalence was 2:1,000. Acute symptoms are rare, however, and in major academic medical centers in New York, new cases are seen less often than once a year. All races seem to be affected. In most series, women are more often affected than men. Symptoms are rare in childhood and are most likely to affect adolescents or young adults.

SYMPTOMS AND SIGNS

Asymptomatic individuals with acute porphyria or variegate porphyria are identified by biochemical tests. Symptoms of either disease occur in attacks that may be induced by commonly used drugs; these are described below. Many attacks cannot be linked to a clear provocation in diet or physical activity. International air travel seems to be hazardous for some patients. The symptoms of an attack are most commonly gastrointestinal (attributed to autonomic neuropathy), psychiatric, and neurologic (Table 92.1). Abdominal pain is most common and may occur alone or with a neurologic or psychiatric disorder. There is usually no abdominal rigidity, but fever, leukocytosis, and diarrhea or constipation often lead to laparotomy. Patients with acute porphyria may actually have appendicitis or some other visceral emergency. The psychiatric disorder may suggest conversion reaction, acute delirium, mood change, or an acute or chronic psychosis. Symptoms of the neuropathy are like those of any peripheral neuropathy except that the signs may be purely motor and are almost always associated with abdominal pain. In one series, 18% of the cases with neuropathy were fatal, 25% recov-

▶ **TABLE 92.1 Clinical Manifestations of Acute Intermittent Porphyria**

	% of Patients
Abdominal pain	85–95
Vomiting	52–75
Constipation	46–70
Diarrhea	9–11
Abdominal surgery	22–46
Paresis	42–72
Myalgia	53
Convulsions	10–16
Sensory loss	9–38
Transient amaurosis	4–6
Diplopia	3
Delirium	18–52
Mood change	28
Psychosis	12
Hypertension	40–55
Tachycardia	28–60
Fever	12–37
Azotemia	6–27

From 352 reported cases in three series cited by Rowland, 1961.

ered completely, and the others were left with some neurologic disability. Survivors may have recurrent attacks. Cerebral manifestations are unusual except for the syndrome of inappropriate secretion of antidiuretic hormone. Unexplained transient amblyopia has been reported. Autonomic abnormalities include hypertension and tachycardia.

LABORATORY DATA

Routine laboratory tests usually give normal results, including cerebrospinal fluid. EMG shows signs of denervation, but motor and sensory nerve velocities are normal or only slightly slow.

Even between attacks, affected individuals can be identified by a qualitative test for PBG in the urine. The Watson-Schwartz test depends on the reaction of the monopyrrole with diaminobenzaldehyde to form a reddish compound that is soluble in chloroform. The test can be performed in a few minutes, and there are few false-positive or false-negative results. Quantitative measurement of urinary PBG and ALA by column chromatography is available in commercial laboratories in the United States. The most reliable test is assay of PBG-deaminase activity in red blood cell membranes, which is about 50% of control values in affected individuals with AIP, between and during attacks. The assay also identifies family members who are at risk even if they are asymptomatic, and DNA analysis is even more accurate.

Variegate porphyria cannot be distinguished from AIP clinically unless there is a rash, which may be lacking in almost half of symptomatic individuals. The acute attacks are virtually identical to those of AIP. The difference is biochemical; excretion of PBG and ALA is increased during attacks but not between attacks. In contrast to AIP, there is increased fecal excretion of protoporphyrin, but even this may be normal, and measurement of the porphyrin in bile seems more accurate. The affected enzyme is protoporphyrinogen oxidase.

DIAGNOSIS

Clinical diagnosis is not difficult if there is a family history of the disease, but the condition is so rare in the United States that physicians often do not recognize the source of unexplained abdominal pain and personality disorder. If peripheral neuropathy is added to the syndrome, however, and the appropriate biochemical tests are made, the diagnosis is ascertained. These tests are more important than looking for red urine or measurement of porphyrins in urine. Neurologically, the major disorder to be considered is the Guillain-Barré syndrome, but the characteristic rise in CSF protein content of that disease is not found in AIP; the CSF protein level rises so rarely in AIP that when this is found, it may be a sign of the Guillain-Barré syndrome in a person with porphyria.

TREATMENT

The fundamental biochemical abnormality cannot be corrected, but the autonomic manifestations of an acute attack may be reversed by propanolol. Doses up to 100 mg every 4 hours may reverse tachycardia, abdominal pain, and anxiety.

The neuropathy and abdominal symptoms may respond dramatically to hematin given intravenously in amounts from 200 to 1,000 mg in attempts to suppress the activity of ALA dehydratase. The optimal dosage is uncertain; one recommendation is to use 4 mg hematin/kg body weight twice daily for 3 days. Although expensive, this may be the most effective treatment, but some advocate the use of cimetidine orally, 800 mg daily.

Treatment of seizures is a problem because most commonly used anticonvulsants have been held responsible for porphyric attacks in human patients or they are porphyrogenic in experimental animals or cultured hepatic cells. In acute attacks of porphyria, seizures may be treated with diazepam or paraldehyde, whereas hematin and propanolol are used to abort the attacks. Between attacks, conventional anticonvulsants may be evaluated cautiously, monitoring urinary excretion of ALA and PBG. Gabapentin is said to be safe and effective.

Other drugs that are suitable for symptomatic relief include codeine and meperidine for pain, chlorpromazine and other psychoactive drugs, and almost all antibiotics. The major drugs to avoid are barbiturates in any form, including pentobarbital for general anesthesia (Table 92.2). Barbiturates may be especially hazardous when given for sedation or anesthesia in the early stages of an attack. It is otherwise difficult to prevent attacks, but some women have symptoms only and regularly in relation to menses; both suppression of ovulation and prophylactic use of hematin have been reported to be effective. In case of accident, patients should wear warning bracelets to identify the drug problem. Prophylactic care requires identification of gene carriers so that they can avoid drugs that precipitate attacks in susceptible people. Liver transplantation was effective in one severely symptomatic patient.

▶ **TABLE 92.2 Porphyrogenic Drugs in Acute Porphyria**[a]

Drugs	Number of Exposures	Only Precipitant
Barbiturate	81	31
Analgesics	16	5
Sulfonamides	16	5
Nonbarbiturate hypnotics	15	4
Unidentified sedatives	14	10
Miscellaneous drugs	12	3
Anticonvulsants	10	5
Hormonal	6	5

[a]153 acute episodes in 138 patients.
From Eales, 1979.

SUGGESTED READINGS

Becker DM, Kramer S. The neurological manifestations of porphyria: a review. *Medicine (Baltimore)* 1977;56:411–423.

Brezis M, Ghanem J, Weiler-Ravell O, et al. Hematin and propanolol in acute intermittent porphyria. Full recovery from quadriplegic coma and respiratory failure. *Eur Neurol* 1979;18:289–294.

Bylesjo I, Brekke OL, Prytz J, et al. Brain magnetic resonance imaging white matter lesions and cerebrospinal fluid findings in acute intermittent porphyria. *Europ Neurol* 2004;51(1):1–5.

Dean G. *The Porphyrias. A Story of Inheritance and the Environment.* 2nd ed. London: Pitman, 1971.

Eales L. Porphyria and the dangerous life-threatening drugs. *S Afr Med J* 1979;2:914–917.

Flugel KA, Druschky KF. EMG and nerve conduction in patients with acute intermittent porphyria. *J Neurol* 1977;214:267–279.

Grandchamp B. Acute intermittent porphyria. *Semin Liver Dis* 1998;18:17–24.

Herick AL, McColl KEL, Moore MR, et al. Controlled trial of haem arginate in acute hepatic porphyria. *Lancet* 1989;1:1295–1297.

Hindmarsh JT. Variable pheotypic expression of genotypic abnormalities in the porphyrias. *Clin Chim Acta* 1993;217:29–38.

Kauppinen R. Molecular diagnostics of acute intermittent porphyria. *Expert Rev Mol Diagn* 2004 Mar;4(2):243–249.

King PH, Bragdon AC. MRI reveals multiple reversible lesions in an attack of acute intermittent porphyria. *Neurology* 1991;41:1300–1302.

Laiwah ACY, Moore MR, Goldberg A. Pathogenesis of acute porphyria. *Q J Med* 1987;63:377–392.

Lee JS, Anvret M. Identification of the most common mutation within the porphobilinogen deaminase gene in Swedish patients with acute intermittent porphyria. *Proc Natl Acad Sci USA* 1991;88:10912–10915.

Llewellyn DH, Smyth SJ, Elder GH, et al. Homozygous acute intermittent porphyria: compound heterozygosity for adjacent base transitions in the same codon of the porphobilinogen deaminase gene. *Hum Genet* 1992;89:97–98.

Loftus CS, Arnold WN. Vincent Van Gogh's illness: acute intermittent porphyria? *Br Med J* 1991;303:1585–1591.

McEneaney D, Hawkins S, Trimble E, et al. Porphyric neuropathy—a rare and often neglected differential diagnosis of Guillain-Barré syndrome. *J Neurol Sci* 1993;114:231–233.

Meyer UA, Schuurmans MM, Lindberg RL. Acute porphyrias: pathogenesis of neurological manifestations. *Semin Liv Dis* 1998;18:43–52.

Moore MR. The biochemistry of heme synthesis in porphyria and in the porphyrinurias. *Clin Dermatol* 1998;16:203–223.

Moore MR, Disler PB. Drug induction of the acute porphyrias. *Adverse Drug React Acute Poison Rev* 1983;2:149–189.

Mustajoki P, Desnick RJ. Genetic heterogeneity in acute intermittent porphyria: characterisation and frequency of porphobilinogen deaminase mutations in Finland. *Br Med J* 1985;291:505–509.

Muthane UB, Vengamma B, Bharathi KC, et al. Porphyric neuropathy: prevention of progression using haeme-arginate. *J Intern Med* 1993;234:611–613.

Peters TJ, Deacon AC. International air travel: a risk factor for attacks of acute intermittent porphyria. *Clin Chim Acta* 2003;335:59–63.

Pierach CA, Weimer MK, Cardinal RA, et al. Red blood cell porphobilinogen deaminase in the evaluation of acute intermittent porphyria. *JAMA* 1987;257:60–61.

Reynolds NC, Miska RM. Safety of anticonvulsants in hepatic porphyrias. *Neurology* 1981;31:480–484.

Ridley A. The neuropathy of acute intermittent porphyria. *Q J Med* 1969;38:307–333.

Rogers PD. Cimetidine in the treatment of acute intermittent porphyria. *Ann Pharmacother* 1997;31:365–367.

Rowland LP. Acute intermittent porphyria: search for an enzymatic defect with implications for neurology and psychiatry. *Dis Nerv Sys* 1961;22(Suppl):1–12.

Sadeh H, Blatt I, Martonovits G, et al. Treatment of porphyric convulsions with magnesium sulfate. *Epilepsia* 1991;32:712–715.

Schneider-Yin X, Hergersberg M, Goldgar DE, et al. Ancestral founder of mutation W283X in the porphobilinogen deaminase gene among acute intermittent porphyria patients. *Hum Hered* 2002;54(2):69–81.

Solis C, Martinez-Bermejo A, Naidich TP, Kaufmann WE, Astrin KH, Bishop DF, Desnick RJ. Acute intermittent porphyria: studies of the severe homozygous dominant disease provides insights into the neurologic attacks in acute porphyrias. *Arch Neurol* 2004 Nov;61(11):1764–1770.

Soonawalla ZF, Orug T, Badminton MN, Elder GH, Rhodes JM, Bramhall SR, Elias E. Liver transplantation as a cure for acute intermittent porphyria. *Lancet* 2004 Feb 28;363(9410):705–706.

Suarez JI, Cohen ML, Larkin J, et al. Acute intermittent porphyria: clinicopathologic correlation. Report of a case and review of the literature. *Neurology* 1997;48:1678–1683.

Suzuki A, Aso K, Ariyoshi C, et al. Acute intermittent porphyria and epilepsy: safety of clonazepam. *Epilepsia* 1992;33:108–111.

Thorner PA, Bilbao JM, Sima AAF, et al. Porphyric neuropathy: an ultrastructural and quantitative study. *Can J Neurol Sci* 1981;8:261–287.

Tishler PV, Woodward B, O'Connor J, et al. High prevalence of intermittent acute porphyria in a psychiatric patient population. *Am J Psychiatry* 1985;142:1430–1436.

Yamada M, Kondo M, Tanaka M, et al. An autopsy case of acute porphyria with a decrease of both uroporphyrinogen I synthetase and ferrochetalase activities. *Acta Neuropathol (Berl)* 1984;64:6–11.

Yeung AC, Moore MR, Goldberg A. Pathogenesis of acute porphyria. *Q J Med* 1987;163:377–392.

Chapter 93

Neurological Syndromes with Acanthocytes

K-H. Christopher Min, Timothy A. Pedley, and Lewis P. Rowland

Several neurologic syndromes are associated with abnormal erythrocytes that are called *acanthocytes* because of spiny projections from the cell surface. *Acantho-* is derived from a Greek word meaning thorns. Three hereditary neurological disorders are associated with the presence of acanthocytes: abetalipoproteinemia, neuroacanthocytosis, and McLeod syndrome. Acanthocytes have also been reported in some cases of Hallervorden-Spatz disease.

ABETALIPOPROTEINEMIA

Abetalipoproteinemia (MIM 200100), the *Bassen-Kornzweig syndrome*, is an autosomal recessive disease characterized by inability of the liver and intestine to secret apolipoprotein B (apoB). It is caused by mutations in the gene encoding the microsomal triglyceride transfer protein, not apoB. Abetalipoproteinemia was originally defined clinically as a neurologic disorder resembling Friedreich ataxia in patients with chronic steatorrhea and acanthocytes.

Although autopsies have been few, the neuropathologic findings account for the clinical syndrome, showing demyelination of the posterior columns, spinocerebellar tracts, and corticospinal tracts. Neuronal changes are seen in the Purkinje cells and molecular layer of the cerebellum and the anterior horn cells. Peripheral nerves show mainly axonal loss with focal areas of demyelination, especially in large myelinated nerves. There is no clear explanation, however, for the clinically evident ophthalmoplegia. Interstitial myocardial fibrosis can occur, and muscle shows signs of denervation with accumulation of lipopigment.

Pathogenesis

Abetalipoproteinemia is caused by mutations in the microsomal triglyceride transfer protein (MTP), a 97-kDa protein related to lipovitellin, which is an ancient transport and storage lipoprotein found in egg-laying vertebrates. MTP forms a heterodimeric complex with protein disulfide isomerase, an endoplasmic reticulum resident protein. MTP plays a role in the lipidation of apoB and also in the assembly of very low-density lipoproteins in the endoplasmic reticulum prior to secretion.

Neuropathologic findings and the clinical phenotype result from nearly complete absence of apoB-containing lipoproteins in the plasma, and circulating levels of low-density and very low-density lipoproteins in the plasma are undetectable. Beta-lipoproteins are needed for the transport of lipids from intestinal mucosa and plasma. Patients with mutations in MTP cannot absorb lipids normally from intestinal mucosa, resulting in a drastically reduced lipid content in the serum, including cholesterol, triglycerides, and phospholipids. For example, serum cholesterol levels, normally 135 to 335 mg/dL, are 25 to 61 mg/dL in affected individuals.

As a consequence of the malabsorption, there is severe deficiency of the fat-soluble vitamins, A, D, E, and K. Vitamin A levels are 0 to 37 μg/dL (normal 20 to 87), a deficiency that probably plays a role in causing retinitis pigmentosa. Vitamin E levels are 0.06 to 0.1 μg/mL (normal 0.5 to 1.5), depletion sufficient to cause the spinocerebellar syndrome seen here as well as in other malabsorption states, including cholestatic liver disease and Crohn disease. The abnormal shape of the erythrocytes is also attributed to the hypolipidemia because the red cell membranes show an abnormal distribution of lipid constituents.

Symptoms and Signs

Fatty diarrhea, evident from infancy, is accompanied by abdominal distention and retarded growth. The children are small and underweight, with delayed bone age. The first neurologic abnormality is loss of tendon jerks at about age 5 years. At about age 10, ataxic gait is noted, then limb ataxia, tremor of the head and hands, and evidence of sensorimotor neuropathy: distal limb weakness and acroparesthesias, with glove-stocking cutaneous and proprioceptive sensory loss. Proximal limb weakness and scoliosis are seen in 25% of patients and

pedal abnormalities include pes cavus. Babinski signs are inconsistent.

Eye movements become progressively restricted, but before ophthalmoplegia is complete, nystagmus may be prominent. Concomitantly, as retinitis pigmentosa develops in adolescence, night-blindness (nyctalopia), with constriction of the visual fields and loss of visual acuity, occurs. The fundi show macular degeneration in the midperiphery of the retina, arteriolar narrowing, bone spicules, and angioid streaks. The syndrome is fully developed by age 20.

Vitamin K deficiency may lead to subdural or retroperitoneal hemorrhage, or there may be excessive blood loss after surgery.

Laboratory Data

In addition to the plasma changes, the erythrocyte sedimentation rate is inordinately low; usually 1 mm/hour. Nerve conduction studies and electromyography indicate that the neuropathy is primarily axonal. Sensory evoked potentials imply abnormality in the posterior columns; brainstem auditory responses are normal. Abnormalities of visual evoked potentials and electroretinography reflect the retinal degeneration and optic neuropathy. ECG abnormalities, cardiac enlargement, and murmurs have been described, but heart block and symptomatic congestive heart failure are not part of the picture.

Diagnosis

The neurologic disorder resembles Friedreich ataxia (spinocerebellar degeneration, sensorimotor peripheral neuropathy, retinitis pigmentosa) but differs with the addition of external ophthalmoplegia. The first clue to the diagnosis of abetalipoproteinemia is the finding of low values for serum cholesterol. Identifying acanthocytes usually requires a fresh blood smear (without EDTA) and even then may go unrecognized unless the technician has been asked to look for them specifically. Measurement of serum beta-lipoprotein and plasma lipids confirms the diagnosis.

Treatment

The essential element of treatment is dietary supplementation with vitamin E in doses of 100 mg/kg of alpha tocopherol acetate daily; blood levels should be monitored to avoid liver damage. In addition, adults should be given vitamin K, at least 5 mg daily. Supplemental corn oil has been recommended to correct or prevent deficiency of fatty acids.

With adequate tocopherol therapy, progression of the neurologic and retinal abnormalities ceases, and some patients even improve. Treatment is most effective when given early, preferably before neurologic signs are apparent. Under these circumstances, the neurologic syndrome may be prevented. Replacement therapy in adults with established symptoms is usually only partially successful.

Hypobetalipoproteinemia

Familial hypobetalipoproteinemia (MIM 107730) is an autosomal codominant disorder characterized by extremely low plasma levels of apoB caused by mutations in the gene encoding apoB. Heterozygous individuals are usually asymptomatic and do not have acanthocytes, although levels of apoB-containing lipoproteins are reduced significantly. The clinical phenotype of individuals with mutations in both alleles of apoB is highly variable, and severe cases are indistinguishable from abetalipoproteinemia, with steatorrhea, adult-onset ataxia, retinitis pigmentosa, and neuropathy with acanthocytosis. As for abetalipoproteinemia, treatment involves dietary supplementation with vitamin E. More than 35 mutations in the apoB gene result in premature truncation of the apoB protein and hypobetalipoproteinemia. Most are nonsense or frameshift mutations. An animal model with a similar phenotype has been created by gene targeting.

Several cases of hypobetalipoproteinemia, acanthocytosis, retinitis pigmentosa, and pallidal degeneration (*HARP syndrome*) have been described. Clinical manifestations are similar to those of Hallervorden-Spatz disease (MIM 234200), which is caused by mutations in the gene encoding pantothenate kinase 2. Re-study of the original case of HARP syndrome showed mutations in the pantothenate kinase 2 gene, so there is some interplay between the biochemical defects of familial hypobetalipoproteinemia and Hallervorden-Spatz disease.

NEUROACANTHOCYTOSIS

Neuroacanthocytosis (*Levine-Critchley syndrome* or chorea-acanthocytosis) (MIM 200150) is a multisystem neurodegenerative disorder characterized by acanthocytosis with normal plasma lipids and lipoproteins and variable neurologic manifestations. Onset is usually in the third or fourth decade, but both juvenile and elderly forms are known. The most consistent clinical feature is a hyperkinetic movement disorder (chorea, orofacial dyskinesias, or dystonia), which may gradually evolve to parkinsonism. In many patients, dementia follows psychiatric features, including obsessive-compulsive disorder and personality changes. An axonal neuropathy with muscle wasting, weakness, and loss of tendon reflexes occurs in most patients. About 40% of patients have epileptic seizures. The course is one of progressive disability, with a mean duration of about 14 years. Only symptomatic

therapy is available, but the response of the involuntary movements to drug treatment is usually poor.

The clinical picture correlates with neuronal degeneration and astrocytic proliferation within the basal ganglia and substantia nigra. Despite the dementia and psychiatric symptoms, the cerebral cortex is histologically normal. The axonal neuropathy involves primarily large-diameter myelinated fibers, and muscle biopsy shows findings consistent with denervation. MRI findings are similar to those of Huntington chorea, including prominent atrophy of the caudate nuclei and increased T2 signal within the striatum.

The inheritance of neuroacanthocytosis is typically autosomal recessive, although apparent autosomal dominance has been reported. A mutation in *CHAC*, a gene that maps to chromosome 9q21, was found in patients with neuroacanthocytosis. The protein encoded by *CHAC* is chorein, which has two splice variants with protein products of 3095 and 3175 amino acids. Chorein is expressed ubiquitously and its function is not known, although it may play a role in intracellular trafficking. The known mutations cause a premature stop of the coding sequence, resulting in shortened forms of the protein.

McLEOD SYNDROME

The *McLeod syndrome* (MIM 314850) is an X-linked disorder defined by abnormal expression of the Kell blood group antigens and absence of the Kx erythrocyte antigen. The first cases were found in asymptomatic people who were donating blood and had blood typing carried out. When they were studied hematologically, the acanthocytes were recognized, and so were high serum levels of creatine kinase, high enough to suggest a true myopathy. Later, some people with the condition were found to have a symptomatic myopathy, amyotrophy, or involuntary movements, as well as a permanent hemolytic state (Table 93.1). In some patients, the clinical features are similar to those of neuroacanthocytosis. In one series, 5 of 22 patients had generalized tonic-clonic seizures.

As with neuroacanthocytosis, MRI findings are similar to those found in Huntington chorea, with atrophy of the caudate nucleus and increased T2 signal in the basal ganglia, especially in the lateral putamen. Unlike for neuroacanthocytosis, muscle biopsy shows myopathic changes, and there are often clinical signs of heart involvement, which can progress to severe cardiomyopathy and death. Areflexia is common, and electrophysiologic and nerve biopsy findings are consistent with axonal degeneration. Serum creatine kinase values are abnormally high in virtually all patients at levels 1.3 to 15 times the upper limit of normal.

XK, the gene responsible for McLeod syndrome, has been localized to chromosome Xp21, between the loci of

▶ **TABLE 93.1** Clinical and Laboratory Findings in Abetalipoproteinemia, Neuroacanthocytosis, and McLeod Syndrome

Findings	Frequency (%) in Abetalipoproteinemia[a]	Frequency (%) in Neuroacanthocytosis[b]	Frequency (%) in McLeod Syndrome[c]
Cognitive changes	25	73	54
Psychopathology	—	60	83
Retinopathy	50	0	0
Abnormal eye movements	44	0	0
Lingual atrophy, fasciculation	39	—	—
Limb weakness	22	54	65
Ataxia	47	0	0
Areflexia	72	90	90
Dorsal column sensory loss	86	13	40
Babinski sign	35	—	—
Cardiomyopathy	0	0	65
Seizures	0	42	50
Chorea	0	85	94
Dystonia	0	50	38
Laboratory Findings			
Acanthocytes	100	88	100
Abnormally low cholesterol	100	0	0
Weak Kell antigens	0	0	100
Abnormally low cholesterol	100	0	0
Abnormal EMG	85	67	79

Adapted from [a]Brin MF. Acanthocytosis. *Handb Clin Neurol* 1993;271–299; [b]Rampoldi L, Danek A, Monaco AP. Clinical features and molecular bases of neuroacanthocytosis. *J Mol Med* 2002;80(Aug):475–491; and [c]Danek A, Rubio JP, Rampoldi L, et al. McLeod neuroacanthocytosis: genotype and phenotype. *Ann Neurol* 2001;50(Dec):755–774.

Duchenne muscular dystrophy and chronic granulomatous disease. A contiguous deletion can affect all three genes to produce all three diseases in the same person. The XK protein is 444 amino acid residues in length, and disease-associated mutations cause either complete absence of the protein or severely truncated forms owing to frame-shift, nonsense, or splice-site mutations. The XK protein is predicted to have 10 transmembrane domains. It has sequence homology to *C. elegans* protein CED-8, which may regulate cell death pathways important in embryonic development. In red cells, the XK protein forms a covalent heterodimeric complex through a disulfide bond with Kell protein, a 731 amino acid type II membrane glycoprotein that processes endothelin through its metalloprotease activity. At this time, the role of XK, Kell, and their complex in the molecular mechanisms leading to the McLeod syndrome have been only partially elucidated, although it has been shown that expression of XK is particularly high in affected tissues.

SUGGESTED READINGS

Ching KH, Westaway SK, Gitschier J, et al. HARP syndrome is allelic with pantothenate kinase-associated neurodegeneration. *Neurology* 2002;58:1673–1674.

Danek A, Rubio JP, Rampoldi L, et al. McLeod neuroacanthocytosis: genotype and phenotype. *Ann Neurol* 2001;50:755–774.

Du EZ, Wang SL, Kayden HJ, et al. Translocation of apolipoprotein B across the endoplasmic reticulum is blocked in abetalipoproteinemia. *J Lipid Res* 1996;37:1309–1315.

Feinberg TE, Cianci CD, Morrow JS, et al. Diagnostic tests for choreoacanthocytosis. *Neurology* 1991;41:1000–1006.

Hardie RJ, Pullon HW, Harding AE, et al. Neuroacanthocytosis. A clinical, haematological and pathological study of 19 cases. *Brain* 1991 Feb;114(Pt 1A):13–49.

Jung HH, Haker H. Schizophrenia as a manifestation of X-linked McLeod-Neuroacanthocytosis syndrome. *J Clin Psychiatry* 2004 May;65(5):722–723.

Kaempf-Rotzoll DE, Traber MG, Arai H. Vitamin E and transfer proteins. *Curr Opin Lipidol* 2003;14:249–254.

Kairamkonda V, Dalzell M. Unusual presentation of three siblings with familial heterozygous hypobetalipoproteinaemia. *Eur J Pediatr* 2003;162(Mar):129–131.

Kim E, Cham CM, Veniant MM, et al. Dual mechanisms for the low plasma levels of truncated apolipoprotein B proteins in familial hypobetalipoproteinemia. Analysis of a new mouse model with a nonsense mutation in the Apob gene. *J Clin Invest* 1998;101:1468–1477.

Levy E. The genetic basis of primary disorders of intestinal fat transport. *Clin Invest Med* 1996;19(Oct):317–324.

MacGilchrist AJ, Mills PR, Noble M, et al. Abetalipoproteinaemia in adults: role of vitamin therapy. *J Inherit Metab Dis* 1988;11(2):184–190.

Meenakshi-Sundaram S, Arun Kumar MJ, Sridhar R, Rani U, Sundar B. Neuroacanthocytosis misdiagnosed as Huntington's disease: a case report. *J Neurol Sci* 2004 Apr 15;219(1–2):163–166.

Muller DP, Lloyd JK, Wolff OH. The role of vitamin E in the treatment of the neurological features of abetalipoproteinaemia and other disorders of fat absorption. *J Inherit Metab Dis* 1985;8(Suppl 1): 88–92.

Rampoldi L, Danek A, Monaco AP. Clinical features and molecular bases of neuroacanthocytosis. *J Mol Med* 2002;80:475–491.

Rinne JO, Daniel SE, Scaravilli F, et al. The neuropathological features of neuroacanthocytosis. *Mov Disord* 1994;9(May):297–304.

Ross RS, Gregg RE, Law SW, et al. Homozygous hypobetalipoproteinemia: a disease distinct from abetalipoproteinemia at the molecular level. *J Clin Invest* 1988;81(Feb):590–595.

Runge P, Muller DP, McAllister J, et al. Oral vitamin E supplements can prevent the retinopathy of abetalipoproteinaemia. *Br J Ophthalmol* 1986;70(Mar):166–173.

Saiki S, Sakai K, Kitagawa Y, et al. Mutation in the CHAC gene in a family of autosomal dominant chorea-acanthocytosis. *Neurology* 2003;61:1614–1616.

Sakai T, Iwashita H, Kakugawa M. Neuroacanthocytosis syndrome and choreoacanthocytosis (Levine-Critchley syndrome). *Neurology* 1985;35:1679.

Satya-Murti S, Howard L, Krohel G, et al. The spectrum of neurologic disorder from vitamin E deficiency. *Neurology* 1986;36:917–921.

Schonfeld G. Familial hypobetalipoproteinemia: a review. *J Lipid Res* 2003;44:878–883.

Sharp D, Blinderman L, Combs KA, et al. Cloning and gene defects in microsomal triglyceride transfer protein associated with abetalipoproteinaemia. *Nature* 1993;365(Sep 2):65–69.

Shizuka M, Watanabe M, Aoki M, et al. Analysis of the McLeod syndrome gene in three patients with neuroacanthocytosis. *J Neurol Sci* 1997;150(Sep 10):133–135.

Sokol RJ. Vitamin E and neurologic deficits. *Adv Pediatr* 1990;37:119–148.

Stevenson VL, Hardie RJ. Acanthocytosis and neurological disorders. *J Neurol* 2001;248:87–94.

Ueno S, Maruki Y, Nakamura M, et al. The gene encoding a newly discovered protein, chorein, is mutated in chorea-acanthocytosis. *Nat Genet* 2001;28(Jun):121–122.

Wetterau JR, Aggerbeck LP, Bouma ME, et al. Absence of microsomal triglyceride transfer protein in individuals with abetalipoproteinemia. *Science* 1992;258:999–1001.

Wong P. A basis of the acanthocytosis in inherited and acquired disorders. *Med Hypotheses* 2004;62:966–969.

C h a p t e r   9 4

Cerebral Degenerations of Childhood

Eveline C. Traeger and Isabelle Rapin

CANAVAN DISEASE (SPONGY DEGENERATION OF THE NERVOUS SYSTEM)

This autosomal-recessive illness (MIM 271900) is one of the more common cerebral degenerative diseases of infancy. Although van Bogaert and Bertrand should be credited with the nosologic identification, it is often called Canavan disease in the United States. It affects all ethnic groups but is especially prevalent among Ashkenazi Jews from eastern Poland, Lithuania, and western Russia, and among Saudi Arabians. A characteristic feature that it shares with Alexander disease and some other diseases is megalencephaly. The clinical picture is often sufficiently distinctive to suggest the diagnosis. It is prenatal in onset with variable progression; at least 50% of children with Canavan disease are symptomatic by 4 months of age.

Extremely poor control of the enlarged head, lack of psychomotor development, spasticity, optic atrophy, and hearing loss are the main features. Affected children may achieve smiling, but they are characteristically quiet and apathetic. Few progress far enough to reach for objects or sit, and except for children with a rare protracted variant, none ever walks independently. Seizures occur in more than 50% of patients. By age 2 years, head growth plateaus as progressive parenchymal destruction leads to hydrocephalus ex vacuo. The children eventually become decerebrate and die of intercurrent illness; survival into the second or third decades is not uncommon.

CT and MRI show increased lucency of the white matter, poor demarcation of gray and white matter (Fig. 94.1), and later, severe brain atrophy with ventricular enlargement and gaping sulci. CSF contents and nerve conduction velocities are usually normal. The pathology includes two characteristic abnormalities: intramyelinic vacuolation of the deep layers of the cortex and superficial layers of the white matter, and gigantic abnormal mitochondria containing a dense filamentous granular matrix and distorted cristae in the watery cytoplasm of hypertrophied astrocytes. Sponginess eventually becomes diffuse and involves the centrum semiovale, brainstem, cerebellum, and

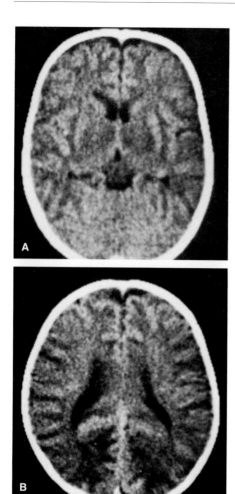

FIGURE 94.1. Axial noncontrast CT in an 11-month-old boy with spongy degeneration. Note the diffuse low density of white matter with occipital preponderance and poor demarcation between gray and white matter. Sulci are mildly widened.

spinal cord. As the disease progresses, the vacuoles enlarge and split the myelin sheath to form cysts that communicate with the extracellular space. This leads to extensive demyelination and tissue destruction with loss of neurons, axons, and oligodendroglia; extensive gliosis follows. Chemical analysis of the brain reveals markedly increased N-acetylaspartic acid (NAA) and water content, as well as nonspecific loss of myelin and other tissue constituents.

Deficiency of aspartoacylase in skin fibroblasts is diagnostic and is associated with elevated levels of NAA in blood and urine, as well as brain. Carrier detection based on aspartoacylase activity in cultured skin fibroblasts is possible; aspartoacylase activity in amniotic fluid, chorionic villi, or amniocytes is unreliable for prenatal diagnosis. The gene for Canavan disease has been cloned and is located on chromosome 17p. Two mutations account for 97% of the alleles in Ashkenazi Jewish patients. In non-Jewish patients, the mutations are different and

more diverse. Carrier detection and prenatal diagnosis by DNA analysis are available in most but not all high-risk families.

Spongy degeneration of the brain also occurs in other conditions, notably intoxication by triethyl tin or hexachlorophene, some neonatal acidurias, some mitochondrial disorders, and the Aicardi-Goutières syndrome (leukodystrophy with CSF lymphocytosis and basal ganglia calcification). In fact, prior to DNA analysis, some cases labeled juvenile spongy degeneration that started in childhood with external ophthalmoplegia and pigmentary degeneration of the retina, with or without other neurologic or systemic abnormalities, may have been Kearns-Sayre syndrome, some other mitochondrial disorder, or a leukodystrophy with either vanishing white matter or subcortical cysts.

INFANTILE NEUROAXONAL DYSTROPHY

Infantile neuroaxonal dystrophy (Seitelberger disease; MIM 256600) is an autosomal-recessive disease of unknown pathophysiology that typically becomes manifest between 6 and 18 months of age and leads to death before the end of the first decade, usually after a variable period of purely vegetative existence. The first symptom is arrest of motor development, followed by loss of skills. The children may be floppy, spastic, or both. Most never achieve independent walking or speaking. In some, the motor disorder progresses from the legs to the arms and finally to the cranial muscles, causing severe dysphagia. There may be loss of sensation in the legs and urinary retention. Ataxia, nystagmus, and optic atrophy are common, but seizures are rare. The degree of dementia is difficult to ascertain because of anarthria; at first, affected children appear alert and seem to understand some language, but intellectual deterioration eventually becomes severe.

A newly described lysosomal storage disease owing to α-N-acetylgalactosaminidase deficiency has been found in patients with a phenotype similar to that of infantile neuroaxonal dystrophy but differing by the presence of prominent generalized or myoclonic seizures. Atypical variants are seen. A few infants are symptomatic from birth, whereas others experience a later onset and more protracted course, some with prominent myoclonus, others with dystonic features.

The relationship of these more chronic cases to Hallervorden-Spatz disease (pantothenate kinase–associated neurodegeneration or PKAN) is controversial. Some authorities consider neuroaxonal dystrophy and PKAN to be the same nosologic entity because spheroid formation is seen in both and because there are clinical similarities. Spheroids, however, are not pathognomonic of either disease, and the distribution of these lesions differs in the two disorders; brown discoloration of the globus pallidus occurs only in PKAN. Discovery of mutations in the PANK2 gene in patients with classic PKAN will resolve the question of the relationship of the two conditions.

The characteristic pathologic picture of neuroaxonal dystrophy is the profusion of axonal spheroids in the brain, spinal cord, and peripheral nerves. Spheroids are eosinophilic, argyrophilic ovoid inclusions that distend axons and myelin sheaths. They may be found anywhere along axons but are especially numerous in axon terminals, including those at the neuromuscular junction. Electron microscopy shows that they contain tubular structures, vesicles, and masses of smooth membranes arranged in stacks or, less often, in circular concentric arrays. The relation of these structures to synaptic vesicles or smooth endoplasmic reticulum is speculative. Spheroids also contain membrane-bound clefts and accumulations of mitochondria. Spheroids are particularly prevalent in the cerebellum, basal ganglia, thalamus, cuneate, gracile, and the brainstem nuclei. The cerebellum is strikingly atrophic because of loss of Purkinje and granular cells. The basal ganglia show neuronal loss and may appear spongy, with demyelinated axons and spheroid deposition. Although lipopigment granules are found in basal ganglia, there is no discoloration visible to the naked eye. The long tracts of the visual system, corticospinal system, spinocerebellar pathways, and posterior columns are degenerated, and there is pallor of the myelin. No characteristic lesions have been described in the viscera. Biochemical changes in the brain are viewed as nonspecific.

Laboratory tests are not helpful. The CSF is usually normal; EEG changes are absent or nonspecific. Nerve conduction velocities may be normal or slow. EMG usually suggests denervation. T2-weighted MRI shows diffuse cerebellar atrophy with hyperintensity of the cerebellar cortex. Definite diagnosis requires autopsy. Nerve, muscle, rectal, or conjunctival biopsy is confirmatory when spheroids are found in nerves or at the neuromuscular junction, but because of sampling problems, normal peripheral nerve or even cortical biopsy does not exclude the diagnosis. There is no chemical or enzymatic test available; intrauterine diagnosis is not feasible. Treatment is limited to symptomatic measures and support and genetic counseling for the child's family.

PANTOTHENATE KINASE-ASSOCIATED NEURODEGENERATION (PKAN) (HALLERVORDEN-SPATZ DISEASE)

PKAN (MIM 234200) is an insidiously progressive autosomal-recessive disease of childhood and adolescence in which motor symptoms predominate. It usually starts with stiffness of gait and is eventually associated with dis-

tal wasting, pes cavus or equinovarus, and toe walking. The arms are held stiffly with hyperextended fingers; the hands may become useless when the child is still ambulatory. The children often have a characteristically frozen, pained expression with risus sardonicus and contracted platysma muscles. They speak through clenched teeth and have difficulty eating. Eventually they become anarthric, although they continue to understand language. Muscle tone is both spastic and rigid, often with painful spasms, yet passive movement with the patient supine reveals an underlying hypotonia. Reflexes are hyperactive, including facial reflexes, and the toes are usually, but not always, upgoing. Some children become dystonic and assume bizarre postures that suggest generalized torsion dystonia (DYT1). Ataxia, tremor, nystagmus, and facial grimacing are seen in some patients, usually early in the illness. Pigmentary degeneration of the retina occurs in some families; in others the eyegrounds are normal or show primary optic atrophy. Assessing intellectual function is difficult; affected children remain alert, and if dementia occurs, it may not be severe. The course of the illness typically spans several decades. Therapy is limited to symptomatic measures.

Once the illness is full-blown, the clinical picture is sufficiently characteristic to suggest the diagnosis. T2-weighted MRI demonstrates striking hypointensity in the globus pallidus, the so-called eye-of-the-tiger sign. Rarely, patients have osmiophilic deposits in lymphocytes and bone marrow macrophages resembling sea-blue histiocytes. Deficiency of the enzyme pantothenate kinase 2 (PANK2), a key regulatory enzyme in the biosynthesis of coenzyme A, has been confirmed in patients with classic disease.

The pathology is restricted in distribution. Olive or golden brown discoloration of the medial segment of the globus pallidus is the macroscopic hallmark of PKAN. Less striking discoloration occurs in the red nucleus and zona reticulata of the substantia nigra. This appearance is owing to granules of an iron-containing lipopigment (similar to neuromelanin) located inside and outside the neurons and hyperplastic astrocytes. Irregular mulberry concretions, some calcified, lie free in the tissue. Increased amounts of iron and other metals (e.g., zinc, copper) and calcium are found in the affected tissue, which contains axonal spheroids identical to those seen in neuroaxonal dystrophy. Neuronal loss and thinning of myelin sheaths are prominent in the globus pallidus, less severe in the rest of the basal ganglia, and uncommon elsewhere, although mild cerebellar atrophy does occur. In contrast to infantile neuroaxonal dystrophy, only a few spheroids are found in the cortex and cerebral white matter.

Variants (Hallervorden-Spatz syndrome) include mid- or late-adult onset. Symptoms include acanthocytosis with or without hypoprebetalipoproteinemia. They lack the typical eye-of-the-tiger MRI except in those with atypical disease who have PANK2 mutations.

PELIZAEUS-MERZBACHER DISEASE

The two clinical forms of Pelizaeus-Merzbacher disease (PMD; MIM 312080) are both X-linked recessive and linked to the proteolipid protein (PLP) gene. One form is present at birth, the so-called connatal variant of Seitelberger, and the other is an infantile variant with a more protracted course, which is the classic form.

A prominent, irregular nystagmus and head tremor or head rolling from birth or the first few months of life are the most striking features of both forms. In the connatal form, these symptoms are associated with floppiness, head lag, grayness of the optic discs, and stridor. Meaningful development does not occur. Boys develop ataxia, severe spasticity, and optic atrophy. Seizures, microcephaly, and failure to thrive supervene, and most infants succumb in the first years of life. Others survive for 8 to 12 years but are mute with limited intellect, despite apparent alertness. In the classic form, slow motor development may enable the children to reach for objects, roll over, crawl, and say a few words. Independent walking is rarely achieved; even these few developmental milestones are lost as increasing ataxia, spasticity with hyperreflexia, and choreoathetotic movements develop. By school age, the affected boy is often mute and confined to a wheelchair.

Patients are likely to develop kyphoscoliosis and joint contractures; they become incontinent. Sensory loss does not occur. Dementia is difficult to assess but may not be profound. Optic atrophy is not severe. Hearing is preserved. Despite severe growth failure and small muscle mass, there is little further deterioration until the patient dies of an intercurrent illness, usually in late adolescence or early adulthood.

Normal nerve conduction velocities and usually normal CSF protein content help differentiate the connatal variant from Krabbe disease and metachromatic leukodystrophy. Prominent nystagmus is the main differentiating symptom from infantile neuroaxonal dystrophy and early-onset PKAN. EEG is normal or mildly slow. CT shows ventricular dilatation, decreased differentiation of gray and white matter, and cerebellar atrophy. MRI shows T_2 prolongation in white matter representing a paucity of myelin.

At autopsy, the brain, cerebellum, brainstem, and spinal cord of children with the connatal variant are essentially devoid of myelin. In the late infantile variant, characteristic changes are limited to brainstem and cerebellar white matter. The hallmark of PMD is a tigroid appearance of the white matter on myelin stains because of perivascular islands of spared myelin against a nonmyelinated background. There is no sparing of U fibers. Axons are spared but are almost devoid of oligodendroglia. The cerebral cortex is preserved, although large pyramids in layer V of the motor cortex (Betz cells) may be lacking in the connatal form. Neuronal dropout is not severe, with the possible exception of granular cell loss in the cerebellum. Areas of cerebral dysgenesis and micropolygyria have been observed too often to be coincidental. Peripheral nerves are characteristically well myelinated.

Duplications, point mutations, insertions, and deletions in the X-linked PLP gene, a component of myelin, have been documented in approximately 75% of patients with PMD. Duplications account for 60% of the mutations. Differences in processing and trafficking of the two PLP gene products, PLP and its smaller isoform DM20, with subsequent oligodendroglial death by apoptosis resulting in deficiency of myelin basic protein, myelin-associated glycoprotein, and cyclic nucleotide phosphodiesterase may explain the pathogenesis. A clinically distinct disease, X-linked spastic paraplegia type 2 (SPG-2), in which demyelination spares most of the central white matter but selectively affects the spinal tracts, is also linked to PLP.

ALEXANDER DISEASE

Three variants of Alexander disease (MIM 203450) affect astrocytes. The first is a rapidly progressive infantile type, beginning in the first 2 years of life with megalencephaly, severe motor and developmental deficits, and seizures. The large head is usually the result of an enlarged brain, but some children develop hydrocephalus owing to an obstruction of the aqueduct of Sylvius by Rosenthal fibers. The children are usually, but not invariably, spastic. Most die in a vegetative state in infancy or during the preschool years. A few children survive into the second decade.

Neuroimaging suggests the diagnosis when there is marked demyelination with frontal predominance, especially if there are enlarged ventricles with a zone of increased density in the subependymal region (Fig. 94.2). Occasionally, the basal ganglia appear necrotic on CT, as in the infantile variant of Leigh disease. The main differential diagnosis is Canavan disease, suggested by the enlarged head, early dementia, and decreased density of white matter, although optic atrophy is not characteristic of Alexander disease.

The juvenile variant becomes evident from around age 4 years to the early teens. The course is more indolent and protracted, with prominent bulbar symptoms and usually without seizures. Alexander disease may also present in adults with signs of bulbar palsy and ataxia with or without intellectual deterioration and spasticity. Alexander disease is defined by the principal histologic characteristic, the so-called Rosenthal fibers, which are hyaline, eosinophilic, and argyrophilic inclusions found exclusively in astrocytic footplates. Rosenthal fibers contain small stress proteins: alpha B-crystallin and heat shock protein 27 (HSP27). Rosenthal fibers are characteristically distributed in subpial, subependymal, and perivascular locations. In some patients, especially infants, the fibers are found diffusely in

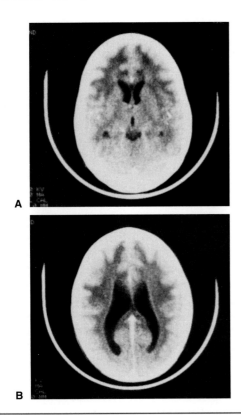

FIGURE 94.2. Axial contrast CT in a 29-month-old girl with Alexander disease. Note the low density of the white matter with frontal-to-occipital gradient and increased periventricular density.

the brain and spinal cord, especially the floor of the fourth ventricle. Rosenthal fibers are not pathognomonic of this illness; they occur in pilocytic astrocytomas, are rarely associated with multiple sclerosis plaques, and have been reported in adolescents and adults without known neurologic symptoms.

Demyelination with loss of oligodendroglia and sparing axons occurs in regions rich in Rosenthal fibers. In infantile cases, demyelination of the centrum semiovale is so severe that it may lead to cavitation; loss of myelin is most severe frontally and has a characteristic frontal-to-occipital gradient. The myelin of peripheral nerves is spared. Neurons are also spared, with the exception of brainstem motor neurons in some juvenile and adult patients with bulbar symptoms, and of basal ganglia neurons in some infantile cases. De novo dominant missense mutations in the coding region of the glial fibrillary acidic protein (GFAP) gene have been identified in most cases of infantile and juvenile onset Alexander disease. There is also confirmation of a GFAP mutation in an adult onset case. Most cases are sporadic, but there are rare reports of affected siblings. Prenatal screening for families whose affected child has an identified mutation is available. Therapy remains purely symptomatic.

COCKAYNE SYNDROME

Cockayne syndrome (MIM 216400) is a progressive multisystem disease with autosomal-recessive inheritance characterized by extreme dwarfing, a characteristic cachectic appearance, and neurologic deterioration. The children are of normal size at birth. Failure to thrive with progressive decrease in height, weight, and head circumference usually becomes apparent before the child reaches age 2 years. These growth measures typically are many standard deviations below the mean by mid-childhood or adolescence. The affected child has an arresting facial appearance with large ears, long aquiline nose, deep-set eyes, thin lips, and jutting chin; the appearance is often accentuated by the loss of severely carious teeth. Some children have atrophic or hyperpigmented skin changes over exposed areas, especially the face. Body proportions, although miniature, are appropriate for the child's age. Signs of maturation, such as the shedding of deciduous teeth and puberty, occur on time, although the penis, testes, and breasts are usually underdeveloped. The children may suffer from carbohydrate intolerance and anomalies of renal function. Most survive at least into the second decade. Rare mild cases survive into adulthood.

Intellectual development is extremely limited, but affected children remain alert and have pleasant personalities. Most do not speak, and many do not walk independently because of progressive spasticity, widespread joint contractures, and deformities of the feet. Some have signs of a demyelinating peripheral neuropathy and are ataxic. Many become deaf, and vision is impaired as the result of variable combinations of corneal opacity, cataract, pigmentary degeneration of the retina, and optic atrophy. The pupils are meiotic and respond poorly to mydriatics. Tearing is reduced or absent. Plain radiographs of the skull and CT typically show stippled calcification in the basal ganglia. Nerve conduction velocities are slow, and CSF protein may be elevated.

The diagnosis is suggested by the clinical features. The main differential diagnosis is Seckel (bird-headed) dwarfism, in which dwarfing is invariably present at birth, with extremely low weights for gestational age. The children do not suffer from progressive physical and neurologic deterioration; they learn to walk and speak, despite their extreme microcephaly; they are less retarded than children with Cockayne syndrome but share similar dysmorphic features. Children with progeria are usually of normal intelligence and have much more prominent signs of premature aging than children with Cockayne syndrome, who do not lose their hair, for example, even though mild, early graying may occur.

The brains of children with Cockayne syndrome (and of Seckel dwarfs) are tiny, weighing 500 to 700 g. A prominent feature is extreme thinness of the white matter, which has a tigroid appearance on myelin stains because of islands of myelinated fibers amid areas without myelin, a pattern reminiscent of that seen in Pelizaeus-Merzbacher disease. Hydrocephalus ex vacuo is typical, but a few have low pressure hydrocephalus and may benefit from shunting. Calcification of the basal ganglia and cerebellar atrophy are typical. Developmental anomalies, seen in some cases, indicate that the disease starts prenatally, despite allegedly normal head circumference and development in infancy. Other pathology features include grotesque dendrites of Purkinje cells and multinucleate astrocytes.

Cockayne fibroblasts and amniocytes are unable to recover their ribonucleic acid synthesis after ultraviolet irradiation. They are defective in the preferential repair of transcriptionally active genes. Cockayne syndrome (CS) is genetically heterogeneous; CSA on chromosome 5q12.1 and CSB to chromosome 10q11. Some mutations of CSB are responsible for the clinically distinct early lethal COFS (cerebro-oculo-facial-skeletal) syndrome of infancy. In addition there are variants with features of xeroderma pigmentosum linked to the xeroderma pigmentosum (XP) XPB, D, and G genes, another disease affecting DNA repair mechanisms resulting in extreme sensitivity to ultraviolet light. There are atypical Cockayne and CS/XP cases, including both neonatal and adult variants.

XERODERMA PIGMENTOSUM NEUROLOGIC DISEASE

Xeroderma pigmentosum is a disease caused by defective DNA repair and is associated with extreme skin sensitivity to sunlight. As a result, skin hyperpigmentation, atrophy, freckling, and innumerable cutaneous carcinomas and melanomas develop from earliest childhood. The variants of xeroderma pigmentosum that affect the nervous system arise from widespread neuronal loss resulting in spasticity, mental retardation, microcephaly in the infantile variants, and in some cases movement disorders, ataxia, dysarthria, progressive hearing loss, and an axonal sensorimotor neuropathy. The severity and course of the disease correlate with age of onset. Infantile variants are severe and may be associated with endocrinopathies (De Sanctis-Cacchione syndrome). This is a genetically heterogeneous syndrome, with some variants causing the XP/CS syndrome. Full understanding of the pathophysiology of these overlapping disorders of DNA repair is still lacking.

RETT SYNDROME

Rett syndrome (MIM 312750) is a clinically defined neurodevelopmental disorder. First described by Professor Andreas Rett in the mid-1960s, it did not come to widespread attention until 1983. It is a common cause of profound mental retardation in girls and women (1 in 10,000 to 15,000 females). The clinical signatures are postnatal deceleration of brain growth between ages 5 months and 4 years, almost continuous stereotypic hand movements, profound cognitive and communicative impairment, respiratory irregularities, and often seizures. Current diagnostic criteria for classic Rett syndrome (75% of cases) and atypical Rett syndrome (25% of cases) are listed in Tables 94.1 and 94.2.

Rett syndrome typically goes through four stages: first, developmental stagnation, then a devastating regression with irritability, loss of purposeful hand use, and loss of psychomotor and communication starting between ages 6 months and 4 years. The period of regression may last months or a few years, sometimes with partial recovery—especially of social skills and mood; and then, cognitive stability. This single period of autisticlike regression followed by stabilization distinguishes Rett syndrome from other developmental and progressive neurologic disorders. The outcome is poor, and most individuals are nonverbal, with almost total lack of adaptive and cognitive skills. Of the 80% who can walk with an apraxic, wide-based gait, about 25% lose the ability to walk during the regressive period. Survival into middle age is common, although sudden unexplained death is prevalent. Treatment is limited to symptomatic measures.

▶ **TABLE 94.1 Diagnostic Criteria for Rett Syndrome**

Necessary criteria
1. Apparently normal prenatal and perinatal history
2. Psychomotor development largely normal through the first 6 months or may be delayed from birth
3. Normal head circumference at birth
4. Postnatal deceleration of head growth rate in the majority, onset 3 months–4 years
5. Loss of achieved purposeful hand skills between ages 6 months and 2½ years
6. Stereotypic hand movements such as hand wringing/squeezing, clapping/tapping, mouthing, and washing/rubbing automatisms emerge between the ages of 1 and 3 years
7. Emerging social withdrawal, communication dysfunction, loss of learned words, and cognitive impairment between ages 9 months and 2½ years
8. Impaired (dyspraxic) or failing locomotion, onset 1–4 years

Supportive criteria
1. Awake disturbances of breathing (hyperventilation, breath holding, forced expulsion of air or saliva, air swallowing)
2. Bruxism
3. Impaired sleep pattern from early infancy
4. Abnormal muscle tone associated with muscle wasting and dystonia
5. Peripheral vasomotor disturbances
6. Scoliosis/kyphosis progressing through childhood
7. Growth retardation
8. Hypotrophic small and cold feet; small, thin hands

> **TABLE 94.2** Delineation of Variant
> Rett Phenotypes

1. Meet at least 3 of 6 main criteria
2. Meet at least 5 of 11 supportive criteria

Six main criteria
1. Absence or reduction of hand skills
2. Reduction or loss of babble speech
3. Monotonous pattern to hand stereotypies
4. Reduction or loss of communication skills
5. Deceleration of head growth from first years of life
6. Rett syndrome profile: a regression stage followed by a recovery of interaction contrasting with slow neuromotor regression

Eleven supportive criteria
1. Breathing irregularities
2. Bloating/air swallowing
3. Bruxism, harsh-sounding type
4. Abnormal locomotion
5. Scoliosis/kyphosis
6. Lower limb amyotrophy
7. Cold, purplish feet, usually growth impaired
8. Sleep disturbances, including night screaming outbursts
9. Laughing, screaming spells
10. Diminished response to pain
11. Intense eye contact, eye pointing

Imaging shows a decrease in brain volume affecting gray matter—especially the frontal cortex and the caudate nucleus—more than white matter. Brain weight is reduced by 14% to 34% compared to controls. Neuropathologic changes are subtle and developmental rather than degenerative: smaller neurons and reduced dendritic arborization resulting in increased cell packing density.

Seventy to eighty percent of patients with Rett syndrome have a mutation in the methyl-CpG binding protein 2 (*MECP2*) gene located on chromosome Xq28. The highest levels of *MECP2*, a widely expressed transcriptional repressor, are found in the brain. Evidence suggests that *MECP2* affects neuronal and synaptic maturation, but the pathogenesis of Rett syndrome is not known. Clinical variability probably results from several factors: the type of mutation, the functional domain affected, and X-chromosome inactivation. Most cases are sporadic, with a high ratio of de novo mutations in the sperm, which explains the extreme paucity of affected males. Skewed X-chromosome inactivation results in unaffected or minimally affected carrier females; this and germ line mosaicism are responsible for recurrence of Rett syndrome in siblings and the birth of the rare severely affected male who dies soon after birth. Prenatal testing for families with an affected child should be considered.

Clinical phenotypes associated with *MECP2* mutations include both classic Rett syndrome and atypical Rett syndrome, as well as an X-linked nonsyndromic mental retardation, X-linked disability with progressive spasticity, an Angelman-like syndrome, and a syndrome characterized by psychosis, pyramidal signs, and macro-orchidism.

SUGGESTED READINGS

Canavan Disease (Spongy Degeneration of the Nervous System)

Banker BQ, Robertson JT, Victor M. Spongy degeneration of the central nervous system in infancy. *Neurology* 1964;14:981–1001.

Cardenas-Mera N, Campos-Castello J, Lucas F, et al. Progressive familial encephalopathy in infancy with calcification of the basal ganglia and cerebrospinal fluid lymphocytosis. *Acta Neuropediatr* 1995;1:207–213.

Feigenbaum A, Moore R, Clarke J, et al. Canavan disease: carrier-frequency determination in the Ashkenazi Jewish population and development of a novel molecular diagnostic assay. *Am J Med Genet* 2004;124A(Jan 15):142–147.

Gascon GG, Ozand PT, Mahdi A, et al. Infantile CNS spongy degeneration—14 cases: clinical update. *Neurology* 1990;40:1876–1882.

Matalon R, Michals-Matalon K. Molecular basis of Canavan disease. *Eur J Paediatr Neurol* 1998;2:69–76.

Matalon R, Michals K, Sebesta D, et al. Aspartoacylase deficiency and N-acetylaspartic aciduria in patients with Canavan disease. *Am J Med Genet* 1988;29:463–471.

McAdams H, Geyer C, Done S, et al. CT and MR imaging of Canavan disease. *AJNR* 1990;11:397–399.

Toft PB, Geiss-Holtorff R, Rolland MO, et al. Magnetic resonance imaging in juvenile Canavan disease. *Eur J Pediatr* 1993;152:750–753.

Traeger EC, Rapin I. The clinical course of Canavan disease. *Pediatr Neurol* 1998;18:207–212.

Van Bogaert L, Bertrand I. *Spongy Degeneration of the Brain in Infancy.* Springfield, IL: Charles C Thomas, 1967.

Infantile Neuroaxonal Dystrophy

Dorfman LJ, Pedley TA, Tharp BR, et al. Juvenile neuroaxonal dystrophy: clinical, electrophysiological, and neuropathological features. *Ann Neurol* 1978;3:419–428.

Gilman S, Barrett RE. Hallervorden-Spatz disease and infantile neuroaxonal dystrophy. *J Neurol Sci* 1973;19:189–205.

Gordon N. Infantile neuroaxonal dystrophy (Seitelberger's disease). *Dev Med Child Neurol* 2002;44:849–851.

Marotti JD, Tobias S, Fratkin JD, et al. Adult onset leukodystrophy with neuroaxonal spheroids and pigmented glia: report of a family, historical perspective, and review of the literature. *Acta Neuropathol* (Berl). 2004;107(Jun):481–488. Epub 2004 Apr 06.

Scheithauer BW, Forno LS, Dorfman LJ, et al. Neuroaxonal dystrophy (Seitelberger's disease) with late onset, protracted course and myoclonic epilepsy. *J Neurol Sci* 1978;36:247–258.

Tanabe Y, Iai M, Ishii M, et al. The use of magnetic resonance imaging in diagnosing infantile neuroaxonal dystrophy. *Neurology* 1993;43:110–113.

Wolfe DE, Schindler D, Desnick RJ. Neuroaxonal dystrophy in infantile alpha-N-acetylgalactosaminidase deficiency. *J Neurol Sci* 1995;132:44–56.

PKAN (Hallervorden-Spatz Disease)

Hayflick SJ, Westaway SK, Levinson B, et al. Genetic, clinical and radiographic delineation of Hallevorden-Spatz syndrome. *N Engl J Med* 2003;348(Jan 2):33–40.

Jankovic J, Kirkpatrick JB, Blomqvist KA, et al. Late-onset Hallervorden-Spatz disease presenting as familial parkinsonism. *Neurology* 1985;35:227–234.

Orrell RW, Amrolia PJ, Heald A, et al. Acanthocytosis, retinitis pigmentosa, and pallidal degeneration: a report of three patients, including the second reported case with hypoprebetalipoproteinemia (HARP syndrome). *Neurology* 1995;45:487–492.

Porter-Grenn L, Silbergleit R, Mehta BA. Hallervorden-Spatz disease with bilateral involvement of globus pallidus and substantia nigra: MR demonstration. *J Comput Assist Tomogr* 1993;17:961–963.

Thomas M, Hayflick SJ, Jankovic J. Clinical heterogeneity of neurodegeneration with brain iron accumulation (Hallervorden-Spatz syndrome) and pantothenate kinase-associated neurodegeneration. *Mov Disord* 2004;19(Jan):36–42.

Wigboldus JM, Bruyn GW. Hallervorden-Spatz disease. In: Vinken PJ, Bruyn GW, eds. *Diseases of the Basal Ganglia. Handbook of Clinical Neurology, vol 6.* New York: Wiley Interscience, 1968:604–631.

Zupane M, Chun R, Gilbert-Barnes E. Osmiophilic deposits in cytosomes in Hallervorden-Spatz syndrome. *Pediatr Neurol* 1990;6:349–352.

Pelizaeus-Merzbacher Disease

Gow A, Lazzarini RA. A cellular mechanism governing the severity of Pelizaeus-Merzbacher disease. *Nat Genet* 1996;13:422–427.

Koeppen AH, Robitaille Y. Pelizaeus-Merzbacher disease. *J Neuropathol Exp Neurol* 2002;61:747–759.

Koeppen AH, Ronca NA, Greenfield EA, et al. Defective biosynthesis of proteolipid protein in Pelizaeus-Merzbacher disease. *Ann Neurol* 1987;21:159–170.

Saugier-Veber P, Munnich A, Bonneau D, et al. X-linked spastic paraplegia and Pelizaeus-Merzbacher disease are allelic disorders at the proteolipid protein locus. *Nat Genet* 1994;6:257–262.

Seitelberger F. Pelizaeus-Merzbacher disease. In: Vinken PJ, Bruyn GW, eds. *Handbook of Clinical Neurology, vol 10.* New York: Elsevier-North Holland, 1970:150–202.

Seitelberger F. Neuropathology and genetics of Pelizaeus-Merzbacher disease. *Brain Pathol* 1995;5:267–273.

Sener RN. Pelizaeus-Merzbacher disease: diffusion MR imaging and proton MR spectroscopy findings. *J Neuroradiol* 2004;31(Mar):138–141.

Alexander Disease

Borrett D, Becker LE. Alexander disease: a disease of astrocytes. *Brain* 1985;108:367–385.

Holland IM, Kendall BE. Computed tomography in Alexander's disease. *Neuroradiology* 1980;20:103–106.

Johnson AB. Alexander disease: a leukodystrophy caused by a mutation in GFAP. *Neurochem Res* 2004;29:961–964.

Li R, Messing A, Goldman JE, et al. GFAP mutations in Alexander disease. *Int J Dev Neurosci* 2002;20:259–268.

Namekawa M, Takiyama Y, Aoki Y, et al. Identification of GFAP gene mutation in hereditary adult-onset Alexander's disease. *Ann Neurol* 2002;52:779–785.

Shah M, Ross J. Infantile Alexander disease: MR appearance of a biopsy-proved case. *AJNR* 1990;11:1105–1106.

Takanashi J, Sugita K, Tanabe Y, et al. Adolescent case of Alexander disease: MR imaging and MR spectroscopy. *Pediatr Neurol* 1998;18:67–70.

Cockayne and Xeroderma Pigmentosum Syndromes

Cockayne EA. Dwarfism with retinal atrophy and deafness. *Arch Dis Child* 1946;21:52–54.

Friedberg EC. Xeroderma pigmentosum, Cockayne syndrome, helicases and DNA repair. *Cell* 1992;128:1233–1237.

Goldstein S. Human genetic disorders which feature accelerated aging. In: Schneider EL, ed. *The Genetics of Aging.* New York: Plenum, 1978.

Kraemer KH, Lee MM, Scotto J. Xeroderma pigmentosum: cutaneous, ocular, and neurologic abnormalities in 830 published cases. *Arch Dermatol* 1987;123:241–250.

Moriwaki S, Stefanini M, Lehmann A, et al. DNA repair and ultraviolet mutagenesis in cells from a new patient with xeroderma pigmentosum group G and Cockayne syndrome resemble xeroderma pigmentosum cells. *J Invest Dermatol* 1996;107:647–653.

Rapin I, Lindenbaum Y, Dickson D, et al. Cockayne syndrome and xeroderma pigmentosum: DNA repair disorders with overlaps and paradoxes. *Neurology* 2000;55:1442–1449.

Robbins JH, Brumback RA, Mendiones M, et al. Neurologic disease in xeroderma pigmentosum: documentation of a late onset type of the juvenile onset form. *Brain* 1991;114:1335–1361.

Seckel HPG. *Birdheaded Dwarfism.* Basel, Switzerland: Karger, 1960.

Shiomi N, Kito S, Oyama M, et al. Identification of the XPG region that causes the onset of Cockayne syndrome by using Xpg mutant mice generated by the cDNA-mediated knock-in method. *Mol Cell Biol* 2004;24:3712–3719.

Sofer D, Grotsky HW, Rapin I, et al. Cockayne syndrome: unusual pathological findings and review of the literature. *Ann Neurol* 1979;6:340–348.

Tian M, Jones DA, Smith M, et al. Deficiency in the nuclease activity of xeroderma pigmentosum G in mice leads to hypersensitivity to UV irradiation. *Mol Cell Biol* 2004;24:2237–2242.

Venema J, Mullenders LH, Natarajan AT, et al. The genetic defect in Cockayne syndrome is associated with a defect in repair of UV-induced DNA damage in transcriptionally active DNA. *Proc Natl Acad Sci U S A* 1990;87:4707–4711.

Rett Syndrome

Amir RE, Van den Veyver IB, Wan M, et al. Rett syndrome is caused by mutations in X-linked *MECP2*, encoding methyl-CpG-binding protein 2. *Nat Genet* 1999;23:185–188.

Christodoulou J, Weaving LS. *MECP2* and beyond: phenotype-genotype correlations in Rett Syndrome. *J Child Neurol* 2003;18:669–674.

Hagberg B, Hanefeld F, Percy A, et al. An update on clinically applicable diagnostic criteria in Rett syndrome. *Eur J Pediatr Neurol* 2002;6(5):293–297.

Naidu S, Bibat G, Kratz L, et al. Clinical variability in Rett syndrome. *J Child Neurol* 2003;18:662–668.

Neul JL, Zoghbi HY. Rett syndrome: a prototypical neurodevelopmental disorder. *Neuroscientist* 2004;10(Apr):118–128.

Percy AK. Rett syndrome current status and new vistas. *Neurol Clin N Am* 2002;20:1125–1141.

Van den Veyver IB, Zoghbi HY. Genetic basis of Rett Syndrome. *MRDD Research Reviews* 2002;8:82–86.

Chapter 95

Diffuse Sclerosis

Marc C. Patterson and Lewis P. Rowland

Some eponyms have lasted for more than 100 years; some come and go. Schilder disease has had its day and seems to be disappearing. Part of the problem was Schilder's genius for recognizing what were then new syndromes. In 1912, 1913, and 1924, he described three patients with diffuse demyelination of the brain. Each of the cases was dramatic, and his contribution was recognized; diffuse sclerosis was called *Schilder disease.*

Unfortunately for the eponym, later advances identified the 1913 description as one of adrenoleukodystrophy, and the 1924 patient had subacute sclerosing panencephalitis. Nevertheless, the 1912 case delineated a clinical and pathologic syndrome that is still seen, even though cases of uncomplicated diffuse sclerosis are so few that each encounter results in a case report. In 1994, Afifi and colleagues counted 12 cases since 1912.

The situation was not helped by the introduction of the term *myelinoclastic* as a tongue-twisting way of denoting demyelination in children; it was intended to distinguish the disorder from *dysmyelination* or loss of myelin because of an inherited biochemical abnormality in the myelin. Schilder disease was and is regarded as a variant of multiple sclerosis, but the etiology and pathogenesis are not known.

At autopsy, there are large areas of demyelination in the centrum ovale (Fig. 95.1), with relative preservation of axons. Subcortical U fibers are often spared. In acute lesions, there is perivascular infiltration by lymphocytes and giant cells. There may be actual necrosis. The lesions are similar to those of multiple sclerosis. In fact, in most cases that include large areas of demyelination, there are also smaller, more typical lesions of multiple sclerosis. For these cases, the term *transitional sclerosis* has been used. It is assumed that the small lesions coalesce to form the large ones.

The clinical syndrome is a leukoencephalopathy, with progressive dementia, psychosis, corticospinal signs, and loss of vision caused by either optic neuritis with papilledema or cerebral blindness. Brainstem signs may include nystagmus and internuclear ophthalmoplegia. The disease is relentlessly progressive, with average survival of about 6 years but sometimes as long as 45 years.

Diagnosis depends on imaging. CT shows large areas of ring-enhancing lucency. MRI shows gadolinium enhancement. There may be CSF pleocytosis with evidence of intrathecal synthesis of gamma globulin and oligoclonal bands. Brain biopsy may be needed to identify the few cases that simulate mass lesions.

The differential diagnosis includes other childhood leukoencephalopathies (see Chapter 96). Most important is the exclusion of adrenoleukodystrophy, a distinction achieved by measurement of very long-chain fatty acids. In areas where measles vaccination has not been practiced, subacute sclerosing panencephalitis must be considered. Steroid therapy is often ineffective, but some reports emphasize the value of steroids in managing acute manifestations; described surgical resection has been used to manage herniation complicating a large lesion.

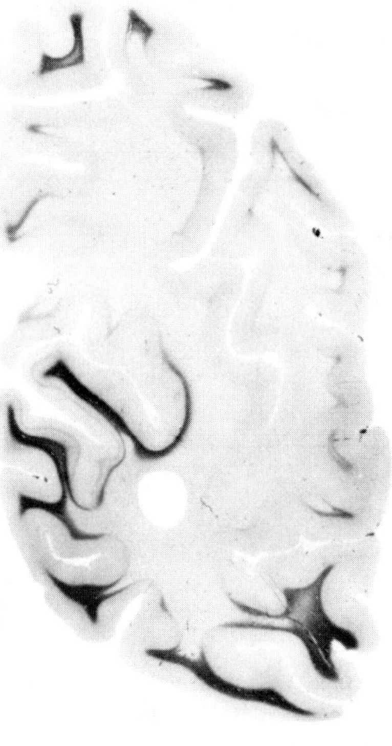

FIGURE 95.1. Diffuse myelinoclastic sclerosis. On myelin sheath staining, there is almost complete loss of myelin in occipital white matter. U fibers are irregularly involved. (Courtesy of Dr. H. Shiraki, Tokyo.)

SUGGESTED READINGS

Afifi AK, Bell WE, Menezs AH, et al. Myelinoclastic diffuse sclerosis (Schilder's disease): report of a case and review of the literature. *J Child Neurol* 1994;9:398–403.

Anselmi G, Masdeu JC, Macaluso C, et al. Disseminated-diffuse sclerosis: a variety of multiple sclerosis with characteristic clinical, neuroimaging, and pathological findings. *J Neuroimaging* 1993;3:143–145.

Censori B, Agostinis C, Partziguian T, et al. Large demyelinating brain lesion mimicking a herniating tumor. *Neurol Sci* 2001;22(Aug):325–329.

Eblen F, Premba M, Grodd W, et al. Myelinoclastic diffuse sclerosis (Schilder's disease): cliniconeuroradiologic correlations. *Neurology* 1991;41:589–591.

Hainfellner JA, Schmidbauer M, Schmitahard E, et al. Devic's neuromyelitis optica and Schilder's myelinoclastic diffuse sclerosis. *J Neurol Neurosurg Psychiatry* 1992;55:1194–1196.

Kotil K, Kalayci M, Koseoglu T, et al. Myelinoclastic diffuse sclerosis (Schilder's disease): report of a case and review of the literature. *Br J Neurosurg* 2002;16(Oct):516–519.

Obara S, Takeshima H, Awa R, et al. Tumefactive myelinoclastic diffuse sclerosis—case report. *Neurol Med Chir* (Tokyo). 2003;43(Nov):563–566.

Poser CM, Foutieres F, Carpentier MA, et al. Schilder's myelinoclastic diffuse sclerosis. *Pediatrics* 1986;77:107–112.

Sastre-Garriga J, Rovira A, Rio J, et al. Clinically definite multiple sclerosis after radiological Schilder-like onset. *J Neurol* 20031;250:871–873.

Schilder P. Zur Kenntnis der sogennanten diffusen Sklerose. *Z Gesamte Neurol Psychiatrie* 1912;10:1–60.

Sewick LA, Lingele TG, Burde RM, et al. Schilder's (1912) disease: total cerebral blindness due to acute demyelination. *Arch Neurol* 1986;43:85–87.

Stachniak JB, Mickle JP, Ellis T, et al. Myelinoclastic diffuse sclerosis presenting as a mass lesion in a child with Turner's syndrome. *Pediatr Neurosurg* 1995;22:266–269.

Chapter 96

▶ Differential Diagnosis

Eveline C. Traeger and Isabelle Rapin

Although most of the degenerative diseases of infancy and childhood are not treatable today, neurologists are obliged to make as definite a diagnosis as possible so they can provide the parents with a prognosis and genetic counseling. Of course, physicians are alert for the few treatable conditions, but there is also responsibility to advance knowledge, and precise diagnosis is the first step toward unraveling the chemical pathology and devising therapy. The clinician's first concern is to determine that the illness is progressive and to review the genetic evidence. Findings on physical and neurologic examination almost always narrow the diagnostic possibilities and guide the selection of laboratory tests.

The most powerful diagnostic resource is Online Mendelian Inheritance in Man (OMIM; http://www.ncbi.nlm.nih.gov/Omim), which can be searched by phenotype and provides an extensive up-to-date differential diagnosis of all currently identified genetic diseases. This database is authored and edited by Dr. Victor A. McKusick and his colleagues at Johns Hopkins University and elsewhere and was developed for the World Wide Web by the National Center for Biotechnology Information. A new resource, the clinician-oriented SimulConsult Neurological Syndromes on the Web at www.simulconsult.com, which also lists diseases by physical findings, has the advantage of providing an estimate of the probability of various diagnoses. Edited by Dr. Michael Segal, it is less comprehensive than OMIM but it is also free and user friendly.

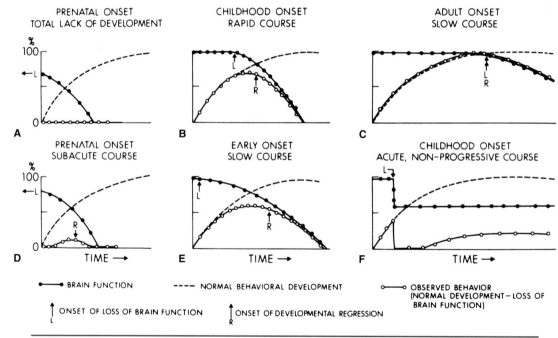

FIGURE 96.1. Theoretical curves show the possible effects of progressive brain dysfunction on behavior, depending on time of onset and rapidity of course. The curve depicting observed behavior ($^\circ$–$^\circ$–$^\circ$) is the difference between the curves indicating expected development (– – –) and brain function (●–●–●). **A.** Prenatal onset with damage at birth so advanced that no development is observed, suggesting a severe static encephalopathy. **B.** Prenatal onset with damage at birth somewhat less severe than in A. Development is minimal and markedly delayed but does appear to take place initially. **C,D.** Onset at birth with a less acute course. **E.** Onset in adulthood. Note that in **B, C,** and **D** loss of milestones may not appear until months or years after the onset of the illness, which therefore does not appear progressive unless it is realized that deceleration of development or developmental standstill implies deteriorating function. When a progressive disease starts after adolescence (**E**), loss of function should be less delayed and the disease recognized as progressive virtually from its start. **F.** A severe static lesion acquired postnatally may produce total regression acutely, but development may be expected to resume until the time of puberty. (From Rapin I. Progressive genetic metabolic diseases. In: Rudolph AM, ed. *Pediatrics,* 16th ed. New York: Appleton-Century-Crofts, 1977; with permission.)

▶ **TABLE 96.1 Pattern of Inheritance Other Than Autosomal Recessive**

Some X-linked recessive diseases	**Some autosomal-dominant diseases**
Adrenoleukodystrophy	Neurofibromatosis
Pelizaeus-Merzbacher disease	Tuberous sclerosis
Fabry disease	Von Hippel-Lindau disease
Hunter syndrome (mucopolysaccharidosis II)	Acute intermittent porphyria
Ornithine transcarbamylase deficiency	Huntington disease
Lesch-Nyhan syndrome	Autosomal-dominant leukodystrophy and
Leber optic atrophy	spheroids
Lowe oculocerebrorenal syndrome	Primary generalized dystonia (DYT1)
Trichopoliodystrophy (Menkes syndrome)	Dentatorubralpallidoluysian atrophy
Duchenne/Becker muscular dystrophy	Spinocerebellar ataxias (SCAs)
Norrie disease	
Fragile X syndrome	**Some mitochondrial cytopathies**
X-linked cortical dysplasias	MERRF (myoclonic epilepsy with red ragged
X-linked mental retardation syndromes	fibers)
	MELAS (mitochondrial encephalomyopathy, lactic
Some X-linked dominant diseases	acidosis, and strokelike episodes)
Incontinentia pigmenti	LHON (Leber hereditary optic neuropathy)
Pseudohypoparathyroidism and	NARP (neuropathy, ataxia, and retinitis
pseudopseudohypoparathyroidism	pigmentosa)
Rett syndrome	Leigh syndrome
Aicardi syndrome	
Subcortical band heterotopia	

Deterioration is usually obvious when a disease affects an adult or adolescent, but in infancy and early childhood, the slope of the developmental curve is so steep that it can mask functional decay, because a child's symptoms represent the net difference between the two opposing trends (Fig. 96.1). An early sign of insidious dementia may be slowing of development rather than loss of milestones. As long as a child continues to acquire new skills, even too slowly, the illness is likely to be misinterpreted as a static condition. When the disease is already advanced at birth, dementia can masquerade as total failure to develop, suggesting an unrecognized intrauterine or perinatal catastrophe. In these situations, the correct diagnosis may not be contemplated until after the birth of an affected sibling.

A family history of similar disease or consanguinity is a strong clue, but neither is frequent. Most of these diseases are recessive, and the birth of the first affected child occurs as a sporadic event. It is important to detect X-linked diseases (Table 96.1) because even in the absence of a specific method for intrauterine diagnosis, sex identification of the fetus can limit the birth of affected children. Knowing that certain diseases are particularly frequent in children of particular ethnic backgrounds is also helpful (Table 96.2).

The age at onset may be a lead to the diagnosis (Table 96.3). Genetically homogeneous syndromes tend to run a predictable course and appear at about the same age, but what is considered to be genetically homogeneous today is likely to prove to be nonhomogeneous tomorrow

▶ **TABLE 96.2 Predominant Ethnic Background in Some Diseases**

Ashkenazi Jews	**Nova Scotia**
Classic Tay-Sachs disease	Type D Niemann-Pick disease
Infantile Niemann-Pick disease	
Primary generalized dystonia (DYT1)	**Japan**
Mucolipidosis IV	Sialidosis with chondrodystrophy
Canavan disease	Dentatorubralpallidoluysian atrophy
Dysautonomia	
Juvenile nonneuronopathic Gaucher disease	**Scandinavia**
	Finnish ceroid lipofuscinos (types 1, 5)
Saudi Arabia	Juvenile neuronopathic Gaucher disease
Canavan disease	Krabbe disease
	Aspartylglucosaminuria
	Baltic myoclonus (Unverricht-Lundborg disease)

▶ TABLE 96.3 Typical Age at Onset

Neonatal or early infantile onset	Sjögren-Larsson syndrome	Kearns-Sayre syndrome
Aminoacidurias and organic acidurias	Canavan disease	Disintegrative psychosis
Urea cycle disorders	Wolman disease	Other autistic regression
Galactosemia	Alexander disease	Leukodystrophy with vanishing white matter
Connatal Pelizaeus-Merzbacher disease	Pelizaeus-Merzbacher disease	
Connatal Alexander disease	Neuroaxonal dystrophy	**Onset in school age or adolescence**
Congenital sialidosis	Alpha-*N*-acetylgalactosaminidase deficiency	Wilson disease
Early-onset mitochondrial cytopathies	Infantile PKAN (Hallervorden-Spatz disease)	Acute intermittent porphyria
Canavan disease	Infantile fucosidosis	Juvenile ceroid lipofuscinosis
Aicardi-Goutières syndrome	Nephrosialidosis	Adrenoleukodystrophy
Infantile Gaucher disease	Sialidosis	Late variants of the gangliosidoses
Infantile adrenoleukodystrophy	Pompe disease	Niemann-Pick type C disease
Zellweger syndrome	Xeroderma pigmentosum neurologic disease	Sialidosis with cherry-red spot myoclonus
Neonatal adrenoleukodystrophy	Cockayne disease	(variants with and without
Chondrodysplasia punctata	Infantile galactosialidosis	chondrodystrophy)
Infantile Refsum disease	Progeria	Fabry disease
GM$_I$ gangliosidosis (infantile variant)	Rett syndrome	Cerebrotendinous xanthomatosis
I-cell disease (mucolipidosis II)		Leigh syndrome (some variants)
Trichopoliodystrophy (Menkes syndrome)	**Onset in preschool years**	Other mitochondrial cytopathies (e.g., MERRF
Cerebro-oculo-facial-skeletal syndrome	Aminoacidurias, organic acidurias, urea cycle	and MELAS syndromes)
(COFS syndrome)	disorders with partial enzyme deficiency	Refsum disease
Neurocutaneous syndromes	Aspartylglucosaminuria	Friedreich ataxia
Progressive spinal muscular atrophy	Marinesco-Sjögren syndrome	Bassen-Kornzweig disease
(Werdnig-Hoffmann disease)	Alexander disease	Other spinocerebellar degenerations
Seckel bird-headed dwarfism	Ataxia telangiectasia	Primary generalized dystonia (DYT1)
	Xeroderma pigmentosum neurologic disease	Juvenile Huntington disease
Infantile onset	Chédiak-Higashi disease	Juvenile parkinsonism
Aminoacidurias, organic acidurias, urea cycle	Metachromatic leukodystrophy	Classic Hallervorden-Spatz disease (PKAN)
disorders with partial enzyme deficiency	Late infantile gangliosidoses	Lafora disease
Many sphingolipidoses,	Niemann-Pick disease, Nova Scotia variant	Baltic myoclonus
mucopolysaccharidoses, mucolipidoses	Late infantile ceroid lipofuscinoses	Subacute sclerosing panencephalitis (SSPE)
Infantile ceroid lipofuscinosis	Sanfilippo syndromes	Cockayne disease (late variants)
Leigh syndrome (early types)	Maroteaux-Lamy disease	Xeroderma pigmentosum neurologic disease
Other mitochondrial cytopathies	Mild Hunter disease	(late variants)
Lesch-Nyhan syndrome	Leigh syndrome and other mitochondrial	
	cytopathies	

because phenocopies are common. As a general rule, the younger a child is when the symptoms appear, the more rapid is the deterioration, but there are exceptions. For example, when Pelizaeus-Merzbacher disease is manifest before age 1 year, the patient may survive into the third decade. Two diseases of mid-childhood or adolescence can progress rapidly to death from liver failure (Wilson disease) or adrenal insufficiency (adrenoleukodystrophy).

The general physical examination may provide helpful clues (Table 96.4). The neurologic symptoms and signs indicate which systems are most affected. Intractable seizures, abnormal involuntary movements, and myoclonus are more typical of diseases of gray matter than of white matter (Table 96.5), whereas spasticity appears early in diseases of white matter. Spasticity may also be the result of diffuse neuronal dropout; it then occurs in later stages of the disease. Hypotonia suggests involvement of the motor unit or cerebellum, or may indicate some global

developmental cerebral dysfunction or even excessive joint laxity (Table 96.6). The combination of hypotonia and increased reflexes suggests that both upper and lower motor neurons are affected. Ataxia and abnormal involuntary movements are particularly useful diagnostic signs. Sensory abnormalities are rarely detectable; lack of sensitivity to pain suggests dysautonomia, infantile neuroaxonal dystrophy, or involvement of both peripheral nerves and CNS.

The eyes are so likely to provide information of diagnostic importance that detailed examination is mandatory (Table 96.7). Dilating the pupil is required to afford an adequate view of the peripheral retina, macula, and disc. The mild corneal haze of some of the mucolipidoses and mucopolysaccharidoses and the detection of early Kayser-Fleischer rings call for slit lamp examination. Electroretinography may disclose pigmentary degeneration of the retina before it is visible with the ophthalmoscope.

▶ TABLE 96.4 Helpful Clues in the Physical Examination

Big head
Tay-Sachs disease
Alexander disease
Canavan disease
Hurler disease
Glutaric aciduria type 1
Other mucopolysaccharidoses
 with hydrocephalus
Leukodystrophy with subcortical
 cysts

Small head
Krabbe disease
Infantile ceroid lipofuscinosis
Some infantile mitochondrial
 cytopathies
Neuroaxonal dystrophy
Incontinentia pigmentia
Cockayne disease
Rett syndrome
Seckel bird-headed dwarfism
Chromosomal abnormalities

Hair abnormalities
 Stiff, wiry
 Trichopoliodystrophy (Menkes
  syndrome)
 Frizzy
 Giant axonal neuropathy
 Hirsutism
 Infantile GM$_1$ gangliosidosis
 Hurler, Hunter, Sanfilippo
  syndromes
 I-cell disease
 Gray
 Ataxia telangiectasia
 Cockayne disease
 Chédiak-Higashi disease
 Progeria

Skin abnormalities
 Telangiectasia
 Ataxia telangiectasia
 Angiokeratoma
 Fabry disease
 Juvenile fucosidosis
 Galactosialidosis
 Adult-onset Alpha-*N*-
  acetylgalactosaminidase
  deficiency
 Ichthyosis
 Refsum disease
 Sjögren-Larsson syndrome
 Hypopigmentation
 Trichopoliodystrophy (Menkes
  syndrome)
 Chédiak-Higashi syndrome
 Tuberous sclerosis (ash leaf
  spots)

Hypomelanosis of Ito
Prader-Willi syndrome
Phenylketonuria
 Hyperpigmentation
 Niemann-Pick disease
 Adrenoleukodystrophy
 Farber disease
 Neurofibromatosis (café au lait
  spots)
 Xeroderma pigmentosum
  neurologic disease
 Incontinentia pigmenti
 Thin atrophic skin
 Ataxia telangiectasia
 Cockayne disease
 Xeroderma pigmentosum
  neurologic disease
 Progeria
 Thick skin
 I-cell disease
 Mucopolysaccharidoses I, II, III
 Infantile fucosidosis
 Subcutaneous nodules
 Farber disease
 Neurofibromatosis
 Cerebrotendinous
  xanthomatosis
 Xanthomas
 Niemann-Pick disease
 Blotching
 Dysautonomia

Enlarged nodes
Farber disease
Niemann-Pick disease
Juvenile Gaucher disease
Chédiak-Higashi disease
Ataxia telangiectasia (lymphoma)

Stridor, hoarseness
Infantile-onset peroxisomal
 disorders
Farber disease
Infantile Gaucher disease
Connatal Pelizaeus-Merzbacher
 disease

Enlarged orange tonsils
Tangier disease

**Severe swallowing problems
 (present late in the course of all
 patients with severe bulbar,
 pseudobulbar, cerebellar, or
 basal ganglia pathology)**
Infantile Gaucher disease
Dysautonomia
Hallervorden-Spatz disease
 (PKAN)

Primary generalized dystonia
 (DYT1)
Zellweger syndrome

Heart abnormalities
Pompe disease
Hurler disease and other
 mucopolysaccharidoses
Fabry disease
Infantile fucosidosis
Refsum disease
Friedreich ataxia
Abetalipoproteinemia
 (Bassen-Kornzweig disease)
Tuberous sclerosis
Progeria
Zellweger syndrome
Disorders of carnitine metabolism
Duchenne muscular dystrophy
Kearns-Sayre syndrome

Strokes
Fabry disease
Trichopoliodystrophy (Menkes
 syndrome)
Progeria
MELAS syndrome
Homocystinuria
Sickle cell diseases

Organomegaly
Mucopolysaccharidoses (most
 types)
Infantile GM$_1$ gangliosidosis
Niemann-Pick disease
Gaucher disease
Generalized peroxisomal
 disorders
Galactosemia
Pompe disease
Mannosidosis

Gastrointestinal problems
 Malabsorption
 Wolman disease
 Bassen-Kornzweig disease
 Nonfunctioning gallbladder
 Metachromatic leukodystrophy
 Infantile fucosidosis
 Jaundice
 Zellweger disease
 Galactosemia
 Niemann-Pick disease
 Vomiting
 Dysautonomia
 Urea cycle defects
 Diarrhea
 Hunter syndrome

Dysmotility
Mitochondrial
 neurogastrointestinal
 encephalomyopathy (MNGIE)

Kidney problems
 Renal failure
 Fabry disease
 Nephrosialidosis
 Some mitochondrial
  cytopathies
 Cysts
 Zellweger syndrome
 Von Hippel-Lindau disease
 Tuberous sclerosis
 Neonatal olivopontocerebellar
  atrophy (OPCA)
 Joubert syndrome
 Stones
 Lesch-Nyhan disease
 Aminoacidurias
 Lowe syndrome
 Wilson disease

Bone and joint abnormalities
 Stiff joints
 Mucopolysaccharidoses
  (all but type I–S)
 Mucolipidoses (most types)
 Fucosidosis
 Farber disease
 Sialidoses (some forms)
 Zellweger syndrome
 Rhizomelic chondrodysplasia
  punctata
 Cockayne disease
 Scoliosis
 Friedreich ataxia
 Ataxia telangiectasia
 Primary generalized dystonia
  (DYT1)
 All chronic diseases with
  muscle weakness
 Rett syndrome
 Kyphosis
 Mucopolysaccharidoses

Endocrine dysfunction
 Adrenals
 Adrenoleukodystrophy
 Wolman disease
 Hypogonadism
 Xeroderma pigmentosum
  neurologic disease
 Ataxia telangiectasia
 Some spinocerebellar
  degenerations
 Diabetes
 Ataxia telangiectasia

(continued)

▶ **TABLE 96.4** Helpful Clues in the Physical Examination (*Continued*)

Dwarfing	**Hypothalamic dysfunction**	Von Hippel-Lindau disease	Cockayne disease
Morquio disease	De Sanctis-Cacchione	Tuberous sclerosis	Kearns-Sayre and Leigh
Other mucopolysaccharidoses	syndrome		syndromes
Cockayne syndrome		**Hearing loss**	Other mitochondrial cytopathies
Progeria	**Neoplasms**	Hunter disease	Some spinocerebellar
Diseases with severe	Ataxia telangiectasia	Other mucopolysaccharidoses	degenerations
malnutrition	Xeroderma pigmentosum	Generalized peroxisomal	Usher syndrome
	neurologic disease	disorders	Olivopontocerebellar atrophy
	Neurofibromatosis	Refsum disease	

▶ **TABLE 96.5** Diseases with Prominent Seizures or Myoclonus

Pyridoxine dependency	Generalized peroxisomal disorders
Acute intermittent porphyria	Infantile Alexander disease
Gangliosidoses (infantile especially)	Krabbe disease
Ceroid lipofuscinoses (late infantile variant especially)	Lafora disease
	Baltic myoclonus
MERRF and MELAS syndromes	Sanfilippo disease
Glucose transporter protein deficiency syndrome (GLUT1)	Juvenile Huntington disease
	Tuberous sclerosis
Trichopoliodystrophy (Menkes)	Juvenile neuronopathic Gaucher disease
Zellweger syndrome	Subacute sclerosing panencephalitis

▶ **TABLE 96.6** Motor Signs Helpful to Diagnosis

Floppiness in infancy	Adrenomyeloneuropathy	Neonatal OPCA
Progressive spinal muscular atrophy	Mucopolysaccharidoses I, II, VI, VII (entrapment)	De Sanctis-Cacchione syndrome
Congenital myopathies		Phosphomannomutase deficiency (CDG-Ia)
Zellweger syndrome	Cockayne syndrome (demyelinating)	
Pompe disease	Xeroderma pigmentosum neurologic disease (axonal)	**Abnormal posture or movements**
Trichopoliodystrophy		Wilson disease
Neuroaxonal dystrophy	Some mitochondrial cytopathies	Lesch-Nyhan disease
Gangliosidoses (early variants)	Giant axonal neuropathy	Hallervorden-Spatz syndrome
Fucosidosis (infantile variant)		Familial striatal necrosis
Infantile ceroid lipofuscinosis	**Prominent cerebellar signs**	Primary generalized dystonia (DYT1)
Canavan disease	Wilson disease	Niemann-Pick disease type C
Leigh syndrome (early variant)	Late infantile ceroid lipofuscinosis	Chronic GM_1 and GM_2 gangliosidoses
Neonatal OPCA	Pelizaeus-Merzbacher disease	Pelizaeus-Merzbacher syndrome
	Neuroaxonal dystrophy	Crigler-Najjar disease
Peripheral neuropathy	Metachromatic leukodystrophy	Ataxia telangiectasia
Acute intermittent porphyria	Ataxia telangiectasia	Juvenile ceroid lipofuscinosis
Metachromatic leukodystrophy	Leigh syndrome	Juvenile Huntington disease
Fabry disease	Niemann-Pick disease type C	Juvenile parkinsonism
Krabbe disease	Some late-onset gangliosidoses	Gilles de la Tourette syndrome
Neuroaxonal dystrophy	Some sialidoses	De Sanctis-Cacchione syndrome (xeroderma
Refsum disease	Friedreich ataxia	pigmentosum with endocrine dysfunction)
Tangier disease	Bassen-Kornzweig disease	Dentatorubralpallidoluysian atrophy
Bassen-Kornzweig disease	Cerebrotendinous xanthomatosis	Glutaric aciduria type 1
Sialidosis (some variants)	Spinocerebellar ataxias (SCAs)	
Mucolipidosis III	Lafora disease	**Spasticity is too common to be discriminating**
Cerebrotendinous xanthomatosis	Baltic myoclonus	
Ataxia telangiectasia	Chédiak-Higashi disease	
	Usher syndrome	

> **TABLE 96.7** Eye Findings

Conjunctival telangiectasia
Ataxia telangiectasia
Fabry disease

Corneal opacity
Wilson disease (Kayser-Fleischer ring)
Mucopolysaccharidoses I, III, IV, VI
Mucolipidoses III, IV
Fabry disease
Galactosialidosis
Cockayne disease
Xeroderma pigmentosum neurologic disease
Zellweger syndrome (inconsistant)

Lens opacity
Wilson disease
Galactosemia
Marinesco-Sjögren syndrome
Lowe disease
Cerebrocutaneous xanthomatosis
Sialidosis (rarely significant clinically)
Mannosidosis
Zellweger syndrome
Cockayne disease

Glaucoma
Mucopolysaccharidosis I (Hurler-Scheie
  syndrome)
Zellweger syndrome (infrequent)

Cherry-red spot
Tay-Sachs disease
Sialidosis (usually)
Infantile Niemann-Pick disease
  (50% of cases)

Infantile GM$_1$ gangliosidosis (50% of cases)
Farber disease (inconsistant)
Multiple sulfatase deficiency (metachromatic
  leukodystrophy variant)

Macular and retinal pigmentary degeneration
Ceroid lipofuscinosis (most types)
Mucopolysaccharidoses I-H and I-S, II, III
Mucolipidosis IV
Bassen-Kornzweig syndrome
  (abetalipoproteinemia)
Peroxisomal disorders
OPCA variant
Refsum disease (all types)
Kearns-Sayre syndrome
Leber congenital amaurosis
Other mitochondrial cytopathies
Hallervorden-Spatz syndrome (some types)
Cockayne disease
Sjögren-Larsson syndrome (not always)
Usher syndrome
Some other spinocerebellar syndromes
Neurocutaneous syndromes

Optic atrophy
Krabbe disease
Metachromatic leukodystrophy
Most sphingolipidoses late in their course
Adrenoleukodystrophy
Alexander disease
Canavan disease
Pelizaeus-Merzbacher disease
Neuroaxonal dystrophy

Neonatal mitochondrial cytopathies
Leber congenital amaurosis
Leber hereditary optic neuropathy
Joubert syndrome
Some spinocerebellar degenerations
Diseases with retinal pigmentary
  degeneration

Nystagmus
Diseases with poor vision (searching
  nystagmus)
Pelizaeus-Merzbacher syndrome
Metachromatic leukodystrophy
Friedreich ataxia
Other spinocerebellar degenerations and
  cerebellar atrophies
Neuroaxonal dystrophy
Ataxia telangiectasia
Joubert syndrome
Leigh syndrome (inconstant)
Marinesco-Sjögren syndrome
Opsoclonus-myoclonus syndrome
Chédiak-Higashi syndrome

Ophthalmoplegia
Leigh syndrome
Kearns-Sayre and Leigh syndromes
Niemann-Pick disease type C
Bassen-Kornzweig syndrome
Ataxia telangiectasia
Infantile Gaucher disease
Tangier disease

Repeated neuropsychologic testing may be needed to document progressive dementia. Lack of dementia, at least early, in the face of motor deterioration suggests a disease that spares the cortex and selectively affects the basal ganglia, brainstem, or cerebellar pathways.

In children with an undiagnosed disease, laboratory investigations are screening devices. How many are used depends partly on accessibility and cost (Table 96.8). "New" diseases are often discovered serendipitously rather than after a directed diagnostic endeavor.

Electrical studies may yield clues (Table 96.9). The plain electroencephalogram rarely provides decisive information. However, photomyoclonus suggests Lafora disease, and action myoclonus suggests sialidosis, ceroid lipofuscinosis, myoclonic epilepsy with ragged-red fibers (MERRF) syndrome, Gaucher disease type III, and Baltic myoclonus.

Radiologic tests are crucial in some cases. Adrenal calcification is virtually pathognomonic of Wolman disease. The diagnostic yield of plain radiographs of the skull is extremely low, in contrast to the efficiency of CT, MRI, or magnetic resonance spectroscopy (MRS). Even if CT or MRI shows only nonspecific atrophy, this is helpful if it is progressive. Adrenoleukodystrophy and Canavan, Alexander, and Krabbe diseases, as well as leukodystrophy with vanishing white matter and subcortical cysts show characteristic patterns of lucency of white matter. A tiger's-eye pattern of the basal ganglia points to pantothenate kinase–associated neurodegeneration (PKAN or Hallervorden-Spatz disease), and lucency of the basal ganglia suggests acute mitochondrial encephalopathy. MRI is critically important in the differential of many nongenetic and genetic malformation syndromes like Arnold-Chiari type I, lissencephaly, Joubert syndrome, Miller-Dieker syndrome, and many others.

The need for biopsy arises when noninvasive tests fail (Table 96.10). A skin biopsy specimen is examined under the electron microscope for abnormal inclusions and is also used for tissue culture. Cultured fibroblasts or leukocytes may yield an enzymatic or DNA diagnosis. Equally important, the cultures can be frozen and kept viable

▌ TABLE 96.8 Useful Laboratory Tests

Urine
Amino acids, organic acids
Galactose, other sugars
Mucopolysaccharides, sialidated
  oligosaccharides
N-acetylaspartic acid
Copper excretion
Porphyrins
Metachromatic granules
Oxalate, cysteine crystals, uric acid

Blood chemistry
Ammonia (urea cycle disorders, some
  mitochondrial encephalopathies, organic
  acidemias)
Lactate-pyruvate ratio (Leigh syndrome, other
  mitochondrial cytopathies)
Amino acids and other special metabolites
C26/C22 very long-chain fatty acid ratio
  (adrenoleukodystrophy, Zellweger disease,
  other peroxisomal diseases)
Phytanic acid
Pipecolic acid
Isoelectrofocusing of serum sialotransferrins
  (congenital disorders of glycosylation)
Long-, medium-, and short-chain fatty acids

White blood cells
Lysosomal enzymes and other enzymatic assays
DNA tests for genetic mutations
Lipid and other inclusions (ceroid lipofuscinoses,
  gangliosidoses)

Red blood cells
Enzymatic assays for galactosemia, porphyria

Cultured skin fibroblasts
Enzymatic assays for most diseases with known
  deficits
Lipid and other inclusions (in mucolipidosis IV,
  I-cell disease, mucopolysaccharidoses,
  Chédiak-Higashi syndrome)
DNA repair after ultraviolet or radiation exposure
  (ataxia telangiectasia, Cockayne disease,
  xeroderma pigmentosum)
DNA tests for genetic mutations

Cerebrospinal fluid
CSF glucose decreased with normal blood
  glucose (GLUT 1 deficiency)
CSF protein (increased in metachromatic
  leukodystrophy, Krabbe disease, infantile
  adrenoleukodystrophy [not always in classic
  variant], Friedreich ataxia, and other
  spinocerebellar degenerations [inconstant],
  Zellweger disease [sometimes], Refsum
  disease, Cockayne disease)
CSF lactate/pyruvate (mitochondrial cytopathies)
CSF neurotransmitter metabolites

Amniotic cells
Enzymatic assays for disease of known
  enzymatic defect
Abnormal inclusion in mucolipidosis IV
Karyotype in X-linked disease
C26/C22 very long-chain fatty acid ratio
DNA tests for genetic mutations

Intradermal histamine test
Dysautonomia

▌ TABLE 96.9 Electrodiagnosis

Electromyography and nerve conduction velocity	To detect neuropathy, anterior horn cell disease, or muscle involvement
Electroretinography	To detect retinal degeneration
Visual evoked responses	Giant potentials in late infantile ceroid lipofuscinosis; delayed latency and decreased amplitude in leukodystrophies or optic atrophy
Otoacoustic emissions and brainstem auditory evoked responses for cochlear vs. retrocochlear disease	Diagnosis of hearing loss; prolonged latency in leukodystrophies; delayed waves with decrease of amplitude in leukodystrophies and other diseases of the brainstem
Somatosensory evoked responses	Giant potentials in sialidosis with cherry-red spot myoclonus; decreased amplitude in peripheral neuropathy; delayed waves with decreased amplitude in diseases of the white matter and peripheral nerves

▶ **TABLE 96.10 Diseases in Which Biopsies for Histology are Likely to Help**

Skin
Ceroid lipofuscinosis
Mucopolysaccharidoses
Mucolipidosis IV
Neuroaxonal dystrophy
Lafora disease

Conjunctiva
Mucopolysaccharidoses
Mucolipidoses
Neuroaxonal dystrophy

Bone marrow
Niemann-Pick disease
Gaucher disease
Mucopolysaccharidoses

Muscle
Glycogenoses
Mitochondrial myopathies (Kearns-Sayre and Leigh syndromes)
Other myopathies
Neuroaxonal dystrophy
Lafora disease

Nerve
Neuroaxonal dystrophy
Metachromatic leukodystrophy
Other diseases with neuropathies

Brain (Rarely needed except possibly for the following)
Neuroaxonal dystrophy
Undiagnosed disease with probable cortical involvement

indefinitely so that tissue will be available when new data suggest further study with new molecular techniques. Cell lines in federally funded repositories provide invaluable resources for future studies. Conjunctival biopsies are helpful when storage in connective tissue is suspected and enzymatic diagnosis is unavailable or when axonal spheroids are being evaluated. Muscle biopsy to identify mitochondrial encephalomyopathies requires special histochemical, biochemical, and DNA studies.

Brain biopsy is rarely needed today and is reserved for patients in whom diagnosis remains elusive despite thorough peripheral investigation. It is imperative to sample the white matter as well as the cortex. Routine histologic examination of the tissue is not sufficient because brain biopsy is reserved for disorders that are biochemical enigmas; therefore, brain biopsy should be carried out in a center that has the resources necessary for many avenues of investigation. Under these conditions, the informational yield of brain biopsy is sufficiently high and its morbidity sufficiently low to make it a rewarding procedure both clinically and scientifically. Biopsy is not a substitute for autopsy because it may not be diagnostic and because some studies can be done only on biopsy tissue or only on autopsy tissue.

When all diagnostic methods have failed, the physician must broach the subject of an autopsy. This can be done when the parents are informed of the likelihood of a fatal outcome. Parents who understand how little is known about their child's illness are likely to want an autopsy; they will also be spared the unnecessary hurt of being pressed for an autopsy when the child actually dies, a time of maximal distress. A planned and speedy autopsy maximizes the probability of obtaining useful data. Viscera, peripheral nerves, muscle, and retina, as well as the brain, must be investigated. Tissue samples should be removed and frozen at $-70°C$ for chemical analysis; other samples are fixed for electron microscopy before the organs are placed in formalin. If autopsy does not yield a diagnosis, brain tissue stored in federally funded brain banks remains available for later diagnosis or research. In the interim, the physician must explain to the parents that the child's illness may be one that is as yet unrecognized and that data of scientific importance may yet emerge from the study of their child, who will thus have made a unique contribution to other children and their families.

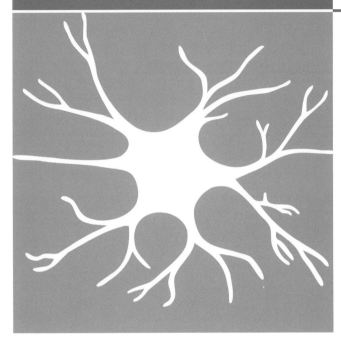

SECTION X

Disorders of
Mitochondrial DNA

Mitochondrial Encephalomyopathies: Diseases of Mitochondrial DNA

Salvatore DiMauro, Eric A. Schon,
Michio Hirano, and Lewis P. Rowland

Mitochondria are uniquely interesting organelles, not only for the variety of functions that they serve but also because they are under the control of two genomes—their own (mtDNA) and that of the nucleus (nDNA). Therefore, mitochondrial diseases, that is, genetic diseases resulting in mitochondrial dysfunction, can be a result of mutations in either genome (Table 97.1). Diseases caused by nDNA mutations are transmitted by Mendelian inheritance: these will be considered in Chapter 99. In this chapter, we con-

▶ **TABLE 97.1 Genetic Classification of Mitochondrial Diseases**

1. **Defects of mitochondrial DNA**
   (A) Single deletions (sporadic)
   (B) Duplications or duplications/deletions (maternal transmission)
   (C) Point mutations (maternal transmission)
2. **Defects of nuclear DNA (mendelian transmission)**
   (A) Mutations in genes encoding enzymes or translocases
       (a) Defects of substrate transport
       (b) Defects of substrate use
       (c) Defects of the Krebs cycle
       (d) Defects of the electron transport chain
       (e) Defects of oxidation/phosphorylation coupling
   (B) Defects of mitochondrial protein importation
   (C) Defects of intergenomic signaling
       (a) Multiple deletions of mtDNA
       (b) Depletion of mtDNA

sider diseases caused by mutations in mtDNA and also a subgroup of disorders (defects of intergenomic signaling, Table 97.1) that, although a result of mutations in nDNA, affect mtDNA integrity or replication.

The ubiquitous nature of mtDNA and the peculiar rules of mitochondrial genetics (more akin to population than to mendelian genetics) contribute to explain the extraordinary clinical heterogeneity of mitochondrial disorders, which, owing to the frequent involvement of brain and muscle tissues, are generally labeled "mitochondrial encephalomyopathies."

HISTORY

The first human disease attributed to mitochondrial dysfunction was a hypermetabolic state in a patient with normal thyroid function and an excessive number of abnormally large mitochondria in skeletal muscle. Biochemical studies showed "loose coupling" of oxidative phosphorylation. The syndrome was named after Rolf Luft, the endocrinologist who led the studies. In the 43 years since then, however, there has been only one other known case of Luft syndrome.

Mitochondrial diseases were brought to prominence by Milton Shy and Nicholas Gonatas in the 1960s, when they set about assigning different myopathies to different organelles. They defined one category by the electron microscopic appearance of overabundant or enlarged mitochondria with paracrystalline inclusions. Soon, Olson and Engel found that these abnormal mitochondria could be identified under the light microscope as *ragged-red fibers* (RRF) with a modified Gomori trichrome stain. For the next two decades, this histological hallmark was the basis for recognizing mitochondrial diseases, while biochemical tests were being developed and applied, eventually leading to a biochemical classification (included in Table 97.1). Throughout this period, there were vigorous debates between those who thought that there were identifiable clinical syndromes and those who thought there was too much overlap of the clinical features (a foreshadow of mitochondrial genetics). *Ophthalmoplegia plus* became a popular term for the lumpers. The splitters, however, recognized the constancy of clinical manifestations in the Kearns-Sayre syndrome (KSS) and noted that it was never familial, in contrast to the often familial nature of two other syndromes, *mitochondrial encephalomyopathy with lactic acidosis and stroke* (MELAS) and *myoclonic epilepsy with ragged-red fibers* (MERRF), both described in the early 1980s. The pattern of inheritance in these disorders was maternal, suggesting mtDNA involvement.

A revolution commenced in 1988, with the demonstration by Holt, Harding, and Morgan-Hughes of mtDNA single deletions in patients with mitochondrial myopathies, and the simultaneous recognition by Wallace and associates of a point mutation in *Leber hereditary optic neuropathy* (LHON). Single deletions were found by Zeviani,

Moraes, and associates to be characteristic of KSS and sporadic progressive external ophthalmoplegia (PEO), but not of familial PEO. In families with autosomal dominant PEO (AD-PEO), Zeviani and associates found multiple rather than single deletions of mtDNA. Soon thereafter, additional point mutations were identified as causes of MELAS and MERRF. In the ensuing years, over 150 pathogenic point mutations and a myriad of rearrangements in mtDNA have been associated with a bewildering array of clinical presentations (Fig. 97.1). A new lexicon was developed to encompass the new acronyms for multisystem diseases and for new concepts to deal with problems of pathogenesis.

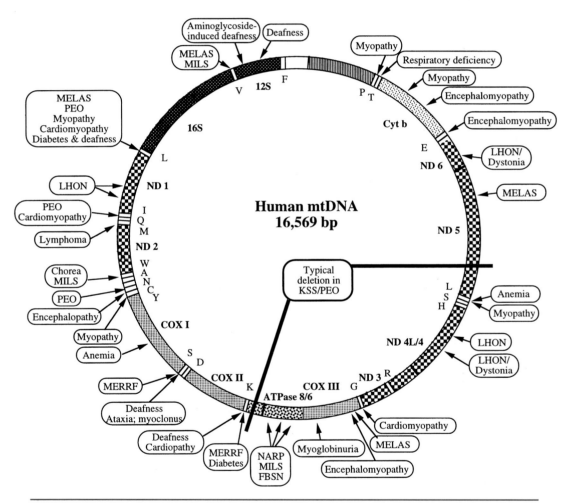

FIGURE 97.1. "Morbidity map" of human mtDNA. The map of the 16.6-kb mtDNA shows differently shaded areas representing the structural genes for the seven subunits of complex I (ND), the three subunits of cytochrome oxidase (COX), cytochrome b (Cyt b), and the two subunits of ATP syntase (ATPase 6 and 8), the 12S and 16S ribosomal RNAs (rRNA), and the 22 transfer RNAs (tRNA), identified by one-letter codes for the corresponding amino acids. LHON, Leber's hereditary optic neuropathy; NARP, neuropathy, ataxia, retinitis pigmentosa; MILS, maternally inherited Leigh syndrome; FBSN, familial bilateral striatal necrosis; MERRF, myoclonus epilepsy with ragged-red fibers; PEO, progressive external ophthalmoplegia; MELAS, mitochondrial encephalomyopathy, lactic acidosis, and stroke. Modified and reproduced with permission from DiMauro and Bonilla, 2004.

PRINCIPLES OF MITOCHONDRIAL GENETICS AND PATHOGENESIS OF MITOCHONDRIAL DISEASES

Human mtDNA is a small (16.6 kb) circle of double-stranded DNA (Fig. 97.1), comprising only 37 genes. Of these, 13 encode polypeptides, all subunits of the respiratory chain: seven subunits of complex I (NADH-ubiquinone oxidoreductase); one subunit of complex III (ubiquinone-cytochrome *c* oxidoreductase); three subunits of complex IV (cytochrome *c* oxidase [COX]); and two subunits of complex V (ATP syntase). The other 24 genes encode 22 transfer RNAs (tRNAs) and two ribosomal RNAs (rRNAs) that are required for translation of messenger RNAs on mitochondrial ribosomes. The subunits of complex II (succinate dehydrogenase–ubiquinone oxidoreductase), and the two small electron carriers, coenzyme Q10 (ubiquinone) and cytochrome *c*, are encoded exclusively by nDNA.

The following main principles distinguish mitochondrial genetics from mendelian genetics and help explain many of the clinical peculiarities of mtDNA-related disorders.

1. *Polyplasmy.* Most cells contain multiple mitochondria and each mitochondrion contains multiple copies of mtDNA, so that there are hundreds or thousands of mitochondrial genomes in each cell.

2. *Heteroplasmy.* When an mtDNA mutation affects some but not all genomes, a cell, a tissue, indeed a whole individual will harbor two populations of mtDNA, normal (or wild type) and mutant, a condition known as heteroplasmy. In normal tissues, all mtDNAs are identical, a situation of homoplasmy. Usually, neutral mutations (or polymorphisms) are homoplasmic. In contrast, most (but not all) pathogenic mtDNA mutations are heteroplasmic.

3. *Threshold effect.* The functional impairment associated with a pathogenic mtDNA mutation is largely determined by the degree of heteroplasmy, and a minimal critical number of mutant genomes has to be present before tissue dysfunction becomes evident (and related clinical signs become manifest), a concept aptly termed "threshold effect." This is, however, a relative concept: Tissues with high metabolic demands, such as brain, heart, and muscle, tend to have lower tolerance for mtDNA mutations than do metabolically less active tissues.

4. *Mitotic segregation.* Both organellar division and mtDNA replication are apparently stochastic events unrelated to cell division: Thus, the number of mitochondria (and mtDNA) can vary not just in space (i.e., among cells and tissues) but also in time (i.e., during development or aging). Moreover, at cell division, the proportion of mutant mtDNAs in daughter cells may drift, allowing for relatively rapid changes in genotype, which, if and when the threshold is crossed, can translate into changes in phenotype, including the clinical picture.

5. *Maternal inheritance.* At fertilization, all mitochondria (and all mtDNA) are contributed to the zygote by the oocyte. Therefore, a mother carrying an mtDNA mutation will pass it on to all her children, males and females, but only her daughters will transmit it to their progeny, in a vertical matrilinear line. When maternal inheritance is evident in a clinical setting, it provides conclusive evidence that an mtDNA mutation must underlie the disease in question. However, the other features of mitochondrial genetics (e.g., heteroplasmy and the threshold effect) often mask maternal inheritance by causing striking intrafamilial clinical heterogeneity. Thus, when suspecting an mtDNA-related disorder, it is crucial to collect the family history meticulously, paying special attention to "soft signs" (such as short stature, hearing loss, or migraine headache) in potentially oligosymptomatic maternal relatives.

Clinical Manifestations

Although specific syndromes can be identified by particular combinations of symptoms and signs (Table 97.2), several clinical manifestations seem to be prevalent among different syndromes, especially short stature, neurosensory hearing loss, and diabetes mellitus. Lactic acidosis, often detected in blood and CSF, is the most common laboratory sign. Perhaps as a result of impaired respiration, mitochondria in muscle proliferate and enlarge, which is the basis for finding RRF (Fig. 97.2). Neuropathologic and neuroradiologic changes fall into four main patterns: (1) microcephaly and ventricular dilatation, sometimes associated with agenesis of the corpus callosum, is seen in infants with severe congenital lactic acidosis; (2) bilateral, symmetrical lesions of basal ganglia, thalamus, brainstem, and cerebellar roof nuclei are the signature of Leigh syndrome; (3) multifocal encephalomalacias, usually involving the cortex of the posterior cerebral hemispheres, correspond to the "strokes" of the MELAS syndrome; (4) spongy encephalopathy, predominantly in the white matter, is characteristic of the KSS. Calcification of the basal ganglia can be seen in all of the disorders but in a minority of patients with any syndrome.

Diagnosis of a mitochondrial disease is based on five crucial elements: recognition of an appropriate clinical syndrome, presence of lactic acidosis in blood or CSF, demonstration of RRF in muscle biopsy, documentation of impaired respiration in biochemical assays of muscle extracts or isolated mitochondria, or identification of a pathogenic mutation in mtDNA (or in nDNA). Not all of

▶ **TABLE 97.2   Classification of Progressive External Ophthalmoplegia**

1. **Mitochondrial**
   (A) Sporadic PEO with single deletions of mtDNA
       (a) PEO with proximal myopathy
       (b) Kearns-Sayre syndrome (KSS)
   (B) Maternally inherited PEO with mtDNA point mutations
       (a) A3243G (MELAS)
       (b) A8344G (MERRF)
       (c) Other mutations
   (C) Autosomal dominant PEO with multiple mtDNA deletions
   (D) Autosomal recessive PEO with multiple mtDNA deletions
       (a) With cardiomyopathy
       (b) With gastrointestinal involvement (MNGIE)
   (E) Autosomal recessive PEO with mtDNA depletion
   (F) Sporadic PEO and late-onset myopathy with multiple mtDNA deletions
2. **Presumably Myopathic**
   (A) Oculopharyngeal muscular dystrophy, autosomal dominant
   (B) Myotubular or centronuclear myopathy
   (C) Congenital myopathic ptosis or PEO, some with muscle fibrosis
   (D) PEO as part of other generalized myopathies
       (a) Myotonic muscular dystrophy
       (a) Myopathic myasthenia gravis
3. **Presumably Neurogenic**
   (A) Congenital PEO and facial diplegia (Möbius syndrome)
   (B) PEO with myelopathy or encephalopathy
       (a) Juvenile onset
       (b) Hereditary ataxia
       (c) Hereditary spastic paraplegia
       (d) Hereditary multisystem disease, including Joseph disease
       (e) Generalized dystonia
       (f) Progressive supranuclear palsy
       (g) Abetalipoproteinemia
   (C) PEO with motor neuron disease
       (a) Infantile spinal muscular atrophy
       (b) Juvenile spinal muscular atrophy
       (c) Amyotrophic lateral sclerosis

these criteria, however, are necessarily present in an individual syndrome. Unfortunately, there is no effective treatment for any of these diseases, although interesting therapeutic strategies are being developed.

We now describe some of the clinical syndromes, more or less following the outline in Table 97.2. References are given at the end of the chapter for these conditions.

PROGRESSIVE EXTERNAL OPHTHALMOPLEGIA

Progressive external ophthalmoplegia (PEO) is defined clinically as a slowly progressive limitation of eye movements until there is complete immobility (*ophthalmoplegia*). PEO is usually accompanied by eyelids droop (*ptosis*)

because they cannot be held up in the normal position by the levator palpebrae. There may or may not be weakness of muscles of face, oropharynx, neck, or limbs.

It is not known whether the ophthalmoplegia is myopathic, neurogenic, or both, because neither EMG of ocular muscles nor autopsy findings suffice to make this determination. This condition is clearly heterogeneous, but several distinct syndromes can be recognized, some related to primary abnormalities of mtDNA (with sporadic single deletions or maternally inherited point mutations) and others related to autosomal genes affecting directly the mtDNA (defects of intergenomic signaling, with multiple deletions of mtDNA). For convenience, a separation can be made into a mitochondrial group; a presumably myopathic group of PEO alone or with myopathic findings in limb muscles; and a third group, presumably neurogenic, associated with disease of the CNS or peripheral neuropathy (Table 97.2).

Sporadic PEO with Single mtDNA Deletions

PEO with or without Limb Weakness

This is a relatively benign condition, often compatible with a normal lifespan. Symptoms usually begin in childhood but may be delayed to adolescence or adult years. Ptosis is often the first symptom, followed by ophthalmoparesis. The disorder is bilateral and symmetric, so diplopia is unusual. Some patients also have pharyngeal and limb weakness.

Kearns-Sayre Syndrome (KSS)

This syndrome is identified by an invariant triad: onset before age 20, PEO, and pigmentary retinopathy. In addition, there must be one of the following: heart block (usually needing a pacemaker), cerebellar syndrome, or CSF protein content of 100 mg/dl or more. Seizures are distinctly infrequent and are usually associated with electrolyte disturbances, as may occur in hypoparathyroidism, one of the several endocrine disorders sometimes associated with KSS. The course is relentlessly downhill, and patients rarely survive past the second decade.

Molecular Genetics

In both sporadic PEO and KSS, patients harbor a single deletion in their mtDNA, which is identical in all tissues in any patient, although the number of deleted genomes varies from tissue to tissue (heteroplasmy). The single mtDNA deletions arise spontaneously early in oögenesis or embryogenesis. Although the molecular defect is the

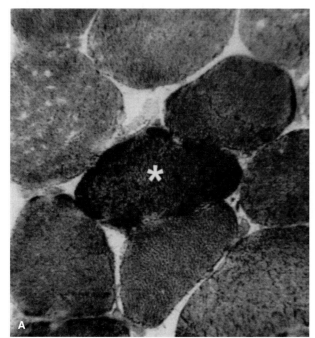
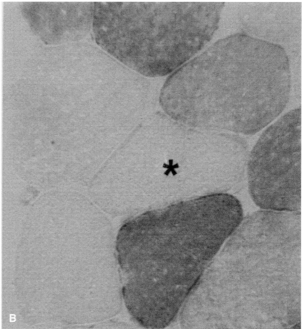

FIGURE 97.2. Histochemistry detects ragged-red fibers in serial sections of human skeletal muscle. **A.** Succinate dehydrogenase enzyme activity shows an intensely staining ragged-red fiber (white asterisk). **B.** Cytochrome c oxidase shows that the ragged-red fiber (black asterisk) as well as other muscle fibers are deficient in this enzyme activity. (Courtesy of Dr. Eduardo Bonilla, Columbia University).

same in both conditions, intermediate cases are surprisingly few.

Laboratory Abnormalities

In both conditions, muscle biopsy shows RRFs that are devoid of histochemically demonstrable COX activity. Raised levels of lactate and pyruvate are usually found in blood both in sporadic PEO and in KSS; in CSF, increased lactate is seen only in KSS. At postmortem examination, typical cases of KSS have spongy degeneration of the brain. The epithelium of the choroid plexus shows oncocytic changes that may explain the very high CSF protein levels. CT or MRI shows leukoencephalopathy, and there may be calcification of basal ganglia.

Treatment

It is crucial to recognize KSS because sudden death as a result of the cardiac conduction disorder is a threat that can be prevented. Episodic coma may result from the combination of diabetes mellitus and encephalopathy. The cerebellar syndrome can be severe enough to be disabling. Because of their severe disabilities and hormonal problems, KSS subjects are not expected to have children, but the few women who have reproduced have had normal children.

However, there are a few reports of maternal transmission of single mtDNA deletions.

Maternally Inherited PEO with Point Mutations of mtDNA

A substantial number of patients with mitochondrial PEO, that is, PEO and RRF in the muscle biopsy, show maternal inheritance of their syndrome, which is dominated by PEO but is often associated with various combinations of other symptoms, including hearing loss, endocrinopathy, heart block, cerebellar ataxia, or pigmentary retinopathy.

The most common mutation in these patients is the typical A3243G MELAS mutation, but other mutations have also been described, including the A8344G mutation typically seen in MERRF. The reason for the appearance of PEO in patients with the MELAS mutation is not known, but it may be related to a selectively high abundance of mutant mtDNA in muscle. There is usually lactic acidosis, and muscle biopsies show RRF.

Autosomal PEO with Multiple Deletions of mtDNA

PEO has been described in numerous families with autosomal dominant (AD) or autosomal recessive (AR) inheritance. Generally, AD-PEO syndromes are dominated by myopathic symptoms, whereas AR-PEO syndromes tend to be multisystemic.

AD-PEO

The clinical syndrome is characterized by ophthalmoplegia, although hearing loss, tremor, cataracts, and psychiatric disorders are variably present and suggest multisystemic involvement. Onset is usually in adult age and there may be weakness of facial, pharyngeal, and respiratory muscles in addition to slowly progressive proximal limb weakness.

AR-PEO with Cardiomyopathy (ARCO)

Severe hypertrophic cardiomyopathy, proximal weakness, and PEO were the clinical hallmarks of two unrelated families from the eastern seaboard of the Arabian peninsula. Onset was in childhood and cardiac transplantation was needed to prevent early death.

Mitochondrial Neurogastrointestinal Encephalomyopathy (MNGIE)

This syndrome starts in childhood or adolescence with chronic intractable diarrhea, loud borborygmi, and recurrent intestinal pseudo-obstruction, causing these patients to appear severely emaciated. There is also PEO, both proximal and distal limb weakness, and sensory neuropathy. MRI shows diffuse leukodystrophy, although patients usually have normal cognition. Death usually occurs in the fourth or fifth decade.

Laboratory Abnormalities

In all conditions described above, muscle biopsy shows RRFs and COX-negative fibers: These are more abundant in AR-PEO than in AD-PEO syndromes. Lactic acidosis is usually present but may not be very marked. In MNGIE, nerve conduction studies and nerve biopsies have shown predominantly demyelinating neuropathy.

Molecular Genetics

Southern blot analysis of muscle mtDNA in these conditions shows multiple bands representing species of mtDNA molecules harboring deletions of different sizes (more abundantly in AR-PEO than in AD-PEO patients). Mutations in three genes have been identified: *ANT1*, which encodes one isoform of the ATP translocator; *Twinkle*, which encodes a mitochondrial protein presumably involved in mtDNA replication; and *POLG*, which encodes polymerase γ, the main catalyst of mtDNA replication. It appears that POLG mutations are the most frequent causes not only of AD-PEO but of some cases of AR-PEO as well. Despite this remarkable progress, in several families with AD-PEO and

AR-PEO (including ARCO) the molecular defects remain unknown.

In MNGIE, numerous mutations have been identified in the gene encoding thymidine phosphorylase (TP). The diagnosis can be established by enzyme assay in leukocytes.

Other Forms of Mitochondrial PEO

Ophthalmoplegia is often seen in patients with the congenital or the infantile myopathic variants of *mtDNA depletion*, which are transmitted as autosomal recessive traits (see below). Ptosis, PEO, or both, can also accompany the *late-onset mitochondrial myopathies*, often associated with multiple mtDNA deletions, which have been described in sporadic elderly individuals and have been interpreted as an exaggerated manifestation of the normal aging process.

Multisystem Neurologic Diseases Without Ophthalmoplegia

MELAS

The distinguishing features of this syndrome are the strokes, with hemiparesis, hemianopia, or cortical blindness, almost invariably occurring before age 40 and often in childhood. Common additional features are focal or generalized seizures, recurrent migrainelike headaches and vomiting, and dementia. The course is one of gradual deterioration.

Laboratory abnormalities include elevated blood and CSF lactate and MRI evidence of encephalomalacic foci, usually involving the occipital cortex and not conforming to the distribution of major vessels. Muscle biopsy shows RRF—which are uncharacteristically COX-positive rather than COX-negative as in most other mtDNA-related diseases—as well as mitochondrial proliferation in the walls of blood vessels (SSVs, strongly SDH-positive vessels).

In about 80% of patients, the molecular defect is a point mutation (A3243G) in the tRNA$^{Leu(UUR)}$ gene of mtDNA. In the remaining patients, a handful of mutations have been described, some of which affect protein-encoding genes rather than tRNA genes—notably ND5, the gene encoding subunit 5 of complex I. The A3243G is the most frequent pathogenic mtDNA mutation and it has been associated not only with MELAS and with maternally inherited PEO but also with diabetes mellitus alone or in combination with deafness.

MERRF

Typical clinical features include myoclonus, generalized seizures, cerebellar ataxia, myopathy, and, in some families, multiple symmetrical lipomas. Onset can be in childhood or in adult life and the course can be slowly progressive or rapidly downhill. As the acronym implies, muscle biopsy shows RRF, which are COX-negative. Most patients with MERRF have a mutation (A8344G) in the tRNA^{Lys} gene of mtDNA.

Neuropathy, Ataxia, Retinitis Pigmentosa (NARP)

This is a maternally transmitted multisystem disorder of young adult life comprising, in various combinations, sensory neuropathy, ataxia, seizures, dementia, and retinitis pigmentosa. Lactic acid in blood may be normal or slightly elevated, and muscle biopsy does not show RRF.

The molecular defect is a point mutation (T8993G) in the gene that encodes ATPase 6. When this mutation approaches homoplasmic levels, onset is in infancy and the clinical and neuropathological features are those of Leigh syndrome (maternally inherited Leigh syndrome or MILS). A different mutation at the very same nucleotide (T8993C) causes a phenotype similar to MILS, but generally milder. A few other mutations in the ATPase 6 gene have been associated with Leighlike syndromes or with familial bilateral striatal necrosis.

Leber hereditary optic neuropathy (LHON) is discussed in Chapter 99.

Depletion of mtDNA

Depletion of mtDNA is the other major defect of intergenomic signaling, together with multiple mtDNA deletions described above. As the name implies, this is a quantitative rather than qualitative mtDNA abnormality, consisting of significantly decreased levels of mtDNA in one or more tissues. The clinical spectrum of mtDNA depletion has been incompletely characterized (and is probably more heterogeneous than was initially thought), but three syndromes stand out, all inherited as autosomal recessive traits:

Congenital Myopathy

At or soon after birth, there is generalized weakness (sometimes including PEO) with lactic acidosis and significantly elevated serum CK. Some children also have renal involvement with Fanconi syndrome. Muscle biopsy shows abundant RRF, which are COX-negative. Due to intractable respiratory failure, these children do not live more than a few months. Southern blot analysis shows a profound defect of mtDNA in muscle (less than 10% of normal).

Infantile Myopathy

In some children, weakness starts a little later but is usually evident by 1 year of age and may cause PEO. Progression is rapid, leading to flaccid paralysis, respiratory insufficiency, and death within 1 or 2 more years. There is only partial mtDNA depletion in muscle (about 30% of normal), with some fibers virtually devoid of mtDNA whereas others look normal. Recognizing this entity is especially difficult because the clinical presentation is nonspecific, lactic acidosis may not be presented initially and is generally mild, and early biopsies may show nonspecific myopathic features rather than mitochondrial proliferation with RRF (which do appear in later biopsies). Notably, some children with the clinical and muscle biopsy features of spinal muscular atrophy (SMA)—but without mutations in the *SMN1* gene—have mtDNA depletion.

Hepatopathy

Infants with severe mtDNA depletion in liver develop intractable liver failure soon after birth and die within months. Liver biopsy shows mitochondrial proliferation in hepatocytes, and biochemical analysis shows very low activities of all respiratory chain complexes containing mtDNA-encoded subunits.

Pathogenic mutations have been identified in two genes, both involved in maintaining the intramitochondrial nucleotide pool. Mutations in *TK2*, encoding the enzyme thymidine kinase, have been associated with the myopathic form (including some children with the SMA phenocopy). Mutations in *DGUOK*, encoding the enzyme deoxyguanosine kinase (DGK), have been associated with the hepatic form. However, other genes must be involved because some patients with mtDNA depletion do not harbor mutations in either *TK2* or *DGUOK*.

Acquired mtDNA Depletion

An iatrogenic form of mtDNA depletion has been recognized in patients with AIDS, who developed a mitochondrial myopathy while treated with zidovudine (AZT). The myopathy is reversible on discontinuation of the drug.

SUGGESTED READINGS

Arnaudo E, Dalakas M, Shanske S, et al. Depletion of muscle mitochondrial DNA in AIDS patients with zidovudine-induced myopathy. *Lancet* 1991;337:508–510.

Berenberg RA, Pellock JM, DiMauro S, et al. Lumping or splitting? "Ophthalmoplegia plus" or Kearns-Sayre syndrome? *Ann Neurol* 1977;1:37–54.

Bohlega S, Tanji K, Santorelli FM, et al. Multiple mtDNA deletions associated with autosomal recessive ophthalmoplegia and severe cardiomyopathy. *Neurology* 1996;46:1329–1334.

Carrozzo R, Hirano M, Fromenty B, et al. Multiple mtDNA deletions features in autosomal dominant and recessive diseases suggest distinct pathogeneses. *Neurology* 1998;50:99–106.

DiMauro S, Hirano M. Mitochondrial DNA deletion syndromes. In: *GeneReviews at Gene Tests: Medical Genetics Information Resource* [database online]. Copyright, University of Washington, Seattle, 1997–2003. Available at http://www.genetests.org. 2005.

DiMauro S, Hirano M, Kaufmann P, et al. Clinical features and genetics of myoclonic epilepsy with ragged-red fibers. In: Fahn S, Frucht SJ, Hallett M, et al., eds. *Myoclonus and Paroxysmal Dyskinesias.* Philadelphia: Lippincott & Wilkins, 2002:217–229.

DiMauro S, Schon EA. Mitochondrial respiratory-chain defects. *New Engl J Med* 2003;348:2656–2658.

DiMauro S, Bonilla E. Mitochondrial Encephalomyopathies. In: Engel AG, Franzini-Armstrong C, eds. *Myology.* New York: McGraw Hill, 2004:1623–1662.

Engel WK, Cunningham CG. Rapid examination of muscle tissue: an improved trichrome stain method for fresh-frozen biopsy specimens. *Neurology* 1963;13:919–923.

Fukuhara N, Tokiguchi S, Shirakawa K, et al. Myoclonus epilepsy associated with ragged red fibers (mitochondrial abnormalities): disease entity or syndrome? *J Neurol Sci* 1980;47:117–133.

Goto YI, Nonaka I, Horai S. A mutation in the tRNA$^{Leu(UUR)}$ gene associated with the MELAS subgroup of mitochondrial encephalomyopathies. *Nature* 1990;348:651–653.

Hirano M, DiMauro S. *ANT1, Twinkle, POLG, and TP*: New genes open our eyes to ophthalmoplegia. *Neurology* 2001;57:2163–2165.

Holt IJ, Harding AE, Morgan-Hughes JA. A new mitochondrial disease associated with mitochondrial DNA heteroplasmy. *Am J Hum Genet* 1990;46:428–433.

Holt IJ, Harding AE, Morgan-Hughes JA. Deletions of muscle mitochondrial DNA in patients with mitochondrial myopathy. *Nature* 1988;331:717–718.

Johnston W, Karpati G, Carpenter, et al. Late-onset mitochondrial myopathy. *Ann Neurol* 1995;37:16–23.

Kearns TP, Sayre G. Retinitis pigmentosa, external ophthalmoplegia, and complete heart block. *Arch Ophthalmol* 1958;60:280–289.

Luft R, Ikkos D, Palmieri G, et al. Severe hypermetabolism of nonthyroidal origin with a defect in the maintenance of mitochondrial respiratory control. *J Clin Invest* 1962;41:1776–1804.

Mancuso M, Salviati L, Sacconi S, et al. Mitochondrial DNA depletion: mutations in thymidine kinase gene with myopathy and SMA. *Neurology* 2002;59:1197–2002.

Mandel H, Szargel R, Labay V, et al. The deoxyguanosine kinase gene is mutated in individuals with depleted hepatocerebral mtDNA. *Nature Genet* 2001;29:337–341.

Marti R, Spinazzola A, Tadesse S, et al. Definitive diagnosis of mitochondrial neurogastrointestinal encephalomyopathy by biochemical assays. *Clin Chem* 2004;50(Jan):120–124.

Moraes CT, Ciacci F, Silvestri G, et al. Atypical presentation associated with the MELAS mutation at position 3243 of human mitochondrial DNA. *Neuromusc Dis* 1993;3:43–50.

Moraes CT, DiMauro S, Zeviani M, et al. Mitochondrial DNA deletions in progressive external ophthalmoplegia and Kearns-Sayre syndrome. *New Engl J Med* 1989;320:1293–1299.

Moraes CT, Shanske S, Tritschler H-J, et al. MtDNA depletion with variable tissue expression: a novel genetic abnormality in mitochondrial diseases. *Am J Hum Genet* 1991;48:492–501.

Olson W, Engel WK, Einaugler R. Oculocraniosomatic neuromuscular disease with ragged red fibers. *Arch Neurol* 1972;26:193–211.

Nishino I, Spinazzola A, Hirano M. Thymidine phosphorylase gene mutations in MNGIE, a human mitochondrial disorder. *Science* 1999;283:689–692.

Nishino I, Spinazzola A, Papadimitriou A, et al. Mitochondrial neurogastrointestinal encephalomyopathy: an autosomal recessive disorder due to thymidine phosphorylase mutations. *Ann Neurol* 2000;47:792–800.

Pavlakis SG, Phillips PC, DiMauro S, et al. Mitochondrial myopathy, encephalopathy, lactic acidosis, and stroke-like episodes. *Ann Neurol* 1984;16:481–487.

Pons R, Andreu AL, Checcarelli N, et al. Mitochondrial DNA abnormalities and autistic spectrum disorders. *J Pediat* 2004;144(Jan):81–85.

Rowland LP. Progressive external ophthalmoplegia. *Handb Clin Neurol* 1992;18:553–593.

Saada A, Shaag A, Mandel H, et al. Mutant mitochondrial thymidine kinase in mitochondrial DNA depletion myopathy. *Nature Genet* 2001;29:342–344.

Salviati L, Sacconi S, Mancuso M, et al. Mitochondrial DNA depletion and *dGK* gene mutations. *Ann Neurol* 2002;52:311–316.

Santorelli FM, Shanske S, Macaya A, et al. The mutation at nt 8993 of mitochondrial DNA is a common cause of Leigh's syndrome. *An Neurol* 1993;34:827–834.

Schon EA, DiMauro S. Medicinal and genetic approaches to the treatment of mitochondrial disease. *CurrMed Chem* 2003;10:2523–2533.

Shy GM, Gonatas NK, Perez M. Childhood myopathies with abnormal mitochondria. I. Megaconial myopathy. II. Pleoconial myopathy. *Brain* 1966;89:133–158.

Tatuch Y, Christodoulou J, Feigenbaum A, et al. Heteroplasmic mtDNA mutation (T−>G) at 8993 can cause Leigh disease when the percentage of mtDNA is high. *Am J Hum Genet* 1992;50:852–858.

Vu TH, Sciacco M, Tanji K, et al. Clinical manifestations of mitochondrial DNA depletion. *Neurology* 1998;50:1783–1790.

Wallace DC, Singh G, Lott MT, et al. Mitochondrial DNA mutation associated with Leber's hereditary optic atrophy. *Science* 1988;242:1427–1430.

Zeviani M, Moraes CT, DiMauro S, et al. Deletions of mitochondrial DNA in Kearns-Sayre syndrome. *Neurology* 1988;38:1339–1346.

Zeviani M, Servidei S, Gellera C, et al. An autosomal dominant disorder with multiple deletions of mitochondrial DNA starting at the D-loop region. *Nature* 1989;339:309–311.

C h a p t e r   9 8

Leber Hereditary Optic Neuropathy

Michio Hirano and Myles M. Behrens

Leber hereditary optic neuropathy (LHON; MIM 535600) is a maternally inherited disorder characterized by loss of central vision and occurring more often in males. It was named for Leber because he reported 15 patients in four families in 1871, following von Graefe's initial description in 1858. Maternal inheritance was recognized in 1970 in a large pedigree residing in Queensland, Australia, with LHON plus other neurologic manifestations. Nikoskelainen studied patients with more typical LHON and in 1984 proposed that mutations in mitochondrial DNA (mtDNA) might be responsible. A major breakthrough came in 1988 when Wallace, Nikoskelainen, and colleagues described the first mtDNA point mutation in a human disease. This accounted for the maternal inheritance, that is, transmission by women to all their progeny (male and female), but not by men.

CLINICAL MANIFESTATIONS

Onset usually occurs in adolescence or early-adult years but may occur from ages 5 to 80 years. Cloudiness of central vision progresses painlessly over weeks, usually first in one eye, to a larger, denser centrocecal scotoma, occasionally breaking out peripherally to a minor extent. Both eyes are usually affected within weeks or months, sometimes simultaneously; it is only rarely unilateral. Color vision is affected, and acuity drops to 20/200 or finger counting. Residual visual loss may be severe and generally remains stationary. Sometimes, there is later improvement, infrequently striking and occasionally sudden, with severity and possibility of improvement varying with the particular mutation. The fundus may appear normal until optic atrophy supervenes, but at onset, as first described by Smith, Hoyt, and Susac (1973), the disc often appears blurred and suggestive of edema, as in papillitis. However, the findings are a result of swelling of the nerve fiber layer around the disc, with circumpapillary telangiectatic microangiopathy and without evidence of abnormal vascular permeability (leakage) on fluorescein angiography. The vascular abnormalities may be seen in presymptomatic and asymptomatic relatives and do not invariably predict imminent visual loss, which may never occur. As the acute stage approaches, vessels dilate and undulate in and out of the thickening peripapillary nerve fiber layer, with increased arteriovenous shunting. This subsides after a few weeks or months. Optic atrophy follows, starting in the temporal portion of the disc, then usually generalized.

In most patients with LHON, visual disturbance is the only symptom, but cardiac pre-excitation is frequently associated. Neurologic examination, however, may reveal subtle neurologic abnormalities, including postural tremor, dystonia, motor tics, parkinsonism with dystonia, or peripheral neuropathy. Several patients (mostly women) with LHON have had multiple sclerosis–like manifestations. The Uhthoff symptom has been reported by a few patients with LHON. Two patients had ataxia and optic neuropathy with an mtDNA point mutation of LHON.

At least five Leber-plus syndromes have been reported: optic neuropathy and dystonia; optic neuropathy and spastic dystonia; optic neuropathy and Leigh-like syndrome optic neuropathy and mitochondrial encephalomyopathy, lactic acidosis and stroke-like episodes (MELAS); and the Queensland variant with optic neuropathy, athetosis, tremor, corticospinal tract signs, posterior column dysfunction, psychiatric disturbances, and acute encephalopathy.

PATHOLOGY AND MOLECULAR GENETICS

Prior to the identification of molecular genetic defects, several autopsy studies of LHON patients revealed atrophy of the retinal ganglion cells, nerve fiber layer, and optic nerve. The clinical manifestations of LHON are similar regardless of the specific genotype, but the molecular genetic features of LHON are complex and unique. First,

there are mtDNA primary mutations that are thought to be pathogenic. Additional mtDNA polymorphisms may be synergistically pathogenic in combination with each other or with primary mutations. Second, at least 90% of patients with LHON harbor primary mutations that are usually homoplasmic, in contrast to the mitochondrial encephalomyopathies, which typically show heteroplasmic mutations.

The first and most common primary mtDNA mutation associated with LHON was found in the gene for subunit 4 of NADH-ubiquinone oxidoreductase, or complex I, of the mitochondrial respiratory chain. The A-to-G transition mutation at nucleotide 11778 (A11778G) in the mtDNA genome changes amino acid 340 in the ND4 gene from arginine to histidine. Two additional common mtDNA mutations in complex I (ND) subunits have been identified: G3460A in ND1 and T14484C in ND6 (Table 98.1). Although the three mtDNA mutations account for >90% of LHON patients, six additional primary mtDNA mutations have been identified in families with LHON. In the North East of England, the prevalence of the common LHON mutations is 11.8 per 100,000 individuals and the prevalence of the symptomatic patients is 3.2 per 100,000. Penetrance rates of the LHON mutations are uncertain; however, some reports estimate that symptoms appear in 20% to 83% of men and 4% to 32% of women at risk. Sixty percent to ninety percent of LHON patients are men. The molecular basis for male predominance is not known. An unknown X-linked factor may interact with a LHON mtDNA mutation, but linkage studies have failed to identify such a locus. Other nuclear DNA and mtDNA polymorphisms may also affect the expression of the LHON mutations. Environmental factors including cigarette smoking and ethanol

▶ **TABLE 98.1 Mitochondrial DNA Mutations Associated with LHON**

Common LHON primary mutations				
Mutation	Gene	Amino acid Substitution	LHON Patients with Mutation (%)	Patients with Visual Recovery (%)
G1178A	ND4	Arg→His	31–89	4
G3460A	ND1	Lys→Pro	8–15	4–20
T14484C	ND6	Met→Val	10–15	37–64

LHON-plus pathogenic mutations			
Phenotype	Mutation	Gene	Amino Acid Substitution
LHON/dystonia	G14459A	ND6	Ala→Val
LHON/spastic dystonia	A11696G	ND4	Val→Ile
	T14596A	ND6	IIE→Met
Queensland LHON variant	T4160C	ND1	Leu→Pro

consumption may increase the risk of developing vision loss, although this has not been proved.

Distinct mtDNA mutations have been associated with LHON-plus phenotypes. In the Queensland LHON-plus variant, two primary coexisting mutations were identified, T4160C in ND1 and T14484C in ND6. Two distinct mitochondrial genotypes have been identified in pedigrees with LHON and dystonia, G14459A in ND6 and a combination of A11696G in ND1 plus T14596A in ND6, which has emerged as a hot spot for LHON mutations. MtDNA mutations in ND5, particularly G13513A, have been associated with LHON/MELAS overlap syndrome.

DIFFERENTIAL DIAGNOSIS

The diagnosis of LHON is usually made when the typical course of visual loss occurs with an appropriate family history or with observation of the typical acute fundus appearance in a patient or compatible fundus changes in close maternal relatives. Now, it can be diagnosed, even without family history and even with optic neuropathy with less typical features, by genetic analysis of a blood sample.

Other forms of bilateral optic neuropathies with centrocecal scotomas include demyelinating, toxic-nutritional optic neuropathy (including tobacco-alcohol amblyopia), other types of hereditary optic atrophy, occasionally glaucoma or ischemic optic neuropathy, and rarely compressive lesions. To help exclude tumors, computed tomography or magnetic resonance imaging includes axial and coronal orbital views with and without contrast to include the optic nerves and chiasm; enlargement and enhancement of the optic nerves and enlargement of the chiasm have been reported in patients with LHON. A retinal basis for central visual defect, which may not be evident on ophthalmoscopy, is cone dystrophy, which may be excluded if multifocal electroretinography is normal.

The dominant variety of hereditary optic atrophy as initially categorized by Kjer (1972) is the most common form of hereditary optic atrophy and must be distinguished from LHON. It is also characterized by centrocecal scotomas, dyschromatopsia, and temporal pallor but is generally milder, usually beginning insidiously between ages 4 and 8 years and slowly progressing with visual acuity from 20/30 to no worse than 20/200, although a minority show more severe defects of acuity. In about 90% of autosomal dominant optic atrophy is caused by mutations in the *OPA1* gene that encodes a dynamin-related GTPase, however, linkage of OPA4 to chromosome 18q12.2-12.3 has demonstrated genetic heterogeneity.

Other forms of hereditary optic atrophy may occur as part of complex neurologic disorders, including the lipidoses, spinocerebellar ataxias, and polyneuropathies including Charcot-Marie-Tooth. Autosomal-recessive *Behr complicated optic atrophy* may be a transitional form between the ataxias and isolated hereditary optic atrophy. Other autosomal-recessive forms of optic atrophy include the rare but severe simple optic atrophy beginning in early infancy and that associated with diabetes insipidus, diabetes mellitus, and hearing defect (DIDMOAD or Wolfram syndrome). Wolfram syndrome is due to mutations in wolframin, an integral membrane glycoprotein primarily localized in endoplasmic reticulum.

A source of confusion in nomenclature is the severe congenital visual loss known as *Leber congenital amaurosis*. This is an autosomal-recessive degeneration of the retina rather than of the optic nerve and is usually characterized by retinal arteriolar narrowing and retinal pigmentary degeneration. Occasionally, the fundus appears normal at first. The electroretinogram is extinguished, whereas it is normal with optic neuropathy. The syndrome has been linked to 10 chromosomal loci and associated with mutations in seven different genes.

TREATMENT

No treatment is of proven value, including corticosteroids, hydroxycobalamin (suggested because of evidence that cyanide toxicity might be a factor), optic nerve sheath fenestration, or craniotomy with lysis of optic nerve chiasm–arachnoidal adhesions. Given the usual sequential involvement of the two eyes, however, it may be possible to prevent loss of vision in the second eye. With the new insights into pathogenesis, it can be hoped that an effective therapy will be found, perhaps one that enhances or preserves mitochondrial respiratory enzyme function. Products that might enhance mitochondrial respiratory enzymes (coenzyme Q10, idebenone, and thiamine) have been used but are not of proven value. Antioxidants have also been used to reduce possible damage from reactive oxygen species generated by the impaired oxidative metabolism. According to consensus, tobacco and alcohol should be avoided in family members at risk. A theoretical molecular therapy is allotopic expression: introduction of a modified gene that can be translated in the cytoplasm into a protein with a mitochondrial targeting signal. In fact, after virally mediated allotopic expression of ND4, cultured cells harboring the G11778A LHON mutation showed improved mitochondrial ATP synthesis.

SUGGESTED READINGS

Alexander C, Votruba M, Pesch UE, et al. OPA1, encoding a dynamin-related GTPase, is mutated in autosomal dominant optic atrophy linked to chromosome 3q28. *Nat Genet* 2000;26:211–215.

Barboni P, Savini G, Valentino ML, et al. Retinal nerve fiber layer evaluation by optical coherence tomography in Leber's hereditary optic neuropathy. *Ophthalmology* 2005;112:120–126.

Brown JJ, Fingert JH, Taylor CM, et al. Clinical and genetic analysis of a family affected with dominant optic atrophy (OPA1). *Arch Ophthalmol* 1997;115:95–99.

Carelli V, Ross-Cisneros FN, Sadun AA. Mitochondrial dysfunction as a cause of optic neuropathies. *Prog Retin Eye Res* 2004;23:53–89.

Delettre C, Lenaers G, Griffoin JM, et al. Nuclear gene OPA1, encoding a mitochondrial dynamin-related protein, is mutated in dominant optic atrophy. *Nat Genet* 2000;26:207–210.

Funalot B, Reynier P, Vighetto A, et al. Leigh-like encephalopathy complicating Leber's hereditary optic neuropathy. *Ann Neurol* 2002;52:374–377.

Guy J, Qi X, Pallotti F, et al. Rescue of a mitochondrial deficiency causing Leber hereditary optic neuropathy. *Ann Neurol* 2002;52:534–542.

Hanein S, Perrault I, Gerber S, et al. Leber congenital amaurosis: comprehensive survey of the genetic heterogeneity, refinement of the clinical definition, and genotype-phenotype correlations as a strategy for molecular diagnosis. *Hum Mutat* 2004;23:306–317.

Harding AE, Sweeney MG, Miller DH, et al. Occurrence of a multiple sclerosis-like illness in women who have a Leber's hereditary optic neuropathy mitochondrial DNA mutation. *Brain* 1992;115:979–989.

Huoponen K, Vilkki J, Aula P, et al. A new mtDNA mutation associated with Leber hereditary optic neuroretinopathy. *Am J Hum Genet* 1991;48:1147–1153.

Johns DR, Neufeld MJ, Park RD. An ND-6 mitochondrial DNA mutation associated with Leber hereditary optic neuropathy. *Biochem Biophys Res Comm* 1992;187:1551–1557.

Kerrison JB, Arnould VJ, Ferraz Sallum JM, et al. Genetic heterogeneity of dominant optic atrophy, Kjer type: identification of a second locus on chromosome 18q12.2-12.3. *Arch Ophthalmol* 1999;117:805–810.

Kerrison JB, Miller NR, Hsu F, et al. A case-control study of tobacco and alcohol consumption in Leber hereditary optic neuropathy. *Am J Ophthalmol* 2000;130:803–812.

Kjer P. Infantile optic atrophy with dominant mode of inheritance. In: Vinken PJ, Bruyn GW, eds. *Neuroretinal degenerations. Handbook of Clinical Neurology, vol 13.* New York: American Elsevier, 1972:111–123.

Kline LB, Glaser JS. Dominant optic atrophy: the clinical profile. *Arch Ophthalmol* 1979;97:1680–1686.

Leber TH. Über hereditäre und congenital-angelegte Sehnervenleiden. *Graefes Archiv Ophthalmol* 1871;17:249–291.

Man PYW, Griffiths PG, Brown DT, et al. The epidemiology of Leber hereditary optic neuropathy in the North East of England. *Am J Hum Genet* 2003;72:333–339.

Man PYW, Turnbull DM, Chinnery PF. Leber hereditary optic neuropathy. *J Med Genet* 2002;39:162–169.

McLeod JG, Low PA, Morgan JA. Charcot-Marie-Tooth disease with Leber optic atrophy. *Neurology* 1978;28:179–184.

Merritt HH. Hereditary optic atrophy (Leber's disease). *Arch Neurol Psychiatry* 1930;24:775–781.

Newman NJ. From genotype to phenotype in Leber hereditary optic neuropathy: still more questions than answers. *J Neuroophthalmol* 2002;22:257–261.

Newman NJ. Hereditary optic neuropathies. In: Miller NR, Newman NJ, eds. *Walsh and Hoyt's Clinical Neuro-Ophthalmology*, 5th ed. Baltimore: Williams & Wilkins, 1998:741–773.

Nikoskelainen EK. New aspects of the genetic, etiologic, and clinical puzzle of Leber's disease. *Neurology* 1984;34:1482–1484.

Nikoskelainen EK, Hoyt WF, Nummelin KU. Ophthalmoscopic findings in Leber's hereditary optic neuropathy. I. Fundus findings in asymptomatic family members. *Arch Ophthalmol* 1982;100:1597–1602.

Nikoskelainen EK, Hoyt WF, Nummelin KU. Ophthalmoscopic findings in Leber's hereditary optic neuropathy. II. The fundus findings in the affected family members. *Arch Ophthalmol* 1983;101:1059–1068.

Nikoskelainen EK, Hoyt WF, Nummelin KU, et al. Fundus findings in Leber's hereditary optic neuropathy. III. Fluorescein angiographic studies. *Arch Ophthalmol* 1984;102:981–989.

Nikoskelainen EK, Marttila RJ, Huoponen K, et al. Leber's "plus": neurological abnormalities in patients with Leber's hereditary optic neuropathy. *J Neurol Neurosurg Psychiatry* 1995;59:160–164.

Novotny EJ, Singh G, Wallace DC, et al. Leber's disease and dystonia: a mitochondrial disease. *Neurology* 1986;36:1053–1060.

Payne M, Yang Z, Katz BJ, et al. Dominant optic atrophy, sensorineural hearing loss, ptosis, and ophthalmoplegia; a syndrome caused by a missense mutation in OPA1. *Am J Opthal* 2004;138:749–755.

Phillips PH, Vaphiades M, Glasier CM, et al. Chiasmal enlargement and optic nerve enhancement on magnetic resonance imaging in leber hereditary optic neuropathy. *Arch Ophthalmol* 2003;121:577–579.

Pulkes T, Eunson L, Patterson V, et al. The mitochondrial DNA G13513A transition in ND5 is associated with a LHON/MELAS overlap syndrome and may be a frequent cause of MELAS. *Ann Neurol* 1999;46:916–919.

Scolding NJ, Keller-Wood HF, Shaw C, et al. Wolfram syndrome: hereditary diabetes mellitus with brainstem and optic atrophy. *Ann Neurol* 1996;39:352–360.

Shoffner JM, Brown MD, Stugard C, et al. Leber's hereditary optic neuropathy plus dystonia is caused by a mitochondrial DNA point mutation. *Ann Neurol* 1995;38:163–169.

Smith JL, Hoyt WF, Susac JO. Ocular fundus in acute Leber optic neuropathy. *Arch Ophthalmol* 1973;90:349–354.

Strom TM, Hortnagel K, Hofmann S, et al. Diabetes insipidus, diabetes mellitus, optic atrophy and deafness (DIDMOAD) caused by mutations in a novel gene (wolframin) coding for a predicted transmembrane protein. *Hum Mol Genet* 1998;7:2021–2028.

Vaphiades MS, Newman NJ. Optic nerve enhancement on orbital magnetic resonance imaging in Leber's hereditary optic neuropathy. *J Neuroophthalmol* 1999;19:238–239.

Von Graefe A. Ein ungewöhnlicher Fall von hereditären Amaurose. *Arch Ophthalmol* 1858;4:266–268.

Votruba M, Fitzke FW, Holder GE, et al. Clinical features in affected individuals from 21 pedigrees with dominant optic atrophy. *Arch Ophthalmol* 1998;116:351–358.

Wallace DC. A new manifestation of Leber's disease and a new explanation for the agency responsible for its unusual pattern of inheritance. *Brain* 1970;93:121–132.

Wallace DC, Singh G, Lott MT, et al. Mitochondrial DNA mutation associated with Leber's hereditary optic neuropathy. *Science* 1988;242:1427–1430.

C h a p t e r 9 9

Mitochondrial Diseases with Mutations of Nuclear DNA

Darryl C. De Vivo and Michio Hirano

The vast majority of polypeptides in mitochondria are encoded in nuclear deoxyribonucleic acid (nDNA); therefore, nDNA mutations are likely to be the cause of many mitochondrial diseases. Most of these disorders are autosomal recessive and lack ragged-red fibers (RRFs) or other structural abnormalities of mitochondria. Exceptions include defects of intergenomic signaling (see Chapter 98) and an X-linked form of pyruvate dehydrogenase deficiency. These diseases can be classified biochemically (Table 99.1) and are being defined at the molecular genetic level. As a rule, symptoms begin in infancy or childhood, when the metabolic demands of growth and development are the

▶ **TABLE 99.1** **Classification of Mitochondrial Diseases Associated with Mutations of Nuclear DNA**

Biochemical Abnormality	Clinical Example	MIM[a]
Substrate transport	Carnitine deficiency	212140
Substrate use	Pyruvate dehydrogenase deficiency	312170
Citric acid cycle	Fumarase deficiency	136850
Respiratory chain	Cytochrome *c* oxidase deficiency	220110
Oxidation-phosphorylation	Luft disease (molecular basis not known)	238800
Protein importation	Mohr-Tranebjaerg (deafness-dystonia) syndrome	304700
Intergenomic signaling	Depletion of mtDNA	251880
Membrane lipid milieu	Barth syndrome, coenzyme Q deficiency	302060
Mitochondrial motility	Spastic paraplegia 4	182601
Metal metabolism	Friedreich ataxia	229300

[a] MIM numbers are from McKusick VA. *Mendelian inheritance in man,* 12th ed. Baltimore: Johns Hopkins University Press, 1998.

greatest. Clinical manifestations may be tissue specific or generalized. Diagnosis depends on the clinical syndrome plus biochemical and DNA analyses.

DISORDERS OF SUBSTRATE TRANSPORT AND USE

Abnormalities of *fatty acid oxidation* provide examples of both substrate transport defects (e.g., carnitine disorders) and substrate use defects (e.g., abnormalities of *β*-oxidation). These conditions are discussed in Chapter 90.

Impaired fatty acid oxidation leads to periods of metabolic decompensation during fasting. Liver, myocardium, and limb muscle are particularly vulnerable; the brain is affected secondarily, a result of nonketotic hypoglycemia and increased fatty acid levels in serum. In infants, the disorder may mimic Reye syndrome (see Chapter 33) and may cause sudden infant death. The most common disorders of fatty acid metabolism are *medium-chain acyl-CoA dehydrogenase deficiency* and *carnitine palmitoyltransferase 2 deficiency* (DiMauro syndrome) usually manifesting as recurrent myoglobinuria.

Impaired substrate use is best illustrated by *pyruvate carboxylase deficiency,* which interferes with the synthesis of oxaloacetate. The syndrome includes congenital hypotonia, psychomotor retardation, failure to thrive, seizures, and metabolic acidosis. About 50% of all reported cases

have what is called the French phenotype, with lactic acidosis, citrullinemia, hyperlysinemia, and hyperammonemia. Aspartate depletion impairs urea cycle activity, and oxaloacetate depletion limits Krebs cycle activity. Ketoacidosis, a prominent metabolic feature, results from the accumulation of acetyl-CoA. A North American phenotype may seem less severe at first but is ultimately fatal in late infancy or early childhood. The two phenotypes parallel the amount of residual enzyme activity.

Deficiencies of *pyruvate dehydrogenase* (PDH) *complex* account for most cases of congenital lactic acidosis. The PDH complex comprises five enzymes encoded by at least nine nuclear genes. Most patients have an abnormality in the E1 *α* subunit with a gene mutation on the short arm of the X chromosome, which accounts for the male predominance. Female involvement is determined by the random pattern of inactivation of the X chromosome. The disorder may be symptomatic in the newborn period with hypotonia, convulsions, episodic apnea, weak sucking, dysmorphic features, low birth weight, failure to thrive, and coma. The distinctive neuropathology includes cystic degeneration of subcortical white matter, basal ganglia, and brainstem. Less common features include agenesis of the corpus callosum, ectopic olivary nuclei, hydrocephalus, optic atrophy, spongy degeneration, and other nonspecific abnormalities. A similar phenotype may become symptomatic later in life. In addition, girls and women may manifest as carriers with mental retardation and ataxia. In these milder forms, lactic acidosis may be minimal.

DISORDERS OF THE CITRIC ACID CYCLE

Congenital lactic acidosis can be a result of defects in enzymes of the Krebs cycle including: dihydrolipoyl dehydrogenase, *α*-ketoglutarate dehydrogenase, or fumarase. Symptoms begin at birth or in early infancy with failure to thrive, hypotonia, seizures, microcephaly, and optic atrophy. Diagnosis can be made by analysis of urinary organic acids, with patterns distinctive for each condition.

DISORDERS OF THE RESPIRATORY CHAIN

These conditions are another cause of congenital lactic acidosis. In contrast to the previously cited autosomal or X-linked conditions, respiratory enzyme disorders can result from mutations of either nDNA or mtDNA. Pathogenic mutations in nDNA-encoded structural subunits of complexes I and II have been identified, and RRFs are typically seen with severe infantile or childhood neurological disorders such as Leigh syndrome or leukoencephalopathy. Mutations in complex II subunits have also been associated with paragangliomas and pheochromocytomas. In contrast, autosomal deficiencies of complex III, IV, or V have not been linked to mutations in nDNA-encoded subunits, but rather to defects of nDNA genes encoding ancillary proteins required for enzyme assembly or insertion of cofactors. These disorders generally manifest as severe encephalopathies with variable involvement of visceral organs. For example, mutations in the complex IV or cytochrome *c* oxidase (COX) assembly factor, Sco2, cause a lethal autosomal recessive cardioencephalomyopathy. In addition, COX deficiency has been associated with a fatal infantile myopathy or a reversible infantile myopathy.

LEIGH SYNDROME

The most common form of complex IV (COX) deficiency is *subacute necrotizing encephalomyelopathy (Leigh syndrome)*. The condition was first described in 1951 in a 7-month-old infant who showed necrotizing lesions in the brainstem that resembled those of Wernicke encephalopathy. The lesions are found in the periaqueductal region of the midbrain and pons and in the medulla adjacent to the fourth ventricle (Table 99.2). Other parts of the central nervous system and peripheral nerves may also be affected. The lesions are a combination of cell necrosis, demyelination, and vascular proliferation. The topology and vascular lesions are distinctive (Fig. 99.1). Pathologically, the condition differs from Wernicke disease because the hypothalamus and mammillary bodies are spared in Leigh syndrome.

The condition may be inherited in an autosomal-recessive, X-linked, or maternal pattern. In adults, it is usu-

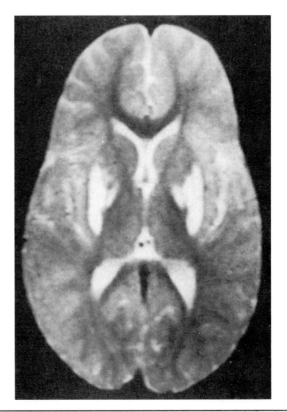

FIGURE 99.1. A 2-year-old girl with cytochrome *c* oxidase deficiency and Leigh syndrome. Heavily T2-weighted MRI shows prominent signal abnormality with bilaterally symmetric involvement of basal ganglia. Putamenal involvement is characteristic of Leigh syndrome.

ally sporadic. Infants may develop normally for months; others may show signs of encephalopathy in early infancy. Poor feeding, feeble crying, and respiratory difficulty may be early symptoms. These are followed by impaired vision and hearing, ataxia, limb weakness, intellectual deterioration, and seizures. Nystagmus is common. In patients with later onset, there may be progressive external ophthalmoplegia, dystonia, or ataxia. Once affected, the child may die in infancy or childhood; some live until adulthood.

Laboratory Abnormalities

CSF protein content is mildly elevated in 25% of patients. Lactate and pyruvate levels are almost always increased in CSF and, to a lesser degree, in blood and urine. These findings and the histopathology lead to a search for an abnormality of oxidative metabolism. EEG changes and abnormal evoked responses are nonspecific. CT may show symmetric lucencies in basal ganglia and the thalamus; the ventricles may be enlarged. MRI demonstrates the distinctive topography in detail (see Fig. 99.1).

▶ **TABLE 99.2 Comparison of Distribution of Brain Lesions in Subacute Necrotizing Encephalomyelopathy (SNE) and Wernicke Disease (WD)**

	SNE (%)	WD (%)
Brainstem	98	85
Midbrain	90	72
Tegmentum	78	—
Substantia nigra	62	5
Medulla	84	58
Spinal cord	74	33
Cerebellum	58	19
Cerebrum	92	97
Cortex	10	33
Basal ganglia	65	11
Thalamus	51	68
Hypothalamus	27	97

Pathogenesis

The biochemical lesions are diverse but impair cerebral oxidative metabolism. Affected enzymes include PDH, biotinidase, or complex I, II, IV, or IV (COX)V of the respiratory chain. In autosomally inherited cases, the mutations are in nDNA-encoded subunits of the enzymes; however, in COX-deficient Leigh syndrome, the first pathogenic mutations were identified in SURF1, a putative assembly or maintenance factor for COX. Point mutations of mtDNA, particularly the T8993G mutation in ATPase 6, have been associated with maternally inherited Leigh syndrome (see Chapter 98). There are no RRFs in any of these conditions. Leigh syndrome is usually fatal before age 1 year when associated with the neuropathy, ataxia, and retinitis pigmentosa (NARP) mutation or PDH complex deficiency.

ALPERS SYNDROME

In 1931, Bernard Alpers described an infant girl with progressive poliodystrophy. The disorder had anoxic features, but in retrospect some authorities have ascribed the changes to status epilepticus and hypoxia-ischemia. Later, Huttenlocher described an autosomal-recessive condition with the same neuropathology and hepatic cirrhosis. Depletion of mtDNA and pathogenic mutations in the mtDNA-encoded polymerase γ gene have been identified in some patients with Alpers syndrome.

IMPAIRED MITOCHONDRIAL TRANSPORT

Proteins encoded in nDNA and destined for mitochondria have targeting signals that are recognized by the mitochondrial importation system, which processes and directs the proteins to the proper compartment within the organelle. Mutations in these peptide signals have caused diseases owing to mistargeting of mitochondrial proteins to other cell compartments. In addition, mutations in the *TIMM8A* gene, which encodes one of the mitochondrial importation proteins, cause X-linked recessive deafness–dystonia syndrome (Mohr-Tranebjaerg syndrome) as well as opticoacoustic nerve atrophy with dementia (Jensen syndrome).

ABNORMAL MITOCHONDRIAL MEMBRANE MILIEU

Virtually all of the components of the respiratory chain are located within the inner mitochondrial membrane. Coenzyme Q10 is a vital mitochondrial constituent that shuttles electrons between complexes I and II to complex III, stabilizes membranes, and is an antioxidant. Primary *coen-*

zyme Q10 deficiency is presumed to be an autosomal recessive condition with a spectrum of syndromes ranging from mainly myopathy with recurrent myoglobinuria and RRF to prominent encephalomyopathy with severe ataxia and variable mental retardation and seizures. The disorder responds to replacement therapy. Another major component of the inner mitochondrial membrane is cardiolipin, an integral part of some respiratory-chain enzymes. Deficiency of cardiolipin has been observed in Barth syndrome, an X-linked mitochondrial myopathy, cardiomyopathy, leucopenia, and growth retardation. The disorder is caused by mutations in tafazzin, an acyl-coenzyme A synthetase, that contributes to cardiolipin synthesis.

DEFECTS OF MITOCHONDRIAL MOTILITY

Mitochondria are mobile organelles driven by energy-activated kinesins along microtubules within cells. Mitochondrial movement is also disrupted in the most common form of hereditary spastic paraparesis caused by mutations in spastin, a protein that is thought to sever microtubules. Another autosomal dominant hereditary spastic paraparesis is due to mutation in the neural kinesin heavy chain gene KIFSI.

DEFECTS OF METAL METABOLISM

Mitochondria contain numerous metalloenzymes; therefore, mitochondrial functions are susceptible to defects of metal metabolism. Friedreich ataxia (see Chapter 108) is a result of mutations (usually abnormal expansions of GAA trinucleotide repeats) in the gene encoding frataxin, a mitochondrial protein involved in iron homeostasis. Wilson disease (see Chapter 91) is a result of mutations in the ATP7B gene, which encodes a copper-transporting ATPase, one isoform of which is localized in mitochondria.

SUGGESTED READINGS

Alexander C, Votruba M, Pesch UE, et al. OPA1, encoding a dynamin-related GTPase, is mutated in autosomal dominant optic atrophy linked to chromosome 3q28. *Nat Genet* 2000;26:211–215.

Alpers BJ. Diffuse progressive degeneration of the grey matter of the cerebrum. *Arch Neurol Psychiatry* 1931;25:469–505.

Astuti D, Latif F, Dallol A, et al. Gene mutations in the succinate dehydrogenase subunit SDHB cause susceptibility to familial pheochromocytoma and to familial paraganglioma. *Am J Hum Genet* 2001;69:49–54.

Atkin BM, Buist NR, Utter MF, et al. Pyruvate carboxylase deficiency and lactic acidosis in a retarded child without Leigh's disease. *Pediatr Res* 1979;13:109–116.

Barth PG, Wanders RJ, Vreken P, et al. X-linked cardioskeletal myopathy and neutropenia (Barth syndrome) (MIM 302060). *J Inherit Metab Dis* 1999;22:555–567.

Baysal BE, Ferrell RE, Willett-Brozick JE, et al. Mutations in SDHD, a mitochondrial complex II gene, in hereditary paraganglioma. *Science* 2000;287:848–851.

Bourgeron T, Rustin P, Chretien D, et al. Mutation of a nuclear succinate dehydrogenase gene results in mitochondrial respiratory chain deficiency. *Nat Genet* 1995;11:144–149.

Delettre C, Lenaers G, Griffoin JM, et al. Nuclear gene OPA1, encoding a mitochondrial dynamin-related protein, is mutated in dominant optic atrophy. *Nat Genet* 2000;26:207–210.

de Lonlay P, Valnot I, Barrientos A, et al. A mutant mitochondrial respiratory chain assembly protein causes complex III deficiency in patients with tubulopathy, encephalopathy and liver failure. *Nat Genet* 2001;29:57–60.

De Meirleir L, Seneca S, Lissens W, et al. Respiratory chain complex V deficiency due to a mutation in the assembly gene ATP12. *J Med Genet* 2004;41:120–124.

De Vivo DC. Complexities of the pyruvate dehydrogenase complex. *Neurology* 1998;51:1247–1249.

De Vivo DC, Haymond MW, Leckie MP, et al. The clinical and biochemical implications of pyruvate carboxylase deficiency. *J Clin Endocrinol Metab* 1977;45:1281–1296.

De Vivo DC, Hirano M, DiMauro S. Mitochondrial disorders. In: Moser H, ed. *Neurodystrophies and neurolipidoses.* Amsterdam: Elsevier Science, 1997:389–446.

Di Donato S, Taroni F. Disorders of lipid metabolism. In: Rosenberg RN, Prusiner SB, DiMauro S, et al., eds. *The Molecular and Genetic Basis of Neurologic and Psychiatric Disease.* Philadelphia: Butterworth-Heinemann, 2003:591–601.

DiMauro S, Hirano M, Bonilla E, et al. *Cytochrome Oxidase Deficiency: Progress and Problems.* Oxford, UK: Butterworth-Heinemann, 1994;1:91–115.

DiMauro S, Schon EA. Mitochondrial respiratory-chain diseases. *N Engl J Med* 2003;348:2656–2668.

Feigin I, Wolf A. A disease in infants resembling chronic Wernicke's encephalopathy. *J Pediatr* 1954;45:243–263.

Fink JK. The hereditary spastic paraplegias: nine genes and counting. *Arch Neurol* 2003;60:1045–1049.

Gellera C, Uziel G, Rimoldi M, et al. Fumarase deficiency is an autosomal-recessive encephalopathy affecting both the mitochondrial and the cytosolic enzymes. *Neurology* 1990;40:495–499.

Harding BN. Progressive neuronal degeneration of childhood with liver disease (Alpers-Huttenlocher syndrome): a personal review. *J Child Neurol* 1990;5:273–289.

Lamperti C, Naini A, Hirano M, et al. Cerebellar ataxia and coenzyme Q10 deficiency. *Neurology* 2003;60:1206–1208.

Leigh D. Subacute necrotizing encephalomyelopathy in an infant. *J Neurol Neurosurg Psychiatry* 1951;14:216–221.

Lutsenko S, Cooper MJ. Localization of the Wilson's disease protein product to mitochondria. *Proc Natl Acad Sci U S A* 1998;95:6004–6009.

McDermott CJ, Grierson AJ, Wood JD, et al. Hereditary spastic paraparesis: disrupted intracellular transport associated with spastin mutation. *Ann Neurol* 2003;54:748–759.

McKusick VA. *Mendelian inheritance in man,* 12th ed. Baltimore: Johns Hopkins University Press, 1998.

Naviauk RK, Nguyen KV. POLG mutations associated with Alper's syndrome and mitochondrial DNA depletion. *Ann Neurol* 2004;55:706–712.

Ogasahara S, Engel AG, Frens D, Mack D. Muscle coenzyme Q deficiency in familial mitochondrial encephalomyopathy. *Proc Nat Acad Sci U S A* 1989;86:2379–2382.

Online Mendelian Inheritance in Man, OMIM(TM). Baltimore: Johns Hopkins University and Bethesda: National Center for Biotechnology Information, National Library of Medicine. World Wide Web URL: http://www.ncbi.nlm.nih.gov/omim/. Accessed 1/18/05

Pandolfo M. Friedreich ataxia. *Semin Pediatr Neurol* 2003;10:163–172.

Papadopoulou LC, Sue CM, Davidson MM, et al. Fatal infantile cardioencephalomyopathy with cytochrome *c* oxidase (COX) deficiency and mutations in *SCO2*, a human COX assembly gene. *Nature Genet* 1999;23:333–337.

Roesch K, Curran SP, Tranebjaerg L, et al. Human deafness dystonia syndrome is caused by a defect in assembly of the DDP1/TIMM8a-TIMM13 complex. *Hum Mol Genet* 2002;11:477–486.

Schlame M, Kelley RI, Feigenbaum A, et al. Phospholipid abnormalities in children with Barth syndrome. *J Am Coll Cardiol* 2003;42:1994–1999.

Stanley CA, De Leeuw S, Coates PA, et al. Chronic cardiomyopathy and weakness or acute coma in children with a defect in carnitine uptake. *Ann Neurol* 1991;30:709–716.

Sue CM, Karadimas C, Checcarelli N, et al. Differential features of patients with mutations in two COX assembly genes, SURF-1 and SCO2. *Ann Neurol* 2000;47:589–595.

Tiranti V, Hoertnagel K, Carrozzo R, et al. Mutations of SURF-1 in Leigh disease associated with cytochrome *c* oxidase deficiency. *Am J Hum Genet* 1998;63:1609–1621.

Van Coster R, Fernhoff PM, De Vivo DC. Pyruvate carboxylase deficiency: a benign variant with normal development. *Pediatr Res* 1991;30:1–4.

Vogel R, Nijtmans L, Ugalde C, et al. Complex I assembly: a puzzling problem. *Curr Opin Neurol* 2004;17:179–186.

Zhu S, Yao J, Johns T, et al. *SURF1*, encoding a factor involved in the biogenesis of cytochrome *c* oxidase, is mutated in Leigh syndrome. *Nat Genet* 1998;20:337–343.

Zinn AB, Kerr DS, Hoppel CL. Fumarase deficiency: a new cause of mitochondrial encephalomyopathy. *N Engl J Med* 1986;315:469–475.

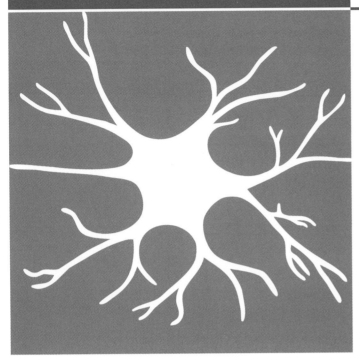

Neurocutaneous Disorders

Neurofibromatosis

Arnold P. Gold and
Marc C. Patterson

Several genetic diseases involve both the skin and nervous system. These are called *neurocutaneous disorders* or *neuroectodermatoses*. In the past, they were referred to as the "phakomatoses" (*phakos* is the Greek word for lentil, flat plate, or spot). Retinal lesions are seen in tuberous sclerosis and sometimes in neurofibromatosis. Other distinct disorders are Sturge-Weber-Dimitri syndrome, linear nevus sebaceous, and incontinentia pigmenti.

Any portion of the central and peripheral nervous system may be affected by these hereditary diseases, and different portions may be involved in various combinations. Some families breed true and show a remarkable consistency with regard to location and extent of the pathologic changes; other families demonstrate great discrepancies among individual members of the family. The clinical spectrum ranges from frequent abortive forms (*formes frustes*) to a severe, potentially lethal condition with highly protean clinical manifestations.

Neurofibromatosis (NF) was first described by von Recklinghausen in 1882; it is one of the most common single-gene disorders of the CNS. The two cardinal features are multiple hyperpigmented marks on the skin (*café au lait spots*) and multiple neurofibromas; other symptoms may result from lesions in bone, the CNS, the peripheral nervous system, or other organs. Two forms are recognized. Neurofibromatosis type 1 (NF-1) is also known as *von Recklinghausen disease* or *peripheral NF* (MIM 162200). It is one of the most common hereditary diseases, with a prevalence of 1 per 3,000 population. Neurofibromatosis type 2 (NF-2) is also known as *central NF* or *bilateral acoustic neuroma syndrome* (MIM 101000). The two conditions differ genetically, pathogenetically, and clinically.

Many of the clinical features, neurofibromas, and CNS lesions affect structures that originate in the neural crest. Other disorders include altered synthesis and secretion of melanin, disturbed cellular organization with hamartomatous collections, and abnormal production and distribution of nerve growth factors. In both syndromes, gene products seem to act as oncogenes.

GENETICS AND INCIDENCE

Both NF-1 and NF-2 are autosomal-dominant conditions; penetrance of NF-1 is almost 100%, but expressivity varies. Mutations are thought to account for 50% of new cases. Both sexes are affected equally, and the condition is found worldwide in all racial and ethnic groups. Incidence figures must be a minimal estimate because abortive cases are often unrecognized clinically.

MOLECULAR GENETICS AND PATHOGENESIS

The NF1 gene has been mapped to chromosome 17q11.2. The gene product is called neurofibromin. Because individuals with NF-1 are at increased risk for benign and malignant tumors, neurofibromin is considered a tumor-suppressor gene. Five different types of NF1 gene mutations are known: translocations, large megabase deletions, large internal deletions, small rearrangements, and point mutations. Although the genotypes differ, the phenotypes are indistinguishable. The marked clinical variability within families having an identical NF1 gene mutation equals the variability among families with different NF1 gene mutations. The only exception is the syndrome of large megabase deletions, in which affected people are typically mentally retarded. Mutation inactivates the gene, and, by analogy with other oncogenes, loss of the allelic gene later in life could result in tumor formation. It is not known, however, how the other manifestations of the disease arise. Neurofibromin is expressed in neurons, but it is not known why some affected people have neurologic disorders and others do not. Modifying genes in other locations may play a role. Differential expression of matrix metalloproteinase 13 (MMP13), platelet-derived growth factor receptor alpha (PDGFRA), and fibronectin (FN1) has been reported in neurofibromas and malignant peripheral nerve sheath tumors, suggesting these genes as potential NF1 modifiers.

The NF2 gene maps to chromosome 22q12. The gene product is similar to that of the moezin-ezrin-radixin-like protein gene; for this reason, it is called *merlin*. Deletions of the gene have been found in schwannoma and meningioma cells, the major tumors in NF-2 patients. NF2 inhibits the Rac/CDC42-dependent Ser/Thr kinase PAK1, which activates both Ras transformation and neurofibromatosis type 1 (NF-1), through two separate domains. Specific inhibitors of PAK1 selectively inhibit the growth of NF2-deficient cancer cells, suggesting that PAK1 is essential for the malignant growth of NF2-deficient cells. Inhibitors of PAK1 might have a future role as therapies for these tumors.

NEUROPATHOLOGY

The neuropathologic changes result from changes in neural supporting tissue with resultant dysplasia, hyperplasia, and neoplasia. These pathologic changes may involve the central, peripheral, and autonomic nervous systems. Visceral manifestations result from hyperplasia of the autonomic ganglia and nerves within the organ. In addition to neural lesions, dysplastic and neoplastic changes affect skin, bone, endocrine glands, and blood vessels. Developmental anomalies include thoracic meningocele and syringomyelia. Patients affected by NF are more likely than others to have neoplastic disorders, including neuroblastoma, Wilms tumor, leukemia, pheochromocytoma, and sarcomas.

Neoplasms involving the peripheral nervous system and spinal nerve roots include schwannomas and neurofibromas. Intramedullary spinal cord tumors include ependymomas (especially of the conus medullaris and filum terminale) and, less often, astrocytomas. The most common intracranial tumors are hemispheral astrocytomas of any histologic grade from benign to highly malignant. Pilocytic astrocytic gliomas of the optic nerve and optic chiasm are also characteristic. Bilateral acoustic neuromas and solitary or multicentric meningiomas commonly occur in adults with NF-2.

SYMPTOMS AND SIGNS

There are at least four forms of NF. *Peripheral NF* (NF-1) as described by von Recklinghausen is most commonly encountered. *Central NF* (NF-2) is manifest by bilateral acoustic neuromas at about age 20 years. Cutaneous changes are mild, and there are only a few café au lait spots or neurofibromas. Antigenic activity of nerve growth

factor is increased. *Segmental NF* probably arises from a somatic cell mutation; it is characterized by café au lait spots and neurofibromas that are limited, usually affecting an upper body segment. The lesions extend to the midline and include the ipsilateral arm but spare the head and neck. *Cutaneous NF* is limited to pigmentary changes; there are numerous café au lait spots but no other clinical manifestations.

NF-1 has protean and progressive manifestations. Not uncommonly, once the diagnosis is established, a fate like that of the grotesque Joseph Merrick (the Elephant Man, who almost certainly had the Proteus syndrome, not NF-1) is anticipated by parents or physicians. In reality, many patients with this disease are functionally indistinguishable from normal. Often, they have only cutaneous lesions and are diagnosed when they see a physician because of a learning disability, scoliosis, or another problem.

Cutaneous Symptoms

The café au lait macule is the pathognomonic lesion, being present in almost all patients (Fig. 100.1). Six or more café au lait spots larger than 5 mm in diameter before puberty and greater than 15 mm in diameter after puberty are diagnostic. The spots are usually present at birth but may not appear until age 1 or 2 years. Increasing in both size and number during the first decade of life, the macules tend to be less evident after the second decade because they blend into the surrounding hyperpigmented skin. These discrete, tan macules involve the trunk and limbs in a random fashion but tend to spare the face.

Other cutaneous manifestations may include freckles over the entire body, but freckles usually involve the axilla and other intertriginous areas. Larger, darker hyperpigmented lesions are often associated with an underlying plexiform neurofibroma (Fig. 100.2); if this involves the midline, it may indicate the presence of a spinal cord tumor.

Ocular Symptoms

Pigmented iris hamartomas (*Lisch nodules*), when present, are pathognomonic and consist of small translucent yellow or brown elevations on slit lamp examination. The nodules increase in number with age and are present in almost all patients older than 20 years. They are observed only in NF-1 and are not seen in the normal eye.

Neurologic Symptoms

Neurofibromas are highly characteristic lesions and usually become clinically evident at ages 10 to 15 years. They always involve the skin, ultimately developing into sessile, pedunculated lesions. The nodules are found on deep peripheral nerves or nerve roots and on the autonomic

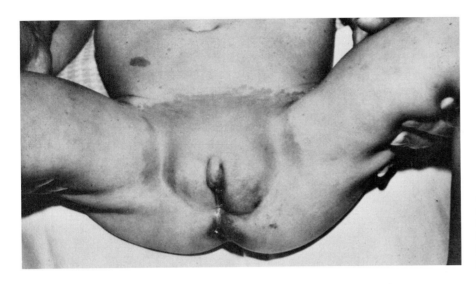

FIGURE 100.1. Neurofibromatosis. Café au lait macule (abdomen) and larger pigmented lesion in the perineal area associated with an underlying plexiform neuroma and elephantiasis of the left labia.

nerves that innervate the viscera and blood vessels. The lesions increase in size and number during the second and third decades. There may be a few or many thousands. These benign tumors consist of neurons, Schwann cells, fibroblasts, blood vessels, and mast cells. They rarely give rise to any symptoms other than pain as a result of pressure on nerves or nerve roots, but may undergo sarcomatous degeneration in the third and fourth decades of life (Fig. 100.3) Neurofibromas involving the terminal distribution of peripheral nerves form vascular plexiform neurofibromas that result in localized overgrowth of tissues or segmental hypertrophy of a limb (*elephantiasis neuromatosa*). Spinal root or cauda equina neurofibromas are often asymptomatic when they are small, but large tumors may compress the spinal cord, causing the appropriate clinical signs.

Optic gliomas, astrocytomas, acoustic neuromas, neurilemmomas, and meningiomas have a combined frequency of 5% to 10% in all patients with NF. Optic nerve gliomas and other intracranial neoplasms are often evident

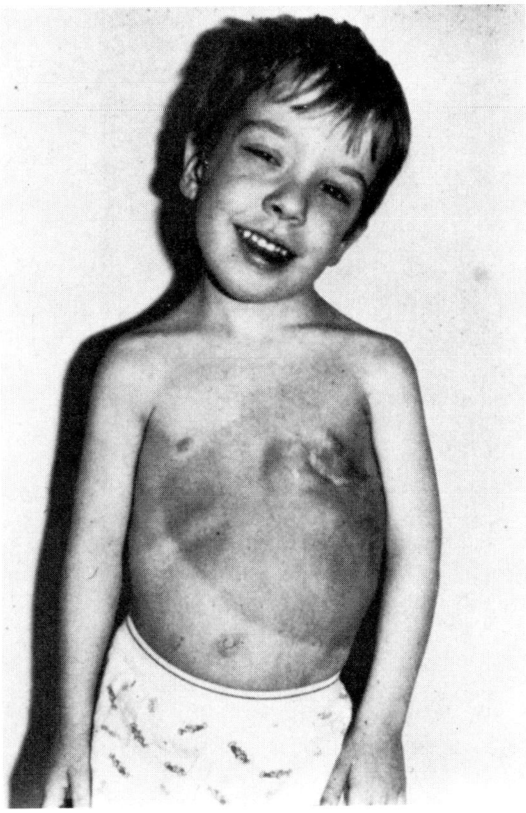

FIGURE 100.2. Neurofibromatosis. Large pigmented lesion with associated progressive scoliosis.

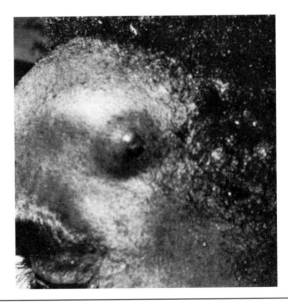

FIGURE 100.3. Neurofibromatosis. Sarcomatous degeneration of a neurofibroma at 35 years.

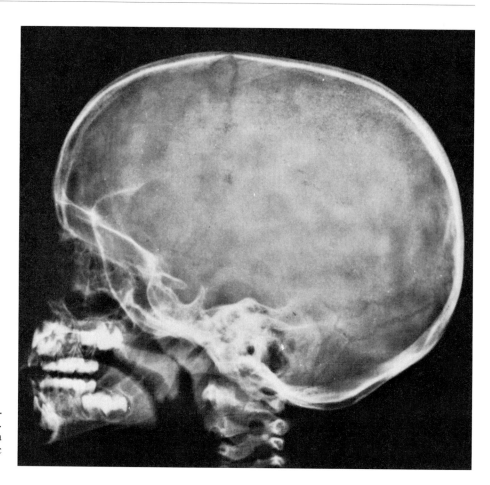

FIGURE 100.4. Neurofibromatosis. Lateral skull radiograph shows a J-shaped sella secondary to an optic chiasm glioma.

before age 10; acoustic neuromas become symptomatic at about age 20. When optic glioma is associated with NF, it commonly involves the optic nerve or is multicentric; less frequently, it involves the chiasm (Figs. 100.4 and 100.5). Optic nerve glioma must be distinguished from the commonly observed non-neoplastic optic nerve hyperplasia. The optic glioma of NF is slowly progressive and has a better prognosis than similar tumors without this association.

NF-2 is clinically evident at about age 20; symptoms include hearing loss, tinnitus, imbalance, and headache. Only a few café au lait spots and neurofibromas are seen. Intracranial and intraspinal neoplasms include meningiomas, schwannomas, and gliomas.

CNS involvement in NF is highly variable. Macrocephaly, a common clinical manifestation of postnatal origin, is an incidental finding with no correlation with academic performance, seizures, or neurologic function. Specific learning disabilities or attention deficit disorder, with or without impaired speech, is the most common neurologic complication of NF. Intellectual retardation or convulsive disorders each occur in about 5% of the patients. Brainstem tumors associated with NF-1 have a more indolent course than those without NF.

Occlusive cerebrovascular disease is rare but is sometimes seen in children, resulting in acute hemiplegia and convulsions. MRA or conventional angiography may demonstrate occlusion of the supraclinoid portion of the internal carotid artery at the origin of the anterior and middle cerebral arteries with associated telangiectasia (moyamoya disease).

Symptoms of the Skull, Spine, and Limbs

Skeletal anomalies characteristic of NF include (1) unilateral defects in the posterosuperior wall of the orbit, with pulsating exophthalmos; (2) a defect in the lambdoid with underdevelopment of the ipsilateral mastoid; (3) dural ectasia with enlargement of the spinal canal and scalloping of the posterior portions of the vertebral bodies (also seen in connective tissue disorders such as Marfan and Ehlers-Danlos syndromes); (4) kyphoscoliosis, seen in 2% to 10% of patients with NF, most commonly involving the cervicothoracic vertebrae; unless corrected, it can be rapidly progressive, characterized by a short-segment angular scoliosis that typically involves the lower thoracic vertebrae; (5) pseudarthrosis, especially involving the tibia and

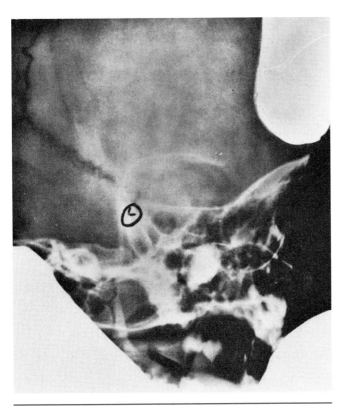

FIGURE 100.5. Neurofibromatosis. Optic canal view shows an enlarged optic foramen secondary to an optic nerve glioma.

radius; (6) "twisted ribbon" rib deformities; and (7) enlargement of long bones.

Miscellaneous Symptoms

Pheochromocytoma, an unusual complication of NF, is never seen in children. Hypertension may be due to a pheochromocytoma or a neurofibroma of a renal artery. Malignant tumors not uncommonly complicating NF include sarcoma, leukemia, Wilms tumor, ganglioglioma, and neuroblastoma. Medullary thyroid carcinoma and hyperparathyroidism rarely occur. Precocious puberty and, less commonly, sexual infantilism result from involvement of the hypothalamus by glioma or hamartoma. Cystic lesions, malignancy, and interstitial pneumonia are pulmonary complications.

DIAGNOSIS

Diagnosis of NF-1 or NF-2 is based on clinical, radiologic, and pathologic findings, as well as the family history. Diagnostic criteria have been established by the National Institutes of Health Consensus Conference (Table 100.1).

▶ **TABLE 100.1 Diagnostic Criteria for Neurofibromatosis**

Neurofibromatosis 1 (any two or more)
Six or more café au lait macules
Before puberty >5 mm diameter
After puberty >15 mm diameter
Freckling in the axillary or inguinal areas
Two or more neurofibromas or one plexiform neurofibroma
A first-degree relative with NF-1
Two or more Lisch nodules (iris hamartomas)
Bone lesion
Sphenoid dysplasia
Thinning of the cortex of long bones with or without pseudarthrosis

Neurofibromatosis 2
Bilateral eighth nerve tumor (MRI, CT, or histologic confirmation)
A first-degree relative with NF-2 and a unilateral eighth nerve tumor
A first-degree relative with NF-2 and any two of the following:
Neurofibroma, meningioma, schwannoma, glioma, or juvenile
    posterior subcapsular lenticular opacity

Modified from Conference statement, National Institutes of Health consensus development conference: neurofibromatosis. *Arch Neurol* 1988;45:575–578.

LABORATORY DATA

Molecular genetic studies are now available but are not always specific or diagnostic. Therefore, all patients and those at risk should receive an extensive clinical evaluation aimed at diagnosis and identification of possible complications. Ancillary laboratory studies, however, should be individualized, determined by the clinical manifestations. Complete evaluation may include psychoeducational and psychometric testing; electroencephalogram; ophthalmologic and audiologic testing; cranial CT, including orbital views; CT of the spine and internal auditory foramina; MRI of brain and spine; and quantitative measurement of 24-hour urinary catecholamines.

Focal areas of high signal intensity on T2-weighted MR images correlate with fine motor and cognitive skills in children with NF-1.

TREATMENT

There is no specific treatment for NF, but complications may be ameliorated with early recognition and prompt therapeutic intervention. Learning disabilities should be considered in all children with NF and may be complicated by behavioral problems (hyperkinesis or attention deficit disorder) that warrant educational therapy or behavioral modification, psychotherapy, and pharmacotherapy. Speech problems require a language evaluation and formal speech therapy, and seizures indicate the need for anticonvulsant medication. Progressive kyphoscoliosis usually requires surgical intervention. Surgery may be necessary for removal of pheochromocytomas and intracranial or spinal neoplasms; cutaneous neurofibromas require extirpation when they compromise function or are disfiguring. Preliminary data suggest that thalidomide might have a role in treating neurofibromas. Radiation therapy is reserved for some CNS neoplasms, including optic glioma. Genetic counseling and psychotherapy with family counseling are important.

SUGGESTED READINGS

Arun D, Gutmann DH. Recent advances in neurofibromatosis type 1. *Curr Op Neurol* 2004;17:101–105.

Cohen MM Jr. Further diagnostic thoughts about the Elephant Man. *Am J Med Genet* 1988;29:777–782.

Crowe FW, Schull WJ, Neel JV. *A Clinical, Pathological and Genetic Study of Multiple Neurofibromatosis*. Springfield, IL: Charles C Thomas, 1956.

Easton DF, Ponder MA, Huson SM, et al. Analysis of variation in expression of neurofibromatosis (NF1): evidence for modifying genes. *Am J Hum Genet* 1993;53:305–313.

Es SV, North KN, McHugh K, et al. MRI findings in children with neurofibromatosis type I: a prospective study. *Pediatr Radiol* 1996:26;478–487.

Evans DGR, Huson SM, Donnai D, et al. A genetic study of type 2 neurofibromatosis in the United Kingdom. II. Guidelines for genetic counseling. *J Med Genet* 1992;29:847–852.

Feldmann R, Denecke J, Grenzebach M, et al. Neurofibromatosis type 1: motor and cognitive function and T2-weighted MRI hyperintensities. *Neurology* 2003;61:1725–1728.

Gupta A, Cohen BH, Ruggieri P, et al. Phase I study of thalidomide for the treatment of plexiform neurofibroma in neurofibromatosis 1. *Neurology* 2003;60(Jan 14):130–132.

Gutmann DH. Recent insights into neurofibromatosis type 1: clear genetic progress. *Arch Neurol* 1998;55:778–780.

Gutmann DH, Collins FS. The neurofibromatosis type 1 gene and its protein product, neurofibromin. *Neuron* 1993;10:335–343.

Hirokawa Y, Tikoo A, Huynh J, et al. A clue to the therapy of neurofibromatosis type 2: NF2/merlin is a PAK1 inhibitor. *Cancer J* 2004;10 (Jan-Feb):20–26.

Holtkamp N, Mautner VF, Friedrich RE, et al. Differentially expressed genes in neurofibromatosis 1-associated neurofibromas and malignant peripheral nerve sheath tumors. *Acta Neuropathol (Berl)* 2004;107(Feb):159–168.

Karmes PS. Neurofibromatosis: a common neurocutaneous disorder. *Mayo Clin Proc* 1998;73:1071–1076.

Korf BR. Neurocutaneous syndromes: neurofibromatosis 1, neurofibromatosis 2, and tuberous sclerosis. *Curr Opin Neurol* 1997;10:131–136.

Levinsohn PM, Mikahel MA, Rothman SM. Cerebrovascular changes in neurofibromatosis. *Dev Med Child Neurol* 1978;20:789–792.

Listernick R, Louis DN, Packer RJ, et al. Optic pathway gliomas in neurofibromatosis I. Optic Pathway Glioma Taskforce. *Ann Neurol* 1997;41:143–149.

Mulvihill JJ, Pavory DM, Sherman JL, et al. Neurofibromatosis 1 (Recklinghausen disease) and neurofibromatosis 2 (bilateral acoustic neurofibromatosis): an update. *Ann Intern Med* 1990;113:39–52.

Neurofibromatosis. Conference Statement. National Institutes of Health Consensus Development Conference. *Arch Neurol* 1988;45:575–578.

North K. *Neurofibromatosis Type 1 in Childhood*. London: MacKeith, 1997.

Riccardi VM. *Neurofibromatosis: Phenotype, Natural History, and Pathogenesis*. 2nd Ed. Baltimore: Johns Hopkins University Press, 1992.

Romanowski CA, Cavallin LI. Neurofibromatosis types I and II: radiological appearance. *Hosp Med* 1998;59:134–139.

Smirniotopoulos JG, Murphy FM. The phakomatoses: neurofibromatosis. *AJNR* 1992;13:737–744.

Stern HJ, Saal HM, Lee JS, et al. Clinical variability of type 1 neurofibromatosis: is there a neurofibromatosis-Noonan syndrome? *J Med Genet* 1992;29:184–187.

Tibbles JAR, Cohen MM. The proteus syndrome: the Elephant Man diagnosed. *BMJ* 1986;293:683–685.

Trofatter JA, MacCollin MM, Rutter JL, et al. A novel moesin-, ezrin-, radixin-like gene is a candidate for neurofibromatosis 2 tumor suppressor. *Cell* 1993;72:1–20.

Upadhyaya M, Han S, Consoli C, et al. Characterization of the somatic mutational spectrum of the neurofibromatosis type 1 (NF1) gene in neurofibromatosis patients with benign and malignant tumors. *Hum Mutat* 2004;23(Feb):134–146.

Chapter 101

Encephalotrigeminal Angiomatosis

Arnold P. Gold and Marc C. Patterson

Encephalotrigeminal angiomatosis (*Sturge-Weber-Dimitri syndrome*; MIM 185300) is manifested by a cutaneous vascular port-wine nevus of the face, contralateral hemiparesis and hemiatrophy, glaucoma, seizures, and mental retardation. In 1847, Sturge described the clinical picture and attributed the neurologic manifestations to a nevoid lesion of the brain similar to the facial lesion. In 1923, Dimitri showed the gyriform pattern of calcification. Weber described the radiographic findings of intracranial calcification. Encephalotrigeminal angiomatosis is attributed to partial persistence of a primitive embryonal vascular plexus that develops around the cephalic portion of the neural tube 6 weeks after conception and under the ectoderm in the region destined to become facial skin. In encephalotrigeminal angiomatosis, the vascular plexus persists beyond the ninth week, when it normally regresses. Variability in this process accounts for unilateral or bilateral involvement, and also for an incomplete syndrome characterized by leptomeningeal angiomatosis without facial involvement.

GENETICS

Most cases are sporadic, but affected siblings suggest autosomal-recessive inheritance in some families. Other cases suggest an autosomal-dominant pattern. Although no consistent genetic locus is known, mutations in RASA1, whose gene product is involved in multiple signaling pathways, have been described in families with both atypical capillary malformations and encephalotrigeminal angiomatosis. This gene may be a susceptibility factor.

NEUROPATHOLOGY

The occipital lobe is most often affected, but lesions may involve the temporal and parietal lobes or the entire cerebral hemisphere. Atrophy is characteristically unilateral and ipsilateral to the facial nevus. Leptomeningeal angiomatosis with small venules fills the subarachnoid space. Calcification of the arteries on the surface of the brain and intracerebral calcifications of small vessels are seen. The trolley-track or curvilinear calcifications seen on skull radiographs are due to calcification of the outer cortex rather than of blood vessels.

SYMPTOMS AND SIGNS

Facial nevus and a neurologic syndrome of seizures, hemiplegia, retardation, and glaucoma are characteristic. Typically, other than the facial nevus, the child has normal function for months or years. The subsequent clinical course is highly variable; a clinical classification was proposed by Roach (Table 101.1).

Cutaneous Symptoms

The port-wine facial nevus flammeus is related to the cutaneous distribution of the trigeminal nerve (Fig. 101.1). Most commonly involving the forehead, the nevus may involve one-half of the face and may extend to the neck. The nevus may cross or fall short of the midline. Rarely, bilateral facial lesions are seen.

Only when the entire ophthalmic sensory area (forehead and upper eyelid) is covered by the nevus flam-

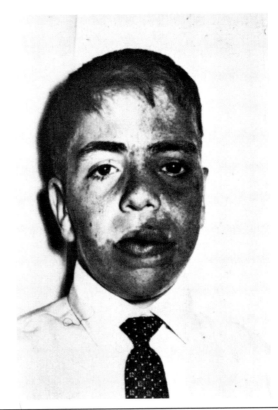

FIGURE 101.1. Encephalotrigeminal angiomatosis. Facial nevus flammeus involves the cutaneous distribution of all three branches of the trigeminal nerve on one side and the mandibular branch on the contralateral side.

meus (with or without involvement of the maxillary and mandibular areas) is there a high risk of glaucoma or neurologic complications. Neuro-ocular disease is rare when only part of the ophthalmic area has a port-wine stain. There is little or no risk when the nevus is localized to the maxillary or mandibular trigeminal sensory areas without involving the ophthalmic area.

Neurologic Symptoms

Epilepsy is the most common neurologic manifestation, usually starting in the first year of life with focal motor, generalized major motor, or partial complex convulsions. Often refractory to anticonvulsants, the focal motor seizures, hemiparesis, and hemiatrophy are contralateral to the facial nevus. Onset of seizures before age 2 years and refractory epilepsy have prognostic significance; these patients are more likely to be intellectually impaired. Intellectual retardation often becomes more marked with age.

Ophthalmologic Symptoms

Raised intraocular pressure with glaucoma and buphthalmos occurs in approximately 30% of patients. Buphthalmos, which is more common than glaucoma, is a

▶ **TABLE 101.1 Encephalofacial Angiomatosis**

Type 1	Both facial and leptomeningeal angiomas; may have glaucoma (Sturge-Weber syndrome)
	Intracranial angioma should be documented histologically or by typical radiographic findings
	Epileptic seizures or EEG findings permit presumptive diagnosis in a child with typical nevus
Type 2	Facial angioma but no evidence of intracranial disease; may have glaucoma
Type 3	Leptomeningeal angioma but no facial nevus; may have glaucoma

Modified from Roach, 1992.

result of antenatal intraocular hypertension. Homonymous hemianopia, a common visual-field complication, is invariable when the occipital lobe is affected. Other congenital anomalies include coloboma of the iris and deformity of the lens.

LABORATORY DATA

The highly characteristic calcifications are rarely seen on radiographs before age 2 years (Fig. 101.2). They appear as paired (trolley-track) curvilinear lines that follow the cerebral convolutions. Cerebral atrophy may be implied by asymmetry of the calvarium, with elevated petrous pyramid, thickening of the calvarial diploë, and enlargement of the paranasal sinuses and mastoid air cells on the side of the lesion. CT documents the intracranial calcification and unilateral cerebral atrophy (Fig. 101.3). MRI with contrast enhanced FLAIR sequences is the most sensitive noninvasive technique to identify leptomeningeal disease. FDG-PET studies are helpful in predicting seizure control and cognitive outcome. Cerebral angiography may demonstrate capillary and venous abnormalities. The capillaries over the affected hemisphere are homogeneously increased, the superficial cortical veins are markedly decreased, and the superior sagittal sinus may be diminished or not seen.

EEG shows a wide area of low potentials over the affected areas, and this electrical silence correlates with the degree of intracranial calcification. The remainder of the hemisphere may show epileptiform activity. Visual-field studies document the homonymous hemianopia.

DIAGNOSIS

The diagnosis is based on the facial vascular portwine nevus flammeus and one or more of the following: seizures, contralateral hemiparesis and hemiatrophy, mental retardation, and ocular findings of glaucoma or buphthalmos. The appearance of calcifications on skull radiographs or CT reinforces the diagnosis. Rarely, Sturge-Weber-Dimitri syndrome may occur with the neurologic syndrome and the typical intracranial calcifications but without the facial nevus. Encephalotrigeminal angiomatosis must be distinguished from other vascular malformation syndromes, including Klippel-Trenaunay and Parkes Weber syndrome, both of which feature combined vascular malformations, in contrast to the pure capillary lesions of encephalotrigeminal angiomatosis. Cohen proposes detailed criteria to separate these disorders.

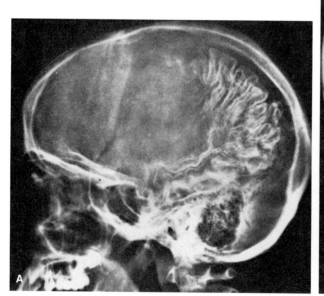
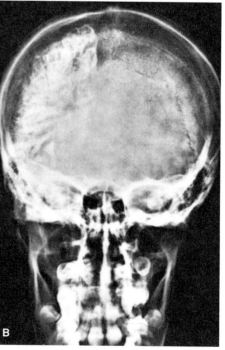

FIGURE 101.2. Encephalotrigeminal angiomatosis. **A.** Lateral skull radiograph shows characteristic calcifications consisting of paired curvilinear lines localized mostly to the occipital and parietal lobes. **B.** Posteroanterior view shows calcifications outlining an atrophic right cerebral hemisphere.

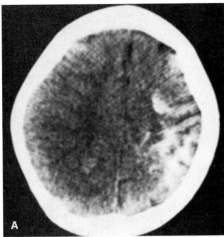

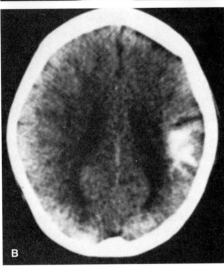

FIGURE 101.3. Noncontrast CT shows subcortical calcification conforming to the gyral pattern of calcification in the Sturge-Weber-Dimitri syndrome. (Courtesy of Dr. S. K. Hilal and Dr. M. Mawad.)

TREATMENT

The facial nevus rarely requires early cosmetic therapy. Later, this blemish can be covered with cosmetics or permanently treated with laser therapy. Seizures may be difficult to control with anticonvulsants. Children with medically intractable seizures often respond to hemispherectomy, even when surgery is delayed. Physical and occupational therapy are indicated for the hemiparesis. Educational therapy and placement in a special school are important in the learning-disabled or intellectually impaired patient; vocational training is essential in affected older children and young adults. Behavioral problems are common and may include attention deficit disorder or overt psychopathology that warrants psychotropic drug therapy and psychotherapy. Prophylactic daily low-dose aspirin to prevent venous thrombosis is controversial but can be considered if there are recurrent TIAs. Yearly monitoring for glaucoma is recommended for all patients and, if present, should be treated aggressively.

SUGGESTED READINGS

Aicardi J, Arzimanoglou A. Sturge-Weber syndrome. *Int Pediatr* 1991; 6:129–134.

Alexander GL. Sturge-Weber syndrome. In: Vinken PJ, Bruyn GW, eds. *The phakomatoses. Handbook of clinical neurology, vol 14.* New York: American Elsevier, 1972:223–240.

Eerola I, Boon LM, Mulliken JB, et al. Capillary malformation-arteriovenous malformation, a new clinical and genetic disorder caused by RASA1 mutations. *Am J Hum Genet* 2003;73:1240–1249.

Feller L, Lemmer J. Encephalotrigeminal angiomatosis. *SADJ* 2003; 58(Oct):370–373.

Griffiths PD, Coley SC, Romanowski CA, et al. Contrast-enhanced fluid-attenuated inversion recovery imaging for leptomeningeal disease in children. *AJNR Am J Neuroradiol* 2003;24:719–723.

Kossoff EH, Buck C, Freeman JM. Outcomes of 32 hemispherectomies for Sturge-Weber syndrome worldwide. *Neurology* 2002;59:1735–1738.

Lee JS, Asano E, Muzik O, et al. Sturge-Weber syndrome: correlation between clinical course and FDG PET findings. *Neurology* 2001;57 (Jul 24):189–195.

Roach ES. Encephalofacial angiomatosis. *Pediatr Clin North Am* 1992; 39:606–613.

Sturge WA. A case of partial epilepsy, apparently due to a lesion of one of the vaso-motor centres of the brain. *Trans Clin Soc Lond* 1879;12:162–167.

Sujansky E, Conradi S. Outcome of Sturge-Weber syndrome in 52 adults. *Am J Med Genet* 1995;57:35–45.

Sujansky E, Conradi S. Sturge-Weber syndrome: age of onset of seizures and glaucoma and the prognosis for affected children. *J Child Neurol* 1995;10:49–53.

Tallman B, Tan OT, Morelli JG, et al. Location of port-wine stains and the likelihood of ophthalmic and/or central nervous system complications. *Pediatrics* 1991;87:323–327.

Vogl J, Stemmler J, Bergman C, et al. MRI and MR angiography of Sturge-Weber syndrome. *AJNR* 1993;14:417–425.

Weber FP. Right-sided hemi-hypertrophy resulting from right-sided congenital spastic hemiplegia, with a morbid condition of the left side of the brain, revealed by radiograms. *J Neurol Psychopathol* 1922;3:134–139.

Chapter 102

Incontinentia Pigmenti

Arnold P. Gold and Marc C. Patterson

INCONTINENTIA PIGMENTI

Incontinentia pigmenti (IP; MIM 308300), described by Bloch and Sulzberger, is a genetic disorder affecting the skin in a characteristic manner and also involving the brain, eyes, nails, and hair.

Genetics

IP is an X-linked dominant condition that is lethal in males. Mutations in the NEMO/IKKγ gene at Xq28 cause the disease. NEMO/IKKγ is an essential component of the newly discovered nuclear factor κB (NF-κB) signaling pathway. When activated, NF-κB controls the expression of multiple genes, including cytokines and chemokines, and protects cells against apoptosis. NEMO/IKKγ deficiency causes the phenotypical expression of the disease via the NF-κB pathway.

Sporadic disease has also appeared in girls with no family history of the disease. In these cases, there is a translocation with a breakpoint at Xp11.21. Some patients and some families do not map to either site, so there must be *locus heterogeneity*, with still more gene loci to be discovered.

Incontinentia pigmenti achromians (IPA, hypomelanosis of Ito; MIM 146150) resembles IP in that the pigmentary changes respect the lines of Blaschko, but is otherwise an unrelated syndrome. A pregnant woman with incontinentia pigmenti runs a 25% risk of a spontaneous miscarriage (the affected male); 50% of her female children will be affected and will have the disease. Daughters are likely to be more severely affected than their mothers.

Neuropathology

The neuropathologic findings are nonspecific and include cerebral atrophy with microgyria, focal necrosis with formation of small cavities in the central white matter, and focal areas of neuronal loss in the cerebellar cortex.

Symptoms and Signs

Cutaneous Symptoms

One half of affected infants have the initial linear vesicobullous lesions at birth, and most of the remaining children show the lesions in the first 2 weeks of life. About 10% are delayed, appearing as late as age 1 year. The skin lesions can recur and ultimately may undergo a characteristic change to linear verrucous and dyskeratotic growth, usually between the second and sixth weeks of life; pigmentary changes appear between 12 and 26 weeks. Some infants may show the pigmentary lesions at birth without further cutaneous progression. The pigmentation involves the trunk and extremities, is slate gray-blue or brown, and is distributed in irregular marbled or wavy lines. With age, the pigmentary lesions fade and become depigmented with atrophic skin changes.

Neurologic, Ophthalmic, and Other Symptoms

About 20% of affected children have a neurologic syndrome that may include slow motor development; pyramidal tract dysfunction with spastic hemiparesis, quadriparesis, or diplegia; mental retardation; and convulsive disorders.

Strabismus, cataracts, and severe visual loss occur in about 20% of affected children. Retinal vascular changes may result in blindness with ectasia, microhemorrhages, avascularity, and later, retinal pigmentation and atrophy.

Partial or total anodontia and peg-shaped teeth are characteristic of incontinentia pigmenti. Partial or complete diffuse alopecia with scarring and nail dystrophy may also occur.

Laboratory Data

Eosinophilia as high as 65% is often seen in infants younger than 1 year, together with an associated leukocytosis. Eosinophils are also found in the vesicobullous lesions and in affected dermis.

Treatment

There is no specific treatment for incontinentia pigmenti, and management is directed at complicating problems, such as anticonvulsants for seizures. Awareness of the ocular manifestations is essential because laser coagulation in retinal ectasia prevents blindness.

INCONTINENTIA PIGMENTI ACHROMIANS (IPA, HYPOMELANOSIS OF ITO)

IPA is a syndrome of regions of cutaneous hypopigmentation that conform to the lines of Blaschko. It is associated with variable involvement of other body systems, particularly the nervous system.

Etiology

The pathogenesis of this disease is similar to that of other neurocutaneous disorders. Migration of neural cells to the brain and melanoblasts to the skin from the neural crest occurs between 3 and 6 months' gestational age. A disturbance of this migration results in both brain and cutaneous pigmentary disease.

Genetics

Incontinentia pigmenti achromians is found in all races and sexes and is a syndrome with multiple etiologies.

The lines of Blaschko, first described by the German dermatologist in 1901, define the cutaneous distribution of many hereditary dermatoses and acquired inflammatory disorders. The pattern is believed to result from functional autosomal mosaicism transmittable through the action of retrotransposons. Most cases of IPA with an identifiable cause are associated with somatic mosaicism for chromosomal trisomies. Families with IPA have been reported linked to Xp11, but most cases are sporadic.

Clinical Manifestations

In infancy, hypopigmented skin lesions appear as whorls or streaks that follow the lines of Blaschko (Fig. 102.1). This lesion is the negative image of incontinentia pigmenti. In later childhood, affected areas tend to return to normal skin color. The cutaneous lesion is often associated with developmental and neurologic abnormalities with hypotonia, pyramidal tract dysfunction, mental retardation (approximately 80%), and seizures. Ophthalmologic disorders, including strabismus, optic atrophy, microophthalmia, tessellated fundus, eyelid ptosis, and heterochromia iridis, are also present. The hair, teeth, and musculoskeletal system may be affected.

Pathology

The hypopigmented skin lesions are characterized by a decrease in the number of dopa-positive melanocytes and decreased pigment production in the basal layer of the epidermis.

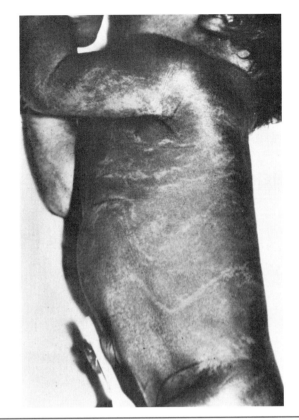

FIGURE 102.1. Incontinentia pigmenti achromians. Hypopigmented skin lesions show streaks or whorls.

Diagnosis and Laboratory Data

Because there is no pathognomonic laboratory test, diagnosis is clinical. Investigation for chromosomal mosaicism, with karyotyping of blood, fibroblasts, and hair bulbs should be considered in all cases.

Treatment

The whorled, marble-cake hypopigmented skin lesions do not require any treatment. Therapy is directed toward the associated complications, such as anticonvulsants for seizures and specialized educational facilities for the learning-disabled or retarded child.

SUGGESTED READINGS

Aydingoz U, Midia M. Central nervous system involvement in incontinentia pigmenti: cranial MRI of two siblings. *Neuroradiology* 1998;40: 364–366.

Berlin AL, Paller AS, Chan LS. Incontinentia pigmenti: a review and update on the molecular basis of pathophysiology. *J Am Acad Dermatol* 2002;47(Aug):169–187.

Donat JF, Walsworth DM, Turk LL. Focal cerebral atrophy in incontinentia pigmenti achromians. *Am J Dis Child* 1980;134:709–710.

Hadj-Rabia S, Froidevaux D, Bodak N, et al. Clinical study of 40 cases of incontinentia pigmenti. *Arch Dermatol* 2003;139(Sep):1163–1170.

Happle R. Dohi Memorial Lecture. New aspects of cutaneous mosaicism. *J Dermatol* 2002;29:681–692.

Hyden-Gramskog C, Salonen R, von Koskull H. Three Finnish incontinentia pigmenti (IP) families with recombinations with the IP loci at Xq28 and Xp11. *Hum Genet* 1993;91:185–189.

Koiffmann CP, deSouza DH, Diament A, et al. Incontinentia pigmenti achromians (hypomelanosis of Ito, MIM 146150): further evidence of localization at Xp11. *Am J Med Genet* 1993;46:529–533.

Landy SJ, Domani D. Incontinentia pigmenti (Bloch-Sulzberger syndrome). *J Med Genet* 1993;30:53–59.

Larsen R, Ashwal S, Peckham N. Incontinentia pigmenti: association with anterior horn cell degeneration. *Neurology* 1987;37:446–450.

Lee AG, Goldberg MF, Gillard JH, Barker PB, Bryan RN. Intracranial assessment of incontinentia pigmenti using magnetic resonance imaging, angiography, and spectroscopic imaging. *Arch Pediatr Adolesc Med* 1995;149;573–580.

O'Brien JE, Feingold M. Incontinentia pigmenti: a longitudinal study. *Am J Dis Child* 1985;139:711–712.

Pascual-Castroviejo I, Roche C, Martinez-Bermejo A, et al. Hypomelanosis of Ito: a study of 76 infantile cases. *Brain Dev* 1998;20:36–43.

Ruggieri M, Pavone L. Hypomelanosis of Ito: clinical syndrome or just phenotype? *J Child Neurol* 2000;15:635–644.

Sulzberger MB. Incontinentia pigmenti (Bloch-Sulzberger): report of an additional case, with comment on possible relation to a new syndrome of familial and congenital anomalies. *Arch Dermatol* 1938;38:57–69.

Wald KJ, Mehta MC, Katsumi O, et al. Retinal detachments in incontinentia pigmenti. *Arch Ophthalmol* 1993;111:614–617.

Chapter 1 0 3

Tuberous Sclerosis Complex

Arnold P. Gold and Marc C. Patterson

Tuberous sclerosis complex (TSC) was first described by von Recklinghausen in 1863. In 1880, Bourneville coined the term *sclérose tubéreuse* for the potato-like lesions in the brain. In 1890, Pringle described the facial nevi, or *adenoma sebaceum*. Vogt later emphasized the classic triad of seizures, mental retardation, and adenoma sebaceum. TSC is called *Pringle disease* when there are only dermatologic findings, *Bourneville disease* when the nervous system is affected, and *West syndrome* when skin lesions are associated with infantile spasms, hypsarrhythmia, and mental retardation. TSC (MIM 191100) is a hereditarily determined progressive disorder characterized by the development in early life of hamartomas, malformations, and congenital tumors of the nervous system, skin, and viscera.

GENETICS AND INCIDENCE

Tuberous sclerosis is inherited as an autosomal-dominant trait, with a high incidence of sporadic cases and protean clinical expressivity. These features are attributed to modifier genes, for which the homozygous condition results in a phenotypically normal individual despite the presence of the gene for tuberous sclerosis; when heterozygous, the modifier gene results in a mildly affected patient. The defective gene has been mapped to chromosome 9q34 (TSC1) in some families and to chromosome 16p13.3 (TSC2) in others. *Hamartin* is the gene product for TSC1, and *tuberin* is the gene product for TSC2. Children with TSC2 mutations tend to have more serious neurologic manifestations when compared with TSC1. Both are involved in the regulation of cell growth and are considered tumor suppressor genes. Hamartin and tuberin form a complex that functions as a negative regulator of the insulin receptor/phosphoinositide 3-kinase/S6 kinase pathway, which suppresses tumorigenesis. Understanding this pathway may lead to targeted drug therapies.

Incidence figures are considered minimal because milder varieties are often unrecognized. Autopsy data gave an incidence of 1 in 10,000 people; clinical surveys gave a prevalence between 1 in 10,000 and 1 in 170,000. Although all races are affected, the disease is thought to be uncommon in blacks, and there may be a greater frequency in males. Pulmonary lymphangiomyomatosis, progressive and often fatal, is present only in young women.

PATHOLOGY AND PATHOGENESIS

The pathologic changes are widespread and include lesions in the nervous system, skin, bones, retina, kidney, lungs, and other viscera. Tuberous sclerosis is a migrational disorder. Multiple small nodules often line the ventricles.

TSC is characterized by the presence of hamartias and hamartomas. Hamartias (from the Greek for "tragic flaw") are malformations in which cells native to a tissue show abnormal architecture and morphology. These lesions do not grow disproportionately for the tissue or organ in which they are found. Hamartomas have the same characteristics, but grow excessively for their site of origin. This old concept is valuable in recognizing the proliferative potential of lesions found in TSC. Thus, cortical tubers are hamartias and do not grow excessively, whereas angiomyolipomas are hamartomas that grow disproportionately and may produce symptoms as a consequence.

The brain is usually normal in size, but variable numbers of hard nodules occur on the surface of the cortex. These nodules are smooth, round, or polygonal and project slightly above the surface of the neighboring cortex. They are white, firm to the touch, and of various sizes. Some

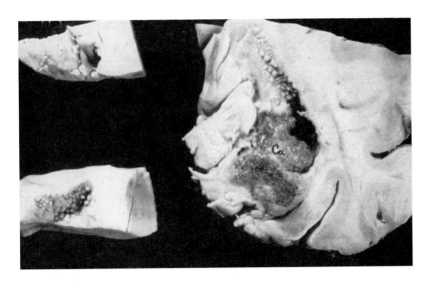

FIGURE 103.1. Tuberous sclerosis. Nodules (candle gutterings) on the surface of ventricles. (Courtesy of Dr. Leon Roizin.)

involve only a small portion of one convolution; others encompass the convolutions of one whole lobe or a major portion of a hemisphere. In addition, there may be developmental anomalies of the cortical convolutions in the form of pachygyria or microgyria. On sectioning of the hemispheres, sclerotic nodules may be found in the subcortical gray matter, the white matter, and the basal ganglia. The lining of the lateral ventricles is frequently the site of numerous small nodules that project into the ventricular cavity (*candle gutterings*; Fig. 103.1). Sclerotic nodules are less frequently found in the cerebellum. The brainstem and spinal cord are rarely involved.

Histologically, the nodules are characterized by a cluster of atypical glial cells in the center and giant cells in the periphery. Calcifications are relatively frequent.

Other features include heterotopia, vascular hyperplasia (sometimes with actual angiomatous malformations), disturbances in the cortical architecture, and occasionally, development of subependymal giant cell astrocytomas. Intracranial giant aneurysm and arterial ectasia are uncommon findings.

The skin lesions are multiform and include the characteristic facial nevi (*adenoma sebaceum*) and patches or plaques of skin fibrosis, typically localized to the frontal area. The facial lesions are not adenomas of the sebaceous glands, but rather, small hamartomas arising from nerve elements of the skin combined with hyperplasia of connective tissue and blood vessels (Fig. 103.2). In late childhood, lesions similar to those on the face are found around or underneath the fingernails and toenails (*ungual*

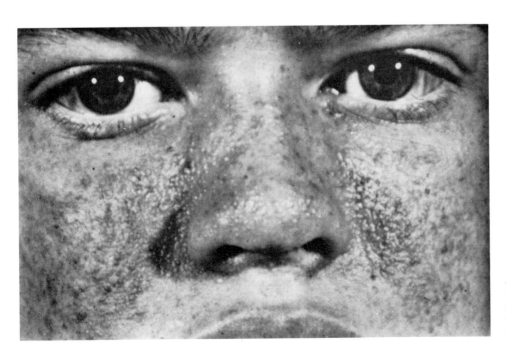

FIGURE 103.2. Tuberous sclerosis. Facial adenoma sebaceum over the butterfly area of the face spares the upper lip.

fibroma). Circumscribed areas of hypomelanosis or depigmented nevi are common in tuberous sclerosis and are often found in infants. Although these depigmented nevi are less specific than the adenoma sebaceum, they are important in raising suspicion for the diagnosis in infants with seizures. Histologically, the skin appears normal except for the loss of melanin, but ultrastructural studies show that melanosomes are small and have reduced content of melanin.

The retinal lesions are small congenital tumors (*phakomas*) composed of glia, ganglion cells, or fibroblasts. Glioma of the optic nerve has been reported.

Other lesions include cardiac rhabdomyoma; renal angiomyolipoma, renal cysts, and, rarely, renal carcinoma; cystic disease of the lungs and pulmonary lymphangioleiomyomatosis; hepatic angiomas and hamartomas; skeletal abnormalities with localized areas of osteosclerosis in the calvarium, spine, pelvis, and limbs; cystic defects involving the phalanges; and periosteal new bone formation confined to the metacarpals and metatarsals.

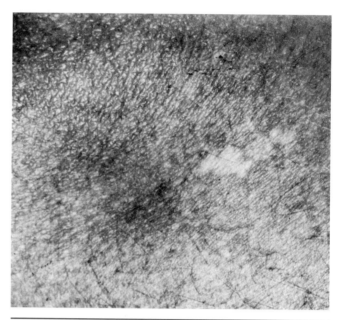

FIGURE 103.3. Tuberous sclerosis. Hypomelanotic or ash leaf macules on the skin.

SYMPTOMS AND SIGNS

The cardinal features of tuberous sclerosis are skin lesions, convulsive seizures, and mental retardation. The disease is characterized by variability and expressivity of the clinical manifestations and is often age related: the symptomatic neonate with cardiac rhabdomyoma and heart failure, the infant with hyphomelanotic macules and infantile spasms; preschool and school age children with adenoma sebaceum, developmental delay, learning disability or retardation, and seizures; and adults with migrational dermatological lesions, subungual fibromas, seizures, and often retardation.

CUTANEOUS SYMPTOMS

Depigmented or hypomelanotic macules are the earliest skin lesion (Fig. 103.3). They are present at birth, persist through life, and may be found only with a Wood lamp examination. The diagnosis is suggested if there are three or more macules measuring 1 cm or more in length. Numerous small macules sometimes resemble confetti or depigmented freckles. Most macules are leaf shaped, resembling the leaf of the European mountain ash tree and sometimes following a dermatomal distribution. Facial adenoma sebaceum (*facial angiofibroma*) is never present at birth but is clinically evident in more than 90% of affected children by age 4. At first, the facial lesion is the size of a pinhead and red because of the angiomatous component. It is distributed symmetrically on the nose and cheeks in a butterfly distribution. The lesions may involve the forehead and chin but rarely involve the upper lip. They gradually increase in size and become yellowish and glistening. *Shagreen patches,* connective tissue hamartomas, are also characteristic. Rarely present in infancy, the patches become evident after age 10. Usually found in the lumbosacral region, shagreen plaques are yellowish-brown elevated plaques that have the texture of pig skin (from which the name originated in French). Other skin lesions include *café au lait spots,* small fibromas that may be tiny and resemble coarse gooseflesh, and ungual fibromas that appear after puberty.

Neurologic Symptoms

Seizures and mental retardation indicate a diffuse encephalopathy. Infantile myoclonic spasms with or without hypsarrhythmia are the characteristic seizures of young infants and, when associated with hypopigmented macules, are diagnostic of tuberous sclerosis. The older child or adult has generalized tonic-clonic or partial complex seizures. There is a close relationship between the onset of seizures at a young age and mental retardation. Mental retardation rarely occurs without clinical seizures, but intellect may be normal, despite seizures. Other than a delayed acquisition of developmental milestones, intellectual impairment, or nonspecific language or coordinative deficiencies, a formal neurologic examination is typically nonfocal. TSC is a major cause of autism and is related to cortical and subcortical dysfunction.

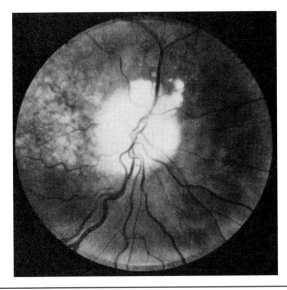

FIGURE 103.4. Tuberous sclerosis. Central calcified hamartoma, or so-called mulberry phakoma, at the optic nerve.

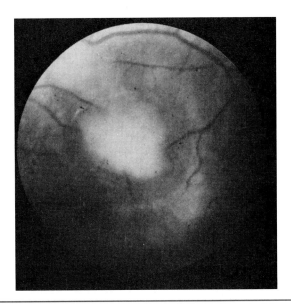

FIGURE 103.5. Tuberous sclerosis. Phakoma or retinal hamartoma involving the peripheral retina.

Ophthalmic Symptoms

Hamartomas of the retina or optic nerve are observed in about 50% of patients. Two types of retinal lesions are seen on funduscopic examination: first, the easily recognized calcified hamartoma near or at the disc with an elevated multinodular lesion that resembles mulberries, grains of tapioca, or salmon eggs (Fig. 103.4); and second, the less distinct, relatively flat, smooth-surfaced, white or salmon-colored, circular or oval lesion located peripherally in the retina (Fig. 103.5). Nonretinal lesions may range from the specific depigmented lesion of the iris (Fig. 103.6) to non-specific, nonparalytic strabismus; optic atrophy; visual-field defects; or cataracts.

Visceral Symptoms

Renal lesions include hamartomas (angiomyolipomas) and hamartias (renal cysts). Typically, both are multiple, bilateral, and usually innocuous and silent. Renal angiomyolipomas grow and occasionally bleed, but most can be followed with annual CT scans. Renal cell carcinoma is a rare complication in the older child or adult. In one series, there was a 50% incidence of tuberous sclerosis in patients

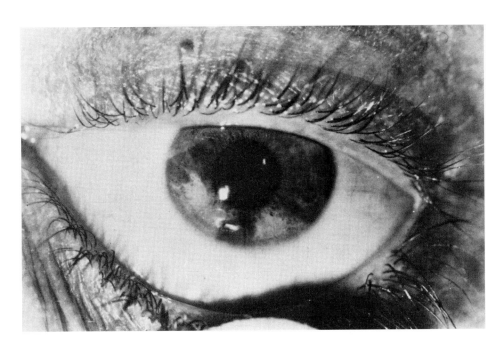

FIGURE 103.6. Tuberous sclerosis. Depigmented or hypomelanotic lesions of the iris.

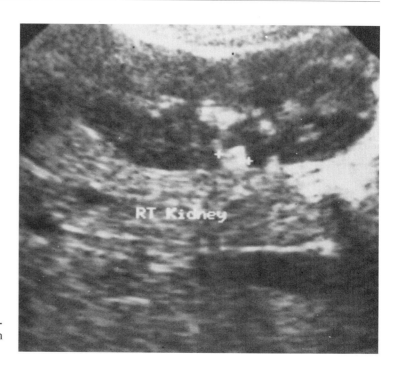

FIGURE 103.7. Tuberous sclerosis. Renal sonogram demonstrates a renal angiomyolipoma.

with cardiac rhabdomyoma. Often asymptomatic, this cardiac tumor may be symptomatic at any age and in infancy can result in death. PET often reveals hypometabolic regions that are not noted on MRI, indicating a more extensive disturbance of cerebral function.

Pulmonary hamartomatous lesions consisting of multifocal alveolar hyperplasia associated with cystic lymphangioleiomyomatosis occur in fewer than 1% of patients. These become symptomatic (often with a spontaneous pneumothorax) in females in the third or fourth decade and are progressive and often fatal. Sclerotic lesions of the calvarium and cystic lesions of the metacarpals and pha-

langes are asymptomatic. Hamartomatous hemangiomas of the spleen and racemose angiomas of the liver are rare and usually asymptomatic. Enamel pitting of the deciduous teeth may aid in diagnosis.

LABORATORY DATA

Unless renal lesions are present, routine laboratory studies are normal. Renal angiomyolipomas are usually asymptomatic and rarely cause gross hematuria, but they may show albuminuria and microscopic hematuria.

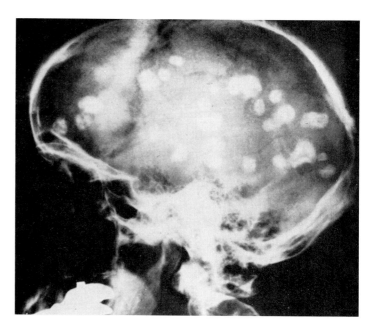

FIGURE 103.8. Tuberous sclerosis. Calcified nodules in the cerebrum. (Courtesy of Dr. P. I. Yakovlev.)

Sonography (Fig. 103.7), angiography, and CT are often diagnostic. Multiple or diffuse renal cysts may be associated with albuminuria or azotemia and hypertension. Intravenous pyelography is diagnostic.

Chest radiographs may reveal pulmonary lesions or rhabdomyoma with cardiomegaly. Electrocardiogram findings are variable, but the echocardiogram is diagnostic.

Skull radiographs usually reveal small calcifications within the substance of the cerebrum (Fig. 103.8). The CSF is normal, except when a large intracerebral tumor is present. The EEG is often abnormal, especially in patients with clinical seizures. Abnormalities include slow-wave activity and epileptiform discharges such as hypsarrhythmia, focal or multifocal spike or sharp-wave discharges, and generalized spike-and-wave discharges. CT is diagnostic when calcified subependymal nodules encroach on the lateral ventricle (often in the region of the foramen of Monro); there may also be calcified cortical or cerebellar nodules (Fig. 103.9). A few nodules appear isodense on CT and are better visualized on MRI. FLAIR MRI images allow more accurate delineation of cortical and subcortical tubers. Calcified periventricular and cortical lesions have been visualized shortly after birth. The number of cortical tubers often correlates with the severity of cortical dysfunction. There is enough variation in clinical outcome that prognosis cannot be based on cortical tuber count alone. PET often reveals hypometabolic regions that are not noted on MRI, indicating a more extensive disturbance of cerebral function.

DIAGNOSIS

Clinical diagnosis is possible at most ages. In infancy, three or more characteristic depigmented cutaneous lesions suggest the diagnosis, and this is reinforced in the presence of infantile myoclonic spasms. In the older child or adult, the diagnosis is made by the triad of tuberous sclerosis: facial adenoma sebaceum, epilepsy, and mental retardation. Retinal or visceral lesions may be diagnostic. The disease, however, is noted for protean manifestations, and a family history may be invaluable in establishing the diagnosis, which is often reinforced by CT or MRI lesions.

The differential diagnosis includes other neurocutaneous syndromes that are differentiated by their characteristic skin lesions. Multisystem involvement may complicate the diagnosis of tuberous sclerosis. The National Tuberous Sclerosis Association has developed a classification of diagnostic criteria (Table 103.1), and the Tuberous Sclerosis Complex Consensus Conference (Table 103.2) provided an additional classification. Prenatal diagnosis is available for both TSC1 and TSC2.

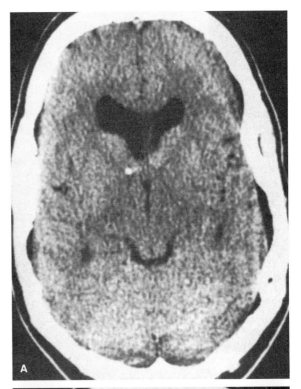

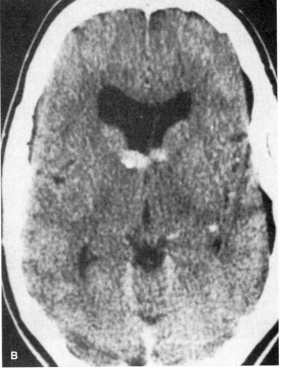

FIGURE 103.9. Tuberous sclerosis. **A.** Noncontrast axial CT demonstrates a calcific density adjacent to the right foramen of Monro, a typical location for tubers. **B.** Postcontrast, this lesion enhances, as do additional noncalcified lesions on the contralateral side. (Courtesy of Dr. J. A. Bello and Dr. S. K. Hilal.)

▶ **TABLE 103.1** Diagnostic Criteria for Tuberous Sclerosis Complex (TSC)

Primary features
Facial angiofibromas[a]
Multiple ungual fibromas[a]
Cortical tuber (histologically confirmed)
Subependymal nodule or giant cell astrocytoma (histologically confirmed)
Multiple calcified subependymal nodules protruding into the ventricle (radiographic evidence)
Multiple retinal astrocytomas[a]
Secondary features
Affected first-degree relative
Cardiac rhabdomyoma (histologic or radiographic confirmation)
Other retinal hamartoma or achromic patch[a]
Cerebral tubers (radiographic confirmation)
Noncalcified subependymal nodules (radiographic confirmation)
Shagreen patch[a]
Forehead plaque[a]
Pulmonary lymphangiomyomatosis (histologic confirmation)
Renal angiomyolipoma (radiographic or histologic confirmation)
Renal cysts (histologic confirmation)
Tertiary features
Hypomelanotic macules[a]
"Confetti" skin lesions[a]
Renal cysts (radiographic evidence)
Randomly distributed enamel pits in deciduous or permanent teeth
Hamartomatous rectal polyps (histologic confirmation)
Bone cysts (radiographic evidence)
Pulmonary lymphangiomyomatosis (radiographic evidence)
Cerebral white matter "migration tracts" or heterotopias (radiographic evidence)
Gingival fibromas
Hamartoma of other organs (histologic confirmation)
Infantile spasms

Definite TSC	One primary feature, two secondary features; or one secondary plus two tertiary features
Probable TSC	Either one secondary plus one tertiary feature or three tertiary features
Suspect TSC	Either one secondary feature or two tertiary features

[a]Histologic confirmation is not required *if* the lesion is clinically obvious. Developed by the National Tuberous Scelerosis Association Professional Advisory Board (Roach ES, Smith M, Huttenlocher P, Alcorn DN).

COURSE AND PROGNOSIS

Mild or solely cutaneous involvement often follows a static course, whereas patients with the full-blown syndrome have a progressive course with increasing seizures and dementia. The child with infantile myoclonic spasms is at great risk of later intellectual deficit. Brain tumor, status epilepticus, renal insufficiency, cardiac failure, or progressive pulmonary impairment can lead to death.

▶ **TABLE 103.2** Diagnostic Criteria—Tuberous Sclerosis Complex Consensus Conference (1998)

Major Features	Minor Features
Facial angiofibromas or forehead plaques	Multiple randomly distributed pits in dental enamel
Nontraumatic ungula or periungual fibroma	Hamartomatous rectal polyps
Hypomelanotic macules (three or more)	Bone cysts
Shagreen patch (connective tissue nevis)	Cerebral white matter radial migration lines
Multiple retinal nodular hamartomas	Gingival fibromas
Cortical tuber	Nonrenal hamartoma
Subependymal nodule	Retinal achromic patch
Subependymal giant cell astrocytoma	"Confetti" skin lesions
Cardiac rhabdomyoma, single or multiple	Multiple renal cysts
Angiomyolipoma	

Diagnosis of tuberous sclerosis complex is established when two major features or one major plus two minor features can be demonstrated.

TREATMENT

There is no specific treatment. The cutaneous lesions do not compromise function, but cosmetic surgery may be indicated for facial adenoma sebaceum or large shagreen patches. Infantile myoclonic spasms respond to corticosteroid or corticotropin therapy; currently vigabatrin is the drug of choice. Focal and generalized seizures are treated with anticonvulsants. Patients with unilateral seizures and minimal developmental delay may experience long-term seizure control following surgical resection of epileptogenic tubers. Progressive cystic renal disease often responds to surgical decompression, but with renal failure, dialysis or renal transplantation may be necessary. Intramural cardiac rhabdomyoma and complicating congestive heart failure are managed medically with cardiotonics, diuretics, and salt restriction. Whole obstructive intracavity tumors and congestive heart failure require surgical extirpation of the tumor. Progressive pulmonary involvement is an indication for respiratory therapy, but response is poor and most patients die a few years after the onset of this complication.

SUGGESTED READINGS

Asano E, Chugani DC, Muzik O, et al. Autism in tuberous sclerosis complex is related to both cortical and subcortical dysfunction. *Neurology* 2001;9;57:1269–1277.

Bourneville DM. Sclerose tubereuse des circonvolutions cerebrales: idotie et epilepsie hemiplegique. *Arch Neurol* 1880;1:81–91.

Curatolo P, ed. *Tuberous Sclerosis Complex: From Basic Science to Clinical Phenotypes*. London: MacKeith, 2003.

Gold AP, Freeman JM. Depigmented nevi: the earliest sign of tuberous sclerosis. *Pediatrics* 1965;35:1003–1005.

Gomez MR, Sampson JR, Whittemore VH, eds. *Tuberous Sclerosis Complex*. 3rd Ed. New York: Oxford University Press, 1999.

Harabayashi T, Shinohara N, Katano H, et al. Management of renal angiomyolipomas associated with tuberous sclerosis complex. *J Urol* 2004;171(Jan):102–105.

Inoue Y, Nemoto Y, Murata R, et al. CT and MR imaging of cerebral tuberous sclerosis. *Brain Dev* 1998;20:209–221.

Jarrar RG, Buchhalter JR, Raffel C. Long-term outcome of epilepsy surgery in patients with tuberous sclerosis. *Neurology* 2004;62 (Feb 10):479–481.

Kandt RS, Gebarski SS, Geotting MG. Tuberous sclerosis with cardiogenic cerebral embolism: magnetic resonance imaging. *Neurology* 1985;35:1223–1225.

Kwiatkowska J, Wigowska-Sowinska J, Napierala D, et al. Mosaicism in tuberous sclerosis as a potential cause of the failure of molecular diagnosis. *N Engl J Med* 1999;340:703–707.

Lucchese NJ, Goldberg MF. Iris and fundus pigmentary changes in tuberous sclerosis. *J Pediatr Ophthalmol Strabismus* 1981;18:45–46.

Nixon JR, Houser OW, Gomez MR, Okazaki H. Cerebral tuberous sclerosis: MR imaging. *Radiology* 1989;170:869–873.

Roach ES. Tuberous sclerosis. *Pediatr Clin North Am* 1992;39:591–620.

Roach ES, DiMario FJ, Kandt RS, et al. Tuberous Sclerosis Consensus Conference; revised clinical diagnostic evaluation. *J Child Neurol* 1999;14:401–407.

Roach ES, Smith M, Huttenlocher P, et al. Diagnostic criteria: tuberous sclerosis complex. Report of the diagnostic criteria committee of the National Tuberous Sclerosis Association. *J Child Neurol* 1992;7:221–224.

Sampson JR. TSC1 and TSC2: genes that are mutated in the human genetic disorder tuberous sclerosis. *Biochem Soc Trans* 2003;31 (Pt 3):592–596.

Weiner DM, Ewalt DH, Roach ES, et al. The tuberous sclerosis complex: a comprehensive review. *J Am Coll Surg* 1998;187:548–561.

Wiederholt WC, Gomez MR, Kurland LT. Incidence and prevalence of tuberous sclerosis in Rochester, Minnesota, 1950 through 1982. *Neurology* 1985;35:600–603.

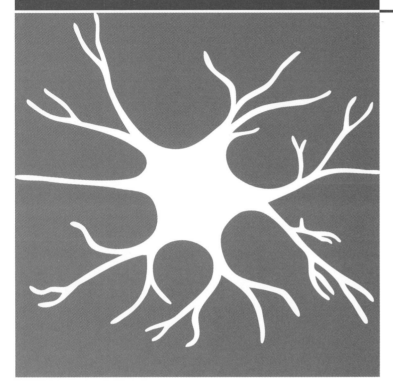

Peripheral Neuropathies

General Considerations

Norman Latov

The peripheral nervous system is composed of multiple cell types and elements that subserve diverse motor, sensory, and autonomic functions. The clinical manifestations of neuropathies depend on the severity, distribution, and functions affected. *Peripheral neuropathy* and *polyneuropathy* are terms that describe syndromes resulting from diffuse lesions of peripheral nerves, usually manifested by weakness, sensory loss, and autonomic dysfunction. *Mononeuropathy* indicates a disorder of a single nerve and is often a result of a local cause such as trauma or entrapment. *Mononeuropathy multiplex* signifies focal involvement of two or more nerves, usually as a result of a generalized disorder such as diabetes mellitus or vasculitis. *Neuritis* is typically reserved for inflammatory disorders of nerves resulting from infection or autoimmunity.

SYMPTOMS AND SIGNS

Polyneuropathy may occur at any age, although particular syndromes are more likely to occur in certain age groups. Charcot-Marie-Tooth (CMT) disease, for example, often begins in childhood or adolescence, whereas neuropathy associated with paraproteinemia is seen more frequently with increasing age. The onset and progression differ; the Guillain-Barré syndrome (GBS), tick paralysis, and porphyria begin acutely and may remit. Others, such as vitamin B_{12} deficiency or carcinomatous neuropathy, begin insidiously and progress slowly. Still others, such as chronic inflammatory demyelinating polyneuropathy, may begin acutely or insidiously and then progress with remissions and exacerbations.

The myelin sheaths or the motor or sensory axons themselves may be predominantly affected, or the neuropathy may be mixed, axonal, or demyelinating. Most polyneuropathies, especially those with primary demyelination, affect both motor and sensory functions. A predominantly motor polyneuropathy is seen in lead toxicity, dapsone or hexane intoxication, tick paralysis, porphyria, some cases of GBS, and in association with multifocal conduction block or anti-GM_1 antibodies. Sensory neuropathy, sometimes with concomitant autonomic dysfunction, is seen in thallium poisoning, ganglioneuritis, pyridoxine (vitamin B_6) deficiency, and occasionally, with diabetes mellitus, amyloidosis, carcinoma, or lepromatous leprosy. Predominant involvement of the autonomic system can be seen in acute or chronic autonomic neuropathy or in amyloidosis.

Symptoms of polyneuropathy include acral (distal) pain, paresthesia, weakness, and sensory loss. Pain may be spontaneous (paresthesias) or elicited by stimulation of the skin (dysesthesias) and may be sharp or burning. Paresthesia is usually described as numbness (a dead sensation), tingling, buzzing, stinging, burning, or a feeling of constriction. Lack of pain perception may result in repeated traumatic injuries with degeneration of joints (*arthropathy* or *Charcot joints*) and in chronic ulcerations.

Weakness is greatest in distal limb muscles in most neuropathies; there may be paralysis of the intrinsic foot and hand muscles with footdrop or wristdrop. Tendon reflexes are often lost, especially in demyelinating neuropathy. In severe polyneuropathy, the patient may become quadriplegic and respirator dependent. The cranial nerves may be affected, particularly in GBS and diphtheritic neuropathy. Cutaneous sensory loss appears in a stocking-and-glove distribution. All modes of sensation may be affected, or there may be selective impairment of "large" myelinated fiber functions (position and vibratory sense) or "small" unmyelinated fiber functions (pain and temperature perception). Often, there is a rise in the threshold of perception of painful stimuli, but with a delayed and greater than normal reaction.

Involvement of autonomic nerves may cause miosis (small pupil), anhidrosis (impaired sweating), orthostatic hypotension, sphincter symptoms, impotence, and vasomotor abnormalities; these may occur without other evidence of neuropathy, but autonomic neuropathy is more commonly seen in association with symmetric distal polyneuropathy. The most common cause of predominantly autonomic neuropathy in the United States is diabetes mellitus. Amyloidosis is another cause. Tachycardia, rapid alterations in blood pressure, flushing and sweating, and abnormalities in gastrointestinal motility are sometimes prominent in thallium poisoning, porphyria, or GBS.

In mononeuropathy or mononeuropathy multiplex, focal motor, sensory, and reflex changes are restricted to areas innervated by specific nerves. When multiple distal subcutaneous nerves are affected in mononeuropathy multiplex, the stocking-and-glove pattern of symmetric distal sensory loss may suggest polyneuropathy. The most frequent causes of mononeuropathy multiplex are diabetes mellitus, periarteritis nodosa, human immunodeficiency virus type 1 infection, rheumatoid arthritis, brachial neuropathy, leprosy, nerve trauma, or sarcoid. Asymmetric neuropathy is also seen in multifocal motor neuropathy with conduction block, sometimes with increased titers of anti-GM$_1$ antibodies, or in multifocal demyelinating sensory and motor neuropathy.

Superficial cutaneous nerves may be thickened and visibly enlarged secondary to Schwann cell proliferation and deposition of collagen as a result of repeated episodes of segmental demyelination and remyelination or to deposition of amyloid or polysaccharides

▶ **TABLE 104.1** Neuropathy Diagnosis and Laboratory Tests

Cause or Diagnosis	*Manifestations*[a]	*Laboratory Tsets*
Vitamin Deficiencies	**S, SM, SYM**	***Vitamins B$_{12}$, B$_6$, B$_1$***
Infectious		
Lyme disease	S, SM, SYM, MF, CN	Serology, PCR
HIV-1	S, SM, SYM, MF, CN	Serology, PCR
Hepatitis C	S. SM, SYM, MF, CN	Serology, PCR
Herpes zoster	S, radicular	Serology, PCR
Cytomegalovirus	SM, M, SYM, MF	Serology, PCR, culture
Immune Mediated		
Guillain-Barré and variants	SM, S, M, SYM, MF, CN	IgG antiganglioside antibodies (GM1,GD1a,GQ1b, GD1b), urine porphyrins
IgM antibody associated	M, MF	IgM anti-GM$_1$, GD1a
	S, SM, SYM	IgM anti-MAG, sulfatide, GD1b, GQ1b
Monoclonal gammopathy	M, S, SM, SYM, MF	Serum immunofixation electrophoresis, quantitative immunoglobulins
Autonomic neuropathy	Autonomic dysfunction	Antinicotinic acetylcholine receptor antibodies
Vasculitis	SM, S, MF, SYM	ESR, cryoglobulins, hepatitis C serology, or PCR
Sacroid	SM, S, MF, SYM	ACE, chest radiograph
Celiac disease	S, SM, MF, SYM	Antigliadin, endomysial, transglutaminase antibodies
Rheumatological diseases	SM, S, MF, SYM	SSA-Ro, SSB-La antibodies
Sjögren syndrome		ANA, ANCA (PR3, myeloperoxidase), dsDNA Ab, RNP, rheumatoid factor
Lupus		
Wegener granulomatosis		
Rheumatoid arthritis		
Paraneoplastic		
Lung cancer	S, SYM	Anti-Hu Ab, Chest radiograph
Waldenström syndrome	SM, S, M, SYM, MF	Serum immunofixation electrophoresis
Myeloma	SM, M, SYM, MF	Serum and urine immunofixation electrophoresis, skeletal survey
Hereditary		
CMT1-1	Demyelinating, SM, SYM, MF	DNA tests for PMP-22, MPZ, EGR2, Cx32
CMT-2	Axonal, SM, SYM	DNA tests for NF-L, Cx32, MPZ
Mitochondrial	NARP, SM, MF	Serum lactate, thymidine phosphorylase, DNA testing
Other	Axonal S, SM, amyloid, porphyria	DNA tests for transthyretin, periaxin; urine porphyrins
Metabolic/Toxic		
Diabetes	S, SM, SYM, MF, CN	Chem 7, HgbA1c, glucose tolerance test
Renal failure	S, SM, SYM	Chem 7
Thyroid disease	S, SM, SYM, MF	TSH, T4
Heavy metal toxicity	S, SM, SYM	Urine lead, mercury, arsenic

[a]MF, male-female, occurs in men and women; NARP, neuropathy, ataxia, retinitis pigmentosa; PCR, polymerace chain reaction; GM$_1$, GD1a, ganglioside components of myelin; SSA, SSB, antigens for Sjögren syndrome severe antibodies; RNP, ribonucleo protein; PMP, peripheral myelin protein; MPZ, myelin protein zero; EGR, early growth response protein; Cx32, connexin; NF-L, neurofilament light chain; S, sensory; SM, sensorimotor; SYM, symmetric; MF, multifocal; M, motor; CN, cranial nerves.

in the nerves. Hypertrophic nerves may be observed in the demyelinating form of CMT disease (type I), Dejerine-Sottas neuropathy, Refsum disease, von Recklinghausen disease (neurofibromatosis), leprous neuritis, amyloidosis, chronic demyelinative polyneuritis, sarcoid, and acromegaly.

Fasciculations, or spontaneous contractions of individual motor units, are visible twitches of limb muscles under the skin and may be seen in the tongue. They are characteristic of anterior horn cell diseases but are also seen in motor neuropathy with multifocal motor conduction block and occasionally in chronic motor neuropathies involving axons.

ETIOLOGY AND DIAGNOSIS

Peripheral nerve disorders may be divided into hereditary and acquired forms. The most common hereditary disorder is CMT syndrome type 1A (peroneal muscular atrophy), associated with duplication of the peripheral myelin protein 22 (PMP22) gene region on chromosome 17. A deletion in the same region is seen in hereditary neuropathy with a liability to pressure palsies. The most common acquired neuropathies in the United States are associated with diabetes mellitus and alcoholism; other causes of polyneuropathy are listed in Table 104.1. Trauma and entrapment are considered in the differential diagnosis of mononeuropathies, particularly if the median nerve is affected at the wrist, the ulnar nerve at the elbow, or the peroneal nerve at the knee. Patients with any form of polyneuropathy seem to be more vulnerable to mechanical injury of nerves; in cachectic or immobile patients, neuropathy may result from pressure or trauma rather than from underlying disease.

In the evaluation of a patient with peripheral neuropathy, a detailed family, social, and medical history; neurologic examination; and electrodiagnostic, laboratory, and skin or nerve biopsy studies are usually necessary for diagnosis. A classification of the most common acquired and hereditary polyneuropathies and their laboratory evaluation are presented in Table 104.1.

TREATMENT

Treatment of patients with peripheral nerve disorders can be divided into two phases: removal or treatment of the condition responsible for the disorder and symptomatic therapy. Specific treatments will be considered in discussions of the individual disorders.

Symptomatic treatment of polyneuropathy consists of general supportive measures, amelioration of pain, and physiotherapy. Tracheal intubation and respiratory support may be needed in GBS. The corneas are protected if there is weakness of eye closure. The bed is kept clean and the sheets are kept smooth to prevent injury to the anesthetic skin; a special mattress can be used to prevent pressure sores. Chronic compression of vulnerable nerves (ulnar at the elbow and common peroneal at the knee) is avoided. Paralyzed limbs are splinted to prevent contractures. Physical therapy includes massage of all weak muscles and passive movement of all joints. When voluntary movement begins to return, muscle training exercises are done daily. Patients should not attempt to walk before muscle testing indicates that they are ready. In chronic polyneuropathy with footdrop, an orthosis for the foot often helps the patient's gait. Patients with postural hypotension are instructed to rise gradually. Treatment includes the use of body stockings to minimize blood pooling in the legs and, if necessary, dietary salt supplementation or mineralocorticoid therapy to expand blood volume.

COURSE

The polyneuropathy may be progressive or remitting, and the prognosis is affected by the extent of destruction of nerves before treatment begins. With removal or treatment of the cause of the neuropathy, recovery is more rapid if macroscopic continuity of the nerves has not been interrupted. Conversely, recovery may be delayed for months if axons are destroyed. Axonal regeneration proceeds at a rate of 1 to 2 mm per day and may be delayed where the axons have to penetrate focally damaged segments of nerve. Aberrant growth of axonal sprouts may lead to formation of persistent neuromas. After severe wallerian degeneration, there may be permanent weakness, muscular wasting, diminution of reflexes, and sensory loss. In demyelinating neuropathies, recovery may sometimes be more rapid and complete.

SUGGESTED READINGS

Dyck PJ, Thomas PK, Griffin JW, et al., eds. *Peripheral Neuropathy.* 3rd Ed. Philadelphia: WB Saunders, 1993.

Latov N, Wokke JHJ, Kelly JJ Jr, eds. *Immunological and Infectious Diseases of the Peripheral Nerves.* New York: Cambridge University Press, 1998.

Mendell JR, Kissel JT, Cornblath DR. *Diagnosis and Management of Peripheral Nerve Disorders.* New York: Oxford University Press, 2001.

Stewart JD. *Focal Peripheral Neuropathies.* 3rd Ed. Philadelphia: Lippincott Williams & Wilkins, 1999.

Chapter 105

Hereditary Neuropathies

Michael E. Shy

Inherited neuropathies, often known as Charcot-Marie-Tooth (CMT) disorders, were described by Charcot and Marie in France and, independently, by Tooth in England in the late 1800s. Although early investigators recognized the weakness and atrophy of muscles innervated by the peroneal nerve, the characteristic foot abnormalities, and the familial nature of the disease, it was also soon recognized that inherited disorders of the peripheral nerve comprised a heterogenous group. Dejerine and Sottas described cases that were more severe and began in infancy, and Roussy and Lévy described cases associated with tremor, ataxia, areflexia, and pes cavus. Studies beginning in the 1960s suggested that most CMT patients had autosomal dominant disorders that could be divided into one group with slow nerve conduction velocities and pathological evidence of a hypertrophic demyelinating neuropathy (CMT type 1), and a second group with relatively normal nerve conduction velocities and axonal degeneration (CMT type 2). Most patients had both weakness and sensory loss, predominantly in the distal legs, and atrophy of the weakened muscles; in most subjects, symptoms began within the first two decades of life.

Despite the clinical similarities among CMT patients, the group is genetically heterogeneous. Initial linkage studies demonstrated CMT1 loci on both chromosome 1 and chromosome 17. In 1991, two groups found that CMT1A, the most common form of CMT1, was associated with a 1.4 Mb duplication within chromosome 17p11.2 in the region containing the *PMP22* gene (*p*eripheral *m*yelin *p*rotein 22). Reports of other genetic defects associated with hereditary neuropathies soon followed. CMT1B, linked to chromosome 1, was associated with mutations in the myelin protein zero glycoprotein (*MPZ*), and an X-linked neuropathy, CMTX1, was caused by mutations in the gap junction beta one (*GJB1*) gene that encodes the protein connexin 32 (Cx32). Deletion, instead of duplication of the CMT1A 1.4 Mb region on chromosome 17, causes hereditary neuropathy with liability to pressure palsies (HNPP). At present, mutations have been identified in more than 30 genes in the inherited neuropathies (Table 105.1; see also http://molgenwww.uia.ac.be/CMTMutations/DataSource/MutByGene.cfm). Last accessed 1/05. The focus of this chapter is on the major forms of inherited neuropathy.

EPIDEMIOLOGY

The overall prevalence of CMT is about 1:2500, without ethnic predisposition. The 17p11.2 duplication causing CMT1A causes 60% to 70% of CMT patients, CMTX1 accounts for approximately 10% to 20% of CMT cases, and CMT1B accounts for less than 5% of patients. Point mutations in *PMP22* or *EGR2* are less frequent. Remarkably, point mutations have frequently been identified as de novo or sporadic events without clear family histories; these are presumably new mutations. The overall prevalence of HNPP is not known, but 84% of 115 unrelated patients with clinical evidence of HNPP were found to have the chromosome 17p11.2 deletion. Fourteen of 63 families with dominantly inherited neuropathies were found to have features consistent with CMT2 in the series of Ionasescu et al.

CLASSIFICATION OF INHERITED NEUROPATHIES

The current classification system of inherited neuropathies is based on the landmark studies of Dyck and Lambert in 1968 (Table 105.2). These authors also introduced the term *hereditary motor and sensory neuropathy* (HMSN), which is used interchangeably with CMT. The system separates CMT1 and CMT2 patients into demyelinating and neuronal groups. CMT3, or HMSN III, designates recessively inherited neuropathies; these patients often have a severe demyelinating neuropathy with onset in infancy, and the eponym is Dejerine-Sottas neuropathy (DSN).

Dyck and Lambert also recognized other unusual forms of inherited neuropathies and used HMSN IV to identify patients we now diagnose with Refsum disease; HMSN V includes patients with hereditary spastic paraplegia (HSP) with amyotrophy, and HMSN V includes patients with distal hereditary purely motor neuropathies.

Although this classification proved invaluable to clinicians and the investigators who subsequently identified the genetic causes of many of these neuropathies, the discovery of the causal genes also led to a need to modify the classification system for several reasons. First, different mutations in the same gene, such as *MPZ* or *PMP22*, were found to cause either typical CMT I phenotypes or severe early-onset neuropathies. Many of these early-onset cases appear sporadically, with no family history of the disease, and would have previously been diagnosed as CMT 3 or DSN. Second, X-linked CMT does not fit easily into the original Dyck-Lambert classification both because of the X-linked inheritance and because nerve conduction velocity (NCV) is intermediately slowed. Finally, different mutations in the same gene, such as *MPZ*, may cause the slow NCV characteristic of CMT1 or nearly normal velocities more characteristic of CMT2. With this in mind, the classification scheme has been

◗ TABLE 105.1

Disorder	Locus/Gene	Inheritance	Protein	Mutation (Frequency)	Testing Method	Type of Testing
Hereditary Motor and Sensory Neuropathies						
CMT1A	17p11.2/PMP22	AD	Peripheral myelin protein 22	Duplication (98%)	Pulse-field gel electrophoresis, FISH, Southern blot	Clinical
				Point mutation (2%)	Sequencing, mutation scanning, mutation analysis	
HNPP	17p11.2/PMP22	AD	Peripheral myelin protein 22	Deletion (80%)	Mutation analysis, FISH, Long PCR-RFLP, Southern blot	Clinical
				Point mutation/small deletion (20%)	Sequencing	
CMT1B	1q22/MPZ	AD	Myelin protein zero	Point mutation	Sequencing, mutation scanning, mutation analysis	Clinical
CMT1C	16p13.1-p12.3/LITAF	AD	SIMPLE			Research
CMT1D	10q21.1-q22.1/EGR2	AD	Early growth response protein 2	Point mutation	Sequencing, mutation scanning	Clinical
CMT2A	1p36.2/MFN2	AD	Mitofusion 2	Point mutation	Sequencing, mutation analysis	Research
CMT2B	3q21/RAB7	AD	Ras-related protein Rab-7	Point mutation	Sequencing, mutation analysis	Research
CMT2C	12q23-24/unknown	AD	Unknown		Direct DNA, linkage analysis	
CMT2D	7p15/GARS	AD	Glycyl-tRNA synthetase	Point mutation	Sequencing, mutation analysis	Research
CMT2E	8p21/NEFL	AD	Neurofilament light		Sequencing	Clinical
CMT2F	7q11-21/HSP27	AD	Heat shock protein 27	Point mutation	Sequencing, mutation analysis	Research
CMT4A	8q13-q21.1/GDAP1	AR	Ganglioside-induced differentiation protein 1	Point mutation	Sequencing, mutation analysis	Clinical
CMT4B1	11q22/MTMR2	AR	Myotubularin-related protein 2	Point mutation	Sequencing, mutation analysis	Research
CMT4BB2	11p15/CMT4B2	AR	SET binding factor 2	Point mutation	Sequencing, mutation analysis	Research
CMT4C	5q32/KIAA1985	AR	Unknown			Research
CMT4D	8q24.3/NDRG1	AR	NDRG1 protein	Point mutation	Sequencing, mutation analysis	Research
CMT4E	10q21.1-q22.1/EGR2	AR	Early growth response protein 2	Point mutation	Mutation analysis, sequencing	Clinical
CMT4F	19q13.1-q13.2/PRX	AR	Periaxin	Point mutation	Mutation analysis, sequencing	Clinical
CMTX	Xq13.1/GJB1	X linked	Gap junction beta-1 protein (Connexin 32)	Point mutations, deletions (rare)	Sequencing, mutation scanning, mutation analysis	Clinical

(continued)

TABLE 105.1 (Continued)

Disorder	Locus/Gene	Inheritance	Protein	Mutation (Frequency)	Testing Method	Type of Testing
Distal Hereditary Motor Neuropathies						
dHMN I	Unknown	AD	Unknown			Research
dHMN II	12q24.3/HSP22	AD	Heat shock protein 22	Point mutation	Sequencing, mutation analysis	Research
dHMN III	1q21-23/Unknown	AR	Unknown			Research
dHMN V	7p15/GARS	AD	Glycul-tRNA synthetase	Point mutation	Sequencing, mutation analysis	Research
dHMN VI	Unknown	AR	Unknown			Research
dHMN VII	2q14/Unknown	AD	Unknown			Research
dHMN Jerash	9p21.1-p12/Unknown	AR	Unknown			Research
ALS4	9q34/SETX	AD	Senataxin	Point mutation	Sequencing, mutation analysis	Research
HMN Dynactin	2p13/DCTN1	AD	Dynactin	Point mutation	Sequencing, mutation analysis	Research
Hereditary Sensory and Autonomic Neuropathies						
HSAN I	9q22.1-q22.3/SPTLC1	AD	Serine palmitoyltransferase light chain 1	Point mutations	Sequencing, mutation analysis	Research
HSAN II	12p13.3/HSN2	AR	Heriditary sensory neuropathy 2	Point mutation	Sequencing, mutation analysis	Research
HSAN III (Riley Day)	9q31/IKBKAP	AR	IkappaB kinase complex-associated protein	2 mutations account for 99% of affected patients of Ashkenazi Jewish descent	Mutation analysis, quantitative PCR	Research
HSAN IV	1q21-q22/NTRK1	AR	tyrosine kinase for nerve growth factor	Point mutation	Sequencing, mutation analysis	Research

CMT, Charcot-Marie-Tooth disease; HNPP, hereditary neuropathy with liability to pressure palsies; DHMN, distal hereditary motor neuropathy; HSAN, hereditary sensory and autonomic neuropathy.

> **TABLE 105.2** **Dyck and Lambert Classification of Hereditary Motor and Sensory Neuropathies**

Type	Features
HMSN Type I A and B (dominantly inherited hypertrophic neuropathy)	Slow nerve conduction velocities Distal weakness, mild sensory loss Palpable nerves Decreased reflexes Pathology demonstrating segmental demyelination, remyelination, onion bulb formation, and axonal loss Autosomal dominant
HMSN Type II (neuronal type of peroneal muscular atrophy)	Normal nerve conduction velocities Distal weakness, mild sensory loss Nonpalpable nerves Pathology demonstrating degeneration of motor and sensory nerves Autosomal dominant
HMSN Type III (hypertrophic neuropathy of infancy; Dejerine and Sottas)	Delayed motor development Severe motor-sensory loss Slow nerve conduction velocities Autosomal recessive
HMSN Type IV Hypertrophic neuropathy (Refsum; associated with phytanic acid excess)	Refsum disease
HMSN Type V (associated with spastic paraplegia)	Spastic paraplegia present
HMSN Type VI (with optic atrophy)	Optic atrophy present
HMSN Type VII	Retinitis pigmentosa present

modified to that in Table 105.1, which is based on the genetic cause of the neuropathy and the inheritance pattern.

Neuropathies caused by genes expressed in Schwann cells, which are the myelinating cells of the peripheral nervous system (PNS) and inherited as dominant disorders are classified as CMT 1 whereas dominantly inherited neuropathies caused by mutations in neuronally expressed genes are classified as CMT 2. CMT 3 is not used in this classification because DSN, previously classified as CMT 3, is now used regardless of whether a gene is expressed in Schwann cells or neurons and regardless of dominant or recessive inheritance. CMT 4 now designates the recessive forms of CMT, regardless of demyelinating or axonal pathology. However, even this genetically based classification system has limitations. For example, certain mutations in the *PMP22* gene (Thr118Met, for example) may cause recessively inherited neuropathies whereas most other *PMP22* mutations are autosomal dominant. In

the end, it may not be possible to classify the various types of CMT perfectly because of the many different genetic causes of these neuropathies and the phenotypic variability conveyed by different mutations of the same gene.

BIOLOGY OF CMT

What makes CMT research appealing to many investigators is that it provides a window into the molecular workings of the peripheral nervous system (PNS). PMP22, MPZ, and Cx32, causes of CMT1 and CMTX1, are all integral myelin proteins whose functions are under investigation by basic myelin biologists. Similarly, neurofilament light chain (NF-L), kinesin KIF1Bβ, and dynactin are investigated for their roles in regulating the axonal cytoskeleton and axonal transport. Mutations in these proteins cause axonal forms of CMT. LITAF/SIMPLE, the myotubulin-related proteins 2 and 13, and RAB7 are proteins involved in intracellular trafficking; determining how they cause CMT will facilitate research into the role of intracellular trafficking in neuropathy. Finally, investigations of disability in CMT1 have demonstrated the importance of Schwann cell–axonal interactions in demyelinating disease, because disability typically correlates better with secondary axonal degeneration rather than demyelination itself. In many ways, CMT serves as a living microarray system for myelinating and neuronal cells; it identifies molecules that are essential for the normal function of the PNS. An illustration of many of the proteins causing CMT and their localization in the PNS is shown in Fig. 105.1.

Specific Genetic Types of CMT
CMT1

CMT1A is the most common form of CMT, probably because of a homologous repeat sequence flanking the duplicated region (CMT1A-REP). Several lines of evidence suggest that the duplication of *PMP22* within the 1.4 Mb domain causes CMT1A: (1) Missense mutations in *PMP22* cause the Trembler (Tr) and Trembler J (Tr^J), naturally occurring mouse models of CMT; (2) transgenic mice and rats bearing extra copies of *PMP22* develop a CMT1A-like neuropathy; and (3) some patients with missense mutations in *PMP22* also develop a similar phenotype to CMT1A.

A deletion of exactly the same 1.4 Mb region, containing *PMP22*, was subsequently found in most cases of HNPP, an entirely different disorder and usually characterized by episodes of focal weakness or sensory loss rather than a length-dependent neuropathy. Missense mutations in *MPZ*, the major PNS myelin protein gene, on chromosome 1, causes CMT1B. MPZ is a member of the

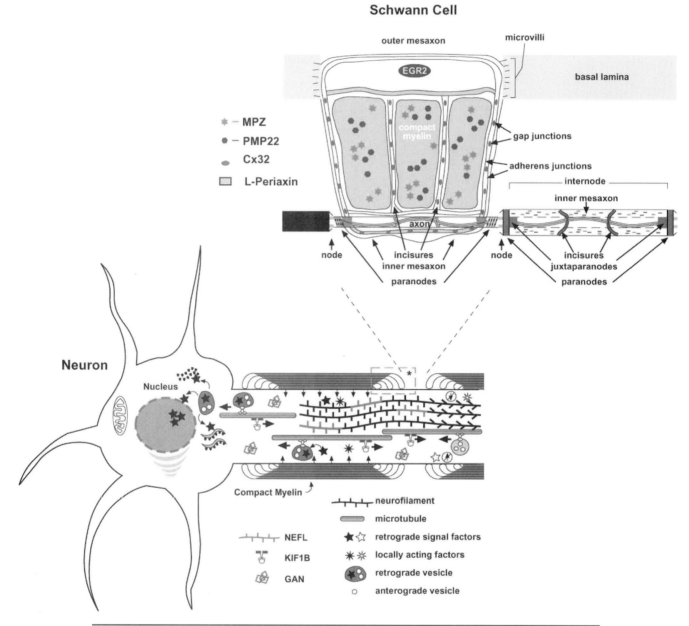

FIGURE 105.1. Schematic view of an axon and its myelinating Schwann cell. Proteins mutated in inherited peripheral neuropathies are shown in color at their cellular location. In the upper part of the panel, the myelinating Schwann cell has been unraveled, showing the nucleus and regions of both compact myelin and noncompact myelin. Cytoskeletal elements within the axon are also illustrated. (Modified from Shy ME, et al., *Lancet Neurology* 2002). (See color insert).

immunoglobulin gene superfamily, has a single transmembrane domain, and is necessary for the adhesion of concentric myelin wraps in the PNS internode. Missense mutations in the early growth response 2 (*EGR2*, also called *Krox20*), on chromosome 10, cause CMT1D. EGR2 is a transcription factor that is involved in the regulations of as yet unspecified genes in the myelinating Schwann cell. Finally, the genetic cause of CMT1C includes point mutations in the gene encoding the putative protein degradation gene *LITAF/SIMPLE*.

CMT2

Molecular genetic studies show that CMT2 is as genetically heterogeneous as CMT1. At least six subtypes of CMT2 (CMT2A, B, C, D, E, F) have been identified by linkage analysis (as listed in Online Mendelian Inheritance in Man (OMIM). CMT2A patients have classic CMT sensorimotor neuropathies. The locus of CMT2A is at chromosome 1p36. Most cases of CMT2A are caused by mutations in the nuclear encoded mitochondrial GTPase mitofusin 2 (*MFN2*) which cause about 10–20% of CMT2 cases. MFN2 is necessary for mitochondrial fusion. A single family has mutations in the kinesin gene KIFIB $\tilde{\beta}$; the protein encoded by this gene plays a fundamental role in anterograde axonal transport in myelinated axons. CMT2B is a predominantly sensory disorder and there is debate as to whether cases should be considered examples of pure sensory neuropathies. CMT2B is caused by mutations in the small GTPase late endosomal protein *RAB7* on chromosome 3q21. CMT2C is a rare disorder in which patients have paresis of the diaphragm and vocal cords in addition to other characteristics of CMT2. Although vocal cord and diaphragm paresis are not unique to CMT2C (CMT4A for example), linkage has been established to chromosome 12 in CMT2C, suggesting that it is genetically distinct. CMT2D is somewhat confusing because some patients have sensorimotor neuropathies whereas others have pure motor syndromes and are classed as hereditary motor neuropathy type V (HMNV). The genetic cause of CMT2D (and therefore HMNV) is mutation in the glycyl tRNA synthetase (*GARS*) gene. The GARS protein is involved in the ligation of glycine to its cognate tRNAs. An additional locus for CMT2 was detected with linkage to chromosome 8p21. Mutations in the neurofilament light (*NEFL*) gene also cause this neuropathy, now known as CMT2E. Because the NEFL protein is an important constituent of the neurofilaments used in axonal transport systems, and neurofilament phosphorylation is abnormal in demyelinating forms of CMT, CMT2E may provide important clues into mechanisms of axonal damage not only in CMT2 but also in CMT1. CMT2F has been reported in a multigenerational Russian family. Linkage studies have localized the causal gene to 7q11-21.

CMT4

CMT4, the autosomal recessively inherited neuropathies, is also a heterogeneous group of disorders. CMT4 cases are rare, usually more severe than the autosomal-dominant disorders, and many patients have systemic symptoms, such as cataracts and deafness. CMT4A is linked to a 5 cM region of 8q13-q21.1. The disorder was first described in four highly inbred families in Tunisia. Symptom onset began in the first 2 years of life, with delayed developmental milestones such as sitting or walking. Pathological studies from sural nerve biopsies revealed a loss of large-diameter myelinated fibers, and hypomyelination, but no abnormalities of myelin folding. So called basal lamina onion bulbs, characterized by concentric layers of basal lamina without intervening regions of Schwann cell cytoplasm, have been described in biopsies. Mutations in a gene encoding a protein of unknown function, ganglioside-induced-differentiation–associated protein1 (GDAP1), cause CMT4A. The mutations can cause either demyelinating or axonal neuropathies. Patients with the axonal form also have vocal cord paralysis in addition to other manifestations of severe sensorimotor neuropathies. Whether mutations in GDAP1 cause neuropathy by disrupting Schwann cell or neuronal function, or a combination of the two, is not known. A likely scenario is that *GDAP1* mutations disrupt signaling between Schwann cells and axons.

CMT4B1 is a recessively inherited disorder characterized clinically by a unique pathological feature: the presence of focally folded myelin sheaths in nerve biopsy. The genetic locus is on chromosome 11q23 and encodes a gene called myotubularin-related protein2 *(MTMR2)*. Affected patients become symptomatic early with an average age of onset of 34 months, and unlike most other forms of CMT, proximal as well as distal weakness is prominent. Motor conduction velocities are severely reduced with temporal dispersion. The amplitude of the compound muscle action potential (CMAP) is reduced, and sensory nerve action potentials (SNAPs) are frequently absent. Segmental demyelination is also found in nerve biopsies.

Four children in a Turkish inbred family were identified with neuropathies characterized by focally folded myelin, a characteristic of CMT4B as cited above. However, homozygosity mapping demonstrated linkage to a distinct locus on chromosome 11p15, leading to the designation of the locus as CMT4B2. Mutations have been identified in a large, novel gene named SET binding factor 2 *(SBF2)* that lies within the interval on 11p15 and segregates with the neuropathy in affected families, suggesting that the mutations are responsible for the disease. SBF2 is a member of the pseudophosphatase branch of myotubularins with striking homology to myotubularin-related protein 2 *(MTMR2)*.

Still another autosomal recessive form of demyelinating CMT is hereditary motor and sensory neuropathy-Russe (HMSNR). Patients develop primarily severe sensory loss, though motor NCVs are moderately reduced (on average, 31.9 m/s for ulnar and median nerves). The locus of HMSNR is positioned to 10q23.2, a small interval telomeric to the EGR2 gene.

Kalaydjieva and colleagues described a separate disorder with linkage to chromosome 8q24 in a Gypsy population with autosomal recessive inheritance; it is recognized as CMT4D. The neuropathy causes distal muscle wasting and weakness, sensory loss, both foot and hand deformities, and loss of tendon reflexes. Deafness is invariant and usually develops by the third decade. Brainstem auditory evoked responses (BAERs) are markedly abnormal with prolonged interpeak latencies. NCV is severely reduced in younger patients and unobtainable after age 15 years.

Mutations are found in the N-myc downstream-regulated gene (*NDRG1*); how the gene abnormality leads to the disorder is unknown.

CMT4C is a childhood-onset demyelinating form of hereditary motor and sensory neuropathy associated with an early-onset scoliosis and a distinct Schwann cell pathology. CMT4C is inherited as an autosomal recessive trait and is caused by homozygous or compound heterozygous mutations in the previously uncharacterized KIAA1985 gene. Scoliosis is prominent early on and may precede weakness or sensory loss. Mean median motor NCV was 22.6 m/s, and nerve biopsy, when obtained, showed demyelination, onion bulb formation, and most typically, large cytoplasmic extensions of Schwann cells. The translated protein defines a new protein family of unknown function with putative orthologues in vertebrates. Comparative sequence alignments indicate that members of this protein family contain multiple SH3 and TPR domains that are likely involved in the formation of protein complexes.

Finally, a novel, severe form of recessive CMT has been designated CMT4F and defined in a large Lebanese family in which mutations have been found in the periaxin (*PRX*) gene on chromosome 19. PRX, expressed in Schwann cells, encodes two proteins that contain PDZ domains that usually interact with other PDZ domain bearing proteins in intracellular signal transduction pathways. Binding partners for PRX in Schwann cells have not yet been identified, nor have the signal transduction pathways involving PRX been delineated. NCV in patients with PRX mutations is markedly slowed and onion bulbs are present in sural nerve biopsies.

DSN and Congenital Hypomyelination

DSN refers to severe genetic neuropathies that begin in infancy. Early motor milestones, such as walking, are frequently delayed and the ultimate course is more severe than described above, though patients may still ambulate independently as adults with appropriate aids. However, occasionally DSN patients die from the neuropathy, particularly if pulmonary sequelae are present. Clinical criteria for DSN include (1) onset by age 2 years with delayed motor milestones; (2) severe motor, sensory, and skeletal deficits with frequent extension to proximal muscles, sensory ataxia, and scoliosis; (3) very abnormal NCV with either slowing in the range of 10 m/sec or severe reductions in motor and sensory amplitudes; and (4), evidence of severe demyelination or axonal loss on nerve biopsy.

Congenital hypomyelination (CH) is a pathologically based term originally used to describe peripheral nerves that so are abnormal they suggest a developmental failure of PNS myelination. Patients with CH are usually hypotonic in the first year of life, have developmental delays in walking, and, in some cases, have swallowing or respiratory difficulties. CH patients often appear as

"floppy" infants. Patients classified as having CH or DSN have shown the same severe pathological changes on sural nerve biopsies and are both associated with very slow NCV (<10 m/sec). In fact, one patient was diagnosed as having CH in one publication and DSN in another. Taken together, these data suggest that it is difficult to distinguish between DSN and CH.

COURSE AND OUTCOME

Phenotypic variability occurs within given genotypes, and natural history studies of most forms of CMT are lacking. Nevertheless, generalizations can be provided about the course of CMT1 and CMT2.

Most patients with CMT, particularly CMT1A, have a classic phenotype in which early developmental milestones are normal and weakness and sensory loss gradually appear in the first two decades of life. Affected children are often slow runners, and activities requiring balance (skating, walking across a log) are particularly difficult. Ambulation aids for ankle support are frequently required in adulthood. Fine movements of the hands for activities such as turning a key or using buttons and zippers are also frequently problems, although the hands are rarely as impaired as feet. Most patients remain ambulatory throughout life and life span is not typically shortened. Some patients do not develop symptoms until adult years. Although usually milder, occasionally these late-onset cases can progress fairly rapidly to require wheelchair use.

ELECTROPHYSIOLOGY

Because NCV is easily measured and provides important information about whether neuropathies are primarily demyelinating or axonal processes, this measure is frequently used alone in classifying CMT as demyelinating or axonal, particularly because sural nerve biopsies are invasive techniques.

In the early 1980s, Lewis and Sumner demonstrated that most cases of inherited demyelinating neuropathies had uniformly slow NCV, whereas acquired demyelinating neuropathies, such as chronic inflammatory demyelinating polyradiculoneuropathy (CIDP), had asymmetric slowing. Thus, NCVs may be used, along with a patient's pedigree, to distinguish inherited and acquired neuropathies. In the past decade, however, this approach has had to be qualified. Most CMT1 patients, particularly those with CMT1A, do have uniformly slow NCV of about 20 m/sec, although values as high as 42 m/sec have been reported and are sometimes used as a cutoff value. However, asymmetric slowing is characteristic of HNPP, and may be found in patients with missense mutations in PMP22, MPZ, EGR2, and GJβ1. Because all of these disorders may appear without a clear family history of neuropathy, caution is needed in using NCV to distinguish acquired from inherited demyelinating neuropathies.

The use of NCV to distinguish between demyelinating and axonal neuropathies is also important. Virtually all forms of CMT1 show both axonal loss and demyelination, and it is likely that the axonal loss correlates better than demyelination with the patient's actual disability. Thus reductions in CMAP and SNAP amplitudes are found in most CMT1 patients; in one series of 43 CMT1A patients, 34 had unobtainable peroneal CMAPs and 41 had unobtainable sural SNAPs.

The distinction between demyelinating and axonal features of NCV is particularly confusing in CMTX1 and CMT1B. NCVs in CMTX1 patients are intermediately slow, and therefore are faster than in most patients with CMT1. These patients often also have prominent reductions in CMAP and SNAP amplitudes. Thus, CMTX1 has even been described as an axonal neuropathy. However, careful analysis of the conductions will reveal the primary demyelinating features of the neuropathy. The conduction velocities are usually not normal, but usually between 30 and 40 m/sec, values that would be considered an intermediate range between CMT1 and CMT2. Moreover, distal motor latencies and F-wave latencies are usually prolonged. In distinguishing between the demyelinating and axonal features of CMTX1, it is important to remember that the disease is caused by mutations in the Cx32 protein, which is expressed in the myelinating Schwann cell. Similar issues occur in some patients with mutations in the MPZ gene. For example, the Thr124Met mutation often has NCVs suggestive of an axonal neuropathy, and it is only through careful evaluation of the studies that evidence of the primary demyelinating features can be detected.

PATHOLOGY

Segmental demyelination, remyelination, and axonal loss are characteristic features of the various demyelinating forms of CMT. In cases of DSN, demyelination is severe. Onion bulbs of concentric Schwann cell lamellae are often found in nerve biopsies. In adults, the presence of onion bulbs may dominate the pathology. Axonal loss varies with individual patients. There is a loss of both small- and large-diameter myelinated fibers in nerve biopsies of CMT1 patients. Some fibers have relatively thickened myelin sheaths, resulting in lowered mean g ratios (axon diameter/fiber diameter). Focal sausage-like thickenings of the myelin sheath (tomacula) are characteristic of HNPP, but may also be found in other forms of CMT1, particularly CMT1B. Pathologic findings from sural nerve biopsies of CMT2 patients typically demonstrate axonal loss without evidence of demyelination.

DISTAL HEREDITARY MOTOR NEURONOPATHIES (HMN)

Distal HMNs comprise about 10% of all HMNs and have been tentatively classified into seven subtypes based on clinical manifestations, age at onset, and mode of inheritance. Genetic loci for several subtypes of distal HMN have been identified.

Distal HMN II has been linked in a large Belgian family to chromosome 12q24.3. Patients typically develop weakness in foot dorsiflexion by their late teens and some, but not all, become wheelchair bound in later years. Occasionally patients have been described with decreased vibratory sensation. NCVs are normal although needle EMG demonstrates evidence of chronic denervation. Recently, mutations in the α-crystallin domain of the small heat shock protein HSP22 were shown to cause dHMN type II. Moreover, mutations in a second sHSP, HSP27, cause either still another form of dHMN or a novel form of CMT2. Mutations in other sHSP family members have also been shown to cause myopathies and congenital cataracts. HSP22 and HSP27 have chaperone-like properties, suggesting that they may participate in the processing of proteins for intracellular trafficking. However, they have also been shown to inhibit apoptosis and to stabilize cytoskeletal systems.

Distal HMNV has been localized to chromosome 7p. It is the same disorder as CMT2D and is caused by mutations in the glycyl tRNA synthetase gene on chromosome 7p15. In a Bulgarian family with 30 affected members, hand weakness and wasting usually occur in the late teenage years. Although foot weakness ultimately develops in 40% of cases, this was usually mild and patients were still walking by age 60. One branch of the family had mild pyramidal features including Babinski signs. NCVs were normal except for reduced CMAP amplitudes in wasted muscles.

A recessive distal HMN has been termed the *Jerash type* based on a large Jordanian family with a locus mapped to chromosome 9p21.1-p12. Patients develop gait instability and footdrop prior to the age of 10 and a few years later develop wasting and weakness of hand muscles. Occasionally, milder phenotypes have been identified in patients over the age of 50. Initially, patients have presented with upper motor neuron signs including hyperreflexia, spasticity, and upgoing toes. Subsequently, ankle reflexes are lost and plantar responses were described as downgoing. The ultimate course of this disorder is relatively benign, with the oldest affected patient ambulatory at age 80.

An additional distal motor syndrome has been mapped to 9q34 and has been classified as an autosomal-dominant form of amyotrophic lateral sclerosis (ALS) (ALS4) because most patients have both upper and lower motor neuron signs including brisk reflexes and upgoing toes. However, the clinical course of these patients is much milder than typical ALS. Patients typically develop difficulties walking in adolescence, proximal weakness in the fourth or fifth decade, and many ultimately become wheelchair bound. Useful hand function is often not lost until the sixth decade. Patients have lived into the 80s. An autopsy on one patient, who died of a myocardial infarction, revealed atrophy of both ventral and dorsal roots, chromatolysis and axonal swelling in both ventral and dorsal roots, and a loss of anterior horn cells. NCV studies revealed decreased CMAP amplitudes in weak wasted muscles, and needle EMG demonstrated changes of chronic denervation and partial reinnervation. The disorder is caused by missense mutations in the senataxin gene (SETX). The function of SETX is unknown but the gene product contains a DNA/RNA helicase domain with strong homology to RNA processing proteins.

Puls and colleagues showed linkage of a lower motor neuron disorder to a region of 4 Mb at chromosome 2p13. Mutation analysis of a gene in this interval that encodes the largest subunit of the axonal transport protein, dynactin, showed a single base-pair change resulting in an amino acid substitution that is predicted to distort the folding of dynactin's microtubule-binding domain. Binding assays show decreased binding of the mutant protein to microtubules, suggesting that dysfunction of dynactin-mediated transport caused the motor neuron degeneration.

HEREDITARY SENSORY AND AUTONOMIC NEUROPATHIES (HSAN)

Rare cases of heritable sensory neuropathies, occasionally with autonomic features, have been described. The specific genetic causes of three of these unusual disorders have been identified.

HSAN type 1 has been shown to be caused by mutations in the serine palmitoyltransferase subunit 1 (SPTLC1) gene on 9q22, which encodes the rate limiting enzyme in ceramide synthesis. Patients with HSAN1 develop symptoms of small sensory fiber dysfunction between the second and fourth decades of life. Typically these symptoms include the development of neuropathic pain, plantar ulcers, loss of pain and temperature sensation, and, in some cases, autonomic problems. Occasionally, large fiber modalities such as vibration sensation and proprioception have also been abnormal. Tendon reflexes are decreased in the legs and patients may have atrophy of distal muscles with pes cavus. NCVs are normal but SNAP amplitudes are reduced. Pathological studies reveal neuronal loss in DRGs and sympathetic ganglia, with subsequent length-dependent degeneration of small fiber axons, although all sizes of sensory axons are affected to some degree. Cases have been described with associated deafness or weakness; whether these are the same disorder is not yet known.

HSAN II is a recessive disorder with an early severe onset. Fingers as well as toes are involved, and patients develop paronychia, whitlows, and ulcerations of their fingers in addition to foot ulcerations. Sensory loss affects both small and large fiber modalities. Sweating is reduced although patients do not develop orthostatic hypotension, sphincter dysfunction, or (in males) impotence. NCVs reveal absent SNAPs, and sural nerve biopsies demonstrate both an absence of myelinated fibers and reduction of nonmyelinated fibers. Recently, a novel gene called HSN2 has been found to be the cause of HSAN type II in five families from Newfoundland and Quebec.

Familial dysautonomia (HSAN III), also known as the Riley-Day syndrome, has been shown to be caused by mutations in the IKAP gene on chromosome 9q31. Although the intronic mutation is present in all cells, it appears to disrupt splicing in a tissue-specific manner in DRG and sympathetic neurons, leading to a truncated protein. The role of IKAP is unknown, but it may play a role in regulating transcription of several genes even though it is not a transcription factor in its own right. HSAN III is particularly frequent in the Ashkenazi Jewish population. Some estimates have placed the frequency of carriers in Israel as high as 18 per 100,000. Clinically, patients display abnormalities from birth, including an absence of fungiform papilla on the tongue, poor sucking, difficulties swallowing, alacrima (loss of overflow tears), and blotching of the skin with emotions. Autonomic abnormalities include labile blood pressure with severe postural hypotension and both excesses and decreases of seating. Intradermal injections of histamine fail to produce the characteristic histamine flare. Tendon reflexes are typically decreased. Most patients have loss of pain and temperature sensation. Corneal reflexes are absent, consistent with trigeminal nerve involvement. Vibration and position sense are also abnormal in some patients. Motor NCVs can be mildly slow and SNAPs reduced. Morphologic studies show a loss of neurons in both cervical and thoracic sympathetic ganglia. Decreased numbers of small, unmyelinated fibers have been reported in sural nerve biopsies.

Congenital insensitivity to pain with anhydrosis (CIPA) has been classified as HSAN IV. Patients present with a congenital insensitivity to painful stimuli and anhydrosis despite normal-appearing sweat glands on skin biopsy. Temperature sensation is also defective, and 20% of patients die owing to hyperpyrexia, usually before the age of three. Body temperatures up to 109°F have been reported. Patients have been known to bite off the tips of their tongue when they develop dentition and self-mutilate their lips and tips of their fingers. Most children are also mentally retarded with IQs between 41 and 78. Sural nerve biopsies reveal a loss of myelinated and nonmyelinated axons. Mice in which the nerve growth factor receptor, TrkA, has been deleted also have insensitivity to pain, and missense mutations in the human homologue of TrkA, NTRK1, deletions of NTRK1, and splice site abnormalities of NTRK1 have all been detected in patients with the disease.

TREATMENT

Traditional Therapies

Because no specific cures are available for the inherited neuropathies, the physician's role is to provide clinical and genetic counseling and to suggest symptomatic and rehabilitative treatment. Advice about the nature of the inheritance and the prognosis is best given only after knowing the kinship history, which in some cases means that available relatives will need to be evaluated.

Genetic counseling should not be based on phenotype, but on information obtained from study of the family history. Because CMT can be transmitted as an autosomal-dominant, autosomal-recessive, X-linked dominant, and X-linked recessive trait, the physician must be familiar with how to recognize the pattern of inheritance.

Appropriate orthotics and bracing may be helpful for many patients. However, in our experience, foot surgery is often not needed. Foot surgery to correct excessively inverted feet, for severe degrees of pes cavus and hammertoes may improve walking and alleviate pain over pressure points and prevent plantar ulcers. The patient must be given realistic objectives for the operation, because obviously it is not a panacea for such other manifestations of the disorder as weakness and sensory loss.

New Therapeutic Approaches

An antagonist to progesterone improves the neuropathy in the transgenic rat model of CMT1A. Administration of the selective progesterone receptor antagonist reduced overexpression of Pmp22 and improved the CMT phenotype, without obvious adverse effects. It is not yet known whether side effects from a progesterone antagonist will limit this therapy in humans. Similarly, it is not known whether this therapy will be effective once the full-blown neuropathy has developed because the rats were treated from a young age. Nevertheless, these data suggest that the progesterone receptor of myelin-forming Schwann cells is a promising pharmacologic target for therapy of CMT-1A.

Similarly, recent studies have demonstrated that high doses of ascorbic acid can limit or improve the neuropathy of a mouse model of CMT1A. This strategy was based on the knowledge that co-cultures of rodent DRGs and Schwann cells require ascorbic acid to myelinate. Currently clinical trials are being developed to assess potential benefits of high dose ascorbic acid in patients with CMT1A.

A small percentage of patients with inherited neuropathy may respond to immunomodulatory therapy, such as prednisone or IVIG. Usually, these patients have had features atypical for CMT1 and findings that mimic CIDP. However, these patients are probably the exception rather than the rule, and it is unlikely that immunomodulatory therapy will be effective in most patients with CMT.

Finally, new treatments are being developed to take advantage of ever-expanding technologies. A mouse model of CMT1A has been developed in which disease severity can be modified a tetracycline responsive element in the Pmp22 promoter. Viral vectors are being used to introduce genes into myelin and neurons to develop gene therapy strategies. Many animal models of CMT have now been developed that can serve as test systems for future therapeutics. It is hoped that the future era of molecular therapeutics will become as exciting and fruitful and exciting as the present era of molecular diagnosis.

ACKNOWLEDGEMENT

The author thanks Karen Krajewski for her help with Table 105.1.

SUGGESTED READINGS

Antonellis A, Ellsworth RE, Sambuughin N, et al. Glycyl tRNA synthetase mutations in Charcot-Marie-Tooth disease type 2D and distal spinal muscular atrophy type V. *Am J Hum Genet* 2003;72:1293–1299.

Arroyo EJ, Scherer SS (2000). On the molecular architecture of myelinated fibers. *Histochem Cell Biol* 2000;113(Jan):1–18.

Bergoffen J, Scherer SS, Wang S, et al. Connexin mutations in X-linked Charcot-Marie-Tooth disease. *Science* 1993;262:2039–2042.

Dyck PJ, Lambert EH. Lower motor and primary sensory neuron diseases with peroneal muscular atrophy. I. Neurologic, genetic, and electrophysiologic findings in hereditary polyneuropathies. *Arch Neurol* 1968a;18:603–618.

Dyck PJ, Lambert EH. Lower motor and primary sensory neuron diseases with peroneal muscular atrophy. II. Neurologic, genetic, and electrophysiologic findings in various neuronal degenerations. *Arch Neurol* 1968b;18:619–625.

Harding AE, Thomas PK. The clinical features of hereditary motor and sensory neuropathy types I and II. *Brain* 1980;103(Jun):259–280.

Harding AE, Thomas PK. Genetic aspects of hereditary motor and sensory neuropathy (types I and II). *J Med Genet* 1980;17:329–336.

Krajewski KM, Lewis RA, Fuerst DR, et al. Neurological dysfunction and axonal degeneration in Charcot-Marie-Tooth disease type 1A. *Brain* 2000;123(Pt 7):1516–1527.

Lewis RA, Sumner AJ, Shy ME. Electrophysiological features of inherited demyelinating neuropathies: a reappraisal in the era of molecular diagnosis. *Muscle Nerve* 2000;23:1472–1487.

Li J, Krajewski K, Lewis RA, et al. Loss of function phenotype of hereditary neuropathy with liability to pressure palsies. *Muscle Nerve* 2004;29(Feb):205–210.

Lupski JR, de Oca-Luna RM, Slaugenhaupt S, et al. DNA duplication associated with Charcot-Marie-Tooth disease type 1A. *Cell* 1991;66 (Jul 26):219–232.

Nelis EC, Van Broeckhoven C, De Jonghe P, et al. Estimation of the mutation frequencies in Charcot-Marie-Tooth disease type 1 and hereditary neuropathy with liability to pressure palsies: a European collaborative study. *Eur J Hum Genet* 1996;4(1):25–33.

Puls I, Jonnakuty C, LaMonte BH, et al. Mutant dynactin in motor neuron disease. *Nat Genet* 2003;33::455–456.

Raeymaekers P, Timmerman V, Nelis E, et al. Duplication in chromosome 17p11.2 in Charcot-Marie-Tooth neuropathy type 1a (CMT 1a). The HMSN Collaborative Research Group. *Neuromuscul Disord* 1991;1(2):93–97.

Shy ME, Garbern J, Kamholz J. Hereditary motor and sensory neuropathies: a biological perspective. *Lancet Neurology* 2002;1:110–118.

Shy ME, Jani A, Krajewski KM, et al. Phenotypic clustering in MPZ mutations. *Brain* 2004;127:371–384

Suter U, Scherer SS. Disease mechanisms in inherited neuropathies. *Nat Rev Neurosci* 2003;4:714–726.

Chapter 106

Acquired Neuropathies

Thomas H Brannagan III, Louis H. Weimer, and Norman Latov

GUILLAIN-BARRÉ SYNDROME AND VARIANTS

The Guillain-Barré syndrome (GBS; acute inflammatory demyelinating neuropathy) is characterized by acute onset of peripheral and cranial nerve dysfunction. Viral respiratory or gastrointestinal infection, immunization, or surgery often precedes neurologic symptoms by 5 days to 3 weeks. Symptoms and signs include rapidly progressive symmetric weakness, loss of tendon reflexes, facial diplegia, oropharyngeal and respiratory paresis, and impaired sensation in the hands and feet. The condition worsens for several days to 3 weeks, followed by a period of stability and then gradual improvement to normal or nearly normal function. Early plasmapheresis or intravenous infusion of human gamma globulins (IVIG) accelerates recovery and diminishes the incidence of long-term neurologic disability.

Etiology

The cause of GBS is unknown. It is thought to be immune mediated because a disease with similar clinical features (i.e., similar pathologic, electrophysiologic, and CSF alterations) can be induced in experimental animals by immunization with whole peripheral nerve, peripheral nerve myelin, or, in some species, peripheral nerve myelin P2 basic protein or galactocerebroside. Although there is no evidence of sensitization to these antigens in humans with spontaneous GBS, activity of the disease seems to correlate with the appearance of serum antibodies to peripheral nerve myelin. When GBS is preceded by a viral infection, there is no evidence of direct viral infection of peripheral nerves or nerve roots.

Electrophysiology and Pathology

Nerve conduction velocities are reduced in GBS, but values may be normal early in the course. Distal sensory and motor latencies are prolonged. As a result of demyelination of nerve roots, F-wave conduction velocity is often slowed or the responses absent. Conduction slowing may persist

for months or years after clinical recovery. In general, the severity of neurologic abnormality is not related to the degree of conduction slowing, but is related to the extent of conduction block or axonal loss. Long-standing weakness is most apt to occur when there are reduced compound motor action potential (CMAP) amplitudes less than 20% of normal.

Histologically, GBS is characterized by focal segmental demyelination (Fig. 106.1) with perivascular and endoneurial infiltrates of lymphocytes and monocytes or macrophages (Fig. 106.2). These lesions are scattered throughout the nerves, nerve roots, and cranial nerves. In particularly severe lesions, there is both axonal degeneration and segmental demyelination. During recovery, remyelination occurs, but the lymphocytic infiltrates may persist.

Incidence

GBS is the most frequent acquired demyelinating neuropathy, with an incidence of 0.6 to 1.9 cases per 100,000 population. The incidence increases gradually with age, but the disease may occur at any age. Men and women are affected equally. The incidence increases in patients with Hodgkin disease, as well as with pregnancy or general surgery.

Symptoms and Signs

GBS often appears days to weeks after symptoms of a viral upper respiratory or gastrointestinal infection. Usually, the first neurologic symptoms are a result of symmetric limb weakness, often with paresthesia. In contrast to most other neuropathies, proximal muscles are sometimes affected more often than distal muscles at first. Occasionally, facial, ocular, or oropharyngeal muscles may be affected first; more than 50% of patients have facial diplegia, and dysphagia and dysarthria develop in a similar number. Some patients require mechanical ventilation. Tendon reflexes may be normal for the first few days but are then lost. The degree of sensory impairment varies. In some patients, all sensory modalities are preserved; others have marked diminution in perception of joint position, vibration, pain, and temperature in stocking-and-glove distribution. Patients occasionally exhibit papilledema, sensory ataxia, and transient extensor plantar responses. Autonomic dysfunction, including orthostatic hypotension, labile blood pressure, tachyarrhythmia and bradyarrhythmia, or resting tachycardia is frequent in more severe cases and an important cause of morbidity and mortality. Many have muscle tenderness, and the nerves may be sensitive to pressure, but there are no signs of meningeal irritation such as nuchal rigidity.

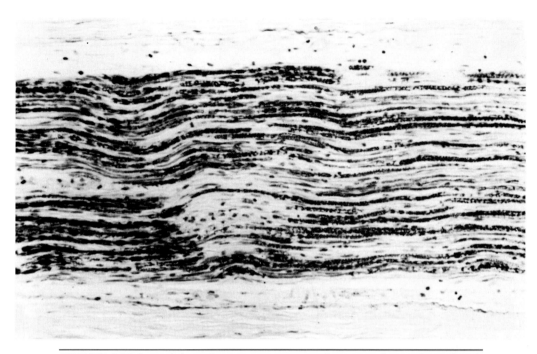

FIGURE 106.1. Focal demyelination in acute GBS. (Courtesy of Dr. Arthur Asbury.)

Variants

Acute motor axonal neuropathy (AMAN) is a variant of GBS. There is motor axonal degeneration and little or no demyelination or inflammation. Despite the axonal involvement, recovery is similar to the demyelinating form.

AMAN may follow infection with *Campylobacter jejuni* or parenteral injection of gangliosides.

The *Miller-Fisher syndrome* is characterized by gait ataxia, areflexia, and ophthalmoparesis; pupillary abnormalities are sometimes present. It is considered a variant of

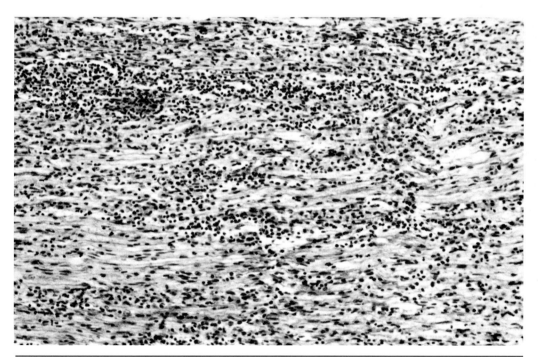

FIGURE 106.2. Diffuse mononuclear infiltrate in peripheral nerve in GBS. (Courtesy of Dr. Arthur Asbury.)

GBS because it is often preceded by respiratory infection, it progresses for weeks and then improves, and CSF protein content is increased. There is no limb weakness, however, and nerve conductions are generally normal; however, H-reflexes may be affected. In some cases, MRI shows brainstem hyperintense lesions.

Other GBS variants include *acute motor and sensory axonal neuropathy, acute sensory neuropathy or neuronopathy,* and *acute autonomic neuropathy* or *pandysautonomia* (Chap 138).

Laboratory Data

The CSF protein content is elevated in most patients with GBS but may be normal in the first few days after onset. The CSF cell count is usually normal, but some patients with otherwise typical GBS have 10 to 100 mononuclear cells/μL of CSF. Antecedent infectious mononucleosis, cytomegalovirus (CMV) infection, viral hepatitis, HIV infection, or other viral diseases may be documented by serologic studies. Increased titers of immunoglobulin (Ig) G or IgA antibodies to GM_1 or GD_{1a} gangliosides may be found in the axonal form of GBS; anti-GQ_{1b} antibodies are closely associated with the Miller-Fisher syndrome.

Course and Prognosis

Symptoms are usually most severe within 1 week of onset but may progress for 3 weeks or more. Death is uncommon but may follow aspiration pneumonia, pulmonary embolism, intercurrent infection, or autonomic dysfunction. The rate of recovery varies. In some, it is rapid, with restoration to normal function within a few weeks. In most, recovery is slow and not complete for many months. Recovery is accelerated by early institution of plasmapheresis or intravenous immunoglobulin therapy. In untreated series, about 35% of patients have permanent residual hyporeflexia, atrophy, and weakness of distal muscles or facial paresis. A biphasic illness, with partial recovery followed by relapse, is present in fewer than 10% of patients. Recurrence after full recovery occurs in about 2%.

Diagnosis and Differential Diagnosis

The characteristic history of subacute development of symmetric motor or sensorimotor neuropathy after a viral illness, delivery, or surgery, together with compatible electrophysiology and an elevated CSF protein content with normal cell count, define GBS.

In the past, the principal diseases to be differentiated from GBS were diphtheritic polyneuropathy and acute poliomyelitis. Both are now rare in the United States. Diphtheritic polyneuropathy can usually be distinguished by the long latency period between the respiratory infection and onset of neuritis, the frequency of paralysis of accommodation, and the relatively slow evolution of symptoms. Acute anterior poliomyelitis was distinguished by asymmetry of paralysis, signs of meningeal irritation, fever, and CSF pleocytosis. Acute West Nile viral infection, however, can lead to a similar picture. Acute encephalitis is the most common West Nile neurologic manifestation, but an acute paralytic syndrome is the next most frequent. Asymmetric or monomelic weakness is characteristic, but some cases develop in a GBS-like manner. Some cases have a flulike prodrome without notable encephalitis. Occasionally, patients with HIV infection have a disorder identical to GBS. Porphyric neuropathy resembles GBS clinically but is differentiated by normal CSF protein, recurrent abdominal crisis, mental symptoms, onset after exposure to barbiturates or other drugs, and high urinary levels of δ-aminolevulinic acid and porphobilinogen. Development of a GBS-like syndrome during prolonged parenteral feeding should raise the possibility of hypophosphatemia-induced neural dysfunction. Toxic neuropathies caused by n-hexane inhalation or thallium or arsenic ingestion may begin acutely or subacutely. Botulism may be difficult to discriminate on clinical grounds from purely motor forms of GBS, but ocular muscles and the pupils are frequently affected. Electrophysiologic tests in botulism reveal normal nerve conduction velocities and a facilitating response to repetitive nerve stimulation. Tick paralysis, which occurs almost exclusively in children, should be excluded by careful examination of the scalp.

Treatment

Early plasmapheresis has proved useful in patients with GBS. IVIG therapy is also reported to be beneficial. Glucocorticoid administration does not shorten the course or affect the prognosis. Mechanically assisted ventilation is sometimes necessary, and precautions against aspiration of food or stomach contents must be taken if oropharyngeal muscles are affected. Exposure keratitis must be prevented in patients with facial diplegia.

CHRONIC INFLAMMATORY DEMYELINATING POLYNEUROPATHY

Chronic inflammatory demyelinating polyneuropathy (CIDP) may begin insidiously or acutely, as in GBS, and then follow a chronic progressive or relapsing course. It often follows nonspecific viral infections, although less often than in GBS. Segmental demyelination and lymphocytic infiltrates are present in peripheral nerves, and a similar disease can be induced in experimental animals by immunization with peripheral nerve myelin. The CSF protein content is often increased but less consistently than in GBS. An infantile form of CIDP begins with hypotonia and delayed motor development. Optic neuritis has been noted in some patients. Nerves may become enlarged because of Schwann cell proliferation and collagen deposition after recurrent segmental demyelination and remyelination.

In contrast to GBS, glucocorticoid therapy is often beneficial. CIDP is also responsive to plasmapheresis or IVIG, and immunosuppressive drug therapy may be effective in resistant cases. Research criteria for the diagnosis of CIDP have been recommended, but there is no specific test, and the diagnosis is often made on clinical grounds. A predominantly sensory form of CIDP and an axonal form have been described; it is likely that CIDP is heterogeneous, including several different chronic immune-mediated diseases that affect peripheral nerves. Tests for HIV-1, monoclonal paraproteins, antibodies to myelin-associated glycoprotein (MAG) and, occasionally, Charcot-Marie-Tooth disease type 1 or hereditary neuropathy with liability to pressure palsy are carried out in suspected patients to evaluate possible causes of demyelinating neuropathy.

MULTIFOCAL MOTOR NEUROPATHY

Multifocal motor neuropathy (MMN) is manifested by a clinical syndrome restricted to signs of a lower motor neuron disorder. Typically, there is weakness, wasting, and fasciculation with preserved or absent tendon reflexes. The findings are often asymmetric and affect the arms and hands more than the legs. Electrophysiologic evidence of denervation is accompanied by the defining abnormality, physiologic evidence of multifocal motor conduction block, at sites other than typical compression sites. Other signs of demyelination are also described. MMN is associated with increased titers of IgM anti-GM_1 in about one-third of the patients; less frequently, anti-GD_{1a} antibodies are found. It is important to recognize these patients and to distinguish them from patients with typical motor neuron disease because the weakness of MMN is reversible with IVIG or immunosuppressive drug therapy.

SENSORY NEURONOPATHY AND NEUROPATHY

Sensory neuropathy may result from primary involvement of the sensory root ganglia, as in ganglioneuritis or sensory neuronitis, or the nerve may be directly affected as in distal sensory neuropathy. *Ganglioneuritis* may be acute or subacute in onset and is characterized by numbness, paresthesia, and pain that can be distal or radicular or involve the entire body including the face. Ataxia and autonomic dysfunction may be evident. Small- or large-fiber sensation or both may be affected to varying degrees. Ten-

don reflexes may be present or absent, and strength is normal. The disease may be self-limiting or chronic, with relapses or slow progression. Motor nerve conduction velocities are normal or near normal, but sensory potentials are reduced in amplitude or absent. Routine electrophysiologic studies may be normal if the disease is mild or if only small fibers are affected. CSF protein content is normal or slightly elevated. Response to glucocorticoids or immunosuppressive therapy is variable. Pathologic studies of spinal root ganglia show inflammatory infiltrates with a predominance of T cells and macrophages. Some patients have sicca or Sjögren syndrome with anti-Ro and anti-La antibodies.

Several autoantibodies to peripheral nerve antigens have been reported to be associated with sensory neuropathy. Some patients with sensory axonal neuropathies have monoclonal or polyclonal IgM antisulfatide antibodies, and monoclonal IgM autoantibodies with anti-GD_{1b} and disialosyl ganglioside antibody activity have been associated with large-fiber sensory neuropathy. Other causes of sensory neuropathy include HIV-1 infection, vitamin B_6 deficiency or toxicity, celiac disease, paraneoplastic neuropathy, amyloidosis, and toxic neuropathy.

IDIOPATHIC AUTONOMIC NEUROPATHY

This condition is characterized by acute or subacute sympathetic or parasympathetic nerve dysfunction. Symptoms include postural syncope, diminished tear and sweat production, marked gastrointestinal dysmotility, impaired bladder function, and impotence. The autonomic preganglionic or postganglionic efferent neurons are affected. Antibodies to the nicotinic acetyl choline receptor alpha 3 subunit are seen in 41% of patients. It may follow viral infection, as in GBS. The disease is usually monophasic, and gradual but usually incomplete recovery occurs. IVIG treatment has shown anecdotal benefit in small series.

VASCULITIC AND CRYOGLOBULINEMIC NEUROPATHIES

Vasculitic neuropathy is manifested as mononeuritis multiplex or distal symmetric polyneuropathy. Nerve conduction studies may show electrical inexcitability of nerve segments distal to an infarct caused by vascular occlusion. If some fascicles in the nerves are spared, they conduct at a normal rate, but the amplitude of the evoked response is diminished. The diagnosis of peripheral nerve involvement may be established by nerve and muscle biopsies (Fig. 106.3), which typically show inflammatory cell infiltrates and necrosis of the walls of blood vessels. The biopsy

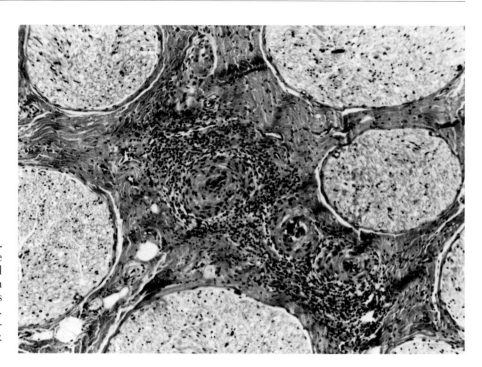

FIGURE 106.3. Polyarteritis in large proximal nerve trunk. Three small epineurial arteries show inflammation in the vessel wall and adventitia, as well as luminal narrowing and fibrosis. Surrounding nerve fascicles are not involved in this section. (Courtesy of Dr. Arthur Asbury.)

specimen, however, may show only axonal degeneration if vasculitis has caused a nerve infarct that is proximal to the site of biopsy, or if no affected vessels are encountered in the specimen.

The vasculitis may be confined to the peripheral nerves or may be associated with systemic disease, such as polyarteritis or cryoglobulinemia. The most common systemic cause of vasculitic neuropathy is polyarteritis nodosa, which may cause purpuric skin lesions, renal failure, Raynaud phenomenon, constitutional symptoms, and sometimes, mixed polyclonal cryoglobulinemia; hepatitis B or C virus (HBV or HCV) or HIV infection may be found. Cryoglobulins are immunoglobulins that precipitate in the cold and are classified as types I through III. Type I contains a monoclonal immunoglobulin only, type II contains both monoclonal and polyclonal immunoglobulins, and type III contains mixed polyclonal immunoglobulins. Types I and II are associated with plasma cell dyscrasia, and type III may be associated with polyarteritis nodosa and HBV or HCV infection.

Other causes of vasculitic neuropathy include the Churg-Strauss syndrome with asthma and eosinophilia; Sjögren syndrome with xerophthalmia, xerostomia, and anti-Ro and anti-La antibodies; and Wegener granulomatosis with necrotizing granulomatous lesions in the upper or lower respiratory tracts, glomerulonephritis, and antineutrophilic cytoplasmic antigen antibodies. Less commonly, vasculitic neuropathy is seen in rheumatoid arthritis, systemic lupus erythematosus, and systemic sclerosis. Vasculitis may respond to therapy with prednisone and cyclophosphamide. Plasmapheresis is also useful in the treatment of cryoglobulinemia.

NEUROPATHIES ASSOCIATED WITH MYELOMA AND NONMALIGNANT IgG OR IgA MONOCLONAL GAMMOPATHIES

Peripheral neuropathy is found in approximately 50% of patients with osteosclerotic myeloma and IgG or IgA monoclonal gammopathies. Some patients have the POEMS syndrome (polyneuropathy, organomegaly, endocrinopathy, myeloma, and skin changes or Crow-Fukase syndrome) with hyperpigmentation of skin, edema, excessive hair growth, hepatosplenomegaly, papilledema, elevated CSF protein content, hypogonadism, and hypothyroidism. POEMS syndrome is sometimes associated with nonosteosclerotic myeloma or with nonmalignant monoclonal gammopathy. The IgG or IgA light-chain type is almost always lambda. Electrophysiologic and pathologic abnormalities are consistent with demyelination and axonal degeneration; the patterns may resemble CIDP.

Malignant or nonmalignant IgG or IgA monoclonal gammopathy may also be associated with neuropathy in primary amyloidosis, in which fragments of the monoclonal light chains are deposited as amyloid in peripheral nerve, and in types I and II cryoglobulinemia, in which the monoclonal immunoglobulins are components of the cryoprecipitates.

The significance of IgG or IgA monoclonal gammopathies is uncertain in the absence of myeloma, POEMS syndrome, amyloidosis, or cryoglobulinemia. Nonmalignant monoclonal gammopathies are found more frequently in patients with neuropathy of otherwise unknown etiology; however, they are also present in approximately 1% of normal adults, and the frequency increases with age or in chronic infections or inflammatory diseases, so the association with neuropathy in some cases could be coincidental. Other causes of neuropathy, particularly inflammatory conditions such as CIDP, should be considered. In cases of myeloma, irradiation, chemotherapy, or bone marrow transplantation may be beneficial.

NEUROPATHIES ASSOCIATED WITH IgM MONOCLONAL ANTIBODIES THAT REACT WITH PERIPHERAL NERVE GLYCOCONJUGATE ANTIGENS

In several syndromes, peripheral neuropathy is associated with polyclonal or monoclonal IgM autoantibodies that react with glycoconjugates in peripheral nerve. IgM antibodies that react with MAG are associated with a chronic demyelinating sensorimotor neuropathy. Pathologic studies show deposits of the monoclonal IgM and complement on affected myelin sheaths, and passive transfer of the autoantibodies in experimental animals reproduces the neuropathy. Treatment consisting of plasmapheresis and chemotherapy to reduce autoantibody concentrations, or IVIG, frequently results in clinical improvement.

Increased titers of polyclonal or monoclonal anti-GM$_1$ ganglioside antibodies are associated with a clinical syndrome of motor neuropathy. Typically, there is weakness, wasting, and fasciculation with active or absent tendon reflexes. The condition is associated with electrophysiologic evidence of denervation and conduction block. Conduction block is not always present, however, in patients with increased antibody titers. The same clinical syndrome may also occur in patients with normal titers of anti-GM$_1$ antibodies. It is important to recognize these patients and to distinguish them from patients with typical motor neuron disease because the weakness may be reversed by immunosuppressive chemotherapy or IVIG.

Other syndromes associated with monoclonal or polyclonal IgM autoantibodies include the following: multifocal motor neuropathy or lower motor neuron syndrome–associated anti-GD$_{1a}$ ganglioside antibodies, large-fiber sensory neuropathy with anti-GD$_{1b}$ and disialosyl ganglioside antibodies, and axonal sensory neuropathy associated with antisulfatide antibodies. Antisulfatide antibodies typically are associated with small-fiber or small- and large-fiber neuropathy, but 25% of cases demonstrate a CIDP-like demyelinating neuropathy.

AMYLOID NEUROPATHY

Amyloid is an insoluble extracellular aggregate of proteins that forms in nerve or other tissues when any of several proteins is produced in excess. The two principal forms of amyloid protein that cause neuropathy are immunoglobulin light chains in patients with primary amyloidosis and plasma cell dyscrasias, and transthyretin in hereditary amyloidosis. The syndrome is often that of a painful, small-fiber sensory neuropathy with progressive autonomic failure, symmetric loss of pain and temperature sensations with spared position and vibratory senses, carpal tunnel syndrome, or some combination of these symptoms. The diagnosis of amyloid neuropathy can be established by histologic demonstration of amyloid in nerve (Fig. 106.4), followed by immunocytochemical characterization of the deposits with the use of antibodies to immunoglobulin light chains or transthyretin. Mutation of the transthyretin gene is detected by DNA analysis. Other hereditary amyloidosis causes, such as apolipoprotein A1 and gelsolin lead to less severe and less frequent neuropathy. Electrophoresis of serum and urine with immunofixation can assist in the diagnosis of primary amyloid neuropathy. Prognosis is generally poor. Liver transplantation has been reported to be beneficial for hereditary amyloidosis, and high-dose chemotherapy followed by bone marrow transplantation has been reported to help some patients with primary amyloidosis.

NEUROPATHY ASSOCIATED WITH CARCINOMA (PARANEOPLASTIC NEUROPATHY)

Both direct and indirect effects of malignant neoplasms on the peripheral nervous system are recognized. In some patients, the nerves or nerve roots are compressed or infiltrated by neoplastic cells. In others, there is no evidence of damage to the nerves by the neoplasm, and dietary deficiency or metabolic, toxic, or immunologic factors may be responsible.

The most characteristic paraneoplastic disorder is a sensory neuropathy of subacute onset, associated with small cell carcinoma of the lung. Electrodiagnostic studies reveal loss of sensory evoked responses. Autoantibodies against the Hu antigen (antineuronal nuclear or ANNA) are characteristic, and postmortem studies show loss of neurons, deposition of antibodies, and inflammatory cells in dorsal root ganglia.

Less consistently associated with carcinoma is a distal sensorimotor polyneuropathy without specific features. Nerve biopsy may reveal infiltration by tumor cells, axonal degeneration, or demyelination. A primarily motor syndrome of subacute onset occurs in Hodgkin disease and other lymphomas. In these patients, the predominant lesion is degeneration of anterior horn cells, but demyelination, perivascular mononuclear cell infiltrates, and alterations in Schwann cell morphology in ventral roots are also observed. Some patients also have probable or definite upper motor neuron signs in life, and corticospinal tract degeneration is found at autopsy; that is, they have clinical

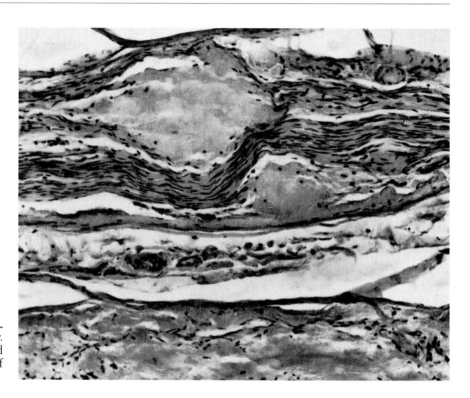

FIGURE 106.4. Amyloid neuropathy. Massive deposits of endoneurial amyloid compress nerve fiber bundles. (Courtesy of Dr. Arthur Asbury.)

and pathologic evidence of amyotrophic lateral sclerosis (ALS).

The diagnosis of malignancy should be suspected in a middle-aged or elderly patient with a subacute sensory neuropathy or polyradiculopathy of obscure cause, particularly with weight loss. The course is usually progressive until the primary malignancy is cured or until it causes death. CSF examination for malignant cells is valuable in the diagnosis of infiltration of the meninges by cancer. In some instances of meningeal infiltration, radiotherapy or intrathecal chemotherapy may be valuable.

HYPOTHYROID NEUROPATHY

Entrapment neuropathies are relatively common in patients with hypothyroidism, probably because acid mucopolysaccharide protein complexes (mucoid) are deposited in the nerve. Painful paresthesia in the hands and feet is the most common symptom of hypothyroidism. Weakness is not a feature. Tendon reflexes are reduced or absent, and, when present, may show the characteristic delayed or "hung-up" response. Direct percussion of muscle produces transient mounding of the underlying skin and muscle (myoedema). Nerve conduction studies show mild slowing of motor nerve conduction and decreased amplitude of the sensory evoked response. Morphologic studies show evidence of demyelination, axonal loss, and excessive glycogen within Schwann cells. CSF protein content is often more than 100 mg/dL. Rarely, dysfunction of cranial

nerves IX, X, and XII causes hoarseness and dysarthria, probably as a result of local myxedematous infiltration of the nerves. The peripheral neuropathy may occur before there is laboratory evidence of hypothyroidism. Once identified, thyroid replacement causes clinical, electrophysiologic, and morphologic improvement.

ACROMEGALIC NEUROPATHY

Entrapment neuropathy is also relatively common in patients with acromegaly. Rarely, acromegalic patients note distal paresthesia, but in contrast to myxedematous patients, weakness may be severe and peripheral nerves may be palpable. There is a significant correlation between total exchangeable body sodium and the severity of the neuropathy. The nerves are enlarged because there is increased endoneurial and perineurial connective tissue, perhaps stimulated by increased levels of somatomedin C (insulinlike growth factor). Tendon reflexes are reduced. Nerve conduction velocities are mildly slow with low evoked response amplitudes.

HYPERTHYROID NEUROPATHY

Hyperthyroidism can produce a syndrome consisting of diffuse weakness and fasciculations with preserved or hyperactive tendon reflexes, resembling ALS. However, the symptoms and signs disappear with treatment of the toxic state. GBS is also seen with hyperthyroidism. No convincing pathologic studies have established the presence of chronic sensorimotor neuropathy with hyperthyroidism.

CELIAC NEUROPATHY

Celiac disease is a chronic inflammatory enteropathy with a prevalence of 1:250. Peripheral neuropathy is the most common neurological condition associated with celiac disease. It is not thought to be a result of nutritional deficiency. In over half of patients with celiac neuropathy, gastrointestinal complaints are absent. Celiac disease is caused by exposure to ingested gluten, the storage proteins of wheat, and similar proteins found in barley and rye. Patients have specific HLA-DQ2 and HLA-DQ8 alleles.

The neuropathy is usually predominantly sensory. Multifocal involvement is frequent, with early involvement of the hands and face, although some have a length-dependent pattern. A small-fiber neuropathy is more commonly initially, but a sensorimotor polyneuropathy is also seen. Diagnosis is suspected with elevated gliadin or transglutaminase antibodies and confirmed by a duodenal biopsy demonstrating inflammation, crypt hyperplasia, and villous atrophy in the small intestine mucosa. Gastrointestinal symptoms improve with a gluten-free diet. The symptoms of peripheral neuropathy have improved in some, but not all, patients after initiating a gluten-free diet. Only small amounts of gluten exposure can result in an ongoing immune response.

UREMIC NEUROPATHY

Peripheral neuropathy is only one of the neuromuscular syndromes associated with chronic renal failure. Restless legs, cramps, and muscle twitching may be early manifestations of peripheral nerve disease. Peripheral neuropathy is present in 70% of patients with chronic renal failure, but most are subclinical and are identified only by nerve conduction studies. Symptoms include painful dysesthesia and glove-stocking loss of sensation, as well as weakness of distal muscles. Electrodiagnostic studies show a sensorimotor neuropathy with axonal features. Pathologic studies confirm the axonopathy. Secondary demyelination may result from axonal loss. Dialysis rarely reverses the neuropathy but may stabilize symptoms; peritoneal dialysis is more effective than hemodialysis. Serial nerve conduction studies can measure the effectiveness of hemodialysis. Renal transplantation often resolves the neuropathy shortly after surgery.

Mononeuropathy, particularly the carpal tunnel syndrome, often appears distal to an implanted arteriovenous fistula, suggesting ischemia as a possible mechanism. Distal ischemia from implanted bovine shunts may cause a more severe ischemic neuropathy in the median, ulnar, and radial nerves, possibly from excessive arteriovenous shunting. Chronic hemodialysis (more than 10 years) causes excessive accumulation of β_2-microglobulin (generalized amyloidosis), another possible cause of carpal tunnel syndrome and peripheral uremic neuropathy.

The cause of uremic neuropathy is uncertain. An accumulation of a toxic metabolite is most likely, but its identity is unknown. A 2- to 60-kDa molecular weight compound in the plasma of uremic patients induced an axonal neuropathy in experimental animals.

NEUROPATHY ASSOCIATED WITH HEPATIC DISEASE

Peripheral neuropathy is rarely associated with primary diseases of the liver. A painful sensory neuropathy is seen with primary biliary cirrhosis, probably caused by xanthoma formation in and around nerves. Electrodiagnostic studies may be normal, or the amplitude of the sensory evoked response may be low or absent. Nerve biopsy shows loss of small-diameter nerve fibers. Sudanophilic material is seen in cells of the perineurium. Treatment is directed at pain control. Tricyclic antidepressants or anticonvulsants may relieve paresthesia.

Infectious diseases of the liver may also be associated with peripheral neuropathy. Viral hepatitis (especially hepatitis C associated with cryoglobulinemia), HIV or cytomegalovirus (CMV) infection, and infectious mononucleosis may be associated with acute demyelinating neuropathy (GBS), chronic demyelinating neuropathy, or mononeuropathy multiplex. Immunologically mediated diseases such as polyarteritis and sarcoidosis may also cause liver abnormalities and mononeuropathy multiplex.

Peripheral neuropathy is often seen with toxic liver disease or hepatic metabolic diseases such as acute intermittent porphyria (see Chapter 92) and abetalipoproteinemia (see Chapter 93).

NEUROPATHIES ASSOCIATED WITH INFECTION

Neuropathy of Leprosy

Direct infiltration of small-diameter peripheral nerve fibers by *Mycobacterium leprae* causes the neuropathy of leprosy. It was formerly the most common neuropathy in the world, although now overtaken by diabetic neuropathy. In the United States, the disease is less endemic but is seen in immigrants from India, Southeast Asia, and Central Africa.

Peripheral nerves are affected differently in tuberculoid and lepromatous forms. In tuberculoid leprosy, there

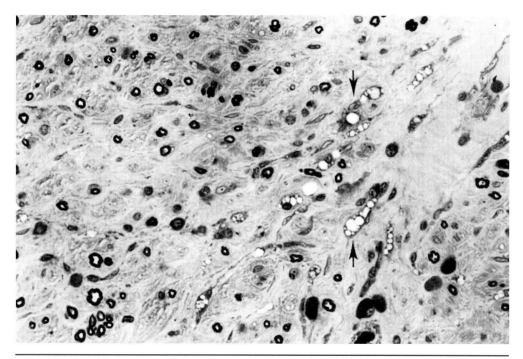

FIGURE 106.5. Lepromatous leprous neuritis. Few myelinated fibers are scattered in fibrotic endoneurium. Abundant foam cells *(arrows)* contain *M. leprae* bacilli when viewed at higher magnification. (Courtesy of Dr. Arthur Asbury.)

are small hypopigmented areas with superficial sensory loss, and the underlying subcutaneous sensory nerves may be visibly or palpably enlarged. Large nerve trunks, such as the ulnar, peroneal, facial, and posterior auricular nerves, may be enmeshed in granulomas and scar tissue. Endoneurial caseation necrosis may occur. The clinical picture is one of mononeuritis or mononeuritis multiplex.

In lepromatous leprosy, Hansen bacilli proliferate in large numbers within Schwann cells and macrophages in the endoneurium and perineurium of subcutaneous nerve twigs (Fig. 106.5), particularly in cool areas of the body (pinnae of the ears and dorsum of the hands, forearms, and feet). Loss of cutaneous sensibility is observed in affected patches; these may later coalesce to cover large parts of the body. Position sense may be preserved in affected areas, whereas pain and temperature sensibility is lost, a dissociation similar to that in syringomyelia. Tendon reflexes are preserved.

Acute mononeuritis multiplex may appear during chemotherapy of lepromatous leprosy in conjunction with erythema nodosum. This complication is treated with thalidomide.

Treatment is designed to eradicate the bacterium using dapsone and to prevent secondary immune reactions that may damage nerves. Because of the dense sensory loss, painless and inadvertent traumatic injuries, such as self-inflicted burns, may occur without extreme caution to avoid trauma to the anesthetic areas.

Diphtheritic Neuropathy

Although diphtheria itself is rare, diphtheritic neuropathy is seen in approximately 20% of infected patients. *Corynebacterium diphtheriae* infects the larynx and pharynx, as well as cutaneous wounds. The organisms release an exotoxin that causes myocarditis and, later, symmetric neuropathy. The neuropathy often begins with impaired visual accommodation and paresis of ocular and oropharyngeal muscles, and quadriparesis follows. Nerve conduction velocities are slow, reflecting the underlying demyelinating neuropathy. Diphtheria may be prevented by immunization, and if infection occurs, antibiotic therapy may be used. Recovery may be slow, and physiologic measures resolve after the clinical syndrome.

HIV-Related Neuropathies

Several neuropathies afflict patients infected with HIV, depending on the stage of the illness and the immunocompetence of the patient. An acute demyelinating neuropathy indistinguishable from sporadic GBS may occur early in the course of infection, often with no signs of immunodeficiency or at the time of seroconversion, as well as once AIDS develops. Sometimes a CSF pleocytosis is present, which is not typical of GBS in non–HIV-infected patients.

Subacute demyelinating neuropathy, clinically indistinguishable from idiopathic CIDP, is usually found in

HIV-positive patients before there is evidence of immunodeficiency (AIDS). The CSF protein content is increased in both idiopathic CIDP and HIV-associated demyelinating neuropathy. Steroids, plasmapheresis, and intravenous Ig therapy have been reported to be effective treatments.

In patients who fulfill diagnostic criteria for AIDS, there is frequently a distal sensorimotor polyneuropathy with axonal features. The syndrome is dominated by severe painful paresthesia affecting the feet first and most intensely. This painful neuropathy can be the most functionally disabling manifestation of AIDS. Nerve conduction studies may be normal, but reduced intraepidermal nerve fiber density is seen on skin biopsy. The exact mechanism is uncertain. HIV infection of dorsal root ganglion neurons has been demonstrated. Because of the scarcity of neuronal infection, other causes such as toxicity of activated macrophages and cytokines and viral protein toxicity have been considered. No treatment reverses the symptoms, but symptomatic medications, such as lamotrigine or gabapentin may help. One form of neuropathy in HIV-infected patients is the diffuse infiltrative lymphocytosis syndrome, a hyperimmune reaction to HIV infection.

Mononeuropathy multiplex occurs in HIV-infected patients at any stage of the disease, sometimes with hepatitis. When CD4 cells number fewer than 50/mm^3, the likely cause of the mononeuropathy is CMV, and prompt treatment with ganciclovir sodium (Cytovene) may be life saving. CMV infection is also associated with polyradiculopathy.

The dideoxynucleotide antiretroviral medications used to treat HIV infection may cause neuropathy. These drugs can cause a painful sensory neuropathy, which is difficult to separate from the painful HIV sensory neuropathy.

Neuropathy of Herpes Zoster

Varicella-zoster virus infection of the dorsal root ganglion produces radicular pain that may precede or follow the appearance of the characteristic skin eruption. Although primarily a sensory neuropathy, weakness from motor involvement occurs in 0.5% to 5% of infected patients. Herpes zoster (shingles) is a common phenomenon most frequent in elderly patients, malignancy, or on immunosuppression. Postrash pain (postherpetic neuralgia) usually in the same myotomal distribution as the dermatomal rash, occurs in a minority, but risk increases significantly with age (50% over 70 years). For diagnosis, pain should persist for 1 to 6 months after the rash disappears. Severe acute pain, more intense rash, scarring, sensory loss, and fever increase the risk of postherpetic neuralgia. Zoster infections are also associated with GBS and CSF pleocytosis. Zoster infection often occurs in patients with HIV infection; the combination of herpes infection and focal weakness in a young person should alert the clinician to the possibility of HIV infection.

Herpes zoster may affect any level of the neuraxis, but it most often involves thoracic dermatomes and cranial nerves with sensory ganglia (V and VII). Ophthalmic herpes infection characteristically involves the gasserian ganglion and the first division of the trigeminal nerve. There may be weakness of ocular muscles and ptosis. Infection of the geniculate ganglion of the facial (VII) nerve causes a vesicular herpetic eruption in the external auditory meatus, vertigo, deafness, and facial weakness (Ramsay Hunt syndrome). Pain is constant, burning, and may include paroxysms of very severe pain. Treatment with acyclovir (Zovirax), 4 g/day in five doses for 5 days, decreases the incidence of segmental motor neuritis and sensory axonopathy but does not reduce the incidence of postherpetic neuralgia. Tricyclic antidepressants, opioids, anticonvulsants (gabapentin), and lidocaine patches may show symptomatic benefit, some verified in randomized clinical trials.

SARCOID NEUROPATHY

Neurologic symptoms appear in 4% of patients with sarcoidosis. Most commonly, there are single or multiple cranial nerve palsies that fluctuate in intensity. Of the cranial nerves, the seventh is most commonly affected, and, as in diabetes mellitus, the facial nerve syndrome in sarcoidosis is indistinguishable from idiopathic Bell palsy. Some cranial neuropathies in sarcoidosis result from basilar meningitis. One distinguishing feature of sarcoid mononeuropathy is a large area of sensory loss on the trunk.

Patients with sarcoidosis occasionally experience symmetric polyneuropathy months or years after the diagnosis is established. The neuropathy may be the first manifestation before the diagnosis of sarcoidosis is made. The clinical syndromes may include GBS, lumbosacral plexopathy, mononeuritis multiplex, pure sensory neuropathy, and small-fiber and autonomic neuropathy. Almost all patients, however, have cranial nerve symptoms.

Nerve biopsy shows a mixture of Wallerian degeneration and segmental demyelination with sarcoid granulomas in endoneurium and epineurium. Sarcoid neuropathy may respond to steroid therapy.

POLYNEUROPATHY ASSOCIATED WITH DIETARY STATES

Thiamine deficiency may cause two clinical syndromes: *wet beriberi,* in which congestive heart failure is the predominant syndrome, and *dry beriberi,* in which peripheral neuropathy is the predominant symptom. Patients with thiamine deficiency have severe burning dysesthesia in the feet more than the hands, weakness and wasting of distal more than proximal muscles, trophic changes (shiny skin, hair loss), and distal sensory loss. EMG and nerve conduction studies reveal the presence of a diffuse sensorimotor peripheral neuropathy that is axonal. Axonal degeneration is also the principal finding seen on nerve biopsy specimens. Treatment of both beriberis should include parenteral B-complex vitamins followed by oral thiamine. Recovery is slow; there may be residual muscular weakness and atrophy.

Niacin (nicotinic acid) deficiency causes pellagra characterized by hyperkeratotic skin lesions. Peripheral neuropathy is usually present in niacin deficient patients, but the neuropathy does not improve solely with niacin supplementation, likely because of multivitamin deficiency. Symptoms usually improve when additional thiamine and pyridoxine are added to the diet.

Vitamin B$_{12}$ deficiency causes the classic clinical syndrome of subacute combined degeneration of the spinal cord. Separation of the peripheral neuropathic symptoms from spinal cord involvement is difficult. Painful paresthesias are present but sensory ataxia with loss of vibration and joint position sense is most severe. Despite the myelopathy, tendon reflexes are often diminished or absent. B$_{12}$ deficiency neuropathy may be present with low normal B$_{12}$ levels and can be established with measurement of the elevated metabolites methylmalonic acid and homocysteine.

Nitrous oxide also irreversibly inactivates cobalamin, producing the same syndrome. A single anesthetic dose in a vulnerable individual or chronic exposure usually with abuse of dental or medical sources or commercial propellants (whipped cream) may result in B$_{12}$ deficiency. Hematologic abnormalities are usually absent in abuse cases.

Vitamin B$_6$ (pyridoxine) deficiency produces a peripheral neuropathy, and the most common cause of pyridoxine deficiency is ingestion of the antituberculous drug, isoniazid. Isoniazid increases the excretion of pyridoxine. The resulting neuropathy affects sensory more than motor fibers and is caused by axonal loss. Treatment consists of supplemental pyridoxine to compensate for the added excretion. The neuropathy can be prevented by prophylactic pyridoxine administration. Pyridoxine excess can lead to severe sensory neuropathy as well.

Vitamin E deficiency contributes to neuropathy in fat malabsorption syndromes—including abetalipoproteinemia, congenital biliary atresia, pancreatic dysfunction, and surgical removal of large portions of the small intestine. The clinical syndrome of vitamin E deficiency resembles spinocerebellar degeneration with ataxia, severe sensory loss of joint position and vibration, and hyporeflexia. Motor nerve conduction studies are normal, but sensory evoked responses are of low amplitude or absent. Somatosensory evoked responses show a delay in central conduction. EMG is usually normal. Serum vitamin E levels can be measured. Repletion with large oral doses is often sufficient if initiated early in the disease course.

Strachan syndrome includes visual loss, oral ulcers, skin changes, and painful neuropathy. The syndrome was originally described in Jamaican sugar workers and caused an epidemic in Cuba in 1991. A nutrient-poor diet with deficient B vitamins has been implicated.

Gastric bypass surgery is associated with subacute and sometimes severe axonal neuropathy that accompanies the rapid postoperative weight loss. Vitamin deficiency of various types is presumed to play a crucial role.

CRITICAL ILLNESS POLYNEUROPATHY

Severe sensorimotor peripheral neuropathy is seen in many patients who are critically ill, suffering from sepsis and multiple organ failure. The diagnosis may arise when a patient experiences difficulty being weaned from a ventilator after a bout of sepsis. Electrodiagnostic studies show a severe sensorimotor axonal neuropathy, but conventional studies may be unable to distinguish this entity from the more common critical illness myopathy, discussed in detail in Chapter 125. Recovery of neuronal function may occur if the underlying cause of multiple organ failure is treated successfully. Mononeuritis or mononeuritis multiplex occurs in 2% of patients with bacterial endocarditis because of septic emboli to peripheral nerves.

NEUROPATHIES CAUSED BY HEAVY METALS

Arsenic

Neuropathy may follow chronic exposure to small amounts of arsenic or ingestion or parenteral administration of a large amount. Chronic exposure may occur in industries in which arsenic is released as a byproduct, such as in copper or lead smelting. Because of the prevalence of these byproducts, arsenic neuropathy is the most common of all heavy metal–induced neuropathies. Acute gastrointestinal symptoms, vomiting, and diarrhea occur when a toxic quantity of arsenic is ingested, but these symptoms may be absent if the arsenic is given parenterally or taken in small amounts over long periods. Acute exposure may lead to encephalopathy or coma. The evolution of polyneuropathy is much slower in chronic arsenic poisoning. Sensory symptoms are prominent in the early stages. Pain and paresthesia in the legs may be present for several days or weeks before onset of weakness. The weakness may progress to complete flaccid paralysis of the legs and sometimes the arms, depending on the dosage. Cutaneous sensation is impaired in a stocking-and-glove distribution, with vibration and position sensation being most affected. Tendon reflexes are lost. Pigmentation and hyperkeratosis of the skin and changes in the nails (*Mees lines*) are frequently present. Arsenic is present in the urine in the acute stages of poisoning but is quickly cleared; levels persist in the hair and nails. Nerve conduction velocities may be normal or mildly diminished; the amplitude of sensory and motor evoked responses may be reduced. Pathologic examination of nerves shows axonal degeneration. Arsenic polyneuropathy is generally treated with a chelating agent, but the effectiveness is uncertain given the rapid clearance in most patients.

Lead

Most toxic neuropathies cause symmetric weakness and loss of sensation in distal more than proximal regions, feet worse than legs. Lead neuropathy is atypical because of motor predominance and arm involvement.

Lead neuropathy occurs almost exclusively in adults. Infants poisoned with lead usually experience encephalopathy. Lead may enter the body through the lungs, skin, or gut. Occupational lead poisoning was common in earlier eras, notably in silver miners, but rarely is encountered in battery workers, painters, and pottery glazers. Accidental lead poisoning follows ingestion of lead in food or beverages, or occurs in children who ingest lead paint. Lead poisoning may cause abdominal distress (lead colic). The classic description is focal wristdrop in a radial neuropathy pattern; however, weakness is not generally limited to one nerve and produces bilateral arm weakness and wasting and lesser or later leg involvement. Footdrop is the most common leg sign. Sensory symptoms and signs are usually absent. Rarely, upper motor neuron signs occur with the lower motor neuron disorder and mimic ALS. Laboratory findings include anemia with basophilic stippling of the red cells, increased serum uric acid, and slight elevation of CSF protein content. Urinary lead excretion is elevated, particularly after administration of a chelating agent. Urinary porphobilinogen excretion is also elevated, but δ-aminolevulinic acid is normal. Primary therapy is prevention of further exposure to lead. With termination of exposure and use of chelation therapy, recovery is gradual over several months.

Mercury

Mercury is used in the electrical and chemical industries. There are two forms of mercury: elemental and organic. The organic form of mercury (methyl and ethyl mercury) is most toxic to the CNS, although distal paresthesia and sensory ataxia are prominent (presumably secondary to dorsal root ganglion degeneration). Ventral roots and motor function are spared. Inorganic mercury may be absorbed through the gastrointestinal tract, and elemental mercury may be absorbed directly through the skin or lungs (it is volatile at room temperature). Elemental mercury expo-

sure is a rare cause of weakness and axonal motor and sensory fiber loss.

Thallium

This element is used as a rodenticide and in other industrial processes. Children exposed to thallium, as with lead, are more likely to experience encephalopathy, whereas neuropathy develops in adults. In contrast to lead poisoning, however, thallium neuropathy is primarily sensory and autonomic. Severe disturbing dysesthesia appears acutely, and diffuse alopecia is a characteristic feature of thallium poisoning. Signs of cardiovascular autonomic neuropathy are sometimes delayed and recover slowly. Electrophysiologic findings are consistent with an axonal neuropathy.

Other Chemicals

Acrylamide monomer is used to prepare polyacrylamide. It is used in chemical laboratories and for the treatment of liquid sewerage. Exposure to the monomer produces a distal sensorimotor neuropathy that may be associated with trophic skin changes and a mild organic dementia. Polyacrylamides, however, are not neurotoxic. Carbon disulfide (CS_2) is rarely inhaled in industrial settings. Exposure may lead to sensorimotor axonal neuropathy. CS_2 is also a metabolite of disulfiram.

Many organophosphates, used in insecticides and rodenticides, are acetylcholinesterase inhibitors and may cause neuropathy. The clinical and electrophysiologic features are similar to those of neuropathies caused by chemotherapeutics. Some, however, affect the CNS, as well as peripheral nerves, and some have certain specific features. *Triorthocresyl phosphate* (Jamaica ginger or jake), an adulterant used in illegal liquor (moonshine) and as a cooking oil contaminant, has been responsible for neuropathy epidemics. *Dimethylaminopropionitrile*, which is used to manufacture polyurethane foam, causes urologic dysfunction and sensory loss localized to sacral dermatomes. Exposure to *methylbromide*, an insecticide, results in a mixture of pyramidal tract, cerebellar, and peripheral nerve dysfunction. Accidental ingestion of *pyriminil*, a rat poison marketed under the name Vacor, gives rise to an acute severe distal axonopathy with prominent autonomic involvement accompanied by acute diabetes mellitus secondary to necrosis of pancreatic beta cells.

Drugs of abuse may lead to neuropathy, notably n-hexane and methyl N butyl ketone, found in widely available household solvents, fuels, and cleaning agents. Inhalation through the nose or mouth (huffing) of these materials is not rare in teens and young adults. Axonal degeneration with sensory and motor impairment is seen, but focal conduction block associated with giant axonal swellings is also characteristic. The phenomenon is similar to the rare hereditary entity, giant axonal neuropathy, linked to a defect in the gigaxonin gene.

Ingested neurotoxins from various sea creatures harboring toxins can induce nerve dysfunction, mostly through sodium channel blockade and block in nerve conduction, mostly producing sensory neuropathy, cramps, diarrhea, and vomiting. Examples include ciguatera from reef fish exposed to a ciguatoxin producing dinoflagellate, saxitoxin (paralytic shellfish poisoning), brevetoxin B (neurotoxic shellfish poisoning), and tetrodotoxin (puffer fish [fugu]). A number of insect venoms are also neurotoxins. Most cause neuromuscular junction blockade, but some, including tick paralysis and frog skin toxins, block sodium channels and peripheral nerve conduction.

NEUROPATHIES CAUSED BY THERAPEUTIC DRUGS

Many medications have been suspected of causing neuropathy, but relatively few have convincing clinical features, laboratory support, and reproduction in animal models. Different aspects of the problem are discussed in Chapters 165, 166, and 167. Most of these neuropathies are dose related, presenting with predominantly sensory symptoms and signs or with a combination of sensory, motor, and autonomic involvement. Most cause toxicity by targeting the axon or dorsal root ganglion neurons directly, but toxicity to Schwann cells and myelin occurs with some agents as well. Pathogenic mechanisms are agent specific and varied. Identification of a toxic effect is most simple when symptoms occur soon after drug exposure or a change in dosage. Most patients fall into this category. In contrast, it is problematic to diagnose a slowly progressive neuropathy starting many months or years on a chronic agent. For example, statin drugs provide a case in point and are discussed later. "Coasting" is a phenomenon in which neuropathy may continue to progress, usually for 2 to 3 weeks, despite drug discontinuation. Improvement after drug cessation helps support the toxic effect, but recovery may be delayed for many months or be incomplete when significant axonal degeneration occurs. Discussion of all of the numerous substances temporally linked to neuropathy is outside the scope of this chapter, and the interested reader should consult comprehensive reviews cited in the suggested readings. Some of the more important and best established causes are discussed.

Chemotherapy is an area in which at this time some toxicity is tolerable assuming the agent is efficacious. The most commonly used antineoplastic agents linked with neuropathy are *vincristine, cisplatin* (Platinol), and *taxoids* (paclitaxel, docetaxel). Vincristine causes a dose-dependent symmetric progressive sensorimotor distal neu-

ropathy that begins in the legs and is associated with arreflexia. Charcot-Marie-Tooth type 1A patients are especially vulnerable, and treatment may unmask subclinical cases. In contrast, cisplatin neuropathy is a purely sensory distal neuropathy with paresthesia, impaired vibration sense, and loss of ankle jerks, likely owing to toxicity and drug access to dorsal root ganglia but not alpha motor neurons. The drug binds to and alters DNA and may trigger apoptosis if DNA repair fails.

Paclitaxel (Taxol) is used to treat cancers of the breast, ovary, and lung. It causes a predominantly sensory neuropathy, but administration of a single high dose may affect motor fibers as well. Disordered arrays of microtubules are induced. Neuropathy is also a prominent feature in chemotherapy with suramin (axonal or demyelinating), bortezomib (Velcade), misonidazole, and thalidomide (sensory). Many chemoprotectant agents to blunt the neurotoxic effects have been studied; none are routinely used in humans but some show promise. Use of numerous other therapeutic drugs may produce neuropathy, including colchicine (myoneuropathy), gold salts, hydralazine, isoniazid (without B_6), metronidazole, nitrofurantoin, and podophyllotoxin resin. Amiodarone (Cordarone) may cause a severe symmetric distal sensorimotor neuropathy, an autonomic or demyelinating neuropathy resembling CIDP. Phenytoin (Dilantin) may produce minor distal sensory impairment and arreflexia, but mostly after long-standing high dosage and is likely overdiagnosed. The major toxicity of some nucleoside analog antiretroviral medications (didanosine [ddI], zalcitabine [ddC], and stavudine [d4T]) is peripheral neuropathy, which may be difficult to distinguish from HIV neuropathy. Others, such as azidothymidine (AZT), are not linked to neuropathy. A predominantly motor neuropathy has been related to disulfiram (Antabuse) or to dapsone. Statin use was associated with idiopathic neuropathy in one large study, especially in those with definite neuropathy and longer-term exposure. The effect is probably rare, but may be important because so many people are exposed.

ALCOHOLIC NEUROPATHY

Peripheral neuropathy in alcohol abusers is well known, but the cause is still debated. A widely held belief is that the neuropathy of alcoholism is owing entirely to nutritional deficiency, particularly vitamin B_1 (thiamine). Koike and colleagues, however, provide the best support for a direct toxic effect of ethanol. Alcoholics with normal thiamine levels develop predominantly small-fiber sensory neuropathy, the most frequent clinical type. More subacute onset with motor involvement is also seen in alcoholics with thiamine deficiency and nondrinkers with primary thiamine deficiency. Symptoms of small-fiber neuropathy, such as burning and pain, are common in chronic alcohol drinkers. Later, loss of vibration sense, proprioception, and tendon reflexes may occur. Sensory ataxia may be problematic to separate from alcoholic cerebellar degeneration. Abstinence can lead to meaningful recovery; vitamin supplements alone are not clearly effective but advised.

DIABETIC NEUROPATHY

The broad diversity of neurologic complications in patients with diabetes mellitus can be considered to consist of two distinct types. In one form, the symptoms and signs are transient; in the other, they progress steadily. The transient category includes acute painful neuropathies, mononeuropathies, and radiculopathies. The painful type starts abruptly with a disabling and continuous pain, often a burning sensation in a stocking distribution. Sometimes, the pain is localized to the thighs as a femoral neuropathy. The pain may last for months. Recovery from severe pain, however, is usually complete within 1 year, and the disorder does not necessarily progress to a conventional sensory polyneuropathy.

The progressive type comprises sensorimotor polyneuropathies with or without autonomic symptoms and signs. Although the actual cause of diabetic neuropathies is unknown, focal nerve involvement is considered to be immune mediated; and progressive symmetric polyneuropathy is probably owing to microvascular disease, resulting from hyperglycemia. There may be as many causal factors as there are clinical pictures. There is evidence of oxidative damage and activation of protein kinase C beta activation in endothelial cells. However, it seems that hyperglycemic hypoxia is mainly responsible for the conduction changes seen in damaged diabetic nerves. Dysfunction of ion conductances, especially voltage-gated ion channels, could contribute to abnormalities in the generation and conduction of action potentials.

Impaired glucose tolerance is also associated with peripheral neuropathy. A 2-hour glucose tolerance test is the preferred method to screen for diabetes or impaired glucose tolerance in patients with neuropathy, being preferable to a fasting glucose or a hemoglobin A1c.

A syndrome recognized by a triad of pain, severe asymmetric muscle weakness, and wasting of the iliopsoas, quadriceps, and adductor muscles is named *diabetic amyotrophy*. Onset is usually acute, but it may evolve over weeks. It occurs primarily in older non–insulin-dependent diabetics and is often accompanied by severe weight loss and cachexia (diabetic neuropathic cachexia). Knee jerks are absent, but there is little or no sensory loss. Although long described as involving the proximal leg muscles, this syndrome can also involve the arms and even respiratory system. The condition resolves spontaneously, but may last 1 to 3 years with incomplete recovery.

Mononeuropathies

It is generally believed but has never been proved that focal neuropathies are more frequent in diabetic patients than in the general population. The syndromes are usually localized to the common sites of nerve entrapment or external compression and may imply an increased liability to pressure palsies. This applies to the median nerve at the carpal tunnel, the ulnar at the elbow, and the peroneal at the fibular head. The electrophysiologic features are similar to those seen in nondiabetic patients with pressure palsies, except that abnormalities outside the clinically affected areas sometimes indicate that the palsies are superimposed on a generalized neuropathy. Cranial nerve palsies are most often localized to the third and sixth nerves. They start abruptly and usually spontaneously resolve completely within 6 months; relapses are rare.

Generalized Polyneuropathies

The most common diabetic neuropathy is a diffuse distal symmetric and predominantly sensory neuropathy with or without autonomic manifestations. Distal limb weakness is usually minimal. The neuropathy develops slowly and is related to the duration of the diabetes, but not all patients are so afflicted. Once present, it does not resolve or significantly recover. Intensive glucose control limited complications including peripheral neuropathy in the diabetes control and complication trial (DCCT) with significant differences in nerve conduction values between intensive and standard glucose control groups. Most evidence suggests that small nerve fibers, both myelinated and unmyelinated, are affected first. Thus, pain and temperature sensation transmitted through the smallest fibers may be affected before the large-fiber modalities (vibration, light touch, position sense). Small-fiber function can be evaluated by determining thresholds for warming and cooling or by a pinprick threshold technique using weighted needles. Perception of cooling and pinprick is conveyed by small myelinated fibers; the sense of warming is carried by unmyelinated fibers. Most patients with diabetic neuropathy do not have pain, but do have numb or anesthetic feet. Diabetic neuropathy is the major predictor of foot ulcers and amputations.

The prevalence of diabetic autonomic neuropathy may be underestimated because nonspecific symptoms are undiagnosed or the condition may be asymptomatic. Symptoms appear insidiously, long after the onset of diabetes. They progress slowly and are usually irreversible. Diabetic autonomic neuropathy (DAN) is an important prognostic indicator with a mortality rate in diabetics without other initial complications of 23% at 8 years compared to 3% in 8 years in diabetics without DAN and similar disease duration. Noninvasive autonomic screening batteries can be performed, and dedicated autonomic testing laboratories are becoming widely available (Chapter 138).

Mild slowing of motor and sensory conduction is a common finding in diabetics, even among those without overt neuropathy. It is generally attributed to axonal degeneration with secondary demyelination. Therapeutic attempts, including continuous subcutaneous insulin infusion to correct hyperglycemia to prevent the diabetic complications, have been unsuccessful in most instances. Although combined pancreas and kidney transplantation may halt the progression of diabetic polyneuropathy, the long-term effect is still doubtful. Patients with pain may benefit from amitriptyline or gabapentin, but side effects may preclude treatment.

BRACHIAL NEURITIS

This syndrome, also known as *neuralgic amyotrophy* or the Parsonage-Turner syndrome is characterized by acute onset of severe pain localized to the shoulder region and followed shortly by weakness of the shoulder girdle or arm muscles ipsilateral to the pain. It may be bilateral and asymmetric. Paresthesia and sensory loss may also be noted. An isolated sensory form is also proposed. In about 50% of patients, the clinical pattern is a mononeuropathy multiplex, followed by mononeuropathy in 33% and plexopathy in 20%. Autoimmune or infectious causes have been suggested, but the etiology is obscure. Some cases have occurred in small epidemics, and the disorder may follow intravenous heroin, HIV seroconversion, surgery, and delivery.

The typical EMG findings, including motor and sensory nerve studies, are consistent with a predominantly focal axonal neuropathy, but demyelination occasionally plays a role. The diversity of physiologic disorders in different nerves or even within the same nerve is attributed to involvement of the terminal nerve twigs or to patchy damage of discrete bundles of fibers within the cords or trunks of the brachial plexus or its branches. The long thoracic and anterior interosseous nerves are commonly affected. A hereditary form that is frequency recurrent and bilateral is rarely encountered. Lumbosacral plexitis also occurs but much less frequently. Recovery depends on the severity of the initial insult. It is considered good in about 66%, fair in 20%, and poor in 14%. Clinical recovery may take 2 months to 3 years.

RADIATION NEUROPATHY

Irradiation for carcinoma may damage nervous tissue, especially since the introduction of high-voltage therapy. Lesions of the brachial plexus are seen after radiotherapy for breast cancer; caudal roots and lumbosacral plexus are sometimes affected by radiation therapy for testicular cancer or Hodgkin disease. The first symptom is usually severe pain, followed by paresthesia and sensory loss. There may be a latent period of 12 to 20 months; in milder cases, several years may elapse before symptoms appear. Limb weakness peaks many months later. Latency intervals of up to 20 years have been reported. The damage may affect a single peripheral nerve initially and then progress slowly to involve others. Clinically, tendon reflexes disappear before weakness and atrophy become obvious; fasciculation and myokymia may be prominent. EMG and conduction studies reveal changes consistent with axonal damage; myokymic discharges are thought to be helpful in differentiating plexopathy caused by radiation from plexopathy caused by tumor infiltration.

LYME NEUROPATHY

Lyme disease is commonly diagnosed in the United States and Europe. It is caused by a tick-borne spirochete, *Borrelia burgdorferi*. The most common clinical feature of neuroborreliosis is a painful sensory radiculitis, which may appear about 3 weeks after the erythema migrans. Pain intensity varies from day to day and is often severe, jumping from one area to another and often associated with patchy areas of unpleasant dysesthesia. Onset may be subacute potentially simulating Guillain-Barré syndrome (GBS), but with significant CSF pleocytosis and without clear signs of demyelination. Focal neurologic signs are common and may present as cranial neuropathy (61%), limb paresis (12%), or both (16%), but detailed electrodiagnostic signs often point to a mononeuropathy multiplex. The clinical pattern may appear as a mononeuropathy, plexopathy, mononeuropathy multiplex or distal symmetric polyneuropathy. The facial nerve is frequently affected; involvement is unilateral twice as often as bilateral. Ophthalmoparesis occasionally occurs. Myeloradiculitis and chronic progressive encephalomyelitis are rare. In some, the disorder is associated with dilated cardiomyopathy. Arthralgia is common among patients in the United States but rare among Europeans (6%). The triad of painful radiculitis, predominantly cranial mononeuritis multiplex, and lymphocytic pleocytosis in the CSF is known as *Bannwarth syndrome* in Europe. Peripheral nerve biopsy shows perineurial and epineurial vasculitis and axonal degeneration, consistent with the electrophysiologic findings. The diagnosis of neuroborreliosis is based on the presence of inflammatory CSF changes and specific intrathecal *B. burgdorferi* antibodies. In some infected patients, however, no free antibodies are detectable. Antigen detection in CSF could then be helpful. Polymerase chain reaction technique for detecting spirochetes or spirochetal DNA turned out to be less specific. The prognosis is good after high-dose penicillin or ceftriaxone treatment. Disabling sequelae are rare and occur mainly in patients with previous CNS lesions.

IDIOPATHIC NEUROPATHY

Patients with a peripheral neuropathy of undiagnosed cause may be later found to have an immune-mediated or hereditary neuropathy with more intensive evaluation. Even then, however, 10 to 35% of patients remain undiagnosed. Among those with painful sensory neuropathy involving the feet, this percentage is even higher. Although no cure is available for the neuropathy, treatment may include management of pain, physical therapy, and counseling related to prognosis. When there is no identifiable cause of a symmetrical predominantly sensory neuropathy, after a thorough evaluation, the neuropathy rarely progresses to loss of ambulation or disability. Persistent pain is sometimes a problem.

SUGGESTED READINGS

General

Dyck PJ, Thomas PK, Griffin JW, eds. *Peripheral Neuropathy*. Philadelphia: WB Saunders, 1993.
Maravilla KR, Bowen BC. Imaging of the peripheral nervous system: evaluation of peripheral neuropathy and plexopathy. *AJNR* 1998;19:1011–1023.

Guillain-Barré Syndrome and Variants

Al-Shekhlee A, Katirji B. Electrodiagnostic features of acute paralytic poliomyelitis associated with West Nile virus infection. *Muscle Nerve* 2004;29:376–380.
Feasby TE, Gilbert JJ, Brown WP, et al. An acute axonal form of Guillain-Barré polyneuropathy. *Brain* 1986;109:1115–1126.
Feasby TE, Hughes RAC. *Campylobacter jejuni*, antiganglioside antibodies, and Guillain-Barré syndrome. *Neurology* 1998;51:340–342.
Hadden RDM, Cornblath DR, Hughes RAC, et al. Electrophysiological classification of Guillain-Barré syndrome: clinical associations and outcome. *Ann Neurol* 1998;44:780–788.
Hainfellner JA, Kristoferitsch W, Lassman H, et al. T-cell mediated ganglioneuritis associated with acute sensory neuronopathy. *Ann Neurol* 1996;39:543–547.
Hartung HP, Pollard JD, Harvey GK, et al. Immunopathogenesis and treatment of the Guillain-Barré syndrome—Part I. *Muscle Nerve* 1995;18:137–153.
Hartung HP, Pollard JD, Harvey GK, et al. Immunopathogenesis and treatment of the Guillain-Barré syndrome—Part II. *Muscle Nerve* 1995;18:154–164.
Ho TW, Willison HJ, Nachamkin I, et al. Anti-GD1a antibody is associated with axonal but not demyelinating forms of Guillain-Barré syndrome. *Ann Neurol* 1999;45:168–173.
Latov N. Antibodies to glycoconjugates in neuropathy and motor neuron disease. *Prog Brain Res* 1993;101:295–303.
Li J, Loeb JA, Shy ME, et al. Asymmetric flaccid paralysis: a neuromuscular presentation of West Nile virus infection. *Ann Neurol* 2003;53:703–710.
McKhann GM, Cornblath DR, Griffin JW, et al. Acute motor axonal neuropathy: a frequent cause of acute flaccid paralysis in China. *Ann Neurol* 1993;33:333–342.

Ogino M, Nobile-Orazio E, Latov N. IgG anti-GM1 antibodies from patients with acute motor axonal neuropathy are predominantly of the IgG1 and IgG3 subclass. *J Neuroimmunol* 1995;58:77–80.
Plomp JJ, Molenaar PC, O'Hanlon GM, et al. Miller Fisher anti-GQ1b antibodies: latrotoxin-like effects on motor end plates. *Ann Neurol* 1999;45:189–199.
Ropper AH, Wijdicks EF, Truax BT. *Guillain-Barré Syndrome*. Philadelphia: FA Davis, 1991.
Smit AA, Vermeulen M, Koelman JH, et al. Unusual recovery from acute panautonomic neuropathy after immunoglobulin therapy. *Mayo Clin Proc* 1997;72:333–335.
Trojaborg W. Acute and chronic neuropathies: new aspects of Guillain-Barré syndrome and chronic inflammatory demyelinating polyneuropathy, an overview and an update. *Electroencephalogr Clin Neurophysiol* 1998;107:303–316.
Van Koningsveld R, Schmitz PIM, van der Meché FGA, et al. Effect of methylprednisolone when added to standard treatment with intravenous immunoglobulin for Guillain-Barré syndrome. *Lancet* 2004;373:192–196.

Chronic Inflammatory Demyelinating Polyneuropathy

Berger AR, Bradley WG, Brannagan TH, et al. Guidelines for the diagnosis and treatment of chronic inflammatory demyelinating polyneuropathy. *J Periph Nerv Sys* 2003;8:282–284.
Bouchard C, Lacroix C, Plante V, et al. Clinicopathologic findings and prognosis of chronic inflammatory demyelinating polyneuropathy. *Neurology* 1999;52:498–503.
Brannagan TH, Pradhan A, Heiman-Patterson T, et al. High-dose cyclophosphamide without stem-cell rescue for refractory CIDP. *Neurology* 2002;58:1856–1858.
Briani C, Brannagan TH, Trojaborg W, et al. Chronic inflammatory demyelinating polyneuropathy. *Neuromuscul Disord* 1996;6:311–325.
Chroni E, Hall SM, Hughes RAC. Chronic relapsing axonal neuropathy: a first case report. *Ann Neurol* 1995;37:112–115.
Dyck PJ, Lais AC, Ohta M, et al. Chronic inflammatory polyradiculoneuropathy. *Mayo Clin Proc* 1975;50:621–637.
Good JL, Chehrenama M, Mayer RF, et al. Pulse cyclophosphamide therapy in chronic inflammatory demyelinating polyneuropathy. *Neurology* 1998;51:1735–1738.
Gorson KC, Allam G, Ropper AH. Chronic inflammatory demyelinating polyneuropathy: clinical features and response to treatment in 67 consecutive patients with and without a monoclonal gammopathy. *Neurology* 1997;48:321–328.
Hahn AF, Bolton CF, Zochodne D, et al. Intravenous gammaglobulin treatment in chronic inflammatory demyelinating polyneuropathy: a double blind, placebo-controlled, cross-over study. *Brain* 1996;119:1067–1077.
Research criteria for diagnosis of chronic inflammatory demyelinating polyneuropathy (CIDP). Report from an ad hoc subcommittee of the American Academy of Neurology AIDS Task Force. *Neurology* 1991;41:617–618.
Van Dijk GW, Notermans NC, Franssen H, et al. Response to intravenous immunoglobulin treatment in chronic inflammatory demyelinating polyneuropathy with only sensory symptoms. *J Neurol* 1996;243:318–322.

Multifocal Motor Neuropathy

Chaudhry V. Multifocal motor neuropathy. *Semin Neurol* 1998;18:73–81.
Chaudhry V, Corse AM, Cornblath DR, et al. Multifocal motor neuropathy: response to human immune globulin. *Ann Neurol* 1993;33:237–242.
Jaspert A, Claus D, Grehl H, et al. Multifocal motor neuropathy: clinical and electrophysiological findings. *J Neurol* 1996;243:684–692.
Kinsella L, Lange D, Trojaborg T, et al. The clinical and electrophysiologic correlates of anti-GM1 antibodies. *Neurology* 1994;44:1278–1282.
Pestronk A. Motor neuropathies, motor neuron disorders, and antiglycolipid antibodies. *Muscle Nerve* 1991;14:927–936.

Idiopathic Sensory Neuronopathy or Ganglioneuritis

Asahina N, Kuwabara S, Asahina M, et al. D-penicillamine treatment for chronic sensory ataxic neuropathy associated with Sjögrens syndrome. *Neurology* 1998;51:1451–1453.

Griffin JW, Cornblath DR, Alexander E, et al. Ataxic sensory neuropathy and dorsal root ganglioneuritis associated with Sjögren's syndrome. *Ann Neurol* 1990;27:304–315.

Quattrini A, Corbo M, Dhaliwal SK, et al. Anti-sulfatide antibodies in neurological disease: binding to rat dorsal root ganglia neurons. *J Neurol Sci* 1992;112:152–159.

Sobue G, Yasuda T, Kachi T, et al. Chronic progressive sensory ataxic neuropathy: clinicopathological features of idiopathic and Sjögren's syndrome associated cases. *J Neurol* 1993;240:1–7.

Windebank AJ, Blexrud MD, Dyck PJ, et al. The syndrome of acute sensory neuropathy. *Neurology* 1990;40:584–589.

Idiopathic Autonomic Neuropathy

Mericle RA, Triggs WJ. Treatment of acute pandysautonomia with intravenous immunoglobulin. *J Neurol Neurosurg Psychiatry* 1997;62:529–531.

Vernino S, Vernino S, Low PA, et al. Autoantibodies to ganglionic receptors in autoimmune autonomic neuropathies. *N Engl J Med* 2000;343:847–855.

Vasculitic and Cryoglobulinemic Neuropathies

Brannagan TH. Retroviral-associated vasculitis of the nervous system. *Neurol Clin* 1997;15:927–944.

Collins MP, Periquet MI, Mendell JR, et al. Nonsystemic vasculitic neuropathy: insights from a clinical cohort. *Neurology* 2003;61:623–630.

Dyck PJ, Benstead TJ, Conn DL, et al. Nonsystemic vasculitic neuropathy. *Brain* 1987;110:845–854.

Ferri C, La Civita L, Longombardo R, et al. Mixed cryoglobulinaemia: a cross-road between autoimmune and lymphoproliferative disorders. *Lupus* 1998;7:275–279.

Nemni R, Corbo M, Fazio R, et al. Cryoglobulinemic neuropathy: a clinical, morphological and immunocytochemical study of 8 cases. *Brain* 1988;111:541–552.

Said G, Lacroix-Ciaudo C, Fujimura H, et al. The peripheral neuropathy of necrotizing arteritis: a clinicopathological study. *Ann Neurol* 1988;23:461–466.

Neuropathies Associated With Myeloma and Nonmalignant IgG or IgA Monoclonal Gammopathies

Kelly JJ Jr, Kyle RA, Latov N. *Polyneuropathies Associated With Plasma Cell Dyscrasias.* Boston: Martinus-Nijhoff, 1987.

Latov N. Neuropathic syndromes associated with monoclonal gammopathies. In: Waksman BH, ed. *Immunologic Mechanisms in Neurologic and Psychiatric Disease.* New York: Raven, 1989.

Motor, Sensory, and Sensorimotor Neuropathies Associated with IgM Monoclonal or Polyclonal Autoantibodies to Peripheral Nerve

Carpo M, Pedotti R, Lolli F, et al. Clinical correlates and fine specificity of anti-GQ1b antibodies in peripheral neuropathy. *J Neurol Sci* 1998;155:186–191.

Chassande B, Leger JM, Younes-Chennoufi AB, et al. Peripheral neuropathy associated with IgM monoclonal gammopathy: correlations between M-protein antibody activity and clinical/electrophysiological features in 40 cases. *Muscle Nerve* 1998;21:55–62.

Elle E, Vital A, Steck A, et al. Neuropathy associated with benign anti-myelin-associated glycoprotein IgM gammapathy: clinical immunological, neurophysiological, pathological findings and response to treatment in 33 cases. *J Neurol* 1996;243:34–43.

Latov N. Pathogenesis and therapy of neuropathies associated with monoclonal gammopathies. *Ann Neurol* 1995;37(Suppl 1):S32–42.2.

Pedersen SF, Pullman SL, Latov N, et al. Physiological tremor analysis of patients with anti-myelin-associated glycoprotein associated neuropathy and tremor. *Muscle Nerve* 1997;20:38–44.

Quattrini A, Corbo M, Dhaliwal SK, et al. Anti-sulfatide antibodies in neurological disease: binding to rat dorsal root ganglia neurons. *J Neurol Sci* 1992;112:152–159.

Renaud S, Gregor M, Fuhr, P, et al. Rituximab in the treatment of polyneuropathy associated with anti-MAG antibodies. *Muscle Nerve* 2003;27:611–615.

Amyloid Neuropathy

Benson MD. Familial amyloidotic polyneuropathy. *Trends Neurosci* 1989;12:88–92.

Kelly JJ Jr, Kyle RA, O'Brien PC, et al. The natural history of peripheral neuropathy in primary systemic amyloidosis. *Ann Neurol* 1979;6:1–7.

Quattrini A, Nemni R, Sferrazza B, et al. Amyloid neuropathy simulating lower motor neuron disease. *Neurology* 1998;51:600–602.

Neuropathy Associated with Carcinoma (Paraneoplastic Neuropathy)

Camdessanche JP, Antoine JC, Honnorat J, et al. Paraneoplastic peripheral neuropathy associated with anti-Hu antibodies. A clinical and electrophysiologic study of 20 patients. *Brain* 2002;125:166–175.

Dalmau J, Graus F, Rosenblum MK, et al. Anti-Hu associated paraneoplastic encephalomyelitis/sensory neuropathy: a clinical study of 71 patients. *Medicine* 1992;71:59–72.

Eggers C, Hagel C, Pfeiffer G. Anti-Hu-associated paraneoplastic sensory neuropathy with peripheral nerve demyelination and microvasculitis. *J Neurol Sci* 1998;155:178–181.

Schold SC, Cho ES, Somasundaram M, et al. Subacute motor neuronopathy: a remote effect of lymphoma. *Ann Neurol* 1979;5:271–287.

Hypothyroid Neuropathy

Dyck PJ, Lambert EH. Polyneuropathy associated with hypothyroidism. *J Neuropathol Exp Neurol* 1970;9:631–658.

Misiunas A, Niepomniszcze H, Ravera B, et al. Peripheral neuropathy in subclinical hypothyroidism. *Thyroid* 1995;5:283–286.

Nemni R, Bottacchi E, Fazio R, et al. Polyneuropathy in hypothyroidism: clinical, electrophysiological and morphological findings in four cases. *J Neurol Neurosurg Psychiatry* 1987;50:1454–1460.

Acromegalic Neuropathy

Jamal GA, Kerr DJ, McLellaan AR, et al. Generalized peripheral nerve dysfunction in acromegaly: a study by conventional and novel neurophysiological techniques. *J Neurol Neurosurg Psychiatry* 1987;50:885–894.

Khaleeli AA, Levy RD, Edwards RHT, et al. The neuromuscular features of acromegaly: a clinical and pathological study. *J Neurol Neurosurg Psychiatry* 1984;47:1009–1015.

Low PA, McLeod JG, Turtle JR, et al. Peripheral neuropathy in acromegaly. *Brain* 1974;97:139–152.

Pickett JBE III, Layzer RB, Levin SR, et al. Neuromuscular complications of acromegaly. *Neurology* 1975;25:638–645.

Celiac Neuropathy

Chin RL, Sander HW, Brannagan TH, et al. Celiac Neuropathy. *Neurology* 2003;60:1581–1585.
Cicarelli G, Della Rocca G, Amboni M, et al. Clinical and neurological abnormalities in adult celiac disease. *J Neurol Sci* 2003:24:311–317.
Cooke WT, Smith WE. Neurological disorders associated with adult coeliac disease. *Brain* 1966;89:683–722.
Kaplan JG, Pack D, Horoupian D, et al. Distal axonopathy associated with chronic gluten enteropathy: a treatable disorder. *Neurology* 1988;38:642–645.

Uremic Neuropathy

Bolton CF. Peripheral neuropathies associated with chronic renal failure. *Can J Neurol Sci* 1980;7:89–96.
Cantaro S, Zara G, Battaggia C, et al. *In vivo* and *in vitro* neurotoxic action of plasma ultrafiltrate from uraemic patients. *Nephrol Dial Transplant* 1998;13:2288–2293.

Neuropathy Associated with Hepatic Disease

Inoue A, Tsukada M, Koh CS, et al. Chronic relapsing demyelinating polyneuropathy associated with hepatitis B infection. *Neurology* 1987;37:1663–1666.
Taukada N, Koh CS, Inoue A, et al. Demyelinating neuropathy associated with hepatitis B virus infection: detection of immune complexes composed of hepatitis B virus antigen. *Neurol Sci* 1987;77:203–210.
Thomas PK, Walker JC. Xanthomatous neuropathy in primary biliary cirrhosis. *Brain* 1965;88:1079–1088.
Zaltron S, Puoti M, Liberini P, et al. High prevalence of peripheral neuropathy in hepatitis C virus infected patients with symptomatic and asymptomatic cryoglobulinaemia. *J Gastroenterol Hepatol* 1998;30:391–395.

Neuropathy of Leprosy

Nations SP, Katz JS, Lyde CB, et al. Leprous neuropathy: an American perspective. *Semin Neurol* 1998;18:113–124.
Pedley JC, Harman DJ, Waudby H, et al. Leprosy in peripheral nerves: histopathological findings in 119 untreated patients in Nepal. *J Neurol Neurosurg Psychiatry* 1980;43:198–204.
Rosenberg RN, Lovelace RE. Mononeuritis multiplex in lepromatous leprosy. *Arch Neurol* 1968;19:310–314.
Thomas PK. Tropical neuropathies. *J Neurol* 1997;244:475–482.

Diphtheritic Neuropathy

Kurdi A, Abdul-Kader M. Clinical and electrophysiological studies of diphtheritic neuritis in Jordan. *J Neurol Sci* 1979;42:243–250.
Solders G, Nennesmo I, Persson A. Diphtheritic neuropathy: an analysis based on muscle and nerve biopsy and repeated neurophysiological and autonomic function tests. *J Neurol Neurosurg Psychiatry* 1989;52:876–880.

HIV-Related Neuropathies

Behar R, Wiley C, McCutchan JA. Cytomegalovirus polyradiculopathy in AIDS. *Neurology* 1987;37:557–561.
Brannagan TH, Nuovo GJ, Hays AP, et al. Human immunodeficiency virus infection of dorsal root ganglion neurons detected by polymerase chain reaction in situ hybridization. *Ann Neurol* 1997;42:368–372.
Brannagan TH, Zhou Y. HIV associated Guillain Barré Syndrome. *J Neurol Sci* 2003;208:39–42.
Cornblath DR, McArthur JC, Kennedy PGE, et al. Inflammatory demyelinating peripheral neuropathies associated with human T-cell lymphotropic virus type III infection. *Ann Neurol* 1987;21:32–40.
Gherardi RK, Chretien F, Delfau-Larue MH, et al. Neuropathy in diffuse infiltrative lymphocytosis syndrome. *Neurology* 1998;50:1041–1044.
Luciano CA, Pardo CA, McArthur JC. Recent developments in the HIV neuropathies. *Curr Opin Neurol* 2003;16:403–409.
Polydefkis M, Yiannoutsos CT, Cohen BA, et al. Reduced intraepidermal nerve fiber density in HIV-associated sensory neuropathy. *Neurology* 2002;58:115–119.
Said G, Lacroix C, Chemouli P, et al. Cytomegalovirus neuropathy in acquired immunodeficiency syndrome: a clinical and pathological study. *Ann Neurol* 1991;29:139–195.
So YT, Holtzman DM, Abrams DI, et al. Peripheral neuropathy associated with AIDS: prevalence and clinical features from a population-based survey. *Arch Neurol* 1988;45:945–948.

Neuropathy of Herpes Zoster

Denny-Brown D, Adams RD, Brady PJ. Pathologic features of herpes zoster: a note on "geniculate herpes." *Arch Neurol Psychiatry* 1944;51:216–231.
Gottschau P, Trojaborg W. Abdominal muscle paralysis associated with herpes zoster. *Acta Neurol Scand* 1991;84:344–347.
Mondelli M, Romano C, Passero S, et al. Effects of acyclovir on sensory axonal neuropathy, segmental motor paresis and postherpetic neuralgia in herpes zoster patients. *Eur Neurol* 1996;36:288–292.
Raja SN, Haythornthwaite JA, Pappagallo M, et al. Opioids versus antidepressants in postherpetic neuralgia; a randomized placebo-controlled trial. *Neurology* 2002;59:1015–1021.
Schmader K. Postherpetic neuralgia in immunocompetent elderly people. *Vaccine* 1998;16:1768–1770.
Watson CP, Vermich L, Chipman M, et al. Nortriptyline versus amitriptyline in postherpetic neuralgia: a randomized trial. *Neurology* 1998;51:1166–1171.

Bacterial Endocarditis

Pruitt AA, Rubin RH, Karchmer AW, et al. Neurologic complications of bacterial endocarditis. *Medicine* 1978;57:329–343.

Tick Paralysis

Swift TR, Ignacio OJ. Tick paralysis: electrophysiologic signs. *Neurology* 1975;25:1130–1133.
Vedanarayanan VV, Evans OB, Subramony SH. Tick paralysis in children; electrophysiology and possibility of misdiagnosis. *Neurology* 2002;59:1088–1090.

Sarcoid Neuropathy

Hoitsma E, Marziniak M, Faber CG, et al. Small fibre neuropathy in sarcoidosis. *Lancet* 2002;359:2085–2086.
Luke RA, Stem BJ, Krumholz A, et al. Neurosarcoidosis: the long-term clinical course. *Neurology* 1987;37:461–463.
Nemni R, Galassi G, Cohen M, et al. Symmetric sarcoid polyneuropathy: analysis of a sural nerve biopsy. *Neurology* 1981;31:1217–1223.
Zuniga G, Ropper AH, Frank J. Sarcoid peripheral neuropathy. *Neurology* 1991;41:1558–1561.

Polyneuropathy Associated with Dietary States

Green R, Kinsella LJ. Current concepts in the diagnosis of cobalamin deficiency. *Neurology* 1995;45:1435–1440.

Lossos A, River Y, Eliakim A, et al. Neurologic aspects of inflammatory bowel disease. *Neurology* 1995;45:416–421.

Parry GJ, Bredeson DE. Sensory neuropathy with low-dose pyridoxine. *Neurology* 1985;35:1466–1468.

Saperstein DS, Wolfe GI, Gronseth GS, et al. Challenges in the identification of cobalamin-deficiency polyneuropathy. *Arch Neurol* 2003;60:1296–1301.

Schaumburg H, Kaplan J, Windebank A, et al. Sensory neuropathy from pyridoxine abuse. A new megavitamin syndrome. *N Engl J Med* 1983;309:445–448.

Sokol RJ, Guggenheim MA, Iannaccone ST, et al. Improved neurologic function after long-term correction of vitamin E deficiency in children with chronic cholestasis. *N Engl J Med* 1985;313:1580–1586.

Victor M, Adams RD, Collins GH. *The Wernicke-Korsakoff Syndrome.* Philadelphia: FA Davis, 1971.

Critical Illness Polyneuropathy

Bolton CF, Laverty DA, Brown JD, et al. Critically ill polyneuropathy: electrophysiological studies and differentiation from Guillain-Barré syndrome. *J Neurol Neurosurg Psychiatry* 1986;49:563–573.

Hirano M, Ott BR, Raps EC, et al. Acute quadriplegic myopathy: a complication of treatment with steroids, nondepolarizing blocking agents, or both. *Neurology* 1992;42:2082–2087.

Rich MM, Raps EC, Bird SJ. Distinction between acute myopathy syndrome and critical illness polyneuropathy. *Mayo Clin Proc* 1995;70:198–200.

Zifko UA, Zipko HT, Bolton CF. Clinical and electrophysiological findings in critical illness polyneuropathy. *J Neurol Sci* 1998;159:186–193.

Neuropathy Produced by Metals, Toxins, and Therapeutic Agents

Buchthal F, Behse F. Electromyography and nerve biopsy in men exposed to lead. *Br J Ind Med* 1979;36:135–147.

Chang AP, England JD, Garcia CA, et al. Focal conduction block in n-hexane polyneuropathy. *Muscle Nerve* 1998;21:964–969.

Chaudhry V, Cornblath DR, Corse A, et al. Thalidomide-induced neuropathy. *Neurology* 2002;59:1872–1875.

Chu CC, Huang CC, Ryu SJ, et al. Chronic inorganic mercury-induced peripheral neuropathy. *Acta Neurol Scand* 1998;98:461–465.

Dalakas MC. Peripheral neuropathy and antiretroviral drugs. *J Periph N Syst* 2001;6:14–20.

Davis LE, Standefer JC, Kornfeld M, et al. Acute thallium poisoning: toxicological and morphological studies of the nervous system. *Ann Neurol* 1981;10:38–44.

Gaist D, Jeppesen U, Andersen M, et al. Statins and risks of polyneuropathy: a case-control study. *Neurology* 2002;58:1333–1337.

Gignoux L, Cortinovis-Tourniaire P, Grimaud J, et al. A brachial form of motor neuropathy caused by lead poisoning. *Rev Neurol (Paris)* 1998;154:771–773.

Goebel HH, Schmidt PF, Bohl J, et al. Polyneuropathy due to acute arsenic intoxication: biopsy studies. *J Neuropathol Exp Neurol* 1990;49:137–149.

Hillbom M, Weinberg A. Prognosis of alcoholic peripheral neuropathy. *J Neurol Neurosurg Psychiatry* 1984;47:699–703.

Iñiguez C, Larrodé P, Mayordomo JI, et al. Reversible peripheral neuropathy induced by a single administration of high-dose paclitaxel. *Neurology* 1998;51:868–870.

Jain KK. Drug-induced peripheral neuropathies. In: Jain KK, ed. Drug-Induced Neurological Disorders. 2nd Ed. Seattle: Hogrefe & Huber, 2001,263–294.

Koike H, Iijima M, Sugiura M, et al. Alcoholic neuropathy is clinicopathologically distinct from thiamine deficiency neuropathy. *Ann Neurol* 2003;54:19–29.

Krarup-Hansen A, Reitz B, Krarup C, et al. Histology and platinum content of sensory ganglia and sural nerves in patients treated with cisplatin and carboplatin: an autopsy study. *Neuropath Appl Neurobiol* 1999;25:29–40.

Laquery A, Ronnel A, Vignolly B, et al. Thalidomide neuropathy: an electrophysiologic study. *Muscle Nerve* 1986;9:837–844.

Lehning EJ, Persuad A, Dyer KR, et al. Biochemical and morphologic characterization of acrylamide peripheral neuropathy. *Toxicol Appl Pharmacol* 1998;151:211–221.

Molloy FM, Floeter MK, Syet NA, et al. Thalidomide neuropathy in patients treated for metastatic prostate cancer. *Muscle Nerve* 2001;24:1050–1057.

Nordentoft T, Andersen EB, Mogensen PH. Initial sensorimotor and delayed autonomic neuropathy in acute thallium poisoning. *Neurotoxicology* 1998;19:421–426.

Oh S. Electrophysiological profile in arsenic neuropathy. *J Neurol Neurosurg Psychiatry* 1991;54:1103–1105.

Quasthoff S, Hartung HP. Chemotherapy-induced peripheral neuropathy. *J Neurol* 2002;249:9–17.

Sahenk Z, Barohn R, New P, et al. Taxol neuropathy: electrodiagnostic and sural nerve biopsy findings. *Arch Neurol* 1994;51:726–729.

Tredici G, Minazzi M. Alcohol neuropathy: an electron-microscopic study. *J Neurol Sci* 1975;25:333–346.

Weimer LH. Medication-induced peripheral neuropathy. *Curr Neurol Neurosci Reports* 2003;3:86–92.

Diabetic Neuropathy

Abbott CA, Vileikyte L, Williamson S, et al. Multicenter study of the incidence of predictive risk factors for diabetic neuropathic foot ulceration. *Diabetes Care* 1998;21:1071–1075.

Asbury AK. Proximal diabetic neuropathy. *Ann Neurol* 1977;2:179–180.

Asbury AK, Aldredge H, Hershberg R, et al. Oculomotor palsy in diabetes mellitus: a clinicopathological study. *Brain* 1970;93:555–566.

Behse F, Buchthal F, Carlsen F. Nerve biopsy and conduction studies in diabetic neuropathy. *J Neurol Neurosurg Psychiatry* 1977;10:1072–1082.

Brannagan TH, Promisloff RA, McCluskey LF, et al. Proximal diabetic neuropathy presenting with respiratory weakness. *J Neurol Neurosurg Psychiatry* 1999;67:539–541.

The Diabetes Control and Complications Trial Research Group. The effect of intensive diabetes therapy on the development and progression of neuropathy. *Ann Intern Med* 1995;122:561–568.

Dyck PJ, Giannini C. Pathologic alterations in the diabetic neuropathies of humans: a review. *J Neuropathol Exp Neurol* 1996;55:1181–1193.

Dyck PJ, Thomas PK. *Diabetic Neuropathy.* 2nd Ed. Philadelphia: WB Saunders, 1999.

Dyck PJB, Windebank AJ. Diabetic and nondiabetic lumbosacral radiculoplexus neuropathies: New insights into pathophysiology and treatment. *Muscle Nerve* 2002;25:477–491.

Feldman EL. Oxidative stress and diabetic neuropathy: a new understanding of an old problem. *J Clin Investigation* 2003;111:431–433.

Lauria G, McArthur JC, Hauer PE, et al. Neuropathological alterations in diabetic truncal neuropathy: evaluation by skin biopsy. *J Neurol Neurosurg Psychiatry* 1998;65:762–766.

Llewelyn JG, Thomas PK, King RH. Epineurial microvasculitis in proximal diabetic neuropathy. *J Neurol* 1998;245:159–165.

Low PA, Walsh JC, Huang CY, et al. The sympathetic nervous system in diabetic neuropathy: a clinical and pathological study. *Brain* 1975;98:341–356.

Navarro X, Sutherland DE, Kennedy WR. Long-term effects of pancreatic transplantation on diabetic neuropathy. *Ann Neurol* 1998;44:149–150.

Quasthoff S. The role of axonal ion conductances in diabetic neuropathy: a review. *Muscle Nerve* 1998;21:1246–1255.

Report of the Expert Committee on the Diagnosis and Classification of Diabetes Mellitus. *Diabetes Care* 1997;20:1183–1197.

Said G, Elgrably F, Lacroix C, et al. Painful proximal diabetic neuropathy: inflammatory nerve lesions and spontaneous favorable outcome. *Ann Neurol* 1997;41:762–770.

Singleton JR, Smith AG, Russell JW, et al. Microvascular complications of impaired glucose tolerance. *Diabetes* 2003:2867–2873.

Brachial Neuritis

Beghi E, Kurland LT, Mulder DW, et al. Brachial plexus neuropathy in the population of Rochester, Minnesota, 1970–1981. *Neurology* 1985;18:320–323.

Evans BA, Stevens JC, Dyck PJ. Lumbosacral plexus neuropathy. *Neurology* 1981;31:1327–1330.

Seror P. Isolated sensory manifestations in neuralgic amyotrophy: report of eight cases. *Muscle Nerve* 2004;29:134–138.

Tsairis P, Dyck PJ, Mulder DW. Natural history of brachial plexus neuropathy: report on 99 patients. *Arch Neurol* 1972;27:109–117.

Radiation Neuropathy

Foley KM, Woodruff JM, Ellis FT, et al. Radiation-induced malignant and atypical peripheral nerve sheath tumors. *Ann Neurol* 1980;7:311–318.

Giese WL, Kinsella TJ. Radiation injury to peripheral and cranial nerves. In: Gulin PH, Leibel SH, eds. *Injury to the Nervous System*. New York: Raven, 1991:383–406.

Gutmann L, Gutmann L. Myokymia and neuromyotonia 2004. *J Neurol* 2004;251:138–142.

Lalu T, Mercier B, Birouk N, et al. Pure motor neuropathy after radiation therapy: 6 cases. *Rev Neurol (Paris)* 1998;154:40–44.

Lamy C, Mas JL, Varet B, et al. Postradiation lower motor neuron syndrome presenting as monomelic amyotrophy. *J Neurol Neurosurg Psychiatry* 1991;54:648–649.

Stoll BA, Andrews JT. Radiation-induced peripheral neuropathy. *BMJ* 1966;1:834–837.

Lyme Neuropathy

Coyle PK, Deng Z, Schutzer SE, et al. Detection of *Borrelia burgdorferi* antigens in cerebrospinal fluid. *Neurology* 1993;43:1093–1098.

Halperin J, Luft BJ, Volkman DJ, et al. Lyme neuroborreliosis. Peripheral nervous system manifestations. *Brain* 1990;11:1207–1221.

Halperin JJ. Lyme disease and the peripheral nervous system. *Muscle Nerve* 2003;28:133–143.

Hansen K, Lebech AM. The clinical and epidemiological profile of Lyme neuroborreliosis in Denmark 1985–1990: a prospective study of 187 patients with *Borrelia burgdorferi* specific intrathecal antibody production. *Brain* 1992;115:399–423.

Pachner AR, Steere AC. The triad of neurologic manifestations of Lyme disease: meningitis, cranial neuritis, and radiculoneuritis. *Neurology* 1985;35:47–53.

Wulff CH, Hansen K, Strange P, et al. Multiple mononeuritis and radiculitis with erythema, pain, elevated CSF protein and pleocytosis (Bannwarth's syndrome). *J Neurol Neurosurg Psychiatry* 1983;46:485–490.

Idiopathic Neuropathy

Chia L, Fernandez A, Lacroix C, et al. Contribution of nerve biopsy findings to the diagnosis of disabling neuropathy in the elderly. A retrospective review of 100 consecutive patients. *Brain* 1996;119:1091–1098.

Dyck PJ, Oviatt KF, Lambert EH. Intensive evaluation of referred unclassified neuropathies yields improved diagnosis. *Neurology* 1981;10:222–226.

Notermans NC, Wokke JHJ, Franssen H, et al. Chronic idiopathic polyneuropathy presenting in middle or old age: a clinical and electrophysiological study of 75 patients. *J Neurol Neurosurg Psychiatry* 1993;56:1066–1071.

Periquet MI, Novak V, Collins MP, et al. Painful sensory neuropathy: prospective evaluation using skin biopsy. *Neurology* 1999;53:1641–1647.

Wolfe GI, Baker NS, Amato AA, et al. Chronic cryptogenic sensory polyneuropathy: clinical and laboratory characteristics. *Arch Neurol* 1999;56:540–547.

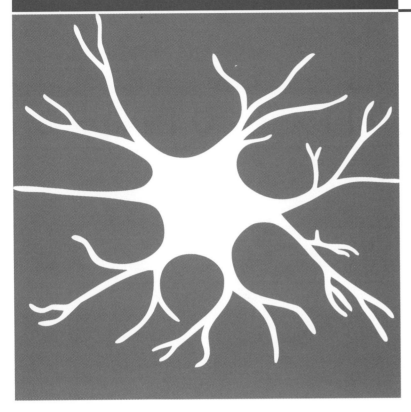

SECTION XIII

Dementias

Alzheimer Disease and Related Dementias

Scott A. Small and Richard Mayeux

The defining features of dementia have evolved since the term was first introduced over 300 years ago. In this era of standardized criteria, those of the *Diagnostic and Statistical Manual of Mental Disorders*, 4th edition (DSM-IV), are most commonly used. According to DSM-IV, the diagnosis of dementia requires "the development of multiple cognitive deficits that are sufficiently severe to cause impairment in occupational or social functioning." The impairments must include memory and other cognitive domains, must represent a decline from premorbid function, and must not be attributable to delirium or confusion (see Chapter 1).

The cellular and molecular mechanisms underlying the pathogenesis of various forms of dementia have been elaborated in the last decade. Although there are many similarities, there are also important differences in the various forms of dementia. Thus, the need for a classification system remains. Dementia can be grouped into four major categories: degenerative, vascular, infectious, and metabolic diseases.

DEGENERATIVE DISEASES

Alzheimer Disease

Kraepelin named the most frequently encountered dementia after Alois Alzheimer, who had described the clinical features and the pathologic manifestations of dementia in a 51-year-old woman at the beginning of the twentieth century. For many years Alzheimer disease was considered a presenile form of dementia, limited to individuals with symptoms beginning before the age of 65. However, subsequent clinical, pathologic, ultrastructural, and biochemical analyses indicated that Alzheimer disease is identical to the more common senile dementia beginning after age 65.

Clinical Syndrome

The manifestations of Alzheimer disease evolve uniformly from the earliest signs of impaired memory to severe cognitive loss. The course is a progressive one, terminating inevitably in complete incapacity and death. Plateaus sometimes occur in which cognitive impairment does not change for a year or two, but progression usually resumes.

Memory impairment for newly acquired information is the usual initial complaint, whereas memory for remote events is relatively unimpaired at the beginning of the illness. As the disease progresses, impairment in language, abstract reasoning, and executive function or decision making may be reported on specific questioning. Depression with insomnia or anorexia occurs in 5% to 8% of patients with Alzheimer disease unrelated to severity, and depressed mood can occur in parallel with the onset of memory decline. Delusions and psychotic behavior increase with progression of Alzheimer disease and are persistent in 20%. Agitation may coexist in up to 20%, increasing with advanced disease. Hallucinations occur with similar frequency and may be either visual or auditory.

Except for the mental state, the neurologic examination is usually normal, but extrapyramidal signs, including rigidity, bradykinesia, shuffling gait, and postural change, are relatively frequent in the disease. Primary motor and sensory functions are otherwise spared. Oculomotor, cerebellar, or peripheral nerve abnormalities on physical examination strongly raise the possibility of some other form of dementia.

Diagnosis

Criteria for the clinical diagnosis of Alzheimer disease were established by a joint effort of the National Institute of Neurological and Communicative Disorders and Stroke and the Alzheimer's Disease and Related Disorders Association in 1984 and are referred to as the NINCDS-ADRDA criteria. These include a history of progressive deterioration in cognitive ability in the absence of other known neurologic or medical problems. Psychological testing, brain imaging, and other criteria establish three levels of diagnostic certainty. The designation of "definite" Alzheimer disease is reserved for autopsy-confirmed disease. If there is no associated illness, the condition is called "probable" Alzheimer disease; "possible" refers to these who meet criteria for dementia but have another illness that may contribute, such as hypothyroidism or cerebrovascular disease. Comparing the clinical with the pathologic diagnosis, the NINCDS-ADRDA criteria provide 90% sensitivity for the diagnosis of probable or possible Alzheimer disease and 60% specificity. In 2001, the American Academy of Neurology endorsed and extended these criteria as the standard of care for practicing physicians.

There are no specific changes in routine laboratory examinations. CSF is normal, but there may be a slight increase in protein content. The measurement of tau protein in the CSF has been used in the differential diagnosis of Alzheimer disease. Tau is required for the stabilization of microtubules in the axons of neurons. In Alzheimer disease, tau becomes hyperphosphorylated and is detected in higher CSF concentrations than in healthy individuals or those with other forms of dementia. In contrast, a species of the amyloid β peptide, Aβ42, a constituent of the neuritic plaques present in brain, is of lower concentration in Alzheimer CSF than in healthy individuals or those with other dementias. These measurements are commercially available but not widely used because lumbar puncture is considered invasive and the tests, individually or combined, lack sufficient sensitivity and specificity for clinical practice.

Other procedures include the EEG, in which generalized slowing without focal features is typically observed. Spectral EEG, cerebral evoked potentials, and other neurophysiologic methods have been explored as diagnostic tools but without consistent results. Neuropsychologic testing is still the most reliable method to detect minimal or subtle cognitive impairment early in the disease. These tests can be used to document the degree of impairment in following the course of the disease (Chapter 20).

Brain imaging has the potential to become important in the diagnosis and management of dementia. MRI or CT typically reveals dilatation of the lateral ventricles and widening of the cortical sulci, particularly in temporal regions. Mild cortical atrophy, however, is seen in some older individuals who function normally by clinical and psychologic testing. During the last decade, MRI approaches have been developed to measure precise volumetric changes in the brain. When applied to Alzheimer disease, volumetric MRI uniformly shows shrinkage in vulnerable brain regions, in particular the entorhinal cortex and hippocampus.

Functional brain imaging techniques include PET, SPECT, and most recently, functional magnetic resonance imaging (fMRI). Although using different technologies, functional imaging techniques are unified in sensitivity to brain metabolism—either glucose uptake in the case of flurodeoxyglucose (FDG) PET, or hemodynamic correlates of oxygen metabolism in the case of O^{15}PET, SPECT, or fMRI. Early studies using PET or SPECT revealed a characteristic pattern of hypometabolism in the posterior parietal lobes. With the use of more sophisticated SPECT and PET approaches, and with the superior spatial resolution afforded by fMRI, studies have begun to map metabolic deficits in smaller brain regions, such as the entorhinal cortex and hippocampus.

Radioligands can now bind amyloid, which can then be visualized with PET. It is possible to detect the amyloid burden in patients with Alzheimer disease.

Although an MRI or CT is recommended as part of the initial workup of patients suspected to have Alzheimer disease, these tests are ordered to rule out other causes of dementia. As of yet, brain imaging cannot, by itself, diagnose Alzheimer disease. Nevertheless, a functional imaging scan is occasionally useful, particularly in distinguishing frontotemporal dementia (see below) from Alzheimer disease. Large-scale studies are in progress, and within the next few years it is expected that some form of brain imaging, individually or in combination, will emerge as reliable in identifying Alzheimer disease. Because the sensitivity of diagnosing Alzheimer disease in a demented patient is already quite high, brain imaging could contribute in the following ways: to improve diagnostic specificity when confronted with a demented patient; to enhance our ability to detect the earliest predementia stages of Alzheimer disease; and to map the clinical course of the disease.

Genetic tests are generally not recommended as diagnostic tests for Alzheimer disease. However, selected testing may be useful in the diagnosis in families with the rare early-onset autosomal-dominant forms of Alzheimer disease. For sporadic or familial late-onset Alzheimer disease, the ϵ4 polymorphism of the apolipoprotein E gene is associated with a higher risk of the disease but does not provide sufficient sensitivity or specificity to be used for diagnosis and is not recommended.

Pathology

Two major features characterize Alzheimer disease: extracellular plaques consisting of the 42 amino-acid amyloid β (Aβ) peptide and intracellular neurofibrillary tangles. At autopsy, the cerebral atrophy owing to widespread neuronal loss is diffuse but more pronounced in the frontal, parietal, and temporal lobes (Fig. 107.1). On microscopic examination, there is loss of both neurons and neuropil in the cortex; sometimes secondary

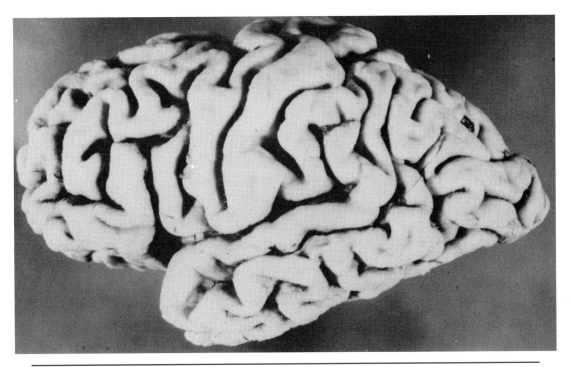

FIGURE 107.1. Alzheimer disease. Diffuse atrophy of brain, especially severe in frontal, temporal, and parietal lobes with sparing of precentral and postcentral gyri. (Courtesy of Dr. Robert Terry.)

demyelination is seen in subcortical white matter. Quantitative morphometry suggests that the earliest cell loss occurs in the entorhinal region of the medial temporal lobe.

The senile neuritic plaques are spherical microscopic lesions with a core of extracellular Aβ surrounded by enlarged axonal endings (neurites). The Aβ peptide is derived from the amyloid precursor protein (APP), a transmembrane protein present in most tissues. A region of the APP resides within an intramembranous domain of intracellular organelles in neurons, and it is believed that proteases, termed *secretases*, are responsible for cleavage of a site residing within a membranous domain. This protein undergoes proteolysis by α, β, and γ secretase enzymes. When cleaved by α secretase a soluble peptide derivative of amyloid is formed, but when cut by β secretase first γ secretase generates two peptides, Aβ40 and Aβ42. The Aβ peptide monomer binds other peptides, forming oligomers, ultimately leading to the accumulation of amyloid in all forms of the disease. Whether oligomeric or monomeric Aβ is the basic neurotoxic element in Alzheimer disease is still matter of debate. In Alzheimer disease, amyloid is deposited around meningeal and cerebral vessels and in gray matter. The gray matter deposits are multifocal, coalescing into miliary structures known as plaques (Fig. 107.2). Parenchymal Aβ plaques are distributed in brain in a characteristic fashion, differentially affecting the various cerebral and cerebellar lobes and cortical laminae.

Neurofibrillary tangles are fibrillary intracytoplasmic structures within the neurons. Electron microscopy shows paired helical filaments of a protein called *tau*. Microtubule proteins provide support for neurons and transport nutrients through a microtubule assembly held together by tau, which binds to a support protein called *tubulin*. In Alzheimer disease, tau aggregates owing to hyperphosphorylation, presumably owing to the aggregation of extracellular Aβ. Once tau aggregates, it forms twisted paired-helical filaments, recognized as neurofibrillary tangles. Although neurofibrillary tangles are not specific to Alzheimer disease, they occur first in the hippocampal formation; later, neurofibrillary tangles may be seen throughout the cerebral cortex (Table 107.1).

Other features of Alzheimer disease include granulovacuolar degeneration of pyramidal cells of the hippocampus and amyloid angiopathy. The Hirano body, a rodlike body containing actin in a paracrystalline array, was first described in the Guamanian Parkinsonism-dementia complex; these neuronal inclusions are also found in Alzheimer disease. Some investigators believe that cognitive decline correlates, not with increased number of plaques but with a decrease in the density of presynaptic boutons from the pyramidal neurons in lamina III and IV, especially in the midfrontal neocortex. Atherosclerotic changes are absent or inconspicuous in most cases.

Biochemically, the most consistent change is a 50% to 90% reduction of the activity of choline acetyltransferase, the biosynthetic enzyme for acetylcholine, in the

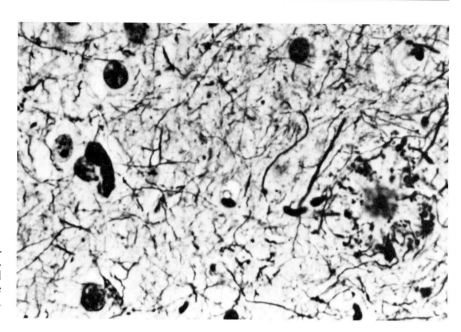

FIGURE 107.2. Alzheimer disease. **Left.** Prominent senile plaques. **Right.** Several neurons with neurofibrillary tangles. Note also disruption of cortical organization. (Courtesy of Dr. Robert Terry.)

cerebral cortex and hippocampus. This enzyme is found in cholinergic neurons, and there is a selective loss of cholinergic neurons, particularly of the cholinergic projection pathway, from deep nuclei in the septum near the diagonal band of Broca to the hippocampus and from the nearby basal nucleus of Meynert to the cerebral cortex. Among the cholinergic receptor subtypes, M2—a presynaptic muscarinic receptor—displays decreased binding in the brains of Alzheimer patients. The severity of cognitive loss is roughly proportional to the loss of choline acetyltransferase. There is decreased content of corticotropin-releasing factor and somatostatin, both of which are found within degenerating neurites of the neuritic plaque. Glutaminergic neurons account for many large neurons lost in the cerebral cortex and hippocampus, and there is variable loss of ascending and descending serotoninergic and adrenergic systems.

▶ **TABLE 107.1 Pathologic Changes in Alzheimer Disease**

Cell loss, plaques, and tangles occur regularly in
Neocortex, especially association areas
Hippocampus, including entorhinal cortex
Amygdala
Basal nucleus of Meynert
Sometimes in
Medial nucleus of thalamus
Dorsal tegmentum
Locus coeruleus
Paramedian reticular area
Lateral hypothalamic nuclei

Epidemiology

Before age 65, the prevalence, or proportion, of individuals with Alzheimer disease is less than 1%, but this rapidly increases to between 5% and 10% at age 65 years and to as high as 30% to 40% at age 85 and older. The age-specific incidence, or the number of new cases arising over a specific period of time, also rises steeply from less than 1% per year before age 65 years to 6.0% per year for individuals aged 85 and older. The average duration of symptoms until death may be 10 years, with a range of 4 to 16 years. Women survive longer with the disease than men. The incidence rates for Alzheimer disease are also slightly higher in women, especially after age 85 years. In families with at least one affected individual, women who are first-degree relatives have a higher lifetime risk of developing Alzheimer disease than men.

Genetic Basis of Alzheimer Disease

Many families with autosomal dominant Alzheimer disease have been described. Siblings of patients have twice the expected lifetime risk of developing the disease. Also, monozygotic twins have significantly higher concordance of Alzheimer disease than do dizygotic twins. Mutations in three genes, the *APP* gene on chromosome 21, the presenilin I (*PSEN1*) on chromosome 14, and the presenilin 2 (*PSEN2*) on chromosome 1, result in an autosomal dominant form of the disease beginning as early as the third decade of life. The existence of 135 different mutations in *PSEN1* suggests that this may be the most common form of familial early-onset Alzheimer disease. *APP* mutations can lead to enhanced generation or aggregation of the amyloid-β peptide, indicating a pathogenic role. *PSEN* I and II are

▶ TABLE 107.2 Genes and Chromsomal Loci Related to Alzheimer Disease

Chromosome	Gene	Age at Onset	Pattern	Variants or Mutations
ch21q21.3	APP	30–60 years	AD	20 (exons 16, 17)
ch14q24.13	PS1	30–50 years	AD and familial	135 (exons 4 + 12)
ch1q31.42	PS2	50–70 years	AD	10 (exons 4, 5, 7)
ch19q13.2	APOE	50–80+ years	Familial and sporadic	3 isoforms
ch12p[a]	?	>65 years	Familial	Unknown
ch10q[a]	?	>65 years	Familial	Unknown
ch9p[a]	?	>65 years	Familial	Unknown

[a]Established by linkage analysis only.
Abbreviations: AD, autosomal dominant; APP, amyloid precursor protein; APOE, apolipoprotein E;
PS1, presenelin-1.

distinct from the immediate regulatory and coding regions of APP and are thought to lead to aggregation of Aβ by interfering with γ-secretase processing. Mutations in these three genes account for about half of the familial forms of early-onset Alzheimer's disease and may be considered deterministic because of nearly complete correspondence between the genotype and phenotype.

The ε4 polymorphism of the apolipoprotein E (*APOE*) gene on chromosome 19 has been associated with the more typical sporadic and familial forms of Alzheimer disease, usually beginning after age 65. In contrast to the disease-causing mutations in the *APP* and *PSEN* I and II genes, the ε4 polymorphism of *APOE* is a normally occurring variant of the gene that appears to significantly increase susceptibility to the disease. In some families with late-onset Alzheimer disease, in a few families with mutations in the *APP* gene, and in patients with Down syndrome, each APOE ε4 allele can lower the age at onset of dementia. The association between the *APOE* ε4 polymorphism and Alzheimer disease is weaker among African Americans and Caribbean Hispanics. Consistent with other genes involved in Alzheimer disease, *APOE* may also act through a complex and poorly understood relationship with amyloid. The apolipoprotein E protein is an obligatory participant in amyloid accumulation, and different apolipoprotein E protein isoforms corresponding to polymorphisms exert at least some of their effects by controlling accumulation.

APOE has been called a "susceptibility" gene because possession of the ε4 allele, a polymorphism, does not always lead to Alzheimer disease. One *APOE-ε4* allele is associated with a twofold to threefold increased risk whereas having two copies is associated with a fivefold increase, and each *APOE-ε4* allele lowers the age at onset in a dose-dependent fashion. The population attributable risk associated with *APOE-ε4* is approximately 20%, making it one of the most important risk factors for the disease.

Over the past five years, genetic linkage and association studies have provided evidence for additional loci producing susceptibility to Alzheimer disease. There appears to be strong consensus for linkage on chromosomes 10q21-22 and 12p11-12. An additional locus on chromosome 9p

has been linked to Alzheimer disease that was confirmed by postmortem examination. A number of case-control studies and a genetic linkage study have associated variant alleles in the chromosome 6p21 region of the major histocompatibility complex. Polymorphisms in HLA-2A and tumor necrosis factor-α have been associated with disease, but inconsistently and without an identified mechanism (Table 107.2).

Other Risk Factors

Though inconsistent, Alzheimer disease has also been associated with traumatic head injury, lower educational achievement, parental age at the time of birth, smoking, and Down syndrome in a first-degree relative. In several observational studies, the use of estrogen replacement therapy in postmenopausal women and the regular use of anti-inflammatory agents in both men and women were associated with lower risks of Alzheimer disease. Clinical trials have not confirmed a protective effect for estrogen, but clinical trials are currently being conducted to determine whether or not nonsteroidal anti-inflammatory agents are effective in preventing the disease (Table 107.3).

▶ TABLE 107.3 Risk Factors Most Consistently Associated With Alzheimer Disease

Risk Factor or Antecedent	Direction	Presumed Mechanism
Head injury	Risk increased	Aβ and APP in brain
Parental age	Risk increased	Advanced physiologic aging
Depression	Risk increased	Neurotransmitter alterations
Education	Risk decreased	Cognitive reserve
Anti-inflammatories	Risk decreased	Prevents complement activation
Estrogen	Risk decreased	Throphic; Aβ APP metabolism
Smoking	Risk increased	Unknown

APP, amyloid precursor protein.

Treatment

Cholinesterase inhibitors are currently the most prominent U.S. Food and Drug Administration–approved treatments for Alzheimer disease and, at present, are considered the standard of care for mild to moderate disease. These medications decrease the hydrolysis of acetylcholine released from the presynaptic neuron into the synaptic cleft by inhibiting acetylcholinesterase, resulting in stimulation of the cholinergic receptor. Four cholinesterase inhibitors are now available: tacrine, donepezil, rivastigmine, and galantamine. The use of tacrine is limited by its hepatotoxicity. The other cholinesterase inhibitors have shown modest effects on cognitive performance at their maximum recommended dosages for periods of up to 2 years. The efficacy of these medications on the functional consequences of the disease is less obvious.

Memantine was the first N-methyl-D-aspartate antagonist used to treat moderate to severe Alzheimer disease. The drug may interfere with glutamatergic excitotoxicity and enhance hippocampal function in the remaining neurons. Both α-tocopherol and selegiline are said to delay the appearance of later stages of Alzheimer disease. Unlike selegiline, α-tocopherol does not interact with other medications, allowing it to be used in most patients without concern. Psychotropic drugs are frequently used to treat agitation, delusions, and psychosis in Alzheimer disease. For depression, nearly all drugs are similar in efficacy, but there are only a handful of randomized controlled studies on which to make therapeutic decisions.

Frontotemporal Dementias

Pick disease is a progressive form of dementia characterized by personality change, speech disturbance, inattentiveness, and sometimes extrapyramidal signs. In contrast to Alzheimer disease, Pick disease is rare. The disease can be familial. Atrophy of the frontal and temporal poles and argyrophilic round intraneuronal inclusions (Pick bodies) are the characteristic morphologic changes. Glial reaction is often pronounced in affected cerebral gray and white matter. Tau-immunoreactive glial inclusions and neuritic changes are recognized. Biochemical and immunocytochemical studies demonstrate that abnormal tau proteins are the major structural components of Pick bodies and differ from those seen in Alzheimer disease. As with other frontotemporal dementias, Pick disease shows filamentous tau pathology that has been associated with mutations in tau protein. Tau is a microtubule-associated protein found mainly in axons; it is involved in microtubule assembly and stabilization.

Frontotemporal dementias other than Pick disease are also rare and have been associated with mutations on chromosome 17 in the tau (τ) gene. Several different mutations account for a diverse array of clinical manifestations in

▶ **TABLE 107.4** **Degenerative Diseases Associated With Dementia and With Specific Tau Mutations**

Familial frontotemporal dementia and parkinsonism
Progressive supranuclear palsy
Familiar progressive subcortical gliosis
Corticobasal ganglionic degeneration
Familial multiple system tauopathy with presenile dementia

addition to contributing to a characteristic pathologic change observed in Alzheimer disease: the neurofibrillary tangle. Table 107.4 lists the diseases associated with mutation in tau. Frontotemporal dementias are also characterized by personality change, deterioration of memory and executive functions, and stereotypical behavior. Extrapyramidal signs are usually prominent. Standard neuropsychologic tests and conventional brain imaging such as MRI and SPECT may not be sensitive to the early changes in the ventromedial frontal cortex. This suggests difficulty in distinguishing this form of dementia from other dementias early in the illness. Over time, however, there are abnormalities on SPECT, frontal atrophy on MRI, or a neuropsychologic profile more typical of frontotemporal dementia.

Although there is clinical and neuropathologic variability among and within families, the consistency of the syndrome led investigators to name the disease *frontotemporal dementia and parkinsonism linked to chromosome 17*. The pathologic changes include atrophy of frontal and temporal cortex and the basal ganglia and substantia nigra. In most cases, these features are accompanied by neuronal loss, gliosis, and deposits of microtubule-associated protein tau in both neurons and glial cells. The distribution and structural and biochemical characteristics of the tau deposits differentiate them from those of Alzheimer disease, corticobasal degeneration, progressive supranuclear palsy, and Pick disease. No β-amyloid deposits are present.

Other degenerative diseases that may include dementia and are associated with tau mutations include progressive supranuclear palsy, familial progressive subcortical gliosis, and corticobasal ganglionic degeneration. Familial multiple-system tauopathy with presenile dementia shows abundant filamentous tau protein pathology.

Parkinson Disease and Lewy Body Dementia

The prevalence of dementia in patients with Parkinson disease may be as high as 40% (see Chapter 115). The risk of dementia with Parkinson disease is about four times that of other people of the same age and increases with age at diagnosis of Parkinson disease and with the presence of depression, visual hallucinations early in the disease, or advanced motor manifestations such as bradykinesia or rigidity. Neither computed tomography nor MRI reliably distinguishes demented from nondemented patients with Parkinson disease. Compared with patients with Parkinson disease who are not demented, those with dementia may show hypometabolism in the frontal lobes and the basal ganglia on PET or SPECT. Dementia associated with Parkinson disease is the third most common form of dementia overall. In addition, the presence of dementia limits the usefulness of nearly all forms of treatment for the motor manifestations because adverse effects such as delusions are more frequent.

Dementia is often superimposed on a mild degree of cognitive loss that is specific to Parkinson disease. Impairment in mental speed and visuospatial functions are impaired in most patients with Parkinson disease in the absence of dementia. With the onset of dementia, impaired memory, verbal fluency, and language compound these manifestations. New dementia occurs at the rate of 7% per year among patients with Parkinson disease. With increasing age, the cumulative risk of dementia by age 85 may be over 65%, suggesting that dementia is an inevitable consequence of Parkinson disease.

Three distinct neuropathologic changes are associated with dementia in Parkinson disease: coincident Alzheimer disease (senile plaques and neurofibrillary tangles) and vascular disease, Lewy bodies (in cortical and subcortical structures) accompanied by Lewy neurites, and primary nigral degeneration. Rarely, there is tau pathology, such as tangle formation, or spongiform change. Both Lewy bodies and neuritis contain α-synuclein, which is expressed in brain, particularly in the substantia nigra. The extracellular plaque containing amyloid in patients with Alzheimer's disease also contains α-synuclein. Similar to other natively unfolded proteins, α-synuclein undergoes a folded confirmation in Parkinson disease. A key pathologic feature of Parkinson disease with dementia, diffuse Lewy body disease, and Alzheimer disease is the presence of ubiquitinated cytoplasmic inclusions as Lewy bodies in the cerebral cortex. Whether these inclusions are involved directly or indirectly in the pathogenesis of these disorders has not been established.

Dementia associated with Lewy bodies is considered clinically distinct from dementia associated with Parkinson disease and Alzheimer disease. Features include persistent cognitive decline with fluctuations in mental ability, recurrent and persistent visual hallucinations, parkinsonism, repeated falls, and sensitivity to neuroleptic medications. A "Lewy body variant" of Alzheimer disease characterized by a greater degree of impairment in attention, verbal fluency, and visuospatial function than typically seen in Alzheimer disease has been described in retrospective postmortem studies. Although criteria for dementia associated with cortical Lewy bodies have been proposed, they require the presence of parkinsonism, which is an inconsistent finding. Some patients with cortical Lewy bodies and dementia have no history or clinical evidence of rigidity, tremor, bradykinesia, or postural change. A fluctuating decline in cognitive function, characterized by episodes of confusion and lucid intervals, is believed by some to distinguish between senile dementia of the Lewy body type and Alzheimer disease. Depression, complex visual hallucinations, and delusions are also part of the clinical spectrum. Yet none of these clinical manifestations is specific for any single form of dementia.

Huntington Disease

This disorder is described in Chapter 109. In addition to chorea and other motor manifestations, memory loss and difficulty performing complex or sequential mental activities are seen early in the disease. After several years, chorea, postural instability, and frank dementia are evident, contributing to functional decline. In a mildly impaired patient, metabolic activity is reduced in the striatum and frontoparietal areas bilaterally. With progression, glucose metabolism is reduced at the junction of temporal and occipital regions. The severity of chorea correlates with subcortical metabolic activity, and the severity of dementia is linked to cortical metabolic rates.

The pathologic correlates of dementia in Huntington disease have not been established. Nonetheless, the expansion of polyglutamine tracts in the huntingtin protein is toxic to neurons resulting in degeneration in the striatum and the cerebral cortex. Later in the disease the hypothalamus and the hippocampus are involved. There is atrophy of the caudate nucleus and putamen with extensive nerve cell loss and astrocytosis. Neurons containing γ-aminobutyric acid, enkephalin, substance P, and dynorphin are reduced in number, with low brain concentrations of γ-aminobutyric acid and glutamic acid decarboxylase.

VASCULAR DISEASES

Cerebrovascular Disease and Dementia

Dementia in association with stroke is the second most frequent cause of dementia overall. As many as 15% to 20% of patients with acute ischemic stroke over age 60 years have dementia at the time of the stroke, and 5% per year become demented thereafter. Risk factors include advancing age, diabetes, history of prior stroke, and the size and location of the stroke. There is a complex interaction between stroke, vascular risk factors, and Alzheimer disease, although the exact nature of this interaction remains unknown.

Dementia and intellectual impairment can result from brain injury caused by stroke, either hemorrhagic or ischemic. The manifestations of dementia after stroke include loss of memory and impairment in at least two other cognitive domains: orientation, attention, language-verbal skills, visuospatial abilities, calculation, executive functions, motor control, praxis, abstraction, and judgment. The impairment must be severe enough to impair "functioning in daily living" or "to interfere broadly with the conduct of the patient's customary affairs of life."

Although stroke increases the risk of dementia, the definition of vascular dementia remains unsettled despite numerous attempts at clarification. There are four major sets of criteria for the clinical diagnosis of "vascular dementia," and they vary depending on the temporal relationship between the stroke and the onset of dementia. Dementia after stroke may be predominantly of the mixed type, a combination of Alzheimer disease and stroke, and the cause is likely to be multifactorial. High blood pressure is associated with dementia after stroke and can be associated with leukoaraiosis found on brain imaging. Severe leukoaraiosis, cerebral hypoperfusion, fluctuations in systemic blood pressure, hypotension induced by medication or systemic conditions, ischemia, carotid atherosclerosis, and diabetes may each increase the risk of dementia after stroke.

Different clinical subtypes of cerebrovascular dementia are described. A cortical syndrome is generally characterized by repeated atherothrombotic or cardioembolic strokes, obvious focal sensorimotor signs, more severe aphasic disturbance when present, and an abrupt onset of cognitive failure. A subcortical syndrome accompanied by deep white matter lesions is characterized by pseudobulbar signs, isolated pyramidal signs, depression or emotional lability, "frontal" behavior, mildly impaired memory, disorientation, poor response to novelty, restricted field of interest, decreased ability to make associations, difficulty passing from one idea to another, inattention, and perseveration.

Cerebral autosomal-dominant arteriopathy with subcortical infarcts and leukoencephalopathy (CADASIL) is an autosomal-dominant form of cerebrovascular dementia with onset in the third and forth decades of life and has been related to mutations in the *notch3* gene on chromosome 19. In patients with multiple deep infarcts resulting in état lacunaire, pseudobulbar palsy is often a central feature with emotional and urinary incontinence, dysarthria, bilateral pyramidal signs, and gait imbalance with marche à petit pas. Regardless of the clinical syndrome, the survival of patients with cerebrovascular dementia is less than that of other forms of dementia, including Alzheimer disease.

Control of hypertension reduces the risk of recurrent cerebral infarction and may secondarily reduce the risk of subsequent dementia. Any effective measure that prevents stroke recurrence could be applied to patients with vascular dementia: antiplatelet therapy, anticoagulants, carotid endarterectomy, and, for most patients, aspirin.

INFECTIOUS DISEASES

Prion-Related Diseases

Prion diseases are rare, fatal neurodegenerative disorders often with dementia as the most prominent manifestation, as discussed also in Chapter 34. The worldwide incidence of sporadic Creutzfeldt-Jakob disease, the most common prion disease, is 0.5 to 1.5 per million population per year and less than one death per million per year. There are no established risk factors for contracting the disease. Prion disorders are characterized by similar histopathology consisting of spongy degeneration, neuronal loss, and astrocytic proliferation. In all prion disorders, there is posttranslational conversion of a normal glycosylphosphatidylinositol anchored glycoprotein, the cellular prion protein, PrPc, to an abnormal isoform, PrPSc.

There are several forms of prion diseases in humans (Table 107.5): sporadic and familial Creutzfeldt-Jakob and a more recently described variant form, Gerstmann-Sträussler-Scheinker, fatal familial insomnia, and kuru. The most common form is sporadic Creutzfeldt-Jakob disease. The diagnosis is usually made in individuals aged 50 to 70 years. A progressive dementia with myoclonus, pyramidal signs, periodic sharp waves on EEG, and cerebellar or extrapyramidal signs suffices for the diagnosis of sporadic Creutzfeldt-Jakob disease. Progression is rapid, with significant decline noted in weeks or months; most die within 6 months or a year of onset. Raised cerebrospinal fluid content of 14-3-3 protein and signal changes in the basal ganglia on magnetic resonance imaging are both helpful in the diagnosis, although neither is specific for the disease. Atypical features such as cerebellar ataxia, cortical blindness, and amyotrophy can occur in some patients. There are no mutations in the gene encoding the prion protein (*PRNP*), also called the prion-related protein gene, although most affected individuals are homozygous at codon 129 for either a methionine or valine.

▶ **TABLE 107.5 Prion-Related Dementias**

Prion-related Diseases	*Markers on PrP Gene, Chromosome 20*
Creutzfeldt-Jakob disease	
Familial	Mutation in codon 200
	88% homozygotes for polymorphism at codon 129[a]
Sporadic	100% homozygotes for polymorphism at codon 129[a]
New variant	
Gerstmann-Sträussler-Scheinker	Mutation in codon 102
Fatal familial insomnia	Mutation in codon 179

[a] Compared with 48% homozygotes among healthy control subjects.

Fifteen percent to 20% of persons with Creutzfeldt-Jakob disease have an autosomal-dominant inheritance pattern on family history. Point mutations, deletions, or insertions between codons 51 and 91 are found in the *PRNP* gene on chromosome 20. In contrast to the sporadic form, these patients typically have a younger age at onset and a more protracted course; they are less likely to have the periodic EEG findings. These mutations are thought to cause prion disease by promoting the conversion of PrPc to the PrPSc isoform. This process alters the folding pattern of the mutated protein to produce a β-pleated configuration that polymerizes into amyloid fibrils. As mentioned previously, the other familial forms of prion disease include Gerstmann-Sträussler-Scheinker and fatal familial insomnia.

Variant Creutzfeldt-Jakob disease begins before age 40 years, and the course is more prolonged than the familial form. These patients are more likely to have psychiatric manifestations, to have paresthesias and sensory loss, and to develop cerebellar ataxia. Psychiatric features such as dysphoria, anxiety, insomnia, or apathy can be prominent. They usually lack the periodic complexes on EEG, and the cerebrospinal fluid 14-3-3 protein is not elevated. However, the presence of thalamic and periaqueductal hyperintensities on magnetic resonance imaging can be useful. In addition, all variant forms are homozygous for a methionine in the *PRNP* gene at codon 129.

Gerstmann-Sträussler-Scheinker disease is a familial form of prion disease with autosomal dominant ataxia, spastic paraplegia, and dementia. Multicentric amyloid plaques are found in the cerebellar and cerebral hemispheres that are immunoreactive for PrP is most marked in this form of prion disease. Four distinct mutations have been found in the *PRNP* gene.

Fatal familial insomnia is associated with a mutation in the *PRNP* gene at codon 178. The same asparagine for aspartic acid substitution has also been observed in familial Creutzfeldt-Jakob disease. The average age at onset varies from 20 to 60 years, and the duration is less than 2 years. Severe loss of weight, insomnia, autonomic dysfunction, and motor abnormalities can be present. The cerebrospinal fluid 14-3-3 protein is not elevated and conventional brain imaging is not specific. Polysomnographic recordings show evidence of marked disorganization of sleep patterns and loss of the normal sleep stages. The brain shows widespread cortical astrogliosis, but degeneration is confined to the thalami and inferior olivary nuclei. Deposition of the PrP in the form of plaques is found in the cerebellum and brainstem.

Kuru is a sporadic prion disease that was associated with cannibalism among natives of New Guinea. The disease has virtually disappeared once cannibalism was halted. Methonine homozygosity at codon 129 in *PRNP* is the major susceptibility determinant.

HIV Type 1-Associated Dementia Complex

HIV type 1 dementia complex is characterized by apathy, memory loss, and cognitive slowing, and may appear before there are other neurologic abnormalities (see also Chapter 25). Diagnosis is established by clinical features and laboratory tests. The differential diagnosis includes cerebral toxoplasmosis, cerebral lymphoma, progressive multifocal leukoencephalopathy, neurosyphilis, cytomegalovirus encephalitis, and cryptococcal and tuberculous meningitis. Examination of the CSF and brain imaging are essential to rule out these treatable diseases. Subcortical hypermetabolism on PET characterizes the early stages of the dementia. There is predominantly frontotemporal atrophy; multinucleated giant cells, microglial nodules, and perivascular infiltrates are evident microscopically.

INHERITED METABOLIC DISEASES

These disorders rarely cause dementia in adults but are important because some are potentially treatable. Young onset of dementia or involvement of other areas of the nervous system (e.g., cerebellar, visual, peripheral nerve, muscle) and body (e.g., skin, skeletal, and visceral organs) should prompt and guide investigation into these disorders (Table 107.6). Most of these diseases are described

▶ **TABLE 107.6 Laboratory Investigations of Inherited Metabolic Dementias**

Disease	Laboratory Tests
Wilson disease	Serum ceruloplasmin, urinary copper
Adrenoleukodystrophy and adrenomyeloneuropathy	Very long-chain fatty acids
Cerebrotendinous xanthomatosis	Serum cholestanol
Kufs disease	Urinary dolichols, skin or brain biopsy
Membranous lipodystrophy	Hand radiographs, bone biopsy
MERRF, MELAS	Lactic acid, muscle biopsy
Metachromatic leukodystrophy	Leukocyte arylsulfatase A
Mucopolysaccaridosis III	Alpha-*N*-acetyl-glucosaminidase
Gaucher disease	Glucocerebrosidase
Niemann-Pick type C	Sphingomyelinase
Krabbe disease	Leukocyte galactocerebroside β-galactosidase
GM$_2$-gangliosidosis	Leukocyte hexosaminidase A
GM$_1$-gangliosidosis	Leukocyte β-galactosidase
Adult polyglucosan body disease	Sural nerve biopsy
Lafora disease	Muscle biopsy

elsewhere in this book. Wilson disease, Hallervorden-Spatz disease, Fabry disease and the Fahr syndrome are dementias associated with abnormal metal metabolism. X-linked adrenoleukodystrophy and adrenomyeloneuropathy are a result of a defect in the peroxisomal enzyme, lignoceroyl-CoA ligase gene. Dementia is one of several manifestations in late-onset forms of these diseases. Cerebrotendinous xanthomatosis, Kufs disease, and membranous lipodystrophy are disorders of lipid metabolism that can cause dementia in adults. Several mitochondrial disorders are associated with dementia, especially MELAS and MERRF (see Chapter 97).

Lysosomal disorders can cause dementia in adults. The most common lysosomal disease with adult-onset dementia is metachromatic leukodystrophy. Other rare lysosomal diseases include mucopolysaccharidosis III (Sanfilippo disease) with α-N-acetyl-glucosaminidase deficiency, Gaucher disease with glucocerebrosidase (glucosylceramide- β-glucosidase) deficiency, Niemann-Pick disease type C with sphingomyelinase deficiency, Fabry disease with α-galactosidase deficiency, Krabbe disease (globoid cell leukodystrophy) with galactocerebrosidase deficiency, GM$_2$ gangliosidosis with hexosaminidase A deficiency, and GM$_1$ gangliosidosis with β-galactosidase deficiency.

Adult polyglucosan body disease and Lafora disease are disorders of carbohydrate metabolism associated with dementia. Neuronal intranuclear hyaline inclusion disease, an autosomal-dominant adult-onset leukodystrophy of unknown origin, Alexander disease, and Mast syndrome are rare causes of dementia.

SUGGESTED READINGS

American Psychiatric Association. *Diagnostic and Statistical Manual of Mental Disorders.* 4th Ed. Washington, DC: American Psychiatric Association, 1994:143–147.

Braak H, Braak E. Staging of Alzheimer's disease related neurofibrillary changes. *Neurobio Aging* 1995;16:271–284.

Breteler MM. Vascular risk factors for Alzheimer's disease: an epidemiologic perspective. *Neurobiol Aging* 2000;21:153–160.

Collins SJ, Lawson VA, Masters CL. Transmissible spongiform encephalopathies. *Lancet* 2004;363:51–61.

Cummings JL. Alzheimer's disease. *N Engl J Med* 2004;351:56–67.

Dickson DW. Neuropathology of Alzheimer's disease and other dementias. *Clin Geriatr Med* 2001;17:209–228.

Diesing TS, Swindells S, Gelbard H, et al. HIV-1-associated dementia: a basic science and clinical perspective. *AIDS Read* 2002;12:358–368.

Hebert LE, Beckett LA, Scherr PA, et al. Annual incidence of Alzheimer disease in the United States projected to the years 2000 through 2050. *Alzheimer Dis Assoc Disord* 2001;15:169–173.

in t' Veld BA, Ruitenberg A, Hofman A, et al. Nonsteroidal antiinflammatory drugs and the risk of Alzheimer's disease. *N Engl J Med* 2001;345:1515–1521.

Jellinger KA. The pathology of Parkinson's disease. *Adv Neurol* 2001;86:55–72.

Kamboh MI. Molecular genetics of late-onset Alzheimer's disease. *Ann Hum Genet* 2004;68:381–404.

Kivipelto M, Helkala EL, Hanninen T, et al. Midlife vascular risk factors and late-life mild cognitive impairment: a population-based study. *Neurology* 2001;56:1683–1689.

Knopman DS, DeKosky ST, Cummings JL, et al. Practice parameter: diagnosis of dementia (an evidence-based review). Report of the Quality Standards Subcommittee of the American Academy of Neurology. *Neurology* 2001;56:1143–1153.

Kotzbauer PT, Trojanowsk JQ, Lee VM. Lewy body pathology in Alzheimer's disease. *J Mol Neurosci* 2001;17:225–232.

Levy G, Schupf N, Tang MX, et al. Combined effect of age and severity on the risk of dementia in Parkinson's disease. *Ann Neurol* 2002;51:722–729.

Levy G, Tang MX, Cote LJ, et al. Motor impairment in PD: relationship to incident dementia and age. *Neurology* 2000;55:539–544.

Li S-H, Li X-J. Huntingtin-protein interactions and the pathogenesis of Huntington's disease. *Trends in Genetics* 2004;20:146–154.

Lim KL, Dawson VL, Dawson TM. The genetics of Parkinson's disease. *Curr Neurol Neurosci Rep* 2002;2:439–446.

Lindsay J, Laurin D, Verreault R, et al. Risk factors for Alzheimer's disease: a prospective analysis from the Canadian study of health and aging. *Am J Epidemiol* 2002;156:445–453.

Mayeux R. Apolipoprotein-E and the epidemiology of Alzheimer's disease. In: Khoury MJ, Little J, Burke W. *Human Genome Epidemiology: Scientific Basis for Using Genetic Information to Improve Health and Prevent Disease.* Oxford, UK: Oxford University Press, 2003:365–382.

McKeith KG, Mosimann UP. Dementia with Lewy bodies and Parkinson's disease. *Parkinsonism and Related Disorders* 2004;10:S15–S18.

McKhann G, Drachman D, Folstein M, et al. Clinical diagnosis of Alzheimer's disease: report of the NINCDS-ADRDA Work Group. *Neurology* 1984;34:939–944.

Recchia A, Debetto P, Negro A, et al. Alpha-synuclien and Parkinson's disease. *FASEB* 2004;18:617–626.

Rogaeva EA, Fafel KC, Song YQ, et al. Screening for PS1 mutations in a referral-based series of AD cases: 21 novel mutations. *Neurology* 2001;57:621–625.

Roman GC, Tatemichi TK, Erkinjuntti T, et al. Vascular dementia: diagnostic criteria for research studies. Report of the NINDS-AIREN international workshop. *Neurology* 1993;43:250–260.

Sampson EL, Warren JD, Rossor MN. Young onset dementia. *Postgrad Med J* 2004;80:125–139.

Taylor JP, Hardy J, Fischbeck KH. Toxic proteins in neurodegenerative disease. *Science* 2002;296:1991–1995.

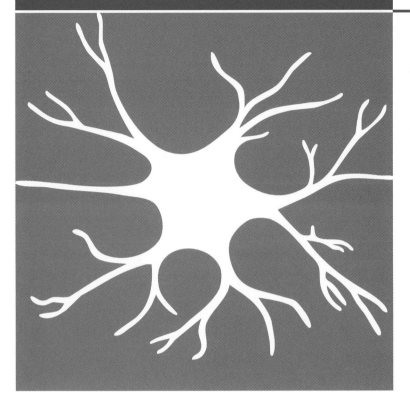

Ataxias

Chapter 108

Hereditary Ataxias

Susan B. Bressman,
Rachel J. Saunders-Pullman,
and Roger N. Rosenberg

CLASSIFICATION

The hereditary ataxias comprise heterogeneous disorders that share three features: ataxia, pathology involving the cerebellum or its connections, and heritability. The pathology usually affects more than the cerebellum, including also the posterior columns, pyramidal tracts, pontine nuclei, and basal ganglia, with corresponding neurologic signs. Within a family, clinical and pathologic features may differ and the heterogeneity creates problems for classification.

In this chapter we concentrate on genetic causes of ataxia, excluding inborn errors of metabolism that are discussed in Sections IX and X. We classify by mode of inheritance, focusing first on the autosomal-recessive ataxias and then the autosomal-dominant ataxias (Table 108.1). However, the mode of inheritance is not always clear. Although cases with parent–child transmission are either dominant or (if maternally inherited) owing to mitochondrial mutations, those with only an affected sibling may be recessive, dominant, or mitochondrial. Also, not all individuals with hereditary ataxia have a family history of ataxia, and hereditary ataxias should be considered in apparently sporadic cases. Because of variable penetrance, anticipation, new mutations, and nonpaternity, apparently sporadic cases may actually be autosomal dominant or recessive.

Recessive ataxias are often of early onset, and dominant ataxias are of later onset. However, as many of one-third of individuals with Friedreich ataxia (FRDA), the most common recessive ataxia, may have late-onset disease, and many people with autosomal dominant spinocerebellar

ataxia (ADCA) have early-onset disease. Dominant ataxias are more often associated with DNA trinucleotide repeats, but FRDA is also a trinucleotide repeat disorder. Nongenetic causes of ataxia including neoplasm, paraneoplastic disorder, multiple sclerosis, vitamin E deficiency, hypothyroidism, alcohol abuse, and vascular disease are also in the differential diagnosis.

EPIDEMIOLOGY

The frequency and most common causes of hereditary ataxias vary with the ethnicity and geographic origin of the population studied. For example, FRDA, with a prevalence of 1 to 2 per 50,000 in the United States and Europe, is the most common form of hereditary ataxia in these populations, and constitutes approximately half of all hereditary ataxia. In contrast, early-onset cerebellar ataxia with hypoalbuminemia is the most common recessive ataxia in Japan.

Among the autosomal dominant ataxias, the most common in the United States is SCA3, followed by SCA-2 and SCA6, then SCA7 and SCA1 and SCA8. SCA3 is more common in Japan and Germany than the United Kingdom. Dentatorubralpallidoluysian atrophy (DRPLA) accounts for 20% of autosomal-dominant SCA in Japan, but is rare in the United States. SCA12, rare elsewhere, is common in Eastern India.

AUTOSOMAL-RECESSIVE ATAXIAS

Friedreich Ataxia (MIM 229300)

Friedreich ataxia (FRDA), described in 1863, is an autosomal-recessive disorder and the most common early-onset ataxia. The typical clinical features are juvenile onset (between puberty and age 25) with progressive ataxia of gait and limbs, absent or hypoactive tendon reflexes in the legs, and extensor plantar responses. Other common features are dysarthria, corticospinal tract clumsiness, proprioceptive and vibratory sensory loss in the legs, and scoliosis. Approximately 25% have hypertrophic cardiomyopathy, and 10% have diabetes mellitus. With the identification of the FRDA gene (see below), it has become

▶ **TABLE 108.1 Hereditary Ataxias by Mode of Inheritance**

Autosomal-recessive ataxias (onset usually before age 20, although some have late-onset forms)	**X linked**
Friedreich ataxia (FRDA)	Fragile X-tremor ataxia
Ataxia telangectasia (AT)	X-linked sideroblastic anemia with ataxia
Ataxia with vitamin E deficiency (AVED)	Uncomplicated ataxia
Abetalipoproteinemia and hypobetalipoproteinemia	Ataxia with spasticity
Ataxia with oculomotor apraxia 1 (AOA1)	With mental retardation
Ataxia with oculomotor apraxia 2 (AOA2)	With deafness
Autosomal recessive spastic ataxia of Charlevoix-Saguenay (ARSACS)	**Autosomal-Dominant Ataxias**
Infantile onset cerebellar ataxia (IOSCA)	SCA1
Ataxia-telangiectasia variant (ATV1)/Nijmegen breakage syndrome	SCA2
Spinocerebellar ataxia with neuropathy	SCA3/Machado-Joseph Disease
Other recessive ataxias	SCA4
With hypogonadism	SCA5
With myoclonus	SCA6
With optic atrophy and mental retardation	SCA7
With deafness	SCA8
With cataracts and mental retardation (Marinesco-Sjögren)	SCA10
Childhood ataxia with CNS hypomyelination/vanishing white matter (CACH)	SCA11
	SCA12
Carboxylase deficiencies	SCA13
Urea cycle defects	SCA14
Aminoacidurias	SCA15
Biotinidase deficiency	SCA16
Wilson disease	SCA17
Hypoceruloplasminemia with ataxia and dysarthria (onset in 40s)	SCA18
Sialidosis	SCA20
Refsum	SCA21
Ceroid lipofuscinosis	SCA25
Leukodystrophies	DRPLA
Cerebrotendinous xanthomatosis	EA1
Hexosaminidase deficiency	EA2
Xeroderma pigmentosum	**Mitochondrial Inheritance**
Cockayne syndrome	Co-Q10 deficiency
Leigh (also mitochondrial inheritance)	Mitochondrial encephalomyopathies (MERRF, NARP, KSS)
	Leigh Syndrome

clear that manifestations may be atypical in 25% of the cases with later age at onset, preserved tendon reflexes, or slower course.

FRDA is not only the most common inherited ataxia in the United States, but it is also the most common autosomal-recessive ataxia. The prevalence of FRDA in North America and Europe is about 1 to 2 per 50,000, with a carrier frequency of about 1:60 to 1:120. Boys and girls are equally affected. Because the disorder is autosomal recessive, parents are asymptomatic, and consanguinity is found in 5.6% to 28% of families. The risk for siblings to be affected is 25% and, in small families, only one person may be affected.

Genetics

The gene for FRDA (X25) maps to 9q and encodes a highly conserved protein, frataxin. Ninety-six percent of FRDA patients are homozygous for an expansion of a GAA triplet repeat in the first intron of X25. About 4% are compound heterozygotes, with a GAA intronic expansion in one allele and an inactivating mutation in the other allele. Some, but not all, compound heterozygotes have milder disease.

Normal chromosomes have fewer than 34 triplets, and disease chromosomes have 66 to more than 1,700 repeats. Repeats in normal chromosomes are stable when transmitted from parent to child, but expanded GAA repeats show meiotic instability, usually contracting after paternal transmission and either expanding or contracting with maternal transmission. Repeats of 34 to 60 are termed *premutation alleles* because they do not cause symptoms but may expand during parental transmission to produce causal mutations. Mitotic instability of the expansion varies in different tissues, including different brain regions.

FRDA is a result of a deficiency of frataxin. The expansion interferes with frataxin transcription and is associated in great reduction of normally spliced FRDA mRNA. Larger repeats more profoundly inhibit frataxin transcription and cause earlier onset and more severe symptoms.

Neuropathology

The pathology in FRDA is attributed to the lack of functional frataxin. Tissues with high levels of frataxin expression, such as heart, liver, skeletal muscle, pancreas, and spinal cord, are affected. Frataxin localizes to the inner mitochondrial membrane, hence the absence of normal frataxin causes defects of mitochondrial oxidative phosphorylation with accumulation of free radicals. Iron deposits have been demonstrated in the hearts of FRDA patients, but this is considered secondary to defective responses to oxidative stress, including damage to iron-sulfur cluster respiratory enzymes.

In FRDA patients, the spinal cord may be thinner than normal. Degeneration and sclerosis are seen in the posterior columns, spinocerebellar tracts, and corticospinal tracts. Nerve cells are lost in the dorsal root ganglia and Clarke column. Peripheral nerves are involved, with fewer large myelinated axons. The brainstem, cerebellum, and cerebrum are normal except for mild degenerative changes of the pontine and medullary nuclei, optic tracts, and Purkinje cells in the cerebellum. Cardiac muscle, nerves, and ganglia are also involved.

Clinical Expression and Genotype–Phenotype Correlations

Clinical features vary by age at onset, and can be divided into early-onset FRDA, late-onset FRDA (LOFA), and very late-onset FRDA (VLOFA). Symptoms usually begin between ages 8 and 15 years, but may start in infancy or after age 50. Like other triplicate repeat disorders, there is a correlation between the GAA repeat size and clinical features, particularly age at onset and rate of progression. However, the age at onset correlates with the shorter of the two alleles because FRDA, unlike other triplicate repeat disorders, is recessive (with expanded repeats in both alleles) and a result of loss of frataxin function. The GAA size, however, does not entirely account for the variability in age at onset or clinical progression; somatic mosaicism and other genetic or environmental modifiers must play a role.

In typical early-onset FRDA, gait ataxia is the most common symptom and is usually the first. Although the gait disorder may be seen in children who have been walking normally, more commonly, children are slow to walk, the gait is clumsy and awkward, and they are less agile than other children. Within a few years, ataxia appears in the arms and trunk, a combination of cerebellar asynergia and loss of proprioceptive sense. Movements are jerky, awkward, and poorly controlled. Intention tremor, most common in the arms, may affect the trunk. Frequent repositioning or

pseudoathetosis and true generalized chorea may occur. Speech becomes explosive or slurred and finally unintelligible. Limb weakness is common, sometimes leading to paraplegia.

Vibratory loss is an early sign. Frequently, position sense is impaired in the legs and later in the arms. Loss of two-point discrimination, partial astereognosis, and impaired appreciation of pain, temperature, or tactile sensation are occasionally seen. Loss of leg reflexes and the presence of Babinski signs were once considered necessary for diagnosis; and almost all patients with typical recessive or sporadic early-onset ataxia with these features have the X25 hyperexpansion.

Ocular movements are usually abnormal; fixation instability and square wave jerks are the most common abnormalities. Also frequent are jerky pursuit, ocular dysmetria, and failure of fixation suppression of the vestibular ocular reflexes. Nystagmus and optic atrophy are each seen in about 25% of patients, but severely reduced visual acuity is rare. Sensorineural hearing loss occurs in about 10%. Sphincter impairment occasionally occurs when patients are bedridden; dementia and psychosis are unusual, and the condition is not incompatible with a high degree of intellectual development.

Skeletal abnormalities are common. Scoliosis or kyphosis, usually in the upper thoracic region, affects more than 75%. Pes cavus and equinovarus deformities occur in more than 50%. Heart disease is found in more than 85%, with cardiomyopathy in two-thirds of patients. The electrocardiogram most commonly shows ST segment changes and T-wave inversions. Congestive heart failure occurs late and may be precipitated by atrial fibrillation. Diabetes mellitus is found in 10% to 20%.

The course is progressive; most patients cease walking by 15 years after onset of symptoms. The mean age at death is in the mid-30s and results from infection or cardiac disease.

Late-Onset FRDA and Very late-Onset FRDA

With the advent of FRDA testing in large populations, it has become evident that the spectrum of FRDA includes late-onset (after age 25 years), retained tendon reflexes, slowly progressive disease, spastic paraparesis without ataxia, and FRDA without cardiomyopathy. In one study of ataxic subjects who were clinically thought not to have FRDA, 10% of those with recessive disease and 5% with sporadic disease had homozygous GAA hyperexpansions. To some extent this variability, especially between families, is explained by the length of the GAA expansion. However, GAA expansion does not account for all the variation, particularly with repeat sizes above 500. For example, Acadian FRDA patients descend from a single founder and have the typical homozygous hyperexpansion with repeat lengths similar to those of other FRDA patients but they have milder symptoms and cardiopathy is rare.

Diagnostic and Laboratory Testing

Clinical testing is currently available to screen for the GAA expansions, which in the homozygous form, account for 96% of cases. In cases with only a single expanded allele, further screening may identify deleterious mutations (nonsense or frameshift mutations that result in premature termination of translation or missense mutations in the highly conserved carboxy terminus) on the other allele.

Laboratory findings include characteristic electrocardiogram changes and ECG evidence of concentric ventricular hypertrophy or, less commonly, asymmetric septal hypertrophy. Normal peripheral nerve conduction studies with absent or markedly reduced sensory nerve action potentials distinguish FRDA from Charcot-Marie-Tooth disease. Other common abnormalities are reduced amplitude of visual evoked responses and small or absent somatosensory evoked potentials recorded over the clavicle and delayed dispersed potentials at the sensory cortex. CT and MRI of the brain are usually normal, but may show mild cerebellar atrophy. Cervical spinal cord atrophy can often be detected on MRI. The CSF is normal. Vitamin E levels should be assessed, as vitamin E deficiency is an important and treatable differential diagnosis and may mimic FRDA.

Treatment

Based on frataxin effects on mitochondrial respiration and production of oxygen free radicals, antioxidant therapies including coenzyme Q10 (CoQ10), vitamin E, and idebenone, a short-chain CoQ10 analog, are being evaluated. Although no medical treatment has yet been truly effective, trials with idebenone show promising results in ameliorating cardiac hypertrophy. In another study, idebenone reduced levels of 8-hydroxy-2′-deoxyguanosine, a marker of oxidative DNA damage. Treatment with CoQ10 and vitamin E improved ATP production in skeletal and cardiac muscle. Supportive treatment includes physical therapy and walking aids, speech therapy, psychological support treatment of associated cardiac disease (cardiac arrhythmia is a major cause of death) and diabetes. Genetic counseling should be offered.

Autosomal-Recessive Ataxias with Prominent Oculomotor Apraxia

Three syndromes with oculomotor ataxia have been described: ataxia telangiectasia (AT), ataxia with oculomotor apraxia (AOA) 1, and AOA2. Although they are also childhood-onset disorders with prominent ataxia, they differ from FRDA in several ways: (1) the presence of prominent oculomotor apraxia in all three conditions, but not in FRDA; (2) prominent movement disorders—particularly

dystonia and chorea in these syndromes; (3) upper motor neuron features in FRDA but not in the other three, except rarely in AOA2; and (4) normal α-fetoprotein (AFP), immunoglobulin, chorioembryonic antigen (CEA), and albumin in FRDA.

Ataxia Telangiectasia

AT (MIM208900) is an early onset autosomal-recessive ataxia caused by defective DNA repair. It is characterized by progressive cerebellar ataxia starting at ages 1 to 4 years, oculomotor apraxia, and slurred speech. Later onset is uncommon. Clinical symptoms and signs vary, but typically there is truncal ataxia in infancy, and this becomes more obvious when the child learns to walk. Later the ataxia becomes more appendicular as well. Prominent oculomotor abnormalities include difficulty generating saccades, dependence on head thrusts to fixate, ocular dysmetria, and nystagmus, as well as slurred speech. Facial hypomimia, chorea, dystonia, drooling, dysarthria, dystonia, myoclonus, and peripheral neuropathy may appear in later childhood or in adolescence. Cutaneous telangiectasias are characteristic but are not always present and generally do not appear in the first years of life. Telangectasias involve the conjunctivae, face, ears, and flexor creases (Fig. 108.1). Growth retardation and delayed sexual development may occur and occasionally there is mild mental retardation. Immune dysfunction is typical and includes recurrent respiratory and cutaneous infections, lymphopenia, and decreased concentrations of IgA and IgG. There may be progeria and premature graying. About 38% of patients develop malignancies, most frequently leukemia or lymphoma. The rate of cancer in heterozygote carriers is also increased.

The disease is progressive; with supportive care most now live beyond 20, and some live to the fifth or sixth decade. In 10% of cases, patients may have a milder phenotype with later onset and slower course, or they may not have all the features of AT. This syndrome is attributed to mutations that permit residual ATM kinase activity. Therefore, AT could account for progressive ataxia of adult onset.

Pathologically, loss of Purkinje cells is seen in the cerebellum with less prominent changes in the granule cell layer, dentate and inferior olivary nuclei, ventral horns, and spinal ganglia. Laboratory abnormalities include an elevation in α-fetoprotein (observed in >90% of patients), decreased serum concentrations of IgA and IgG, cytogenetic abnormalities with a 7;14 chromosome translocation, abnormal sensitivity to ionizing radiation (colony survival assay), and decreased serine-protein kinase ATM AT (mutated) on Western blot.

The gene maps to chromosome 11 and is named ATM (Table 108.1). Typical AT is usually caused by null ATM alleles that truncate or severely destabilize the ATM

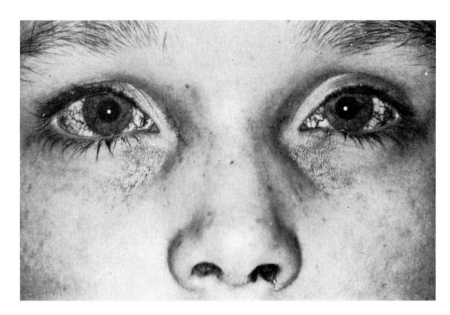

FIGURE 108.1. Ataxia telangiectasia. Telangiectases in the bulbar conjunctiva. (Courtesy of Dr. G. Gaull.)

protein. The ATM protein belongs to a family of protein kinases. ATM is a key regulator of multiple signaling cascades that respond to DNA strand breaks induced by damaging agents or by normal processes, such as meiotic recombination. The altered responses involve failure to activate cell checkpoints and repair DNA. One percent of the population is heterozygous for ATM. Population screening for the mutation is difficult because the gene is large and there are many different mutations; however, among different ethnic groups, a small number of alleles account for most causal mutations, facilitating molecular genetic testing.

Although no treatment is curative, supportive treatment including caution about doses of ionizing radiation used, physical therapy, monitoring for malignancy and treatment of infection, and genetic counseling is beneficial. Antioxidant treatment with vitamin E is often given empirically.

Ataxia with oculomotor apraxia (AOA) resembles AT and can be divided into two subtypes, AOA1 and AOA 2. AOA1 is characterized by slowly progressive childhood-onset ataxia, oculomotor apraxia, and areflexia, followed by motor neuropathy and sometimes quadriplegia. The mean age at onset is 4.7 years. Chorea is common and may regress. This form is most common in Japan (more frequent than FRDA) and Portugal. Mental function is initially normal, but there may be late cognitive decline.

Hypoalbuminemia and hypercholesterolemia are present in 70% of patients with duration of 10 to 15 years. The causative gene, APTX, encodes aprataxin, which may play a role in DNA repair, similar to the protein in AT, but pathology is limited to the nervous system.

A second form of AOA, AOA2, is associated with elevated AFP, like AT, but the increases are moderate (five-fold) compared to AT (tenfold increase). AOA2 symptoms begin later than AT and primarily affect the nervous system. AOA2 is characterized by ataxia, oculomotor apraxia, and elevated α-fetoprotein levels, with sensorimotor neuropathy in 90% and dystonia or chorea in 40%. Movement disorders, particularly arm dystonia, chorea, and head or arm tremor, are common and, unlike AOA1, they do not improve. Axonal sensory neuropathy with pes cavus is frequent but moderate in severity, leading to less disability than in AOA1. AOA2 is secondary to mutations in the gene encoding senataxin, an ortholog of yeast RNA helicase. In Europe, it may be the second most frequent AR ataxia after FRDA.

Other Autosomal-Recessive Ataxias (Tables 108.1 and 108.2)

Autosomal recessive spastic ataxia of Charlevoix-Saguenay is an early childhood–onset disorder (12 to 18 months) characterized by ataxia, spasticity, dysarthria, distal muscle wasting, distal sensorimotor neuropathy mainly in the legs, and horizontal gaze nystagmus. Yellow streaks of hypermyelination, known as retinal striations, are noted in Quebec-born patients. The gene encodes a novel protein, sacsin, which is similar to heat shock chaperone proteins. Although initially described in Eastern Canada, families in Japan, Italy, and Tunisia have now been reported, and the gene may be responsible for more cases of childhood-onset ataxia than previously recognized.

Ataxia with vitamin E deficiency (AVED, MIM 277460) is an autosomal-recessive disorder that mimics FRDA clinically. However, later onset, prominent titubation in 28%, and dystonia are more common than with FRDA. Deleterious mutations are found in the α-tocopherol transfer protein gene, which maps to chromosome 8q13 and impairs

▶ **TABLE 108.2 Clinical Features in Selected Autosomal-Recessive Ataxias**

Disorder	Chromosome	Gene	Gene Product	Age Onset-Typical (range in years)	Clinical Features (all have ataxia)
Friedreich ataxia (FRDA)	9q13	X25	Frataxin	Childhood-teens (infant–40)	Hyporeflexia, position sense loss, sensory loss, dysarthria, Babinksi signs, cardiomyopathy, scoliosis; may be manifest by late-onset spastic paraparesis without much or any ataxia
Ataxia telangectasia (AT)	11q22.3	ATM	Serine protein kinase ATM	Early childhood (infant–27)	Oculocutaneous telangectasia, immunodeficiency, elevated α-fetoprotein, malignancy
Ataxia with oculomotor apraxia type 1 (AOA1)	9p13.3	APTX	Aprataxin	7 (2–16)	Dysarthria, dysmetria, axonal neuropathy with areflexia, chorea, dystonia, decreased serum albumin and total cholesterol
Ataxia with oculomotor apraxia type 2 (AOA2)	9q34	SEXT	Senataxin	15 (10–25)	Sensory motor neuropathy, oculomotor apraxia, chorea, dystonia, increased α-fetoprotein
Autosomal-recessive spastic ataxia of Charlevoix-Saguenay (ARSACS)	13q12	SACS	Sacsin	Childhood	Retinal striations, spasticity, peripheral neuropathy
Infantile onset spinocerebellar ataxia (IOSCA)	10q24	IOSCA		Infancy	Peripheral neuropathy, chorea, optic atrophy, hearing loss
Marinesco- Sjögren		MSS		Infancy	Cataracts, mental retardation, hypotonia, myopathy
Ataxia with vitamin E deficiency (AVED)	8q13.1–3	TTPA	α-tocopherol transferase protein	Child to teen (2–52)	FRDA-like head titubation

the incorporation of α-tocopherol into very low-density lipoprotein (VLDL), which is needed for the efficient recycling of vitamin E. Abetalipoproteinemia (Bassen-Kornzweig) and cholestatic liver disease are also associated with vitamin E deficiency.

One rare infantile-onset autosomal-recessive disorder (*infantile-onset spinocerebellar ataxia*, or IOSCA) in Finnish families was mapped to chromosome 10q24. Affected children develop ataxia, athetosis, and loss of tendon reflexes before age 2. This is followed by hypotonia, optic atrophy, ophthalmoplegia, deafness, and sensory neuropathy.

Another early-onset recessive ataxia is the *Marinesco-Sjögren syndrome,* characterized by ataxia, bilateral cataracts, mental retardation, and short stature. Other rare autosomal recessive conditions include ataxia with pigmentary retinopathy, ataxia with deafness, and ataxia with hypogonadism.

The *Ramsay Hunt syndrome* is an etiologically heterogeneous syndrome characterized by myoclonus and progressive ataxia. It is most commonly a result of the

mitochondrial syndrome MERRF (mitochondrial encephalomyopathy with ragged red fibers).

The autosomal-recessive disorder Unverricht-Lundborg disease, or progressive myoclonus epilepsy (PME) type 1, which maps to chromosome 2lq (MIM 254800), may also cause Ramsay Hunt syndrome. The PME type 1 gene encodes cystatin B, which acts within cells to block the action of cathepsins, proteases that degrade other cell proteins.

Additional etiologies of autosomal recessive ataxias are listed in Table 108.1.

Diagnostic Evaluation of Early-Onset Recessive Ataxia

The diagnostic workup of a patient with early-onset recessive ataxia depends on the constellation of clinical features in the family. If FRDA genetic testing is negative, other causes of sporadic or recessive ataxia need to be considered (Table 108.3). Evaluation includes blood lipids,

▶ TABLE 108.3 Clinical Features in Selected Autosomal-Dominant Ataxias

Disorder	Chromosome	Gene (and trinucleotide repeat, if any)	Gene Product	Age Onset (years, range)	Distinguishing Clinical Features (ataxia including dysarthria is common for all)
SCA1	6p23	SCA1 (CAG)	Ataxin-1	30s (childhood–>60)	Pyramidal, signs, dysphagia, opthalmoparesis, neuropathy
SCA2	12q24	SCA2 (CAG)	Ataxin-2	20s–30s (infant–67)	Slow saccades, neuropathy, hyporeflexia, dementia
SCA3	14q24.3-q31	MJD (CAG)	Machado-Joseph disease protein 1	30s (6–70)	Opthalmoparesis, pyramidal and extrapyramidal signs, amyotrophy, sensory loss
SCA4	16q22.1	SCA4		30s (19–59)	Sensory neuropathy, pyramidal signs
SCA5	11p11-q11	SCA5		30s (10–68)	Slowly progressive,
SCA6	19p13	CACNA1A (CAG)	Voltage-dependent calcium channel alpha1-A subunit	48 (19–75)	Slowly progressive, sometimes episodic, downbeat nystagmus
SCA7	3p21.1-p12	SCA7 (CAG)	Ataxin-7	30s (infant–60s)	Visual loss with optic atrophy and pigmentary retinopathy, opthalmoparesis, pyramidal signs, extreme anticipation
SCA8	13q21	SCA8 (CTG)		39 (18–65)	Hyperreflexia, decreased vibratory sense, maternal bias for transmission
SCA10	22q13	SCA10 (ATTCT)	Ataxin-10	36	Seizures, polyneuropathy
SCA11	15q14-q21.3	SCA11		30 (15–70)	Slowly progressive, hyperreflexia, vertical nystagmus
SCA12	5q31-q33	PPP2R2B (CAG)	Serine/threonine protein phosphatase	33 (8–55)	Early tremor, bradykinesia, dystonia, dementia, dysautonomia, hyperreflexia
SCA13	19q13.3-q13.4	SCA13		Child	Mental retardation, short stature
SCA14	19q13.4-qter	PRKCG	Protein kinase C gamma	28 (12–42)	Early axial myoclonus
SCA15	3p24.2-3pter	SCA15		Childhood to teens	Dysarthria (pure ataxia)
SCA16	8q22.1-q24.1	SCA16		39 (20–66)	Head tremor, nystagmus, dysarthria
SCA17	6q27	TBP (CAG)	TATA-box binding protein/transcription initiation factor (TFIID)	6–34	Dementia, parkinsonism, dystonia, chorea, seizures, cerebral and cerebellar atrophy on MRI
SCA18	7q22-q32			Teens	Motor/sensory neuropathy
SCA19	1p21-q21				Tremor, myoclonus, cognitive impairment
SCA20	11cen			46 (19–64)	Palatal tremor/myoclonus, dysarthria, hypermetric saccades, pyramidal signs, dentate calcification on CT
SCA21	7p21-15			6–30	Akinesia, rigidity, tremor, cognitive impairment
SCA22	1p21-q23			10–46	Slowly progressive
SCA25	2p15.21			1–39	Sensory neuropathy
DRPLA	12p13.31	DRPLA (CAG)	Atrophin-1 related protein	30s (child–70)	Early-onset myoclonus and epilepsy, late-onset chorea; dementia in both
EA1	12p13	KCNA 1	Voltage-gated potassium channel protein Kv1.1	Child (2–15)	Exercise- or startle-induced ataxia, myokymia (attack duration: seconds–minutes), no vertigo
EA2	19p13	CACNA1A	Voltage-dependent P/Q type calcium channel subunit	Child (3–52)	Stress- or fatigue-induced episodic ataxia (attack duration: minutes–hours), later permanent ataxia, acetazolamide responsive
	2q22-q23	CACNB4	Dihydropyridine-sensitive calcium channel subunit		

vitamin E, α-fetoprotein, hexosaminidase A, very long-chain fatty acids, immunoglobulins, lactate and pyruvate, ceruloplasmin, and thyroid function. Additional studies including screens for amino and organic acids, biotinidase, ammonia level, phytanic acid, EM for curvilinear bodies, and mitochondrial mutation screening may be indicated depending on clinical features. Abetalipoproteinemia and AVED, in particular, can mimic the spinocerebellar findings of FRDA and may respond well to treatment. Finally, clinical molecular genetic testing is available for AVED, AOA, and autosomal recessive spastic ataxia of Charlevoix-Saguenay, as well as the autosomal dominant cerebellar ataxias (ADCA), which can occasionally present as sporadic or recessive disease.

X-Linked Hereditary Ataxias

X-linked inherited ataxias are rare except for the fragile X-tremor ataxia syndrome associated with premutation expansions (55-200 CCG repeats) in the fragile X mental retardation gene (FMR1). This disorder of adult male carriers of premutation alleles includes ataxia and intention tremor. Additionally, there may be short-term memory loss, executive functional deficits, parkinsonism, peripheral neuropathy, proximal leg weakness, and autonomic dysfunction. Penetrance is age related with 75% of carriers older than 80 years expressing signs.

Rare syndromes of pure ataxia and spastic paraparesis with ataxia beginning in childhood, adolescence, or early adult years have an X-linked recessive pattern. An infant-onset X-linked form includes ataxia, deafness, optic atrophy, and hypotonia.

Mitochondrial Disorders with Ataxia

Mitochondrial disorders also account for progressive ataxia, particularly in children. MERRF is characterized by ataxia, myoclonus, seizures, myopathy, and hearing loss. Maternal relatives may be asymptomatic or have partial syndromes, including a characteristic "horse collar" distribution of lipomas. Other mitochondrial disorders are described in Chapter 97.

AUTOSOMAL-DOMINANT ATAXIAS

In 1893, Marie applied the term *hereditary cerebellar ataxia* to syndromes that differed from FRDA in later-onset autosomal-dominant inheritance, hyperactive tendon reflexes, and frequently, ophthalmoplegia. Classification has been the subject of controversy because nosology was based on pathology, leading to eponyms named for Marie, Menzel, and Holmes, but with poor clinical-pathologic correlation, even within a single family. Harding challenged these confusing pathology-based schemes, lumping ADCA and then dividing them into clinical groups. With the mapping and cloning of autosomal-dominant ataxia genes, emphasis has shifted to a genetic classification, leading to a sequential numbering system of autosomal spinocerebellar ataxia (SCA) loci, with 20 SCA loci (SCA 1-8, 10-18, 20, 21, 25) and 10 known genes (SCA 1-3, 6-8, 10, 12, 14, 17). This classification has the advantage of defining a group based on a genetic mode of transmission (Table 108.1). However, the numbering is based on the temporal order when SCA numbers were assigned and does not have clinical or pathologic significance. Some advocate classification by pathogenesis, such as CAG repeat toxicity or channelopathies. But many of the SCA genes are still undetermined. Furthermore, many SCAs have overlapping clinical features.

In this description, we bridge the clinical-genetic gap, emphasize prominent and distinguishing clinical features of each major SCA class, and will describe the ADCAs in order of the Human Genome Organization (HUGO) SCA designation.

Although distinct features can be discerned, most SCAs share clinical features. Symptoms usually begin in early or midadult years, but the age at onset varies from childhood to the eighth decade (Table 108.3). The first and generally most prominent sign is gait ataxia, occasionally starting with sudden falls. Limb ataxia and dysarthria are also early symptoms. Hyperreflexia may be present initially, but tendon reflexes may later be depressed and vibration and proprioception may be lost. Eye signs include nystagmus, slow saccades, and abnormal pursuit. Dementia, dystonia, parkinsonism, tremor, facial fasciculations, neuropathy, and distal wasting may occur, although the frequency of these features differs among the various SCAs. Anticipation and potentiation, earlier onset, and more severe symptoms in succeeding generations are observed in most of the SCAs (most dramatically in SCA7 and DRPLA but not in SCA6), and the majority are severely disabled 10 to 20 years after symptom onset (Table 108.3).

All identified ADCA genes except SCA8, 10, 12 and 14 share the same type of mutation, unstable expansions of a CAG trinucleotide repeat in the protein-coding region of the gene. SCA10 is a result of an untranslated pentanucleotide repeat, SCA12 of an untranslated CAG repeat, and SCA 14 appears to be a result of missense mutations. As in other dominant disorders with trinucleotide expansions (e.g., Huntington disease, dentatorubropallidoluysian atrophy), there is an inverse relation between repeat size and age at onset. Another feature of the trinucleotide expansion in ADCA is meiotic instability. In a parent–child transmission, the size of the repeat may change, either expanding or contracting. In all SCAs, paternal and maternal transmissions differ. In all but SCA8, there is a greater tendency for an increase in repeat size in paternally transmitted disease chromosomes. As a result, anticipation is more pronounced in paternally transmitted disease. In SCA8, most expansions occur during maternal transmission.

The CAG expansions result in an expanded polyglutamine tract, because CAG codes for glutamine. Unlike the FRDA triplet expansion, which causes disease by inducing frataxin deficiency, the dominant SCA triplet expansions cause disease by altering the protein, a toxic gain of function. The disease mechanisms of the polyglutamine proteins are not yet fully clarified, but impaired protein clearance and transcriptional dysregulation are two proposed mechanisms. However, each polyglutamine disorder has distinctive clinical-pathologic features, so some other feature, in addition to the polyglutamine, must play a role.

SCA1 (MIM 164400)

Genetics

The first ADCA locus, SCA1, was mapped to the short arm of chromosome 6 in 1974, based on linkage to the human leukocyte antigen. In 1991, highly polymorphic DNA markers flanking the SCA1 gene were identified, and in 1993, the SCA1 mutation was identified. A trinucleotide expansion was specifically sought because of the known anticipation in SCA1 families and the earlier identification of expanded trinucleotide repeats and anticipation in Huntington disease. Normal alleles have 6 to 44 CAG repeats, and the repeat configuration is interrupted by 1 to 3 CAT repeats when the allele contains 21 or more repeats. Abnormal alleles have 39 or more repeats without the CAT interruption. Intermediate alleles are those with 36 to 38 CAG repeats without the CAT interruption. Intermediate alleles appear to have no associated clinical signs, but on transmission to offspring can expand to the abnormal range. The CAT repeats serve to stabilize the repeat from expanding.

The protein encoded by SCA1 is called *ataxin-1*, a protein of unknown function. It is expressed ubiquitously. Mutated ataxin-1 accumulates in the nucleus into a single aggregate. These aggregates include ubiquitin, chaperones, and proteasomal subunits that are important for protein refolding and degradation. Protein clearance appears then to be important to SCA1 pathogenicity.

Epidemiology

The prevalence of SCA1 is estimated at 1 to 2 per 100,000, varying in different populations. In North America the proportion is estimated at 6%, whereas in Italy and England the number is 30%, and even more in South Africa. In all series, SCA1 rarely if ever accounts for ataxia in singleton or apparently recessive cases.

Clinical and Pathologic Features

Typically, SCA1 starts in the fourth decade, but the range at onset is 6 to 60 years. Gait ataxia predominates and is often the first sign, usually with mild dysarthria, hypermetric saccades, nystagmus, and hyperreflexia. With progression, nystagmus may disappear and saccadic abnormalities and opthalmoparesis (particularly upgaze) develop. Worsening limb, gait, and speech ataxia evolve. Hypotonia with decreased tendon reflexes and sensory loss are common later. Late in the disease, bulbar manifestations include lingual atrophy, fasciculations, and severe dysphagia. Optic atrophy, dementia, personality change, dystonia, and chorea are less common.

The pathology includes neuronal loss in the cerebellum, brainstem, spinocerebellar tracts, and dorsal columns with rare involvement of the substantia nigra and basal ganglia. Purkinje cell loss and severe neuronal degeneration in the inferior olive are seen; degeneration is also seen in the cranial nerve nuclei, restiform body, brachium conjunctivum, dorsal and ventral spinocerebellar tracts, posterior columns, and rarely the anterior horn cells. MRI shows atrophy of the brachia pontis and anterior lobe of the cerebellum and enlargement of the fourth ventricle.

SCA2 (MIM 183090)

This autosomal dominant locus was mapped to chromosome 12q23-24 in 1993, in a study of ataxic patients originating from the Holguin province of Cuba and descended from an Iberian founder. Subsequently, SCA2 families were found in Italy, Germany, French Canada, Tunisia, and Japan. In 1996, three independent groups identified the SCA2 gene.

Normal individuals have <30 CAG repeats (with most containing 22), interrupted by one to three CAAs within the CAG repeat. SCA2 patients have CAG expansions of 36 or more and no CAAs within the repeat. Reduced penetrance is about 33%. These individuals may or may not develop clinical signs. There is an inverse correlation between age at onset and CAG number. When the CAG expansion is large, manifestations are likely to include dementia, chorea, myoclonus, and dystonia. The function of *ataxin-2*, the protein encoded by SCA2, is not known, but in normal and SCA2 brains it is localized in the cytoplasm of neurons, especially Purkinje cells. In transgenic mouse models, *ataxin-2* accumulates in the cytoplasm and intranuclear aggregates are not observed. In cellular models, expression of full-length *ataxin-2* with the expanded repeat disrupts normal morphology of the Golgi apparatus and colocalization with Golgi markers is lost.

Epidemiology

SCA2 is a relatively frequent cause of ADCA worldwide, varying from 14% to 18% in German and U.S. families to 37% to 47% in Italian and English families and more than 30% of families from Eastern India. Rarely, it is a cause in families with apparent recessive inheritance (i.e., siblings but not parents affected) or in sporadic cases.

Clinical and Pathologic Features

The disease usually begins in the fourth decade, but onset ranges from infancy to the seventh decade. The most common clinical features are gait and limb ataxia and dysarthria. Other common features include depressed or absent tendon reflexes, slow saccades, kinetic or postural arm tremor, fasciculations, ophthalmoplegia, and vibratory and position sensory loss. Less common features are cramps, staring gaze, dementia, leg hyperreflexia, chorea, dystonia, and levodopa-responsive parkinsonism. Nystagmus may be present at onset but tends to disappear as slow saccades emerge. Although other SCA subtypes include these features, patients with SCA2 are most likely to have slow saccades and hyporeflexia. Many show electrophysiologic evidence of axonal neuropathy with severe involvement of sensory fibers. The highly variable phenotype occasionally seems to "breed true" in families (e.g., kindreds with dementia and extrapyramidal signs, or with moderate ataxia, facial fasciculations, prominent eye signs that include lid lag, and retinitis).

Pathology, like clinical signs, varies. Usually there is olivopontocerebellar atrophy with severe neuronal loss in the inferior olive, pons, and cerebellum. However, there may also be degeneration of the substantia nigra, dorsal columns, and anterior horn cells. Rarely, degeneration is restricted to the cerebellum.

SCA3/Machado-Joseph Disease (MIM 109150)

Genetics and Clinical–Genetic Correlation

Machado-Joseph disease (MJD) was first described in families of Azorean Portuguese descent. Common signs, regardless of age at onset, include gait and limb ataxia, dysarthria, and progressive ophthalmoplegia. Findings more dependent on age at onset include pyramidal signs, dystonia and rigidity, amyotrophy, facial and lingual fasciculations, and lid retraction with bulging eyes. Four clinical subclasses were proposed:

1. Adolescent or young adult onset: rapidly progressive with spasticity, rigidity, bradykinesia, weakness, dystonia, and ataxia;
2. Midadult onset (ages 30 to 50): moderate progression of ataxia;
3. Late adult onset (ages 40 to 70): slower progression of ataxia, prominent peripheral nerve signs, and few extrapyramidal findings;
4. Adult onset: parkinsonism and peripheral neuropathy.

The pathology was considered distinct with primarily spinopontine atrophy and involvement of pontine nuclei, spinocerebellar tracts, Clarke column, anterior horn cells, substantia nigra, and basal ganglia; the inferior olives and cerebellar cortex were spared. With mutation screening, however, it is now evident that the olives and cerebellar cortex may be involved.

In addition to the Portuguese families, a similar disorder was described in German, Dutch, African American, and Japanese people. In 1993, Takiyama and colleagues mapped a gene in several Japanese families to chromosome 14q24.3-32. This locus then was confirmed in MJD families of Azorean descent. In 1994, linkage to the same region was found in French families that were clinically similar to SCA1 or SCA2, and the locus was numbered SCA3. Because these French families were not of Azorean descent and because of several clinical differences (lack of dystonia and facial fasciculation), it was uncertain whether MJD and SCA3 were owing to different genes, different mutations in the same gene, or the varying phenotypic expressions of the same mutation in individuals with different ancestry. In 1994, an expanded and unstable CAG repeat was found in the coding region of the MJD gene. Subsequently, all 14q-linked families have been found to have the same unstable CAG repeat within the SCA3/MJD gene, so that SCA3 and MJD are a single genetic disorder with a wide clinical spectrum. As with the other ADCA genes, there may be intrafamilial genetic modifiers (including differences within the SCA3/MJD gene) that influence the phenotype.

The normal repeat number is up to 47, and disease alleles range from 53 to 89. Mutable normal (or intermediate) allele size is between 48 and 51 repeats. There is no evidence that a phenotype or reduced penetrance is associated with this intermediate range, but it is associated with meiotic instability and pathologic expansion in subsequent generations. As in other CAG repeat diseases, there is a strong inverse correlation between the length of the repeat and age at onset. Greater instability in paternal meioses seems to be true for SCA3, as in the other ADCA genes. Some, but not all, homozygous SCA3 individuals have early-onset severe disease, suggesting a gene dosage effect.

The SCA3/MJD gene encodes *ataxin-3*, a protein of unknown function that is not related to ataxin-1 or -2. It is ubiquitously expressed in the cytoplasm of cell bodies and processes. In SCA3/MJD brain, there is aberrant nuclear localization and accumulation of ubiquitinated nuclear inclusions.

Epidemiology

SCA3 is a common cause of ADCA in many but not all populations. In the United States, about 21% of families with ataxia have SCA3; in a study of mixed populations,

41% were SCA3, but this dropped to 17% when Portuguese families were excluded. SCA3 seems to be common in Germany (accounting for 50% of ADCA cases), China, and Japan but rare in Italy and uncommon in England.

SCA4 (MIM 600223)

SCA4 maps to chromosome 16q. The phenotype consists of late-onset (19 to 59 years) ataxia, prominent sensory axonal neuropathy, normal eye movements in most, and pyramidal tract signs. The gene is not yet identified. The earliest symptom is unsteadiness of gait. Dysarthria is present in 50%, absent ankle jerks in 100%, decreased sensation in 100%, extensor plantar responses in 20%, and saccadic pursuit eye movements in only 15%. Nerve conduction studies indicate an axonal sensory neuropathy.

SCA5 (MIM 600224)

This locus was mapped to the pericentromeric region of chromosome llq in a kindred descended from the paternal grandparents of President Abraham Lincoln. Symptoms of this relatively benign, slowly progressive, cerebellar syndrome appear at 10 to 68 years, with anticipation (Table 108.3). All four juvenile-onset patients (10 to 18 years) resulted from maternal transmission rather than the paternal pattern seen in the other SCA syndromes. The juvenile-onset patients showed cerebellar and pyramidal tract signs, as well as bulbar dysfunction. The gene is not yet identified.

SCA6 (MIM 183086)

The SCA6 gene maps to chromosome 19p13 and encodes for an alpha IA voltage-dependent calcium channel subunit (CACNA1A). There are three distinct phenotypes associated with different CACNA1A mutations. The SCA6 symbol is reserved for an adult-onset cerebellar syndrome with CAG repeat expansions. SCA6 CAG repeats are 20 to 33, with an average disease-causing length of 22. Normal expansions are 4 to 18, and 19 repeats are considered intermediate (not associated with a phenotype but known to expand to the pathologic range). A severe SCA6 phenotype has also been observed with a CACNA1A missense mutation, G293R.

The two other phenotypes associated with CACNAIA mutations are familial hemiplegic migraine (FHM) and episodic ataxia type 2 (EA2). EA2 is caused by CACNA1A mutations that predict protein truncation, abnormal splicing, or rarely, missense mutations, and about 50% of FHM is associated with CACNA1A missense mutations. Although most families "breed true" as SCA6, FHM, or EA2, phenotypic overlap may occur. Not uncommonly, SCA6 patients have episodes of ataxia, and one family with

CAG expansions had members with episodic ataxia and others with progressive ataxia. One family with EA2 had members with hemiplegia or migraine during episodes of ataxia. The correlation between number of SCA6 repeats and age at onset is quite loose; 22 repeats, the most common expansion, is associated with range of age onset, even within sibships. Unlike the other ADCA repeat disorders, the repeat is stable during transmission and anticipation is generally not observed. Like MJD, the phenotype is more severe in homozygous individuals. New mutations underlie some sporadic cases.

The molecular basis of disease is unknown, and SCA6 may differ from the other repeat ataxias. First, the expansion in SCA6 is small; as few as 20 repeats can cause disease. Second, clinical overlap is seen between episodic ataxia type 2 and SCA6. This suggests that these different mutations share pathogenic mechanisms that are likely to involve impaired calcium channel function.

Clinical and Pathologic Features

The clinical picture of SCA6 is fairly uniform. The average age at onset is somewhat older than other SCAs, about 45 to 50 years (range, 20 to 75). The first symptom is usually unsteady gait. Dysarthria, leg cramps, and diplopia can also be early symptoms. Occasionally, patients describe positional vertigo or nausea. Cerebellar signs include gait and limb ataxia (especially leg), cerebellar dysarthria, saccadic pursuit, and dysmetric saccades. Horizontal and downbeat nystagmus (most prominent on lateral gaze) are common eye signs, but very slow saccades are not observed. Noncerebellar signs occur with less frequency and usually less clinical impact than in other SCA disorders but include hyperreflexia, decreased vibration and position sense, impaired upgaze, and parkinsonism. Onset of ataxia may be episodic or apoplectic and resembles episodic ataxia type 2 with attacks of unsteadiness, vertigo, and dysarthria that last for hours; between attacks there are few if any symptoms or signs. The attacks may occur for years before progressive cerebellar signs emerge.

The course is slowly progressive, but after 10 to 15 years most affected individuals are no longer able to walk without assistance. MRI shows cerebellar atrophy but little brainstem or cortical atrophy. Pathologically, there is cerebellar atrophy with loss of Purkinje and granule cells and limited involvement of the inferior olives.

Epidemiology

In the United States and Germany, SCA6 accounts for 10% to 15% of ADCA families. It is more common in Japan (30%) and is uncommon in France, where only 1% of ADCA families harbor the mutation. Five percent to 6% of sporadic ataxia patients demonstrate SCA6 expansions. Some are new mutations, but it is also likely that some appear sporadic because of the late age at onset and relatively indolent course.

SCA7 (MIM 164500)

This type was first distinguished from other forms of ADCA by the associated retinal degeneration. The locus mapped to chromosome 3p in 1995, and the gene was cloned in 1997. SCA7 is a result of the expansion of a coding sequence CAG repeat. Normal alleles have up to 29 repeats. Abnormal alleles have from 36 to >450 repeats. Mutable normal (intermediate) repeats are between 30 and 35. Alleles in this range are considered to be unstable, producing an increased risk to having a child with an abnormal repeat length, but are not convincingly associated with a phenotype. Dramatic examples of anticipation, especially with paternal transmission, is due to repeat instability, which exceeds any other CAG repeat SCA, and is related to age at onset, rate of progression, and clinical signs. The function of ataxin-7 is unknown.

SCA7 age at onset ranges from infancy to the seventh decade and averages around 30 years. The course varies with age at onset. A severe infantile form occurs with large expansions (>200) that are paternally inherited. These infants have hypotonia, dysphagia, visual loss, cerebellar and cerebral atrophy, and congestive heart failure with cardiac anomalies. This differs from childhood and adult forms, which are marked by early visual loss, moderately progressive limb and gait ataxia, dysarthria, opthalmoparesis, and Babinski signs. In late-onset cases (fourth to sixth decade), ataxia may occur in isolation or it may precede visual symptoms (Table 108.3). Affected individuals all have abnormal yellow–blue color discrimination (which in the mildest forms may be asymptomatic), and clinically there is often optic disc pallor with granular and atrophic changes in the macula.

Pathology

Degeneration affects the cerebellum, basis pontis, inferior olive, and retinal ganglion cells. Neuronal intranuclear inclusions containing the expanded polyglutamine tract are found in many brain regions, most frequently in the inferior olive.

Epidemiology

SCA7 accounts for almost all families with both ADCA and retinal degeneration and about 5% of all ADCA families.

SCA8 (MIM 608768)

SCA8 has a slowly progressive course that begins at a mean of 39 years (range 1 to 65 years). The common initial findings include limb and gait ataxia and dysarthria, and compared to other SCAs, severe scanning dysarthria, truncal titubation, and leg ataxia are more common. Severely affected individuals are not able to walk by the fourth decade. Hyperreflexia, Babinski signs with spasticity, and ophthalmoplegia may also occur.

SCA8 is unique among the ataxia trinucleotide repeat disorders for several reasons: (1) The trinucleotide repeat is a CTG repeat rather than a CAG repeat, (2) the repeat length does not necessarily correlate with severity, (3) abnormal allele length has been reported in other ataxias as well as normal controls, (4) allele expansion occurs with maternal transmission and contraction with paternal transmission, and (5) the gene product is a noncoding RNA. Abnormal CTG expansions (>44 repeats) have been reported in healthy and disease controls. Hence, it has been postulated that the trinucleotide expansion is a polymorphism genetically linked to an unidentified disease-causing gene. However, initial studies with transgenic mice suggest that CTG expansions produce an ataxic phenotype.

SCA10 (MIM 603516)

In 1999, two independent groups mapped this locus to chromosome 22q. The phenotype is marked by pure cerebellar signs and seizures, and most families are of Mexican or Brazilian ancestry suggesting a common, possibly native American, founder population. Age at onset ranges from 12 to 48 years with evidence of anticipation. There is slowly progressive ataxia with eventual difficulty sitting. Scanning dysarthria, dyscoordination of oral muscles, upper limb incoordination, and abnormal tracking eye movements also develop in most patients. Although seizures may be infrequently associated with SCA2 and SCA17, they are a prominent feature in SCA10: between 20% and 100% of patients have recurrent partial complex and generalized motor seizures. Seizures usually start after the gait ataxia, and are well controlled with anticonvulsants. Mild cognitive disorders, mood disorders, mild pyramidal signs, behavioral disturbances, and peripheral neuropathy may occur. Furthermore, non-neurologic features of hepatic failure, anemia, and/or thrombocytopenia were reported in one family. MRI demonstrates progressive pancerebellar atrophy, and interictal EEG shows evidence of cortical dysfunction with or without focal epileptiform discharges in some.

SCA10 is caused by a large ATTCT pentanucleotide repeat expansion in intron 9 of *ataxin-10,* a new type of dynamic repeat expansion. Although the normal repeat range is 10 to 22 alleles, affected individuals have 800 to 4,500 repeats. The expanded repeat alleles are unstable with paternal transmission, and there is an inverse correlation between the repeat number and age at onset. An association between ataxia or seizure phenotype and allele size has not been established.

SCA11 (MIM 604432)

In 1999, two British families were reported with benign slowly progressive gait and limb ataxia, mapping to chromosome 15q14-21. It is a pure cerebellar syndrome except for mild pyramidal signs. The average age of onset is approximately 25 years, with a normal life expectancy.

SCA12 (MIM 604326)

SCA12 has been described in American European and Indian Asian families. It starts between ages 8 and 55, usually in the midthirties. It differs clinically from other ADCAs with its frequent action tremor. The slowly progressive ataxia may not be disabling. Other features include hyperreflexia, subtle parkinsonism, focal dystonia, dysautonomia, dementia, and psychiatric features. MRI shows cerebral as well as cerebellar atrophy. The CAG repeat expansion is not translated and does not involve polyglutamine toxicity. Normal repeat length is 7 to 28 repeats, whereas it is greater than 65 repeats in affected individuals.

SCA13 (MIM 605250)

A single family with childhood onset ataxia, dysarthria, moderate mental retardation and delayed motor development with linkage to chromosome 19q was reported. Nystagmus and pyramidal features were also noted. Most individuals had mild progression.

SCA14 (MIM 605361)

Initially described in a single Japanese family, individuals with early- (<27 years) and late-onset ataxia were described; those with early onset also have intermittent axial myoclonus, whereas those with late onset had pure ataxia. The gene was mapped to 19q13, and later a U.S. family with overlapping linkage, but without any members demonstrating axial myoclonus, was reported. Mutations affect the protein kinase C gamma gene in American and Japanese families.

SCA15 (MIM 606658)

SCA15 was initially characterized by pure cerebellar ataxia and slow progression in a large Australian kindred and was mapped to 3p26. No trinucleotide repeat expansion was identified. MRI predominantly demonstrated atrophy of the superior vermis. Two Japanese families with postural and action tremor and slow progression of ataxia also linked to 3p26.

SCA16 (MIM 606364)

SCA16 was reported in a single Japanese family with pure cerebellar ataxia. One-third had head tremor and some family members also had dysarthria, horizontal gaze–evoked nystagmus, and impaired pursuit. The range of age of onset is 20 to 66 years, with an average of 40 years. Linkage to chromosome 8q22-24 was reported.

SCA17 (MIM 607136)

Initially described in a Japanese patient with childhood onset ataxia and no family history, SCA17 has now been reported in Japanese and European kindreds. Age at onset ranges from 19 to 48 years, starting with gait ataxia and dementia; psychiatric features sometimes precede the motor disorder. Limb ataxia, hyperreflexia, chorea, dystonia, myoclonus, parkinsonism (including tremor, bradykinesia, postural instability, and rigidity), as well as epilepsy have also been reported. MRI is notable for both cerebral and cerebellar atrophy. SCA17 is secondary to a CAG repeat expansion in the TATA binding protein (TBG) gene, a transcription-initiating factor, (TFIID). Normal repeat length is 29 to 42, and patients have 44 to 63 CAG repeats. Neuropathology demonstrates Purkinje cell loss and intranuclear inclusions with polyglutamine expansions.

SCA18

SCA18 is a syndrome of ataxia and hereditary sensorimotor neuropathy reported in an American family of Irish ancestry. Onset is usually in adolescence, and all developed gait ataxia, dysmetria, and nystagmus. This condition exemplifies the overlap between hereditary sensory neuropathies and the SCAs, because sensory loss, pyramidal tract signs, and muscle weakness were also seen. In some patients, nerve conduction studies showed sensory axonal neuropathy, and muscle biopsy revealed neurogenic atrophy. MRI demonstrated mild cerebellar atrophy. Linkage to 7q22-32 was demonstrated.

SCA19 (MIM 607346) and SCA22

This locus was mapped in a Dutch family with mild ataxia, nystagmus, cognitive impairment, myoclonus, sensory neuropathy, and irregular postural tremor. Age of onset ranged from 20 to 45 years. MRI showed marked cerebellar hemispheric atrophy with mild vermian and cerebral atrophy. The syndrome linked to chromosome 1p21-q21. Subsequently, linkage to the same region was described in a Chinese family. Variable dysarthria and hyporeflexia were noted and MRI demonstrated homogeneous cerebellar atrophy. Because their linked regions overlap, these two families may have a single disorder and the Chinese family may be a second SCA 19 family.

SCA20 (MIM 608687)

This syndrome was identified in an Australian family of Anglo Celtic descent. Age at onset is 9 to 64 with a mean of 47 years. Slowly progressive dysarthria or gait ataxia were typical. Most patients have a 2-Hz palatal tremor with some spread to lips and pharynx as well as dysphonia. Mild pyramidal features and hypermetric saccades are seen. MRI demonstrates dentate nucleus calcification. Two of nine individuals with imaging also had pallidal calcification and two had olivary calcification. Hence pathology in the Mollaret triangle may account for the palatal tremor. No calcium metabolic etiology has been identified, and the syndrome differs from familial idiopathic brain calcification. It links to chromosome 11, and the gene has not been identified.

SCA21 (MIM 607454)

SCA21 is mapped to 7p15-21 and has been described in one French family. Age of onset ranged from 6 to 30 years with an average of 17 years. It is characterized by slowly progressive gait and limb ataxia and hyporeflexia, as well as parkinsonian features of akinesia, rigidity, tremor, or mild cognitive impairment.

SCA25 MIM 608703

Localized to chromosome 2p, SCA 25 was reported in a French family with ataxia and sensory neuropathy. Age at onset was 17 months to 39 years. Most patients had prominent ataxia, but some had a purely sensory neuropathy with minimal cerebellar involvement. The condition may mimic FRDA. Linkage to chromosome 2p was identified.

DRPLA (MIM 125370)

DRPLA is most common in Japan where it constitutes 10% to 20% of ADCA families. Rare cases have been described in other groups. The pathology involves the dentate, red nucleus, subthalamic nucleus, and the external globus pallidus; the posterior columns may be involved. The phenotype includes ataxia and dementia but varies in other features depending on age at onset. Early-onset cases (before age 20) tend to show severe and rapid progression of myoclonus, epilepsy, and cognitive decline, whereas later-onset cases display ataxia, chorea, dementia, and psychiatric problems (resembling Huntington disease; Table 108.3). Anticipation is evident, and paternal transmission is associated with more severe early-onset disease. One clinical variant, the *Haw River syndrome*, was described in an African American family in North Carolina. This variant includes all the above symptoms except for myoclonic seizures, and additional features include basal ganglia calcification, neuroaxonal dystrophy, and

demyelination of the central white matter. MRI may show atrophy of the cerebral cortex, cerebellum, and pontomesencephalic tegmentum, with high signal in white matter of the cerebrum and brainstem.

The disorder is a result of an expansion of a CAG repeat in the DRPLA gene, which maps to chromosome 12p. There is an inverse relationship between repeat size and age at onset; normal subjects have up to 35 repeats and disease alleles have 48 or more (Table 108.3). The gene is expressed in all tissues, including brain. The DRPLA gene product, *atrophin-1*, is found in neuronal cytoplasm. Ubiquinated intranuclear inclusions are seen in neurons and to a lesser extent in glia. The neuronal inclusions are concentrated in the striatum, pontine nuclei, inferior olive, cerebellar cortex, and dentate.

Other Unmapped Autosomal-Dominant Cerebellar Ataxias

The mapped and cloned SCA genes account for 60% to 90% of ADCAs. Other loci for ADCA remain to be identified.

Genetic Testing for Autosomal-Dominant Disorders

Genetic testing for a SCA is usually considered if the family history is consistent with dominant inheritance. Rarely sporadic cases, especially SCA6 and SCA2, may be due to a SCA. Before embarking on SCA screening in a sporadic case, however, imaging and evaluation of acquired causes should be done; if these are unrevealing, FRDA should be screened first as this is a more likely cause than any SCA.

Genetic testing is the patient's decision, and counseling is part of the testing process so that patients and family members can learn the complexities of both positive and negative results. For example, comprehensive commercial ataxia testing does not screen for about 40% of genetic causes of ataxia; a negative result does not exclude genetic causation.

Molecular genetic clinical testing is now available for SCA1, SCA2, SCA3, SCA6, SCA7, SCA8, SCA10, SCA12, SCA17, and DRPLA. Because testing all genes is expensive, clinicians may choose to prioritize tests on the basis of clinical features, such as retinopathy for SCA7, action tremor for SCA12, seizures for early-onset DRPLA or SCA10, and on ethnicity (Table 108.3). However, there are often no distinguishing features to help choose the most likely SCA. Whole-panel testing may then be a reasonable alternative.

EPISODIC OR PAROXYSMAL ATAXIAS

Episodes of ataxia can be the first manifestation of metabolic disorders such as multiple carboxylase deficiencies or aminoacidurias. However, the term episodic or paroxysmal ataxia is generally applied when the major manifestations are self-limited episodes of cerebellar dysfunction with little fixed or progressive neurologic dysfunction. Two major clinical-genetic subtypes are described: episodic ataxia with myokymia (EA1/myokymia) and episodic ataxia with nystagmus (EA2/nystagmus). EA3 and EA4 are reserved loci for single families excluded from known loci.

In EA1/myokymia, the attacks usually last a few minutes; they can occur spontaneously but are also provoked by startle, sudden movement, or change in posture and exercise (especially if the subject is excited, anxious, or fatigued). Usually, these are one or a few attacks each day. Onset is in childhood or adolescence; the disorder is not associated with neurologic deterioration, but myokymia appears around the eyes and in the hands. The Achilles tendon may be shortened and there may be a tremor of the hands. The attacks are often heralded by an aura of weightlessness or weakness; an attack comprises ataxia, dysarthria, shaking tremor, and twitching. In some families, acetazolamide reduces the frequency of attacks; phenytoin and other anticonvulsants may reduce myokymia. This disorder is caused by missense point mutations in the potassium voltage-gated channel gene KCNA1 on chromosome 12p (Table 108.3).

EA2/nystagmus attacks last longer, usually hours or even days. Attacks are provoked by stress, exercise, fatigue, caffeine, fever, alcohol, and phenytoin. They do not generally occur more than once per day. Age at onset varies from infancy to 40 years and typically starts in childhood or adolescence. Unlike EA1/myokymia, the cerebellar syndrome may progress with increasing ataxia and dysarthria. Even when there is no progressive cerebellar syndrome, interictal nystagmus is often seen (Table 108.3). During an attack, associated symptoms include headache, diaphoresis, nausea, vertigo, ataxia, dysarthria, tinnitus, ptosis, and ocular palsy. Acetazolamide is usually effective in reducing attacks. Most families with EA2 are associated with mutations in the gene for brain-specific (CACNA1A). In one family, the dihydropyridine-sensitive L-type calcium channel β-4 subunit was involved.

Different mutations in CACNA1A can also produce SCA6 or hemiplegic migraine, and some families have overlapping phenotypes. Most EA2 mutations are nonsense changes that result in truncated proteins and reduction in P/Q channel activity.

SPORADIC CEREBELLAR ATAXIA OF LATE ONSET

Many patients with ataxia beginning after age 40 have no affected relatives. Some apparent sporadic cases with late-onset ataxia are a result of SCA mutations. Compared with ADCA, sporadic cases begin later (in the sixth decade), have a more rapid course, and are less likely to have ophthalmoplegia, amyotrophy, retinal degeneration, or optic atrophy. However, many of these patients have parkinsonism and upper motor neuron signs. Some also have autonomic dysfunction and are classified as having multisystem atrophy of the olivopontocerebellar type.

CONGENITAL AND ACQUIRED CEREBELLAR ATAXIAS

The cerebellum and spinocerebellar tracts are the primary sites involved in several developmental, metabolic, infectious, neoplastic, and vascular disorders. Most of these syndromes are discussed elsewhere in this book. Two acquired cerebellar syndromes are common causes of subacute and chronic ataxia in adults, paraneoplastic (see Chapter 153) and alcohol-related cerebellar degeneration (see Chapter 163).

MANAGEMENT OF HEREDITARY ATAXIAS

No specific treatments benefit the hereditary ataxias, except that vitamin E replacement can prevent or improve the ataxia of familial isolated vitamin E deficiency. In FRDA, orthopedic procedures are indicated for the relief of foot deformity and antioxidant therapies may slow progression, especially cardiac manifestations. In the SCAs, especially MJD/SCA3, SCA2, and other subtypes with parkinsonism, levodopa may bring symptomatic relief of rigidity, tremor, and bradykinesia; Lioresal or tizanidine may help spasticity. Acetazolamide can control the attacks of the episodic paroxysmal cerebellar ataxias (EA1 and EA2), and phenytoin ameliorates the facial and hand myokymia associated with EA1. Amantadine and buspirone may improve different forms of cerebellar ataxia, but any effect is moderate at best. We can hope for novel specific therapies based on our increasing knowledge of the molecular mechanisms underlying the hereditary ataxias.

SUGGESTED READINGS

Early-Onset Inherited Ataxias

Friedreich Ataxia

Berciano J, Mateo I, De Pablos C, et al. Friedreich ataxia with minimal GAA expansion presenting as adult-onset spastic ataxia. *J Neurol Sci* 2002;194:75–82.

Buyse G, Mertens L, Di Salvo G, et al. Idebenone treatment in Friedreich's ataxia: neurological, cardiac, and biochemical monitoring. *Neurology* 2003;60:1679–1678.

Campuzano V, Montermini L, Molto MD, et al. Friedreich's ataxia: autosomal recessive disease caused by an intronic triplet repeat expansion. *Science* 1996;271:1374–1375.

De Castro M, Garcia-Planells J, Monros E, et al. Genotype and phenotype analysis of Friedreich's ataxia compound heterozygous patients. *Hum Genet* 2000;106:86–92.

Durr A, Cossee M, Agid Y, et al. Clinical and genetic abnormalities in patients with Friedreich's ataxia. *N Engl J Med* 1996;335:1222–1224.

Friedreich N. Uber Ataxic mit besonderer Berucksichtigung der hereditaren Formen. *Virchows Arch Pathol Anat* 1863;26:391–419, 433–459; 27:1–26.

Harding AE. Clinical features and classification of inherited ataxias. *Adv Neurol* 1993;61:1–14.

Harding AE. Friedreich's ataxia: a clinical and genetic study of 90 families with an analysis of early diagnostic criteria and intrafamilial clustering of clinical features. *Brain* 1981;104:589–620.

Hausse AO, Aggoun Y, Bonnet D, et al. Idebenone and reduced cardiac hypertrophy in Friedreich's ataxia. *Heart* 2002;87:346–349.

Jauslin ML, Meier T, Smith RA, et al. Mitochondria-targeted antioxidants protect Friedreich ataxia fibroblasts from endogenous oxidative stress more effectively than untargeted antioxidants. *FASEB J* 2003;17:1972–1974.

Lhatoo SD, Rao DG, Kane NM, et al. Very late onset Friedreich's presenting as spastic tetraparesis without ataxia or neuropathy. *Neurology* 2001;56:1776–1777.

Lodi R, Hart PE, Rajagopalan B, et al. Antioxidant treatment improves in vivo cardiac and skeletal muscle bioenergetics in patients with Friedreich's ataxia. *Ann Neurol* 2001;49:590–596.

Mariotti C, Solari A, Torta D, et al. Idebenone treatment in Friedreich patients: one-year-long randomized placebo-controlled trial. *Neurology* 2003;60:1676–1679.

Montermini L, Richter A, Morgan K, et al. Phenotypic variability in Friedreich ataxia: role of the associated GAA triplet repeat expansion. *Ann Neurol* 1997;41:675–682.

Monticelli A, Giacchetti M, De Biase I, et al. New clues on the origin of the Friedreich ataxia expanded alleles from the analysis of new polymorphisms closely linked to the mutation. *Hum Genet* 2004;114:458–463.

Priller J, Scherzer CR, Faber PW, et al. Frataxin gene of Friedreich's ataxia is targeted to mitochondria. *Ann Neurol* 1997;42:265–269.

Sakamoto N, Larson JE, Iyer RR, et al. GGA*TCC-interrupted triplets in long GAA*TTC repeats inhibit the formation of triplex and sticky DNA structures, alleviate transcription inhibition, and reduce genetic instabilities. *J Biol Chem* 2001;276:27178–27187.

Schols L, Amoiridis G, Przuntek H, et al. Friedreich ataxia: revision of the phenotype according to molecular genetics. *Brain* 1997;120:2131–2140.

Other Early-Onset Ataxias

Apak S, Yuksel M, Ozmen M, et al. Heterogeneity of X-linked recessive (spino) cerebellar ataxia with or without spastic diplegia. *Am J Med Genet* 1989;34:155–158.

Ben Hamida C, Doerflinaer N, Belal S, et al. Localization of Friedreich ataxia phenotype with selective vitamin E deficiency to chromosome 8q by homozygosity mapping. *Nat Genet* 1993;5:195–200.

Barbot C, Coutinho P, Chorao R, et al. Recessive ataxia with ocular apraxia: review of 22 Portuguese patients. *Arch Neurol* 2001;58:201–205.

Bouchard JP, Richter A, Mathieu J, et al. Autosomal recessive spastic ataxia of Charlevoix-Saguenay. *Neuromuscul Disord* 1998;8:474–479.

Cavalier L, Ouahchi K, Kayden HJ, et al. Ataxia with isolated vitamin E deficiency: heterogeneity of mutations and phenotypic variability in a large number of families. *Am J Hum Genet* 1998;62:301–310.

Cellini E, Piacentini S, Nacmias B, et al. A family with spinocerebellar ataxia type 8 expansion and vitamin E deficiency ataxia. *Arch Neurol* 2002;59:1952–1953.

Date H, Onodera O, Tanaka H, et al. Early-onset ataxia with ocular motor apraxia and hypoalbuminemia is caused by mutations in a new HIT superfamily gene. *Nat Genet* 2001;29:184–188.

Engert JC, Berube P, Mercier J, et al. ARSACS, a spastic ataxia common in northeastern Quebec, is caused by mutations in a new gene encoding an 11.5-kb ORF. *Nat Genet* 2000;24:120–125.

Gatti RA, Berkel L, Boder E, et al. Localization of an ataxia-telangiectasia gene to chromosome I lq-22-23. *Nature* 1988;336:577–580.

Gotoda T, Arita M, Arai H, et al. Adult-onset spinocerebellar dysfunction caused by a mutation in the gene for the alpha tocopheral transfer protein. *N Engl J Med* 1995;333:1313–1318.

Lamperti C, Naini A, Hirano M, et al. Cerebellar ataxia and coenzyme Q10 deficiency. *Neurology* 2003;60:1206–1208.

Le Ber I, Moreira MC, Rivaud-Pechoux S, et al. Cerebellar ataxia with oculomotor apraxia type 1: clinical and genetic studies. *Brain* 2003;126:2761–2672.

Moreira MC, Barbot C, Tachi N, et al. The gene mutated in ataxia-ocular apraxia 1 encodes the new HIT/Zn-finger protein aprataxin. *Nat Genet* 2001;29:189–193.

Moreira MC, Klur S, Watanabe M, et al. Senataxin, the ortholog of a yeast RNA helicase, is mutant in ataxia-ocular apraxia 2. *Nat Genet* 2004;36:225–227.

Raskind WH, Wijsman E, Pagon RA, et al. X-linked sideroblastic anemia and ataxia: linkage to phosphoglycerate kinase at Xq13. *Am J Hum Genet* 1991;48:335–341.

Richter A, Rioux JD, Bouchard JP, et al. Location score and haplotype analyses of the locus for autosomal recessive spastic ataxia of Charlevoix-Saguenay, in chromosome region 13q11. *Am J Hum Genet* 1999;64:768–775.

Sutton IJ, Last JI, Ritchie SJ, et al. Adult-onset ataxia telangiectasia due to ATM 5762ins137 mutation homozygosity. *Ann Neurol* 2004;891–895.

Yokota T, Shicjiri T, Gotoda T, et al. Friedreich-like ataxia with retinitis pigmentosa caused by the His101 Gln mutation of the alpha-tocopherol transfer protein gene. *Ann Neurol* 1997;41:826–832.

Late-Onset Autosomal-Dominant Cerebellar Ataxia

Abele M, Burk K, Schols L, et al. The aetiology of sporadic adult-onset ataxia. *Brain* 2002;125:961–968.

Benton CS, de Silva A, Rutledge SL, et al. Molecular/clinical studies in SCA 7 define a broad clinical spectrum and infantile phenotype. *Neurology* 1998;51:1081–1085.

Bird T. Hereditary Ataxia Overview. www.genetests.org.

Brkanac Z, Bylenok L, Fernandez M, et al. A new dominant spinocerebellar ataxia linked to chromosome 19q13. 4-qter. *Arch Neurol* 2002;59:1291–1295.

Brkanac Z, Fernandez M, Matsushita M, et al. Autosomal dominant sensory/motor neuropathy with ataxia (SMNA): linkage to chromosome 7q22-q32. *Am J Med Genet* 2002;114:450–457.

Brusco A, Gellera C, Cagnoli C, et al. Molecular genetics of hereditary spinocerebellar ataxia: mutation analysis of spinocerebellar ataxia genes and CAG/CTG repeat expansion detection in 225 Italian families. *Arch Neurol* 2004;61:727–733.

Bryer A, Krause A, Bill P, et al. The hereditary adult-onset ataxias in South Africa. *J Neurol Sci* 2003;216:47–54.

Chen DH, Brkanac Z, Verlinde CL, et al. Missense mutations in the regulatory domain of PKC gamma: a new mechanism for dominant nonepisodic cerebellar ataxia. *Am J Hum Genet* 2003;72:839–849.

Chen DH, Cimino PJ, Ranum L, et al. Prevalence of SCA 14 and spectrum of PKCy mutations in a large panel of ataxia patients. *Am J Hum Genet* 2003;73(Suppl):546.

Chung MY, Lu YC, Cheng NC, et al. A novel autosomal dominant spinocerebellar ataxia (SCA22) linked to chromosome 1p21-q23. *Brain* 2003;126:1293–1299.

Chung MY, Soong BW. Reply to: SCA-19 and SCA-22: evidence for one locus with a worldwide distribution. *Brain* 2004;127:E7.

Day JW, Schut LJ, Moseley ML, et al. Spinocerebellar ataxia type 8: clinical features in a large family. *Neurology* 2000;55:649–657.

De Michele G, Maltecca F, Carella M, et al. Dementia, ataxia, extrapyramidal features, and epilepsy: phenotype spectrum in two Italian families with spinocerebellar ataxia type 17. *Neurol Sci* 2003;24:166–167.

Devos D, Schraen-Maschke S, Vuillaume I, et al. Clinical features and genetic analysis of a new form of spinocerebellar ataxia. *Neurology* 2001;56:234–238.

Fujigasaki H, Martin J-J, De Deyn PP, et al. CAG repeat expansion in the TATA box-binding protein gene causes autosomal dominant cerebellar ataxia. *Brain* 2001;124:1939–1947.

Fujigasaki H, Tardieu S, Camuzat A, et al. Spinocerebellar ataxia type 10 in the French population. *Ann Neurol* 2002;51:408–409.

Giunti P, Sabbadini M, Sweeney MG, et al. The role of SCA2 trinucleotide repeat expansion in 89 autosomal dominant ataxia families. *Brain* 1998;121:459–467.

Grewal RP, Tayag E, Figueroa KP, et al. Clinical and genetic analysis of a distinct autosomal dominant spinocerebellar ataxia. *Neurology* 1998;51:1423–1426.

Herman-Bert A, Stevanin G, Netter JC, et al. Mapping of spinocerebellar ataxia 13 to chromosome 19q13.3-q13.4 in a family with autosomal dominant cerebellar ataxia and mental retardation. *Am J Hum Genet* 2000;67:229–2235.

Ikeuchi T, Koide R, Tanaka H, et al. Dentatorubral-pallidoluysian atrophy: clinical features are closely related to unstable expansions of trinucleotide (CAG) repeat. *Ann Neurol* 1995;37:769–775.

Jodice C, Mantuano E, Veneziano L, et al. Episodic ataxia type 2 (EA2) and spinocerebellar ataxia type 6 (SCA6) due to CAG repeat expansion in the CACNA I A gene on chromosome l9p. *Hum Mol Genet* 1997;11:1973–1978.

Johansson J, Forsgren L, Sandgren O, et al. Expanded CAG repeats in Swedish spinocerebellar ataxia type 7 (SCA7) patients: effect of CAG repeat length on the clinical manifestation. *Hum Mol Genet* 1998;7:171–176.

Juvonen V, Hietala M, Paivarinta M, et al. Clinical and genetic findings in Finnish ataxia patients with the spinocerebellar ataxia 8 repeat expansion. *Ann Neurol* 2000;48:354–361.

Klockgether T, Ludtke R, Kramer B, et al. The natural history of degenerative ataxia: a retrospective study in 466 patients. *Brain* 1998;121 (Pt 4):589–600.

Knight, MA, Gardner RJM, Bahlo M, et al. Dominantly inherited ataxia and dysphonia with dentate calcification: spinocerebellar ataxia type 20. *Brain* 2004;127:1172–1181.

Knight MA, Kennerson ML, Anney RJ, et al. Spinocerebellar ataxia type 15 (sca15) maps to 3p24.2-3pter: exclusion of the ITPR1 gene, the human orthologue of an ataxic mouse mutant. *Neurobiol Dis* 2003;13:147–157.

Knight MA, Kennerson M, Nicholson GA, et al. A new spinocerebellar ataxia, SCA15. *Am J Hum Genet* 2001;69(Suppl):509.

Margolis RL. The spinocerebellar ataxias: order emerges from chaos. *Curr Neurol Neurosci Rep* 2002;5:447–456.

Maruyama H, Izumi Y, Morino H, et al. Difference in disease-free survival curve and regional distribution according to subtype of spinocerebellar ataxia: a study of 1,286 Japanese patients. *Am J Med Genet* 2002;114:578–583.

Matsumura R, Futamura N, Ando N, et al. Frequency of spinocerebellar ataxia mutations in the Kinki district of Japan. *Acta Neurol Scand* 2003;107:38–41.

Matsuura T, Ranum LP, Volpini V, et al. Spinocerebellar ataxia type 10 is rare in populations other than Mexicans. *Neurology* 2002;58:983–984.

Matsuura T, Yamagata T, Burgess DL, et al. Large expansion of the ATTCT pentanucleotide repeat in spinocerebellar ataxia type 10. *Nat Genet* 2000;26:191–194.

Meijer IA, Hand CK, Grewal KK, et al. A locus for autosomal dominant hereditary spastic ataxia, SAX1, maps to chromosome 12p13. *Am J Hum Genet* 2002;70:763–769.

Miyoshi Y, Yamada T, Tanimura M, et al. A novel autosomal dominant spinocerebellar ataxia (SCA16) linked to chromosome 8q22.1-24.1. *Neurology* 2001;57:96–100.

Moreira MC, Klur S, Watanabe M, et al. Senataxin, the ortholog of a yeast RNA helicase, is mutant in ataxia-ocular apraxia 2. *Nat Genet* 2004;36:225–227.

Nakamura K, Jeong SY, Uchihara T, et al. SCA17, a novel autosomal dominant cerebellar ataxia caused by an expanded polyglutamine in TATA-binding protein. *Hum Mol Genet* 2001;10:1441–1448.

Nagaoka U, Takashima M, Ishikawa K, et al. A gene on SCA4 locus causes dominantly inherited pure cerebellar ataxia. *Neurology* 2000;54:1971–1975.

Nance MA. Seeking clarity through the genetic lens: a work in progress. *Ann Neurol* 2003;54:5–7.

O'Hearn E, Holmes SE, Calvert PC, et al. SCA-12: tremor with cerebellar and cortical atrophy is associated with a CAG repeat expansion. *Neurology* 2001;56:299–303.

Paulson HL, Perez MK, Trottier PY, et al. Intranuclear inclusions of expanded polyglutamine protein in spinocerebellar ataxia type 3. *Neuron* 1997;19:333–344.

Potter NT, Nance MA. Genetic testing for ataxia in North America. *Mol Diagn* 2000;5:91–99.

Pulst SM. Inherited ataxias. In: Pulst SM, ed. *Genetics of Movement Disorders*. Amsterdam: Academic Press, 2002:19–34.

Ranurn LP, Schut LJ, Lundgren JK et al. Spinocerebellar ataxia type 5 in a family descended from the grandparents of President Lincoln maps to chromosome 11. *Nat Genet* 1994;8:280–284.

Rosenberg RN, Nyhan WL, Bay C, et al. Autosomal dominant striatonigral degeneration: a clinical, pathologic and biochemical study of a new genetic disorder. *Neurology* 1976;26:703–714.

Rosenberg R, Paulson H. The inherited ataxias. In: Rosenberg RN, Prusiner SB, DiMauro S, et al., eds. *The Molecular and Genetic Basis of Neurologic and Psychiatric Disease*. Philadelphia: Butterworth-Heineman, 2003:369–382.

Saleem Q, Choudhry S, Mukerji M, et al. Molecular analysis of autosomal dominant hereditary ataxias in the Indian population: high frequency of SCA2 and evidence for a common founder mutation. *Hum Genet* 2000;106:179–187.

Schelhaas HJ, Ippel PF, Hageman G, et al. Clinical and genetic analysis of a four-generation family with a distinct autosomal dominant cerebellar ataxia. *J Neurol* 2001;248:113–120.

Schelhaas HJ, Verbeek DS, Van de Warrenburg BP, et al. SCA19 and SCA22: evidence for one locus with a worldwide distribution. *Brain* 2004;127:E6.

Schols L, Bauer P, Schmidt T, et al. Autosomal dominant cerebellar ataxias: clinical features, genetics, and pathogenesis. *Lancet Neurol* 2004;3:291–304.

Schols L, Bauer I, Zuhlke C, et al. Do CTG expansions at the SCA8 locus cause ataxia? *Ann Neurol* 2003;54:110–115.

Silveira I, Miranda C, Guimaraes L, et al. Trinucleotide repeats in 202 families with ataxia: a small expanded (CAG)n allele at the SCA17 locus. *Arch Neurol* 2002;59:623–629.

Stevanin G, Bouslam N, Thobois S, et al. Spinocerebellar ataxia with sensory neuropathy (SCA25) maps to chromosome 2p. *Ann Neurol* 2004;55:97–104.

Swartz BE, Burmeister M, Somers JT, et al. A form of inherited cerebellar ataxia with saccadic intrusions, increased saccadic speed, sensory neuropathy, and myoclonus. *Ann N Y Acad Sci* 2002;956:441–444.

Tachi N, Kozuka N, Ohya K, et al. Hereditary cerebellar ataxia with peripheral neuropathy and mental retardation. *Eur Neurol* 2002;43:82–87.

Takashima H, Boerkoel CF, John J, et al. Mutation of TDP1, encoding a topoisomerase I-dependent DNA damage repair enzyme, in spinocerebellar ataxia with axonal neuropathy. *Nat Genet* 2002;32:267–272.

Tan EK, Ashizawa T. Genetic testing in spinocerebellar ataxias: defining a clinical role. *Arch Neurol* 2001;58:191–195.

Yabe I, Sasaki H, Chen DH, et al. Spinocerebellar ataxia type 14 caused by a mutation in protein kinase C gamma. *Arch Neurol* 2003;60:1749–1751.

van Swieten JC, Brusse E, de Graaf BM, et al. A mutation in the fibroblast growth factor 14 gene is associated with autosomal dominant cerebral ataxia. *Am J Hum Genet* 2003;72:191–199.

Vuillaume I, Devos D, Schraen-Maschke S, et al. A new locus for spinocerebellar ataxia (SCA21) maps to 7p21.3-p15.1. *Ann Neurol* 2002;52:666–670.

Episodic Ataxia

Bomont P, Watanabe M, Gershoni-Barush R, et al. Homozygosity mapping of spinocerebellar ataxia with cerebellar atrophy and peripheral neuropathy to 9q33-34, and with hearing impairment and optic atrophy to 6p21-23. *Eur J Hum Genet* 2000;8:986–990.

Brunt EP, Van Weerden TW. Familial paroxysmal ataxia and continuous myokymia. *Brain* 1990;113:1361–1382.

Jen J, Kim GW, Baloh RW. The clinical spectrum of episodic ataxia type 2. *Neurology* 2004;62:17–22.

Mantuano E, Veneziano L, Jodice C, et al. Spinocerebellar ataxia type 6 and episodic ataxia type 2: differences and similarities between two allelic disorders. *Cytogenet Genome Res* 2003;100:147–153.

Ophoff RA, Terwindt GM, Vergouwe MN, et al. Familial hemiplegic migraine and episodic ataxia type 2 are caused by mutations in the CA^{2+} channel gene CACNLIA4. *Cell* 1996;87:543–552.

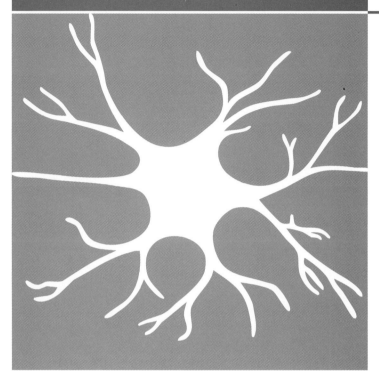

Movement Disorders

Chapter 109

Huntington Disease

Stanley Fahn

Huntington disease (HD; MIM 143100) is a progressive hereditary disorder that usually appears in adult life. It is characterized by a movement disorder (usually chorea), dementia, and personality disorder. It was first recognized clinically by Waters in 1842 and became accepted as a clinical entity with the comprehensive description and interpretation of the mode of transmission by George Huntington in 1872.

PATHOLOGY

At postmortem examination, the brain is shrunken and atrophic; the caudate nucleus is the most affected structure (Fig. 109.1). Histologically, the cerebral cortex shows loss of neurons, especially in layer 3. The caudate nucleus and putamen are severely involved, with loss of neurons, particularly the medium-sized spiny neurons, and their GABA-ergic striatal efferents. Those lost earliest are the efferents (containing GABA and enkephalin) projecting to the lateral globus pallidus, which is thought to account for chorea. With progression of the disease, the striatal efferents projecting to the medial pallidum are lost; their loss is thought to account for the later developing rigidity and dystonia. Dementia is attributed to changes in both the cerebral cortex and deep nuclei (i.e., subcortical dementia).

Less marked changes occur in other structures, such as the thalamus and brainstem. A reactive gliosis is apparent in all affected areas. In advanced cases, the striatum may be completely devoid of cells and replaced by a gliotic process, at which time choreic movements abate and are replaced by dystonia and an akinetic-rigid state. Progressive striatal atrophy is the basis for staging the severity of the disease. The age at onset is inversely correlated to the severity of striatal degeneration.

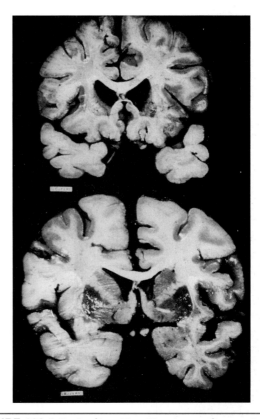

FIGURE 109.1. Brain slices. **Top.** Huntington disease. Atrophy of caudate nucleus and lentiform nuclei with dilatation of lateral ventricle. **Bottom.** Normal brain.

BIOCHEMISTRY

There is loss of striatal and nigral GABA and its synthesizing enzyme glutamic acid decarboxylase, whereas the cholinergic and somatostatin striatal interneurons are relatively spared. The receptors for dopamine and acetylcholine are decreased in the striatum. N-methyl-D-aspartate receptors are reduced severely in the striatum and cerebral cortex. These defects can be duplicated experimentally in animals by striatal injection of excitotoxins, such as kainic acid, and an excitotoxic hypothesis has been proposed as the pathogenesis of the disease. The neurochemical changes have not yet been translated into effective therapy because trials with GABA and acetylcholine agonists have not been beneficial. A defect in mitochondrial energy metabolism is considered to be present in HD.

This in turn can lead to oxidative stress, which has been measured in the vulnerable regions of brain of caudate and putamen.

PREVALENCE

HD occurs worldwide and in all ethnic groups, especially whites. The prevalence rate in the United States and Europe ranges from 4 to 8 per 100,000, whereas in Japan the rate is 10% of this figure. The highest prevalence rates have been reported from geographically somewhat isolated regions where affected families have resided for many generations (e.g., the Lake Maracaibo region in Venezuela and Moray Firth in Scotland).

GENETICS

A major discovery in 1983 was the identification and characterization of the HD gene near the tip of the short arm of chromosome 4 (4p16.3). Studies on HD families of different ethnic origins and countries found that despite the marked variability in phenotypic expression, there does not seem to be any genetic heterogeneity. The abnormal gene contains extra copies in exon 1 of trinucleotide repeats of CAG (cytosine-adenine-guanine) that codes for glutamine. Normal individuals have 10 to 29 repeats; those with HD have 36 to 121 repeats. This trinucleotide repeat is unstable in gametes; change in the number of repeats is transmitted to the next generation, sometimes with a decrease in number but more often with an increase. Spontaneous mutations occur from expansion of repeats from parents who have repeat lengths of 30 to 35 units, which span the gap between the normal and HD distributions, the so-called intermediate alleles. Spontaneous mutations in HD previously were considered rare, but this concept has changed as more sporadic (simplex) cases are evaluated by DNA analysis.

Affected mothers tend to transmit the abnormal gene to offspring in approximately the same number of trinucleotide repeats, plus or minus about three repeats. Affected fathers often transmit a greater increase in the length of trinucleotide repeats to offspring, thus resulting in many more juvenile cases of HD when an individual inherits the gene from the father. The trinucleotide repeat is stable over time in lymphocyte DNA but is unstable in sperm DNA. This characteristic may account for the occasional marked increase in the number of trinucleotide repeats in offspring of affected fathers, leading to a 10:1 ratio of juvenile HD when the affected parent is the father. This arises because of an inverse correlation between the number of trinucleotide repeats and the age at onset of symptoms. Knowing the number of repeats in an at-risk offspring helps fairly well in predicting the age at onset of symptoms. The rate of pathologic degeneration also correlates with the number of repeats.

HD is an autosomal dominant disease. Although the age at onset is similar in both homozygotes and heterozygotes, the homozygous double dose leads to a more severe clinical course. The toxic gain of function could be increased by doubling the cellular load of mutated proteins and aggregates thereof. The protein product of the normal gene is called *huntingtin*. The increase in polyglutamine seems to prevent the normal turnover of the protein, resulting in aggregation of the protein with accumulation in the cytoplasm and the nucleus. Other genetic disorders with expanded trinucleotide repeats of CAG include the Kennedy syndrome (X-linked spinal and bulbar muscular atrophy), myotonic dystrophy, many of the spinocerebellar atrophies, and dentatorubropallidoluysian atrophy. A similar pathogenesis for all these disorders has been proposed, but there is uncertainty whether aggregation of protein is a toxic cause of cell death or a protective mechanism.

One-third of individuals with HD share a common haplotype, thus implying a common ancestor. The other two-thirds appear to derive HD through a spontaneous mutation in the distant or near past. A diagnosis of HD can be established by testing for the gene, but genetic counseling should be carried out prior to and after the test result is revealed. Preclinical and prenatal testing can also be carried out, but appropriate genetic counseling is required. Diagnosis is still uncertain in those with a borderline number of trinucleotide repeats (i.e., between 30 and 35); for them, the diagnosis is "inconclusive."

Disclosure of positive results of the HD gene in asymptomatic individuals often leads to transient symptoms of depression, but suicidal ideation has been rare. Because of the ethical and legal implications that arise with DNA identification of a gene carrier, predictive testing must be performed by a team of clinicians and geneticists who not only are knowledgeable about the disease and the genetic techniques but also are sensitive to the psychosocial issues and counseling that precede and follow testing.

SIGNS AND SYMPTOMS

Symptoms usually appear between 35 and 40 years of age. The range of age at onset is broad, however, with cases recorded as early as age 5 and as late as age 70. The three characteristic manifestations of the disease are movement disorder, personality disorder, and mental deterioration. The three may occur together at onset or one may precede the others by a period of years. In general, the onset of symptoms is insidious, beginning with clumsiness, dropping of objects, fidgetiness, irritability, slovenliness, and neglect of duties, progressing to frank choreic movements and dementia. Overt psychotic episodes, depression, and irresponsible behavior may occur. Weight loss is common. The disease tends to run its course over a period of 15 years, more rapidly in those with an earlier age at onset.

Choreic Movements

The most striking and diagnostic feature of the disease is the appearance of involuntary movements that seem purposeless and abrupt but less rapid and lightning-like than those seen in myoclonus. The somatic muscles are affected in a random manner, and choreic movements flow from one part of the body to another. Proximal, distal, and axial muscles are involved. In the early stages and in the less severe form, there is slight grimacing of the face, intermittent movements of the eyebrows and forehead, shrugging of the shoulders, and jerking movements of the limbs. Pseudopurposeful movements (*parakinesia*) are common in attempts to mask the involuntary jerking. As the disease progresses, walking is associated with more intense arm and leg movements, which cause a dancing, prancing, stuttering type of gait, an abnormality that is particularly characteristic of HD. Motor impersistence or inhibitory pauses during voluntary contraction probably account for "milkmaid grips," dropping of objects, and inability to keep the tongue steadily protruded. Ocular movements become impaired with reduced saccades and loss of smooth pursuit. The choreic movements are increased by emotional stimuli, disappear during sleep, and become superimposed on voluntary movements to the point that they make volitional activity difficult. With increased severity, the routine daily activities of living become difficult, as do speech and swallowing. Terminally, choreic movements may disappear and be replaced by muscular rigidity and dystonia.

Mental Symptoms

Characteristically, there is an organic dementia with progressive impairment of memory, loss of intellectual capacity, apathy, and inattention to personal hygiene. Early in the disease, less profound abnormalities consist of irritability, impulsive behavior, and bouts of depression or fits of violence; these are not infrequent. In some patients, frank psychotic features that are schizophrenic predominate, and the underlying cause is not evident until choreic movements develop. The dementing and psychotic features of the disease usually lead to commitment to a mental institution.

Other Neurologic Manifestations

Cranial nerves remain intact except for rapid eye movements, which are impaired in a large percentage of patients. Patients often blink during the execution of a sac-

cadic eye movement. Sensation is usually unaffected. Tendon reflexes are usually normal but may be hyperactive; the plantar responses may be abnormal.

Muscle tone is hypotonic in most patients except for those with the so-called akinetic-rigid variety (*Westphal variant*). With childhood onset (approximately 10% of cases), the akinetic-rigid state usually occurs instead of chorea and in conjunction with mental abnormalities and convulsive seizures. This form of the disease is rapidly progressive with a fatal outcome in less than 10 years. The observation that 90% of all patients with childhood onset inherit the disease from their father stems from the greater likelihood of a large increase in the number of CAG repeats in sperm cells. In the terminal stages of the more classic form of HD, muscular rigidity and dystonia tend to replace chorea, and seizures are not unusual.

LABORATORY DATA

Routine studies of blood, urine, and cerebrospinal fluid show no abnormalities. Diffuse abnormalities are seen in the electroencephalogram. Radiographs of the skull are normal, but computed tomography and magnetic resonance imaging show enlarged ventricles with characteristic butterfly appearance of the lateral ventricles, a result of degeneration of the caudate nucleus (Fig. 109.2). Patients with the akinetic-rigid form of HD are likely to show striatal hyperintensity on T2-weighted magnetic resonance imaging. PET using fluorodeoxyglucose has shown hypometabolism in the caudate and the putamen in

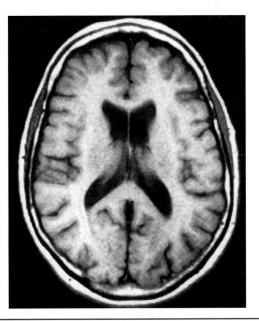

FIGURE 109.2. T1-weighted MRI of Huntington disease brain showing ventricular enlargement with atrophy of the head of the caudate nucleus.

affected patients. Abnormalities in striatal metabolism may precede caudate atrophy, but positron emission tomography is not sufficiently sensitive to detect the disease in presymptomatic persons.

DIAGNOSIS AND DIFFERENTIAL DIAGNOSIS

Even prior to the availability of DNA testing, HD could be diagnosed without difficulty in an adult with the clinical triad of chorea, dementia, and personality disorder and family history of the disease. Difficulties arose when the family history was lacking. The patient may be ignorant of the family history or may deny that history. Direct DNA testing of the HD gene is the most accurate diagnostic test.

Other conditions in which choreic movements are a major manifestation can often be excluded on clinical grounds. The most common other adult-onset choreic disorder is neuroacanthocytosis. It is manifested by mild chorea, tics, tongue biting, peripheral neuropathy, feeding dystonia, increased serum creatine kinase, and red cell acanthocytes. It is also common for these patients to have had a few seizures. Dentatorubralpallidoluysian atrophy can also mimic HD. Besides chorea, it can present with myoclonus, ataxia, seizures, and dementia. Three genetic disorders, referred to as Huntington disease–like (HDL), have been identified, in which there are clinical similarities to HD, but with previously unrecognized gene mutations. For instance, HDL2 (MIM 606438) maps to 16q24.3; CTG triplet repeats expand in a manner similar to those of HD itself. Differentiation of all these phenotypically similar disorders is by gene testing.

Sydenham chorea has an earlier age at onset, is self-limited, and lacks the characteristic mental disturbances. Chorea and mental disturbances occurring as manifestations of lupus erythematosus are usually more acute in onset, the chorea is more localized and often periodic, and there are characteristic serologic and clinical abnormalities. Involuntary movements occurring in psychiatric patients on long-term treatment with neuroleptic agents (the so-called *tardive dyskinesia*) occasionally pose a diagnostic problem. Such movements, however, are usually repetitive (stereotypy), in contrast to the nonrepetitive and random nature of chorea. Oral-lingual-buccal dyskinesia is the most common feature of tardive dyskinesia. Gait is usually normal in tardive dyskinesia and is abnormal in HD (see Table 117.1 for more distinguishing differences). The presenile dementias (Alzheimer and Pick diseases) are similar in the mental disorder, but language is more often involved; aphasic abnormalities are not seen early in HD. Myoclonus, rather than chorea, occasionally occurs. The peculiarities of the childhood disorder with rigidity, convulsive seizures, and mental retardation require differentiation from other heritable disorders, such as the leukodystrophies and gangliosidosis. Tics, particularly those of the Gilles de la Tourette syndrome, usually pose little problem in view of the complex nature of the involuntary movements, the characteristic vocalizations, and their suppressibility. Hereditary nonprogressive chorea begins in childhood, does not worsen, and is not associated with dementia or with personality disorder.

TREATMENT

There are no known means of altering the disease process or the fatal outcome. Attempts to replace the deficiency in GABA by using GABA-mimetic agents or inhibitors of GABA metabolism have been unsuccessful. Symptomatic treatment of depression and psychosis can be achieved with antidepressants and typical or atypical (i.e., clozapine and quetiapine) antipsychotic agents. The choreic movements can be controlled by the use of neuroleptic agents including dopamine receptor blockers, such as haloperidol and perphenazine, and presynaptic dopamine depleters, such as reserpine and tetrabenazine. Use of dopamine receptor blockers is less desirable than the depleters because of the risk of developing tardive dyskinesia. Using these drugs combined with supervision of the patient's daily activities allows management at home during the early stages of the disorder. As the disease advances, however, confinement to a psychiatric facility is often necessary.

SUGGESTED READINGS

Albin RL, Reiner A, Anderson KD, et al. Striatal and nigral neuron subpopulations in rigid Huntington's disease: implications for the functional anatomy of chorea and rigidity-akinesia. *Ann Neurol* 1990;27:357–365.

Alford RL, Ashizawa T, Jankovic J, et al. Molecular detection of new mutations, resolution of ambiguous results and complex genetic counseling issues in Huntington disease. *Am J Med Genet* 1996;66:281–286.

Aylward EH, Sparks BF, Field KM, et al. Onset and rate of striatal atrophy in preclinical Huntington disease. *Neurology* 2004;63:66–72.

Bamford KA, Caine ED, Kido DK, et al. A prospective evaluation of cognitive decline in early Huntington's disease: functional and radiographic correlates. *Neurology* 1995;45:1867–1873.

Bates G. Huntingtin aggregation and toxicity in Huntington's disease. *Lancet* 2003;361:1642–1644.

Beal MF, Ferrante RJ. Experimental therapeutics in transgenic mouse models of Huntington's disease. *Nat Rev Neurosci* 2004;5:373–384.

Brandt J, Bylsma FW, Gross R, et al. Trinucleotide repeat length and clinical progression in Huntington's disease. *Neurology* 1996;46:527–531.

Brinkman RR, Mezei MM, Theilmann J, et al. The likelihood of being affected with Huntington disease by a particular age, for a specific CAG size. *Am J Hum Genet* 1997;60:1202–1210.

Browne SE, Bowling AC, MacGarvey U, et al. Oxidative damage and metabolic dysfunction in Huntington's disease: selective vulnerability of the basal ganglia. *Ann Neurol* 1997;41:646–653.

Davies SW, Beardsall K, Turmaine M, et al. Are neuronal intranuclear inclusions the common neuropathology of triple-repeat disorders with polyglutamine-repeat expansions? *Lancet* 1998;351:131–133.

Djousse L, Knowlton B, Cupples LA, et al. Weight loss in early stage of Huntington's disease. *Neurology* 2002;59:1325–1330.

Duyao M, Ambrose C, Myers R, et al. Trinucleotide repeat length instability and age of onset in Huntington's disease. *Nat Genet* 1993;4:387–392.

Huntington's Disease Collaborative Research Group. A novel gene containing a trinucleotide repeat that is expanded and unstable on Huntington's disease chromosomes. *Cell* 1993;72:971–983.

Marder K, Sandler S, Lechich A, et al. Relationship between CAG repeat length and late-stage outcomes in Huntington's disease. *Neurology* 2002;59:1622–1624.

Myers RH, MacDonald ME, Koroshetz WJ, et al. De novo expansion of a (CAG)n repeat in sporadic Huntington's disease. *Nat Genet* 1993;5:168–173.

Myers RH, Vonsattel JP, Stevens TJ, et al. Clinical and neuropathologic assessment of severity in Huntington's disease. *Neurology* 1988;38:341–347.

Penney JB, Vonsattel JP, MacDonald ME, et al. CAG repeat number governs the development rate of pathology in Huntington's disease. *Ann Neurol* 1997;41:689–692.

Penney JB, Young AB, Shoulson I, et al. Huntington's disease in Venezuela: 7 years of follow-up on symptomatic and asymptomatic individuals. *Mov Disord* 1990;5:93–99.

Squitieri F, Gellera C, Cannella M, et al. Homozygosity for CAG mutation in Huntington disease is associated with a more severe clinical course. *Brain* 2003;126:946–955.

Chapter 110

Sydenham and Other Forms of Chorea

Stanley Fahn

▶ **TABLE 110.1 Common Causes of Chorea**

Hereditary
Huntington disease
Huntington disease–like syndromes (HDL1, HDL2, HDL3)
Hereditary nonprogressive chorea
Neuroacanthocytosis
Dentatorubralpallidoluysian atrophy
Spinocerebellar atrophy 17 (SCA17)
Wilson disease
Ataxia telangiectasia
Lesch-Nyhan syndrome

Secondary
  Infections/immunologic
  Sydenham chorea
  Encephalitis
  Systemic lupus erythematosus
  Antiphospholipid syndrome
  Drug-induced
  Levodopa
  Anticonvulsants
  Anticholinergics
  Antipsychotics
  Metabolic and endocrine
  Chorea gravidarum
  Hyperthyroidism
  Birth control pills
  Hyperosmolar nonketotic hyperglycemic encephalopathy
  Vascular
  Hemichorea/hemiballism with subthalamic nucleus lesion
  Postpump choreoathetosis after cardiac surgery
  Periarteritis nodosa

Unknown etiology
Senile chorea
Essential chorea

For a complete listing of causes of chorea, see Shoulson I. *Clin Neuropharmacol* 1986;9[Suppl 2]:585–599.

Choreic movements can be associated with many disorders; the most common are listed in Table 110.1.

SYDENHAM CHOREA

In 1686, Thomas Sydenham described the chorea now known by his name but originally called St. Vitus dance. His description was of children with a halting gait and jerky movements.

Sydenham chorea (acute chorea, St. Vitus dance, chorea minor, rheumatic chorea) is a disease of childhood characterized by rapid, irregular, aimless, involuntary movements of the muscles of the limbs, face, and trunk that resemble continuous restlessness. There is also muscular weakness, hypotonia, and emotional lability. Behavioral and mental changes may occur and persist. Once common, it now is encountered infrequently in developed countries.

The chorea, with some exceptions, is self-limited and fatalities are rare except as a result of cardiac complications.

Etiology and Pathology

Sydenham chorea is considered an autoimmune disorder, a consequence of infection with group A beta-hemolytic streptococcus. Unlike arthritis and carditis, which occur soon after the infection, chorea may be delayed for 6 months or longer. The incidence of Sydenham chorea had fallen dramatically with the introduction of antibiotics and with better sanitary conditions. The streptococcus is thought to induce antibodies that cross-react with neuronal cytoplasmic antigens of caudate and subthalamic nuclei, which apparently account for the symptoms characteristic of rheumatic chorea. These antineuronal antibodies are found in nearly all patients with Sydenham chorea. Antibodies to cardiolipin, which have been found in chorea associated with lupus erythematosus, have not been found in Sydenham chorea. Pathologic studies are rare in this nonfatal disease. Postmortem changes in fatal cases can be attributed to embolic phenomena and terminal changes. A mild degree of inflammatory reaction has been found in a few patients.

Knowledge of the etiology and immunology of Sydenham chorea has spawned the concept of other "*pediatric autoimmune neuropsychiatric disorders associated with streptococcal infection*" (PANDAS). This diagnostic appellation is being applied to children or adolescents who develop tic disorders or obsessive-compulsive disorder after group A beta-hemolytic streptococcal infections.

Incidence

Acute chorea is almost exclusively a disease of childhood; over 80% of the cases occur in patients between the ages of 5 and 15. Onset before the age of 5 is rare, and the occurrence of the first attack after the age of 15 is uncommon, except during pregnancy or the use of oral contraceptives in the late teens and early twenties. All races are affected. Girls are affected more than twice as frequently as boys. The disease occurs at all times of the year but is less common in summer.

Symptoms and Signs

In addition to the choreic movements and accompanying motor impersistence, Sydenham chorea is associated with irritability, emotional lability, obsessive-compulsive symptoms, attention deficit, and anxiety. Neurologic manifestations other than chorea are speech impairment and, more rarely, encephalopathy, reflex changes, weakness, gait disturbance, headache, seizures, and cranial neuropathy. Chorea is generalized in about 80% and unilateral in 20% of cases.

The clinical features of the chorea in Sydenham chorea differ from those of Huntington disease. In Sydenham, the chorea is usually more flowing with a restless-appearing quality. In Huntington, the chorea tends to be more individualistic and jerky and becomes more flowing when the chorea worsens. Physiologic recordings in Sydenham chorea reveal the bursts of electromyographic activity to last more than 100 ms and to occur asynchronously in antagonistic muscles. These findings are in contrast to Huntington chorea, in which more frequent bursts of 10 to 30 ms and 50 to 100 ms occur.

Complications

Other manifestations of the rheumatic infection may occur during the course of the chorea or may precede or follow it. Cardiac complications, usually endocarditis, occur in approximately 20% of patients. Myocarditis and pericarditis are less common. Vegetative endocarditis and embolic phenomena may occur but are rare. A previous history of rheumatic polyarthritis is common, but involvement of the joints during the course of the chorea is rare. Other infrequent complications include subcutaneous rheumatic nodules, erythema nodosum, and purpura. Persistent mental and behavioral effects can also result from Sydenham chorea.

Diagnosis

The diagnosis is made without difficulty from the appearance of the characteristic choreic movements in a child. Helpful for diagnosis are the presence of behavioral changes and diffuse slowing on the EEG. Often, a history of prior streptococcal infection is not elicited, and tests for rheumatoid factor, antinuclear antibodies, antistreptolysin titers, and CSF oligoclonal bands are often negative. The CSF is usually normal, but pleocytosis has been reported in a few cases. MRI is usually normal except for selective enlargement of the caudate, putamen, and globus pallidus. In contrast to many other types of choreic disorders, PET reveals striatal hypermetabolism that returns to normal when the symptoms abate.

Some other causes of symptomatic chorea in childhood are presented in Table 110.2; some are reviewed here. The *withdrawal emergent syndrome*, occurring in children when neuroleptic agents are suddenly discontinued, closely resembles the type of chorea seen in Sydenham, but a history of having taken these drugs should enable this diagnosis to be made. Some patients labeled as having chronic Sydenham chorea may actually have the withdrawal emergent syndrome instead.

▶ **TABLE 110.2 Other Causes of Symptomatic Chorea in Childhood**

Adrenal insufficiency
Anoxic encephalopathy
Antiphospholipid antibody
Benign hereditary chorea
Cardiopulmonary bypass, complication of
Encephalitis, e.g., ECHO virus type 25, mononucleosis, HIV infection, bacterial endocarditis, typhoid fever, Lyme disease
GM_1 gangliosidosis
Human immunodeficiency virus
Huntington disease, juvenile
Hypocalcemia, hypercalcemia
Hypothermia, deep
Lesch-Nyhan syndrome
Moyamoya disease
Systemic lupus erythematosus
Wilson disease
Withdrawal emergent syndrome (a form of tardive dyskinesia)

Other dyskinesias in childhood also could be considered in differential diagnosis, but the distinctions between these and choreic movements should lead to the correct diagnosis. Tics may offer some difficulty, but these movements are stereotyped and localized always to the same muscle or groups of muscles.

Idiopathic torsion dystonia often begins in childhood, but the sustained and twisting movements are quite distinct from choreic movements. On the other hand, some dystonic movements are more rapid, but repetitive and twisting, and have been mislabeled as chorea. Dystonic movements affect the same body parts repetitiously, so-called patterning, in contrast to chorea. Also, childhood dystonia persists and does not have the self-limiting characteristic of Sydenham chorea. Essential hereditary myoclonus can begin in childhood and sometimes could be difficult to distinguish from chorea. Athetosis in childhood often is seen with static encephalopathy or some metabolic diseases and usually occurs in the first few years of life, not at the ages commonly encountered with Sydenham chorea.

Course and Prognosis

Sydenham chorea often is a benign disease, and complete recovery is the rule in uncomplicated cases. The mortality rate of approximately 2% is a result of cardiac complications. The duration of symptoms varies; they generally persist for 3 to 6 weeks but may last for several months. It is not unusual for involuntary movements of mild degree to persist for many months after the more severe movements subside. Recurrences after months or several years are reported in approximately 35% of the cases.

Rarely, a patient may have persistent chorea throughout life. Residual behavioral and EEG changes, however, are not uncommon in Sydenham chorea. Susceptibility to *chorea gravidarum*, chorea from oral contraceptives and topical vaginal creams containing estrogen, and even increased sensitivity to levodopa-induced chorea are sequelae of Sydenham chorea. The end of pregnancy and the discontinuation of oral contraceptives or estrogen provide relief from the involuntary movements. A postmortem examination of a case of chorea gravidarum revealed neuronal loss and astrocytosis in the striatum.

Treatment

There is no specific treatment for the disease. Symptomatic therapy may be of great value in the control of the movements. In the mild form, bed rest during the period of active movements is sufficient. The room should be quiet, and all external stimuli should be reduced to a minimum. When the severity of the movements interferes with proper rest, sedatives in the form of barbiturates, chloral hydrate, or paraldehyde may be needed. If further treatment is necessary, a benzodiazepine, valproate, or corticosteroids may be effective. Although antidopaminergic drugs can suppress choreic movements, a dopamine-receptor blocking agent, such as a phenothiazine, should not be administered because of its potential to produce tardive dyskinesia or tardive dystonia. A dopamine-depleting drug, such as reserpine or tetrabenazine, could be used if milder drugs are ineffective. Prophylactic administration of penicillin for at least 10 years is recommended to prevent other manifestations of rheumatic fever, of which Sydenham chorea may be its sole manifestation.

OTHER IMMUNE CHOREAS

Chorea in *systemic lupus erythematosus* (SLE) has been associated with the presence of antiphospholipid antibodies (lupus anticoagulant), a heterogeneous group of antibodies that can cause platelet dysfunction and result in thrombosis. Chorea is intermittent in SLE. PET has not found caudate hypometabolism in SLE in contrast to many other choreas. Treatment with antidopaminergic agents has been successful.

The *primary antiphospholipid antibody syndrome* also includes chorea, particularly in young women. Systemically, patients have migraine, spontaneous abortions, venous and arterial thromboses, thickened cardiac valves, livedo reticularis, and Raynaud phenomenon. The CNS is involved with strokes, multi-infarct dementia, and chorea. Activated partial thromboplastin time is prolonged because of the presence of lupus anticoagulant, and high titers of anticardiolipin antibodies exist. Anticoagulation, immunosuppressive drugs, and plasmapheresis have had variable success; it is difficult to interpret the effectiveness of therapeutic interventions because spontaneous remission occurs frequently. Striatal hypermetabolism is seen in PET. Some cases of chorea gravidarum may have anti–basal ganglia antibodies, supporting an immunological basis in those situations.

VASCULAR CHOREA AND BALLISM

Choreic movements confined to the arm and leg on one side of the body (hemichorea, hemiballism) may develop abruptly in middle-aged or elderly patients. Ballistic movements are a more violent form of chorea and are characterized by large-amplitude uncoordinated activity of the proximal appendicular muscles, so vigorous that the limbs are forcefully and aimlessly thrown about. Padding of the limbs is necessary to prevent injury. The movements are present at rest and may be suppressed during voluntary limb movement.

The sudden onset suggests a vascular basis; indeed, it may be preceded by hemiplegia or hemiparesis. In such instances, the choreic or ballistic movements appear when return of motor function occurs. This type of movement disorder is the result of a destructive lesion of the contralateral subthalamic nucleus or its connections. It has also been seen with scattered encephalomalacic lesions involving the internal capsule and basal ganglia. Vascular lesions, hemorrhagic or ischemic, are the most common cause, but hemiballism has been found with tumors or plaques from multiple sclerosis in the subthalamic nucleus and has occasionally followed attempted thalamotomy when the target was missed. In general, the movements tend to diminish over time, but they may be persistent and require treatment. The agents noted above for the control of choreic movements in general have proved effective.

Hemiballism or hemichorea is seen in patients with AIDS and a toxoplasmosis lesion involving the subthalamic nucleus; these movements also respond to antidopaminergic medication. Chorea-ballism is a common feature of hyperosmolar hyperglycemic nonketotic syndrome, which appears related to hypoperfusion in the striatum (see Chapter 52). Choreoathetosis as a sequela to surgery for congenital heart disease appears to be associated with prolonged time on pump, deep hypothermia, and circulatory arrest. In most cases of postpump syndrome, the chorea persists and fewer than 25% improve with antidopaminergic therapy.

NEUROACANTHOCYTOSIS

Perhaps the most common hereditary chorea after Huntington disease is neuroacanthocytosis (MIM 100500), formerly called chorea-acanthocytosis, which is also described in Chapter 93. The chorea is typically less severe than that seen with Huntington disease but occasionally is just as severe. In addition to chorea, patients with neuroacanthocytosis usually have tics, occasional seizures, amyotrophy, absent tendon reflexes, high serum creatine kinase, feeding dystonia (tongue pushes food out of the mouth), and self-mutilation with lip and tongue biting. Age at onset is typically in adolescence and young adulthood, but the range is wide (8 to 62 years). As with Huntington disease, a young age at onset is more likely to produce parkinsonism or dystonia rather than chorea. The diagnosis depends on finding more than 15% spiky erythrocytes (acanthocytes) in blood smears. Some authorities have proposed that detection of acanthocytes can be enhanced if a wet smear of blood is diluted 1:1 with normal saline.

The cerebral pathology is similar to that of Huntington disease, with striatal degeneration causing caudate atrophy and hypometabolism in the caudate nucleus in the PET. PET also reveals reduced fluorodopa uptake and decreased dopamine receptor binding in the striatum. Erythrocyte membrane lipids are altered. Tightly bound palmitic acid (C16:0) is increased, and stearic acid (C18:0) is decreased. Choline acetyltransferase and glutamic acid decarboxylase are normal in basal ganglia and cortex, substance P levels are low in the substantia nigra and striatum, and norepinephrine is elevated in the putamen and pallidum.

Neuroacanthocytosis has been found to be a result of various mutations on the CHAC (chorea-acanthocytosis) gene on chromosome 9q-21-q22, coding for the protein named chorein. A rare patient may have the McLeod phenotype, an X-linked (Xp21) form of acanthocytosis associated with chorea, seizures, neuropathy, liver disease, hemolysis, and elevated creatine kinase.

DENTATORUBRALPALLIDOLUYSIAN ATROPHY (DRPLA; MIM 125370)

Once thought to be found mainly in the Japanese population, this autosomal dominant disorder is now known to be more widespread, thanks to discovery of an expanded CAG repeat on a gene on chromosome 12p12. It has been called the Haw River syndrome in African American families. Dentatorubralpallidoluysian atrophy clinically overlaps with Huntington disease and manifests combinations of chorea, myoclonus, seizures, ataxia, and dementia. The phenotype varies according to triplet (CAG) repeat length, and anticipation and excess of paternal inheritance in younger onset cases with longer repeat lengths are seen. The neuropathologic spectrum is centered in the cerebellofugal and pallidofugal systems, but neurodegenerative changes can be found in many nuclei.

HUNTINGTON DISEASE–LIKE (HDL) SYNDROMES

In addition to neuroacanthocytosis and DRPLA, other syndromes that resemble Huntington Disease (HD) have been linked to other gene markers. When the HD gene test is normal, one should consider these less-common conditions. HDL1 (MIM 603218), an autosomal-dominant disorder, maps to chromosome 20p and has an octapeptide repeat in the prion protein. The autosomal-dominant HDL2 (606438) seems to affect exclusively or predominantly people of African origin. It is a result of CTG and CAG repeat expansions of the gene on chromosome 16q23, encoding junctophilin-3, a protein of the junctional complex that connects the plasma membrane and the endoplasmic reticulum. HDL3 (MIM 604802), although labeled as such, is an autosomal-recessive neurodegenerative disease beginning at 3 to 4 years of age. It is manifested by chorea, dystonia, ataxia, gait disorder, spasticity, seizures, mutism, intellectual impairment, and bilateral frontal and caudate atrophy. HDL3 has been linked to 4p15.3. Although labeled as a spinocerebellar degeneration, SCA17 can present with chorea and manifest with other features of HD. SCA17 is a result of an expanded CAG repeat in the gene on chromosome 6q27 for the TATA-binding protein, which has a transcription initiation function.

HEREDITARY NONPROGRESSIVE CHOREA (MIM 118700)

This rare disorder is not associated with dementia or other neurologic problems aside from chorea, which is nonprogressive and usually lessens in severity over time. The glucose PET shows striatal hypometabolism. It follows an autosomal-dominant transmission pattern and usually begins in childhood. It has been linked to a marker on chromosome 14q13.1-q21.1. A single nucleotide substitution in the ITF-1 gene has been identified in one family. In the absence of a family history, a benign nonprogressive chorea without other neurologic features can be rarely encountered, so-called essential chorea.

SENILE CHOREA

Senile chorea is characterized by late-onset generalized chorea with no family history and no dementia. As a rule, the movements begin insidiously, are mild, and usually involve the limbs. More complex movements of the lingual-facial-buccal regions, however, are on occasion encountered. Slow progression in the intensity and extent of the movements may occur. With DNA testing, half the patients show the CAG expansion in the HD gene. Most other cases have been shown to have other diagnoses, such as the antiphospholipid antibody syndrome, hypocalcemia, tardive dyskinesia, and basal ganglia calcification. Still, rarely, a patient can remain undiagnosed despite extensive investigation and is left with the diagnosis of senile chorea. In such a case, pathologic changes are found in the caudate nucleus and putamen but not to the degree seen in Huntington disease. Significantly, degenerative changes in the cerebral cortex are absent. In general, the symptoms are mild and there is little need to resort to therapeutic measures. In those instances in which oral-facial and neck muscle involvement occurs, however, drugs used to control chorea as indicated previously may prove useful.

SUGGESTED READINGS
Sydenham Chorea

Aron AM, Freeman JM, Carter S. The natural history of Sydenham's chorea. *Am J Med* 1965;38:83–95.

Cardoso F, Eduardo C, Silva AP, et al. Chorea in fifty consecutive patients with rheumatic fever. *Mov Disord* 1997;12:701–703.

Chatterjee A, Frucht SJ. Tetrabenazine in the treatment of severe pediatric chorea. *Mov Disord* 2003;18:703–706.

Church AJ, Cardoso F, Dale RC, et al. Anti-basal ganglia antibodies in acute and persistent Sydenham's chorea. *Neurology* 2002;59:227–231.

Garvey MA, Giedd J, Swedo SE. PANDAS: The search for environmental triggers of pediatric neuropsychiatric disorders. Lessons from rheumatic fever. *J Child Neurol* 1998;13:413–423.

Giedd JN, Rapoport JL, Kruesi MJP, et al. Sydenham's chorea: magnetic resonance imaging of the basal ganglia. *Neurology* 1995;45:2199–2202.

Ichikawa K, Kim RC, Givelber H, et al. Chorea gravidarum. Report of a fatal case with neuropathological observations. *Arch Neurol* 1980;37:429–432.

Singer HS, Loiselle CR, Lee O, et al. Anti-basal ganglia antibody abnormalities in Sydenham chorea. *J Neuroimmunol* 2003;136(Mar):154–161.

Weindl A, Kuwert T, Leenders KL, et al. Increased striatal glucose consumption in Sydenham's chorea. *Mov Disord* 1993;8:437–444.

Other Immune Choreas

Cervera R, Asherson RA, Font J, et al. Chorea in the antiphospholipid syndrome: clinical, radiologic, and immunologic characteristics of 50 patients from our clinics and the recent literature. *Medicine (Baltimore)* 1997;76:203–212.

Furie R, Ishikawa T, Dhawan V, et al. Alternating hemichorea in primary antiphospholipid syndrome: evidence for contralateral striatal hypermetabolism. *Neurology* 1994;44:2197–2199.

Miranda M, Cardoso F, Giovannoni G, et al. Oral contraceptive induced chorea: another condition associated with anti-basal ganglia antibodies. *J Neurol Neurosurg Psychiat* 2004;75:327–328.

Vascular Chorea-Ballism

Holden KR, Sessions JC, Cure J, et al. Neurologic outcomes in children with postpump choreoathetosis. *J Pediatr* 1998;132:162–164.

Lai PH, Tien RD, Chang MH, et al. Choreaballismus with nonketotic hyperglycemia in primary diabetes mellitus. *Am J Neuroradiol* 1996;17:1057–1064.

Oh S-H, Lee K-Y, Im J-H, Lee M-S. Chorea associated with non-ketotic hyperglycemia and hyperintensity basal ganglia lesion on T1-weighted brain MRI study: a meta-analysis of 53 cases including four present cases. *J Neurol Sci* 2002;200:57–62.

Vidakovic A, Dragasevic N, Kostic VS. Hemiballism: report of 25 cases. *J Neurol Neurosurg Psychiatry* 1994;57:945–949.

Neuroacanthocytosis

Dobson-Stone C, Danek A, Rampoldi L, et al. Mutational spectrum of the CHAC gene in patients with chorea-acanthocytosis. *Eur J Human Genet* 2002;10:773–781.

Dobson-Stone C, Velayos-Baeza A, Filippone LA, et al. Chorein detection for the diagnosis of chorea-acanthocytosis. *Ann Neurol* 2004;56(Aug):299–302.

Hardie RJ, Pullon HWH, Harding AE, et al. Neuroacanthocytosis—a clinical, haematological and pathological study of 19 cases. *Brain* 1991;114:13–49.

Saiki S, Sakai K, Kitagawa Y, et al. Mutation in the CHAC gene in a family of autosomal dominant chorea-acanthocytosis. *Neurology* 2003;61:1614–1616.

Tanaka M, Hirai S, Kondo S, et al. Cerebral hypoperfusion and hypometabolism with altered striatal signal intensity in chorea-acanthocytosis: a combined PET and MRI study. *Mov Disord* 1998;13:100–107.

Ueno S, Maruki Y, Nakamura M, et al. The gene encoding a newly discovered protein, chorein, is mutated in chorea-acanthocytosis. *Nat Genet* 2001;28:121–122.

Dentatorubralpallidoluysian Atrophy

Becher MW, Rubinsztein DC, Leggo J, et al. Dentatorubral and pallidoluysian atrophy (DRPLA): clinical and neuropathological findings in genetically confirmed North American and European pedigrees. *Mov Disord* 1997;12:519–530.

Burke JR, Wingfield MS, Lewis KE, et al. The Haw River syndrome: dentatorubropallidoluysian atrophy in an African-American family. *Nature Genet* 1994;7:521–524.

Ikeuchi T, Koide R, Tanaka H, et al. Dentatorubral-pallidoluysian atrophy: Clinical features are closely related to unstable expansions of trinucleotide (CAG) repeat. *Ann Neurol* 1995;37:769–775.

Huntington Disease–Like Syndromes

Holmes SE, O'Hearn E, Rosenblatt A, et al. A repeat expansion in the gene encoding junctophilin-3 is associated with Huntington disease-like 2. *Nat Genet* 2001;29:377–378.

Kambouris M, Bohlega S, Al-Tahan A, et al. Localization of the gene for a novel autosomal recessive neurodegenerative Huntington-like disorder to 4p15.3. *Am J Hum Genet* 2000;66:445–452.

Moore RC, Xiang F, Monaghan J, et al. Huntington disease phenocopy is a familial prion disease. *Am J Hum Genet* 2001;69:1385–1388.

Stevanin G, Camuzat A, Holmes SE, et al. CAG/CTG repeat expansions at the Huntington's disease-like 2 locus are rare in Huntington's disease patients. *Neurology* 2002;58:965–967.

Stevanin G, Fujigasaki H, Lebre AS, et al. Huntington's disease-like phenotype due to trinucleotide repeat expansions in the *TBP* and *JPH3* genes. *Brain* 2003;126:1599–603.

Toyoshima Y, Yamada M, Onodera O, et al. SCA17 homozygote showing Huntington's disease-like phenotype. *Ann Neurol* 2004;55:281–286.

Hereditary Nonprogressive Chorea

Breedveld GJ, Percy AK, MacDonald ME, et al. Clinical and genetic heterogeneity in benign hereditary chorea. *Neurology* 2002;59:579–584.

Kleiner-Fisman G, Rogaeva E, Halliday W, et al. Benign hereditary chorea: clinical, genetic, and pathological findings. *Ann Neurol* 2003;54:244–247.

Kuwert T, Lange HW, Langen KJ, et al. Normal striatal glucose consumption in 2 patients with benign hereditary chorea as measured by positron emission tomography. *J Neurol* 1990;237:80–84.

Senile Chorea

Friedman JH, Ambler M. A case of senile chorea. *Mov Disord* 1990;5:251–253.

Ruiz PJG, Gomez-Tortosa E, Delbarrio A, et al. Senile chorea: a multicenter prospective study. *Acta Neurol Scand* 1997;95:180–183.

Warren JD, Firgaira F, Thompson EM, et al. The causes of sporadic and "senile" chorea. *Aust N Z J Med* 1998;28:429–431.

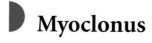

C h a p t e r   1 1 1

Myoclonus

Stanley Fahn

Myoclonus refers to brief lightning-like muscle jerks owing to brief electromyographic bursts of 10 to 50 ms, rarely more than 100 ms in duration. The jerks are usually a result of positive muscle contractions but can also be a result of sudden brief lapses of contraction (i.e., so-called negative myoclonus) such as is seen in *asterixis*. Asterixis is a tremorlike phenomenon of the extended wrists owing to brief lapses of muscle contraction. It is usually encountered in the metabolic encephalopathies that accompany severe hepatic, renal, and pulmonary disorders. Agonists and antagonists usually fire (or are inhibited in negative myoclonus) synchronously. Myoclonus is common, with a prevalence rate of 8.6 per 100,000.

Clinically, there is a wide expression of myoclonus. The jerks are simple, unlike the complex movements seen in tics, and the burst duration is less than 100 msec. This fast speed allows it to be differentiated from other abnormal movements, and polymyography is a useful diagnostic tool that can often localize the CNS origin of the bursts and also help differentiate the disorder from psychogenic myoclonus. Myoclonic jerks may occur singly or repetitively. They may be focal, segmental, or generalized. The amplitude ranges from mild contractions that do not move a joint to gross contractions that move limbs, the head, or the trunk. Myoclonic jerks range in frequency from rare isolated events to many events each minute; they may occur at rest, with action, or with intention movements. Commonly, myoclonic jerks are stimulus sensitive (reflex myoclonus); they can be induced by sudden noise, movement, light, visual threat, or pinprick. Most often, myoclonic jerks occur irregularly and unpredictably. But some occur in bursts of oscillations, and some are rhythmic, as in palatal myoclonus. Myoclonus can resemble tremor when rhythmic. Rhythmical myoclonus almost always denotes a segmental origin, either brainstem or spinal cord. An uncommon rhythmical form, called *cortical tremor*, originates in the cerebral cortex.

Usually, however, myoclonus arising from the cerebral cortex (cortical myoclonus) is focal and reflex induced. *Epilepsia partialis continua* can be considered within the cortical myoclonus family. The cortical origin can be ascertained by enlarged somatosensory evoked potentials or by spikes in the EEG associated with electromyographic correlated jerks that are revealed by a back-averaging technique. *Rasmussen encephalitis* is a disorder of childhood and adolescence in which there is a unilateral focal seizure disorder, including epilepsia partialis continua, and a progressive hemiplegia owing to focal cortical inflammation and destruction.

Myoclonus originating from the brainstem can be either generalized (reticular myoclonus) or segmental (e.g., *ocular-palatal-pharyngeal myoclonus*). Palatal myoclonus is rhythmical (approximately 2 Hz) and can be primary or secondary. The secondary form is more common and results from a lesion within the Guillain-Mollaret triangle encompassing the dentate, red, and inferior olivary nuclei. This results in an interruption of the dentato-olivary pathway, leading to denervation of the olives, which become hypertrophic and visualized by MRI. Vascular lesions and multiple sclerosis are common causes of secondary palatal myoclonus that persists during sleep. This disorder is commonly associated with vertical rhythmical ocular movements, also occurring at 2 Hz, so-called ocular myoclonus. Primary palatal myoclonus is of unknown cause and is often associated with annoying constant clicking sounds in the ear caused by contractions of the tensor veli palatini muscles, which open the eustachian tubes. Primary palatal myoclonus disappears during sleep.

Myoclonus arising from the spinal cord is of two clinical types. *Spinal segmental myoclonus* is rhythmic and persists during sleep, whereas *propriospinal myoclonus* causes truncal flexion jerks, usually triggered by a stimulus, such as when eliciting the knee jerk. In propriospinal myoclonus, the first muscles activated are usually from the thoracic cord, with slow upward and downward spread. Myoclonic jerks can sometimes arise from a peripheral nerve, plexus, or spinal root.

Myoclonus can be classified into the following etiologic categories: physiologic myoclonus, essential myoclonus, epileptic myoclonus, and symptomatic dystonia, which seems to be the same entity as myoclonus-dystonia. Epileptic myoclonus occurs in patients whose main complaint is epilepsy but who also have myoclonus. Examples of physiologic myoclonus include sleep jerks and hiccough. Essential myoclonus may be familial or sporadic, is not associated with other neurologic abnormalities, and does not have a progressive course. Some patients with essential myoclonus have features of dystonia.

Symptomatic myoclonus is the largest etiologic group. In this category, myoclonus occurs as part of a more widespread encephalopathy, including storage diseases, spinocerebellar degenerations, dementias, infectious encephalopathies, metabolic encephalopathies, toxic encephalopathies, physical encephalopathies (e.g., posthypoxic and posttraumatic), and with focal brain damage. The infectious encephalopathy of Whipple disease features a facial myoclonus referred to as oculofacial-masticatory myorhythmia; other common features include supranuclear vertical gaze palsy and cognitive changes.

Encephalomyelitis with rigidity is a severe sudden-onset variant of the stiff-person syndrome and is denoted by stiffness and excessive startle and stimulus-triggered myoclonic jerks; it often responds to steroid therapy. Degenerative disorders include Lafora disease and dentatorubropallidoluysian atrophy, as well as the dementias of Creutzfeldt-Jakob and Alzheimer disease. Among the toxic encephalopathies is the *serotonin syndrome* owing to medications that produce excessive serotonergic stimulation; along with myoclonus there is diaphoresis, flushing, rigidity, hyperreflexia, shivering, confusion, agitation, restlessness, coma, and autonomic instability.

Thus, myoclonus is classified by three different approaches (Table 111.1). What was previously called "nocturnal myoclonus" is now referred to as periodic movements of sleep, which accompanies the restless-legs syndrome.

An uncommon form of myoclonus is *polyminimyoclonus*, in which the jerks are of small amplitude, resembling irregular tremor that is continuous and generalized. The eyes are often involved with spontaneous, irregular, chaotic saccades. Because the dancing eyes are known as *opsoclonus*, the term *opsoclonus-myoclonus syndrome* is sometimes applied. First described as part

▶ TABLE 111.1 Classification of Myoclonus

Clinical	*Anatomic*	*Etiology*
1. At rest action reflex	1. Cortical Focal Multifocal Generalized Epilepsia partialis continua	1. Physiologic
		2. Essential
2. Focal axial multifocal generalized	2. Thalamic	3. Epileptic
		4. Symptomatic Storage diseases
3. Irregular oscillatory rhythmic	3. Brainstem Reticular Startle Palatal	Cerebellar degenerations Basal ganglia degenerations Dementias Infectious encephalopathy
	4. Spinal Segmental Propriospinal	Metabolic encephalopathy Toxic encephalopathy
	5. Peripheral	Hypoxia Focal damage

Myoclonus can be classified according to clinical features, by anatomic origin of the pathophysiology of the jerks, and by etiology.

of an encephalopathic picture in infants, particularly in association with a neuroblastoma, it also has been found in adults, usually as a paraneoplastic or postviral syndrome. The latter disorder is self-limiting after months or years. The paraneoplastic syndrome is associated with antineuronal antibodies and may remit on removal of the tumor.

Exaggerated startle syndromes, related to the myoclonias and of brainstem origin, consist of a sudden jump to an unexpected auditory, tactile, or visual stimulus. Included are a blink, contraction of the face, flexion of the neck and trunk, and abduction and flexion of the arms. The motor reaction can be either a short or a prolonged complex motor act; falling can result. Known as *hyperekplexia* (MIM 244100), this disorder can result from a brainstem disorder or can be primary and inherited as an autosomal dominant trait with mutations on chromosome 5q coding the α_1 subunit of the inhibitory glycine receptor. When hyperekplexia appears in infancy, it is sometimes called the stiff-baby syndrome because prolonged tonic spasms occur when the infant is handled. Apnea can occur during these spasms; the dibenzodiazepine, clobazam, has been reported to be an effective treatment. Certain excessive startle syndromes may be culturally related and also can manifest echolalia and automatic obedience. These syndromes are known by colorful regional names, such as *jumping Frenchmen of Maine* (Quebec), myriachit (Siberia), latah (Indonesia, Malaysia), and ragin' Cajun (Louisiana). Myoclonus and hyperekplexia can sometimes be controlled with the anticonvulsants clonazepam and valproic acid and with the serotonin precursor 5-hydroxytryptophan.

Treatment of myoclonus usually requires polypharmacy. The most successful medications have been sodium valproate, clonazepam, levetiracetam, and primidone.

SUGGESTED READINGS

Antel JP, Rasmussen T. Rasmussen's encephalitis and the new hat. *Neurology* 1996;46:9–11.

Asmus F, Zimprich A, Tezenas Du, et al. Myoclonus-dystonia syndrome: epsilon-sarcoglycan mutations and phenotype. *Ann Neurol* 2002;52:489–492.

Bodner RA, Lynch T, Lewis L, Kahn D. Serotonin syndrome. *Neurology* 1995;45:219–223.

Brown P. Myoclonus: a practical guide to drug therapy. *CNS Drugs* 1995;3:22–29.

Brown P, Rothwell JC, Thompson PD, et al. The hyperekplexias and their relationship to the normal startle reflex. *Brain* 1991;114:1903–1928.

Caviness JN. Myoclonus. *Mayo Clin Proc* 1996;71:679–688.

Caviness JN, Alving LI, Maranganore DM, et al. The incidence and prevalence of myoclonus in Olmsted County, Minnesota. *Mayo Clin Proc* 1999;74:565–569.

Caviness JN, Forsyth PA, Layton DD, et al. The movement disorder of adult opsoclonus. *Mov Disord* 1995;10:22–27.

Chan EM, Ackerley CA, Lohi H, et al. Laforin preferentially binds the neurotoxic starch-like polyglucosans, which form in its absence in progressive myoclonus epilepsy. *Hum Mol Genet* 2004;13:1117–1129.

Cockerell OC, Rothwell J, Thompson PD, et al. Clinical and physiological features of epilepsia partialis continua: cases ascertained in the UK. *Brain* 1996;119:393–407.

Deuschl G, Toro C, Vallssole J, et al. Symptomatic and essential palatal tremor. 1. Clinical, physiological and MRI analysis. *Brain* 1994;117:775–788.

Fahn S, Marsden CD, Van Woert NH, eds. Myoclonus. *Adv Neurol* New York: Raven Press, 1986.

Fahn S, Sjaastad O. Hereditary essential myoclonus in a large Norwegian family. *Mov Disord* 1991;6:237–247.

Frucht SJ, Louis ED, Chuang C, et al. A pilot tolerability and efficacy study of levetiracetam in patients with chronic myoclonus. *Neurology* 2001;57:1112–1114.

Frucht SJ, Trost M, Ma Y, et al. The metabolic topography of posthypoxic myoclonus. *Neurology* 2004;62:1879–1881.

Hallett M. Electrodiagnosis in movement disorders. In: Levin KH and Lüders HO, eds. *Comprehensive Clinical Neurophysiology*. Philadelphia: WB Saunders, 2000:281–294.

Hammer MS, Larsen MB, Stack CV. Outcome of children with opsoclonus-myoclonus regardless of etiology. *Pediatr Neurol* 1995;13:21–24.

Ikeda A, Kakigi R, Funai N, et al. Cortical tremor: a variant of cortical reflex myoclonus. *Neurology* 1990;40:1561–1565.

Lance JW, Adams RD. The syndrome of intention or action myoclonus as a sequel to hypoxic encephalopathy. *Brain* 1963;86:111–136.

Louis ED, Lynch T, Kaufmann P, et al. Diagnostic guidelines in central nervous system Whipple's disease. *Ann Neurol* 1996;40:561–568.

Magaudda A, Gelisse P, Genton P. Antimyoclonic effect of levetiracetam in 13 patients with Unverricht-Lundborg disease: clinical observations. *Epilepsia* 2004;45:678–681.

Marsden CD, Hallett M, Fahn S. The nosology and pathophysiology of myoclonus. In: Marsden CD, Fahn S, eds. *Movement Disorders*. London: Butterworths, 1982:196–248.

Marsden CD, Harding AE, Obeso JA, et al. Progressive myoclonic ataxia (the Ramsay Hunt syndrome). *Arch Neurol* 1990;47:1121–1125.

Obeso JA, Artieda J, Burleigh A. Clinical aspects of negative myoclonus. *Adv Neurol* 1995;67:1–7.

Rio J, Montalban J, Pujadas F, et al. Asterixis associated with anatomic cerebral lesions: a study of 45 cases. *Acta Neurol Scand* 1995;91:377–381.

Scarcella A, Coppola G. Neonatal sporadic hyperekplexia: a rare and often unrecognized entity. *Brain Dev* 1997;19:226–228.

Shiang R, Ryan SG, Zhu YZ, et al. Mutations in the alpha 1 subunit of the inhibitory glycine receptor cause the dominant neurologic disorder, hyperekplexia. *Nat Genet* 1993;5:351–358.

Tijssen MA, Vergouwe MN, van Dijk JG, et al. Major and minor form of hereditary hyperekplexia. *Mov Disord* 2002;17:826–30.

Chapter 112

▶ Gilles de la Tourette Syndrome

Stanley Fahn

The Gilles de la Tourette syndrome (MIM 137580), commonly shortened to *Tourette syndrome*, is a neurobehavioral disorder consisting of both multiple motor and phonic tics that change in character over time, beginning before 21 years of age, and with symptoms that wax and wane but last more than 1 year. Many patients have a behavioral component of obsessive-compulsive, attention deficit disorder or poor impulse control. Although the definition is a useful criterion for research on the disorder, it excludes chronic motor tics or an onset beyond the age of 21 years. It is likely that these situations represent milder expressions of Tourette syndrome. Tourette syndrome is the most common cause of tics; other causes include neuroacanthocytosis, encephalitis, neuroleptics, and head trauma.

Tics range from intermittent simple brief jerks to a complex pattern of rapid, coordinated, involuntary movements, often preceded by an unpleasant sensation that is relieved by the movement. Although tics usually can be suppressed for short periods of time, the inner sensation builds up, consequently leading to a burst of tics when the patient stops suppressing them. Tics usually begin in the face (eye blinking, grimacing) and neck (head shaking). They may spread to involve the limbs and may be accompanied by sounds (sniffing, throat clearing, barking, words, or parts of words) and sometimes by foul utterances (coprolalia). Repeating sounds (echolalia) or movements (echopraxia) are sometimes seen. The speed of tics ranges from very fast (clonic tics) to sustained contractions (dystonic tics). Simple clonic tics resemble essential myoclonus, and the two conditions are difficult to distinguish. Dystonic tics need to be differentiated from primary torsion dystonia. Sydenham chorea is distinct in manifesting as a continuous restless type of movement pattern, and it is self-limited. Premonitory sensations, intermittency, and suppressibility help distinguish tics from most other movement disorders. On average, tics begin around age 5 years and increase in severity, reaching their most intense period around age 10. After the most severe period, there is usually a steady decline in tic severity. By age 18 years, nearly half of the patients are virtually free from tics.

Estimates of prevalence rates of tics have varied broadly, depending on clinical definitions and how the study was carried out. One conservative result provides prevalence in adolescents of about 5 per 10,000 in males and 3 per 10,000 in females. Volumetric MRI has shown inconsistent asymmetries in the basal ganglia. In patients who have come to necropsy, no specific morphologic changes in the brain have been noted. Because dopamine receptor blocking drugs can suppress tics, supersensitive dopamine receptors had long been suspected, but postmortem binding studies of dopamine receptors failed to provide support for this hypothesis. PET studies, however, suggest there is increased dopamine storage and release in striatum.

An immune hypothesis proposes that the Tourette syndrome is sometimes owing to infection with β-hemolytic streptococcus, as seen in children who develop Sydenham chorea. Known as a pediatric autoimmune neuropsychiatric disorder associated with streptococcus infections (PANDAS), this proposal for Tourette syndrome has been controversial, and there have been conflicting results from studies testing antistriatal antibodies. The search for genetic mutations, fruitless for years, eventually led to finding linkage in a large French Canadian family to chromosome 11q23 and to finding susceptibility loci in Afrikaner families to chromosomes 2p11, 8q22, and 11q23-24.

When tics are mild and not socially disabling, no treatment is required. When they are more severe, motor and phonic tics can sometimes be reduced with clonidine or clonazepam. Dopamine antagonists and depletors are more effective but often have more adverse effects. The antagonists can cause the more serious complication of tardive dystonia and thus should be reserved as a last resort. Attention deficit and obsessive-compulsive disorders are usually a greater social problem than are the tics.

SUGGESTED READINGS

Albin RL, Koeppe RA, Bohnen NI, et al. Increased ventral striatal monoaminergic innervation in Tourette syndrome. *Neurology* 2003; 61:310–315.

Church AJ, Dale RC, Lees AJ, et al. Tourette's syndrome: a cross sectional study to examine the PANDAS hypothesis. *J Neurol Neurosurg Psychiatry* 2003;74:602–607.

Cohen DJ, Jankovic J, Goetz CG, eds. *Tourette Syndrome, Adv Neurol*, Vol. 85, Philadelphia: Lippincott Williams & Wilkins, 2001.

Comings DE, Himes JA, Comings BG. An epidemiologic study of Tourette's syndrome in a single school district. *J Clin Psychiatry* 1990; 51:463–469.

Diaz-Anzaldua A, Joober R, Riviere JB, et al. Tourette syndrome and dopaminergic genes: a family-based association study in the French Canadian founder population. *Molec Psychiat* 2004;9(Mar):272–277.

Fahn S. Motor and vocal tics. In: Kurlan R, ed. *Handbook of Tourette's Syndrome and Related Tic and Behavioral Disorders*. New York: Marcel Dekker, 1993.

Kurlan R, ed. *Handbook of Tourette's Syndrome and Related Tic and Behavioral Disorders*. New York: Marcel Dekker, 1993.

Leckman JF, Zhang HP, Vitale A, et al. Course of tic severity in Tourette syndrome: the first two decades. *Pediatrics* 1998;102:14–19.

Loiselle CR, Lee O, Moran TH, et al. Striatal microinfusion of Tourette syndrome and PANDAS sera: failure to induce behavioral changes. *Mov Disord* 2004;19:390–396.

Loiselle CR, Wendlandt JT, Rohde CA, et al. Antistreptococcal, neuronal, and nuclear antibodies in Tourette syndrome. *Pediatr Neurol* 2003;28:119–125.

Merette C, Brassard A, Potvin A, et al. Significant linkage for Tourette syndrome in a large French Canadien family. *Am J Hum Genet* 2000;67:1008–1013.

Peterson BS. Neuroimaging studies of Tourette syndrome: a decade of progress. *Adv Neurol* 2001;85:179–196.

Simonic I, Nyholt DR, Gericke GS, et al. Further evidence for linkage of Gilles de la Tourette syndrome (GTS) susceptibility loci on chromosomes 2p11, 8q22, and 11q23-24 in South African Afrikaners. *Am J Med Genet* 2001;105:163–167.

Singer HS. Current issues in Tourette syndrome. *Mov Disord* 2000;15: 1051–1063.

Singer HS, Loiselle CR, Lee O, et al. Anti-basal ganglia antibodies in PANDAS. *Mov Disord* 2004;19:406–415.

Singer HS, Szymanski S, Giuliano J, et al. Elevated intrasynaptic dopamine release in Tourette's syndrome measured by PET. *Am J Psychiatry* 2002;159:1329–1336.

Tourette Syndrome Classification Study Group. Definitions and classification of tic disorders. *Arch Neurol* 1993;50:1013–1016.

Chapter 113

Dystonia

Stanley Fahn and Susan B. Bressman

After parkinsonism, dystonia is the movement disorder most commonly encountered in movement disorder clinics. The term *dystonia* was coined by Oppenheim in 1911 to indicate that the disorder he was describing manifested hypotonia at one occasion and tonic muscle spasms at another, usually but not exclusively elicited on volitional movements. Although the term *dystonia* has undergone various definitions since 1911, today it is defined as a syndrome of sustained muscle contractions, frequently causing twisting and repetitive movements or abnormal postures. Limb, axial, and cranial voluntary muscles can all be affected by dystonia. The involuntary movements are often exacerbated during voluntary movements, so-called *action dystonia*. If the dystonic contractions appear only with a specific action, it is referred to as *task-specific dystonia* (e.g., writer's cramp and musician's cramp). As the dystonic condition progresses, voluntary movements in parts of the body not affected with dystonia can induce dystonic movements of the involved body part, so-called *overflow*. Talking is the most common activity that causes overflow dystonia in other body parts. With further worsening, the affected part can develop dystonic movements while at rest. Thus, dystonia at rest is usually more severe

than pure action dystonia. Sustained abnormal postures of affected body parts may be the eventual outcome.

Dystonic movements tend to increase with fatigue, stress, and emotional states; they tend to be suppressed with relaxation, hypnosis, and sleep. Dystonia often disappears during deep sleep, unless the movements are extremely severe. A characteristic and almost unique feature of dystonic movements is that they can be diminished by tactile or proprioceptive "sensory tricks" (geste antagoniste). For example, patients with cervical dystonia (torticollis) often place a hand on the chin or side of the face to reduce nuchal contractions, and orolingual dystonia is often helped by touching the lips or placing an object in the mouth. Lying down may reduce truncal dystonia; walking backward or running may reduce leg dystonia.

Rapid muscle spasms that occur in a repetitive pattern may be present in torsion dystonia; when rhythmic, the term *dystonic tremor* is applied. Rarely, some children and adolescents with primary or secondary dystonia may experience a crisis, a sudden increase in the severity of dystonia, which has been called *dystonic storm* or *status dystonicus*. It can cause myoglobinuria with a threat of death by renal failure. Placing the patient in an intensive care unit for barbiturate narcosis is usually necessary for relief.

CLASSIFICATION OF TORSION DYSTONIA

To emphasize the twisting quality of the abnormal movements and postures, the term *torsion* is often placed in front of the word dystonia. Torsion dystonia is classified in three ways: age at onset, body distribution of abnormal movements, and etiology (Table 113.1). Age at onset is the most important factor related to prognosis of primary dystonia. As a general rule, the younger the age at onset, the more likely the dystonia will become severe and spread to multiple parts of the body. In contrast, the older the age at

▶ **TABLE 113.1 Classifications of Torsion Dystonia**

By age at onset
Childhood onset, 0–12 yr
Adolescent onset, 13–20 yr
Adult onset, >20 yr

By distribution
Focal
Segmental
Multifocal
Generalized
Hemidystonia

By etiology
Primary (also known as idiopathic) dystonia
Dystonia plus
Secondary dystonia
Heredodegenerative diseases (usually presents as dystonia plus)

onset, the more likely dystonia will remain focal. Onset of dystonia in a leg is the second most important predictive factor for a more rapidly progressive course.

Because dystonia usually begins in a single body part, and because dystonia either remains focal or spreads to other body parts, it is useful to classify dystonia according to anatomic distribution. *Focal dystonia* affects only a single area. Frequently seen types of focal dystonia have specific labels: blepharospasm, torticollis, oromandibular dystonia, spastic dysphonia, writer's cramp, or occupational cramp. If dystonia spreads, it usually affects a contiguous body part. When dystonia affects two or more contiguous parts of the body, it is *segmental dystonia*. *Generalized dystonia* is a combination of leg involvement plus some other area. *Multifocal dystonia* fills a gap in the preceding designations, describing involvement of two or more noncontiguous parts. Dystonia affecting one half of the body is *hemidystonia*, which is usually symptomatic rather than primary. Adult-onset dystonia is much more often focal than generalized.

The most common focal dystonia is cervical dystonia (torticollis), followed by dystonias of cranial muscles: blepharospasm, spasmodic dysphonia, or oromandibula dystonia. Less common is arm dystonia, such as writer's cramp. The most common segmental dystonia involves the cranial muscles (Meige syndrome) or cranial and neck muscles (cranial-cervical dystonia).

The etiologic classification identifies four major categories: primary, dystonia-plus syndromes, secondary (environmental causes), and heredodegenerative diseases. *Primary dystonia* (familial or sporadic) is a pure dystonia (except that tremor may be present). *Dystonia-plus* syndromes are related to the primary dystonias in this classification scheme because neither type is neurodegenerative. Dystonia-plus syndromes include symptoms and signs in addition to dystonia; for instance, dopa-responsive dystonia includes parkinsonism and myoclonus-dystonia includes myoclonus. *Secondary dystonias* are owing to environmental insult. *Heredodegenerative dystonias* are neurodegenerative diseases usually inherited; these conditions usually have other neurologic features in addition to dystonia. Known genetic causes of dystonia can be found in primary, dystonia-plus, and heredodegenerative forms (Table 113.2).

▶ **TABLE 113.2 Gene Nomenclature for the Dystonias**

Name	Locus	Inheritance Pattern	Phenotype	Protein
DYT1	9q34	AD	Young, limb onset (Oppenheim)	torsinA
DYT2	?	AR	Early onset	?
DYT3	Xq13.1	XR	Filipino, dystonia/parkinsonism (lubag)	Multiple transcript system
DYT4	?	AD	Whispering dysphonia	?
DYT5	14q22.1	AD	DRD/parkinsonism (Segawa)	GCH-1
DYT6	8p	AD	Mixed type, Mennonite/Amish	?
DYT7	18p	AD	Adult cervical	?
DYT8	2q33-q35	AD	PNKD (FDP1) (Mount-Rebak)	?
DYT9	1p21	AD	CSE, episodic choreoathetosis with spasticity	?
DYT10	16	AD	PKD (EKD1 and 2)	?
DYT11	7q21	AD	Myoclonus-dystonia	ε-Sarcoglycan
DYT12	19q	AD	Rapid-onset dystonia-parkinsonism	?
DYT13	1p36	AD	Cervical/cranial/brachial	?
DYT14	14q13	AD	DRD	?
DYT15	18p11	AD	Myoclonus-dystonia	?

Genetic nomenclature is presented in the chronologic order named. The DYT1 gene has a deletion of one of a sequential pair of GAG triplets. DYT2 was set aside for any possible autosomal recessive forms, and two families are considered possible. DYT3 is for changes in the multiple transcript system that is associated with X-linked dystonia-parkinsonism, also known as lubag, and encountered in Filipino males. DYT4 was labeled for an Australian family with dystonia, including a whispering dysphonia. DYT5 is for the GCHI gene mutations causing DRD. DYT6 is the gene causing an adult- and childhood-onset dystonia of both limbs and cranial structures ("mixed"), so far seen in a large Mennonite/Amish kindred. DYT7 is for familial torticollis in a family from northwest Germany. DYT8–10 are for paroxysmal dyskinesias; 8 is for nonkinesigenic type, known as the Mount-Rebak syndrome; 9 is for a family with episodic choreoathetosis and spasticity; 10 is reserved for what appear to be two genes for paroxysmal kinesigenic dyskinesia on chromosome 16. DYT11 has been named for mutations in the ε-sarcoglycan gene that cause myoclonus-dystonia. DYT12 is for a gene mapped to chromosome 19q causing rapid-onset dystonia-parkinsonism. DYT13 is for a gene mapped to 1p36 causing cervical-cranial-brachial dystonia in a family in Italy. DYT14 is for a family with DRD linked to 14q13. DYT15 is for a myoclonus-dystonia family mapped to 18p11.

AD, autosomal dominant; AR, autosomal recessive; XR, X-linked recessive; DRD, dopa-responsive dystonia; PKND, paroxysmal nonkinesignic dyskinesia; FDP1, familial paroxysmal dyskinesia type 1; CSE, choreoathetosis/spasticity episodic; PKD, paroxysmal kinesignic dyskinesia; RDP, rapid-onset dystonia parkinsonism.

PRIMARY TORSION DYSTONIAS

Primary torsion dystonias (PTD) comprise familial and nonfamilial (sporadic) types. Neurologic abnormality is restricted to dystonic postures and movements except that there may be a tremor resembling essential tremor. Within the primary dystonias are several identified genetic disorders and four gene loci (DYT1, DYT6, DYT7, and DYT13). But the causes of most primary dystonias still unknown.

Oppenheim Dystonia (DYT1)

The gene at the DYT1 locus has been identified and causes the dystonia described by Oppenheim. In most patients with DYT1 dystonia, symptoms begin in childhood or adolescence, and the mean age at onset is 13 years. Symptoms rarely begin after age 26 years, although onset as late as 64 may occur. In most patients, first symptoms involve an arm or leg, with rare cases beginning in the cervical or cranial muscles. About 65% of all DYT1 patients progress to a generalized or multifocal distribution, but the proportion progressing is even higher for those with childhood onset. About 10% have segmental dystonia and 25% only focal involvement. Most of those with focal dystonia have writer's cramp, but isolated cervical (torticollis) and upper facial (blepharospasm) dystonia have been reported. In terms of body regions ultimately involved, one or more limbs are affected in the vast majority, with over 95% having an affected arm. The trunk and neck are affected in 25% to 35%, and they may be the regions producing the greatest disability; the cranial muscles are less likely to be involved. Also, there may be great intrafamilial variability, ranging for no dystonia (70% of gene carriers have no dystonia) to mild writer's cramp to severe generalized dystonia. When dystonia begins in a leg, it usually starts as an action dystonia resulting in a peculiar twisting of the leg when the child walks forward, even though walking backward, running, or dancing may still be normal. Bizarre stepping or a bowing gait may be noted when the dystonic movements affect proximal muscles of the leg. Difficulty in placing the heel on the ground is evident when distal muscles are affected (Fig. 113.1). As the disorder progresses, the movements may appear when the leg is at rest; the foot may be plantar flexed and ankle everted or inverted; the knee and hip often assume a flexed posture.

With arm involvement, action dystonia may interfere with writing; the fingers curl, the wrist flexes and pronates, the triceps contracts, and the elbow elevates. Dystonic tremor of the arm is common, with features of both postural and action tremors. With progression, other activities of the arm are impaired; the arm often moves backward behind the body when the patient walks. Later, dystonia may be present when the arm is at rest.

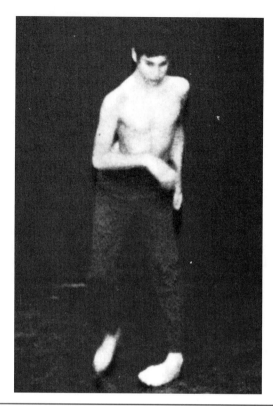

FIGURE 113.1. Generalized dystonia with involvement of the legs, trunk, and arms. Patient is still able to walk.

As the dystonia becomes worse, the contractions become constant so that instead of moving, the body part remains in a fixed twisted posture. The trunk may develop wiggling movements and fixed scoliosis, lordosis, and tortipelvis. The neck may become involved with torticollis, anterocollis, retrocollis, or head tilt and shift. Facial grimacing and difficulties in speech may occur but are much less common. Although muscle tone and power seem normal, the involuntary movements interfere and make voluntary activity extremely difficult. In general, mental activity is normal, and there are no alterations in tendon reflexes or sensation. The rate of progression of this type is extremely variable; in most cases generalized spread occurs within the first 5 to 10 years followed by a static phase, but late worsening, especially more forceful contractions in a body region already affected, may occur. The continuous spasms result in marked distortion of the body to a degree rarely seen in any other disease (Fig. 113.2). With active treatment, it is now uncommon to encounter the severe deformities seen before the 1980s.

Oppenheim dystonia is an autosomal dominant disorder with markedly reduced penetrance of 30% to 40%. The DYT1 gene is localized to chromosome 9q34.1 and encodes the protein torsinA. There is only one DYT1 mutation that has been associated oligomeric complexes with dystonia

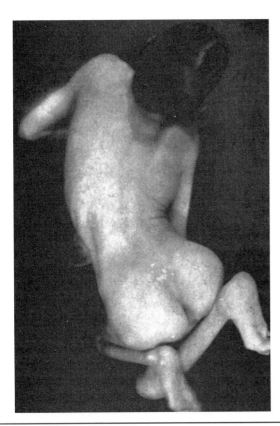

FIGURE 113.2. An advanced state of generalized dystonia with fixed postures: torticollis, scoliosis, tortipelvis, and limb dystonia.

a 3-bp (GAG) deletion resulting in the loss of a glutamic acid. TorsinA shows homology to the AAA+ superfamily of ATPases. Typically, AAA+ proteins form oligomeric complexes and may have roles in protein folding and degradation, cytoskeletal dynamics, membrane trafficking and vesicle fusion, and response to stress. The function of torsinA remains unknown. Both the message and protein are widely distributed in neurons throughout the brain, with most intense expression in substantia nigra compacta dopamine neurons.

Oppenheim dystonia affects most ethnic groups, but is particularly prevalent in the Ashkenazi Jewish population, in which the prevalence is about 1 per 6,000. The increased prevalence is attributed to a founder mutation that was introduced into the population living in Lithuania and Byelorussia about 350 to 400 years ago.

Because all DYT1 cases, Jewish and non-Jewish, are owing to one recurring mutation, screening for the mutation is straightforward. Genetic testing is recommended for all patients with primary dystonia and an onset before age 26 years, regardless of family history. It is also advised for those with later onset who have a relative with early onset as well as those with writer's cramp and those whose age at onset is difficult to ascertain. Genetic counseling should accompany testing; DYT1 has low penetrance and variable expression and does not account for all genetic causes of primary dystonia; these complex issues require discussion with patients and their family members.

Other Early-Onset Non-DYT1 Primary Dystonias

DYT1 accounts for most childhood- and adolescent-onset primary dystonia in Ashkenazi Jews and about 30% to 50% in non-Jews. Therefore, DYT1 has been excluded in a significant proportion of early-onset primary dystonia patients and families. Although some families are clinically similar to DYT1, other families have autosomal-dominant inheritance of a somewhat different family phenotype. Dystonia begins on average several years later with a higher proportion having adult onset, there is greater involvement of muscles in the cranial-cervical region, and there is a greater likelihood of dystonia remaining localized as focal and segmental. In two large related Amish or Mennonite families with this phenotype, a gene called DYT6 was mapped to chromosome 8p21-q22. Many affected individuals in this kindred were disabled by dysphonia, dysarthria, and cervical dystonia. Another locus, DYT13, was mapped to 1p36 in an Italian family with autosomal-dominant inheritance. In this family dystonia usually started with jerky movements of the neck and shoulder, there was variable spread to cranial and brachial muscles, and in most disability was mild.

ADULT ONSET PRIMARY DYSTONIA

Most primary dystonias are of adult onset. The precise prevalence is not known, but it is about 30 per 100,000 population in Rochester, Minnesota. These dystonias usually remain localized to the muscles (and immediately contiguous muscles) first involved (i.e., focal and segmental dystonia). Common sites are neck (cervical dystonia), face (blepharospasm), jaw (oromandibular dystonia), vocal cords (spastic dysphonia), and arm (writer's cramp).

Family studies have demonstrated an increased rate of dystonia among family members, suggesting a genetic etiology. With equal rates in parents, offspring, and siblings, the pattern of transmission is consistent with autosomal dominant inheritance; however, it seems to be much less penetrant than childhood-onset dystonia, with penetrance rates of only 10% to 15% rather than 30% to 40% and few with higher penetrance. In one such family with cervical dystonia, a locus, DYT7 on chromosome 18p, was mapped. This locus has been excluded in other adult-onset families, so its role in primary dystonia is not known. Association studies to assess the role of candidate genes have implicated the D5 dopamine receptor gene. Other possible causes of adult-onset PTD include dysfunction of mitochondrial complex I and copper metabolism.

Cervical dystonia, commonly known as *spasmodic torti-collis* or *wry neck*, is the most common focal dystonia. It occurs at any age, usually beginning between ages 20 and 60, and is more frequent in women. Any combination of neck muscles can be involved, especially the sternocleido-mastoid, trapezius, splenius capitus, levator scapulae, and scalenus muscles. Sustained turning, tilting, flexing, or ex-tending the neck or shifting the head laterally or anteriorly can result (Fig. 113.3). The shoulder is usually elevated and anteriorly displaced on the side to which the chin turns. Instead of sustained deviation of the head, some patients have jerking movements of the head. Neck pain occurs in about two-thirds of patients with cervical dystonia and usually responds successfully to injections of botulinum toxin at the site of the pain. A common sensory trick to relieve cervical dystonia is the placement of one hand on the back of the head or on the chin. About 10% of patients with cervical dystonia have a remission, usually within a year of onset; most remissions are followed by a relapse years later.

Some patients with torticollis have a horizontal head tremor that may be impossible to distinguish from es-sential tremor. Other considerations in the differential di-agnosis of dystonic torticollis are congenital contracture of the sternocleidomastoid muscle, which can be treated with surgical release. In young boys after a full meal, ex-treme head tilt may be caused by gastroesophageal reflux (*Sandifer syndrome*), which can be treated by plication

surgery. Other diagnostic considerations are trochlear nerve palsy; Arnold-Chiari malformation; malformations of the cervical spine, such as Klippel-Feil fusion or at-lantoaxial subluxation; cervical infections; and spasms from cervical muscle shortening.

Blepharospasm is caused by contraction of the orbic-ularis oculi muscles. It usually begins with increased fre-quency of blinking, followed by closure of the eyelids, then more firm and prolonged closure of the lids, which may produce functional blindness if untreated. Blinking and lid closure can be intermittent and are often temporarily sup-pressed by talking, humming, singing, or looking down. The condition is worsened by walking and by bright light. A common sensory trick that relieves contractions is plac-ing of a finger just lateral to the orbit. Blepharospasm is usually accompanied by cocontraction of lower facial mus-cles, such as the platysma and risorius. This type of focal dystonia sometimes becomes segmental by spreading to other cranial targets, such as the jaw, tongue, vocal cords, or cervical muscles. The combination of blepharospasm with other cranial dystonias is called *Meige syndrome*. Blepharospasm occurs more often in women than in men, usually beginning after age 50, although younger people may be affected. Abnormalities of the blink reflex have been found with blepharospasm and with other cranial or cervical dystonias.

The differential diagnosis of blepharospasm includes *hemifacial* spasm, which is unilateral. Rarely, hemifacial spasm is bilateral, but the contractions on the two sides of the face are not synchronous as they are in blepharospasm. *Blinking tics* can resemble blepharospasm, but tics almost always begin in childhood. *Sjögren syndrome* of dry eyes often causes the eyelids to close, but testing for tear pro-duction usually distinguishes this disorder. Injections of botulinum toxin are effective in >80% of patients with blepharospasm.

Writer's cramp of adult onset usually remains limited to one limb, usually the dominant side. In about 15% of cases, it spreads to the other arm. When it affects only writing, the patient may learn to write with the nondominant hand. For bilateral involvement or for dystonia that affects other activities (buttoning, shaving, or playing a musical instru-ment), carefully placed injections of botulinum toxin may be effective.

Dystonia of the vocal cords occurs in two forms. The more common type is *spastic (spasmodic) dysphonia* in which the vocalis muscles contract, bringing the vocal cords together and causing the voice to be restricted, strangled, and coarse, often broken up with pauses. *Breathy (whispering) dysphonia* is caused by contractions of the posterior cricoarytenoids (abductor muscles of the vocal cords), so that the patient cannot talk in a loud voice and tends to run out of air while trying to speak. Spas-tic dysphonia is often associated with tremor of the vo-cal cords. Essential tremor (with vocal cord tremor) is an

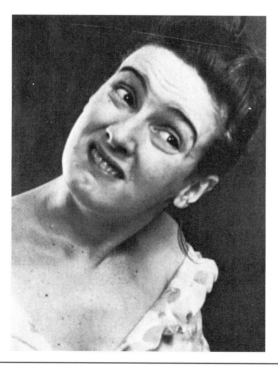

FIGURE 113.3. Spasmodic torticollis with some dystonia of facial muscles (segmental dystonia).

important differential diagnosis; the presence of tremor in the hands or neck leads to such diagnosis. Injections of botulinum toxin can be dramatically effective for spastic dysphonia, but are less certain for breathy dysphonia. For each type, a physician must be experienced with the procedure of injecting the correct muscle.

Pathology and Pathophysiology of Primary Dystonia

The pathology of the primary torsion dystonias is unknown. Gross examination of the brain and histologic studies by light microscopy do not reveal any consistent morphologic changes; thus, these disorders are not considered progressively degenerative. Yet striatal and dopamine dysfunction have long been suspected to play an important role in causation based on the pathologies and causes of nonprimary dystonias. For example, pathology involving the lentiform nucleus occurs in neurodegeneration with brain iron accumulation, Wilson disease, glutaric aciduria, and infarction resulting in dystonia. Dystonia may also be caused by conditions that perturb normal dopamine transmission, such as acute and tardive dystonia owing to dopamine blocking agents, levodopa-induced dyskinesias in Parkinson disease, and dopa-responsive dystonia owing to enzyme defects in the biosynthesis of dopamine.

Recently there has been some pathological support for striatal abnormalities in primary dystonia. A study of DYT1 brains did not show degeneration but did find evidence for increased turnover of dopamine. Transcranial sonography of primary dystonia patients identified hyperechogenic changes in the lenticular nucleus, and pathological studies of the brains of a small number of patients with adult-onset focal dystonia found increased lentiform copper and abnormalities of proteins involved in copper metabolism. There is, however, a paucity of pathological studies in primary dystonia, and further studies are needed.

The electromyogram in the dystonias shows cocontraction of agonist and antagonist muscles with prolonged bursts and overflow to extraneous muscles. Spinal and brainstem reflex abnormalities, including reduced reciprocal inhibition and protracted blink reflex recovery, indicate a reduced presynaptic inhibition of muscle afferent input to the inhibitory interneurons as a result of defective descending motor control. The sensorimotor cerebral cortex shows an increased region of activation related to the affected body part. PET studies found increased metabolic activity in the lentiform nuclei. In DYT1 dystonia, two patterns of abnormal metabolic activity have been found. In nonmanifesting carriers and in affected carriers who are asleep, there is hypermetabolism of the lentiform, cerebellum, and supplementary motor cortex. On the other hand, in DYT1 patients having active muscle contractions,

metabolic activity is increased in the thalamus, cerebellum, and midbrain.

DYSTONIA-PLUS SYNDROMES

This category includes nondegenerative disorders in which parkinsonism (dopa-responsive dystonia and rapid-onset dystonia-parkinsonism) or myoclonus (myoclonus-dystonia) coexists with the dystonia.

Dopa-Responsive Dystonia

About 10% of patients with childhood-onset dystonia have the autosomal-dominant disorder *dopa-responsive dystonia* (DRD), sometimes called *Segawa disease*. Distinguishing DRD from PTD is important because DRD responds so well to treatment. It differs from primary dystonia by the signs of parkinsonism, which may be subtle. These include bradykinesia, cogwheel rigidity, and impaired postural reflexes. Other distinguishing features include: diurnal fluctuations with improvement after sleep and worsening as the day wears on; a peculiar "spastic" straight-legged gait, with a tendency to walk on the toes; hyperreflexia, particularly in the legs and sometimes with Babinski signs; and a remarkable therapeutic response to low doses of levodopa or anticholinergic drugs.

DRD usually begins between ages 6 and 16, but can appear at any age. When it begins in infants, it resembles cerebral palsy. When it begins in adults, it usually manifests as pure parkinsonism, mimicking Parkinson disease, responding to levodopa, and having a generally benign course. DRD affects girls more often than boys, has a worldwide distribution, and is not known to have a higher prevalence in any specific ethnic group. Mutations in the gene for GTP cyclohydrolase I (GCHI) located at 14q22.1 are responsible for the majority of DRD. In some patients other genetic etiologies can be found (e.g., recessively inherited mutations in tyrosine hydroxylase), but in others no genetic cause can be identified.

GCHI catalyzes the first and rate-limiting step in the biosynthesis of tetrahydrobiopterin (BH4), the cofactor required for the enzymes tyrosine hydroxylase, phenylalanine hydroxylase, and tryptophan hydroxylase. These hydroxylase enzymes add an $-OH$ group to the parent amino acid and are required for the synthesis of biogenic amines. The genetic label for DRD owing to GCH1 mutations is DYT5. A family with clinical and pathological features identical to DYT5 but linked to a different locus on chromosome 14q has been described and assigned DYT14.

Pathologic investigations of DRD revealed no loss of neurons within the substantia nigra pars compacta, but the cells are immature with little neuromelanin. Neuromelanin synthesis requires dopamine (or other monoamines) as the initial precursor. Biochemically, there is marked

▶ **TABLE 113.3** Differential Features Between Dopa-Responsive Dystonia (DRD), Oppenheim Torsion Dystonia (DYT1), and Juvenile Parkinson Disease (JPD)

	DRD	*DYT1*	*Juvenile PD/Parkin*
Average age at onset (range)	6 yr (infancy–6th decade)	13 years (4 yr–7th decade)	Adolescence (7 yr–6th decade)
Gender	Female > male	Female = male	Male = female
Initial signs	Leg > arm or trunk action dystonia, abnormal gait (scissoring, toe walking)	Arm or leg action dystonia, occasionally trunk or neck	Foot/leg > hand/arm dystonia, rest tremor (esp legs), akinesia/ridigity
Diurnal fluctuations	Often prominent	Rare	May occur
Bradykinesia	Yes (may be mild)	No	Yes
Postural instability	Occurs	No	Occurs
Response to l-dopa	Excellent to very low to low dose	Inconsistent and usually not dramatic	Excellent at low to moderate dose
Initial	Excellent		Dyskinesias, may fluctuate
Long term			
CSF			
HVA	⇓	=	⇓
Biopterin	⇓	=	⇓
Neopterin	⇓⇓	=	⇓
F-DOPA PET	Normal	Normal	Decreased
Inheritance	AD, reduced penetrance	AD, reduced penetrance	AR
Gene	Heterozygous mutations in GCH1 in many, rarely recessive GCH1 or TH	Heterozygous GAG deletion in DYT1	Homozygous or compound heterozygous parkin mutations
Testing	Screening for GCH1 mutations in select labs	Commercially available	Screening for parkin mutations in select labs
Prognosis	Return to near normal with RX in most	Progresses at first, then stabilizes	Slow to moderate progression

reduction of dopamine concentration and tyrosine hydroxylase activity within the striatum in DRD.

Aside from mutations in GCH1, DRD can rarely be caused by mutations in other enzymes involved in dopamine synthesis including tyrosine hydroxylase and pterin synthesis deficiencies. DRD owing to tyrosine hydroxylase deficiency is an autosomal-recessive disorder that begins in infancy or early childhood. The phenotype may mimic DRD, but clinical features range from a mild syndrome of spastic paraparesis to severe parkinsonism, dystonia, and oculogyric crises. Other features include ptosis, miosis, rigidity, hypokinesia, chorea, myoclonus, seizures, temperature disturbance, and hypersalivation. These latter features represent deficiencies of norepinephrine and serotonin in addition to dopamine; hyperphenylalaninemia is present, and the disorder may respond partially to levodopa.

Another disorder of infants is the autosomal-recessive deficiency of the enzyme aromatic L-amino acid decarboxylase, which catalyzes the transformation of levodopa to dopamine. Levodopa is ineffective in this disorder, but patients respond partially to dopamine agonists coupled with a monoamine oxidase inhibitor.

The most important differential diagnosis of DRD is juvenile parkinsonism, a progressive nigral degenerative disorder usually caused by homozygous or compound heterozygous mutations in the parkin gene. In this disorder, dystonia often precedes the parkinsonian features that become the major clinical feature. Distinguishing laboratory tests include fluorodopa PET and beta-CIT SPECT, which are normal in DRD but abnormal in juvenile parkinsonism, showing marked reduction of uptake in the striatum. A phenylalanine loading test has also been proposed; in DRD, there is a slower conversion to tyrosine. Other differential features of DRD from juvenile parkinsonism and Oppenheim dystonia are listed in Table 113.3.

One may also suspect DRD if a young patient with dystonia responds dramatically to low doses of anticholinergic agents. However, the most effective agent is levodopa. The suggested starting dose of carbidopa/levodopa for DRD is 12.5/50 mg two or three times a day, a dose low enough to avoid dyskinesias. The usual maintenance dose is 25/100 mg two or three times a day.

Rapid-Onset Dystonia-Parkinsonism

Rapid-onset dystonia-parkinsonism is an autosomal dominant disease; the gene has been mapped to 19q. Affected individuals develop dystonia and parkinsonism between ages 14 and 45 years, reaching maximum involvement of dystonia with parkinsonism in hours or days, usually associated with physical or emotional stress. Some affected family members have rapid worsening of baseline mild dystonia, paroxysmal attacks of dystonia, and seizures. The cerebrospinal fluid homovanillic acid concentration is low, there are no imaging abnormalities, and in the one autopsy no neurodegeneration was detected. There is no effective treatment.

Myoclonus-Dystonia

Although lightning-like movements occasionally occur in Oppenheim dystonia, they are a prominent feature in a distinct autosomal-dominant disorder known as myoclonus-dystonia (M-D). In families with M-D, affected individuals have myoclonus as the primary sign, and it may occur with or without dystonia; rarely, dystonia is the only feature as writer's cramp or torticollis. Symptom onset is usually in the first or second decade; males and females are equally affected in most families, and the pattern of inheritance is autosomal dominant with reduced penetrance that is dependent on the transmitting parent. That is, most affected individuals inherit the disorder through their father, indicating maternal imprinting of the disease gene. The neck and arms are involved most commonly, followed by the trunk and bulbar muscles, with less common involvement of the legs. The disorder tends to plateau in adulthood, and the muscle jerks respond dramatically to alcohol. Also, there appears to be an excess of psychiatric symptoms, including obsessive-compulsive disorder, in family members, even those not affected with motor signs of M-D.

A large proportion of familial M-D is owing to mutations in the ε-sarcoglycan gene mapped to chromosome 7q21 (DYT11). The sarcoglycans are a family of genes that encode components of the dystrophin-glycoprotein complex and mutations in alpha, beta, gamma, and delta sarcoglycan produce recessive muscular limb-girdle dystrophy. ε-sarcoglycan, however, is expressed widely in brain and is imprinted; its function and how the mutated protein produces M-D are still obscure.

Although many M-D families have mutations in ε-sarcoglycan, some families and sporadic cases do not appear to have mutations in this gene. Recently, a second locus on 18p, DYT15, was mapped in an M-D family.

SECONDARY DYSTONIA

Secondary dystonia is defined as a dystonic disorder that develops mainly as the result of environmental factors that affect the brain. Spinal cord injury and peripheral injury are also recognized causes of dystonia. Examples include levodopa-induced dystonia in the treatment of parkinsonism; acute and tardive dystonia owing to dopamine receptor blocking agents; and dystonias associated with cerebral palsy, cerebral hypoxia, cerebrovascular disease, cerebral

infectious and postinfectious states, brain tumor, and toxicants such as manganese, cyanide, and 3-nitroproprionic acid. Other causes include psychogenic disorders, peripheral trauma followed by focal dystonia in the affected region, head injury, and delayed-onset dystonia after cerebral infarct or other cerebral insult. Prior history of one of these insults suggests the correct diagnosis, as does neuroimaging that shows a lesion in the basal ganglia or their connections.

A more complete listing of secondary dystonias is presented in Table 113.4. A number of disorders in this group, such as the infectious and toxicant-induced neurodegenerations, are not limited to pure dystonia but show a mixture of other neurologic features, often the parkinsonian features bradykinesia and rigidity. *Tardive dystonia*, a persistent complication of agents that block dopamine receptors, is the most common form of secondary dystonia. Tardive dystonia is usually focal or segmental, affecting the cranial

▶ **TABLE 113.4 Causes of Secondary Dystonia**

Secondary dystonia
1. Perinatal cerebral injury
   a. Athetoid cerebral palsy
   b. Delayed onset dystonia
   c. Pachygyria
2. Encephalitis, infections, and postinfections
   a. Reye syndrome
   b. Subacute sclerosing leukoencephalopathy
   c. Wasp sting
   d. Creutzfeldt-Jakob disease
   e. HIV infection
3. Head trauma
4. Thalamotomy
5. Primary antiphospholipid syndrome
6. Focal cerebral vascular injury
7. Arteriovenous malformation
8. Hypoxia
9. Brain tumor
10. Multiple sclerosis
11. Brainstem lesion, including pontine myelinolysis
12. Posterior fossa tumors
13. Cervical cord injury or lesion
14. Lumbar canal stenosis
15. Peripheral injury
16. Electrical injury
17. Drug induced
    a. Levodopa
    b. Dopamine D2 receptor blocking agents
       1. Acute dystonic reaction
       2. Tardive dystonia
    c. Ergotism
    d. Anticonvulsants
18. Toxins—Mn, CO, carbon disulfide, cyanide, methanol, disulfiram, 3-nitroproprionic acid
19. Metabolic—hypoparathyroidism
20. Psychogenic

▶ TABLE 113.5 Clues Suggestive of Symptomatic Dystonia

1. History of possible etiologic factor, e.g., head trauma, peripheral trauma, encephalitis, toxin exposure, drug exposure, perinatal anoxia
2. Presence of neurologic abnormality, e.g., dementia, seizures, ocular, ataxia, weakness, spasticity, amyotrophy, parkinsonism
3. Onset of rest (instead of action) dystonia
4. Early onset of speech involvement
5. Leg involvement in an adult
6. Hemidystonia
7. Abnormal brain imaging
8. Abnormal laboratory workup
9. Presence of false weakness or sensory exam, or other clues of psychogenic etiology (see Table 113.6)

▶ TABLE 113.6 Clues Suggestive of Psychogenic Dystonia

Clues relating to the movements
1. Abrupt onset
2. Inconsistent movements (changing characteristics over time)
3. Incongruous movements and postures (movements do not fit with recognized patterns or with normal physiologic patterns)
4. Presence of additional types of abnormal movements that are not consistent with the basic abnormal movement pattern or are not congruous with a known movement disorder, particularly rhythmical shaking, bizarre gait, deliberate slowness carrying out requested voluntary movement, bursts of verbal gibberish, and excessive startle (bizarre movements in response to sudden unexpected noise or threatening movement)
5. Spontaneous remissions
6. Movements disappear with distraction
7. Response to placebo, suggestion, or psychotherapy
8. Present as a paroxysmal disorder
9. Dystonia beginning as a fixed posture
10. Twisting facial movements that move the mouth to one side or the other (Note: organic dystonia of the facial muscles usually does not move the mouth sideways)

Clues relating to the other medical observations
1. False weakness
2. False sensory complaints
3. Multiple somatizations or undiagnosed conditions
4. Self-inflicted injuries
5. Obvious psychiatric disturbances
6. Employment in the health profession or in insurance claims field
7. Presence of secondary gain, including continuing care by a "devoted" spouse
8. Litigation or compensation pending

structures in adults; in children, however, it can be generalized, involving the trunk and limbs. It often is associated with features of tardive dyskinesia, especially oral-buccal-lingual movements (see Chapter 117). Clues suggesting a secondary dystonia are listed in Table 113.5.

Psychogenic dystonia can be considered within the secondary dystonia category. For many decades, Oppenheim dystonia was considered psychogenic because of the bizarre nature of the symptoms, exaggeration in periods of stress, variability, and suppression by sensory tricks. This misdiagnosis often led to a long delay in identification of the nature of the disorder and to prolonged periods of needless psychotherapy. Awareness of the capricious nature of the disorder and serial observation of patients can avoid this pitfall. On the other hand, psychogenic dystonia does occur, but in less than 5% of patients who otherwise would be considered to have primary torsion dystonia. Clues suggestive of psychogenic dystonia are listed in Table 113.6.

HEREDODEGENERATIVE DYSTONIA

In this category, neurodegenerations produce dystonia as a prominent feature. Usually other neurologic features, especially parkinsonism, are also present and can predominate. In some patients with these disorders, dystonia may fail to appear, and other neurologic manifestations may be the presenting feature, for example, chorea in Huntington disease, in which dystonia may be a late-stage feature. Tremor or juvenile parkinsonism may be the mode of onset of Wilson disease, and dystonia may fail to appear in such patients. Because many of these neurodegenerations are a result of genetic abnormalities, the term *heredodegenerative* is applied to this category. However, some of the diseases listed here are of unknown etiology, and it is not clear what the role of genetics might be. For convenience, we place all the neurodegenerations in this category. These

are listed in Table 113.7 in which heredodegenerative disorders are organized by the nature of their genetics whenever the genes are known, followed by other neurodegenerations in which the etiology remains unknown.

An X-linked recessive disorder causing dystonia and parkinsonism affects young adult Filipino men. The Filipino name for the condition is *lubag*. It has been designated as DYT3. It can begin with dystonia in the feet or cranial structures; lingual and oromandibular dystonia are common, sometimes with stridor. With progression, generalized dystonia often develops. Many patients develop parkinsonism; in some patients, the sole manifestation may be progressive parkinsonism. The abnormal gene is localized to the centromeric region of the X chromosome, and disease-specific mutations have been identified in a system that involves the transcription of multiple genes. Pathologic study reveals a mosaic pattern of gliosis in the striatum. Patients respond only partially to levodopa, anticholinergics, baclofen, clonazepam, or zolpidem.

▶ **TABLE 113.7** Heredodegenerative diseases (typicaley not pure dystonia)

1. **Autosomal dominant**
   Huntington disease
   Machado-Joseph disease (SCA3)
   Other SCA subtypes (eg, SCA 2, 6, 17)
   Familial basal ganglia calcification (Fahr disease)
   Frontotemporal dementia (FTD)
   Dentatorubropallidoluysian atrophy (DRPLA)
   Neuroferritinopathy

2. **Autosomal recessive**
   Juvenile parkinsonism (parkin gene)
   Wilson disease
   Glutaric academia
   NBIA/PKAN (Hallervorden-Spatz disease)
   Gangliosidoses (GM1, GM2)
   Dystonic lipidosis/Niemann Pick type C (NPC1)
   Juvenile neuronal ceroid-lipofuscinosis
   Metachromatic leukodystrophy
   Homocystinuria
   Propionic acidemia
   Methylmalonic aciduria
   Hartnup disease
   Ataxia telangiectasia
   Ataxia with vitamin E deficiency
   Recessive ataxia with ocular apraxia
   Neuroacanthocytosis
   Neuronal intranuclear inclusion disease

3. **X-linked recessive**
   Lubag (X-linked dystonia-parkinsonism; DYT3)
   Pelizaeus-Merzbacher disease
   Deafness/dystonia syndrome
   Lesch-Nyhan syndrome

4. **Mitochondrial**
   Leigh disease
   Leber disease
   MERRF/MELAS

5. **Complex etiology (multifactorial)**
   Parkinson disease
   Progressive supranuclear palsy
   Multiple system atrophy
   Cortical-basal ganglionic degeneration

Adapted from Fahn et al. (1998).

OTHER DYSKINESIA SYNDROMES WITH DYSTONIA

Dystonia can appear in disorders not ordinarily considered to be part of torsion dystonia (Table 113.8). These include dystonic tics that are more conveniently classified with tic disorders (see Chapter 112), paroxysmal dyskinesias more conveniently classified with paroxysmal dyskinesias (see Chapter 9), and hypnogenic dystonia that can be either paroxysmal dyskinesias or seizures (see Chapter 9).

▶ **TABLE 113.8** Other Movement Disorders in Which Dystonia May be Present

Tic disorders with dystonic tics
Paroxysmal dyskinesias with dystonia
   Paroxysmal kinesigenic dyskinesia
   Paroxysmal nonkinesigenic dyskinesia
   Paroxysmal exertional dyskinesia
   Benign infantile paroxysmal dyskinesias
Hypnogenic dystonia
   (sometimes these are seizures)

PSEUDODYSTONIA

To complete the classification, Table 113.9 lists disorders that can mimic torsion dystonia but are not generally considered to be true dystonias. These disorders typically manifest themselves as sustained muscle contractions or abnormal postures, which is why they are often mistaken for dystonia. However, these contractions are secondary to either a peripheral or reflex mechanism or as a reaction to some other problem. For example, Sandifer syndrome is a result of gastroesophageal reflux, with apparent reduction of the gastric contractions when the head is tilted to the side; Isaacs syndrome is a result of continuous peripheral neural firing; orthopedic disease causes a number of postural changes; and seizures can result in sustained twisting postures.

▶ **TABLE 113.9** Pseudodystonias (not classified as dystonia but can be mistaken for dystonia because of sustained postures)

Sandifer syndrome
Stiff-person syndrome
Isaacs syndrome
Satoyoshi syndrome
Rotational atlantoaxial subluxation
Soft tissue nuchal mass
Bone disease
Ligamentous absence, laxity, or damage
Congenital muscular torticollis
Congenital postural torticollis
Juvenile rheumatoid arthritis
Ocular postural torticollis
Congenital Klippel-Feil syndrome
Posterior fossa tumor
Syringomyelia
Arnold-Chiari malformation
Trochlear nerve palsy
Vestibular torticollis
Seizures manifesting as sustained twisting postures
Inflammatory myopathy

TREATMENT

After levodopa therapy has been tested to be certain that DRD has not been overlooked, other oral medications may be effective and should be tried in people with dystonia not amenable or not adequately responding to botulinum toxin injections. The following drugs have been reported to be effective in dystonia: high-dose anticholinergics (e.g., trihexyphenidyl), high-dose baclofen, benzodiazepines (clonazepam, diazepam), and antidopaminergics (reserpine, dopamine receptor blockers).

For focal dystonias, such as blepharospasm, torticollis, oromandibular dystonia, and spastic dysphonia, local injections of botulinum toxin are beneficial. This agent also can be used to treat generalized dystonia, with injections limited to the most severely affected focal site. This muscle-weakening agent can be effective for about 3 months before a repeat injection is needed. About 5% of patients develop antibodies to botulinum toxin, thus rendering that particular strain of toxin ineffective.

Surgical procedures used for dystonia patients include the following: intrathecal baclofen, which may be especially helpful in patients with spasticity and dystonia; peripheral denervation of cervical muscles for patients with torticollis not responding to botulinum toxin injections; and central surgery including thalamotomy, pallidotomy, and deep brain stimulation of the globus pallidus interna for disabling dystonia unresponsive to other therapies. Bilateral deep brain stimulation of the pallidum appears to provide moderate to marked improvement for generalized primary dystonia without the high risk for dysarthria that occurs after bilateral thalamotomy.

SUGGESTED READINGS

Asmus F, Zimprich A, duMontcel ST, et al. Myoclonus-dystonia syndrome: epsilon-sarcoglycan mutations and phenotype. *Ann Neurol* 2002;52:489–492.

Augood SJ, Hollingsworth Z, Albers DS, et al. Dopamine transmission in DYT1 dystonia: a biochemical and autoradiographical study. *Neurology* 2002;59:445–448.

Berardelli A, Rothwell JC, Hallett M, et al. The pathophysiology of primary dystonia. *Brain* 1998;121:1195–1212.

Brandfonbrener AG, Robson C. Review of 113 musicians with focal dystonia seen between 1985 and 2002 at a clinic for performing artists. *Adv Neurol* 2004;94:255–256.

Bressman SB, de Leon D, Brin MF, et al. Idiopathic torsion dystonia among Ashkenazi Jews: evidence for autosomal dominant inheritance. *Ann Neurol* 1989;26:612–620.

Burke RE, Fahn S, Marsden CD. Torsion dystonia: a double-blind, prospective trial of high-dosage trihexyphenidyl. *Neurology* 1986;36:160–164.

Chuang C, Fahn S, Frucht SJ. The natural history and treatment of acquired hemidystonia: report of 33 cases and review of the literature. *J Neurol Neurosurg Psychiatry* 2002;72:59–67.

Curtis ARJ, Fey C, Morris CM, et al. Mutation in the gene encoding ferritin light polypeptide causes dominant adult-onset basal ganglia disease. *Nat Genet* 2001;28:345–349.

Dauer WT, Burke RE, Greene P, et al. Current concepts on the clinical features, aetiology and management of idiopathic cervical dystonia. *Brain* 1998;121:547–560.

Doheny DO, Morrison CE, Smith CJ, et al. Phenotypic features of myoclonus-dystonia in three kindreds. *Neurology* 2002;59:1187–1196.

Eidelberg D, Moeller JR, Antonini A, et al. Functional brain networks in DYT1 dystonia. *Ann Neurol* 1998;44:303–312.

Fahn S. The varied clinical expressions of dystonia. *Neurol Clin* 1984;2:541–552.

Fahn S, Bressman SB, Marsden CD. Classification of dystonia. *Adv Neurol* 1998;78:1–10.

Fahn S, Hallett M, DeLong MR, eds. Dystonia 4. *Adv Neurol* 2004;94.

Fahn S, Marsden CD, Calne DB, eds. Dystonia 2. *Adv Neurol* 1988;50.

Fahn S, Marsden CD, DeLong MR, eds. Dystonia 3. *Adv Neurol* 1998;78.

Frucht SJ, Fahn S, Greene PE, et al. The natural history of embouchure dystonia. *Mov Disord* 2001;16:899–906.

Grattan-Smith PJ, Wevers RA, Steenbergen-Spanjers GC, et al. Tyrosine hydroxylase deficiency: clinical manifestations of catecholamine insufficiency in infancy. *Mov Disord* 2002;17:354–359.

Greene P, Kang UJ, Fahn S. Spread of symptoms in idiopathic torsion dystonia. *Mov Disord* 1995;10:143–152.

Grimes DA, Han F, Lang AE, et al. A novel locus for inherited myoclonus-dystonia on 18p11. *Neurology* 2002;59:1183–1186.

Grotzsch H, Pizzolato GP, Ghika J, et al. Neuropathology of a case of dopa-responsive dystonia associated with new genetic locus, DYT14. *Neurology* 2002;58:1839–1842.

Hayflick SJ, Westaway SK, Levinson B, et al. Genetic, clinical, and radiographic delineation of Hallervorden-Spatz syndrome. *N Engl J Med* 2003;348(Jan 2):33–40.

Khan NL, Wood NW, Bhatia KP. Autosomal recessive, DYT2-like primary torsion dystonia: a new family. *Neurology* 2003;61:1801–1803.

Kuoppamaki M, Bhatia KP, Quinn N. Progressive delayed-onset dystonia after cerebral anoxic insult in adults. *Mov Disord* 2002;17:1345–1349.

Kupsch A, Klaffke S, Kuhn AA, et al. The effects of frequency in pallidal deep brain stimulation for primary dystonia. *J Neurol* 2003;250:1201–1205.

Lozano AM, Abosch A. Pallidal stimulation for dystonia. *Adv Neurol* 2004;94:301–308.

Manji H, Howard RS, Miller DH, et al. Status dystonicus: the syndrome and its management. *Brain* 1998;121:243–252.

Marsden CD, Obeso JA, Zarranz JJ, et al. The anatomical basis of symptomatic hemidystonia. *Brain* 1985;108:463–483.

Muller J, Wissel T, Masuhr F, et al. Clinical characteristics of the geste antagoniste in cervical dystonia. *J Neurol* 2001;248:478–482.

Nolte D, Niemann S, Muller U. Specific sequence changes in multiple transcript system DYT3 are associated with X-linked dystonia parkinsonism. *Proc Natl Acad Sci USA* 2003;100:10347–10352.

Nutt JG, Muenter MD, Aronson A, et al. Epidemiology of focal and generalized dystonia in Rochester, Minnesota. *Mov Disord* 1988;3:188–194.

Nygaard TG, Trugman JM, de Yebenes JG, et al. Dopa-responsive dystonia: the spectrum of clinical manifestations in a large North American family. *Neurology* 1990;40:66–69.

Opal P, Tintner R, Jankovic J, et al. Intrafamilial phenotypic variability of the DYT1 dystonia: From asymptomatic TOR1A gene carrier status to dystonic storm. *Mov Disord* 2002;17:339–345.

Oppenheim H. Über eine eigenartige Krampfkrankheit des kindlichen und jugendlichen Alters (Dysbasia lordotica progressiva, Dystonia musculorum deformans). *Neurol Centrabl* 1911;30:1090–1107.

Ozelius LJ, Hewett JW, Page CE, et al. The early-onset torsion dystonia gene (DYT1) encodes an ATP binding protein. *Nat Genet* 1997;17:40–48.

Saunders-Pullman R, Shriberg J, Heiman G, et al. Myoclonus dystonia—Possible association with obsessive-compulsive disorder and alcohol dependence. *Neurology* 2002;58:242–245.

Trost M, Carbon M, Edwards C, et al. Primary dystonia: is abnormal functional brain architecture linked to genotype? *Ann Neurol* 2002;52:853–856.

Zweig RM, Hedreen JC, Jankel WR, et al. Pathology in brainstem regions of individuals with primary dystonia. *Neurology* 1988;38:702–706.

Chapter 114

Essential Tremor

Elan D. Louis

Essential tremor (ET) is a chronic, progressive neurological disease. The hallmark motor feature is a 4- to 12-Hz tremor that may involve several regions of the body, including the arms and cranial structures (neck, voice, chin) but rarely the legs. The tremor is present during movement (touching finger to nose, writing) and often has an intentional component; it may also be present with sustained posture (arms extended in front of the body). Tremor at rest, without other cardinal features of parkinsonism, occurs in about 20% of patients with essential tremor attending a specialty clinic. Mild gait ataxia, eye movement abnormalities, and nonmotor features including mild cognitive impairment and impaired smell can also occur, although with the exception of the ataxia, these are signs rather than symptoms.

As with other progressive neurological disorders of later life, ET may be a family of diseases rather than a single condition; neurologic manifestations in a patient may depend on the localization of pathology within the nervous system. For instance, the kinetic tremor in ET may be the result of an abnormality in an olivo-cerebellar-thalamic pathway. However, signs may indicate more widespread cerebellar involvement (intention tremor, ataxia, eye motion abnormalities), or involvement of the basal ganglia (rest tremor) or cortex (cognitive deficits). In a population study based on direct neurologic examination, the prevalence of essential tremor was estimated to be 4% after age 40 and 6% after age 65.

The disorder is partly genetic. Many large kindreds show an autosomal-dominant pattern, and in a few, linkage has been demonstrated to regions on chromosomes 2p and 3q. However, the existence of sporadic cases, variability in age at onset in familial cases, and lack of complete disease concordance in monozygotic twins argues for nongenetic environmental causes as well. PET and MRS show metabolic abnormalities in the cerebellum, but published autopsy studies are scant and it is not known whether the disease is the result of a progressive loss of selected neuronal populations.

Symptoms begin at any age, and about 5% of cases begin in childhood, although the incidence increases markedly with advancing age and most prevalent cases are age 60 or older. Initially, the tremor may be mild and asymptomatic and it may not worsen for years. However, most patients note a gradual increase in tremor severity, and in 30% to 50% of patients, the tremor may spread to the neck (head). Isolated neck tremor is rare. Many patients note that tremor is temporarily suppressed by drinking alcoholic beverages, but a rebound exacerbation sometimes follows. Alcoholism is rare.

TREATMENT

The tremor may be severe enough to result in embarrassment and functional disability. In up to 15% of patients, the tremor leads to early retirement. Beta-blockers and primidone, alone or in combination, are the most effective pharmacologic therapies. Propranolol has been used in doses up to 360 mg daily, and primidone in doses of up to 1500 mg daily, although lower doses are often effective. These drugs reduce the amplitude of tremor in 30% to 70% of patients, but they do not abolish it unless the tremor is mild. Other agents that have been used include gabapentin, benzodiazepines (alprazolam or clonazepam), topiramate, and clozapine. High-frequency thalamic stimulation markedly reduces the severity of the tremor and has replaced stereotactic thalamotomy as the treatment of choice for severe tremor.

DIFFERENTIAL DIAGNOSIS

Essential tremor is frequently misdiagnosed as parkinsonism, particularly in the elderly and especially when a tremor at rest is seen. Differentiation may readily be made, however, by the absence of muscular rigidity or bradykinesia and the presence of large, irregular, and tremulous handwriting in contrast to the tremulous micrographia of parkinsonism. Dystonic tremor, which can affect the limbs or neck, can be distinguished from essential tremor by dystonic posturing, muscle hypertrophy, and pain. Absence of dysdiadochokinesia, dysmetria, or cerebellar speech distinguishes essential tremor from the spinocerebellar ataxias. Hyperthyroidism or the use of medications such as lithium or valproate are usually excluded by clinical history. The most difficult differential is between a mild case of essential tremor and enhanced physiologic tremor.

SUGGESTED READINGS

Cohen O, Pullman S, Jurewicz E, et al. Rest tremor in essential tremor patients: prevalence, clinical correlates, and electrophysiological characteristics. *Arch Neurol* 2003;60:405–410.

Deuschl G, Wenzelburger R, Loffler K, et al. Essential tremor and cerebellar dysfunction. Clinical and kinematic analysis of intention tremor. *Brain* 2000;123:1568–1580.

Dogu O, Sevim S, Camdeviren H, et al. Prevalence of essential tremor: door-to-door neurological exams in Mersin Province, Turkey. *Neurology* 2003;61:1804–1807.

Gasparini M, Bonifati V, Fabrizio E., et al. Frontal lobe dysfunction in essential tremor. A preliminary study. *J Neurol* 2001;248:399–402.

Gulcher JR, Jonsson P, Kong A, et al. Mapping of a familial essential tremor gene, FET1, to chromosome 3q13. *Nat Genet* 1997;17:84–87.

Helmchen C, Hagenow A, Miesner J, et al. Eye movement abnormalities in essential tremor may indicate cerebellar dysfunction. *Brain* 2003;126:1319–1332.

Higgins JJ, Pho LT, Nee LE. A gene (ETM) for essential tremor maps to chromosome 2p22-p25. *Mov Disord* 1977;12:859–864.

Jenkins IH, Bain PG, Colebatch JG, et al. A positron emission tomography study of essential tremor: evidence for overactivity of cerebellar connections. *Ann Neurol* 1993;34:82–90.

Louis ED, Bromley SM, Jurewicz EC, et al. Olfactory dysfunction in essential tremor: a deficit unrelated to disease duration or severity. *Neurology* 2002;59:1631–1633.

Louis ED, Ford B, Frucht S, et al. Risk of tremor and impairment from tremor in relatives of patients with essential tremor: a community-based family study. *Ann Neurol* 2001;49:761–769.

Louis ED, Ottman R, Hauser WA. How common is the most common adult movement disorder? Estimates of the prevalence of essential tremor throughout the world. *Mov Disord* 1998;13:5–10.

Louis ED, Shungu D, Chan S, et al. Metabolic abnormality in patients with essential tremor: a proton magnetic resonance spectroscopic imaging study. *Neurosci Lett* 2002;333:17–20.

Louis ED, Zheng W, Jurewicz EC, et al. Elevation of blood β-carboline alkaloids in essential tremor. *Neurology* 2002;59:1940–1944.

Rajput AH, Offord KP, Beard CM, et al. Essential tremor in Rochester, Minnesota: a 45-year study. *J Neurol Neurosurg Psychiatry* 1984;47:466–470.

Zesiewcz TA, Hauser S, Louis ED, et al. Practice parameter: therapies for essential tremor (an evidence-based review). The Quality Standards Subcommittee of the American Academy of Neurology. *Neurology* In press, 2004.

▶ TABLE 115.1   Classification of Major Parkinsonian Syndromes

Primary parkinsonism
Parkinson disease—sporadic and familial

Secondary parkinsonism
Drug-induced: dopamine antagonists and depletors
Hemiatrophy-hemiparkinsonism
Hydrocephalus; normal-pressure hydrocephalus
Hypoxia
Infectious; postencephalitic
Metabolic; parathyroid dysfunction
Toxin: Mn, CO, MPTP, cyanide
Trauma
Tumor
Vascular; multi-infarct state

Parkinson-plus syndromes
Cortical-basal ganglionic degeneration
Dementia syndromes
  Alzheimer disease
  Diffuse Lewy body disease
  Frontotemporal dementia
Lytico-Bodig (Guamanian parkinsonism-dementia-ALS)
Multiple system atrophy syndromes
  Striatonigral degeneration
  Shy-Drager syndrome
  Sporadic olivopontocerebellar degeneration (OPCA)
  Motor neuron disease–parkinsonism
Progressive pallidal atrophy
Progressive supranuclear palsy

Heredodegenerative diseases
Hallervorden-Spatz disease
Huntington disease
Lubag (X-linked dystonia-parkinsonism)
Mitochondrial cytopathies with striatal necrosis
Neuroacanthocytosis
Wilson disease

MPTP, 1-methyl-4-phenyl-1,2,3,6-tetrahydropyridine; ALS, amyotrophic lateral sclerosis.

Chapter 115

▶ Parkinsonism

Stanley Fahn and Serge Przedborski

In 1817, James Parkinson described the major clinical features of what today is recognized as a symptom complex manifested by any combination of six cardinal features: tremor at rest, rigidity, bradykinesia-hypokinesia, flexed posture, loss of postural reflexes, and the freezing phenomenon. At least two of these features, with at least one being either tremor at rest or bradykinesia, must be present for a diagnosis of definite parkinsonism. The many causes of parkinsonism (Table 115.1) are divided into four categories—idiopathic, symptomatic, Parkinson-plus syndromes, and various heredodegenerative diseases in which parkinsonism is a manifestation.

The core biochemical pathology in parkinsonism is decreased dopaminergic neurotransmission in the basal ganglia. In most of the diseases in Table 115.1, degeneration of the nigrostriatal dopamine system results in marked loss of striatal dopamine content. In some, degeneration of the striatum with loss of dopamine receptors is characteristic. Drug-induced parkinsonism is the result of blockade of dopamine receptors or depletion of dopamine storage. It is not known how hydrocephalus or abnormal calcium metabolism produces parkinsonism. Physiologically, the decreased dopaminergic activity in the striatum leads to disinhibition of the subthalamic nucleus and the medial globus pallidus, which is the predominant efferent nucleus in the basal ganglia. Understanding the biochemical pathology led to dopamine replacement therapy; understanding the physiologic change led to surgical interventions, such as pallidotomy, thalamotomy, and subthalamic nucleus stimulation.

The clinical features of tremor, rigidity, and flexed posture are referred to as *positive phenomena* and are reviewed first; bradykinesia, loss of postural reflexes, and freezing are *negative phenomena*. In general, the negative phenomena are the more disabling. *Rest tremor* at a frequency of 4 to 5 Hz is present in the extremities, almost always distally; the classic "pill-rolling" tremor involves the thumb and forefinger. Rest tremor disappears with action but reemerges as the limbs maintain a posture. Rest tremor is also common in the lips, chin, and tongue. Rest tremor of the hands increases with walking and may be an early sign when others are not yet present. Stress worsens the tremor.

Rigidity is an increase of muscle tone that is elicited when the examiner moves the patient's limbs, neck, or trunk. This increased resistance to passive movement is equal in all directions and usually is manifest by a ratchety "give" during the movement. This so-called cogwheeling is caused by the underlying tremor even in the absence of visible tremor. Cogwheeling also occurs in patients with es-

sential tremor. Rigidity of the passive limb increases while another limb is engaged in voluntary active movement.

The *flexed posture* commonly begins in the arms and spreads to involve the entire body (Fig. 115.1). The head is bowed, the trunk is bent forward, the back is kyphotic, the arms are held in front of the body, and the elbows, hips, and knees are flexed. Deformities of the hands include ulnar deviation of the hands, flexion of the metacarpophalangeal joints, and extension of the interphalangeal joints (striatal hand). Inversion of the feet is apparent, and the big toes may be dorsiflexed (striatal toe). Lateral tilting of the trunk commonly develops, and extreme flexion of the trunk (camptocormia) is sometimes seen.

Akinesia is a term used interchangeably with bradykinesia and hypokinesia. *Bradykinesia* (slowness of movement, difficulty initiating movement, and loss of automatic movement) and *hypokinesia* (reduction in amplitude of movement, particularly with repetitive movements, so-called decrementing) are the most common features of parkinsonism, although they may appear after the tremor. Bradykinesia has many facets, depending on the affected body parts. The face loses spontaneous expression (masked facies, *hypomimia*) with decreased frequency of blinking. Poverty of spontaneous movement is

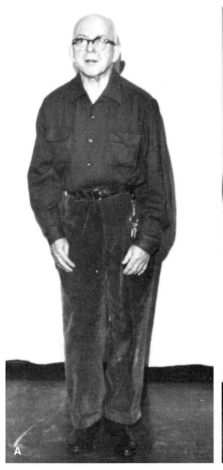
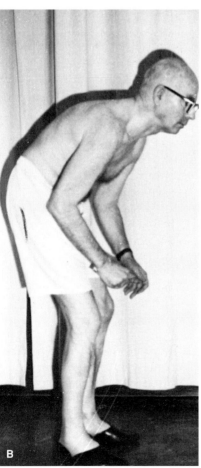

FIGURE 115.1. Parkinson patient body posture. **A.** Front view. **B.** Side view.

characterized by loss of gesturing and by the patient's tendency to sit motionless. Speech becomes soft (*hypophonia*), and the voice has a monotonous tone with a lack of inflection (*aprosody*). Some patients do not enunciate clearly (*dysarthria*) and do not separate syllables clearly, thus running the words together (*tachyphemia*). Bradykinesia of the dominant hand results in small and slow handwriting (*micrographia*) and in difficulty shaving, brushing teeth, combing hair, buttoning, or applying makeup. Playing musical instruments is impaired. Walking is slow, with a shortened stride length and a tendency to shuffle; arm swing decreases and eventually is lost. Difficulty rising from a deep chair, getting out of automobiles, and turning in bed are symptoms of truncal bradykinesia. Drooling saliva results from failure to swallow spontaneously, a feature of bradykinesia, and is not caused by excessive production of saliva. The patients can swallow properly when asked to do so, but only constant reminders allow them to keep swallowing. Similarly, arm swing can be normal if the patient voluntarily and, with effort, wishes to have the arms swing on walking. Pronounced bradykinesia prevents a patient with parkinsonism from driving an automobile; foot movement from the accelerator to the brake pedal is too slow.

Bradykinesia is commonly misinterpreted by patients as weakness. Fatigue, a common complaint in parkinsonism, particularly in the mild stage of the disease before pronounced slowness appears, may be related to mild bradykinesia or rigidity. Subtle signs of bradykinesia can be detected even in the early stage of parkinsonism if one examines for slowness in shrugging the shoulders, lack of gesturing, decreased arm swing, and decrementing amplitude of rapid successive movements. With advancing bradykinesia, slowness and difficulty in the execution of activities of daily living increase. A meal normally consumed in 20 minutes may be only half eaten in an hour or more. Swallowing may become impaired with advancing disease, and choking and aspiration are concerns.

Loss of postural reflexes leads to falling and eventually to inability to stand unassisted. Postural reflexes are tested by the *pull-test*, which is performed by the examiner, who stands behind the patient, gives a sudden firm pull on the shoulders, and checks for retropulsion. With advance warning, a normal person can recover within one step. The examiner should always be prepared to catch the patient when this test is conducted; otherwise, a person who has lost postural reflexes could fall. As postural reflexes are impaired, the patient collapses into the chair on attempting to sit down (sitting *en bloc*). Walking is marked by festination, whereby the patient walks faster and faster, trying to move the feet forward to be under the flexed body's center of gravity and thus prevent falling.

The *freezing* phenomenon (motor block) is transient inability to perform active movements. It most often affects the legs when walking but also can involve eyelid opening (known as *apraxia of lid opening* or levator inhibition), speaking (*palilalia*), and writing. Freezing occurs suddenly and is transient, lasting usually no more than several seconds with each occurrence. The feet seem as if "glued to the ground" and then suddenly become "unstuck," allowing the patient to walk again. Freezing typically occurs when the patient begins to walk (start hesitation), attempts to turn while walking, approaches a destination, such as a chair in which to sit (destination hesitation), and is fearful about inability to deal with perceived barriers or time-restricted activities, such as entering revolving doors, elevator doors that may close, and crossing heavily trafficked streets (sudden transient freezing). Freezing is often overcome by visual clues, such as having the patient step over objects, and is much less frequent when the patient is going up steps than when walking on level ground. The combination of freezing and loss of postural reflexes is particularly devastating. When the feet suddenly stop moving forward, the patient falls because the upper part of the body continues in motion as a result of the inability to recover an upright posture. Falling is responsible for the high incidence of hip fractures in parkinsonian patients. Likely related to the freezing phenomenon is the difficulty for parkinsonian patients to perform two motor acts simultaneously.

PARKINSON DISEASE (PRIMARY PARKINSONISM)

Pathology

The pathology of Parkinson disease (PD) is distinctive. Degeneration of the neuromelanin-containing neurons in the brainstem occurs, especially in the ventral tier of the pars compacta in the substantia nigra and in the locus ceruleus; many of the surviving neurons contain eosinophilic cytoplasmic proteinacious inclusions known as *Lewy bodies*, the pathologic hallmark of the disease. By the time symptoms appear, the substantia nigra already has lost about 60% of dopaminergic neurons and the dopamine content in the striatum is about 80% less than normal.

Epidemiology

PD makes up approximately 80% of cases of parkinsonism listed in Table 115.1. The age at onset assumes a bell-shaped curve with a mean of 55 years in both sexes and a wide range in age from 20 to 80 years. Onset at younger than 20 years is known as *juvenile parkinsonism*; when primary, it is usually familial and without Lewy bodies in the degenerating substantia nigra. Juvenile parkinsonism is not always primary and can be owing to heredodegenerative diseases such as Huntington disease and Wilson disease. Onset of primary parkinsonism between 20 and 40 years is known as young-onset PD. PD is more common in men, with a male-to-female ratio of 3:2. The prevalence of PD is approximately 160 per 100,000, and the incidence is about 20 per 100,000/year. Prevalence and incidence increase with age. At age 70, the prevalence is approximately 550 per 100,000, and the incidence is 120 per 100,000/year.

Symptoms and Signs

The clinical motor features of PD are the six cardinal features described for parkinsonism in general. The onset is insidious; tremor is the symptom first recognized in 70% (Table 115.2). Symptoms often begin unilaterally, but as the disease progresses, it becomes bilateral. The disease can remain confined to one side, although steadily worsening for several years before the other side becomes involved. The disease progresses slowly, and if untreated, the patient eventually becomes wheelchair bound and bedridden. Despite severe bradykinesia with marked immobility, patients with PD may rise suddenly and move normally for a short burst of motor activity, so-called *kinesia paradoxica*.

In addition to the motor signs that are used to define parkinsonism, most patients with PD have behavioral signs as well. Attention span is reduced, and there is visuospatial impairment. The personality changes; the patient slowly becomes more dependent, fearful, indecisive, and passive. The spouse gradually makes more of the decisions and becomes the dominant partner. The patient speaks less spontaneously. The patient eventually sits much of the day and is inactive unless encouraged to exercise. Passivity and lack of motivation are common and are expressed by the patient's aversion to visiting friends. Depression is frequent in patients with PD, developing at a rate of about 2% per year.

Cognitive decline is another common feature, but is usually not the severe type of dementia seen in Alzheimer disease. Memory impairment is not a feature of PD; rather, the patient is just slow in responding to questions, so-called *bradyphrenia*. The correct answer can be obtained if the patient is given enough time. Subtle signs of bradyphrenia, such as the inability to change mental set rapidly, may be present early in the disease. Fifteen percent to 20% of patients with PD have a more profound dementia, similar to that in Alzheimer disease. These patients are usually elderly and have developed concurrent Alzheimer disease or diffuse Lewy body disease, in which Lewy bodies are present in cortical neurons. These disorders are not always distinguishable, but Lewy body disease is often characterized by fluctuating hallucinations.

Sensory symptoms are fairly common, but objective sensory impairment is not seen in PD. Symptoms of pain, burning, and tingling occur in the region of motor involvement. A patient may have dull pain in one shoulder as an early symptom of the disease, which often is misdiagnosed as arthritis or bursitis, and even before clear-cut signs of bradykinesia appear in that same arm. *Akathisia* (inability to sit still, restlessness) and the *restless legs syndrome* occur in some patients with PD. In both syndromes, uncomfortable sensations disappear with movement, and sometimes the two conditions are difficult to distinguish. Akathisia is usually present most of the day; it may respond to levodopa but otherwise has not been treated successfully. The restless legs syndrome develops late in the day with crawling sensations in the legs and may be associated with periodic movements in sleep, thereby disturbing sleep. This problem can be treated successfully with opioids, such as propoxyphene, oxycodone, and codeine. Other sleep problems are fragmented sleep and REM sleep behavior disorder; the latter is usually successfully treated with clonazepam. Other sleep problems are encountered with dopaminergic medications including excessive daytime sleepiness and sudden attacks of sleep without warning.

Autonomic disturbances also are encountered. The skin is cooler, constipation is a major complaint, bladder emptying is inadequate, erection may be difficult to achieve, and blood pressure may be low. A major diagnostic consideration is the Shy-Drager syndrome, also called multiple system atrophy (MSA). Seborrhea and seborrheic dermatitis are common, but can be controlled with good hygiene.

Tendon reflexes are usually unimpaired in PD; an abnormal extensor plantar reflex suggests a Parkinson-plus

▶ **TABLE 115.2 Initial Symptoms in Parkinson Disease**

	No. of Cases (n = 183)	Percent
Tremor	129.1	70.5
Stiffness or slowness of movement	36	19.7
Loss of dexterity and/or handwriting disturbance	23	12.6
Gait disturbance	21	11.5
Muscle pain, cramps, aching	15	8.2
Depression, nervousness, or other psychiatric disturbance	8	4.4
Speech disturbance	7	3.8
General fatigue, muscle weakness	5	2.7
Drooling	3	1.6
Loss of arm swing	3	1.6
Facial masking	3	1.6
Dysphagia	1	0.5
Paresthesia	1	0.5
Average number of initial symptoms per patient	1.4	

syndrome. An uninhibited glabellar reflex (*Myerson sign*), snout reflex, and palmomental reflexes are common, even early in the disease.

Etiology, Pathogenesis, and Genetics

The cause of PD in the vast majority of patients is unknown. Research has concentrated on genetics, exogenous toxins, and endogenous toxins from cellular oxidative reactions. Based on twin studies, onset of PD before age 50 has a higher likelihood of a genetic cause.

Several genes have been identified, usually causing young-onset parkinsonism (Table 115.3). The first (PARK1) is owing to mutations in the gene for the protein, *α-synuclein*, located on chromosome 4q21.3. *α*-Synuclein is an abundant presynaptic protein of unclear function. The resulting parkinsonism transmits in an autosomal-dominant pattern. It is rare, being seen only in a few families in Greece, Italy, Germany, and Spain. After the discovery of this genetic defect, however, *α*-synuclein was found to be present in Lewy bodies (even in patients with PD without this genetic mutation). It is believed that the mutant protein aggregates and accumulates in cells, causing neuronal death. Yet, triplication of the *α*-synuclein gene also causes familial parkinsonism (PARK4), suggesting that overexpression of the normal protein may suffice to provoke dopaminergic neurodegeneration.

The most commonly occurring gene defect causing familial parkinsonism is PARK2 on chromosome 6q25.2–q27, coding for a previously unknown protein named *parkin*. This protein is an E2-dependent E3 ubiquitin-protein ligase, which is abundantly expressed in the substantia nigra. Mutations in the parkin gene result in an autosomal-recessive parkinsonism that is slowly progressive, with onset usually before the age of 40 years and with sleep benefit; rest tremor is not prominent. There is degeneration of substantia nigra neurons, but in most instances no Lewy body inclusions are found. Some typical adult-onset PD patients have been found to have a single mutation of the parkin gene and with Lewy bodies at autopsy.

Three additional known gene defects causing familial parkinsonism are PARK5 (on 4p14), PARK6 (on 1p35-p36) and PARK7 (on 1p36). PARK5 results from a mutation in the gene encoding ubiquitin carboxy-terminal hydrolase L1. PARK6 is the result of a mutation in PINK1, a mitochondrial protein with unknown function. PARK7 results from mutations in the gene encoding DJ-1.

Rare families with PD seem to exhibit a maternal mode of inheritance, suggesting a mitochondrial DNA defect. Dopa-responsive dystonia may present during adulthood as PD. It tends to be benign, responding to relatively low doses of levodopa and not progressing. This disorder is discussed in Chapter 113.

The discovery that the chemical agent 1-methyl-4-phenyl-1,2,3,6-tetrahydropyridine (MPTP) can cause parkinsonism raised the possibility that PD might be caused by an environmental toxin. No single environmental factor has emerged as essential, but growing up in a rural environment was disproportionately frequent in some studies. Because aging is associated with a loss of catecholamine-containing neurons and an increase in monoamine oxidase (types A and B) activity, an endogenous toxin hypothesis has emerged. Cellular oxidation reactions (such as enzymatic oxidation and autooxidation of dopamine and other monoamines) result in the formation of reactive oxygen species (ROS) such as hydrogen peroxide and dopamine quinone, and if not removed properly, these molecules can damage the monoamine neurons. Substantia nigra in patients with PD shows severe depletion of reduced glutathione, the major substrate required for the elimination of ROS. This change is also seen in brains with incidental Lewy bodies and therefore could be the earliest biochemical abnormality of PD. It is not known, however, if this change causes oxidative stress (increasing oxyradicals) or is the result of oxidative stress (because reduced glutathione is oxidized under conditions of oxidative stress). Iron in the substantia nigra may also play a critical role because it can catalyze the formation of the highly reactive hydroxyl radical from hydrogen peroxide.

Postmortem biochemical observations showed that complex I activity of mitochondria is reduced in substantia nigra of patients with PD (MPP^+ also affects complex I). This reduction could be the result of an exogenous toxin, oxidative stress, or a genetic defect stemming from the mitochondrial DNA. On the other hand, a primary defect of complex I would decrease the synthesis of ATP and also lead to the buildup of free electrons, thereby increasing oxyradicals and accentuating oxidative stress.

Based on these postmortem investigations and on studies of toxic models of PD and of the functions of genes implicated in inherited forms of PD, two major pathogenic hypotheses have been suggested. One hypothesis proposes that misfolding and aggregation of proteins are instrumental in the PD neurodegenerative process, whereas the other suggests that mitochondrial dysfunction and oxidative stress are the culprits. These two hypotheses are not mutually exclusive, and interactions among these pathogenic factors could be key to the demise of dopaminergic neurons in PD.

Differential Diagnosis

The diagnosis of PD is based on the clinical features of parkinsonism, insidious asymmetric onset, slow progression, and the lack of other findings in the history, examination, or laboratory tests that would point to some other cause of parkinsonism. One of the most common disorders mistaken for PD is essential tremor (see Chapter 114),

▶ **TABLE 115.3 Genetic Forms of Parkinson Disease**

Name and Locus	Gene	Mode of Inheritance; Pathological and Clinical Features	Protein Function	Where Found	Pathogenic Mutations
PARK1 4q21.3	α-Synuclein	Autosomal dominant; Lewy bodies; young onset; dementia occurs	Possibly synaptic vesicle trafficking; elevated in bird song learning	Families in Germany, Italy-U.S. (Contoursi kindred), Greece, Spain	A53T and A30P, may promote aggregation; Lewy body and Alzhemer plaque component; protofibrils (toxic) accumulation
PARK2 6q25.2–q27	Parkin	Autosomal recessive (also dominant?); often juvenile onset w/o Lewy bodies; slowly progressive	Ubiquitin E3 ligase, attaches short ubiquitin peptide chains to a range of proteins, likely to mark degradation	Ubiquitous, originally in Japan, very common in juvenile onset	Over 70 mutations identified; mostly likely loss of function mutations
PARK3 2p13	Unknown	Autosomal dominant; Lewy bodies, indistinguishable from idiopathic PD		4 families in southern Denmark and northern Germany, probable common ancestor	
PARK4 4q	Multiple copies of wild-type α-synuclein	Autosomal dominant; wide range of symptoms from idiopathic PD to dementia with Lewy bodies	See PARK1	Spellman-Muenter and the Waters-Miller families with common ancestor in the United States, European families	Duplications/ triplications of chromosomal region that contains wild-type α-synuclein gene
PARK5 4p14	Ubiquitin-C-terminal hydrolase L1	Possibly autosomal dominant	Removes polyubiquitin	1 family in Germany	
PARK6 1p35-p36	PINK-1	Autosomal recessive; juvenile onset	Mitochondrial protein; provides protection against multiple stress factors	1 family in Sicily	
PARK7 1p36	DJ-1	Autosomal recessive; early onset	Sumoylation pathway	Families in Holland, Italy, Uruguay	L166P, M261, and a variety of other candidates
PARK8 12p11.2-q13.1	Unknown	Autosomal dominant; nigral degeneration, no Lewy bodies		1 family in Japan	
PARK9 1p36	Unknown	Autosomal recessive; Kufor-Rakeb syndrome, a Parkinson-plus disorder		1 family in Jordan	
PARK10 1p32	Unknown	Autosomal recessive; typical late onset		Families in Iceland	
PARK11 2q36-q37	Unknown	Autosomal dominant		Families in the U.S.	

▶ **TABLE 115.4 Clues Indicates the Likely Type of Parkinsonism**

Clinical		
Never responded to levodopa	Psychotic sensitivity to levodopa	Upper motor neuron findings
Other than PD	Diffuse Lewy body disease; AD	Multiple system atrophy
Predominantly unilateral	Early loss of postural reflexes	Laboratory
PD; HP-HA syndrome; CBGD	Progressive supranuclear palsy	Fresh blood smear: acanthocytes
Symmetric onset	Impaired downgaze	Neuroacanthocytosis
PD; most forms of parkinsonism	Progressive supranuclear palsy	Grossly elevated creatine kinase
Presence of rest tremor	Deep nasolabial folds	Neuroacanthocytosis
PD; secondary parkinsonism	Progressive supranuclear palsy	MRI: many lacunes
Lack of rest tremor	Furrowed forehead and eyebrows	Vascular parkinsonism
Parkinson-plus syndromes	Progressive supranuclear palsy	MRI: "tiger's eye" in pallidum
History of encephalitis	Nuchal dystonia	Hallervorden-Spatz disease
Postencephalitic parkinsonism	Progressive supranuclear palsy	MRI: caudate atrophy
History of toxin exposure	Abducted arms when walking	HD; neuroacanthocytosis
Parkinsonism caused by the toxin	Progressive supranuclear palsy	MRI: decreased T2 signal in striatum
Taking neuroleptics	Square wave jerks	Multiple system atrophy
Drug-induced parkinsonism	Progressive supranuclear palsy	MRI: midbrain atrophy
Severe unilateral rigidity	Pure freezing	Progressive supranuclear palsy
CBGD	Progressive supranuclear palsy	MRI: huge ventricles
Cortical sensory signs	Meaningful orthostatic hypotension	Normal pressure hydrocephalus
CBGD	Shy-Drager syndrome	Abnormal autonomic function tests
Unilateral cortical myoclonus	Urinary or fecal incontinence	Shy-Drager syndrome
CBGD	Shy-Drager syndrome	Denervation on sphincter EMG
Unilateral apraxia	Cerebellar dysarthria and dysmetria	Shy-Drager syndrome
CBGD	Olivopontocerebellar degeneration	
Alien limb	Laryngeal stridor (vocal cord paresis)	
CBGD	Striatonigral degeneration	
Early dementia	Lower motor neuron findings	
CBGD	Multiple system atrophy	

CBGD, cortical–basal ganglionic degeneration; HP-HA, hemiparkinsonism-hemiatrophy syndrome; AD, Alzheimer disease; HD, Huntington disease; PD, Parkinson disease.

which is characterized by postural and kinetic tremor, not rest tremor.

Several clinical clues suggest that a patient with parkinsonism has some form of the syndrome other than PD itself (Table 115.4). In general, PD often appears with symptoms on only one side of the body, whereas patients with symptomatic parkinsonism or Parkinson-plus syndromes almost always have symmetric symptoms and signs (notable exceptions are cortical-basal ganglionic degeneration and parkinsonism resulting from a focal brain injury, such as head trauma). Similarly, a rest tremor almost always indicates PD because it rarely is seen in symptomatic parkinsonism or Parkinson-plus syndromes, except in drug-induced and MPTP-induced parkinsonism, which do include rest tremor. The patient who does not have unilateral onset or rest tremor, however, still can have PD that begins symmetrically and without tremor. Perhaps the most important diagnostic aid is the response to levodopa. Patients with PD almost always have a satisfactory response to this drug. If a patient never responds to levodopa, the diagnosis of some other form of parkin-

sonism is likely. A response to levodopa, however, does not confirm the diagnosis of PD because many cases of symptomatic parkinsonism (e.g., MPTP, postencephalitic, reserpine induced) and many forms of Parkinson-plus syndromes in their early stages (e.g., Shy-Drager syndrome, striatonigral degeneration, olivopontocerebellar atrophy) also respond to levodopa. Table 115.4 provides a list of some helpful clues. Below are short clinical descriptions of other parkinsonian disorders, other than progressive supranuclear palsy, which is covered in Chapter 116.

Drug-induced Parkinsonism

Drugs that block striatal dopamine D2 receptors (e.g., phenothiazines and butyrophenones) or deplete striatal dopamine (e.g., reserpine, tetrabenazine) can induce a parkinsonian state (see also Chapter 117). This condition is reversible when the offending agent is withdrawn, but it may require several weeks. Parkinsonism that persists longer than 6 months is attributed to underlying PD that becomes evident during exposure to these antidopaminergic drugs. Anticholinergic drugs can ameliorate the parkinsonian signs and symptoms. The atypical antipsychotic agents, clonazapine and quetiapine, are the least likely antipsychotics to induce or worsen parkinsonism.

Hemiparkinsonism-Hemiatrophy Syndrome

This relatively benign syndrome consists of hemiparkinsonism in association with ipsilateral body hemiatrophy or contralateral brain hemiatrophy. The parkinsonism usually begins in young adults and often remains as hemiparkinsonism, sometimes with hemidystonia. It tends to be nonprogressive or slowly progressive compared with PD. The disorder is thought to be the result of brain injury early in life, possibly even perinatally. It usually responds poorly to medications.

Normal Pressure Hydrocephalus

The gait disorder in normal pressure hydrocephalus (see Chapter 49) resembles that of parkinsonism, with shuffling short steps and loss of postural reflexes and sometimes freezing. Features of urinary incontinence and dementia occur later. Tremor is rare. The grossly enlarged ventricles lead to the correct diagnosis, with the symptoms improving on removal or shunting of cerebrospinal fluid. The gait disorder is in striking contrast to the lack of parkinsonism in the upper part of the body. The major differential diagnosis for *lower body parkinsonism* includes vascular parkinsonism and the idiopathic gait disorder of the elderly.

Postencephalitic Parkinsonism

Although rarely encountered today, postencephalitic parkinsonism was common in the first half of the last century. Parkinsonism was the most prominent sequela of the pandemics of *encephalitis lethargica (von Economo encephalitis)* that occurred between 1919 and 1926. Although the causative agent was never established, it affected mainly the midbrain, thus destroying the substantia nigra. The pathology is distinctive because of the presence of neurofibrillary tangles in the remaining nigral neurons and absence of Lewy bodies. In addition to slowly progressive parkinsonism, with features similar to those of PD, oculogyric crises often occur in which the eyes deviate to a fixed position for minutes to hours. Dystonia, tics, behavioral disorders, and ocular palsies may be present. Patients with postencephalitic parkinsonism are more sensitive to levodopa, with limited tolerance because of the development of dyskinesias, mania, or hypersexuality at low dosages. Anticholinergics are tolerated well, however, and are also effective against oculogyria.

1-Methyl-4-Phenyl-1,2,3,6-Tetrahydropyridine-Induced Parkinsonism

Although rare, this disorder is important because this toxin selectively destroys the dopamine nigrostriatal neurons, and its mechanism has been investigated intensively for possible clues to the cause and pathogenesis of PD. MPTP is a protoxin, being converted to MPP$^+$ by the action of the enzyme monoamine oxidase type B. MPP$^+$ is taken up selectively by dopamine neurons and terminals via the dopamine transporter system. MPP$^+$ inhibits complex I in the mitochondria, depletes ATP, and increases the content of superoxide ion radicals. Superoxide in turn can react with nitric oxide to form the oxyradical peroxynitrite. MPTP-induced parkinsonism has occurred in drug abusers who used it intravenously and possibly also in some laboratory workers exposed to the toxin. The clinical syndrome is indistinguishable from PD and responds to levodopa. PET indicates that a subclinical exposure to MPTP results in a reduction of fluorodopa uptake in the striatum, thereby making the person liable to future development of parkinsonism.

Vascular Parkinsonism

Vascular parkinsonism resulting from lacunar disease is not common, but can be diagnosed by neuroimaging with magnetic resonance imaging evidence of hyperintense T2-weighted signals compatible with small infarcts. Hypertension is usually required for the development of this disorder. The onset of symptoms, usually with a gait disorder, is insidious, and the course is progressive. A history of a major stroke preceding the onset of parkinsonism is rare, although a stepwise course is sometimes seen. Gait is profoundly affected (lower body parkinsonism), with freezing and loss of postural reflexes. Tremor is rare. Response to the typical antiparkinsonian agents is poor.

Cortical-Basal Ganglionic Degeneration

Initially reported as *corticodentatonigral degeneration*, this disorder is characterized pathologically by enlarged achromatic neurons in cortical areas (particularly parietal and frontal lobes) along with nigral and striatal neuronal degeneration. The onset is insidious and typically unilateral, with marked rigidity-dystonia on the involved arm. Cortical signs of apraxia, *alien limb phenomena*, cortical sensory loss, and cortical reflex myoclonus of that limb are also seen. Speech is hesitant, gait is poor, and occasionally action tremor is evident. The disease usually spreads slowly to involve both sides of the body, and supranuclear gaze difficulties often occur late. It can resemble progressive supranuclear palsy, and both conditions accumulate *tau* protein. Medications have been ineffective.

Lytico-Bodig (Parkinson–Dementia–Amyotrophic Lateral Sclerosis Complex of Guam)

A combination of parkinsonism, dementia, and motor neuron disease occurred among the Chamorro natives on Guam in the Western Pacific. The incidence has declined gradually. Epidemiologic evidence supports a probable environmental cause, with exposure occurring during adolescence or adulthood. One hypothesis is that environmental exposure to the neurotoxin found in the seed of the plant *Cycas circinalis* was responsible for the neuronal degeneration. Natives on Guam used this seed to make flour in World War II. But this hypothesis has been questioned. Besides parkinsonism, dementia, and motor neuron disease in various combinations, supranuclear gaze defects also appear. A characteristic pathologic finding is the presence of neurofibrillary tangles in the degenerating neurons, including the substantia nigra. Lewy bodies and senile plaques are absent.

Other Parkinson–Dementia Syndromes

Although bradyphrenia is common in PD, dementia also occurs in about one-fifth of patients. The incidence of dementia increases with age, and those with dementia have a higher mortality rate. The two most common pathologic substrates for dementia in parkinsonism are the changes typical of Alzheimer disease and the presence of Lewy bodies diffusely in the cerebral cortex. It is not known if the Alzheimer changes are coincidental because of the elderly population of affected individuals or whether Alzheimer and PD are somehow related. Similarly, it is not known whether the spread of Lewy bodies into the cortex is a feature of progression of PD or a distinct entity. The presence of dementia limits the tolerance of antiparkinsonian agents because they tend to increase confusion and produce psychosis.

Multiple System Atrophy

MSA has been applied to a group of four syndromes previously considered as distinct and separate entities: striatonigral degeneration, Shy-Drager syndrome, olivopontocerebellar atrophy, and parkinsonism-amyotrophy syndrome (Table 115.5). The full pathologic spectrum consists of neuronal loss and gliosis in the neostriatum, substantia nigra, globus pallidus, cerebellum, inferior olives, basis pontine nuclei, intermediolateral horn cells, anterior horn cells, and corticospinal tracts. A common pathologic feature is the presence of widespread glial cytoplasmic inclusions, particularly in oligodendroglia. The

▶ **TABLE 115.5** Different Clinical Entities of Multiple System Atrophy

Characteristic Feature	Nosology
Pure parkinsonism	Striatonigral degeneration
Autonomic dysfunction	Shy-Drager syndrome
Ataxia	Olivopontocerebellar atrophy
Amyotrophy	Amyotrophy-parkinsonism

presence of these argyophilic α-synuclein-positive perinuclear structures, which are primarily composed of straight microtubules containing ubiquitin and *tau* protein, in this tetrad of syndromes supports the concept that these conditions are variations of the same disease process.

Patients with MSA have with parkinsonism one of the other clinical features listed in Table 115.5; each entity can be identified by its characteristic clinical feature. Corticospinal tract findings may be present as well. MSA may account for 10% of patients with parkinsonism. In striatonigral degeneration, nerve cell loss and gliosis are found predominantly in the substantia nigra and neostriatum. The symptoms are those of parkinsonism, without tremor. Also, the beneficial response to levodopa is slight because striatal neurons containing dopamine receptors are lost. Dystonic reactions commonly follow low-dosage levodopa therapy. Laryngeal stridor may be caused by paresis of one or both vocal cords. Occasionally, degeneration is seen in the cerebellum, but the presence of cerebellar symptoms classifies the disorder as olivopontocerebellar atrophy.

In the Shy-Drager syndrome, the preganglionic sympathetic neurons in the intermediolateral horns are lost. In addition, other areas may be affected, particularly the substantia nigra (to produce parkinsonism), the cerebellum (to cause ataxia), and the striatum (to cause lack of response to levodopa). Less often, the anterior horn cells are involved (to cause amyotrophy). Because the postganglionic sympathetic neuron is intact in Shy-Drager syndrome, plasma norepinephrine is normal when the patient is supine but fails to rise when the patient stands. Orthostatic hypotension is a major disabling symptom, but other dysautonomic symptoms are also troublesome, including impotence and bladder and bowel dysfunction. Sometimes the striatum is spared, thus allowing a response to levodopa therapy. Levodopa, however, can exaggerate orthostatic hypotension. Measures to overcome this problem include wearing support hose, ingesting salt, and taking fludrocortisone or midodrine, but this approach can result in supine hypertension, which is partially offset if the patient sleeps at an incline instead of in a recumbent position. If the striatum becomes more involved, with presumed loss of dopamine receptors, the benefit of levodopa as an antibradykinetic drug diminishes.

Many disorders make up the complex known as olivopontocerebellar atrophy. Familial olivopontocerebellar atrophy appears as a cerebellar syndrome, whereas sporadic olivopontocerebellar atrophy is characterized by a mixture of parkinsonism and cerebellar syndrome. In addition to degeneration of the olives, pons, and cerebellum, neuronal loss in the striatum and substantia nigra occurs. Some patients respond to levodopa therapy if the striatum is not severely degenerated.

The least common part of the spectrum of MSA involves just the anterior horn cells (to cause amyotrophy) and the nigrostriatal complex (to cause parkinsonism). Only a few of these cases have been described.

Helpful in diagnosing MSA is fluorodeoxyglucose PET showing hypometabolism in the striatum and the frontal lobes.

Treatment of MSA, like other Parkinson-plus syndromes, requires testing levodopa to the maximum tolerated dose or up to 2 g/day (in the presence of carbidopa) to determine whether any therapeutic response can be obtained. In most situations, dopamine replacement therapy is of limited value. Anticholinergics may provide some mild benefit, however.

Treatment

Treatment of parkinsonism in general is based on the treatment of PD, which is the focus of this section. At present, treatment is aimed at controlling symptoms because no drug or surgical approach unequivocally prevents progression of the disease. Treatment is individualized because each patient has a unique set of symptoms, signs, response to medications, and a host of social, occupational, and emotional needs that must be considered. The goal is to keep the patient functioning independently as long as possible. Practical guides are the symptoms and degree of functional impairment and the expected benefits and risks of therapeutic agents.

Drug Therapy

Although pharmacotherapy is the basis of treatment, physiotherapy is also important. It involves patients in their own care, promotes exercise, keeps muscles active, and preserves mobility. This approach is especially beneficial as parkinsonism advances because many patients tend to remain sitting and inactive. Psychiatric assistance may be required to deal with depression and the social and familial problems that may develop with this chronic disabling illness. Electroconvulsive therapy may have a role in patients with severe intractable depression.

Table 115.6 lists the drugs useful in parkinsonism according to mechanisms of action. It also lists some of the surgical approaches available. Selection of the most suitable drugs for the individual patient and deciding when

> **TABLE 115.6 Therapeutic Choices for Parkinson Disease**

Medications

Dopamine precursor: levodopa ± carbidopa; standard and slow release

Dopamine agonists: bromocriptine, pergolide, pramipexole, ropinirole, lisuride, apomorphine, cabergoline

Catecholamine-O-methyltransferase inhibitors: tolcapone and entacapone

Dopamine releaser: amantadine

Glutamate antagonist: amantadine

Monoamine oxidase type B inhibitors: selegiline and rasagiline

Anticholinergics: trihexyphenidyl, benztropine, ethopropazine, biperiden, cycrimine, procyclidine

Anitihistaminics: diphenhydramine, orphenadrine, phenindamine, chlorphenoxamine

Antidepressants: amitriptyline and other tricyclics, fluoxetine and other serotonin-uptake inhibitors

Muscle relaxants: cyclobenzaprine, diazepam

Peripheral antidopaminergic: domperidone

  Antipsychotic: clozapine, quetiapine

Antianxiety agents: benzodiazepines

Surgery
  Ablative surgery
  Thalamotomy
  Pallidotomy
  Restorative surgery
  Embryonic dopaminergic tissue transplantation
  Deep brain stimulation
  Thalamic stimulation
  Pallidal stimulation
  Subthalamic stimulation

to use them in the course of the disease are challenges for the treating clinician. In many Parkinson-plus disorders, the response to treatment is not satisfactory, but the principles for treating PD are used in treating these disorders as well. Because PD is chronic and progressive, treatment is lifelong. Medications and their doses change with time as adverse effects and new symptoms are encountered. Tactical strategy is based on the severity of symptoms.

In Table 115.6, *carbidopa* is listed as the peripheral dopa decarboxylase inhibitor, but in many countries *benserazide* is also available. These agents potentiate the effects of levodopa, thus allowing about a fourfold reduction in dosage to obtain the same benefit. Moreover, by preventing the formation of peripheral dopamine, which can act at the area postrema (vomiting center), they block the development of nausea and vomiting. *Domperidone* is a dopamine receptor antagonist that does not enter the CNS, it is used to prevent nausea, not only from levodopa but also from dopamine agonists. Domperidone is not available in the United States. Of the listed dopamine agonists, bromocriptine, pergolide, pramipexole, ropinirole, and apomorphine are available in the United States; they are reviewed in a following section. Because it is water soluble, apomorphine is used as an injectable, rapidly acting dopaminergic to overcome "off" states. Cabergoline has the longest half-life. Catecholamine-O-methyltransferase (COMT) inhibitors extend the elimination half-life of levodopa.

Amantadine, selegiline, and the anticholinergics are reviewed in following sections. Because the anticholinergics can cause forgetfulness and even psychosis, they should be used cautiously in patients most susceptible (those older than 70 years). The antihistaminics, tricyclics, and cyclobenzaprine have milder anticholinergic properties that make them useful in PD, particularly in the older patient who should not take the stronger anticholinergics.

Antidepressants are needed for treating depression. Because of its anticholinergic and soporific effects, amitriptyline can be useful for these properties as well as for its antidepressant effect. The serotonin uptake inhibitors are also effective in treating depression of PD but may aggravate parkinsonism if antiparkinsonian drugs are not given concurrently. Diazepam and other benzodiazepines are usually well tolerated without worsening parkinsonism and can help to lessen tremor by reducing the reaction to stress that worsens tremor. Clozapine, a selective dopamine D4 receptor antagonist, can ameliorate levodopa-induced psychosis without worsening parkinsonism, but weekly monitoring of white blood cells is necessary to prevent irreversible agranulocytosis. The drug is discontinued if the white blood cell count declines. Quetiapine, a related drug, does not need hematologic monitoring and therefore can more conveniently be tried first to overcome psychosis.

Surgery

The surgical approaches listed in Table 115.6 are not considered in the early stages of PD but are reserved for patients who have failed to respond satisfactorily to drugs. Stereotaxic lesions have been largely replaced by high-frequency electrical stimulation at the same targets because of safety concerns. *Thalamotomy and thalamic stimulation* (target for both is the ventral intermediate nucleus) are best for contralateral intractable tremor. Tremor can be relieved in at least 70% of cases. Although a unilateral lesion carries a small risk, bilateral operations result in dysarthria in 15% to 20% of patients. Thalamic stimulation seems to be safer and can be equally effective against tremor, but it runs the risks associated with foreign bodies and thin electronic wires that can break. *Pallidotomy* (target is the posterolateral part of the globus pallidus interna) is most effective for treating contralateral dopa-induced dystonia and chorea but also has some benefit for bradykinesia and tremor. The target in the globus pallidus interna is believed to be the site of afferent excitatory glutamatergic fibers coming from the subthala-

> **TABLE 115.7** **Five Major Outcomes After More Than 5 Years of Levodopa Therapy ($N = 330$ Patients)[a]**

Smooth good response, $n = 83$ (25%)
Troublesome fluctuations, $n = 142$ (43%)
Troublesome dyskinesias, $n = 67$ (19%)
Toxicity at therapeutic or subtherapeutic dosages, $n = 14$ (4%)
Total or substantial loss of efficacy, $n = 27$ (8%)

[a]Thirty-six patients had both troublesome fluctuations and troublesome dykinesias. From Fahn S. Adverse effects of levodopa. In: Olanow CW, Lieberman AN, eds. *The Scientific Basis for the Treatment of Parkinson's Disease.* Carnforth, England: Parthenon, 1992.

mic nucleus, which is overactive in PD. *Lesions of the subthalamic nucleus,* although effective in relieving parkinsonism in animal models, are hazardous in humans because hemichorea or hemiballism may result. Instead, *stimulation of the subthalamic nucleus* is used and appears to be the most promising in reducing contralateral bradykinesia and tremor. Subthalamic nucleus stimulation in a patient reduces symptoms of PD that respond to levodopa in that patient. It is not effective against symptoms that do not respond to levodopa (with the exception of intractable tremor, which can respond to stimulation). This type of surgery often allows a marked reduction of levodopa dosage, thereby reducing dopa-induced dyskinesias as well as treating parkinsonian symptoms. Controlled surgical trials of *fetal dopaminergic tissue implants* have found the benefits to be less efficacious than initially reported in open-label investigations and have also led to the development of persistent dyskinesias. Until this problem can be solved, transplantation surgery is not a useful option.

Levodopa is uniformly accepted as the most effective drug available for symptomatic relief of PD. If it were uniformly and persistently successful and also free of complications, new strategies for other treatment would not be needed. Unfortunately, 75% of patients have serious complications after 5 years of levodopa therapy (Table 115.7).

STAGES OF PARKINSON DISEASE

Early Stage

It is debated whether early use of levodopa is responsible for later response fluctuations and other complications (Table 115.7). Authorities generally agree, however, that in the early stage of PD when symptoms are noticed but not troublesome, symptomatic treatment is not necessary. All symptomatic drugs can induce side effects, and if a patient is not troubled socially or occupationally by mild symptoms, drug therapy can be delayed until symptoms become more pronounced.

The major decision is when to introduce levodopa, the most effective drug. All patients are likely to develop complications associated with long-term use. Younger patients, in particular, are more likely to show response fluctuations, so other antiparkinsonian drugs should be used first to delay the introduction of levodopa; when deemed necessary, levodopa should be administered at the lowest effective dose. This approach is known as the *levodopa-sparing strategy*. On the other hand, clinicians who doubt that levodopa is responsible for these complications might choose to use levodopa first because the therapeutic response is greater. No long-term controlled clinical trials have been carried out to determine the eventual effect of high-dosage levodopa, and opinions differ about retrospective studies.

Selegiline delays the need for levodopa therapy by an average of 9 months. Because this monoamine oxidase (MAO) type B inhibitor provides a mild symptomatic effect, it has not been possible to conclude that selegiline also exerts a neuroprotective effect. However, a controlled study evaluating selegiline in the presence of levodopa therapy showed that those on selegiline performed better than subjects receiving placebo, lending evidence that selegiline likely provides some neuroprotection and thus should be considered as therapy when the diagnosis of PD is made. Selegiline has few adverse effects when given without levodopa, but when given concurrently with levodopa, it can increase the dopaminergic effect, allows a lower dose of levodopa, and contributes to dopaminergic toxicity. *Rasagiline*, another propargylamine MAO-B inhibitor, also provides mild symptomatic effect, and one controlled study suggests it might have some neuroprotective effect as well.

The antioxidant *tocopherol* (vitamin E) was tested at a dose of 2,000 U/day in mild PD as part of a controlled clinical trial and had no effect in delaying the need for levodopa or providing any slowing of progression. *Coenzyme Q10*, an antioxidant and mitochondrial-active agent, at 1200 mg/day showed some reduction of parkinsonism in a controlled pilot study but failed to delay the need of levodopa therapy.

Stage When Symptoms and Signs Require Symptomatic Treatment

Eventually, PD progresses and symptomatic treatment must be used. The most common problems that clinicians consider important in deciding to use symptomatic agents are the following: threat to employment; threat to ability to handle domestic, financial, or social affairs; threat to handle activities of daily living; and appreciable worsening of gait or balance. In clinical practice, a global judgment for initiating such therapy is made in discussions between the patient and the treating physician.

The choice now is whether to introduce levodopa or some other antiparkinsonian drug, such as amantadine,

an anticholinergic, or a dopamine agonist. Levodopa is superior in relieving symptoms. Patients and clinicians who prefer a levodopa-sparing strategy, however, select other agents.

Amantadine

Amantadine is a mild indirect dopaminergic agent that acts by augmenting dopamine release for storage sites and possibly blocking reuptake of dopamine into the presynaptic terminals. It also has some anticholinergic and antiglutamatergic properties. In the early stages of PD, it is effective in about two-thirds of patients. A major advantage is that benefit, if it occurs, is seen in a couple of days. The effect can be substantial. Unfortunately, its benefit in more advanced PD is often short lived, with patients reporting a fall-off effect after several months of treatment. After dopamine stores are depleted, the effect of amantadine is exhausted. A common adverse effect is livedo reticularis (a reddish mottling of skin) around the knees; other adverse effects are ankle edema and visual hallucinosis. Sometimes, when the drug is discontinued, a gradual worsening of parkinsonian signs may follow, thus indicating that the drug has been helpful. The usual dose is 100 mg two times per day, but sometimes a higher dose (up to 200 mg two times per day) may be required. Amantadine can be useful not only in the early phases of symptomatic therapy by forestalling use of levodopa or reducing the required dosage of levodopa but also in the advanced stages as an adjunctive drug to levodopa and the dopamine agonists. It can also reduce the severity of levodopa-induced dyskinesias, probably by its antiglutamatergic mechanism of action.

Anticholinergic (Antimuscarinic) Drugs

As a general rule, anticholinergic agents are less effective antiparkinsonian agents than are the dopamine agonists. The anticholinergic drugs are estimated to improve parkinsonism by about 20%. Many clinicians find that when tremor is not relieved by an agonist or levodopa, addition of an anticholinergic drug can be effective. Because the anticholinergic agent sometimes can lessen tremor severity even without levodopa, many clinicians use such an agent as monotherapy for tremor. If not helpful, continual use of the drug can be beneficial while a dopamine agonist or levodopa is added. Later, if tremor is relieved by the dopaminergic agent, the anticholinergic drug may be discontinued.

Trihexyphenidyl is a widely used anticholinergic agent. A common starting dose is 2 mg three times per day. It can be gradually increased to 20 mg or more per day.

Adverse effects from anticholinergic drugs are common, particularly in the age range of most patients with PD. Adverse cerebral effects are predominantly forgetfulness and decreased short-term memory. Occasionally, hallucinations and psychosis occur, particularly in the elderly patient; these drugs should be avoided in patients older than 70 years. If tremor is not relieved by dopaminergic drugs and one wishes to add an anticholinergic agent to the therapy for an elderly patient, amitriptyline, diphenhydramine, orphenadrine, or cyclobenzaprine are sometimes beneficial, without the central side effects of more potent agents. Diphenhydramine and amitriptyline can cause drowsiness and can be used as a hypnotic. For tremor control, the dose is increased gradually to 50 mg three times per day. A similar dose schedule is useful for orphenadrine. Cyclobenzaprine can be increased gradually until 20 mg three times per day is reached.

Peripheral side effects are common and are often the reason for discontinuing or limiting the dosage of anticholinergic drugs. These adverse effects, however, can usually be overcome by adding pilocarpine eye drops if blurred vision occurs or if glaucoma is present. Pyridostigmine, up to 60 mg three times per day, can help to overcome dry mouth and urinary difficulties.

Dopamine Agonists

Dopamine agonists can be used as conjunctive therapy with levodopa to potentiate an antiparkinsonian effect, to reduce the dosage needed for levodopa alone, and to overcome some of the adverse effects of long-term use of levodopa or as monotherapy in the early stage of the disease to delay introduction of levodopa. It is likely that early use of dopamine agonists, by delaying the introduction of levodopa, reduces the time to develop complications from chronic levodopa therapy.

The agonists are less effective than levodopa as antiparkinsonian agents, and most patients require the addition of levodopa within a couple of years. Bromocriptine, pergolide, lisuride, and cabergoline are ergot derivatives. As such, they could induce red inflamed skin (St. Anthony's fire), but this side effect is rare and is reversible on discontinuing the drug. Retroperitoneal, pleural, and pericardial fibrosis are more serious adverse, but also rare, events. Restrictive fibrotic cardiac valvulopathy may occur in up to one-third of patients taking pergolide (detected by echocardiography), thought to be owing to its ergot effect, thus raising the specter that the ergot dopamine agonists may prove more dangerous than previously thought. The valvulopathy was reversed in some patients by withdrawal of pergolide, and careful monitoring should be undertaken in patients on the ergolines. The nonergoline agonists, pramipexole and ropinirole, are also associated with drowsiness and ankle edema (with redness of the skin). Sleep attacks, including falling asleep without warning when driving a vehicle, are infrequent problems with dopamine agonists, and drivers need to be cautioned about such a serious possibility. Observing sleep attacks at home when just sitting in a chair is a warning sign not to drive. Defensive methods, such as delaying a dose of agonist or taking the antinarcoleptic drug modafinil before a long drive may be reasonable, but studies on whether these approaches are effective have not been carried out. Besides sleep effects and ankle edema, dopamine agonists are more prone than levodopa to induce hallucinations, particularly in the elderly who already may have some cognitive impairment.

All agonists tend to induce orthostatic hypotension, particularly when the drug is first introduced. Afterward, this complication is much less common. Therefore, the best starting regimen is a small dose at bedtime for the first 3 days (bromocriptine 1.25 mg, pergolide 0.05 mg, pramipexole 0.125 mg, ropinirole 0.25 mg) and then switch from bedtime to daytime regimens at this dose for the next few days. The daily dose can be increased gradually at weekly intervals to avoid adverse effects (bromocriptine 1.25 mg, pergolide 0.25 mg, pramipexole 0.25 mg, ropinirole 0.75 mg) until a benefit or a plateau dosage is reached (bromocriptine 5 mg three times per day, pergolide and pramipexole 0.5 mg three times per day, ropinirole 1 mg three times per day). If this plateau is not satisfactory, the dose either can be increased gradually until it is quadrupled or can be held constant while beginning carbidopa/levodopa. If the agonists alone still are not effective, carbidopa/levodopa is needed.

Besides the adverse effects listed above, there are subtle differences among the dopamine agonists. Cabergoline has the longest pharmacologic half-life and theoretically could be taken in once-a-day dosing. Pergolide acts at both the D1 and D2 dopamine receptors (Table 115.8). Bromocriptine is a partial D1 antagonist. All act at the D2 receptor, which may account for most, if not all, of their anti-PD activity. Pergolide, pramipexole, and ropinirole also act at the D3 dopamine receptor, but it is not clear what effect this has clinically. All three appear to be equally effective against PD; bromocriptine appears to have the weakest anti-PD effect. It also seems to be more likely to induce psychosis and confusion, whereas the other three agonists are more likely to induce dyskinesias. Dopamine agonists, when used in the absence of levodopa, rarely induce dyskinesias. Whether this is because of their longer half-life and possibly more continuous dopaminergic receptor stimulation, or because they exert a different receptor effect than that of levodopa, is unknown. Their longer half-lives make them useful to reduce the severity of "off" states in patients on levodopa therapy.

Levodopa

Some clinicians prefer to begin therapy with carbidopa/levodopa for early symptomatic treatment and to add an agonist after a small dose has been reached (e.g., 25/100 mg three times per day). This approach is

▶ TABLE 115.8 Effect on Receptors by Dopamine Agonists

Agonist	D1	D2	D3	D4	D5	5HT Receptor
Bromocriptine	−	+	++	+	+	0
Pergolide	+	++	+++	?	+	?
Pramipexole	−	++	++++	++	?	?
Ropinirole	−	++	++++	+	−	?
Cabergoline	−	+++	?	?	?	?
Lisuride	+	++	?	?	?	+

+, activates; −, inhibits; 0, no effect; ?, uncertain.

particularly useful if a patient already has some disability. The advantage of using levodopa at this stage in preference to a dopamine agonist is that a therapeutic response is virtually guaranteed. Nearly all patients with PD respond to levodopa and do so quickly. In contrast, only some benefit adequately from a dopamine agonist alone, and it may take months to discover this because of a slower buildup of dosage. Therefore, if a definite response is needed quickly (e.g., to remain at work or to be self-sufficient), levodopa is preferable. On the other hand, if there is no particular urgency for a rapid clinical response and if the patient has no cognitive problems and is younger than 70 years of age, then beginning with a dopamine agonist allows one to use the levodopa-sparing strategy. Patients older than 70 are less likely to develop response fluctuations with levodopa and more likely to develop confusion and hallucinations with dopamine agonists, so in this population, carbidopa/levodopa would be a good choice as a starting drug. In controlled trials comparing levodopa and agonists as initial therapy, levodopa produced a superior clinical response but more fluctuations and dyskinesias.

Stage When Symptoms and Signs Require Treatment with Levodopa

When other antiparkinsonian medications are no longer bringing about a satisfactory response, levodopa is required to reduce the severity of parkinsonism. Levodopa is the most potent anti-PD drug. In treating patients with PD, the rule of thumb has been to use the lowest dosage that can bring about adequate symptom reversal, not the highest dosage that the patient can tolerate. As previously mentioned, the longer the duration of levodopa therapy and the higher the dose, the greater the likelihood motor complications will occur. After 5 years of levodopa therapy, about 75% of patients with PD have some form of troublesome complication (Table 115.7). On the other hand, a dose-response study showed a clear-cut dose-related clinical benefit, which is an advantage with higher dosages.

Most clinicians prefer to use levodopa with a peripheral dopa decarboxylase inhibitor (e.g., carbidopa) to increase therapeutic potency and to avoid gastrointestinal adverse effects. Slow-release forms of carbidopa/levodopa (Sinemet CR) and benserazide/levodopa (Madopar HBS) provide a longer half-life and a lower peak plasma level of levodopa. In the early stage of levodopa therapy, when complications have not yet developed, use of slow-release carbidopa/levodopa had not proven advantageous over use of the standard preparation in a controlled trial because it did not delay motor fluctuations. However, that study design may have been flawed, and it may be useful to start treatment with such a sustained-release preparation in elderly patients to avoid too high a brain concentration of levodopa that might induce drowsiness.

Once response fluctuations have developed, the slow-release preparation could reduce mild wearing off. Also, a bedtime dose often allows more mobility during the night. Disadvantages are a delay in the response with each dose and the possibility of a late-in-the-day excessive dyskinesia response that can be prolonged. For a quick response on awakening, patients often take the standard preparation as the first morning dose in addition to the slow-release form. Some patients need a combination of standard and sustained-release preparations of levodopa throughout the day to obtain a smoother response and minimize their motor complications.

The slow-release tablets of carbidopa/levodopa are available in two strengths: scored (50/200 mg, which can be broken in half) and unscored (25/100 mg). Neither should be crushed because the matrix of the tablet that delays solubilization would no longer be effective. When added to a dopamine agonist, a dose of 25/100 mg three to four times per day often suffices. When used alone, a starting dose of 25/100 mg three times per day often is necessary and can be increased as needed to 50/200 mg three or four times per day. For those desiring to produce a continuous dopaminergic stimulation effect, multiple dosings a day should be considered. If greater relief is required, a dopamine agonist or standard carbidopa/levodopa should be added.

It should be noted that the entire content of the slow-release formulation is not absorbed before the tablet passes the duodenum, so that an equivalent dose needs to be approximately 1.3 times greater than a dose of standard carbidopa/levodopa.

Inadequate Response to Levodopa Treatment

As a general rule, the single most important piece of information to help the differential diagnosis of PD and other forms of parkinsonism is the response to levodopa. If the response is nil or minor, the disorder probably is not PD. An adequate response, however, does not ensure the diagnosis of PD. All presynaptic disorders (e.g., reserpine-induced, MPTP-induced, postencephalitic parkinsonism) respond to levodopa. Also, a response to levodopa can occur in the early stages of MSA and progressive supranuclear palsy; only later, when striatal dopamine receptors are lost, is the response lost.

Before concluding that levodopa is without effect in a given patient, an adequate dose must be tested. Not every symptom has to respond, but bradykinesia and rigidity respond best, whereas tremor can be resistant. Therefore, if rest tremor is the only symptom, lack of improvement does not exclude the diagnosis of PD. Tremor may never respond satisfactorily, even if adjunctive antiparkinsonian drugs are also used. Before concluding that carbidopa/levodopa is ineffective, a reasonable test dose of up to 2,000 mg levodopa/day should be given. If anorexia, nausea, or vomiting prevent attainment of a therapeutic dosage, the addition of extra carbidopa (additional 25 mg four times per day) or domperidone (10 to 20 mg before each levodopa dose) is usually effective in overcoming the adverse effect. If other adverse effects (drug-induced dystonia, psychosis, confusion, sleepiness, postural hypotension) prevent attainment of an effective dose, uncertainty about the diagnosis of PD will continue. In particular, dystonia induced by low doses of levodopa suggests a diagnosis of MSA. Similarly, drug-induced psychosis suggests diffuse Lewy body disease or accompanying Alzheimer disease. Using clozapine or quetiapine may suppress psychosis and allow the use of levodopa.

COMPLICATIONS OF LONG-TERM LEVODOPA THERAPY

Response fluctuations, dyskinesias, and behavioral effects are the major problems encountered with long-term levodopa therapy (Tables 115.9 and 115.10).

Fluctuations

When levodopa therapy is initiated, the benefit from levodopa is usually sustained, with general improvement throughout the day and no dose-timing variations; this is the long-duration benefit. Skipping a dose is usually without loss of effect, and the response is evident on arising in the morning despite the lack of medication throughout the night. The pharmacokinetics of levodopa show a short initial distribution phase with a half-life of 5 to 10 minutes, a peak plasma concentration in about 30 minutes,

▶ **TABLE 115.9 Major Fluctuations and Dyskinesias as Complications of Levodopa**

Fluctuations ("offs")	Dyskinesias
Slow "wearing-off"	Peak-dose chorea and dystonia
Sudden "off"	Diphasic chorea and dystonia
Random "off"	"Off" dystonia
Yo-yoing	Myoclonus
Episodic failure to respond (dose failures)	
Delayed "on"	
Weak response at end of day	
Varied response in relationship to meals	
Sudden transient freezing	

and an elimination phase of about 90 minutes. Brain levels follow plasma levels. This long-duration benefit of levodopa is attributed to a combination of prolonged storage of dopamine from exogenous levodopa in residual nigrostriatal nerve terminals and a prolonged postsynaptic effect on dopamine receptors.

With chronic levodopa therapy, most patients, including all patients with onset before age 40, begin to experience fluctuations. At first, fluctuations take the form of *wearing off* (also known as end-of-dose deterioration), which is defined as a return of parkinsonian symptoms in less than 4 hours after the last dose. Gradually, the duration of benefit shortens further and the "off" state becomes more profound. Eventually these fluctuations become more abrupt in onset and random in timing; the condition is then the "on–off" effect and cannot be related to the timing of the levodopa intake. Motor "offs" are often accompanied by changes in mood (depression, dysphoria), anxiety, thought (more bradyphrenia), and sensory symptoms (pain). Such behavioral and sensory "offs" can occur in the absence of motor "offs."

Loss of striatal storage sites of dopamine by itself is not the sole cause of this problem. Treatment with direct-acting agonists does not eliminate the fluctuations but does

▶ **TABLE 115.10 Behavioral Adverse Effects with Levodopa**

Drowsiness
Delusions
Reverse sleep–wake cycle
Paranoia
Vivid dreams
Confusion
Benign hallucinations
Dementia
Malignant hallucinations
Behavioral "offs":
Depression, anxiety, panic, pain, akathisia, dysphoria

make the depths of the "off" state less severe. It seems that both the central effects on dopamine receptors and the peripheral pharmacokinetics of levodopa are involved. The dopamine receptor becomes more sensitive to levodopa in patients with fluctuations, thus affecting both the antiparkinsonian and the dyskinetic effects. Simultaneously, the duration of response is shorter.

The brief peripheral half-life of levodopa, by itself, is not likely to be responsible for fluctuations. The half-life, present from the beginning of treatment, does not change. Also, no difference exists in the pharmacokinetics in patients with early disease who show a stable response and in those with advanced disease and fluctuations.

One hypothesis is that intermittent (compared with continuous) administration of levodopa contributes to the development of motor complications. These peaks and valleys of brain dopamine levels are thought to alter the striatal dopaminoceptive medium spiny neurons, with a potentiation of glutamate receptors (of the *N*-methyl-D-aspartate subtype) on these GABAergic striatal efferents. This increased glutamatergic activity then produces the motor complications. Another potential mechanism is that dopamine can lead to the formation of free radicals by autoxidation or by enzymatic oxidation, and these oxyradicals could be the culprits attacking and altering the dopamine receptors.

Once established, motor complications are seemingly irreversible. Substituting dopamine agonists for levodopa therapy or maintaining plasma concentrations at a constant therapeutic level by chronic infusion of levodopa diminishes the severity of the complications but does not eliminate them. In research centers, jejunal infusions of levodopa, subcutaneous infusions of apomorphine, and hourly oral administration of liquefied levodopa have been used. But these methods of treatment are often not practical. Selegiline, rasagiline, and COMT inhibitors are partially effective in treating mild wearing-off problems, probably by prolonging dopamine levels at the synapse. The addition of these drugs to patients taking levodopa, however, may lead to dopaminergic toxicity, including dyskinesias, confusion, and hallucinations. Another approach is to substitute the slow-release forms of carbidopa/levodopa (Sinemet CR) for the standard form. Again, this approach is effective mainly on wearing-off problems and not on complicated "on–off" fluctuations. Furthermore, the sustained-release formulation results in less predictable plasma levels of levodopa and often increases dyskinesias. Standard carbidopa/levodopa can be given alone by shortening the interval between doses. For the more severe state of "on–off" phenomenon, a more rapid and more predictable response sometimes can be achieved by dissolving the levodopa tablet in carbonated water or ascorbic acid solution because an acidic solvent is required to dissolve levodopa and to prevent auto-oxidation of the drug. Liquid levodopa enters the small intestine faster, is absorbed faster, and can be used to fine-tune dosing. Patients with fluctuations also usually have delayed "ons" and dose failures resulting from delayed entry of the tablet into the small intestine. Liquefying levodopa can help to resolve this problem.

Direct-acting dopamine agonists, with a biologic half-life longer than that of levodopa, can be used in combination with standard or slow-release forms of levodopa. The agonists are useful for treating both wearing-off and "on–off" by reducing both the frequency and the depth of the "off" states. In yet another approach to treating "on–offs," the patients inject themselves with apomorphine subcutaneously to quickly return the "on" state. Trimethobenzamide or the peripheral dopamine receptor antagonist domperidone can be used to block nausea and vomiting from apomorphine.

Some patients report that high-protein meals tend to produce "off" states. Levodopa is absorbed from the small intestine by the transport system for large neutral amino acids and thus competes with these other amino acids for this transport. Patients with this problem may benefit from special diets that contain little protein for the first two meals of the day, followed by a high-protein meal at the end of the day when they can afford to be "off."

Dyskinesias

Dyskinesias are commonly encountered with levodopa therapy but are often mild enough to be unnoticed by the patient. Severe forms, including chorea, ballism, dystonia, or combinations of these, can be disabling. The incidence and severity increase with duration and dosage of levodopa therapy, but they may appear early in patients with severe parkinsonism. Dyskinesias are divided into the following categories according to the timing of levodopa dosing:

1. Peak-dose dyskinesias appear at the height of antiparkinsonian benefit (20 minutes to 2 hours after a dose).
2. Diphasic dyskinesias, usually affecting the legs, appear at the beginning and end of the dosing interval.
3. "Off" dystonia, which can be painful sustained cramps, appear during "off" states and may be seen at first as early-morning dystonia presenting as foot cramps; these are relieved by the next dose of levodopa.

Dyskinesias are usually seen in patients who have fluctuations, and some patients may move rapidly from severe dyskinesias to severe "offs"; this process is known as *yo-yoing*. These patients may have only a brief "on" state. More commonly, they have good "ons" for parts of the day but are intermittently disabled by dyskinesias or "offs." These diurnal variations are major problems; patients with this combination have a narrow therapeutic window for levodopa. The mechanisms for dyskinesias and fluctuations are not thought to be identical or even linked. For example, sensitivity to dyskinesias is not altered by chronic infusion of levodopa, whereas fluctuations are suppressed. Because dopamine agonists are much less likely to cause dyskinesias, which have much less activation of the D1 receptor, increased sensitivity and response of the D1 receptor by dopamine derived from levodopa is thought to play a role in the production of dyskinesias.

Amantadine can reduce the severity of dyskinesias, but a dosage of at least 400 mg/day is required, and it is not known how long the benefit may last. Treatment of peak-dose dyskinesias also includes reducing the size of each dose of levodopa. If doing so results in more wearing off, the drug is given more frequently, a switch is made to the slow-release form, or a dopamine agonist or inhibitor of MAO-B or COMT is added with the reduced dose of levodopa. Diphasic dyskinesias are more difficult to treat. Increasing the dosage of levodopa can eliminate this type of dyskinesia, but peak-dose dyskinesia usually ensues. A switch to a dopamine agonist as the major antiparkinsonian drug is more effective; low doses of levodopa are used as an adjunctive agent. The principle of treating "off dystonia" is to try to keep the patient "on" most of the time. Here again, using a dopamine agonist as the major antiparkinsonian drug, with low doses of levodopa as an adjunct, can often be effective.

Freezing

The freezing phenomenon is often listed as a type of fluctuation because of transient difficulty in initiating movement. But this phenomenon should be considered as distinct from the other types of fluctuations. "Off-freezing" must be distinguished from "on-freezing." Off-freezing, best considered a feature of parkinsonism itself, was encountered before levodopa was discovered. The treatment goal of off-freezing is to keep the patient from getting "off." On-freezing remains an enigma; it tends to be aggravated by increasing the dosage of levodopa or by adding direct-acting dopamine agonists or selegiline without reducing the dosage of levodopa. Rather, it is lessened by reducing the dosage of levodopa. Both on- and off-freezing seem to correlate with both the duration of illness and the duration of levodopa therapy.

Patients with a combination of complicated fluctuations, dyskinesias, and off-freezing may respond to subthalamic nucleus stimulation.

SURGICAL THERAPY

Prior to the introduction of levodopa therapy, stereotactic surgery producing lesions in the thalamus or pallidum was common, resulting in reduction of tremor more than relief of other features of PD. Such surgery faded away after levodopa became available. But with the problems of motor complications from levodopa, there has been renewed interest in surgical therapy, mainly to treat these motor complications. The most common type of surgery today is to use electrical stimulation of the subthalamic nucleus. Such deep brain stimulation (DBS) provides a reduction of not only tremor but also bradykinesia and rigidity, allowing a reduction of dosage of dopaminergic medication. The antiparkinsonian effect is never better than the best levodopa effect (except for tremor, in which surgery seems superior). Therefore, DBS can be useful in patients with a very good anti-PD response to levodopa but with uncontrollable response fluctuations. DBS has the potential to smooth out these fluctuations. The best results are seen with younger patients. The presence of cognitive problems or lack of benefit from levodopa are contraindications. Cognitive problems worsen with surgical penetration in the brain. DBS produces levodopalike benefits probably by restoring the physiological balance in the basal ganglia circuitry, bypassing the need to restore dopamine levels. In this concept, DBS could be considered like an electronic levodopa. Adverse effects from the surgery include brain hemorrhage (rare), infection from a foreign body, speech impairment, dystonia, and breakage of the wires. Exposure of the metallic stimulators to diathermy can result in permanent brain injury.

MENTAL AND BEHAVIORAL CHANGES

The adverse effects of confusion, agitation, hallucinosis, hallucinations, delusions, paranoia, and mania are probably related to activation of dopamine receptors in nonstriatal regions, particularly cortical and limbic structures. Elderly patients and those with diffuse Lewy body disease or concomitant Alzheimer disease are sensitive to small doses of levodopa. But all patients with PD, regardless of age, can develop psychosis if they take excessive amounts of levodopa to overcome "off" periods. Patients with pronounce sensory offs tend to take more and more levodopa. Psychosis can often be treated without worsening parkinsonism by adding quetiapine or clozapine, antipsychotic agents that block the dopamine D4 and serotonin receptors. These drugs easily induce drowsiness, and they should be given at bedtime, starting with a dose of 12.5 mg. The dose can be gradually increased if necessary. Start with quetiapine to avoid the biweekly blood counts required with clozapine. If quetiapine is not effective, use clozapine instead. Because clozapine induces agranulocytosis in 1% to 2% of patients, patients must have blood counts monitored biweekly, and the drug must be discontinued if leukopenia develops. If clozapine is not tolerated, other drugs, including small doses of olanzapine, molindone, pimozide, or other relatively weak antipsychotic drugs, can be used. If the antipsychotic drugs increase the parkinsonism, lowering the dosage of levodopa to avoid the psychosis is preferable to maintaining the antipsychotic agent at high dosage. Levodopa cannot be discontinued suddenly because the abrupt cessation may induce a neuroleptic malignantlike syndrome.

COURSE

The degenerative forms of parkinsonism, including PD, worsen with time. Before the introduction of levodopa, PD caused severe disability or death in 25% of patients within 5 years of onset, in 65% in the next 5 years, and in 89% in those surviving 15 years. The mortality rate from PD was three times that of the general population matched for age, sex, and racial origin. Although no definite evidence indicates that levodopa alters the underlying pathologic process or stems the progressive nature of the disease, indications exist of a major impact on survival time and functional capacity. The mortality rate has dropped 50%, and longevity is extended by several years.

The hemiparkinsonism-hemiatrophy syndrome progresses more slowly and may never cause the severe disability seen with PD. In these patients, fluorodeoxyglucose PET studies reveal hypometabolism in the contralateral striatum and frontal cerebral cortex. Another relatively benign form of parkinsonism is adult-onset dopa-responsive dystonia (see Chapter 113). In that disorder, features of PD appear, but the patients continue to respond to low-dosage levodopa treatment and never develop the complications encountered so frequently with PD.

A debated point in the treatment of PD is the cause of declining efficacy from continuing treatment with levodopa seen in many patients. End-stage PD is denoted when the response to levodopa is inadequate to allow patient-assisted activities of daily living. Progression of the illness with further loss of dopamine storage sites in the presynaptic terminals cannot be the explanation for this outcome because loss of these structures in postencephalitic parkinsonism results in greater, not lower, sensitivity to levodopa. Perhaps as PD progresses, it is associated with loss of striatal dopamine receptors and loss of the presynaptic dopaminergic neuron.

SUGGESTED READINGS

Bonifati V, Rizzu P, van Baren MJ, et al. Mutations in the DJ-1 gene associated with autosomal recessive early-onset parkinsonism. *Science* 2003;299:256–259.

Chase TN. The significance of continuous dopaminergic stimulation in the treatment of Parkinson's disease. *Drugs* 1998;55:1–9.

Dauer W, Przedborski S. Parkinson's disease: mechanisms and models. *Neuron* 2003;39:889–909.

Dawson TM, Dawson VL. Rare genetic mutations shed light on the pathogenesis of Parkinson disease. *J Clin Invest* 2003;111:145–151.

Dooneief G, Chen J, Mirabello E, et al. An estimate of the incidence of depression in idiopathic Parkinson's disease. *Arch Neurol* 1992;49:305–307.

Eidelberg D, Takikawa S, Moeller JR, et al. Striatal hypometabolism distinguishes striatonigral degeneration from Parkinson's disease. *Ann Neurol* 1993;33:518–527.

Elble RJ, Hughes L, Higgins C. The syndrome of senile gait. *J Neurol* 1992;239:71–75.

Fahn S. The freezing phenomenon in parkinsonism. *Adv Neurol* 1995;67:53–63.

Fahn S, Sulzer D. Neurodegeneration and neuroprotection in Parkinson disease. *NeuroRx* 2004;1:139–154.

FitzGerald PM, Jankovic J. Lower body parkinsonism: evidence for vascular etiology. *Mov Disord* 1989;4:249–260.

Freed CR, Greene PE, Breeze RE, et al. Transplantation of embryonic dopamine neurons for severe Parkinson's disease. *N Engl J Med* 2001;344:710–719.

Friedman J, Lannon M, Comella C, et al. Low-dose clozapine for the treatment of drug-induced psychosis in Parkinson's disease. *N Engl J Med* 1999;340:757–763.

Friedman JH, Feinberg SS, Feldman RG. A neuroleptic malignant-like syndrome due to levodopa therapy withdrawal. *JAMA* 1985;254:2792–2795.

Gibb WRG, Luthert PJ, Janota I, et al. Cortical Lewy body dementia: clinical features and classification. *J Neurol Neurosurg Psychiatry* 1989;52:185–192.

Gibb WRG, Luthert PJ, Marsden CD. Corticobasal degeneration. *Brain* 1989;112:1171–1192.

Giladi N, Burke RE, Kostic V, et al. Hemiparkinsonism-hemiatrophy syndrome: clinical and neuroradiological features. *Neurology* 1990;40:1731–1734.

Giladi N, McDermott MP, Fahn S, et al. Freezing of gait in PD: Prospective assessment in the DATATOP cohort. *Neurology* 2001;56:1712–1721.

Hughes AJ, Daniel SE, Ben-Shlomo Y, et al. The accuracy of diagnosis of parkinsonian syndromes in a specialist movement disorder service. *Brain* 2002;125(Pt 4):861–870.

Hughes AJ, Daniel SE, Kilford L, et al. Accuracy of clinical diagnosis of idiopathic Parkinson's disease—a clinicopathological study of 100 cases. *J Neurol Neurosurg Psychiatry* 1992;55:181–184.

Kitada T, Asakawa S, Hattori N, et al. Mutations in the parkin gene cause autosomal recessive juvenile parkinsonism. *Nature* 1998;392:605–608.

Krack P, Batir A, Van Blercom N, et al. Five-year follow-up of bilateral stimulation of the subthalamic nucleus in advanced Parkinson's disease. *N Engl J Med* 2003;349:1925–1934.

Mayeux R, Denaro J, Hemenegildo N, et al. A population-based investigation of Parkinson's disease with and without dementia: relationship to age and gender. *Arch Neurol* 1992;49:492–497.

Metman LV, Deldotto P, van den Munckhof P, et al. Amantadine as treatment for dyskinesias and motor fluctuations in Parkinson's disease. *Neurology* 1998;50:1323–1326.

Metman LV, Konitsiotis S, Chase TN. Pathophysiology of motor response complications in Parkinson's disease: Hypotheses on the why, where, and what. *Mov Disord* 2000;15:3–8.

Parkinson Study Group. A controlled, randomized, delayed-start study of rasagiline in early Parkinson disease. *Arch Neurol* 2004;61:561–566.

Parkinson Study Group. Pramipexole versus levodopa as the initial treatment for Parkinson's disease: a randomized controlled trial. *JAMA* 2000;284:1931–1938.

Przedborski S, Giladi N, Takikawa S, et al. The metabolic topography of the hemiparkinsonism-hemiatrophy syndrome. *Neurology* 1994;44:1622–1628.

Rascol O, Brooks DJ, Korczyn AD, et al. A five-year study of the incidence of dyskinesia in patients with early Parkinson's disease who were treated with ropinirole or levodopa. *N Engl J Med* 2000;342:1484–1491.

Shoulson I, Oakes D, Fahn S, et al., Parkinson Study Group. Impact of sustained deprenyl (selegiline) in levodopa-treated Parkinson's disease: a randomized placebo-controlled extension of the deprenyl and tocopherol antioxidative therapy of parkinsonism trial. *Ann Neurol* 2002;51:604–612.

Shults CW, Oakes D, Kieburtz K, et al. Effects of coenzyme Q10 in early Parkinson disease: evidence of slowing of the functional decline. *Arch Neurol* 2002;59:1541–1550.

Tanner CM, Goldman SM. Epidemiology of Parkinson's disease. *Neuroepidemiology* 1996;14:317–335.

Tanner CM, Ottman R, Goldman SM, et al. Parkinson disease in twins: an etiologic study. *JAMA* 1999;281:341–346.

Valente EM, Abou-Sleiman PM, Caputo V, et al. Hereditary early-onset Parkinson's disease caused by mutations in PINK1. *Science* 2004; 304:1158–1160.

Van Camp G, Flamez A, Cosyns B, et al. Treatment of Parkinson's disease with pergolide and relation to restrictive valvular heart disease. *Lancet* 2004;363:1179–1183.

Wooten GF, Currie LJ, Bennett JP, et al. Maternal inheritance in Parkinson's disease. *Ann Neurol* 1997;41:265–268.

Zijlmans JC, Daniel SE, Hughes AJ, et al. Clinicopathological investigation of vascular parkinsonism, including clinical criteria for diagnosis. *Mov Disord* 2004;19:630–640.

Chapter 116

▶ Progressive Supranuclear Palsy

Paul E. Greene

Olszewski, Steele, and Richardson reviewed autopsies of patients who had a syndrome of pseudobulbar palsy, supranuclear ocular palsy (chiefly affecting vertical gaze), extrapyramidal rigidity, gait ataxia, and dementia. They found a consistent pattern of neuronal degeneration and neurofibrillary tangles, chiefly affecting the pons and midbrain. This condition became known as *progressive supranuclear palsy* (PSP), or the Steele-Richardson-Olszewski syndrome.

PATHOLOGY

Atrophy of the dorsal midbrain, globus pallidus, and subthalamic nucleus; depigmentation of the substantia nigra; and mild dilatation of the third and fourth ventricles and aqueduct are seen on gross visual inspection of the postmortem brain in typical PSP. Light microscopy shows neuronal loss with gliosis, numerous neurofibrillary tan-

gles (NFTs), and neurophil threads in many subcortical structures, including the subthalamic nucleus, pallidum, substantia nigra, locus ceruleus, periaqueductal gray matter, superior colliculi, nucleus basalis, and vestibular, red, and oculomotor nuclei. Less severe neuronal loss, gliosis, and deposition of NFTs are usually found in the cerebral cortex, especially the prefrontal and precentral cortices.

The NFTs are argyrophilic and appear as skeins of fine fibrils, globose in shape in the brainstem and coil-shaped in the cortex. Ultrastructurally, they are composed of short straight 12- to 15-nm tubules arranged in circling and interlacing bundles. They react with antisera to several antigens on neurofilaments and to the neurotubule-associated protein tau. The histologic features in typical PSP are similar to those found in postencephalitic (von Economo) parkinsonism and Guamanian amyotrophic lateral sclerosis–Parkinson–dementia syndrome (Lytico-Bodig). New histologic techniques have demonstrated hyperphosphorylated, insoluble tau in cases of PSP, Alzheimer Disease (AD), corticobasal ganglionic degeneration, Pick disease (PD), and frontotemporal dementia–parkinsonism. The significance of this overlap is not known. Immunohistochemical analysis demonstrates differences in the tau found in these disorders: In PSP, inclusion of exon 10 of tau creates a predominance of four repeated microtubule binding domains, compared to three repeated domains in most cases of Pick disease and a mixture of three and four repeated domains in AD.

SYMPTOMS AND SIGNS

Patients with PSP have an akinetic rigid parkinsonlike syndrome; rest tremor is uncommon. Balance difficulty and falling are early symptoms. Unlike PD, axial rigidity exceeds limb rigidity, and the posture may be erect. Patients have marked facial dystonia with deep nasolabial folds and furrowed brow (Procerus sign), an appearance of surprise or concern (Fig. 116.1). When the patient walks, the neck may be extended; the arms are abducted at the shoulders and flexed at the elbows. Dysphagia and dysarthria are usually severe. The voice is slurred and hoarse, and some patients become anarthric as the disease progresses. "Freezing" may be prominent; transient arrest of motor activity interrupts walking, speaking, or other actions.

The first visual symptoms are failure to maintain eye contact in social interactions and difficulty with tasks requiring downgaze, such as reading, eating, or descending stairs. The patients often complain of diplopia, blurred vision, or difficulty reading. Disturbances of eyelid motility are common, including blepharospasm and apraxia of eyelid opening or closing.

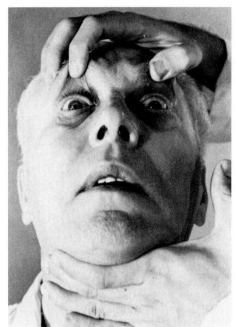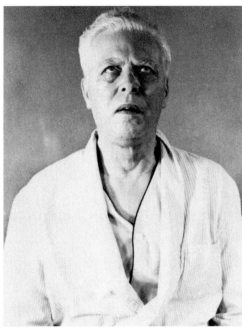

FIGURE   116.1.   Progressive supranuclear palsy. Oculocephalic maneuver demonstrates intact reflex downgaze in a patient unable to look down voluntarily.

The cognitive impairment of PSP has been considered the archetype of *subcortical dementia*. The striking features are severe bradyphrenia, impaired verbal fluency, and difficulty with sequential actions or shifting from one task to another. Cognitive tests that depend on visual performance are especially affected. Dementia is less severe than might be suggested by the dysarthria, bradyphrenia, poor eye contact, and loss of facial expression. Apathy and disinhibition are common. Emotional incontinence is dominated by inappropriate weeping or, less frequently, laughing.

The course is aggressive; at 3 to 4 years after onset, patients cannot walk without assistance, and at a median of 5 years after onset they are confined to bed and chair. They succumb to infection (from aspiration or pressure ulcers) or the sequelae of falls. The course is one of inexorable deterioration, culminating in death in 6 to 10 years.

LABORATORY DATA

Routine laboratory investigations are normal. The EEG may show some slowing and disorganization without localizing features. Atrophy of the pons, midbrain, and anterior temporal lobes may be noted on CT or MRI. Rostral midbrain atrophy may produce a CT or MRI appearance resembling the beak of a hummingbird. PET with [18F]fluoro-l-dopa shows equal loss of uptake in caudate and putamen; PET using [18F]fluorodeoxyglucose shows

global reduction in metabolism, most severe in the frontal lobes. Neither of these PET findings is specific for PSP. CSF is unremarkable.

DIAGNOSIS

Levodopa-unresponsive parkinsonism with abnormal gait, loss of postural reflexes, and supranuclear ophthalmoplegia suggest the diagnosis of PSP. Clinical criteria for possible, probable, and definite PSP have been proposed by the National Institute of Neurological Disorders and Stroke (Table 116.1). These criteria are specific but will exclude some patients with PSP who are mild or have unusual clinical features. The chief differential diagnoses are PD, corticobasal ganglionic degeneration, cerebral multi-infarct disease, frontotemporal dementia–parkinsonism and diffuse Lewy body disease. Differentiation from olivopontocerebellar atrophy (OPCA) with ophthalmoplegia may also be difficult; but the ocular palsy in OPCA preferentially affects horizontal movements. In the absence of the characteristic ocular palsy, diagnosis is difficult.

Examination of ocular and eyelid motility is crucial to the clinical diagnosis of PSP. Eyelid opening and closing apraxias are far more common in PSP than in any other extrapyramidal disorder. Fixation instability with coarse square-wave jerks and faulty suppression of the vestibulo-ocular reflex are helpful features. Hesitation on voluntary downgaze is one of the earliest signs. Loss of vertical opticokinetic nystagmus on downward movement of the target confirms that finding. The demonstration

▶ **TABLE 116.1 Diagnostic Criteria for Progressive Supranuclear Palsy**

Possible PSP
Gradually progressive parkinsonism
Onset after age 40 yr
Vertical supranuclear palsy or slow vertical saccades with early falling
Absence of each of these: history of encephalitis; focal cortical deficits (e.g., alien limb syndrome, cortical sensory deficits, focal cortical myoclonus); cortical dementia of the Alzheimer type; prominent early cerebellar symptoms; unexplained dysautonomia (e.g., hypotension, urinary disturbances); severe asymmetric parkinsonian signs; neuroradiologic evidence of relevant structural abnormality (e.g., lobar atrophy, basal ganglia, or brainstem infarcts); evidence of Whipple disease (confirmed by polymerase chain reaction, if indicated)

Probable PSP
Possible PSP with vertical supranuclear palsy and early falling

Definite PSP
Possible PSP or *probable PSP* and histopathologic evidence of typical PSP

Supportive criteria
Symmetric akinesia or rigidity, proximal more than distal
Abnormal neck posture, especially retrocollis
Poor or absent response of parkinsonian symptoms to levodopa therapy
Early dysphagia and dysarthria
Early onset of cognitive impairment, including at least two of the following:
    Apathy
    Impairment in abstract thought
    Decreased verbal fluency use or imitation behavior
    Frontal release signs

Modified from Litvan I, Agid Y, Calne D, et al. Clinical research criteria for the diagnosis of progressive supranuclear palsy (Steele-Richardson-Olszewski syndrome). *Neurology* 1996;47:1–9.

of greater impairment of voluntary than of pursuit movements and of preservation of reflex ocular movements supports the diagnosis. Similar abnormalities, however, are occasionally seen in corticobasal ganglionic degeneration, cerebral multi-infarct disease, and diffuse Lewy body disease.

TREATMENT

The etiology of PSP is unknown, and there is no specific treatment. Levodopa/carbidopa and other antiparkinson medications are usually ineffective, although they are rarely helpful in alleviating the parkinsonian features of rigidity and bradykinesia. When they are helpful, benefit is short lived or limited by toxic psychic effects, which tend to become prominent when dementia develops. Tricyclic antidepressants may suppress inappropriate crying or laughing. Anticholinergic drugs administered in modest doses may be useful in controlling drooling. Apraxia of eyelid opening and painful neck or limb dystonia may improve with botulinum toxin injections. Some patients and families choose to use an enteric feeding tube when dysphagia becomes severe.

SUGGESTED READINGS

Aarsland D, Litvan I, Larsen JP. Neuropsychiatric symptoms of patients with progressive supranuclear palsy and Parkinson's disease. *J Neuropsychiatry Clin Neurosci* 2001;13:42–49.

Burn DJ, Lees AJ. Progressive supranuclear palsy: where are we now? *Lancet Neurology* 2002;1:359–369.

Friedman DI, Jankovic J, McCrary III JA. Neuro-ophthalmic findings in progressive supranuclear palsy. *J Clin Neruo-ophthalmol* 1992;12:104–109.

Josephs KA, Dickson DW. Diagnostic accuracy of progressive supranuclear palsy in the Society for Progressive Supranuclear Palsy brain bank. *Mov Disord* 1003;18:1018–1026.

Kato N, Arai K, Hattori T. Study of the rostral midbrain atrophy in progressive supranuclear palsy. *J Neurol Sci* 2003;210:57–60.

Litvan I, Agid Y, eds. *Progressive Supranuclear Palsy: Clinical and Research Approaches.* New York: Oxford University Press, 1992.

Litvan I, Agid Y, Calne D, et al. Clinical research criteria for the diagnosis of progressive supranuclear palsy (Steele-Richardson-Olszewski syndrome). *Neurology* 1996;47:1–9.

Nath U, Ben-Shlomo Y, Thomson RG, et al. Clinical features and natural history of progressive supranuclear palsy. *Neurology* 2003;60:910–916.

Pastor P, Tolosa E. Progressive supranuclear palsy: clinical and genetic aspects. *Curr Opin Neurol* 2002;15:429–437.

Piccini P, de Yebenez J, Lees AJ, et al. Familial progressive supranuclear palsy: detection of subclinical cases using ^{18}F-dopa and ^{18}fluorodeoxyglucose positron emission tomography. *Arch Neurol* 2001;58:1846–1851.

Pierrot-Deseilligny C, Gaymard B, Mun R, et al. Cerebral ocular motor signs. *J Neurol* 1997;244:65–70.

Riley DE, Fogt N, Leigh RJ. The syndrome of "pure akinesia" and its relationship to progressive supranuclear palsy. *Neurology* 1994;44:1025–1029.

Steele JC, Richardson JC, Olszewski J. Progressive supranuclear palsy: a heterogenous degeneration involving the brain stem, basal ganglia and cerebellum with vertical gaze and pseudobulbar palsy, nuchal dystonia and dementia. *Arch Neurol* 1964;10:333–359.

Thobois S, Guillouet S, Broussolle E. Contributions of PET and SPECT to the understanding of the pathophysiology of Parkinson's disease. *Neurophysiol Clin* 2001;31:321–340.

Chapter 117

Tardive Dyskinesia and Other Neuroleptic-Induced Syndromes

Stanley Fahn and Robert E. Burke

The most widely used drugs that block dopamine D2 receptors are the antipsychotic agents, such as the phenothiazines and the butyrophenones; others include metoclopramide, flunarizine (Sibelium), and cinnarizine. These D2 receptor blocking agents can cause the following adverse neurologic effects:

Acute dystonic reaction
Oculogyric crisis
Acute akathisia
Drug-induced parkinsonism
Neuroleptic malignant syndrome
Withdrawal emergent syndrome
Persistent dyskinesias (tardive dyskinesia syndromes)
    Classic orobuccolingual dyskinesia
    Tardive dystonia
    Tardive akathisia
    Tardive tics
    Tardive myoclonus
    Tardive tremor

The atypical neuroleptic clozapine (Clozaril), a drug that predominantly blocks the D4 receptor, is free of these complications, except for acute akathisia. The related drug quetiapine is also relatively free from the adverse effects listed above. Other drugs, also commonly called atypical neuroleptics, such as olanzapine (Zyprexa) and risperidone (Risperdal), more readily induce the above adverse effects. The dopamine-depleting drugs reserpine and tetrabenazine can induce acute akathisia and drug-induced parkinsonism but have never been convincingly implicated in causing the other complications listed, other than acute dystonic reactions from tetrabenazine.

Acute dystonic reactions tend to occur within the first few days of exposure to the dopamine-receptor blocker and predominantly affect children and young adults and males more than females. Severe twisting and uncomfortable postures of limbs, trunk, neck, tongue, and face are dramatic. *Oculogyric crisis* is a form of dystonia in which the eyes are deviated conjugately in a fixed posture for minutes or hours. Dystonic reactions are easily reversible with parenteral administration of antihistamines (e.g., diphenhydramine, 50 mg intravenously), anticholinergic drugs (e.g., benztropine mesylate [Cogentin], 2 mg intramuscularly), or diazepam (5 to 7.5 mg intramuscularly).

Acute akathisia occurs within the first few months of drug use; it may appear as the dosage is being increased. Akathisia consists of a *subjective* sense of restlessness or aversion to being still. The *motor* features of restlessness include frequent and repetitive stereotyped movements, such as pacing, repeatedly caressing the scalp, or crossing and uncrossing the legs. It can occur in subjects of any age. The β-adrenergic blocker propranolol may be helpful in doses of 20 to 80 mg/day. Anticholinergic agents occasionally help. Acute akathisia disappears on discontinuance of the offending drug.

Drug-induced parkinsonism resembles idiopathic parkinsonism in manifesting all the cardinal signs of the syndrome. Levodopa is not effective in reversing this complication, probably because the dopamine receptors are blocked and occupied by the antipsychotic agent. Oral anticholinergic drugs and amantadine are effective. On withdrawal of the offending antipsychotic drug, the symptoms slowly disappear in weeks or months.

The *neuroleptic malignant syndrome* is characterized by a triad of fever, signs of autonomic dysfunction (e.g., pallor, diaphoresis, blood pressure instability, tachycardia, pulmonary congestion, tachypnea), and a movement disorder (e.g., akinesia, rigidity, or dystonia). The level of consciousness may be depressed, eventually leading to stupor or coma; death may occur. Withdrawal of antipsychotic medication and supportive therapy, including intravenous hydration and cooling, are recommended. Although controlled trials have not been conducted, numerous reports suggest that dantrolene sodium (Dantrium), a muscle relaxant, or bromocriptine (Parlodel), a direct-acting dopamine agonist, may be beneficial. Carbamazepine (Tegretol) is also effective. In most patients, the antipsychotic medication can be restarted later without recurrence of the syndrome.

The *withdrawal emergent syndrome* may be a variant of tardive dyskinesia. "Emergent" implies that the symptoms emerge after abrupt cessation of the chronic use of an antipsychotic drug. The syndrome is primarily one of children. The choreic movements resemble those of Sydenham chorea because the movements are flowing rather than repetitive, as seen in classic tardive dyskinesia. The withdrawal emergent syndrome is self-limiting but may take weeks to resolve. Reintroducing the antipsychotic drug and then slowly tapering the dosage can eliminate the choreic movements.

The *persistent dyskinesia syndromes* are the most feared complications of antipsychotic medications because the symptoms are long lasting and often permanent. *Classic tardive dyskinesia* consists of repetitive (stereotypic) rapid movements. The lower part of the face is most often involved; this orobuccolingual dyskinesia resembles continual chewing movements, with the tongue intermittently darting out of the mouth ("fly-catcher" tongue). Movements of the trunk may cause a repetitive pattern of flexion and extension (body rocking). The distal parts of the limbs may show incessant flexion-extension movements ("piano-playing" fingers and toes). The proximal muscles are usually spared, but respiratory dyskinesias are not. The patient may not be aware of the dyskinesia.

The prevalence of classic tardive dyskinesia increases with age; it is more severe among elderly women and more likely to occur with longer duration of exposure to antipsychotic drugs. The time of onset is difficult to discern because these drugs mask the movements. Reducing the dosage or discontinuing the offending drug can unmask the disorder, and reinstituting the drug can suppress the movements.

Not all cases of *oral dyskinesia* are classic tardive dyskinesia. There are many other choreic and nonchoreic causes. Essential to the diagnosis of tardive dyskinesia is a history of exposure to dopamine D2 receptor blocking drugs. For this diagnosis, the symptoms should have started while the patient was still taking the drug or less than 3 months after discontinuing the drug. If oral dyskinesia is induced by other types of drugs, it is not, by definition, tardive dyskinesia. The following list outlines the classification of movement disorders affecting the face:

Chorea and stereotypies
  Encephalitis lethargica; postencephalitic
  Drug-induced
    Tardive dyskinesia (antipsychotics)
    Levodopa
    Anticholinergic drugs
    Phenytoin intoxication
    Antihistamines
    Tricyclic antidepressants
  Huntington disease
  Hepatocerebral degeneration
  Cerebellar and brainstem infarction
  Edentulous malocclusion
  Idiopathic
Dystonia
  Meige syndrome
    Complete: oromandibular dystonia plus
      blepharospasm
    Incomplete syndromes
      Mandibular dystonia
      Orofacial dystonia
      Lingual dystonia
      Pharyngeal dystonia
      Essential blepharospasm
  Bruxism
    As part of a segmental or generalized dystonic
      syndrome

Myoclonus and tics
  Facial tics
  Facial myoclonus of central origin
  Facial nerve irritability
    Hemifacial spasm
    Myokymia
    Faulty regeneration; synkinesis
Tremor
  Essential tremor of neck and jaw
  Parkinsonian tremor of jaw, tongue, and lips
  Idiopathic tremor of neck, jaw, tongue, or lips
  Cerebellar tremor of neck

Huntington disease and oromandibular dystonia are the major differential diagnoses of the oral dyskinesias. Oromandibular dystonia is probably the most common form of spontaneous oral dyskinesia. Clinical features differentiating these disorders from classic tardive dyskinesia are presented in Table 117.1. Patients with Huntington disease are frequently treated with antipsychotic drugs; a resulting tardive dyskinesia may be superimposed on the chorea. The presence of akathisia or repetitive (stereotyped) involuntary movements suggests the additional diagnosis of tardive dyskinesia. Often, oromandibular dystonia takes the appearance of a repetitive opening and closing of the jaw as the patient attempts to overcome the muscle pulling. By asking the patient not to fight the involuntary movement but to let it "do what it wants to do," one can usually discern whether the oral dystonia is of the jaw-closing or jaw-opening form.

Several important forms of tardive dyskinesia syndrome are now recognized. Unlike classic oral dyskinesia, these forms are frequently quite disabling. *Tardive dystonia* is a chronic dystonia resulting from exposure to dopamine D2 receptor blockers. Individuals of all ages are susceptible to tardive dystonia, and younger individuals are more likely to have a more severe generalized form. Tardive dystonia usually begins in the face or neck, and may remain confined to these regions or may spread to the arms and trunk. The legs are infrequently affected. Often, neck involvement consists of retrocollis and the trunk arches backward. The arms are typically rotated internally, the elbows extended, and the wrists flexed. The differential diagnosis includes all the many causes of dystonia. Wilson disease, in particular, must be excluded specifically in any patient with psychiatric symptoms and dystonia.

Tardive akathisia is another important disabling variant of tardive dyskinesia. It is a chronic akathisia consisting of a subjective aversion to being still. Motor signs of restlessness include frequent, repeated, stereotyped movements, such as marching in place, crossing and uncrossing the legs, and repetitively rubbing the face or hair with the hand. Patients may not use the word "restless" to describe their symptoms; instead they may use expressions such as "going to jump out of my skin" or "jittery" or "exploding

▶ **TABLE 117.1** Clinical Features of Classic Tardive Dyskinesia (TD), Oromandibular Dystonia (OMD), and Huntington Disease (HD)

Clinical Signs	*TD*	*OMD*	*HD*
Type of Involuntary Movements	*Stereotypic*	*Dystonic*	*Choreic*
Flowing movements	0	0	+++
Repetitive movements	+++	+	±
Sustained contractions	+	+++	±
Movements of mouth	+++	+++	+
Blepharospasm	+	+++	+
Forehead chorea	±	±	++
Platysma	±	+++	±
Masticatory muscles	+++	+++	±
Nuchal muscles	+	++	±
Trunk, legs	++	0	+++
Akathisia	++	0	0
Marching in place	++	0	0
Truncal rocking	++	0	+
Motor impersistence (tongue, grip)	0	0	+++
Stuttering, ataxic gait	±	0	+++
Postural instability	0	0	+++
Effect of			
Antidopaminergics	Decrease	Decrease	Decrease
Anticholinergics	Increase	Decrease	±
Effect on			
Talking, chewing	±	+++	+
Swallowing	0	++	+++

0, not seen; ±; may be seen; +, occasionally seen; ++, usually seen; +++, almost always seen.

inside." Akathisia can appear as focal discomfort, such as pain, or as moaning sounds. It can be a distressing symptom. In contrast to acute akathisia, the delayed type tends to become worse when antipsychotic medication is withdrawn, similar to the worsening of classic tardive dyskinesia on discontinuance of these drugs. As with other types of tardive dyskinesia syndrome, tardive akathisia tends to persist. Usually, tardive akathisia is associated with classic oral dyskinesia. Classic tardive dyskinesia, tardive dystonia, and tardive akathisia may occur together. Less common variants of tardive dyskinesia include *tardive tics, tardive myoclonus,* and *tardive tremor.*

Efforts should be made to avoid the tardive dyskinesia syndromes. Antipsychotic drugs should be given only when indicated, namely, to control psychosis or a few other conditions where no other effective agent has been helpful, as in some choreic disorders or tics. These drugs should not be used indiscriminately, and when they are used, the dosage and duration should be as low and as brief as possible. If the psychosis has been controlled, the physician should attempt to reduce the dosage and even try to eliminate the drug, if possible. Once a tardive dyskinesia syndrome has appeared, treatment depends on eliminating the causative agents, the dopamine D2 receptor blocking drugs. Unfortunately, psychosis may no longer be under

control if these drugs are withdrawn; if the medication is required, increasing the dosage or adding reserpine may suppress the dyskinesia and akathisia. If the antipsychotic drug can be tapered and discontinued safely, the dyskinesia and akathisia may slowly subside in months or years. If the dyskinetic or akasthitic symptoms are too distressful, treatment with dopamine-depleting drugs, such as reserpine, may suppress them. The dosage of reserpine should be increased gradually to avoid the side effects of postural hypotension and depression. A dosage of 6 mg/day or more may be required. Addition of α-methyltyrosine may be necessary to relieve symptoms, but this combination is more likely to cause postural hypotension and parkinsonism. With time, these dopamine-depleting drugs may eventually be tapered and discontinued. Tardive dystonia may be treated by dopamine depletion, but unlike oral tardive dyskinesia and akathisia, it may be treated with anticholinergic drugs. Clozapine may be helpful in some patients with tardive dystonia.

The pathogenesis of the tardive dyskinesia syndromes is unknown. No one hypothesis is able to explain the disorder, and more than one factor may be necessary. These factors include the development of dopamine receptor supersensitivity, activation of dopamine D1 receptors, and loss of γ-aminobutyric acid activity in the subthalamic nucleus.

SUGGESTED READINGS

Andersson U, Haggstrom JE, Levin ED, et al. Reduced glutamate decarboxylase activity in the subthalamic nucleus in patients with tardive dyskinesia. *Mov Disord* 1989;4:37–46.

Burke RE, Kang UK, Jankovic J, et al. Tardive akathisia: an analysis of clinical features and response to open therapeutic trials. *Mov Disord* 1989;4:157–175.

Correll CU, Leucht S, Kane JM. Lower risk for tardive dyskinesia associated with second-generation antipsychotics: a systematic review of 1-year studies. *Am J Psychiatry* 2004;161:414–425.

Dolder CR, Jeste DV. Incidence of tardive dyskinesia with typical versus atypical antipsychotics in very high risk patients. *Biol Psychiatry* 2004;53:1142–1145.

Fahn S. A therapeutic approach to tardive dyskinesia. *J Clin Psychiatry* 1985;46:19–24.

Ford B, Greene P, Fahn S. Oral and genital tardive pain syndromes. *Neurology* 1994;44:2115–2119.

Friedman J, Feinberg SS, Feldman RG. A neuroleptic malignant-like syndrome due to l-dopa withdrawal. *Ann Neurol* 1984;16:126–127.

Henderson VW, Wooten GF. Neuroleptic malignant syndrome: a pathogenetic role for dopamine receptor blockade? *Neurology* 1981;31:132–137.

Kane JM, Woerner M, Borenstein M, et al. Integrating incidence and prevalence of tardive dyskinesia. *Psychopharmacol Bull* 1986;22:254–258.

Kang UJ, Burke RE, Fahn S. Natural history and treatment of tardive dystonia. *Mov Disord* 1986;1:193–208.

Kiriakakis V, Bhatia KP, Quinn NP, et al. The natural history of tardive dystonia: a long-term follow-up study of 107 cases. *Brain* 1998;121:2053–2066.

Oosthuizen PP, Emsley RA, Maritz JS, et al. Incidence of tardive dyskinesia in first-episode psychosis patients treated with low-dose haloperidol. *J Clin Psychiatry* 2003;64:1075–1080.

Paulsen JS, Caligiuri MP, Palmer B, et al. Risk factors for orofacial and limb-truncal tardive dyskinesia in older patients: a prospective longitudinal study. *Psychopharmacology* 1996;123:307–314.

Seeman P, Tallerico T. Antipsychotic drugs which elicit little or no parkinsonism bind more loosely than dopamine to brain D2 receptors, yet occupy high levels of these receptors. *Mol Psychiatry* 1998;3:123–134.

Smith JM, Baldessarini RJ. Changes in prevalence, severity and recovery in tardive dyskinesia with age. *Arch Gen Psychiatry* 1980;37:1368–1373.

Thomas P, Maron M, Rascle C, et al. Carbamazepine in the treatment of neuroleptic malignant syndrome. *Biol Psychiatry* 1998;43:303–305.

Van Harten PN, Kamphuis DJ, Matroos GE. Use of clozapine in tardive dystonia. *Prog Neuropsychopharmacol Biol Psychiatry* 1996;20:263–274.

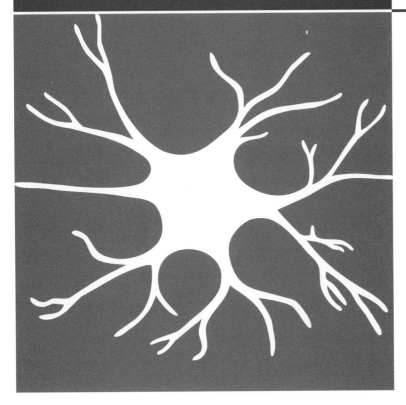

Spinal Cord Diseases

Hereditary and Acquired Spastic Paraplegia

*Lewis P. Rowland and
Paul H. Gordon*

Several different diseases are evident solely or primarily by spastic gait disorder (spastic paraparesis), which may progress to spastic paralysis of the legs (paraplegia). Autopsy usually reveals degeneration of the corticospinal tracts with or without involvement of other motor, sensory, or cerebellar systems. Among both heritable and acquired diseases, there is heterogeneity of pathogenesis.

HEREDITARY SPASTIC PARAPLEGIA

Harding (1993) divided hereditary spastic paraplegia (HSP) syndromes into pure and complicated types, depending on the clinical manifestations. The complications include epilepsy, mental retardation, dementia, parkinsonism, ataxia, amyotrophy, peripheral neuropathy, and blindness or deafness. One multisystem syndrome, spastic paraplegia (SPG1), gained the acronym CRASH (corpus callosum hypoplasia, retardation, adducted thumbs, spasticity, and hydrocephalus). Even in pure HSP, sensory evoked responses may be abnormal, and the spinocerebellar tracts were affected at autopsy in Strumpell's original description in 1890.

Genetics

The syndrome is genetically heterogeneous; most families show autosomal-dominant inheritance, but some are autosomal recessive and others are X linked (Table 118.1). Locus heterogeneity is evident because X-linked forms map to chromosome Xq28, Xq21, or Xq11. Autosomal-dominant families map to ten different loci (Table 118.2).

Families mapped to 16q24.3 have homozygous mutations in the gene for *paraplegin*, a mitochondrial ATPase. Mutations have also been found in the genes for spastin, heat shock protein 60, kinesin heavy chain, atlastin, spartin, prion protein, presenilin, or a triplet nucleotide expansion; anticipation is seen in some families. In one X-linked family, the mutation affected the gene for proteolipid protein,

TABLE 118.1   Classification of the Hereditary Spastic Paraplegias

MIM no.		SPG No
Pure spastic paraplegia		
182600	Autosomal dominant (AD)	3
182601	Autosomal dominant	4
600363	Autosomal dominant	6
607152	Autosomal dominant	19
603563	Autosomal dominant	8
605280	Autosomal dominant	13
604805	Autosomal dominant	12
270800	Autosomal recessive (AR)	5
Complicated spastic paraplegia with		
604187	Distal atrophy or uncomplicated, AD	10
270685	Amyotrophy of hands, AD, Silver syndrome	
605229	Mental retardation, motor neuropathy, AR	
604360	Thin corpus callosum, mental retardation, dysarthria, AR	
270700	Retinal degeneration, AR	
312920	CNS white matter abnormality or uncomplicated, X-linked	
248900	Spastic dysarthria and pseudobulbar signs, AR	
607259	Mitochondrial abnormalities or uncomplicated, AR	
275900	Amyotrophy of hands, AR, Troyer syndrome	
270805	Myoclonic epilepsy	
248900	Dementia, Mast syndrome	
600361	Peroneal muscular atrophy, AD	
303350	Mental retardation, aphasia, adducted thumbs, X-linked	
300266	Aphasia, poor vision, mental retardation, X-linked	
606353	Amyotrophy, juvenile primary lateral sclerosis, AR	
300100	Adrenomyeloneuropathy	
270200	Ichthyosis, mental retardation, retinopathy (Sjögren-Larsson syndrome)	
270550	Ataxia, Charlevoix-Sageunay syndrome, AR	
270950	Pigmentary macular degeneration, mental retardation	
182830	Optic atrophy	
270750	Hypopigmentation	
182690	Deafness, nephropathy	

▶ TABLE 118.2 Familial Spastic Paraplegia

Locus	Chromosome	Protein
Autosomal dominant		
SPG4	2p22	Spastin
SPG13	2q24-q34	Heat shock protein 60 mitochondrial chaperonin
SPG8	8q23-q24	
SPG9	10q23.3-q24.2	
SPG17	11q12-q14	
SPG10	12q13	Kinesin heavy chain
SPG3A	14q11-q21	Atlastin
SPG6	15q11	NIPA1
SPG12	19q13	
SPG19	9q33-q34	
Autosomal recessive		
SPG14	3q27-28	
SPG5	8q	
SPG11	15q	
SPG7	16q	Paraplegin
SPG15	14q	
SPG20	13q	Spartin
SPG21	13q14	
X-linked Recessive		
SPG1	Xq28	L1 cell adhesion molecule
SPG2	Xq21	Proteolipid protein
SPG16	Xq11.2	

Adapted from Fink JK. The hereditary spastic paraplegias. *Arch Neurol* 2003;60:1045–1049.

which is also involved in Pelizaeus-Merzbacher disease. Not all familial forms are inherited because infection with human T-cell lymphotropic virus type I (HTLV-I) can affect more than one person in a family.

Clinical Manifestations

The syndrome is also clinically heterogeneous. Some cases start early, others after age 35 years. Some are mild and some are severe. The complicated forms differ in the nature of the clinical associations. All are usually slowly progressive. The spastic gait disorder is one of coordination; there may be no weakness in manual muscle tests. Tendon reflexes are overactive, and Babinski signs and clonus are often evident. Sensation is usually normal on routine examination, but quantitative studies may show an abnormality. Sphincter symptoms may appear in late-onset forms. Manifestations often differ in members of the same family.

Laboratory Data

Laboratory studies, including MRI of the brain or spinal cord, are usually unrevealing. However, one family showed white matter lesions in the brain, and some show promi-

nent thinning of the corpus callosum. Sensory evoked potentials may be abnormal even without clinically evident sensory loss. Magnetic stimulation usually shows an abnormality of central motor conduction; responses are either absent or delayed. The CSF is not diagnostic.

Diagnosis and Treatment

Diagnosis is usually evident from the clinical and family data. Sporadic cases could be the result of new mutations, but most prove to be multiple sclerosis, as reviewed later in the differential diagnosis of primary lateral sclerosis. Definite diagnosis can be made in some by identification of the causative gene.

Management is primarily symptomatic. Physical therapy and conditioning exercise may help patients remain mobile. Baclofen (Lioresal), either oral or intrathecal, dantrolene, and tizanidine (Zanaflex) may reduce spasticity, but there have been no controlled trials in HSP. Oxybutynin (Ditropan) may relieve urinary urgency.

TROPICAL MYELONEUROPATHIES

The term *tropical myeloneuropathies* refers to several syndromes encountered in equatorial countries around the world. The syndromes are manifestations of lesions in the spinal cord and peripheral nerves, separately or together. These disorders have been long-standing public health problems. Some have been traced to specific causes, including infection with HTLV-I, or the chronic ingestion of cassava beans or lathyrogenic agents. Other exogenous toxins may play a role. In the past and perhaps still today, similar syndromes have been ascribed to nutritional deprivation.

Among the numerous names for these disorders are *Strachan syndrome, Jamaican neuropathy, tropical spastic paraparesis* (TSP), *tropical ataxic neuropathy* (TAN), *konzo*, and *lathyrism*. TSP has generated other acronyms: RAM (for retrovirus-associated myelopathy) and HAM (for HTLV-I-associated myelopathy).

History, Clinical Manifestations, and Pathology

Because the symptoms and signs of these disorders are similar and the modes of pathogenesis are only now being identified with precision, it seems reasonable to describe the several conditions together.

Strachan Syndrome (Nutritional Neuropathy)

Strachan (1897) is credited with the first description of these syndromes when he reported his observations of a disorder found on the Caribbean island of Jamaica. The symptoms included numbness and burning in the limbs, girdling pains, impairment of vision and hearing, muscle weakness and wasting, hyporeflexia, and sensory ataxia. Mucocutaneous lesions included angular stomatitis, glossitis, and scrotal dermatitis. Scott later described similar manifestations in Jamaican sugarcane workers; identical cases were reported in World War II prisoner-of-war camps in the Middle East and Asia; in the malnourished populations of Africa, India, and Malaya; and among those besieged in Madrid in the Spanish Civil War. Most patients so afflicted with *Strachan syndrome* have a predominantly sensory neuropathy, presumably a consequence of nutritional depletion. Neuropathologic studies have demonstrated symmetric ascending (secondary) degeneration in the posterior columns, spinocerebellar tracts, optic nerves, and peripheral nerves.

Jamaican Neuropathies: Tropical Ataxic Neuropathy and Tropical Spastic Paraparesis

Montgomery and colleagues (1964) described another group of patients in Jamaica. The dominant signs were spasticity and other evidence of corticospinal tract disease, sometimes with the peripheral manifestations of Strachan syndrome.

Two seemingly distinct varieties have been identified. Both are primarily diseases of adults. The *ataxic* form seems less common in Jamaica (but is more common in Nigeria). It evolves slowly and is generally less severe than the *spastic* type. Manifestations include sensory ataxia, numbness and burning sensations in the feet, deafness, visual impairment with optic atrophy and a central or paracentral scotoma, mild spasticity with Babinski signs, and wasting and weakness of the legs, sometimes with footdrop. Patients appear undernourished but without stigmata of nutritional disorder.

TSP is the more common variety of Jamaican neuropathy. It is a subacute condition in which pyramidal tract signs predominate and are accompanied by impairment of posterior column sensibility, bladder dysfunction, and girdling lumbar pain (Table 118.3). In both varieties, histamine-fast gastric achlorhydria and positive serologic tests for syphilis are frequent; in the more common subacute form, protein elevation and lymphocytic pleocytosis are found in the CSF. Myopathy, peripheral neuropathy, and leukoencephalopathy have been seen in some patients with HTLV-I infection. Antibodies to HTLV-I have been found in more than 80% of patients with TSP, and the virus has been isolated from CSF. The serologic abnormalities are similar in tropical countries throughout the world—Colombia, the Seychelles, Martinique, and the southernmost part of Japan around the city of Kagoshima.

The pathologic basis of *TAN* is not clear; it is presumed to be a myelopathy, and the ataxia is attributed to sensory loss. The pathology of TSP also needs more study, but descriptions include symmetric and severe degeneration of the pyramidal tracts and posterior columns. The

▶ **TABLE 118.3** Neurologic Signs in Tropical Spastic Paraparesis

Abnormal Signs	Affected (%)
Corticospinal	
Legs	100
Arms	60–90
Jaw jerk	30–70
Bladder dysfunction	70–90
Impaired position, vibration sense	10–60
Root or cord sensation	20–65
Optic atrophy	2–20
Cerebellar	3–10

Modified from Rodgers-Johnson et al., 1990.

spinocerebellar and spinothalamic pathways are affected in some patients. Nerve cell loss is evident in the Clarke column and in the anterior horns. Demyelination appears in the posterior spinal roots and in the optic and auditory nerves. In more acute cases, inflammatory exudates are seen in cord and spinal roots. The immune response to the virus may be an important cause of the nervous system abnormalities.

Lathyrism

The clinical manifestations of lathyrism are similar to those of TSP. It is mainly a disease of adults, and the manifestations are primarily those of pyramidal tract dysfunction. It is slowly progressive but may ultimately cause paraplegia. Descriptions of the disease extend back to ancient Hindu writings and to Hippocrates. Lathyrism was once probably prevalent in Europe, as well as tropical countries, but now seems restricted to India, Bangladesh, and Ethiopia.

Etiology

Malnutrition

Nutritional deprivation has long been recognized as a cause of peripheral neuropathy, optic neuropathy, and myelopathy. Avitaminosis and lack of other dietary necessities may account for some of the original cases of TSP and TAN, but other causes are now likely.

Persistent Viral Infection

The evidence of widespread HTLV-I infection in patients with TSP has had a major impact. Theoretically, it again shows that chronic viral infection can cause chronic human disease. The pathogenesis has not been elucidated, but transmission has been linked to blood transfusion, venereal contacts, contaminated needles of intravenous drug users, and the milk of nursing mothers. People with serologic evidence of syphilis, yaws, or HIV infection have a higher frequency of antibodies to HTLV-I. The disease may occur in more than one person in a family and could be confused with hereditary spastic paraparesis.

Dietary Toxins

The cause of lathyrism has long been ascribed to chronic ingestion of the chickling pea or vetch. *Lathyrus sativus* is a nourishing and inexpensive food that has been popular in impoverished countries. The active agent, isolated by Spencer and Schaumberg (1983), is a simple amino acid: β-(*N*)-oxalyl-amino-l-alanine.

Another dietary constituent has been implicated in the African ataxic disorder TAN. Among patients in Nigeria, ingestion of the cassava plant seems to be important. Although the essential ingredient has not been identified, some investigators suspect compounds that can generate cyanide.

Other Toxins and Nutritional Deprivation

No other toxins have been shown to be important in TSP or TAN. However, another myelopathy closely resembling TSP clinically was encountered in Japan until corrective measures were taken. That condition, called *subacute myelopathy-neuropathy,* was attributed to use of iodochlorhydroxyquinoline to treat traveler's diarrhea. The drug was withdrawn, and the syndrome seems to have disappeared.

Vernant disease is seen in the French West Indies and is characterized by the triad of optic neuritis, cervical myelopathy, and hypothalamic-hypophyseal abnormalities. The cause is not known. In Cuba, an epidemic of optic neuritis has been ascribed to nutritional deficiency.

Prevention and Treatment

These tropical diseases are widespread and have been called the "hidden endemias." Prevention seems more likely to have an impact than treatment. Malnutrition ought to be preventable. Venereal transmission is amenable to control (though not easily). Exogenous toxins can be excluded from the environment. Blood intended for transfusion must be monitored for HTLV-I.

Once neurologic damage exists, however, the task is more difficult. Prednisone therapy seems to be effective in TSP; however, it seems more likely to benefit motor function in Japan and Colombia and to help bladder symptoms in Jamaica. Antiviral drug therapy remains a goal. Even replacement therapy with vitamins may not restore function to normal. Rehabilitation and adaptation remain important.

PRIMARY LATERAL SCLEROSIS (PLS)

In theory, primary lateral sclerosis (PLS) should be the pure upper motor neuron component of amyotrophic lateral sclerosis (ALS), just as adult-onset progressive muscular atrophy is the purely lower motor neuron version of that disease. That assumption has not been proved, however, and the condition is still a diagnosis of exclusion. Before the introduction of MRI, many clinicians eschewed the clinical diagnosis of PLS because some other condition often turned up at autopsy. Now, however, MRI plays a key role in the clinical diagnosis, which concerns the differential diagnosis of spastic paraparesis of middle life.

Information about the prevalence of this condition is not available, but the syndrome accounts for less than 5% of all cases of motor neuron disease.

Clinical Manifestations

PLS commences after age 40 with a spastic gait disorder that is slowly progressive and becomes stable. In our experience, patients rarely lose the ability to walk with a cane or other assistance. No paresthesias or findings of sensory loss are evident on examination. Most patients with PLS have no sphincter symptoms.

Laboratory Data

The CSF is usually normal, but the protein content may be increased, without a rise in gamma globulin values or oligoclonal bands. Although EMG should not show signs of denervation, it sometimes does so without uniformly predicting the later appearance of lower motor neuron disease. MRI with or without gadolinium shows no consistent abnormality, but after age 40 years many asymptomatic people show small white matter lesions in the brain; PLS patients are not more likely to show these changes. However, there may be MRI evidence of atrophy of the motor cortex or high signal in the corticospinal tract. We and others have found MR spectroscopy more reliable in identifying pathology of the upper motor neuron in both PLS and ALS. Because PLS is likely to be heterogeneous in pathology, some cases may involve subcortical structures primarily, and MR spectroscopy may therefore be normal. Magnetic stimulation of the motor cortex may show delayed conduction of the corticospinal tracts. Sensory evoked potentials should be normal.

Diagnosis

The clinical diagnosis is made only after other possible causes of adult-onset progressive spastic paraparesis have been excluded. This process can be done with a reasonable dependence on modern imaging and a few blood tests (Table 118.4).

▶ **TABLE 118.4** Differential Diagnosis of Primary Lateral Sclerosis

Disease	Tests
Multiple sclerosis	MRI of brain and cervical spical cord with gadolinium; CSF examination with oligoclonal bands and gamma globulin synthesis; visual, somatosensory, brainstem auditory-evoked responses
Cervical cord compression 　Cervical spondylosis 　Chiari malformation 　Foramen magnum tumors 　Arteriovenous malformations	MRI with gadolinium
Amyotrophic lateral sclerosis	EMG
Adrenoleukodystrophy	Very long chain fatty acids in plasma
Tropical spastic paraparesis	HTLV-I antibody titer
HIV-associated myelopathy	HIV antibody titer
Paraneoplastic myelopathy	Evidence of primary neoplasm
Combined system disease	Serum vitamin B_{12} level

Modified from Younger et al., 1988.

No reliable figures exist for the relative frequency of the different diseases that cause spastic paraparesis. Most observers agree, however, that the main cause is the chronic and progressive form of spinal multiple sclerosis (MS). That diagnosis can be excluded with more than 90% certainty if none of the characteristic abnormalities of MS shows on all three modern tests: MRI with gadolinium to examine the brain and upper cervical cord, CSF examination including oligoclonal bands and gamma globulin, and evoked responses. Prominent bladder symptoms are more likely to be found in MS.

In the process of evaluating for MS, MRI also excludes other possible causes, such as cervical spondylotic myelopathy, Chiari malformation or other hindbrain anomaly, arteriovenous malformation, or tumor at the foramen magnum. Exclusion of cervical spondylosis may be difficult because the MRI findings of that condition are so prevalent in asymptomatic people. MRI also evaluates the possibility of multi-infarct brain disease. In theory, ALS sometimes should start first as a purely upper motor neuron disorder, but that seems truly exceptional. Clinical evidence of fasciculation implicates the lower motor neurons and, by definition, excludes PLS. However, PLS is truly a diagnosis of exclusion and conversion to ALS has been reported after 20 years of PLS. Clinical signs of parkinsonism, cerebellar disorder, or orthostatic hypotension imply a multisystem CNS disease, such as the Machado-Joseph syndrome or multiple system atrophy (Shy-Drager syndrome). One patient with PLS proved to have Lewy body disease, and we have seen one who proved to have Friedreich ataxia by DNA analysis. Rare causes of paraparesis are HTLV-I infection, HIV myelopathy, or adrenoleukodystrophy, which can be detected by appropriate tests. In time, some of these adult-onset cases are likely to be sporadic examples of one of the hereditary spastic paraparesis syndromes, but that possibility awaits better delineation of the specific mutations so that they can be tested. The condition is age-related, with almost all cases starting after age 40 years, so similar findings in children are likely to be owing to some other disease. In Tunisia and Saudi Arabia, juvenile PLS is familial, with mutations in the ALSIN gene.

SUGGESTED READINGS

Hereditary Spastic Paraplegia

Casali C, Valente EM, Bertini E, et al. Clinical and genetic studies in hereditary spastic paraplegia with thin corpus callosum. *Neurology* 2004;62:262–268.

Casari G, De Fusco M, Ciarmatori S, et al. Spastic paraplegia and OXPHOS impairment caused by mutations in paraplegin, a nuclear-encoded mitochondrial metalloprotease. *Cell* 1998;93:973–983.

Claus D, Waddy HM, Harding AE, et al. Hereditary motor and sensory neuropathies and hereditary spastic paraplegia: a magnetic stimulation study. *Ann Neurol* 1990;28:43–49.

Crook R, Verkkoniemi A, Perez-Tur J, et al. A variant of Alzheimer's disease with spastic paraparesis and unusual plaques due to deletion of exon 9 of presenilin 1. *Nat Med* 1998;4:452–455.

Fink JK. The hereditary spastic paraplegias. *Arch Neurol* 2003;60:1045–1049.

Gutmann DH, Fischbeck KH, Kamholz J. Complicated spastic paraparesis with cerebral white matter lesions. *Am J Med Genet* 1990;36:251–257.

Harding AE. Hereditary spastic paraplegia. *Semin Neurol* 1993;13:333–336.

Kitamoto T, Amano N, Terao Y, et al. A new inherited prion disease (PrP-P105L mutation) showing spastic paraparesis. *Ann Neurol* 1993;34:808–813.

Ueda M, Katayama Y, Kamiya T, et al. Hereditary spastic paraplegia with a thin corpus callosum and thalamic involvement in Japan. *Neurology* 1998;6:1751–1754.

Wilkinson PA, Simpson MA, Bastaki L, et al. A new locus for autosomal recessive complicated hereditary spastic paraplegia (SPG26) maps to chromosome 12p11.1–12q14. *J Med Genet* 2005 Jan;42(1):80–82.

Winner B, Uyanik G, Gross C, et al. Clinical progression and genetic analysis in hereditary spastic paraplegia with thin corpus callosum in spastic gait gene 11 (SPG11). *Arch Neurol* 2004;61:117–121.

Tropical Myeloneuropathies

Achiron A, Pinlas-Hamiel OP, Doll L, et al. Spastic paraparesis associated with human T-lymphotropic virus type 1: clinical, serological, and genomic study in Iranian-born Mashhadi Jews. *Ann Neurol* 1993;34:670–675.

Berger JR, Sabet A. Infectious myelopathies. *Semin Neurol* 2002;22:133–142.

Cruickshank EK. Neuromuscular disease in relation to nutrition. *Fed Proc* 1961;20([Suppl 7):345–360.

Cuetter AC. Strachan's syndrome. A nutritional disorder of the nervous system. *Proc Wkly Semin Neurol* 1968;18(Jan):20–27.

Denny-Brown D. Neurological conditions resulting from prolonged and severe dietary restriction. *Medicine* 1947;26:41–113.

Domingues RB, Muniz MR, Jorge ML, et al. Human T-cell lymphotropic virus type-1-associated myelopathy/tropical spastic paraparesis in Sao Paulo, Brazil: association with blood transfusion. *Am J Trop Med Hyg* 1997;57:56–59.

Douen AG, Pringle CE, Guberman A. Human T-cell lymphotropic virus type 1 myositis, peripheral neuropathy, and cerebral white matter lesions in the absence of spastic paraparesis. *Arch Neurol* 1997;54:896–900.

Fisher CM. Residual neuropathological changes in Canadians held prisoners of war by the Japanese. *Can Service Med J* 1955;11:157–199.

Gessain A, Gout O. Chronic myelopathy associated with human T-lymphotropic virus type 1 (HTLV-1). *Ann Intern Med* 1992;117:933–946.

Izumo S, Umehara F, Kashio N, et al. Neuropathology of HTLV-1-associated myelopathy (HAM/TSP). *Leukemia* 1997;11(Suppl 3):82–84.

Janssen RS, Kaplan JE, Khabbaz RF, et al. HTLV-1-associated myelopathy/tropical spastic paraparesis in the United States. *Neurology* 1991;41:1355–1357.

Kira J, Fujihara K, Itoyama Y, et al. Leucoencephalopathy in HTLV-1-associated myelopathy/tropical spastic paraparesis: MRI analysis and two-year follow-up study after corticosteroid therapy. *J Neurol Sci* 1991;106:41–49.

Montgomery RD, Cruickshank EK, Robertson WB, et al. Clinical and pathological observations on Jamaican neuropathy. *Brain* 1964;87:425–462.

Nagai M, Osame M. Human T-cell lymphotropic virus type I and neurological diseases. *J Neurovirol* 2003;9:228–235.

Osuntokun BO. An ataxic neuropathy in Nigeria: a clinical, biochemical and electrophysiological study. *Brain* 1965;91:215–248.

Roman GC. Tropical myeloneuropathies revisited. *Curr Opin Neurol* 1998;11:539–544.

Roman GC, Vernant JC, Osame M, eds. *HTLV-1 and the Nervous System.* New York: Alan R Liss, 1989.

Salazar-Grueso EF, Holzer TJ, et al. Familial spastic paraparesis syndrome associated with HTLV-1 infection. *N Engl J Med* 1990;108:732–737.

Smith CR, Dickson D, Samkoff L. Recurrent encephalopathy and seizures in a U.S. native with HTLV-1 associated myelopathy/tropical spastic paraparesis: clinicopathologic study. *Neurology* 1992;42:658–661.

Spencer PS, Schaumberg HH. Lathyrism: a neurotoxic disease. *Neurobehav Toxicol Teratol* 1983;5:625–629.

Strachan H. On a form of multiple neuritis prevalent in the West Indies. *Practitioner* 1897;59:477.

Tylleskar T, Howlett WP, Rwiza HT, et al. Konzo: a distinct disease entity with selective upper motor neuron damage. *J Neurol Neurosurg Psychiatry* 1993;56:638–643.

Umehara F, Nagatomo S, Yoshishige K, et al. Chronic progressive cervical myelopathy with HTLV-I infection: Variant form of HAM/TSP? *Neurology* 2004; 12;63(7):1276–1280.

Vernant JC, Maurs L, Gesain A, et al. Endemic tropical spastic paraparesis associated with human T-lymphotropic virus type I: a clinical and seroepidemiological study of 25 cases. *Ann Neurol* 1987;21:123–131.

Primary Lateral Sclerosis

Brown WF, Ebers GC, Hudson AJ, et al. Motor-evoked responses in primary lateral sclerosis. *Muscle Nerve* 1992;15:626–629.

Forsyth PA, Dalmau J, Graus F, et al. Motor neuron syndromes in cancer patients. *Ann Neurol* 1997;41:722–730.

Grignani G, Gobbi PG, Piccolo G, et al. Progressive necrotic myelopathy as a paraneoplastic syndrome: report of a case and some pathogenetic considerations. *J Intern Med* 1992;231:81–85.

Hainfellner JA, Pliz P, Lassmann H, et al. Diffuse Lewy body disease as substrate of primary lateral sclerosis. *J Neurol* 1995;242:59–63.

Le Forestier N, Maisonobe T, Piquard A, et al. Does primary lateral sclerosis exist? A study of 20 patients and a review of the literature. *Brain* 2001;124:1989–1999.

Mochizuki A, Komatsuzaki Y, Iwamoto H, Shoji S. Frontotemporal dementia with ubiquitinated neuronal inclusions presenting with primary lateral sclerosis and parkinsonism: clinicopathological report of an autopsy case. *Acta Neuropathol (Berl)* 2004 Apr; 107(4):377–380.

Pringle CE, Hudson AJ, Ebers GC. Primary lateral sclerosis: the clinical and laboratory definition of a discrete syndrome. *Can J Neurol Sci* 1990;17:235–236.

Pringle CE, Hudson AJ, Munoz DG, et al. Primary lateral sclerosis: clinical features, neuropathology, and diagnostic criteria. *Brain* 1992;115:495–520.

Rowland LP. Diagnosis of amyotrophic lateral sclerosis. *J Neurol Sci* 1998;160(Suppl 1);S6–S24.

Rowland LP. Paraneoplastic primary lateral sclerosis and amyotrophic lateral sclerosis. *Ann Neurol* 1997;41:703–705.

Rowland LP. Primary lateral sclerosis: disease, syndrome, both, or neither? *J Neurol Sci* 1999;170:1–4.

Swash M, Desai J, Misra VP. What is primary lateral sclerosis? *J Neurol Sci* 1999;170:5–10.

Tan CF, Kakita A, Piao YS, et al. Primary lateral sclerosis: a rare upper-motor-predominant form of amyotrophic lateral sclerosis often accompanied by frontotemporal lobar degeneration with ubiquitinated neuronal inclusions? Report of an autopsy case. *Acta Neuropath* 2003;105:615–620.

Younger DS, Chou S, Hays AP, et al. Primary lateral sclerosis: a clinical diagnosis reemerges. *Neurology* 1988;45:1304–1307.

Zhai P, Pagan F, Statland J, et al. Primary lateral sclerosis. A heterogeneous disorder composed of different subtypes? *Neurology* 2003;60:1258–1265.

Baclofen Therapy

Dario A, Tomei G. A benefit-risk assessment of baclofen in severe spinal spasticity. *Drug Saf* 2004;27(11):799–818.

McLean BN. Intrathecal baclofen in severe spasticity. *Br J Hosp Med* 1993;49:262–267.

Van Schaeybroeck P, Nuttin B, Lagae L, et al. Intrathecal baclofen for intractable cerebral spasticity: a prospective placebo-controlled, double-blind study. *Neurosurgery* 2000;46:603–609.

Zahavi A, Geertzen JH, Middel B, Staal M, Rietman JS. Long term effect (more than five years) of intrathecal baclofen on impairment, disability, and quality of life in patients with severe spasticity of spinal origin. *J Neurol Neurosurg Psychiatry* 2004 Nov;75(11):1553–1557.

Chapter 119

Hereditary and Acquired Motor Neuron Diseases

Lewis P. Rowland, Hiroshi Mitsumoto, and Darryl C. De Vivo

DEFINITIONS AND CLASSIFICATIONS

Several different diseases are characterized by progressive degeneration and loss of motor neurons in the spinal cord with or without similar lesions in the motor nuclei of the brainstem or the motor cortex, and by replacement of the lost cells by gliosis. All these can be considered *motor neuron diseases* (plural). The term *motor neuron disease* (singular) however, is used to describe an adult disease, *amyotrophic lateral sclerosis* (ALS), in which both upper and lower motor neurons are affected. (The terms *motor neuron disease* and *ALS* have become equivalent in the United States.)

The term *spinal muscular atrophy* (SMA) refers to syndromes characterized solely by lower motor neuron signs. By conventional usage, the term SMA is reserved for the childhood form, which is heritable. In adults, some patients also show only lower motor neuron signs in life (*progressive muscular atrophy* [PMA]). In five autopsy series, however, 53 of 70 patients with adult-onset PMA showed degeneration of the corticospinal tracts (Table 119.1). For that reason, adult-onset PMA is considered a form of ALS. Almost all adult-onset cases are sporadic, not familial.

A *motor neuropathy of adults* is also evident by lower motor neuron signs alone, with no sensory loss, and therefore resembles PMA. The condition is considered a neuropathy rather than a disease of the perikaryon because nerve conduction measurements show evidence of diffuse demyelination, focal demyelination (conduction block), or axonal neuropathy (see Chapter 15). Rarely, the diagnosis of motor neuropathy might depend on histologic changes in nerve rather than on physiologic criteria.

SPINAL MUSCULAR ATROPHIES OF CHILDHOOD

Three major syndromes of SMA occur in children. They differ in age at onset and severity of symptoms. All are autosomal recessive and map to the same locus, chromosome 5q11-q13. They are therefore regarded as examples of

▶ **TABLE 119.1** Autopsy Findings in Clinical Syndromes of Motor Neuron Disease: Degeneration of Pyramidal Tracts

	Clinical State		
	LMN Alone	**LMN + UMN**	**Total (%)**
Authors			
Brownell et al.	11/17	16/18	27/35
Lawyer-Netsky	6/8	45/45	51/53
Leung et al.	8/12	50/53	58/65
Shaw et al.	5/10	55/63	60/73
Piao et al.	23/23	59/59	82/82
Total	53/70	225/238	278/308
	(75.7)	(94.5)	(90.2)

In five autopsy series, the corticospinal tracts were affected in 75.7% of cases of the purely lower motor neuron syndrome, progressive muscular atrophy (PMA), and in 94.5% of cases in which there were both upper and lower motor neuron signs in life. Therefore, PMA is considered a form of ALS. References are listed in Suggested Reading.

allelic heterogeneity; that is, mutations of the same gene. In theory, there ought to be some locus heterogeneity, with some families showing the same or similar phenotype but mapping to different chromosomes; in fact, however, families throughout the world map to the same locus.

The gene is called *survival motor neurons gene* (SMN); SMN has two almost identical copies on chromosome 5, one telomeric (SMN1) and one centromeric (SMN2). If there were a conversion from the telomeric to the centromeric, SMN1 would seem to have been deleted, but there would be extra copies of SMN2, as is actually found in the less severe forms of the disease. The phenotypic variability of SMA correlates directly with the SMN2 copy number. SMN1 gene mutation is embryonic lethal in the absence of SMN2 gene. A quantitative study of SMN2 copy number in 375 patients with SMA Types 1, 2, and 3 showed that 80% of SMA1 patients had one or two SMN2 copies, 82% of SMA2 patients had three SMN2 copies, and 96% of SMA3 patients had three or four SMN2 copies. In theory, SMA carriers have approximately 50% SMN protein. A mouse model for SMA was made by knocking out the SMN1 gene and introducing the human SMN2 trans gene. The murine SMA phenotype is mitigated by increasing the SMN2 copy number, confirming observations in humans. These findings have become the basis for attempted treatment to increase SMN2 expression in children with SMA.

In 98% of children with the severe infantile SMA type I, there is a deletion of SMN1, and point mutations are found in the few who lack a deletion. Direct deletion analysis has high sensitivity and specificity and can be used for diagnosis without muscle biopsy in suspected cases; it is also effective in antenatal diagnosis in an at-risk fetus. The SMN protein is depleted in the spinal cords of patients.

How absence of SMN leads to the disease, however, still has to be elucidated.

Infantile SMA type I (Werdnig-Hoffmann syndrome; MIM 253300) is evident at birth or soon thereafter, always before age 6 months. Mothers may notice that intrauterine movements are decreased. In the neonatal period, nursing problems may occur and limb movements are feeble and decreased; this is one of the most common forms of the *floppy infant syndrome*. Proximal muscles are affected before distal muscles, but ultimately complete flaccid quadriplegia results. The tongue is often seen to fasciculate, but twitching is seen only rarely in limb muscles, presumably because of the ample subcutaneous fat. Sooner or later, respiration is compromised and paradoxical movements of the chest wall are seen; the sternum may be depressed with inspiration. Tendon reflexes are absent. The condition is devastating, and most infants die before age 2 years. The others may survive but never sit; their condition may remain stable for many years with respiratory assistance.

SMA type II (MIM 253550) patients have clinical onset from 6 months to 1 year and learn to sit but never walk. Respiratory insufficiency and scoliosis are dreaded complications.

With the introduction of EMG after World War II, Kugelberg and Welander noted physiologic evidence of denervation in adolescents with proximal limb weakness. The essentials of that disorder were delineated in the title of their paper, "Juvenile Spinal Muscular Atrophy Simulating Muscular Dystrophy;" the condition described is now called the *Kugelberg-Welander Syndrome*, or *SMA type III* (MIM 253400). These patients learn to walk but have varying degrees of weakness. Symptoms begin with a slowly progressive gait disorder in late childhood or adolescence. The onset is followed by symptoms of proximal arm weakness and wasting; tendon reflexes are lost. Unlike the Werdnig-Hoffmann syndrome, fasciculation of limb muscles, as well as of the tongue, and a tremor of the outstretched limb may be visible. This condition is relatively benign; many patients continue to function socially with a normal life span. Others may be handicapped with scoliosis, but serious dysphagia or respiratory compromise is rare. Sensation is spared, and no other organ systems are affected.

Laboratory Data

Electrodiagnostic studies show evidence of denervation with normal nerve conductions. Muscle biopsy similarly shows evidence of denervation. The CSF shows no characteristic changes. Serum levels of sarcoplasmic enzymes, such as creatine kinase, may be increased; in the Kugelberg-Welander Type, the increase may be 20 times normal, in the range of many myopathies. The electrocardiogram is normal.

Diagnosis now depends on DNA analysis. Muscle biopsy and even EMG are not necessary if a deletion or mutation of SMN is found.

Treatment

There are some promising leads for specific therapy. Classical gene therapy experiments now can target the SMN1 and SMN2 genes; splice-site enhancers can focus on SMN2 trying to increase the percentage of wild-type transcript, and pharmacological strategies may upregulate the SMN2 transcripts. Histone deacetylase inhibitors are a promising class of compounds that increase SMN protein in vitro. Treatment of survivors is analogous to that described for children with muscular dystrophy, using rehabilitative measures, bracing, attention to scoliosis, and assistance in education and social adaptation. Some authorities believe that children with SMA are characteristically of high intelligence; education programs are important.

FOCAL MUSCULAR ATROPHIES OF CHILDHOOD AND ADOLESCENCE

These syndromes do not map to 5q11 and differ in the focal distribution of symptoms and signs. Most are autosomal recessive, but some families show dominant inheritance.

Fazio-Londe Syndrome

In contrast to the sparing of cranial nerve functions in most juvenile SMA, selective dysarthria and dysphagia in Fazio-Londe syndrome (MIM 211500) begin in late childhood or adolescence. Wasting of the tongue with visible fasciculation occurs. Symptoms may be restricted for years, but weakness of the arms and legs may occur later, and respiration may be affected. There have been few documented cases and fewer autopsy-proven cases.

Scapuloperoneal and Facioscapulohumeral Forms of Spinal Muscular Atrophy

Scapuloperoneal (MIM 271220, 181400) and facioscapulohumeral (FSH; MIM 182970) forms of SMA have been reported. Some may actually have had FSH muscular dystrophy with ambiguous results on EMG and biopsy that led to incorrect classification as a neurogenic disorder. The distinction now depends on DNA analysis.

Childhood Spinal Muscular Atrophy with Known Biochemical Abnormality

Hexosaminidase deficiency (MIM 272800) may cause a syndrome of SMA starting in childhood or adolescence. The pattern of inheritance is autosomal recessive. Some patients also have upper motor neuron signs, as in ALS. Associated psychosis, dementia, or cerebellar signs may appear. Other rare biochemical abnormalities seen with SMA are lysosomal diseases, phenylketonuria, hydroxyisovaleric aciduria, mutations of mitochondrial DNA, peroxisomal disease, and ceroid lipofuscinosis.

Diagnosis

Most of the childhood SMAs can be identified by the history and clinical examination. They must be differentiated from muscular dystrophies by EMG, muscle biopsy, or DNA analysis; the family history aids in classification. Hexosaminidase deficiency is suspected in families of Ashkenazi Jewish background, especially if there are known cases of Tay-Sachs disease in the family or if some family members are known to be carriers of the gene. Kennedy syndrome is recognized by onset after age 40 years, distribution of weakness, and gynecomastia.

MOTOR NEURON DISEASES OF ADULT ONSET

X-linked Recessive Spinobulbar Muscular Atrophy (Kennedy Disease)

Symptoms of X-linked recessive spinobulbar muscular atrophy (Kennedy disease; MIM 313200) usually begin after age 40 years with dysarthria and dysphagia; limb weakness is delayed for years. The tongue fasciculates and movements of the lips exacerbate fasciculation in the mentalis muscle; also, twitching of limb muscles is often visible. Limb weakness is usually more severe proximally. Tendon reflexes are lost, and upper motor neuron signs are never evident. Although the condition is purely motor in life, nerve conduction studies suggest a large-fiber sensory peripheral axonopathy; sensory evoked potentials may be abnormal and sensory tracts in the spinal cord may be affected at autopsy. Exceptional cases have shown upper motor neuron signs or dementia. Gynecomastia is present in most but not all patients; reproductive fitness is only slightly decreased.

Diagnosis is aided by the characteristic distribution of signs, lack of upper motor neuron signs, slow progression, and a family history suggesting X linkage. Nevertheless, 2% of patients clinically diagnosed with ALS show the Kennedy mutation, so diagnosis is not always straightforward. Careful screening and appropriate genetic testing should be able to reduce such misdiagnosis.

The gene maps to Xq11-12, the site of the androgen receptor. The mutation is an expansion of a CAG repeat. At autopsy, immunochemical studies show the presence of both normal and mutant gene products, including nuclear inclusions that contain androgen receptor. It is not known how these abnormalities cause the disease. There are no reports of a neurologic disorder in people with the testicular feminizing syndrome, which is the major clinical manifestation of a mutation in the gene for the androgen receptor. This and other evidence suggests that, with the expanded polyglutamine repeat, the disease results from a toxic gain of function. Kennedy syndrome was one of the first to be associated with an expansion of a trinucleotide repeat and, as in others of this class, there is an inverse relationship between the number of repeats and the severity of the disorder.

Amyotrophic Lateral Sclerosis
Definition

ALS is a disease of unknown cause and pathogenesis. It is defined pathologically as one in which there is degeneration of both upper and lower motor neurons. Charcot made the key clinical and pathologic description, and the disease is named for him in Europe. In the United States, the disease is colloquially called "Lou Gehrig's disease" after a famous baseball player who had the disease. The PMA form is deduced from clinical observations, but few patients show only lower motor neuron changes at autopsy. In life, the disease is defined by finding evidence of both lower motor neuron disease (weakness, wasting, and fasciculation) and upper motor neuron disease (hyperactive tendon reflexes, Hoffmann signs, Babinski signs, or clonus) in the same limbs. The accuracy of clinical diagnosis is assumed to be more than 95%, but that figure has not been formally tested. Nevertheless, the reliability of clinical diagnosis suffices to make the findings in the history and examination part of the definition. Problems in diagnosis are reviewed below.

Epidemiology

The disease is found worldwide in roughly the same prevalence (about 50×10^{-6}). In 1945, however, about 50 times that number was found on the island of Guam, where the findings of ALS were frequently associated with parkinsonism and dementia. With modernization of the island, the disease seems to have declined in frequency to levels found elsewhere. (Some authorities believe dementia has replaced ALS as Guamanian people now live longer, creating a different form of the same basic disease.) A few other areas of unexplained high incidence have surfaced. Apparent clusters in a building or a small community have not yet led to identification of an etiologic agent. Similarly, case-control studies have not identified consistent risk factors related to occupation, trauma, diet, or socioeconomic status. Controversial data have implicated exposure to lead, smoking cigarettes, diets of high glutamate or fat

▶ **TABLE 119.2 Inherited Motor Neuron Diseases**

Name	OMIM	Site	Gene	Inheritance	Comment
ALS1	105400	21q22.1	SOD1	AD	Adult
ALS2	205100	2q33	Alsin	AR	Juvenile; may resemble PLS. Alsin a GTPase regulator protein?
ALS3	606640	Unknown			
ALS4	602433	9q34	Senataxin (DNA/RNA helicase)	AD	Juvenile; allelic to CMT2
ALS5	602099	15q		AR	Juvenile
ALS6	606640	18q21		AD	Adult
ALS–no number		20q13.33		AD	Adult
ALS-FTD	105550	9q21-q22		AD	Adult
FTD-PD-17 amyotrophy	600274	17q21-q22	Tau	AD	Adult
ALS-X				XR	Juvenile
PMA		2p13	Dynactin	AD	Adult
GM2 gangliosidosis		15q23-23	Hexosaminidase	AR	
SMA		5q11.2-13.3	SMN	AR	Infantile (Werdnig-Hoffmann); juvenile (Kugelberg-Welander)
CMT2A	605995	1p36	Mitochondrial Kinesin KIF1Bβ	AD	Axonal CMT2A
XBSMA		Xq21-22	Androgen Receptor	XR	Kennedy disease
3A syndrome	231550	12q13		AR	Allgrove syndrome: alacrima, achalasia, adrenal insufficiency, amyotrophy

Abbreviations: AD, autosomal dominant; AR, autosomal recessive; ALS, amyotrophic lateral sclerosis; FTD, frontotemporal dementia; FTDP17, frontotemporal dementia with parkinsonism (and amyotrophy), Wilhelmsen-Lynch syndrome; OMIM, Online Mendelian Inheritance in Man; PLS, primary lateral sclerosis; SMN, survival motor neuron; XBSMA, X-linked bulbospinal muscular atrophy; XR, x-linked, recessive.

content, or serving in Gulf War. Participation in varsity athletics increased the risk of later ALS in one study but not in another. An "epidemic" among soccer players in Italy led to a study by a national commission and the results are awaited.

The disease is one of middle and late life. Only 10% of cases begin before age 40 years; 5% begin before age 30. An increase in age-adjusted incidence is seen in succeeding decades, except for a decrease after age 80. In most series, men are affected one to two times more often than women. There is no known ethnic predilection.

About 5% of cases are familial in an autosomal dominant pattern (MIM 105400). About 20% of familial cases map to chromosome 21, where there are mutations in the gene for superoxide dismutase (SOD). The evidence suggests no deficiency in normal SOD; rather, the mutant protein exerts a toxic effect on motor neurons. The essential elements of the disease have been reproduced in transgenic mice bearing the mutant protein, providing the first clue to the pathogenesis of motor neuron disease. The familial cases that do not map to this locus are taken as evidence of locus heterogeneity. For example, mutations in the gene for "alsin" cause a juvenile and predominantly upper motor neuron disease (ALS2), found in Tunisia and Kuwait (Table 119.2). Mutations in the gene for dynactin, a "motor" protein associated with axonal transport, cause a lower motor neuron disease in young adults. Mutations in other motor proteins have also been linked to motor neuron disease, among them kinesins, dynein, and spastin. The occurrence of dementia and parkinsonism seems to increase in first-degree relatives of patients with ALS, implying a common susceptibility to the neurodegenerative diseases of aging.

Pathogenesis

The cause of sporadic ALS is not known. Because of the high incidence in Guam, environmental factors have been suspected, but none have emerged there or anywhere else. Lead and mercury intoxication may cause similar syndromes but are no longer seen in modern societies. HIV and other retroviral infections are unproven possible causes. Excitotoxic amino acids, especially glutamate, are now held suspect, but there is no indication how the condition might arise or why the same theory should be considered for Alzheimer disease or Parkinson disease. Some authorities believe that an autoimmune disorder is present in all patients; others think there is a higher than expected frequency of monoclonal gammopathy or lymphoproliferative disease, but, together, these abnormalities are found in less than 10%. Among the sporadic cases, fewer than 5% are new SOD mutations.

Information from the transgenic mice has reinforced the theory that both sporadic and familial ALS result from excitotoxic effects. Accumulating data also suggest that motor neuron degeneration results from apoptosis, which may be triggered by oxidative stress, mitochondrial dysfunction, and overloaded endoplasmic reticulum. Furthermore, proinflammatory cytokines are increased in degenerating motor neurons, which also triggers microglial inflammation. In sporadic ALS, evidence of these complex neurodegenerative processes is accumulating, and drugs with antiglutamate, antiapoptotic, antioxidative, and antineuroinflammatory effects have been tested in humans and transgenic mice.

Whether there is a paraneoplastic form of ALS has long been debated. An increased frequency of malignancy has been difficult to prove in a case-control study of patients with ALS. Several reports, however, have described ALS syndromes that improved or disappeared when a lung or renal cancer was cured. In addition, the frequency of association of ALS and lymphoma seems to be disproportionately high.

The pathology of ALS implies selective vulnerability of motor neurons, which show several neuronal inclusions that include ubiquitinated skeins or Lewy-like formations and Bunina bodies. These structures are found in most patients with sporadic ALS. In familial forms, a different form is the "hyaline conglomerate," which includes neurofilaments and does not contain ubiquitin. Determination of the nature of these structures could elucidate which pathogenesis. Authorities believe the cellular abnormalities identify a common basic mechanism for the syndromes of ALS, PMA, primary lateral sclerosis (PLS), and ALS-dementia.

The clinical syndrome of ALS can be induced by several known agents, including radiotherapy, lead poisoning, and lightning stroke. Less dramatic environmental effects could bring on more typical sporadic ALS in a person who is genetically susceptible. APOE, SMN, ALSIN, TAU, and VEGF are among the genes that may confer ALS susceptibility. The search is on for both genetic factors and environmental agents.

Clinical Manifestations

Weakness may commence in the legs, hands, proximal arms, or oropharynx (with slurred speech or dysarthria, or difficulty swallowing). Often, the hands are affected first, usually asymmetrically. Painless difficulty with buttons or turning a key is an ominous symptom in midlife. Gait is impaired because the muscles are weak, and footdrop is characteristic, although proximal muscles are sometimes affected first. Alternatively, a spastic gait disorder may ensue. Slowly, the weakness becomes more severe, and more areas of the body are affected, leading to an increasing state of dependency. Muscle cramps (attributed to the hypersensitivity of denervated muscle) and weight loss (resulting from the combination of muscle wasting and dysphagia) are characteristic symptoms. Respiration is usually affected late but, occasionally, may be an early or even the first manifestation; breathing is compromised by paresis of intercostal muscles and diaphragm, or the dysphagia may lead to aspiration and pneumonitis, which can be the terminal event. Sensation is not clinically affected; pain and paresthesia are impermissible with this diagnosis, unless there is a complicating disease (e.g., diabetic neuropathy) and bladder function is spared. The eye muscles are affected only exceptionally. Pain is not an early symptom but may occur later when limbs are immobile.

Lower motor neuron signs must be evident if the diagnosis is to be considered valid. Fasciculation may be seen in the tongue, even without dysarthria. If there is weakness and wasting of limb muscle, fasciculation is almost always seen. Tendon reflexes may be increased or decreased; the combination of overactive reflexes with Hoffmann signs in arms with weak, wasted, and fasciculating muscles is virtually pathognomonic of ALS (except for the syndrome of motor neuropathy, which is discussed later). Unequivocal signs of upper motor neuron disorder are Hoffmann or Babinski signs and clonus. If a spastic gait disorder is seen without lower motor neuron signs in the legs, weakness in the legs may not be found, but incoordination is evident by clumsiness and slowness in the performance of alternating movements.

The cranial nerve motor nuclei are implicated by dysarthria, lingual wasting and fasciculation, and impaired movement of the uvula. Facial weakness and wasting can be discerned, especially in the mentalis muscle, but is usually not prominent. Dysarthria and dysphagia caused by upper motor neuron disease (*pseudobulbar palsy*) is made evident by movements of the uvula that are more vigorous on reflex innervation than on volition; that is, the uvula does not move well (or at all) on phonation, but a vigorous response is seen in the pharyngeal or gag reflex. A common manifestation of pseudobulbar palsy is *emotional lability* with inappropriate laughing or, more often, crying, and that can be regarded erroneously as a reactive depression because of the diagnosis. Emotional lability is better regarded as a release phenomenon of the complex reflexes involved in emotional expression.

The course is relentless and progressive without remissions, relapses, or even stable plateaus. Death results from respiratory failure, aspiration pneumonitis, or pulmonary embolism after prolonged immobility. The mean duration of symptoms is about 4 years; 20% of patients live longer than 5 years. Once a tracheostomy has been placed, the patient may be kept alive for years, although totally paralyzed and unable to move anything other than the eyes; this condition can be a locked-in state. Exceptional patients die in the first year or live longer than 25 years.

About 10% of patients have associated dementia. The most common pathology is that of frontotemporal dementia; some show changes of Alzheimer disease and some show nonspecific pathology. The chromosome 17–related dementia, a tauopathy, has included amyotrophy in a few cases.

Clinical Classification

In addition to the terms *PMA* and *ALS*, two other labels have been used. *Progressive bulbar palsy* implies prominent dysarthria and dysphagia. This term, however, is falling into disfavor because almost all patients with bulbar symptoms already have fasciculations in arms and legs or display upper motor neuron signs; that is, the signs are not restricted to the cranial nerves and the syndrome is clearly ALS. *PLS* refers to a syndrome causing only upper motor neuron signs in life. At autopsy, cases of this nature are found in 5% or fewer of patients, and it is difficult to prove that the condition is really a form of ALS rather than a separate disease. PLS is described in Chapter 118 in the differential diagnosis of spastic paraparesis. PMA (lower motor neuron signs alone) also accounts for fewer than 5% of cases at autopsy. At a meeting in El Escorial, Spain, ALS experts formulated a classification of suspected, possible, probable, and definite ALS (Table 119.3) The classification was designed to ensure uniform populations in therapeutic trials but has become widely used in clinical practice.

Laboratory Data

There is no pathognomonic laboratory abnormality, but the clinical diagnosis should be confirmed by EMG evidence of active denervation in at least three limbs. Nerve conduction velocities should be normal or nearly so; conduction block is rare in patients with frank upper motor neuron signs. CSF protein content is increased above 50 mg/dL in about 30% of patients and above 75 mg/dL in about 10%; the higher values seem more likely to occur in the presence of monoclonal gammopathy or

▶ **TABLE 119.3 Original and Revised El Escorial Criteria (EEC) For the Diagnosis of ALS**

- Suspected ALS: a pure LMN syndrome (based on the original EEC)
- Possible ALS: UMN and LMN signs present together in 1 region, or UMN signs alone in 2 or more regions, or UMN signs caudal to LMN signs
- Laboratory-supported ALS: UMN and LMN signs in 1 region, or UMN signs alone in 1 region with LMN signs identified by EMG in 2 limbs
- Probable ALS: UMN and LMN signs in more than 2 regions, but some UMN signs must be rostral to LMN signs
- Definite ALS: UMN and LMN signs in more than 3 regions

Abbreviations: ALS, amyotrophic lateral sclerosis; EEC, El Escorial Criteria; LMN, lower motor neuron; UMN, upper motor neuron.

lymphoma. Gammopathy is found by sensitive methods, such as immunofixation electrophoresis, in 5% to 10% of patients. Bone marrow examination is reserved for patients with monoclonal gammopathy. Magnetic resonance spectroscopy (MRS) and transcranial magnetic stimulation are emerging as effective measures of upper motor neuron dysfunction in patients who have few or no clinical corticospinal signs. Antibodies to the neuronal ganglioside GM_1 are demonstrable in 10% or less. No evidence supports the notion that ALS may be a manifestation of Lyme disease. A few cases have been found in patients with serologic evidence of human immunodeficiency virus or human T-cell lymphotrophic virus type I infection.

Diagnosis

In adults, the finding of widespread lower motor neuron signs is virtually diagnostic of motor neuron disease, especially if Babinski signs or clonus appear. Even if these definite upper motor neuron signs are lacking, the diagnosis is similarly secure if inappropriately active tendon reflexes or Hoffmann signs are found in arms with weak, wasted, and twitching muscles. The accuracy of clinical diagnosis has not been formally determined but, from clinical experience, is probably better than 95%. The World Federation of Neurology established the ALS Diagnostic Criteria for defining the diagnostic certainty for clinical trials in patients with ALS (Table 119.1). Rarely, some other condition, such as polyglucosan body disease, turns up at autopsy in a patient with clinical signs of ALS. The combination of ALS and dementia has been associated with several different pathologic changes (including Pick disease, Lewy body disease, or nonspecific subcortical gliosis).

Although clinical diagnosis can be considered reliable, several common diagnostic problems occur:

1. The most important disorder, because it is treatable, is *multifocal motor neuropathy with conduction block* (MMNCB), which is defined by finding conduction block in more than one nerve and not at sites of entrapment neuropathy. Strict criteria include more than 50% decline in amplitude between proximal and distal sites of stimulation with less than 50% increase in duration of the response. As described, MMNCB primarily affects the hands, is asymmetric, affects men much more often than women, and is "predominantly lower motor neuron." None of these features, however, clearly distinguishes the disorder from ALS. MMNCB progresses more slowly than ALS, so that relatively little disability after 5 years of symptoms would favor the diagnosis; however, that criterion is not applicable if a patient is seen soon after onset. More of a problem is the fact some patients with MMNCB have had active tendon jerks in limbs with clear lower motor neuron signs. Regardless of the clinical similarities to ALS, the finding of conduction block is an indication for immunosuppressive drug therapy or intravenous immunoglobulin therapy because many patients with MMNCB show a good response. Patients who have clinical signs compatible with motor neuropathy but normal conduction studies may nevertheless respond to intravenous immunoglobulin therapy. In the few autopsies of patients with MMNCB, there has been loss of motor neurons, suggesting that both motor neuron and peripheral nerve are affected in some cases.

2. *Myasthenia gravis* (MG) is a common cause of dysarthria and dysphagia in people who are in the age range of those afflicted with ALS. If there is concomitant ptosis or ophthalmoparesis, if diurnal fluctuation in severity is marked, or if remissions have occurred, MG is more likely. If the syndrome is compatible and if there is an unequivocal response to edrophonium chloride, high titer of antibodies to acetylcholine receptor, or evidence of thymoma on computed tomography, the diagnosis is MG. If fasciculations are evident and the patient is not taking pyridostigmine bromide, or if upper motor neuron signs appear, the syndrome cannot be caused by MG.

3. The differential diagnosis of spastic paraplegia in middle life includes multiple sclerosis (MS), ALS, cervical spondylosis, tropical spastic paraplegia, vitamin B_{12} deficiency, and adrenoleukodystrophy. The appropriate tests are described in Chapter 118. Because MRI evidence of spondylosis is so common in asymptomatic people, the findings can be seen coincidentally in patients with ALS. The differentiation of ALS from spondylotic myelopathy can therefore be vexing; the diagnosis of spondylotic myelopathy should be made cautiously if unequivocal lower motor neuron signs are found in the hands without sensory symptoms or signs. The presence of fasciculations in legs or tongue is incompatible with cervical spondylosis. In contrast, neck pain and persistent paresthesia with unequivocal sensory loss are incompatible with ALS, unless there is an additional condition. MRS and transcranial magnetic stimulation of the motor cortex may be helpful in identifying PLS.

4. *Pseudobulbar palsy* is seen in ALS and MS and after bilateral strokes. MRI is especially useful in identifying the causes other than motor neuron disease. Clinically, lower motor neuron signs are found in all patients with ALS, and they are incompatible with MS or stroke. In a patient with ALS, the liability to weeping should not be construed as a reactive depression.

5. Some authorities carry out tests for monoclonal gammopathy, conduction block, antibodies to GM_1 ganglioside and myelin-associated glycoprotein (MAG), and lymphoproliferative disease in patients with ALS.

6. ALS is differentiated from myopathies by finding fasciculations or upper motor neuron signs on examination. If these are lacking, the differential diagnosis depends on EMG evidence of denervation.

7. The *postpolio syndrome* is important for theoretic reasons (because persistent infection by the virus might cause ALS) and for practical reasons (because survivors of acute poliomyelitis have feared that the virus might be revived and attack again). No evidence suggests that survivors of acute childhood polio are at increased risk of ALS. The postpolio syndrome takes three forms: loss of ability to compensate for residual paresis with increasing age; addition of arthritis or some other physical condition that impedes adaptation and compensation; or, decades after the original paralysis, new weakness of muscles thought not to have been affected in the childhood attack. These developments are accompanied by evidence of acute and chronic denervation on EMG, but conduction velocities are normal; the consensus is that this syndrome is a residual effect in previously paralyzed muscles and that it is not a new motor neuron disease. Progression is slow and is limited to previously paralyzed muscles. No upper motor neuron signs appear, and clinically evident fasciculations are exceptional.

8. *Monomelic muscular atrophy* (Hirayama syndrome) affects men 10 times more often than women, starts at about age 20 years, and is restricted to one limb, usually an arm and hand rather than a leg. Although first reported in Japan, it has been seen in other countries. Many of those affected seem to be athletes, but the syndrome is not overtly related to cervical trauma. The condition progresses slowly for 1 or 2 years and then seems to become arrested in most cases. The origin of this disorder is not known; Hirayama attributes the myelopathy to compression by the dural sac on flexing the neck, but others believe it is a focal motor neuron disorder. The patient must be observed for some months to be certain that other signs of motor neuron disease do not appear.

9. *Reversible motor neuron* disease is the hope of diagnosis, but cases of spontaneous recovery are so rare that it is difficult to mention the possibility to a patient with ALS. The reversible syndrome may be one of lower motor neurons alone or may include the full picture of ALS. Many patients are younger than 30, but some are older.

10. The syndrome of *benign fasciculation and cramps* is virtually restricted to medical students, physicians, and other medical workers because they are the only people in society who know the malignant implications of fasciculating muscles. The syndrome can be called the *Denny-Brown, Foley syndrome* after the discoverers. The condition has been rediscovered several times and given other names. The origin is not known, but because neither weakness nor wasting occurs, it is not ALS. In theory, ALS should sometimes start with this syndrome. For reasons unknown, however, it almost never does; only one case has been reasonably documented.

Treatment

Sadly, there is no effective drug therapy for ALS. Therapeutic trials have shown no benefit from immunosuppression, immunoenhancement, plasmapheresis, lymph node irradiation, glutamate antagonists, nerve growth factors, antiviral agents, and numerous other categories of drugs. Riluzole (Rilutek), a glutamate inhibitor, is the only drug approved by the U.S. Food and Drug Administration for the treatment of ALS. It is said to prolong life by a few months but has no visible effect on function or quality of life. Treatment is therefore symptomatic, and emotional support is vitally important; management may be carried out most efficiently in an ALS center.

Early in the course, patients should try to continue to perform routine activities as long as they can. There is difference of opinion about exercising weak muscles, but physical therapy can help maintain function as long as possible. Drooling of saliva (sialorrhea) may be helped by atropine sulfate, glycopyrrolate (Robinul), or amitriptyline. Antispasticity agents have not been helpful in the spastic gait disorder, but intrathecal administration of baclofen (Lioresal) might be considered in some patients. Dysphagia leads to percutaneous gastrostomy to maintain nutrition; it does not prevent aspiration. Communication devices can ameliorate severe dysarthria. Noninvasive positive pressure ventilation has been used with increasing frequency to improve nocturnal dyspnea, insomnia, and overall respiratory discomfort; it may prolong life. The long-term care of patients with ALS has been addressed by evidence-based medicine recommendations made by a committee of the American Academy of Neurology.

The major decision concerns the use of tracheostomy and chronic mechanical ventilation, which can be done at home. In making the decision, patients should be in-formed fully about the long-term consequences of life without movement; they must decide whether they want to be kept alive or made as comfortable as possible—two choices that are not identical. Palliative care (relief of symptoms but not prolonging life) is becoming a standard option (see Chapter 171).

Immunosuppressive therapy, starting with IVIG is used for the few patients with lymphoproliferative disease, monoclonal gammopathy, conduction block, or high titers of antibodies to GM_1 or MAG. Chronic therapy with cyclophosphamide or fludarabine may follow. Favorable responses, however, are few.

In familial ALS, the question of presymptomatic diagnosis raises other ethical questions.

SUGGESTED READINGS
Spinal Muscular Atrophy

Brzustowicz LM, Lehner T, Castilla LH, et al. Genetic mapping of chronic childhood-onset spinal muscular atrophy to chromosome 5q11.2-13.3. *Nature* 1990;344:540–541.

Crawford TO. Spinal muscular atrophies. In: Jones HR Jr, De Vivo DC, Darras BT, eds. *Neuromuscular Disorders of Infancy, Childhood and Adolescence, A Clinician's Approach.* New York: Butterworth-Heinemann, 2003:145–166.

Dubowitz V. Chaos in classification of the spinal muscular atrophies of childhood. *Neuromuscul Disord* 1991;1:77–80.

Feldkotter M, Schwarzer V, Wirth R, et al: Quantitative analyses of SMN1 and SMN2 based on real-time lightCycler PCR: fast and highly reliable carrier testing and prediction of severity of spinal muscular atrophy. *Am J Hum Genet* 2002;70:358–368.

Gilliam TC, Brzustowicz LM, Castilla LH, et al. Genetic homogeneity between acute and chronic forms of spinal muscular atrophy. *Nature* 1990;345:823–825.

Gubitz AK, Feng W, Dreyfuss G. The SMN complex. *Exp Cell Res* 2004;296(May 15):51–56.

Iannaccone ST, Smith SA, Simard LR. Spinal muscular atrophy. *Curr Neurol Neurosci Rep* 2004 Jan;4(1):74–80.

Lefebvre S, Burglen L, Frezal J, et al. The role of the SMN gene in proximal spinal muscular atrophy. *Hum Mol Genet* 1998;7:1531–1536.

McShane MA, Boyd S, Harding B, et al. Progressive bulbar paralysis of childhood: a reappraisal of Fazio-Londe disease. *Brain* 1992;115:1889–1900.

Melki J, LeFebvre S, Burglen L, et al. De novo and inherited deletions of the 5q13 region in spinal muscular atrophies. *Science* 1994;264:1474–1476.

Monani UR, Sendtner M, Coovert DD, et al. The human centromeric survival motor neuron gene (SMN2) rescues embryonic lethality in Smn(-/-) mice and results in a mouse with spinal muscular atrophy. *Hum Mol Genet* 2000;12:333–339.

Moulard B, Salachas F, Chassande B, et al. Association between centromeric deletions of the SMN gene and sporadic adult-onset lower motor neuron disease. *Ann Neurol* 1998;43:640–644.

Ogino S, Wilson RB. Spinal muscular atrophy: molecular genetics and diagnostics. *Expert Rev Mol Diagn* 2004 Jan;4(1):15–29.

Rowland LP. Molecular basis of genetic heterogeneity: role of the clinical neurologist. *J Child Neurol* 1998;13:122–132.

Rubi-Gozalbo ME, Smeitink JAM, Ruitenbeck W, et al. Spinal muscular atrophy-like picture, cardiomyopathy, and cytochrome-c-oxidase deficiency. *Neurology* 1999;52:383–386.

Stewart H, Wallace A, McGaughran J, et al. Molecular diagnosis of spinal muscular atrophy. *Arch Dis Child* 1998;78:531–535.

Sumner CJ, Huynh TN, Markowitz JA, et al: Valproic acid increases SMN levels in spinal muscular atrophy patient cells. *Ann Neurol* 2003;54:647–654.

Kennedy Disease

Fischbeck KH. Kennedy disease. *J Inherit Metab Dis* 1997;20:152–158.

Harding AE, Thomas PK, Baraister M, et al. X-linked bulbospinal neuronopathy: report of 10 cases. *J Neurol Neurosurg Psychiatry* 1982;45:1012–1019.

La Spada AR, Wilson EM, Lubahn DB, et al. Androgen receptor gene mutation in X-linked spinal and bulbar muscular atrophy. *Nature* 1991;352:77–79.

Li M, Miwa S, Kobayashi Y, et al. Nuclear inclusions of the androgen receptor protein in spinal and bulbar muscular atrophy. *Ann Neurol* 1998;44:249–254.

Merry DE, Kobayashi Y, Bailey CK, et al. Cleavage, aggregation and toxicity of the expanded androgen receptor in spinal and bulbar muscular atrophy. *Hum Mol Genet* 1998;7:693–701.

Paraboosingh JS, Figlwicz DA, Krizus A, et al. Spinobulbar muscular atrophy can mimic ALS: the importance of genetic testing in male patients with atypical ALS. *Neurology* 1997;49:568–572.

Sinnreich M, Klein CJ. Bulbospinal muscular atrophy: Kennedy's disease. *Arch Neurol* 2004 Aug;61(8):1324–1326.

Sopher BL, Thomas PS Jr, LaFevre-Bernt MA, et al. Androgen receptor YAC transgenic mice recapitulate SBMA motor neuronopathy and implicate VEGF164 in the motor neuron degeneration. *Neuron* 2004;41:687–699.

Sperfeld AD, Karitzky J, Brummer D, et al. X-linked bulbospinal neuronopathy: Kennedy disease. *Arch Neurol* 2002;59:1921–1926.

Trojaborg W, Wulff CH. X-linked bulbospinal neuronopathy (Kennedy's syndrome): a neurophysiological study. *Acta Neurol Scand* 1994;89:214–219.

Amyotrophic Lateral Sclerosis

Armon C. An evidence-based medicine approach to the evaluation of the role of exogenous risk factors in sporadic amyotrophic lateral sclerosis. *Neuroepidemiology* 2003;22:217–28.

Ashworth N, Satkunam L, Deforge D. Treatment for spasticity in amyotrophic lateral sclerosis/motor neuron disease. *Cochrane Database Syst Rev* 2004(1):CD004156.

Ben Hamida M, Hentati F, Hamida CB. Hereditary motor system disease (chronic juvenile amyotrophic lateral sclerosis). *Brain* 1990;113:347–363.

Blexrud MD, Windebank AJ, Daube JR. Long-term follow-up of 121 patients with benign fasciculations. *Ann Neurol* 1993;34:622–625.

Bonduelle M. Amyotrophic lateral sclerosis. In: Vinken PJ, Bruyn GW, de Jong JMBV, eds. *System Disorders and Atrophies. Handbook of Clinical Neurology, vol 22.* Amsterdam: North-Holland, 1975:281–338.

Brownell B, Trevor-Hughes J. Central nervous system in motor neuron disease. *J Neurol Neurosurg Psychiatry* 1970;33:338–357.

Chan S, Kaufmann P, Shungu DC, et al. Amyotrophic lateral sclerosis and primary lateral sclerosis: evidence-based diagnostic evaluation of the upper motor neuron. *Neuroimag Clin N Am* 2003;13:307–26.

Chen Y-Z, Bennett CL, Huy M, et al. DNA/RNA helicase gene mutations in a form of juvenile amyotrophic lateral sclerosis (ALS4). *Am J Hum Genet* 2004;74;1128–1135.

Chiò A, Galletti R, Finocchiaro C, et al. Percutaneous radiological gastrostomy: a safe and effective method of nutritional tube placement in advanced ALS. *J Neurol Neurosurg Psychiatry* 2004;75:645–647.

Dalakas MC, Elder G, Hallet M, et al. A long-term follow-up study of patients with post-poliomyelitis neuromuscular symptoms. *N Engl J Med* 1986;314:959–963.

DeCarolis P, Montagna P, Cipiuli M, et al. Isolated lower motor neuron involvement following radiotherapy. *J Neurol Neurosurg Psychiatry* 1986;48:718–719.

de Carvalho M, Swash M. Cramps, muscle pain, and fasciculations: not always benign? *Neurology* 2004 Aug 24;63(4):721–723.

Evans BK, Fagan C, Arnold T, et al. Paraneoplastic motor neuron disease and renal cell carcinoma. *Neurology* 1990;40:960–963.

Forsyth PA, Dalmau J, Graus F, et al. Motor neuron syndromes in cancer patients. *Ann Neurol* 1997;41:722–730.

Gordon PH, Rowland LP, Younger DS, et al. Lymphoproliferative disorders and motor neuron disease. *Neurology* 1997;48:1671–1678.

Henkel JS, Engelhardt JI, Siklos L, et al. Presence of dendritic cells, MCP-1, and activated microglia/macrophages in amyotrophic lateral sclerosis spinal cord tissue. *Ann Neurol* 2004;55(Feb):221–35.

Horner RD, Kamins KG, Feussner JR, et al. Occurrence of amyotrophic lateral sclerosis among Gulf War veterans. *Neurology* 2003;61:742–749.

Ince PG, Evans J, Knopp M, et al. Corticospinal tract degeneration in the progressive muscular atrophy variant of ALS. *Neurology* 2003;60:1252–1258.

Jubelt B. Motor neuron diseases and viruses: poliovirus, retroviruses, and lymphomas. *Curr Opin Neurol Neurosurg* 1992;5:655–658.

Kuroda Y, Sugihara H. Autopsy report of HTLV-1-associated myelopathy presenting with ALS-like manifestations. *J Neurol Sci* 1991;106:199–205.

Lawyer T, Netsky MG. Amyotrophic lateral sclerosis: clinico-anatomic study of 53 cases. *Arch Neurol Psychiatry* 1953;69:171–192.

Lomen-Hoerth C, Anderson T, Miller B. The overlap of amyotrophic lateral sclerosis and frontotemporal dementia. *Neurology* 2002;59:1077–1079.

Lomen-Hoerth C, Murphy J, Langmore S, et al. Are amyotrophic lateral sclerosis patients cognitively normal? *Neurology* 2003;60:1094–1097.

Mackenzie IR, Feldman H. Extrapyramidal features in patients with motor neuron disease and dementia; a clinicopathological correlative study. *Acta Neuropathol (Berl)* 2004;107:336–340.

Malapert D, Brugieres P, Degos JD. Motor neuron syndrome in the arms after radiation treatment. *J Neurol Neurosurg Psychiatry* 1991;54:1123–1124.

Matherson L, Barrau K, Blin O. Disease management: the example of amyotrophic lateral sclerosis. *J Neurol* 1998;245(Suppl 2):S20–S28.

Mitsumoto H, Chad DA, Piro EP, eds. *Amyotrophic Lateral Sclerosis.* Philadephia: FA Davis, 1998.

Moss AH, Case P, Stocking CB, et al. Home ventilation for amyotrophic lateral sclerosis patients: outcomes, costs, and patient, family, and physician attitudes. *Neurology* 1993;43:438–443.

Munsat TL. *Post-Polio Syndrome.* New York: Butterworth-Heinemann, 1991.

Nishimura AL, Mitne-Neto M, Silva HCA, et al. A novel locus for late onset amyotrophic lateral sclerosis/motor neurone disease variant at 20q13. *J Med Genet* 2004;41;315–320.

Piao YS, Wakabayashi K, Kakita A, et al. Neuropathology with clinical correlations of sporadic amyotrophic lateral sclerosis: 102 autopsy cases examined between 1962 and 2000. *Brain Pathol* 2003;13(Jan):10–22.

Piazza O, Siren A-L, Ehrenreich H. Soccer, neurotrauma and amyotrophic lateral sclerosis: is there a connection? *Curr Med Res Op* 2004;20:505–508.

Przedborski S. Programmed cell death in amyotrophic lateral sclerosis: a mechanism of pathogenic and therapeutic importance. *Neurologist* 2004;10(Jan):1–7.

Przedborski S, Mitsumoto H, Rowland LP. Recent advances in amyotrophic lateral sclerosis research. *Curr Neurol Neurosci Rep* 2003;3:70–77.

Rosen DR, Siddique T, Patterson D, et al. Mutations in Cu/Zn superoxide dismutase gene are associated with familial amyotrophic lateral sclerosis. *Nature* 1993;362:59–62.

Rosenfeld MR, Posner JB. Paraneoplastic motor neuron disease. *Adv Neurol* 1991;56:445–463.

Rothstein JD, Martin LJ, Kuncl RW. Decreased glutamate transport by the brain and spinal cord in amyotrophic lateral sclerosis. *N Engl J Med* 1992;326:1464–1468.

Rowland LP, ed. *Amyotrophic Lateral Sclerosis and Other Motor Neuron Diseases.* New York: Raven, 1991.

Rowland LP. Diagnosis of amyotrophic lateral sclerosis. *J Neurol Sci* 1998;160(Suppl 1):S6–S24.

Rowland LP. Surgical treatment of cervical spondylotic myelopathy: time for a controlled trial. *Neurology* 1992;42:5–13.

Rowland LP, Shneider NA. Amyotrophic lateral sclerosis. *N Engl J Med* 2001;344:1688–1700.

Shaw PJ, Strong MJ, eds. *Motor Neuron Disorders.* Philadelphia: Elsevier, Butterworth-Heinemann, 2003.

Smith RG, Henry YK, Mattson MP, et al. Presence of 4-hydroxynonenal in cerebrospinal fluid of patients with sporadic amyotrophic lateral sclerosis. *Ann Neurol* 1998;44:696–699.

Smith RG, Siklos L, Alexianu ME, et al. Autoimmunity and ALS. *Neurology* 1996;47 (Suppl 2):S40–S46.

Tucker T, Layzer RB, Miller RG, et al. Subacute reversible motor neuron disease. *Neurology* 1991;41:1541–1544.

van den Berg-Vos RM, Visser J, Franssen H, et al. Sporadic lower motor neuron disease with adult onset: classification of subtypes. *Brain* 2003;126:1036–1047.

Veldink JH, Wokke JH, van der Wal G, et al. Euthanasia and physician assisted suicide among patients with amyotrophic lateral sclerosis in the Netherlands. *N Engl J Med* 2002;346:1638–1644.

Wilhelmsen KC, Forman MS, Rosen HJ et al. 17q-linked frontotemporal dementia-amyotrophic lateral sclerosis without tau mutations with tau and alpha-synuclein inclusions. *Arch Neurol* 2004;61:398–406.

Yamanaka K, Vande Velde C, Eymard-Pierre E, et al. Unstable mutants in the peripheral endosomal membrane component ALS2 cause early-onset motor neuron disease. *Proc Nat Acad Sci USA* 2003;100:16041–16046.

Yokota T, Miyagishi M, Hino T, et al. siRNA-based inhibition specific for mutant SOD1 with single nucleotide alternation in familial ALS, compared with ribozyme and DNA enzyme. *Biochem Biophys Res Comm* 2004;314(1):283–291.

Yoshida M. Amyotrophic lateral sclerosis with dementia: the clinico-pathological spectrum. *Neuropathology* 2004;24(Mar):87–102.

Multifocal Motor Neuropathy with Conduction Block

Lange DJ, Trojaborg W, Latov N, et al. Multifocal motor neuropathy with conduction block: is it a distinct clinical entity? *Neurology* 1992;42:497–505.

Nagale SV, Bosch EP. Multifocal motor neuropathy with conduction block: current issues in diagnosis and treatment. *Semin Neurol* 2003;23:325–334.

Nobile-Orazio E, Terenghi F, Carpo M, et al. Treatment of multifocal motor neuropathy. *Neurol Sci* 2003;24(Suppl 4):S251–255.

Olney RK, Lewis RA, Putnam TD, et al. Consensus criteria for the diagnosis of multifocal motor neuropathy. *Muscle Nerve* 2003;27(Jan):117–121.

Pestronk A, Cornblath DR, Ilyas AA, et al. A treatable multifocal motor neuropathy with antibodies to GM1 ganglioside. *Ann Neurol* 1988;24:73–78.

Vucic S, Black KR, Chong PS, Cros D. Multifocal motor neuropathy: decrease in conduction blocks and reinervation with long-term IVIg. *Neurology* 2004 Oct 12;63(7):1264–1269.

Focal Amyotrophies

Chen CJ, Hsu HL, Tseng YC, et al. Hirayama flexion myelopathy: neutral-position MR imaging findings—importance of loss of attachment. *Radiology* 2004;231(Apr):39–44.

Gourie-Devi M, Nalini A. Madras motor neuron disease variant, clinical features of seven patients. *J Neurol Sci* 2003;209(May 15):13–17.

Hirayama K, Tokumaru Y. Cervical dural sac and spinal cord in juvenile muscular atrophy of distal upper extremity. *Neurology* 2000;54:1922–1926.

Chapter 120

Syringomyelia

Elliott L. Mancall

Cavitation within the spinal cord was first described by Esteinne in 1546 in *La dissection du corps humain.* Ollivier D'Angers applied the term *syringomyelia* in 1827. This term connotes a chronic, progressive disorder that most often involves the spinal cord. The exact incidence of syringomyelia is not known, but it is rare. It occurs more frequently in men than in women. Familial cases have been described. The disease usually appears in the third or fourth decade of life, with a mean age at onset of about 30 years. It is rare in childhood or late-adult years. Syringomyelia usually progresses slowly; the course extends over many years. An acute course may be evident when the brainstem is affected (*syringobulbia*). Kyoshima and Bogdanov recorded spontaneous resolution.

Syringomyelia rarely occurs de novo or in isolation, but usually arises as a result of an associated anomaly. Over two-thirds of cases of syringomyelia are associated with the Arnold-Chiari type 1 malformation. (Type 2 is associated with myelomeningocoele and hydrocephalus, not syringomyelia.) Less commonly, a variably sized syringomyelic cavity, or syrinx, is found within or adjacent to an intramedullary tumor, generally a glioma. Syringomyelia may also be a late consequence of spinal cord trauma, arising ex vacuo after absorption of an intramedullary hematoma (*hematomyelia*). In about 5% of patients with spinal cord injury, the delayed onset of an ascending spinal cord syndrome is caused by an expanding syrinx. CSF circulation may be impaired by dense arachnoiditis at the site of the trauma, thereby causing the delayed formation of a syrinx on an ischemic basis.

CLINICAL MANIFESTATIONS

Symptoms depend primarily on the location of the lesion. Milhorat and his colleagues have isolated several individual cavitary patterns, each producing a more or less distinctive clinical appearance. The syrinx is most commonly encountered in the lower cervical region, particularly at the base of the posterior horn, extending into the central gray matter and anterior commissure. The cyst interrupts the decussating spinothalamic fibers that mediate pain and temperature sensibility, resulting in loss of these sensations; light touch, vibratory sense, and position sense are relatively preserved, at least early in the disease, by virtue of sparing of the posterior columns. This pattern of loss of cutaneous sensibility with preservation of posterior column sensory modalities is commonly referred to as *dissociated sensory loss*. Pain and temperature sensations are typically impaired in the arm on the involved side, sometimes in both arms or in a shawl-like distribution (*en cuirasse*) across the shoulders and upper torso, front and back. When the cavity enlarges to involve the posterior columns, there is loss of position and vibratory sense in the feet, and astereognosis may be noted in the hands. Extension of the lesion into the anterior horns with loss of motor neurons causes amyotrophy that begins in the small muscles of the hands (*brachial amyotrophy*), ascends to the forearms, and ultimately affects the shoulder girdle. The hand may be strikingly atrophied, with the development of a claw-hand deformity (*main en griffe*). Weakness appears in the hands, forearms, and shoulder girdle, and fasciculations may be seen. Because the syrinx is asymmetrically placed early in its development, manifestations in the arms and hands tend to be similarly asymmetric. Muscle stretch reflexes in the arms are characteristically lost early. As the syrinx extends into the lateral columns, spasticity appears in the legs, with paraparesis, hyperreflexia, and extensor plantar responses. Impairment of bowel and bladder functions may be a late manifestation. A Horner syndrome may appear, reflecting damage to the sympathetic neurons in the intermediolateral cell column.

Pain, generally deep and aching, is sometimes experienced and may be severe. It involves the neck and shoulders or follows a radicular distribution in the arms or trunk.

The syrinx sometimes ascends into the medulla. Syringobulbia is evidenced by dysphagia, pharyngeal and palatal weakness, asymmetric weakness and atrophy of the tongue, sensory loss involving primarily pain and temperature sense in the distribution of the trigeminal nerve, and nystagmus. Signs of cerebellar dysfunction may appear. Rarely, the syrinx extends even higher in the brainstem or into the centrum semiovale as a *syringocephalus*.

Many other clinical abnormalities are evident. Scoliosis is characteristically seen, and neurogenic arthropathies (*Charcot joints*) may affect the shoulder, elbow, or wrist. Acute painful enlargement of the shoulder may appear and is associated with destruction of the head of the humerus. Painless ulcers of the hands are frequent. The hands are occasionally the site of remarkable subcutaneous edema and hyperhidrosis (*main succulente*), presumably caused by interruption of central autonomic pathways.

A cyst sometimes develops in the lumbar cord either in association with or independent of a cervical syrinx. Lumbar syringomyelia is characterized by atrophy of proximal and distal leg muscles with dissociated sensory loss in lumbar and sacral dermatomes. Stretch reflexes are lost in the legs; impairment of sphincter function is common. The plantar responses are ordinarily flexor. Women with syringomyelia are at risk because symptoms may start or worsen in childbirth.

PATHOLOGY AND PATHOGENESIS

As emphasized by Greenfield, syringomyelia may be defined as a tubular cavitation of the spinal cord, usually beginning within the cervical cord and generally extending over many segments. Syringomyelia should be regarded as distinct from simple cystic expansion of the central canal of the cord; the term *hydromyelia* is more appropriately applied to that condition. The syrinx may communicate with the central canal, and ependymal cells occasionally line the wall of the syrinx. The fluid within the cyst is similar to, if not identical with, CSF. The syrinx may be limited to the cervical cord or may extend the length of the cord; it tends to vary in transverse diameter from segment to segment, usually achieving maximal extent in the cervical and lumbosacral enlargements. Originally confined to the base of a posterior horn or to the anterior commissure, the cyst slowly enlarges to involve much of both gray and white matter; at times, only a narrow rim of cord parenchyma can be identified histologically. The cyst itself is surrounded by a dense glial fibril wall. Extension of the cavity into the medulla or, rarely, higher within the neuraxis may be noted. Developmental abnormalities in the cervical spine and at the base of the skull, such as platybasia, are common. Features of the Arnold-Chiari malformation, such as displacement of the cerebellar tonsils into the cervical canal, are often identified. Hydrocephalus is frequent, and cerebellar hypoplasia may be found. In a few patients, ependymoma or astrocytoma of the spinal cord is encountered, usually in juxtaposition with the syrinx itself.

The pathogenesis of syringomyelia is uncertain. Following Gardner, it is widely held that most cases of syringomyelia are of a "communicating" variety. Dilatation of the central canal is attributed to CSF pulsations directed downward from the fourth ventricle because the foramina of exit are occluded by a developmental defect in the rhombic roof or other anomalies of the cervico-medullary junction. According to this hydrodynamic theory, obstruction or atresia of the normal outlets of the fourth ventricle is essential; in most cases, the ventricular obstruction is associated with features of the Arnold-Chiari malformation and, often, with hydrocephalus. As a modification of Gardner's theory, Boulay and associates emphasized systolic excursions of CSF in the basal cisterns in the formation of the cystic cavity.

Alternatively, Williams proposed that the Arnold-Chiari malformation is an acquired anomaly that results from excessive molding of the head during difficult, usually high forceps, delivery. A ball-valve effect of the cerebellar tonsils in the foramen magnum could create a dissociation between cranial and spinal CSF pressures, particularly during Valsalva maneuvers, which in turn could lead to syrinx formation. Both the Gardner and Williams hypotheses are challenged by the evidence cited by Milhorat and associates to the effect that most syrinx cavities do not in fact communicate with the fourth ventricle; caudal flow of CSF from the fourth ventricle into the central canal cannot therefore be considered the explanation for the appearance of a syrinx with a lesion of the hindbrain.

In the traditional nomenclature of Greenfield, distention of the central canal is therefore designated *hydromyelia*, with the term *syringomyelia* reserved for a noncommunicating cyst. From this perspective, and in keeping with the observations of Milhorat, the syringomyelic cavity cannot be considered part of the ventricular system in what is essentially a persistent embryonic configuration; rather, it is an independent development. As already stressed, noncommunicating syrinx has been attributed to several factors, including extension of CSF under pressure along the Virchow-Robin spaces, cystic degeneration of an intramedullary glioma, and ischemia with cyst formation secondary to arachnoiditis caused by meningitis or subarachnoid hemorrhage with resultant insufficiency of blood flow in the anterior spinal artery. A syrinx may also develop after spinal cord trauma either soon after resorption of an intramedullary hematoma (*hematomyelia*) or as a delayed phenomenon after cord contusion or compression with microcystic cavitation. Birth trauma may be important in the development of syringomyelia.

The debates continue. Levine proposed a theory whereby standing erect, coughing, and pulsatile changes in CSF pressure with the cardiac cycle increase intracranial pressure above the subarachnoid obstruction at the foramen magnum. This increases transmural venous and capillary pressures to dilate vessels below the block and collapse those above the block. Mechanical stress below the block disrupts the blood–spinal cord barrier, allowing exudation of protein-poor fluid, initiating the syrinx.

In the last analysis, the distinction between communicating and noncommunicating forms of syringomyelia may be artificial; the term *syringohydromyelia* has been suggested as a more inclusive term. Most instances of syringomyelia do seem to fall into the Gardner communicating variety, although the precise pathogenetic mechanisms remain incompletely understood. In some individuals, the original communication with the fourth ventricle may have been obliterated with time, resulting in the spurious appearance of a noncommunicating configuration.

LABORATORY DATA

CSF ordinarily demonstrates few abnormalities. CSF pressure is sometimes elevated, and complete subarachnoid block may be noted. The cell count is only rarely more than $10/mm^3$. A mild elevation of CSF protein content occurs in 50% of patients; in presence of subarachnoid block, CSF protein may exceed 100 mg/dL.

MRI is the diagnostic procedure of choice for the diagnosis and evaluation of syringomyelia. Cystic enlargement of the spinal cord extends over several segments (Fig. 120.1). The signal intensity of the cyst is generally similar to that of CSF. The cyst margins are often irregular and may demonstrate periodic folds or septations that may result from turbulent flow within the cavity. If syringomyelia is identified on MRI, further evaluation should include MRI of the brain and

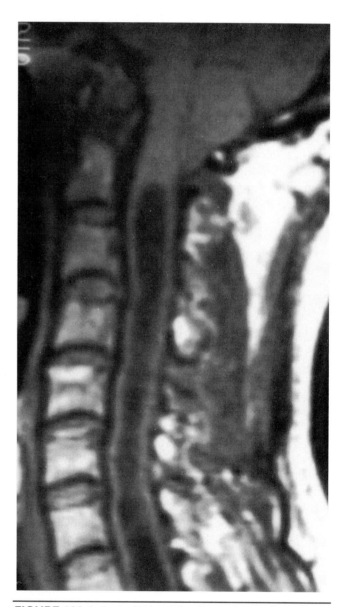

FIGURE 120.1. Sagittal T1-weighted MRI shows a large syrinx. Note the associated Arnold-Chiari malformation with cerebellar tonsillar herniation below the foramen magnum. Decompression of the foramen magnum usually results in resolution of the syrinx.

craniovertebral junction to identify associated anomalies, such as hydrocephalus or an Arnold-Chiari malformation. If syringomyelia occurs without an Arnold-Chiari malformation or prior spinal cord injury, a complete spinal MRI with gadolinium is performed to rule out an intramedullary spinal cord tumor. Myelography and CT are rarely used for the diagnosis or evaluation of syringomyelia. CT is useful for delineating the bony anomalies that occur at the craniovertebral junction in patients with hindbrain abnormalities. Continuous motor unit activity and other forms of spontaneous activity in the EMG are attributed to neuronal hyperexcitability.

DIFFERENTIAL DIAGNOSIS

Amyotrophic lateral sclerosis (ALS) commonly causes weakness, atrophy, and reflex loss in the arms that is often asymmetric, with heightened reflexes and extensor-plantar responses in the legs. Sensory loss, however, does not occur in ALS. Multiple sclerosis (MS) may mimic syringomyelia. Early atrophy of hand muscles, however, does not occur in MS, and the lack of evidence of dissemination of lesions elsewhere argues against this diagnosis. MRI of brain and spinal cord separates MS and syringomyelia. Intrinsic tumors of the spinal cord may produce clinical signs similar to those of syringomyelia. Again, MRI generally distinguishes the two. MRI also differentiates syringomyelia from cervical spondylosis. Anomalies of the craniovertebral junction and cervical ribs may also cause symptoms reminiscent of syringomyelia; because both may be associated with true syringomyelia, identification of these abnormalities is not sufficient to exclude cavitation within the spinal cord.

TREATMENT

The treatment of syringomyelia consists of either drainage of the syrinx cavity or correction of the abnormal dynamics that allowed the syrinx to develop. In tumor-associated syringomyelia, for example, removal of the mass nearly always results in resolution of the syrinx. Syringomyelia arising as a late consequence of spinal cord trauma usually requires direct drainage because the dense arachnoiditis at the level of the trauma generally cannot be corrected. Simple drainage can consist of either percutaneous needle aspiration or open syringotomy. These maneuvers provide temporary relief at best, and the cavity usually re-expands because of spontaneous closure of the syringotomy and persistence of the filling mechanism. Prolonged successful drainage usually requires the insertion through laminectomy of a small Silastic tube directly into the syrinx cavity. The other end of the catheter is placed in either the pleural or the peritoneal space, thereby allowing continuous drainage of the syrinx into a cavity of lower pressure.

Management of syringomyelia that occurs in association with an Arnold-Chiari malformation is more complicated. Ventriculoperitoneal shunting is generally performed initially if significant hydrocephalus is present. In the absence of hydrocephalus or if the ventriculoperitoneal shunt fails to relieve symptoms, a posterior fossa decompression with or without simultaneous shunting of the syrinx can be performed. The posterior fossa decompression consists of a wide suboccipital craniectomy and cervical laminectomy with duraplasty to enlarge the foramen magnum effectively. Plugging of the obex with muscle or the placement of a Silastic stent into the fourth ventricle to improve the CSF outflow into the basal cisterns and subarachnoid space may also be performed, but each is controversial. In most patients, adequate posterior fossa decompression results in shrinkage or even resolution of the syrinx. In refractory cases, a direct syrinx shunt may be placed.

SUGGESTED READINGS

Asgari S, Engelhorn T, Bschor M, et al. Surgical prognosis in hindbrain related syringomyelia. *Acta Neurol Scand* 2003;107(Jan):12–21.

Barnett HJM, Foster JB, Hudgson P. *Syringomyelia*. Philadelphia: WB Saunders, 1973.

Batzdorf U, Klekamp J, Johnson JP. A critical appraisal of syrinx cavity shunting procedures. *J Neurosurg* 1998;89:382–388.

Berry RG, Chambers RA, Lublin FD. Syringoencephalomyelia (syringocephalus). *J Neuropathol Exp Neurol* 1981;40:633–644.

Bogdanov EI, Heiss JD, Mendelevich EG, Mikhaylov IM, Haass A. Clinical and neuroimaging features of "idiopathic" syringomyelia. *Neurology* 2004 Mar;62(5):791–794.

Del Bigio MR, Deck JHN, MacDonald JK. Syrinx extending from conus medullaris to basal ganglia: a clinical, radiological, and pathological correlation. *Can J Neurol Sci* 1993;20:240–246.

Dyste GN, Menezes AH, VanGilder JC. Symptomatic Chiari malformations: an analysis of presentation, management, and long-term outcome. *J Neurosurg* 1989;71:159–168.

Fischbein NJ, Dillon WP, Cobbs C, et al. The "presyrinx state": a reversible myelopathic condition that may precede syringomyelia. *AJNR* 1999;20:7–20.

Gardner WH, McMurry FG. "Non-communicating" syringomyelia: a nonexistent entity. *Surg Neurol* 1976;6:251–256.

Gardner WJ. Hydrodynamic mechanism of syringomyelia: its relationship to myelocele. *J Neurol Neurosurg Psychiatry* 1965;28:247–259.

Goldstein JH, Kaptain GJ, Do HM, et al. CT-guided percutaneous drainage of syringomyelia. *J Comput Assist Tomogr* 1998;22:984–988.

Haponik EF, Givens D, Angelo J. Syringobulbia-myelia with obstructive sleep apnea. *Neurology* 1983;33:1046–1049.

Hodge C, Jones M. Syringomyelia and spinal cord tumors. *Curr Opin Neurol Neurosurg* 1991;4:597–600.

Isu T, Susaki H, Takamura H, et al. Foramen magnum decompression with removal of the outer layer of the dura as treatment for syringomyelia occurring with Chiari I malformation. *Neurosurgery* 1993;33:844–849.

Jones J, Wolf S. Neuropathic shoulder arthropathy (Charcot joint) associated with syringomyelia. *Neurology* 1998;50:825–827.

Keung YK, Cobos E, Whitehead RP, et al. Secondary syringomyelia due to intramedullary spinal cord metastasis: case report and review of literature. *Am J Clin Oncol* 1997;20:577–579.

Kyoshima K, Bogdanov GI. Spontaneous resolution of syringomyelia:

report of two cases and review of the literature. *Neurosurgery* 2003;53:762–769.

Levine DN. The pathogenesis of syringomyelia associated with lesions at the foramen magnum: a critical review of existing theories and proposal of a new hypothesis. *J Neurol Sci* 2004;220(May 15): 3–21.

Mariani C, Cislaghi MG, Barbieri S, et al. The natural history and results of surgery in 50 cases of syringomyelia. *J Neurol* 1991;238:433–438.

Milhorat TH, Capocelli, AL, Anzil, AP, et al. Pathological basis of spinal cord cavitation in syringomyelia: analysis of 105 autopsy cases. *J Neurosurg* 1995;82:802–812.

Milhorat TH, Miller JI, Johnson WD, et al. Anatomical basis of syringomyelia occurring with hindbrain lesions. *Neurosurgery* 1993;32:748–754.

Nalini A, Ravishankar S. "Dropped head syndrome" in syringomyelia: report of two cases. *J Neurol Neurosurg Psychiatry* 2005 Feb;76(2):290–291.

Nogues MA, Stalberg E. Electrodiagnostic findings in syringomyelia. *Muscle Nerve* 1999;22:1653–1659.

Oldfield EH, Muraszko K, Shawker TH, et al. Pathophysiology of syringomyelia associated with Chiari I malformation of the cerebellar tonsils: implications for diagnosis and treatment. *J Neurosurg* 1994;80:3–15.

Parker JD, Broberg JC, Napolitano PG. Maternal Arnold-Chiari type I malformation and syringomyelia: a labor management dilemma. *Am J Perinatol* 2002;19:445–450.

Pillay PK, Awad IA, Hahn JF. Gardner's hydrodynamic theory of syringomyelia revisited. *Cleve Clin J Med* 1992;59:373–380.

Poser CM. *The Relationship Between Syringomyelia and Neoplasm.* Springfield, IL: Charles C Thomas, 1956.

Sackellares JC, Swift TR. Shoulder enlargement as the presenting sign in syringomyelia. *JAMA* 1976;236:2878–2879.

Schurch B, Wichmann W, Rossier AB. Post-traumatic syringomyelia (cystic myelopathy): a prospective study of 449 patients with spinal cord injury. *J Neurol Neurosurg Psychiatry* 1996;60:61–67.

Vassilouthis J, Papandreou A, Anagnostaras S, et al. Thecoperitoneal shunt for syringomyelia: report of three cases. *Neurosurgery* 1993;33:324–327.

Williams B. On the pathogenesis of syringomyelia: a review. *J R Soc Med* 1980;73:798–806.

Williams B. Post-traumatic syringomyelia, an update. *Paraplegia* 1990;28:296–313.

Williams B. Syringomyelia. *Neurosurg Clin N Am* 1990;1:653–685.

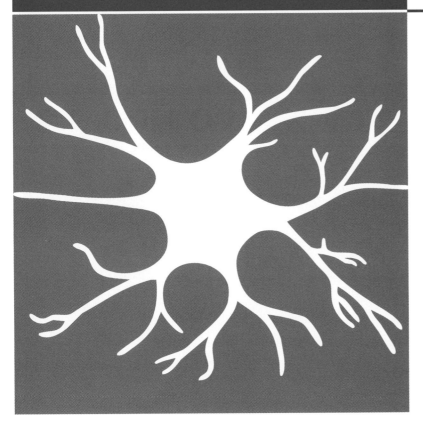

Disorders of the Neuromuscular Junction

Chapter 121

▶ Myasthenia Gravis

Audrey S. Penn and Lewis P. Rowland

Myasthenia gravis (MG) is caused by a defect of neuromuscular transmission owing to antibody-mediated attack on nicotinic acetylcholine receptors (AChR) at neuromuscular junctions. It is characterized by fluctuating weakness that is improved by inhibitors of cholinesterase.

ETIOLOGY AND PATHOGENESIS

The pathogenesis of MG is related to the destructive effects of autoantibodies to AChR, as indicated by several lines of evidence:

1. In several species of animals, experimental immunization with AChR purified from the electric organ of the torpedo, an electric fish, induced high titers of antibody to the receptor. Overt evidence of weakness varies but may be uncovered by small doses of curare. Many animals also showed the essential electrophysiologic and pathologic features of human MG. This was first found in rabbits by Patrick and Lindstrom (1973).
2. Serum antibodies that react with human AChR are found in humans with MG.
3. Toyka and colleagues (1975) found that the electrophysiologic features of MG were reproduced by passive transfer of human immunoglobulin (IgG) to mice. By analogy, human transient neonatal MG could then be explained by transplacental transfer of maternal antibody.
4. Pinching found that plasmapheresis reduced plasma levels of anti-AChR and ameliorated MG symptoms and signs.

The polyclonal IgG antibodies to AChR are produced by plasma cells in peripheral lymphoid organs, bone marrow, and thymus. These cells are derived from B cells that have been activated by antigen-specific T-helper (CD4+) cells. The T cells have also been activated, in this case by binding to AChR antigenic peptide sequences (epitopes) that rest within the histocompatibility antigens on the surface of antigen-presenting cells.

The AChR antibodies react with multiple determinants, and enough antibody circulates to saturate up to 80% of all AChR sites on muscle. A small percentage of the anti-AChR molecules interfere directly with the binding of ACh, but the major damage to end plates seems to result from actual loss of receptors owing to complement-mediated lysis of the membrane and to acceleration of normal degradative processes (internalization, endocytosis, lysosomal hydrolysis) with inadequate replacement by new synthesis. As a consequence of the loss of AChR and the erosion and simplification of the end plates, the amplitude of miniature end plate potentials is about 20% of normal, and patients are abnormally sensitive to the competitive antagonist curare. The characteristic decremental response to repetitive stimulation of the motor nerve reflects failure of end plate potentials to reach threshold so that progressively fewer fibers respond to arrival of a nerve impulse.

How the autoimmune disorder starts is not known. In human disease, in contrast to experimental MG in animals, the thymus gland is almost always abnormal; there are often multiple lymphoid follicles with germinal centers ("hyperplasia of the thymus"), and in about 15% of patients, there is an encapsulated benign tumor, a thymoma. These abnormalities are impressive because the normal thymus is responsible for the maturation of T-cells that mediate immune protection without promoting autoimmune responses. AChR antibodies are synthesized by B cells in cultures of hyperplastic thymus gland. The hyperplastic glands contain all the elements needed for antibody production: class II HLA-positive antigen-presenting cells, T-helper cells, B cells, and AChR antigen; that is, messenger ribonucleic acid for subunits of AChR has been detected in thymus, and "myoid cells" are found in both normal and hyperplastic thymus. The myoid cells bear surface AChR and contain other muscle proteins. When human myasthenic thymus was transplanted into severely congenitally immunodeficient mice, the animals produced antibodies to AChR that bound to their own motor end plates, even though weakness was not evident.

Excessive and inappropriately prolonged synthesis of thymic hormones that normally promote differentiation of T-helper cells may contribute to the autoimmune response. Still another possible initiating factor is immunogenic alteration of the antigen, AChR, at end plates, because penicillamine therapy in patients with rheumatoid arthritis may initiate a syndrome that is indistinguishable from MG except that it subsides when administration of the drug is stopped.

There are few familial cases of the acquired autoimmune disease, but disproportionate frequency of some HLA haplotypes (B8, DR3, DQB1) in MG patients suggests that genetic predisposition may be important. Other autoimmune diseases also seem to occur with disproportionate frequency in patients with MG, especially hyperthyroidism and other thyroid disorders, systemic lupus erythematosus, rheumatoid arthritis, pernicious anemia, and pemphigus.

Most AChR antibodies are directed against antigenic determinants on the extracellular portion of the protein farthest out from the membrane rather than the ACh binding site. The summed effects of the polyclonal anti-AChR antibodies, especially those that fix complement, result in destruction of the receptors. Physiologic studies indicate impaired postsynaptic responsiveness to ACh, which accounts for the physiologic abnormalities, clinical symptoms, and beneficial effects of drugs that inhibit acetylcholinesterase. If binding or blocking antibodies are absent, tests can be done for "modulating" antibodies that enhance degradation of the receptors in cultured cells, bringing the number of positive tests to 90%, according to Howard et al.

SPECIAL FORMS OF MYASTHENIA GRAVIS

Juvenile and Adult Forms

Typical MG may begin at any age, but it is most common in the second to fourth decades. It is less frequent before age 10 or after age 65 years. Circulating AChR antibodies are demonstrated in 85% to 90% of patients with generalized MG and 50% to 60% of those with restricted ocular myasthenia. Patients without antibodies do not differ clinically or in response to immunotherapy; this seronegative MG may be more common in patients who are symptomatic before puberty. These are the typical forms of MG; other forms are rare.

Neonatal Myasthenia

About 12% of infants born to myasthenic mothers have a syndrome characterized by impaired sucking, weak cry, limp limbs, and, exceptionally, respiratory insufficiency. Symptoms begin in the first 48 hours and may last several days or weeks, after which the children are normal. The mothers are usually symptomatic but may be in complete remission; in either case, AChR antibodies are demonstrable in both mother and child. Symptoms disappear as the antibody titer in the infant declines. Severe respiratory insufficiency may be treated by exchange transfusion, but the natural history of the disorder is progressive improvement and total disappearance of all symptoms within days or weeks. Respiratory support and nutrition are the key elements of treatment. Rare instances of arthrogryposis multiplex congenita have been attributed to transplacental transfer of antibodies that inhibit fetal AChR.

Congenital Myasthenia

Children with congenital MG, although rarely encountered, show several characteristics. The mothers are asymptomatic and do not have circulating anti-AChR in the blood. Usually, no problem occurs in the neonatal period; instead, ophthalmoplegia is the dominant sign in infancy. Limb weakness may be evident. The condition is often familial. Antibodies to AChR are not found, but there are decremental responses to repetitive stimulation. Ultrastructural and biochemical examination of motor end plates, microelectrode analysis, and identification of mutations have delineated a series of disorders that include both presynaptic and postsynaptic proteins. Disorders of the ion channel formed by the AChR molecule include the *slow-channel syndrome*, in which the response to ACh is enhanced because the opening episodes of the channel are abnormally prolonged. Forearm extensors tend to be selectively weak. More than 11 different mutations have been identified in different AChR subunits. Quinidine shortens the prolonged openings and gives therapeutic benefit. A *fast-channel syndrome*, with impaired response to ACh, has been reported in rare patients with mutations of the ε-subunit. Another mutation in the same subunit leads to *abnormal kinetics of AChR activation* so that the channel opens more slowly and closes more rapidly than normal. The 37 known mutations in the ε-subunit are inherited recessively and result in severe *lack of AChR in the end plates*. One syndrome results from mutations in the collagen tail subunit of the enzyme, creating *deficiency of acetylcholinesterase*. These landmark observations were made at the Mayo Clinic by Andrew G. Engel and his colleagues. Anticholinesterase drugs may help in some of these disorders, but parents should be warned that sudden apneic spells may be induced by mild infections.

The British team led by Vincent and Newsom-Davis found clinical differences between those with mutations in the AChR ε-subunit and those with mutations in rapsyn, the end plate AChR clustering protein. The receptor mutations caused congenital ophthalmoplegia, bulbar symptoms, and limb weakness. The rapsyn mutations caused an early-onset syndrome with arthrogryposis and life-threatening crises in childhood or a late-onset syndrome beginning in adolescence or later and resembling seronegative myasthenia.

Drug-induced Myasthenia

The best example of this condition occurs in patients treated with penicillamine for rheumatoid arthritis, scleroderma, or hepatolenticular degeneration (Wilson disease). The clinical manifestations and AChR antibody titers are similar to those of typical adult MG, but both disappear when drug administration is discontinued. Cases attributed to trimethadione (Tridione) have been less thoroughly studied.

PATHOLOGY

The Overt pathology of MG is found primarily in the thymus gland. About 70% of thymus glands from adult patients with MG are not involuted and weigh more than normal. The glands show lymphoid hyperplasia: In normal individuals, germinal centers are numerous in lymph nodes and spleen but are sparse in the thymus. Immunocytochemical methods indicate that these thymic germinal centers contain B cells, plasma cells, HLA class II DR-positive T cells, and interdigitating cells.

Another 10% of myasthenic thymus glands contain thymomas of the lymphoepithelial type. The lymphoid cells in these tumors are T cells; the neoplastic elements are epithelial cells. Benign thymomas may nearly replace the gland, with only residual glandular material at the edges, or they may rest within a large hyperplastic gland. Thymomas tend to occur in older patients, but in Castleman's series, 15% were found in patients between ages 20 and 29 years. They may invade contiguous pleura, pericardium, or blood vessels, or seed onto more distant thoracic structures, including the diaphragm; however, they almost never spread to other organs. In older patients without thymoma, the thymus gland appears involuted, often showing hyperplastic foci within fatty tissue on microscopic examination of multiple samples.

In about 50% of cases, muscles contain *lymphorrhages*, which are focal clusters of lymphocytes near small necrotic foci without perivascular predilection. In a few cases, especially in patients with thymoma, there is diffuse muscle fiber necrosis with infiltration of inflammatory cells; similar lesions are rarely encountered in the myocardium. Lymphorrhages are not seen near damaged neuromuscular junctions (although inflammatory cells may be seen in necrotic end plates in rat experimental autoimmune MG), but morphometric studies have shown loss of synaptic folds and widened clefts. Some nerve terminals are smaller than normal, and multiple small terminals are applied to the elongated, simplified postsynaptic membrane; others are absent. Other end plates appear normal. On residual synaptic folds, immunocytochemical methods show Y-shaped antibodylike structures, IgG, complement components 2 and 9, and complement membrane attack complex.

INCIDENCE

MG is a common disease. An apparent increase in the incidence of the disease in recent years is probably owing to improved diagnosis. According to Phillips and Torner (1996), the prevalence rate is 14 per 100,000 (or about 17,000 cases) in the United States. Before age 40 years, the disease is three times more common in women, but at older ages both sexes are equally affected.

Familial cases are rare; single members of pairs of fraternal twins and several sets of identical twins have been affected. Young women with MG tend to have HLA-B8, -DR3, and -DQB1* 0102 haplotypes; in young Japanese women HLA-A12 is prominent. These observations imply the presence of a linked immune response gene that encodes a protein involved in the autoimmune response. First-degree relatives show an unusual incidence of other autoimmune diseases (systemic lupus erythematosus, rheumatoid arthritis, thyroid disease) and HLA-B8 haplotype.

SYMPTOMS

The symptoms of MG have three general characteristics that, together, provide a diagnostic combination. Formal diagnosis depends on demonstration of the response to cholinergic drugs, electrophysiologic evidence of abnormal neuromuscular transmission, and demonstration of circulating antibodies to AChR.

The fluctuating nature of myasthenic weakness is unlike any other disease. The weakness varies in the course of a single day, sometimes within minutes, and it varies from day to day or over longer periods. Major prolonged variations are termed *remissions* or *exacerbations;* when an exacerbation involves respiratory muscles to the point of inadequate ventilation, it is called a *crisis.* Variations sometimes seem related to exercise; this and the nature of the physiologic abnormality have long been termed "excessive fatigability," but there are practical reasons to deemphasize fatigability as a central characteristic of MG. Patients with the disease almost never complain of fatigue or symptoms that might be construed as fatigue except when there is incipient respiratory muscle weakness. Myasthenic symptoms are *always* owing to weakness and not to rapid tiring. In contrast, patients who complain of fatigue, if they are not anemic or harboring a malignant tumor, almost always have emotional problems, usually depression.

The second characteristic of MG is the distribution of weakness. Ocular muscles are affected first in about 40% of patients and are ultimately involved in about 85%. Ptosis and diplopia are the symptoms that result. Other common symptoms affect facial or oropharyngeal muscles, resulting in dysarthria, dysphagia, and limitation of facial movements. Together, oropharyngeal and ocular weakness cause symptoms in virtually all patients with acquired MG. Limb and neck weakness is also common, but in conjunction with cranial weakness. Almost never are the limbs affected alone.

Crisis is most likely to occur in patients with oropharyngeal or respiratory muscle weakness. It seems to be provoked by respiratory infection in many patients or by surgical procedures, including thymectomy, although it may occur with no apparent provocation. Both emotional stress and systemic illness may aggravate myasthenic weakness for reasons that are not clear; in patients with oropharyngeal weakness, aspiration of secretions may occlude lung passages to cause rather abrupt onset of respiratory difficulty. Major surgery may be followed by respiratory weakness without aspiration, however, so this cannot be the entire explanation. Spontaneous crisis seems to be less common now than it once was.

The third characteristic of myasthenic weakness is the clinical response to cholinergic drugs. This occurs so uniformly that it has become part of the definition, but it may be difficult to demonstrate in some patients, especially those with purely ocular myasthenia.

Aside from the fluctuating nature of the weakness, MG is not a steadily progressive disease. The general nature of the disease, however, is usually established within weeks or months after the first symptoms. If myasthenia is restricted to ocular muscles for 2 years, certainly if it is restricted after 3 years, it is likely to remain restricted, and only in rare cases does it then become generalized. Distinguishing solely ocular myasthenia from generalized myasthenia soon after onset is challenging. Solely ocular myasthenia differs serologically from generalized myasthenia because AChR antibodies are found in lower frequency—50%—and in low titer. Additionally, single-fiber EMG is more likely to be normal. Current debate centers on ability to predict generalized spread after ocular onset. Some suggest that early immunosuppression will suppress/retard generalization. However, there have been no reports of successful weaning from these medications followed by complete remission. Spontaneous remissions occur in about 25% of all patients and are also more likely to occur in the first 2 years.

Before the advent of intensive care units and the introduction of positive pressure respirators in the 1960s, crisis was a life-threatening event, and the mortality of the disease was about 33%. With improved respiratory care, however, patients rarely die of MG, except when cardiac, renal, or other disease complicates the picture.

SIGNS

The vital signs and general physical examination are usually within normal limits, unless the patient is in crisis. The findings on neurologic examination depend on the distribution of weakness. Weakness of the facial and levator palpebrae muscles produces a characteristic expressionless facies with drooping eyelids. Weakness of the ocular muscles may cause paralysis or weakness of isolated muscles, paralysis of conjugate gaze, complete ophthalmoplegia in one or both eyes, or a pattern resembling internuclear ophthalmoplegia. Weakness of oropharyngeal or limb muscles, when present, can be shown by appropriate tests. Respiratory muscle weakness can be detected by pulmonary function tests, which should not be limited to measurement of vital capacity but should also include inspiratory and expiratory pressures, the measurements of which may be abnormal even before overt symptoms exist. Muscular wasting of variable degree is found in about 10% of patients, but is not focal and is usually encountered only in patients with malnutrition owing to severe dysphagia. Fasciculations do not occur, unless the patient has received excessive amounts of cholinergic drugs. Sensation is normal and the reflexes are preserved, even in muscles that are weak.

For the purpose of rating clinical status and for use in clinical trials, new classifications of severity and of response to therapy have been developed by Jaretzki and the Medical Advisory Board of the Myasthenia Gravis Foundation.

LABORATORY DATA

Routine examinations of blood, urine, and CSF are normal. The characteristic electrodiagnostic abnormality is progressive decrement in the amplitude of muscle action potentials evoked by repetitive nerve stimulation at 3 or 5 Hz. In generalized MG, the decremental response can be demonstrated in about 90% of patients, if at least three neuromuscular systems are used (median-thenar, ulnar-hypothenar, accessory-trapezius). In microelectrode study of intercostal muscle, the amplitude of miniature end plate potentials is reduced to about 20% of normal. This is caused by a decrease in the number of AChR available to agonists applied by microiontophoresis. In single-fiber EMG, a small electrode measures the interval between evoked potentials of the muscle fibers in the same motor unit. This interval normally varies, a phenomenon called *jitter*, and the normal temporal limits of jitter have been defined. In MG, the jitter is increased, and an impulse may not appear at the expected time; this is called *blocking*, and the number of blockings is increased in myasthenic muscle. All these electrophysiologic abnormalities are characteristic of MG, but blocking and jitter are also seen in disorders of ACh release. The standard EMG is usually normal, occasionally shows a myopathic pattern, and almost never shows signs of denervation unless some other condition supervenes. Similarly, nerve conduction velocities are normal.

Antibodies to AChR are found in 85% to 90% of patients of all ages with generalized MG if human muscle is used as the test antigen. There have been no false-positive results except for rare patients with Lambert-Eaton syndrome or thymoma without clinical or provocable MG, or in remission; these may be considered unusual forms of MG. Antibodies may not be detected in patients with strictly ocular disease, in some patients in remission (or after thymectomy), or even in some patients with severe symptoms. The titer does not match the severity of symptoms; patients in complete clinical remission may have high titers. Antibodies to myofibrillar proteins (titin, myosin, actin, actomyosin) are found in 85% of patients with thymoma and may be the first evidence of thymoma in some cases. In the first report of seronegative myasthenia, Soliven et al. found no clinical differences between patients who had or lacked AChR antibodies. Subsequently, more than half of these seronegative patients were found to have antibodies to muscle specific receptor tyrosine kinase (MuSK). More recent reports are divided. Some find no difference in response to thymectomy whereas others believe that the clinical picture is almost always one of generalized MG and predominant bulbar signs, as well as poor and inconsistent responses to pyridostigmine, immunosuppressants, and thymectomy but excellent response to plasmapheresis.

The different forms of congenital MG can be identified only in a few special centers that are prepared to perform microelectrode and ultrastructural analyses of intercostal muscle biopsies for miniature end plate potentials, AChR numbers, and determination of bound antibodies. It seems likely that deoxyribonucleic acid analysis may soon suffice for diagnosis.

Other serologic abnormalities are encountered with varying frequency, but in several studies, antinuclear factor, rheumatoid factor, and thyroid antibodies were encountered more often than in control populations. Laboratory (and clinical) evidence of hyperthyroidism occurs at some time in about 5% of patients with MG. Radiographs of the chest (including 10° oblique films) provide evidence of thymoma in about 15% of patients, especially in those older than 40 years. CT of the mediastinum demonstrates all but microscopic thymomas. MRI is not more sensitive than CT.

DIAGNOSIS

The diagnosis of MG can be made without difficulty in most patients from the characteristic history and physical examination. The dramatic improvement that follows the injection of neostigmine bromide (Prostigmin) or edro-

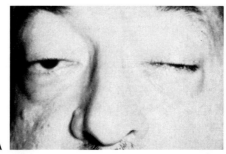
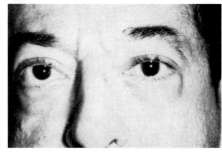

FIGURE 121.1. Myasthenia gravis. **A.** Severe ptosis of the lids. **B.** Same patient 1 minute after intravenous injection of edrophonium (10 mg). (From Rowland LP, Hoefer PFR, Aranow H Jr. Myasthenic syndromes. *Res Publ Assoc Res Nerv Ment Dis* 1961;38; with permission.)

phonium (Tensilon) makes the administration of these drugs essential. Return of strength in weak muscles occurs uniformly after the injection of neostigmine or edrophonium (Fig. 121.1); if no such response occurs, the diagnosis of MG can be doubted. Demonstration of the pharmacologic response is sometimes difficult; however, if the clinical features are suggestive, the test should be repeated, perhaps with a different dosage or rate of administration. Withholding anticholinesterase medication overnight may be helpful. False-positive responses to edrophonium are exceptional but have been recorded with structural lesions, such as a brainstem tumor. (MG can also coexist with other diseases, such as Graves ophthalmopathy or the Lambert-Eaton syndrome.)

The diagnosis of MG is buttressed by the finding of high titers of antibodies to AChR, but a normal titer does not exclude the diagnosis. Somnier found that the test had a specificity of more than 99.9%; sensitivity was 88% because of the negative tests.

Responses to repetitive stimulation and single-fiber EMG also help. If a thymoma is present, the diagnosis of MG (rather than some other neuromuscular disease) is likely. In the past, clinicians used the increased sensitivity to curare as a test to prove that a syndrome simulating MG was actually psychasthenia or something else; however, the test was inconvenient and, if done without proper precautions, was even hazardous. Since the advent of the antibody test, the curare test has virtually disappeared.

In the neostigmine test, 1.5 to 2 mg of the drug and atropine sulfate, 0.4 mg, are given intramuscularly. Objective improvement in muscular power is recorded at 20-minute intervals up to 2 hours. Edrophonium is given intravenously in a dose of 1 to 10 mg. The initial dose is 2 mg followed in 30 seconds, if necessary, by an additional 2 mg and in another 15 to 30 seconds by 5 mg to a maximum of 10 mg. Improvement is observed within 30 seconds and lasts a few minutes. Most responses are seen with doses <5.0 mg. Because of the immediate and dramatic nature of the response, edrophonium is preferred for evaluation of ocular and other cranial muscle weakness, and neostigmine is generally reserved for evaluation of limb or respiratory weakness, which may require more time. Placebo injections are sometimes useful in evaluating limb weakness, but placebos are not necessary in evaluating cranial muscle weakness because that abnormality cannot be simulated. For all practical purposes, a positive response is diagnostic of MG.

DIFFERENTIAL DIAGNOSIS

The differential diagnosis includes all diseases that are accompanied by weakness of oropharyngeal or limb muscles, such as the muscular dystrophies, amyotrophic lateral sclerosis, progressive bulbar palsy, ophthalmoplegias of other causes, and the asthenia of psychoneurosis or hyperthyroidism. There is usually no difficulty in differentiating these conditions from MG by the findings on physical and neurologic examination and by the failure of symptoms in these conditions to improve after parenteral injection of neostigmine or edrophonium. Occasionally, blepharospasm is thought to mimic ocular myasthenia, but the forceful eye closure in that condition involves both the upper and lower lids; the narrowed palpebral fissure and signs of active muscle activity are distinctive.

The only other conditions in which clinical improvement has been documented after use of edrophonium are other disorders of neuromuscular transmission: botulinum intoxication, snake bite, organophosphate intoxication, or unusual disorders that include features of both MG and the Lambert-Eaton syndrome. Denervating disorders, such as motor neuron disease or peripheral neuropathy, do not show a reproducible or unequivocal clinical response to edrophonium or neostigmine. The response should be unequivocal and reproducible. If a structural lesion of the third cranial nerve seems to respond, the result should be photographed (and published).

TREATMENT

Clinicians must choose the sequence and combination of five kinds of therapy: Anticholinesterase drug therapy and plasmapheresis are symptomatic treatments, whereas thymectomy, steroids, and other immunosuppressive drugs may alter the course of the disease.

It is generally agreed that anticholinesterase drug therapy should be given as soon as the diagnosis is made. Of the three available drugs—neostigmine, pyridostigmine bromide, and ambenonium (Mytelase)—pyridostigmine is the most popular but has not been formally assessed in controlled comparison with the other drugs. The muscarinic side effects of abdominal cramps and diarrhea are the same for all three drugs but are least severe with pyridostigmine; none has more side effects than another. The usual starting dose of pyridostigmine is 60 mg given orally every 4 hours while the patient is awake. Depending on clinical response, the dosage may be increased, but incremental benefit is not to be expected in amounts greater than 120 mg every 2 hours. If patients have difficulty eating, doses can be taken about 30 minutes before a meal. If patients have special difficulty on waking in the morning, a prolonged-release 180-mg tablet of pyridostigmine (Mestinon Timespan) can be taken at bedtime. Muscarinic symptoms can be ameliorated by preparations containing atropine (0.4 mg) with each dose of pyridostigmine. Excessive doses of atropine can cause psychosis, but the amounts taken in this regimen have not had this effect. Other drugs may be taken if diarrhea is prominent. There is no evidence that any one of the three drugs is more effective than the others in individual patients, and there is no evidence that combinations of two drugs are better than any one drug alone.

Although cholinergic drug therapy sometimes gives impressive results, there are serious limitations. In ocular myasthenia, ptosis may be helped, but some diplopia almost always persists. In generalized MG, patients may improve remarkably, but some symptoms usually remain. Cholinergic drugs do not return function to normal, and the risk of crisis persists because the disease is not cured. Therefore, usually, one of the other treatments is used promptly to treat generalized MG.

Thymectomy was originally reserved for patients with serious disability because the operation had a high mortality. With advances in surgery and anesthesia, however, the operative mortality is now negligible in major centers. About 80% of patients without thymoma become asymptomatic or go into complete remission after thymectomy; although there has been no controlled trial of thymectomy, these results seem to diverge from the natural history of the untreated disease. Thus, thymectomy is now recommended for most patients with generalized MG. Decisions made for children or patients older than 65 must be individualized. Although it is safe, thymectomy is a major operation and is not usually recommended for patients with ocular myasthenia unless there is a thymoma. The beneficial effects of thymectomy are usually delayed for months or years. It is never an emergency measure, and other forms of therapy are usually needed in the interim.

Mantegazza et al. found a remission rate of about 50% 6 years after surgery with either the standard transsternal operation or a minimally invasive thorascopic operation.

Prednisone therapy is used by some authorities to prepare patients for thymectomy, but that function is also served by plasmapheresis or by IVIG therapy. Exchanges of about 5% of calculated blood volume may be given several times before the day of surgery to be certain that the patient is functioning as well as possible and to ameliorate or avoid a postoperative respiratory crisis. Plasmapheresis is also used for other exacerbations; the resulting improvement, seen in most patients, may be slight or dramatic and may last only a few days or several months. Plasmapheresis is safe but expensive and is not convenient for many patients. Indwelling catheters may lead to misplacement, bleeding, or infection. IVIG is easier to administer but is even more expensive. It is preferred over plasmapheresis in those with poor venous access, including children.

IVIG therapy is usually given in five daily doses to a total of 2 g/kg body weight. Side effects include headache, aseptic meningitis, and a flulike syndrome that can be alarming but subsides in 1 or 2 days. Thromboembolic events, including stroke, have occurred but are not clearly related to the treatment, which is generally regarded as safe, less cumbersome than plasmapheresis, and less dependent on technical staff who may not be available on weekends. Both treatments are also available for management of exacerbations.

If a patient is still seriously disabled after thymectomy, most clinicians use prednisone, 60 to 100 mg every other day, to achieve a response within a few days or weeks. An equally satisfactory response can be seen with a lower dosage, but it takes longer; for instance, if the dose is 25 to 40 mg, benefit may be seen in 2 to 3 months. Once improvement is achieved, the dosage should be reduced gradually to 20 to 35 mg every other day. This has become a popular form of treatment for disabled patients, but there has been no controlled trial. If the patient does not improve in about 6 months, treatment with azathioprine (Imuran) or cyclophosphamide would be considered, in doses up to 2.5 mg/kg daily for an adult. The dosage should be increased gradually and may have to be taken with food to avert nausea. A popular immunosuppressive drug is mycophenolate mofetil (CellCept). In one report, 73% of 85 patients improved; adverse effects led to discontinuation of treatment in 6%. Whether steroids and immunosuppressive drugs have additive effects is uncertain, and the relative risks are difficult to assess. The numerous side effects of prednisone must be weighed against the possibilities of marrow suppression, susceptibility to infection, or delayed malignancy in patients who are taking immunosuppressive drugs. The use of immunosuppressive drugs often assists in lowering the dose of prednisone.

Prednisone, 20 to 35 mg on alternate days, is also recommended by some clinicians for ocular myasthenia, weighing risks against potential benefit. For some patients in sensitive occupations, the risks of prednisone therapy may be necessary (e.g., actors, police officers, roofers or others who work on heights, or those who require stereoscopic vision). Ocular myasthenia is not a threat to life; however, pyridostigmine may alleviate ptosis. An eye patch can end diplopia, and prisms help some patients with stable horizontal diplopia. Thymectomy has become so safe that it might be considered for ocular myasthenia that is truly disabling.

Patients with thymoma are likely to have more severe MG and are less likely to improve after thymectomy; nevertheless, many of these patients also improve if the surrounding thymus gland is excised in addition to the tumor.

Myasthenic crisis is defined as the need for assisted ventilation, a condition that arises in about 10% of myasthenic patients. It is more likely to occur in patients with dysarthria, dysphagia, and documented respiratory muscle weakness, presumably because they are liable to aspirate oral secretions, but crisis may also occur in other patients after respiratory infection or major surgery (including thymectomy). The principles of treatment are those of respiratory failure in general. Cholinergic drug therapy is usually discontinued once an endotracheal tube has been placed and positive pressure respiration started; this practice avoids questions about the proper dosage or cholinergic stimulation of pulmonary secretions. Crisis is viewed as a temporary exacerbation that subsides in a few days or weeks. The therapeutic goal is to maintain vital functions and to avoid or treat infection until the patient spontaneously recovers from the crisis. Cholinergic drug therapy need not be restarted unless fever and other signs of infection have subsided, there are no pulmonary complications, and the patient is breathing without assistance.

To determine whether plasma exchange or IVIG actually shortens the duration of crisis would require a controlled trial, but that has not been done. Even so, pulmonary intensive care is now so effective that crisis is almost never fatal and many patients go into a remission after recovery from crisis. Because of advances in therapy, MG is still serious, but not so grave.

SUGGESTED READINGS

Bever CT Jr, Chang HW, Penn AS, et al. Penicillamine-induced myasthenia gravis: effects of penicillamine on acetylcholine receptor. *Neurology* 1982;32:1077–1082.

Bufler J, Pitz R, Czep M, et al. Purified IgG from seropositive and seronegative patients with myasthenia gravis reversibly blocks currents through nicotinic acetylcholine receptor channels. *Ann Neurol* 1998;43:458–464.

Burke G, Cossins J, Maxwell S, et al. Distinct phenotypes of congenital acetylcholine receptor deficiency. *Neuromusc Disord* 2004;14:356–364.

Ciafaloni E, Massey JM. Myasthenia gravis and pregnancy. *Neurol Clin* 2004 Nov;22(4):771–782.

Donaldson JO, Penn AS, Lisak RP, et al. Antiacetylcholine receptor antibody in neonatal myasthenia gravis. *Am J Dis Child* 1981;135:222–226.

Eaton LM, Lambert EH. Electromyography and electric stimulation of nerves in diseases of motor unit: observations in myasthenic syndrome associated with malignant tumors. *JAMA* 1957;163:1117–1120.

Engel AG, ed. *Myasthenia Gravis and Myasthenic Disorders.* New York: Oxford University Press, 1999.

Engel AG, Ohno K, Sine SM. Sleuthing molecular targets for neuromuscular diseases at the neuromuscular junction. *Nat Rev Neurosci* 2003;4:339–352.

Erb W. Zur Causistik der bulbären Lächmungen: über einem neuen, wahrscheinlich bulbären Symptomencomplex. *Arch Psychiatr Nervenkr* 1879;336–350.

Evoli A, Tonali PA, Padua L, et al. Clinical correlates with anti-MuSK antibodies in generalized seronegative myasthenia gravis. *Brain* 2003;126:2304–2311.

Goldflam S. Über einen scheinbar heilbaren bulbärparalytischen Symptomencomplex mit Beteiligungen der Extremitäten. *Dtsch Z Nervenheilk* 1893;4:312–352.

Guillermo GR, Téllez-Zenteno JF, Weder-Cisneros N, et al. Response of thymectomy: clinical and pathological characteristics among seronegative and seropositive myasthenia gravis patients. *Acta Neurol Scand* 2004;109:217–221.

Harper CM, Engel AG. Quinidine sulfate therapy for the slow-channel congenital myasthenic syndrome. *Ann Neurol* 1998;43:480–484.

Hoff JM, Daltveit AK, Gihus NE. Myasthenia gravis. Consequences for pregnancy, delivery, and the newborn. *Neurology* 2003;61:1362–1366.

Hohlfeld R, Wekerle H. The immunopathogenesis of myasthenia gravis. In: Engel AG, ed. *Myasthenia Gravis and Myasthenic Disorders.* Oxford, UK: Oxford University Press, 1999:87–100.

Howard FM, Lennon VA, Finley J, et al. Clinical correlations of antibodies that bind, block, or modulate human acetylcholine receptors in myasthenia gravis. *Ann N Y Acad Sci* 1987;505:526–538.

Jaretzki A 3rd, Barohn RJ, Ernstoff RM, et al. Myasthenia gravis: recommendations for clinical research standards. Task Force of the Medical Scientific Advisory Board of the Myasthenia Gravis Foundation of America. *Neurology* 2000;55(Jul 12):16–23.

Jaretzki A 3rd, Penn AS, Younger DS, et al. "Maximal" thymectomy for myasthenia gravis: results. *J Thorac Cardiovasc Surg* 1988;95:747–757.

Jaretzki A, Steinglass KM, Sonett JR. Thymectomy in the management of myasthenia gravis. *Semin Neurol* 2004 Mar;24(1):49–62.

Jolly F. Über Myasthenia Gravis pseudoparalytica. *Berl Klin Wochenschr* 1895;1:1–7.

Juel VC, Massey JM. Autoimmune Myasthenia Gravis: Recommendations for Treatment and Immunologic Modulation. *Curr Treat Options Neurol* 2005 Jan;7(1):3–14.

Kaminski HJ, ed. *Myasthenia Gravis and Related Disorders.* Totowa, NJ: Humana, 2002.

Kawaguchi N, Kuwabara S, Nemoto Y, et al. Treatment and outcome of myasthenia gravis: retrospective multi-center analysis of 470 Japanese patients, 1999–2000. *J Neurol Sci* 2004 Sep 15;224(1–2):43–47.

Kondo K, Monden Y. Thymoma and myasthenia gravis: a clinical study of 1,089 patients from Japan. *Ann Thorac Surg* 2005 Jan;79(1):219–224.

Kupersmith MJ. Does early treatment of ocular myasthenia gravis with prednisone reduce progression to generalized disease? *J Neurol Sci* 2004;217:123–124.

Lindner A, Schalke B, Toyka KV. Outcome in juvenile onset myasthenia gravis: a retrospective study with long-term follow-up of 79 patients. *J Neurol* 1997;244:515–520.

Lindstrom J, Seybold M, Lennon VA, et al. Antibody to acetylcholine receptor in myasthenia gravis: prevalence, clinical correlates, and diagnostic value. *Neurology* 1976;26:1054–1059.

Mantegazza R, Baggi F, Bernasconi P, et al. Video-assisted thorascopic extended thymectomy and extended transsternal thymectomy (T-3b) in non-thymomatous myasthenia gravis patients: remission after 6 years of follow-up. *J Neurol Sci* 2003;212:31–36.

McConville J, Farrugia ME, Beeson D, et al. Detection and characterization of MuSK antibodies in seronegative myasthenia gravis. *Ann Neurol* 2004;55:580–584.

Meriggioli MN, Ciafaloni E, Al-Hayk KA, et al. Mycophenolate mofetil for myasthenia gravis. An analysis of efficacy, safety, and tolerability. *Neurology* 2003;61:1438–1440.

Miller RG, Filler-Katz A, Kiprov D, et al. Repeat thymectomy in chronic refractory myasthenia gravis. *Neurology* 1991;41:923–924.

Myasthenia Gravis Clinical Study Group. Randomised clinical trial comparing prednisone and azathioprine in myasthenia gravis. Results of the second interim analysis. *J Neurol Neurosurg Psychiatry* 1993;56:1157–1163.

Odel JG, Winterkorn JMS, Behrens MM. The sleep test for myasthenia gravis. *J Clin Neuroophthal* 1991;11:288–292.

Ohno K, Engel AG, Sine S. The spectrum of congenital myasthenic syndromes. *Mol Neurobiol* 2002;26:47–67.

Oosterhuis HJ. The natural course of myasthenia gravis: a long-term follow-up study. *J Neurol Neurosurg Psychiatry* 1989;52:1121–1127.

Palace J, Newsom-Davis J, Lecky B, and the Myasthenia Gravis Study Group. A randomized double-blind trial of prednisolone alone or with azathioprine in myasthenia gravis. *Neurology* 1998;50:1778–1783.

Patrick J, Lindstrom J. Autoimmune response to acetylcholine receptor. *Science* 1973;180:871–872.

Qureshi AJ, Choudry MA, Akbar MS, et al. Plasma exchange versus intravenous immunoglobulin treatment in myasthenic crisis. *Neurology* 1999;52:629–632.

Romi F, Gilhus NE, Varhaug JE, et al. Disease severity and outcome in thymoma myasthenia gravis: a long-term observation study. *Eur J Neurol* 2003;10:701–706.

Rowland LP. Controversies about the treatment of myasthenia gravis. *J Neurol Neurosurg Psychiatry* 1980;43:644–659.

Rowland LP, Hoefer PFR, Aranow H Jr. Myasthenic syndromes. *Res Publ Assoc Res Nerv Ment Dis* 1961;38:548–600.

Rowland LP, Hoefer PF, Aranow H Jr, et al. Fatalities in myasthenia gravis: a review of 39 cases with 26 autopsies. *Neurology* 1956;6:307–326.

Sanders DB, El-Salem K, Massey JM, et al. Clinical aspects of MuSK antibody positive seronegative MG. *Neurology* 2003;60:1978–1980.

Soliven B, Lange DJ, Penn AS, et al. Seronegative myasthenia gravis. *Neurology* 1988;38:514–517.

Soleimani A, Moayyeri A, Akhondzadeh S, et al. Frequency of myasthenic crisis in relation to thymectomy in generalized myasthenia gravis: a 17-year experience. *BMC Neurol* 2004 Sep 11;4(1):12.

Somnier FE, Engel PJH. The occurrence of anti-titin antibodies and thymomas. A population survey of MG 1970–1999. *Neurology* 2002;59:92–98.

Thomas CE, Mayer SA, Gungor Y, et al. Myasthenic crisis: clinical features, mortality, complications, and risk factors for intubation. *Neurology* 1997;48:1253–1260.

Toyka KV, Drachman DB, Pestronk A, et al. Myasthenia gravis: passive transfer from man to mouse. *Science* 1975;190:397–399.

Vincent A, McConville J, Farrugia ME, Newsom-Davis J. Seronegative myasthenia gravis. *Semin Neurol* 2004 Mar;24(1):125–133.

Wang ZU, Karachunski PI, Howard JF, et al. Myasthenia in SCID mice grafted with myasthenic patient lymphocytes: role of CD4 and CD8 cells. *Neurology* 1999;52:484–497.

Watanabe A, Watanabe T, Obama T, et al. Prognostic factors for myasthenic crisis after transsternal thymectomy in patients with myasthenia gravis. *J Thorac Cardiovasc Surg* 2004 Mar;127(3):868–876.

Chapter 122

Lambert-Eaton Syndrome

Audrey S. Penn

The Lambert-Eaton myasthenic syndrome (LEMS) is an autoimmune disease of peripheral cholinergic synapses. Antibodies are directed against voltage-gated calcium channels in peripheral nerve terminals. A disease of adults, LEMS is found in 60% of patients with small cell carcinoma of the lung. The neurologic symptoms almost always precede those of the tumor; the interval may be as long as 5 years. Other tumors have also been implicated, but about 33% of cases are not associated with tumor. Tumor-free individuals tend to show the HLA B8, DR 3 haplotype, which are not found in those with neoplasms. Cell lines derived from the lung cancer bear voltage-gated calcium channels displaying the antigenic sites. If tumor cells are grown in the presence of immunoglobulin (IgG) from a patient with LEMS, the number of functional channels declines. Similar antigens are found on voltage-gated calcium channels from neuroendocrine tumors. The cultured carcinoma cells also bear receptors for dihydropyridines.

The abnormality of neurotransmission is attributed to inadequate release of acetylcholine (ACh) from nerve terminals at both nicotinic and muscarinic sites and is related to *abnormal voltage-dependent calcium channels*. When IgG from affected patients is injected into mice, the number of ACh quanta released by nerve stimulation is reduced, and there is disarray of the active zone particles that can be detected by freeze-fracture ultrastructural analysis.

Purified calcium channel proteins can be directly radiolabeled. An alternative label can be generated by the use of specific ligand, omega-conotoxin, which is prepared from a marine snail (*Conus magus*) and has been used to identify P/Q-type calcium channels in extracts of small cell carcinoma, neuroblastoma, and other neuroendocrine cell lines. A diagnostic test for the autoantibodies is based on radiolabeled preparations, but it is not fully specific. In the series of Motomura and associates (1997), 92% of 72 patients had a positive reaction. There have been a few positive tests in paraneoplastic cerebellar disorders. Some patients have both LEMS and a cerebellar syndrome.

LEMS may be suspected in patients with symptoms of proximal limb weakness who have lost knee and ankle jerks and complain of dry mouth or myalgia. Other, less common autonomic symptoms include impotence, constipation, and hypohidrosis. LEMS differs clinically from myasthenia gravis (MG) because diplopia, dysarthria, dysphagia, and dyspnea are lacking. Autonomic symptoms are more common in LEMS than in MG.

The disease is defined, and the diagnosis made, by the characteristic incremental response to repetitive nerve stimulation, a pattern that is the opposite of MG. The first evoked potential has an abnormally low amplitude, which decreases even further at low rates of stimulation. At rates greater than 10 Hz, however, there is a marked increase in the amplitude of evoked response (2 to 20 times the original value). This incremental response results from facilitation of release of transmitter at high rates of stimulation; at low rates the number of quanta released per impulse (quantal content) is inadequate to produce end plate potentials that achieve threshold. Similar abnormalities are found in preparations exposed to botulinum toxin or to a milieu low in calcium or high in magnesium.

Some patients with LEMS have ptosis with antibodies to ACh receptor. This combined syndrome may be an example of multiple autoimmune diseases in the same individual.

Treatment is directed to the concomitant tumor. The neuromuscular disorder is treated with drugs that facilitate release of ACh. A combination of pyridostigmine bromide and 3,4-diaminopyridine improves strength, but other aminopyridines may be hazardous. 4-Aminopyridine causes convulsions. Other drugs that facilitate release of ACh have had adverse effects. Guanidine hydrochloride (20 to 30 mg/kg per day) may depress bone marrow or cause severe tremor and cerebellar syndrome. Plasmapheresis is often helpful, but the effects are transient. Cytotoxic drugs should be used cautiously because a risk of malignancy is already present, even in patients who do not seem to have one already. IVIG therapy is another alternative.

SUGGESTED READINGS

Agius MA, Richman DP, Fairclough RH, et al, eds. Myasthenia gravis and related disorders: biochemical basis for disease of the neuromuscular junction. Conference proceedings, May 29-June 1, 2002. *Ann N Y Acad Sci* 2003;998:1–552.

Fetell MR, Shin HS, Penn AS, et al. Combined Eaton-Lambert syndrome and myasthenia gravis. *Neurology* 1978;28:398 (abstract).

Katz JS, Wolfe GI, Bryan WW, et al. Acetylcholine receptor antibodies in the Lambert-Eaton myasthenic syndrome. *Neurology* 1998;50:470–475.

Lambert EH, Rooke ED, Eaton LM, et al. Myasthenic syndrome occasionally associated with bronchial neoplasm: neurophysiologic studies. In: Viets HR, ed. *Myasthenia Gravis.* Springfield, IL: Charles C Thomas, 1961:362–410.

Lang B, Newsom-Davis J, Wray D, et al. Autoimmune etiology for myasthenic (Eaton-Lambert) syndrome. *Lancet* 1981;2:224–226.

Lennon VA, Kryzer TJ, Griesmann GE, et al. Calcium-channel antibodies in the Lambert-Eaton syndrome and other paraneoplastic syndromes. *N Engl J Med* 1995;332:1467–1474.

Leys K, Lang B, Johnston I, et al. Calcium channel autoantibodies in the Lambert-Eaton myasthenic syndrome. *Ann Neurol* 1991;29:307–314.

Lund H, Nilsson O, Rosen I. Treatment of Lambert-Eaton syndrome: 3,4-diaminopyridine and pyridostigmine. *Neurology* 1984;34:1324–1330.

Mareska M, Gutmann L. Lambert-Eaton myasthenic syndrome. *Semin Neurol* 2004 Jun;24(2):149–153.

Mason WP, Graus F, Lang B, et al. Small-cell lung cancer, paraneoplastic cerebellar degeneration, and the Lambert-Eaton myasthenic syndrome. *Brain* 1997;120:1279–1300.

Motomura M, Lang B, Johnston I, et al. Incidence of serum anti-P/Q-type and anti-N-type calcium channel autoantibodies in the Lambert-Eaton myasthenic syndrome. *J Neurol Sci* 1997;147:35–42.

Newsom-Davis J. Antibody-mediated channelopathies at the neuromuscular junction. *Neuroscientist* 1997;3:337–346.

Newsom-Davis J. Therapy in myasthenia gravis and Lambert-Eaton myasthenic syndrome. *Semin Neurol* 2003;23:191–198.

Newsom-Davis J, Leys K, Vincent A, et al. Immunological evidence for the co-existence of the Lambert-Eaton myasthenic syndrome and myasthenia gravis in two patients. *J Neurol Neurosurg Psychiatry* 1991;54:452–453.

Nudler S, Piriz J, Urbano FJ, et al. Ca²⁺ channels and synaptic transmission at the adult, neonatal, and P/Q-type deficient neuromuscular junction. *Ann N Y Acad Sci* 2002;998:11–17.

Raymond C, Walker D, Bichet D, et al. Antibodies against the beta subunit of voltage-dependent calcium channels in Lambert-Eaton myasthenic syndrome. *Neuroscience* 1999;90:269–277.

Roberts A, Perera S, Lang B, et al. Paraneoplastic myasthenic syndrome IgG inhibits ⁴⁵Ca²⁺ flux in a small cell carcinoma line. *Nature* 1985;2:737–739.

Sanders DB, Massey JM, Sanders LL, et al. A randomized trial of 3,4-diaminopyridine in Lambert-Eaton myasthenic syndrome. *Neurology* 2000;54:603–607.

Verschuuren JJ, Dalmau J, Tunkel R, et al. Antibodies against the calcium channel beta subunit in Lambert-Eaton myasthenic syndrome. *Neurology* 1998;50:475–479.

Vincent A. Antibodies to ion channels in paraneoplastic disorders. *Brain Pathol* 1999;9:285–291.

Waterman SA, Lang B, Newsom-Davis J. Effect of Lambert-Eaton myasthenic syndrome antibodies on autonomic neurons in the mouse. *Ann Neurol* 1997;42:147–156.

Wirtz PW, Bradshaw J, Wintzen AR, Verschuuren JJ. Associated autoimmune diseases in patients with the Lambert-Eaton myasthenic syndrome and their families. *J Neurol* 2004 Oct;251(10):1255–1259.

Chapter 123

Botulism and Antibiotic-induced Neuromuscular Disorders

Audrey S. Penn

BOTULISM

Botulism is a disease in which nearly total paralysis of nicotinic and muscarinic cholinergic transmission is caused by botulinum toxin, which acts on presynaptic mechanisms for release of acetylcholine (ACh) in response to nerve stimulation. The heavy chain of the toxin mediates binding of the toxin to surface receptors on motor nerve terminals. This allows the toxin molecule to be internalized via endocytosis, and the light chain is then translocated into the cytoplasm. The light chain functions as a zinc-dependent protease that cleaves different components of synaptic vesicles depending on the serotype of the toxin. Toxin types A and E cleave SNAP-25; type B, synaptotagmin and type B, synaptobrevin so that exocytosis of vesicles is blocked. The toxins are produced by spores of *Clostridium botulinum*, which may contaminate foods grown in soil (types A, B, F, and G) or by fish (type E). Intoxication results if contaminated food is inadequately cooked and the spores are not destroyed, or if fish are not eviscerated before drying or salt curing. Toxin can be produced in anaerobic wounds that have been contaminated by organisms and spores. Ingestion or inhalation of spores by infants may cause botulism when toxin type A is then produced in the gastrointestinal tract during periods of constipation. An analogous syndrome may occur in adults with persistent growth of *C. botulinum* in the intestine after surgery, from gastric achlorhydria, or from antibiotic therapy. The toxin does not cause cell death although it disrupts exocytosis. The effects slowly disappear over several months.

Electrophysiologic evidence of severely disturbed neuromuscular transmission includes an abnormally small single-muscle action potential evoked in response to a supramaximal nerve stimulus. When the synapse is driven by repetitive stimulation at high rates (20 to 50 Hz), the evoked response is potentiated up to 400%. In affected infants, muscle action potentials are unusually brief, of low amplitude, and overly abundant. This is presumably related to involvement of terminal nerve twigs in endings of many motor units. In patients who have been treated for blepharospasm or other movement disorders by intramuscular injections of botulinum toxin, single-fiber EMG shows increased jitter in muscles remote from those injected, and the jitter is maximally increased at low firing rates. These abnormalities are not symptomatic but imply an effect of circulating toxin.

C. botulinum toxin may be the "most poisonous poison" (the lethal dose for a mouse is 10^{-12} g/kg body weight). If the patient survives and reaches a hospital, symptoms include dry, sore mouth and throat, blurred vision, diplopia, nausea, and vomiting. Signs include hypohidrosis, total external ophthalmoplegia, and symmetric descending facial, oropharyngeal, limb, and respiratory paralysis. Pupillary paralysis, however, is not invariable. Not all patients are equally affected, suggesting variable toxin intake or variable individual responses. When cases occur in clusters, the diagnosis is usually suspected immediately.

Isolated cases in children and adolescents may be thought to be Guillain-Barré syndrome, myasthenia gravis, or even diphtheria. Ptosis has responded to intravenous edrophonium chloride in a few patients, but response to anticholinesterase drugs is neither sufficiently extensive nor sufficiently prolonged to be therapeutic. Infants with botulism are usually younger than 6 months. They show generalized weakness, which is manifest by reduced spontaneous movements, lethargy, poor sucking, and drooling. Sucking and gag reflexes are decreased or absent. There is facial diplegia, ptosis, and ophthalmoparesis. Diagnosis is made by the following characteristics: symmetry of signs, dry mouth or absence of saliva, pupillary paralysis, and the characteristic incremental response to repetitive nerve stimulation. The Centers for Disease Control and Prevention (CDC; with a dedicated emergency 24-hour telephone number) or appropriate state laboratories should be notified so that the toxin can be identified in refrigerated samples of serum, stool, or residual food samples. In suspected infantile botulism, feces should be evaluated for the presence of *C. botulinum*, as well as toxin.

Patients should be treated in intensive care facilities for respiratory care. Specific therapy includes antitoxin (a horse serum product that may cause serum sickness or anaphylaxis), available from the CDC, and guanidine hydrochloride, which promotes release of transmitter from residual spared nerve endings but may depress bone marrow.

ANTIBIOTIC-INDUCED NEUROMUSCULAR BLOCKADE

Aminoglycoside antibiotics (neomycin sulfate, streptomycin sulfate, kanamycin sulfate, gentimicin, and amikacin) and polypeptide antibiotics (colistin sulfate and polymyxin B sulfate) may cause symptomatic block in neuromuscular transmission in patients without any known neuromuscular disease. Antibiotics occasionally aggravate myasthenia gravis. The problem surfaces when blood levels are excessively high, which usually occurs in patients with renal insufficiency, but levels may be within the therapeutic range. Studies of bath-applied streptomycin in neuromuscular preparations disclosed inadequate release of ACh; the effect was antagonized by an excess of calcium ion. In addition, the sensitivity of the postjunctional membrane to ACh was reduced. Different compounds varied in relative effects on presynaptic and postsynaptic events. Neomycin and colistin produced the most severe derangements. The effects of kanamycin, gentamicin sulfate, streptomycin, tobramycin sulfate, and amikacin sulfate were moderate; tetracycline, erythromycin, vancomycin hydrochloride, penicillin G, and clindamycin had negligible effects. Patients who fail to regain normal ventilatory effort after anesthesia or who show delayed depression of respiration after extubation and are receiving one of the more potent agents should receive ventilatory support until the agent can be discontinued or another antibiotic substituted.

SUGGESTED READINGS

Cherington M. Botulism: update and review. *Semin Neurol* 2004 Jun;24(2):155–163.

Davis LE, Johnson JK, Bicknell JM, et al. Human type A botulism and treatment with 3,4-diaminopyridine. *Electromyogr Clin Neurophysiol* 1992;32:379–383.

DeJesus PV, Slater R, Spitz LK, et al. Neuromuscular physiology of wound botulism. *Arch Neurol* 1973;29:425–431.

Griffin PM, Hathaway CL, Rosenbaum RB, et al. Endogenous antibody production to botulinum toxin in an adult with intestinal colonization botulism and underlying Crohn's disease. *J Infect Dis* 1997;175:633–637.

Jankovic J. Botulinum toxin in clinical practice. *J Neurol Neurosurg Psychiatry* 2004:75:951–957.

MacDonald KL, Rutherford GW, Friedman SM, et al. Botulism and botulism-like illness in chronic drug abusers. *Ann Intern Med* 1985;102:616–618.

Maselli RA, Ellis W, Mandler RN, et al. Cluster of wound botulism in California: clinical, electrophysiological, and pathologic study. *Muscle Nerve* 1997;20:1284–1295.

Pichler M, Wang Z, Grabner-Weiss C, et al. Block of P/Q-type calcium channels by therapeutic concentrations of aminoglycoside antibiotics. *Biochemistry* 1996;35:14659–14664.

Pickett J, Berg B, Chaplin E, et al. Syndrome of botulism in infancy: clinical and electrophysiologic study. *N Engl J Med* 1976;295:770–772.

Rowland LP. Stroke, spasticity, and botulinum toxin. *N Engl J Med* 2002;347:382–383.

Sanders DB. Clinical neurophysiology of disorders of the neuromuscular junction. *J Clin Neurophysiol* 1993;10:167–180.

Schiavo G, Matteoli M, Montecucco C. Neurotoxins affecting neuroexocytosis. *Physiol Rev* 2000;80:717–766.

Simpson LL. Identification of the characteristics that underlie botulinum toxin potency: implications for designing novel drugs. *Biochemie* 2000;82:943–953.

Terranova W, Palumbo JN, Breman JG. Ocular findings in botulism type B. *JAMA* 1979;241:475–477.

Woodrull BA, Griffin PM, McCroskey LM, et al. Clinical and laboratory comparison of botulism from toxin types A, B, and E in the United States, 1975–1988. *J Infect Dis* 1992;166:1281–1286.

Chapter 124

Acute Quadriplegic Myopathy

Michio Hirano and Louis H. Weimer

In 1977, MacFarlane and Rosenthal described an acute myopathy after high-dose steroid therapy. Since then, hundreds of cases of acute quadriplegic myopathy (AQM) in critically ill patients have been reported and there is growing evidence that this phenomenon may affect a high percentage of critically ill patients to variable degrees (Table 124.1). Corticosteroids, nondepolarizing neuromuscular blocking agents, or both are considered the prime inciting factors; however, this entity, also called critical illness myopathy (CIM), develops in individuals who received neither agent. Patients undergoing treatment for status asthmaticus, organ transplantation, and severe trauma appear to be particularly vulnerable.

Severe quadriplegia and muscle atrophy commence 4 to 105 days after initiation of intensive care therapy. The weakness may be primarily distal or proximal but is usually diffuse; many patients lose tendon reflexes. Ophthalmoparesis and facial muscle weakness are occasionally present. Persistent respiratory muscle weakness complicates weaning patients from mechanical ventilation and frequently raises initial diagnostic suspicions of AQM/CIM. Improvement is generally evident in 1 to several months in most individuals who survive their critical illness, but protracted recovery or persistent deficits are common.

Laboratory studies have shown normal or elevated serum creatine kinase levels. Nerve conduction studies demonstrate absent or low amplitude compound motor action potentials. Sensory nerve action potentials are normal, reduced, or absent but frequently hampered by technical constraints in the ICU environment and local limb edema. EMG studies variably show signs of denervation from muscle necrosis and myogenic or normal motor unit action potentials; however, motor unit and recruitment analysis are frequently suboptimal owing to severe weakness, encephalopathy, sedation, or other confounding factors. Direct muscle stimulation has shown a loss of muscle fiber excitability, which has been attributed to voltage-gated sodium channel fast inactivation, based on animal models of steroid-treated denervated muscle. Serum from AQM/CIM patients also affects murine muscle fiber excitability and rest potential. Enhanced ex-

TABLE 124.1 Clinical and Laboratory Features of 213 Reported Cases of Acute Quadriplegic Myopathy

Features	Cases (No./Total)	%
Corticosteroids	178/213	84
Hydrocortisone (1–4 g/d)		
Prednisone (50–75 mg/d)		
Methylprednisolone (500–1,440 mg/d)		
Dexamethasone (40–80 mg/d)		
Nondepolarizing neuromuscular blocking agent	190/211	91
Presenting illness		
Asthma	87/213	41
Post-organ transplant	42/213	20
Sepsis	35/213	16
Trauma	23/213	11
COPD	23/213	11
Pneumonia	22/213	10
ARDS	16/213	8
Other	55/213	26
Weakness (onset, 4–105 days)	213/213	100
Diffuse	117/147	80
Proximal	27/117	23
Distal		2
Opthalmoparesis	11/147	7
Areflexia	64/120	53
Creatine kinase		
Normal	27/105	26
Elevated (from 4 to 410 × control)	78/105	74
EMG/NCS		
Myopathic	95/162	59
Neuropathic	39/162	24
Normal	5/162	3
Muscle biopsy		
Myopathy	133/159	84
Neuropathy	16/159	10
Normal	1/159	1
Outcome		
Died (10 of the primary illness, 57 unknown)	67/159	42
Improved	92/159	58
Normal	29/159	18

pression of ubiquitin, lysosomal enzymes, and calcium-activated proteases (calpains) have been observed and postulated to play a pathogenic role. These catabolic pathways appear to be activated in muscle by induction of transforming growth factor-β/mitogen activated protein kinase pathways. Immune activation by cytokines may also contribute to the myopathy. These changes possibly trigger apoptosis as a final mechanism.

Muscle biopsies demonstrate myopathic changes. Three distinct histologic features have been described in skeletal muscle biopsies; the abnormalities may be present in isolation or in variable combinations. Muscle fiber atrophy, often more prominent in type 2 fibers, is routinely seen. In patients with markedly elevated creatine kinase levels, necrosis of muscle fibers has been observed. The most striking feature revealed by electron microscopy is loss of thick (myosin) filaments, corroborated by antimyosin-antibody stains and reduced mRNA levels.

Thus, acute myopathy must be distinguished from the persistent weakness that may follow administration of nondepolarizing blocking agents to a person with impaired hepatic metabolism, reduced renal excretion, or both. *Critical-illness polyneuropathy,* an axonal neuropathy in the setting of gram-negative sepsis, multiorgan failure, or both, is an alternative cause of weakness in intensive care unit patients and may coexist with AQM/CIM, but appears in most recent series to be less common.

SUGGESTED READINGS

Bird SJ, Rich MM. Critical illness myopathy and polyneuropathy. *Curr Neurol Neurosci Rep* 2002;2:527–533.

De Letter MA, van Doorn PA, Savelkoul HF, et al. Critical illness polyneuropathy and myopathy (CIPNM): evidence for local immune activation by cytokine-expression in the muscle tissue. *J Neuroimmunol* 2000;106:206–213.

Di Giovanni S, Molon A, Broccolini A, et al. Constitutive activation of MAPK cascade in acute quadriplegic myopathy. *Ann Neurol* 2004;55:195–206.

Friedrich O, Hund E, Weber C, et al. Critical illness myopathy serum fractions affect membrane excitability and intracellular calcium release in mammalian skeletal muscle. *J Neurol* 2004;251:23–65.

Helliwell TR, Wilkinson A, Griffiths RD, et al. Muscle fibre atrophy in critically ill patients is associated with the loss of myosin filaments and the presence of lysosomal enzymes and ubiquitin. *Neuropathol Appl Neurobiol* 1998;24:507–517.

Hirano M, Ott BR, Raps EC, et al. Acute quadriplegic myopathy: a complication of treatment with steroids, nondepolarizing blocking agents, or both. *Neurology* 1992;42:2082–2087.

Hoke A, Rewcastle NB, Zochodne DW. Acute quadriplegic myopathy unrelated to steroids or paralyzing agents; quantitative EMG studies. *Can J Neurol Sci* 1999;28:325–329.

Lacomis D, Petrella JT, Giuliani MJ. Causes of neuromuscular weakness in the intensive care unit: a study of ninety-two patients. *Muscle Nerve* 1997;1998:610–617.

Lacomis D, Zochodne DW, Bird SJ. Critical illness myopathy. *Muscle Nerve* 2000;23:1785–1788.

MacFarlane IA, Rosenthal FD. Severe myopathy after status asthamaticus [Letter]. *Lancet* 1977;2:615.

Minetti C, Hirano M, Morreale G, et al. Ubiquitin expression in acute steroid myopathy with loss of myosin thick filaments. *Muscle Nerve* 1996;19:94–96.

Rich MM, Pinter MJ. Crucial role of sodium channel fast inactivation in muscle fibre inexcitability in a rat model of critical illness myopathy. *J Physiol* 2003;547:555–566.

Rich MM, Teener JW, Raps EC, et al. Muscle is electrically inexcitable in acute quadriplegic myopathy. *Neurology* 1996;46:731–736.

Segredo V, Caldwell JE, Matthay MA, et al. Persistent paralysis in critically ill patients after long-term administration of vecuronium. *N Engl J Med* 1992;327:524–527.

Showalter CJ, Engel AG. Acute quadriplegic myopathy: analysis of myosin isoforms and evidence for calpain-mediated proteolysis. *Muscle Nerve* 1997;20:316–322.

Trojaborg W, Weimer LH, Hays AP. Electrophysiologic studies in critical illness associated weakness: myopathy or neuropathy—a reappraisal. *Clin Neurophysiol* 2001;112:1586–1593.

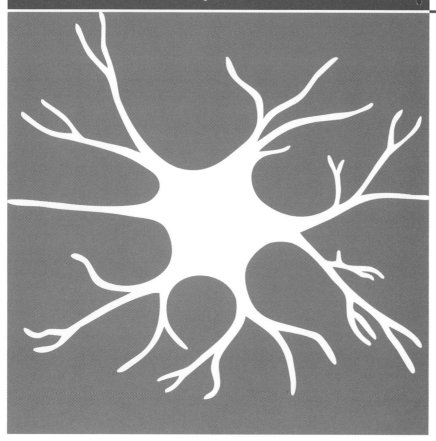

Myopathies

Chapter 125

Identifying Disorders of the Motor Unit

Lewis P. Rowland

Muscle weakness may result from lesions of the corticospinal tract or the motor unit. Central disorders are accompanied by the distinctive and recognizable signs of upper motor neuron dysfunction. However, lesions of the motor unit (which includes the anterior horn cell, peripheral motor nerve, and muscle) are all manifested by flaccid weakness, wasting, and depression of tendon reflexes. Because the abnormalities are so similar, there may be problems identifying disorders that affect one or another of the structures of the motor unit. As a result, there has been controversy about the classification of individual cases, as well as about some of the criteria used to distinguish the disorders.

Nevertheless, for many reasons, it is still convenient to separate diseases of the motor unit according to the signs, symptoms, and laboratory data, as indicated in Table 125.1. It is necessary to oversimplify to prepare such a table; there are probably exceptions to each of the statements made in the table, and individual cases may be impossible to define because of ambiguities or incongruities in clinical or laboratory data. However, there is usually a satisfactory consistency between the different sets of findings. Some syndromes can be recognized clinically without recourse to laboratory tests, including typical cases of Duchenne dystrophy, Werdnig-Hoffmann disease, peripheral neuropathies, myotonic dystrophy, myotonia congenita, periodic paralysis, dermatomyositis, myasthenia gravis, inclusion body myositis, and the myoglobinurias, to name a few. Controversies are mostly limited to syndromes of proximal limb weakness without clear signs of motor neuron disease (fasciculation) or peripheral neuropathy (sensory loss and high cerebrospinal fluid protein content).

LABORATORY DATA

The essential laboratory tests have been described in detail in other chapters: EMG and nerve conduction velocity in Chapter 15, and biopsy of muscle and nerve in Chapter 19. EMG is essential in identifying neurogenic or myopathic disorders. Measurement of nerve conduction velocities helps distinguish axonal and demyelinating sensorimotor peripheral neuropathy; slow conduction implies demyelination. In motor neuron diseases, conduction is typically normal or only slightly delayed. However, conduction velocity is also normal in axonal forms of peripheral neuropathy. Therefore, slow conduction indicates the presence of a peripheral neuropathy, but normal values can be seen in either an axonal peripheral neuropathy or a motor neuron disease (spinal muscular atrophy).

Muscle Biopsy

Muscle biopsy helps distinguish neurogenic and myopathic disorders. Evidence of degeneration and regeneration involves fibers in a random pattern in a myopathy. Some fibers are unusually large, and fiber splitting may be evident. In chronic diseases, there is usually little or no inflammatory cellular response; however, infiltration by white blood cells may be prominent in dermatomyositis and polymyositis. Some authorities use histologic patterns rather than clinical findings in identifying dermatomyositis and polymyositis (as discussed in chapters 132 and 133).

In the dystrophies, there may be infiltration by fat and connective tissue, especially as the disease advances. In denervated muscle, the major fiber change is simple atrophy, and groups of small fibers are typically seen adjacent to groups of fibers of normal size. In histochemical stains, fibers of different types are normally intermixed in a random checkerboard pattern, but in denervated muscle, fibers of the same staining type are grouped, presumably because of reinnervation of adjacent fibers by one motor neuron. In denervated muscle, angular fibers may be the earliest sign. In other conditions, histochemical stains may give evidence of storage products, such as glycogen or fat, or may indicate structurally specific abnormalities, such as nemaline rods, central cores, or other unusual structures.

▶ TABLE 125.1 Identification of Disorders of the Motor Unit

	Anterior Horn Cell	Peripheral Nerve	Neuromuscular Junction	Muscle
Clinical				
Symptoms				
Persistent weakness	Yes	Yes	Yes	Yes
Variable weakness	No	No	Yes	Yes
Painful cramps	Often	Rare	No	Rare
Myoglobinuria	No	No	No	No
Paresthesia	No	Yes	No	No
Bladder disorder	Rare	Occasional	No	No
Signs				
Weakness	Yes	Yes	Yes	Yes
Wasting	Yes	Yes	No	Yes
Reflexes lost	Yes	Yes	No (MG)	Yes
Reflexes increased	Yes (ALS)	No	No	No
Babinski	Yes (ALS)	No	No	No
Acral sensory loss	No	Yes	No	No
Fasciculation	Common	Rare	No	No
Laboratory				
Serum enzymes	No or mild	No	No	Yes
CSF protein	Yes or mild	Yes	No	No
Motor nerve conduction				
Velocity slow	No or mild	Often	No	No
or ↓amplitude (repetitive stimulation)	No	No	Yes	No
EMG				
Denervation	Yes	Yes	No	No
Myopathic	No	No	No	Yes
Biopsy				
Neurogenic features	Yes	Yes	No	No
Myopathic features	No	No	No	Yes

ALS, amyotrophic lateral sclerosis; MG, myasthenia gravis.

Serum Enzymes

Serum enzyme determination is another important diagnostic aid. Creatine kinase (CK) is the most commonly used enzyme for diagnostic purposes; it is present in high concentration in muscle and is not significantly present in liver, lung, or erythrocytes. To this extent, it is specific, and high serum content of CK usually indicates disease of the heart or skeletal muscle. The highest values are seen in Duchenne dystrophy, dermatomyositis, polymyositis, and attacks of myoglobinuria. In these conditions, other sarcoplasmic enzymes are also found in the serum, including aspartate transaminase (SGOT), alanine transaminase (SGPT), and lactate dehydrogenase. CK may also be increased in neurogenic diseases, especially Werdnig-Hoffmann disease, Kugelberg-Welander syndrome, and amyotrophic lateral sclerosis, although not to the same extent as in the myopathies named. For instance, with the normal maximum value for CK at 50 U/L, values of about 3,000 U/L are common in Duchenne dystrophy or dermatomyositis and may reach 50,000 U/FL in myoglobinuria. In the denervating diseases, CK values greater than 500 U/L are unusual but do occur. In some individuals, CK may be inexplicably increased with no other evidence of any muscle disease. Cardiologists have used isoenzyme analysis of CK to help differentiate between skeletal muscle and heart as the source of the increased serum activity. However, in the differential diagnosis of muscle disease, isoenzyme study has not been helpful, and the appearance of the "cardiac" isoenzyme of CK does not necessarily implicate the heart when there is limb weakness.

DEFINITIONS

It is useful to define some terms. *Atrophy* is used in three ways: to denote wasting of muscle in any condition, to denote small muscle fibers under the light microscope, and to name some diseases. By historical accident, all the diseases in which the word atrophy has been used in the name proved to be neurogenic (e.g., peroneal muscular atrophy or spinal muscular atrophy). Therefore, it seems prudent to use the word *wasting* in clinical description of limb muscles, unless it is known that the disorder is neurogenic. *Myopathies* are conditions in which the symptoms are owing to dysfunction of muscle and in which there is no evidence of causal emotional disorder or of denervation on clinical grounds or in laboratory tests. The symptoms of myopathies are almost always a result of weakness, but other symptoms include impaired relaxation (myotonia), cramps or contracture (McArdle disease), or myoglobinuria. *Dystrophies* are myopathies with five special characteristics: (1) They are inherited, (2) all symptoms are owing to weakness, (3) the weakness is progressive, (4) symptoms result from dysfunction in voluntary muscles, and (5) there are no histologic abnormalities in muscle other than degeneration and regeneration or the reaction to those changes in muscle fibers (infiltration by fat and connective tissue). There is no storage of abnormal metabolic products. Some heritable myopathies are not called dystrophies because weakness is not the dominant symptom (e.g., familial myoglobinurias) or the syndrome is not usually progressive (e.g., periodic paralysis or static, presumably congenital myopathies), and other names are assigned.

SUGGESTED READINGS

Engel AG, Franzini-Armstrong C, eds. *Myology.* 3rd Ed. New York: McGraw-Hill, 2004.

Karpati G, Hilton Jones D, Griggs RC, eds. *Disorders of Voluntary Muscle.* 7th Ed. Cambridge, UK: Cambridge University Press, 2001.

Mendell JR, Kissel JT, Cornblath DR, eds. *Diagnosis and Management of Peripheral Nerve Disorders* (Contemporary Neurology Series, 59) Oxford, UK: Oxford University Press, 2001.

Royden Jones H, De Vivo DC, Darras BT, eds. *Neuromuscular Disorders of Infancy and Childhood: A Clinician's Approach.* New York: Butterworth-Heinemann, 2002.

Chapter 126

Progressive Muscular Dystrophies

Petra Kaufmann, Louis H. Weimer, and Lewis P. Rowland

DEFINITION

A muscular dystrophy has five essential characteristics:

1. It is a myopathy, as defined by clinical, histologic, and EMG criteria. No signs of denervation or sensory loss are apparent unless there is a concomitant and separate disease.
2. All symptoms are effects of limb or cranial muscle weakness. (The heart and visceral muscles may also be involved.)
3. Symptoms become progressively worse.
4. Histologic changes imply degeneration and regeneration of muscle, but no abnormal storage of a metabolic product is evident.
5. The condition is recognized as heritable, even if there are no other cases in a particular family.

Although not part of the definition, there are two further characteristics, which we hope will be reversed in the future:

1. It is incompletely understood why muscles are weak in any of these conditions, even when the affected gene product is known.
2. As a result, there is no curative therapy for any of the dystrophies, and gene therapy has not yet been successful.

Therefore, prevention is often the best help that can be offered. The current acceleration of research progress may change this state of affairs.

The definition requires qualifications. For instance, some familial myopathies manifest by symptoms other than limb weakness, but those conditions are not called dystrophies. Familial recurrent myoglobinuria, for example, is considered a metabolic myopathy. The several forms of familial periodic paralysis do not qualify as dystrophies even if there is progressive limb weakness, because the attacks of weakness are the dominant manifestation in most patients. Syndromes that include

▶ **TABLE 126.1** Features of the Most Common Muscular Dystrophies

	Duchenne (DMD)	Facioscapulohumeral (FSHD)	Myotonic Dystrophy (DM 1) and Proximal Myotonic Myopathy (PROMM, DM 2)
MIM Number	310200	158900	DM1 16090; DM2 60268
Incidence estimates	1 in 3,500 live male births	1 in 20,000 births	1 in 8,000 births
Mode of Inheritance	X-linked recessive	Autosomal-dominant	Autosomal dominant
Gene Defect	Deletion or point mutation in gene for dystrophin	Reduced number of tandem repeats in D4Z4: 1–8 repeats (normal 10 to >100 repeats)	**DM 1:** CTG expansion in protein kinase gene; 50 to >2000 repeats (normal 5–37 repeats) **DM 2:** CCTG repeat expansion in zinc finger protein 9 gene
Gene Location	Xp21.2	4q35	**DM1** 19q13; **DM2:** 3q21
Expressivity	Complete	Variable	Variable
Age of Onset	Childhood	Adolescence, rarely childhood	**DM 1:** broad range (infancy to adult life) **DM 2:** adolescence to adult life
Site of Onset	Pelvic girdle	Shoulder girdle	**DM 1:** face and distal limbs; **congenital form:** hypotonia, club feet, dysphagia, dysmorphism, respiratory distress, mental retardation. **DM 2:** pelvic girdle, neck flexors **DM 1 compared to PROMM** patients usually have more: facial weakness, dysphagia, and distal weakness and wasting.
Calf Hypertrophy	Common	Never	**DM 1:** never **DM 2:** some
Rate of Progression	Relatively rapid	Slow	Variable
Facial Weakness	Rare and mild	Common	Common
Contractures	Common	Rare	Rare
Cardiac disease	Usually late (cardiomyopathy)	None	Common (conduction defect)
Other clinical features	Respiratory insufficiency; scoliosis; cognitive function variably impaired (sometimes high function)	High-frequency hearing loss and retinal vasculopathy (rare)	Cataracts, endocrine dysfunction.
Genetic heterogeneity	Duchenne and Becker allelic. Becker resembles Duchenne, but onset later and less severe	Not all FSH phenotypes linked to 4q35	Some PROMM patients not linked to 3q21

myotonia incorporate that word in the name of the disease, as in myotonia congenita, but are called muscular dystrophy only when there is progressive limb weakness, as in myotonic muscular dystrophy. In addition, static conditions, such as congenital myopathies, are not called dystrophies because the weakness does not become progressively more severe. This distinction allows some exceptions: A slowly progressive dystrophy may seem static, and some congenital myopathies slowly become more severe. Another exception is the term *congenital muscular dystrophy*, which may be severe and static from birth.

CLASSIFICATION

The classification of muscular dystrophies is based on both clinical and genetic characteristics, starting with three main types: Dudrenne Muscular Dystrophy (DMD), Facioscapulohumeral Muscular Dystrophy (FSHD), and Myotonic Muscular Dystrophy (MMD). Each type differs from the others in age at onset, distribution of weakness, rate of progression, presence or absence of calf hypertrophy or high serum levels of sarcoplasmic enzymes, such as CK, and pattern of inheritance (Table 126.1).

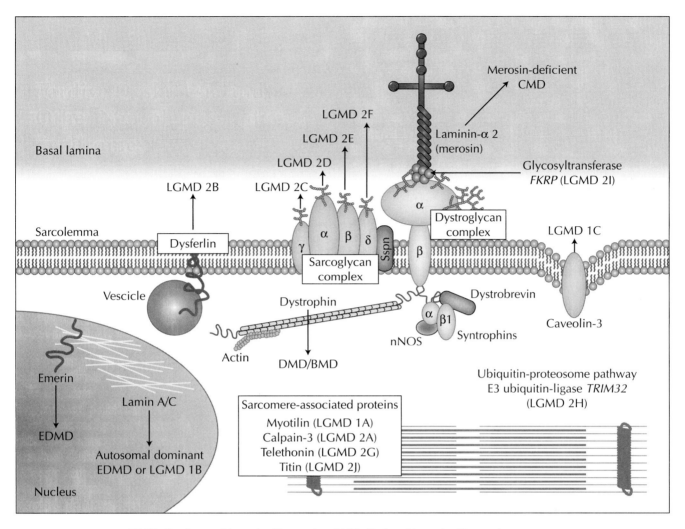

DMD: Duchenne Muscular Dystrophy; BMD: Bedeer Muscular Dystrophy;
CMD: Congenital Muscular Dystrophy; EDMD: Emery Dreifuss Muscular Dystrophy.

FIGURE 126.1. Skeletal muscle proteins and muscular dystrophies. The dystrophin-glycoprotein complex (DGC) comprises dystrophin, the dystroglycans (α, β), the sarcoglycans (α, β, γ, δ), sarcospan, the syntrophins (α, β_1), and dystrobrevin (α). The complex stabilizes the sarcolemma and protects surface membranes in muscle contraction. Nitric oxide synthetase (nNOS) interacts with the syntrophin complex and laminin2, one of many extracellular ligands of α-dystroglycan. Disease-causing mutations are cited in the text and Table 126.3. (Reproduced with permission from Mathews KD, Moore SA, Limb-girdle muscular dystrophy. *Curr Neurol Neurosci Rep* 2003;3:78–85. (See color insert).

Early investigators recognized that these three types did not include all muscular dystrophies, so they included a fourth type, limb-girdle muscular dystrophy (LGMD). That class has been depleted with the improved diagnosis of metabolic, congenital, and inflammatory myopathies and refined with the discovery of new mutations.

Progressive muscular dystrophies result from diverse defects in muscle proteins associated with the extracellular matrix (collagen VI, merosin), cell membrane and associated proteins (dystrophin, sarcoglycans, caveolin-3, dysferlin, integrins), cellular enzymes (calpain-3), organelle or sarcomere function (telethonin, myotilin, titin), and nuclear envelope (lamins, emerin; Fig. 126.1).

LABORATORY DIAGNOSIS

It had long been conventional practice to perform EMG and muscle biopsy for each new patient in a family. DNA analysis in white blood cells, however, now often obviates the need for biopsy. DNA studies are available for Duchenne, Becker, facioscapulohumeral, scapuloperoneal, and myotonic dystrophy, and about half of the LGMDs. Some DNA tests are commercially available whereas others are currently performed only in research laboratories. If no deletion is found in a patient with presumed Duchenne or Becker dystrophy, the diagnosis can be confirmed by immunohistochemistry or Western blotting of muscle tissue or sequencing white blood cell DNA. In addition, muscle biopsy can improve prognostic accuracy in some syndromes. If no defining mutation is found in a limb-girdle syndrome, muscle biopsy is needed for histochemical and electrophoretic studies of dystrophin, the associated glycoproteins, and other possibly abnormal proteins. If unique features are encountered in the biopsy, a regional research center can be consulted. Muscle biopsy is needed to characterize most congenital and metabolic myopathies. Serum CK determination and ECG are included for all patients with any kind of myopathy.

X-LINKED MUSCULAR DYSTROPHIES

Definitions

Duchenne and Becker dystrophies (MIM 310200) are defined by clinical features (see Table 126.1) and also by particular mutations. Both diseases are caused by mutations in the gene for dystrophin at Xp21. Neither disease can be diagnosed without an abnormality of the dystrophin gene or the gene product and they are therefore considered dystrophinopathies. Nondystrophin diseases that map to the same position are called Xp21 myopathies.

Prevalence and Incidence

The incidence of DMD is about 1 in 3,500 male births, with no geographic or ethnic variation. Approximately one-third of the cases are caused by new mutations; the others are more clearly familial. Because the life span of patients with DMD is shortened, the prevalence is less—about 1 in

18,000 males. Becker Muscular Dystrophy (BMD) is much less common, with a frequency of about 1 in 20,000.

Duchenne and Becker Muscular Dystrophies

Duchenne Muscular Dystrophy

The condition may become evident at birth if serum enzymes are coincidentally measured, for example, for an incidental respiratory infection. Authorities often state that symptoms do not begin until age 3 to 5 years, but that view may be a measure of the crudeness of muscle evaluation in infants. Walking may be delayed, and the boys probably never run normally; there is much commotion but little forward progression because they cannot raise their knees properly. Soon, toe walking and waddling gait are evident. Then, the condition progresses to overt difficulty in walking, climbing stairs, and rising from chairs. An exaggerated lordosis is assumed to maintain balance. The boys tend to fall easily if jostled, and then they have difficulty rising from the ground. In doing so, they use a characteristic maneuver called the *Gowers sign* (Fig. 126.2). They roll over to kneel, push down on the ground with extended forearms to raise the rump and straighten the legs, then move the hands to the knees and push up to a standing position. The process has been called "climbing up himself." It is also seen in other conditions that include proximal limb and trunk weakness, such as spinal muscular atrophy. At this stage, the knee jerks may be lost, whereas ankle jerks are still present; this discrepancy is a measure of the proximal accentuation of weakness.

As the disease progresses, the arms and hands are affected. Slight facial weakness may be seen, but speech, swallowing, and ocular movements are spared. Iliotibial contractures limit hip flexion; heel cord contractures are partly responsible for toe walking. At ages 9 to 12 years, the boys no longer walk and use a wheelchair. Scoliosis may then become serious and may compromise limb and respiratory function. Elbow and knee contractures contribute to disability. Respiratory muscle weakness causes

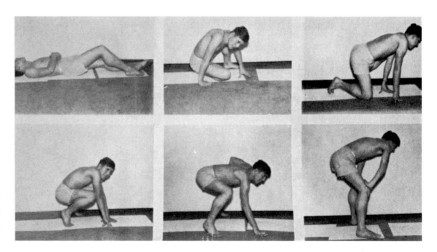

FIGURE 126.2. Gowers sign in a patient with Duchenne or Becker MD. Postures assumed in attempting to rise from the supine position.

progressive decline in lung capacity beginning at about age 8 years. Nocturnal hypoventilation may occur and cause morning headaches and daytime fatigue if untreated. By about age 20, respiration is so compromised that respiratory support is needed. Life expectancy in DMD has improved greatly in the last three decades, probably because of better coordinated medical care and home nocturnal ventilation. Some attribute the improvement to prednisone therapy.

The heart is usually spared clinically until late in the disease, when congestive heart failure (CHF) and arrhythmias may develop. The ECG is abnormal in most patients, with increased QRS amplitude in lead V_1 and deep, narrow Q waves in left precordial leads. Echocardiography shows progressively diminished contractility. Signs of cardiomyopathy may not be apparent because of the inability to exercise, but may supervene in a few cases. The gastrointestinal system is usually spared, but intestinal hypomotility and acute gastric dilatation are uncommon complications, probably related to dystrophin deficiency in smooth muscle. Osteoporosis begins in the ambulatory years, is more severe in the legs, and may contribute to fractures. Intellectual impairment is seen in one-third of boys with DMD, and the average intelligence quotient is shifted approximately one standard deviation below normal. Therefore, some boys with DMD have average or above average intelligence.

Anesthetic catastrophes may occur with hyperkalemia, extremely high CK levels (even more than 20 times the normal maximum), acidosis, cardiac failure, hyperthermia, and rigidity. The risk can be decreased by avoiding inhaled general anesthetics and depolarizing muscle relaxants, especially succinylcholine. This vulnerability can be considered a form of malignant hyperthermia, as discussed in Chapter 129.

Becker Muscular Dystrophy

This condition resembles DMD in essential characteristics. It is X-linked, calf hypertrophy is present, weakness is greatest proximally, and serum CK levels are high. EMG and muscle histology are the same. The two differences are age at onset (typically after age 10) and rate of progression (still walking after age 20, often later). Cognitive impairment is less common than in DMD. Cardiopathy usually develops later but may overshadow limb weakness. Cardiac complications contribute to 50% of BMD deaths compared to 20% with DMD. However, some patients have severe cardiomyopathy and mild muscle weakness. Another allelic disorder, X-linked dilated cardiomyopathy, demonstrates little to no skeletal muscle weakness.

Intermediate Phenotype

Some patients show an intermediate phenotype that can be considered either severe BMD or mild DMD. They remain ambulatory after age 12, but become wheelchair bound before age 16. They have preserved antigravity strength in the neck flexors longer than typical DMD patients.

Manifesting Carriers: DMD is an X-linked recessive trait. Female mutation carriers are usually asymptomatic but "manifesting carriers" can have limb weakness, calf hypertrophy, cardiomyopathy, or high serum CK levels.

Diagnosis

The diagnosis of Duchenne dystrophy is usually evident from clinical features. In sporadic and atypical cases, spinal muscular atrophy might be mistaken for DMD. Fasciculations and EMG evidence of denervation, however, identify the neurogenic disorder. High CK values are sometimes encountered in screening blood chemistry analysis done for some other purpose; regardless of the clinical findings, this may lead to the erroneous diagnosis of Duchenne dystrophy. However, typical DMD or BMD CK values are at least 20 times normal; few other conditions attain these values, not even interictal phosphorylase deficiency or acid maltase deficiency. Similarly, when a child with an incidental infection has routine blood tests, increased serum liver enzyme values may lead to a diagnosis of hepatitis; serum CK should then be assayed, and if it is elevated, a myopathy should be suspected, not a liver disease. In DMD, serum CK levels are highest in the presymptomatic years and then gradually decrease with age.

Increased CK levels are also seen in Xp21 gene carriers, in some patients with spinal muscular atrophy, and, for unknown reasons, in some otherwise asymptomatic people (idiopathic or asymptomatic hyperCKemia). Even before myopathic symptoms start, high CK values are seen in the dysferlinopathies (Miyoshi myopathy or LGMD), which are discussed later. Similarly, caveolin-3 mutations may cause hyperCKemia before symptoms of that limb-girdle dystrophy are evident.

Molecular Genetics

The dystrophin gene is involved in both Duchenne and Becker dystrophies, which are allelic diseases. Dystrophin is a cytoskeletal protein located at the plasma membrane. Brain and other organs contain slightly different isoforms. In muscle, dystrophin is associated with membrane glycoproteins that link the cytoskeleton with membrane proteins and then to laminin and the extracellular matrix (Fig. 126.1). The protein probably plays an essential role in maintaining muscle fiber integrity. If dystrophin is absent, as in Duchenne dystrophy, or abnormal, as in Becker dystrophy, the sarcolemma becomes unstable in contraction and relaxation, and the damage results in excessive calcium influx, thereby leading to muscle cell necrosis. If

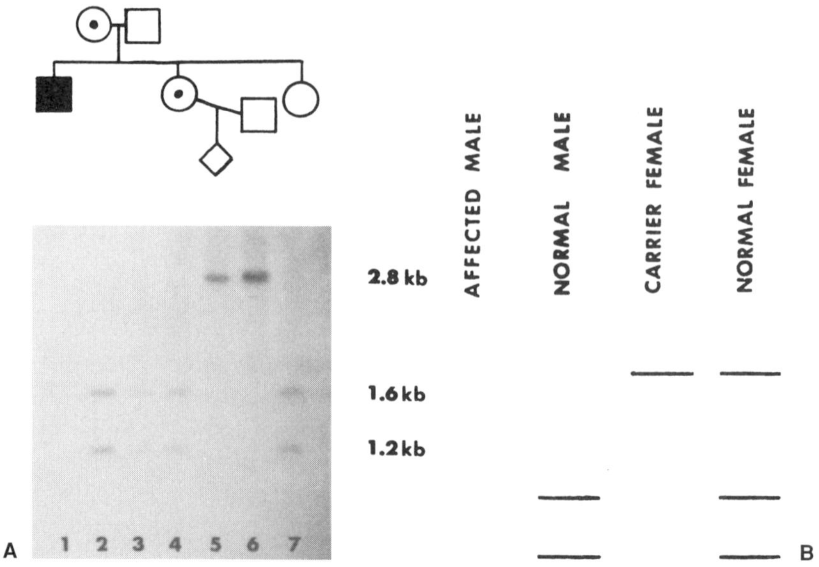

FIGURE 126.3. Prenatal diagnosis in DMD. **A.** Autoradiograph of Southern blot of 1% agarose gel with DNA samples from each individual digested with the restriction enzyme Xmnl and probed with pERT87-15. The affected male is deleted (no signal). His sister who was pregnant has a deleted X and an X chromosome with the 1.6/1.2 allele. Her husband's X chromosome contains the 2.8 allele. The fetus contains the husband's X and the deleted X. **B.** Diagram of the four possible outcomes of the prenatal diagnosis. The fetus is a carrier female. (Courtesy A. D. Roses.)

specific glycoproteins are abnormal or missing, the same problems arise, as in some LGMDs (described later).

These findings have been put to practical use in the diagnosis of Duchenne and Becker dystrophies and in genetic counseling. DNA analysis demonstrates a deletion or duplication at Xp21 in about 65% of DMD and 85% of BMD patients. Point mutations account for the remainder and can be detected by gene sequencing. The presence of a deletion or point mutation in a patient with compatible clinical findings is diagnostic. Carriers can be similarly identified, and the test can be used for prenatal diagnosis (Fig. 126.3).

If blood DNA testing and the clinical phenotype are diagnostic, muscle biopsy is not needed. In general, mutations that interfere with the expression of dystrophin cause DMD and those that lead to abnormal quality or quantity of dystrophic cause BMD. Muscle biopsy is sometimes performed in sporadic cases of unclear phenotype, even when a deletion has been identified, because immunocytochemistry for dystrophin and Western blot for quantitative dystrophin analysis can confirm and refine the diagnosis in these questionable cases. If no deletion is found and if dystrophin sequencing is not available, muscle biopsy is needed.

In Duchenne dystrophy, dystrophin staining is absent by both cytochemistry and Western blot. In Becker dystrophy, immunocytochemistry shows an interrupted pattern of staining on the surface membrane on and the Western blot shows decreased dystrophin levels or abnormal protein size. Carriers show a mosaic pattern; some fibers contain normal dystrophin staining and others show none at all. However, it is not known why the lack of dystrophin results in either the clinical syndrome or high serum CK values, or why decreased amount or abnormal structure of

dystrophin leads to the Becker type. In the X-linked mdx mouse model, dystrophin is also absent and serum CK levels are high, but weakness is not evident and histologic changes are meager.

Gene expression profiling has not yet indicated which genes, other than dystrophin, are important in degeneration or regeneration of muscle in patients or in the mdx mouse.

Treatment

Prednisone therapy improved function and strength in placebo-controlled trials, but the side effects of chronic administration—in particular, weight gain, growth retardation, and behavioral changes—often limit the practical use of steroids. If not prohibited by side effects, prednisone is usually offered to ambulatory patients over 5 years of age and may be continued until the patient becomes wheelchair bound. Data on the use of prednisone before age 5 years or during the wheelchair years are insufficient.

Experimental attempts at gene replacement through implanted myoblasts were unsuccessful. The experiments were limited by inefficiency of the process; too few transplanted myoblasts fused into the host myofibers, and only about half of those that did fuse produced normal dystrophin. In another approach, gentamicin is under investigation as possible treatment for the minority of DMD patients with a point mutation resulting in a premature stop codon, because aminoglycosides may aid "reading through" nonsense mutations.

Supportive management is aimed at maintaining function and independence, avoiding complications, and improving quality of life.

Orthopedic and rehabilitation measures include stretching exercises and ankle-foot orthoses during sleep to prevent contractures. Later, standing and walking can be maintained with ankle-foot orthoses or knee-ankle-foot orthoses combined with standing devices or walkers. Surgical release of contractures is occasionally used to maintain ambulation. During the wheelchair years, surgical scoliosis stabilization can help maintaining a comfortable sitting position and may reduce the risk of atelectasis and pneumonia.

Pulmonary function should be monitored regularly in patients with respiratory symptoms and in those who are nonambulatory to detect declines in respiratory muscle strength or ability to cough. Reduced cough strength increases the risk of atelectasis and respiratory infections. Patients may find mechanical exsufflators helpful. When symptoms of sleep-disordered breathing are suspected, overnight oximetry can confirm nocturnal hypoventilation. Noninvasive nighttime mechanical ventilation should then be considered. Later in the disease when respiratory muscle weakness progresses, a delicate decision must be confronted, whether to do a tracheostomy for chronic mechanical ventilation.

Cardiac function should be assessed prior to any major surgery, in those with respiratory insufficiency or cardiac symptoms, and in the late stages of the disease. Cardiac transplantation has been used for some BMD patients.

Other measures include precautions with general anesthesia, influenza and pneumococcal vaccinations, weight control, neuropsychologic evaluation to guide in educational issues, and social support to aid emotionally and financially. Genetic counseling for families is crucial.

Other Xp21 Myopathies
Dystrophinopathies

A deletion in a neighboring gene can extend into the dystrophin gene and produce myopathy. The resulting syndrome may be dominated by congenital adrenal insufficiency or glycerol kinase deficiency, but myopathy may range from mild to severe. These syndromes are customarily called "Becker variants" if appropriate dystrophin abnormalities are found. This nomenclature may be confusing, however, because the original definition of Becker dystrophy was based on clinical criteria and these syndromes are clinically different. Among them are myopathies that affect girls or women, not only manifesting carriers but also girls with Turner syndrome or balanced translocations that involve Xp21, as well as syndromes of atypical distributions of weakness, such as distal myopathy or quadriceps myopathy. Some syndromes lack limb weakness but are manifested by other symptoms, such as recurrent myoglobinuria or X-linked cramps without

weakness. The appearance of any of these atypical syndromes warrants studies of dystrophin.

Non-dystrophin-related Xp21 Myopathies

One of the mysteries of molecular genetics is the McLeod syndrome, a disorder first discovered in blood banks because the donors lacked a red cell antigen, the Kell antigen. These people were found to have abnormally shaped red blood cells (acanthocytes), and serum CK values were often 29 times normal or higher. In addition, some had myopathic limb weakness and the condition mapped to Xp21. Therefore, this condition, too, was expected to be a dystrophinopathy. In fact, however, dystrophin is normal. How the myopathy arises is unknown. It is also described in Chapter 93 (acanthocytes).

EMERY-DREIFUSS MUSCULAR DYSTROPHY

Emery-Dreifuss muscular dystrophy (EDMD) is a muscular dystrophy with several distinct manifestations:

1. The characteristic humeroperoneal distribution of weakness is unusual. That is, the biceps and triceps are affected rather than shoulder girdle muscles, and distal muscles are affected more than proximal muscles in the legs. The limb weakness may be mild or severe.
2. Contractures are disproportionately severe and are evident before much weakness is noted. The contractures affect the elbows, knees, ankles, fingers, and spine. A rigid spine develops, and neck flexion is limited.
3. Heart block, atrial paralysis, and atrial fibrillation are found in 95% of patients by age 30 years and lead to placement of a pacemaker. Dilated cardiomyopathy occurs in about 35% of all cases.

EDMD is characteristically an X-linked recessive disease (MIM 310300) and is linked to mutations in the EMD or *emerin* gene on Xq28. Emerin is localized to the nuclear membrane in muscle and other organs. Occasionally, the phenotype is inherited in an autosomal-dominant (MIM 181350) or recessive pattern (MIM 604929) linked to the LMNA gene on 1q21, encoding lamin A/C. Lamin A/C is located in the inner nuclear lamina and has also been linked to several allelic disorders, discussed later.

Symptoms of EDMD usually start before age 5 with difficulty walking. Examination typically shows symmetric contractures and weakness without pseudohypertrophy. Tendon reflexes are hypoactive or absent, and there may be mild facial weakness. Serum CK activity is often mildly elevated to levels less than 10 times normal. The diagnosis is usually confirmed by DNA testing. Absence of emerin can be demonstrated by immunocytochemical study of a muscle biopsy. Emerin staining is absent not only in muscle nuclei but also in circulating white blood cells and skin. As a result, skin biopsy, leukocytes, or inner cheek swabs for exfoliated mucosal cells can be examined diagnostically instead of muscle biopsy. However, DNA or gene product analysis is preferred for precise diagnosis. Cardiac surveillance (including 24-hour ECG and echocardiography) is crucial.

EDMD must be distinguished from other conditions. The rigid spine syndrome includes vertebral and limb contractures, but not cardiopathy or muscle wasting. Because the cardiac abnormality may not be evident in childhood, some patients with a rigid spine might be expected to have EDMD. Bethlem myopathy (MIM 158810) includes contractures and myopathy, but not cardiopathy, as discussed later.

Management is symptomatic and may include physical therapy and surgical tendon release for contractures. Pacemaker implantation and treatment of cardiomyopathy is often crucial. Female carriers are at risk of arrhythmias and should have regular cardiac evaluations.

FACIOSCAPULOHUMERAL MUSCULAR DYSTROPHY

Definition

Facioscapulohumeral muscular dystrophy (FSHD; MIM 158900) is defined by clinical and genetic features that differ from those of DMD in all particulars. Inheritance is autosomal dominant. The name designates the characteristic distribution of weakness, which causes symptoms that differ from those of DMD. The face is almost always affected. Severity varies, and some of those affected are asymptomatic but show diagnostic signs. Progression is slow. Symptoms usually begin in adolescence, but signs may be evident in children. Serum CK levels are normal or minimally elevated.

Molecular Genetics

The disease is autosomal dominant with nearly complete penetrance. Almost all FSHD patients have deletions of the subtelomeric repeat array, termed D4Z4, on chromosome 4q35. Normal individuals have 11 to 150 repeats; FSHD patients usually have fewer than 11. The deletions do not seem to interrupt any identifiable gene. Instead, they move the telomere closer to the centromere and seem to act indirectly, increasing the expression of neighboring genes. The pathogenesis of the disease is unknown but may result from inappropriate chromatin interactions at the nuclear envelope. Somatic mosaicism may be common in de novo cases.

Clinical Manifestations

The following features are characteristic of FSHD:

1. Facial weakness is evident not only by limitation of lip movements but also in the slightly everted lips and wide palpebral fissures. Patients may state that they have never been able to whistle or blow up a balloon. Some are said by relatives to sleep with eyes open.
2. Scapular winging is prominent. Protrusion of the scapulae is more evident when the patient tries to push against a wall with elbows extended and hands at shoulder level. The winging becomes more evident when the patient tries to raise the arms laterally. The patient cannot raise the arms to shoulder level even though there is no weakness of the deltoids on manual testing. This limitation is caused by inadequate fixation of the scapulae to the chest wall.
3. The shoulder girdle has a characteristic appearance. Viewed from the front, the clavicles seem to sag and the tips of the scapulae project above the supraclavicular fossa. This abnormality becomes more marked when the subject tries to raise the arms laterally to shoulder level. Smallness of the pectoral muscles affects the anterior axillary fold, which is ordinarily diagonal but assumes a vertical position. Abdominal muscle weakness may cause asymmetric abdominal protrusion. The limb muscle weakness is often asymmetric.
4. Leg weakness may affect proximal muscles or, more often, the anterior tibials and peroneals, resulting in footdrop.

In family studies, asymptomatic individuals can be identified by mild versions of these signs. Within a single family, the condition may vary markedly. Progression is slow, however, and the condition may not shorten longevity. About 20% of patients eventually use a wheelchair. Respiratory insufficiency is rare. Men may be more severely affected than women.

Associated Disorders

Mild sensorineural hearing loss and vascular retinopathy are occasionally seen in children with FSHD, as well as oropharyngeal symptoms, Coats disease (exudative telangiectasia of the retina), and, possibly, mental retardation. However, these findings are not consistent and it is not known how they relate to the genetic abnormality. Cardiac arrhythmias are rarely seen in FSHD.

Laboratory Studies

In most cases, the diagnosis can be confirmed by leukocyte DNA testing for a contraction of the subtelomeric repeat array on 4q35. Presymptomatic diagnosis is possible in families with more than one affected member, but testing should be done only with appropriate counseling. EMG and muscle biopsy, by definition, should show a myopathic pattern. The histologic changes are mild and nonspecific. Inflammatory cells are found in some patients, raising the question of polymyositis, but immunosuppressive therapy has always failed in these patients. DNA diagnosis resolves this possible confusion and may obviate muscle biopsy. Some patients with typical manifestations do not show the characteristic mutation, which may imply locus heterogeneity (mutation at some other locus) or could exceed the limits of sensitivity of current tests for the mutation.

Differential Diagnosis

The differential diagnosis includes uncommon myogenic and neurogenic scapuloperoneal syndromes, especially when facial weakness is lacking. Additionally, EDMD is sometimes confused with FSHD, but the essential clinical features are different. The increasing availability of genetic testing for FSHD, LGMD, and EDMD is likely to clarify these diagnostic problems. Infantile onset of FSHD is rare, but facial weakness may be severe enough to simulate the Möbius syndrome of congenital facial diplegia.

Management

Albuterol, a β2-agonist sympathomimetic drug, was evaluated in an open label pilot study followed by a randomized clinical trial of 90 FSHD patients for 12 months comparing two dose levels (8 mg and 16 mg of albuterol twice daily) to placebo. The primary end point, a difference in global strength, was not reached, but albuterol increased two of the secondary end points: grip strength and muscle mass.

Supportive treatment includes physical therapy, analgesics for joint pain, and ankle-foot orthoses for footdrop. Wiring the scapulae to the chest wall has been used to facilitate use of the arms, but the data seem insufficient to warrant widespread use.

MYOTONIC MUSCULAR DYSTROPHY (DM 1) AND PROXIMAL MYOTONIC MYOPATHY (PROMM, DM 2)

Definition

Myotonic dystrophy (MIM 160900, DM 1) is an autosomal dominant, multisystem disease of unique distribution that includes muscular dystrophy, myotonia, cardiomyopathy, cataracts, and endocrinopathy. Proximal myotonic myopathy (MIM 602668, DM 2) shares many characteristics with DM 1, but differs genetically.

Epidemiology

Myotonic dystrophy is compatible with long life, and gene penetrance is almost 100%. Because of these characteristics, myotonic dystrophy is a disease of high prevalence, about 5 per 100,000 throughout the world, with no specific geographic or ethnic variation. It is probably the most common form of muscular dystrophy. The incidence is about 13.5 per 100,000 live births.

Clinical Manifestations

In DM 1, as in many other autosomal-dominant diseases, variation in age at onset and severity are characteristic. Some affected people are asymptomatic but show signs of the disease on examination. The myopathy is distinctive in distribution (Fig. 126.4). Unlike any of the other major forms of muscular dystrophy, it affects several cranial muscles. Ptosis is common; eye movements may be impaired, and dysarthria and dysphagia may be problems. The temporal muscles are small and the resulting appearance is distinctive, with a long lean face and ptosis. In men, frontal baldness contributes to the impression. Insensitive clinicians perpetuate unkind words to describe this facial appearance. The sternomastoid muscles are characteristically small and weak. Limb weakness is most

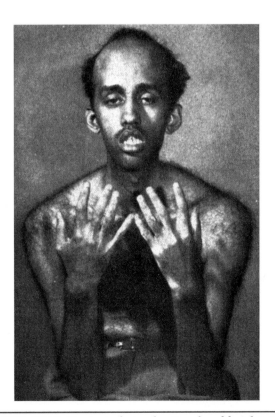

FIGURE 126.4. Myotonic dystrophy. Atrophy of facial, temporal, neck and hand muscles.

pronounced distally and affects the hands and feet equally. This dystrophy is one of the few neuromuscular disorders in which weakness of the finger flexors is prominent. Distal leg weakness may cause a footdrop or steppage gait. Most patients are generally thin, and focal wasting is not prominent. The tendon jerks are lost in proportion to the weakness.

Muscles of respiration may be affected even before there is much limb weakness; this symptom may contribute to the hypersomnia seen in MMD. Sensitivity to general anesthesia may be increased, with prolonged hypoventilation in the postoperative period. MMD, however, is not a muscle disease likely to cause alveolar hypoventilation. The rate of progression is slow and longevity may not be affected, but variation is evident; some people are almost asymptomatic, and some become disabled.

Myotonia has a dual definition. First, clinically, it is a phenomenon of impaired relaxation. Second, the EMG shows a distinctive pattern of waxing and waning high-frequency discharges that continue after relaxation begins, thus prolonging and impeding the effort. The EMG pattern is essential to the definition because there are other forms of impaired relaxation (see Chapter 130). Myotonia is most evident in the hands. Symptomatically, it may impair skilled movements or may embarrass the patient by complicating the attempt to shake hands or turn a doorknob because it is difficult to let go. As a sign on examination, the slow relaxation can be elicited by tapping the thenar eminence or, in the forearm, the bellies of the extensors of the fingers. Eliciting percussion myotonia in other limb muscles may be difficult for reasons unknown, but lingual myotonia may be present. Myotonia can also be evoked by asking the patient to grasp forcefully and then relax, which a normal person can do rapidly. In someone with myotonia, however, the grasp is followed by slow relaxation. The abnormal activity arises in the muscle because the response to percussion persists in curarized muscle of these patients; that is, the activity persists after neuromuscular transmission has been blocked.

Cataracts are almost universal but take years to appear. Early findings include characteristic iridescent opacities and posterior opacities.

Endocrinopathy is most readily seen in men. Frontal baldness is almost universal, and testicular atrophy is common; fertility is little diminished, however, so that the disease continues to be propagated in the family. Menstrual irregularities and ovarian failure are not nearly so frequent, and fertility is little decreased in women. Diabetes mellitus may be more common than in the general population, but otherwise no specific endocrine abnormalities are encountered.

The *cardiac disorder* is manifested by conduction disturbances, atrial fibrillation and flutter, and ventricular tachyarrhythmias. More than half of the adult patients have abnormalities in the ECG. However, these are often asymptomatic and pacemakers are needed in only about 5% of patients. CHF and syncope or sudden death may be more common in affected individuals.

Gastrointestinal disorders include impaired swallowing, pseudo-obstruction, or megacolon. *Cognitive impairment* is common in the congenital form of DM 1, but many patients with adult-onset DM 1 are socially well adjusted. However, mild cognitive and neuropsychiatric impairment with avoidant personality traits may be evident. *Excessive daytime somnolence* is attributed to nocturnal hypoventilation and may be helped by treatment with modafinil or methylphenidate. *Respiratory difficulties* may occur owing to diaphragmatic and intercostal muscle weakness as well as impaired respiratory drive.

Congenital Myotonic Dystrophy

About 5% of children born to a person with DM 1 have symptoms at birth, a condition termed *congenital myotonic dystrophy*. It affects children of either sex who are born to a woman with the usual adult form of the disease, which is often so mild that the woman may be asymptomatic but shows signs of the condition; the mother is the affected parent in almost all cases, but paternal transmission has been reported. The infants have difficulty feeding and breathing in the newborn period, develop slowly, are often mentally retarded, and show developmental anomalies of the face and jaws, as well as severe limb weakness and clubfeet. The genetic basis for the syndrome is discussed below. The clinical syndrome can be confused with other congenital anomalies, and identification of the disease in the mother is therefore essential; this may be difficult because the mother may be asymptomatic or mildly affected. The child may not show EMG evidence of myotonia, but the mother does.

Proximal Myotonic Myopathy (PROMM, DM2)

When the mutation causing DM1 was discovered in 1992, it became evident that some patients do not show the mutation. Their symptoms and signs are similar to those of DM1 in many respects, including autosomal-dominant myopathy, myotonia, cataracts, and weakness of the sternomastoids. It differs in the distribution of limb weakness, because DM1 is primarily a distal myopathy, and in DM2 weakness of pelvic girdle muscles is more pronounced than the distal leg weakness. Other differences are less conspicuous. For instance, myotonia is more difficult to elicit, symptoms are less severe, and there may be calf hypertrophy. Congenital myotonic dystrophy has not been reported in DM2 families. Most important, the syndrome does not map to chromosome 19, but maps to chromosome 3q.

Laboratory Studies

EMG shows evidence of myopathy and the characteristic myotonic discharges. Muscle biopsy shows mild and non-specific changes. Serum CK level may be normal or slightly increased. DNA analysis is now obligatory for precise diagnosis but may raise sensitive questions in a family, and individuals at risk may not wish to be tested. When tested, they should be offered adequate genetic counseling and psychosocial support.

Molecular Genetics and Pathophysiology

The gene for *DM 1* maps to 19q13.2. The mutation is an expansion of a CTG triplet repeat within the DMPK gene. Unaffected people have 5 to 30 CTG repeats; affected individuals have more than 50. Infants with congenital myotonic dystrophy have more than 800 repeats, but there is otherwise no strict relation between the number of repeats and clinical severity. Two patients with the same number of repeats may differ in severity. However, the larger the number of repeats, the younger the age at onset, a phenomenon referred to as anticipation, and the more severe the syndrome is likely to be (potentiation).

It is not known how the repeat expansion causes the disease. There is no deficiency of the DMPK gene but mutant mRNA, may be retained in the nucleus in structures called ribonuclear inclusions. This may reduce the expression of DMPK, but knockout mice do not show a myopathy or myotonia. It has therefore been suggested that the mutant mRNA itself may be toxic, a suspicion confirmed by transgenic mice that show expanded CUG repeats and show ribonuclear inclusions and myotonia. The mutant mRNA may bind essential proteins, such as "muscleblind," which is found in the inclusions of patient's cells. The knockout mouse lacking that gene shows muscle, eye, and RNA splicing abnormalities characteristic of DM.

Locus heterogeneity implies that a different gene must be involved in *DM2*, which maps to chromosome 3q21. An expanded CCTG repeat has been found in the gene for a zinc finger protein, ZNF9, which is an RNA-binding protein.

Whatever the fundamental fault in these diseases, it must explain how the mutation could cause such a *pleiotropic* disorder, with manifestations in so many different organs.

Diagnosis

The clinical features of DM 1 are so characteristic that the diagnosis is often evident at a glance by noting the long lean face, baldness in men, small sternomastoids, distal myopathy, and myotonia. Early footdrop may lead to con-fusion with Charcot-Marie-Tooth disease, but EMG patterns distinguish the two. Noting an autosomal-dominant familial pattern is helpful in general, and diagnosing the mother is especially important in congenital myotonic dystrophy, which can be mistaken for other causes of mental retardation or chromosome abnormalities. DNA analysis can confirm the diagnosis in most cases.

"Nondystrophic myotonias" are described in other chapters: hyperkalemic periodic paralysis and paramyotonia congenita in Chapter 127, and myotonia congenita and the Schwartz-Jampel syndrome in Chapter 130. "Pseudomyotonia," or impaired relaxation without true myotonic discharges, is seen in the Isaacs syndrome or neuromyotonia (see Chapter 130). Myotoniclike discharges but not clinical myotonia are seen in patients with acid maltase deficiency. However, none of these other myotonic syndromes have characteristic myopathy of myotonic dystrophy and rarely cause diagnostic confusion.

Management and Genetic Counseling

Myotonia can be ameliorated with mexiletine, phenytoin sodium (Dilantin), or other anticonvulsant drugs. However, myotonia is only rarely a bothersome symptom in contrast to other myotonic syndromes; it is the weakness that is disabling. Rehabilitation measures are helpful in keeping the muscles functioning as best they can and in assisting the patient in the activities of daily living. Orthoses help the footdrop. Ocular and cardiac symptoms are treated as they would be in any patient. An ECG should be recorded annually for adults, and slit lamp examination is also carried out periodically. General anesthesia should be avoided if possible because of increased postoperative pulmonary complications. In congenital DM 1, respiratory support and feeding tubes are often needed, and early intervention is indicated to address the problems associated with global developmental delay. The families are educated about the nature of the disease, inheritance, and the availability of DNA diagnosis for adults and for prenatal testing.

LIMB-GIRDLE MUSCULAR DYSTROPHY

History and Definition

Limb-girdle muscular dystrophy (LGMD) is a term originally conceived to separate progressive muscular dystrophies that were not X-linked (Duchenne/Becker) or otherwise clinically distinct, such as FSHD or myotonic dystrophy. The group comprises a heterogeneous collection of other progressive muscular dystrophies primarily involving shoulder and hip girdle muscles, autosomal-dominant or -recessive inheritance, and a normal dystrophin gene product. Metabolic myopathies have been

▶ **TABLE 126.2** **Conditions Simulating Limb-Girdle Muscular Dystrophy**

Acquired disease
Inflammatory
  Polymyositis, dermatomyositis, inclusion body myositis, sarcoidosis
Toxic myopathies
  Chloroquine, steroid myopathy, vincristine, lovastatin, ethanol abuse, phenytoin
Endocrinopathies
  Hyperthyroidism, hypothyroidism, hyperadrenocorticism (Cushing syndrome), hyperparathyroidism, hyperaldosteronism
Vitamin deficiency
  Vitamin D and vitamin E malabsorption
Paraneoplastic
  Lambert-Eaton syndrome, carcinomatous myopathy

Heritable diseases
Becker muscular dystrophy
Manifesting carrier of Duchenne or Becker gene
Emery-Dreifuss muscular dystrophy
Facioscapulohumeral or scapulohumeral dystrophy
Myotonic muscular dystrophy
Congenital myopathies (centronuclear, central core, emaline, tubular aggregates, cytoplasmic body)
Metabolic myopathies: glycogen storage diseases (phosphorylase deficiency, acid maltase deficiency, debrancher deficiency), lipid storage diseases (carnitine deficiences), mitochondrial myopathies
Myopathy of periodic paralysis

Modified from Jerusalem and Sieb, 1992.

separated, especially acid maltase and debrancher enzyme deficiencies; other limb-girdle syndromes proved to be Becker dystrophy, mitochondrial myopathies, polymyositis, inclusion body myositis, or other diseases (Table 126.2). The remaining group was expected to have diverse genetic causes, and in the last 10 years, specific gene defects or locations have been discovered for most of the remaining entities; the count currently stands at 17. The disorders are usually not clinically distinguishable, because of marked variability in severity and age onset, even in a single family. However, some characteristic features are seen with specific defects (Table 126.3). The identification of new gene defects has led not only to refinement of this category, but has also advanced the understanding of basic muscle cellular biology. The newly identified proteins include many not previously known to play a role in normal muscle function.

Clinical Manifestations

The diseases are separated into autosomal-dominant (type 1) and autosomal-recessive (type 2) groups. Individual protein defects are given an additional letter designation in order of discovery. In general, recessive forms are more common, more severe, and of earlier onset. Some have characteristic manifestations, but none can be conclusively diagnosed on clinical grounds alone. All of the disorders are characterized by proximal weakness of the pelvic or shoulder girdle muscles and dystrophic signs on muscle biopsy; some include cardiomyopathy. Disorders with primarily distal myopathic weakness are grouped separately as *distal myopathies*. Onset may occur in children, adolescents, or adults; infantile onset is considered congenital muscular dystrophy as described in chapter 128. Severity may vary between and within families. Difficulty with stair climbing and rising from a chair are common early symptoms. A waddling gait then develops. Difficulty raising the arms and scapular winging may be seen. Knee jerks tend to be lost before ankle jerks. Cranial muscles are usually spared. Serum CK levels are almost always high in recessive types and are often elevated in dominant forms. Progression is slow. EMG and muscle biopsy show nondiagnostic myopathic and dystrophic changes.

Molecular Genetics

Availability of specific protein antibody markers for muscle biopsy immunohistochemistry and molecular genetic analysis varies for each LGMD, but some are commercially available. A nonprofit federally supported database for both current commercial and research testing can be found at http://www.genetests.org. Many of the entities, especially dominant ones, have one or more allelic disorders, in some cases with identical gene defects with multiple manifestations (Table 126.3). Allelic disorders include several with isolated hyperCKemia without muscular weakness (CAV3, calpain3, dysferlin), some with neurogenic weakness (lamin A/C), and others with other muscle disorders such as rippling muscle disease (CAV3), autosomal dominant EDMD (lamin A/C), and distal myopathy (dysferlin). The functions of the altered proteins span far wider than maintenance of the sarcolemma as initially postulated. Correlation of genetic defects and clinical manifestations is still in progress.

Autosomal-Recessive LGMD

Now that specific proteins are recognized with varying manifestations, disorders based on the proteins rather than phenotype may emerge, as in the dystrophinopathies. Currently the following LGMD classification is still in use (Table 126.3).

LGMD2A

Mutations in the calpain-3 (CAPN3) gene are probably the most common cause of LGMD, and nearly 100 distinct mutations spanning numerous countries are known. In some populations, these mutations account for 28%

▶ **TABLE 126.3 Limb-Girdle Muscular Dystrophies**

MIM No.		Map Position	Gene Product	Features & Allelic Neurologic Disorders	Other Allelic Disorders	Comment/ Diagnosis Method
AUTOSOMAL DOMINANT						
159000	LGMD1A	5q31	Myofilin	Nasal speech	Myofibrillar myopathy	Rare
159001	LGMD1B	1q11–21	Lamin A/C	AD-EDMD; CMT2B	Familial liposdystrophy; cardiomyopathy; mandibuloacral dysplasia; Hutchinson Gilford progeria	Uncommon DNA
607801	LGMD1C	3p25	Caveolin-3	HyperCKemia; rippling muscle disease; distal myopathy		Muscle
602067	LGMD1D	6q23	Unknown	Familial dilated cardiomyopathy with conduction disease and myopathy		
603511	LGMD1E	7q	Unknown			
	Other		Unknown			
AUTOSOMAL RECESSIVE						
253600	LGMD2A	15q15	Calpain-3	HyperCKemia	—	Most common DNA*
253601	LGMD2B	2p13	Dysferlin	Miyoshi myopathy; distal myopathy; high CK		Blood*; muscle & DNA
253700	LGMD2C	13q12	γ-sarcoglycan	Early onset, severe		Muscle & DNA
608099	LGMD2D	17q12–21	α-sarcoglycan (adhalin)	[~10% of LGMD are Sarcoglycanopathies]		Muscle & DNA
604286	LGMD2E	4q12	β-sarcoglycan			Muscle & DNA
601287	LGMD2F	5q33–34	δ-sarcoglycan			Muscle & DNA
601954	LGMD2G	17q11–12	Telethonin	Rimmed vacuoles		Rare
254110	LGMD2H	9q31–34	TRIM32	Manitoba Hutterites	—	Rare
607155	LGMD2I	19q13.4	Fukutin-related protein	Congenital MD1C		Blood*
	LGMD2J	2q	Titin	Tibial muscular dystrophy		

LGMD, limb-girdle muscular dystrophy; hyperCKemia, asymptomatic increased creatine kinase; AD-EDMD, autosomal dominant Emery-Dreifuss muscular dystrophy; CMT2B, Charcot-Marie-Tooth type 2B; TRIM32, Tripartite motif protein 32 (E3-ubiquitin ligase); Muscle, diagnostic muscle biopsy immunostaining, DNA, genetic screening needed; blood, lymphocyte immunoblot analysis; *commercially available.

to 50% of LGMD cases, if sarcoglycanopathies and dystrophinopathies are excluded. The protein is a calcium-sensitive protease that is activated through autolysis. Calpain-3 is a muscle cytoskeletal regulator through cleavage of titin and filamin C. Disease severity varies from asymptomatic hyperCKemia to severe weakness. Onset ranges from 2 to 45 years; some have predominantly distal myopathy. Pelvic weakness sparing hip abductors, scapular winging, abdominal laxity, and frequent contractures are characteristic. CK is moderately elevated. At present, muscle biopsy immunostaining is not reliable, and Western blot screening, genetic testing, or both are needed for diagnosis.

LGMD2B

Dysferlin mutations are seen in LGMD but more commonly in distal Miyoshi myopathy with an identical gene defect. Both forms prominently affect the gastrocnemius muscles, but the LGMD form progresses proximally. Onset is later than most recessive LGMDs, usually after age 15. CK is elevated more than most LGMDs, likely because dysferlin appears to play an important role in muscle membrane repair. Muscle cell injury induces membrane patches enriched in dysferlin. Muscle immunostaining or blood immunoblot for dysferlin is commercially available; DNA confirmation is more accurate, but is not generally available.

LGMD2C Through LGMD2F

Sarcoglycans are dystrophin-associated glycoproteins (DAGs) integral to sarcolemmal stability. The four primary protein subunits ($\alpha,\beta,\gamma,\delta$) form a complex that provides support and signaling functions for the muscle membrane. These four DAGs have been implicated in specific forms of LGMD. A distinct epsilon subunit replaces α-sarcoglycan in smooth muscle and in some striated muscle cells; ε mutations lead to a myoclonus-dystonia syndrome, not LGMD. A mutation in any of the four main subunits typically disrupts the complex as a whole leading to decreased function and typically loss of muscle immunostaining. Alpha sarcoglycan (adhalin) is most commonly screened on muscle biopsy, but DNA analysis is needed to confirm the mutant subunit. Cases with complete complex loss manifest from 3 to 15 years of age and are typically wheelchair bound by age 15. Partial loss delays onset until the teens or early adulthood. Gamma subunit defects are more severe, often with congenital onset. Duchenne dystrophy can result in secondary DAG deficiency, and dystrophin must be proved normal before a sarcoglycanopathy can be diagnosed by muscle biopsy. Combined mutations in these four subunits represent roughly only 10% of teen- or adult-onset cases; LGMD2D (α-sarcoglycanopathy) is most common. Associated cardiomyopathy is seen, more in β and γ and less in α forms, likely due to vascular smooth muscle disease that causes vascular constrictions and ischemia. The LGMD, however, appears to be a primary myopathy and not a vasculopathy.

LGMDG-J

The remaining known recessive forms are considerably rarer. *LGMD2G* is a very rare disorder linked to defects in *telethonin*, which is a muscle-specific protein localized to the Z-disk, associated with *titin*, and likely affects sarcomere structure. *LGMD2H* is a relatively mild LGMD seen only in Canadian Hutterites owing to a defect in *TRIM32*, which is likely involved in targeting proteins for proteasome degradation. *LGMD2I* is one of a growing number of dystrophies caused by abnormal α-dystroglycan glycosylation and disruption of the link between dystroglycan and laminin. This form is a result of a defect in the fukutin-related protein (FKRP), which also causes congenital muscular dystrophy 2C, discussed later, but can cause LGMD of variable severity and age of onset. Accurate prevalence data are not yet known. Muscle hypertrophy and cardiomyopathy may be present. *LGMD2J* is a rare form of LGMD also known as *tibial muscular dystrophy*; it is caused by defects in the very large *titin* gene. This sarcomeric protein has multiple proposed roles and directly interacts with numerous other proteins discussed in this section. Distal myopathy and familial dilated cardiomyopathy are other titinopathies.

Autosomal-Dominant LGMD

Dominant forms are less common (<10% of LGMD), but are associated with greater clinical heterogeneity.

LGMD1A

LGMD1A is rare and linked to defects in *myotilin*, localized to the Z-disc near *telethonin*. Affected members are described as having a distinctive, dysarthric speech pattern.

LGMD1B

LGMD1B is a result of mutations in the LMNA gene that encodes both lamin A and lamin C, which are alternative splice forms. Mutations in this gene lead to multiple distinct phenotypes, including autosomal-dominant EDMD, hypertrophic cardiomyopathy, familial partial lipodystrophy, mandibuloacral dysplasia, Hutchinson Gilford progeria, as well as LGMD. Lamins A and C are found on the inner nuclear membrane and interact with integral nuclear membrane proteins including *emerin*, discussed earlier. The LGMD phenotype is relatively mild, but often has significant cardiomyopathy and cardiac conduction disease similar to X-linked EDMD; some also have contractures, but less severely than EDMD. To add to the heterogeneity and confusion, this gene is also mutated in a form of axonal Charcot-Marie-Tooth disease (2C).

LGMD1C

Caveolins are plasma membrane vesicular invaginations important in cellular trafficking and signaling. Caveolin-3 (CAV3) is a muscle-specific caveolin-related protein in skeletal, smooth, and cardiac muscle. In addition to LGMD, mutations of this gene can produce nondystrophic rippling muscle disease, idiopathic and familial asymptomatic hyperCKemia, and a form of distal myopathy. LGMD often begins around age 5 with cramping, mild weakness, and calf hypertrophy, but mild cases without clinical weakness are also seen. Caveolin-3 appears to interact with dysferlin, and in some patients with limb-girdle muscular dystrophy 2B (dysferlin) there is a secondary reduction in CAV3 levels.

LGMD1D Through LGMD1F

These disorders are chromosomally mapped forms awaiting gene identification. LGMD1D (6q) was previously named *familial dilated cardiomyopathy with conduction disease and myopathy*.

Oculopharyngeal muscular dystrophy (OPMD) is a late-onset autosomal-dominant disorder with progressive ptosis, dysphagia, and late-onset proximal limb weakness. Autosomal recessive forms are known. Although originally recognized in French Canadian families, cases have been recognized worldwide. The bulbar onset, however, is usually confused more often with myasthenia gravis than other myopathies. Muscle filamentous intranuclear inclusions are a pathologic hallmark, but rimmed vacuoles are also prominent. The CK is normal or mildly elevated. The disease maps to 14q11.2-q13 and is caused by an expanded GCG repeat in the polyadenylation binding protein 2 (PABP2). The disease-producing repeat number is unusually short. The normal repeat length is 6 and disease results from lengths of 7 to 13, with 9 and 10 repeats being most common. A more severe phenotype with earlier onset is described in homozygous patients. *Oculodistal muscular dystrophy* is even less common than OPMD and differs in the distribution of limb weakness but has not yet been mapped.

Bethlem myopathy (MIM 158810) is an autosomal dominant muscular dystrophy form inconsistently considered to be a LGMD or a discrete entity, but not given a letter designation. The disorder is progressive, with onset in infancy or childhood. Contractures are prominent, but CK is only mildly elevated and, in contrast to EDMD, cardiopathy is not seen. Defects have been found in three different α-subunits of the collagen VI gene and in a more severe congenital form—Ulrich disease (sclerotonic muscular dystrophy). Skin biopsy analysis for collagen VI may be diagnostic.

Other Rare Dystrophies

Several forms of scapuloperoneal weakness with dystrophic muscle pathology are not linked to the FSHD site, but await gene identification from identified loci. Some show hyaline bodies. Both dominant and recessive inheritance patterns are described. A similar phenotype is neurogenic (scapuloperoneal muscular atrophy). Other rare discrete entities include Epidermolysis bullosa simplex with late-onset muscular dystrophy linked to plectin gene mutations and desmin-related myopathy, one with a defect in the alpha-beta crystalline gene on 11q as well as dominant and recessive forms linked to the desmin gene

on 2q. Despite all of the identified genetic defects, additional forms of LGMD will be linked to yet unidentified chromosomal loci and novel pathogenic genes.

CONGENITAL MUSCULAR DYSTROPHIES

These conditions are discussed in Chapter 128.

DISTAL MYOPATHIES (DISTAL MUSCULAR DYSTROPHIES)

Distal myopathies (distal muscular dystrophies) are defined by clinical manifestations in the feet and hands before proximal limb muscles are affected. As heritable diseases with features of myopathy and slow progression, they are properly considered muscular dystrophies. The distinction from hereditary neuropathies is supported by spared sensation and histologic and electrodiagnostic features of myopathy. Most distal myopathies have been assigned to different map positions, confirming the clinical differences in patterns of inheritance, onset in leg or hands, predominant leg weakness in anterior or posterior compartments, presence or absence of vacuoles, and rise in serum CK (Table 126.4).

The most common form is *Welander distal myopathy* (MIM 604454), which was first described in Sweden; inheritance is autosomal dominant. Symptoms begin in adolescence or adult years and progress slowly. The legs are affected before the hands. Histologic changes are mild, but filamentous inclusions may resemble those seen in oculopharyngeal dystrophy or inclusion body myositis. Serum CK is only slightly elevated. The gene maps to chromosome 2p13, but may not be owing to the nearby dysferlin gene.

In the autosomal-recessive *Nonaka* variant (MIM 605820), a vacuolar myopathy is seen, the gastrocnemius

▶ **TABLE 126.4 Distal Myopathies**

Type	Heritance	Map/Gene Product	Site	CK	Vacuoles	MIM No.
Onset after age 40 yr						
Welander	AD	2p13	Hands	Normal	Sometimes	604454
Markesberry-Griggs-Udd	AD	2q31, Titin	AC	Normal	Yes	600334
Onset before age 40 yr						
Nonaka	AR	9p1–q1, GNE	AC	<5X	Yes	605820
Miyoshi	AR	2p13, dysferlin	PC	10–150X	No	254130
Laing	AD	14q	AC	<3X	No	160500

AC, anterior compartment of legs; AD, autosomal dominant; AR, autosomal recessive; CK, creatine kinase; MIM, Mendelian Inheritance in Man (McKusick); PC, posterior compartment, GNE, UDP-N-acetylglucosamine-2-epimerase/N-acetylmannosamine kinase muscles are spared, and serum enzyme values are only slightly increased. Nonaka distal myopathy and hereditary inclusion body myopathy share clinical and morphologic similarities; both conditions are a result of defects in the UDP-N-acetylglucosamine 2-epimerase/N-acetylmannosamine kinase (GNE) gene. *Miyoshi* (MIM 254130) distal myopathy is also autosomal recessive but differs from Nonaka in that the histologic changes are nonspecific (without vacuoles), the gastrocnemius muscles are affected first, and serum CK values are notably high; hyperCKemia may be noted before symptomatic weakness. The Miyoshi variety and LGMD type 2B (proximal limb weakness) are allelic, map to 2p17, and are associated with mutations in dysferlin (Fig. 126.1). Some Miyoshi families do not link to this position, which implies locus heterogeneity. Other variants of distal myopathies have been described and more are likely to be identified.

SUGGESTED READINGS

Ahlberg G, von Tell D, Borg K, et al. Genetic linkage of Welander distal myopathy to chromosome 2p13. *Ann Neurol* 1999;46:399–404.

Alias L, Gallanoi P, Moreno D, et al. A novel mutation in the caveolin-3 gene causing familial isolated hyperCKaemia. *Neuromuscul Disord* 2004;14:321–324.

Angelini C, Fanin M, Freda P, et al. The clinical spectrum of sarcoglycanopathies. *Neurology* 1999;52:176–179.

Bachinski LL, Udd B, Meola G et al. Confirmation of the type 2 myotonic dystrophy (CCTG)n expansion mutation in patients with proximal myotonic myopathy/proximal myotonic dystrophy of different European origins: a single shared haplotype indicates an ancestral founder effect. *Am J Hum Genet* 2003;73:835–848.

Bansal D, Miyake K, Vogel SS, et al. Defective membrane repair in dysferlin-deficient muscular dystrophy. *Nature* 2003;423:168–172.

Beltran-Valero de Bernabe D, Currier S, Steinbrecher A, et al. Mutations in the O-mannosyltransferase gene POMT1 give rise to the severe neuronal migration disorder Walker-Warburg syndrome. *Am J Hum Genet* 2002;71:1033–1043.

Betz RC, Schoser BGH, Kasper D, et al. Mutations in CAV3 cause mechanical hyperirritability of skeletal muscle in rippling muscle disease. *Nat Genet* 2001;28:218–219.

Bonne G, Di Barletta MR, Varnous S, et al. Mutations in the gene encoding lamin A/C cause autosomal dominant Emery-Dreifuss muscular dystrophy. *Nat Genet* 1999;21:285–288.

Brais B, Rouleau GA, Bouchard JP, et al. Oculopharyngeal muscular dystrophy. *Semin Neurol* 1999;19:59–66.

Brockington M, Yuva Y, Prandini P, et al. Mutations in fukutin-related protein gene (FKRP) identify limb-girdle muscular dystrophy 2I as a milder allelic variant of congenital muscular dystrophy MDC1C. *Hum Mol Genet* 2001;10:2851–2859.

Brown SC, Torelli S, Brockington M, et al. Abnormalities in alpha-dystroglycan expression in MDC1C and LGMD2I muscular dystrophies. *Am J Pathol* 2004;164:727–737.

Bushby K, Muntoni F, Bourke JP. 107th ENMC international workshop: the management of cardiac involvement in muscular dystrophy and myotonic dystrophy. 7th-9th June 2002, Naarden, the Netherlands. *Neuromuscul Disord* 2003;13:166–172.

Campbell C, Sherlock R, Jacob P, et al. Congenital myotonic dystrophy; assisted ventilation duration and outcome. *Pediatrics* 2004;113:811–816.

Campbell KP. Adhalin gene mutations and autosomal recessive limb-girdle muscular dystrophy. *Ann Neurol* 1995;38:353–354.

Carbone I, Bruno C, Sotgia F, et al. Mutation in the CAV3 gene causes partial caveolin-3 deficiency and hyperCKemia. *Neurology* 2000;54:1373–1376.

Chaouch M, Allal Y, De Sandre-Giovannoli A, et al. The phenotypic manifestations of autosomal recessive axonal Charcot-Marie-Tooth due to a mutation in Lamin A/C gene. *Neuromuscul Disord* 2003;13(Jan):60–67.

Chou FL, Angelini C, Daentl D, et al. Calpain III mutation analysis of a heterogeneous limb girdle muscular dystrophy population. *Neurology* 1999;52:1015–1020.

De Sandre-Giovannoli A, Chaouch M, Kozlov S, et al. Homozygous defects in LMNA, encoding lamin A/C nuclear-envelope proteins, cause autosomal recessive axonal neuropathy in human (Charcot-Marie-Tooth disorder type 2) and mouse. *Am J Hum Genet* 2002;70:726–736.

Eagle M, Baudouin SV, Chandler C, et al. Survival in Duchenne muscular dystrophy: improvements in life expectancy since 1967 and the impact of home nocturnal ventilation. *Neuromuscul Disord* 2002;12:926–929.

Fanin M, Pegoraro E, Matsuda-Asada C, et al. Calpain-3 and dysferlin protein screening in patients with limb-girdle dystrophy and myopathy. *Neurology* 2001;56:660–665.

Fatkin D, MacRae C, Sasaki T, et al. Missense mutations in the rod domain of the lamin A/C gene as causes of dilated cardiomyopathy and conduction-system disease. *N Engl J Med* 1999;341:1715–1724.

Fischer D, Aurino S, Nigro V, et al. On symptomatic heterozygous alpha-sarcoglycan gene mutation carriers. *Ann Neurol* 2003;54:674–678.

Flanigan KM, von Niederhausern A, Dunn DM, et al. Rapid direct sequence analysis of the dystrophin gene. *Am J Hum Genet* 2003;72:931–939.

Frosk P, Weiler T, Nylen E, et al. Limb-girdle muscular dystrophy type 2H associated with mutation in TRIM32, a putative E3-ubiquitin-ligase gene. *Am J Hum Genet* 2002;70:663–672.

Gamez J, Navarro C, Andreu AL, et al. Autosomal dominant limb-girdle muscular dystrophy. A large kindred with evidence for anticipation. *Neurology* 2001;56:450–454.

Gordon ES, Hoffman EP. The ABC's of limb-girdle muscular dystrophy: alpha-sarcoglycanopathy, Bethlem myopathy, calpainopathy and more. *Curr Opin Neurol* 2001;14:567–573.

Gussoni E, Blau HM, Kunkel LM. The fate of individual myoblasts after transplantation into muscles of DMD patients. *Nat Med* 1997;3:970–977.

Harper PS. *Myotonic Dystrophy.* 3rd Ed. London, UK: W.B. Saunders, 2001.

Hayashi YK. Membrane-repair machinery and muscular dystrophy. *Lancet* 2003;362:843–844.

Illarioshkin SN, Ivanova-Smolenskaya IA, Greenberg CR, et al. Identical dysferlin mutation in limb-girdle muscular dystrophy type 2B and distal myopathy. *Neurology* 2000:55:1931–1933.

Jobsis GJ, Boers JM, Barth PG, et al. Bethlem myopathy: a slowly progressive congenital muscular dystrophy with contractures. *Brain* 1999;122:649–655.

Kanadia RN. Johnstone KA. Mankodi A, et al. A muscleblind knockout model for myotonic dystrophy. *Science* 2003;302:1978–1980.

Katz JS, Rando TA, Barohn RJ, et al. Late-onset distal muscular dystrophy affecting the posterior calves. *Muscle Nerve* 2003;28:443–448.

Kissel JT, McDermott MP, Mendell JR, et al. FSH-DY Group. Randomized, double-blind, placebo-controlled trial of albuterol in facioscapulohumeral dystrophy. *Neurology* 2001;57:1434–1440.

Lemmers RJ, van der Wielen MJ, Bakker E, et al. Somatic mosaicism in FSHD often goes undetected. *Ann Neurol* 2004;55:845–850.

Logigian EL, Moxley RT 4th, Blood CL, et al. Leukocyte CTG repeat length correlates with severity of myotonia in myotonic dystrophy type 1. *Neurology* 2004;62:1081–1089.

Mankodi A, Teng-Umnuay P, Krym M, et al. Ribonuclear inclusions in skeletal muscle in myotonic dystrophy types 1 and 2. *Ann Neurol* 2003;54:760–768.

Mankodi A, Thornton CA. Myotonic syndromes. *Curr Op Neurol* 2002;15:545–552.

Masny PS, Bengtsson U, Chung SA, et al. Localization of 4q35.2 to the nuclear periphery: Is FSHD a nuclear envelope disease? *Hum Mol Genet* In press 2004.

Mathews KD, Moore SA. Limb-girdle muscular dystrophy. *Curr Neurol Neurosci Rep* 2003;3:78–85.

Meola G, Sansone V, Marinou K, et al. Proximal myotonic myopathy: a syndrome with a favourable prognosis? *J Neurol Sci* 2002;193: 89–96.

Meola G, Sansone V, Perani D, et al. Executive dysfunction and avoidant personality trait in myotonic dystrophy type 1 (DM-1) and in proximal myotonic myopathy (PROMM/DM-2). *Neuromuscul Disord* 2003;13:813–821.

Mercuri E, Poppe M, Quinlivan R, et al. Extreme variability of phenotype in patients with an identical missense mutation in the lamin A/C gene: from congenital onset with severe phenotype to milder classic Emery-Dreifuss variant. *Arch Neurol* 2004;61:690–694.

Minetti C, Sotgia F, Bruno C, et al. Mutations in the caveolin-3 gene cause autosomal dominant limb-girdle muscular dystrophy. *Nat Genet* 1998;18:365–368.

Miske LJ, Hickey EM, Kolb SM, et al. Use of the mechanical in-exsufflator in pediatric patients with neuromuscular disease and impaired cough. *Chest* 2004;125:1406–1412.

Moreira ES, Wiltshire TJ, Faulkner G, et al. Limb-girdle muscular dystrophy type 2G is caused by mutations in the gene encoding the sarcomeric protein telethonin. *Nat Genet* 2000;24:163–166.

Muchir A, Bonne G, van der Kooi AJ, et al. Identification of mutations in the gene encoding lamins A/C in autosomal dominant limb girdle muscular dystrophy with atrioventricular conduction disturbances (LGMD1B). *Hum Mol Genet* 2000;9:1453–1459.

Muntoni F, Fisher I, Morgan JE, et al. Steroids in Duchenne muscular dystrophy: from clinical trials to genomic research. *Neuromuscul Disord* 2002;12(Suppl 1):S162–165.

Muntoni F, Valero de Bernabe B, Bittner R, et al. 114th ENMC International Workshop on Congenital Muscular Dystrophy (CMD) 17-19 January 2003, Naarden, The Netherlands: (8th Workshop of the International Consortium on CMD; 3rd Workshop of the MYO-CLUSTER project GENRE). *Neuromuscul Disord* 2003;13:579–588.

Nishino I, Noguchi S, Murayama K, et al. Distal myopathy with rimmed vacuoles is allelic to hereditary inclusion body myopathy. *Neurology* 2002;59:1689–1693.

Rando TA. The dystrophin-glycoprotein complex, cellular signaling, and the regulation of cell survival in the muscular dystrophies. *Muscle Nerve* 2001;24:1575–1594.

Takahashi T, Aoki M, Tateyama M, et al. Dysferlin mutations in Japanese Miyoshi myopathy: relationship to phenotype. *Neurology* 2003;60:1799–1804.

Takeda S, Kondo M, Sasaki J, et al. Fukutin is required for maintenance of muscle integrity, cortical histiogenesis and normal eye development. *Hum Mol Genet* 2003;12:1449–1459.

Talbot K, Stradling J, Crosby J, et al. Reduction in excess daytime sleepiness by modafinil in patients with myotonic dystrophy. *Neuromuscul Disord* 2003;13:357–364.

Tawil R. Facioscapulohumeral muscular dystrophy. *Curr Neurol Neurosci Rep* 2004;4:51–54.

Tonini MM, Passos-Bueno MR, Cerqueira A, et al. Asymptomatic carriers and gender differences in facioscapulohumeral muscular dystrophy (FSHD). *Neuromuscul Disord* 2004;14:33–38.

Tupler R, Gabellini D. Molecular basis of facioscapulohumeral muscular dystrophy. *Cell Mol Life Sci* 2004;61:557–566.

von Tell D, Bruder CE, Anderson LV, et al. Refined mapping of the Welander distal myopathy region on chromosome 2p13 positions the new candidate region telomeric of the DYSF locus. *Neurogenetics* 2003;4:173–177.

Wallgren-Pettersson C, Bushby K, Mellies U, et al.; ENMC. 117th ENMC workshop: ventilatory support in congenital neuromuscular disorders—congenital myopathies, congenital muscular dystrophies, congenital myotonic dystrophy and SMA (II) 4–6 April 2003, Naarden, The Netherlands. *Neuromuscul Disord* 2004;14:56–69.

Wohlgemuth M, van der Kooi EL, van Kesteren RG, et al. Ventilatory support in facioscapulohumeral muscular dystrophy. *Neurology* 2004;63:176–178.

Woodman SE, Sotgia F, Galbiati F, et al. Caveolinopathies: mutations in caveolin-3 cause four distinct autosomal dominant muscular diseases. *Neurology* 2004;62:538–543.

Yan J, Feng J, Buzin CH, et al. Three-tiered noninvasive diagnosis in 96% of patients with Duchenne muscular dystrophy (DMD). *Hum Mutat* 2004;23:203–204.

Zatz M, de Paula F, Starling A, et al. The 10 autosomal recessive limb-girdle muscular dystrophies. *Neuromuscul Disord* 2003;13(Sep):532–544.

Chapter 127

Familial Periodic Paralysis

Lewis P. Rowland and Paul H. Gordon

Familial periodic paralysis comprises diseases characterized by episodic bouts of limb weakness. On clinical grounds, there are three main types: hypokalemic periodic paralysis (HoPP; MIM 170400), hyperkalemic (HyPP; MIM 170500), and Andersen syndrome, or periodic paralysis with cardiac arrhythmia (MIM 170390). HyPP maps to the gene for the alpha subunit of the sodium channel, SCN4A, on chromosome 17q13. HoPP most often maps to the gene for the dihydropyridine-sensitive L-type calcium channel of muscle, CACNL1A3, at 1q32, but may also map to the SCN4A gene. Andersen syndrome maps to the gene for the inwardly rectifying potassium channel, KCNJ2, on chromosome 17q23. Locus heterogeneity validates the clinical classification, although many investigators now lump the conditions as channelopathies, including paramyotonia congenita and other nondystrophic myotonias.

Attacks are similar in all three conditions but differ somewhat in severity and duration (Table 127.1). The two main types were first separated by the level of serum potassium during a spontaneous or induced attack. Provocative tests can be performed by intravenous administration of glucose and insulin to drive the potassium level down or by administration of potassium salts to increase the serum level, although these tests are used much less frequently due to the rare induction of cardiac arrhythmia and because of the increasing availability of DNA testing.

The greatest uncertainty concerns paramyotonia congenita, which, like HyPP, maps to the SCN4A gene. Most investigators consider this a separate syndrome that is

▶ **TABLE 127.1**   Clinical Features of Low- and High-Serum Potassium Periodic Paralysis and Paramyotonia

	Low-serum Potassium Periodic Paralysis	*High-serum Potassium Periodic Paralysis*	*Paramyotonia Congenita*
Age of onset	Usually second or latter part of first decade	First decade	First decade
Sex	Male preponderance	Equal	Equal
Incidence of paralysis	Interval of weeks or months	Interval of hours or days	May not be present; otherwise, interval of weeks or months
Degrees of paralysis	Tends to be severe	Tends to be mild but can be severe	Tends to be mild but can be severe
Effect of cold	May induce an attack	May induce an attack	Tends to induce an attack
Effect of food (especially glucose)	May induce an attack	Relieves an attack	Relieves an attack
Serum potassium	Low	High	Tends to be high
Oral potassium	Prevents an attack	Precipitates an attack	Precipitates an attack
Onset	During sleep	After precipitants	After precipitants
Precipitants	Food, cold	Fasting, stress, rest after exercise, K rich foods	Fasting, stress, rest after exercise
Myotonia	Absent	Present	Present

Modified from Hudson AJ. *Brain* 1963;86:811.

manifest by only myotonia, with no attacks of paralysis. Some authorities believe that there are disease-specific mutations within the sodium channel gene. The word *paramyotonia* is used because the condition is thought to differ from ordinary myotonia in two ways: Paramyotonia is brought on by cold (but so are other forms of myotonia), and it is paradoxic in that it becomes more severe with exercise, whereas the myotonia of other diseases is ameliorated by exercise. In families with HyPP, many individuals have myotonia, and in presumed families with paramyotonia congenita, some individuals have attacks of paralysis (including the original families described by Eulenberg in Germany and Rich in the United States). Some people with paramyotonia congenita are susceptible to attacks induced by administration of potassium. The diseases are allelic, mapping to the same gene. Similarly, the same SCN4A gene accounts for paramyotonic variants, such as myotonia fluctuans, acetazolamide-responsive myotonia, and painful myotonia.

The third type of familial periodic paralysis, *Andersen syndrome*, was first thought to be normokalemic, then hyperkalemic. In fact, spontaneous attacks have been associated with high, low, or normal potassium levels. Nevertheless, patients are sensitive to administered potassium, which always induced an attack before the provocative test was deemed dangerous. The hazard is feared because affected children are likely to have cardiac arrhythmias that lead to the need for a pacemaker. The syndrome was named after Andersen because she described a dysmorphic boy; since then dysmorphism has become one of five criteria for diagnosis; the others are periodic paralysis, potassium sensitivity, myotonia (usually mild), and cardiac arrhythmia.

The dysrhythmia may be preceded by an asymptomatic prolonged QT interval on the ECG.

Vacuoles are found in the muscles in the early stages of both HoPP and HyPP. These vacuoles seem to arise both from the terminal cisterns of the sarcoplasmic reticulum and from proliferation of the T tubules. In the later stage, there may be degeneration of the muscle fibers, possibly related to persistent weakness in the intervals between attacks.

HYPOKALEMIC PERIODIC PARALYSIS

In HoPP, the potassium content decreases in a spontaneous attack to values of 3.0 mEq/L or lower. Attacks may be induced by the injection of insulin, epinephrine, fluorohydrocortisone, or glucose, or they may follow ingestion of a meal high in carbohydrates. The potassium content of the urine is also decreased in an attack. It is not clear why potassium shifts into muscle to cause the attack.

Incidence

The disease is rare. There are no large series reported in the literature, and only one or two new patients are seen each year in any of the large neurologic centers in the United States. Penetrance is complete in males but reduced in females; as a result, men are affected more often in a ratio of 2:1. The first attack usually occurs at about the time of puberty, but it may occur as early as age 4 years or be delayed until the sixth decade.

Symptoms and Signs

An attack usually begins after a period of rest. It commonly develops during the night or is present on waking in the morning, especially after ingestion of a high-carbohydrate meal before retiring on the previous night. The extent of the paralysis varies from slight weakness of the legs to complete paralysis of all the muscles of the trunk and limbs. The oropharyngeal and respiratory muscles are usually spared, even in severe attacks. There may be retention of urine and feces during a severe attack. The duration of an individual attack varies from a few hours to 24 or 48 hours. According to some patients, strength improves if they keep active or "walk it off." The interval between attacks may be as long as 1 year, or one or more attacks of weakness may occur daily.

In the interval between attacks, patients are usually strong and the potassium content of the serum is normal. In some patients, mild proximal limb weakness persists. In a mild attack, tendon reflexes and electrical reactions of the muscles are diminished in proportion to the degree of weakness. In severe attacks, tendon and cutaneous reflexes are absent and the muscles do not respond to electrical stimulation. Cutaneous sensation is not disturbed.

Course

Familial HoPP is not accompanied by any impairment of general health. As a rule, the frequency of the paralytic attacks decreases with the passage of years, and they may cease altogether after age 40 or 50. Fatalities are rare, but death may occur from respiratory paralysis. The fixed myopathy, usually mild, may be severe and disabling.

Diagnosis

The diagnosis can usually be made without difficulty on the basis of the familial occurrence of transient attacks of weakness. The diagnosis is usually confirmed by finding low potassium and high sodium content in the serum during an attack or by inducing an attack with an intravenous infusion of glucose (100 g) and regular insulin (20 U). Now, the provocative test can be avoided by DNA testing. However, if a patient is in the hospital during a spontaneous attack, it is important to determine which type of periodic paralysis is to be treated.

In sporadic cases, the first attack must be differentiated from other causes of hypokalemia (Table 127.2). Persistent hypokalemia from any cause may manifest as an acute attack of paralysis or persistent limb weakness with high levels of serum creatine kinase. Sometimes, there are attacks of myoglobinuria.

Repeated attacks of HoPP, identical clinically to the familial form, occur in patients with hyperthyroidism, particularly those of Japanese and Chinese ancestry, and have

▶ TABLE 127.2 **Potassium and Paralysis: Noninherited Forms**

Hypokalemic
  Excessive urinary loss
    Hyperaldosteronism
    Drugs: glycyrrhizate (licorice), thiazides, furosemide, chlorthalidone, ethacrynic acid, amphotericin, duogastrone
    Pyelonephritis, renal tubular acidosis
    Recovery from diabetic acidosis
    Ureterocolostomy
  Excessive gastrointestinal loss
    Melabsorption syndrome
    Laxative abuse
    Diarrhea
    Fiseulas, vomiting, villous adenoma
    Pancreatic tumor, diarrhea
  Thyrotoxicosis
Hyperkalemia
  Uremia
  Addison disease
  Spironolactone excess
  Excessive intake
    Iatrogenic
    Geophagia

been linked to the potassium channel beta subunit gene, KCNE3. The paralytic attacks cease when the thyroid disorder has been successfully treated.

Treatment

Acute attacks, spontaneous or induced, may be safely and rapidly terminated by ingestion of 20 to 100 mEq of potassium salts. Intravenous administration of potassium is usually avoided because of the hazard of inducing hyperkalemia.

The basis of prophylactic therapy is oral administration of the carbonic anhydrase inhibitor acetazolamide (Diamox), 250 to 1,000 mg daily. This regimen prevents attacks in about 90% of patients with HoPP and also improves the interictal weakness attributed to the vacuolar myopathy. The mechanism of action of acetazolamide is uncertain; the beneficial effect may be related to the mild metabolic acidosis it induces. For those not helped by acetazolamide, other effective agents include triamterene (Dyrenium) or spironolactone (Aldactone), which promote retention of potassium. Another carbonic anhydrase inhibitor of value is dichlorphenamide (Daranide). Dietary controls are usually not accepted by patients and are not effective.

Treatment of other forms of HoPP depends on the nature of the underlying renal disease, diarrhea, drug ingestion, or thyrotoxicosis. Patients with thyrotoxic periodic paralysis are susceptible to spontaneous or induced attacks during the period of hyperthyroidism. When the patients become euthyroid, spontaneous attacks cease and they are no longer sensitive to infusion of glucose and insulin. Glucose and insulin are useful in the interim between treatment of hyperthyroidism by drugs or radioiodine, before the euthyroid state returns. Repeated attacks can be prevented by either acetazolamide or propranolol.

HYPERKALEMIC PERIODIC PARALYSIS

In 1951, Frank Tyler recognized a form of familial periodic paralysis in which attacks were not accompanied by a decrease in the serum potassium content. In 1957, Gamstorp and colleagues drew attention to several other features of these cases that separated them from the usual cases of periodic paralysis. The disease is transmitted by an autosomal-dominant gene with almost complete penetrance. In addition to the absence of hypokalemia in the attacks, the syndrome is characterized by an early age of onset (usually before age 10). The attacks tend to occur in the daytime and are likely to be shorter and less severe than those in HoPP. Myotonia is usually demonstrable by EMG, but abnormalities of muscular relaxation are rarely symptomatic. Myotonic lid lag (Fig. 127.1) and lingual myotonia may be the sole clinical evidence of the trait. Serum potassium content and urinary excretion of potassium may be increased during an attack, possibly the result of leakage of potassium from muscle. The attacks tend to be precipitated by hunger, rest after exercise, or cold, or by administration of potassium chloride.

Attacks may be terminated by administration of calcium gluconate, glucose, and insulin. Acetazolamide, 250 mg to 1 g orally daily, has been effective in reducing the number of attacks or in abolishing them altogether. Other diuretics that promote urinary excretion of potassium are also effective. If acetazolamide therapy fails, thiazides or fludrocortisone acetate (Florinef) may be beneficial. In addition, beta-adrenergic drugs may be effective prophylactic agents. Epinephrine, salbutamol, and metaproterenol have been used. They presumably act by increasing the activity of Na+, K+ -ATPase.

Pathophysiology

The pathophysiology of the HyPP has been analyzed by the team of Rudel, Ricker, and Lehmann-Horn (1993); their findings led to the suspicion that a sodium channel protein would be a good candidate gene. First, using microelectrode studies of intercostal muscle, they confirmed that muscle isolated from patients with HyPP is partially depolarized at rest. The abnormal depolarization was blocked by tetrodotoxin, which specifically affects the alpha subunit of the sodium channel. Patch clamp experiments showed faulty inactivation, leading to the conclusion that excessive sodium influx causes repetitive firing of action potentials (myotonia) and eventual inactivation of the membrane (weakness). Cloning and analysis of the gene encoding the voltage-gated Na+ channel have identified more than 20 missense mutations in the SCN4A gene. Some mutations exhibit both interfamilial and intrafamilial phenotypic variability.

In contrast, the calcium channel gene for HoPP was found not by physiology but by a genome-wide search. The pathophysiology of HoPP is not clear, but may include an indirect effect on a sarcolemmal ATP-sensitive potassium channel.

The challenge now is to determine just how the single amino acid substitutions result in the altered function. Alternatively, as in myotonic muscular dystrophy and other autosomal-dominant diseases, there could be pleiotropic expression of the mutation, which is expressed by four abnormalities: paralytic attacks, myotonia, potassium sensitivity, and cold sensitivity. In a family, one or more of these manifestations may be dominant in different individuals.

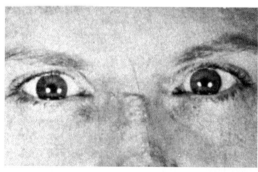
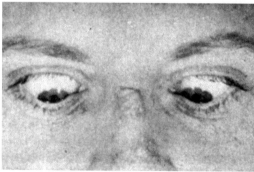

FIGURE 127.1. Paramyotonia congenita. Myotonia of muscles of the upper eyelids on looking downward. (Courtesy of Dr. Robert Layzer.)

SUGGESTED READINGS

Hypokalemic Periodic Paralysis

Cannon SC. An expanding view for the molecular basis of familial periodic paralysis. *Neuromuscul Disord* 2002;12:533–543.

Comi G, Testa D, Cornelio F, et al. Potassium depletion myopathy: a clinical and morphological study of six cases. *Muscle Nerve* 1985;8:17–21.

Dias Da Silva MR, Cerutti JM, Arnaldi LA, et al. A mutation in the KCNE3 potassium channel gene is associated with susceptibility to thyrotoxic hypokalemic periodic paralysis. *J Clin Endocrinol Metab* 2002;87:4881–4884.

Engel AG, Lambert EH, Rosevear JW, et al. Clinical and electromyographic studies in a patient with primary hypokalemic periodic paralysis. *Am J Med* 1965;38:626–640.

Griggs RC, Engel WK, Resnik JS. Acetazolamide treatment of hypokalemic periodic paralysis: prevention of attacks and improvement of persistent weakness. *Ann Intern Med* 1970;73:39–48.

Holtzapple GE. Periodic paralysis. *JAMA* 1905;45:1224–1231.

Jurkat-Rott K, Lehmann-Horn F. Periodic paralysis mutation MiRP2-R83H in controls: Interpretations and general recommendation. *Neurology* 2004 Mar 23;62(6):1012–1015.

Layzer RB, Goldfield E. Periodic paralysis caused by abuse of thyroid hormone. *Neurology* 1974;24:949–952.

Lehmann-Horn F, Jurkat-Rott K, Rudel R. Periodic paralysis: understanding channelopathies. *Curr Neurol Neurosci Rep* 2002;2:61–69.

Minaker KL, Menelly GS, Flier JS, et al. Insulin-mediated hypokalemia and paralysis in familial hypokalemic periodic paralysis. *Am J Med* 1988;84:1001–1006.

Roadma JS, Reidenberg MM. Symptomatic hypokalemia resulting from surreptitious diuretic ingestion. *JAMA* 1981;246:1687–1689.

Striessnig J, Hoda JC, Koschak A, et al. L-type Ca^{2+} channels in Ca^{2+} channelopathies *Biochem Biophys Res Commun* 2004 Oct 1; 322(4):1341–1346.

Venance SL, Jurkat-Rott K, Lehmann-Horn F, Tawil R. SCN4A-associated hypokalemic periodic paralysis merits a trial of acetazolamide. *Neurology* 2004 Nov 23;63(10):1977.

Vicart S, Sternberg D, Fournier E, Ochsner F, Laforet P, Kuntzer T, Eymard B, Hainque B, Fontaine B. New mutations of SCN4A couse a potassium-sensitive normokalemic periodic paralysis. *Neurology* 2004 Dec 14;63(11):2120–2127.

Vroom FQ, Jarrell MA, Maren TH. Acetazolamide treatment of hypokalemic periodic paralysis: probable mechanisms of action. *Arch Neurol* 1975;32:385–392.

Yazaki K, Kuribayashi T, Yamamura Y, et al. Hypokalemic myopathy associated with 17 α-hydroxylase deficiency: a case report. *Neurology* 1982;32:94–97.

Lisak RP, Lebeau J, Tucker SH, et al. Hyperkalemic periodic paralysis and cardiac arrhythmia. *Neurology* 1972;22:810–815.

McArdle B. Adynamia episodica hereditaria and its treatment. *Brain* 1962;85:121–148.

Miller TM, Dias da Silva MR, Miller HA, et al. Correlating phenotype and genotype in the periodic paralyses. *Neurology* 2004 Nov 9;63(9):1647–1655.

Moxley RT, Ricker KM, Kingston WJ, et al. Potassium uptake in muscle during paramyotonic weakness. *Neurology* 1989;39:952–955.

Ponce SP, Jennings AE, Madias NE, et al. Drug-induced hyperkalemia. *Medicine* 1985;64:357–370.

Ptacek LJ, Fu YH. Channels and disease: past, present, and future. *Arch Neurol* 2004;61(11):1665–1668.

Ptacek LJ, Timmer JS, Agnew WS, et al. Paramyotonia congenita and hyperkalemic periodic paralysis map to the same sodium channel locus. *Am J Hum Genet* 1991;49:851–854.

Rich EC. A unique form of motor paralysis due to cold. *Med News* 1894;65:210–213.

Ricker K, Bohlen R, Rohkamm R. Different effectiveness of tocainide and hydrochlorothiazide in paramyotonia congenita with hyperkalemic episodic paralysis. *Neurology* 1983;33:1615–1618.

Riggs JE, Griggs RC, Moxley RT. Acetazolamide-induced weakness in paramyotonia congenita. *Ann Intern Med* 1977;86:169–173.

Rudel R, Ricker K, Lehmann-Horn F. Genotype-phenotype correlations in human skeletal muscle sodium channel diseases. *Arch Neurol* 1993;50:1241–1248.

Sansone V, Griggs RC, Meola G, et al. Andersen's syndrome: a distinct periodic paralysis. *Ann Neurol* 1997;42:305–312.

Streib EW. Hypokalemic paralysis in two patients with paramyotonia congenita and known hyperkalemic/exercise-induced weakness. *Muscle Nerve* 1989;12:936–937.

Tricarico D, Servidei S, Tonali P, et al. Impairment of skeletal muscle adenosine triphosphate-sensitive K+ channels in patients with hypokalemic periodic paralysis. *J Clin Invest* 1999;103:675–682.

Tristani-Firouzi M, Jensen JL, Donaldson MR, et al. Functional and clinical characterization of KCNJ2 mutations associated with LQT7 (Andersen syndrome). *J Clin Invest* 2002;110:381–388.

Hyperkalemic Periodic Paralysis

Bendahhou S, Donaldson MR, Plaster NM, Tristani-Firouzi M, Fu YH, Ptacek LJ. Defective potassium channel Kir2.1 trafficking underlies Andersen-Tawil syndrome. *J Biol Chem* 2003 Dec 19;278(51):51779–51785.

Bendheim PE, Reale EO, Berg BO. Beta-adrenergic treatment of hyperkalemic periodic paralysis. *Neurology* 1985;35:746–749.

Benstead TJ, Camfield PR, Ding DB. Treatment of paramyotonia congenita with acetazolamide. *Can J Neurol Sci* 1987;14:156–158.

Borg K, Hovmoller M, Larsson L, et al. Paramyotonia congenita (Eulenberg): clinical, neurophysiological and muscle biopsy observations in a Swedish family. *Acta Neurol Scand* 1993;87:37–42.

Christopher GA, Johnson JP, Palevsky PM, et al. Hyperkalemia in hospitalized patients. *Arch Intern Med* 1998;158:917–924.

Donaldson MR, Yoon G, Fu YH, Ptacek LJ. Andersen-Tawil syndrome: a model of clinical variability, pleiotropy, and genetic heterogeneity. *Ann Med* 2004;36 (Suppl 1):92–97.

Eulenberg A. Über einer familiäre, durch 6 Generationen verfolgbare Form congenitaler Paramyotonie. *Neurol Centralbl* 1886;5:265–272.

Evers S, Engelien A, Karsch V, et al. Secondary hyperkalemic paralysis. *J Neurol Neurosurg Psychiatry* 1998;64:249–252.

Gamstorp I. Adynamia episodica hereditaria. *Acta Pediatr (Uppsala)* 1956;45(Suppl 108):1–126.

Hanna MF, Stewart J, Schapira AH, et al. Salbutamol treatment in a patient with hyperkalaemic periodic paralysis due to a mutation in the skeletal muscle sodium channel gene (SCN4A). *J Neurol Neurosurg Psychiatry* 1998;65:248–250.

Hoffman EH, Wang J. Duchenne-Becker muscular dystrophy and the nondystrophic myotonias. *Arch Neurol* 1993;50:1227–1237.

Jurkat-Rott K, Lerche H, Lehmann-Horn F. Skeletal muscle channelopathies. *J Neurol* 2002;249:1493–1502.

Layzer RB, Lovelace RE, Rowland LP. Hyperkalemic periodic paralysis. *Arch Neurol* 1967;16:455–472.

Congenital Disorders of Muscle

Olajide Williams

Primary muscle diseases are evident at birth or are thought to begin soon after birth because motor milestones are delayed. The conditions are grouped into several categories: congenital myotonic dystrophy and congenital muscular dystrophies, which share muscle biopsy features characterized by muscle destruction and replacement by fat and connective tissue; congenital myopathies, defined by disease-specific structural abnormalities in muscle fibers; myotonia congenita, a disorder of muscle contractility

▶ **TABLE 128.1** **Morphological Classification of Congenital Myopathies**

Chief Structure Involved	Myopathy
Sarcomere	Central core, multicore, trilaminar, hyaline body (lysis of myofibrils)
Z Disc	Nemaline rod, desmin related
Nuclear abnormalities, inclusions	Myotubular, centronuclear, fingerprint, reducing body
Organelle	Tubular aggregate myopathy
Abnormality of fiber size/number	Congenital fiber type disproportion; uniform type 1 fiber myopathy

Adapted from Bodensteiner J B. *Muscle Nerve* 1994;17:133.

characterized by myotonia with little or no weakness; and chondrodystrophic myotonia (Schwartz-Jampel syndrome), which combines myotonia and severe dysmorphic features.

The distinction between congenital muscular dystrophies and congenital myopathies is artificial, because the term *muscular dystrophy* was once ascribed to progressively more severe weakness, whereas *myopathy* was reserved for a static, not progressive, condition. In fact, both conditions may be static or slowly progressive. Advances in genetic and histochemical features reveal overlap of congenital muscular dystrophies and congenital myopathies. Congenital muscular dystrophy is discussed in Chapter 126.

CONGENITAL MYOPATHIES

Congenital myopathies have been historically defined by distinctive structural and histochemical features on muscle biopsy (Tables 128.1 and 128.2). Some muscular dystrophies are the result of protein deficiencies ("protein-minus myopathies") whereas congenital myopathies are often marked by aggregation of defective, mutant proteins. This observation has led to a gene- and protein-oriented nosology of these disorders (Table 128.3). As the name implies, congenital myopathies are evident in infancy

▶ **TABLE 128.2** **Congenital Myopathies Awaiting Confirmation by More Investigators**

Congenital Myopathy With	Number of Patients
Broad A-bands	2
Hexagonal tubular arrays	2
Apoptotic changes	1
Muscle spindle excess	3
Tubulin-reactive crystalline inclusions	1
Tubofilamentous tubular aggregates	3

Adapted from Goebel HH. Congenital myopathies at their molecular dawning. *Muscle Nerve* 2003;27:542.

because milestones are delayed or because the child moves less than expected in the neonatal period ("floppy baby syndrome"); the onset of symptoms is sometimes delayed until adult years when muscle biopsy shows structures usually found in children. Most are familial but sporadic cases are seen. Clinical features are not restricted to skeletal muscle, and the heart may be affected occasionally, as in nemaline or desmin-related myopathies. Weakness may progress slowly or not at all. Serum creatine kinase (CK) is normal or mildly elevated, and EMG usually reveals mild myopathic features but may also be normal. Treatment of congenital myopathies is symptomatic.

Central Core Disease

Central core myopathy (CCM) was the congenital myopathy to be described, as reported by Shy and Magee in 1956. It is typically autosomal dominant with variable penetrance, although an autosomal-recessive form is suggested by sporadic cases. Clinical features include proximal limb weakness, hypotonia, absent tendon reflexes, and delayed motor milestones, but up to one-third of individuals with central cores have no abnormalities on clinical examination. Less commonly, dysmorphic features include club feet, scoliosis, hip dislocation, or contractures of the fingers. Muscle cramps may occur, especially after exercise. In general, the absence of severe muscle atrophy, short stature, and relative sparing of bulbar muscles may suggest CCM.

Patients with CCM are at increased risk for malignant hyperthermia (MH), even in the absence of clinical weakness. Up to 80% of CCM and 50% of MH cases map to 19q13.1. This chromosome contains the ryanodine receptor gene (RYR1), which encodes the key channel that mediates calcium release of the skeletal muscle sarcoplasmic reticulum. Mutations in the RYR1 gene may also be responsible for cases of CCM presenting with rods as a secondary feature on muscle biopsy. Cases of CCM with hypertrophic cardiomyopathy, but not MH, associated with a mutation in the beta-myosin heavy chain gene on chromosome 14 have been described, confirming that CCM is genetically heterogeneous.

The serum CK level of patients with CCM is usually normal or slightly elevated, and EMG may be normal or reveal myopathic features. The average number of fibers innervated by a single anterior horn cell may be increased in CCM (increased terminal innervation ratio) accounting for single-fiber EMG abnormalities.

Muscle biopsy reveals circumscribed circular regions in the center of most type 1 fibers; in these lesions, oxidative enzyme activity is lacking, as are mitochondria and sarcoplasmic reticulum. Altered T-tubule systems are present, streaming of the Z-disc is often seen, and little glycogen is found within the core. These cores are of two types: structural cores with preserved myofibrillar architecture; and unstructured cores, in which the organization of

▶ TABLE 128.3 Molecular Genetics of Congenital Myopathies

Myopathy	Gene Locus	Protein Product
Nemaline myopathy	1q21–23	α-Tropomyosin [TPM3]
	2q21.2–22	Nebulin [NEB]
	1q42. 1	Sarcomeric actin [ACTA]1
		β–Tropomyosin [TPM2]
	9p13.2	Troponin T1 [TNNT1]
	19q13.4	Ryanodine receptor 1
Central core disease	19q13.1	[RYR1]
	14q11.2	Cardiac β–myosin
		[MYH7]
		Heavy chain
Myotubularin myopathy	X28q	Myotubularin [MTMX]
Desminopathy	2q35	Desmin [DES]
α B-crystallinopathy	11q22	αB-crystallin [CRYAB]
Desmin-related myopathies		Unknown
	2q21	Unknown
	10q22.3	Unknown
	12	Unknown
	15q22	

From Goebel HH. Congenital myopathies at their molecular dawning. *Muscle Nerve* 2003;27:528.

contractile elements in myofibrils is lost. Both types may be present in the same patient, and no evolution from structured to unstructured has been identified. The pathophysiology of core formation is unknown. However, type 1 fiber predominance and single-fiber EMG abnormalities suggest a neurogenic basis, a possibility also raised by and the resemblance of cores to target fibers.

Nemaline Myopathy

Nemaline myopathy was described by Gonatas and Shy in 1963. It was named after the Greek word *nema*, which means thread, because of the presence of rodlike structures that stain red with a modified trichrome stain of affected muscle. At least five gene loci and corresponding protein products cause the disease (Table 128.2). Autosomal-dominant, autosomal–recessive, and sporadic disease occur. Six clinical forms range from the floppy infant with dysmorphism to an adult-onset that may cause the dropped head sign. Skeletal abnormalities are not uncommon, and infants may present with congenital dislocation of the hip. A few patients show arthrogryposis congenita multiplex with flexion contractures of the limbs; others have cardiomyopathy, ophthalmoplegia, or rigid spine. Susceptibility to MH has also been described in nemaline myopathy. Routine laboratory studies, including serum creatine kinase, are usually unrewarding. EMG may be myopathic, and as the disease progresses, may reveal neuropathic features that are attributed to active degeneration and regeneration of muscle fibers. Muscle biopsy (using a modified trichrome stain) reveals dark red staining material in type 1 fibers that look like short rods on longitudinal sections. Ultrastructurally, the rods are usu-

ally found in the cytoplasm. The structures originate from the Z discs and are composed of alpha actinin and actin. Focal aggregation of desmin may be seen around nuclei and rod regions. Weakness correlates more with the degree of type 1 fiber predominance, and not with the number of fibers showing rods or the number of rods in each fiber. The mechanism of rod formation is unknown; some experts speculate that they may be a nonspecific reaction of an altered Z disc, perhaps as a result of abnormal or deficient activity of the protease dipeptidyl peptidase 1 enzyme. Rods have also been described in myopathies associated with HIV infection.

Myotubular Myopathy

The first case of myotubular myopathy, reported by Spiro and Shy in 1966, was observed in a 12-year-old boy with external ophthalmoplegia, facial diplegia, areflexia, and progressive proximal limb weakness. A second family of two sisters and mother followed. The girls had delayed motor milestones with slowly progressive weakness, ophthalmoplegia, ptosis, and facial weakness. Inheritance was autosomal dominant in those cases, but an X-linked form is probably the most severe of all congenital myopathies, with a 90% fatality rate in the 1st year. It is caused by mutations in the myotubularin (MTM1) gene on chromosome Xq28 that encodes a tyrosine phosphatase, myotubularin, which dephosphorylates the lipid second messenger phosphatidyl inositol 3-phosphate, which may impede myogenesis.

Researchers have described 141 disease-associated mutations. Muscle specimens may reveal undifferentiated or differentiated fiber types with type 1 hypotrophy.

Severe hypotonia, weakness, poor suck and swallow, and prominent respiratory failure are often present at birth. Despite the nonprogressive nature of this X-linked form, it is so severe that survival is not possible without ventilatory support. There is often a history of maternal polyhydramnios and previous perinatal deaths. Female carriers are usually asymptomatic, but some exhibit mild proximal limb weakness and kyphoscoliosis, which are attributed to abnormal expression or distribution of myotubularin rather than X-inactivation patterns. In affected infants, CK levels are usually normal. The EMG shows myopathic potentials plus spontaneous activity that may include bizarre high-frequency potentials and myotonia. Pathologically small myofibers with central nuclei resembling fetal myotubes are seen, raising the possibility that this disease arises from arrest of development or maturation of the primitive myotube. Centronuclear myopathy was originally called myotubular myopathy. It is now recognized as a distinct and uncommon entity consisting of non-X-linked autosomal and sporadic forms of myotubular myopathy characterized by central nuclei in approximately 35% to 90% of type 1 fibers.

Multiminicore Myopathy

Multiminicore myopathy (MMM) is usually nonprogressive and inherited in an autosomal-recessive pattern. Four homogenous phenotypes have been described: one with axial weakness, scoliosis, respiratory insufficiency, and distal joint laxity. A second type is characterized by ophthalmoplegia with severe facial and limb weakness. Other syndromes include an early-onset form with arthrogryposis and a slowly progressive form with weakness and hand amyotrophy. Cardiomyopathy, septal cardiac defects. and malignant hyperthermia also occur. Histopathologically, the cores of MMM, unlike those of CCM, do not extend the full length of the fiber. Like CCM, they consist of small areas of sarcomeric disruption that lack mitochondria. They affect both fiber types with type 1 predominance and hypotrophy.

A mutation in the selenoprotein gene (SEPN1) was recently described in a subset of patients with the severe classic form of MMM known as rigid spine syndrome.

Desmin-Related Myopathies

Desmin-related myopathy (DRM; also known as myofibrillar myopathy) includes cytoplasmic body myopathy, sarcoplasmic body myopathy, spheroid body myopathy, Mallory body–like myopathy, and granulofilamentous myopathy. These myopathies have been recently categorized under the term *surplus protein myopathies*. DRM inheritance may be autosomal dominant or autosomal recessive. Mutations and defects in the desmin gene

may disrupt the α helix and impair desmin filament assembly in muscle. Muscle biopsy of these disorders is characterized by aggregation of desmin into inclusion bodies or granulofilamentous material. Immunohistochemical techniques show that a heterogenous group of proteins congregate with desmin. These proteins include vimentin, dystrophin, nebulin, β-amyloid, emerin, α B-crystallin, calpain, and certain cyclin-dependent kinases. The clinical spectrum of DRM is broad: distal muscle weakness, cardiomyopathy, smooth muscle involvement, respiratory failure, and asymptomatic hyperCKemia may be seen in affected children.

Congenital Muscle Fiber Type Disproportion

Congenital muscle fiber type disproportion (CFTD) is characterized by a morphologic pattern in muscles in which there are a predominance of type 1 fibers that are more than 12% smaller (mean difference) than type 2 fibers. Type 1 fiber predominance is seen in most congenital muscle diseases and certain neuropathies. Some experts regard CFTD as a histochemical syndrome rather than a distinct congenital myopathy. Clinical features of CFTD are usually evident in the neonatal period with weakness, hypotonia, dysmorphism, and contractures dominating the picture. The presence of these contractures suggests intrauterine weakness. CFTD has also been associated with rigid spine syndrome, respiratory insufficiency, and severe insulin-resistant diabetes.

Myopathies with Abnormal Inclusions of Unknown Origin

Other myopathies with abnormal inclusions include hyaline, reducing, fingerprint, zebra, and cylindrical body myopathies. These are rare disorders that need further biochemical and genetic characterization.

Hyaline body myopathy is a disorder that affects both children and adults. It may be inherited in an autosomal-dominant fashion or may occur sporadically. Weakness often takes on a scapuloperoneal distribution. Pathologically, subsarcolemmal hyaline granules are seen in type 1 fibers lacking glycogen and oxidative reactivity.

Reducing body myopathy is a nonprogressive myopathy affecting infants, children, or adults. Clinically severe hypotonia, proximal weakness, joint contractures, and ptosis may be seen. Reducing bodies have also been found with the rigid spine syndrome. Pathologic features include intracytoplasmic inclusions with reducing activity that do not react to nicotinamide adenine dehydrogenase-tetrazolium reductase, but react strongly with menadione-linked α-glycerophosphate dehydrogenase. Ultrastructurally, the bodies consist of masses of granules or tubular filaments.

Fingerprint body myopathy is also nonprogressive. Clinical manifestations include proximal limb weakness, sparing the oculofacial muscles, with absent tendon reflexes and, often, subnormal intelligence. Pathologically, the fingerprint bodies appear as dense bodies under the sarcolemma. Fingerprint inclusions have also been seen in patients with myotonic dystrophy or dermatomyositis.

The existence of *zebra body myopathy* is controversial. Zebra bodies are nonspecific findings in normal extraocular muscle and at the myotendinous junction.

Cylindrical spiral myopathy has been reported in a few families and eight sporadic cases. Most had prominent cramps or myalgia. Like zebra body myopathy, it may not be a distinct clinical entity.

MYOTONIA CONGENITA

Myotonia congenita was first described by a Danish physician in 1876. He described the autosomal-dominant form in his family (Thomsen disease). An autosomal-recessive form (Becker-type generalized myotonia) was described much later in 1966. Although distinguishing features are recognized, there is overlap in manifestations in the two forms. Becker myotonia is more common than the Thomsen type, and symptoms usually begin early and more severely. Myotonia affects the face, jaw, tongue, pharynx, and arms more than the legs, and is generally more severe than that in myotonic muscular dystrophy. Respiratory muscles are spared. Muscle hypertrophy is attributed to the constant activity of myotonia. These patients lack the pleiotropic manifestations of myotonic muscular dystrophy (cataracts, endocrinopathy, and cardiac abnormalities).

Myotonia is a result of electrical instability of the sarcolemma causing repetitive electrical discharges of affected muscle fibers leading to muscle stiffness. Characteristically, myotonia is worse on the initiation of exercise and is ameliorated by gradually increasing the vigor of movements by warming up. In the Becker form, repeated exercise may lead to transient weakness. Although patients with these disorders do not develop profound sensitivity to cold or weakness, myotonia may worsen in cold environments. Careful preoperative screening of muscular symptoms and family history is vital, because life-threatening muscular spasms may follow administration of depolarizing muscle relaxants (suxamethonium). The EMG in both forms reveals profuse myotonic discharges, and muscle biopsy may demonstrate tubular aggregates and absence of type 2b fibers.

Myotonia congenita is one of the best understood genetic diseases caused by dysfunction of ion channels. The skeletal muscle voltage-gated chloride channel CLCN1 is expressed in mammalian skeletal muscle and mediates muscle chloride conductance. Missense or nonsense mutations in the CLCN1 are responsible for both forms of myotonia congenita. As chloride conductance is essential for repolarization following each action potential, the diminished chloride ion conductance seen with this disease allows sequential membrane depolarizations that are manifest clinically as myotonia or persistent muscle contraction. A rarer form of myotonia congenita, responsive to acetazolamide, is caused by sodium channel mutations in the SCN4A gene. In contrast to the chloride channel myotonias, this form is often associated with periodic paralysis and is grouped under with hyperkalemic periodic paralysis or nondystrophic myotonias. A novel animal model for myotonia congenita has been developed without mutations in the CLCN or SCN4A genes. Treatment of myotonia depends on phenytoin, quinine, and mexiletine. Procainamide is effective but is avoided because its can induce systemic lupus erythematosus. Acetazolamide is sometimes effective.

CHONDRODYSTROPHIC MYOTONIA (SCHWARTZ-JAMPEL SYNDROME)

Chondrodystrophic myotonia was first described by Schwartz and Jampel in 1962. It is a rare disorder characterized by skeletal dysplasia and myotonia. Increased prevalence in Middle Eastern and South African families is related to parental consanguinity in these regions. Mutations in the gene *perlecan* (HSPG2) encoding the protein heparin sulfate proteoglycan are responsible. Three forms have been described: type 1A is associated with moderate bone dysplasia and is recognized in childhood; type 1B is associated with more prominent bone dysplasia and is evident at birth; type 2 is the least common, most severe, and potentially fatal neonatal form, a genetically distinct disorder, the Stuve-Wiedemann syndrome.

Although the more common autosomal-recessive type 1 form is caused by mutations in perlecan at 1p36.1, type 2 does not show linkage to this locus. Children with type 1 have a distinct facial appearance that is recognizable at birth because of blepharophimosis, low-set ears, pinched nose, pursed lips, micrognathia, and a high arched palate. Other skeletal anomalies include dwarfism, short neck, kyphosis, and flexion contractures of the limbs. The prevalence of mental retardation has been estimated at 25%, but the mechanism behind this remains unclear. Generalized stiffness of limb muscles is present, often accompanied by hypertrophy, and associated with severe voluntary and percussion myotonia. This stiffness is the result of almost continuous muscle fiber activity, which manifests itself as myotonia on EMG and resembles the neuromyotonic discharges seen in the Isaacs syndrome (chapter 130). Like other forms of myotonia, these discharges persist after nerve block, curare, or nerve degeneration. CK may be mildly elevated, and muscle biopsy may reveal myopathic and neurogenic features. Current treatment is symptomatic, and a multidisciplinary approach includes orthopedic surgeons, physiatrists, and neurologists. Ophthalmologic intervention may facilitate normal vision. Malignant hyperthermia may occur during anesthesia. Myotonia can be treated with phenytoin, carbamazepine, procainamide, or mexiletine.

SUGGESTED READING

Congenital Myopathies

Avila G. Intracellular Ca (2+) dynamics in malignant hyperthermia and central core disease: established concepts, new cellular mechanisms involved. *Cell Calcium* 2005 Feb;37(2):121–127.

Bruno C, Minetti C. Congenital myopathies. *Curr Neurol Neurosci Rep* 2004 Jan;4(1):68–73.

Deconinck N, Laterre EC, Van den Bergh PY. Adult-onset nemaline myopathy and monoclonal gammopathy: a case report. *Acta Neurol Belg* 2000;100(Mar):34–40.

Ferreiro A, Quijano-Roy S, Pichereau C, et al. Mutations of the selenoprotein N gene, which is implicated in rigid spine muscular dystrophy, cause the classical phenotype of multiminicore disease: reassessing the nosology of early-onset myopathies. *Am J Hum Genet* 2002;71:739–749.

Fujii J, Otsu K, Zorato F, et al. Identification of a mutation in porcine ryanodine receptor associated with malignant hyperthermia. *Science* 1991;253:448–451.

Goebel H. Central core disease. In: Karpati G, ed. *Pathology and Genetics: Structural and Molecular Basis of Skeletal Muscle Diseases.* Basel, Switzerland: ISN Neuropath Press, 2002:65–67.

Goebel H, Warlo IA. Surplus protein myopathies. *Neuromuscul Disord* 2001;11:3–6.

Goebel HH. Congenital myopathies at their molecular dawning. *Muscle Nerve* 2003;27:527–548.

Gonatas NK, Shy GM, Godfrey EH. Nemaline myopathy. The origin of nemaline structures. *N Engl J Med* 1966;274:535–539.

Guis S, Figarella-Branger D, Monnier N, et al. Multiminicore disease in a family susceptible to malignant hyperthermia. *Arch Neurol* 2004;61:106–113.

Jungbluth H, Sewry CA, Buj-Bello A, et al. Early and severe presentation of X-linked myotubular myopathy in a girl with skewed X-inactivation. *Neuromusc Disord* 2003;13(1):55–59.

Lomen-Hoerth C, Simmons ML, DeArmond SJ, et al. Adult-onset nemaline myopathy: another cause of dropped head. *Muscle Nerve* 1999;22:1146–1150.

Mancuso M, Ferraris S, Nishigaki Y, et al. Congenital or late-onset myopathy in patients with the T14709C mtDMA mutation. *J Neurol Sci* 2005 Jan 15;228(1):93–97.

Mathews KD, Moore SA. Multiminicore myopathy, central core disease, malignant hyperthermia susceptibility, and RYR1 mutations: one disease with many faces? *Arch Neurol* 2004 Jan;61(1):27–29.

Messina S, Hartley L, Main M, Kinali M, Jungbluth H, Muntoni F, Mercuri E. Pilot trial of salbutamol in central core and multi-minicore diseases. *Neuropediatrics* 2004 Oct;35(5):262–266.

McCarthy TV, Quane KA, Lynch PJ. Ryanodine receptor mutations in malignant hyperthermia and central core disease. *Hum Mutat* 2000;15:410–417.

Sanoudou D, Frieden LA, Haslett JN et al. Molecular classification of nemaline myopathies: "nontyping" specimens exhibit unique patterns of gene expression. *Neurobiol Dis* 2004;15:590–600.

Scacheri PC, Hoffman EP, Fratkin JD, et al. A novel ryanodine receptor gene mutation causing both cores and rods in congenital myopathy. *Neurology* 2000;55:1689–1696.

Selcen D, Ohno K, Engel AG. Myofibrillar myopathy: clinical, morphological and genetic studies in 63 patients. *Brain* 2004;127(Pt 2):439–451.

Shy GM, Engel WK, Somers JE, et al. Nemaline myopathy. A new congenital myopathy. *Brain* 1963;79:793–810.

Shy GM, Magee KR. A new congenital non-progressive myopathy. *Brain* 1956;79:610–621.

Spiro AJ, Shy GM, Gonatas NK. Myotubular myopathy. *Arch Naeurol* 1966;14:1–14.

Taratuto AL. Congenital myopathies and related disorders. *Curr Opin Neurol* 2002;15:553–561.

Wallegren-Pettersson C. Nemaline and myotubular myopathies. *Semin Pediatr Neurol* 2002;9:132–144.

Myotonia Congenita

Becker PE. Zur Genetik der Myotonien. In Kuhn E, ed. *Progressive Muskeldystrophie, Myotonie, Myasthenie.* Berlin: Springer-Verlag, 1966:247–255.

Chen L, Schaerer M, Lu ZH, et al. Exon 17 skipping in CLCN1 leads to recessive myotonia congenita. *Muscle Nerve* 2004;29(5):670–676.

Duno M, Colding-Jorgensen E, Grunnet M, Jespersen T, Vissing J, Schwartz M. Difference in allelic expression of the CLCN1 gene and the possible influence on the myotonia congenita phenotype. *Eur J Hum Genet* 2004 Sep;12(9):738–743.

Farbu E, Softeland E, Bindoff LA. Anesthetic complications associated with myotonia congenital: case study and comparison with other myotonic disorders. *Acta Anaesthesiologica Scandinavica* 2003;47:630–634.

Koch MC, Steinmeyer K, Lorenz C, et al. The skeletal muscle chloride channel in dominant and recessive human myotonia. *Science* 1992;257:797–800.

Ptacek LJ, Tawil R, Griggs RC, et al. Sodium channel mutations in acetazolamide-responsive myotonia congenital, paramyotonia congenital and hyperkalemic periodic paralysis. *Neurolgy* 1994;44:1500–1503.

Shirakawa T, Sakai K, Kitagawa Y, et al. A novel murine myotonia congenital without molecular defects in the CLC-1 and the SCN4A. *Neurology* 2002;59:1091–1094.

Thomsen J. Tonische Krampfe in willkurlich beweglichen Muskulen in Folge von ererbter psychischer Disposition (Ataxia muscularis?). *Arch Psychiatrie* 1876;6:702–718.

Chondrodystrophic Myotonia (Schwartz-Jampel Syndrome)

Arikawa-Hirasawa E, Le AH, Nishino I, et al. Structural and functional mutations of the perlecan gene cause Schwartz-Jampel syndrome, with myotonic myopathy and chondrodysplasia. *Am J Hum Genet* 2002;70:1368–1375.

Ho NC, Sandusky S, Madike V, et al. Clinico-pathogenetic findings and management of chondrodystrophic myotonia (Schwartz-Jampel syndrome): a case report. *BMC Neurology* 2003;3:3.

Nicole S, Davoine C-S, Topaloglu H, et al. Perlecan, the major proteoglycan of basement membranes, is altered in patients with Schwartz-Jampel syndrome (chondrodystrophic myotonia). *Nat Genet* 2000;26:480–483.

Reed UC, Reimao R, Espindola AA, et al. Schwartz-Jampel syndrome: a report of five cases. *Arq Neuropsiquitr* 2002;60:734–738.

Schwartz O, Jampel RS. Congenital blepharophimosis associated with a unique generalized myopathy. *Arch Opthal* 1962;68:52–57.

Squires LA, Prangley J. Neonatal diagnosis of Schwartz-Jampel syndrome with dramatic response to carbamazepine. *Ped Neurol* 1996;15:172–174.

Yapicioglu H, Satar M, Yildizdas D, et al. Schwartz-Jampel syndrome: three pediatric case reports. *Genet Couns* 2003;14:353–358.

Myoglobinuria

Lewis P. Rowland

When necrosis of muscle is acute, myoglobin escapes into the blood and then into the urine. In the past, the term *myoglobinuria* was reserved for grossly pigmented urine, but modern techniques can detect amounts of this protein so minute that discoloration may not be evident. (Determination of serum myoglobin content by radioimmunoassay has the same diagnostic significance as measurement of serum creatine kinase [CK] activity.) The clinically important syndromes, however, are associated with gross pigmenturia. Sometimes, the disorder can be recognized without direct demonstration of myoglobin in the urine, for instance, in cases of acute renal failure with very high levels of serum CK activity. Inexplicably, *rhabdomyolysis* has become the official (*Index Medicus*) term for these syndromes, although it is really a synonym for the syndrome of myoglobinuria. Myoglobin is the visible pigment in the urine, and myoglobin is the toxin that injures the kidney; the syndrome originates with muscle necrosis, which does not need a new name.

No classification of myoglobinuria is completely satisfactory, but Table 129.1 lists the most important causes. Sporadic cases are often associated with traumatic muscle injury, and even some cases of inherited recurrent myoglobinuria are of unidentified cause. In six forms, however, the genetic defect has been recognized: lack of phosphorylase (McArdle), phosphofructokinase (Tarui), carnitine palmitoyltransferase (CPT; DiMauro-Bank), phosphoglyceraldehyde kinase (DiMauro), phosphoglycerate mutase (DiMauro), and lactate dehydrogenase (Kanno). CPT is important in lipid metabolism; the others are involved in glycogenolysis or glycolysis and are reviewed in Chapter 85. In all these conditions, there is a disorder in the metabolism of a fuel necessary for muscular work; in all six, exercise is limited by painful cramps after exertion, and myoglobinuria occurs after especially strenuous activity. There may be a subtle difference in the kinds of activity that provoke attacks, which are more prolonged in CPT deficiency than in the glycogen disorders. The glycogen disorders can be identified by a simple clinical test: A cramp is induced by ischemic exercise of forearm muscles for less than 1 minute, and venous lactate fails to rise as it does in normal individuals or those with CPT deficiency. Specific diagnosis can be made by DNA analysis on blood or

by muscle histochemistry or biochemistry. Five of the conditions are inherited in autosomal-recessive pattern; phosphoglycerate kinase deficiency is X linked. Mutations in mitochondrial DNA also account for some cases of recurrent myoglobinuria (Table 129.1).

The relative frequency of all causes of *recurrent* myoglobinuria differed in two studies. In the United States, samples were sent to an active referral laboratory, and almost 50% had an identifiable cause. Phosphorylase, phosphorylase kinase, phosphofructokinase, CPT, and myoadenylate deaminase deficiencies accounted for almost all in the report of Tonin and colleagues (1990). In Finland, however, only 23% of 22 patients with recurrent myoglobinuria had an identifiable cause, and none had CPT deficiency or myoadenylate deaminase deficiency. Lofberg and associates (1998) gave two explanations of recurrent myoglobinuria without an enzyme defect: disappearance of some genes from the genetically isolated population in Finland and an increase in recreational distance running or bodybuilding.

Another important form of inherited myoglobinuria occurs in *malignant hyperthermia* (MIM 180901, 145600), which is considered an aberrant reaction to succinylcholine, halothane, or both together. The characteristic syndrome includes widespread muscular rigidity, a rapid rise in body temperature, myoglobinuria, arrhythmia, and metabolic acidosis. In some cases, muscular rigidity is lacking. The pathogenesis is uncertain, but the offending drugs may interact with a defective protein in the muscle sarcoplasmic reticulum that fails to bind calcium. The muscle, flooded with calcium, shortens to create the stiff muscles and attendant muscle necrosis.

The syndrome is often familial in an autosomal-dominant pattern, but many cases are sporadic. In some families, the gene mapped to chromosome 19q12-13.2, the site of the gene for the *ryanodine receptor*, which is the calcium release channel and also the locus for central core disease, a congenital myopathy that seems to increase the risk of malignant hyperthermia. A similar syndrome in pigs maps to the same gene product. However, there is evidence of locus heterogeneity because only 50% of all families with malignant hyperthermia map to that locus. Another calcium-binding protein of the sarcoplasmic reticulum is the dihydropyridine receptor, but the disease does not map to the locus for that candidate gene product. Yet another sign of heterogeneity is the occurrence of the syndrome in children with Duchenne muscular dystrophy or myotonia congenita. A closely related disorder is the *neuroleptic malignant syndrome*, which is similar in clinical manifestations, although the offending drugs are different and the disorder has not yet appeared in a family with malignant hyperthermia (Chapter 117).

Most attacks of *acquired myoglobinuria* occur in nonathletic individuals who are subjected to extremely vigorous exercise, a hazard faced primarily by military

▶ **TABLE 129.1 Classification of Human Myoglobinuria**

Hereditary myoglobinuria
Myophosphorylase deficiency (McArdle; MIM 232600)
Phosphofructokinase deficiency (Tarui; MIM 171840)
Carnitine palmitoyl transferase deficiency (DiMauro; MIM 255110, 255120)
Phosphoglycerate kinase (DiMauro; MIM 311800)
Phosphoglycerate mutase (DiMauro; MIM 261670)
Lactate dehydrogenase (Kanno; MIM 150000)
Incompletely characterized syndromes
    Excess lactate production (Larsson)
Uncharacterized
    Familial; biochemical defect unknown
        Provoked by diarrhea or infection
        Provoked by exercise
Malignant hyperthermia (MIM 180901, 145600)
Repeated attacks in an individual; biochemical defect unknown
 	
Sporadic myoglobinuria
  Exertion in untrained individuals
  "Squat-jump" and related syndromes
  Anterior tibial syndrome
  Convulsions
  High-voltage electric shock, lightning stroke
  Agitated delirium, restraints
  Status asthmaticus
  Prolonged myoclonus or acute dystonia
  Crush syndrome
  Compression by fallen weights
  Compression by body in prolonged coma
  Ischemia
  Arterial occlusion
  Cardioversion
  Coagulopathy in sickle-cell disease or disseminated intravascular coagulation
  Ischemia in compression and anterior tibial syndromes
  Laparoscopic nephrectomy
  Ligation of vena cava
  Surgery on morbidly obese people, including bariatric surgery
	Metabolic abnormalities
	Mitochondrial myopathies
	Cytochrome oxidase-1 mutation.
	Mitochondrial tRNA mutation
	Trifunctional protein deficiency
	Metabolic depression
	Barbiturate, carbon monoxide, narcotic coma
	Cold exposure
	Diabetic acidosis
	General anesthesia
	Hyperglycemic, hyperosmolar coma
	Hypothermia
	Exogenous toxins and drugs
	Alcohol abuse
	Amphotericin B
	Carbenoxolone
	Clopidogrel (and heart transplant)
	Gemfibrozil (plus statin)
	Glycyrrhizate
	Haff disease
	Heat stroke
	Heroin
	Hypokalemia, chronic, any cause
	Interferon alpha 2B
	Isoretinoin
	Malayan sea-snake bite poison
	Malignant neuroleptic syndrome
	Plasmocid
	Phenylpropanolamine
	Statin drugs
	Succinylcholine
	Toxic shock syndrome
	Wasp stings
	Progressive muscle disease
	Alcoholic myopathy
	Dystrophinopathy
	Polymyositis or dermatomyositis
	Cause unknown

recruits. These individuals are otherwise normal. Even trained runners may experience myoglobinuria in marathon races. If muscle is compressed, as occurs in the crush syndrome of individuals pinned by fallen timber after bombing raids, or after prolonged coma in one position, myoglobinuria may ensue. Ischemia after occlusion of large arteries may also lead to necrosis of large amounts of muscle. Depression of muscle metabolism, especially after drug ingestion, may also be responsible in some cases. Hypokalemia from any cause may predispose to myoglobinuria, but especially after chronic licorice ingestion or abuse of thiazide diuretics. Alcoholics seem especially prone to acute attacks of myoglobinuria, which may punctuate or initiate a syndrome of chronic limb weakness (alcoholic myopathy). In children, as in adults,

the attacks may be precipitated by exercise (often with an identifiable enzymatic defect); in contrast to adults, however, myoglobinuria in children seems more often associated with a nonspecific viral infection and fever.

Heat cramps arise after heavy sweating during vigorous exercise if water is replaced but not salt; the hyponatrenia is usually benign, but contracture tests point to susceptibility for malignant hyperthermia in some subjects. *Heat exhaustion* is a syndrome of salt or water depletion after exercise in hot environments; it is manifested by malaise and collapse, but there is no tissue damage. *Heat stroke* is a killer disorder and shares similarities with malignant hyperthermia. Two major forms are seen; the first is essentially described above, exercise-induced myoglobinuria in hot weather, which is sometimes fatal in athletes—especially football players. The second form occurs during heat waves and is likely to affect young children or the elderly and the poor who do not have air conditioning. The key abnormalities are increased core temperature and cerebral symptoms that range from inappropriate behavior to delirium, seizures, encephalopathy, coma, and death. About 30% of patients have renal failure, often a consequence of myoglobinuria, but no organ is spared and coagulopathies are serious; it is considered a multiorgan-dysfunction syndrome. Death rates have not changed much in decades, ranging from 10% to 50%.

Another major contemporary cause of myoglobinuria is *statin myopathy* because millions of people are now taking these drugs. Among the muscle-related abnormalities are cramps; abnormal CK values, sometimes more than 10 times the upper limit of normal; and frank attacks of myoglobinuria, sometimes with renal failure. Because attacks of myoglobinuria were fatal in those taking cerivastatin (Baycol) and were encountered 16 to 80 times more often than with any of the other five statins, the drug was withdrawn in August 2001.

It is difficult to determine how often overt myoglobinuria occurs in patients taking a statin, because the word *rhabdomyolysis* is often used as a synonym for asymptomatic hyperCKemia. The incidence of deaths is 0.04 per one million prescriptions. Among 83,858 patients in a controlled trial of statin therapy, 7 patients and 5 placebo controls had "rhabdomyolysis." In another trial, equal numbers of patients (33%) taking a statin and their controls had "muscle complaints." It seems reasonable to conclude that hyperCKemia occurs in people taking statins, that myoglobinuria occurs more frequently in people taking statins (but not how much more frequently), and attacks of myoglobinuria may be fatal (but we do not know how often). Some of these uncertainties arise from the use of "rhabdomyolysis" instead of myoglobinuria.

The mechanism of statin-induced myopathy is uncertain. It seems to be related more to mevalonate metabolism than cholesterol. Mitochondrial damage may play a role because ubiquinone (coenzyme Q10) levels decrease in blood and perhaps in muscle.

Whatever the cause, the clinical syndrome of myoglobinuria is similar: widespread myalgia, weakness, malaise, renal pain, and fever. Pigmenturia usually ceases within a few days, but the weakness may persist for weeks, and high concentrations of serum enzymes may not return to normal for even longer. The main hazard of the syndrome is heme-induced nephropathy with anuria, azotemia, and hyperkalemia. Hypercalcemia occurs in a few patients after anuria. Occasionally, respiratory muscles are symptomatically weakened.

Treatment of an acute episode of myoglobinuria is directed primarily toward the kidneys. Promotion of diuresis with mannitol seems desirable whenever there is oliguria. Dialysis and measures to combat hyperkalemia may be necessary. In recurrent cases owing to defects of glycolytic enzymes or to unknown cause, various therapeutic regimens have been tried, but patients usually learn the limits of exercise tolerance.

The treatment of malignant hyperthermia is unsatisfactory because the rigidity is not abolished by curare. Intravenous infusions of dantrolene sodium (Dantrium) are given because this drug inhibits the release of calcium from the sarcoplasmic reticulum, relaxing the hypercontracted muscle. The average dose in successfully treated patients is 2.5 mg/kg body weight. Emergency treatment includes stopping the administration of the offending agent, cooling, and correcting acidosis or arrhythmias.

Once a person has been identified with malignant hyperthermia, the clinician must determine whether other family members are at risk. With the mapping of the gene to chromosome 19, it was hoped that a DNA test would be available. Locus heterogeneity, however, means that other, still unidentified genes are sometimes responsible. An alternative test to identify susceptibility is the caffeine contracture test, during which bundles of fibers from a muscle biopsy are exposed to the drug and tension is measured. Individuals are deemed susceptible if the response is significantly greater than normal. Unfortunately, the test is not completely reliable. Nevertheless, the condition is now so well known to anesthesiologists that offending volatile and neuromuscular blocking agents are avoided in people who may be at risk, and the frequency of attacks has fallen.

For the malignant neuropletptic syndrome, bromocriptine mesylate (Parlodel) and carbamazepine (Tegretol) have reportedly been beneficial (see Chapter 117).

For statin-induced hyperCKemia, cardiologists recommend cessation of statin therapy if CK levels are sustained at more than 10 times normal; this seems prudent even though there is no evidence that these high levels imply incipient myoglobinuria. Monitoring CK levels to provide a baseline also seems prudent. Ezetimibe, an inhibitor of intestinal cholesterol absorption, lowers serum levels of cholesterol and is being used to reduce statin levels or to substitute for statins.

SUGGESTED READINGS

Bank WJ, DiMauro S, Bonilla E, et al. A disorder of lipid metabolism and myoglobinuria: absence of carnitine palmityl transferase. *N Engl J Med* 1975;292:443–449.

Bouchanna A, Knochel JP. Heat stroke. *N Engl J Med* 2002;346:1978–88.

Bristow MF, Kohen D. How "malignant" is the neuroleptic malignant syndrome? *BMJ* 1993;307:1223–1224.

Britt BA, Kalow W. Malignant hyperthermia: a statistical review. *Can Anaesth Soc J* 1970;17:293–315.

Corpier CL, Jones PH, Suki WN, et al. Rhabdomyolysis and renal injury with lovastatin use: report of two cases in cardiac transplant patients. *JAMA* 1988;260:239–241.

Denborough M. Malignant hyperthermia. *Lancet* 1998;352:1131–1136.

DiMauro S, Dalakas M, Miranda AF. Phosphoglycerate kinase deficiency: another cause of recurrent myoglobinuria. *Ann Neurol* 1983;13: 11–19.

DiMauro S, DiMauro PMM. Muscle carnitine palmityl transferase deficiency and myoglobinuria. *Science* 1973;182:929–931.

Duthie DJR. Heat-related illness. *Lancet* 1998;352:1329–1330.

Ebadi M, Pfeiffer RF, Murrin LC. Pathogenesis and treatment of neuroleptic malignant syndrome. *Gen Pharmacol* 1990;21:367–386.

Editorial. How a statin might destroy a drug company. *Lancet* 2003; 361:793.

Gabow PA, Kaehny WD, Kelleher SP. The spectrum of rhabdomyolysis. *Medicine* 1982;61:141–152.

Girard T, Treves S, Voronkov E, et al. Molecular genetic testing for malignant hyperthermia susceptibility. *Anesthesiology* 2004;100: 1076–80.

Grogan H, Hopkins PM. Heat stroke: implications for critical care and anesthesia. *Brit J Anaesth* 2002;88:700–707.

Guis S, Figarella-Branger D, Monnier N, et al. Multiminicore disease in a family susceptible to malignant hyperthermia: histology, in vitro contracture tests, and genetic characterization. *Arch Neurol* 2004;61(Jan):106–113.

Hogan K. The anesthetic myopathies and malignant hyperthermias. *Curr Opin Neurol* 1998;11:469–476.

Hollander AS, Olney RC, Blackett PR, et al. Fatal malignant hyperthermia-like syndrome with rhabdomyolysis complicating the presentation of diabetes mellitus in adolescent males. *Pediatrics* 2003;111(Pt 1):1447–1452.

Lofberg M, Jankala H, Paetau A, et al. Metabolic causes of recurrent rhabdomyolysis. *Acta Neurol Scand* 1998;98:268–275.

Manning BM, Quane KA, Ording H, et al. Identification of novel mutations in the ryanodine-receptor gene (RYR1) in malignant hyperthermia: genotype-phenotype correlation. *Am J Hum Genet* 1998;62:599–609.

Melamed I, Romen Y, Keren G, et al. March myoglobinuria: a hazard to renal function. *Arch Intern Med* 1982;142:1277–1279.

Penn AS, Rowland LP, Fraser DW. Drugs, coma, and myoglobinuria. *Arch Neurol* 1972;26:336–343.

Perkoff GT. Alcoholic myopathy. *Annu Rev Med* 1971;22:125–132.

Quane KA, Healy JMS, Keating KE, et al. Mutations in the ryanodine receptor gene in central core disease and malignant hyperthermia. *Nat Genet* 1993;5:51–55.

Reuter DA, Anestseder M, Muller R, et al. The ryanodine contracture test may help diagnose susceptibility to malignant hyperthermia. *Canad J Aneasth* 2003;50:643–648.

Robinson RL, Anetseder MJ, Brancadoro V, et al. Recent advances in the diagnosis of malignant hyperthermia susceptibility: how confident can we be of genetic testing? *Europ J Hum Genet* 2003;11(Apr):342–348.

Rowland LP. Myoglobinuria. *Can J Neurol Sci* 1984;11:1–13.

Tein I, DiMauro S, Rowland LP. Myoglobinuria. In: Vinken PJ, Bruyn GW, Klawans HL, et al., eds. *Myopathies. Handbook of Clinical Neurology*, rev ser, vol 62(18). New York: Elsevier Science, 1992:479–526.

Thompson PD. Statin-associated myopathy. *JAMA* 2003;289:1681–1690.

Tonin P, Lewis P, Servidei S, et al. Metabolic causes of myoglobinuria. *Ann Neurol* 1990;27:181–185.

Ueda M, Hamamoto M, Nagayama H, et al. Susceptibility to neuroleptic malignant syndrome in Parkinson's disease. *Neurology* 1999;52:777–781.

Wedel DJ. Malignant hyperthermia and neuromuscular disease. *Neuromuscul Disord* 1993;3:157–164.

Yaqub B, Al Deeb S. Heat strokes: aetiopathogenesis, neurological characteristics, treatment and outcome. *J Neurol Sci* 1998;156:144–151.

Chapter 130

Muscle Cramps and Stiffness

Robert B. Layzer and Lewis P. Rowland

The term *muscle stiffness* implies a state of continuous muscle contraction at rest; *cramps* or *spasms* are transient, involuntary contractions of a muscle or group of muscles. Table 130.1 lists some of the many disorders that cause muscle stiffness or cramps.

ORDINARY MUSCLE CRAMPS

The common *muscle cramp* is a sudden, forceful, often painful muscle contraction that lasts from a few seconds to several minutes. Cramps are provoked by a trivial movement or by contracting a shortened muscle. They may occur during vigorous exercise, but are more likely to occur after exercise ceases. Unusually frequent cramps tend to accompany pregnancy, hypothyroidism, uremia, profuse sweating or diarrhea, hemodialysis, and lower motor neuron disorders, especially anterior horn cell diseases. Benign fasciculations or myokymia may be associated with frequent muscle cramps in apparently healthy people.

Nocturnal cramps typically cause forceful flexion of the ankle and toes, but cramps can affect almost any voluntary muscle. A cramp often starts with fasciculations, after which the muscle becomes intermittently hard and knot-like as the involuntary contraction waxes and wanes, passing from one part of the muscle to another. EMG shows brief, periodic bursts of motor unit potentials discharging at a frequency of 200 to 300 Hz, appearing irregularly and intermingling with similar discharges from adjacent motor units. Several foci within the same muscle may discharge independently. This electrical activity clearly arises within the lower motor neuron; whether it occurs in the soma, in the peripheral nerve, or in the intramuscular nerve terminals is still debated, but cramps can be induced by electrical stimulation of a motor nerve trunk distal to a complete block, and such cramps can be terminated by stretching the muscle, favoring a nerve terminal site of origin.

Stretching the affected muscle usually terminates a cramp. Information about prophylactic therapy is largely anecdotal, and no single agent appears to be uniformly effective. For nocturnal leg cramps, a bedtime dose of

▶ **TABLE 130.1 Motor Unit Disorders Causing Cramps and Stiffness**

Location of Abnormality	Name of Disorder	Principal Manifestations	Treatment
Spinal cord and brainstem	Stiff-man syndrome	Rigidity and reflex spasms	Diazepam
	Tetanus	Rigidity and reflex spasms	Diazepam
	Progressive encephalomyelitis with rigidity and spasms	Rigidity and reflex spasms, focal neurologic deficits	None
	Myelopathy with alpha rigidity	Extensor rigidity	None
	Spinal myoclonus	Segmental repetitive myoclonic jerks	Clonazepam
Peripheral nerves	Tetany	Carpopedal spasm	Correction of calcium, magnesium, or acid–base derangement
	Neuromyotonia	Stiffness, myokymia, delayed relaxation	Phenytoin, carbamazepine
Muscle	Myotonic disorders	Delayed relaxation, percussion myotonia	Phenytoin, carbamazepine, procainamide
	Schwartz-Jampel syndrome	Stiffness and myotonia	Phenytoin, carbamazepine
	Phosphorylase deficiency, phosphofructokinase deficiency	Cramps during intense or ischemic exercise	None
	Malignant hyperthermia	Rigidity during anesthesia	Dantrolene
Unknown	Ordinary muscle cramps	Cramps during sleep or ordinary activity	Quinine, phenytoin, carbamazepine

quinine, phenytoin (Dilantin), carbamazepine (Tegretol), or diazepam may be used. The beneficial effects of quinine have been demonstrated by controlled trials. Serious adverse effects are uncommon; tinnitus is relieved by interrupting treatment. However, thrombocytopenia has been reported and over-the-counter sales are no longer permitted. The conventional dosage is 300 or 600 mg at bedtime. Frequent daytime cramps sometimes respond to maintenance therapy with carbamazepine or phenytoin.

Most people have cramps at some time, but a few people have inordinately frequent cramps, often accompanied by fasciculations. The syndrome of *benign fasciculation with cramps* is disproportionately more frequent among physicians and other medical workers because they are more likely to know the ominous implications of fasciculations for the diagnosis of motor neuron disease. In fact, however, motor neuron disease almost never starts with fasciculations alone. If neither weakness nor wasting is seen, motor neuron disease is essentially excluded. The syndrome of benign fasciculation has been reported many times with variations on the name. Because the syndrome and the physiologic analysis were completely described by Denny-Brown and Foley, a reasonable eponym is the *Denny-Brown, Foley syndrome.*

True cramps must be distinguished from cramplike muscle pain unaccompanied by spasm. The cramps of McArdle disease occur only during intense or ischemic exercise. Because no electrical activity is evident in the EMG during the painful shortening of muscle affected by McArdle disease, the term *contracture* is used. The origin of the contracture is not known; depletion of adenosine triphosphate has long been suspected (because of the block of

glycogen metabolism) but has not been proved, even by magnetic resonance spectroscopy.

Mild dystrophinopathies, with little or no clinical weakness, may be manifested by exertional muscle pain and even myoglobinuria. These symptoms have been referred to as muscle cramps, but actual muscle spasm has not been described in such cases; the pain may simply be a measure of muscle injury.

Myalgia and cramps are believed to be especially common in *myoadenylate deaminase deficiency* (MIM 102770), but that state is common in asymptomatic people (found in 1% to 3% of all muscle biopsies). Therefore, the association is difficult to confirm. Moreover, in affected families, a poor correlation exists between the muscle enzyme deficiency and clinical symptoms. An autosomal-dominant cramp syndrome is seen without known biochemical abnormality (MIM 158400).

NEUROMYOTONIA (ISAACS SYNDROME)

Isaacs first described this disorder as a state of "continuous muscle fiber activity." The invariable clinical manifestation is *myokymia* (clinically visible and continuous muscle twitching that may be difficult to distinguish from vigorous fasciculation). The word has two meanings, one clinical and the other electromyographic. Physiologically, spontaneous activity takes one of two forms. In electrical myokymia, grouped discharges fire at rates up to 60 Hz. In electrical *neuromyotonia*, on the other hand, continuous discharges occur at rates of 150 to 300 Hz and tend to start or stop abruptly. In Isaacs syndrome, both the clinical and the EMG features are present, but myokymia may be found in the EMG of some individuals without any clinically visible twitching.

As a result of the continuous activity, a second characteristic of the syndrome is the finding of *abnormal postures* of the limbs, which may be persistent or intermittent and are identical to carpal or pedal spasm. A third characteristic is *pseudomyotonia*, which resembles the difficulty in relaxing in true myotonia; here, however, the characteristic EMG pattern—waxing and waning of myotonic bursts—is not seen. Instead, continuous motor unit activity interferes with relaxation. In addition, there is no percussion myotonia. The fourth characteristic is *liability to cramps. Hyperhidrosis,* or increased sweating, is variable.

The syndrome affects children, adolescents, or young adults and begins insidiously, progressing slowly for months or a few years. Slow movement, clawing of the fingers, and toe-walking are later joined by stiffness of proximal and axial muscles; occasionally, oropharyngeal or respiratory muscles are affected. The stiffness and myokymia are seen at rest and persist in sleep. Voluntary contraction may induce a spasm that persists during attempted relaxation.

▶ **TABLE 130.2 Manifestations of Isaacs Syndrome in 28 Patients**

	Patients (n)		
	Present	**Absent**	**Not Mentioned**
Clinical			
Myokymia	28	0	0
Cramps	15	2	11
Pseudomyotonia	15	3	10
Carpopedal spasm	12	2	14
Sweating	15	3	10
Chvostek sign	1	2	25
Trousseau sign	1	2	25
Response to hyperventilation	0	0	28
Electromyography			
Multiplets	18	0	10
After discharge	6	1	21
Ischemia augments	3	0	16
Ischemia decreases	9	0	16
Hyperventilation increases	0	1	27
Activity decreased by			
Sleep	0	18	10
General anesthesia	0	6	22
Spinal anesthesia	1	4	23
Nerve block	9	7	12
Curare	7	0	21
Diazepam	1	12	15
Carabamazepine	14	2	12
Phenytoin	16	5	7
Evidence of peripheral neuropathy			
Paresthesia	3	7	18
Cutaneous sensory loss	4	14	10
Limb weakness	7	16	5
Knee jerks	16	12	0
Ankle jerks	13	15	0
CSF protein 50–100 mg/dL	1	13	12
> 100 mg/dL	2	13	12
MNCV slow	9	11	8
SNCV slow	4	8	16
Denervation, muscle biopsy	5	13	10
Abnormal nerve biopsy	2	1	25
Neuropathy clear	4	22	—
Neuropathy possible	2	22	—

MNCV, motor nerve conduction velocity; SNCV, sensory nerve conduction velocity.
Modified from Rowland, 1985.

The EMG recorded from stiff muscles reveals prolonged myokymic or neuromyotonic discharges. Voluntary effort triggers more intense discharges that persist during relaxation, accounting for the myotonialike aftercontraction. The condition is often attributed to a peripheral neuropathy because acral sensory loss is noted in some patients, nerve conduction may be slow, or abnormality may appear on sural nerve biopsy. The EMG activity may persist after nerve block by injection of local anesthetic but is abolished by botulinum toxin, implying that the activity arises distal to the nerve block and proximal to the neuromuscular junction; the generator must be in the nerve terminals. In an analysis of 28 reported cases, however, only four patients had definite evidence of peripheral neuropathy (Table 130.2).

Many of the advances have come from a group of investigators centered at Oxford University. They now classify these conditions as variants of autoimmune peripheral nerve hyperexcitability. Hart et al. compared the clinical characteristics of two groups of patients with fasciculations, myokymia, or cramps. One group showed myokymic doublets or multiplets in the EMG; the other did not. In both groups, compared to normal populations, there were VGKC antibodies and other autoantibodies (especially to the acetyl choline receptor); thymoma with or without myasthenia gravis and myasthenia gravis with or without thymoma, insulin-dependent diabetes mellitus, and carcinomas of breast or lung. Cerebral symptoms are evident in some patients who have sleep disorders and personality change as well as VGKC antibodies; the name for this condition is Morvan syndrome. The same antibodies are found in limbic encephalitis. The possibility of paraneoplastic or autoimmune disorder should therefore be considered in the differential diagnosis of Foley, Denny-Brown or neuromyotonia.

Treatment with carbamazepine or phenytoin usually controls the symptoms and signs. Plasmapheresis and intravenous immunoglobulin therapy have been effective in some patients.

TETANY

Tetany is a clinical syndrome characterized by convulsions, paresthesia, prolonged spasms of limb muscles, or laryngospasm; it is accompanied by signs of hyperexcitability of peripheral nerves. It occurs in patients with hypocalcemia, hypomagnesemia, or alkalosis; it is occasionally a primary neural abnormality. Hyperventilation may unmask latent hypocalcemic tetany, but respiratory alkalosis itself only rarely causes outright tetany.

Intense circumoral and digital paresthesia generally precedes the typical carpopedal spasms, which consist of adduction and extension of the fingers, flexion of the metacarpophalangeal joints, and equinovarus postures of the feet. In severe cases, the spasms spread to the proximal and axial muscles, eventually causing opisthotonus. In all forms of tetany, the nerves are hyperexcitable, as manifested by the reactions to ischemia (Trousseau sign) and percussion (Chvostek sign). The spasms are owing to spontaneous firing of peripheral nerves, starting in the proximal portions of the longest nerves. EMG shows individual motor units discharging independently at a rate of 5 to 25 Hz; each discharge consists of a group of two or more identical potentials.

The treatment of tetany consists of correcting the underlying metabolic disorder. In hypomagnesemia, tetany does not respond to correction of the accompanying hypocalcemia unless the magnesium deficit is also corrected.

STIFF MAN SYNDROME (MOERSCH-WOLTMAN SYNDROME)

The catchy name for this syndrome was coined by two senior clinicians at the Mayo Clinic in 1956. The name has been perpetuated since, but the titles have sometimes been awkward (e.g., stiff man syndrome in a woman, stiff man syndrome in a boy, stiff baby syndrome, or stiff person syndrome). We now strive for gender-neutral language; the masculine version is especially inappropriate for a syndrome that occurs equally often in women and men. The eponym seems apropos.

Clinical Manifestations

The Moersch-Woltman syndrome is defined clinically, with progressive muscular rigidity and painful spasms that resemble a chronic form of tetanus. The symptoms develop over several months or years and may either increase slowly or become stable. Aching discomfort and stiffness tend to predominate in the axial and proximal limb muscles, causing awkwardness of gait and slowness of movement. Trismus does not occur, but facial and oropharyngeal muscles may be affected. The stiffness diminishes during sleep and under general anesthesia. Later, painful reflex spasms occur in response to movement, sensory stimulation, or emotion. The spasms may lead to joint deformities and are powerful enough to rupture muscles, rip surgical sutures, or fracture bones. Passive muscle stretch provokes an exaggerated reflex contraction that lasts several seconds. Whether any of the findings in Table 130.3 must be present to make the diagnosis is not clear. For instance, the response to diazepam may not be complete, or the spinal deformity may not be present. And some investigators have noted that findings on examination and EMG activity are compatible with those of voluntary behavior. A psychogenic cause has been mentioned, however, only to be derided because the tin-soldier appearance of the patient is so dramatic and because the spasms may cause physical injury. However, when the motor disorder is severe, 44% of patients in one

▶ **TABLE 130.3** Defining Characteristics of the
Moersch-Woltman Syndrome

Prodromal stiffness of axial muscles
Slow progress to proximal limbs; walking awkward
Fixed deformity of the spine; lordosis; "permanent shrug"
   (neck drawn down to shoulder girdle)
Spasms precipitated by startle, jarring, noise, emotional upset
Otherwise normal findings on motor and sensory examination
Normal intellect and affect
Continuous motor activity in affected muscles relieved by intravenous
   or oral diazepam

Modified from Lorish et al., 1989.

series had task-specific phobia, fearing open spaces or trying to cross a street. Psychogenic movement disorder may be the most difficult alternate diagnosis.

Laboratory Data

EMG recordings from stiff muscles show a continuous discharge of motor unit potentials resembling normal voluntary contraction. As in tetanus, the activity is not inhibited by voluntary contraction of the antagonist muscles; however, a normal silent period is present during the stretch reflex, indicating that there is no impairment of recurrent spinal inhibition. The rigidity is abolished by spinal anesthesia, by peripheral nerve block, or by selective block of gamma motor nerve fibers. Some authors have postulated that both alpha and gamma motor neurons are rendered hyperactive by excitatory influences descending from the brainstem. The electroencephalogram is normal. Routine CSF analysis is also normal, but the IgG concentration may be increased and oligoclonal immunoglobulin G (IgG) bands may be present.

Administration of diazepam is the most effective symptomatic treatment; high doses may be required. Additional benefit can be obtained in some cases from administration of baclofen, phenytoin, clonidine (Catapres), or tizanidine (Zanaflex). Intrathecal baclofen (Lioresal) has been used. The long-term prognosis is still uncertain.

The pathogenesis may involve autoimmunity. Antibodies to glutamate decarboxylase have been found in both serum and CSF, with evidence of intrathecal synthesis in more than half the cases. Diabetes mellitus occurs in 30% of Moersch-Woltman patients; similarly, nearly all patients with insulin-dependent diabetes have serum antibodies to glutamic acid decarboxylase, although the titers are much lower than in the Moersch-Woltman syndrome.

Treatment with intravenous human immunoglobulin is beneficial in most patients, and other types of immunosuppressive therapy are sometimes helpful. The Moersch-Woltman syndrome is sometime paraneoplastic; cases associated with breast cancer are usually accompanied by antibodies to amphiphysin rather than glutamic acid decarboxylase.

Differential Diagnosis

Evidence of corticospinal tract disease or abnormality of the CSF implies an anatomic disorder of the CNS, but in postmortem examination of typical cases, no CNS histopathology is revealed. Patients with similar physical findings may show CSF pleocytosis or Babinski signs. In autopsies of those patients, however, inflammation has been sufficient to warrant the term *encephalomyelitis*. Stiffness of the arms in some patients with cervical lesions is attributed to spontaneous activity of alpha motor neurons isolated from synaptic influences. That combination is best regarded as *stiff encephalomyelitis*, because the pathogenesis ought to differ in the two categories with or without clear evidence of CNS disease. However, antibodies to glutamate decarboxylase have also been found in patients with myelitis. A related disorder has been called the *stiff limb syndrome*.

The main distinction between Moersch-Woltman and Isaacs syndromes is the distribution of the symptoms, which affect the distal arms and legs in Isaacs and the trunk in Moersch-Woltman. Myokymia is seen only in Isaacs. Many of the features of Isaacs syndrome are similar to those of tetany, as are the painful tonic spasms multiple sclerosis (MS). MS, however, is identified by other signs of disseminated CNS lesions. These tonic spasms, like other paroxysmal symptoms in MS, are thought to originate as ectopic activity in demyelinated CNS nerve tracts. They usually last less than 1 minute but occur many times a day. The attacks usually respond promptly to treatment with carbamazepine or phenytoin. The startle reactions of Moersch-Woltman syndrome are similar to those in the autosomal-dominant condition *hyperekplexia* or *startle disease* (MIM 149400). Hyperekplexia, however, lacks axial rigidity and has been mapped to a subunit of an inhibitory glycine receptor on chromosome 5. It is relieved by the τ-aminobutyric acid agonist clonidine. The Moersch-Woltman syndrome itself is rarely autosomal dominant (MIM 184850). The fixed postures of the limbs in Isaacs syndrome can be simulated by the Schwartz-Jampel syndrome (SJS) (see Chapter 126). However, SJS is characterized by a unique facial appearance (blepharophimosis), short stature, and bony abnormalities. In SJS, the more frequent EMG pattern is that of myotonia, but there may be continuous motor activity with both myokymic and neuromyotonic discharges.

SUGGESTED READINGS

Cramps and Related Disorders

Blexrud MD, Windebank AJ, Daube JR. Long-term follow-up of 121 patients with benign fasciculations. *Ann Neurol* 1993;34:622–625.
Connolly PS, Shirley EA, Wasson JH, et al. Treatment of nocturnal leg cramps: crossover trial of quinine versus vitamin E. *Arch Intern Med* 1992;152:1877–1880.

Dressler D, Thompson PD, Gledhill RF, et al. The syndrome of painful legs and moving toes. *Mov Disord* 1994;9:13–21.

Layzer RB. Motor unit hyperactivity states. In: Engel AG, Franzini-Armstrong C, eds. *Myology.* 3rd Ed. London: Churchill Livingstone, 2004.

Layzer RB. The origin of muscle fasciculations and cramps. *Muscle Nerve* 1994;17:1243–1249.

Man-Son Hing M, Wells G, Lau A. Quinine for nocturnal leg cramps: a meta-analysis including unpublished data. *J Gen Intern Med* 1998;13:600–606.

Rose MR, Ball JA, Thompson PD. Magnetic resonance imaging in tonic spasms of multiple sclerosis. *J Neurol* 1993;241:115–117.

Rowland LP. Cramps, spasms, and muscle stiffness. *Rev Neurol (Paris)* 1985;4:261–273.

Rowland LP, Trojaborg W, Haller RG. Muscle contracture: physiology and clinical classification. In: Serratrice G, Pouget J, Azulay J-Ph, eds. *Exercise Intolerance and Muscle Contracture.* Paris: Springer, 1999:161–170.

Neuromyotonia

Arimura K, Sonoda Y, Watanabe O, et al. Isaacs syndrome as a potassium channelopathy of the nerve. *Muscle Nerve* 2002 (Suppl);11:S55–58.

Deymeer F, Oge AE, Serdaroglu P, et al. The use of botulinum toxin in localizing neuromyotonia to the terminal branches of the peripheral nerve. *Muscle Nerve* 1998;21:643–646.

Eunson LH, Rea R, Zuberi SM, et al. Clinical, genetic, and expression studies of mutations in potassium channel gene KCNA1 reveal a new phenotypic variability. *Ann Neurol* 2000;48:647–656.

Hart IK, Maddison P, Newsom-Davis J, et al. Phenotypic variants of autoimmune peripheral nerve hyperexcitability. *Brain* 2002;125:1887–1895.

Karpati G, Charuk J, Carpenter S, et al. Myopathy caused by a deficiency of Ca2+-adenosine triphosphatase in sarcoplasmic reticulum (Brody's disease). *Ann Neurol* 1986;20:38–49.

Liguori R, Vincent A, Clover L, et al. Morvan's syndrome: peripheral and central nervous system and cardiac involvement with antibodies to voltage-gated potassium channels. *Brain* 2001;124;2417–2426.

Newsom-Davis J, Buckley C, Clover I, et al. Autoimmune disorders of neuronal potassium channels. *Ann N Y Acad Sci* 2003;998:202–210.

Newsom-Davis J, Mills KR. Immunological associations of acquired neuromyotonia (Isaacs' syndrome). *Brain* 1993;116:453–469.

Taylor RG, Layzer RB, Davis HS, et al. Continuous muscle fiber activity in the Schwartz-Jampel syndrome. *Electroencephalogr Clin Neurophysiol* 1972;33:497–509.

Torbensen T, Stalberg E, Brautaset NJ. Generator sites for spontaneous activity in neuromyotonia: an EMG study. *Electroencephalogr Clin Neurophysiol* 1996;101:69–78.

Stiff Man Syndrome (Moersch-Woltman Syndrome)

Barker RA, Revesz T, Thom M, et al. Review of 23 patients affected by the stiff man syndrome: clinical subdivision into stiff trunk (man) syndrome, stiff limb syndrome, and progressive encephalomyelitis with rigidity. *J Neurol Neurosurg Psychiatry* 1998;65:633–640.

Dalakas MC, Fujii M, Lufti B, et al. High dose intravenous immune globulin for stiff-person syndrome. *N Engl J Med* 2001;345:1870–1876.

Dalakas MC, Li M, Fujii M, et al. M. Stiff person syndrome. Quantification, specificity, and intrathecal synthesis of GAD$_{65}$ antibodies. *Neurology* 2001;57:780–784.

Floeter MK, Valla-Sole J, Toro C, et al. Physiologic studies of spinal inhibitory circuits in patients with stiff-person syndrome. *Neurology* 1998;51:85–93.

Henningsen P, Meinck HM. Specific phobia is a frequent non-motor feature in stiff man syndrome. *J Neurol Neurosurg Psychiatry* 2003;74:462–465.

Lorish TR, Thorsteinsson G, Howard FH Jr. Stiff-man syndrome updated. *Mayo Clin Proc* 1989;64:629–636.

McEvoy KM. Stiff-man syndrome. *Mayo Clin Proc* 1991;66:303–304.

Meinck H-M, Thompson PD. Stiff man syndrome and related conditions. *Movement Dis* 2002;17:853–866.

Moersch FP, Woltman HW. Progressive fluctuating muscular rigidity and spasm (stiff-man syndrome): report of a case and some observations in 13 other cases. *Proc Staff Meet Mayo Clin* 1956;31:421–427.

Penn RD, Mangieri EA. Stiff-man syndrome treated with intrathecal baclofen. *Neurology* 1993;43:2412.

Petzold GC, Marcucci M, Butler MH, et al. Rhabdomyolysis and paraneoplastic stiff-man syndrome with amphiphysin autoimmunity. *Ann Neurol* 2004;55:286–290.

Solimena M, Folli F, Aparisi R, et al. Autoantibodies to GABA-ergic neurons and pancreatic beta cells in stiff man syndrome. *N Engl J Med* 1990;322:1555–1560.

▶ Dermatomyositis

Lewis P. Rowland

Dermatomyositis, a disease of unknown cause, is characterized by inflammatory changes in skin and muscle.

PATHOLOGY AND PATHOGENESIS

Dermatomyositis is thought to be an autoimmune disease, but there has been no consistent evidence of either antibodies or lymphocytes directed against specific muscle antigens. However, muscle histologists have agreed that dermatomyositis is humorally mediated, characterized by more B cells than T cells in the muscle infiltrates, and a vasculopathy with deposits of complement in intramuscular blood vessels. This contrasts with the predominance of T cells in polymyositis, which is attributed to a disorder of lymphocyte regulation. Some authorities believe that the pathogenesis of dermatomyositis differs in adults and children.

The acute changes of both skin and muscle are marked by signs of degeneration, regeneration, edema, and infiltration by lymphocytes. The inflammatory cells are found around small vessels or in the perimysium rather than within the muscle fiber itself. In muscle biopsies, however, lymphocytic infiltration may be lacking in 25% of patients; this probably depends on the time of sampling, as well as on the distribution and severity of the process. The lymphocytes are predominantly B cells, with some CD4 (T-helper) cells. Capillaries often show endothelial hyperplasia; deposits of immunoglobulin (Ig) G, IgM, and complement (the membrane attack complex) may be found within and occluding these vessels. Evidence of muscle degeneration and regeneration is multifocal and may be most marked at the periphery of muscle bundles (*perifascicular atrophy*), where the capillaries are occluded. Increasingly, investigators have come to believe that the primary attack is on blood vessels. A similar myopathy without skin lesions can be induced in animals by immunization with muscle extracts. Viruslike particles have been seen in some cases, but no virus has been cultured from muscle. Some authorities make the diagnosis from the perifasciular atrophy and other histologic changes rather than the clinical features, but Greenberg and Amato (2004) provide a healthy skepticism about the holes in modern theories.

INCIDENCE

Dermatomyositis is rare. Together with polymyositis, the incidence has been estimated to be about seven cases each year for a population of 1 million. That figure may be too low; in our 1,200-bed hospital, we see about five new cases of dermatomyositis and 10 cases of polymyositis each year.

Dermatomyositis occurs in all decades of life, with peaks of incidence before puberty and at about age 40 years. In young adults, women are more likely to be affected. Familial cases are rare. It is generally believed that about 10% of cases starting after age 40 are associated with malignant neoplasms, most often carcinoma of lung or breast. Typical findings, including the rash, have also been seen in patients with agammaglobulinemia, graft-versus-host disease, toxoplasmosis, hypothyroidism, sarcoidosis, ipecac abuse, hepatitis B virus infection, penicillamine reactions, or vaccine reactions. Cases have even been ascribed to azathioprine (Imuran). Most cases are idiopathic but the diverse causes indicate that dermatomyositis is a syndrome, not necessarily a unique condition.

SYMPTOMS AND SIGNS

The first manifestations usually involve both skin and muscle at about the same time. The rash may precede weakness by several weeks, but weakness alone is almost never the first symptom. Sometimes, the rash is so typical that the diagnosis can be made even without evidence of myopathy (amyopathic dermatomyositis), and sometimes weakness is not evident but there is EMG, biopsy, or serum creatine kinase (CK) evidence of myopathy.

The rash may be confined to the face in a butterfly distribution around the nose and cheeks, but the edema and erythema are especially likely to affect the eyelids, periungual skin, and extensor surfaces of the knuckles, elbows, and knees. The upper chest is another common site. The initial redness may be replaced later by brownish pigmentation. The Gottron sign is denoted by red-purple scaly macules on the extensor surfaces of finger joints. Fibrosis of subcutaneous tissue and thickening of the skin may lead to the appearance of scleroderma. Later, especially in children, calcinosis may involve subcutaneous tissues and fascial planes within muscle. The calcium deposits may extrude through the skin.

Affected muscles may ache and are often tender. Weakness of proximal limb muscles causes difficulty in lifting, raising the arms overhead, rising from low seats, climbing stairs, or even walking on level ground. The interval from onset of weakness to most severe disability is measured in weeks. Cranial muscles are spared, except that dysphagia is noted by about one-third of patients. Some patients have difficulty in holding the head up because neck muscles are weak. Sensation is preserved, tendon reflexes may or may not be lost, and there is no fasciculation.

Systemic symptoms are uncommon. Fever and malaise may characterize the acute stage in a minority of patients. Pulmonary fibrosis is encountered, and rarely there are cardiac symptoms. Arthralgia may be prominent, but deforming arthritis and renal failure have never been documented.

In about 10% of patients, the cutaneous manifestations have features of both scleroderma and dermatomyositis, warranting the name *sclerodermatomyositis*. These cases have sometimes been designated as *mixed connective tissue disease*, with a high incidence of antibody to extractable nuclear antigen; however, it now seems unlikely that the mixed syndrome is unique in any way.

DIAGNOSIS

The characteristic rash and myopathy usually make the diagnosis clear at a glance. Problems may arise if the rash is inconspicuous; in those cases the differential diagnosis is that of polymyositis (see Chapter 132). Other collagen-vascular diseases may cause both rash and myopathy at the same time, but systemic lupus erythematosus is likely to affect kidneys, synovia, and the CNS in patterns that are never seen in dermatomyositis. Similarly, there has never been a documented case of typical rheumatoid arthritis with typical dermatomyositis. The diagnosis of dermatomyositis is therefore clinical, based on the rash and myopathy. There is no pathognomonic laboratory test.

Except for the presence of lymphocytes and perifascicular atrophy in the muscle biopsy and increased serum CK (and other sarcoplasmic enzymes), there are no characteristic laboratory abnormalities. The EMG shows myopathic abnormalities and, often, evidence of increased irritability of muscle. CT and MRI show nonspecific changes in muscle but are useful in evaluating pulmonary fibrosis. Nonspecific serologic abnormalities include rheumatoid factor and several different kinds of antinuclear antibodies, none consistently present in patients with dermatomyositis. For instance, anti-Jo antibodies (against histidyl transfer RNA synthetase) are present in about 50% of patients with pulmonary fibrosis, but only 20% of all patients with inflammatory myopathies.

Once the diagnosis is made, many clinicians set off on a search for occult neoplasm. In preimaging days, Callen (1982) showed that in most cases a tumor was already evident or that there was an abnormality in some simple routine test (blood count, erythrocyte sedimentation rate, test for heme pigment in stool, chest film) or in findings on physical examination including pelvis and rectum. However, investigations have not yet evaluated the impact of CT or MRI of the chest, abdomen, and pelvis on the discovery of tumors in patients with dermatomyositis. PET has gained in popularity in seeking an occult tumor. Sometimes, no matter how exhaustive the search, the tumor is not discovered until autopsy is performed.

PROGNOSIS

The natural history of dermatomyositis is now unknown because patients are automatically treated with steroids. The disease may become inactive after 5 to 10 years. Although the mortality rate 50 years ago was given as 33% to 50%, it is not appropriate to use those ancient figures for current comparison; antibiotics and respirators affect outcome as much as any presumably specific immunotherapy. Even so, in reviews published after 1982, mortality rates were 23% to 44%. Because few fatalities have occurred in children, many of the deaths are caused by the associated malignancy. Other causes of death are myocarditis, pulmonary fibrosis, or steroid-induced complications. The myopathy may also be severe. In an analysis of survivors of childhood dermatomyositis, 83% were capable of self-care, almost all were working, and 50% were married; 33% had persistent rash or weakness, and a similar number had calcinosis.

TREATMENT

The standard therapy for dermatomyositis is administration of prednisone. The recommended dose for adults is at least 60 mg daily; higher dosages are often given for severe cases. For children, the recommended dose is higher: 2 mg/kg body weight. The basic dosage is continued for at least 1 month, perhaps longer. If the patient has improved by then, the dosage can be reduced slowly. If there has been no improvement, choices include prolonging the trial of prednisone in the same or a higher dosage with or without the addition of an immunosuppressive drug chosen according to local usage.

In the past decade, improvement was reported in 80% of all steroid-treated patients in one series, but only 50% or fewer patients benefited in other studies. Apparent response to treatment of individual patients with relapses on withdrawal of medication has been reported anecdotally many times. In one retrospective analysis, favorable outcome of childhood dermatomyositis seemed to be linked to early treatment (less than 4 months after onset) and use of high doses of prednisone. Dubowitz (1984), however, reported just the reverse: better outcome and fewer steroid complications with low doses of prednisone (1 mg/kg body weight).

The value of steroid treatment is still unproved, however, because there has never been a prospectively controlled study. In one retrospective analysis, untreated patients were seen many years before treated patients. In another study, there was no difference in outcome of patients treated with prednisone alone or with both prednisone and azathioprine. Moreover, it is not clear whether immunosuppressive drugs are more or less dangerous than steroids, and there is no evidence that any single immunosuppressive drug is superior to others. Azathioprine, methotrexate, cyclophosphamide, and cyclosporine have all been championed.

Plasmapheresis was of no value in a controlled trial, but IVIG therapy was uniformly beneficial in eight patients with steroid-resistant dermatomyositis, in contrast to no improvement in seven blinded, control patients who were given placebo. IVIG therapy may therefore be the procedure of choice for acute therapy of seriously ill patients. Some long-term immunosuppressive therapy, however, would have to be added. IVIG therapy is also useful in adults or children who do not respond to other agents. Mycophenolate is increasingly popular. Therapy is clearly not optimal because cyclophosphamide is still being used for children, with relative safety.

Some clinicians worry that exercising a weak muscle may be harmful, but formal tests in dermatomyositis and polymyositis have shown benefit.

SUGGESTED READINGS

Andrews A, Hickling P, Hutton C. Familial dermatomyositis. *Br J Rheumatol* 1998;37:231–232.

Banker BQ, Victor M. Dermatomyositis (systemic angiopathy) in childhood. *Medicine* 1966;45:261–289.

Bohan A, Peter JB, Bowman RL, et al. A computer-assisted analysis of 153 patients with polymyositis and dermatomyositis. *Medicine* 1977;56:255–286.

Callen JP. The value of malignancy evaluation in patients with dermatomyositis. *J Am Acad Dermatol* 1982;6:253–259.

Chalmers A, Sayson R, Walters K. Juvenile dermatomyositis: medical, social and economic status in adulthood. *Can Med Assoc J* 1982;126: 31–33.

Dalakas MC, Hohlfeld R. Polymyositis and dermatomyositis. *Lancet* 2003;362;971–982.

Dalakas MC, Illa I, Dambrosia JM, et al. A controlled trial of high-dose intravenous immune globulin infusions as treatment for dermatomyositis. *N Engl J Med* 1993;329:1993–2000.

Dalakas MC. Inflammatory disorders of muscle: progress in polymyositis, dermatomyositis and inclusion body myositis. *Curr Opin Neurol* 2004;17(5):561–567.

Dubowitz V. Prognostic factors in dermatomyositis [Letter]. *J Pediatr* 1984;105:336–337.

Esmie-Smith AM, Engel AG. Microvascular changes in early and advanced dermatomyositis: a quantitative study. *Ann Neurol* 1990;27:343–356.

Euwer RL, Sontheimer RD. Amyopathic dermatomyositis (dermatomyositis sine myositis): six new cases. *J Am Acad Dermatol* 1991;24: 959–966.

Fathi M, Dastmalchi M, Rasmussen E, et al. Interstitial lung disease, a common manifestation of newly diagnosed polymyositis and dermatomyositis. *Ann Rheum Dis* 2004;63(Mar):297–301.

Greenberg SA, Amato A. Uncertainties in the pathogenesis of adult dermatomyositis. *Curr Op Neurol* 2004;17:359–364.

Hengstman GJ, van den Hoogen FH, van Engelen BG. Treatment of dermatomyositis and polymyositis with anti-tumor necrosis factor-alpha: long-term follow-up. *Eur Neurol* 2004;52(1):61–63.

Hochberg MC. Mortality from polymyositis and dermatomyositis in the United States, 1968–1978. *Arthritis Rheum* 1983;26:1465–1472.

Hochberg MC, Feldman D, Stevens MB. Adult-onset polymyositis/dermatomyositis: an analysis of clinical and laboratory features and survival of 76 patients. *Semin Arthritis Rheum* 1986;15:168–178.

Kissel JT, Halterman RK, Rammohan KW, et al. The relationship of complement-mediated microvasculopathy to the histologic features and clinical duration of disease in dermatomyositis. *Arch Neurol* 1991;48:26–30.

Maugars YM, Berthelot JMM, Aabbas AA, et al. Long-term prognosis of 69 patients with dermatomyositis or polymyositis. *Clin Exp Rheumatol* 1996;14:263–274.

Mease PJ, Ochs HD, Wedgwood RJ. Successful treatment of echovirus meningoencephalitis and myositis-fasciitis with intravenous immune globulin therapy in a patient with X-linked agammaglobulinemia. *N Engl J Med* 1981;304:1278–1281.

Mendez EP, Lipton R, Ramsey-Goldman R, et al. US incidence of juvenile dermatomyositis, 1995–1998: results from the National Institute of Arthritis and Musculoskeletal and Skin Diseases Registry. *Arthritis Rheum* 2003;49:300–305.

Nimmelstein SH, Brody S, McShane D, et al. Mixed connective tissue disease: a subsequent evaluation of the original 25 patients. *Medicine* 1980;59:239–248.

Ollivier I, Wolkenstein P, Gheradi R, et al. Dermatomyositis-like graft-versus-host disease. *Br J Dermatol* 1998;138:358–359.

Pachman LM, Hayford JR, Chung A, et al. Juvenile dermatomyositis at diagnosis: clinical characteristics of 79 children. *J Rheumatol* 1998;25:1198–1204.

Riley P, Maillard SM, Wedderburn LR, et al. Intravenous cyclophosphamide pulse therapy in juvenile dermatomyositis. A review of efficacy and safety. *Rheumatology (Oxford)* 2004;43(Apr):491–496.

Rowland LP, Clark C, Olarte MR. Therapy for dermatomyositis and polymyositis. *Adv Neurol* 1977;17:63–97.

Sigurgeirsson B, Lindelof B, Edhag O, et al. Risk of cancer in patients with dermatomyositis or polymyositis: a population-based study. *N Engl J Med* 1992;326:363–367.

Van der Meulen MFG, Bronner IM, Hoogendijk JE, et al. Polymyositis: an overdiagnosed entity. *Neurology* 2003;61:316–321.

Vasconcelos OM, Campbell WW. Dermatomyositis-like syndrome and HMG-CoA reductase inhibitor (statin) intake. *Muscle Nerve* 2004 Dec;30(6):803–807.

Wiesinger GF, Quittan M, Graninger M, et al. Benefit of 6 months' long-term physical training in polymyositis/dermatomyositis patients. *Br J Rheumatol* 1998;37:1338–1342.

C h a p t e r   1 3 2

Polymyositis, Inclusion Body Myositis, and Related Myopathies

Lewis P. Rowland

DEFINITION OF POLYMYOSITIS

Polymyositis is a disorder of skeletal muscle of diverse causes. It is characterized by acute or subacute onset and possible intervals of improvement of symptoms; typically, muscle biopsy shows infiltration of myofibers by lymphocytes. Polymyositis is one of the three major categories of inflammatory myopathy; each differs from the others clinically and in muscle pathology. The other two conditions are dermatomyositis and inclusion body myositis (IBM).

This definition is insufficiently precise, however, because there is no pathognomonic clinical syndrome, laboratory test, or combination of the two. The problem arises because lymphocytic infiltration of muscle may be lacking in an individual case or the typical pattern may not be seen; also, lymphocytic infiltration can be seen in other conditions. Additionally, polymyositis may occur alone or as part of a systemic disease, especially a collagen-vascular disease. The vagaries of definition have generated vigorous debates about the frequency of polymyositis compared to the other inflammatory myopathies or even whether it is more than a mythical unicorn.

CLINICAL MANIFESTATIONS

The symptoms are those of a myopathy that primarily affects proximal limb muscles: difficulty climbing stairs or rising from low seats, lifting packages or dishes, or working with the arms overhead. Weakness of neck muscles may result in difficulty holding the head erect, the dropped head or floppy head syndrome. Distal muscles are usually affected later, so difficulty using the hands is not encountered at first. Eyelids and ocular movements are spared; the only cranial symptom is dysphagia, usually without dysarthria. Respiration is only rarely affected as a consequence of muscle weakness (but pulmonary fibrosis may occur).

Symptoms of systemic disease, malaise, or even weight loss are not evident. In many cases, arthralgia is symptomatic without objective change in the joints. Raynaud symptoms may be prominent, but by definition, there is no rash of dermatomyositis. No visceral lesions appear, other than interstitial lung disease and pulmonary fibrosis in some patients. Myocarditis may also occur. The syndrome is usually subacute in onset, reaching a nadir in months rather than weeks or years, but both acute and chronic forms are seen. Symptoms may persist for years, and then the condition seems to become quiescent.

LABORATORY DATA

The findings are those of a myopathy, with characteristic EMG findings of small-amplitude short-duration potentials and full recruitment. Signs of muscle "irritability" may be noted, with fibrillations and positive waves but no fasciculations. Nerve conduction studies give normal values. Serum levels of creatine kinase (CK) and other sarcoplasmic enzymes are often increased to values 10 times normal or even more. Serum enzyme levels may be normal, however, probably depending on the stage of the disease.

A definite diagnosis requires characteristic changes in the muscle biopsy, especially infiltration around healthy muscle fibers by cells that have the immunocytochemical characteristics of CD8+ T lymphocytes. Signs of muscle necrosis and regeneration are apparent, but the pattern differs from that of dermatomyositis because neither vascular lesions nor perifascicular atrophy are seen. The pattern differs from IBM because vacuoles or the defining inclusions are not evident. Dalakas has advocated evidence of infiltration by CD8 lymphocytes and expression of the MHC-1 antigen. Some rheumatologists still depend on criteria proposed by Bohan and Peters a half century ago; neurologists interested in neuromuscular disease never embraced those criteria, which essentially define a myopathy, nothing more.

PATHOGENESIS

Polymyositis is considered an autoimmune disease of disordered cellular immunity (in contrast to the presumed humoral abnormalities of dermatomyositis). The nature of the antigen is not known, however, and the nature of the immunologic aberration is not known. The association with collagen-vascular disease increases the likelihood of autoimmune disorder, as does the association of polymyositis with other autoimmune diseases, including Crohn disease, biliary cirrhosis, sarcoidosis, myasthenia gravis with thymoma and candidiasis, or graft-versus-host disease. HIV and human T-cell lymphotropic virus type I are viral diseases associated with polymyositis; it is not known whether this kind of polymyositis is a viral infection of muscle or an autoimmune reaction. In contrast to

dermatomyositis, myopathy without rash is uncommon in patients with concomitant malignant neoplasms.

Fibers adjacent to the T cells express the class 1 major histocompatibility complex, an antigen that is lacking in normal fibers and is a recognition factor for the activation of T cells. Circulating T cells may be cytotoxic to cultures of the patient's myotubes.

In the past decade, interest has been directed to antibodies to cytoplasmic ribonucleoproteins. Because they are not disease specific, however, they neither help to explain pathogenesis nor provide a reliable diagnostic tool. Anti-Jo antibodies are found in about half of all patients with both polymyositis and pulmonary fibrosis.

DIAGNOSIS

In the past, polymyositis was regarded as dermatomyositis without a rash. The histologic differences are now recognized, but the clinical problem remains: How can we identify the qualities of polymyositis that are similar to those of dermatomyositis while distinguishing polymyositis from other myopathies with which it might be confused, such as muscular dystrophies, metabolic myopathies, or disorders of the neuromuscular junction? The following criteria are suggested:

1. There is no family history of similar disease, and onset is usually after age 35. No familial limb-girdle dystrophy starts so late. Cases of younger onset are few, unless there is some associated collagen-vascular or other systemic disease. If there is no family history, it may be necessary to test for the sarcoglycanopathies.
2. Progression from onset to peak weakness is measured in weeks or months, not years as in the muscular dystrophies.
3. Symptoms may improve spontaneously or concomitantly with the administration of immunosuppressant therapy, unlike any adult-onset muscular dystrophy.
4. In addition to proximal limb weakness, there may be dysphagia or weakness of neck flexors, but other cranial muscles are not affected. (If eyelids or ocular muscles are involved, it would be difficult or impossible to distinguish the disorder from myasthenia gravis.)
5. Arthralgia, myalgia, and Raynaud symptoms help to make the diagnosis, but lack of these symptoms does not exclude the diagnosis.
6. Muscle biopsy usually shows the abnormalities described above, especially early in the course. As in patients with dermatomyositis, however, lymphocytic infiltration may be lacking in muscle biopsies in polymyositis. Typical histologic changes help to make the diagnosis; lack of these changes does not exclude the diagnosis because the changes may be focal in the muscle (skip lesions) or transient and not present in

the muscle at the site and time of the biopsy. In histochemical stains, there must be no evidence of excess lipid or glycogen storage and there should be no signs of denervation.

7. In addition to conventional EMG signs of myopathy, increased irritability of muscle may be evident.

The problem of diagnosis is exemplified by a patient with limb weakness at age 40 when EMG and muscle biopsy indicate that the disorder is a myopathy. Search must then be made for known causes of myopathy (Table 132.1). If none is found, the diagnosis of exclusion is idiopathic polymyositis.

It seems unlikely that this residual group is all owing to one disease because there is clinical heterogeneity, such as differences in rapidity of progression, distribution of weakness, or severity of disorder. In addition, if there are so many known causes of similar syndromes, it is likely

▶ **TABLE 132.1 Differential Diagnosis of Polymyositis**

Etiology unknown: Idiopathic polymyositis
Collagen-vascular diseases
SLE, rheumatoid arthritis, periarteritis nodosa, systemic sclerosis, giant cell arteritis, Sjögren syndrome
Infections
Toxoplasmosis, trichinosis, schistosomiasis, cysticercosis, Chagas disease, Legionnaire disease, candidiasis, acne fulminans, microspiradosis, AIDS, influenza virus, rubella, hepatitis B, Behçet, Kawasaki, mycoplasma, coxsackie, Echovirus
Immunization
Drugs
Systemic: ethanol penicillamine, clofibrate, steroids, emetine, chloroquine, kaluretics, aminocaproic acid, rifampicin, ipecac, zidovudine
Intramuscular: meperidine, pentazocine
Systemic diseases
Carcinoma, thymoma, sarcoid, amyloid, psoriasis, hyperglobulinemia (plasma cell dyscrasia), celiac disease, papular mucinosis, graft-vs.-host disease after transplantation, alcoholism
Endocrine diseases
Hyperthyroidism, hypothyroidism, hyperadrenocorticism, hyperparathyroidism, Hashimoto thyroiditis
Metabolic diseases
Therapeutic starvation, total parenteral nutrition, anorexia nervosa
Hypocalcemia, osteomalacia, chronic renal disease
Chronic K^+ depletion
Carnitine deficiency in muscle
Lack of acid maltase, phosphorylase, phosphofructokinase
Iron overload on maintenance hemodialysis
Toxins
Contaminated tryptophan (eosinophilia-myalgia syndrome), contaminated rapeseed oil (toxic oil syndrome)

that still more remain to be identified. A restricted concept of idiopathic polymyositis will emerge only when more is known about the disordered immunology of dermatomyositis itself.

If there is no family history of similar disease and especially if there are no inflammatory cells in the muscle biopsy, a form of limb-girdle muscular dystrophy must be considered. Sometimes polymyositis is the suspected diagnosis, but muscle biopsy shows glycogen or lipid accumulation or mitochondrial disease.

RELATION OF POLYMYOSITIS TO DERMATOMYOSITIS

These conditions are usually considered together because of the similarities in course and muscle disease. There are, however, important differences, as follows:

1. Dermatomyositis is most often a seemingly homogeneous condition, only rarely associated with a known cause other than carcinoma. Polymyositis is associated with some other systemic disease in about half the cases.
2. Polymyositis is often a manifestation of a specific collagen-vascular disease, such as systemic lupus erythematosus, systemic sclerosis, or different forms of vasculitis. Dermatomyositis, however, is rarely if ever associated with evidence of collagen-vascular disease other than scleroderma. When polymyositis occurs in a patient with lupus erythematosus, for instance, it can be regarded as a manifestation of lupus, not a combination of two different disorders (or an overlap syndrome).
3. Dermatomyositis occurs at all ages, including childhood. Polymyositis is rare before puberty.
4. As assessed by inability to walk, the myopathy of dermatomyositis is severe more often than the myopathy of polymyositis.
5. Dermatomyositis is far more likely to be associated with malignant neoplasm than is myopathy without rash.

RELATION OF POLYMYOSITIS TO INCLUSION BODY MYOSITIS

The attempt to link polymyositis to a viral infection led Chou (1986) to find tubular filaments in nuclear and cytoplasmic vacuoles in some patients with other pathologic features of polymyositis. Yunis and Samaha coined the name in 1971. These histologic findings were then related to a characteristic clinical syndrome (Table 132.2).

Polymyositis and IBM are similar in that they are inflammatory myopathies, lack a rash, and rarely affect children. IBM is slower in progression. Dysphagia is common

▶ **TABLE 132.2 Defining Features of Inclusion Body Myositis in 48 Patients**

	Patients (%)
Histology	
Fibers with rimmed vacuoles	100.00
Non-necrotic cells invaded	89.6
Necrotic fibers	79.2
Groups of atrophic fibers	91.7
Eosinophilic inclusions	58.3
Inflammation	
Endomysial	95.8
Perivascular	87.5
Perimysial	37.5
EM filaments (40/43 cases)	93.3
Symptoms	
Limb weakness	100.0
Age >50 year	83.7
Family history of same disease	0.0
Dysphagia	33.3
Myalgia	16.7
Signs	
Distal limb weakness	50.0
Distal weakness ≥proximal	35.0
KJs and AJs absent	27.1
Brisk tendon jerks	4.2
EMG	
Insertion activity increased	100.0
Fibrillation potentials	100.0
Fasciculation potentials	10.0
Short-duration potentials	100.0
Long-duration potentials	77.5
Both short and long in same muscle	75.0
Laboratory test	
Increased sedimentation rate	17.5
Creatine kinase level increased	80.0
Blood glucose increased	35.0
Antinuclear antibody	18.8

KJs, knee jerks; AJs, ankle jerks.
Modified from Lotz BP, Engel AG, Nishino H, et al. Inclusion body myositis. Observations in 40 patients. *Brain* 1989;112:727–747.

in both. Neither IBM nor polymyositis, in contrast to dermatomyositis, is often a paraneoplastic disorder. The two conditions differ clinically and histologically.

Clinically, IBM affects proximal limb muscles but, in contrast to polymyositis, is much more likely to affect distal muscles of the legs, and IBM is one of the few myopathies that causes weakness of the long finger flexors, an early and prominent symptom and sign in most IBM patients. IBM characteristically affects men after age 50; polymyositis affects younger adults as well and women more often than men. IBM more often shows mixed neurogenic and myopathic features in conventional EMG. In contrast to polymyositis, IBM is less often seen with

collagen-vascular or other autoimmune disorders. Serum CK values are normal or only slightly increased in IBM. A major distinction is the failure of IBM to respond to steroid therapy.

IBM and polymyositis differ pathologically because IBM is characterized by rimmed vacuoles, with the defining cellular inclusions and vacuoles. The pathogenesis of IBM is not known. Originally, IBM was thought to be a variant of polymyositis because, in addition to the inclusions, muscle is often infiltrated by lymphocytes in distribution, number, and T-cell characteristics similar to those of polymyositis. However, the vacuoles give immunochemical stains for proteins seen in the brain of patients with Alzheimer disease (β-amyloid precursor protein and others), which leads some investigators to regard IBM as a degenerative disease rather than an autoimmune disorder. Formally, the diagnosis should not be made without proof by biopsy. However, the clinical picture is so characteristic and rimmed vacuoles are so often lacking that clinical diagnosis is accepted as reliable, with implications about the lack of response to immunotherapy.

Yet another peculiar facet of IBM is the presence of ragged fibers and cytochrome *c* oxidase negative fibers, findings that imply abnormalities of mitochondria, which prove to be multiple deletions of mitochondrial DNA. How this arises or what it means in the pathogenesis of the disorder is still uncertain.

IBM may be familial with little inflammation and vacuolar histologic characteristics similar to those of autosomal-dominant Welander distal muscular dystrophy or oculopharyngeal muscular dystrophy; these syndromes differ clinically, but the similarities may cause problems in classification. Familial IBM is called inclusion body "myopathy" not "myositis." Originally described as an autosomal-recessive disease in Iranian Jews, it maps to 9p12-13 and is caused by mutations of the gene for UDP-N-acetylglucosamine-2-epimerase kinase (GNE). Clinically it differs from sporadic IBM in that the quadriceps is spared and, usually but not always, little inflammation is seen in the biopsy. A founder effect is evident and, in Israel, Muslims are affected as well as Jews. Some people carry the mutation without clinical symptoms. An autosomal-dominant form has been mapped to chromosome 9, so there is locus heterogeneity.

RELATION OF POLYMYOSITIS TO EOSINOPHILIC MYOSITIS

Rarely, a myopathy is associated with infiltration of muscle by eosinophils in addition to or instead of lymphocytes. One is the eosinophilic myositis of trichinosis or other parasitic infestation. Another form was seen in an epidemic in Spain of the toxic oil syndrome that was attributed to ingestion of denatured rapeseed oil. In addition to rash, fever, adenopathy, and other symptoms, some patients had prominent myalgia, but serum CK values were normal. In 1989, an epidemic in the United States of similar symptoms was finally attributed to ingestion of a contaminated preparation of L-tryptophan as a sedative. As many as 10,000 cases of that eosinophilia-myalgia syndrome may have occurred. Arthralgia, limb swelling, and evidence of myopathy or sensorimotor peripheral neuropathy were prominent. Muscle biopsy showed fascitis, perimyositis, and inflammatory microangiopathy. Eosinophilic myositis was found in some cases. The neuropathy had physiologic features of axonal damage in most patients, but some had conduction block. The condition seems to have disappeared.

MYOPATHY IN AIDS

Myopathy may appear in patients with AIDS. Intense debate has ensued about the pathogenesis of the disorder. Some believe it is an autoimmune polymyositis or the result of viral invasion of muscle. Others believe it is virtually restricted to those taking zidovudine; in those cases most show ragged-red fibers, and depletion of mitochondrial DNA has been documented. DNA levels return to normal when the drug therapy is interrupted.

RELATION OF POLYMYOSITIS TO POLYMYALGIA RHEUMATICA

In polymyalgia rheumatica, no symptomatic weakness or elevation of serum CK levels occurs. If overt weakness or high CK levels were evident, the syndrome would be impossible to distinguish from polymyositis. Polymyalgia can be defined as a syndrome in which a person older than age 65 has joint pains, myalgia, malaise, and a high erythrocyte sedimentation rate as described in Chapter 155.

THERAPY

Polymyositis is treated with steroids and immunosuppressive drugs, as described for dermatomyositis in Chapter 131. The advantages and risks must be balanced against the patient's disability. In controlled trials, plasmapheresis and leukapheresis had no effect, but IVIG therapy has been beneficial, at least temporarily.

IBM characteristically does not respond to steroid therapy; this feature has led to the diagnosis of IBM in patients originally thought to have polymyositis. IBM does not respond to plasmapheresis, but benefit was found in a few patients participating in a trial of intravenous immunoglobulin. Favorable results have been few. The eosinophilia-myalgia syndrome has not responded to conventional immunosuppression, steroids, or plasmapheresis.

SUGGESTED READINGS

Polymyositis (Also Refer to Suggested Readings in Chapter 131)

Amato AA, Griggs RC. Unicorns, dragons, polymyositis, and other mythological beasts. *Neurology* 2003;61:288–290.

Arahata K, Engel AG. Monoclonal antibody analysis of mononuclear cells in myopathies. V: T8+ cytotoxic and suppressor cells. *Ann Neurol* 1988;23:493–499.

Bautista J, Gil-Necija E, Castilla J, et al. Dialysis myopathy. Report of 13 cases. *Acta Neuropathol (Berl)* 1983;61:71–75.

Bronner IM, Linssen WH, van der Meulen MF, Hoogendijk JE, de Visser M. Polymyositis: an ongoing discussion about a disease entity. *Arch Neurol* 2004;1(1):132–135.

Cohen O, Steiner I, Argov Z, et al. Mitochondrial myopathy with atypical subacute presentation. *J Neurol Neurosurg Psychiatry* 1998;410–411.

Crennan JM, Van Scoy RE, McKenna CH, et al. Echovirus polymyositis in patients with hypogammaglobulinemia: failure of high-dose intravenous gamma globulin therapy. *Am J Med* 1986;81:35–42.

Dalakas MC, Hohlfeld R. Polymyositis and dermatomyositis. *Lancet* 2003;362;971–982.

Dewberry RG, Schneider BF, Cale WF, et al. Sarcoid myopathy presenting with diaphragm weakness. *Muscle Nerve* 1993;16:832–835.

Fujisawa T, Suda T, Nakamura Y, et al. Differences in clinical features and prognosis of interstitial lung diseases between polymyositis and dermatomyositis. *J Rheumatol* 2005 Jan;32(1):58–64.

Gheradi RK, Coquet M, Cherin P, et al. Macrophagic myofasciitis: an emerging entity. *Lancet* 1998;352:347–352.

Hopkinson ND, Shawe DJ, Gumpel JM. Polymyositis, not polymyalgia rheumatica. *Ann Rheum Dis* 1991;50:321–322.

Kaufman LD, Kephart GM, Seidman RJ, et al. The spectrum of eosinophilic myositis. *Arthritis Rheum* 1993;36:1014–1024.

Lange DJ. Neuromuscular diseases associated with HIV infection. *Muscle Nerve* 1994;7:16–30.

Layzer RB, Shearn MA, Satya-Murti S. Eosinophilic polymyositis. *Ann Neurol* 1977;1:65–71.

Moskovic E, Fisher C, Wetbury G, et al. Focal myositis: a benign inflammatory pseudotumor: CT appearance. *Br J Radiol* 1991;64:489–493.

Navarro C, Bragado FG, Lima J, et al. Muscle biopsy findings in systemic capillary leak syndrome. *Hum Pathol* 1990;21:297–301.

Phillips BA, Zilko P, Garlepp MJ, et al. Frequency of relapses in patients with polymyositis and dermatomyositis. *Muscle Nerve* 1998;21:1668–1672.

Pickering MC, Walport MJ. Eosinophilic myopathic syndromes. *Curr Opin Rheumatol* 1998;10:504–510.

Ringel SP, Thorne EG, Phanuphak P, et al. Immune complex vasculitis, polymyositis, and hyperglobulinemic purpura. *Neurology* 1979;29:682–689.

Rowland LP, Clark C, Olarte M. Therapy for dermatomyositis and polymyositis. In: Griggs RC, Moxley RT, eds. *Treatment of Neuromuscular Disease.* New York: Raven, 1977.

Spuler S, Emslie-Smith A, Emgel AG. Amyloid myopathy: an underdiagnosed entity. *Ann Neurol* 1998;43:719–728.

Symmans WA, Beresford CH, Bruton D, et al. Cyclic eosinophilic myositis and hyperimmunoglobulin-E. *Ann Intern Med* 1986;104:26–32.

Vaish AK, Mehrotra S, Kushwaha MRS. Proximal muscle weakness due to amyloid deposition. *J Neurol Neurosurg Psychiatry* 1998;409–410.

Drug-Induced Myopathies

Arnaudo E, Dalakas M, Shanske S, et al. Depletion of muscle mitochondrial DNA in AIDS patients with zidovudine-induced myopathy. *Lancet* 1991;337:508–510.

Batchelor TT, Taylor LP, Thaler HT, et al. Steroid myopathy in cancer patients. *Neurology* 1997;48:1234–1238.

Choucair AK, Ziter FA. Pentazocine abuse masquerading as familial myopathy. *Neurology* 1984;34:524–527.

Doyle DR, McCurley TL, Sergent JS. Fatal polymyositis in D-penicillamine-induced nephropathy and polymyositis. *N Engl J Med* 1983;308:142–145.

Giordano N, Senesesi M, Mattii G, et al. Polymyositis associated with simvastatin. *Lancet* 1997;349:1600–1601.

Haller RG, Knochel JP. Skeletal muscle disease in alcoholism. *Med Clin North Am* 1984;68:91–103.

Kalkner KM, Ronnblom L, Karlsson Parra AK, et al. Antibodies against double-stranded DNA and development of polymyositis during treatment with interferon. *QJM* 1998;91:393–399.

Koumis T, Nathan JP, Rosenberg JM, Cicero LA. Strategies for the prevention and treatment of statin-induced myopathy: is there a role for ubiquinone supplementation? *Am J Health Syst Pharm* 2004 Mar 1; 61(5):515–519.

Miller FW, Rider LG, Plotz PH, et al. Diagnostic criteria for polymyositis and dermatomyositis [Letter]. Response by Dalakas MC, Hohlfeld R. *Lancet* 2003;362:1762–1763.

Ojeda VJ. Necrotizing myopathy associated with steroid therapy. Report of two cases. *Pathology* 1982;14:435–438.

Rosenson RS. Current overview of statin-induced myopathy. *Am J Med* 2004 Mar 15;116(6):408–416.

Schultz CE, Kincaid JC. Drug-induced myopathies. In: Biller J, ed. *Iatrogenic Neurology*. Boston: Butterworth-Heinemann, 1998:305–318.

Simpson DM, Citak KA, Godfrey E, et al. Myopathies associated with HIV and zidovudine. Can their effects be distinguished? *Neurology* 1993;43:971–976.

Simpson DM, Slasor P, Dafni U, et al. Analysis of myopathy in a placebo-controlled zidovudine trial. *Muscle Nerve* 1997;20:382–385.

Takahasi K, Ogita T, Okudaira H, et al. Penicillamine-induced polymyositis in patients with rheumatoid arthritis. *Arthritis Rheum* 1986;29:560–564.

Inclusion Body Myositis

Amato AA, Gronseth GS, Jackson CE, et al. Inclusion body myositis: clinical and pathological boundaries. *Ann Neurol* 1996;40:581–586.

Argov Z, Eisenberg I, Grabov-Nardini G, et al. Hereditary inclusion body myopathy: the Middle Eastern genetic cluster. *Neurology* 2003;60:1519–1523.

Askanas V. New developments in hereditary inclusion body myositis. *Ann Neurol* 1997;41:421–422.

Askanas V, Serratrice G, Engel WK, eds. *Inclusion-Body Myositis*. Cambridge, UK: Cambridge University Press, 1998.

Brannagan TH, Hays AP, Lange DJ, et al. The role of quantitative electromyography in inclusion body myositis. *J Neurol Neurosurg Psychiatry* 1997;63:776–779.

Chou SM. Inclusion body myositis: a chronic persistent mumps myositis? *Hum Pathol* 1986;17:765–777.

Dabby R, Lange DJ, Trojaborg W, et al. Inclusion body myositis mimicking motor neuron disease. *Arch Neurol* 2001;58:1253–1256.

Dalakas MC. Inflammatory disorders of muscle: progress in polymyositis, dermatomyositis and inclusion body myositis. *Curr Opin Neurol* 2004;17(5):561 567.

Eisenberg I, Grabov-Nardini G, Hochner H, et al. Mutations spectrum of GNE in hereditary inclusion body myopathy sparing the quadriceps. *Hum Mutat* 2003;21(Jan):99.

Griggs RC, Askansas V, DiMauro S, et al. Inclusion body myositis and myopathies. *Ann Neurol* 1995;38:705–713.

Lotz BP, Engel AG, Nishino H, et al. Inclusion body myositis. Observations in 40 patients. *Brain* 1989;112(Pt 3):727–747.

Moslemi A-R, Lindberg C, Oldfors A. Analysis of multiple mitochondrial DNA deletions in inclusion body myositis. *Hum Mutat* 1997;10:381–386.

Sadeh M, Gadoth N, Hadar H, et al. Vacuolar myopathy sparing the quadriceps. *Brain* 1993;116:217–232.

Watts GD, Thorne M, Kovach MJ, et al. Clinical and genetic heterogeneity in chromosome 9p associated hereditary inclusion body myopathy: exclusion of GNE and three other candidate genes. *Neuromusc Disord* 2003;13:559–567.

Chapter 133

▶ Myositis Ossificans

Lewis P. Rowland

The identifying characteristic of myositis ossificans (MIM 135100), a rare disorder, is the deposition of true bone in subcutaneous tissue and along fascial planes in muscle. McKusick (1974) believed that the primary disorder is in connective tissue and preferred the term *fibrodysplasia ossificans* rather than its traditional name, which implies a disease of muscle. Nevertheless, in some cases myopathic changes occur in muscle biopsy or electromyogram, and occasionally serum creatine kinase levels are increased.

Symptoms usually start in the first or second year of life. Transient and localized swellings of the neck and trunk are the first abnormality. Later, minor bruises are followed by deposition of solid material beneath the skin and within

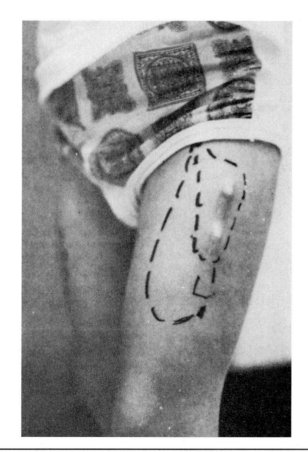

FIGURE 133.1. Ossification of muscle biopsy scar in boy with myositis ossificans. The outer border of marks indicates extent of spontaneous ossification.

muscles. Plates and bars of material may be seen and felt in the limbs (Fig. 133.1), paraspinal tissues, and abdominal wall. These concretions are readily visible on radiographic examination, MRI, or CT; when they cross joints, a deforming ankylosis results. The cranial muscles are spared, but the remainder of the body may be encased in bone. The extent of disability depends on the extent of ossification, which varies considerably. No abnormality of calcium metabolism has been detected.

Almost all cases are sporadic, but it is suspected that the disease is inherited because minor skeletal abnormalities occur in almost all patients, and these abnormalities seem to be transmitted in the family in an autosomal-dominant pattern. Familial cases map to 4q27-31. Bone morphogenetic proteins (BMP-4) may play a role, and an antagonist called *noggin* might offer therapy. The most common congenital deformities are a short great toe (*microdactyly*) and curved fingers (*clinodactyly*); other digital variations are also seen. Most cases are attributed to new mutations because reproductive fitness is much reduced. The gene locus has not been mapped yet. Restricted ossification at the site of single severe injury may also occur in otherwise normal adults with no apparent genetic risk.

Treatment is symptomatic. Excision of ectopic bone is fruitless because local recurrence is invariable and disability may become worse. Surgery sometimes helps to refix a joint in a functionally better position. Treatment with diphosphonates inhibits calcification of new ectopic matrix but does not block production of the fibrous material and may have adverse effects on normal skeleton.

SUGGESTED READINGS

Blaszczyk M, Majewski S, Brzezinska-Wcislo L, et al. Fibrodysplasia ossificans progressiva. *Eur J Dermatol* 2003;13(May–Jun):234–237.

Cohen RB, Hahn GV, Tabas JA, et al. The natural history of heterotopic ossification in patients who have fibrodysplasia ossificans progressiva. A study of forty-four patients. *J Bone Joint Surg Am* 1993;75:215–219.

Connor JM, Skirton H, Lunt PW. A three-generation family with fibrodysplasia ossificans progressiva. *J Med Genet* 1993;30:687–689.

Debene-Bruyerre C, Chikhami L, Lockhart R, et al. Myositis ossificans progressiva: five generations where the disease was exclusively limited to the maxillofacial region. *Int J Oral Maxillofac Surg* 1998;27:299–302.

De Smet AA, Norris MA, Fisher DR. Magnetic resonance imaging of myositis ossificans: analysis of seven cases. *Skeletal Radiol* 1992;21:503–507.

Feldman G, Li M, Martin S, et al. Fibrodysplasia ossificans progressiva, a heritable disorder of severe heterotopic ossification, maps to human chromosome 4q27-31. *Am J Hum Genet* 2000;66(Jan):128–135.

Kaplan FS, Tabas JA, Gauman FH, et al. The histopathology of fibrodysplasia ossificans progressiva. *J Bone Joint Surg Am* 1993;75:220–230.

McKusick VA. *Heritable Diseases of Connective Tissue.* 4th Ed. St Louis, MO: CV Mosby, 1972.

Olmsted EA, Kaplan FS, Shore EM. Bone morphogenetic protein-4 regulation in fibrodysplasia ossificans progressiva. *Clin Orthop* 2003;408:331–343.

Semonin O, Fontaine K, Daviaud C, et al. Identification of three novel mutations of the noggin gene in patients with fibrodysplasia ossificans progressiva. *Am J Med Genet* 2001 Sep 1;102:314–317.

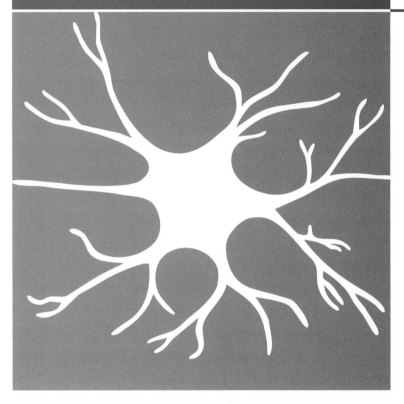

Demyelinating Diseases

Chapter 134

Multiple Sclerosis

Saud A. Sadiq

DEFINITION

Multiple sclerosis (MS) is a chronic disease that usually begins in young adults. Patholigcally, it is characterized by multiple areas of CNS white matter inflammation, demyelination, and glial scarring (sclerosis). The lesions are therefore multiple in space. The clinical course of MS varies from a benign, largely symptom-free disease to a rapidly progressive and disabling disorder. At first, it is usually a relapsing and remitting illness and recovery from relapses is almost complete. Later, permanent neurologic disabilities accrue gradually. The lesions are therefore multiple in time. If effective treatment is introduced early in the disease, the natural hisotry may be altered favorably. The cause remains elusive, but autoimmune mechanisms, possibly triggered by environmental factors in genetically susceptible individuals, are probably important.

INCIDENCE AND EPIDEMIOLOGY

Age at onset follows a unimodal distribution with a peak between ages 20 and 30 years; onset is rarely before age 10 or after age 60. In a series of 660 patients, Bauer and Hanefeld found that almost 70% of patients had symptoms at ages 21 to 40, 12.4% at ages 16 to 20, and 12.8% at 41 to 50. The youngest patient had symptoms at age 3 and the oldest at 67 years. Younger and older cases have been reported.

MS is more common among women than men, with an incidence of 1.4 to 3.1 times as many women than men affected. In patients with later onset of MS, the sex ratio tends to be equal.

The geographic distribution is uneven. In general, the disease increases in frequency with latitude in both the northern and southern hemispheres, although the rates tend to decrease above 65° north or south. Because of differences in methods of case-finding and the need to rely on subjective clinical criteria in identifying cases of MS in large populations, the absolute numbers in any given area are uncertain. The distribution of MS is best considered in terms of zones. High-prevalence areas are those with cases equal to or more than 30/100,000 population, medium-prevalence areas have rates between 5 and 30/100,000 population, and low-prevalence areas have rates less than 5/100,000 population. Most of northern Europe, northern United States, southern Canada, and southern Australia and New Zealand are areas of high prevalence. Southern Europe, southern United States, Asia Minor, the Middle East, India, parts of northern Africa, and South Africa have medium prevalence rates. Low-prevalence areas are Japan, China, and Latin and South America. MS is virtually unknown among native Inuit in Alaska and among the indigenous people of equatorial Africa.

Although latitude may be an independent variable affecting MS prevalence rates, racial differences may explain some of the geographic distribution. This is illustrated by comparing the prevalence rate for MS in Britain (85 per 100,000) and Japan (1.4 per 100,000); although both countries lie at the same latitude, the difference is striking. When racial differences are correlated with prevalence rates for MS worldwide, white populations are at greatest risk and both Asian and black populations have a low risk.

Studies of migrant populations provide evidence of environmental changes in risk of MS while keeping genetic factors constant. Children born in Israel of immigrants from Asian and North African countries showed relatively higher incidence rates of MS—like those of European immigrants, rather than the low rates characteristic of their parents. This finding implies that an environmental factor is critically important in pathogenesis. Similar differences were noted among the native-born South African whites, who had a lower incidence than among immigrants from Great Britain. Age at time of immigration played an important role; a person leaving the country of origin before age 15 had nearly the same risk of acquiring MS as that of the native-born Israeli or South African. Individuals migrating after age 15 had the risk of the country of origin. These studies were confirmed by studies of people migrating to Great Britain from the Indian subcontinent or the West Indies. The data suggest that an infectious agent of long latency is acquired at the time of puberty.

Epidemics of MS provide further evidence of an environmental factor. The most impressive wave occurred in the Faroe Islands when cases appeared shortly after the islands were occupied by British troops in World War II. Similar "epidemics" of cases have been seen in Iceland, in the Orkney and Shetland Islands, and in Sardinia. Rigorous epidemiologic scrutiny failed to prove, however, that these cases were true point-source epidemics. Therefore, other plausible explanations cannot be excluded.

MS is reported to occur more frequently in higher socioeconomic classes and in urban areas, but these assertions are unproved.

ETIOLOGY AND PATHOGENESIS

The cause of MS is unknown. It is postulated that in genetically susceptible hosts, an initial trigger early in life (probably a virus) leads over time to autoimmune mechanisms causing demyelination.

Genetic Susceptibility

Compelling data indicate that susceptibility to MS is inherited. The epidemiologic studies summarized above reveal a racial susceptibility to MS. Whites are at greatest risk. Within this group are regional trends; the highest rates are in areas where Nordic invasions took place. Alternatively, genetic resistance to MS in Asians and African Americans helps to explain racial variations in prevalence rates. Because racial prevalence of MS changes with migration, however, definite conclusions of genetic predisposition cannot be drawn.

Studies of families and twins provide more support for genetic susceptibility. In high-prevalence regions, the lifetime risk of developing MS is about 0.00125% in the general population. Siblings of MS patients have a risk of about 2.6%, parents a risk of about 1.8%, and children a risk of about 1.5%. First-, second-, and third-degree relatives also have a higher risk. Overall, about 15% of patients with MS have an affected relative. Data from twin studies indicate a concordance rate of about 25% in monozygotic twins and of only 2.4% for same-sex dizygotic twins. These studies suggest a substantial genetic component. Rather than a single dominant gene, however, multiple genes probably confer susceptibility.

Pedigree data from families with more than one affected member are consistent with the hypothesis that multiple unlinked genes predispose to MS. The major histocompatibility complex (MHC) on chromosome 6 has been identified as one genetic determinant for MS. The MHC en-

codes the genes for the histocompatibility antigens (the HLA system) involved in antigen presentation to T cells. Of the three classes of HLA genes, the strongest association is with the class II alleles, particularly the DR and DQ regions. In whites, the class II haplotype DR15, DQ6, Dw2 is associated with increased risk of MS. Delineation of this haplotype in patients with MS and in normal people, however, revealed no significant differences, thus suggesting that the genetic susceptibility to MS may reside in functional aspects of these genes. The roles of other genes in MS, including the T-cell receptor and immunoglobulin heavy chain genes, are reviewed later in the chapter.

Immunology

Substantial evidence from peripheral blood abnormalities, CSF findings, and CNS pathology in MS and animal models of demyelination suggests that autoimmune mechanisms are involved in the pathogenesis of MS. In the peripheral blood, several nonspecific changes are seen, particularly in secondary progressive MS. These changes are similar to those encountered in other autoimmune diseases, such as systemic lupus erythematosus (SLE). Reduction occurs in activity of suppressor CD8+ T cells and also in the autologous mixed lymphocyte reaction (AMLR). The AMLR seems to be an important indication of autoreactive cell suppression. In MS, as in SLE, there are a decreased number of CD4+CD45RA+ suppressor-inducer T cells in the peripheral blood. An increase in activated T cells in MS is unlikely, because cell surface molecules associated with T-cell activation are not abundant and lymphokine levels are normal.

CSF pleocytosis is common, particularly in the acute phases of MS. T cells that are helper-inducers (CD4+CDw29+ cells) constitute most of the cells and are found in higher ratios in CSF than in the peripheral circulation. By contrast, the number of CD4+CD45RA T cells, which induce suppressor cells, is decreased. Although some T lymphocytes in the CSF of patients with MS are activated, the antigenic stimulus is unclear. T-cell reactivity is found against several epitopes of myelin basic protein (MBP) and proteolipid protein (PLP). Analysis of the T-cell receptor (TCR) gene, which is unique to each T-cell clone, suggests that the immune response is polyclonal and thus likely to have multiple antigenic specificities. Furthermore, sequencing of the variable regions of these cells reveals a high degree of somatic hypermutations, as is seen in chronic stimulation in vivo.

Antibody-secreting B cells are also activated in MS. The amount of IgG in the CSF and the rate of IgG synthesis are increased. Because only a few clones of CSF cells are activated, the response is oligoclonal. This seems to be a restricted response to stimulation within the neuraxis because similar oligoclonal IgGs are either not found at all or found in lower concentrations in the serum than in CSF. Oligoclonal IgG is found in other inflammatory or infectious conditions, such as viral encephalitis or CNS syphilis. In these situations, however, the oligoclonal IgGs are antibodies directed against the agents of the infecting agent. In MS, an antigen for most of the oligoclonal IgG has not been identified. Therefore, the CSF IgG may be a secondary effect, possibly a result of the decrease in CD4+CD45RA+ suppressor-inducer cells, which allows a few clones of antibody-producing cells to escape suppression.

Perivascular lymphocyte and macrophage infiltration is characteristic of the CNS immunopathology. The predominant lymphocytes in MS lesions are helper-inducer cells (CD4+CDw29+). Interleukin-2 (IL-2) receptors are demonstrable on many of the T cells, thereby indicating that these cells are secreting cytokines and are immunologically activated. Also, astrocytes, which normally do not express MHC molecules, express class II molecules in active lesions. This pattern suggests that astrocytes are involved in antigen presentation to T cells. In more chronic lesions, γ/δ T cells are present around the edges of the plaque. Oligoclonal IgG is also present in MS plaques. Overall, the types of immunologically active cells and IgGs in the CNS lesions are similar to those found in CSF.

The cytokines produced by activated T cells and macrophages may play a role in tissue damage. The cytokine called tissue necrosis factor (TNF) is toxic to oligodendroglial cells and myelin and can be found in MS plaques. Furthermore, CSF levels of TNF may correlate with MS disease activity.

Further evidence of an immunologic basis comes from experimental allergic encephalomyelitis (EAE), which is induced in genetically susceptible animals by immunization with normal CNS tissue and an adjuvant. The chronic relapsing-remitting form of EAE is pathologically similar to that of MS. EAE can also be induced by immunization with MBP or immunodominant peptide regions of MBP, thus suggesting that MBP is the putative antigen in EAE. T cells reactive against MBP and PLP mediate the CNS inflammation, as shown by "adoptive transfer"; sensitized T cells from an animal with EAE can transfer disease to a healthy syngeneic recipient. The T-cell response in EAE seems to be genetically restricted to a few families on the TCR gene, however, and removal or suppression of these T-cell lines leads to immunity from EAE. This response contrasts with the findings in human MS where the TCR gene response is more heterogeneous

Although current understanding of MS pathogenesis derives mainly from consideration of the EAE and chronic EAE models, many features of the clinical disease are still not fully understood and not entirely explained by this animal model. We do not know the precipitant antigens or even if autoimmunity is the primary process. There are differences in the pathology of the experimental and human disorder, and there may be differences in the relative roles of cytokine activation, antibody-mediated immunity, and macrophage activity. A healthy skepticism about theories of pathogenesis is appropriate.

Viruses

The epidemiologic data previously reviewed imply a role for environmental exposure in MS. Viral encephalitis in children may be followed by demyelination. In animals, the most widely studied model of viral-induced demyelinating disease is created by the Theiler virus, a murine picornavirus. Infection with some Theiler strains results in an infection of oligodendrocytes with multifocal perivascular lymphocytic infiltration and demyelination. Genetic factors influence susceptibility to development of demyelination and clinical disease; this susceptibility is linked to the immune response generated in the animals against viral determinants. Therefore, in MS, demyelination could be precipitated by a viral infection. Measles, rubella, mumps, coronavirus, parainfluenza, herpes simplex, vaccinia, and HTLV-I viruses all have been reported to be present in patients with MS. None of these agents, however, has been reproducibly and uniformly detected. The two virus candidates most consistently implicated in the pathogenesis of MS are Epstein-Barr virus (EBV) and human herpes virus 6 (HHV6). The evidence is indirect, but it is postulated that after early infection, the viruses persist in latent form and clinical relapses are caused by periods of viral reactivation. Causality has not been determined, and therapeutic trials of antiviral agents have not reduced the frequency of episodes in MS patients.

Other Factors

Other mechanisms have been suggested as precipitating the onset of MS or relapses. In many cases, physical trauma has been invoked as precipitating or aggravating the disease. In a population-based cohort study, however, Siva and colleagues found no association between MS and head injuries in 819 patients. Other studies also failed to show any causal correlation between trauma and MS. The effect of pregnancy is difficult to evaluate because MS is most common in women of childbearing age. If the pregnancy year is considered, however, exacerbations seem to cluster in the postpartum period rather than during pregnancy. Whether this clustering is related to hormonal changes or other factors is unclear. In any event, no convincing evidence has revealed that MS is worsened by pregnancy. Therefore, interruption of pregnancy in women with MS is not indicated on this basis alone.

Vaccination is also cited frequently as a precipitating event, although the evidence is anecdotal. One study with influenza vaccine found no relationship. Another with hepatitis B vaccine suggested increased risk. In the absence

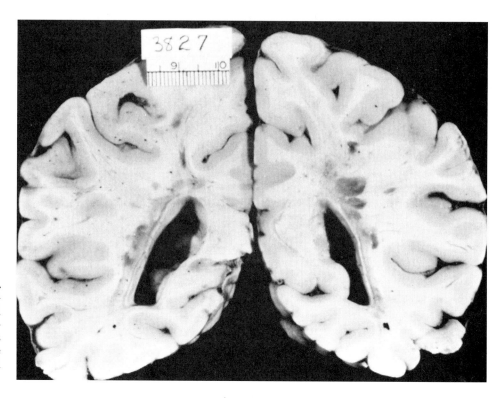

FIGURE 134.1. Gross appearance, coronal section, occipital lobe. Note extensive periventricular lesions. Several small lesions are scattered elsewhere in the white matter. (Courtesy of Dr. Daniel Perl.)

of definitive studies, patients with MS should be advised against routine casual vaccination, especially if previous exacerbations have been preceded by vaccination. However, medically indicated inoculations should not be withheld. Surgery, anesthesia, and lumbar punctures also have been invoked in MS, but controlled studies failed to show any relationship.

PATHOLOGY

The gross appearance of the external surface of the brain is usually normal. Frequently in long-standing cases there is evidence of atrophy and widening of cerebral sulci with enlargement of the lateral and third ventricles. Brain sections reveal numerous small irregular grayish areas in older

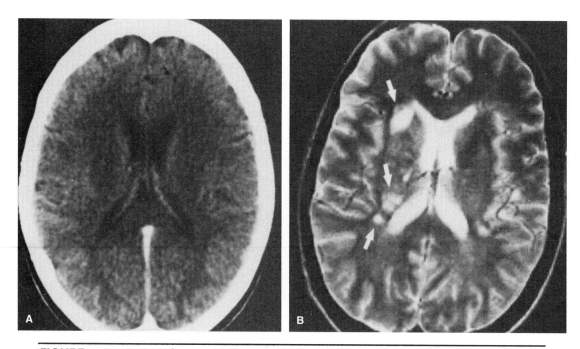

FIGURE 134.2. A. Normal contrast-enhanced CT scan. **B.** The axial T2-weighted MRI scan in the same patient during the same period shows multiple white matter lesions, the largest designated by *arrows*.

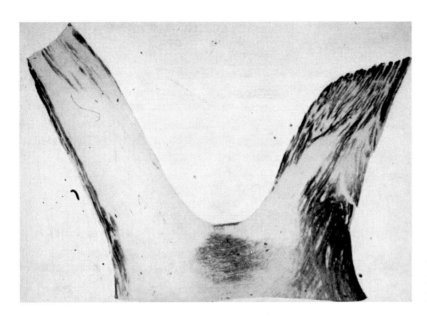

FIGURE 134.3. Multiple sclerosis. Demyelinization of optic nerves and chiasm. (Courtesy of Dr. Abner Wolf.)

lesions and pink areas in acute lesions in the cerebral hemispheres, particularly in the white matter and in periventricular regions (Fig. 134.1). The white matter that forms the superior lateral angle of the body of the lateral ventricles is frequently and characteristically affected. Similar areas of discoloration are also found in the brainstem and cerebellum. These are the plaques of MS.

The external appearance of the spinal cord is usually normal. In a few cases, the cord is slightly shrunken and the pia arachnoid may be thickened. The cord is occasionally swollen over several segments if death follows soon after the onset of an acute lesion of the cord. Plaques similar to those seen in the cerebrum are seen occasionally on the external surface of the cord, but they are recognized most easily on cross section. The optic nerves may be shrunken, but the external appearance of the other cranial nerves is usually normal.

Myelin sheath stains of CNS sections show areas of demyelination in the regions that were visibly discolored in the unstained specimen. In addition, many more plaques are apparent. These plaques are sharply circumscribed and are diffusely scattered throughout all parts of the brain and spinal cord (Fig. 134.2). The lesions in the brain tend to be grouped around the lateral and third ventricles. Lesions in the cerebral hemispheres vary from the size of a pinhead to large areas that encompass the major portion of one lobe of the hemisphere. Small lesions may be found in the gray matter and in the zone between the gray and white matter. Plaques of varying size may be found in the optic nerves, chiasm, or tracts (Fig. 134.3). Lesions in the corpus callosum are not uncommon (Fig. 134.4). The lesions in the brain stem are usually numerous (Fig. 134.5), and sections from this area when stained by the Weigert method have a characteristic Holstein cow appearance (Fig. 134.6).

In sections of the spinal cord, the areas of demyelination vary from small lesions involving a portion of the posterior or lateral funiculi to almost complete loss of myelin in an entire cross section of the cord (Figs. 134.7 and 134.8).

Lesions are usually characterized by sharp delimitation from the surrounding normal tissue. Within the lesion is variable destruction of the myelin and to a lesser degree damage to the neurons, proliferation of the glial cells, changes in the blood vessels, and relatively good preservation of the ground structure. Only rarely is the damage

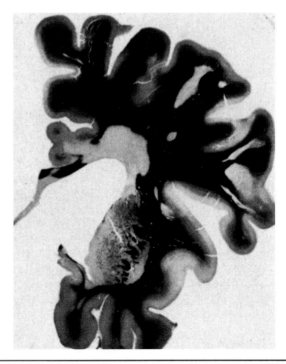

FIGURE 134.4. Myelin sheath stain of right cerebral hemisphere in multiple sclerosis (celloidin). Note lesions in corpus callosum and superior lateral angle of the ventricle, and several plaques in the subcortical white matter. (Courtesy of Dr. Charles Poser.)

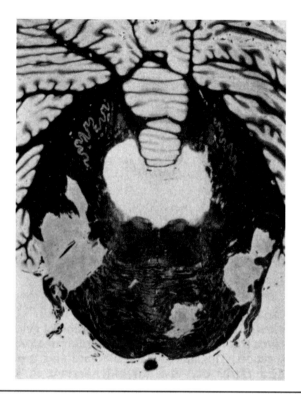

FIGURE 134.5. Multiple sclerosis. Myelin sheath stain. Lesions in pons, middle cerebellum peduncle, and cerebellar white matter, typically near the dentate nuclei. (Courtesy of Dr. Charles Poser.)

severe enough to affect the ground substance and produce a cyst (Fig. 134.6).

Most myelin sheaths within a lesion are destroyed, and many of those that remain show swelling and fragmentation. The degree of damage to the neurons varies. In the more severe lesions, axons may be entirely destroyed, but more commonly only a few are severely injured and the remainder appear normal or show only minor changes. How-

ever, loss of axons is found in even the earliest MS plaques. Secondary degeneration of long tracts occurs when the axons have been significantly destroyed. Axonal loss and resulting brain atrophy, rather than the number or size of plaques, are probably more closely correlated with irreversible clinical dysfunction. When the lesion involves gray matter, nerve cells are less affected than is myelin, but some cells may be destroyed and show degenerative changes.

In the early or acute lesion, there is marked hypercellularity, with macrophage infiltration and astrocytosis accompanied by perivenous inflammation with lymphocytes and plasma cells. Myelin sheaths disintegrate and chemical breakdown of myelin occurs. It is not yet established whether the cellular response leads to, or occurs as a result of, the myelin breakdown. These acute lesions may remain active for several months with continued macrophage and astrocytic hyperactivity and breakdown of myelin. Phagocytic cells are laden with lipid degradation products of myelin. In these active but nonacute plaques, the inflammatory cell response is minimal centrally. At the edges, however, myelin disintegration is still active and numbers of macrophages, lymphocytes, and plasma cells are increased. With time, the plaques become inactive. Demyelination is prominent, almost total oligodendrocyte cell loss occurs, and gliosis is extensive. Inactive lesions are hypocellular and devoid of myelin breakdown products.

Remyelination in MS plaques, particularly following the early acute phase, is thought to result from the differentiation of a precursor cell that is common to type II astrocytes and oligodendrocytes. This remyelination, however, is usually aberrant and incomplete. Uniform areas of incomplete myelination (*shadow plaques*) are evident in some chronic lesions; it is not known whether these regions result from partial demyelination or incomplete remyelination.

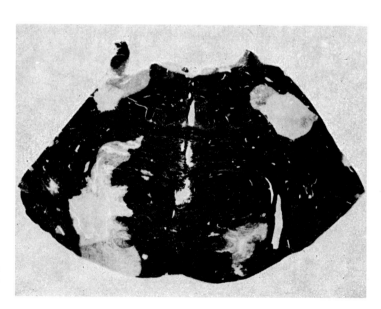

FIGURE 134.6. Myelin sheath stain of brain stem in multiple sclerosis. Note sharp demarcation of lesions.

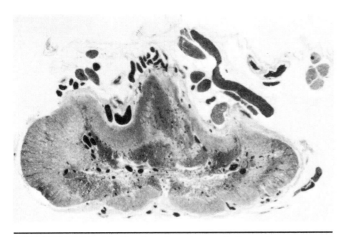

FIGURE 134.7. Myelin sheath stain: tenth thoracic segment of spinal cord. Almost complete demyelination of the entire section. The gray matter is severely involved, and cystic degeneration causes obliteration of normal architecture.

Electron microscopy reveals different aspects of myelin disorder in MS, including widening of the outer myelin lamellae, splitting and vacuolation of myelin sheaths, vesicular dissolution of myelin, myelin sheath fragmentation, ball and ovoid formation, filamentous accumulations in sheath, thin myelin sheaths, and macrophage-associated pinocytosis and actual peeling of layers of myelin by the processes of these microglial cells.

The peripheral nerves are usually normal. Subtle changes, however, in sural nerve biopsies include endothelial pinocytosis, expansion of the endoneurial space, mononuclear cell infiltration, or demyelination. In addition, hypertrophic neuropathy and chronic inflammatory demyelinating polyneuropathy (CIDP) have been reported in patients with MS.

Biochemical analysis of MS lesions reveals a decrease in both the protein and the lipid components of normal myelin. Thus, by immunocytochemistry, a decrease in staining results for the MBP and myelin-associated glyco-protein (MAG), as well as a decrease in cholesterol, glycolipids, phosphoglycerides, and sphingomyelins. Because of phagocytosis and lysosomal activation, myelin breakdown products, including polypeptides, glycerol, fatty acids, and triglycerides, are abundant, particularly in active lesions.

Although inflammatory-mediated demyelination is a central event in all cases of MS, pathologic heterogeneity does occur. Based largely on immunohistologic analysis of cell types in lesions, four patterns of pathology are described: a macrophage/T-cell inflammatory type; an antibody-dependent/complement-driven pattern; an oligodendroglial/myelin-associated glycoprotein-directed inflammatory subtype; and a degenerative form with a lack of perivascular demyelination and an absence of remyelination. In general, there is a tendency for only one pattern of immunopathology to exist in a single patient.

SYMPTOMS AND SIGNS

In the typical relapsing-remitting (RR) form of MS, exacerbations and remissions occur and in addition, signs and symptoms usually indicate more than one lesion. Clinical manifestations may be transient and some may seem bizarre. The patient may experience unusual sensations that are difficult to describe and impossible to verify objectively. Over time and untreated, most patients with RRMS will evolve into a secondary progressive course (SPMS). From the onset of symptoms, 15% of patients have a primary progressive (PPMS) course, with a steady decline in neurologic function.

The symptoms and signs (Tables 134.1 and 134.2) are diverse and seem to include all the symptoms that can result from injury to any part of the neuraxis from the spinal cord to the cerebral cortex. The chief characteristics are multiplicity and tendency to vary in nature and severity with time. Complete remission of the first symptoms frequently occurs, but with subsequent attacks, remissions tend not to occur or are incomplete. The clinical course

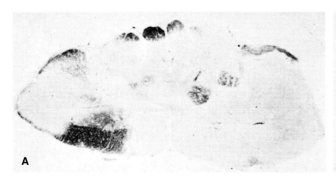
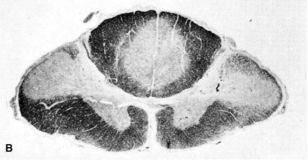

FIGURE 134.8. Multiple sclerosis. **A.** Almost complete loss of myelin in transverse section of cord. **B.** Symmetric lesions in the posterior and lateral funiculi simulating distribution of lesions in combined system disease. (From Merritt HH, Mettler FA, Putnam TJ. *Fundamentals of Clinical Neurology.* Philadelphia: Blakiston, 1947.)

▶ **TABLE 134.1 Common Symptoms and Signs in Chronic Multiple Sclerosis**

Functional System	% Frequency[a]
Motor	
Muscle weakness	65–100
Spasticity	73–100
Reflexes (hyperreflexia,Babinski, absent abdominals)	62–98
Sensory	
Impairment of vibratory/position sense	48–82
Impairment of pain, temperature, or touch	16–72
Pain (moderate to severe)	11–37
Lhermitte sign	1–42
Cerebellar	
Ataxia (limb/gait/truncal)	37–78
Tremor	36–81
Nystagmus (brainstem or cerebellar)	54–73
Dysarthria (brainstem or cerebellar)	29–62
Cranial nerve/brainstem	
Vision affected	27–55[b]
Ocular disturbances (excluding nystagmus)	18–39
Cranial nerves V, VII, VIII	5–52
Bulbar signs	9–49
Vertigo	7–27
Autonomic	
Bladder dysfunction	49–93
Bowel dysfunction	39–64
Sexual dysfunction	33–59
Others (sweating and vascular abnormalities)	38–43
Psychiatric	
Depression	8–55
Euphoria	4–18[c]
Cognitive abnormalities	11–59
Miscellaneous	
Fatigue	59–85

[a]Frequency values derived from the lowest and highest published rates. The higher frequency values are obtained mostly from studies with older patients with long-standing disease.
[b]Visual-evoked response abnormalities not included in these figures.
[c]Earlier studies suggested a much higher frequency, but these rates are not reproducible using current psychometric tests and therefore are excluded.

▶ **TABLE 134.2 Symptoms and Signs Seen Infrequency in Multiple Sclerosis**

Well-Recognized Associations	Rare Associations
Generalized seizures	Aphasia
Tonic seizure	Anosmia
Headache	Hiccoughs
Trigeminal neuralgia	Deafness
Paroxysmal dysarthria/ataxia	Horner syndrome
Paroxysmal itching	
Chorea/athetosis	Cardiac arrhythmias
Myoclonus	Acute pulmonary edema
Facial hemispasm	Hypothalamic dysfunction
Myokymia	Narcolepsy
Spasmodic torticollis/focal dystonia	
Lower motor neuron signs—wasting, decreased tone, areflexia	
Restless legs	
Hysteria	

extends for one or many decades in most cases, but a rare few are fatal within a few months of onset.

The clinical manifestations depend on the areas of the CNS involved. Although no classic form of MS exists, for unknown reasons the disease frequently involves some areas and systems more than others. The optic chiasm, brainstem, cerebellum, and spinal cord, especially the lateral and posterior columns, are commonly involved (Table 134.1). Some clinicians have therefore classified MS into spinal, brainstem, cerebellar, and cerebral forms. These "forms" are often combined, and this classification is of no clinical value. In fact, the combination of anatomically unrelated symptoms and signs forms the basis for the clinical diagnosis of MS.

Visual symptoms include diplopia, blurred vision, diminution or loss of visual acuity on one or both sides, and visual field defects ranging from a unilateral scotoma or field contraction (Fig. 134.9) to homonymous hemianopsia. These symptoms characteristically begin over hours or days. Patients may also complain of a curious and quite distinctive problem in recognizing objects or faces, often stated as blurry vision. This symptom is caused by optic nerve lesions that result in loss of contrasts of shade and colors. In early or mild optic or retrobulbar neuritis, color vision may be decreased whereas black and white vision remains normal. Rarely, when color vision is affected in both eyes, either transient or permanent red-green color blindness may result. Examination of the visual fields with a red or green test object may uncover a central scotoma or field contraction that is not apparent with the usual white test object. Optic neuritis must be differentiated from papilledema, because the fundoscopic appearance of both may be similar if the plaque is near the nerve head. Optic neuritis, however, is characterized by early impairment of visual acuity, which is a late manifestation of papilledema. A central or cecocentral scotoma is the most characteristic field loss. Retrobulbar neuritis, a common manifestation of MS, may not be associated with any fundoscopic abnormality but is revealed only by loss of visual acuity. An important and almost always present clinical feature of optic neuritis is orbital or retro-orbital pain precipitated by movement of the affected eye.

The sudden onset of optic neuritis, without any other CNS signs or symptoms, is often interpreted as the first symptom of MS. Optic neuritis may also result, however, from a postinfectious or postvaccinal reaction or other conditions. The frequency with which MS follows a single isolated episode of optic neuritis is difficult to determine; published figures range from 15% to 85%. This spread is

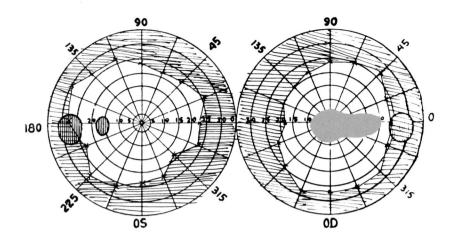

FIGURE 134.9. Cecocentral scotoma in patient with acute right optic neuropathy: MS of 3 years' duration.

probably the result of differences of follow-up periods or of diagnostic and assessment measures. More accurate prediction of whether an initial episode of optic neuritis heralds MS is possible by considering brain MRI scan activity. If optic neuritis is associated with a normal brain MRI, there is a less than 10% probability of MS. On the other hand, with three or more typical lesions on brain MRI, an initial optic neuritis episode will evolve into full-blown MS in more than 80% of patients.

The most common pupillary abnormalities are irregularities in the outline of the pupil, partial constriction, and partial loss of the light reflex. Diplopia may follow lesions in the medial longitudinal fasciculus (MLF) that cause *internuclear ophthalmoplegia*. In young adults, this syndrome is uncommon in any other condition and is therefore an important sign in the diagnosis of MS. It is characterized by paresis of one medial rectus with failure of the eye to adduct on the side of the lesion and by nystagmus and weakness of the lateral rectus on the other side. This impairment of gaze may be seen on attempts to look to one or both sides. In uncomplicated lesions of the MLF, action of the medial rectus is preserved in reflex convergence, thus implying a supranuclear lesion. Mild diplopia may be reported as blurred vision. The true nature of the complaint is discovered only if the patient shuts one eye and vision improves.

Involvement of the descending root of the fifth cranial nerve may impair pain sensation in the face, and the corneal reflex may be diminished or lost. Paroxysmal pain is sometimes identical to that of cryptogenic trigeminal neuralgia and often responds to carbamazepine therapy. MS should be considered whenever a young adult develops trigeminal neuralgia.

Weakness of the facial muscles of the lower half of one side of the face is common, but complete peripheral facial palsy is rare. On the other hand, *hemifacial spasm* (consisting of spasmodic contractions of facial muscles) is a rare but characteristic paroxysmal disorder of MS. True vertigo, which often lasts several days and may be severe,

is seen with new lesions of the floor of the fourth ventricle but is seldom a chronic symptom. Dysarthria and, rarely, dysphagia are seen in advanced MS because of cerebellar lesions or bilateral demyelination of corticobulbar tracts that cause pseudobulbar palsy, which is also characterized by emotional lability and forced laughing or crying without the accompanying affect.

Limb weakness is the most common sign, almost always present in advanced cases as monoparesis, hemiparesis, or tetraparesis—most often, asymmetric paraparesis. Direct testing of muscle strength alone often does not correlate with the degree of difficulty in walking. Concomitant spasticity and ataxia augment the gait disturbance. Gait ataxia is caused by a combination of lesions in the cerebellar pathways and loss of proprioception resulting from lesions in the posterior columns of the spinal cord.

In some patients, particularly those with late-onset symptoms, there may be a slowly progressive spastic paraparesis or monoparesis, with no abnormality except corticospinal signs (spasticity, hyperreflexia, bilateral Babinski signs) and slight impairment of proprioceptive sensation. The cerebellum and its connections with the brainstem are usually involved, thereby causing dysarthria, gait ataxia, tremor, and incoordination of the trunk or limbs. Tremor of the head and body is occasionally almost continuous when the patient is awake. The characteristic scanning speech of MS is a result of cerebellar incoordination of the palatal and labial muscles combined with dysarthria of corticobulbar origin. (The so-called *Charcot triad* of dysarthria, tremor, and ataxic gait is a combination of cerebellar symptoms.)

Urinary symptoms are also common, including incontinence and frequency or urgency of urination, and must be differentiated from manifestations of urinary tract infections or local conditions. Fecal incontinence or urgency is less common than urinary disturbances, but constipation is not unusual, especially in established cases. Loss of libido and erectile impotence are common problems in men. Almost invariably these are associated with sphincter disturbances or corticospinal tract dysfunction, but psychologic problems may compound the problem. Sexual dysfunction in women is also frequent. Lack of lubrication and failure to reach orgasm are the major problems, but sensory dysesthesias are also significant.

Paresthesias and sensory impairment are common. When they are symptoms of an acute relapse, they tend to resolve completely in 6 to 8 weeks. In advanced disease, vibratory perception is commonly affected. Frequently, patients feel tingling or numbness in the limbs, trunk, or face. The *Lhermitte symptom* is a sensation of "electricity" down the back after passive or active flexion of the neck. It indicates a lesion of the posterior columns in the cervical spinal cord and may be seen in other diseases. The Lhermitte symptom is rarely elicited by flexion of the trunk. Pain is increasingly recognized as a frequent and disabling symptom. Pain may be associated with the Lhermitte phenomenon, trigeminal neuralgia, or retrobulbar neuritis. Other types of pain include painful flexor-extensor spasms; painful tonic spasms of the limbs; such local pain syndromes as constricting pain around a limb, burning pain, or pseudoradicular pain, foreign body sensation; headache; pain with pressure sores; pain caused by joint contractures and osteoporosis; pseudorheumatic pain with myalgia and arthralgia; or neuralgic pain shooting down the legs or around the abdomen, as in tabetic pain.

Psychiatric mood disorder symptoms are frequent. Depression is common. Whether it is directly related to MS lesions or a psychologic response to the disease is unclear. Both mechanisms are likely. Euphoria was once considered characteristic of MS patients. Even when this symptoms exists, it appears more likely to be a frontal lobe dysinhibition syndrome, and underlying depression is often found. Hypomanic or bipolar disorders may be more common than expected by chance. This does not appear to be part of the disease, because the lifestyle is apparent long before neurologic symptoms occur. A genetic linkage has been suggested, but without epidemiologic support.

Some have commented on a tendency of patients to exaggerate and extend symptoms that have an obvious anatomic basis. Thus, diplopia may be transformed into triplopia, quadriplopia, or monocular double vision. However, because even the most obvious sensory symptoms often lack distinct correlates in the neurologic examination, it is dangerous to assume that unexplained sensory phenomena are psychogenic.

Cognitive, judgment, and memory disorders are common features in MS and may be more important than physical disorders in disability outcome. These changes may range from the very obvious to subtle, and even sophisticated psychometric studies may not detect early changes. Remedial training for memory problems may be helpful. Awareness of these potential difficulties may help relatives and friends as well as patients cope with otherwise difficult behavior. Aphasic disorders may occur and occasionally are the major feature of an exacerbation.

Fatigue is another common symptom. It may appear as persistent fatigue, easy fatigability related to physical activity, or fatigue related to minor degrees of mental exertion. It is often a prodromal symptom of an impending exacerbation. Fatigue is not related to age, because it is noted with the same frequency by patients younger than 30 and older than 50. Also, fatigue is not related to the amount of physical disability, because it is noted in more than 50% of patients with early MS. It is important to analyze the symptom, as fatigue associated with depression or lack of sleep, for example because of nocturia, may play an important role in the complaint. Often the fatigue associated with MS responds to brief naps. As may be seen from Table 134.1, most of these symptoms occur in more than 50% of patients with MS at some time. The clinical features of MS, however, are protean; almost any part of the CNS may be affected (Table 134.2).

One of the characteristics of symptoms of MS is that they may be evanescent. Diplopia may last for seconds. Paresthesias may last for seconds or hours; diminution of visual acuity may be equally short lived. Transient loss of color vision may presage the onset of optic neuritis. Because of the transient and bizarre nature of these symptoms, they are frequently deemed hysterical, before clearer manifestations arise. There may also be paroxysmal limb spasms, incoordination syndromes, or neuralgias. Trigeminal neuralgia in young people is most clearly associated with MS, but similar pains in other distributions may occur.

Other transient disorders may be precipitated by exercise, exposure to heat, or other stimuli. Transient dysesthesias, visual blurring (*Uhtoff phenomenon*), or diplopia or weakness following hot showers or exercise may occur. These episodes appear to represent derangements of the neurologic signal through previously damaged pathways and not an increase in the inflammatory process. They invariably disappear soon after the provoking activity is stopped.

Remissions are also characteristic, but clinicians have difficulty agreeing on the nature or duration of some remissions. If a remission is defined only by the complete or almost complete disappearance of a major symptom, such as loss of vision, marked weakness of a limb, or diplopia, clinical remissions occur in about 70% of all patients early in the course of the disease.

Mode of Onset

In RRMS, the onset is usually acute or subacute within days and is only rarely apoplectic. There is no characteristic mode of onset, but some symptoms and signs are more common (Table 134.3). Monosymptomatic onset is most

▶ **TABLE 134.3** **Common Symptoms and Signs at the Onset of Disease in Patients with Clinically Definite Multiple Sclerosis**

Clinical Feature	% Frequency
Monosymptomatic	45–79
Polysymptomatic	21–55
Weakness	10–40
Parasthesias	21–40
Sensory loss	13–39
Optic neuritis[a]	14–29
Diplopia	8–18
Ataxia	2–18
Bladder dysfunction	0–13
Vertigo	2–9

[a] Optic neuritis is more common in Japanese series (approximately 40%).

common, but when onset is polysymptomatic, the clinical features often help to establish the diagnosis. Frequently, however, review of the past history reveals remote or recent episodes of other manifestations that had been ignored or not considered significant by the patient or physician. Such dismissal is particularly true of transient paresthesias, mild urinary disturbances, and mild ocular manifestations, such as blurring of vision or transient diminution of monocular visual acuity. In the less common PPMS, onset of symptoms (often monoparesis) is usually imperceptible and patients have difficulty in dating the initial event.

LABORATORY DATA

No pathognomonic test for MS exists, but MRI, CSF examination, and evoked potential studies are of greatest diagnostic value (Table 134.4). The most valuable laboratory aid is MRI, which shows multiple white matter lesions in 90% of patients (Fig. 134.10) and is the imaging procedure of choice in the diagnosis of MS. T2-weighted imaging has been the standard for demonstrating areas of involvement. Subsequently, proton density images and now fluid inversion recovery (FLAIR) technique have enhanced

▶ **TABLE 134.4** **Laboratory Findings in Multiple Sclerosis (MS)**

MRI

Appropriate T2-weighted scans abnormal in approximately 90% of patients.

MRI interpretation should be conservative and correlate with the clinical findings.

Typically, at least four white matter areas of increased signal of >3 mm diameter or three areas if at least one is periventricular should be seen.

False-positive scans are common in patients with one or two white matter lesions, particularly in patients older than age 50 yrs

Cerebrospinal fluid findings

Protein	Normal or mildly increased in 50%
Glucose	Normal
Lymphocytes	Normal in 66%; in remainder, range from 5 to 20 cells/mm^3; T/B lymphocyte ratio is 80:20 CD4$^+$/CD8$^+$ is 2:1
IgG	Increased in about 70%
Increased IgG synthesis	3.3 mg/day in 90% of patients
High IgG index	0.7 in 90% of patients
Oligoclonal IgG bands	90% of cases immunoelectrophoresis and silver staining
Light chains	Increased ratio of kappa/lambda and free kappa light chains
Myelin basic protein	Normally <1 ng/mL; increased in acute relapses to 4 ng/mL in 80% of cases

Evoked potentials

Visual-evoked responses	Very sensitive for detecting plaques in optic nerves, chiasm, or tracts
	Abnormal responses in 85% of those with definite and 58% of those with probable MS
	Interocular P$_{100}$ latency difference is common feature
Brainstem auditory	Most useful in detecting suspected pontine lesions
	Abnormal responses in 67% of patients with definite and 41% of those with probable MS
Somatosensory	Useful to document sensor abnormalities in patients with MS who have normal clinical sensory examinations
	Abnormal in 77% of patients with definite and 67% of patients with probable MS

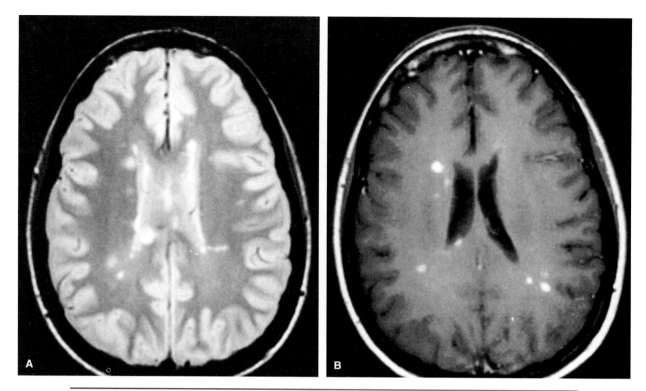

FIGURE 134.10. A. Proton-density axial MRI scan shows multiple hyperintense lesions within the periventricular white matter and corona radiata that are suggestive of demyelinating plaques. **B.** T1-weighted axial MRI scan after gadolinium enhancement shows that some of these lesions exhibit contrast enhancement. (Precontrast T1-weighted images showed no hyperintense lesions.) Contrast enhancement of demyelinating plaques suggests active demyelination, and acute exacerbation of multiple sclerosis was evident clinically in this patient. (Courtesy of Dr. S. Chan.)

the ability to detect lesions, particularly in periventricular distribution.

The distribution and morphology of plaques on T2-weighted MRI may be strongly suggestive of MS (Fig. 134.11), but occasionally it is difficult to distinguish from other lesions, particularly vascular disease. The MS plaques are found in the white matter in a periventricular distribution; the posterior poles of the lateral ventricles and the area of the centrum semiovale are most frequently involved. Corpus callosum lesions are very characteristic of MS and are brought out best with sagittal proton density or FLAIR images. The most common appearance is of homogeneously hyperintense lesions; less commonly, ring or cystic lesions may occur. T1 imaging is not sensitive for lesion detection. However, occurrence of hypodense areas ("black holes") may be observed. Although these can be seen superimposed on active lesions, in the context of stable disease they correlate with frank tissue necrosis and glial scarring. Gadolinium is useful in defining areas undergoing active inflammation, particularly when done with magnetic transfer sequences. Triple-dose gadolinium is more sensitive than the standard dose, and delay in scanning after injection also enhances detection of inflammation. Because nonspecific white matter abnormalities are commonly seen, particu-

larly in patients older than 50 years, a careful approach is still advisable when interpreting MRI studies despite the improvement in techniques (Table 134.4). Correlation of the MRI and the clinical history is of paramount importance.

Although MRI has been extremely useful diagnostically, correlation of standard techniques with clinical findings and disability is disappointing. First, MRI involvement is only an indirect measure of the actual lesions, and histologic damage may be far less than the size of scan abnormality. This amplification factor is useful diagnostically, but reduces the correlation with functional loss. Second, much of observed motor dysfunction in MS is based on spinal cord lesions that are notoriously difficult to image and unobserved if only brain scans are obtained. Volumetric MRI can demonstrate cerebral atrophy even early in the course, when obvious lesions are sparse. This atrophy apparently results from axonal and neuronal loss and correlates better with disability than earlier scanning techniques, particularly with cognitive and memory dysfunction. Unfortunately, volumetric techniques may be unavailable for routine clinical use.

Magnetic resonance spectroscopy is useful for analyzing the parenchyma involved in MS lesions. Changes in tissue components may antedate even the earliest observable

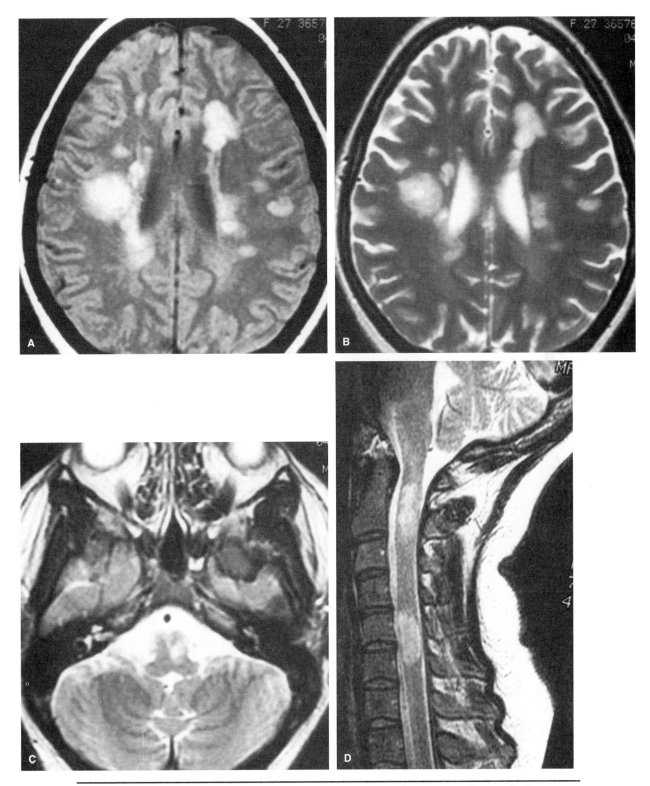

FIGURE 134.11. A and **B.** Proton-density and T2-weighted axial MRI scans show multiple periventricular hyperintense lesions, many of which abut the ependymal lining of the lateral ventricles. **C.** T2-weighted axial MRI scan shows single hyperintense lesion within inferior left pons. **D.** T2-weighted sagittal MRI scan shows two hyperintense lesions within cervical cord. This distribution of lesions is highly suggestive of multiple sclerosis. (Courtesy of Dr. S. Chan and Dr. A. G. Khandji.)

MRI finding of gadolinium-enhancement and blood-brain barrier breakdown by more than a week.

Examination of the CSF frequently provides supportive information for the diagnosis (Table 134.4). The characteristic changes in CSF gamma globulins (IgG) are the most useful findings. The presence of oligoclonal IgG bands by electrophoretic analysis of CSF is the most frequent abnormality. A few antibody-producing plasma cell clones may proliferate within the neuraxis in MS. The IgG production of these clones stands out in the electrophoretic analysis of the CSF as distinct, oligoclonal bands (OCBs). This pattern is not seen in normal people, in whom the CSF IgGs are passively derived from the serum and appear as diffuse broad bands in electrophoretic gels. For OCBs to be diagnostically useful, two or more bands must be seen, and these bands should be either absent from the serum or present in lower concentrations than in CSF, implying primary intrathecal synthesis of the IgG. More than 90% of patients with clinically definite MS have CSF OCBs, but they are also detected in patients with other CNS inflammatory or infectious diseases. The other conditions, however, often reveal serum bands of at least equal intensity, thus indicating the systemic nature of the illness. For reasons unknown, OCBs are found in about 5% of patients with other (noninflammatory) neurologic problems.

The first abnormality of CSF IgG reported in MS was a relative increase in concentration of IgG compared to CSF total protein. This increase is found in only 70% of patients with clinically definite MS. Refinements of technique now compare the concentration of CSF IgG to serum IgG and take into account the relative concentrations of serum and CSF albumin, thereby increasing the sensitivity of the measurement. By accounting for the relative albumin concentrations, these techniques also allow consideration of cases in which the CSF total protein content is elevated, indicating breakdown of the blood-brain barrier and passive diffusion of antibody into the CSF from the serum. Formulas have been derived to estimate *intrathecal IgG synthetic rate*, which is elevated in MS. The sensitivity of these measurements now approaches the frequency of detection of CSF OCBs by electrophoresis.

The recording of cortical evoked responses from visual, auditory, and somatosensory stimulation is also of great value in demonstrating clinically unsuspected lesions (Table 134.4). Visual evoked responses (VERs) to both flash and pattern reversal stimuli demonstrate abnormalities in many patients without symptoms or signs of visual impairment. Somatosensory evoked potentials may be helpful in some situations, but are usually normal unless there are distinct clinical symptoms or findings. Brainstem auditory evoked responses are even less sensitive in detecting abnormalities in asymptomatic patients. They may be useful, however, in confirming the presence of abnormalities in patients with brainstem dysfunction. These procedures are simple, noninvasive, and harmless and may be quite useful in providing evidence of anatomic abnormalities in unclear clinical circumstances. Magnetically evoked motor potentials are sensitive in detecting lesions of the motor pathways from the cortex to spinal cord.

DIAGNOSIS

Because no specific test for MS is available, diagnosis rests on the multiple signs and symptoms with characteristic remissions and exacerbations. Diagnosis can rarely be made with assurance at the time of the first attack. The diagnosis of MS is based on evidence from the history, neurologic examination, and laboratory tests that there are lesions in different parts of the CNS. A careful history, designed to bring out mild transient past events, and a detailed examination, for example, testing for monocular color vision, may be needed to confirm dissemination of lesions in time and space as required to diagnose MS with confidence.

The advent of technologically based laboratory tests (Table 134.4) has added a new dimension to the documentation of multiple lesions. MRI findings are integrated with other clinical and paraclinical diagnostic methods to objectively reach a diagnostic decision (Tables 134.5, 134.6, and 134.7). These criteria take into the distinct clinical entities of typical relapsing-remitting disease, early non-symptomatic cases, and insidious slowly progressive disease without relapses.

Finally, when the diagnosis of MS cannot be made with certainty, the clinician should re-evaluate the patient rather than make a hasty diagnostic decision. In some cases, however, MS may remain asymptomatic, and a firm diagnosis may be made only at autopsy.

Differential Diagnosis

In young adults with characteristic manifestations (Table 134.3) and laboratory abnormalities (Table 134.4), the diagnosis is easily made. Although the complete list of diagnostic possibilities may seem endless, only a few disorders have similar clinical or laboratory features that lead to diagnostic difficulties (Table 134.8).

It is difficult, if not impossible, to differentiate between the first attack of MS and acute disseminated encephalomyelitis (ADEM). ADEM follows infection or vaccination and occurs most commonly in children. A clear distinction between the two conditions may not be possible because about 25% of patients diagnosed as having ADEM later develop MS. Furthermore, the pathologic lesions of MS and ADEM are difficult to distinguish.

In endemic areas, Lyme disease is an important consideration because chronic CNS infection with *Borrelia burgdorferi* can cause spastic paraparesis, cerebellar signs, and cranial nerve palsies. The MRI and CSF abnormalities of MS can also be seen in Lyme disease, so the diagnosis of

▶ TABLE 134.5 Diagnostic Criteria

Clinical Manifestations	Additional Data Needed for MS Diagnosis
Two or more attacks; objective clinical evidence of 2 or more lesions	None[a]
Two or more attacks; objective clinical evidence of 1 lesion	Dissemination in space, demonstrated by MRI[b] or Two or more MRI-detected lesions consistent with MS plus positive CSF[c] or Await further clinical attack implicating a different site
One attack; objective clinical evidence of 2 or more lesions	Dissemination in time, demonstrated by MRI[d] or Second clinical attack
One attack; objective clinical evidence of 1 lesion (monosymptomatic presentation; clinically isolated syndrome)	Dissemination in space, demonstrated by MRI[b] or Two or more MRI-detected lesions consistent with MS plus Positive CSF[c] and Dissemination in time, demonstrated by MRI[d] or Second clinical attack
Insidious neurologic progression suggestive of MS	Positive CSF[c] and Dissemination in space, demonstrated by (1) Nine or more T2 lesions in brain *or* (2) two or more lesions in spinal cord, *or* 3) 4–8 brain plus 1 spinal cord lesion or abnormal VEP[e] associated with 4–8 brain lesions, or with fewer than 4 brain lesions plus 1 spinal cord lesion demonstrated by MRI and Dissemination in time, demonstrated by MRI[d] or Continued progression for 1 year

If criteria indicated are fulfilled, the diagnosis is MS; if the criteria are not completely met, the diagnosis is "possible MS"; if the criteria are fully explored and not met, the diagnosis is "not MS."

[a]No additional tests are required; however, if tests MRI, CSF are undertaken and are *negative*, extreme caution should be taken before making a diagnosis of MS. Alternative diagnoses must be considered. There must be no better explanation for the clinical picture.

[b]MRI demonstration of space dissemination must fulfill the criteria derived from Barkhof et al.[6] and Tintoré et al.[7] (see Table 134-6).

[c]Positive CSF determined by oligoclonal bands detected by established methods (preferably isoelectric focusing) different from any such bands in serum or by a raised IgG index.

[d]MRI demonstration of time dissemination must fulfill the criteria listed in Table 134-7.

[e]Abnormal visual evoked potential of the type seen in MS (delay with a well-preserved wave form).

▶ TABLE 134.6 MRI Criteria for Brain Abnormality

Three of the four following:
1. One gadolinium-enhancing lesion or nine T2-hyperintense lesions if there is no gadolinium-enhancing lesion
2. At least one infratentorial lesion
3. At least one juxtacortical lesion
4. At least three periventricular lesions

Note: One spinal cord lesion can be substituted for one brain lesion.
Data from Barkhof et al. and Tintoré et al.

Lyme disease must rest on a history of characteristic acute symptoms and rash of Lyme disease, with demonstration of antibodies to *Borrelia* antigens in high titer and in both CSF and serum.

Because other infections may mimic MS, serologic tests for HIV, HTLV-I, and syphilis are required. Progressive multifocal leukoencephalopathy should be considered in immunosuppressed individuals.

Several autoimmune diseases have CNS manifestations and particularly MRI changes that can resemble MS. SLE,

▶ **TABLE 134.7   MRI Criteria for Dissemination of Lesions in Time**

1. If a first scan occurs 3 months or more after the onset of the clinical event, the presence of a gadolinium-enhancing lesion is sufficient to demonstrate dissemination in time, provided that it is not at the site implicated in the original clinical event. If there is no enhancing lesion at this time, a follow-up scan is required. The timing of this follow-up scan is not crucial, but 3 months is recommended. A new T2- or gadolinium-enhancing lesion at this time then fulfills the criterion for dissemination in time.
2. If the first scan is performed less than 3 months after the onset of the clinical event, a second scan done 3 months or more after the clinical event showing a new gadolinium-enhancing lesion provides sufficient evidence for dissemination in time. However, if no enhancing lesion is seen at this second scan, a further scan not less than 3 months after the first scan that shows a new T2 lesion or an enhancing lesion will suffice.

polyarteritis nodosa, Sjögren syndrome, Behçet disease, and sarcoidosis are the most notable. The non-CNS features of these diseases usually distinguish them from MS, but if diagnostic difficulties are encountered, specific serum antibody tests, such as anti-DNA antibodies in SLE, or a biopsy of an appropriate site, such as in sarcoidosis, are sufficient to clinch the diagnosis.

Paraneoplastic syndromes with cerebellar signs may cause diagnostic problems, particularly in older patients. Serum antibodies to Purkinje cells are useful in making the diagnosis.

Subacute combined degeneration should be excluded in all cases of spinal MS by measuring serum vitamin B_{12} levels. Similarly, women with progressive spastic paraparesis should have a test for the plasma content of very long-chain fatty acids to exclude the heterozygous carrier state of adrenomyeloneuropathy. Subacute myelo-optic neuritis (SMON) is an adverse reaction to chlorhydroxyquinoline; relapses of sensory symptoms, limb weakness, and optic neuritis may occur. SMON is restricted almost exclusively to Japanese people, and no further cases should be seen because the drug has been withdrawn.

Hereditary spinocerebellar ataxia syndromes can cause diagnostic dilemmas. If the syndrome is Friedreich ataxia, differentiation is easily made on clinical grounds, but if only cerebellar and pyramidal signs develop, diagnosis may be difficult. The most vexing problem is to separate slowly progressive spastic paraparesis of MS from hereditary spastic paraplegia or primary lateral sclerosis, especially if CSF studies and MRI are normal.

Vascular disease, arteriovenous malformations, tumors of brain or spinal cord, and arachnoid cysts can have relapsing-remitting signs. MRI is usually defining. The effects of an Arnold-Chiari malformation can simulate MS clinically, but MRI findings are usually diagnostic. Cervical spondylotic myelopathy may simulate spinal MS; MRI of the brain and CSF changes may indicate MS.

Common neurologic conditions, including cerebrovascular disease or cervical spondylosis, may be found in a patient who also has MS. Determination of whether new symptoms are caused by relapse of MS or by the coexisting condition may be challenging. History, examination, and MRI are of greatest use in determining the cause.

COURSE AND PROGNOSIS

The clinical course of MS varies. Exceptional cases are clinically silent for a lifetime; the typical pathologic findings are discovered only at autopsy. At the other extreme, some cases are so rapidly progressive or malignant (Marburg variant) that only a few months elapse between onset and death.

Clinical observation of the course of MS has led to the description of different types. *Relapsing-remitting* MS is is usually present at the outset and is characterized by exacerbations followed by a variable extent of improvement, ranging from complete resolution of neurologic deficit to significant residual dysfunction. About 10% of patients have relatively few attacks throughout their life and accrue minimal disability. This is referred to as *benign MS*. Relapsing-remitting MS frequently (about 85% of the time) evolves into a situation in which the course progresses slowly in between or in lieu of discrete attacks. This is referred to as *secondary progressive MS*. Various subsets have also been described. These descriptions have limitations because a relapsing-remitting course may last several years to be followed by a chronic-progressive illness. Also, no universal agreement has been reached about the definition of *relapse* or *remission*. Determining if a patient is having a relapse may be difficult, especially in mild cases, and the assessment is often made in retrospect.

There is no discernible difference in MRI scan activity between the relapsing-remitting and secondary progressive MS, and the change of course does not necessarily imply a change in the inflammatory process. Primary progressive MS has some characteristics that differ from the other types, as discussed below.

The diagnostic use of evoked potentials, CSF oligoclonal bands, and MRI has changed concepts about the course of MS. Patients previously thought to have a mild neurologic disorder of undetermined cause are now included as having probable or definite MS, thereby altering the incidence and prevalence data of clinical subtypes.

The question most frequently asked by patients is that of prognosis. Unfortunately, no reliable prognostic indicators are available, and the generalizations that follow may not be applicable in individual cases. The characteristics of a good prognosis in order of usefulness are the following: minimal disability 5 years after onset; complete and rapid remission of initial symptoms; age 35 years or less at onset; only one symptom during the first year; acute onset of first

▎ TABLE 134.8 Differential Diagnosis of MS

Disorder	Distinguishing Clinical/Laboratory Features
Acute disseminated encephalomyelitis	Follows infections or vaccination in children; fever, headaches, and meningism common
Lyme disease	Antibodies to *Borrelia* antigens in serum and CSF by ELISA and Western blotting
HIV-associated myelopathy	HIV serology
HTLV-I myelopathy	HTLV-I serology in serum/CSF
Neurosyphilis	Serum/CSF serology
Progressive multifocal leukoencephalopathy	Immunosuppressed patients; biopsy of lesions demonstrates virus by electron microscopy
Systemic lupus erythematosus	Non-CNS manifestations of lupus; antinuclear antibodies, anti-dsDNA and anti-Sm antibodies
Polyarteritis nodosa	Systemic signs; angiography shows microaneuryms; biopsy of involved areas shows vasculitis
Sjögren syndrome	Dry eyes and mouth; anti-Ro and anti-La antibodies; lower lip biopsy helpful
Behçet disease	Oral/genital ulcers, antibodies to oral mucosa
Sarcoidosis	Non-CNS signs; increased protein in CSF; biopsy shows granuloma
Paraneoplastic syndromes	Older age group; anti-Yo antibodies; identify neoplasm
Subacute combined degeneration of cord	Peripheral neuropathy; vitamin B_{12} levels
Subacute meylooptic neuritis	Mainly in Japanese; adverse reaction to chlorhydroxyquinoline
Adrenomyeloneuropathy	Adrenal dysfunction; neuropathy; plasma very-long-chain fatty acids increased
Spinocerebellar syndromes	Familial; pes cavus; scoliosis; absent reflexes; normal CSF IgG and no bands
Hereditary spastic paraparesis/primary lateral sclerosis	Normal CSF studies
Miscellaneous	Strokes, tumors, arteriovenous malformations, arachnoid cysts, Arnold-Chiari malformations, and cervical spondylosis all may lead to diagnostic dilemmas on occasion. These conditions may coexist; differentiation based on history, clinical follow-up and MRI features.

symptoms; and brief duration of the most recent exacerbation. In general, onset of disease with sensory symptoms or mild optic neuritis is also associated with a good prognosis. Poor prognostic indicators include polysymptomatic onset, such cerebellar signs as ataxia or tremor, vertigo, or corticospinal tract signs. Finally, effective treatments for MS have been available for only about a decade, and the prognosis of early treated cases awaits to be fully defined.

Disability and work capacity are important concerns in any chronic disease with onset from 15 to 55 years (Table 134.9). Although there is overall only a modest effect on life expectancy in MS, disability is a major issue; after 10 years, 70% of MS patients are not working full time. Major causes of disability include cognitive and memory disorders, spastic paraparesis, poor coordination, and sphincter dysfunction.

▎ TABLE 134.9 Working Capacity and Survival in 800 Patients with MS

Duration	1–5 yr (%)	6–10 yr (%)	11–15 yr (%)	16–20 yr (%)	21 yr (%)
Working	71	50	31	30	28
Disabled	29	49	63	57	52
Dead	—	1	6	13	20

From Bauer HJ. *Neurology* 1978;28:8–20.

Death from MS itself is rare. Bronchopneumonia as a result of either aspiration or progressive respiratory insufficiency is the most common cause of death. Other causes include cardiac failure, malignancies (as would be expected in older patients regardless of MS), septicemia (decubitus ulcers, urinary infections), and suicide. In the last few decades, average survival has increased from about 25 years to 35 years after onset, probably as a result of better management of infection and decubitus ulcers.

Variants of Multiple Sclerosis

Several variants of MS appear to exist. The typical form of relapsing-remitting disease, which often evolves into more progressive disease, is called the *Charcot variant*. Primary progressive MS differs from the more common form in that the progressive nature is seen from the outset and distinct exacerbations do not occur. It accounts for about 10% of all MS cases and is more common in older men. Brain MRI lesions tend to be sparse or absent, and this appears to be mainly a spinal cord syndrome. Not infrequently, optic neuropathy is present as demonstrated by VERs. The pathology tends to show a less exuberant immune inflammatory component than in more typical disease. Oligoclonal bands are, however, found in the CSF in over 50% of patients. It appears to have a more relentless course than typical MS.

A more rapidly progressive disease with severe deficits and frequently death occurring in the first year has been designated the *Marburg variant*. The pathology shows more exuberant inflammation and axonal loss than the Charcot variant. Some patients have a fulminant myelitic picture associated closely if not simultaneously with optic neuritis that is frequently bilateral, the *Devic syndrome*. Some consider this a separate disease because of the severely necrotic lesions and a relative paucity of immune active cells as well as the absence of lesions in the brain on MRI. *Schilder disease* (Chapter 95) is sometimes considered fulminant multiple sclerosis of childhood. The pathology is similar to that seen in MS, but confluent lesions involving both hemispheres are typical. The *concentric sclerosis of Balo* also occurs primarily in children. The course is often similar to that of typical MS but the pathology is strikingly different, characterized by concentric rings of inflammation and demyelination. It is unknown how this pattern comes about. Although all these variants are unusual, without clear knowledge of etiology and pathogenesis, it is impossible to know whether they should be considered as separate diseases or forms of MS.

Finally, some paroxysmal inflammatory CNS disorders in adults are equivocally related to MS. Cases of recurrent optic neuritis without any evidence of other neuraxis involvement are known. Similarly, recurrent episodes of myelitis occur in isolation. The CSF may be inflammatory, but oligoclonal bands are often absent. ADEM may be clinically indistinguishable from an attack of MS. Lesions tend to be more inflammatory and less demyelinating than MS plaques. ADEM is characteristically monophasic and may be more of a cognate for EAE than ME. Recurrences have been reported, but that pattern should be more properly classified as MS.

MANAGEMENT

MS is a major challenge for the physician. The fact that no known cure exists often leads to neglect of symptoms and complications that are amenable to prevention and treatment. Although no cure is in sight, the results of controlled therapeutic trials with a number of agents suggest that the natural history of MS can be favorably altered.

Before making specific recommendations about treatment, some general guidelines should be considered:

1. The patient and family should be informed of the diagnosis by specific name when it is firmly established, so they can begin to accept the diagnosis and can avail themselves of all available services.
2. The disease should be explained in understandable terms, with a realistic but best possible prognosis.
3. At first, the patient should be re-evaluated at short intervals for counseling and support, and then at regular intervals to monitor possible complications and to evaluate progress.
4. The patient should be given realistic information about the goals of therapy and should participate in decisions.
5. Patients with MS have complex problems, and many benefit from care at MS centers, where a team approach provides comprehensive service.
6. The patient should be informed about local and national MS societies that provide educational material, support groups, and other services.

Therapeutic regimens are either disease specific (immunosuppressive or immunomodulatory) or symptomatic.

For acute attacks, methylprednisolone is given in a dose of 1 g by intravenous infusion daily for 7 to 10 days. This is followed by oral prednisone in a tapering schedule. A typical tapering regimen follows: prednisone 80 mg daily for 4 days; followed by 60 mg, 40 mg, 20 mg, 10 mg, and 5 mg each for 4 days; and then 4 doses of 5 mg on alternate days. Tapering schedules are arbitrary and are often empiric or based on speculative theoretical considerations. They may be considerably longer or shorter than the one described.

In controlled trials, steroid therapy hastens recovery from acute attacks, but it is not clear that it affects the eventual outcome. Both CSF pleocytosis and MRI abnormalities diminish in patients who receive intravenous high-dose steroid therapy. A shorter (3-day) high-dose intravenous methylprednisolone treatment was compared to oral steroids and placebo over a 2-year period in patients with an initial episode of only optic neuritis. Accelerating recovery without influencing eventual outcome was confirmed. Retrospective data analysis suggested that the development of MS was delayed in the intravenous methylprednisolone group. The 3-day course of intravenous high-dose corticosteroids appears to be a matter of convenience and has never been demonstrated to be as effective as longer courses.

In the short term, adverse effects of corticosteroids are usually minimal or transitory. Psychologic agitation is perhaps most common and should be treated appropriately. Avascular necrosis of joints is rare, but can occur regardless of the steroid dose. Patients who have frequent relapses and are treated repeatedly with steroids, however, are at risk of serious adverse effects. To minimize these effects, the steroid dosage should be tapered and calcium carbonate supplements (650 mg two times per day) should be given to forestall osteoporosis. Chronic oral steroid use has no merit, either daily or on alternate days, because this treatment does not alter the course of the disease.

In 1993 the first practical treatments for use in early MS that altered the course of the disease became available. Four classes of medications are now FDA approved for use in MS. β-interferons are available in three preparations. The first was β-interferon-1b (Betaseron) a chemical modification of naturally occurring human β-interferon. This is given on alternate days subcutaneously in a dose of 0.250 mg. Unaltered β-interferon-1a (Avonex) is given intramuscularly once a week in a dose of 30 mcg. Another presparation of β-interferon-1a (Rebif) is given 44 mcg subcutaneously three times a week. In placebo-controlled studies, all three forms of β-interferon gave similar results. They all seem to reduce the frequency of attacks in the relapsing-remitting phase by about 30%. The severity of attacks was also reduced, and effects on MRI lesions were favorable. Most important, long-term disability has been less. However, a beneficial effect for progressive forms of MS with this class of therapy has not been demonstrated.

The β-interferons are tolerated well. Early in treatment a flulike syndrome may occur following each injection, rarely lasting longer than 24 hours. It may include myalgia, arthralgia, headache, and fever. These symptoms usually dissipate in a few weeks. Taking the medication in the evening and with acetaminophen or a nonsteroidal anti-inflammatory drug often ameliorates the syndrome. Low doses of corticosteroids at the outset of treatment have also been advocated. On rare occasions these symptoms may persist and force discontinuation of treatment. Patients with severe weakness and spasticity may find that their function decreases the day after an injection, and this may also necessitate discontinuation. Hepatic abnormalities and bone marrow depression may occur, but only rarely lead to discontinuation. Periodic blood studies are advisable, especially during the first 2 years of administration. With Betaseron and Rebif, injection site reactions are occasionally severe enough to stop treatment. Although there is no known danger to the fetus, manufacturers have indicated pregnancy (including the period of conception

and breast-feeding as a contraindication to the use of the β-interferons. Depression is commonly thought to be worsened by β-interferons, but there is no firm scientific support for this contention.

All these medications can be self-administered, if neurologic function permits. Neutralizing antibodies against β-interferon may occur during the course of treatment and may render it ineffective. Development of antibodies appears to be more frequent with Betaseron (about 30%), intermediate with Rebif (24%), and least frequent with Avonex (5%). The subcutaneous route for injection may be a factor in antibody development. The medication should probably be stopped if antibodies are found and alternative treatment considered.

The second class of disease-specific therapy currently available is glatiramer acetate (Copaxone or copolymer-I), a mixture of polymers of four amino acids. One of the sequences is a nonencephalitogenic peptide fragment of myelin basic protein. It has been demonstrated to have effects similar to the β-interferons on the frequency of exacerbations and the severity of attack. However, effects on lesions in brain MRI and development of disability are less well established. Some experts consider this the drug of choice in early mild cases, and controlled studies suggest that this group might benefit the most from glatiramer acetate, which is given subcutaneously on a daily basis. It is not associated with systemic symptoms or abnormalities, but some patients report anginalike chest pressure without evidence of cardiac ischemia. Although glatiramer is the best tolerated of all the FDA-approved medications, injection site reactions occur. Acutely intense itching associated with local inflammation may arise, subsiding in a few weeks. Long-term fat necrosis at site reactions in about 40% of patients is cosmetically disfiguring and irreversible. Self-inspection of injection sites helps prevent this complication, and treatment should be switched to an alternate agent.

As evidence has accrued that these medications have a favorable effect on disease progression, the importance of early initiation of treatment has become more apparent. A committee of the National Multiple Sclerosis Society recommends treatment with a disease modifier for all patients with clinically definite exacerbating disease.

Mitoxantrone (Novantrone) is the third class of FDA-approved medications for MS. It is indicated for severe and frequent relapsing or progressive MS. It is a synthetic antineoplastic anthracenedione that is given as an intravenous infusion at a dose of 12 mg/m^2 body surface area every 3 months. Because of cumulative cardiac toxicity, this therapy is limited to about 8 to 10 cycles over a lifetime. Before starting therapy, an echocardiogram is warranted to ensure a left ventricular ejection fraction of greater than 50%. Reversible hair loss, menstrual irregularities, leucopenia, and asthenia are other infrequent complications. Acute, fatal leukemia is the most serious complication and occurs in the first 5 years post-therapy in about 1% of cases.

The fourth class of FDA-approved medications for MS is natalizumab (Tysabri), a selective adhesion molecule inhibitor. Natalizumab acts by preventing trafficking of lymphocytes across the blood brain barrier (BBB). Lymphocytes express a $\alpha4$-$\beta1$-integrin molecule that binds to the vascular adhesion cell molecule (VCAM)-1 on the endothelial cell resulting in lymphocyte arrest and migration across the BBB. Natalizumab is a recombinant monoclonal antibody directed against the $\alpha4$-$\beta1$-integrin receptor and thus it blocks binding of the lymphocyte to VCAM-1. In placebo-controlled studies, natalizumab reduced the rate of clinical relapses by about 66% (approximately twice as effective as any of the other class of medications for MS) and decreased gadolinium-enhancing brain MRI lesions by over 90%. In a related combination study of natalizumab with β-interferon 1-a, patients on combination therapy had a 53% reduction of clinical relapses over patients taking β-interferon 1-a alone. In the one-year data analysis, there are no serious adverse effects of natalizumab therapy although patients should be monitored for allergic reactions. It is given as a monthly infusion at dose of 300 mgs over one hour. Although these early results are very promising, long-term safety, sustained efficacy, and effect on disease progression will need to be established before natalizumab is considered the standard first line treatment for MS.

A few patients continue to have disease activity and clinical progression despite the above treatments. These patients have no response to high-dose intravenous steroids or, more often, have a modest initial response and minimal responses with subsequent cycles of therapy. If a β-interferon is being administered, it is appropriate to determine the neutralizing antibody level.

Alternative treatments that may be used are mainly immunosupressants. Cyclophosphamide has been used in monthly pulse doses of 800 to 1,000 mg/m²s.a. in 500 mL of 0.9% sodium chloride solution infused over 2 to 4 hours. Patients are given 3 L of fluid over 24 hours to maintain adequate urinary output. Sodium 2-mercaptoethane sulfonate, also generically known as mesna (Uromitexan) can be added to the cyclophosphamide in equal amounts to reduce bladder irritation. Ondansetron 10 mg and dexamethasone 10 mg can reduce nausea and vomiting. Whether cyclophosphamide is beneficial is uncertain because clinical trials have given conflicting results. Many clinicians use it based on anecdotal experience and believe it stabilizes the disease without improvement. Another agent with conflicting results in the literature is cladribine (Leustatin). This is relatively specific for T$_4$ helper cells, and some consider this a theoretical advantage. Azathioprine taken orally in a dose of 1 to 2 mg/kg of body weight merits mention. Methotrexate taken in doses similar to those used in rheumatoid arthritis (7.5–15 mg orally once a week) has been demonstrated to be modestly effective in progressive disease.

It should be considered in situations when prophylactic agents or more intensive chemotherapy is not indicated. High-dose (1 gm/kg) gamma globulin given intravenously once a month is also used and has shown to be efficacious in relasping-remitting MS. Plasmapheresis may be used for acute attacks when neurologic deterioration does not respond to high-dose methylprednisolone. It is anticipated that drug combination therapy will increasingly be used for single-drug treatment–resistant MS. Commonly used combinations include β-interferon or glatiramer acetate in combination with pulsed monthly methylprednisolone or IVIG or mitoxantrone.

In a disease that cannot be prevented or cured, symptomatic therapy is important to minimize functional deficit and discomfort. Spasticity with stiffness, painful flexor or extensor spasms, and clonus are major causes of disability. If untreated, contractures may develop, thereby increasing disability. Baclofen is the most commonly used drug at a dose of 40 to 80 mg per day in divided doses. If tolerated, higher doses may be used in severe cases. Diazepam or dantrolene may be added or substituted if necessary. Tizanidine in doses up to 24 mg daily may also be considered. It supposedly does not cause as much weakness as the other antispasticity agents. Unfortunately, sedation is a major problem with tizanidine and slow titration is required. For localized adductor spasms, injections of botulinum toxin may be useful. However, the large muscle groups involved require large doses of medication and antibody production rapidly develops. In resistant cases, baclofen may be given intrathecally with an indwelling catheter and implantation of a reservoir pump. Only patients who have a beneficial effect with an intrathecal test bolus dose of 50 to 100 mcg of baclofen should have the pump implanted. Adverse effects are not common. Cracks in the tubing may develop and should be considered if effect is rapidly lost. In addition to relief of spasticity, patients with bladder symptoms frequently improve. The dosage of all antispastic agents must be closely monitored and titrated with the clinical response; flaccidity, unmasked weakness, or changes in mentation may result in functional deterioration.

Bladder management is important to prevent debilitating and life-threatening infections and stone formation and to allow for maximum functional independence. The basic problem may be failure to retain urine, excessive urinary retention, or a combination of the two. In all these problems, the symptoms of urgency, frequency, and incontinence are similar. The most important measures are postvoiding residuals, urine cultures, and, occasionally, urodynamic studies or renal ultrasound studies. The atonic bladder with a residual volume over 100 mL is best managed by a program of clean intermittent self-catheterization. Cholinergic drugs, such as bethanechol, carbachol, and pyridostigmine, are marginally and transiently effective in aiding bladder emptying. For acute urinary retention during a relapse of MS, phenoxybenzamine is the drug of choice because it induces relaxation of the bladder neck. Patients with bladder atony are susceptible to urinary infections. Some authorities routinely use urine acidifiers, such as vitamin C, and urinary antiseptics, such as methenamine hippurate, for all such patients.

Detrusor muscle hyperexcitability that causes the spastic bladder is the most common cause of urinary urgency and incontinence in patients with MS. Oxybutynin is the most effective agent in relieving symptoms, but other anticholinergic medications include propantheline, hycosamine, and imipramine. A sustained release form of oxybutynin is also used and has fewer anticholineric adverse effects. Tolterodine (Detrol), a long-acting anticholinergic, has been released, which decreases the frequency of dosing. The synthetic antidiuretic hormone (vasopressin), desmopressin acetate (DDAVP), has been used with success as an intranasal spray, particularly for patients with nocturia. The usual dose is 10 to 40 μg at night. Serum osmolality and electrolytes should be measured weekly for the first month and then monthly as a precaution in these patients. Some patients find a morning-after rebound effect, which is unacceptable. DDAVP is also available in oral form.

In patients with long-standing bladder disease, indwelling catheters may have to be used even though the risk of infection increases. Disposable catheters, periodic irrigation, weekly catheter renewal, and urine acidifiers minimize infections. Bladder augmentation with a section of bowel has been helpful when bladder size has diminished because of spasticity. A continent port may be placed on the abdominal wall to facilitate catheterization in appropriate situations. In late stages, suprapubic cystostomy or urinary diversion procedures may be appropriate. In all patients with urinary symptoms, a urine culture should be obtained, because treatment of infection alone may suffice to relieve new symptoms.

Cerebellar symptoms are generally resistant to therapy. An occasional patient with disabling intention tremor may respond to propranolol or clonazepam. Cryothalamotomy may be effective, but should be reserved for severe cases.

Painful radiculopathy or neuralgia and painful paresthesias may respond to carbamazepine or, if not tolerated, to phenytoin or amitriptyline. Gabapentin is also used. Less specific pain syndromes may respond to nonsteroidal anti-inflammatory agents. Occasionally with MS, an intractable neurogenic pain syndrome may be seen and relief may be obtained only with intrathecal narcotic therapy.

Fatigue may respond to amantadine or pemoline, as well as to a change in work schedule. Modafinil (Provigil), a novel waking agent used in narcolepsy, has become the drug of first choice in MS. Methylphenidate is used to control fatigue in resistant cases. Depression may contribute to fatigue and usually responds to SSRI antidepressants. Whether these drugs might have an effect on fatigue independent of depression is conjectural. For fatigue associated with endurance, 4-aminopyridine, a potassium channel blocking agent may be used. Its use is limited despite controlled studies showing benefit because of increased seizure risk. It is not approved by the FDA, but is available in other countries and through special-order pharmacies in this country.

Constipation responds best to changes in diet, bulk-providing substances, and stool softeners. Laxatives are reserved for resistant cases. Bowel incontinence is less common and is generally unresponsive to medication. Regularization of bowel habits seems the most useful approach. Anticholinergic drugs may be useful adjuncts.

Sexual dysfunction should be treated with counseling for both partners, and treatments may alleviate the problems. In the past, erectile dysfunction was treated with papaverine injections, alprostadil intracavernosal injections, intraurethral suppositories, or vacuum devices designed to increase penile blood flow. Although often successful, few patients continue to use these treatments because sildenafil (Viagra) has been so successful in patients with MS. Its ease of use makes it more likely to be of continuing benefit. In women, lubricating agents may be of use. Sildenafil is being evaluated for restoring orgasmic capability and lubrication. Vardenafil (Levitra) and tadalafil (Cialis) await formal evaluation for MS.

When paraparesis is severe, skin care to prevent decubitus ulcers is essential. Physical therapy and nursing care with adequate nutrition and hydration are valuable in preventing painful, disabling complications, such as decubitus ulcers, renal and bladder calculi, contractures, and intercurrent infections. When these complications occur, aggressive attempts to relieve them often give gratifying results.

Diet therapy and vitamin supplements are frequently advocated, but no special supplementation or elimination diet has proved to be more beneficial than a well-balanced diet that maintains correct body weight and provides sufficient roughage for bowel management. Other therapies, such as hyperbaric oxygen, neurostimulation, cobra or bee sting venom, and acupuncture, are unproven, and any response to these treatments is usually a result of coincidental spontaneous remission so often seen early in the disease.

Physical therapy should be applied judiciously with the goals of maintaining mobility in ambulatory patients or avoiding contractures in bedridden patients. Excessive active exercise may exhaust the patient, and the increase in body temperature may cause transient symptoms. Swimming in cool water is the best active physical therapy. Occupational therapy is important to assist patients in activities of daily living. MS is one of the few diseases for which a cure is unavailable, yet a comprehensive therapeutic regimen supervised by an experienced and sympathetic physician can give rewarding results.

SUGGESTED READINGS

Ablashi D, Lapps W, Kaplan M, et al. Human herpesvirus-6 (HHV-6) infection in multiple sclerosis: a preliminary report. *Multiple Sclerosis* 1998;4:490–496.

Baranzini SE, Oksenberg JR, Hauser SL. New insights into the genetics of multiple sclerosis. *J Rehabil Res Dev* 2002;39(Mar-Apr):201–209.

Beck RW, Cleary PA, Anderson MM, et al. A randomized, controlled trial of corticosteroids in the treatment of acute optic neuritis. *N Engl J Med* 1992;326:581–588.

Beck RW, Cleary PA, Trobe JD, et al. The effects of corticosteroids for acute optic neuritis on the subsequent development of multiple sclerosis. *N Engl J Med* 1993;329:1764–1769.

Benedict RH, Carone DA, Bakshi R. Correlating brain atrophy with cognitive dysfunction, mood disturbances, and personality disorder in multiple sclerosis. *J Neuroimaging* 2004;14(Suppl 3):36S–45S.

Bielekova B, Martin R. Development of biomarkers in multiple sclerosis. *Brain* 2004 Jul;127(Pt 7):1463–1478.

Billiau A, Kieseier BC, Hartung HP. Biologic role of interferon beta in multiple sclerosis. *J Neurol* 2004 Jun;251 suppl 2:II10–II14.

Borras C, Rio J, Porcel J, et al. Emotional state of patients with relapsing-remitting MS treated with interferon beta-1b. *Neurology* 1999;52:1636–1639.

Compston A, Ebers G, Lassman H, et al., eds. *McAlpine's Multiple Sclerosis.* Edinburgh, Scotland: Churchill-Livingston, 1998.

Confavreux C, Hutchinson M, Hours MM, et al. Rate of pregnancy-related relapse in multiple sclerosis. Pregnancy in Multiple Sclerosis Group [see comments]. *N Engl J Med* 1998;339:285–291.

Dyment DA, Ebers GC, Sadovnick AD. Genetics of multiple sclerosis. *Lancet Neurology* 2004;3(Feb):104–110.

Edan G, Morrissey S, Le Page E. Rationale for the use of mitoxantrone in multiple sclerosis. *J Neurol Sci* 2004 Aug 15;223(1):35–39.

Fazekas F, Deisenhammer F, Strasser-Fuchs S, et al. Randomized placebo-controlled trial of monthly intravenous immunoglobulin therapy in relapsing-remitting multiple sclerosis. *Lancet* 1997;349:589–593.

Filippi M, Iannucci G, Tortorella C, et al. Comparison of MS clinical phenotypes using conventional and magnetization transfer MRI. *Neurology* 1999;52:588–594.

Flachenecker P, Rieckmann P. Health outcomes in multiple sclerosis. *Curr Opin Neurol* 2004 Jun,17(Jun).257–61.

Garell PC, Menezes AH, Baumbach G, et al. Presentation, management and follow-up of Schilder's disease. *Pediatr Neurosurg* 1998;29(Aug):86–91.

Goodin DS, Arnason BG, Coyle PK, et al. The use of mitoxantrone (Novantrone) for the treatment of multiple sclerosis: report of the Therapeutics and Technology Assessment Subcommittee of the American Academy of Neurology. *Neurology* 2003;61:1332–1338.

Haegert DG, Francis GS. HLA-DQ polymorphisms do not explain HLA class II associations with multiple sclerosis in two Canadian patient groups. *Neurology* 1993;43:1207–1210.

Hartung HP, Gonsette R, Konig N, et al. Mitoxantrone in progressive multiple sclerosis. *Lancet* 2002;260:2018–2025.

Hernan MA, Jick SS, Olek MJ, et al. Recombinant hepatitis B vaccine and the risk of multiple sclerosis. *Neurology* 2004;63:838–842.

Hohlfeld R, Wekerle H. Autoimmune concepts of multiple sclerosis as a basis for selective immunotherapy: from pipe dreams to (therapeutic) pipelines. *Proc Natl Acad Sci U S A* 2004 Oct 5;101 Suppl 2:14599–14606.

Interferon beta-1b is effective in relapsing-remitting multiple sclerosis. I. Clinical results of a multicenter, randomized, double-blind, placebo-controlled trial. The IFNB Multiple Sclerosis Study Group. *Neurology* 1993;43:655–661.

Jacobs LD, Cookfair DL, Rudick RA, et al. Intramuscular interferon beta-1a for disease progression in relapsing multiple sclerosis. *Ann Neurol* 1996;39:285–294.

Johnson KP, Brooks BR, Cohen JA, et al. Copolymer 1 reduces relapse rate and improves disability in relapsing-remitting multiple sclerosis: results of a phase III multicenter, double-blind placebo-controlled trial. The Copolymer 1 Multiple Sclerosis Study Group [see comments]. *Neurology* 1995;45:1268–1276.

Johnson KP, Brooks BR, Cohen JA, et al. Extended use of glatiramer acetate (Copaxone) is well tolerated and maintains its clinical effect on multiple sclerosis relapse rate and degree of disability. Copolymer 1 Multiple Sclerosis Study Group. *Neurology* 1998;50:701–708.

Kalman B, Leist TP. Familial multiple sclerosis and other inherited disorders of the white matter. *Neurologist* 2004 Jul;10(4):201–215.

Kieseier BC, Hartung HP. Current disease-modifying therapies in multiple sclerosis. *Sem Neurol* 2003:23(Jun):133–146.

Kim MO, Lee SA, Choi CG, et al. Balo's concentric sclerosis: a clinical case study of brain MRI, biopsy, and proton magnetic resonance spectroscopic findings. *J Neurol Neurosurg Psychiatry* 1997;62:655–658.

Leuzzi V, Lyon G, Cilio MR, et al. Childhood demyelinating diseases with a prolonged remitting course and their relation to Schilder's disease: report of two cases. *J Neurol Neurosurg Psychiatry* 1999;66(Mar):407–408.

Mandler RN, Davis LE, Jeffery DR, et al. Devic's neuromyelitis optica: a clinicopathological study of 8 patients. *Ann Neurol* 1993;34(Aug):162–168.

Marrie RA. Environmental risk factors in multiple sclerosis aetiology. *Lancet Neurol* 2004 Dec;3(12):709–718.

Matthews PM. An update on neuroimaging of multiple sclerosis. *Curr Opin Neurol* 2004 Aug;17(4):453–458.

McDonald WI, Compston A, Edan G, et al. Recommended diagnostic criteria for multiple sclerosis: guidelines from the International Panel on the diagnosis of multiple sclerosis. *Ann Neurol* 2001;50:121–127.

Miller DH, Filippi M, Fazekas F, et al. Role of magnetic resonance imaging within diagnostic criteria for multiple sclerosis. *Ann Neurol* 2004 Aug;56(2):273–278.

Miller DH, Khan OA, Shremata WA, et al. A controlled trial of natalizumab for relapsing multiple sclerosis. *N Engl J Med* 2003;348:68–72.

Miller JR, Burke AM, Bever CT. Occurrence of oligoclonal bands in multiple sclerosis and other CNS diseases. *Ann Neurol* 1983;13:53–56.

Munari L, Lovati R, Boiko A. Therapy with glatiramer acetate for multiple sclerosis. *Cochrane Database Systematic Rev* 2004;(1):CD004678.

Nelson RF. Ethical issues in multiple sclerosis. *Semin Neurol* 1997;17:227–234.

Noseworthy JH. Multiple sclerosis clinical trials: old and new challenges. *Semin Neurol* 1998;18:377–388.

O'Connor PW, Goodman A, Willmer-Hulme AJ, et al. Randomized multicenter trial of natalizumab in acuate MS relapses: clinical and MRI effects. *Neurology* 2004;62:2038–2043.

Paty DW, Li DK. Interferon beta-1b is effective in relapsing-remitting multiple sclerosis. II. MRI analysis results of a multicenter, randomized, double-blind, placebo-controlled trial. UBC MS/MRI Study Group and the IFNB Multiple Sclerosis Study Group [see comments]. *Neurology* 1993;43:662–667.

Placebo-controlled multicentre randomised trial of interferon beta-1b in treatment of secondary progressive multiple sclerosis. European Study Group on interferon beta-1b in secondary progressive MS. *Lancet* 1998;352:1491–1497.

Rammohan KW, Rosenberg JH, Lynn DJ, et al. Efficacy and safety of modafinil (Provigil) for the treatment of fatigue in multiple sclerosis: a two centre phase 2 study. *J Neurol Neurosurg Psychiatry* 2002;72:179–183.

Randomised double-blind placebo-controlled study of interferon beta-1a in relapsing/remitting multiple sclerosis. PRISMS (Prevention of Relapses and Disability by Interferon beta-1a Subcutaneouly in Multiple Sclerosis) Study Group. *Lancet* 1998;352:1498–1504.

Rudick RA. Impact of disease-modifying therapies on brain and spinal cord atrophy in multiple sclerosis. *J Neuroimaging* 2004; 14(3 Suppl):54S–64S.

Rudick RA, Goodkin DE, Jacobs LD, et al. Impact of interferon beta-1a on neurologic disability in relapsing multiple sclerosis. The Multiple Sclerosis Collaborative Research Group (MSCRG). *Neurology* 1997;49:358–363.

Sadovnick AD, Ebers GC, Wilson RW, et al. Life expectancy in patients attending multiple sclerosis. *Neurology* 1992;42:991–994.

Sibley WA. *Therapeutic Claims in Multiple Sclerosis.* New York: Demos, 1992.

Siva A, Radhaskrishnan K, Kurland LT, et al. Trauma and multiple sclerosis: a population based cohort study from Olstead County, Minnesota. *Neurology* 1993;43:1878–1881.

Sotgiu S, Pugliatti M, Fois ML, et al. Genes, environment, and susceptibility to multiple sclerosis. *Neurobiol Dis* 2004; Nov;17(2):131–143.

Steinman L, Martin R, Bernard C, et al. Multiple sclerosis: deeper understanding of the pathogenesis reveals new targets for therapy. *Ann Rev Neurosci* 2002;25:491–505.

Trapp BD, Peterson J, Ransohoff RM, et al. Axonal transection in the lesions of multiple sclerosis. *N Engl J Med* 1998;338:278–285.

Weiner HL, Mackin GA, Orav EJ, et al. Intermittent cyclophosphamide pulse therapy in progressive multiple sclerosis: final report of the Northeast Cooperative Multiple Sclerosis Treatment Group. *Neurology* 1993;43:910–918.

Weinshenker BG, Issa M, Baskerville J. Long-term and short-term outcome of multiple sclerosis: a 3-year follow-up study. *Arch Neurol* 1996;53(Apr):353–358.

Wekerle H, Hohlfeld R. Molecular mimicry in multiple sclerosis. *New Engl J Med* 2003;349:185–186.

Wingerchuk DM, Lucchinetti CF, Noseworthy JH. Multiple sclerosis: current pathophysiological concepts. *Lab Invest* 2001;81(Mar):263–268.

Wolinsky JS. Glatiramer acetate for the treatment of multiple sclerosis. *Expert Opin Pharmacother* 2004;5:875–891.

Chapter 135

Marchiafava-Bignami Disease

Lewis P. Rowland

Primary degeneration of the corpus callosum is clinically characterized by altered mental status, seizures, and multifocal neurologic signs. Demyelination of the corpus callosum without inflammation is the primary pathologic feature, but other areas of the CNS may be involved. The disease was first described by Marchiafava and Bignami in 1903.

ETIOLOGY

The cause is not known. The disease was first noted in middle-aged and elderly Italian men who consumed red wine. It has been described worldwide, however, and is not confined to drinkers of red wine. In some cases, alcohol consumption was not a factor. Nutritional deficiencies also have been implicated. The syndrome is rare, however, even in severe malnutrition. Toxic factors have been suggested, but no agent has been implicated.

PATHOLOGY

The sine qua non is necrosis of the medial zone of the corpus callosum. The dorsal and ventral rims are spared. The necrosis varies from softening and discoloration (Fig. 135.1) to cavitation and cyst formation. Usually, all stages of degeneration are found. In most cases, the rostral position of the corpus callosum is affected first. The lesions arise as small symmetric foci that extend and become confluent. Although medial necrosis of the corpus callosum is the principal finding, there also may be degeneration of the anterior commissure (Fig. 135.2), the posterior commissure, centrum semiovale, subcortical white matter, long association bundles, and middle cerebellar peduncles. All these lesions have a constant bilateral symmetry. Usually spared are the internal capsule, corona radiata, and subgyral arcuate fibers. The gray matter is not grossly affected.

Few diseases have such a well-defined pathologic picture. The corpus callosum may be infarcted as a result of

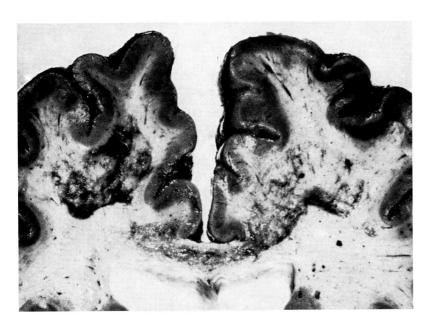

FIGURE 135.1. Marchiafava-Bignami disease. Acute necrosis of corpus callosum and neighboring white matter of the frontal lobes. (From Merritt HH, Weisman AD. *J Neuropathol Exp Neurol* 1945;4:155–163.)

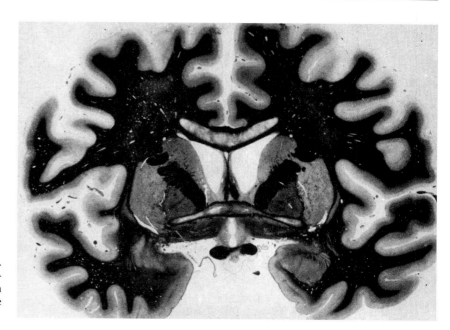

FIGURE 135.2. Marchiafava-Bignami disease. Medial necrosis of the corpus callosum and anterior commissure with sparing of the margins. (Courtesy of Dr. P. I. Yakovlev.)

occlusion of the anterior cerebral artery, but the symmetry of the lesions, sparing of the gray matter, and occurrence of similar lesions in the anterior commissure, long association bundles, and cerebellar peduncles are found only in Marchiafava-Bignami disease.

The microscopic alterations are the result of a sharply defined necrotic process with loss of myelin but relative preservation of axis cylinders in the periphery of the lesions. There is usually no evidence of inflammation aside from a few perivascular lymphocytes. In most cases, fat-filled phagocytes are common. Gliosis is usually not well advanced. Capillary endothelial proliferation may be present in the affected area, but no thrombi are seen. The disease has been reported with central pontine myelinolysis or Wernicke encephalopathy in alcoholics and in nonalcoholic persons, thus suggesting a possible common pathogenesis.

INCIDENCE

More than 100 cases have been reported, but the disease is probably more common. Before the advent of modern imaging, however, the diagnosis was rarely made before death because the symptoms and findings are nonspecific. Genetic predisposition has been suspected because of the frequent reports in Italian men. The onset is usually in middle age or late life.

SYMPTOMS AND SIGNS

The onset is usually insidious, and the first symptoms are so nonspecific that the time of onset is difficult to determine. There is a mixture of focal and diffuse signs of cerebral disease. In addition to memory loss and confusion, manic, paranoid, or delusional states may occur. Depression and extreme apathy are typical.

DIAGNOSIS

Marchiafava-Bignami disease is suspected when insidiously developing dementia, multifocal neurologic signs, and seizures occur in elderly men, particularly alcohol abusers. CT and MRI are accurate in diagnosis, but MRI is preferred in showing the callosal lesions and symmetric demyelinating lesions in subcortical white matter. In the original reports, status epilepticus was prominent and, in modern times, an acute form may be seen. The differential diagnosis includes Wernicke encephalopathy, which may occur simultaneously, manifested by ataxia, ophthalmoplegia, and nystagmus as well as dementia or delirium.

COURSE

The disease is usually slowly progressive and results in death within 3 to 6 years. There is a rare acute fever lasting days or weeks. In an occasional patient there is a temporary remission. Some reports of reversibility exist, but the diagnosis has been only by imaging studies.

TREATMENT

Generally, the outlook for recovery is poor. However, spontaneous recovery has been reported, and some patients improve with thiamine or corticosteroid therapy. Metabolic recovery may be documented by MR spectroscopy.

SUGGESTED READINGS

Arbelaez A, Pajon A, Castillo M. Acute Marchiafava-Bignami disease: MR findings in two paitents. *AJNR Am J Neuroradiol* 2003;24:1955–1957.

Berek K, Wagner M, Chemelli AP, et al. Hemispheric disconnection in Marchiafava-Bignami disease: clinical, neuropsychological and MRI findings. *J Neurol Sci* 1994;123:2–5.

Gambini A, Falini A, Moiola L, et al. Marchiafava-Bignami disease: longitudinal MR imaging and MR spectroscopy study. *AJNR Am J Neuroradiol* 2003;24:249–253.

Gass A, Birtsch G, Olster M, et al. Marchiafava-Bignami disease: reversibility of neuroimaging abnormality. *J Comput Assist Tomogr* 1998;22:503–504.

Hatashi T, Tanohata K, Kunimoto M, et al. Marchiafava-Bignami disease with resolving symmetrical putaminal lesion. *J Neurol* 2002;249:227–228.

Heinrich A, Runge U, Khaw AV. Clinicoradiologic subtypes of Marchiafava-Bignami disease. *J Neuro* 2004 Sep;251(9):1050–1059.

Ironside R, Bosanquet FD, McMenemey WH. Central demyelination of the corpus callosum (Marchiafava-Bignami disease). *Brain* 1961;84:212–230.

Kawarabuki K, Sakakibara T, Hirai M, et al. Marchiafava-Bignami disease: magnetic resonance imaging findings in corpus callosum and subcortical white matter. *Europ J Radiol* 2003;48(Nov):175–177.

Marchiafava E, Bignami A. Sopra un'alterazione del corpo calloso osservata in soggetti alcoolisti. *Riv Patol Nerve* 1903;8:544–549.

Yamashita K, Kobayashi S, Yamaguchi S, et al. Reversible corpus callosum lesions in a patient with Marchiafava-Bignami disease: serial changes on MRI. *Eur Neurol* 1997;37:192–193.

Chapter 136

Central Pontine Myelinolysis

Gary L. Bernardini and Elliott L. Mancall

In 1959, Adams, Victor, and Mancall described a distinctive, previously unrecognized disease characterized primarily by the symmetric destruction of myelin sheaths in the basis pontis. They called it *central pontine myelinolysis*. The general term *myelinolysis* may be more appropriate, because the condition affects extrapontine brain areas as well.

Most patients who develop pontine myelinolysis have had documented hyponatremia, and serum sodium levels were corrected rapidly to normal or supranormal levels. Chronic alcoholism and undernutrition are frequently associated with this condition. Pontine myelinolysis has been seen, however, in hyponatremic nonalcoholic patients, including some with dehydration resulting from vomiting, diarrhea, or diuretic therapy; with postoperative overhydration; or with psychogenic water intoxication. Severe malnutrition, including that resulting from extensive burn injuries, may be a predisposing condition. The main underlying factor to the development of pontine myelinolysis in these cases seems to be too rapid correction of serum sodium levels. Correction after hypernatremia rather than hyponatremia has also been encountered. The condition has been described with increasing frequency in patients undergoing orthotopic liver transplantation. Pontine myelinolysis is found in 0.28% to 9.8% of these cases. A more benign form of pontine myelinolysis may occur without hyponatremia in alcoholic binge drinkers or some with anorexia nervosa. This syndrome has a good clinical outcome, and the MRI abnormalities disappear. In addition, central pontine myelinolysis occurs in chronic alcohol users with profound hypophosphatemia.

The clinical manifestations vary from asymptomatic to comatose, although there may be signs of a generalized encephalopathy associated with low levels of serum sodium. Neurologic signs and symptoms of myelinolysis usually appear within 2 to 3 days after rapid correction of sodium levels. Findings include dysarthria or mutism, behavioral abnormalities, ophthalmoparesis, bulbar and pseudobulbar palsy, hyperreflexia, quadriplegia, seizures, and coma. Typically, a rapidly progressive corticobulbar and corticospinal syndrome may be noted in a debilitated patient, often during an acute illness with associated electrolyte imbalance and correction or overcorrection of hyponatremia. Although the patients are mute, coma is unusual. The patients may be "locked in," and communication by eye blinking can sometimes be established. The course is rapid, and death generally ensues within days or weeks after onset of symptoms.

Extrapontine myelinolysis is seen in about 10% of all cases of pontine myelinolysis. Clinically, extrapontine myelinolysis can cause ataxia, irregular behavior, visual field deficits, or parkinsonism, choreoathetosis, dystonia, or paroxysmal kinesigenic dyskinesias. The movement disorders can appear with or without radiographic evidence of extrapontine myelinolysis. In extrapontine myelinolysis, bilateral symmetric involvement may affect the white matter of the cerebellum, putamen, thalamus, corpus callosum, subcortical white matter, claustrum, caudate, hypothalamus, lateral geniculate bodies, amygdala, subthalamic nuclei, substantia nigra, or medial lemnisci.

Although most cases have been diagnosed only at autopsy, the syndrome can be diagnosed in life. The clinical diagnosis is supported by radiologic studies. CT may be normal, especially early in the course, but CT abnormalities include symmetric areas of hypodensity in the basis pontis and extrapontine regions without associated mass effect. MRI is more sensitive and typically shows symmetric increased signal intensity in the central pons on T2-weighted and fluid attenuation inversion recovery (FLAIR) images; lesions are hypointense on T1-weighted images

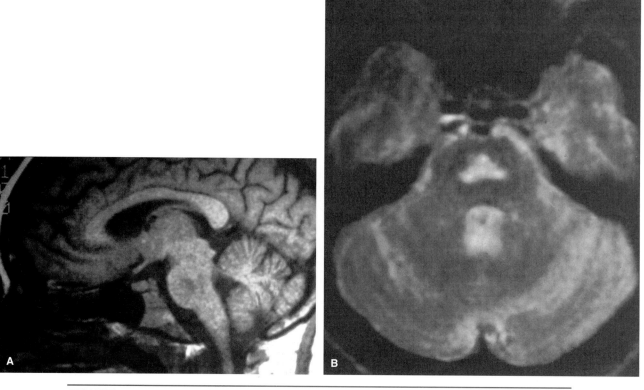

FIGURE 136.1. A. T1-weighted sagittal MR image in a 21-year-old alcoholic woman after rapid correction of severe hyponatremia, showing a hypointense area in the basis pons consistent with the lesion of pontine myelinolysis. **B.** T2-weighted axial MR image in the same patient demonstrating the characteristic centrally located hyperintense areas consistent with demyelination within the pons. (Courtesy of Dr. L. A. Heier.)

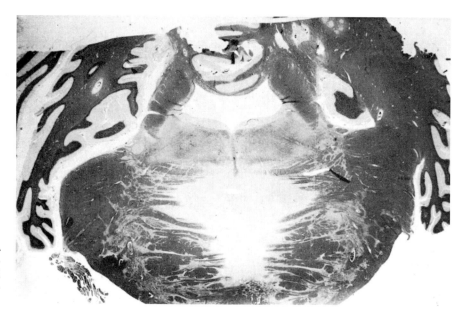

FIGURE 136.2. Central pontine myelinolysis. Histologic section through rostral pons showing characteristic lesion. (Courtesy of Dr. J. Kepes.)

and typically do not enhance (Fig. 136.1). MRI diffusion-weighted imaging (DWI) demonstrates restricted diffusion of water in the central pons within 24 hours of onset of symptoms of myelinolysis, and lesions appear hyperintense. Although conventional imaging with CT and MRI may lag behind clinical manifestations by up to 2 weeks, MRI DWI may be the most sensitive technique for early diagnosis. Brainstem auditory evoked responses may demonstrate prolonged III-V and I-V latencies consistent with bilateral pontine lesions. An EEG may show slowing and low voltage. CSF levels of protein and myelin basic protein may be elevated.

The principal pathologic change is demyelination; within affected areas, nerve cells and axon sheaths are spared, blood vessels are unaffected, and there is no inflammation. The pathophysiology seems caused by physiologic imbalance of osmoles in the brain. Apoptosis may deplete the supply of energy to glial cells and Na^+/K^+-ATPase pumps, thus impairing cellular adaptation to osmotic stress. In animal studies, the initial event after administration of hypertonic saline in hypotonic rats seems to be opening of the blood-brain barrier, followed sequentially by swelling of the inner loop of the myelin sheath, oligodendrocyte degeneration, and release of macrophage-derived factors leading to the eventual breakdown of myelin. Histologically, the lesion begins in the median raphe and may involve all or part of the base of the pons (Fig. 136.2). The lesion may spread into the pontine tegmentum or superiorly into the mesencephalon or involve bilateral extrapontine areas with or without concurrent basis pontis lesions. Microscopically, the lesions resemble those of Marchiafava-Bignami disease.

The exact cause of pontine myelinolysis is uncertain. In those with hyponatremia that has been rapidly corrected to normal or supranormal levels, it is not clear whether the low sodium, the rate of correction, or the absolute change in the serum sodium content is the causative factor. Symptoms are, however, more likely to develop with rapid correction of chronic (more than 48 hours) rather than acute hyponatremia. In experimental animals, pontine myelinolysis developed in hyponatremic rats, rabbits, or dogs treated rapidly with hypernatremic saline. Animals left with untreated hyponatremia did not develop neuropathologic changes. Therefore, attention has focused on the rate of correction of the hyponatremia rather than on the hyponatremia itself as the inciting mechanism of myelinolysis.

Prevention of myelinolysis includes judicious correction of hyponatremia with normal saline and free water restriction, discontinuation of diuretic therapy, and correction of associated metabolic abnormalities and medical complications. Hyponatremic patients who are asymptomatic may not require saline infusion; those with agitated confusion, seizures, or coma should be treated with normal saline until the symptoms improve. Caution should be used in giving hypertonic saline to patients with symptomatic hyponatremia; frequent laboratory evaluations of serum sodium can be used as a guide to avoid too rapid correction of low sodium levels. Based on clinical data and animal studies, there is a low incidence of myelinolysis if the increase in serum sodium is less than or equal to 12 mmol/L in 24 hours. Late appearance of tremor, dystonia, or cognitive and behavioral changes have been reported in survivors. Full recovery has also been seen.

SUGGESTED READINGS

Adams RD, Victor M, Mancall EL. Central pontine myelinolysis: a hitherto undescribed disease occurring in alcoholic and malnourished patients. *Arch Neurol Psychiatry* 1959;81:154–172.

Ashrafian H, Davey P. A review of the causes of central pontine myelinolysis: yet another apoptotic illness? *Eur J Neurol* 2001;8:103–109.

Ayus JC, Krothpalli RK, Arieff AI. Treatment of symptomatic hyponatremia and its relation to brain damage. *N Engl J Med* 1987;317:1190–1195.

Baba Y, Wszolek ZK, Normand MM. Paroxysmal kinesigenic dyskinesia associated with central pontine myelinolysis. *Parkinsonism Relat Disord* 2003;10:113.

Brunner JE, Redmond JM, Haggar AM, et al. Central pontine myelinolysis and pontine lesions after rapid correction of hyponatremia: a prospective magnetic resonance imaging study. *Ann Neurol* 1990;27:61–66.

Donahue SP, Kardon RH, Thompson HS. Hourglass-shaped visual fields as a sign of bilateral lateral geniculate myelinolysis. *Am J Ophthalmol* 1995;119:378–380.

Hadfield MG, Kubal WS. Extrapontine myelinolysis of the basal ganglia without central pontine myelinolysis. *Clin Neuropathol* 1996;15:96–100.

Harris CP, Townsend JJ, Baringer JR. Symptomatic hyponatremia: can myelinolysis be prevented by treatment? *J Neurol Neurosurg Psychiatry* 1993;56:626–632.

Kleinschmidt-Demasters BK, Norenberg MD. Rapid correction of hyponatremia causes demyelination: relation to central pontine myelinolysis. *Science* 1981;211:1068–1071.

Lee TM, Cheung CC, Lau EY, et al. Cognitive and emotional dysfunction after central pontine myelinolysis. *Behav Neurol* 2003;14:103–107.

Martin RJ. Central pontine and extrapontine myelinolysis: the osmotic demyelination syndromes. *J Neurol Neurosurg Psychiatry* 2004 Sep;75 Suppl 3:iii22–28.

Mitchell AW, Burn DJ, Reading PJ. Central pontine myelinolysis temporally related to hypophosphatemia. *J Neurol Neurosurg Psychiatry* 2003;74:820.

Morlan L, Rodriguez E, Gonzales J, et al. Central pontine myelinolysis following correction of hyponatremia: MRI diagnosis. *Eur Neurol* 1990;30:149–152.

Rojiani AM, Cho ES, Sharer L, et al. Electrolyte-induced demyelination in rats. 2. Ultrastructural evolution. *Acta Neuropathol* 1994;88:293–299.

Ruzek KA, Campeau NG, Miller GM. Early diagnosis of central pontine myelinolysis with diffusion-weighted imaging. *AJNR* 2004;25:210–213.

Salerno SM, Kurlan R, Joy SE, et al. Dystonia in central pontine myelinolysis without evidence of extrapontine myelinolysis. *J Neurol Neurosurg Psychiatry* 1993;56:1221–1223.

Schrier RW. Treatment of hyponatremia. *N Engl J Med* 1985;312:1121–1122.

Thompson DS, Hutton JT, Stears JC, et al. Computerized tomography in the diagnosis of central and extrapontine myelinolysis. *Arch Neurol* 1981;38:243–246.

Uchino A, Yuzuriha T, Murakami M, et al. Magnetic resonance imaging of sequelae of central pontine myelinolysis in chronic alcohol abusers. *Neuroradiology* 2003;45:877–880.

Wright DG, Laureno R, Victor M. Pontine and extrapontine myelinolysis. *Brain* 1979;102:361–385.

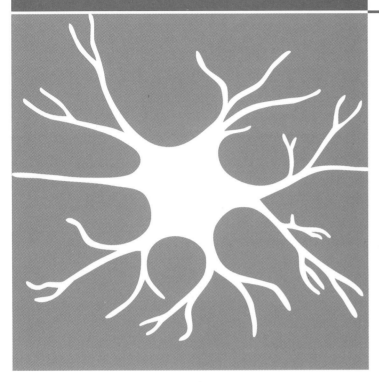

Autonomic Disorders

Chapter 137

▶ # Neurogenic Orthostatic Hypotension and Autonomic Failure

Louis H. Weimer

Postural or orthostatic hypotension (OH) is a clinical sign seen in numerous and diverse neurologic and non-neurologic conditions. One consensus agreement defined OH as a fall in systolic blood pressure (SBP) of 20 mmHg or 10 mmHg diastolic within 3 minutes of standing or similar orthostatic challenge, such as $\geq 60°$ upright tilt, although some require a 30 mmHg decline. OH, however, may be asymptomatic, especially in the elderly, and varies according to underlying conditions or confounding factors (Table 137.1). The sign is one marker of advanced autonomic failure and may be secondary to disease of central autonomic pathways or peripheral autonomic neuropathy. Pathogenic mechanisms are numerous including degenerative, immune-mediated, toxic, hereditary, and others. Some more severe and important causes are discussed; others are listed in Table 137.2.

PARKINSONIAN SYNDROMES AND PURE AUTONOMIC FAILURE

Marked autonomic failure (AF) including OH in patients with multiple system atrophy (MSA), previously known as Shy-Drager syndrome, is frequent. However, other autonomic symptoms often predate OH, including impotence or ejaculatory dysfunction, decreased sweating, and urinary and less commonly fecal incontinence. MSA is a group of disorders with overlapping neuropathology and may have autonomic, parkinsonian, or cerebellar symptoms at onset or later, as discussed in Chapter 116. Other common manifestations include sleep apnea, incon-

tinence, impotence, dystonia, inspiratory stridor, hoarseness, and lack of rest tremor or effective or sustained L-dopa response. The condition is recognized with increasing frequency. Virtually all MSA patients eventually show autonomic signs or symptoms, regardless of initial manifestations. Demonstration of argyrophilic glial cytoplasmic inclusions in oligodendroglia (GCIs) is a pathologic MSA hallmark; however, the same inclusions are occasionally seen in other disorders. GCIs are prominent in sites of central autonomic control and correlate better with clinical findings than do areas of neuronal loss.

Many patients with idiopathic Parkinson disease (IPD) also have autonomically mediated complaints, most commonly constipation, but measurable OH is often asymptomatic. Exacerbation or inducement of OH from medications such as L-dopa is recognized, but the actual significance is uncertain in cases without autonomic failure. Some patients with otherwise typical Parkinson disease (PD) have more severe autonomic failure including symptomatic OH and are designated PD with autonomic failure. A separate disorder known as pure autonomic failure (PAF) or idiopathic orthostatic hypotension was first described by Bradbury and Eggleston in 1925; this is a profound, slowly progressive disorder with disabling OH and usually

▶ **TABLE 137.1 Factors Affecting Orthostatic Hypotension**

Aggravating factors
Warm environment, hot bath
Postexercise
Prolonged motionless standing
Large meals (carbohydrate load)
Early morning
Valsalva maneuver, isometric exercise
Volume depletion
Rising after prolonged bed rest
Rapid postural change
Space flight
Alcohol
Medications (Table 137.2)

Beneficial maneuvers
Squatting, leg crossing
Abdominal and leg compression
Nighttime slight upright tilt
Isotonic exercise

▶ **TABLE 137.2 Selected Disorders of Autonomic Function (Pure Autonomic Failure—PAF, Bradbury-Eggleston Syndrome)**

Multisystem disorders
  Multiple system atrophy (MSA)
  Parkinson disease with autonomic failure
  Machado-Joseph disease

Central
  Brain tumors (posterior fossa, third ventricle, hypothalamus), syringobulbia, MS, tetanus,
    Wernicke-Korsakoff syndrome, fatal familial insomnia

Spinal cord
  MS, syringomyelia, transverse myelitis, trauma, mass lesion

Peripheral
  Immune mediated
    Guillain-Barré syndrome (Chapter 106), acute and subacute autonomic neuropathy, acute cholinergic
      neuropathy, Sjögren disease, SLE, rheumatoid arthritis, Holmes-Adie syndrome
  Metabolic
    Diabetes, vitamin B_{12} and thiamine deficiency, uremia
  Paraneoplastic
    Paraneoplastic autonomic neuropathy and paraneoplastic syndromes with autonomic neuropathy
      (ANNA-1, α3-AChR, CRMP-5, PCA-2 antibodies), enteric neuropathy, Lambert-Eaton myasthenic
      syndrome [cholinergic]
  Infectious
    Chagas disease (cholinergic), syphilis, leprosy, HIV, Lyme disease, diphtheria
  Hereditary
    Familial amyloidosis, hereditary sensory and autonomic neuropathies (Chapter 105), dopamine
      β-hydroxylase deficiency, porphyria, Fabry disease, norepinephrine transporter deficiency, fragile X
      premutation–associated tremor/ataxia syndrome
  Toxins and medications
    Botulism, vincristine, cisplatin, taxol, amiodarone, pyriminil (Vacor), hexacarbon, carbon disulfide,
      heavy metals, podophyllin, alcohol
  Drug and medication effects
    Anticholinergics: tricyclic antidepressants, atropine, oxybutynin
    β-Adrenergic blockers: propranolol and others
    α_2-Agonists: clonidine, prazosin, alpha methyl dopa, terazosin, doxazosin
    α_1-Antagonists: phentolamine, phenoxybenzamine, guanabenz
    Ganglionic blockers: guanethidine, hexamethonium, mecamylamine
    Other: hydralazine, nitrates, diuretics, calcium channel blockers, ACE inhibitors, antihistamines,
      antipsychotics, Sinemet, narcotics, sildenafil, tadalafil
  Reduced orthostatic tolerance
    Neurocardiogenic syncope, orthostatic intolerance syndrome (POTS), mitral valve prolapse syndrome,
      prolonged bed rest or weightlessness, ? Chiari malformation
  Other
    Acquired amyloidosis, chronic idiopathic autonomic neuropathies, small-fiber neuropathy, idiopathic
      hyperhidrosis, idiopathic anhidrosis, Ross syndrome

SLE, systemic lupus erythematosus; POTS, postural orthostatic tachycardia syndrome; PCA-2, Purkinje cell
cytoplasmic antibody type 2; CRMP-5, collapsing response mediator protein-5.

starts after age 50. Autonomic testing abnormalities, including OH, are marked. By definition no other neurologic impairment is seen, and the ultimate diagnosis is often delayed 3 to 5 years to ensure that MSA or parkinsonism does not emerge. Autopsies show a similar pattern of classic Lewy bodies in peripheral autonomic and enteric ganglia in both PD with AF and PAF. Similarities between PD and PAF are further supported by cardiac fluorodopamine PET studies demonstrating loss of cardiac sympathetic innerva-

tion in both, but not in MSA. The relationship between idiopathic PD (IPD) and PAF is not clear, but some shared neurodegenerative mechanisms are suggested.

Dopamine β-hydroxylase deficiency is a rare but treatable entity with severe OH, syncope, and nearly undetectable norepinephrine and epinephrine leading to a failure of blood pressure to increase when the subject stands. The norepinephrine precursor L-threo-dihydroxyphenylserine (L-DOPS) can be beneficial for these patients and in patients with other forms of autonomic failure, but the drug is not yet FDA approved. Numerous other common and uncommon disorders affecting the brain and spinal cord affect autonomic function but less commonly cause symptomatic OH (Table 137.2). Additionally, some processes may be pathway specific such as predominantly cholinergic, adrenergic, regional, or organ-specific processes.

CHRONIC AUTONOMIC NEUROPATHIES

Many of the scores of different peripheral neuropathies include autonomic involvement, often limited to distal sweating and vasomotor control, especially those disproportionately affecting small diameter fibers. Dysfunction is generally insufficient to impair peripheral vasoconstriction or postural reflexes enough to produce symptomatic OH. A few, however, lead to severe or targeted autonomic dysfunction, which can produce frank autonomic failure and symptomatic OH. Particularly noteworthy causes include diabetes, amyloidosis, paraneoplastic neuropathies, selected hereditary and toxic neuropathies, and rare hereditary conditions. Some of the more prominent examples are listed in Table 137.2.

Diabetic autonomic neuropathy (DAN) is the most common and important cause of autonomic neuropathy and the most extensively examined. Somatic peripheral neuropathy is usually concurrent. Much attention has focused on the impact of diabetic autonomic dysfunction on long-term survival. Ewing et al. found 56% of 73 patients with DAN died within 5 years, many owing to nonautonomic complications such as renal failure. Later studies showed an increased but less ominous DAN mortality rate in diabetics without other initial complications (23% at 8 years) compared with diabetics without DAN and similar disease duration (3% at 8 years). The added autonomic dysfunction risk is also independent of coronary perfusion deficits. Upper GI dysmotility, bladder complaints, impotence, sudomotor loss, constipation, episodic diarrhea, and gustatory sweating are a few common manifestations in addition to OH that aid in diagnosis and may require symptomatic treatment.

Amyloidosis, including both hereditary and acquired forms, is another important consideration in patients with severe autonomic failure. Mutations in transthyretin (TTR) are associated with more severe autonomic neuropathy than mutations in apolipoprotein A1 or gelsolin. Hepatic and bone marrow transplantation have been performed in some patients.

Immune-mediated and paraneoplastic forms discussed in Chapter 138 are potentially treatable and often begin subacutely. A chronic form is also seen in isolation or in association with other autoimmune disorders, including

Sjögren disease. Idiopathic small-fiber neuropathy often affects autonomic function, but rarely causes symptomatic OH. Other forms of autonomic neuropathy are listed in Table 137.2.

Diagnosis

Nonautonomic conditions can produce OH as well; most important are adrenal failure and pheochromocytoma. Asymptomatic OH is a prevalent sign in the elderly, and causes are often multifactorial. Symptoms of dysautonomia are numerous, span many organ systems, and are often nonspecific is isolation. Thus, objective support for autonomic dysfunction is desirable in many cases. Formal laboratory evaluation of autonomic disorders is becoming widely available, in part owing to reliable noninvasive techniques. Unlike somatic peripheral nerves, autonomic function is not assessed directly, but responses of complex reflex loops are measured after controlled perturbations. Numerous techniques are described, but cardiovagal heart rate testing, Valsalva maneuver analysis, orthostatic stress from standing or controlled tilt, and sudomotor testing are suitable for clinical application (Table 137.3).

Treatment of autonomic failure is directed at symptomatic relief and improved quality of life, especially for generally the most disabling symptom—OH. Numerous pharmacologic and nonpharmacologic interventions are used to lessen OH and improve orthostatic tolerance. Asymptomatic hypotension on standing usually does not require treatment; adequate precautions and avoidance of precipitating factors may be adequate. However, lesser indicators of hypoperfusion such as postural "coat-hanger" pattern shoulder fatigue and headache (local muscle ischemia), pure vertigo, postprandial fatigue, and cognitive slowing should be considered as possible indicators of OH. Supplemental water intake and salt (0.5-2g/day) have been

▌ **TABLE 137.3 Well-Established Tests of Autonomic Function**

Cardiovagal (Parasympathetic)
HR variability to cyclic deep breathing
HR response to the Valsalva maneuver (Valsalva ratio)
HR response to standing (30:15 ratio)
Adrenergic (Sympathetic)
BP response to the Valsalva maneuver (phases IV and late II)
BP response to orthostatic stress
Head-up tilt
Standing
Sudomotor
Quantitative sudomotor axon reflex test (QSART)
Thermoregulatory sweat test
Silastic sweat imprint testing
Sympathetic skin responses

HR, heart rate; BP, blood pressure.

independently shown to be beneficial and lessen need for medications. Raising the head of the bed 4 inches stimulates baroreceptors and decreases nocturnal diuresis. Useful postural and physical measures to attempt and others to avoid are listed in table 137.1. Cumbersome compressive garments with abdominal compression are mildly effective in reducing venous pooling but are problematic for many with neurologic disorders; abdominal binders alone may help to a lesser degree. Small, frequent meals low in carbohydrates lessen postprandial hypotension. Re-evaluation of the need for prescribed blood pressure (BP) lowering and autonomically active agents should be considered (Table 137.2).

If these measures are insufficient, first-line medications include fludrocortisone (starting at 0.1 mg/day) or the α-adrenergic agonist midodrine or both. Midodrine is short acting, and the dosage must cover vulnerable periods, especially early morning, and is not given after 6 PM. Excessive fluid retention and heart failure are concerns, especially in the elderly. Relative anemia will exacerbate OH. Correcting iron deficiency or erythropoietin treatment may be beneficial. Supine hypertension is a concern in some, and long-term consequences are controversial and unresolved. Second-line agents are numerous and are sometimes effective if earlier agents have failed. Concomitant treatment of urinary dysfunction, gastric and intestinal dysmotility, impotence, and secretomotor dysfunction is often necessary. In MSA, inspiratory stridor may lead to tracheostomy, and nocturnal positive pressure ventilation may be needed for sleep apnea.

Exacerbating factors are important considerations for both patient and physician to take appropriate precautions or avoid certain situations (Table 137.1). Arising in stages can minimize an exercise-induced reflex, in part responsible for the immediate BP drop on standing. Patients with chronic, symptomatic OH may learn to recognize these conditions but often need physician instruction. Chronic OH also results in optimized cerebral autoregulation and relative tolerance of low BP, but provides a narrow window between an asymptomatic state and syncope.

SUGGESTED READINGS

Assessment: clinical autonomic testing report of the Therapeutics and Technology Assessment Subcommittee of the American Association of Neurology. *Neurology* 1996;46:873–880.

Consensus statement on the definition of orthostatic hypotension, pure autonomic failure, and multiple system atrophy. The Consensus Committee of the American Autonomic Society and the American Academy of Neurology. *Neurology* 1996;46:1470.

Ejaz AA, Haley WE, Wasiluk A, Meschia JF, Fitzpatrick PM. Characteristics of 100 consecutive patients presenting with orthostatic hypotension. *Mayo Clin Proc* 2004 Jul;79(7):890–894.

Ewing DJ, Campbell IW, Clarke BF. The natural history of diabetic autonomic neuropathy. *Q J Med* 1980;49:95–108.

Gerritsen J, Dekker JM, TenVoorde BJ, et al. Impaired autonomic function is associated with increased mortality, especially in subjects with diabetes, hypertension, or a history of cardiovascular disease: the Hoorn Study. *Diabetes Care* 2001;24:1793–1798.

Goldstein DS, Holmes CS, Dendi R, et al. Orthostatic hypotension from sympathetic denervation in Parkinson's disease. *Neurology* 2002;58:1247–1255.

Hague K, Lento P, Morgello S, et al. The distribution of Lewy bodies in pure autonomic failure: autopsy findings and review of the literature. *Acta Neuropathol (Berl)* 1997;94:192–196.

Klein CM, Vernino S, Lennon VA, et al. The spectrum of autoimmune autonomic neuropathies. *Ann Neurol* 2003;53:752–758.

Low PA, Vernino S, Suarez G. Autonomic dysfunction in peripheral nerve disease. *Muscle Nerve* 2003;27:646–661.

Magalhães M, Wenning GK, Daniel SE, et al. Autonomic dysfunction in pathologically confirmed multiple system atrophy and idiopathic Parkinson's disease—a retrospective comparison. *Acta Neurol Scand* 1995;91:98–102.

Mathias CJ. Orthostatic hypotension: causes, mechanisms, and influencing factors. *Neurology* 1995;45(Suppl 5):S6–S11.

Papp MI, Lantos PL. The distribution of oligodendroglial inclusions in multiple system atrophy and its relevance to clinical symptomatology. *Brain* 1994;117:235–243.

Ravits J, Hallett M, Nilsson J, et al. Electrophysiological tests of autonomic function in patients with idiopathic autonomic failure syndromes. *Muscle Nerve* 1996;19:758–763.

Shi SJ, South DA, Meck JV. Fludrocortisone does not prevent orthostatic hypotension in astronauts after spaceflight. *Aviat Space Environ Med* 2004;75(Mar):235–239.

Shy GM, Drager GA. A neurological syndrome associated with orthostatic hypotension: a clinical-pathologic study. *Arch Neurol* 1960;2:511–527.

Vagaonescu TD, Saadia D, Tuhrim S, et al. Hypertensive cardiovascular damage in patients with primary autonomic failure. *Lancet* 2000;355:725–726.

Weimer LH. Postural hypotension. In: *Manual of Neurologic Practice.* Evans R, ed. Philadelphia: WB Saunders, 2003:916–920.

Weimer LH, Williams O. Syncope and orthostatic intolerance. *Med Clin N Am* 2003;87:835–865.

Chapter 138

Acute Autonomic Neuropathy

Louis H. Weimer

Acute or subacute autonomic neuropathy (AAN) or *acute pandysautonomia*, is an unusual but notably distinct entity, which primarily affects peripheral autonomic nerves. Roughly half are preceded by a viral prodrome similar to Guillain-Barré syndrome (GBS). Patients typically develop generalized autonomic failure including orthostatic hypotension, anhidrosis, parasympathetic failure, and gastrointestinal dysfunction, although predominantly adrenergic and cholinergic variants are seen. The illness is monophasic with acute or subacute onset over several weeks. Recovery generally occurs but is often slow and incomplete. Acute signs such as ileus may develop into lesser degrees of dysmotility including bloating, early satiety, nausea, vomiting, and alternating diarrhea and constipation. Antecedent viruses include herpes simplex, mononucleosis, rubella, and nondescript febrile illnesses. Roughly 25% have a restricted cholinergic form (*acute cholinergic neuropathy*) characterized by dry eyes and mouth, ileus, and other signs of gastrointestinal dysmotility, bladder dysfunction, hypohidrosis, unreactive pupils, fixed heart rate, and sexual dysfunction but without significant orthostatic hypotension (OH). Abnormalities on formal autonomic testing are prominent in the involved systems. Nerve conduction studies are typically normal or show minor sensory abnormalities. The lack of OH in cholinergic cases makes laboratory support especially valuable for diagnosis. Mononuclear cell infiltrates have been seen in sural nerve biopsies with concomitant decreases in small myelinated and unmyelinated fibers.

Demonstration of antibodies to nicotinic ganglionic AChR α-3 subunits, which are similar but distinct from those at the neuromuscular junction (α-1 subunits), supports an immune-mediated basis. A paraneoplastic form, which develops in a similar time course is indistinguishable on clinical or laboratory grounds, may appear before the tumor is discovered. In screening patients with autonomic disorders and controls, Vernino et al. found that 41% of patients with idiopathic autonomic neuropathy had high antibody titers and paraneoplastic neuropathy patients were frequently positive as well. A smaller percentage of patients with orthostatic intolerance and idiopathic gastrointestinal dysmotility were positive; none with degenerative autonomic disorders such as multiple system atrophy, pure autonomic failure, or gastric symptoms with normal motility studies had elevated titers. Knockout mouse models of the α-3 subunit gene, rabbits immunized against the subunit, and passive antibody transfer to other animals all induce signs of autonomic failure supporting the assertion that the antibodies are causative. Antibody titers also correlate with disease severity.

Exaggerated orthostatic tachycardia may be evident in some cases without significant cardiac denervation. This led to the proposal that some patients with the common syndrome of idiopathic orthostatic intolerance without OH (postural orthostatic tachycardia syndrome) may have an attenuated form of acute autonomic neuropathy. This assertion is supported by abnormalities of sudomotor and other autonomic systems in one-third to one-half of cases and an over-representation of antecedent viral infection in these patients. Orthostatic intolerance symptoms include postural lightheadedness, fatigue, cognitive changes, and presyncope despite minimal changes in blood pres-

sure. Mechanisms are multiple, including excessive venous pooling, idiopathic hypovolemia, adrenergic hypersensitivity, and altered cerebrovascular autoregulation. An indistinguishable hereditary form resulting from a mutation in a norepinephrine transporter gene is known. This syndrome is the most common cause of consultation in many autonomic centers.

Subacute autonomic neuropathy or predominantly enteric neuropathy is also seen in isolation or with somatic sensory neuropathy and other underlying antibodies, especially type 1 antineuronal nuclear antibodies (ANNA-1, anti-Hu) usually in patients with small cell lung cancer. Paraneoplastic neuropathy is also associated with other paraneoplastic antibodies including Purkinje cell cytoplasmic antibody type 2 (PCA-2) and collapsing response mediator protein-5 (CRMP-5). Botulism (cholinergic), acute intermittent porphyria, and toxic neuropathy are other diagnostic considerations. A chronic form analogous to chronic inflammatory demyelinating polyneuropathy is known. Rare cases with acute autonomic neuropathy (AAN) and myasthenia gravis have both types of AChR antibodies. Some patients have thymoma without myasthenia. Autonomic involvement is common in typical GBS, especially in more severe cases, and is a prominent cause of morbidity and mortality, as discussed in more detail in Chapter 106.

A range of outcomes is expected. One-third make a good functional recovery, one-third have a partial recovery with substantial deficits including symptomatic OH, and the remainder do not improve. Gastrointestinal dysfunction and OH are usually the most debilitating manifestations.

Supportive care and management of the orthostatic hypotension and system-specific problems are the mainstays of treatment. Several anecdotal reports of a more impressive improvement than historical descriptions after IVIG make this treatment a reasonable first step.

SUGGESTED READINGS

Camdessanche JP, Antoine JC, Honnorat J, et al. Paraneoplastic peripheral neuropathy associated with anti-Hu antibodies. A clinical and electrophysiological study of 20 patients. *Brain* 2002;125:166–175.

Fagius J, Westerburg CE, Olsson Y. Acute pandysautonomia and severe sensory deficit with poor recovery. A clinical, neurophysiological and pathological case study. *J Neurol Neurosurg Psychiatry* 1983;46:725–733.

Heafield MTE, Gammage MD, Nightingale S, et al. Idiopathic dysautonomia treated with intravenous gammaglobulin. *Lancet* 1996;347:28–29.

Jacob G, Biaggioni I. Idiopathic orthostatic intolerance and postural tachycardia syndromes. *Am J Med Sci* 1999;317:88–101.

Lennon VA, Ermilov LG, Szurszewski JH, et al. Immunization with neuronal nicotinic acetylcholine receptor induces neurological autoimmune disease. *J Clin Invest* 2003;111:64–65.

Low PA, Dyck PJ, Lambert EH, et al. Acute panautonomic neuropathy. *Ann Neurol* 1983;13:412–417.

Sandroni P, Vernino S, Klein CM, et al. Idiopathic autonomic neuropathy: comparison of cases seropositive and seronegative for ganglionic acetylcholine receptor antibody. *Arch Neurol* 2004;61:44–48.

Schondorf R, Low PA. Idiopathic postural orthostatic tachycardia syndrome. An attenuated form of acute pandysautonomia? *Neurology* 1993;43:132–137.

Shannon JR, Flattem NL, Jordan J, et al. Orthostatic intolerance and tachycardia associated with norepinephrine-transporter deficiency. *N Engl J Med* 2000;342:541–549.

Suarez GA, Fealey RD, Camilleri M, et al. Idiopathic autonomic neuropathy: clinical, neurophysiologic and follow-up studies on 27 patients. *Neurology* 1994;44:1675–1682.

Vernino S, Low PA, Fealey RD, et al. Autoantibodies to ganglionic acetylcholine receptors in autoimmune autonomic neuropathies. *N Engl J Med* 2000;343:847–855.

Xu W, Gelber S, Orr-Urtreger A, et al. Megacystitis, mydriasis, and ion channel defect in mice lacking the alpha3 neuronal nicotinic acetylcholine receptor. *Proc Natl Acad Sci U S A* 1999;96:5746–5751.

Young RR, Asbury AK, Corbett JL, et al. Pure pandysautonomia with recovery. *Brain* 1975;98:613–636.

Zochodne DW. Autonomic involvement in Guillain-Barré syndrome: A review. *Muscle Nerve* 1994;17:1145–1155.

Chapter 139

▶ Familial Dysautonomia

Alan M. Aron

OVERVIEW

Familial dysautonomia (FD) was described by Riley et al. in 1949. Autonomic symptoms are prominent, but the condition also affects other parts of the nervous system and general somatic growth. It is a rare autosomal recessive disease; more than 650 cases have been reported. Virtually all patients are of Eastern European (Ashkenazi) Jewish descent where the carrier rate may be as high as 1 in 27.

The causative gene has been identified as IKBKAP (I kappa B kinase complex–associated protein) and mapped to chromosome 9q31-q33. Two mutations in the gene IKBKAP are responsible. The major FD mutation is a splice defect that displays tissue-specific expression. It causes aberrant tissue-specific mRNA splicing. The second infrequent mutation is a missense mutation. The end result is a congenital sensory and autonomic neuropathy. In the past, linkage analyses using closely related markers have permitted reliable prenatal diagnosis in families with a previously affected child. More recently, specific assays for mutations of IKBKAP have facilitated carrier screening for FD.

The condition can be diagnosed in the perinatal period. Clinical manifestations tend to increase with age.

Biochemical alterations point to decreased synthesis of noradrenaline. Hypersensitivity to sympathomimetic drugs suggests a denervation type of supersensitivity. The exact pathophysiology has yet to be explained.

CLINICAL MANIFESTATIONS

The dysautonomic infant frequently shows low birth weight and breech presentation. Neurologic abnormalities detected in the neonatal period include decreased muscle tone, diminished or absent deep tendon reflexes, absent corneal responses, poor Moro response, and weak cry and suck. The tongue tip lacks fungiform papillae and appears smooth. Uncoordinated swallowing with resultant regurgitation may cause aspiration and pneumonia. Some infants require tube feeding, gastrostomy, and fundoplication because of gastroesophageal reflux. Absence of overflow tears, which may be normal for the first 3 months, persists thereafter and becomes a consistent feature. Corneal ulceration can occur.

During the first 3 years of life, affected children show delayed physical and developmental milestones, episodic vomiting, excessive sweating, excessive drooling, blotchy erythema, and breath-holding spells. Dysautonomic crises occur after age 3, with irritability, self-mutilation, negativistic behavior, diaphoresis, tachycardia, hypertension, and thermal instability. One most outstanding symptom is episodic vomiting, which can be cyclic and require hospitalization for stabilization with parenteral hydration.

The school-aged dysautonomic child tends to have short stature, awkward gait, and nasal speech. School performance may be poor. As a group, patients score in the average range on intelligence tests, but they are frequently 20 or more points below unaffected siblings. Scoliosis is frequent and can begin in childhood and progress rapidly during preadolescence. The prevalence of spinal deformity in FD patients older than 20 years approaches 83%. Some poorly developed patients show delayed puberty. Vomiting and vasomotor crises tend to decrease during adolescence when more frequent symptoms center on decreased exercise tolerance, poor general coordination, emotional difficulties, and postural hypotension. Vasovagal responses may occur after micturition or during laryngeal intubation for anesthesia. Up to one-third of patients have seizures during early life. These are usually associated with fever, breath-holding spells, or hypoxia. Less than 10% of patients have subsequent long-standing seizure disorders.

Patients show abnormal responses to altered atmospheric air. Hypercapnia and hypoxia do not produce expected increases in ventilatory effort. Drownings have occurred, presumably because air hunger did not develop when submerged. Coma has occurred in patients at high altitudes.

DIAGNOSIS

The diagnosis should be made on the constellation of clinical symptoms and genetic background. A most distinctive sign is the absence or paucity of overflow tearing. Low doses of methacholine may restore transient tearing. Other cardinal clinical features include hyporeflexia, absent corneal responses, and the absence of the fungiform tongue papillae. This is associated with impaired taste sensation. There is relative indifference to pain, poor temperature control, and postural hypotension.

Intradermal histamine phosphate in a dosage of 1:1,000 (0.03–0.05 mL) normally produces pain and erythema. Within minutes, a central wheal forms and is surrounded by an axon flare that is a zone of erythema measuring 2 to 6 cm in diameter. The flare lasts for several minutes. In dysautonomic patients, the pain is greatly reduced and there is no axon flare. In infants, a saline solution of 1:10,000 histamine should be used. The methacholine test involves installation of one drop of 2.5% methacholine into the eye. (One drop of dilute pilocarpine [0.0625%] is equivalent to 2.5% methacholine.) The other eye serves as control. The pupils are compared at 5-minute intervals for 20 minutes. The normal pupil remains unchanged in size; the dysautonomic pupil develops miosis. The pupillary responses to light and accommodation in FD appear normal.

The combination of absent axon flare response to intradermal histamine, miosis with methacholine or pilocarpine, and absent glossal fungiform pupillae are diagnostic. Frequently, there is an elevated urinary homovanillic acid–vanilylmandelic acid ratio. This assay is not required for diagnosis.

BIOCHEMICAL AND PATHOLOGIC DATA

The neuronal abnormality is probably present at birth, but subsequent degenerative changes seem to occur. The primary metabolic defect is unknown. Fibroblast study has shown normal mitochondrial DNA and respiratory chain activity. Mitochondrial dysfunction owing to glycosphingolipid accumulation, changes in mitochondrial DNA, or mutation of chromosome 9 genetic material in mitochrondial functions have not been demonstrated.

Serum levels of both norepinephrine and dopamine are markedly elevated during dysautonomic crises. Vomiting coincides with high dopamine levels; hypertension correlates with increased norepinephrine levels. Pathologic data reveal hypoplastic cervical sympathetic ganglia with diminished volume and neuronal counts. Sympathetic preganglionic spinal cord neurons seem to be reduced in number. Patients are deficient in type C fibers. The parasympathetic sphenopalatine ganglia have shown the most depleted neuronal populations with only minimal reductions in the ciliary ganglia. The lingual submucosal neurons and sensory axons are reduced. Tastebuds are scant; circumvallate papillae are hypoplastic.

PATHOPHYSIOLOGY

Gastroesophageal dysfunction, manifested by prolonged esophageal transit time, gastroesophageal reflux, and delayed gastric emptying, has been demonstrated by scintigraphic analysis, cineradiography, pH monitoring, and endoscopy. There is severe oropharyngeal incoordination.

Cardiovascular instability is a prominent manifestation. Prolonged QT intervals greater than 440 milliseconds without shortening during exercise demonstrate a defect in autonomic regulation of cardiac conduction. Renal insufficiency, common in adult patients, can be assessed by noninvasive Doppler techniques to detect changes in renal blood flow.

Sympathetic denervation may increase the responsiveness to regulators of cardiovascular integrity such as atrial natriuretic peptide. Medication can also influence circulating atrial natriuretic peptide and cathecholamines.

Excessive drooling and swallowing difficulties are common and can be attributable to salivary gland denervation hypersensitivity. Hypersalivation may account for the low caries rate and increased plaque formation.

Postural hypotension can be explained by peripheral sympathetic denervation. Skin blotching and hypertension are attributed to denervation supersensitivity at the sympathetic effector sites. Lack of overflow tears correlates with the diminution of neurons in the sphenopalatine ganglia. Other symptoms can be explained as manifestations of a diffuse sensory deficit and autonomic insufficiency with hypersensitivity to acetylcholine and possibly to catecholamines. In addition, there may be decreased or dysfunctional adrenoceptors and decreased denervation.

PROGNOSIS

Long-term survival has been documented. Surviving patients include women whose pregnancies terminated in the birth of normal infants. Infant and childhood fatalities may be a result of aspiration pneumonia, gastric hemorrhage, or dehydration. A second cluster of fatalities between the ages of 14 and 24 years showed pulmonary complications, sleep deaths, and cardiopulmonary arrests. The oldest patients are now in their fifth decade.

TREATMENT

Laparoscopic surgery for performing a modified Nissen fundoplication and gastrostomy has modified gastroesophageal reflux and the resultant pulmonary complications associated with aspiration. The use of epidural anesthesia has been advocated for surgical procedures such as Nissen fundoplication and cesarean section. This is to avoid intubation and the sometimes fatal complications of general anesthesia. Use of deep sedation with midazolam followed by propofol for endoscopy has proven to be a safe management.

Midodrine, a peripheral α-adrenergic agonist, may be useful in the management of orthostatic hypotension in a dose of 0.25 mg/kg per day. Symptomatic treatment is indicated for dysautonomic crises with parenteral fluids, diazepam, sedation, and antiemetic therapy. Midazolam and clonidine have also been used with effectiveness for symptomatic control of crises.

With the identification of the specific gene defect, definitive treatment can be anticipated in the future. Tocotrienols may elevate IKBKAP gene expression and cause increased functional IKBKAP protein produced in FD patients. Growth hormone treatment in selected patients with FD may also have the potential to increase growth velocity. Preimplantation genetics can offer an alternative for couples at risk who would be unwilling to accept prenatal diagnosis and pregnancy termination.

SUGGESTED READINGS

Alvarez E, Ferrer T, Perez-Conde C, et al. Evaluation of congenital dysautonomia other than Riley-Day syndrome. *Neuropediatrics* 1996;27: 26–31.

Anderson SL, Coli R, Daly IW, et al. Familial dysautonomia is caused by mutations of the IKAP gene. *Am J Hum Genet* 2001;3:753–758. Epub 2001 Jan 22.

Anderson SL, Qui J, Rubin BY. EGCG corrects aberrant splicing of IKAP mRNA in cells from patients with familial dysautonomia. *Biochem Biophys Res Commun* 2003;2:627–633.

Anderson SL, Qui J, Rubin BY. Tocotrienols induce IKBKAP expression: a possible therapy for familial dysautonomia. *Biochem Biophys Res Commun* 2003;1:303–309.

Axelrod FB. Familial dysautonomia. *Muscle Nerve* 2004 Mar;29(3):352–363.

Axelrod FB. Familial dysautonomia: a 47-year perspective. How technology confirms clinical acumen. *J Pediatr* 1998;132(3 Pt 2):S2–S5.

Axelrod FB, Goldberg, JD, Ye XY, et al. Survival in familial dysautonomia: impact of early intervention. *J Pediatr* 2002;2:518–523.

Axelrod FB, Goldstein DS, Holmes C, et al. Genotype and phenotype in familial dysautonomia. *Adv Pharmacol* 1998;42:925–928.

Axelrod FB, Krey L, Glickstein JS, et al. Atrial natriuretic peptide response to postural change and medication in familial dysautonomia. *Clin Auton Res* 1994;4:311–318.

Axelrod FB, Porges RF, Seir ME. Neonatal recognition of familial dysautonomia. *J Pediatr* 1987;110:969–948.

Blumenfeld A, Slaugenhaupt SA, Axelrod FB. Localization of the gene for familial dysautonomia on chromosome 9 and definition of DNA markers for genetic diagnosis. *Nat Genet* 1993;4:160–164.

Cuajungco MP, Leyne M, Mull J, et al. Tissue-specific reduction in splicing efficiency of IKBKAP due to the major mutation associated with familial dysautonomia. *Am J Hum Genet* 2003;3:749–758.

Dong J, Edelmann L, Bajwa AM, et al. Familial dysautonomia: detection of the IKBKAPIVS20(+6T≥ C) and R696P mutations and frequencies among Ashkenazi Jews. *Am J Med Genet* 2002;3:253–257.

Eng CM, Slaugenhaupt SA, Blumenfeld A, et al. Prenatal diagnosis of familial dysautonomia by analysis of linked CA-repeat polymorphisms on chromosome 9q31-q33. *Am J Med Genet* 1995;59:349–355.

Kamboj MK, Axelrod FB, David R, et al. Growth treatment in children with familial dysautonomia. *J Pediatr* 2004;1:63–67.

Korczyn AD, Rubenstein AE, Yahr MD, et al. The pupil in familial dysautonomia. *Neurology* 1981;31:628–629.

Marthol H, Tutaj M, Brys M, et al. Clonidine improves postprandial baroreflex control in familial dysautonomia. *Eur J Clin Invest* 2003;10:912–918.

Pearson J, Pytel B. Quantitative studies of ciliary and sphenopalatine ganglia in familial dysautonomia. *J Neurol Sci* 1978;39:123–130.

Pearson J, Pytel B. Quantitative studies of sympathetic ganglia and spinal cord intermediolateral gray columns in familial dysautonomia. *J Neurol Sci* 1978;39:47–59.

Riley CM, Day RL, Greely DM, et al. Central autonomic dysfunction with defective lacrimation. I. Report of five cases. *Pediatrics* 1949;3:468–478.

Slaugenhaupt SA, Gusella JF. Familial dysautonomia. *Curr Opin Gen Dev* 2002;3:307–311.

Smith AA, Dancis J. Responses to intradermal histamine in familial dysautonomia—a diagnostic test. *J Pediatr* 1963;63:889–894.

Strasberg P, Bridge P, Merante F, et al. Normal mitochondrial DNA and respiratory chain activity in familial dysautonomia fibroblasts. *Biochem Mol Med* 1996;59:20–27.

Szald A, Udassin R, Maayan C, et al. Laparoscopic modified Nissen fundoplication in children with familial dysautonomia. *J Pediatr Surg* 1996;31:1560–1562.

Udassin R, Seror D, Vinograd I, et al. Nissen fundoplication in the treatment of children with familial dysautonomia. *Am J Surg* 1992;164:332–336.

Wengrower D, Gozal D, Goldin E. Familial dysautonomia: deep sedation and management in endoscopic procedures. *Am J Gastroenterol* 2002;10:2550–2552.

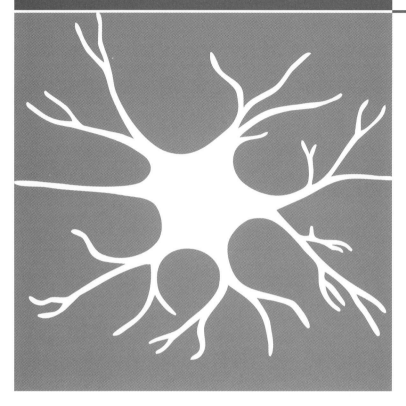

Paroxysmal Disorders

▶ Migraine and Other Headaches

Neil H. Raskin and Mark W. Green

When headache is chronic, recurrent, and unattended by signs of intracranial or systemic disease, the physician confronts a challenging but ultimately gratifying problem. Previously, head pain was thought to originate from either contracted scalp and neck muscles or vascular dilatation. Neither of these mechanisms has achieved scientific support; so central mechanisms of head pain are of current interest. In migraine, the neurologic symptoms are attributed to neuronal dysfunction similar to that of spreading depression; a phase of vasoconstriction and vasodilatation also undoubtedly occurs, as does a final phase that includes secretion of vasoactive peptides. Most recurring headaches are probably caused by impaired central inhibitory mechanisms at varying loci within the brain, likely on a genetic basis.

MIGRAINE

The term *migraine* derives from Galen's usage of *hemicrania* to describe a periodic disorder that comprises paroxysmal and blinding hemicranial pain, vomiting, photophobia, recurrence at regular intervals, and relief by darkness and sleep. Hemicrania was later corrupted into low Latin as *hemigranea* and *migranea*; eventually the French translation, migraine, gained acceptance in the 18th century and has prevailed ever since. This designation is misleading, however, because head pain is lateralized in fewer than 60% of those affected. Furthermore, undue emphasis on the dramatic features of migraine has often led to the illogical conclusion that a periodic headache lack-

ing these characteristics is not migrainous in mechanism. Severe headache attacks, regardless of cause, are more likely to be throbbing and associated with vomiting and scalp tenderness. Milder headaches tend to be nondescript—tight bandlike discomfort often involving the entire head, the profile of "tension headache." These differing clinical patterns of headaches that are not caused by intracranial structural anomalies or systemic disease are probably different points on a continuum rather than disparate clinical entities. Whether a common mechanism underlies the different types of headache remains to be determined.

A working descriptive definition follows. Migraine is a benign recurring headache, recurring neurologic dysfunction, or both; it is usually attended by pain-free interludes and is almost always provoked by stereotyped stimuli. It is far more common in women; those affected have a hereditary predisposition toward attacks; and the cranial circulatory phenomena that attend attacks seem to arise from a primary brainstem disorder.

Clinical Subtypes

The designation *migraine with aura* denotes the syndrome of headache associated with characteristic premonitory sensory, motor, or visual symptoms; *migraine without aura* denotes the syndrome in which no focal neurologic symptoms precede the headache. Focal symptoms, however, occur in only a small proportion of attacks and are more common during headache attacks than as prodromal symptoms. Spreading cortical depression, rather than cerebral ischemia, is the likely mechanism of these focal complaints. Apparently asymptomatic individuals may also experience spreading cortical depression, and the distinction between these two forms of migraine might be artificial. Focal neurologic symptoms without headache or vomiting are called *migraine equivalents* or *accompaniments* and are more common after age 40. The old term *complicated migraine* is generally used to describe migraine with dramatic focal neurologic features, thus overlapping what was designated *classic migraine*. Because the location of the cortical dysfunction leads to the aura symptom, there is no fundamental difference in the pathophysiology or prognosis of a visual, sensory, or hemiplegic aura.

Migraine Without Aura (Common Migraine)

Benign periodic headache lasting several hours and often attributed to tension by its sufferers is the most liberal way of describing common migraine. The fallacy intrinsic to most of the traditionally acceptable definitions is that they define severe attacks but do not include patients with more modest head pain; thus, unilateral pain, attendant nausea or vomiting, positive family history, responsiveness to ergotamine or triptans, and scalp tenderness in varying combinations have been alleged to establish a diagnosis of migraine. Each of these occurs in 60% to 80% of patients, however, and the validity of using these clinical features to diagnose migraine has never been established. Migraine without aura is the most frequent type of headache and includes the now anachronistic concept of periodic "tension headache."

Migraine With Aura (Classic Migraine)

The most common premonitory symptoms are visual, arising from activation and subsequent depression of occipital lobe neurons. Scotomas or hallucinations occur in about one-third of migraineurs with aura and usually appear in the central portion of the visual fields. A highly characteristic syndrome occurs in about 10% of patients; it usually begins as a small paracentral scotoma that slowly expands into a C shape. Luminous angles appear at the enlarging outer edge and become colored as the scintillating scotoma expands and moves toward the periphery of the involved half of the visual field. It eventually disappears over the horizon of peripheral vision; the entire process consumes 20 to 25 minutes. This phenomenon rarely occurs during the headache phase of an attack and is pathognomonic of migraine; it has never been described with a cerebral structural anomaly. It is commonly called a "fortification spectrum" because of the serrated edges of the hallucinated C; Dr. Hubert Airy described his own migrainous visions as resembling a "fortified town with bastions all round it;" "spectrum" is used in the sense of an apparition or specter. Because the auras of migraine are brought about through stimulation of cortical neurons followed by a relative refractoriness of these cells, a positive phenomenon (flashing lights, tingling, muscle tightness) is followed by a negative phenomenon (numbness, scotomata, weakness). This pattern distinguishes migraine auras from transient ischemic attacks with headache.

Basilar Migraine

Symptoms implying altered brainstem function include vertigo, dysarthria, and diplopia; they occur as the only neurologic symptoms of migraine in about 25% of patients. Bickerstaff called attention to a stereotyped sequence of dramatic neurologic events, often with total blindness and sensorial clouding; this is most commonly seen in adolescent women but also occurs in others. The episodes begin with total blindness accompanied or followed by admixtures of vertigo, ataxia, dysarthria, tinnitus, and distal and perioral paresthesia. In about 25% of patients, a confusional state supervenes. The symptoms usually persist for about 30 minutes and are followed by a throbbing occipital headache. This basilar migraine syndrome also occurs in children; after age 50, it is more difficult to diagnose because of the possibility of occlusive vascular disease. Sensorial alterations, including confusional states that may be mistaken for psychotic reactions, may last as long as 5 days. Triptans are contraindicated in patients with basilar migraine, a decision made because people experiencing basilar migraines were excluded from clinical trials; there has been no report of negative outcomes during treated attacks.

Carotidynia

The carotidynia syndrome, sometimes called "lower-half headache" or "facial migraine," is more prominent among somewhat older patients, with peak incidence at ages 30 to 69. Pain is usually located at the jaw or neck and is sometimes periorbital or maxillary. It is often continuous, deep, dull, and aching and episodically becomes pounding or throbbing. Sharp ice pick–like jabs are commonly superimposed. Attacks occur one to several times a week, each lasting minutes to hours. Tenderness and prominent pulsations of the cervical carotid artery and swelling of soft tissues over the carotid are usually present homolateral to the pain; many patients report throbbing ipsilateral headache concurrent with carotidynia and interictally. Dental trauma is a common precipitant. Carotid artery involvement in the more traditional forms of migraine is also common; more than 50% of patients with frequent migraine attacks show carotid tenderness at several points homolateral to the cranial side involved in most of their attacks. Carotid artery dissection must be excluded, although that should not cause the recurrent symptoms of migraine.

Hemiplegic Migraine

Hemiparesis occasionally occurs during the prodromal phase of migraine; like the fortification spectrum, it often resolves in 20 to 30 minutes, and contralateral head pain then commences. The affected side may vary from attack to attack. A more profound form appears as hemiplegia, often affecting the same side, and persisting days or weeks after headache subsides.

A clear autosomal-dominant pattern of attacks may appear within a family. The gene for familial hemiplegic migraine maps to chromosome 19 in one-half of the families. There are mutations within the CACNLIA4 gene, which encodes a P/Q type calcium channel subunit expressed only in brain. Different mutations within the gene are the cause of episodic ataxia, type 2. Alternating hemiplegia of childhood may be another migraine variant, but is not genetically related to familial hemiplegic migraine. Dysarthria and aphasia occur in more than 50% of patients; hemihypesthesia attends hemiparesis in nearly every case. There may be CSF pleocytosis as high as 350 cells/mm^3 or transient CSF protein elevations to 200 mg/dL.

Ophthalmoplegic Migraine

Rarely, patients report infrequent attacks of periorbital pain accompanied by vomiting for 1 to 4 days. As the pain subsides, ipsilateral ptosis appears, and within hours, a complete third nerve palsy occurs, often including pupillary dilatation and loss of the response to light. The ophthalmoplegia may persist for a duration from a few days to 2 months. After many attacks, some ophthalmoparesis may remain. This syndrome usually begins in childhood, in contrast to the Tolosa Hunt syndrome, another painful ophthalmoplegia, which affects adults. Enhancement of the oculomotor nerve is seen with MRI in most cases, suggesting that this is an inflammatory cranial neuropathy rather than a migrainous disorder.

Pathogenesis

Modern orientations toward migraine began with Liveing's 1873 publication, *A Contribution to the Pathology of Nerve Storms*, the first major treatise devoted to migraine. He recognized the similarity of migraine to epilepsy and that the clinically apparent circulatory phenomena of migrainous attacks were caused by cerebral discharges or "nerve storms." In the 1930s, attention was focused on the vascular features of migraine by Graham and Wolff, who found that the administration of ergotamine reduced the amplitude of temporal artery pulsations in patients and that this effect was often, but not consistently, associated with a decrease in head pain. Therefore, authorities believed for many years that the headache phase of migrainous attacks was caused by extracranial vasodilatation and that neurologic symptoms were produced by intracranial vasoconstriction, the "vascular" hypothesis of migraine. A barrage of publications by Wolff and coworkers supported this concept; nonresonant observations during the 1940s were generally ignored. Ergotamine tartrate, a potent arterial vasoconstrictor, had widespread use, whereas dihydroergotamine, a weak arterial vasoconstrictor, was rarely used.

In 1941, K. S. Lashley, a neuropsychologist, was among the first to chart his own migrainous fortification spectrum. He estimated that the scotoma proceeded across the occipital cortex at a rate of 3 mm/min. He speculated that a wave front of intense excitation was followed by a wave of complete inhibition of activity across the visual cortex.

Uncannily, in 1944, the phenomenon of "spreading depression" was described in the cerebral cortex of laboratory animals by the Brazilian physiologist Leão. A slowly moving (2 to 3 mm/min) potassium-liberating depression of cortical activity is preceded by a wave front of increased metabolic activity. Spreading depression can be produced by diverse experimental stimuli, including hypoxia, mechanical trauma, and the topical application of potassium.

These observations, striking in retrospect, could not be incorporated into the vascular model of migraine. Cerebral blood flow studies, however, have rendered untenable a primary vascular mechanism and support the possibility that spreading depression, or more likely a neuronal phenomenon with similar characteristics, is important in the pathogenesis of migraine.

The mechanism of migraine can be partitioned into three phases. The first results from activation of the first-order neuron, the trigeminovascular neuron, a bipolar neuron whose cell body resides in the trigeminal ganglion. A branch innervates the meningeal arteries and another synapses with the trigeminal nucleus caudalis. Early in an attack, pain is experienced within the trigeminal distribution, most commonly V1, and has a pulsatile quality. Should the attack continue, the second-order neuron is activated; the second neuron is located between the trigeminal nucleus caudalis and the thalamus. At this point the brainstem center is activated and sensitized, and if the attack is not aborted, this region will remain activated even if the afferent input from the first-order neuron ceases. Sufferers at this stage describe allodynic symptoms in their scalp and neck; stimuli that are not ordinarily painful cause discomfort. Should the attack continue, the third-order neuron, located between the thalamus and cerebral sensory cortex, is involved; the pain becomes more pervasive and nonpulsatile.

During attacks of migraine with aura, studies of regional cerebral blood flow show a modest cortical hypoperfusion that begins in visual cortex and spreads forward at a rate of 2 to 3 mm/min. The decrease in blood flow averages 25% to 30% (too little to explain symptoms; oligemic rather than ischemic) and progresses anteriorly in a wavelike fashion that is independent of the topography of cerebral arteries. The wave of hypoperfusion persists for 4 to 6 hours, follows the convolutions of the cortex, and does not cross the central or lateral sulcus but progresses to the frontal lobe via the insula. Subcortical perfusion is normal. Contralateral neurologic symptoms appear during the period of temporoparietal hypoperfusion; at times, hypoperfusion persists in these regions after symptoms cease. More often, frontal spread continues as the headache phase begins. A few patients experiencing migraine with aura show no abnormalities of blood flow; rarely, focal ischemia is sufficient to cause symptoms. Focal ischemia, however, does not appear necessary for focal symptoms to occur. In attacks of common migraine, no abnormalities of blood flow have been seen. The changes in cerebral blood flow are attributed to alterations of cerebral neuronal function. The cortical events require a "generator," which has been identified within the brainstem.

Pharmacologic data converge on serotonin receptors. About 35 years ago, methysergide was found to antagonize peripheral actions of serotonin (5-hydroxytryptamine) and was introduced as the first drug capable of preventing migraine attacks by stabilizing the basic fault. Platelet levels of serotonin fall at the onset of headache, and migrainous episodes can be triggered by drugs that release serotonin. These changes in circulating levels proved to be pharmacologically trivial, however, and interest in the role of serotonin declined, only to be revived by the introduction of sumatriptan, which is remarkably effective for migraine attacks. Sumatriptan was the first designer drug synthesized to activate selectively a particular subpopulation of serotonin receptors.

There are seven families of serotonin receptors; within each family are receptor subtypes. Triptans act as agonists of the 5-HT1B and 5-HT1D receptors. Some triptans have variable affinities to the 5-HT1E and the 5-HT1F receptor, but the clinical meaning of this has not been established. All triptans have similar affinities to the relevant serotonin receptor subtypes. In contrast, dihydroergotamine, another drug effective in aborting migraine attacks, is most potent as an agonist of 5-HT1A receptors, but is an order of magnitude less potent at 5-HT1D and 5-HT1B receptors. It has affinity for alpha-adrenergic and dopaminergic receptors that probably do not contribute to migraine relief, as such, but do contribute to side effects. After systemic administration, dihydroergotamine in the brain is found in highest concentrations in the midbrain dorsal raphe. The dorsal raphe contains the highest concentration of serotonin receptors in the brain and could be the generator of migraine and the main site of drug action. Raphe receptors are mainly of 5-HT1A, but 5-HT1D receptors are also present.

Electrical stimulation near dorsal raphe neurons can result in migrainelike headaches. Projections from the dorsal raphe terminate on cerebral arteries and alter cerebral blood flow. The dorsal raphe also projects to visual processing neurons in the lateral geniculate body, superior colliculus, retina, and visual cortex. These projections could provide the anatomic and physiologic bases for the circulatory and visual characteristics of migraine. The dorsal raphe cells cease firing during deep sleep, and sleep ameliorates migraine; antimigraine drugs also stop the firing of the dorsal raphe cells through a direct or indirect agonist effect (Fig. 140.1). The shutdown of an inhibitory system may enhance or stabilize neurotransmission. PET scans have demonstrated an activation of the periaqueductal gray in the region of the dorsal raphe nucleus during attacks of migraine without aura; this region becoming inactive between attacks.

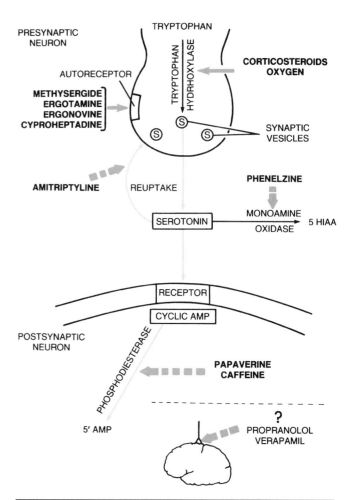

FIGURE 140.1. The actions of the antimigraine drugs at brainstem and forebrain synapses. The *solid arrows* indicate agonist properties; the *segmented arrows* indicate inhibitory properties. (From Raskin NH. *Headache.* 2nd Ed. New York: Churchill Livingstone, 1988.)

Migraine may therefore be considered a hereditary perturbation of central inhibitory mechanisms. Similar perturbations may underlie many types of head pain; "ordinary" periodic headaches may be the "noise" of the normally functioning system. Transcranial magnetic stimulation of the cerebral cortex causes subjects to see phosphenes, but migraineurs see these with far less cortical stimulation, further documenting the fundamental cortical hyperexcitability of migraine.

Treatment

Nonpharmacologic treatments have been advocated, but rigorously controlled trials have shown no benefit without concomitant drug treatment. The mainstay of therapy is the judicious use of one or more of the many drugs.

Acute Treatment

In general, an adequate dose of whichever agent is chosen should be used at the onset of an attack. This is needed to terminate the attack before central sensitization occurs and the brainstem activation is self-sustaining. Drug absorption is impaired during attacks because of reduced gastrointestinal motility. Absorption may be delayed in the absence of nausea, and the delay is related to the severity of the attack but not to the duration. Therefore, when oral agents fail, the major considerations include rectal administration of ergotamine, subcutaneous sumatriptan, intranasal sumatriptan or zolmitriptan, parenteral dihydroergotamine, intravenous chlorpromazine, prochlorperazine, metoclopramide, or a parenterally administered nonsteroidal anti-inflammatory agent.

For patients with a prolonged buildup of headache, oral agents usually suffice. The treatments should be tailored to the historical features of the attacks: those with moderate to severe attacks should start with triptans or ergots; those with milder attacks might be successfully managed with nonsteroidal anti-inflammatory agents, isometheptene, or butalbital combination drugs. Because successful treatment almost always needs to be initiated promptly, it is essential not to save the more potent agents for use only hours after other agents have failed.

Sumatriptan can be given orally, intranasally, or subcutaneously. Zolmitriptan is available for oral or intranasal administration. Rizatriptan, almotriptan, and eletriptan are available as tablets. All of these agents have similar success rates. Naratriptan and frovatriptan appear to have the most favorable side-effect profile of this group and the lowest recurrence rates in successfully treated attacks; but they are less effective than the other triptans in actually terminating an attack. There is no evidence of any difference in cardiovascular safety between brands or forms of triptans. There is also no evidence that recurrent migraines are best treated with triptans with the longest half-lives, possibly because those agents are least effective in terminating attacks. All triptans are effective in reducing the nausea, vomiting, photophobia, and phonophobia that often accompany the pain, assuming that the agent is adequately absorbed in the presence of nausea. In that situation, intranasal or subcutaneous administration is more appropriate.

When ergotamine is used, a subnauseating dose, if possible, should be determined for the individual patient. A dose that provokes nausea—probably a centrally mediated effect—is too high for therapy and may intensify head pain. The average oral dose of ergotamine is 3 mg (three 1-mg ergotamine-caffeine tablets); the average dose of the 2-mg suppository is one-half (1 mg). Many patients use one-fourth of a suppository (0.5 mg) with an optimal result. Dihydroergotamine is available as a parenteral preparation and as a nasal spray. Peak plasma levels of dihy-

droergotamine are achieved 45 to 60 minutes after nasal administration, 45 minutes after subcutaneous administration, 30 minutes after intramuscular administration, and 3 minutes after intravenous administration. If an attack has not already peaked, subcutaneous or intramuscular administration of 1 mg suffices for about 90% of patients. A common intravenous protocol is the mixture of prochlorperazine 5 mg and dihydroergotamine 0.5 mg given over 2 minutes (they are miscible).

When a patient's headache pattern transforms into a chronic daily headache syndrome, opioid or other analgesics should be restricted to 2 days weekly. The mainstay of therapy for these patients is daily amitriptyline or nortriptyline (30–100 mg), divalproex sodium (500–2000 mg daily), topiramate (50–200 mg), or zonisamide (100–200 mg). A beta-blocker can be concomitantly administered if needed. For recalcitrant individuals, monoamine oxidase (MAO) inhibitors or atypical neuroleptics may be necessary. Drugs that have antidepressant effects act independent of such effects in migraine, and the serotonin reuptake inhibitors have failed to demonstrate efficacy for headache in most studies. The choice of these several alternatives is a matter of personal choice for the physician; the data are too scanty for an evidence-based decision.

Prophylactic Treatment

Several drugs can stabilize migraine and prevent attacks; for this purpose, the drugs must be taken daily (Table 140.1). When to implement this approach depends on the frequency of attacks and the efficacy of acute treatment. Comorbid conditions, such as hypertension and bipolar disease, can influence the choice of prophylactic medication. At least two or three attacks a month could signal an indication for this approach. Usually a lag of at least 2 weeks must pass before a beneficial effect is seen; this may be the time needed to downregulate serotonin receptors. The early lack of efficacy coincides with the period of maximal side effects. The major drugs and their daily dose are propranolol (40–320 mg), amitriptyline, nortriptyline, and doxepin (10–175) mg), verapamil (120–480 mg), divalproex (500–2000 mg), topiramate (75–200 mg), and zonisamide (200–500 mg).

Phenelzine is usually reserved for more recalcitrant headaches because of serious adverse effects. Because phenelzine is an MAO inhibitor, concomitant use of tyramine-containing foods and a variety of medications is contraindicated.

The probability of success with any one of the antimigraine drugs is about 50%. With successful prophylaxis, attacks may be more responsive to acute therapy. If one drug is assessed each month, the likelihood is high that stabilization will be achieved within a few months. If chronic daily headaches are not well controlled by 6 months, the prognosis for recovery becomes poor. Therefore, these

▶ **TABLE 140.1** **Drug Stabilization of Migraine**

Drug	Tablet Size (mg)	Daily Dose Range (mg)	Most Common Side Effects
Propranolol	10, 20, 40, 60, 80, 90; sustained release: 60, 80, 120, 160	40–320	Fatigue, insomnia, lightheadedness, impotence
Amitriptyline	10, 25, 50, 75, 100	10–175	Sedation, dry mouth, appetite stimulation
Ergonovine	0.2	0.4–2.0	Nausea, abdominal pain, leg tiredness, diarrhea
Verapamil	40, 80, 120; sustained release: 120, 180, 240	120–480 320–960	Constipation, nausea, fluid retention, lightheadedness, hypotension
Valproate	125, 250, 500	500–2,000	Nausea, tremor, alopecia, appetite stimulation
Phenelzine	15	30–90	Sedation, orthostatic hypotension, constipation, urinary retention
Topiramate	25,100	75–200	

trials need to be conducted systematically and rapidly. Once effective, the drug is continued for about 6 months, and the dose is then tapered slowly to assess continued need. Many patients can discontinue medication and experience fewer and less severe attacks for a long time, thus suggesting that the drugs may alter the natural history of migraine.

CLUSTER HEADACHE

Recognition of this disorder has been retarded by confusing names, including *Raeder syndrome, histamine cephalalgia, and sphenopalatine neuralgia*. Cluster headache is firmly established as a distinct syndrome that is likely to respond to treatment. The episodic type, the most common, is characterized by one to three short-lived attacks of periorbital pain each day for 4 to 8 weeks, followed by a pain-free interval for a mean of 1 year. The chronic form may begin de novo or may appear several years after an episodic pattern has been established. The attacks are similar and there are no sustained periods of remission. Either type may transform into the other.

Men are affected more often than women in a proportion of about 8:1. Hereditary factors are usually absent. The prevalence is 69 cases per 100,000 people. Although headaches usually start between the ages of 20 and 50 years, the syndrome may begin as early as the first decade or as late as the eighth. The cluster syndrome differs from migraine genetically, biochemically, and clinically. Propranolol and amitriptyline are largely ineffective in cluster headache. Lithium, however, is beneficial for the cluster syndrome and ineffective in migraine. Nevertheless, the two disorders may blend into one in occasional patients, suggesting that the mechanisms include some common features.

Clinical Features

Periorbital or, less commonly, temporal or maxillary pain begins without warning and reaches a crescendo within 5 minutes. It is often excruciating in intensity and is deep, nonfluctuating, and relatively explosive in quality; only rarely is it pulsatile. Pain is strictly unilateral and usually affects the same side in subsequent months. Attacks typically last from 30 minutes to 2 hours; the associated symptoms are homolateral lacrimation, reddening of the eye, nasal stuffiness, and lid ptosis. Nausea is uncommon, but may appear in severe attacks. Alcohol provokes attacks in about 70% of patients, but has no effect when the bout remits; this on–off vulnerability to alcohol is nearly pathognomonic of cluster headache. Following an attack, there is a brief refractory period during which time another attack cannot be provoked with alcohol. Only rarely do foods or emotional factors activate the mechanism, in contradistinction to migraine.

Periodicity of attacks is evident in at least 85% of patients. At least one of the daily attacks of pain recurs at about the same hour each day for the duration of a bout. This clock mechanism is set for nocturnal hours in about 50% of patients; in these circumstances, the pain usually wakens patients within 2 hours of falling asleep.

Pathogenesis

No consistent changes in cerebral blood flow attend attacks of pain. Perhaps the strongest evidence pointing to a central mechanism is the periodicity; reinforcing this conclusion are the bilateral autonomic symptoms that accompany the pain and are more severe on the painful side. The hypothalamus is probably the site of activation; activation of the hypothalamic grey has been reported in PET scans of spontaneous attacks, in contradistinction to migraine where the midbrain and pons are activated. The posterior hypothalamus contains cells that regulate autonomic functions, and the anterior hypothalamus contains cells (the suprachiasmatic nuclei) that serve as the principal circadian pacemaker in mammals. Activation of both is necessary to explain the symptoms of cluster headache. The pacemaker is modulated serotonergically through projections of the dorsal raphe. Therefore, both migraine and cluster headache may result from abnormal serotonergic neurotransmission, albeit at different loci.

Treatment

The most satisfactory treatment is the administration of drugs to prevent cluster attacks until the bout is over. The major prophylactic drugs are prednisone, lithium carbonate, topiramate, divalproex, and verapamil. Lithium (600–900 mg daily) appears to be particularly effective for the chronic form. A 10-day course of prednisone, beginning at 60 mg daily for 7 days and rapidly tapering, seems to curtail the bout for many patients. There is weak evidence that early treatment of a new cluster period with corticosteroids may shorten the duration of the new bout. Ergotamine is most effective when given 1 or 2 hours before an expected attack; for patients with a single nocturnal episode, 1 mg ergotamine in suppository formulation taken at bedtime may be all that is necessary. Patients must be educated regarding the early symptoms of ergotism (limb claudication) when ergotamine is used daily; a weekly limit of 14 mg should be followed. Should sumatriptan be used to terminate attacks, ergots cannot be used preventively.

For the attacks themselves, oxygen inhalation (about 10 L/min given with a nonrebreathing mask) is effective; 15 minutes of inhalation of 100% oxygen is often necessary. The self-administration of intranasal lidocaine, either 4% topical or 2% viscous, to the most caudal aspect of the inferior nasal turbinate can deliver a sphenopalatine ganglion block that is often remarkably effective for the termination of an attack, particularly if much of the pain in centered in the lower portions of the face. Sumatriptan, 6 mg subcutaneously, usually shortens an attack to 10 to 15 minutes and is highly effective. The use of sumatriptan within 24 hours of the use of ergotamine is contraindicated.

CHRONIC PAROXYSMAL HEMICRANIA

Chronic paroxysmal hemicrania comprises attacks that are phenomenologically similar to cluster headaches, but attacks are briefer and more frequent. Unlike cluster headaches, there is a female preponderance. Five or more attacks daily are seen and attacks may last 2 to 45 minutes. The pain has a boring quality reaching full intensity very rapidly; it is associated with ipsilateral lacrimation, nasal congestion, eyelid edema, and a partial Horner syndrome. Like cluster, episodic forms can be seen. These attacks are remarkably responsive to indomethacin therapy. Doses of 50 to 250 mg daily are effective. There is a significant and expected morbidity from chronic therapy with indomethacin, although doses can commonly be reduced with prolonged treatment. Additionally, many patients re-

spond to COX-II inhibitors, which have better gastrointestinal tolerability.

SUNCT SYNDROME

Short-lasting unilateral neuralgiform headache with conjunctival injection and tearing (SUNCT) is rare and uncommonly diagnosed. Sufferers tend to be men much more than women. Multiple attacks per hour are experienced, but last only seconds; the pain is described as stabbing or throbbing in quality and moderate to severe in intensity. They are associated with the same autonomic disturbances seen with cluster headaches: conjunctival injection, lacrimation, nasal congestion, rhinorrhea, ptosis, and eyelid edema. Although treatment is difficult, lamotrigine or gabapentin may be effective.

HEMICRANIA CONTINUA

Often confused with chronic migraine or cluster, hemicrania continua causes a continuous unilateral headache, fluctuating in severity and associated with the same autonomic symptoms as cluster headaches. There are no clear precipitating factors, and headaches tend to become chronic de novo rather than representing a transformation from an episodic form. Sufferers tend to respond dramatically and immediately to indomethacin.

COUGH HEADACHE

Another male-dominated (4:1) syndrome is cough headache, which is characterized by transient severe head pain brought on by coughing, bending, lifting, sneezing, or stooping. Head pain persists seconds or a few minutes. Many patients date the origin of the syndrome to a lower respiratory infection accompanied by severe coughing or to strenuous weight-lifting programs. Headache is usually diffuse but is lateralized in about one-third of patients. The incidence of serious intracranial structural anomalies causing this condition is about 25%; the Arnold-Chiari malformation is a common cause. MRI is indicated for these patients. The benign disorder may persist for a few years; it is inexplicably and remarkably ameliorated by indomethacin at doses of 50 to 200 mg daily. A large-volume (40 mL) lumbar puncture dramatically terminates the syndrome for 50% of patients so treated.

Many patients with migraine note that attacks of headache may be provoked by sustained physical exertion, such as during the third mile of a 5-mile run. These headaches build up over hours and therefore differ from the cough headache syndrome. The term "effort migraine" has been used to avoid the ambiguous term "exertional headache."

COITAL HEADACHE

In another male-dominated (4:1) syndrome, headaches occur during coitus, usually close to orgasm. They are abrupt in onset and subside in a few minutes if coitus is interrupted. These headaches are nearly always benign and usually occur sporadically; if a coital headache persists for hours or is accompanied by vomiting, subarachnoid hemorrhage must be evaluated by CT or CSF examination. An unruptured aneurysm may result in a headache during coitus and can be indistinguishable from benign coital headache; therefore, angiography should be considered for the first attack of coital headache. If attacks occur frequently and are brief, however, the disorder is benign.

NOCTURNAL HEADACHES

Migraine is the most common cause of headache awakening one out of sleep. This complicates treatment in that headaches are often well established before medications are initiated. There are a variety of reasons why migraine and cluster headaches are commonly triggered by sleep. Many occur coincident with rapid eye movement (REM) sleep, which is associated with cerebral vasodilation. The sleep apnea syndrome can also trigger migraine, and as attacks become pervasive, a polysomnogram is appropriate to exclude this problem. In many such identified cases, treatment, including positive airway pressure, improves the nocturnal and early morning pain. Habitually sleeping with covers over the head, or "turtling," can lead to morning head pain, possibly through hypercapnia. Hypnic headaches are generally seen in the elderly, with headaches that awaken them nightly and last 15 to 60 minutes. The pain is poorly localized and often throbbing. Autonomic symptoms such as lacrimation and rhinorrhea are not seen. Because this kind of headache is rare and begins in the elderly, intracranial neoplasms and giant cell arteritis need to be excluded. Treatment is generally successful with 150 to 300 mg of lithium carbonate administered at night. A caffeine source at bedtime, if it is tolerated, may suffice.

POSTCONCUSSION HEADACHES

After a seemingly trivial head injury and particularly after a rear-end motor vehicle collision, many people report admixtures of headache, vertigo, mood changes, and impaired memory and concentration for months or years after the injury. Despite the term "postconcussive," loss of consciousness is not a prerequisite for the development of these headaches, and there may actually be an inverse relationship between the severity of headaches and the severity of head injury. The syndrome is usually not associated with an anatomic lesion of the brain and may occur whether or not the person was rendered unconscious by head trauma. In general, this headache is "neurobiologic" rather than "psychologic." The syndrome usually persists long after the settlement of a lawsuit. Some evidence suggests that concussion perturbs neurotransmission within the brain and that restoration of this condition is typically delayed. Understanding this common problem is contingent on clarification of the biology of cerebral concussion. Occasionally, chronic subdural hematomas, herniated cervical discs, or facet joint pathology secondary to the trauma explains the development of symptoms. Treatment is symptomatic, including repeated encouragement that the syndrome eventually remits.

GIANT CELL ARTERITIS

This is a relatively common disorder among the elderly; the average annual incidence is about 25 per 100,000 people after age 50. The cause is unknown, but there may be a genetic predisposition and possibly an infectious origin. Women account for 65% of cases, and the average age at onset is 70 years, with a range of 50 to 85 years. The inflammatory process may result in blindness in 50% of patients if corticosteroid treatment is not instituted; indeed, the ischemic optic neuropathy of giant cell arteritis is the major cause of rapidly developing bilateral blindness after age 60. Additional vascular complications can include thrombosis of any predural artery as well as aortic aneurysm with rupture.

The most common initial symptoms are headache, polymyalgia rheumatica, jaw or tongue claudication, fever, and weight loss (see Chapter 156). Headache is the dominant symptom and usually appears with malaise and myalgia. Head pain may be unilateral or bilateral and is located temporally in 50% of patients, but may involve any and all aspects of the cranium. Pain usually appears gradually over a few hours before peak intensity is reached; occasionally, it is explosive in onset. The quality of pain is only seldom throbbing; it is almost invariably described as dull and boring with superimposed episodic ice pick-like lancinating pains similar to the sharp pains that appear in migraine. Most patients recognize that the origin of the pain is superficial and external to the skull, rather than deep within the cranium (the site of pain in migraine).

The scalp pain may be allodynic as seen in prolonged migraine; scalp tenderness is present, often marked; brushing the hair or resting the head on a pillow may be impossible because of pain. Headache is usually worse at night and is often aggravated by exposure to cold. Reddened tender nodules or red streaking of the skin overlying the temporal arteries is found in many patients with headache, as is tenderness of the temporal or, less commonly, the occipital arteries. The erythrocyte sedimentation rate is often, but not invariably, elevated; a normal erythrocyte sedimentation rate does not exclude giant cell arteritis. Serum viscosity and C-reactive protein levels are often elevated and may prove useful to follow the effects of treatment, particularly in those with normal erythrocyte sedimentation levels. Plasma interleukin-6 (IL-6) measurement may be the most sensitive marker of disease activity.

After temporal artery biopsy, prednisone is promptly initiated at 80 mg daily for the first 4 to 6 weeks, when clinical suspicion is high. Some authorities recommend starting with 3 days of 500 mg of intravenous methylprednisolone. Because patients with migraine and other headaches also report amelioration of headaches with corticosteroid therapy, therapeutic responses are not diagnostic. Contrary to widespread notions, the prevalence of migraine among the elderly population is substantial, considerably higher than that of giant cell arteritis.

IDIOPATHIC INTRACRANIAL HYPERTENSION AND HYPOTENSION

These important causes of headache are discussed in Chapter 50.

LUMBAR PUNCTURE HEADACHE

Headache after lumbar puncture usually begins within 48 hours, but may be delayed for up to 12 days. The mean incidence is about 30%. Initially, head pain is dramatically positional; it begins when the patient sits or stands upright and subsides on reclining or with abdominal compression. The value of prolonged bed rest after lumbar puncture in preventing low-pressure headaches has been questioned. It is worsened by head shaking or jugular vein compression. The pain is usually a dull ache but may be throbbing; the location is occipitofrontal. Nausea and stiff neck often accompany headache, and some patients report blurred vision, photophobia, tinnitus, and vertigo. The symptoms usually resolve over a few days but may persist for weeks or months. Spontaneous intracranial hypotension can occur and may explain some cases of new daily persistent headache. Low CSF pressure is seen and radiologically there may be dural thickening and enhancement on MRI as well as downward displacement of the cerebellar tonsils and subdural effusions. Leaks from head trauma, erosions through the dura from adjacent lesions, and dural root sleeve tears can cause this syndrome. Although meningeal enhancement on MRI is characteristic of intracranial hypotension, dural carcinomatosis or lymphoma, sarcoidosis, and rheumatoid arthritis need to be excluded.

Loss of CSF volume decreases the supportive cushion of the brain; when the patient is erect, vascular dilatation probably results and tension is placed on anchoring intracranial structures, including the pain-sensitive dural sinuses. There is often intracranial hypotension, but the full-blown syndrome may occur with normal CSF pressure.

Treatment is remarkably effective. Intravenous caffeine sodium benzoate given over a few minutes as a 500-mg dose promptly terminates headache in 75% of patients; a second dose 1 hour later brings the total success rate to 85%. In the case of post–lumbar puncture headache, an epidural blood patch accomplished by injection of 15 mL of the patient's blood rarely fails for those who do not respond to caffeine. The explanation for the success of this treatment is not clear because the blood patch has an immediate effect; thus, the occlusion of a dural hole with blood clot is an unlikely mechanism of action. More likely, the patch of blood displaces an engorged lumbar epidural venous plexus, increasing the intracranial pressure.

BRAIN TUMOR HEADACHE

About 30% of patients with brain tumors consider headache their chief complaint. Headaches are more likely to be a symptom of a mass lesion in those with a pre-existing primary headache syndrome. Most characteristic is the progression of headache for weeks to months. The head pain syndrome is nondescript; a deep dull aching quality of moderate intensity occurs intermittently, is worsened by exertion or change in position, and is associated with nausea and vomiting. Patients may note increased severity and frequency of a pre-existing headache type, a pattern that results from migraine far more often than from brain tumor. Headache disturbs sleep in about 10% of patients, but awakenings are far more common in migraine and cluster headaches than in brain tumor headaches. Vomiting that precedes the appearance of headache by weeks suggests a posterior fossa brain tumor. There is little localizing value to the side of the headache. Posterior fossa or intraventricular neoplasms are more likely to cause headache than those above the tentorium.

SUGGESTED READINGS

Breslau N, Rasmussen BK. The impact of migraine: epidemiology, risk factors, and co-morbidities. *Neurology* 2001;56(Suppl 1):S4–S12.

Cutrer FM, Sorensen AG, Weisskoff RM, et al. Perfusion-weighted imaging defects during spontaneous migrainous aura. *Ann Neurol* 1998;43:25–37.

Ferrari MD. Migraine. *Lancet* 1998;351:1043–1051.

Goadsby PJ. A triptan too far? *J Neurol Neurosurg Psychiatry* 1998;64:143–147.

Goadsby PJ, Gundlach AL. Localization of ^{3}H-dihydroergotamine binding sites in the cat central nervous system: relevance to migraine. *Ann Neurol* 1991;29:91–94.

Green MW. The emergency management of headaches. *Neurologist* 2003;9:93–98.

Grimson BS, Thompson HS. Raeder's syndrome. A clinical review. *Surg Ophthalmol* 1980;24:199–210.

Hoskin KL, Kaube H, Goadsby PJ. Sumatriptan can inhibit trigeminal afferents by an exclusively neural mechanism. *Brain* 1996;119:1419–1428.

Kors EE, Melberg A, Vanmolkot KR, et al. Childhood epilepsy, familial hemiplegic migraine, cerebellar ataxia, and a new CACMA1A mutation. *Neurology* 2004 Sep 28;63(6):1136–1137.

Mannix LK, Calhoun AH. Menstrual migraine. *Curr Treat Options Neurol* 2004 Nov;6 (6):489–498.

Nyholt DR, Lea RA, Goadsby PJ, et al. Familial typical migraine. *Neurology* 1998;50:1428–1432.

Olesen J. Cerebral and extracranial circulatory disturbances in migraine: pathophysiological implications. *Cerebrovasc Brain Metab Rev* 1991;3:1–28.

Pietroban D, Striessnig J. Neurological diseases: neurobiology of migraine. *Nat Rev Neurosci* 2003;4:386–398.

Raskin NH. Lumbar puncture headache: a review. *Headache* 1990;30:197–200.

Raskin NH. Short-lived head pains. *Neurol Clin* 1997;15:143–152.

Schraeder PL, Burns RA. Hemiplegic migraine associated with an aseptic meningeal reaction. *Arch Neurol* 1980;37:377–379.

Shields KG, Goadsby PJ. Propranolol modulates trigeminovascular responses in thalamic ventroposteromedial nucleus: a role in migraine? *Brain* 2005 Jan;128 (Pt 1):86–97.

Silberstein SD, ed. *An Atlas of Headache.* London: Taylor & Francis, 2002.

Silberstein SD. Migraine. *Lancet* 2004;363:381–391.

Silberstein SD. The pharmacology of ergotamine and dihydroergotamine. *Headache* 1997;37(Suppl):S15–S25.

Silberstein S, Lipton R, Dalessio D. *Wolff's Headache.* 7th Ed. Oxford, UK: Oxford University Press, 2001.

Silberstein SD, Lipton RD, Goadsby PJ, eds. *Headache in Clinical Practice.* 2nd Ed. London: Taylor & Francis, 2002.

Symonds C. Cough headache. *Brain* 1956;79:557–568.

Weiller C, May A, Limmroth V, et al. Brain stem activation in spontaneous human migraine attacks. *Nat Med* 1995;1:658–660.

Chapter 141

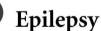

Epilepsy

Carl W. Bazil, Martha J. Morrell, and Timothy A. Pedley

An epileptic seizure is the result of a temporary physiologic dysfunction of the brain caused by a self-limited, abnormal, hypersynchronous electrical discharge of cortical neurons. There are many different kinds of seizures, each with characteristic behavioral changes and electrophysiologic disturbances that can usually be detected in scalp EEG recordings. The particular manifestations of any single seizure depend on several factors: whether most or only a part of the cerebral cortex is involved at the beginning, the functions of the cortical areas where the seizure originates, the subsequent pattern of spread of the electrical ictal discharge within the brain, and the extent to which subcortical and brainstem structures are engaged.

A seizure is a transient epileptic event, a symptom of disturbed brain function. Although seizures are the cardinal manifestation of epilepsy, not all seizures imply epilepsy. For example, seizures may be self-limited in that they occur only during the course of an acute medical or neurologic illness; they do not persist after the underlying disorder has resolved. Some people, for no discoverable reason, have a single unprovoked seizure. These kinds of seizures are not epilepsy.

Epilepsy is a chronic disorder, or group of chronic disorders, in which the indispensable feature is recurrence of seizures that are typically unprovoked and usually unpredictable. About 40 million people are affected worldwide. Each distinct form of epilepsy has its own natural history and response to treatment. This diversity presumably reflects the fact that epilepsy can arise from a variety of underlying conditions and pathophysiologic mechanisms, although most cases are classified as idiopathic (of presumed genetic origin) or cryptogenic (arising from a past injury that is not defined).

CLASSIFICATION OF SEIZURES AND EPILEPSY

Accurate classification of seizures and epilepsy is essential for understanding epileptic phenomena, developing a rational plan of investigation, making decisions about when and for how long to treat, choosing the appropriate antiepileptic drug, and conducting scientific investigations that require delineation of clinical and EEG phenotypes.

Classification of Seizures

The classification used today is the 1981 Classification of Epileptic Seizures developed by the International League Against Epilepsy (ILAE; Table 141.1). This system classifies seizures by clinical symptoms supplemented by EEG data.

Inherent in the classification are two important physiologic principles. First, seizures are fundamentally of two types: those with onset limited to a part of one cerebral hemisphere (*partial* or *focal* seizures) and those that seem to involve the brain diffusely from the beginning (*generalized* seizures). Second, seizures are dynamic and evolving; clinical expression is determined as much by the sequence of spread of electrical discharge within the brain as by the area where the ictal discharge originates. Variations in the seizure pattern exhibited by an individual imply variability in the extent and pattern of spread of the electrical discharge.

▶ **TABLE 141.1 ILAE Classification of Epileptic Seizures**

I. Partial (focal) seizures
A. Simple partial seizures (consciousness not impaired)
1. With motor signs (including jacksonian, versive, and postural)
2. With sensory symptoms (including visual, somatosensory, auditory, olfactory, gustatory, and vertiginous)
3. With psychic symptoms (including dysphasia, dysmensic, hallucinatory, and affective changes)
4. With autonomic symptoms (including epigastric sensation, pallor, flushing, pupillary changes)
B. Complex partial seizures (consciousness is impaired)
1. Simple partial onset followed by impaired consciousness
2. With impairment of consciousness at onset
3. With automatisms
C. Partial seizures evolving to secondarily generalized seizures
II. Generalized seizures of nonfocal origin (convulsive or nonconvulsive)
A. Absence seizures
1. With impaired consciousness only
2. With one or more of the following: atonic components, tonic components, automatisms, autonomic components
B. Myoclonic seizures
Myoclonic jerks (single or multiple)
C. Tonic-clonic seizures (may include clonic-tonic-clonic seizures)
D. Tonic seizures
E. Atonic seizures
III. Unclassified epileptic seizures

ILAE, International League Against Epilepsy.
Adapted from Commission on Classification and Terminology of the International League Against Epilepsy. Proposal for revised clinical and electroencephalographic classification of epileptic seizures. *Epilepsia* 1981;22:489–501.

Both generalized and partial seizures are further divided into subtypes. For partial seizures, the most important subdivision is based on consciousness, which is preserved in *simple* partial seizures or lost in *complex* partial seizures. Simple partial seizures may evolve into complex partial seizures, and either simple or complex partial seizures may evolve into secondarily generalized seizures. In adults, most generalized seizures have a focal onset whether or not this is apparent clinically. For generalized seizures, subdivisions are based mainly on the presence or absence and character of ictal motor manifestations.

The initial events of a seizure, described by either the patient or an observer, are usually the most reliable clinical indication to determine whether a seizure begins focally or is generalized from the moment of onset. Sometimes, however, a focal signature is lacking for several possible reasons:

1. The patient may be amnesic after the seizure, with no memory of early events.

2. Consciousness may be impaired so quickly or the seizure may become generalized so rapidly that early distinguishing features are blurred or lost.

3. The seizure may originate in a brain region that is not associated with an obvious behavioral function. Thus, the seizure becomes clinically evident only when the discharge spreads beyond the ictal onset zone or becomes generalized.

Partial Seizures

Simple partial seizures result when the ictal discharge occurs in a limited and often circumscribed area of cortex, the *epileptogenic focus*. Almost any symptom or phenomenon can be the subjective (aura) or observable manifestation of a simple partial seizure, varying from elementary motor (jacksonian seizures, adversive seizures) and unilateral sensory disturbance to complex emotional, psychoillusory, hallucinatory, or dysmnesic phenomena. Especially common auras include an epigastric rising sensation, fear, a feeling of unreality or detachment, déjà vu and jamais vu experiences, and olfactory hallucinations. Patients can interact normally with the environment during simple partial seizures except for limitations imposed by the seizure on specific localized brain functions.

Complex partial seizures, on the other hand, are defined by impaired consciousness and imply bilateral spread of the seizure discharge, at least to basal forebrain and limbic areas. In addition to loss of consciousness, patients with complex partial seizures usually exhibit automatisms, such as lip-smacking, repeated swallowing, clumsy perseveration of an ongoing motor task, or some other complex motor activity that is undirected and inappropriate. Postictally, patients are confused and disoriented for several minutes, and determining the transition from ictal to postictal state may be difficult without simultaneous EEG recording. Of complex partial seizures, 70% to 80% arise from the temporal lobe; foci in the frontal and occipital lobes account for most of the remainder.

Generalized Seizures

Generalized tonic-clonic (*grand mal*) seizures are characterized by abrupt loss of consciousness with bilateral tonic extension of the trunk and limbs (*tonic phase*), often accompanied by a loud vocalization as air is forcedly expelled across contracted vocal cords (*epileptic cry*), followed by synchronous muscle jerking (*clonic phase*). In some patients, a few clonic jerks precede the tonic-clonic sequence; in others, only a tonic or clonic phase is apparent. Postictally, patients are briefly unarousable and then lethargic and confused, often preferring to sleep. Many patients report inconsistent nonspecific premonitory symptoms (*epileptic prodrome*) for minutes to a few hours before a generalized tonic-clonic seizure. Common symptoms include ill-defined anxiety, irritability, decreased concentration, and headache or other uncomfortable feelings; these are not auras.

Absence (petit mal) seizures are momentary lapses in awareness that are accompanied by motionless staring and arrest of any ongoing activity. Absence seizures begin and end abruptly; they occur without warning or postictal period. Mild myoclonic jerks of the eyelid or facial muscles, variable loss of muscle tone, and automatisms may accompany longer attacks. When the beginning and end of the seizure are less distinct, or if tonic and autonomic components are included, the term *atypical absence* seizure is used. Atypical absences are seen most often in retarded children with epilepsy or in epileptic encephalopathies, such as the Lennox-Gastaut syndrome (defined later).

Myoclonic seizures are characterized by rapid brief muscle jerks that can occur bilaterally, synchronously or asynchronously, or unilaterally. Myoclonic jerks range from isolated small movements of face, arm, or leg muscles to massive bilateral spasms simultaneously affecting the head, limbs, and trunk.

Atonic (astatic) seizures, also called *drop attacks,* are characterized by sudden loss of muscle tone, which may be fragmentary (e.g., head drop) or generalized, resulting in a fall. When atonic seizures are preceded by a brief myoclonic seizure or tonic spasm, an acceleratory force is added to the fall, thereby contributing to the high rate of self-injury with this type of seizure.

Classification of Epilepsy (Epileptic Syndromes)

Attempting to classify the kind of epilepsy a patient has is often more important than describing seizures, because the formulation includes other relevant clinical information of which the seizures are only a part. The other data include historical information (e.g., a personal history of brain injury or family history of first-degree relatives with seizures); findings on neurologic examination; and results of EEG, brain imaging, and biochemical studies.

The ILAE classification separates major groups of epilepsy first on the basis of whether seizures are partial (*localization-related epilepsies*) or generalized (*generalized epilepsies*) and second by cause (*idiopathic, symptomatic,* or *cryptogenic* epilepsy). Subtypes of epilepsy are grouped according to the patient's age and, in the case of localization-related epilepsies, by the anatomic location of the presumed ictal onset zone.

Classification of the epilepsies has been less successful and more controversial than the classification of seizure types. A basic problem is that the classification scheme is empiric, with clinical and EEG data emphasized over anatomic, pathologic, or specific etiologic information. This classification is useful for some reasonably well-defined syndromes, such as *infantile spasms* or *benign partial childhood epilepsy with central-midtemporal spikes,* especially because of the prognostic and treatment implications of these disorders. On the other hand, few epilepsies imply a specific disease or defect. A further drawback to the ILAE classification is that the same epileptic syndrome (e.g., infantile spasms or Lennox-Gastaut syndrome) may be "symptomatic" of a specific disease (e.g., tuberous sclerosis), considered "cryptogenic" on the basis of nonspecific imaging abnormalities, or categorized as "idiopathic." Another biologic incongruity is the excessive detail in which some syndromes are identified, with specific entities culled from what are more likely simply different biologic expressions of the same abnormality (e.g., childhood and juvenile forms of absence epilepsy). As a result, a new classification of epilepsy syndromes has been proposed and is presently under discussion (Engel, 2001).

With the foregoing reservations, there is little question that defining common epilepsy syndromes has practical value. Table 141.2 gives a modified version of the current ILAE classification.

▶ **TABLE 141.2 Modified Classification of Epileptic Syndromes**

I. Idiopathic epilepsy syndromes (focal or generalized)
  A. Benign neonatal convulsions
   1. Familial
   2. Nonfamilial
  B. Benign childhood epilepsy
   1. With central midtemporal spikes
   2. With occipital spikes
  C. Childhood/juvenile absence epilepsy
  D. Juvenile myoclonic epilepsy (including generalized tonic-clonic seizures on awakening)
  E. Idiopathic epilepsy, otherwise unspecified
II. Symptomatic epilepsy syndromes (focal or generalized)
  A. West syndrome (infantile spasms)
  B. Lennox-Gastaut syndrome
  C. Early myoclonic encephalopathy
  D. Epilepsia partialis continua
   1. Rasmussen syndrome (encephalitic form)
   2. Restricted form
  E. Acquired epileptic aphasia (Landau-Kleffner syndrome)
  F. Temporal lobe epilepsy
  G. Frontal lobe epilepsy
  H. Post-traumatic epilepsy
  I. Other symptomatic epilepsy, focal or generalized, not specified
III. Other epilepsy syndromes of uncertain or mixed classification
  A. Neonatal seizures
  B. Febrile seizures
  C. Reflex epilepsy
  D. Other unspecified

SELECTED GENERALIZED EPILEPSY SYNDROMES

Infantile Spasms (West Syndrome)

The term *infantile spasms* denotes a unique age-specific form of generalized epilepsy that may be either idiopathic or symptomatic. When all clinical data are considered, including results of imaging studies, only about 15% of patients are now classified as idiopathic. Symptomatic cases result from diverse conditions, including cerebral dysgenesis, tuberous sclerosis, phenylketonuria, intrauterine infections, or hypoxic-ischemic injury.

Seizures are characterized by sudden flexor or extensor spasms that involve the head, trunk, and limbs simultaneously. The attacks usually begin before 6 months of age. The EEG is grossly abnormal, showing chaotic high-voltage slow activity with multifocal spikes, a pattern termed *hypsarrhythmia*. The treatment of choice is corticotropin or prednisone; spasms are notoriously refractory to conventional antiepileptic drugs. Exceptions are topiramate and zonisamide, which have been shown to be an effective alternative to corticotropin in selected cases. Vigabatrin, a drug not approved for use in the United States, can also be effective, especially in children with tuberous sclerosis. Although treatment with corticotropin, zonisamide, or topiramate usually controls spasms and reverses the EEG abnormalities, it has little effect on long-term prognosis. Only about 5% to 10% of children with infantile spasms have normal or near-normal intelligence, and more than 66% have severe disabilities.

Childhood Absence (Petit Mal) Epilepsy

This disorder begins most often between the ages of 4 and 12 years and is characterized predominantly by recurrent absence seizures, which, if untreated, can occur literally hundreds of times each day. EEG activity during an absence attack is characterized by stereotyped, bilateral, 3-Hz spike-wave discharges. Generalized tonic-clonic seizures also occur in 30% to 50% of cases. Most children are normal, both neurologically and intellectually. Ethosuximide and valproate are equally effective in treating absence seizures, but valproate or lamotrigine are preferable if generalized tonic-clonic seizures coexist. Topiramate and zonisamide may also be effective in generalized-onset seizures.

Lennox-Gastaut Syndrome

This term is applied to a heterogeneous group of childhood epileptic encephalopathies that are characterized by mental retardation, uncontrolled seizures, and a distinctive EEG pattern. The syndrome is not a pathologic entity, because clinical and EEG manifestations result from brain malformations, perinatal asphyxia, severe head injury, CNS infection, or, rarely, a progressive degenerative or metabolic syndrome. A presumptive cause can be identified in 65% to 70% of affected children. Seizures usually begin before age 4 years, and about 25% of children have a history of infantile spasms. No treatment is consistently effective, and 80% of children continue to have seizures as adults. Best results are generally obtained with broad-spectrum antiepileptic drugs, such as valproate, lamotrigine, topiramate, or zonisamide. Despite the higher incidence of severe side effects, felbamate is often effective when these other agents do not result in optimal seizure control. Refractory cases may be considered for vagus nerve stimulation or anterior corpus callosotomy. Both of these are palliative procedures, and complete seizure control is rare.

Juvenile Myoclonic Epilepsy (JME)

The JME subtype of idiopathic generalized epilepsy most often begins in otherwise healthy individuals between the ages of 8 and 20 years. The fully developed syndrome comprises morning myoclonic jerks, generalized tonic-clonic seizures that occur just after waking, normal intelligence, a family history of similar seizures, and an EEG that shows generalized spikes, 4- to 6-Hz spike waves, and multiple spike (polyspike) discharges. The myoclonic jerks vary in intensity from bilateral massive spasms and falls to minor isolated muscle jerks that many patients consider nothing more than "morning clumsiness." Linkage studies have produced conflicting results with different groups reporting susceptibility loci on chromosomes 6p, 5q. and 15q. A mutation in the alpha1 subunit of the $GABA_A$ receptor has been found in a large French Canadian family with JME but not in individuals with the common sporadic form of JME. Valproate is the treatment of choice and controls seizures and myoclonus in more than 80% of cases. Lamotrigine, zonisamide, levetiracetam, and topiramate can be equally effective in many patients, although lamotrigine sometimes exacerbates myoclonus.

SELECTED LOCALIZATION-RELATED EPILEPSY SYNDROMES

Benign Focal Epilepsy of Childhood

Several "benign" focal epilepsies occur in children, of which the most common is the syndrome associated with central-midtemporal spikes on EEG. This form of idiopathic focal epilepsy, also known as *benign rolandic epilepsy*, accounts for about 15% of all pediatric seizure disorders.

Onset is between 4 and 13 years; children are otherwise normal. Most children have attacks mainly or exclusively at night. Sleep promotes secondary generalization, so that parents report only generalized tonic-clonic seizures; any focal manifestations go unobserved. In contrast, seizures that occur during the day are clearly focal with twitching of one side of the face; speech arrest; drooling from a corner of the mouth; and paresthesias of the tongue, lips, inner cheeks, and face. Seizures may progress to include clonic jerking or tonic posturing of the arm and leg on one side. Consciousness is usually preserved.

The interictal EEG abnormality is distinctive and shows stereotyped diphasic or triphasic sharp waves over the central-midtemporal (rolandic) regions. Discharges may be unilateral or bilateral. They increase in abundance during sleep and, when unilateral, switch from side to side on successive EEGs. In about 30% of cases, generalized spike-wave activity also occurs. The EEG pattern is inherited as an autosomal-dominant trait with age-dependent penetrance. The inheritance pattern of the seizures, although clearly familial, is probably multifactorial and less well understood. More than half the children who show the characteristic EEG abnormality never have clinical attacks. Linkage has recently been reported in some families to chromosome 15q14.

The prognosis is uniformly good. Seizures disappear by mid to late adolescence in all cases. Seizures in many children appear to be self-limited, and not all children need antiepileptic drug treatment. Treatment can usually be deferred until after the second or third attack. Because seizures are easily controlled and self-limited, drugs with the fewest adverse effects, such as carbamazepine, oxcarbazepine, or gabapentin, should be used. Low doses, often producing subtherapeutic blood concentrations, are generally effective. Polytherapy should be avoided.

Temporal Lobe Epilepsy

This is the most common epilepsy syndrome of adults. In most cases, the epileptogenic region involves mesial temporal lobe structures, especially the hippocampus, amygdala, and parahippocampal gyrus. Seizures usually begin in late childhood or adolescence, and a history of febrile seizures is common. Virtually all patients have complex partial seizures, some of which secondarily generalize. Auras are frequent; visceral sensations are particularly common. Other typical behavioral features include a motionless stare, loss of awareness that may be gradual, and oral-alimentary automatisms, such as lip smacking. A variable but often prolonged period of postictal confusion is the rule. Interictal EEGs show focal temporal slowing and epileptiform sharp waves or spikes over the anterior temporal region. Antiepileptic drugs are usually successful in suppressing secondarily generalized seizures, but most pa-

tients continue to have partial attacks. When seizures persist, anterior temporal lobe resection is the treatment of choice. The results of a randomized controlled trial comparing seizure outcomes in patients treated either medically or surgically were striking: 58% of surgically treated patients were seizure free at one year compared to 8% of medically treated patients. Other series have shown that temporal lobe resection for refractory medial temporal lobe epilepsy associated with hippocampal sclerosis results in complete seizure control for at least one year in over 80% of patients.

Frontal Lobe Epilepsy

The particular pattern of the many types of frontal lobe seizures depends on the specific location where the seizure discharge originates and on the pathways subsequently involved in propagation. Despite this variability, the following features, when taken together, suggest frontal lobe epilepsy:

1. Brief seizures that begin and end abruptly with little, if any, postictal period;
2. A tendency for seizures to cluster and to occur at night;
3. Prominent, but often bizarre, motor manifestations, such as asynchronous thrashing or flailing of arms and legs, pedaling leg movements, pelvic thrusting, and loud, sometimes obscene, vocalizations, all of which may suggest psychogenic seizures;
4. Minimal abnormality on scalp EEG recordings;
5. A history of status epilepticus.

Frontal lobe epilepsy occurs in some families as an autosomal-dominant syndrome. In these patients, seizures almost always occur during sleep. Most patients respond well to medication.

Post-traumatic Seizures

Seizures occur within 1 year in about 7% of civilian and in about 34% of military head injuries. The differences relate mainly to the much higher proportion of penetrating wounds in military cases. The risk of developing post-traumatic epilepsy is directly related to the severity of the injury and also correlates with the total volume of brain lost as measured by CT. Depressed skull fractures may or may not be a risk; the rate of post-traumatic epilepsy was 17% in one series but not increased above control levels in another. Head injuries are classified as *severe* if they result in brain contusion, intracerebral or intracranial hematoma, unconsciousness, or amnesia for more than 24 hours or in persistent neurologic abnormalities, such as aphasia, hemiparesis, or dementia. *Mild* head injury (brief loss of consciousness, no skull fracture, no focal neurologic signs, no contusion or hematoma) does not increase the risk of seizures significantly above general population rates.

Nearly 60% of those who have seizures have the first attack in the first year after the injury. In the Vietnam Head Injury Study, however, more than 15% of patients did not have epilepsy until 5 or more years later. Post-traumatic seizures are classified as *early* (within the first 1 to 2 weeks after injury) or *late*. Only recurrent late seizures (those that occur after the patient has recovered from the acute effects of the injury) should be considered *post-traumatic epilepsy*. Early seizures, however, even if isolated, increase the chance of developing post-traumatic epilepsy. About 70% of patients have partial or secondarily generalized seizures. *Impact seizures* occur at the time of or immediately after the injury. These attacks are attributed to an acute reaction of the brain to trauma and do not increase the risk of later epilepsy.

Overt seizures should be treated according to principles reviewed later in this chapter. The most controversial issue concerns the prophylactic use of antiepileptic drugs to retard or abort the development of subsequent seizures. Based on the data of Temkin, we recommend treating patients with severe head trauma, as just defined, with phenytoin for the first week after injury to minimize complications from seizures occurring during acute management. Phenytoin, or fosphenytoin, should be given intravenously in a loading dose of about 20 mg/kg; subsequent doses should be adjusted to maintain blood levels of 15 to 20 μg/mL. If seizures have not occurred, we do not continue phenytoin beyond the initial 1 to 2 weeks, because evidence does not show that longer treatment prevents the development of later seizures or of post-traumatic epilepsy. Recent data have also shown that valproate is less effective than phenytoin in suppressing acute seizures and is also ineffective in preventing the development of post-traumatic seizures.

Epilepsia Partialis Continua

Epilepsia partialis continua (EPC) refers to unremitting motor seizures involving part or all of one side of the body. They typically consist of repeated clonic or myoclonic jerks that may remain focal or regional or may march from one muscle group to another, with the extent of motor involvement waxing and waning in endless variation. In adults, EPC occurs in diverse settings, such as with subacute or chronic inflammatory diseases of the brain (Koshevnikov Russian spring-summer encephalitis, Behçet disease) or with acute strokes, metastases, and metabolic encephalopathies, especially hyperosmolar nonketotic hyperglycemia.

The most distinctive form of EPC, known as the *Rasmussen syndrome*, occurs in children; it usually begins before the age of 10 years. The underlying disorder is chronic focal encephalitis, although an infectious agent has not been identified consistently. About two-thirds of patients report an infectious or inflammatory illness 1 to 6 months before onset of EPC. Generalized tonic-clonic seizures are often the first sign and appear before the EPC establishes itself. About 20% of cases begin with an episode of convulsive status epilepticus. Slow neurologic deterioration inevitably follows, with development of hemiparesis, mental impairment, and usually, hemianopia. If the dominant hemisphere is affected, aphasia occurs. EEGs are always abnormal, but findings are not specific and they frequently do not correlate with clinical manifestations. MRI may be normal early but later show unilateral cortical atrophy and signal changes consistent with gliosis. Autoantibodies GluR3 protein of the glutamate receptor have been found in some patients, suggesting that autoimmunity may play a role in the pathogenesis of the disorder in some patients, and immunotherapy is sometimes beneficial. Antiepileptic drugs are usually ineffective in controlling seizures and preventing progression of the disease, as are corticosteroids and antiviral agents. When seizures have not spontaneously remitted by the time there is a severe degree of hemiparesis, functional hemispherectomy can control seizures and leads to substantial intellectual improvement in many patients. Controversy arises in the decision about the best time for hemispherectomy, whether it should be performed earlier, before there is serious motor or language impairment.

EPIDEMIOLOGY

In the United States, about 6.5 persons per 1,000 population are affected with recurrent unprovoked seizures, so-called *active epilepsy*. Based on 1990 census figures, age-adjusted annual incidence rates for epilepsy range from 31 to 57 per 100,000 in the United States (Fig. 141.1). Incidence rates are highest among young children and the elderly; epilepsy affects males 1.1 to 1.5 times more often than females.

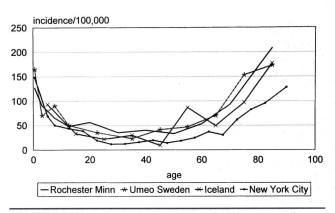

FIGURE 141.1. Age-specific incidence of epilepsy in Rochester, Minnesota, 1935–1984. (From Hauser et al. [1993].)

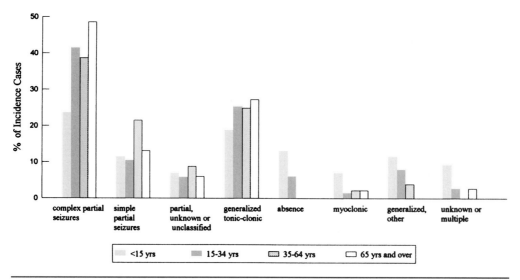

FIGURE 141.2. Proportion of seizure types in newly diagnosed cases of epilepsy in Rochester, Minnesota, 1935–1984. (From Hauser et al. [1993].)

Complex partial seizures are the most common seizure type among newly diagnosed cases, but age-related variability occurs in the proportions of different seizure types (Fig. 141.2). The cause of epilepsy also varies somewhat with age. Despite advances in diagnostic capabilities, however, the "unknown" etiologic category remains larger than any other for all age groups (Fig. 141.3). Cerebrovascular disease, associated developmental neurologic disorders (e.g., cerebral palsy and mental retardation), and head trauma are the other most commonly identified causes.

Although defined genetic disorders account for only about 1% of epilepsy cases, heritable factors are important. Monozygotic twins have a much higher concordance rate for epilepsy than do dizygotic twins. By age 25, nearly 9% of children of mothers with epilepsy and 2.4% of children of affected fathers develop epilepsy. The reason for an increased risk of seizures in children of women with epilepsy is not known.

Some forms of epilepsy are more heritable than others. For example, children of parents with absence seizures have a higher risk of developing epilepsy (9%) than do offspring of parents with other types of generalized seizures or partial seizures (5%). As a general rule, though, even offspring born to a high-risk parent have a 90% or greater chance of being unaffected by epilepsy.

Many persons who experience a first unprovoked seizure never have a second. By definition, these people do not have epilepsy and generally do not require long-term drug treatment. Unfortunately, our ability to identify such individuals with accuracy is incomplete. Treatment decisions must be based on epidemiologic and individual considerations. Some seizure types, such as absence and myoclonic, are virtually always recurrent by the time the patient is seen by a physician. On the other hand, patients

FIGURE 141.3. Etiology of epilepsy in all cases of newly diagnosed seizures in Rochester, Minnesota, 1935–1984 (From Hauser et al. [1993].)

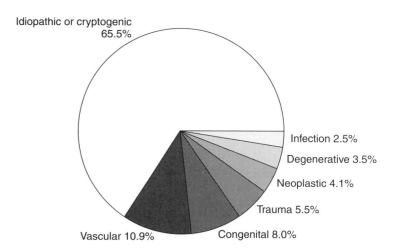

with convulsive seizures may seek medical attention after a first occurrence because of the dramatic nature of the attack. Prospective studies of recurrence after a first seizure indicate a 2-year recurrence risk of about 40%, which is similar in children and adults. The risk is lowest in people with an idiopathic generalized first seizure and normal EEG (about 24%), higher with idiopathic generalized seizures and an abnormal EEG (about 48%), and highest with symptomatic (i.e., known preceding brain injury or neurologic syndrome) seizures and an abnormal EEG (about 65%). Epileptiform, but not nonepileptiform, EEG abnormalities impart a greater risk for recurrence. If the first seizure is a partial seizure, the relative risk of recurrence is also increased. The risk for further recurrence after a second unprovoked seizure is greater than 80%; a second unprovoked seizure is, therefore, a reliable marker of epilepsy.

About 4% of persons living to age 74 have at least one unprovoked seizure. When provoked seizures (i.e., febrile seizures or those related to an acute illness) are included, the likelihood of experiencing a seizure by age 74 increases to at least 9%. The risk of developing epilepsy is about 3% by age 74.

Of persons with epilepsy, 60% to 70% achieve remission of seizures with antiepileptic drug therapy. Factors that favor remission include an idiopathic (or cryptogenic) form of epilepsy, normal findings on neurologic examination, and onset in early to middle childhood (except neonatal seizures). Unfavorable prognostic factors include partial seizures, an abnormal EEG, and associated mental retardation or cerebral palsy (Table 141.3).

Mortality is increased in persons with epilepsy, but the risk is incurred mainly by symptomatic cases in which higher death rates are related primarily to the underlying disease rather than to epilepsy. Accidental deaths, especially drowning, are more common, however, in all patients with epilepsy. Sudden unexplained death is nearly 25 times more common in patients with epilepsy than in the general population; estimates of incidence rates range from 1 in 500 to 1 in 2,000 per year. Severe epilepsy and uncontrolled generalized convulsions are risk factors.

▶ **TABLE 141.3 Predictors of Intractability**

Very young age at onset (<2 yr)
Frequent generalized seizures
Failure to achieve control readily
Evidence of brain damage
A specific cause of the seizures
Severe EEG abnormality
Low IQ
Atonic atypical absence seizures

INITIAL DIAGNOSTIC EVALUATION

The diagnostic evaluation has three objectives: to determine if the patient has epilepsy; to classify the type of epilepsy and identify an epilepsy syndrome, if possible; and to define the specific underlying cause. Accurate diagnosis leads directly to proper treatment and formulation of a rational plan of management. The differential diagnosis is considered in Chapter 3.

Because epilepsy comprises a group of conditions and is not a single homogeneous disorder, and because seizures may be symptoms of both diverse brain disorders and an otherwise normal brain, it is neither possible nor desirable to develop inflexible guidelines for what constitutes a standard or minimal diagnostic evaluation. The clinical data from the history and physical examination should allow a reasonable determination of probable diagnosis, seizure and epilepsy classification, and likelihood of underlying brain disorder. Based on these considerations, diagnostic testing should be undertaken selectively.

History and Examination

A complete history is the cornerstone for establishing a diagnosis of epilepsy. An adequate history should provide a clear picture of the clinical features of the seizures and the sequence in which manifestations evolve; the course of the epileptic disorder; seizure precipitants, such as alcohol or sleep deprivation; risk factors for seizures, such as abnormal gestation, febrile seizures, family history of epilepsy, head injury, encephalitis or meningitis, and stroke; and response to previous treatment. In children, developmental history is important.

In describing the epileptic seizure, care should be taken to elicit a detailed description of any aura. The aura was once considered to be the warning of an impending attack, but it is actually a simple partial seizure made apparent by subjective feelings or experiential phenomena observable only by the patient. Auras precede many complex partial or generalized seizures and are experienced by 50% to 60% of adults with epilepsy. Auras confirm the suspicion that the seizure begins locally within the brain; they may also provide direct clues about the location or laterality of the focus. Information about later events in the seizure usually are obtained from an observer because of the patient's impaired awareness or frank loss of consciousness or because of postictal amnesia even though responses to questions during the seizure indicate preserved responsiveness.

The nature of repetitive automatic or purposeless movements (automatisms), sustained postures, presence of myoclonus, and the duration of the seizure help to delineate specific seizure types or epileptic syndromes. Nonspecific postictal findings of lethargy and confusion must be distinguished from focal neurologic abnormalities, such as

▶ **TABLE 141.4 Risk Factors for Epilepsy**

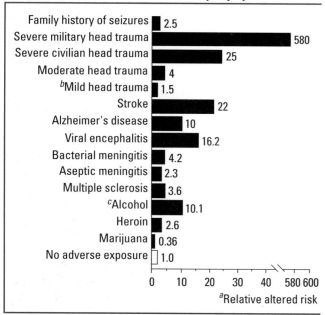

	Relative altered risk
Family history of seizures	2.5
Severe military head trauma	580
Severe civilian head trauma	25
Moderate head trauma	4
[b]Mild head trauma	1.5
Stroke	22
Alzheimer's disease	10
Viral encephalitis	16.2
Bacterial meningitis	4.2
Aseptic meningitis	2.3
Multiple sclerosis	3.6
[c]Alcohol	10.1
Heroin	2.6
Marijuana	0.36
No adverse exposure	1.0

[a]Relative altered risk

[a]Relative to people without these adverse exposures.
[b]Not statistically significant.
[c]One pint of 80 proof, 2.5 bottles of wine.
From Hauser WA, Hesdorffer DC. *Epilepsy: frequency, causes and consequences.* New York: Demos, 1990.

hemiparesis or aphasia, which could point to the hemisphere of seizure onset.

Information about risk factors (Table 141.4) may suggest a particular cause and assist in prognosis. Discussion with parents may be necessary, because children or adults may be uninformed about, or may not recall, early childhood events, such as perinatal encephalopathy, febrile seizures, brain infections, head injuries, or intermittent absence seizures. Age at seizure onset and course of the seizure disorder should be clarified, because these features differ in the various epilepsy syndromes.

Findings on neurologic examination are usually normal in patients with epilepsy but occasionally may provide etiologic clues. Focal signs indicate an underlying cerebral lesion. Asymmetry of the hand or face may indicate localized or hemispheric cerebral atrophy contralateral to the smaller side. Phakomatoses are commonly associated with seizures and may be suggested by café-au-lait spots, facial angioma, conjunctival telangiectasia, hypopigmented macules, fibroangiomatous nevi, or lumbosacral shagreen patches.

Electroencephalography

Because epilepsy is fundamentally a physiologic disturbance of brain function, the EEG is the most important laboratory test in evaluating patients with seizures. The EEG helps both to establish the diagnosis of epilepsy and to characterize specific epileptic syndromes. EEG findings may also help in management and in prognosis.

Epileptiform discharges (spikes and sharp waves) are highly correlated with seizure susceptibility and can be recorded on the first EEG in about 50% of patients. Similar findings are recorded in only 1% to 2% of normal adults and in a somewhat higher percentage of normal children. When multiple EEGs are obtained, epileptiform abnormalities eventually appear in 60% to 90% of adults with epilepsy, but the yield of positive studies does not increase substantially after three or four tests. Prolonged ambulatory or inpatient recordings increase the yield of interictal epileptiform abnormalities both because of the longer sampling times but also because complete waking-sleep cycles are included. It is important to remember, therefore, that 10% to 40% of patients with epilepsy do not show epileptiform abnormalities on routine EEG; a normal or nonspecifically abnormal EEG never excludes the diagnosis. Sleep, hyperventilation, photic stimulation, and special electrode placements are routinely used to increase the probability of recording epileptiform abnormalities. Different and distinctive patterns of epileptiform discharge occur in specific epilepsy syndromes as summarized in Chapter 14.

Brain Imaging

MRI should be performed in all patients over age 18 years and in children with abnormal development, abnormal findings on physical examination, or seizure types that are likely to be manifestations of symptomatic epilepsy. CT will often miss common epileptogenic lesions such as hippocampal sclerosis, cortical dysplasia, and cavernous malformations. Because CT is very sensitive for detecting brain calcifications, a noncontrast CT (in addition to MRI) may be helpful in patients at risk for neurocysticercosis.

Routine imaging is not necessary for children with idiopathic epilepsy, including the benign focal epilepsy syndromes (see later section). Brain MRI, although more costly, is more sensitive than CT in detecting potentially epileptogenic lesions, such as cortical dysplasia, hamartomas, differentiated glial tumors, and cavernous malformations. Both axial and coronal planes should be imaged with both T1 and T2 sequences. Gadolinium injection does not increase the sensitivity for detecting cerebral lesions, but may assist in differentiating possible causes.

Imaging in the coronal plane perpendicular to the long axis of the hippocampus and other variations in technique have improved the detection of hippocampal atrophy and gliosis, findings that are highly correlated with mesial temporal sclerosis (Fig. 141.4) and an epileptogenic temporal lobe. An even more sensitive measure of hippocampal atrophy is MRI measurement of the volume of the hippocampus. Hippocampal volume measurements in an individual patient then can be compared with those of normal control subjects. In patients being considered for surgery, PET scans can add valuable localizing information,

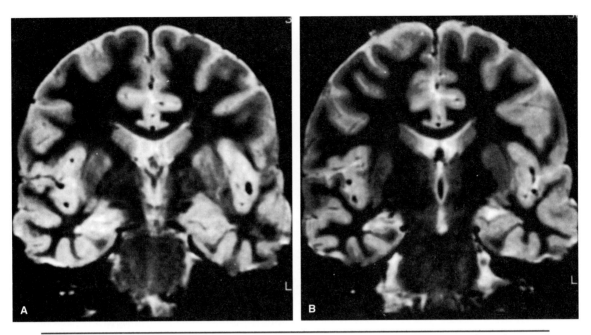

FIGURE 141.4. Mesial temporal sclerosis. **A and B.** Short-tau inversion recovery (STIR) coronal MR images through the temporal lobes show increased signal and decreased size of right hippocampus as compared with left. These findings are characteristic of mesial temporal sclerosis. Note incidental focal dilatation of left choroid fissure, which represents a choroid fissure cyst and is a normal variant. (Courtesy of Dr. S. Chan, Columbia University College of Physicians and Surgeons, New York, NY.)

especially when the MRI scan is negative. SPECT scans are also used; although resolution is less than either MRI or PET. Subtraction of an ictal from an interictal image and coregistration of the findings with an MRI scan of the brain is also helpful in localizing the epileptogenic brain region in some cases.

Other Laboratory Tests

Routine blood tests are rarely diagnostically useful in healthy children or adults. They are necessary in newborns and in older patients with acute or chronic systemic disease to detect abnormal electrolyte, glucose, calcium, or magnesium values or impaired liver or kidney function that may contribute to seizure occurrence. In most patients, serum electrolytes, liver function tests, and a complete blood count are useful mainly as baseline studies before initiating antiepileptic drug treatment.

Any suspicion of meningitis or encephalitis mandates lumbar puncture. Urine or blood toxicologic screens should be considered when otherwise unexplained new-onset generalized seizures occur.

LONG-TERM MONITORING

The most direct and convincing evidence of an epileptic basis for a patient's episodic symptoms is the recording of an electrographic seizure discharge during a typical behavioral attack. This recording is especially necessary if the history is ambiguous, EEGs are repeatedly normal or nonspecifically abnormal, and reasonable treatment has failed. Because most patients have seizures infrequently, routine EEG rarely records an attack. Long-term monitoring permits EEG recording for a longer time, thus increasing the likelihood of recording seizures or interictal epileptiform discharges. Two methods of long-term monitoring are now widely available: simultaneous closed-circuit television and EEG (CCTV/EEG) monitoring and ambulatory EEG. Both have greatly improved diagnostic accuracy and the reliability of seizure classification, and both provide continuous recordings through one or more complete waking-sleep cycles and capture ictal episodes. Each has additional specific advantages and disadvantages. The method used depends on the question posed by a particular patient.

Long-term monitoring using CCTV/EEG, usually in a specially designed hospital unit, is the procedure of choice to document psychogenic seizures and other nonepileptic paroxysmal events. It can also establish electrical-clinical correlations and localize epileptogenic foci for resective surgery. The emphasis in monitoring units is usually on behavioral events, not interictal EEG activity. The availability of full-time technical or nursing staff ensures high-quality recordings and permits examination of patients during clinical events. Antiepileptic drugs can be discontinued safely to facilitate seizure occurrence. Computerized detection programs are used to screen EEG continuously for epileptiform abnormalities and subclinical seizures.

The other method of long-term monitoring is designed for outpatient use in the patient's home, school, or work environment. Ambulatory EEG is often especially helpful in pediatrics, because children are often more comfortable in their familiar and unrestricted home environment. The major limitations of ambulatory monitoring are the limited coverage of cortical areas, variable technical quality resulting from lack of expert supervision, frequent distortion of EEG data by environmental contaminants, and the absence of video documentation of behavioral changes. Ambulatory monitoring is most useful in documenting interictal epileptiform activity when routine EEGs have been repeatedly negative or in recording ictal discharges during typical behavioral events. At present, however, ambulatory EEG is not a substitute for CCTV/EEG monitoring, especially when psychogenic seizures are an issue or when patients are being evaluated for epilepsy surgery.

MEDICAL TREATMENT

Therapy of epilepsy has three goals: to eliminate seizures or reduce their frequency to the maximum extent possible, to avoid the side effects associated with long-term treatment, and to assist the patient in maintaining or restoring normal psychosocial and vocational adjustment. No medical treatment now available can induce a permanent remission ("cure") or prevent development of epilepsy by altering the process of epileptogenesis.

The decision to institute antiepileptic drug therapy should be based on a thoughtful and informed analysis of the issues involved. Isolated infrequent seizures, whether convulsive or not, probably pose little medical risk to otherwise healthy persons. However, even relatively minor seizures, especially those associated with loss or alteration of alertness, have many psychosocial, vocational, and safety ramifications. Finally, the probability of seizure recurrence varies substantially among patients, depending on the type of epilepsy and any associated neurologic or medical problems. Drug treatment, on the other hand, carries a risk of adverse effects, which approaches 30% after initial treatment. Treatment of children raises additional issues, especially the unknown effects of long-term antiepileptic drug use on brain development, learning, and behavior.

These considerations mean that although drug treatment is indicated and beneficial for most patients with epilepsy, certain circumstances call for antiepileptic drugs to be deferred or used for only a limited time. As a rule of thumb, antiepileptic drugs should be prescribed when the potential benefits of treatment clearly outweigh possible adverse effects of therapy.

Acute Symptomatic Seizures

These seizures are caused by, or associated with, an acute medical or neurologic illness. A childhood febrile seizure is the most common example of an acute symptomatic seizure, but other frequently encountered causes include metabolic or toxic encephalopathies and acute brain infections. To the extent that these conditions resolve without permanent brain damage, seizures are usually self-limited. The primary therapeutic concern in such patients should be identification and treatment of the underlying disorder. If antiepileptic drugs are needed to suppress seizures acutely, they generally do not need to be continued after the patient recovers.

The Single Seizure

About 25% of patients with unprovoked seizures come to a physician after a single attack, nearly always a generalized tonic-clonic seizure. Most of these people have no risk factors for epilepsy, have normal findings on neurologic examination, and show a normal first EEG. Only about 25% of these patients later develop epilepsy. For this group, the need for treatment is questionable. For many years, no convincing data indicated any beneficial effect of treatment on preventing recurrence. In 1993, a large multicenter randomized study from Italy convincingly demonstrated that antiepileptic drugs reduce the risk of relapse after the first unprovoked convulsive seizure. Among nearly 400 children and adults, treatment within 7 days of a first seizure was followed by a recurrence rate of 25% at 2 years. In contrast, untreated patients had a recurrence rate of 51%. When patients with previous "uncertain spells" were excluded from the analysis, treatment benefit was still evident, but the magnitude of the effect was reduced to a recurrence rate of 30% in the treated group and 42% in untreated patients.

Although treatment of first seizures reduces the relapse rate even in low-risk patients, there is no evidence that such treatment alters the prognosis of epilepsy. Thus, treatment should not be automatic, and the decision to treat should be made only in consultation with the patient or parents after weighing the unique circumstances posed by that individual. In most patients with idiopathic epilepsy, deferring treatment until a second seizure occurs is a reasonable and often preferable decision.

Benign Epilepsy Syndromes

Several electroclinical syndromes begin in childhood and are associated with normal development, normal findings on neurologic examination, and normal brain imaging studies. They have a uniformly good prognosis for complete remission in mid to late adolescence without long-term behavioral or cognitive problems. The most common and best characterized of these syndromes is benign partial epilepsy of childhood with central-midtemporal sharp waves (rolandic epilepsy). Most seizures occur at night as secondarily generalized convulsions. Focal seizures occur during the day and are characterized by twitching of one side of the face, anarthria, salivation, and paresthesias of the face and inner mouth followed variably by hemiclonic movements or hemitonic posturing. Other benign syndromes include benign partial epilepsy with occipital spike waves and benign epilepsy with affective symptoms.

Because of the good prognosis, the sole goal of treatment in such cases is to prevent recurrence. Because many children, especially those who are older, tend to have only a few seizures, treatment is not always necessary. Antiepileptic drugs are usually reserved for children whose seizures are frequent or relatively severe or whose parents, or the children themselves, are frightened at the prospect of future attacks. With these considerations in mind, only about half the children with benign partial epilepsy require treatment.

> **TABLE 141.5 Drugs Used in Treating Different Types of Seizures**

Type of Seizure	Drugs[a]
Simple and complex partial:	Carbamazepine, valproate; gabapentin, lamotrigine, topiramate, oxcarbazepine, zonisamide, levetiracetam, phenytoin, pregabalin, primidone, phenobarbital
Secondarily generalized:	Carbamazepine, valproate, gabapentin, lamotrigine, topiramate, oxcarbazepine, zonisamide, levetiracetam, phenytoin, pregabalin, phenobarbital, primidone
Primary generalized seizures:	
Tonic-clonic	Valproate, lamotrigine, topiramate, zonisamide, carbamazepine, oxcarbazepine, phenytoin
Absence	Valproate, lamotrigine, ethosuximide, zonisamide
Myoclonic	Valproate, clonazepam, levetiracetam
Tonic	Valproate, felbamate, clonazepam, zonisamide

[a] Not all drugs have FDA approval for listed uses.

Antiepileptic Drugs

Selection of Antiepileptic Drugs

Two nationwide collaborative Veterans Administration Cooperative Studies (1985 and 1992) compared the effectiveness of the then available major antiepileptic drugs. In the 1985 study, carbamazepine, phenytoin, primidone, and phenobarbital were equally effective in controlling complex partial and secondarily generalized seizures. In the 1992 study, carbamazepine was slightly more effective than valproate in treating complex partial seizures, but both drugs were of equal efficacy in controlling secondarily generalized seizures. These studies also demonstrated that despite their relatively uniform ability to suppress seizures, the drugs had different risks of adverse effects. More recently, there have been randomized trials in patients with partial seizures comparing the effectiveness of gabapentin, lamotrigine, topiramate, or oxcarbazepine with that of carbamazepine and phenytoin. None has shown definite superiority, although many have demonstrated that the newer agents have improved tolerability. A survey of epilepsy experts in North America found that carbamazepine remains the drug of first choice for partial seizures when both efficacy and tolerability are considered. Gabapentin, lamotrigine, topiramate, oxcarbazepine, and phenytoin remain reasonable alternatives for many patients.

In general, valproate is the drug of choice for generalized-onset seizures and can be used advantageously as monotherapy when several generalized seizure types coexist (Table 141.5). Lamotrigine and topiramate are suitable alternatives if valproate is ineffective or not tolerated. Levitiracetam and zonisamide may also prove to be effective, but they require further study. Phenytoin, carbamazepine, and oxcarbazepine are useful in suppressing generalized tonic-clonic seizures, but the response is less predictable than that with valproate. Carbamazepine, phenytoin, gabapentin, and sometimes lamotrigine can aggravate myoclonic seizures; all of these except lamotrigine also sometimes exacerbate absence seizures. Tiagabine can aggravate or induce absence seizures. Ethosuximide is as effective as valproate in controlling absence seizures and has fewer side effects. Ethosuximide is ineffective against tonic-clonic seizures, however, so its main use is as an alternative to valproate in patients who have only absence seizures.

Elderly patients with epilepsy require special consideration because of age-related changes in both pharmacokinetic profiles and pharmacodynamic characteristics. Relevant physiologic changes include decreased hepatic metabolism and plasma protein binding, decreased renal clearance, and slower gastrointestinal motility and absorption. There is greater sensitivity to both desirable and undesirable effects on brain function. Additionally, concurrent medical illnesses are common, and as a result, most elderly patients take multiple drugs, which increases the likelihood of clinically significant drug interactions. Several clinical trials involving elderly patients, including a recently completed large VA cooperative study, have found that lamotrigine and gabapentin are better tolerated than carbamazepine, although, as in younger patients, differences in effectiveness, if any, are small.

Adverse Effects of Antiepileptic Drugs

All antiepileptic drugs have undesirable effects in some patients. Although interindividual variation occurs, most adverse drug effects are mild and dose related. Many are common to virtually all antiepileptic drugs, especially when treatment is started. These include sedation, mental dulling, impaired memory and concentration, mood changes, gastrointestinal upset, and dizziness. The incidence of particular adverse effects varies with the individual agent. In general, sedation and cognitive effects are less likely with lamotrigine or gabapentin than with older agents, especially in elderly persons. Some adverse effects are relatively specific for particular drugs.

Dose-Related Side Effects

These typically appear when a drug is first given or when the dosage is increased. They usually, but not always, correlate with blood concentrations of the parent drug or major metabolites (Table 141.6). Dose-related side effects are always reversible on lowering the dosage or discontinuing the drug. Adverse effects frequently determine the limits of treatment with a particular drug and have a major influence on compliance with the prescribed regimen. Because dose-related side effects are broadly predictable, they are often the major differentiating feature in choosing among otherwise equally effective therapies.

Idiosyncratic Side Effects

Idiosyncratic reactions account for most serious and virtually all life-threatening adverse reactions to antiepileptic drugs. All antiepileptic drugs can cause similar serious side effects (Table 141.6), but with the exception of rash, these are fortunately rare. For example, the risk of carbamazepine-induced agranulocytosis or aplastic anemia is about 2 per 575,000; with felbamate, the risk of aplastic anemia may be as high as 1 per 5,000. Idiosyncratic reactions are not dose related; rather they arise either from an immune-mediated reaction to the drug or from poorly defined individual factors, largely genetic, that convey an unusual sensitivity to the drug. An example of the genetic mechanism is valproate-induced fatal hepatotoxicity. Valproate, like most antiepileptic drugs, is metabolized in the liver, but several biochemical pathways are available to the drug. Clinical and experimental data indicate that one of these pathways results in a hepatotoxic compound that may accumulate and lead to microvesicular steatosis with necrosis. The extent to which this pathway is involved in biotransformation is age dependent and promoted by concurrent use of other drugs that are eliminated in the liver. Thus, most patients who have had fatal hepatotoxicity were younger than 2 years of age and treated with polytherapy (Table 141.7). In addition, most

had severe epilepsy associated with mental retardation, developmental delay, or congenital brain anomalies. No hepatic deaths have occurred in persons older than 10 years of age treated with valproate alone.

No laboratory test, certainly not untargeted routine blood monitoring, identifies individuals specifically at risk for valproate hepatotoxicity or any other drug-related idiosyncratic reaction. Clinical data, however, permit identification of groups of patients at increased risk for serious adverse drug reactions, including patients with known or suspected metabolic or biochemical disorders, a history

▶ **TABLE 141.6 Toxicity of Antiepileptic Drugs**

Dose-related adverse effects
  Systemic toxicity
   Gastrointestinal (dyspepsia, nausea, diarrhea; esp. valproate, zonisamide)
   Benign elevation in liver enzymes (esp. valproate, phenobarbital, phenytoin, carbamazepine, oxcarbazepine)
   Benign leukopenia (esp. carbamazepine)
   Gingival hypertrophy (esp. phenytoin)
   Weight gain (esp. valproate, gabapentin)
   Anorexia (esp. felbamate, topiramate, zonisamide)
   Hair loss, change in hair texture (esp. valproate)
   Hirsutism (esp. phenytoin, valproate)
   Hyponatremia (esp. carbamazepine, oxcarbazepine)
   Coarsening of facial features (esp. phenytoin)
   Dupuytren contracture, frozen shoulder
   Osteoporosis (esp. phenytoin, carbamazepine, valproate)
   Impotence (esp. phenobarbital, carbamazepine)

  Neurologic toxicity
   Drowsiness, sedation
   Impaired cognition (memory, concentration)
   Depression and mood changes
   Irritability, hyperactivity
   Insomnia (esp. felbamate)
   Dizziness/vertigo
   Nystagmus, diplopia
   Ataxia
   Tremor, asterixis
   Dyskinesias, dystonia, myoclonus
   Dysarthria
   Headache
   Sensory neuropathy

  Idiosyncratic reactions
   Rash (rare with valproate, gabapentin, levetiracetam)
   Exfoliative dermatitis
   Erythema multiforme
   Stevens-Johnson syndrome
   Agranulocytosis
   Aplastic anemia (esp. felbamate)
   Hepatic failure (esp. felbamate, valproate)
   Pancreatitis
   Connective tissue disorders
   Thrombocytopenia
   Pseudolymphoma syndrome

▶ **TABLE 141.7** **Effect of Age and Treatment on Risk of Developing Fatal Valproate Hepatotoxicity**

Age	Monotherapy	Polytherapy
<2 yr	1/7,000	1/500
>2 yr	1/80,000	1/25,000

Modified from Dreifuss FE, Santilli N, Langer DH, et al. *Neurology* 1987;37:379–385.

of previous drug reactions, and medical illnesses affecting hematopoiesis or liver and kidney function.

Rash can occur with virtually any drug, and rarely this results in Stevens-Johnson syndrome. The frequency of severe rash is about the same with carbamazepine, phenytoin, phenobarbital, and (if started slowly over several weeks) lamotrigine. There is some cross-reactivity among these drugs, so that a patient who develops a rash on one has a slightly increased risk of developing a rash with another. Rash is unusually reported with valproate, gabapentin, or levetiracetam. To date, life-threatening idiosyncratic effects have not been reported with gabapentin, topiramate, oxcarbazepine, tiagabine, or levitiracetam, but total patient exposures to the last two agents are smaller than to the others.

Antiepileptic Drug Pharmacology

Table 141.8 provides summary information about dose requirements, pharmacokinetic properties, and therapeutic concentration ranges for the major antiepileptic drugs available in the United States. Of patients with epilepsy, 60% to 70% achieve satisfactory control of seizures with currently available antiepileptic drugs, but fewer than 50% of adults achieve complete control without drug side effects. Many patients continue to have frequent seizures despite optimal medical therapy.

Therapy should start with a single antiepileptic drug chosen according to the type of seizure or epilepsy syndrome and then be modified, as necessary, by considerations of side effects, required dosing schedule, and cost. Phenytoin, phenobarbital, gabapentin, and levetiracetam can be loaded acutely. In most cases, however, antiepileptic drugs should be started in low dosages to minimize acute toxicity and then increased according to the patient's tolerance and the drug's pharmacokinetics. The initial target dose should produce a serum concentration in the low-to-mid therapeutic range. Further increases can then be titrated according to the patient's clinical progress, which is measured mainly by seizure frequency and the occurrence of drug side effects. A drug should not be judged a failure unless seizures remain uncontrolled at the maximal tolerated dosage, regardless of the blood level.

Dosage changes generally should not be made until the effects of the drug have been observed at steady state concentrations (a time about equal to five drug half-lives). If the first drug is ineffective, an appropriate alternative should be gradually substituted (Table 141.5). Combination treatment using two drugs should be attempted only when monotherapy with primary antiepileptic drugs fails. Combination therapy is sometimes effective, but the price of improved seizure control is often additional drug

▶ **TABLE 141.8** **Antiepileptic Drugs: Dosage and Pharmacokinetic Data**

Drug	Usual Adult Dose 24 hr (mg)	Half-life (hr)	Usually Effective Plasma Concentration (μg/mL)	Time to Peak Concentration (hr)	Bound Fraction (%)
Phenytoin	300–400	22	10–20	3–8	90–95
Carbamazepine	800–1,600	8–22	8–12	4–8	75
Phenobarbital	90–180	100	15–40	2–8	45
Valproate	1,000–3,000	15–20	50–120	3–8	80–90
Ethosuximide	750–1,500	60	40–100	3–7	<5
Felbamate	2,400–3,600	14–23	20–140	2–6	25
Gabapentin	1,800–3,600	5–7	4–16[a]	2–3	<5
Lamotrigine	100–500	12–60[b]	2–16[a]	2–5	55
Topiramate	200–400	19–25[b]	4–10[a]	2–4	9–17
Vigabatrin	1,000–3,000	5–7	NE	1–4	5
Tiagabine	32–56	5–13	NE	1	95
Levetiracetam	1,000–3,000	6–8	5–45[a]	1	<10
Oxcarbazepine	900–2400	8–10[c]	10–35[a]	3–13	40[c]
Zonisamide	100–600	24–60[b]	10–40[a]	2–6	40
Pregabalin	150–600	5–7	NE	1	<5

[a]Not established; corresponds to usual range in patients treated with recommended dose.
[b]Highly dependent on concurrently administered drugs.
[c]Of MHD, the active metabolite.
NE, not established.

toxicity. Sometimes combination therapy with relatively nonsedating drugs (e.g., carbamazepine, lamotrigine, gabapentin, or valproate) is preferable to high-dose monotherapy with a sedating drug (e.g., phenobarbital or primidone). When used together, carbamazepine and lamotrigine result in a pharmacodynamic interaction that often produces neurotoxicity at dosages that are usually well tolerated when either drug is used alone.

Dosing intervals should usually be less than one-third to one-half the drug's half-life to minimize fluctuations between peak and trough blood concentrations. Large fluctuations can result in drug-induced side effects at peak levels and in breakthrough seizures at trough concentrations. Sometimes, however, a drug has a relatively long pharmacodynamic half-life, so that twice a day dosing is reasonable even if the pharmacokinetic half-life is short. This is typically the case with valproate, tiagabine, and, possibly, gabapentin and levetiracetam.

Therapeutic drug monitoring has improved the care of patients with epilepsy, but published therapeutic ranges are only guidelines. Most patients who achieve drug concentrations within a standard therapeutic range usually achieve adequate seizure control with minimal side effects, but notable exceptions occur. Some patients develop unacceptable side effects at "subtherapeutic" concentrations; others benefit from "toxic" concentrations without adverse effects.

Determining serum drug concentrations when seizure control has been achieved or when side effects appear can assist in future management decisions. Drug levels are also useful in documenting compliance and in assessing the magnitude and significance of known or suspected drug interactions. Therapeutic drug monitoring is an essential guide to treating neonates, infants, young children, elderly persons, and patients with diseases (e.g., liver or kidney failure) or physiologic conditions (e.g., pregnancy) that alter drug pharmacokinetics. Although the total blood concentrations that are routinely reported are satisfactory for most indications, unbound (free) concentrations are use-ful when protein binding is altered, as in renal failure, pregnancy, extensive third-degree burns, and combination therapy using two or more drugs that are highly bound to serum proteins (e.g., phenytoin, valproate, tiagabine).

Specific Drugs

Phenytoin is unique among antiepileptic drugs because it exhibits nonlinear elimination at therapeutically useful serum concentrations. That is, hepatic enzyme systems metabolizing phenytoin become increasingly saturated at plasma concentrations greater than 10 to 12 μg/mL, and metabolic rate approaches a constant value at high concentrations. With increasing doses, phenytoin plasma concentrations rise exponentially (Fig. 141.5), so that steady state concentration at one dose cannot be used to predict directly the steady state concentration at a higher dose. Clinically, this requires cautious titration within the therapeutic range, using dose increments of 30 mg to avoid toxic effects.

Carbamazepine induces activation of the enzymes that metabolize it. The process, termed *autoinduction*, is time dependent. When carbamazepine is first introduced, the half-life approximates 30 hours. With increasing hepatic clearance in the first 3 to 4 weeks of therapy, however, the half-life shortens to 11 to 20 hours. As a result, the starting dose should be low, the dosage should be increased gradually, and dosing should be frequent (three or four times daily). Extended-release formulations now permit twice-a-day administration. The principal metabolite is carbamazepine-10,11-epoxide, which is pharmacologically active. Under certain circumstances (e.g., when coadministered with valproate or felbamate), the epoxide metabolite accumulates selectively, thereby producing neurotoxic effects even though the plasma concentration of the parent drug is in the therapeutic range or low.

Valproate is highly bound to plasma proteins, but the binding is concentration dependent and nonlinear. The

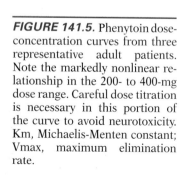

FIGURE 141.5. Phenytoin dose-concentration curves from three representative adult patients. Note the markedly nonlinear relationship in the 200- to 400-mg dose range. Careful dose titration is necessary in this portion of the curve to avoid neurotoxicity. Km, Michaelis-Menten constant; Vmax, maximum elimination rate.

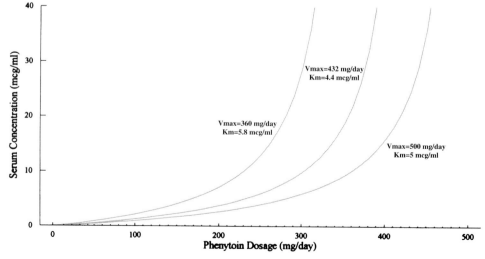

unbound fraction increases at plasma concentrations greater than 75 μg/mL because protein binding sites become saturated. For example, doubling the plasma concentration from 75 to 150 μg/mL can result in a more than sixfold rise in concentration of free drug (from 6.5 to 45 μg/mL). Therefore, as the dose of valproate is increased, side effects may worsen rapidly because of the increasing proportion of unbound drug. Furthermore, adverse effects may vary in the course of a single day or from day to day, because concentrations of unbound drug fluctuate despite seemingly small changes in total blood levels. Additionally, circulating fatty acids displace valproate from protein binding sites. If fatty acid levels are high, the amount of unbound valproate increases. Lamotrigine and felbamate prolong the half-life of valproate; reduced dosage is typically necessary when these drugs are added.

Gabapentin requires an intestinal amino acid transport system for absorption. Because the transporter is saturable, the percentage of drug that is absorbed after an oral dose decreases with increasing dosage. More frequent dosing schedules using smaller amounts may therefore be necessary to increase blood levels. When dosages above 3,600 mg/day are used, blood levels can be helpful in demonstrating that an increase in dosage is reflected in an increased serum concentration. Gabapentin does not interact to any clinically significant degree with any other drugs, which makes it especially useful when antiepileptic drug polytherapy is necessary and in patients with medical illnesses that also require drug treatment. It is not metabolized in the liver, but as it is excreted unchanged by the kidneys, dose adjustment is required in patients with renal failure. Pregabalin is structurally and mechanistically similar to gabapentin, but does not show dose-dependent absorption. It has increased potency compared to gabapentin.

Lamotrigine is sensitive to coadministration of other antiepileptic drugs. Enzyme-inducing agents, such as phenytoin and carbamazepine, decrease the half-life of lamotrigine from 24 to 16 hours (or less) as do oral contraceptive agents. In contrast, enzyme inhibition by valproate increases the half-life of lamotrigine to 60 hours. Therefore, lamotrigine dosing depends very much on whether it is used as monotherapy or in combination with other antiepileptic drugs. Lamotrigine has little or no effect on other classes of drugs. Rash occurs in about 10% of patients; it is more common in children and rarely leads to Stevens-Johnson syndrome. The incidence of rash can be minimized by slow titration schedules.

Levetiracetam, like gabapentin, has no appreciable interactions with other drugs and therefore has advantages in medically complicated patients. The plasma half-life is 6 to 8 hours, but clinical trials support twice-daily dosing, possibly owing to a longer pharmacodynamic half-life. Metabolism occurs in the liver, and there is also renal clearance. Adverse effects are generally mild and self-limited, although mood changes and even psychosis occur in a small subset of patients. No life-threatening idiosyncratic reactions have yet been described.

Oxcarbazepine is structurally similar to carbamazepine, but it is metabolized by a different pathway. As a result, there is no epoxide metabolite that is responsible for some of the adverse effects of carbamazepine. Although individual patients may tolerate oxcarbazepine better than carbamazepine, the overall profiles of the two drugs are similar, including development of leukopenia (usually asymptomatic and benign), mild increase in hepatic enzymes, and hyponatremia. Pharmacologic half-life of the active metabolite, a meta-hydroxy derivative (MHD) is 8 to 10 hours. Clinical studies support twice-daily dosing, although peak toxicity can occur when this is done at higher dosages.

Topiramate is also affected by other antiepileptic drugs taken concurrently. Carbamazepine, phenytoin, and phenobarbital shorten its half-life; valproate has little effect. Topiramate does not affect most other drugs, although phenytoin blood levels may increase by 25%. Adverse cognitive effects, especially word-finding difficulty and impaired memory, frequently limit the dosage patients can tolerate. These are usually dose dependent and can be minimized with slow titration schedules. Cognitive effects are also less common in monotherapy. Glaucoma, anhydrosis, and renal stones occur rarely. Doses above 400 mg/day do not usually lead to better seizure control but are associated with an increasing incidence of side effects.

Tiagabine is highly bound to serum proteins and will therefore displace other drugs (e.g., phenytoin, valproate) that are also protein bound. Other drugs do not affect tiagabine's metabolism significantly. Gastrointestinal side effects usually limit the rate at which the dosage may be increased.

Zonisamide is affected by other drugs that induce hepatic enzymes. Zonisamide's half-life when used as monotherapy is about 60 hours. When coadministered with enzyme-inducing drugs, the half-life can be reduced to 24 hours. In either case, once-daily dosing is appropriate. Although its metabolism occurs primarily in the liver, zonisamide itself does not appear to affect other drugs. Rash, renal stones, and anyhydrosis are rare side effects.

Felbamate has a much higher risk of serious adverse reactions, including aplastic anemia and hepatic failure, than other antiepileptic drugs. The actual risk has been difficult to estimate, but is probably between 1/5,000 and 1/20,000 exposures. For this reason, its use is currently restricted to patients who are refractory to other agents and in whom the risk of continued seizures outweighs the risk of side effects. Use of felbamate is also limited by other common but less serious adverse effects, including anorexia, weight loss, insomnia, and nausea, and by numerous complex drug interactions. Nonetheless, felbamate remains useful in cases of severe epilepsy such as Lennox-Gastaut syndrome.

Discontinuing Antiepileptic Drugs

Epidemiologic studies indicate that 60% to 70% of patients with epilepsy become free of seizures for at least 5 years within 10 years of diagnosis. Similarly, prospective clinical trials of treated patients whose seizures were in remission for 2 years or more showed that a nearly identical percentage of patients remained seizure free after drug withdrawal. These studies also identified predictors that permit patients to be classified as being at low or high risk for seizure relapse after drug therapy ends. The risk of relapse was high if patients required more than one antiepileptic drug to control seizures, if seizure control was difficult to establish, if the patient had a history of generalized tonic-clonic seizures, and if the EEG was significantly abnormal when drug withdrawal was considered. Continued freedom from seizures is favored by longer seizure-free intervals (up to 4 years) before drug withdrawal is attempted, few seizures before remission, monotherapy, normal EEG and examination, and no difficulty establishing seizure control.

All benign epilepsy syndromes of childhood carry an excellent prognosis for permanent drug-free remission. In contrast, juvenile myoclonic epilepsy has a high rate of relapse when drugs are discontinued, even in patients who have been seizure free for years. The prognosis for most other epilepsy syndromes is largely unknown.

Discontinuing antiepileptic drug therapy in appropriate patients is reasonable when they have been seizure free for at least 2 years. The most powerful argument for stopping antiepileptic drugs is concern about long-term systemic and neurologic toxicity, which may be insidious and not apparent for many years after a drug has been introduced. On the other hand, however, is the concern of the patient or family about seizure recurrence. Even a single seizure can have disastrous psychosocial and vocational consequences, particularly in adults. Therefore, the decision to withdraw drugs must be weighed carefully in the light of individual circumstances. If a decision is made to discontinue antiepileptic drugs, we favor slow withdrawal, over 3 to 6 months, but this recommendation is controversial because few studies have been conducted of different withdrawal rates.

REPRODUCTIVE HEALTH ISSUES

Gender-based differences in antiepileptic drug pharmacokinetics, sex steroid hormones, and reproductive life events raise special issues for women with epilepsy. The management of pregnancy in the woman with epilepsy is discussed in detail in Chapter 157. This section focuses on the effects of reproductive hormones on seizures and on the effects of seizures and antiepileptic drugs on reproductive health.

Although the prevalence of epilepsy is not higher in women, epilepsy in women may be specially affected by changes in reproductive steroids. Estrogen is a proconvulsant drug in animal models of epilepsy, whereas progesterone and its metabolites have anticonvulsant effects. Ovarian steroid hormones act at the neuronal membrane and on the genome to produce immediate and long-lasting effects on excitability. Estrogen reduces GABA-mediated inhibition, whereas progesterone enhances GABA effects. Estrogen also potentiates the action of excitatory neurotransmitters in some brain regions and increases the number of excitatory synapses. These dynamic and significant changes in neuronal excitability are observed with changes in estrogen and progesterone concentrations similar to those observed in the human menstrual cycle.

Approximately one-third of women with epilepsy report patterns of seizure occurrence that relate to phases of the menstrual cycle (*catamenial seizures*). Women with catamenial seizures indicate that seizures are more frequent, or more severe, just before menstruation and during the time of menstrual flow. In some women, seizures also increase at ovulation. These are times in the menstrual cycle when estrogen levels are relatively high and progesterone concentration is relatively low. Several small clinical trials have described benefit from chronic progesterone therapy in women with catamenial seizure patterns. Changes in seizures related to puberty and menopause are not well understood.

The pharmacokinetics of some antiepileptic drugs can complicate epilepsy management in women. Antiepileptic drugs that induce activity of the cytochrome P450 enzyme system (carbamazepine, phenytoin, phenobarbital, primidone, and, to a lesser extent, topiramate) interfere with the effectiveness of estrogen-based hormonal contraception. In women taking these drugs, the metabolism and binding of contraceptive steroids is enhanced, thus reducing the biologically active fraction of steroid hormone. The failure rate of oral contraceptive pills exceeds 6% per year in women taking enzyme-inducing antiepileptic drugs, in contrast to a failure rate of less that 1% per year in medication-compliant women without epilepsy. A woman motivated to avoid pregnancy should consider using a contraceptive preparation containing 50 μg or more of an estrogenic compound or using an additional barrier method of contraception. Alternatively, she should discuss with her physician the possibility of selecting an antiepileptic drug that does not alter steroid metabolism or binding.

Reproductive health may be compromised in both women and men with epilepsy. Fertility rates for men and women with epilepsy are one-third to two-thirds those of men and women without epilepsy. Lower birth rates cannot be explained on the basis of lower marriage rates, because marriage rates for women with epilepsy are now similar to those of nonepileptic women. Reduced fertility appears to be the direct result of a disturbance in reproductive physiology.

Men and women with epilepsy show a higher-than-expected frequency of reproductive endocrine disturbances. These include abnormalities both in the cyclic release and concentration of pituitary luteinizing hormone and prolactin and in the concentration of gonadal steroid hormones. Some of these abnormalities are likely to be a consequence of seizure activity. Antiepileptic drugs can also alter concentrations of gonadal steroids by affecting steroid hormone metabolism and binding. Antiepileptic drugs that increase steroid metabolism and binding reduce steroid hormone feedback at the hypothalamus and pituitary. Antiepileptic drugs that inhibit steroid metabolism (e.g., valproate) increase concentrations of steroid hormones, particularly androgens.

The polycystic ovary syndrome (PCOS) is a gynecologic disorder affecting approximately 7% of reproductive-age women. Women with epilepsy are at risk for developing features of this syndrome. Diagnostic requirements for polycystic ovary syndrome are phenotypic or serologic evidence for hyperandrogenism and anovulatory cycles (Morrell, 2003). Phenotypic signs of hyperandrogenism include hirsutism, truncal obesity, and acne. Hirsutism presents as increased facial and body hair, coarsening of pubic hair with extension down the inner thigh, and male pattern scalp hair loss—temporal recession and thinning over the crown. Health consequences of PCOS include infertility, accelerated atherosclerosis, diabetes, and endometrial carcinoma, underscoring the importance of detection and treatment. As many as 30% of cycles in women with epilepsy are anovulatory, and anovulatory cycles appear to be most frequent in women receiving valproic acid (VPA). Women with epilepsy are more likely to have polycystic appearing ovaries and polycystic-appearing ovaries with hyperandrogenism arise in as many as 40% of women with epilepsy receiving VPA. The long-term consequences of polycystic ovary–like syndrome in women with epilepsy are unknown. Data such as these suggest that epilepsy and some antiepileptic drugs (AEDs) individually affect fertility and that these effects may be additive. This implies that the most sophisticated therapy for epilepsy will consider disease-treatment effects on reproductive health.

Sexual dysfunction affects about one-third of men and women with epilepsy. Men report low sexual desire, difficulty achieving or maintaining an erection, or delayed ejaculation. Women with epilepsy can experience painful intercourse because of vaginismus and lack of lubrication. Although there are certainly psychosocial reasons for sexual dysfunction in some people with epilepsy, physiologic causes are demonstrable in others. Physiologic causes of sexual dysfunction include disruption of brain regions controlling sexual behavior by epileptogenic discharges, abnormalities of pituitary and gonadal hormones, and side effects of antiepileptic drugs.

Women with epilepsy who have difficulty conceiving, irregular or abnormal menstrual cycles, midcycle menstrual bleeding, sexual dysfunction, obesity, or hirsutism should be referred for a reproductive endocrine evaluation. Men with sexual dysfunction or difficulty conceiving should also have an endocrine evaluation and semen analysis. All the reproductive disorders seen in people with epilepsy are potentially treatable.

BONE HEALTH

Persons with epilepsy are at greater risk for bone disease, which typically presents as pathologic fracture. Bone biochemical abnormalities described in people with epilepsy include hypocalcemia, hypophosphatemia, elevated serum alkaline phosphatase, elevated parathyroid hormone (PTH) and reduced levels of vitamin D and its active metabolites (Pack and Morrell, 2004). The most severe bone and biochemical abnormalities are found in patients receiving AED polytherapy and in patients who have taken AEDs for a longer time.

SURGICAL TREATMENT

Surgery should be considered when seizures are uncontrolled by optimal medical management and when they disrupt the quality of life. Quantifying these issues, however, has defied strict definition, perhaps deservedly, because intractability is clearly more than continued seizures. Only patients know how their lives differ from what they would like them to be; the concept of *disability* includes both physical and psychologic components. Some patients with refractory seizures suffer little disability; others, for whatever reason, find their lives severely compromised by infrequent attacks. Still others have had their seizures completely cured by surgery but are still disabled and incapable of functioning productively. Determining which patients are "medically refractory" and which are "satisfactorily controlled" can always be argued in the abstract. Fortunately, there is usually general agreement in practice about which patients should be referred for surgical evaluation.

Few patients benefit from further attempts at medical treatment if seizures have not been controlled after two trials of high-dose monotherapy using two appropriate drugs and one trial of combination therapy. These therapeutic efforts can be accomplished within 1 to 2 years; the detrimental effects of continued seizures or drug toxicity warrant referral to a specialized center after that time.

There are few blanket contraindications to epilepsy surgery today, although patients with severe concurrent medical illness and progressive neurologic syndromes are usually excluded. Some centers prefer not to operate on patients with psychosis or other serious psychiatric disorder, those older than 60, and those with an IQ of less than 70. Patients in these categories, however, must be considered individually. Many patients who undergo corpus callosum section for atonic seizures associated with Lennox-Gastaut syndrome have IQs <70. Although surgery for epilepsy is increasingly performed in children, functional resections in infancy remain controversial for several reasons: the uncertain natural history of seizures in many of these patients; the unknown effects of surgery on the immature brain; and the lack of data about long-term neurologic, behavioral, and psychologic outcomes.

Because of technical advances in imaging and electrophysiologic monitoring, epilepsy surgery is no longer automatically contraindicated in patients with multifocal interictal epileptiform abnormalities or even foci near language or other eloquent cortical areas.

Resective Procedures

Focal brain resection is the most common type of epilepsy surgery. Resection is appropriate if seizures begin in an identifiable and restricted cortical area, if the surgical excision will encompass all or most of the epileptogenic tissue, and if the resection will not impair neurologic function. These criteria are met most often by patients with temporal lobe epilepsy, but extratemporal resections are increasingly common.

Anterior Temporal Lobe Resection

This resective procedure is the most common, but the operation varies in what is considered "standard," especially with regard to how much lateral neocortical and mesial limbic structures are removed. At our institution, most patients with unilateral temporal foci undergo Spencer's 1991 anteromedial temporal lobe resection, which includes removal of the anterior middle and inferior temporal gyri, parahippocampal gyrus, 3.5 to 4 cm of hippocampus, and a variable amount of amygdala. For nondominant foci, this approach may be slightly modified to include the anterior superior temporal gyrus as well. Patients with medial temporal lobe epilepsy associated with hippocampal sclerosis are ideal candidates for anterior temporal lobe resection, because over 80% will become seizure free with the remainder having substantial improvement. Results of a large multicenter study in the United States were reported by Spencer et al. in 2003, confirming the high rates of complete seizure control following temporal lobe resection. A randomized controlled Canadian trial has demonstrated a clear superiority for surgery over medical management in patients with medial temporal lobe epilepsy.

Lesionectomy

Well-circumscribed epileptogenic structural lesions (cavernous angiomas, hamartomas, gangliogliomas, and other encapsulated tumors) can be removed by stereotactic microsurgery. The extent to which tissue margins surrounding the lesion are included in the resection depends on how the margins are defined (radiologic, visual, electrophysiologic, or histologic inspection) and the surgeon's preference. Seizures are controlled by this method in 50% to 60% of patients. A lesion involving the cerebral cortex should always be considered the source of a patient's seizures unless compelling EEG evidence suggests otherwise.

Nonlesional Cortical Resections

When a lesion cannot be visualized by MRI, it is difficult to demonstrate a restricted ictal onset zone outside the anterior temporal lobe. This situation almost always requires placement of intracranial electrodes to map the extent of epileptogenic tissue and to determine its relation to functional brain areas. Outcome after nonlesional cortical resections is not as good as with anterior temporal lobectomy or lesionectomy, mainly because the boundaries of epileptogenic cortical areas often cannot be delineated precisely, and removal of all the epileptogenic tissue often is not possible.

Corpus Callosotomy

Section of the corpus callosum disconnects the two hemispheres and is indicated for treatment of patients with uncontrolled atonic or tonic seizures in the absence of an identifiable focus suitable for resection. Most patients referred for corpus callosotomy have severe and frequent seizures of multiple types, usually with mental retardation and a severely abnormal EEG (the Lennox-Gastaut syndrome).

Unlike resective surgery, corpus callosotomy is palliative, not curative. Nonetheless, it can be strikingly effective for generalized seizures, with 80% of patients experiencing complete or nearly complete cessation of atonic, tonic, and tonic-clonic attacks. This outcome is often remarkably beneficial because it eliminates falls and the associated self-injury. The effect on partial seizures, however, is inconsistent and unpredictable. Complex partial seizures are reduced or eliminated in about half the patients, but simple or complex partial seizures are exacerbated in about 25%. Therefore, refractory partial seizures alone are not an indication for corpus callosotomy. Similarly, absence, atypical absence, and myoclonic seizures either do not benefit or show an inconsistent response.

▶ **TABLE 141.9 Outcome After Epilepsy Surgical Procedures**

Procedure	Seizure Free (%)	Improved (%)	Not Improved (%)
Anterior temporal lobectomy ($n = 3,579$)	68.8	22.2	9.0
Lesionectomy ($n = 293$)	66.6	21.5	11.9
Nonlesional extratemporal neocortical resection ($n = 805$)	45.1	35.2	19.8
Hemispherectomy ($n = 190$)	67.4	21.1	11.6
Corpus callosum section ($n = 563$)	7.6	60.9	31.4

Modified from Engel J Jr. *Surgical Treatment of the Epilepsies.* 2nd Ed. New York: Raven, 1993.

Hemispherectomy

Removal or disconnection of large cortical areas from one side of the brain is indicated when the epileptogenic lesion involves most or all of one hemisphere. Because hemispherectomy guarantees permanent hemiplegia, hemisensory loss, and usually hemianopia, it can be considered only in children with a unilateral structural lesion that has already resulted in those abnormalities and who have refractory unilateral seizures. Examples of conditions suitable for hemispherectomy include infantile hemiplegia syndromes, Sturge-Weber disease, Rasmussen syndrome, and severe unilateral developmental anomalies, such as hemimegalencephaly. In appropriate patients, the results are dramatic. Seizures cease, behavior improves, and development accelerates (Table 141.9).

Preoperative Evaluation

The objective in evaluating patients for focal resection is to demonstrate that all seizures originate in a limited cortical area that can be removed safely. This determination requires more extensive evaluation than is necessary in the routine management of patients with epilepsy. The different tests used provide complementary information about normal and epileptic brain functions.

CCTV/EEG monitoring is necessary to record a representative sample of the patient's typical seizures to confirm the diagnosis and classification and also to localize the cortical area involved in ictal onset. Volumetric or other special MRI techniques may demonstrate unilateral hippocampal atrophy or other anatomic abnormalities that may be epileptogenic. PET and ictal SPECT are useful in demonstrating focal abnormalities in glucose metabolism or cerebral blood flow that correspond to the epileptogenic brain region. Neuropsychologic testing is useful in demonstrating focal cognitive dysfunction, especially language and memory. Intracarotid injection of amobarbital (the *Wada test*) to determine hemispheric dominance for language and memory competence is generally considered necessary before temporal lobectomy, but the implications of a failed test are uncertain. Some centers are beginning to supplement this with information from functional MR studies. Although functional MRI (fMRI) reliably lateralizes language, determining memory competence of one temporal lobe has not yet been reliably established.

Intracranial electrodes are necessary if noninvasive methods do not unequivocally localize the epileptogenic area or if different noninvasive tests give conflicting results. Intracranial electrode placement is also necessary when vital brain functions (language, motor cortex) must be mapped in relation to the planned resection.

Vagus Nerve Stimulation

Vagus nerve stimulation is a novel nonpharmacologic treatment for medically refractory partial seizures. Like corpus callosotomy, vagus nerve stimulation is a palliative procedure, because very few patients become seizure free. Vagus nerve stimulation is delivered via a stimulating lead attached to the left vagus nerve. The stimulus generator is implanted in the upper left chest. The device is usually programmed to give a 30-second electrical pulse every 5 minutes, although stimulus parameters can be adjusted to the requirements of an individual patient. In patients with aura, a magnetic wand can be used to deliver vagus nerve stimulation on demand, which may abort seizure progression. About 30% to 35% of patients have at least a 50% reduction in seizure frequency, which compares favorably with the efficacy of new antiepileptic drugs. Chronic adverse effects include hoarseness and difficulty swallowing, both of which increase at the time of stimulation.

STATUS EPILEPTICUS

Convulsive status epilepticus is a medical emergency, and failure to treat the condition in a timely and appropriate manner can result in serious systemic and neurologic morbidity. At least 65,000 cases of status epilepticus occur each year in the United States. It is diagnosed if seizures last longer than 10 minutes or if two or more seizures occur in close succession without recovery of consciousness.

Status epilepticus may be either *convulsive* or *nonconvulsive*. The most life-threatening pattern, and that requiring the most urgent treatment, is convulsive status epilepticus, which, like seizures and epileptic syndromes, may be a manifestation either of idiopathic (i.e., nonfocal) epilepsy or secondary to spread from a localized epileptogenic brain region. Nonconvulsive status epilepticus occurs as a kind of twilight confusional state and is caused by either continuing generalized absence seizures or complex partial seizures.

Status epilepticus is most frequent in infants and young children and in elderly persons, but it occurs at all ages. More than 50% of those affected do not have a history of epilepsy. In about 10% of patients with epilepsy, status epilepticus is the first manifestation, and about 15% of patients with epilepsy have had one or more episodes of status at some time.

In two-thirds of cases of status epilepticus, an acute cause or precipitating factor, such as systemic metabolic derangement, alcohol or other drug abuse, hypoxia, head trauma, infection, or a cerebral lesion, such as a stroke or tumor, can be identified. Therefore, part of the emergency evaluation of patients in status is determining the probable cause (Table 141.10).

Convulsive Status Epilepticus

Convulsive status epilepticus generates metabolic and physiologic stresses that contribute to permanent brain damage, including hyperthermia, hypoxia, lactic acidosis, hypoglycemia, and hypotension. Plasma catecholamine levels are acutely elevated during the attack and may trigger fatal cardiac arrhythmias. Death usually results from the underlying condition rather than from the status epilepticus itself. Nonetheless, death from status epilepticus per se occurs in 2% to 3% of children and in 7% to 10% of adults.

▶ **TABLE 141.10** Causes of Status Epilepticus

Diagnosis	Children (%)	Adults (%)
Stroke	3	25
Drug change/noncompliance	20	20
Alcohol/other drugs	2	15
CNS infection	5	10
Hypoxia	5	10
Metabolic	10	10
Tumor	<1	5
Trauma	3.5	5
Fever/infection	35	2
Congenital	10	<1

Modified from Hauser WA. *Neurology* 1990;40(Suppl 2):9–13; and DeLorenzo RJ, Towne AR, Pellock JM, et al. *Epilepsia* 1992;33(Suppl 4):S15–S25.

▶ **TABLE 141.11** Protocol and Timetable for Treating Status Epilepticus at the Neurological Institute of New York, Columbia-Presbyterian Medical Center

Time (min)	Action
0–5	Diagnose; give O_2; ABCs; obtain i.v. access; begin ECG monitoring; draw blood for chem-7, Mg, Ca, CBC, AED levels, ABG; toxicology screen
6–10	Thiamine 100 mg i.v.; 50 mL of D50 i.v. unless adequate glucose level known Lorazepam (Ativan) 4 mg i.v. over 2 min; repeat once in 8–10 min p.r.n. *Or* Diazepam (Valium) 10 mg i.v. over 2 min; repeat once in 3–5 min p.r.n.
10–20	If status persists or if it was stopped with diazepam, immediately begin fosphenytoin (Cerebyx) 20 mg/kg i.v. at 150 mg/min, with blood pressure and ECG monitoring
20–30	If status persists, give additional 5 mg/kg fosphenytoin two times (total 30 mg/kg)
30+	If status persists, intubate and give one of the following (in order of our preference), preferably with EEG monitoring: 1. Phenobarbital 20 mg/kg i.v. at 50–100 mg/min. Additional 5-mg/kg boluses can be given as needed; *or* 2. Midazolam continuous infusion, 0.2 mg/kg slow bolus, then 0.1–2.0 mg/kg/hr; *or* 3. Propofol continuous infusion, 1–5 mg/kg bolus over 5 min, then 2–4 mg/kg/hr

ABCs, airway, blood pressure, cardiac function; AED, antiepileptic drug; ABG, arterial blood gas; D50, 50% dextrose in water.

The goals of treatment are to eliminate all seizure activity and to identify and treat any underlying medical or neurologic disorder. Initial management is that of any comatose patient: to ensure airway and oxygenation, to access circulation and maintain blood pressure, and to monitor cardiac function (Table 141.11). Blood should be obtained for antiepileptic drug levels, blood count, and routine chemistries. Brain imaging should be done in all adult patients with status epilepticus and in all children with nonfebrile status epilepticus. Patients should be in stable condition, and CT is usually sufficient to exclude an acute brain lesion. MRI should be obtained later if the CT was normal. Lumbar puncture should be performed in any febrile patient, even if signs of meningitis are not present. If brain infection is strongly suspected, the need for lumbar puncture is urgent, and the procedure should be carried out immediately. If signs of increased intracranial pressure are apparent or if a mass lesion is suspected, antibiotics should be given immediately and a CT obtained before lumbar puncture.

If the history is at all uncertain, glucose should be given, preceded by thiamine in adults. Although several antiepileptic drug regimens are effective for treating status epilepticus, we begin with lorazepam, 0.1 mg/kg, followed immediately by fosphenytoin, 20 mg/kg phenytoin equivalent (PE). If there is no response, additional fosphenytoin, 5 mg/kg, should be administered. A large, randomized VA Cooperative Study found that lorazepam was superior to phenytoin alone. Although diazepam plus phenytoin was an equally effective regimen, the authors recommended lorazepam for initial treatment because of its ease of use. The combination of lorazepam and phenytoin was not evaluated. The VA cooperative trial also reinforced the need to control status epilepticus as rapidly as possible; prolonged status became progressively more difficult to treat.

If status persists after initial treatment measures, the patient should be intubated and anesthetized with pentobarbital, midazolam, or propofol with EEG monitoring to ensure complete suppression of all electrical ictal activity. EEG monitoring is necessary because approximately 20% of patients whose motor activity stops completely continue to have electrographic ictal discharges. After the patient has been stabilized and seizures controlled, a rigorous search for an underlying condition should be instituted. Fosphenytoin is a phosphate ester prodrug of phenytoin. Unlike intravenous phenytoin, fosphenytoin is compatible with all intravenous solutions in common use. Because it is much less alkaline, it causes only minimal local irritation and can be infused at much faster rates than phenytoin. After entering the blood, fosphenytoin is converted rapidly to phenytoin by phosphatases in the liver and red blood cells. The pharmacologic properties of phosphenytoin are identical to those of phenytoin, and it is dosed in phenytoin equivalents. Unique side effects are paresthesias in the low back and groin, probably owing to the phosphate load.

Nonconvulsive Status Epilepticus

This condition is difficult to diagnose clinically and is frequently unrecognized. Patients are most often middle-aged or elderly and usually have no past history of seizures. Onset is generally abrupt, and all patients show altered mentation and behavioral changes that typically last for days to weeks. Patients in nonconvulsive status are characteristically alert (although dull), and the absence of stupor or coma contributes to misdiagnosis. A psychiatric diagnosis is often the first consideration if the condition presents as bizarre behavior and change in affect, often with hallucinations, paranoia, or catatonia. When memory loss, disorientation, and mood changes predominate, diagnostic possibilities include dementia, stroke, or metabolic/toxic encephalopathy.

Once the suspicion of nonconvulsive status epilepticus has been raised, diagnosis depends on demonstrating ictal patterns in the EEG while the patient is symptomatic. Nonconvulsive status can be caused by either generalized or focal (usually temporal or frontal) ictal discharges. Diagnosis of nonconvulsive status epilepticus is confirmed by the response to intravenous diazepam (5–10 mg) or lorazepam (1–2 mg): Epileptiform EEG abnormalities disappear, and the patient's mental state improves. Long-term seizure control can be achieved using any of the available agents that are effective for the seizure type, although it is usually advantageous to use a drug that can be rapidly loaded either intravenously (phenytoin, phenobarbital, or valproic acid) or orally (gabapentin or levetiracetam).

Laboratory studies are usually normal, but occasionally they identify a cause for the nonconvulsive status epilepticus, such as nonketotic hyperglycemia, electrolyte imbalance, drug toxicity (e.g., lithium), or a focal cerebral lesion (e.g., frontal lobe infarction).

GENE MUTATIONS IN EPILEPSY

Genetic factors are implicated strongly in several epilepsy syndromes, and twin studies have confirmed important genetic determinants in both localization-related and generalized types of seizure disorders. The concordance rate for monozygotic twins with idiopathic generalized epilepsy is well over 75%. Hereditary aspects are easiest to discern in childhood absence epilepsy, juvenile myoclonic epilepsy, benign rolandic epilepsy, and idiopathic grand mal seizures. Some inherited disorders, such as tuberous sclerosis and neurofibromatosis, are associated with brain lesions that in turn give rise to symptomatic epilepsies. In most cases of epilepsy, however, the role of genetic factors is complex because there are multiple interacting genes that convey varying degrees of seizure susceptibility and also affect the brain's response to environmental influences. In any given patient, the relative contribution from genetic or acquired factors determines whether the epilepsy presents as an idiopathic syndrome or as a symptomatic disorder. In addition, however, there also seems to be some degree of sharing of genetic susceptibilities in both the idiopathic and symptomatic epilepsies, as children of parents with either localization-related or generalized epilepsy develop seizures at increased rates, although the difference is greatest in families with idiopathic generalized epilepsy. Thus, a major challenge facing investigators today is to clarify how different genes alter an individual's susceptibility to seizures and epilepsy in the presence of acquired brain pathology or as a reaction to acute or subacute cerebral dysfunction. This

▶ **TABLE 141.12   Genes Identified in Idiopathic Human Epilepsies**

Gene	Syndrome	Chromosome
Na⁺ Channels		
SCN1A	Generalized epilepsy with febrile seizures plus (GEFS⁺)	2q24
SCN1A	Severe myoclonic epilepsy of infancy	2q
SCN2A	Benign familial neonatal seizures and GEFS⁺	2q24
SCN1B	GEFS⁺	19q13
K⁺ Channels		
KCNQ2	Benign familial neonatal seizures	20q13
KCNQ3	Benign familial neonatal seizures	8q24
Cl⁻ Channels		
CLN2	Idiopathic generalized epilepsy (heterogeneous)	3q26
Ca⁺² Channels		
CACNA1A (P/Q)	Absence epilepsy and cerebellar ataxia	19q
CACNB4	Idiopathic generalized epilepsy (heterogeneous)	2q22–23
Nicotinic ACH-R		
CHRNA4	Autosomal-dominant nocturnal frontal lobe epilepsy	20q13
CHRNB2	Autosomal-dominant nocturnal frontal lobe epilepsy	1q
GABA_A Receptor		
GABRG2	GEFS⁺	5q34
GABRA1	Juvenile myoclonic epilepsy (French-Canadian family)	
Other		
LGI1	Autosomal-dominant partial epilepsy with auditory features	10q22–24

is no easy task, however, because the number of genes that encode molecules that regulate cortical excitability directly through membrane and synaptic functions and the second messenger cascades that indirectly regulate membrane proteins involved in signal transduction is very large.

A number of causative genes have been identified in idiopathic epilepsies with a monogenic mode of inheritance (Table 141.12). Mutations in two voltage-gated potassium channel genes, KCNQ2 (chr 20q13) and KCNQ3, (chr 8q24), cause benign familial neonatal convulsions. Autosomal-dominant frontal lobe epilepsy is caused by mutations in two cholinergic receptor genes, the CHRNA4 (chr 20q13) and CHRNB2 (chr 1q). A syndrome of generalized epilepsy with febrile seizures (GEFS⁺) has been related to mutations in three Na⁺ channel subunits: SCN1B (chr 19q13), SCN1A (2q24), and SCN2A (2q24). A similar syndrome has also been seen in families with mutations in the $\gamma 2$ subunit gene (GABRG2 on chr 5q34) of the GABA_A receptor. De novo mutations in the $\alpha 1$ subunit of the Na⁺ channel also cause severe myoclonic epilepsy of infancy (Dravet syndrome). Mutations in the CLCN2 gene encoding a Cl⁻ channel have recently been described in three families with idiopathic generalized epilepsies of heterogeneous phenotype. An autosomal dominant form of juvenile myoclonic epilepsy occurring in a French Canadian family is associated with a mutation in the $\alpha 1$ subunit of the GABA receptor (GABRA1). A mutation in the leucine-rich glioma inactivated (LCI1) gene on chromosome 10q22-24 causes an autosomal-dominant form of partial epilepsy with auditory features.

PSYCHOSOCIAL AND PSYCHIATRIC ISSUES

The impact of epilepsy on the quality of life is usually greater than the limitations imposed by the seizures alone. The diagnosis of epilepsy frequently carries other consequences that can greatly alter the lives of many patients. For adults, the most important problems are discrimination at work and driving restrictions, which lead to loss of mobility and independence. Children and adults alike may be shunned by uninformed friends. Patients must learn to avoid situations that precipitate seizures, and a change in lifestyle may be necessary. Common factors that increase the likelihood of seizure occurrence include sleep deprivation, alcohol (and other drugs), and emotional stress (Table 141.13). Compliance with antiepileptic drug treatment is often an issue, especially with adolescents. Psychiatric symptoms, especially depression, may complicate management.

Some restrictions are medically appropriate, at least for limited times. For example, when seizures impair consciousness or judgment, driving and certain kinds of employment (working at exposed heights or with power equipment) and a few other activities (swimming alone) should be interdicted. On the other hand, legal prohibitions on driving vary in different states in the United States and in different countries and are often not medically justified. Employers frequently have unrealistic fears about the physical effects of a seizure, the potential for liability, and the impact on insurance costs. In fact, the Americans with Disabilities Act prohibits denying employment to persons

▶ **TABLE 141.13 Factors That Lower the Seizure Threshold**

Common	*Occasional*
Sleep deprivation	Barbiturate withdrawal
Alcohol withdrawal	Hyperventilation
Stress	Flashing lights
Dehydration	Diet and missed meals
Drugs and drug interactions	Specific "reflex" triggers
Systemic infection	
Trauma	
Malnutrition	
Noncompliance	

with disability if the disability does not prevent them from meeting job requirements.

Children have special problems because their seizures affect the entire family. Parents may, with the best of intentions, handicap the child by being overly restrictive. The necessary and special attention received by the "sick" child may encourage passive manipulative behavior and overdependence while unintentionally exacerbating normal sibling rivalries.

The physician must be sensitive to these important quality of life concerns, even when they are not raised spontaneously by the patient or family. In fact, psychosocial issues often become the major focus of follow-up visits after the diagnosis has been made, the initial evaluation completed, and treatment started. We cannot emphasize too much the physician's responsibility to educate society to counter misperceptions and prejudices and to separate myth from medical fact. The Epilepsy Foundation (Landover, Maryland; 1-800-EFA-1000; www.epilepsyfoundation.org) and its nationwide system of affiliates have a wealth of materials about epilepsy suitable for patient, family, and public education.

Compliance

The most common cause of breakthrough seizures is noncompliance with the prescribed therapeutic regimen. Only about 70% of patients take antiepileptic medications as prescribed. For phenytoin or carbamazepine, noncompliance can be inferred when sequential blood levels vary by more than 20%, assuming similarly timed samples and unchanged dosage. Persistently low antiepileptic drug levels in the face of increasing dosage also generally imply poor compliance. Caution is warranted with phenytoin, however, because as many as 20% of patients have low levels as a result of poor absorption or rapid metabolism.

Noncompliance is especially common in adolescents and elderly persons, when seizures are infrequent or not perceived as disabling, when antiepileptic drugs must be taken several times each day, and when toxic effects persist. Compliance can be improved by patient education, by

simplifying drug regimens, and by tailoring dosing schedules to the patient's daily routines. Pill box devices that alert the patient to scheduled doses can be useful.

Depression and Psychosis

In referral centers, depression and suicide are more common in patients with epilepsy than in patients with other neurologic disorders or in disease-free control subjects. Whether this predilection is true for the epilepsy population at large is not known, because few community-based population studies have been conducted. Depression in epilepsy may be influenced by several factors: the type or severity of the seizures, the location of the epileptogenic focus, associated neurologic or medical conditions, the antiepileptic drugs used, and the personal stigma and limitations that accompany the diagnosis. Curiously, depression sometimes follows successful epilepsy surgery.

Treatment of depression begins with optimal treatment of the seizure disorder. Barbiturate and succinimide drugs may adversely affect mood, inducing symptoms that mimic endogenous depression. Topiramate and levetiracetam seem to cause depression in a small minority of patients, whereas lamotrigine can occasionally improve depression. Levetiracetam has also been associated with rare psychosis. Although tricyclic antidepressants reduce the seizure threshold in experimental models of epilepsy, this is not a practical concern because they only rarely trigger seizures or increase seizure frequency in humans. MAO inhibitors neither induce seizures nor increase seizure frequency. Modern electroconvulsive therapy does not worsen epilepsy. We have used all available selective serotonin reuptake inhibitors without exacerbating seizures.

The relation between psychosis and epilepsy is controversial. No convincing evidence shows that interictal psychosis is a manifestation of epilepsy, but some demographic features are over-represented in patients with epilepsy. Postictal psychosis is, however, a well-recognized and self-limited complication of epilepsy. Its cause is unknown, but it may represent a behavioral analog of a Todd's paresis. Symptoms typically appear 24 to 72 hours after a lucid interval following a prolonged seizure or cluster of seizures. Delusions and paranoia are common. The psychosis is self-limited, usually to a few days, although symptoms occasionally last as long as 1 to 2 weeks. Treatment with haloperidol or risperidone is usually effective. In cases where postictal psychosis regularly follows clusters of seizures, chronic treatment with low-dose risperidone can be helpful. Long-term emphasis should be on improving seizure control. Phenothiazines, butyrophenones, and clozapine lower seizure threshold in experimental animals and occasionally seem to induce seizures in nonepileptic patients. Most occurrences have been associated with high drug doses or a rapid increase in dose. With the possible exception of clozapine, however, little evidence supports the notion that reasonable and conservative use of antipsychotic medications increases seizure frequency in patients with epilepsy.

Interictal aggressive behavior is not more common in people with epilepsy. Directed aggression during seizures occurs in less than 0.02% of patients with severe epilepsy; it is almost certainly less common in the general epilepsy population. Undirected pushing or resistance occasionally occurs postictally when attempts are made to restrain confused patients.

SUGGESTED READINGS

Bazil CW. *Living Well with Epilepsy.* HarperCollins, Inc. 2004.

Bazil CW, Malow BA, Sammaritano MR, eds. *Sleep and Epilepsy: The Clinical Spectrum.* New York: Elsevier, 2002.

Bazil CW, Pedley TA. Clinical pharmacology of antiepileptic drugs. *Clin Neuropharmacol* 2003;26:38–52.

Beghi E. Overview of studies to prevent posttraumatic epilepsy. *Epilepsia* 2003;44(Suppl 10):21–26.

Benardo LS. Prevention of epilepsy after head trauma: do we need new drugs or a new approach? *Epilepsia* 2003;44(Suppl 10):27–33.

Berg AT, Shinnar S. The risk of seizure recurrence following a first unprovoked seizure: a quantitative review. *Neurology* 1991;41:965–972.

Brodie MJ, French JA. Management of epilepsy in adolescents and adults. *Lancet* 2000;356:323–329.

Cendes F. Febrile seizures and mesial temporal sclerosis. *Curr Opin Neurol* 2004;17:161–164.

Commission on classification and terminology of the International League Against Epilepsy. Proposal for revised clinical and electroencephalographic classification of epileptic seizures. *Epilepsia* 1981;12:489–501.

DeLorenzo RJ, Pellock JM, Towne AR, et al. Epidemiology of status epilepticus. *J Clin Neurophysiol* 1995;12:316–325.

Engel J Jr. Surgical treatment of the epilepsies, 2nd ed. New York, Raven Press, 1993.

Engel J Jr. A proposed diagnostic scheme for people with epileptic seizures and with epilepsy: report of the ILAE Task Force on Classification and Terminology. *Epilepsia* 2001;42:796–803.

Engel J Jr, Pedley TA, eds. *Epilepsy: A Comprehensive Textbook.* Philadelphia: Lippincott Williams & Wilkins, 1998.

First Seizure Trial Group. Randomized clinical trial on the efficacy of antiepileptic drugs in reducing the risk of relapse after a first unprovoked tonic-clonic seizure. *Neurology* 1993;43:478–483.

French J, Kanner AM, Bautista J. Efficacy and tolerability of the new antiepileptic drugs. I. Treatment of new onset epilepsy. *Neurology* 2004;62:1252–1260.

French J, Kanner AM, Bautista J. Efficacy and tolerability of the new antiepileptic drugs. II. Treatment of refractory epilepsy. *Neurology* 2004;62:1261–1273.

Gourfinkel-An I, Baulac S, Nabbout R, et al. Monogenic idiopathic epilepsies. *Lancet Neurol* 2004;3:209–218.

Granata T, Fusco L, Gobbi G, et al. Experience with immunomodulatory treatments in Rasmussen's encephalitis. *Neurology* 2003;61:1807–1810.

Gutierrez-Delicado E, Serratosa JM. Genetics of the epilepsies. *Curr Opin Neurol* 2004;17:147–133.

Hauser WA. Status epilepticus: epidemiologic considerations. *Neurology* 1990;40(Suppl 2):9–13.

Hauser WA, Hesdorffer DC. *Epilepsy: Frequency,Ccauses and Consequences.* New York: Demos, 1990.

Hauser WA, Rich SS, Lee JR-J, et al. Risk of recurrent seizures after two unprovoked seizures. *N Engl J Med* 1998;338:429–434.

Hirsch LJ, Hauser WA. Can sudden unexplained death in epilepsy be prevented? *Lancet* 2004; Dec 18;364(9452):2157–2158.

Husain AM, Horn CJ, Jacobson MP. Non-convulsive status epilepticus: usefulness of clinical features in selecting patients for urgent EEG. *J Neurol Neurosurg Psychiatry* 2003;74:189–191.

Jackson GD, Berkovic SF, Tress BM, et al. Hippocampal sclerosis can be reliably detected by magnetic resonance imaging. *Neurology* 1990;40:1869–1875.

Karceski S, Morrell M, Carpenter D. The Expert Consensus Guideline Series. Treatment of epilepsy. *Epilepsy Behav* 2001;2:A1–A50.

Kwan P, Brodie MJ. Early identification of refractory epilepsy. *N Engl J Med* 2000;342:314–319.

Lee SI. Non-convulsive status epilepticus. Ictal confusion in later life. *Arch Neurol* 1985;42:778–781.

Lowenstein DH. Treatment options for status epilepticus. *Curr Opin Pharmacol* 2003;3:6–11.

Lowenstein DH, Alldredge BK. Status epilepticus. *N Engl J Med* 1998;338:970–976.

Mattson RH, Cramer JA, Collins JF. Comparison of valproate with carbamazepine for the treatment of complex partial seizures and secondarily generalized tonic-clonic seizures in adults. *N Engl J Med* 1992;327:765–771.

Mattson RH, Cramer JA, Collins JF, et al. A comparison of carbamazepine, phenobarbital, phenytoin, and primidone in partial and secondarily generalized tonic-clonic seizures. *N Engl J Med* 1985;313:145–151.

Medical Research Council Antiepileptic Drug Withdrawal Study Group. Randomised study of antiepileptic drug withdrawal in patients in remission. *Lancet* 1991;337:1175–1180.

Morrell MJ. Reproductive and metabolic disorders in women with epilepsy. *Epilepsia* 2003;44(Suppl 4):11–20.

Morrell MJ, Flynn K, eds. *Women with Epilepsy.* Cambridge, UK: Cambridge University Press, 2003.

Musicco M, Beghi E, Solari A, et al. Treatment of first tonic-clonic seizure does not improve the prognosis of epilepsy. *Neurology* 1997;49:991–998.

Nguyen DK, Spencer SS. Recent advances in the treatment of epilepsy. *Arch Neurol* 2003;60:929–935.

Noebels JL. The biology of epilepsy genes. *Annu Rev Neurosci* 2003;26:599–625.

Ottman R, Winawer MR, Kalachikov S, Barker-Cummings C, Gilliam TC, Pedley TA, Hauser WA. LGI1 mutations in autosomal dominant partial epilepsy with auditory features. *Neurology* 2004 Apr 13; 62(7):1120–1126.

Pack AM, Morrell MJ. Epilepsy and bone health in adults. *Epilepsy and Behavior* 2004;5(Suppl 2):524–529.

Pedley TA, Hauser WA. Sudden death in epilepsy: a wake-up call for management. *Lancet* 2002;359:1790–1791.

Pellock JM, Willmore LJ. A rational guide to routine blood monitoring in patients receiving antiepileptic drugs. *Neurology* 1991;41:961–964.

Salazar AM, Jabbari B, Vance SC, et al. Epilepsy after penetrating head injury. I. Clinical correlates: a report of the Vietnam Head Injury Study. *Neurology* 1985;35:1406–1414.

Scheffer IE, Berkovic SF. The genetics of human epilepsy. *Trends Pharmacol Sci* 2003;24:428–433.

Sheen VL, Walsh CA. Developmental genetic malformations of the cerebral cortex. *Curr Neurol Neurosci Rep* 2003;3:433–441.

Sillanpaa M, Jalava M, Kaleva O, et al. Long-term prognosis of seizures with onset in childhood. *N Engl J Med* 1998;338:1715–1722.

Spencer SS, Berg AT, Vickrey BG, et al. Initial outcomes in the multicenter study of epilepsy surgery. *Neurology* 2003;61:1680–1685.

Sperling MR, Feldman H, Kirman J, et al. Seizure control and mortality in epilepsy. *Ann Neurol* 1999;46:45–50.

Sullivan JE, Dlugos DJ. Idiopathic generalized epilepsy. *Curr Treat Options Neurol* 2004;6:231–242.

Temkin NR, Dikmen SS, Wilensky AJ, et al. A randomized, double blind study of phenytoin for the prevention of post-traumatic seizures. *N Engl J Med* 1990;323:497–502.

Treiman DM, Meyers PD, Walton NY, et al. A comparison of four treatments for generalized convulsive status epilepticus. *N Engl J Med* 1998;339:792–798.

Wiebe S, Blume WT, Girvin JP, et al. A randomized, controlled trial of surgery for temporal-lobe epilepsy. *New Engl J Med* 2001;345:311–318.

Wyllie E, ed. *The Treatment of Epilepsy.* 3rd Ed. Philadelphia: Lippincott Williams & Wilkins, 2001.

Zahn CA, Morrell MJ, Collins SD, et al. Management issues for women with epilepsy: a review of the literature. American Academy of Neurology Practice Guidelines. *Neurology* 1998;51:949–956.

Chapter 142

Febrile Seizures

Linda D. Leary, Douglas R. Nordli, Jr., and Timothy A. Pedley

A febrile seizure is "an event in infancy or childhood, usually occurring between 3 months and 5 years of age, associated with fever, but without evidence of an intracranial infection or defined cause" (National Institutes of Health Consensus Conference, 1980). This definition excludes children who have had previous afebrile seizures.

Febrile seizures are the most common cause of convulsions in children: Between 2% and 5% of all children in the United States and Europe and 6% to 9% of children in Japan have at least one febrile seizure before age 5 years. Hauser (1994) estimated that in 1990, there were 100,000 cases of newly diagnosed febrile seizures in the United States. Genetic predisposition is an important factor. Overall, siblings and offspring of affected probands have a twofold to threefold increased risk of seizures with fever. Based on studies of large families with simple febrile seizures, four genetic loci have been mapped. These loci are referred to as FEB1 (8q13-q21), FEB2 (19p), FEB3 (2q23-q24), and FEB4 (5q14-q15). Some families have a susceptibility to febrile seizures and later epilepsy, and these traits are inherited in an autosomal-dominant fashion. This has been termed generalized epilepsy febrile seizures plus (GEFS+). Mutations in the voltage-gated sodium channel β-1 subunit gene (SCN1B; OMIM 600235) on chromosome 19q13 cause GEFS+ type 1; mutations in the SCN1A gene (OMIM 182389) on 2q24 cause GEFS+ type 2; and mutations in the GABRG2 gene (OMIM 137164) on 5q31.1-q33.1 cause GEFS+ type 3. Mutations in the SCN2A (OMIM 182390) gene cause febrile seizures associated with afebrile seizures. Owing to the overlap between the loci for FEB 3 and GEFS+ type 2, it is uncertain if FEB3 is a unique genetic locus for simple febrile seizures. The role of identified genes in sporadic febrile seizures remains to be determined.

CLINICAL MANIFESTATIONS

About two-thirds of febrile seizures occur early in the febrile illness (that is, within the first 24 hours). In some children, the seizure is the first indication of illness. Febrile seizures are subdivided into *simple* and *complex* types. Simple febrile seizures are most common, representing 80% to 90% of all febrile seizures. Simple febrile seizures are isolated, brief generalized convulsions. Complex febrile seizures are those that are focal or followed by a postictal deficit (Todd paresis), last more than 10 to 15 minutes, or occur more than once within 24 hours.

DIAGNOSIS

Diagnosis is made by excluding other possible causes of the convulsion, such as meningitis, metabolic abnormalities, or structural brain lesions. Depending on the manifestations and the clinician's experience, laboratory tests are not always necessary. Usually, a clinically identifiable illness such as otitis media, upper respiratory infection, or gastroenteritis is present. Fever after immunization may also trigger a febrile seizure. Any suspicion of meningitis, however, mandates lumbar puncture. The typical indicators of meningeal irritation, such as nuchal rigidity and the Brudzinski sign, are not reliable in young infants. Practice guidelines of the American Academy of Pediatrics (1996) recommend that lumbar puncture be strongly considered if the child is younger than 12 months of age or if the child has already been treated with antibiotics regardless of age. Lumbar puncture may be indicated in children between 12 and 18 months. If the seizure has focal features, or if the examination elicits focal neurologic abnormalities, brain imaging is necessary. EEG is not useful, because it does not provide information regarding either the risk for recurrence of febrile seizures or later development of epilepsy.

PROGNOSIS AND TREATMENT

About one-third of children with febrile seizures have more than one attack. Recurrence is highest in infants whose first febrile seizure occurred before the age of 1 year and in children with a family history of febrile seizures. Febrile seizures represent acute symptomatic or reactive seizures, and even when recurrent do not warrant the designation of epilepsy.

Children who have an isolated febrile seizure have a risk of developing epilepsy that is similar to that of the general population. This risk increases if simple febrile seizures recur (2%–3%), and if the febrile seizures are complex, there is a family history of afebrile seizures, or neurological abnormalities were detected before the first febrile convulsion (10%–13%). When all three features of complex febrile seizures are present (prolonged, focal, repeated), the risk of subsequent epilepsy may be as high as 49%. Mortality is not increased in children with febrile seizures who are neurologically normal.

Simple febrile seizures have not been associated with, nor do they lead to, mental retardation, low IQ, poor school achievement, or behavioral problems. Most studies have also failed to demonstrate any cognitive or behavioral consequences of complex febrile seizures, although some differences have been reported. In children with prolonged febrile convulsions, nonverbal intelligence measures may be slightly lower compared with children with simple febrile seizures and normal controls. Children with complex febrile seizures are also more likely to require special schooling than those with simple febrile seizures.

Whether prolonged febrile seizures cause mesial temporal sclerosis and refractory partial seizures is controversial. Large prospective studies have failed to find an association, but experience in adult epilepsy surgical centers suggests otherwise, because many adults with mesial temporal sclerosis have had a prolonged febrile convulsion as a child. Furthermore, MRI in some children with prolonged febrile seizures has shown acute changes in the mesial temporal region that progress over time to mesial temporal sclerosis.

Because most children with febrile seizures have no long-term consequences, prophylactic treatment using antiepileptic drugs should be avoided, even after two or three isolated convulsions. Although both phenobarbital and valproate are effective in reducing recurrence, evidence does not show that treatment alters the risk of later epilepsy. In addition, adverse drug effects occur in as many as 40% of infants and children treated with phenobarbital, and valproate carries a risk of idiosyncratic fatal hepatotoxicity and pancreatitis. Phenytoin and carbamazepine are ineffective.

If treatment is considered at all, it should be reserved for children with a high risk of developing epilepsy or a history of prolonged febrile seizures. A reasonable alternative to chronic drug therapy is intermittent treatment using rectal diazepam. Several studies have shown that rectal administration of diazepam during febrile illnesses is safe and as effective as phenobarbital in reducing seizure recurrence. Although oral diazepam has also been shown to be effective, as many as 30% of children experience adverse effects, including ataxia, lethargy, or irritability. Antipyretics may improve the child's comfort during the febrile illness, but they have not been shown to be effective in preventing the recurrence of febrile convulsions.

Watching their child have a convulsion is a frightening experience for parents. The physician therefore must provide reassurance to dispel any myths the family may have, emphasizing in particular that febrile seizures are neither life threatening nor damaging to the brain. The American Academy of Pediatrics offers copies of its Guidelines and an information sheet for parents through its website (www.aap.org), and the Epilepsy Foundation website (www.epilepsyfoundation.org) provides information about febrile seizures.

SUGGESTED READINGS

American Academy of Pediatrics. Committee on Quality Improvement, Subcommittee on Febrile Seizures. Practice parameter: long-term treatment of the child with simple febrile seizures. *Pediatrics* 1999;103:1307–1309.

American Academy Academy of Pediatrics. Provisional Committee on Quality Improvement, Subcommittee on Febrile Seizures. Practice parameter: the neurodiagnostic evaluation of the child with a first simple febrile seizure. *Pediatrics* 1996;97:769–772.

Annegers JF, Hauser WA, Shirts SB, et al. Factors prognostic of unprovoked seizures after febrile convulsions. *N Engl J Med* 1987;316:493–498.

Baram TZ, Shinnar S, eds. *Febrile Seizures.* San Diego, CA: Academic Press, 2002.

Berg AT, Darefsky AS, Holford TR, et al. Seizures with fever after unprovoked seizures: an analysis in children followed from the time of a first febrile seizure. *Epilepsia* 1998;39:77–80.

Berg AT, Shinnar S, Darefsky AS, et al. Predictors of recurrent febrile seizures. A prospective cohort study. *Arch Pediatr Adolesc Med* 1997;151:371–378.

Berg AT, Shinnar S, Shapiro ED, et al. Risk factors for a first febrile seizure: a matched case-control study. *Epilepsia* 1995;36:334–341.

Hauser WA. The prevalence and incidence of convulsive disorders in children. *Epilepsia* 1994;35(Suppl 2):S1–6.

Hirose S, Mohney RP, Okada M, et al. The genetics of febrile seizures and related epilepsy syndromes. *Brain Dev* 2003;25:304–312.

MacDonald BK, Johnson AL, Sander JWAS, et al. Febrile convulsions in 220 children—neurological sequelae at 12 years follow-up. *Eur Neurol* 1999;41:179–186.

Nelson KB, Ellenberg JH. Prognosis in children with febrile seizures. *Pediatrics* 1978;61:720–727.

Rosman NP, Colton T, Labazzo RNC, et al. A controlled trial of diazepam administered during febrile illnesses to prevent recurrence of febrile seizures. *N Engl J Med* 1993;329:79–84.

Tarkka R, Rantala H, Huhari M, et al. Risk of recurrence and outcome after the first febrile seizure. *Pediatr Neurol* 1998;18:218–220.

VanLandingham KE, Heinz ER, Cavazos JE, et al. MRI evidence of hippocampal injury following prolonged, focal febrile convulsions. *Ann Neurol* 1998;43:413–426.

Verity CM, Greenwood R, Golding J. Long-term intellectual and behavioral outcomes of children with febrile convulsions. *N Engl J Med* 1998;338:1723–1728.

Chapter 143

Transient Global Amnesia

John C. M. Brust

Transient global amnesia (TGA) is characterized by sudden inability to form new memory traces (*anterograde amnesia*) in addition to retrograde memory loss for events of the preceding days, weeks, or even years. During attacks, which affect both verbal and nonverbal memory, there is often bewilderment or anxiety and a tendency to repeat one or several questions (e.g., "Where am I?"). Physical and neurologic examinations, including mental status, are otherwise normal. Immediate registration of events (e.g., serial digits) is intact, and self-identification is preserved. Attacks last minutes or hours, rarely longer than a day, with gradual recovery. Retrograde amnesia clears in a forward fashion, often with permanent loss for events occurring within minutes or a few hours of the attack; there is also permanent amnesia for events during the attack itself. TGA sometimes seems to be precipitated by physical or emotional stress, such as sexual intercourse, driving an automobile, pain, photogenic events, or swimming in cold water. Because amnesia can accompany a variety of neurologic disturbances, such as head trauma, intoxication, partial complex seizures, or dissociative states, criteria for diagnosing TGA should include observation of the attack by others.

Patients are usually middle-aged or elderly and otherwise healthy. Recurrent attacks occur in less than 25% of cases, and fewer than 3% have more than three attacks. Intervals between attacks range from 1 month to 19 years. Permanent memory loss is rare, although subtle defects have been reported after only one attack. The cause of TGA is uncertain. Case-control series and anecdotal reports variably implicate stroke, seizures, or migraine.

In a large series of patients with TGA, the cause was epileptic in 7%. Attacks in this group were nearly always less than 1 hour in duration and tended to occur on awakening; two-thirds had additional seizure types, usually simple or complex partial seizures. Sleep, but not interictal, electroencephalograms revealed temporal lobe epileptiform discharges.

TGA has been anecdotally described in association with carotid artery occlusion and amaurosis fugax, with infarction of the inferomedial temporal lobe, with infarction of the retrosplenial corpus callosum, and with cerebral angiography (especially vertebral). In large series, however, major risk factors for stroke (hypertension, diabetes mel-litus, tobacco, ischemic heart disease, atrial fibrillation, and past stroke or transient ischemic attack) are no more common among patients with TGA than in age-matched controls, and TGA is not a risk factor for stroke. Studies addressing a possible association of TGA with cardiac valvular disease, patent foramen ovale, or jugular valve incompetence have been inconsistent. Patients with amnestic stroke owing to documented posterior cerebral artery occlusion do not report previous TGA; their neurologic signs usually include more than simple amnesia (e.g., visual impairment), and they do not exhibit repetitive queries. Reduced blood flow to the thalamus or temporal lobes has been documented during attacks of TGA but could be secondary to neuronal dysfunction rather than its cause.

Epidemiologic studies confirm an association of TGA with migraine, even though in most migraine patients headache attacks are recurrent, whereas attacks of TGA are not. Sometimes, both amnestic and migrainous attacks (including visual symptoms and vomiting) occur simultaneously or follow one another. A case report described a man with repeated episodes of TGA associated with sexual activity whose spells cleared as long as he took the beta-blocker metoprolol. Spreading depression of Leao (possibly the pathophysiologic basis of cerebral symptoms in migraine) could, by affecting the hippocampus, explain some cases of TGA. Diffusion-weighted MRI during or soon after an attack of TGA in several patients revealed signal abnormalities in one or both temporal lobes that were more suggestive of spreading depression than primary ischemia.

Thus, even when strict diagnostic criteria are applied, TGA probably has diverse origins. In patients in whom epilepsy and migraine can be excluded and who have risk factors for cerebrovascular disease, antiplatelet drugs should be considered, but the benign natural history makes it difficult to evaluate any preventive treatment.

SUGGESTED READINGS

Berlit P. Successful prophylaxis of recurrent transient global amnesia with metoprolol. *Neurology* 2000;55:1937–1938.

Chen ST, Tang LM, Lee TH, et al. Transient global amnesia and amaurosis fugax in a patient with common carotid artery occlusion—a case report. *Angiology* 2000;51:257–261.

Eustache F, Desgranges B, Laville P, et al. Episodic memory in transient global amnesia: encoding, storage, or retrieval deficit? *J Neurol Neurosurg Psychiatry* 1999;66:148–154.

Garji A. spreading depression: a review of the clinical relevance. *Brain Res Rev* 2001;38:33–60.

Gass A, Gaa J, Hirsch J, et al. Lack of evidence of acute ischemic tissue change in transient global amnesia on single-shot echo-planar diffusion-weighted MRI. *Stroke* 1999;30:2070–2072.

Greer DM, Schaefer PW, Schwamm LH. Unilateral temporal lobe stroke causing ischemic transient global amnesia: role for diffusion-weighted imaging in the initial evaluation. *J Neuroimag* 2001;11:317–319.

Guillery B, Desgranges B, de la Sayette V, et al. Transient global amnesia: concomitant episodic memory and positron emission tomography assessment in two additional patients. *Neurosci Lett* 2002;325:62–66.

Hodges JR, Warlow CP. The aetiology of transient global amnesia: a case-control study of 114 cases with prospective follow-up. *Brain* 1990;113:639–658.

Huber R, Aschoff AJ, Ludolph AC, et al. Transient global amnesia: evidence against vascular ischemic etiology from diffusion weighted imaging. *J Neurol* 2002;249:1520–1524.

LaBar KS, Gitelman DR, Parrish TB, et al. Functional changes in temporal lobe activity during transient global amnesia. *Neurology* 2002;58:638–641.

Maalikjy AN, Agosti C, Anzola GP, et al. Transient global amnesia: a clinical and sonographic study. *Eur Neurol* 2003;49:67–71.

Melo TP, Ferro JM, Ferro H. Transient global amnesia: a case-control study. *Brain* 1992;115:261–270.

Rösler A, Mrass GJ, Frese A, et al. Precipitating factors of transient global amnesia. *J Neurol* 1999;246:53–54.

Sander D, Winbeck K, Etgen T, et al. Disturbance of venous flow patterns in patients with transient global amnesia. *Lancet* 2000;356:1982–1984.

Sedlaczek O, Hirsch JG, Grips E, et al. Detection of delayed focal MR changes in the lateral hippocampus in transient global amnesia. *Neurology* 2004 Jun 22;62(12):2165–2270.

Strupp M, Brüning R, Wu RH, et al. Diffusion-weighted MRI in transient global amnesia: elevated signal intensity in the left mesial temporal lobe in 7 of 10 patients. *Ann Neurol* 1998;43:164–170.

Zeman AZJ, Boniface SJ, Hodges JR. Transient epileptic amnesia: a description of the clinical and neuropsychological features in 10 cases and a review of the literature. *J Neurol Neurosurg Psychiatry* 1998;64:435–443.

Zorzon M, Antonutti L, Masè G, et al. Transient global amnesia and transient ischemic attack: natural history, vascular risk factors, and associated conditions. *Stroke* 1995;26:1536–1542.

Chapter 144

Ménière Disease

Ian S. Storper

INTRODUCTION

Ménière disease was described over 140 years ago, but little about it is understood. It affects at least 1 in 500 Americans, and more cases are unrecognized. The condition is often progressive, but with medical and surgical treatment options, disability may be averted or ameliorated.

HISTORICAL REVIEW

The disease was first described by Prosper Ménière in Paris in 1861. He described a number of women who had recurrent attacks of vertigo that lasted from hours to days, with asymptomatic periods in between. With the attacks were episodes of unilateral fluctuating hearing loss and roaring tinnitus. At first, the hearing loss and tinnitus occurred with the attacks, but as the disease progressed, they became permanent. In one patient who died of unrelated causes during an attack, Ménière found hemorrhage in the inner ear, proving that the disease is caused by a disturbance in the inner ear rather than one in the brain.

In 1943, Cawthorne added a fourth symptom: fullness in the affected ear. Often, sudden fullness of the affected ear is the harbinger of an attack, with the other symptoms to follow. The fullness usually abates before the end of an attack.

In 1871, Knapp postulated that symptoms of Ménière disease were caused by dilatation of the endolymphatic compartment of the inner ear. The cochlear and vestibular hair cells, which sense hearing and balance, are located in this compartment, and pressure surges in it can cause attacks of Ménière symptoms. In 1938, Hallpike and Cairns confirmed this experimentally.

Once the condition was attributed to endolymphatic hydrops, treatments emerged; the first were surgical and destructive. Parry, in 1902, sectioned the intracranial division of the eighth nerve. Milligan and Lake, separately in 1904, fenestrated the horizontal semicircular canal and vestibule to control vertigo.

As time progressed, procedures became more conservative. Portmann, in 1926, performed the first endolymphatic sac decompression, in the belief that removal of bone on the sac would reduce pressure surges. McKenzie, in 1936, performed the first vestibular neurectomy, leaving the cochlear nerve intact, to preserve hearing. Schuknecht, in 1957, described the transcanal labyrinthectomy, entering directly through the external auditory canal to destroy the vestibular portion of the membranous labyrinth. House, in 1962, shunted endolymph through the back wall of the sac into the subarachnoid space. Paparella, in 1976, performed an endolymphatic-mastoid shunt to relieve endolymphatic hydrops, instead of shunting the fluid into the subarachnoid space; this is the current surgical technique.

Medical treatment with low-sodium diet and diuretic therapy began in the late 1960s, significantly decreasing the frequency and severity of attacks and progression of the disease.

DEFINITIONS

Ménière disease is defined as the *idiopathic* occurrence of attacks of vertigo, hearing loss, tinnitus, or fullness in the affected ear. If a cause is assumed, the term is Ménière syndrome.

The causes of Ménière syndrome are many. Symptoms begin unilaterally in about 95% of cases. Bilateral symptoms suggest an autoimmune etiology. Ménière syndrome may be posttraumatic, after inner ear concussion or fracture of the temporal bone. Rupture of the inner ear membranes (perilymphatic fistula) and Ménière syndrome may follow exposure to pressure change. The syndrome may be infectious, occurring after labyrinthitis, meningitis, Lyme disease, or otosyphilis. It may be congenital, owing to anatomic abnormality of the inner ear, such as a dilated vestibular aqueduct or aplasia of the inner ear. The syndrome may be caused by tumor—for example, vestibular Schwannoma pressing on the eighth nerves. If it is caused by vertebrobasilar insufficiency, other signs and symptoms are also seen.

Ménière attacks typically last from hours to days. After an attack, the patient often feels "foggy" or tired. At first, only one or two symptoms may be present; for example, a patient may note only episodic vertigo or only episodic fluctuating tinnitus. The hallmark is fluctuation. In the early stages, patients are often asymptomatic between attacks. With progression of the disease, low-frequency hearing loss becomes permanent and may progress to involve all frequencies. The tinnitus is usually loud and roaring, resembling the sound of machinery or the ocean. The vertigo is usually severe, a true spinning sensation of the patient or surroundings. Nausea, vomiting, sweating, and pallor are typical, because the vertigo arises peripherally, in the inner ear rather than in the brain. Some describe a linear motion or feel as though they are on a boat. Rarely, the vertigo is noted only with change of position, mimicking benign paroxysmal positional vertigo. It is distinguishable, however, because positional vertigo of Ménière disease occurs in attacks. If the disease is untreated, disequilibrium may persist between attacks of vertigo.

It is believed that most Ménière sufferers are women, which is attributable to hormonal causes of increased water retention. Symptoms may be exacerbated prior to the menstrual cycle.

Typically, the attacks become less frequent and less severe, with or without medical management. Within about two years of diagnosis, more than half of all patients are better, even with no treatment. Medical treatment decreases the frequency and severity of attacks and minimizes permanent hearing loss or disequilibrium. Only 5% of medically treated patients progress to surgery.

About 10% of patients never experience vertigo; their disorder is termed *cochlear Ménière disease*. Another 10% of patients never experience auditory symptoms. The term "burned out Ménière disease" applies to the unusual patient who has totally lost auditory and vestibular function. Finally, there is no loss of consciousness during Ménière attacks; if loss of consciousness is seen, some other neurologic disease is likely. There may be confusion or panic, however, owing to the emotional stress of the attack. A rare entity associated with Ménière disease is referred to as drop attack or crisis of Tumarkin; the patient suddenly drops to the ground. Head injury may ensue.

DIAGNOSIS

Ménière disease is diagnosed clinically; no test has sufficient sensitivity and specificity to be pathognomonic. Tests are used to rule out other disorders and to help confirm the diagnosis.

Careful history and physical examination are therefore essential. Ménière disease should be considered in any patient without other obvious cause who suffers episodic vertigo, hearing loss, tinnitus, or aural fullness. Ménière disease is not diagnosed unless the symptoms have occurred at least twice.

Between attacks, the examination is often normal, especially early in the disease. During an attack, a patient typically appears acutely vertiginous, with horizontal nystagmus beating toward the affected ear. If the nystagmus is vertical, CNS disease should be considered. Later, between attacks, there may be gaze-induced nystagmus toward the unaffected ear.

Tests that help in the diagnosis of Ménière disease include audiometry, electronystagmography (ENG), and MRI. If the symptoms are bilateral, blood tests for autoimmune inner ear disease and infections are ordered, including CBC, ESR, rheumatoid factor, anti-68-kilodalton protein, ANA, anti–double-stranded DNA, Lyme titer, and fluorescent treponemal antigen. Early in the disease, the audiogram is often normal. Later, low-frequency sensorineural hearing loss can develop. Ultimately, hearing loss may also involve high frequencies. Rarely, the audiometric asymmetries may be in the high frequencies rather than the low frequencies. During an attack, there may be a hearing loss in the affected ear, and this may resolve afterward. Often appreciated on audiometric testing is *recruitment*, so called because an increase in intensity of an applied sound is perceived as abnormally loud by the patient. Acoustic reflex decay is not typical; if it is present, cerebellopontine angle pathology is more likely. If conductive hearing loss or abnormal tympanogram is found, other diagnoses, such as cholesteatoma or glomus tumor, should be considered.

ENG should never be performed on an acutely vertiginous patient because the induced vertigo will be intolerable. Early in Ménière disease, the ENG is usually normal because vestibular function recovers between attacks. As the disease progresses, caloric testing often yields a unilateral vestibular weakness in the affected ear. If testing is inadvertently performed during an attack, hyperfunction of the affected ear is usually seen. In end-stage disease, there is complete weakness (100%) in the affected ear. If central pathology rather than peripheral is present, the caloric test results are usually normal. Gaze and positional testing, as well as optokinetic nystagmus testing, are often abnormal.

MRI is recommended for every patient with recurrent vertigo, asymmetric sensorineural hearing loss, or unilateral constant tinnitus. The study should include the brain and internal auditory canals, with and without gadolinium. This test evaluates intracranial pathology such as vestibular Schwannoma, stroke, or demyelination, which can cause these symptoms.

If symptoms begin after age 60, four-vessel neck and transcranial Doppler examinations are performed to evaluate possible cerebrovascular disease. Electrocochleography is helpful in diagnosing Ménière disease. The test demonstrates abnormally high ratios of the summating potential/action potential in Ménière patients; the sensitivity and specificity, however, are not high enough for routine use. Once other causes are excluded, the most accurate way to establish the diagnosis is to determine whether it responds to treatment.

TREATMENT

The treatment of Ménière disease begins with diet and medication. Approximately 85% of patients respond well, with effective decrease in frequency and severity of symptoms. About 5% of patients find that therapy with diet and medication is not sufficient and ultimately turn to surgical management.

Medical Therapy

The standard of care for medical management is a low-sodium diet and diuretic therapy. First, it should be ascertained that it is safe for the patient by consultation with his or her internist. A new patient should be started on a diuretic regimen only between attacks of vertigo. The diet should be a strict 1500 mg/day sodium regimen, and the patient should be informed that this usually requires checking labels carefully. If patients enjoy eating outside the home, it should be in places where they know the exact amount of sodium in their food. Sodium intake should be even with each meal to avoid surges in pressure. Patients are encouraged to drink copious amounts of water to help flush out the sodium and maintain blood pressure. They are advised to avoid caffeine and alcohol, which are thought to aggravate the symptoms. Emotional stress can also aggravate the symptoms of Ménière Disease, and psychiatric consultation may be necessary.

Because sodium levels are hormonally regulated, adding a diuretic is useful to defeat the mechanism. Typically, the patient is started on hydrochlorothiazide 37.5 mg/triamterene 25 mg once daily. This diuretic sheds sodium well and is required only once daily. Triamterene typically protects the potassium level. Electrolyte levels and renal function should be monitored periodically while this diuretic is being taken. Discontinuation or dose adjustment may be required. Patients should be advised that it can take a few weeks before knowing if this regimen is beneficial.

Vestibular suppressants may help control vertigo during attacks. Anticholinergic drugs are useful because they decrease the intrinsic rate of firing in the vestibular nuclei. The author prefers glycopyrrolate 2 mg orally twice per day during attacks. An alternative is meclizine 12.5, 25, or 50 mg orally up to three times daily. Although meclizine is effective, it is also sedating because it has antihistamine properties. Other medications for vestibular suppression are the benzodiazepines. Diazepam 5 mg orally three times daily during attacks can control vertigo, but is also sedating and habit forming. It should be used with caution if the vertigo does not respond to anticholinergic drugs.

In the event of intractable vertigo with nausea and vomiting, an emergency room visit may be necessary. Intravenous hydration should be given, being careful not to overload the patient with sodium. Promethazine 75 mg intramuscularly or droperidol 0.625 mg intravenously are useful for emergencies, but both are heavily sedating.

Surgical Therapy

Surgical treatments for Ménière disease may be destructive or conservative. In all cases, these operations are performed only if symptoms persist despite medical optimization or a patient cannot tolerate medical therapy.

Conservative Procedures

Endolymphatic Shunts

These procedures are designed to decrease the pressure in the endolymphatic compartment by shunting the fluid out of it. Shunts may be internal or external. For internal shunting, a fistula is created to connect the endolymphatic space to the perilymphatic space. Postoperative results are best with cochleosacculotomy: 70% of patients reported control of vertigo, but 25% of patients suffered hearing loss as a result of the procedure, with complete deafness in 10%. The advantage of the procedure is that it can be done quickly in the office, but it is rarely performed because hearing loss occurs so often.

In external shunts, endolymphatic fluid is shunted out of the sac into either the subarachnoid space or the mastoid. Control of vertigo is roughly the same in both procedures. Because the endolymphatic-subarachnoid shunt has higher risk of meningitis and other CNS complications, the endolymphatic-mastoid shunt is the current procedure of choice.

In the past, endolymphatic shunts were controversial. The controversy arose in the 1980s when a Danish group found similar vertigo control in Ménière patients who had undergone endolymphatic shunts to Ménière patients who had undergone only mastoidectomy ("sham procedures"). However, the same data were re-evaluated in 2000 by Welling and Nagaraja. In comparing the shunt group to the sham group, vertigo control was significantly better in the shunt group, nausea and vomiting was significantly less in the shunt group, and tinnitus was significantly less in the shunt group.

Results of this operation vary with each study. In reviewing the literature, Brackmann found vertigo control in 35% to 91% of patients, hearing improvement in 6% to 44%, and tinnitus improvement in 15% to 57%. Complications of shunt procedures are rare and do not differ significantly from those of complete mastoidectomy. Endolymphatic shunt is a reasonable first procedure for patients with good hearing and mild to moderate symptoms.

Vestibular Neurectomy

The vestibular nerve can be separated from the cochlear nerve and sectioned. Although the vestibular nerve is destroyed, this procedure is generally considered a conservative procedure because hearing is preserved. This operation may be performed via the retrosigmoid, retrolabyrinthine, and middle fossa approaches. The risks of craniotomy must be considered, and the indications are more stringent. Patient selection criteria for vestibular neurectomy include episodic disabling vertigo owing to Ménière disease, serviceable hearing in the affected ear, and failure of medical management. Moreover, there must be unilateral vestibular weakness in the affected ear on caloric testing, but not complete. This procedure should not be performed on the side of an only-hearing or significantly better-hearing ear.

The results of vestibular neurectomy are excellent. Vertigo is controlled in 94% of patients. Hearing loss, tinnitus, and fullness in the ear are unaffected, so the patient must continue on low sodium diet and diuretic. Complications of vestibular neurectomy include sensorineural hearing loss in 2% to 3% of patients, CSF leak in 5% to 12%, temporary unsteadiness in up to 25%, headache in 10%, and tinnitus in 7%.

Although the degree of complexity of this operation is much greater than that of an endolymphatic shunt, it remains the gold standard for vertigo control with serviceable hearing. It should be performed in patients with disabling episodic vertigo or in those who have failed shunt surgery.

Destructive Procedures

Labyrinthectomy

In this operation, the vestibular portion of the inner ear is destroyed and all five end organs are removed via the transmastoid approach. Because the hearing in the operated ear is destroyed, this procedure is limited to patients with no serviceable hearing in the affected ear who suffer from episodic, disabling vertigo, and in whom medical management has failed. This is the gold standard for vertigo control in patients with no hearing. Vestibular weak-ness must be shown in the affected ear on caloric testing, but not complete loss of response.

If performed correctly, labyrinthectomy should eradicate attacks of vertigo about 95% of the time. Aside from temporary postoperative unsteadiness in 10% of patients, the risks of this procedure do not differ significantly from those of complete mastoidectomy.

OTHER METHODS OF TREATMENT

Intratympanic Gentamicin

Middle ear perfusion with gentamicin has been used for over a decade; the aminoglycoside preferentially destroys vestibular hair cells over cochlear hair cells. Gentamicin is instilled into the middle ear, which provides a pathway into the inner ear via the round window. Results vary. Vertigo control is about 80%, but there is a significant incidence of sensorineural hearing loss. In one study, it was found that patients given intratympanic gentamicin had a statistically significant decrease in pure tone average and speech discrimination scores, but that patients undergoing vestibular neurectomy did not. Vertigo control was achieved in 80% of patients given gentamicin and in 95% of patients with neurectomy. In another study, 90% of patients had complete initial control of vertigo after gentamicin, but 29% of them had recurrences after 4 months. In a third recent study, 85% of patients had complete control of vertigo from gentamicin perfusion, but hearing was decreased in 25.6%. Gentamicin perfusion is less effective for vertigo control than surgery. The author prefers to use gentamicin only for patients who are too elderly or medically infirm for surgery.

Meniett Device

The Meniett device delivers micropressure pulses to the inner ear via a tympanostomy tube to set up pressure gradients in the endolymphatic compartment via the round window. The device is worn for 5 minutes three times per day. At the time of publication of this book, there is no clear experimental evidence of benefit from this mode of treatment.

Intramuscular Streptomycin

Streptomycin has been banned by the FDA for decades because of its inner ear toxicity. However, it is useful for end-stage patients with bilateral Ménière disease, who still have attacks of vertigo and no hearing. The drug is administered intramuscularly, in regular doses, until caloric responses disappear. The drug eradicates the remaining vestibular function.

SUGGESTED READINGS

Brackmann DE. Surgical treatment of vertigo. *J Laryngol Otol* 1990; 104:849–859.

Gates GA, Green JD. Intermittent pressure therapy of intractable Meniere's disease using Meniett device: a preliminary report. *Laryngoscope* 2002;112:1489–1493.

Hillman TA, Chen DA, Arriaga MA. Vestibular neurectomy vs intratympanic gentamicin for Meniere's disease. *Laryngoscope* 2004;114:216–222.

Kaplan DM, Nedzelski JM, Chen JM, et al. Intratympanic gentamicin for treatment of unilateral Meniere's disease. *Laryngoscope* 2000;110:1298–1305.

Knapp H. A clinical analysis of the inflammatory affections of the inner ear. *Arch Ophthalmol* 1871;2:204–283.

McKenzie KG. Intracranial division of the vestibular portion of the auditory nerve for Meniere's disease. *CMAJ* 1936;34:369–381.

Ménière P. Memoire sur des lesions de l'orielle interne donnant lieu a des symptoms de congestion cerebrale apoplectiforme. *Gaz Med Paris* 1861;16:597–601.

Paparella MM, Hanson DG. Endolymphatic sac drainage for intractable vertigo (method and experiences). *Laryngoscope* 1976;86:697–703.

Parry RH. A case of tinnitus and vertigo treated by division of the auditory nerve. *J Laryngol Otol* 1904;19:402–406.

Portmann G. Vertigo: surgical treatment by opening the saccus endolymphaticus. *Arch Otolaryngol* 1927;6:309–319.

Schuknecht HF. Cochleosacculotomy for Meniere's disease: theory, technique and results. *Laryngoscope* 1982;92:853–858.

Storper IS, Spitzer JB, Scanlan M. Use of glycopyrrolate in the treatment of Ménière's disease. *Laryngoscope* 1998;108:1442–1445.

Thomsen J, Bretlau P, Tos M, et al. Placebo effect in surgery for Meniere's disease. *Arch Otolaryngol* 1981;107:271–277.

Welling DB, Nagaraja HN. Endolymphatic mastoid shunt: a reevaluation of efficacy. *Otolaryngol Head Neck Surg* 2000;122:340–345.

Wu IC, Minor LB. Long term hearing outcome in patients receiving gentamicin for Meniere's disease. *Laryngoscope* 2003;113:815–820.

Chapter 145

▶ Sleep Disorders

June M. Fry and Bradley V. Vaughn

Sleep, as a function of the brain, offers an opportunity to assess neuronal networks that may not be apparent during wakefulness. Understanding of the physiology of sleep and wakefulness has led to the *i*dentification and *c*lassification of a variety of clinical *s*leep *d*isorders (ICSD 2). These disorders highlight abnormalities in the control of sleep–wake determination or the physiology associated with sleep. Classification of these disorders is based on a combination of clinical and polysomnographic features and underscores the importance of accurate diagnostic interpretation to confirm these clinical syndromes objectively.

SLEEP PHYSIOLOGY

Sleep is an active process that involves numerous distinct neuronal networks, which are ultimately expressed as altered physiological functions. Heart rate, blood pressure, gastrointestinal function, and even kidney function are altered in sleep.

Sleep is classified into stages based on three measures: EEG, eye movement, or electrooculography (EOG), and muscle tone as assessed by EMG of the mentalis muscle. Classic sleep stage scoring uses these techniques to divide the process into wakefulness, four stages of non–rapid eye movement (NREM) sleep, and one stage of rapid eye movement (REM) sleep.

Wakefulness is identified by a low fast EEG, high muscle tone, and rapid eye movements. *Stage 1* sleep is characterized by a low-voltage, mixed-frequency EEG and slow, rolling eye movements. Reactivity to outside stimuli is decreased, and mentation may proceed but is no longer reality oriented. *Stage 2* consists of a moderate low-voltage background EEG with sleep spindles (bursts of 12- to 14-Hz activity lasting 0.5 to 2 seconds) and K complexes (brief high-voltage discharges with an initial negative deflection followed by a positive component). *Stage 3* sleep consists of high-amplitude delta (0 to 2 Hz) frequencies occupying 20% to 50% of the background, as well as interspersed K complexes and sleep spindles. *Stage 4* sleep is similar to stage 3, except that high-voltage delta waves make up at least 50% of the EEG. Stages 3 and 4 are often combined and referred to as *delta sleep, slow-wave sleep,* or *deep sleep.* During this deeper sleep, heart and respiratory rates are slowed and regular. In NREM sleep, the tonic chin EMG is of moderately high amplitude but less than that of quiet wakefulness.

The EEG pattern during REM sleep consists of low-voltage, mixed-frequency activity and is similar to that of stage 1 sleep. Moderately high-amplitude, 3- to 6-Hz triangular waveforms referred to as sawtooth waves are intermittently present and are unique to REM sleep. Intermittent bursts of rapid conjugate eye movements occur. Tonic chin EMG activity is absent or markedly reduced, and phasic muscle discharges occur in irregular bursts. The decreased EMG activity is a reflection of muscle paralysis resulting from active inhibition of muscle activity. During REM sleep, surges of parasympathetic and sympathetic activity are denoted by greater variability in heart and respiratory rates. This stage is also associated with complex vivid imagery, but visual imagery can occur in all stages.

During a normal night, sleep comprises recurring cycles. Within each cycle of 80 to 120 minutes, NREM sleep alternates with REM sleep. The normal healthy adult typically falls asleep within 10 minutes and goes through the sequence of stages 1 through 4, followed by reversion to stage 2 sleep. Afterward, the first REM sleep period occurs 70 to 100 minutes into sleep. The first REM period is usually the shortest, about 10 minutes. This pattern of NREM and REM sleep is repeated three to five times. Typically, most stage 3 and stage 4 sleep is seen in the first two sleep cycles, and REM sleep periods increase in duration and intensity of REM activity as the night progresses. Stage 2 sleep, however, is the most common sleep stage, typically making up half of a normal adult's night.

Anatomically, NREM sleep is expressed when a network of neurons in the anterior and posterior hypothalamus, midbrain, and brainstem create the conditions that decrease the metabolic rate of most of the cortex and promote neuronal synchrony through the thalamus. REM sleep, however, is an activation of cholinergic neurons in the pontine dorsal tegmentum that subsequently excite neurons responsible for REM-associated atonia, rapid eye movements, and other features. REM sleep is inhibited by activation of the dorsal raphe and locus ceruleus. A network of neurons in the hypothalamus and thalamus seems to regulate REM sleep cycling while the cortex is metabolically active.

DIAGNOSTIC PROCEDURES

Clinical polysomnography, the simultaneous recording of sleep and multiple physiologic variables, provides objective documentation of sleep disorders. An all-night polysomnogram includes EEG, EOG, mentalis EMG, surface EMG of the anterior tibial muscles for detection of leg movements in sleep, electrocardiogram, and measurement of nasal and oral airflow, respiratory effort, and oxygen saturation. Polysomnographic tracings are analyzed in detail to determine the subject's sleep pattern, including the possible presence of a sleep disorder.

Patients with excessive daytime sleepiness are also evaluated by the multiple sleep latency test (MSLT), a series of four or five nap opportunities with sleep recordings at 2-hour intervals throughout the day. The nap is terminated 15 minutes after sleep onset. If no sleep occurs, each recording session is terminated after 20 minutes. The sleep latency (the time it takes to fall asleep) is determined for each nap and provides an objective measure of daytime sleepiness. Patients with pathologic daytime sleepiness generally fall asleep in less than 5 minutes on all naps. Normally alert individuals take more than 10 minutes to fall asleep or often remain awake. The MSLT is also used to determine the presence of sleep-onset REM periods that characterize narcolepsy and another condition called REM sleep rebound. The Maintenance of Wakefulness Test, similar to the MSLT, measures the time taken before the patient reaches sleep. However, in this test the patient is instructed to remain awake, and the test may provide more information about the patient's ability to sustain wakefulness.

SPECIFIC DISORDERS OF SLEEP

Sleep is a unique function of the CNS. Nearly all patients with neurologic disorders are at high risk for sleep dysfunction, which may be a direct result of or secondary effect of the neurologic condition. Sleep disorders may exacerbate the symptoms of the underlying neurological disorder and impair quality of life. In this chapter, we describe selected disorders.

Disorders with Insomnia

Insomnia is the combination of difficulty initiating or maintaining sleep combined with adverse daytime sequelae. The daytime symptoms include excessive fatigue, impaired performance, or emotional change. Most people have an occasional night fraught with difficulty falling asleep or trouble maintaining sleep. Transient insomnia of occasional nights to less than 3 weeks might be closely linked to the surrounding events, psychological challenges, or sudden changes in medical condition. Surveys have shown that approximately 35% of individuals complain their sleep is disrupted and that a smaller group of approximately 10% have a more persistent insomnia. Chronic insomnia is usually attributed to multiple factors. The factors may be divided into predisposing, precipitating, and perpetuating, which outline the formation of insomnia as an ongoing process. Characteristics that predispose an individual for insomnia are female gender, older age, psychiatric or chronic medical illness, lower socioeconomic status, poor education, obsessive-compulsive nature, poor coping strategies, and "hyperalert" individuals. Insomnia may be initiated by sudden changes in environment or challenges to the body or mind. These challenges may come in the form of acute medical illness, psychological or psychiatric events, shift in schedule, or changes in medications or supplements. After the start of the insomnia, patients adopt behaviors or rituals that perpetuate the insomnia. Patients may use maladaptive habits that occur during the day or night and include heavy caffeine or alcohol use, watching television or playing video games while in bed, or even eating or exercising during the usual sleep period, or they may become dependent on certain somnogenic substances. Some patients actually fear going to bed.

This expectation of poor sleep promotes the apprehension toward sleep and is a predominant feature of psychophysiologic insomnia.

The symptom complex may indicate an underlying disorder related to primary failure of the sleep mechanism or one in which sleep disruption is the byproduct of another disorder. Patients with obstructive sleep apnea, restless legs syndrome, and even narcolepsy can complain of insomnia. Circadian rhythm disorders can also masquerade as complaints of insomnia or excessive sleepiness. Difficulty with the onset of sleep suggests a potential of delayed sleep phase; early morning arousal raises the possibility of advanced sleep phase. Sleep diaries of bedtime and wake time can be useful in determining potential links to schedule or circadian rhythm issues. Perception of good sleep is an important factor in evaluating the complaint of insomnia. Some patients exaggerate their symptoms, whereas other patients may not perceive they are asleep. These individuals display the normal physiologic parameters of sleep, but do not recognize that they have slept. This *sleep misperception state* is one form of the primary insomnias. Another primary insomnia, *idiopathic insomnia*, is associated with no clear inciting factors. These individuals usually have lifelong difficulty of sleep and may have significant family history.

Insomnia may also be a complaint produced by medical or neurologic disorders. Derangement of almost any system in the body can disrupt sleep. Patients with diseases affecting the nervous system, heart, liver, kidneys, gastrointestinal tract, or lungs commonly complain of insomnia. Musculoskeletal discomfort may become worse with periods of rest. Pain from entrapment neuropathies such as carpal tunnel are typically worse at night, and headaches such as cluster headache and pain related to increased intracranial pressure or brain mass lesions can become more intense during sleep. Arthritis and other rheumatologic disorders frequently can disrupt sleep by increasing nighttime pain and stiffness. Nearly all of the psychiatric illnesses have some link to poor sleep. Patients with depression or anxiety disorders may have insomnia years prior to the presentation of the affective component. Although the cause and effect are still in debate, the association is clear. Insomnia may herald the onset of psychosis or mania.

Treatment of insomnia should be directed toward the underlying cause. Therapy for neurologic and psychiatric disorders should be optimized, and a multipronged approach addressing the patient's behaviors, psychological perspectives, and the potential underlying neurochemistry should be constructed. Behavioral therapy consisting of relaxation therapy, stimulus control, sleep hygiene (Table 145.1), and potentially sleep restriction may provide a solid therapeutic foundation. Substances that promote alertness should be minimized when possible, and

▶ **TABLE 145.1 Principles of Sleep Hygiene**

Regulate the sleep–wake cycle
Wake regularly at a fixed time
Regulate the amount of sleep obtained each night
Exercise daily and regularly but not in the late evening
Sleep in a quiet environment
Avoid caffeinated beverages
Avoid alcohol within 3 hours of bedtime
Avoid hypnotic drugs
Do something relaxing before bedtime

additional medicinal therapy should be directed toward a specific disease process.

Disorders of Excessive Somnolence

Sleepiness is defined as the propensity to enter sleep. This is a normal feeling as one approaches a typical sleep period, but excessive sleepiness occurs when one enters sleep at an inappropriate time or setting. Excessive sleepiness can occur in degrees. In mild sleepiness, one might have only limited impairment falling asleep while reading a book. Greater degrees of sleepiness, however, may be associated with bouts of irresistible sleep or sleep attacks that intrude on such activities as driving, having a conversation, or eating meals. This degree of sleepiness places the patient at significant risk for accidents and has a major impact on the person's well-being.

Clinicians should always question their hypersomnic patients for clues of potential sleep debt, sleep disorders, or other medical or psychiatric causes (Table 145.2). Sleep deprivation is the most common cause of sleepiness. Information regarding sleep habits, schedule during the week and weekends, and environment often discloses other important contributing factors. Excessive sleepiness may result from a wide range of medical disorders and medication. Patients with heart, kidney, or liver failure or rheumatologic or endocrinologic disorders such as hypothyroidism and diabetes may note sleepiness and fatigue. Neurologic disorders such as strokes, tumors, demyelinating diseases epilepsy, and head trauma can evoke

▶ **TABLE 145.2 Differential Diagnosis for Excessive Daytime Sleepiness**

Insufficient sleep syndrome
Sleep apnea syndromes
Narcolepsy and other hypersomnias
Drugs, e.g., antidepressants, hypnotics, and antihistamines
Periodic limb movement disorder
Circadian rhythm disorders
Depression

excessive sleepiness. Sleepiness is frequently the cardinal symptom of many sleep disorders (Table 145.2). Patients with sleep apnea and narcolepsy, restless leg syndrome–periodic limb movements, and even parasomnias may note excessive daytime sleepiness as their main complaint.

Sleep-Related Respiratory Disorders

Control of respiration during sleep is an excellent model of state-dependent neuronal regulation. Respiratory patterns vary with sleep stage. Near sleep onset, occasionally individuals will have normal pauses in breathing. Mild periodicity to breathing can be noted in light sleep but on entrance into slow wave sleep, breathing is very regular and response to high CO_2 and low oxygen levels is blunted. During REM sleep, chest musculature is paralyzed and ventilation occurs only via diaphragmatic movement. REM sleep is also characterized by significant variation in respiratory pattern and the least response to high CO_2 levels and low oxygen. Each of these stages allows for the expression of dysfunction in the regulation of breathing during sleep. Some individuals with brain or cardiac pathology may express dramatic periodic breathing or Cheyne-Stokes respiration in light NREM or REM sleep, whereas others who have impairment of ventilation owing to diaphragmatic impairment or impediment will demonstrate hypoventilation during REM sleep. More commonly, individuals may have obstruction of the upper airway during sleep.

Snoring

Snoring is created by turbulent airflow vibrating upper airway soft tissue. Snoring occurs in approximately 32% of adults and over 3% of children and is more prominent during inspiration. Persistent loud snoring is a classic symptom of obstructive sleep apnea syndrome, but the absence of snoring does not exclude the diagnosis. Some patients' airways do not resonate to produce snoring. This is especially true in patients who have had upper airway surgical procedures that tightened tissue. Other individuals may not generate enough force, such as those with neuromuscular disorders. Regardless, individuals who snore have a greater risk of vascular disease and raise the suspicion of obstructive sleep apnea.

Sleep Apnea

Apnea is the absence of ventilation, and on overnight sleep studies this absence of airflow must persist for 10 seconds. *Hyponeas* are defined as the partial reduction of airflow for a similar time. These respiratory events are accompanied by oxygen desaturation and usually by arousals. Apneas and hyponeas are typically more prevalent during light NREM sleep and REM sleep. An all-night polysomnographic recording is used to diagnose, characterize, and quantify sleep apnea.

Historically, bed partners may describe these events as though the breathing has stopped or the patient is holding his or her breath during sleep. These events may be aborted with a loud gasp, snort, body jerks, or the quiet resumption of breathing. Some patients have hundreds of events per night and are unable to obtain quality sleep. These individuals are typically unaware of any sleep disruption but feel unrefreshed in the morning. Patients with neurologic disorders are also at higher risk for sleep apnea. Sleep apnea is more commonly seen in individuals with CNS disease such as epilepsy, strokes, and head trauma and peripheral disease such as muscular dystrophy and myotonic dystrophy. Sleep apnea is classified in two major forms: obstructive and central.

Obstructive apnea is the most common form of sleep apnea. These apneas occur owing to obstruction or collapse of the upper airway. The obstructive sleep apnea syndrome (OSAS) is the cluster of features including snoring, witnessed apneas, excessive daytime sleepiness, insomnia, impairment of daytime performance, headache, irritability, and depression caused by the repetitive apneas. OSAS is frequently seen in individuals with hypertension, diabetes mellitus, and vascular disease. In adults, OSAS occurs predominantly between the fourth and sixth decades and is about 2.5 times more common in men. The prevalence of OSAS increases with age and is higher in individuals with habitual snoring and obesity. Many patients are obese, yet some have normal body habitus. Common structural abnormalities such as narrow nasal passage, long soft palate, large tonsils, or retroflexed mandible leading to a small airway contribute to airway obstruction.

OSAS also evokes higher risk for development of vascular disease. Recognized systemic complications of OSAS are systemic hypertension, pulmonary hypertension, diabetes mellitus, cardiac enlargement, myocardial infarction, stroke, elevated hematocrit, and an increased risk of sudden death during sleep.

Sleep apnea also occurs in infants and children. In infants, it has been associated with the "acute life-threatening event," as well as familial, congenital, and acquired dysautonomia syndromes and craniofacial disorders. Differential from normal periodic breathing is critical in infants. The peak incidence in children is around age 4 years and is often associated with adenotonsillar hypertrophy. Daytime sequelae of hyperactivity, poor school performance, behavior problems, and limited growth have been documented.

Central apnea is the absence of ventilation owing to an absence of any swings in the intrathoracic pressure. Central apneas cause complaints of frequent awakenings and restless unrefreshing sleep. These respiratory events can be caused by neurologic abnormalities involving respiratory regulatory neuronal networks. Apneas may also follow neurologic events such as nocturnal seizures or acute strokes. One form of periodic breathing, Cheyne-Stokes breathing, can have features of both central and obstructive apnea. This classic pattern is seen in individuals with heart failure, neurologic lesions, and metabolic or toxic encephalopathies. Patients with central apnea need a complete cardiac and neurologic examination.

Treatment for sleep apnea consists primarily of methods of promoting airway patency for obstructive apnea and stimulation of breathing in central apnea. For both forms of apneas, nasal continuous positive airway pressure (CPAP) is the most common and effective treatment. Constant air pressure is generated by a small pump and delivered via tubing to a nasal mask. Each patient must have a treatment trial during polysomnography to determine the pressure required to alleviate airway obstruction during sleep. The pressure for inspiration and expiration can be altered to maximize each breath, using a bilevel positive airway pressure device. In some patients, especially children and young adults, the removal of enlarged tonsils and adenoids relieves the obstruction. The surgical procedure, uvulopalatopharyngoplasty, has been an inconsistently beneficial treatment, and selection criteria are not well established. Genioglossal and mandibular advancement have successfully treated patients with structural abnormalities causing hypopharyngeal obstruction. Other treatments for less severe cases have been sustained weight loss in obese patients and use during sleep of an oral appliance that advances the lower jaw.

Alveolar hypoventilation syndrome, a cause of sleep disruption, is associated with major changes in respiratory function during sleep. In this disorder, patients fail to ventilate adequately, especially during REM sleep, which is associated with recurrent hypoxemia, hypercapnia, and a decreased tidal and minute volume. This syndrome may be idiopathic or associated with other disorders; these include chronic residual poliomyelitis, muscle diseases (e.g., muscular dystrophy, anterior horn cell disease), involvement of thoracic cage bellows action or diaphragmatic muscle weakness, cervical spinal cordotomy, brainstem lesions of structures that control ventilation, dysautonomia syndromes, and massive obesity.

Movement in Sleep

Restless Legs Syndrome and Periodic Limb Movement Disorder

In the *restless legs syndrome* (RLS), the patient feels an irresistible urge to move the legs, especially when sitting or lying down. Patients may complain of unpleasant crawling, deep aching sensation in the legs or arms, which causes the need for them to walk or have continuous movement of their limbs. Some patients note that their legs move involuntarily. The symptoms are worse in the evening, usually interfering with sleep onset, and cause insomnia. Diagnostic criteria focusing on the main symptoms have been established. Patients with RLS may relay that the discomfort can be debilitating at times and even drive some individuals to pursue extreme measures to decrease the symptoms.

Periodic limb movements in sleep (PLMS) are found in most patients with RLS who are studied with polysomnography. Patients or their bed partner may complain of leg or arm movements during sleep. These movements may occur as periodic events or appear random. PLMS are repetitive stereotyped movements of any of the extremities. These most commonly occur in NREM sleep and activate the lower extremities as extension of the great toe with dorsiflexion of the ankle and flexion of the knee and hip. Movements can also occur in the arms and axial muscles. The individual movements are relatively brief, lasting 0.5 to 4.0 seconds, occur at 20- to 120-second intervals, and may continue for minutes to hours. Limb movements may be accompanied by an arousal or awakening. In contrast to most movement disorders, which are diminished by sleep (e.g., cerebellar and extrapyramidal tremors, chorea, dystonia, hemiballism), PLMS are initiated by sleep or drowsiness. They are also different from *hypnic jerks* (sleep starts), which are nonperiodic, isolated myoclonic movements that occur at sleep onset and simultaneously involve the muscles of the trunk and extremities. Hypnic jerks are considered normal.

Some patients with periodic movements of sleep complain of disturbed sleep or daytime sleepiness. The severity of symptoms appears to be related to the frequency of limb movements and associated arousals and awakenings. Similar factors that provoke periodic limb movements increase the likelihood of RLS. Periodic movements of sleep have been associated with uremia, peripheral vascular disease, anemia, arthritis, peripheral neuropathy, spinal cord lesions, antidepressants, and caffeine use.

Investigation of idiopathic RLS has found that in some individuals the deficit may be low iron stores in the posterior hypothalamus. Some familial cases are related to deficiencies in iron transporter proteins.

Treatment for these individuals should be tailored to improving their symptoms. After confirmation that other sleep disorders have been excluded, patients may be treated with one of three classes of medication. Dopamine agonists such as ropinirole, pramipexole, and pergolide have been used most commonly, and the doses required are very much smaller than those used for Parkinson disease. Levodopa plus benzerazide or carbidopa is effective, but patients often experience increased or rebound daytime symptoms when treated only at night; thus this agent is not used frequently. Additionally, gabapentin has proved useful in treating the discomfort and movement at night. Other anticonvulsants such as carbamazepine, zonisamide, and topiramate have been reported to reduce the symptoms, and benzodiazepines such as clonazepam or temazepam may be beneficial. For those individuals who have low iron, iron supplementation should be considered. Opiates are also useful, especially in severe cases.

Dysfunction in the Control of Sleep
Narcolepsy

Narcolepsy is an incurable lifelong neurologic disorder characterized by the tetrad of (1) excessive daytime sleepiness, (2) cataplexy, (3) sleep paralysis, and (4) hypnagogic hallucinations. Estimates of prevalence range between 2 and 10 per 10,000 individuals in North America and Europe. It is about five times more prevalent in Japan, and the incidence is only 1 per 500,000 in Israel. The symptoms of narcolepsy typically present between ages 12 and 30 years, although cases have been reported with onset as early as age 2 years and as late as 76 years. Men and women are equally affected. Recognition that the patient has a medical disorder often takes years.

Narcolepsy is a prototype disorder of loss of control of sleep–wake determination. Patients have bouts of irresistible sleep and frequent arousals during sleep, with episodes of partial intrusion of REM sleep into wakefulness. This last point is most evident in the presence of the symptoms of cataplexy, sleep paralysis, and hypnagogic hallucinations. Each of these symptoms is a portion of REM sleep intruding into wakefulness.

Daytime sleepiness is usually the first and most prominent symptom to appear, but hyperactivity may present in children as attempts to fight off sleep. Patients often complain of attacks of irresistible sleep that occur at inappropriate times, such as during conversation, driving, and eating. Brief naps for some are refreshing. More than 50% of narcoleptic patients have automatic behavior that they describe as memory lapses or blackouts. These episodes are caused by intrusion of sleep into wakefulness. Patients carry out semipurposeful activity but are amnestic for the activity. Patients may recount stories of putting milk containers in the oven, typing or writing gibberish, or even missing an exit on the highway. Automatic behavior also occurs in other disorders of excessive sleepiness. The symptom of excessive daytime sleepiness is disabling and often leads to personal, social, and economic problems.

Cataplexy is the abrupt onset of paralysis or weakness of voluntary muscles without change in consciousness; it is precipitated by strong emotions. Events can be triggered by a joke, surprise, anger, fear, or athletic endeavors. These events last seconds to minutes and patients have clear memory for the complete event with no postictal confusion or deficits. Longer events may be ended with the patient entering sleep. The severity of cataplexy is variable. Some patients may have as few as two or three episodes in a lifetime, whereas others may have several episodes every day. A full range of severity exists between these extremes. Cataplexy may be partial and affect only certain muscles; common examples include dysarthria, drooping of the head, and slight buckling of the knees. Severe global attacks affect all skeletal muscles except muscles of respiration and cause collapse. Examination of the patient during the cataleptic attack will demonstrate paralysis with diffuse hypotonia, absence of deep tendon reflexes, diminished corneal reflexes, preserved pupillary responses, and phasic muscle twitching. Phasic muscle twitching can occur as single jerks or repetitive muscle twitching and is most frequently seen in the face. Most episodes last only seconds, but severe attacks can last minutes.

The combination of excessive daytime sleepiness and cataplexy is nearly always related to narcolepsy. Cataplexy can rarely be seen as an isolated symptom, suggesting an underlying neurologic disorder. The historical feature of clear emotional triggers differentiates cataplexy from vertebral basilar insufficiency and the group of neuromuscular disorders known to produce periodic paralysis.

Sleep paralysis is a global paralysis of voluntary muscles that occurs at the entry into or emergence from sleep. These events may include the feeling of being chased or impending danger. The terror associated with the events can be recounted by patients years later. The events are aborted with a simple touch. The paralysis associated with the event is thought to result from the same motor inhibition that occurs in REM sleep. Sleep paralysis without narcolepsy can occur in an isolated form in sleep-deprived healthy individuals but is also frequently seen in patients with depression.

Hypnagogic hallucinations are vivid dreamlike images that occur during sleep onset or hypnopompic when occurring at sleep offset. They may be simple to complex visual, auditory, or tactile hallucinations. Patients are usually aware of their surroundings and may have difficulty in discerning the hallucinations from reality. The hallucinations can be relatively pleasant or terrifying. Patients may note a feeling of weightlessness, falling, or flying, or have out-of-body–like experiences that may sometimes terminate with a sudden jerk (hypnic jerk). Hypnagogic hallucinations are most likely the result of dissociated CNS processes involved in dreaming during REM sleep. They can be precipitated by sleep deprivation, medications, and alcohol in normal individuals.

Narcolepsy symptoms produce major social, familial, educational, and economic consequences for both the patient and the family. Patients often do not achieve their intellectual potential and suffer frequent failures of occupation, education, and marriage. Family members, friends, and even patients often interpret the symptoms as indicating laziness, lack of ambition, delayed maturation, or psychologic defects. Because these symptoms begin during the crucial period of maturation from puberty to adulthood, misinterpretation and lack of a diagnosis can greatly affect a patient's personality and feelings of self-esteem.

Genetic linkage research shows a gene candidate in the region of the major histocompatibility complex *DQB1 * 602*. Genetic family studies suggest that this gene is not sufficient itself to produce narcolepsy and that an additional gene or genes may be needed for disease expression. Identification of the hypocretin-orexin gene and receptors in mouse models and humans revealed that narcolepsy with cataplexy is caused by loss of hypocretin-orexin–producing neurons in the lateral hypothalamus. Hypocretin-orexin in the CSF is found low in patients with cataplexy. Brains from narcolepsy patients show an absence of hypocretin-orexin–producing neurons.

The current treatment for the sleepiness of narcolepsy is the use of stimulant drugs: modafinil, methylphenidate hydrochloride, and amphetamines. Modafinil, a wakefulness-promoting agent that is chemically and pharmacologically distinct from the amphetamine stimulants, has been shown to be effective in reducing daytime sleepiness in patients with narcolepsy. Use of stimulant drugs should be carefully monitored; patients and physicians should cooperate in adjusting the amount and timing of doses to meet functional daytime needs and scheduling of patients' activities. Cataplexy, when present to a significant degree, is usually well controlled with the serotonin reuptake blockers (paroxetine hydrochloride or fluoxetine hydrochloride) and tricyclic compounds (imipramine hydrochloride, protriptyline hydrochloride, or clomipramine); however, impotence can be an undesirable side effect in men. These medications are thought to treat cataplexy effectively because they suppress REM sleep. γ-Hydroxybutyrate is used for cataplexy; it is given at bedtime and during the night to improve sleep and reduce the frequency and severity of cataplexy. An important adjunctive treatment for narcolepsy is the rational scheduling of daytime naps and the maintenance of proper sleep hygiene. The physician's role in providing the patient with a clear understanding of the nature of the symptoms and with emotional support in coping with the many adaptive difficulties cannot be overemphasized.

Recurrent hypersomnia (*Kleine-Levin syndrome*) consists of recurrent episodes of hypersomnia and binge eating lasting up to several weeks, with an interval of 2 to 12 months between episodes. Neurobehavioral and psychologic changes, such as disorientation, automatic behavior, forgetfulness, depression, depersonalization, hallucinations, irritability, aggression, and sexual hyperactivity, often accompany the episodes of hypersomnia. Onset is typically in early adolescent boys and less common in girls. Episodes decrease in frequency and severity with age and are rarely present after the fourth decade. A definitive treatment for Kleine-Levin syndrome is not known, but there are reports of limited success with stimulant and antidepressant therapy.

Disorders of the Sleep–Wake Schedule

Throughout the 24-hour day, the human body has a symphony of endocrinologic and metabolic variations that are timed to maximize performance during wakefulness and promote quality rejuvenation during sleep. Our evolutionary development on a planet that rotates every 24 hours has led to a delicate neurochemistry cycle that prepares the body for the upcoming sleep–wake state. These circadian cycles are approximately 1 day as captured in the Greek meaning of *circa dian*. Many body functions, including body temperature, plasma and urine hormones, renal functions, psychologic performance measures, and internal sleep-stage organization, participate in this circadian rhythm. Humans have a circadian rhythm that is approximately 24.3 hours and is driven by the suprachiasmatic nucleus. This nucleus is influenced by external time clues to synchronize the body clock with the outside world, including bright light, activity, meals, and social interactions. Evidence for the importance of circadian rhythms comes from studies of acute phase shifts, such as those that occur after jet lag or shift work. Because our internal clock is longer than 24 hours, adaptation is slower after an eastward flight (phase advance) in the laboratory than after a westward flight (phase delay).

Disorders of the circadian sleep–wake cycle are divided into two major categories, transient and persistent. The *transient disorders* include the temporary sleep disturbance following an acute work-shift change and a rapid time-zone change (jet lag). Both sleep deprivation and the circadian phase shift produce symptoms including insomnia, disrupted sleep, and excessive sleepiness. *Persistent* sleep–wake cycle disorders are divided into several major clinical categories. Persons who frequently change their sleep–wake schedule (e.g., shift workers) have a mixed pattern of excessive sleepiness alternating with arousal at inappropriate times of the day or have minimal circadian pattern. Sleep is typically short and disrupted. Waking is associated with a decrease in performance and vigilance. This syndrome often disrupts social and family life.

The *delayed-sleep-phase syndrome* is a specific chronobiologic sleep disorder characterized by going to bed late and waking up late in the morning. Patients are typically unable to fall asleep earlier and go to sleep between 1 and 6 AM. On weekends and vacation days, they sleep until late morning or early afternoon and feel refreshed, but have great difficulty awakening at the required 7 or 8 AM for work or school. These patients have a normal sleep length and internal organization of sleep when clock time of sleep onset and sleep offset coincides with the circadian timing that controls daily sleep.

Successful treatment has been a phase shift of the time of the daily sleep episode by progressive phase delay of the sleep time. By delaying the time of going to sleep and awakening by 2 or 3 hours each day (i.e., a 26- or 27-hour sleep–wake cycle), the patient's sleep timing can be successfully reset to the preferred clock time. Additionally, treatment with bright light and exercise in the morning may help shift the circadian rhythm to a desired schedule.

The *advanced-sleep-phase syndrome* is a condition in which individuals go to bed early in the evening and wake early in the morning. Typical sleep onset is between 6 and 8 PM, with wake times between 1 and 3 PM despite efforts to delay sleep time. This is more likely to occur in elderly persons. Treatment of bright light and mild activity in the evening may help delay the bedtime.

The patient with the *non-24-hour sleep–wake disorder* is completely out of touch with the 24-hour cycle of the rest of society. These rare individuals maintain a 25- to 27-hour biologic day despite all attempts to entrain themselves to a 24-hour cycle. This is in contrast to a person with an *irregular sleep–wake pattern* consisting of considerable irregularity without an identifiable persistent sleep–wake rhythm. There are frequent daytime naps at irregular times and a disturbed nocturnal sleep pattern. A personality disorder or blindness may predispose to this condition. However, most patients with this syndrome have congenital, developmental, or degenerative brain dysfunction, although it does occur rarely in cognitively intact patients. Treatment is difficult but should include regularly scheduled activities and time in bed based on sleep hygiene principles.

Parasomnias

Parasomnias are undesirable physical or behavioral phenomena that occur predominantly during sleep. They include disorders of arousals, such as sleepwalking or night terrors; sleep–wake transition disorders, such as sleep talking, rhythmic movement disorder (e.g., head banging); and REM parasomnias, such as REM sleep behavior disorder. These behavioral events may mimic epileptic seizures or other psychiatric events. Key features of age of onset, time of night of the events, stereotypic behavior, memory for the events, and family history are important in historically distinguishing the etiologies. Although historical features can be useful in distinguishing these disorders, most patients require polysomnographic recording to delineate the cause or other potential sleep disorders provoking the parasomnia.

The classic disorders of arousal include *sleepwalking* and *sleep terrors*, as well as the more recently designated disorder *confusional arousals*. These behaviors are more common in children and are characterized as events occurring as partial arousals from the deeper stages of NREM sleep. These patients are caught in a transition of part of the brain in NREM sleep and another portion in wake. Typically, patients have no memory for the events and the events are not stereotypic. Sleepwalking usually involves a series of complex behaviors, such as sitting up in bed, walking, opening and closing doors, opening a window, climbing stairs, dressing, and even preparing food. Sleep terrors, however, start with a piercing scream or fright with significant sympathetic nervous system output. Patients have tachycardia, pupillary dilation, and sweating and appear wide-eyed and inconsolable. A subgroup of patients may be harmful to themselves or others, such as breaking furniture, throwing objects, and climbing out or walking through a window. These events usually emerge from slow-wave sleep during the first third of the night. Confusional arousals occur following sudden awakening and may be accompanied with disorientation and the patient striking out. These disorders frequently are provoked by other sleep disorders such as obstructive sleep apnea, and thus these patients should be considered for polysomnography. A small nightly dose of a benzodiazepine, such as clonazepam or temazepam, is useful, especially when potential exists for the patient or bed partner to be injured.

REM sleep behavior disorder (RBD), a REM sleep–related parasomnia, is characterized by intermittent loss of REM sleep atonia with dream enactment. Patients usually have clear recall of the dream, and witnesses can relate the activity to the dream mentation. Events are more likely to occur in the later half of the night and do not have stereotypic behavior. Injury to self or bed partner is common. The prevalence of RBD is unknown but appears to be more common in older men and may be a precursor to select degenerative neurologic disorders such as Parkinson disease, multisystem atrophy, or Lewy body dementia. Patients may also develop RBD from structural lesions affecting the REM atonia pathway. Medications such as serotonin reuptake blockers and norepinephrine reuptake blockers have been cited to provoke RBD. The diagnosis is usually suggested by history and confirmed by polysomnography. Recordings show persistent muscle tone and complex behaviors during REM sleep. Most patients respond to clonazepam at bedtime, but success has been reported with melatonin and donepezil.

Sleep Disorders Associated with Neurologic Disorders

Nearly every CNS process has been associated with disruption of sleep. The ubiquity of sleep and the brain makes this dynamic relationship even more important. Sleep may be abnormal because of involvement of brain structures that control and regulate sleep and wakefulness or because of abnormal movements or behaviors that occur during sleep. Additionally, the loss of sleep provokes further dysfunction of the brain. For example, patients with epilepsy have fewer seizures once treated for their sleep disorder. As neurologists, we must be keenly aware that sleep provides another dimension of diagnostic and therapeutic avenues for diseases of the nervous system.

Fatal familial insomnia, a prion disease, is discussed in Chapter 34.

SUGGESTED READINGS

Aharon-Peretz J, Masiah A, Pillar T, et al. Sleep-wake cycles in multi-infarct dementia and dementia of the Alzheimer type. *Neurology* 1991;41:1616–1619.

American Academy of Sleep Medicine. *The International Classification of Sleep Disorders: Diagnostic and Coding Manual* (ICSD2). Rev. Ed. Chicago: American Academy of Sleep Medicine, 2005.

Billiard M. Idiopathic hypersomnia. *Neurol Clin* 1996;14:573–582.

Boeve BF, Silber MH, Parisi JE, et al. Synucleinopathy pathology and REM sleep behavior disorder plus dementia or parkinsonism. *Neurology* 2003;61(Jul 8):40–405.

Bresnitz EA, Goldberg R, Kosinski RM. Epidemiology of obstructive sleep apnea. *Epidemiol Rev* 1994;16:210–227.

Chen S, Ondo WG, Rao S, et al. Genomewide linkage scan identifies a novel susceptibility locus for restless legs syndrome on chromosome 9p. *Am J Hum Genet* 2004;74:876–85.

Chesson A Jr, Hartse K, Anderson WM, et al. Practice parameters for the evaluation of chronic insomnia. An American Academy of Sleep Medicine report. Standards of Practice Committee of the American Academy of Sleep Medicine. *Sleep* 2000;23:237–241.

Chesson AL Jr, Ferber RA, Fry JM, et al. The indications for polysomnography and related procedures. *Sleep* 1997;20:423–487.

Chesson AL Jr, Wise M, Davila D, et al. Practice parameters for the treatment of restless legs syndrome and periodic limb movement disorder. An American Academy of Sleep Medicine Report. Standards of Practice Committee of the American Academy of Sleep Medicine. *Sleep* 1999;22:961–968.

Coleman R, Pollak CP, Weitzman ED. Periodic movements in sleep (nocturnal myoclonus): relation to sleep disorders. *Ann Neurol* 1980;8:416–421.

Connor JR, Boyer PJ, Menzies SL, et al. Neuropathological examination suggests impaired brain iron acquisition in restless legs syndrome. *Neurology* 2003;61:304–309.

Feber R. Childhood sleep disorders. *Neurol Clin* 1996;14:493–511.

Fry JM. Restless legs syndrome and periodic leg movements in sleep exacerbated or caused by minimal iron deficiency. *Neurology* 1986;36(Suppl 1):276.

Fry JM, ed. Current issues in the diagnosis of and management of narcolepsy. *Neurology* 1998;50:(Suppl 1).

Hla KM, Young TB, Bidwell T, et al. Sleep apnea and hypertension: a population study. *Ann Intern Med* 1994;120:382–388.

Kryger MH, Roth T, Dement WC, eds. *Principles and Practice of Sleep Medicine* 3rd Ed. Philadelphia: WB Saunders, 2000.

Littner M, Hirshkowitz M, Kramer M, et al; American Academy of Sleep Medicine; Standards of Practice Committee. Practice parameters for using polysomnography to evaluate insomnia: an update. *Sleep* 2003;26:754–760.

Mahowald MW, Schenck CH. NREM sleep parasomnias. *Neurol Clin* 1996;14:675–696.

Martin TJ, Sanders MH. Chronic alveolar hypoventilation: a review for the clinician. *Sleep* 1995;18:617–634.

Mignot E, Lammers GJ, Ripley B, et al. The role of cerebrospinal fluid hypocretin measurement in the diagnosis of narcolepsy and other hypersomnias. *Arch Neurol* 2002;59:1553–1562.

Obermeyer WH, Benca RM. Effects of drugs on sleep. *Neurol Clin* 1996;14:827–840.

Prinz PN. Sleep and sleep disorders in older adults. *J Clin Neurophysiol* 1995;12:139–145.

Randomized trial of modafinil for the treatment of pathological somnolence in narcolepsy. US Modafinil in Narcolepsy Multicenter Study Group. *Ann Neurol* 1998;43:88–97.

Richardson GS, Malin HV. Circadian rhythm sleep disorders: pathophysiology and treatment. *J Clin Neurophysiol* 1996;13:17–31.

Rosenthal NE, Joseph-Vanderpool JR, Levendosky AA, et al. Phase-shifting effect of bright morning light as treatment for delayed sleep-phase syndrome. *Sleep* 1990;13:354–361.

Schenck CH, Mahowald MW. REM sleep parasomnias. *Neurol Clin* 1996;14:697–720.

Schmidt-Nowara W, Lowe A, Wiegand L, et al. Oral applications for the treatment of snoring and obstructive sleep apnea: a review. *Sleep* 1995;18:501–510.

Shamsuzzaman AS, Gersh BJ, Somers VK. Obstructive sleep apnea: implications for cardiac and vascular disease. *JAMA* 2003;290:1906–1914.

Spielman AJ, Nunes J, Glovinsky PB. Insomnia. *Neurol Clin* 1996;14:513–543.

Srollo PJ, Rogers RM. Obstructive sleep apnea. *N Engl J Med* 1996;334:99–104.

Thorpy MJ, Westbrook P, Ferber R, et al. The clinical use of the Multiple Sleep Latency Test. *Sleep* 1992;15:268–276.

Weitzman ED, Czeisler CA, Zimmerman JC, et al. Biological rhythms in man: relationship of sleep-wake, cortisol, growth hormone and temperature during temporal isolation. In: Martin JB, Reichlin S, Bick K, eds. *Neurosecretion and Brain Peptides.* New York: Raven, 1981:475–499.

Wise MS. Narcolepsy and other disorders of excessive sleepiness. *Med Clin No Am* 2004;88:597–610.

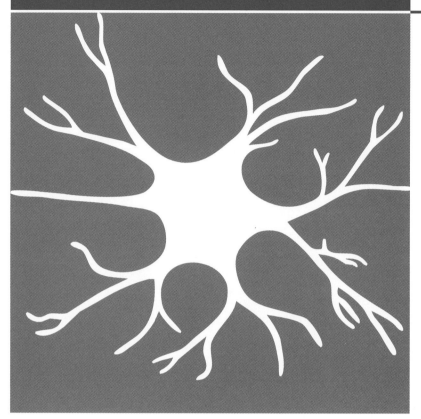

Systemic Diseases and General Medicine

Endocrine Diseases

Gary M. Abrams and Earl A. Zimmerman

Endocrine secretions have a profound influence on the metabolism of the nervous system. Disturbances of consciousness and cognition, along with other neurologic symptoms, may occur with endocrine diseases. This chapter considers the common structural and secretory endocrine disorders that may cause important neurologic symptoms.

PITUITARY

Hypopituitarism

Hypofunction of the pituitary may follow damage to the gland by tumors, inflammatory processes, vascular lesions, or trauma. The location of the lesion may be the pituitary itself, the stalk that connects it with the hypothalamus, or the hypothalamus. Destruction of the hypophyseal portal system in the stalk or the median eminence above by a tumor, such as a craniopharyngioma, or sarcoidosis deprives the anterior pituitary of hypothalamic regulatory hormones. In hypothalamic disease, as in pituitary disease, peripheral blood levels of all the anterior pituitary hormones may be reduced except for prolactin (PRL), which is normally under inhibitory control by hypothalamic dopamine. Undetectable PRL is associated with severe anterior pituitary failure. Diabetes insipidus (DI) (see later), which may result from disruption of neurosecretory pathways terminating in the posterior pituitary, is also a feature of some structural diseases causing hypopituitarism. Additionally, neurologic manifestations of hypopituitarism are owing to "neighborhood effects" resulting from the contiguous location of the pituitary to

the visual pathways and cranial nerves controlling ocular motility.

Secretory and nonsecretory pituitary tumors are the most common causes of neurologic symptoms of hypopituitarism. The size of the lesion usually determines the extent of neurologic symptoms and the degree of hypopituitarism. Headache and visual loss are common when tumors are large and extend into the suprasellar region in the vicinity of the optic chiasm. Lateral extension of masses may produce syndromes involving structures in the cavernous sinus. Growth of tumors superiorly may compress the hypothalamus and obstruct the CSF pathways to cause hydrocephalus.

Vascular lesions of the pituitary may cause dramatic and life-threatening onset of hypopituitarism. In *pituitary apoplexy,* sudden hemorrhage into a pituitary tumor may cause headache, meningismus, visual loss, oculomotor abnormalities, and alteration in the level of consciousness. Hypopituitarism, including acute adrenal insufficiency, may result from a combination of vascular necrosis and compression by the enlarging pituitary mass. Neurosurgical decompression can improve neurologic and endocrine function.

Sheehan syndrome or postpartum necrosis of the pituitary may also cause acute hypopituitarism and local neurologic symptoms. Hypotension or shock from obstetric hemorrhage or infection causes occlusive spasm of pituitary arteries with anoxic–ischemic necrosis of a pituitary gland that has hypertrophied under estrogen stimulation from pregnancy. Acutely, there may be a shocklike syndrome with obtundation, hypotension, tachycardia, and hypoglycemia. Acute and chronic Sheehan syndromes are both characterized by syndromes of anterior pituitary insufficiency, particularly amenorrhea and failure to lactate. Rarely, DI occurs. A neurologic disorder might be suspected if patients complain of lightheadedness or diminished libido.

In adults, hypopituitarism is often recognized first by impaired secretion of gonadotropins with irregular menstrual periods or amenorrhea in women or loss of libido, potency, or fertility in men. The skin is often thin, smooth, and dry; the peculiar pallor (alabaster skin) and inability to tan have been related to loss of melanotropic (melanocyte-stimulating hormone) or adrenocorticotropic (ACTH) hormones. Axillary and pubic hair may be sparse, with relatively infrequent facial shaving. Depending on the severity of the decrease of production of ACTH and thyroid-stimulating hormone (TSH), patients may note lethargy, weakness, fatigability, cold intolerance, and constipation. There may be an acute adrenal crisis with nausea, vomiting, hypoglycemia, hypotension, and circulatory collapse, particularly in response to stress. Hypothalamic hypopituitarism may additionally be accompanied by hyperprolactinemia with galactorrhea.

Evaluation of patients with pituitary insufficiency caused by an intrasellar or hypothalamic lesion depends on measurement of pituitary hormone levels in the peripheral blood, coupled with functional assessment of the target organs. The basic endocrine evaluation includes thyroid functions (tri-iodothyronine [T_3], thyroxine [T_4], and TSH), PRL determination, and assessment of adrenal reserve, such as ACTH stimulation for cortisol responsiveness. Pituitary hormone levels must be interpreted in the context of clinical findings. For example, normal gonadotropin levels (follicle-stimulating hormone, luteinizing hormone) may indicate pituitary insufficiency after menopause, when elevated levels would be expected. Elevated levels of gonadotropin or TSH suggest primary gonadal or thyroid failure but, rarely, may be secreted by pituitary tumors. Dynamic tests of pituitary reserve or stimulation tests with synthetic hypothalamic releasing factors are sometimes needed to detect mild hypopituitarism or to distinguish between pituitary and hypothalamic causes of hypopituitarism.

Pituitary Tumors

Most pituitary tumors are associated with oversecretion of one or more anterior pituitary hormones or their subunits. These tumors produce symptoms related to the metabolic or trophic effect of the secreted hormone. Symptoms may be associated with variable degrees of hypopituitarism, depending on the extent of destruction caused by the tumor. Microadenomas (less than 10 mm) typically cause only symptoms referable to the secreted hormone; macroadenomas (greater than 10 mm) more often cause neural or pituitary dysfunction. Fewer than 10% of microadenomas that secrete PRL show progressive enlargement.

The PRL-secreting adenoma, or *prolactinoma*, is the most common secretory adenoma of the pituitary. It is the most common cause of clinically manifest hyperprolactinemia. In women, there is often a microadenoma with amenorrhea and galactorrhea. In men, the endocrine effects of hyperprolactinemia include impotence, infertility, or, rarely, galactorrhea. In men, prolactinoma is more commonly associated with mass effects of the macroadenoma: headaches, visual-field deficits, and ocular motility problems.

The causes of hyperprolactinemia are listed in Table 146.1. In prolactinoma, serum PRL levels may be <200 μg

> **TABLE 146.1 Causes of Elevated Prolactin Levels**

Normal	Drugs	Diseases
Sleep	Phenothiazines	Pituitary adenoma
Stress	Butyrophenones	Pituitary stalk section
Exercise	Benzamides	Hypothalamic diseases
Coitus	Reserpine	Sarcoidosis
Nipple	Methyldopa	Tumors (e.g.,
stimulation	Morphine	craniopharyngioma)
Pregnancy	Thyrotropin-releasing	Histiocytosis X
Nursing	hormone	Primary hypothyroidism
	Estrogens	Renal failure
		Partial seizures

per liter and must be distinguished from other causes of hyperprolactinemia. Values >200 μg per liter, however, are nearly always associated with a prolactinoma. There is a rough positive correlation between the PRL level and the size of the tumor. Several random PRL levels of >200 μg per liter establish the diagnosis of prolactinoma; more modest elevations may be caused by drugs, hypothalamic disorders, or hypothyroidism (Table 146.1). In primary hypothyroidism, thyrotropin-releasing hormone (TRH) secretion is presumably enhanced in response to the low circulating levels of thyroid hormone; TRH is a potent stimulus for PRL release. The pituitary may be enlarged (Fig. 146.1).

CT or MRI establishes the diagnosis of a sellar or parasellar mass. Prolactinoma does not have specific imaging characteristics; the diagnosis is established by correlation with clinical and laboratory findings. Important diagnostic considerations include carotid aneurysm, inflammatory (e.g., lymphocytic hypophysitis) and hormonal causes of pituitary enlargement (e.g., primary hypothyroidism), and craniopharyngioma.

Treatment of hyperprolactinemia is accomplished with the dopaminergic agonists bromocriptine or cabergoline, which usually reduce serum PRL levels to normal, but treatment of the primary pathology with thyroid hormone replacement is used if the cause is primary hypothyroidism. Return of PRL levels to normal is usually associated with restoration of gonadal function and cessation of galactorrhea. In patients with a prolactinoma, bromocriptine or cabergoline therapy is often accompanied by reduction of tumor size, resolution of neurologic symptoms, and reversal of pituitary insufficiency. Long-term therapy may be required because the tumor may recur when bromocriptine or cabergoline is withdrawn, particularly in the case of macroadenoma. Microadenoma is usually treated with dopamine agonists, particularly bromocriptine if pregnancy is expected. If the drug is not tolerated, the condition is generally cured by trans-sphenoidal adenomectomy. Macroadenomas within the sella can be treated with the dopaminergic drugs, but suprasellar extension requires

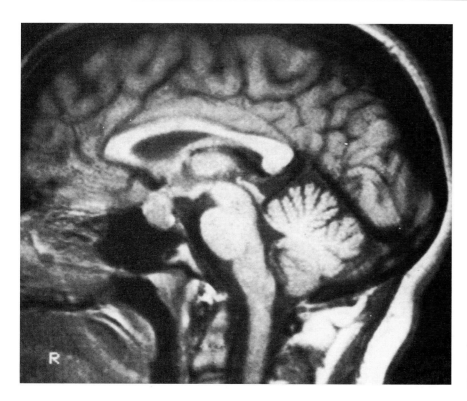

FIGURE 146.1. Pituitary enlargement in association with primary hypothyroidism is shown on MRI.

surgery. "Cure" rates are correlated with tumor size and PRL level, but surgery is most effective for rapid decompression of the optic nerves or chiasm. Surgical cures have been associated with tumor recurrence rates of 20% to 50% after 5 years. Radiotherapy alone or in combination with surgery or pharmacotherapy is also a therapeutic option.

Infertility in women as a result of hyperprolactinemia from a pituitary tumor can be successfully treated with bromocriptine. If pregnancy results, bromocriptine therapy is discontinued, although there has been no evidence of teratogenesis. Estrogen stimulation of prolactinoma during pregnancy causes tumor enlargement, but clinically significant enlargement occurs in only 10% to 15% of macroadenomas. Bromocriptine therapy may be reintroduced with successful control of symptoms; in unusual cases, trans-sphenoidal surgery can be used.

Excessive Growth Hormone and Acromegaly

Growth hormone (GH)–secreting pituitary tumors are the most common cause of *acromegaly* (Figs. 146.2–146.4). When fully developed, acromegaly is easily recognized by excessive skeletal and soft tissue growth. Facial features are coarse, with a large bulbous nose, prominent supraorbital ridges, a protruding mandible, separated teeth, and thick lips. Hands and feet are enlarged, and sweating is frequently increased. These changes are usually slowly progressive. Patients complain of headaches, fatigue, muscular pain, visual disturbances, and impairment of gonadal function. Paresthesia, sometimes with a typical carpal tunnel syndrome, may be present. Generalized arthritis and diabetes mellitus (DM) are frequent components. Mortality is increased with acromegaly because of cardiovascular and respiratory complications. Biventricular hypertrophy occurs independently of hypertension and metabolic complications owing to GH and insulin-like growth factor-I (IGF-I) hypersecretion. In young patients before epiphyseal closure, excessive secretion of GH results in gigantism.

The neuroendocrine regulation of GH secretion is complex. The major releasing factor is *GH-releasing hormone;* the major inhibitory agent is *somatostatin.* GH has a predominantly nocturnal pattern of secretion and is influenced by age and sleep. The diagnosis of acromegaly is most easily established by demonstrating sustained elevation of GH that cannot be suppressed by physiologic stimuli, such as glucose. Paradoxic elevation of GH may occur with glucose or TRH, suggesting hypothalamic dysfunction. Many actions of GH are mediated by IGF-1, which is elevated in acromegaly.

MRI is sensitive in localizing even small GH-secreting adenomas, and surgical removal is the treatment of choice. The cure rate is highest for microadenomas. Surgical decompression and radiation therapy may be the best alternative for larger tumors. Bromocriptine therapy has been useful in some patients. The long-acting somatostatin analog octreotide acetate (Sandostatin) offers specific adjunctive therapy for control of GH secretion and reduces tumor size in most cases. Somatostatin analogs are now the major medical treatment for acromegaly.

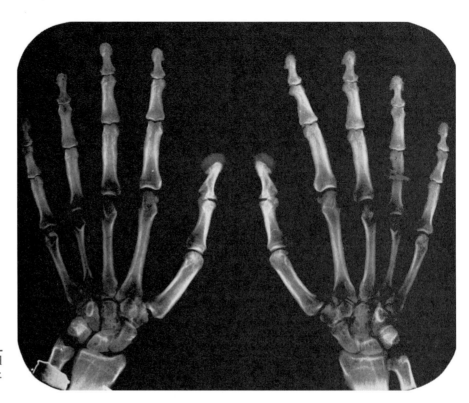

FIGURE 146.2. Tufting of the terminal phalanges in acromegaly. (Courtesy of Dr. Juan Taveras.)

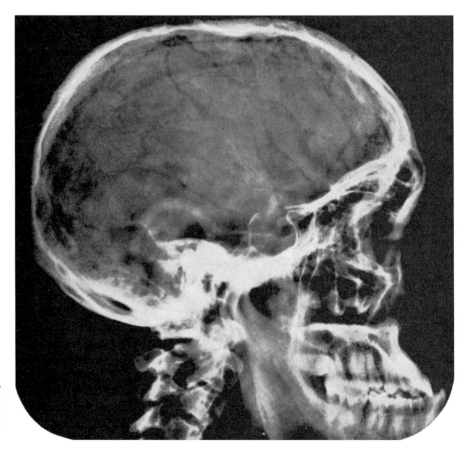

FIGURE 146.3. Pituitary tumor with ballooning of the sella turcica, prognathism, and enlargement of the skull bones. (Courtesy of Dr. Juan Taveras.)

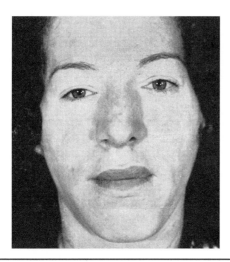

FIGURE 146.4. Prognathism and enlargement of nose in acromegaly secondary to pituitary adenoma. (Courtesy of Dr. E. Herz.)

Excessive Adrenocorticotropic Hormone

Cushing disease results from hypersecretion of ACTH by a pituitary tumor. Such tumors are usually small and often difficult to detect. Cushing disease may be difficult to distinguish from other causes of hyperadrenalism, such as adrenal adenoma or ectopic ACTH production by neoplasms. The symptoms of Cushing disease include plethoric facies, centripetal obesity, hypertension, DM, amenorrhea, hirsutism, acne, and osteoporosis. Mental status changes or myopathy may be prominent.

The differential diagnosis of Cushing syndrome can be challenging. Elevated urinary free cortisol levels and suppressibility of cortisol secretion by dexamethasone are the key tests for establishing the diagnosis of pituitary-dependent Cushing syndrome. Direct assay of plasma ACTH may be helpful; high levels are seen with ectopic ACTH production. The ACTH response to corticotropin-releasing factor may distinguish Cushing disease from other causes of hypercortisolism. Selective sampling of ACTH levels from the petrosal sinuses may help localize an adenoma within the pituitary.

MRI with gadolinium is the most sensitive procedure for detecting these tumors. Trans sphenoidal adenomectomy is the treatment of choice. It is more likely to be curative in microadenomas than in larger tumors or those that invade the cavernous sinuses. Radiation therapy may be helpful in controlling the tumor. In patients treated by bilateral adrenalectomy, an aggressive ACTH-secreting pituitary tumor may develop to cause the hyperpigmentation of Nelson syndrome. The hypothalamus may play a role in the pathogenesis of both Cushing disease and Nelson syndrome. Ketoconazole (Nizoral), an inhibitor of adrenal steroidogenesis, may inhibit the adverse effects of hypercortisolism.

The *empty sella syndrome* rarely poses difficulty in the diagnosis of pituitary tumors. The syndrome develops with herniation of the subarachnoid space through the diaphragm of the sella turcica; the condition may be idiopathic or follow destruction or surgical removal of the pituitary gland. Remodeling and enlargement of the bony sella turcica may occur, and the sella may appear enlarged on skull radiograph. CT or MRI usually clarifies the diagnosis. Pituitary dysfunction is uncommon and, if present, suggests that the apparently empty sella is accompanied by a pituitary tumor. The clinical accompaniments of the empty sella syndrome—obese women with headache—are similar to those of pseudotumor cerebri; chronically increased CSF pressure may precipitate the development of an empty sella.

Diabetes Insipidus

DI is characterized by excessive excretion of urine and an abnormally large fluid intake caused by impaired production of antidiuretic hormone (arginine vasopressin). There are two general groups of patients. In primary DI, there is no known lesion in the pituitary or hypothalamus; secondary DI is associated with lesions in the hypothalamus either in the supraoptic and paraventricular nuclei or in their tracts in the medial eminence or upper pituitary stalk. Among the lesions are tumors (e.g., pituitary adenoma, craniopharyngioma, meningioma), aneurysms, xanthomatosis (Schüller-Christian disease), sarcoidosis, trauma, infections, and vascular disease. Primary DI is rare. Heredity is a factor in some patients. Many different mutations have been found in familial autosomal-dominant DI. Autopsy studies of a few cases revealed loss of neurons in the supraoptic and paraventricular nuclei. Secondary or symptomatic DI is more frequent but still uncommon. It may follow head injury and is present in many patients with xanthomatosis and in some patients with tumors or other lesions in the hypothalamic region. The syndrome is evidence of hypothalamic disease.

Unless complicated by other symptoms associated with the lesion, the symptoms of DI are limited to polyuria and polydipsia. Eight to 20 L or even more of urine are passed in 24 hours, and there is a comparably high level of water intake. The frequent voiding and excessive water intake may interfere with normal activities and disturb sleep. Usually, however, general health is maintained if this is an isolated deficiency of the hypothalamus. The symptoms and signs in patients with tumors or other lesions in the hypothalamic region are those usually associated with these conditions (see Chapter 59). The laboratory findings are normal, except for a low specific gravity of the urine

(1.001 to 1.005) and increased serum osmolality in many patients.

The diagnosis is made, based on polyuria and polydipsia. It is distinguished from DM by the glycosuria and high specific gravity of the urine in DM. A large amount of urine may be passed by patients with chronic nephritis but not the large volumes (>3 L per day) found in DI; the presence of albumin and casts in the urine and other findings should prevent any confusion in recognizing nephritis. Psychogenic polydipsia must be considered (see below).

A rare cause of DI is failure of the kidneys to respond to vasopressin, a hereditary defect in infant boys. Absence of vasopressin is difficult to determine in blood by radioimmunoassay. Therefore, the diagnosis is made by clinical tests that include antidiuretic responses to exogenous vasopressin and dehydration. Administration of five pressor units of aqueous vasopressin rapidly results in a marked decrease in urinary output and an increase in osmolality (specific gravity greater than 1.011) in a patient with DI; there is no response in nephrogenic disease. Psychogenic polydipsia, however, may also show a limited response. In contrast to DI, however, there is a normal response to dehydration in psychogenic polydipsia, although the time required for an increase in urinary concentration may be 12 to 18 hours. Normal subjects dehydrated for 6 to 8 hours reduce urinary volume and concentrate urinary osmolality to roughly twice that of plasma (specific gravity greater than 1.015). Patients with severe DI do not respond and should be observed closely, with care taken to prevent loss of >3% of body weight during the test; otherwise, patients may become severely dehydrated. A useful clinical test, devised by Moses and Miller, combines dehydration with the response to exogenous vasopressin and distinguishes these disorders and also partial DI.

The diagnosis of DI carries with it the necessity of determining the cause. This means a thorough neurologic examination with particular attention to visual acuity and visual fields. MRI is essential. In DI, the normally bright spot outlining the posterior pituitary gland on MRI may be absent or displaced more proximally in the hypothalamic infundibular stalk (ectopic; Fig 146.5). MRI may also show craniopharyngioma, hamartoma, dysgerminoma, or histiocytosis X.

Primary DI may persist for years. DI caused by known lesions in the hypothalamus may also be permanent, but complete remission with reversal of symptoms is not infrequent.

Treatment of DI associated with tumors or other remediable hypothalamic lesions is that appropriate to the lesion (surgical removal or radiation therapy). Symptomatic therapy of the DI, if it persists in these cases and in syndromes of unknown cause, is directed toward suppression of diuresis. No effort is made to limit fluid intake. Aqueous vasopressin (Pitressin) can be administered subcutaneously in five pressor-unit doses one to four times daily;

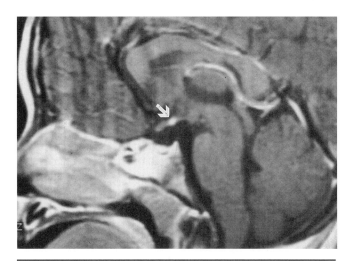

FIGURE 146.5. Hypothalamic hypopituitarism. On MRI, the bright-spot *(arrow)* appearance of the posterior pituitary gland is missing from its normal location in the sella turcica. Instead, it is located in the lower hypothalamus and upper pituitary stalk in this child with congenital GH and TSH deficiency. Damage to the stalk interrupts the hypophyseal portal system and vasopressin fibers. These fibers regenerate, forming a new, usually smaller, posterior pituitary in this location (ectopic). Such patients may recover from or have partial DI. More proximal lesions in the hypothalamic nuclei and tracts to the vasopressin system do not regenerate. Interruption of the releasing-factor pathways and the portal system results in anterior pituitary deficiencies. (From Zimmerman EA. Neuroendocrine disorders. In: Rosenberg R, ed. *Atlas of Clinical Neurology.* Philadelphia: Current Medicine, 1998:3.1–3.15; with permission.)

it may also be sprayed transnasally in the form of lysine vasopressin or placed high in the nasopharynx on cotton pledgets. Vasopressin tannate in oil injected intramuscularly is slowly absorbed and may be effective for several days.

The drug of choice is now the synthetic analog of vasopressin, 1-deamino-8-D-arginine vasopressin (DDAVP). DDAVP has no smooth muscle effects and has no pressor or cardiac complications. It also avoids the nasal irritation associated with administration of lysine vasopressin nasal spray. It is given by nasal instillation or spray and provides good control for about 8 hours. An oral form is also now available; the usual dose is 300 to 600 μg per day in divided doses. Partial DI may require no therapy or may be ameliorated by oral administration of clofibrate or chlorpropamide. Chlorpropamide occasionally causes hypoglycemia and, rarely, water intoxication.

Excessive Secretion of Antidiuretic Hormone

Inappropriate secretion of antidiuretic hormone may occur with injury to the hypothalamohypophyseal system by head injury, infections, tumors, and other causes. It has been reported in association with lung carcinoma and, occasionally, with other tumors that elaborate vasopressin. It may also be associated with lung diseases that may overstimulate afferent pathways to the hypothalamus or with drugs that cause excess secretion of vasopressin, such as carbamazepine (Tegretol). Other drugs associated with the syndrome include vasopressin and its oxytocin analog, nonsteroidal anti-inflammatory medications, antipsychotics, thiazides, and selective serotonin-reuptake inhibitors.

Hyponatremia and natriuresis in patients with intracranial disease may also be owing to "cerebral salt wasting," which is now recognized as different from inappropriate secretion of antidiuretic hormones, as it is associated with the loss of salt and hypovolemia and responds to their replacement. The salient features of the syndrome are hyponatremia and hypotonicity of body fluids, excessive urinary excretion of sodium despite hyponatremia, normal renal and adrenal function, absence of edema, hypotension, azotemia or dehydration, and improvement of the electrolyte disturbance and clinical symptoms on restriction of fluid intake. Evidence of cerebral dysfunction includes headache, confusion, somnolence, coma, seizures, transient focal neurologic signs, and an abnormal EEG. Mild forms clear with simple fluid restriction. Severe cases with seizures or coma are treated with furosemide (Lasix) diuresis and electrolyte replacement (3% sodium chloride). Caution should be used in rapid correction of hyponatremia to avoid central pontine demyelination. Intravenous urea and normal saline have also been used for rapid correction. In the near future, vasopressin antagonists may be useful in diagnosing and treating this condition.

THYROID

Hypothyroidism

Thyroid hormone is important in early growth and development, and the neurologic consequences of hypothyroidism depend on the age of the patient when the deficiency begins. Severe thyroid deficiency in utero or early life results in delayed physical and mental development or *cretinism*. Soon after birth, subcutaneous tissue thickens, the infant's cry becomes hoarse, the tongue enlarges, and the infant has widely spaced eyes, a potbelly, and an umbilical hernia. Neurologically, there is mental retardation, with pyramidal and extrapyramidal signs in a proximal and truncal distribution. Strabismus, deafness, and primitive reflexes are common. In many patients, thyroid hormone therapy administered within the first 2 months of life results in nearly complete restoration of normal physical and mental function. Treatment should begin during the first 2 weeks of life for optimal intellectual development. Despite early treatment, mild hearing and vestibular dysfunction may persist.

Juvenile myxedema is similar to cretinism, with variations that depend on age at onset of thyroid deficiency. The severity of physical and mental retardation is usually less than in infantile myxedema. Precocious puberty also occurs in juvenile hypothyroidism. Pituitary hypertrophy has been seen in juvenile myxedema and other forms of long-standing hypothyroidism, which can be associated with hyperprolactinemia. Adult myxedema is characterized by lethargy, somnolence, or impairment of attention and concentration; weakness; slowness of speech; nonpitting edema of the subcutaneous tissues; coarse, pale skin; dry, brittle hair; thick lips; macroglossia; and increased sensitivity to cold environmental temperatures.

The neurologic complications of hypothyroidism include headache, disorders of the cranial and peripheral nerves, sensorimotor abnormalities, and changes in cognition and level of consciousness. Cranial nerve abnormalities, other than visual and acoustic nerve problems, are unusual. Decreased vision and hearing loss may occur, and vertigo and tinnitus may be present. Visual and auditory evoked potentials have been reported to be abnormal and respond to treatment. The cause of headache is uncertain. Pseudotumor cerebri has been reported in hypothyroidism in children receiving thyroid replacement therapy. Subacute or abrupt encephalopathy (Hashimoto encephalopathy) is discussed in Chapter 158.

Mild polyneuritis is a rare complication characterized mainly by paresthesias in the hands and feet. Entrapment neuropathy of the median nerve (carpal tunnel syndrome) is attributed to the accumulation of acid mucopolysaccharides in the nerve and surrounding tissues. Neuromuscular findings include slowing of voluntary movements and slow relaxation of tendon reflexes, particularly the ankle jerks. Electrically silent mounding of muscles on direct percussion is called *myoedema*. There may be exercise intolerance or myopathic weakness. Creatine kinase levels are elevated. Neuromuscular symptoms improve with thyroid replacement.

In hypothyroid infants, a remarkable generalized enlargement or hypertrophy of muscles constitutes the Kocher-Debré-Sémélaigne syndrome, creating an "infant Hercules" (Fig. 146.6); the muscles decrease in size with replacement therapy. In older children, muscle hypertrophy may result from a mutation in the gene for myostatin. Enlargement of muscles with pain and stiffness in adults produces *Hoffmann syndrome*.

Cerebellar ataxia (*myxedema staggers*) may occur in adults, manifesting as a slow or stiff, unstable gait. In children, cell loss has been detected in the vermis.

Mental status changes may be prominent, with decreased attentiveness, poor concentration, lethargy, and dementia. Psychiatric symptoms—delirium, depression, or frank psychosis (*myxedema madness*)—may appear, depending on the severity and duration of thyroid deficiency. *Myxedema coma* may be accompanied by hypothermia,

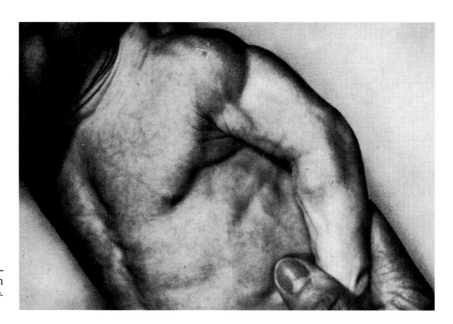

FIGURE 146.6. Enlargement of muscles in Kocher-Debré-Sémélaigne syndrome. (Courtesy of Dr. Arnold Gold.)

hypotension, and respiratory and metabolic disturbances, and, if untreated, has a high mortality rate.

Severe hypothyroidism or myxedema is primarily associated with thyroid failure as opposed to hypothalamic–pituitary disease. The characteristic findings are low circulating T_4 and T_3, elevated TSH, and low radioiodine uptake by the thyroid. The CSF protein content increases; values >100 mg/mL are not exceptional. EEG abnormalities include slowing and generalized decrease in amplitude.

The treatment of hypothyroidism depends on the severity of the deficiency. Myxedema coma should be treated rapidly with intravenous administration of levothyroxine. In other patients, gradually increasing doses of oral levothyroxine are recommended. Angina pectoris or heart failure can be precipitated by too rapid replacement in adults. In secondary hypothyroidism, thyroid replacement should not be started without concomitant corticosteroid replacement. Prophylactic treatment of cretinism is important in goiter districts, where iodine should be given to all pregnant women. Treatment of subclinical thyroid disease (i.e., normal thyroid hormone levels with elevated or depressed TSH levels) is controversial.

Hyperthyroidism

Hyperthyroidism or thyrotoxicosis is associated with an increased metabolic rate, abnormal cardiovascular and autonomic functions, tremor, and myopathy. It may present with minimal clinical signs or as atrial fibrillation in older adults. Mental disturbances range from mild irritability to psychosis. When hyperthyroidism is associated with diffuse goiter, ophthalmopathy, and dermopathy, it is termed *Graves disease,* which is an autoimmune disorder. Immunologic mechanisms play an important role in the thyroid, eye, and skin manifestations. Hyperthyroidism may

be subtle in older patients, with apathy, myopathy, and cardiovascular disease as the most prominent symptoms.

Ocular symptoms are common in thyrotoxicosis. These may be present as infrequent blinking, lid lag, or weakness of convergence and are distinct from the infiltrative ophthalmopathy associated with thyroid disease known as *Graves ophthalmopathy.* The relationship of the eye disorder to thyroid status is unclear; it may appear in hyperthyroid patients, in euthyroid patients after thyroidectomy, or in euthyroid patients with no history of hyperthyroidism.

The pathologic changes are confined to the orbit. There is an increase in the orbital contents with edema, hypertrophy, infiltration, and fibrosis of the extraocular muscles (Fig. 146.7). Onset of symptoms is gradual; exophthalmos is often accompanied by diplopia secondary to paresis of one or more ocular muscles. Clinically, eyelid retraction (*Dalrymple sign*) is the first evidence in 75% of cases, and pain is the most common symptom. Both eyes may be involved simultaneously, or the exophthalmos in one eye may precede the other by several months. Papilledema sometimes occurs, and ulcerations of the cornea may develop secondary to failure of the lid to protect the eye. The symptoms progress rapidly for a few months and may lead to complete ophthalmoplegia. Occasionally, spontaneous improvement occurs; as a rule, the symptoms persist unchanged throughout a patient's life unless relieved by therapy.

Treatment of thyroid ophthalmopathy is controversial and may include immune suppression with corticosteroids, radiotherapy, or surgical decompression of the orbit. Methylcellulose drops, shields, or partial suturing of the lids is recommended to protect the eye. A definitive therapy awaits a better understanding of the pathogenic mechanism.

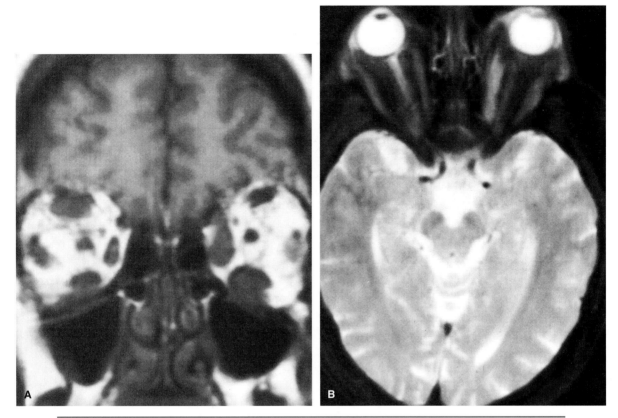

FIGURE 146.7. Graves disease. Coronal T1-weighted **(A)** and axial T2-weighted fat-suppressed **(B)** MR images of the orbits show bilateral proptosis with enlargement of the medial rectus muscles (left greater than right), the left lateral and inferior rectus muscles, and the right superior rectus muscle. Although the most common pattern of extraocular muscle enlargement is symmetric, asymmetric involvement is not uncommon in Graves disease. This patient had known hyperthyroidism secondary to Graves disease. (Courtesy of Dr. S. Chan.)

Limb weakness is common with hyperthyroidism. *Thyrotoxic myopathy* is characterized by painless weakness and wasting of the muscles of the pelvic girdle, particularly the iliopsoas, and, to a lesser extent, the muscles of the shoulder girdle. Tendon reflexes are normal or hyperactive, and sensation is normal. Fasciculations or myokymia may be noted. Thyrotoxic myopathy needs to be distinguished from myasthenia gravis (MG), which may accompany hyperthyroidism. Improvement of the myopathy follows effective treatment of the hyperthyroidism.

The occurrence of hyperthyroidism and periodic paralysis is more common in people of Asian ancestry, predominantly men. *Thyrotoxic periodic paralysis* is similar to hypokalemic periodic paralysis in terms of precipitants and treatment. Propanolol may temporarily reduce the number of attacks. Symptoms disappear when the treated patient becomes euthyroid.

There is an association between hyperthyroidism and MG. About 5% of patients with MG have hyperthyroidism. In most patients, MG precedes or occurs simultaneously with the hyperthyroidism. Differential diagnosis between thyrotoxic myopathy and MG is made primarily on the

myasthenic clinical features, serologic testing, response to edrophonium, and electrophysiologic abnormalities. If there are cranial symptoms (dysarthria, dysphagia, ptosis) in a hyperthyroid patient, MG should be suspected. Interpretation of ocular signs may be complicated by thyrotoxic ophthalmopathy, but even with exophthalmos, the presence of ptosis suggests concomitant MG, which may respond to edrophonium. Orbital imaging will be abnormal in thyroid opthalmopathy.

PARATHYROID

Hypoparathyroidism

Hypoparathyroidism results in a disturbance of calcium and phosphorus metabolism that is manifested especially by tetany. Hypoparathyroidism may be owing to primary deficiency of parathyroid hormone or from lack of peripheral responses to parathyroid hormone. Hypoparathyroidism may follow thyroidectomy or may be part of an idiopathic autoimmune syndrome, which sometimes includes multiple endocrine organ failure.

In *pseudohypoparathyroidism,* symptoms of hypocalcemia result from the ineffective action or antagonism of parathyroid hormone at cellular receptors. Patients have a characteristic habitus, with short stature, stocky physique, rounded face, and shortening of the metacarpal and metatarsal bones. Common clinical features of hypoparathyroidism and pseudohypoparathyroidism include mental deficiency, cataracts, tetany, and seizures (Table 146.2). Lesions of ectodermally derived tissue include scaly skin, alopecia, or atrophic changes in the nails. Other neurologic manifestations are directly related to the effects of hypocalcemia on the nervous system.

Tetany is the most distinctive sign that may be manifested by carpopedal spasm. *Latent tetany* can be demonstrated by contracture of the facial muscles on tapping the facial nerve in front of the ear (*Chvostek sign*), evoking carpal spasm by inducing ischemia in the arm with an inflated blood pressure cuff (*Trousseau sign*), or demonstrating the lowered threshold of electrical excitability of the nerve (*Erb sign*).

Dementia and psychosis occur with variable improvement after correction of hypocalcemia. Convulsions are a symptom of hypocalcemia regardless of cause. Seizures are usually generalized, tend to be frequent, and respond poorly to anticonvulsant drugs. EEG changes are nonspecific and typically revert to normal with correction of the serum calcium levels. Although rare, hypoparathyroidism should be considered when seizures are frequent or bizarre and difficult to control with medication.

Intracranial calcifications are common in hypoparathyroidism (Fig. 146.8). The basal ganglia are the predominant site for calcium deposition, but other regions may be affected. The calcifications are usually not associated with symptoms, but cognitive impairment and a variety of hypokinetic and hyperkinetic movement disorders have been

▶ **TABLE 146.2 Incidence of Signs and Symptoms in Pseudohypoparathyroidism**

Characteristics	Patients (%)
Biochemical	
Hypocalcemia	96
Increased alkaline phosphatase	20
Body habitus	
Short stature	80
Round face	92
Stocky or obese	50
Ocular	
Lenticular opacities	49
Dental	
Hypoplasia, enamel defects	51
Calcification	
Subcutaneous	55
Basal ganglia	50
Skeletal	
Short metacarpals	68
Thickened calvarium	62
Neurologic	
Mental retardation	75
Seizures	59
Muscle cramps, twitches	38

In: Stanbury JB, Wyngaarden JB, Fredrickson DS, eds. Pseudohypoparathyroidism. *The metabolic basis of inherited disease,* 3rd ed. New York: McGraw-Hill, 1983:1508–1527; with permission.

seen in hypoparathyroidism. Symptoms may be reversible with appropriate treatment.

Increased intracranial pressure with papilledema has been reported with hypoparathyroidism. The mechanism is unexplained. CSF pressure returns to normal with correction of serum calcium values. Sensorineural hearing loss and myopathy occur rarely.

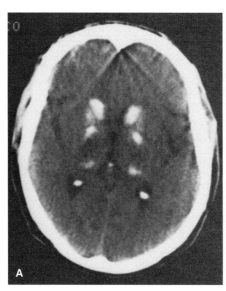 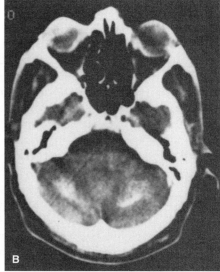

FIGURE 146.8. Pseudohypoparathyroidism. **A.** Dense areas of calcification are evident in the head of the caudate nucleus (anterior putamen and globus pallidus (middle pair) and pulvinar (posterior). The fine densities in the occipital horns are calcifications in the choroid plexus. **B.** Calcification is also seen in subcortical areas of the cerebellar hemispheres. (Courtesy of Dr. S. K. Hilal and Dr. M. Mawad.)

▶ **TABLE 146.3 Clues to the Diagnosis of Hyperparathyroidism in the First 343 Cases at the Massachusetts General Hospital**

Clue	Cases (n)
Bone disease	80
Renal stones	195
Peptic ulcer	27
Pancreatitis	9
Fatigue	10
Hypertension	6
Mental disturbance	3
CNS signs	7
Multiple endocrine abnormalities	3
Lumps in neck	1
No symptoms	2

From Cope, 1966; with permission.

The diagnosis of hypoparathyroidism is made based on clinical symptoms, hypocalcemia, and low or undetectable plasma parathyroid hormone levels. In pseudohypoparathyroidism, parathyroid hormone levels are elevated. Hypocalcemia may be associated with electrocardiogram changes, including prolongation of the QT interval and T-wave changes.

Vitamin D and calcium supplements are the primary therapy for most forms of hypoparathyroidism. They are effective in relieving tetany and in restoring the serum calcium and phosphorus values to normal. Dosage needs to be adjusted to the needs of the patient.

Hyperparathyroidism

Primary hyperparathyroidism is most commonly a result of the oversecretion of parathyroid hormone by a solitary adenoma of the parathyroid glands. The classic syndrome of hyperparathyroidism is hypercalcemia with a combination of renal lithiasis, osteitis, and peptic ulcer disease (Table 146.3). Modern-day hyperparathyroidism, however, is frequently seen with minimal symptoms. The diagnosis of hyperparathyroidism is now often made by automated blood chemistry tests in routine examinations before there are clinical signs. Calcium levels are not as elevated as in the past, and the classic neuromuscular symptoms and signs are less frequently observed. Limb weakness, paresthesia, and muscle cramps may be seen, but neurologic abnormalities are now uncommon.

Common symptoms include fatigue and subjective weakness. Mental status changes include memory loss, irritability, and depression, which improve with return to normal of serum calcium levels. Neuromuscular signs include symmetric proximal limb weakness and muscle wasting. Tendon reflexes may be normal or hyperactive.

EMG and muscle biopsy may show evidence of myopathic or neuropathic disease. These signs and symptoms typically respond to parathyroidectomy. Differential diagnosis includes the conditions that cause hypercalcemia, including secondary hyperparathyroidism.

PANCREAS

Hypoglycemia

The CNS depends almost entirely on glucose for its metabolism; dysfunction develops rapidly when the amount of glucose in the blood falls below critical levels. Hypoglycemia may be associated with an overdose of insulin in the treatment of DM. Spontaneous hypoglycemia is usually the result of *pancreatic hyperinsulinism*. Hypersecretion of insulin by the pancreas may be owing to a tumor of the islet cells or functional overactivity of these cells. Hypoglycemia may also occur when liver function is impaired or when there is severe damage to the pituitary or adrenal glands.

The symptoms of hyperinsulinism are paroxysmal, tending to occur when the blood glucose could be expected to be low (in the morning before breakfast, after a fast, or after heavy exercise). Occasionally, symptoms follow a meal. The duration of symptoms varies from minutes to hours. The severity also varies. There may be only nervousness, anxiety, or tremulousness, which is relieved by the ingestion of food. Severe attacks last for hours, during which the patient may perform automatic activity with complete amnesia for the entire period, or seizures may be followed by coma. The frequency of attacks varies from several per day to infrequent episodes.

Spontaneous hypoglycemia is occasionally seen in infants. Risk factors include immaturity, low birthweight, or severe illness. Infants of diabetic mothers may exhibit hyperinsulinism. A host of genetic or metabolic defects may cause hypoglycemia, including galactosemia, fructose intolerance, or leucine sensitivity. The symptoms of infantile hypoglycemia are muscular twitching, myoclonic jerks, and seizures. Mental retardation results if the condition is not recognized and adequately treated. Hypoglycemic symptoms can be divided into two groups: autonomic and cerebral. Sympathetic symptoms are present in most patients at the onset of hypoglycemia, usually preceding the more serious cerebral manifestations. Autonomic symptoms include lightheadedness, sweating, nausea, vomiting, pallor, palpitations, precordial oppression, headache, abdominal pain, and hunger. In DM with autonomic neuropathy, many of these symptoms may not occur.

Cerebral symptoms usually occur with the sympathetic phenomena but may be the only manifestations. The most common manifestations are paresthesia, diplopia, and blurred vision, which may be followed by tremor, focal neurologic abnormalities, abnormal behavior, or convulsions. After prolonged, severe hypoglycemia, coma may ensue. Confusion and abnormal behavior from episodic hypoglycemia may simulate complex partial seizures, although hyperinsulinism only rarely causes epilepsy. Chronic or repeated hypoglycemia may produce dementia or other behavioral abnormalities. Distal axonal neuropathy has also been observed.

The neurologic examination is usually normal, except during attacks of hypoglycemia when there may be findings as described. The diagnosis is established by documentation of hypoglycemia during a symptomatic episode, but the timing of the specimen is important because homeostatic mechanisms may return the blood glucose level to normal. The level of blood glucose at which symptoms appear varies from person to person, but generally is <30 to 40 mg/dL. The EEG shows focal or widespread dysrhythmia during an attack of hypoglycemia and, in some patients, even in the interval between attacks.

The diagnosis of hyperinsulinism is made by the paroxysmal appearance of signs of autonomic and cerebral dysfunction in association with a low blood glucose level and an inappropriately high circulating insulin level. Factitious hypoglycemia may be caused by self-administration of insulin or inappropriate use of oral hypoglycemic agents. If it is not possible to obtain a blood specimen during an attack, a diagnostic fast should be considered. After 12 to 14 hours, 80% of patients with islet cell tumors have low glucose and high insulin levels. Longer fasts may be needed. The diagnosis of *islet cell adenoma* can be difficult; additional endocrine tests and imaging studies may be needed. Hypoglycemia associated with diseases of the liver, adrenal, or pituitary can usually be distinguished by other signs and symptoms of disease in these organs.

Early, intensive treatment of acute hypoglycemia is important to prevent CNS damage. Sugar can be given orally in conscious patients. Comatose patients should be given glucose intravenously. Functional hyperinsulinism is treated by diet modifications to avoid excessive insulin secretion by the pancreas. Long-term management of hyperinsulinism is directed at identification and correction of the underlying cause.

Diabetes Mellitus

DM is a systemic metabolic disorder characterized by hypoinsulinism or peripheral resistance to the action of insulin. Current classification systems broadly divide DM into two types defined by clinical characteristics and pattern of insulin deficiency. *Type 1 DM* usually occurs in young, nonobese people with insulin deficiency. *Type 2 DM* is generally encountered in older, obese individuals with peripheral resistance to the action of insulin. The neurologic complications in both types of DM are similar; the presence of neurologic disease is roughly correlated with the duration and severity of the disease and is commonly associated with other tissue complications of DM, such as retinopathy and nephropathy.

The primary neurologic complication of DM is peripheral neuropathy. This includes mononeuropathies (peripheral and cranial nerves), polyneuropathy, autonomic neuropathy, radiculopathies, and entrapment neuropathy (median, ulnar, and peroneal; see Chapter 106). The cause of these neuropathies is uncertain; metabolic, vascular, and hypoxic mechanisms have been advanced.

Mononeuropathies are attributed to vascular lesions of peripheral nerves. Onset of symptoms is rapid, and pain is common in both mononeuropathies and radiculopathies caused by DM. Common cranial neuropathies involve the oculomotor and abducens nerves and are also a result of vascular lesions. Pupillary sparing is common but not invariable because of the pattern of vascular damage to the oculomotor nerve. The prognosis for recovery from mononeuropathy or radiculopathy is good.

Distal symmetric polyneuropathy of DM is the one most commonly encountered. There is typically a gradual onset of symptoms, the character of the symptoms depending on the type of peripheral nerve fiber affected. Numbness and burning are common complaints. Rarely, a patient may present with a Charcot joint or skin ulcer if nociceptive fibers have sustained the predominant damage. Distal sensory loss may be accompanied by weakness; tendon reflexes are usually lost. Diagnosis of diabetic polyneuropathy is aided by nerve conduction studies that show a mixed demyelinating and axonal neuropathy. CSF protein content is usually elevated but may be normal.

Autonomic neuropathy may be prominent in DM. Cardiovascular symptoms include arrhythmias or orthostatic hypotension. These may complicate diagnosis and treatment of concurrent myocardial disease. Gastrointestinal motility problems can produce nausea, vomiting, or diarrhea, depending on the severity and distribution of the autonomic neuropathy. Diabetic neuropathy may lead to bladder dysfunction or erectile and ejaculatory failure in men.

CNS complications of DM are primarily owing to the metabolic derangements of hypoinsulinism and hypoglycemia that may follow administration of insulin. Cerebrovascular disease is an important problem in diabetics because of accelerated atherosclerosis of cerebral blood vessels and related cardiovascular disorders of heart failure, hypertension, and coagulation abnormalities. Hyperinsulinism or insulin resistance may also be a secondary feature of other neurologic disorders (e.g., Friedreich ataxia) and may share common etiologic features with some genetic or familial diseases.

ADRENAL

The adrenal gland is composed of two distinct parts: the mesodermally derived cortex and the neuroectodermally derived medulla. The cortex synthesizes and secretes steroid hormones, including mineralocorticoids, glucocorticoids, progestins, estrogens, and androgens. Aldosterone is the principal mineralocorticoid and is involved in sodium and potassium homeostasis by the kidney. Glucocorticoids play an important role in metabolic and immunologic processes. Under normal circumstances, sex steroid production by the adrenal plays a relatively minor role compared with the contribution by the gonads. The adrenal medulla contains chromaffin cells, the most important source of circulating catecholamines. These catecholamines, epinephrine and norepinephrine, have important cardiovascular, metabolic, and neural effects.

Hypoadrenalism

Hypofunction of the adrenal cortex is usually owing to atrophy of the gland of unknown cause. The gland may be destroyed by tuberculosis, neoplasms, amyloidosis, hemochromatosis, or fungal or human immunodeficiency virus infection. *Addison disease*, or chronic insufficiency of the adrenal cortex, is characterized by weakness, weight loss, increased pigmentation of the skin, hypotension, behavioral changes, and hypoglycemia. Chronic adrenal insufficiency may be an autoimmune disorder, occasionally in association with other autoimmune disorders, such as MG. It may also be a feature of the abnormal metabolism of long-chain fatty acids in X-linked adrenoleukodystrophy. It may be the only clinical expression in about 10% of cases, including both the cerebral and adrenomyelopathic forms of the disease. In one study, one-third of young males diagnosed with primary adrenal failure (Addison disease) were found to have adrenoleukodystrophy after measurement of long-chain fatty acids. Secondary adrenal insufficiency follows pituitary failure, in which symptoms are less severe because of the relative preservation of mineralocorticoid function, which is not regulated by ACTH.

CNS manifestations of Addison disease are common, primarily in cognition and behavior. Psychotic symptoms are rare. Elevated CSF pressure is sometimes accompanied by cerebral edema. Autopsy studies of the brain in Addison disease indicate that glucocorticoids play an important trophic function in the CNS, sustaining the granule cells of the hippocampus. (The loss of hippocampal neurons with adrenocortical hormone receptors in aging is accelerated in Alzheimer disease and appears to be associated with hypercortisolism.)

Diagnosis is suggested by the clinical features and is confirmed by low plasma levels of cortisol with elevated ACTH levels (in primary adrenal failure), decreased excretion of 17-hydroxycorticosteroids, and failure of the adrenal cortex to respond to ACTH. Treatment is based on administration of a glucocorticoid preparation and replacement of mineralocorticoids with sodium. The latter may not be needed if the pituitary is the source of adrenal insufficiency.

Hyperadrenalism

Hyperfunction of the adrenal cortex produces *Cushing syndrome*, which was first attributed by Cushing to a basophilic adenoma of the pituitary. The clinical symptoms of Cushing disease can be reproduced by the administration of corticosteroids. Mental status changes, including difficulties with memory, and myopathy are two of the more common neurologic symptoms. The syndrome of idiopathic intracranial hypertension with headache, nausea, vomiting, and papilledema may occur with reduction or withdrawal of corticosteroids being used as therapy. Symptoms resolve with reinstatement of steroid dosage, and withdrawal is accomplished more gradually.

The differential diagnosis of Cushing syndrome may be difficult because there are several potential sources of hyperadrenalism (pituitary, adrenal, or ectopic source of ACTH production) and also because of the effects of common clinical conditions, such as obesity and depression, on the production and suppressibility of corticosteroids. These conditions may make interpretation of diagnostic tests challenging (Table 146.4). Treatment is directed at control of corticosteroid secretion and the underlying pathology.

Primary Hyperaldosteronism

In 1955, Conn described a syndrome caused by production of aldosterone from a tumor of the adrenal cortex. The clinical manifestations include recurrent attacks of muscular weakness simulating periodic paralysis, tetany, polyuria, hypertension, and a striking imbalance of electrolytes with hypokalemia, hypernatremia, and alkalosis. Paresthesia may occur as a result of the alkalosis. Vertigo may be caused by abrupt fluid and electrolyte shifts. Idiopathic intracranial hypertension has been reported. Preliminary diagnosis is made by finding an elevated plasma aldosterone concentration to plasma renin activity. Treatment involves identification and removal of the adrenal tumor coupled with aldosterone inhibition and receptor blockade.

Pheochromocytoma

Hyperfunction of the adrenal medulla as a result of a tumor of the chromaffin cells is accompanied by increased secretion of catecholamines. The tumor may be familial, alone or in conjunction with other endocrine tumors. Pheochromocytoma may be seen with neurofibromatosis,

▶ **TABLE 146.4 Evaluation of Hypercortisolism (Cushing Syndrome)**

Clinical Presentation	Morning Cortisol Level After Overnight Dexamethasone	Urinary Corticosteroids After High-Dose Dexamethasone (8 mg/24 h)	Plasma ACTH
Obesity	Suppress to normal	Suppress	—
Adrenal hyperplasia (Cushing disease)	Does not suppress	Suppress	Often elevated
Adrenal tumor (adenoma or carcinoma)	Does not suppress	Does not suppress	Low
Ectopic ACTH secretion	Does not suppress	Does not suppress	High

von Hippel-Lindau disease, ataxia-telangiectasia, or Sturge-Weber syndrome, consistent with the neuroectodermal origin of the adrenal medulla. Familial pheochromocytoma is associated with bilateral adrenal tumors, whereas sporadic cases are nearly always unilateral.

Hypertension of a moderate or severe degree is characteristic. The hypertension may be paroxysmal or sustained and is associated with palpitations, episodic hyperhidrosis, headaches, and other nonspecific systemic symptoms, such as nausea, emesis, or diarrhea. Anxiety attacks are common. Death may result from cerebral hemorrhage, pulmonary edema, or cardiac failure in one of the acute attacks or as a result of one of these complications from sustained hypertension.

Diagnosis and treatment are directed at establishing the increased excretion of catecholamine metabolites in the urine and localization and removal of the tumor. The tumor may occur in sites other than the adrenal; imaging techniques are helpful in localization.

GONADS

Neurologic disorders associated with diseases of the ovary or testes are not well defined. However, the primary secretions of the gonads—estrogens, progestins, and androgens—have been reported to influence a variety of neurologic symptoms. Cyclic or phasic fluctuations in gonadal secretion (during the menstrual cycle or pregnancy) have been linked to common problems such as migraine headache and epilepsy and to less common disorders such as porphyria. Therapeutic use of estrogen–progestin preparations in oral contraceptives poses potential risks for neurologic complications, notably cerebrovascular disease.

Although migraine has been frequently reported in association with menstrual periods, the true incidence of *catamenial migraine* is difficult to determine. Somerville demonstrated that some women have headaches precip-

itated by the rapid decline in circulating estradiol during the late-luteal phase and that these headaches can be prevented by administration of estrogen, but not progesterone. The mechanism of action is not clear, but the role of estrogens in catamenial migraine may explain the onset and variation of headaches during pregnancy or with the use of oral contraceptives. Although long-term estrogen treatment is said to be useful in catamenial migraine, this is not practical for most women. Premenstrual administration of prostaglandin inhibitors may be helpful. Discontinuation of estrogen-containing oral contraceptives usually relieves the symptoms.

The relation of oral contraceptive use and the occurrence of stroke has been a controversial topic. Numerous epidemiologic studies indicate that age >35 years and cigarette smoking increase the risk of ischemic and hemorrhagic stroke in women using oral contraceptives. Contraceptive preparations with lower doses of synthetic estrogens are thought to be safest. Hypercoagulability associated with estrogens is thought to be an important etiologic factor in arterial strokes, as well as in the syndromes of cerebral venous thrombosis that may complicate pregnancy or contraceptive use.

Direct effects of sex steroids on the CNS may explain the effects of estrogens (epileptogenic) and progestins (anticonvulsant) on seizure frequency in epilepsy. Oral contraceptives or pregnancy may unmask latent chorea (*chorea gravidarum*), and menstrual cyclicity or exogenous administration of estrogen has been reported to be associated with functional changes in parkinsonism, myoclonus, and other movement disorders. Sex steroid receptors on CNS neoplasms may influence growth characteristics of the tumor. Clinically evident enlargement of meningioma may be seen with pregnancy.

The developmental effects of estrogens and androgens on the brain are extensive. Many behavioral characteristics, sexual and otherwise, may be directed by the influence of these hormones on the morphology of neurons and the creation of neural networks. Studies of cognitive function in hypothalamic hypogonadism emphasize the linkages between endocrine and neural function. Clinical interventions may be forthcoming. Similarly, the effect of sex hormones in aging on cognitive performance is an area of active investigation.

SUGGESTED READINGS

Pituitary

Abrams GM, Schipper HM. Neuroendocrine syndromes of the hypothalamus. *Neurol Clin* 1986;4:769–782.

Barzilay J, Heatley GJ, Cushing GW. Benign and malignant tumors in patients with acromegaly. *Arch Intern Med* 1991;151:1629–1632.

Brada M, Ford D, Ashley S, et al. Risk of second brain tumour after conservative surgery and radiotherapy for pituitary adenoma. *BMJ* 1992;304:1343–1346.

Brunner HO, Otten BJ. Precocious puberty in boys. *N Eng J Med* 1999;341:1763–1765.

Cannavo S, Almoto B, Dall'Asta C, et al. Long-term results of treatment in patients with ACTH-secreting pituitary macroadenomas. *Eur J Endocrinol* 2003;149:195–200.

Chan TY. Drug-induced syndrome of inappropriate antidiuretic hormone secretion: causes, diagnosis and management. *Drugs Aging* 1998;11:27–44.

Chanson P, Weinbraub BD, Harris AG. Octreotide therapy for thyroid-stimulating hormone-secreting pituitary adenomas: a follow-up of 52 patients. *Ann Intern Med* 1993;119:236–240.

Colao A, DiSarno A, Cappabianca P, et al. Withdrawal of long-term cabergoline therapy for tumoral and nontumoral hyperprolactinemia. *N Engl J Med* 2003;349:2023–2033.

Colao A, Ferone D, Marzullo P, et al. Systemic complications of acromegaly: epidemiology, pathogenesis, and management. *Endocr Rev* 2004;25:102–152.

Damaraju SC, Rajshekhar V, Chandy MJ. Validation study of a central venous pressure-based protocol for the management of neurosurgical patients with hyponatremia and natriuresis. *Neurosurgery* 1997;40:312–317.

Dash RJ, Gupta V, Suri S. Sheehan's syndrome: clinical profile, pituitary hormone responses and computed sellar tomography. *Aust N Z J Med* 1993;23:26–31.

David SR, Taylor CC, Kinon BJ, et al. The effects of olanzapine, risperidone, and haloperidol on plasma prolactin levels in patients with schizophrenia. *Clin Ther* 2000;22:1085–1096.

DeSouza B, Brunetti A, Fulham MJ, et al. Pituitary microadenomas: a PET Study. *Radiology* 1990;177:39–44.

Findling JW, Raff H, Aron DC. The low-dose dexamethasone suppression test: a reevaluation in patients with Cushing's syndrome. *J Clin Endocrinol Metab* 2004;89:1222–1226.

Glass LC. Pituitary apoplexy. *N Engl J Med* 2003:2034.

Harrigan MR. Cerebral salt wasting syndrome: a review. *Neurosurgery* 1996;38:152–160.

Hirshberg B, Ben-Yehuda A. The syndrome of inappropriate antidiuretic hormone secretion in the elderly. *Am J Med* 1997;103:270–273.

Khaleeli A, Lerg RD, Edwards RHT, et al. The neuromuscular features of acromegaly: a clinical and pathological study. *J Neurol Neurosurg Psychiatry* 1984;47:1009–1015.

Kivela T, Pelkonen R, Heiskanen O. Diabetes insipidus and blindness caused by a suprasellar tumor: Pieter Pauw's observations from the 16th century. *JAMA* 1998;279:48–50.

Kleinberg DL, Noel GL, Frantz AG. Galactorrhea: a study of 235 cases including 48 with pituitary tumors. *N Engl J Med* 1977;296:589–600.

Klibanski A, Zervas NT. Diagnosis and management of hormone-secreting pituitary adenomas. *N Engl J Med* 1991;342:822–830.

Kurosaki M, Luedecke DK, Abe T. Effectiveness of secondary transnasal surgery in GH-secreting pituitary macroadenomas. *Endocr J* 2003;50:635–642.

Lam KS, Wat MS, Choi KL, et al. Pharmacokinetics, pharmacodynamics, long-term efficacy and safety of oral 1-deamino-8-D-arginine va-

sopressin in adult patients with central diabetes insipidus. *Br J Clin Pharmacol* 1996;42:379–385.

Losa M, Mortini P, Barzaghi R, et al. Surgical treatment of prolactin-secreting pituitary adenomas: early reversals and long-term outcome. *J Clin Endocrinol Metab* 2002;87:3180–3186.

Mahmoud-Ahmed AS, Suh JH. Radiation therapy for Cushing's disease: a review. *Pituitary* 2002;5:175–180.

Mangupli R, Lisette A, Ivett C, et al. Improvement of acromegaly after octreotide LAR treatment. *Pituitary* 2003;6:29–34.

Mantello MT, Schwartz RB, Jones KM, et al. Imaging of neurologic complications associated with pregnancy. *AJR* 1993;160:843–847.

Martin JB, Reichlin S. *Clinical Neuroendocrinology.* 2nd Ed. Philadelphia: FA Davis, 1987.

Melmed S. Acromegaly. *N Engl J Med* 1990;322:966–977.

Molitch ME. Pituitary incidentalomas. *Endocrinol Metab Clin North Am* 1997;26;724–740.

Molitch M. Prolactinomas. In: Melmed S, ed. *The Pituitary.* 2nd Ed. Malden, MA: Blackwell, 2002:455–495.

Morris DG, Grossman AB. Dynamic tests in the diagnosis and differential diagnosis of Cushing's syndrome. *J Endocrinol Invest* 2003;26: 64–73.

Moses AM, Notman DD. Diabetes insipidus and syndrome of inappropriate antidiuretic hormone secretion (SIADH). *Adv Intern Med* 1982;27:73–100.

Mukherjee A, Murray RD, Columb B, et al. Acquired prolactin deficiency indicates severe hypopituitarism in patients with disease of the hypothalamic-pituitary axis. *Clin Endocrinol (Oxf)* 2003;59:743–748.

Naidich MJ, Russell EJ. Current approaches to imaging of the sellar region and pituitary. *Endocrinol Metab Clin North Am* 1999;28:45–79.

Oldfield EH, Chrousas GP, Schulte HM. Preoperative lateralization of ACTH-secreting pituitary microadenomas by bilateral and simultaneous inferior petrosal sinus sampling. *N Engl J Med* 1985;312:100–103.

Onesti ST, Wisniewski T, Post KD. Clinical versus subclinical pituitary apoplexy: presentation, surgical management, and outcome in 21 patients. *Neurosurgery* 1990;26:980–986.

Ozbev N, Inanc S, Aral F, et al. Clinical and laboratory evaluation of 40 patients with Sheehan's syndrome. *Isr J Med Sci* 1994;11:826–829.

Paisley AN, Trainer PJ. Medical treatment in acromegaly. *Curr Opin Pharmacol* 2003;3:672–677.

Papastolou C, Mantzoros CS, Evagelopoulou C, et al. Imaging of the sella in the syndrome of inappropriate secretion of antidiuretic hormone. *J Intern Med* 1995;237:181–185.

Plum F, Van Uitert R. Nonendocrine diseases and disorders of the hypothalamus. In: Reichlin S, Baldessarini RJ, Martin JB, eds. *The Hypothalamus.* New York: Raven, 1978.

Randva HS, Schoebel J, Byrne J, et al. Classical pituitary apoplexy: clinical features, management and outcome. *Clin Endocrinol (Oxf)* 1999;51:181–188.

Repaske DR, Phillips JA 3d. The molecular biology of human hereditary central diabetes insipidus. *Prog Brain Res* 1992;93:295–306.

Rittig S, Robertson GL, Siggaard C, et al. Identification of 13 new mutations in the vasopressin-neurophysin II gene in 17 kindreds with familial autosomal dominant neurohypophyseal diabetes insipidus. *Am J Hum Genet* 1996;58:107–117.

Robinson DB, Michaels RD. Empty sella resulting from the spontaneous resolution of a pituitary macroadenoma. *Arch Intern Med* 1992;152:1920–1923.

Ruitshauser J, Boni-Schnetzler M, Boni J, et al. A novel point mutation in the translation initiation codon of the pre-pro-vasopressin-neurophysin II gene: cosegregation with morphological abnormalities and clinical aymptoms in autosomal dominant neurohypophyseal diabetes insipidus. *J Clin Endocrinol Metab* 1996;81:192–198.

Saito T, Ishikawa S, Abe K, et al. Acute aquaresis by the nonpeptide arginine vasopressin (AVP) antagonist OPC-31260 improves hyponatremia in patients with the syndrome of inappropriate secretion of antidiuretic hormone (SIADH). *J Clin Endocrinol Metab* 1997;82:1054–1057.

Schlechte JA. Prolactinoma. *N Engl J Med* 2003;349:2035–2041.

Serri O, Beauregard C, Hardy J. Long-term biochemical status and disease-related morbidity in 53 postoperative patients with acromegaly. *J Clin Endocrinol Metab* 2004;89:658–661.

Singer I, Oster JR, Fishman LM. The management of diabetes insipidus in adults. *Arch Intern Med* 1997;157:1293–1301.

Styne D, Grumbach MM, Kaplan SL, et al. Treatment of Cushing's disease in childhood and adolescence by transsphenoidal microadenomectoma. *N Engl J Med* 1984;310:889–893.

Tanigawa K, Yamashita S, Nagataki S. Acute quadriplegia in acromegaly. *Ann Intern Med* 1992;117:94–95.

Vidal E, Cevallos R, Vidal J, et al. Twelve cases of pituitary apoplexy. *Arch Intern Med* 1992;152:1893–1899.

Woo MH, Smythe MA. Association of SIADH with selective serotonin reuptake inhibitors. *Ann Pharmacother* 1997;31:108–110.

Young WF, Scheithauer BW, Kovacs KT, et al. Gonadotropin adenoma of the pituitary gland: a clinicopathologic analysis of 100 cases. *Mayo Clin Proc* 1996;71:649–656.

Zimmerman EA. Neuroendocrine disorders. In: Rosenberg R, ed. *Atlas of Clinical Neurology.* Philadelphia: Current Medicine, 1998:3.1–3.15.

Thyroid

Anasti JN, Flack MR, Nelson LM, et al. A potential novel mechanism for precocious puberty in juvenile hypothyroidism. *J Clin Endocrinol Metab* 1995;80:276–279.

Atchison JA, Lee PA, Albright AL. Reversible suprasellar pituitary mass secondary to hypothyroidism. *JAMA* 1989;262:3175–3177.

Barnard RD, Campbell MJ, McDonald MI. Pathologic findings in a case of hypothyroidism with ataxia. *J Neurol Neurosurg Psychiatry* 1971;34:755–760.

Bartley GB, Patourechi V, Kadrmas EP, et al. Clinical features of Graves' ophthalmopathy in an incidence cohort. *Am J Ophthalmol* 1996;121:284–290.

Beghi E, Delodovici ML, Bogliun G, et al. Hypothyroidism and polyneuropathy. *J Neurol Neurosurg Psychiatry* 1989;52:1420–1423.

Bellman SC, Davies A, Fuggle PW, et al. Mild impairment of neuro-otological function in early treated congenital hypothyroidism. *Arch Dis Child* 1996;74:215–218.

Bongers-Schokking JJ, Koot HM, Wiersma D, et al. Influence of timing and dose of thyroid hormone replacement on development in infants with congenital hypothyroidism. *J Pediatr* 2000;136:292–297.

Chao T, Wang JR, Hwang B. Congenital hypothyroidism and concomitant anomalies. *J Pediatr Endocrinol Metab* 1997;10:217–221.

Dugbartey AT. Neurocognitive aspects of hypothyroidism. *Arch Int Med* 1998;158:1413–1418.

Fort P, Lipschitz F, Pugliese M, et al. Neonatal thyroid disease: differential expression in three successive offspring. *J Clin Endocrinol Metab* 1988;66:645–647.

Garcia CA, Fleming H. Reversible corticospinal tract disease due to hyperthyroidism. *Arch Neurol* 1977;34:647–648.

Hagberg B, Westphal O. Ataxic syndrome in congenital hypothyroidism. *Acta Paediatr Scand* 1970;59:323–327.

Haggerty JJ Jr, Prange AJ Jr. Borderline hypothyroidism and depression. *Annu Rev Med* 1995;46:37–46.

Halpern JF, Boyages SC, Maberly GF, et al. The neurology of endemic cretinism. A study of two endemias. *Brain* 1991;114:825–841.

Jacobson, DM. Dysthyroid orbitopathy. *Semin Neurol* 2000;20:43–54.

Jordan RM. Myxedema coma. Pathophysiology, therapy, and factors affecting prognosis. *Med Clin North Am* 1995;79:185–194.

Kaminski HJ, Ruff RL. Neurologic complications of endocrine diseases. *Neurol Clin* 1989;7:489–508.

Kelley DE, Gharib H, Kennedy FP, et al. Thyrotoxic periodic paralysis: report of 10 cases and review of electromyographic findings. *Arch Intern Med* 1989;149:2597–2600.

Klein I, Parker M, Shebert R, et al. Hypothyroidism presenting as muscle stiffness and pseudohypertrophy: Hoffmann's syndrome. *Am J Med* 1981;70:891–894.

Kothbauer-Margreiter I, Sturzenegger M, Komor J, et al. Encephalopathy associated with Hashimoto thyroiditis: diagnosis and treatment. *J Neurol* 1996;243:585–593.

Martin FI, Deam DR. Hyperthyroidism in elderly hospitalized patients. Clinical features and treatment outcomes. *Med J Austr* 1996;164:200–203.

Ober KP. Thyrotoxic periodic paralysis in the United States: report of 7 cases and review of the literature. *Medicine* 1992;71:109–120.

Pandit L, Shankar SK, Gayathri N, et al. Acute thyrotoxic neuropathy—Basedow's paraplegia revisited. *J Neurol Sci* 1998;155:211–214.

Perros P, Kendall-Taylor F. Pathogenetic mechanisms in thyroid-associated ophthalmopathy. *J Intern Med* 1992;231:205–211.

Prabhakar BS, Bahn RS, Smith TJ. Current perspective on the pathogenesis of Graves' disease and ophthalmopathy. *Endocrine Rev* 2003;24:802–835.

Reidl S, Frisch H. Pituitary hyperplasia in a girl with gonadal dysgenesis and primary hypothyroidism. *Horm Res* 1997;47:126–130.

Schuelke M, Wagner KR, Stolz LE, et al. Myostatin mutation associated with gross muscle hypertrophy in a child. *N Engl J Med* 2004;350:2682–2688.

Shaw PJ, Bates D, Kendall-Taylor P. Hyperthyroidism presenting as pyramidal tract disease. *BMJ* 1988;297:1395–1396.

Spiro AJ, Hirano A, Beilin RL, et al. Cretinism with muscular hypertrophy (Kocher-Debré-Sémélaigne syndrome). *Arch Neurol* 1970;23:340–349.

Surks MI, Ortiz E, Daniels GH, et al. Subclinical thyroid disease: scientific review and guidelines for diagnosis and management. *JAMA* 2004;291:228–238.

Tallstedt L, Lundell G, Torring O, et al. Occurrence of ophthalmopathy after treatment for Graves' hyperthyroidism. *N Engl J Med* 1992;326:1733–1738.

Van Dop C, Conte FA, Koch TK. Pseudotumor cerebri with initiation of levothyroxine therapy for juvenile hypothyroidism. *N Engl J Med* 1983;308:1076–1080.

Warwar RE. New insights into pathogenesis and potential therapeutic options for Graves orbitopathy. *Curr Opin Ophthalmol* 1999;10:358–361.

Wiersinga WM, Prummel MF. Graves' ophthalmopathy: a rational approach to treatment. *Trends Endocrinol Metab* 2002;13:280–287.

Wise MP, Blunt S, Lane RJ. Neurological presentations of hypothyroidism: the importance of slow-relaxing reflexes. *J R Soc Med* 1995;88:272–274.

Wong PS, Hee FL, Lip GY. Atrial fibrillation and the thyroid. *Heart* 1997;78:623–624.

Yamamoto TJ, Fukuyama J, et al. Factors associated with mortality of myxedema coma: report of eight cases and literature survey. *Thyroid* 1999;12:1167–1174.

Parathyroid

Abe S, Tojo K, Ichida K, et al. A rare case of idiopathic hypoparathyroidism with varied neurological manifestations. *Intern Med* 1996;35:129–134.

Bastepe M, Juppner H. Pseudohypoparathyroidism. New insights into an old disease. *Endocrinol Metab Clin North Am* 2000;29:569–589.

Cogan MG, Covey CM, Arieff AI, et al. Central nervous system manifestations of hyperparathyroidism. *Am J Med* 1978;65:563–630.

Cope O. The story of hyperparathyroidism at the Massachusetts General Hospital. *N Engl J Med* 1966;274:1174–1182.

Kowdley KV, Coull BM. Cognitive impairment and intracranial calcification in chronic hypoparathyroidism. *Am J Med Sci* 1999;317:273–277.

Silverberg SJ, Shane E, Jacobs TP, et al. A 10-year prospective study of primary hyperparathyroidism with or without parathyroid surgery. *New Engl J Med* 1999;341:1249–1255. Erratum in: *N Engl J Med* 2000;342:144.

Tabaee-Zadeh MJ, Frame B, Kappahn K. Kinesigenic choreoathetosis and idiopathic hypoparathyroidism. *N Engl J Med* 1972;286:762–763.

Turken SA, Cafferty M, Silverberg S, et al. Neuromuscular involvement in mild asymptomatic primary hyperparathyroidism. *Am J Med* 1989;87:553–557.

Pancreas

Dyck PJ, Thomas PK, Asbury AK, et al., eds. *Diabetic Neuropathy.* Philadelphia: WB Saunders, 1987.

Field JB. Hypoglycemia. Definition, clinical presentations, classification, and laboratory tests. *Endocrinol Metab Clin North Am* 1989;18:27–43.

Harati Y. Diabetes and the nervous system. *Endocrinol Metab Clin North Am* 1996;25:325–359.

Harrison MJ. Muscle wasting after prolonged hypoglycaemic coma: case report with electrophysiological data. *J Neurol Neurosurg Psychiatry* 1976;39:465–470.

Hefter H, Mayer P, et al. Persistent chorea after recurrent hypoglycemia. A case report. *Eur Neurol* 1993;33:244–247.

Malouf R, Brust JCM. Hypoglycemia: causes, neurological manifestations and outcome. *Ann Neurol* 1985;17:421–430.

Mohseni, S. Hypoglycemic neuropathy. *Acta Neuropathol (Berl)* 2001;102:413–421.

Mooradian A. Pathophysiology of central nervous system complications of diabetes mellitus. *Clin Neurosci* 1997;4:322–326.

Pagliara AS, Karl IE, Haymond M, et al. Hypoglycemia in childhood. *J Pediatr* 1973;82:365–379.

Silas JH, Grant DS, Maddocks JL. Transient hemiparetic attacks due to unrecognized nocturnal hypoglycemia. *BMJ* 1981;282:132–133.

Adrenal

Abbas DH, Schlagenhauff RE, Strong HE. Polyradiculoneuropathy in Addison's disease: case report and review of literature. *Neurology* 1977;27:494–495.

Anagnos A, Ruff RL, Kaminski HJ. Endocrine neuromyopathies. *Neurol Clin* 1997:15:673–696.

Atsumi T, Ishikawa S, Miyatake T, et al. Myopathy and primary aldosteronism: electron microscopic study. *Neurology* 1979;29:1348–1358.

Boscaro ML, Barzon L, Fallo F, et al. Cushing's syndrome. *Lancet* 2001;357:783–791.

Brennemann W, Kohler W, Zierz S, et al. Occurrence of adrenocortical insufficiency in adrenomyeloneuropathy. *Neurology* 1996;47:605.

Condulis N, Germain G, Charest N, et al. Pseudotumor cerebri: a presenting manifestation of Addison's disease. *Clin Pediatr* 1997;36:711–713.

De Kloet ER, Vreugdenhil E, Oitzl MS, et al. Brain corticosteroid receptor balance in health and disease. *Endocr Rev* 1998;19:269–301.

Falorni A, Laureti S, et al. Autoantibodies in autoimmune polyendocrine syndrome type II. *Endocrinol Metab Clin North Am* 2002;31:369–389.

Findling JW, Raff H. Diagnosis and differential diagnosis of Cushing's syndrome. *Endocrinol Metab Clin North Am* 200130:729–747.

Huang YY, Hsu BR, Tsai JS. Paralytic myopathy: a leading clinical presentation for primary aldosteronism in Taiwan. *J Clin Endocrinol Metab* 1997;82:2377–2378.

Jefferson A. A clinical correlation between encephalopathy and papilloedema in Addison's disease. *J Neurol Neurosurg Psychiatry* 1956;19:21–26.

Kandt RS, Heldrich FJ, Moser HW. Recovery from probable central pontine myelinolysis associated with Addison's disease. *Arch Neurol* 1983;40:118–119.

Laureti S, Casucci G, Santeusania F, et al. X-linked adrenoleukodystrophy is a frequent cause of idiopathic Addison's disease in young adult male patients. *J Clin Endocrinol Metab* 1996;81:470–474.

Litchfield WR, Anderson BF, Weiss RJ, et al. Intracranial aneurysm and hemorrhagic stroke in glucocorticoid-remediable aldosteronism. *Hypertension* 1998;31:445–450.

Machlen J, Torvik A. Necrosis of granule cells of hippocampus in adrenocortical failure. *Acta Neuropathol* 1990;80:85–87.

Manger WM. Psychiatric manifestations in patients with pheochromocytoma. *Arch Intern Med* 1985;145:229–230.

Moser HW. Adrenoleukodystrophy: phenotype, genetics, pathogenesis, and therapy. *Brain* 1997;120:1485–1508.

Neumann H, Berger DP, Sigmund G, et al. Pheochromocytomas, multiple endocrine neoplasia type 2, and von Hippel-Lindau disease. *N Engl J Med* 1993;329:1531–1538.

Newman PK, Snow M, Hudgson P. Benign intracranial hypertension and Cushing's disease. *BMJ* 1980;281:113.

Oelkers W. Adrenal insufficiency. *N Engl J Med* 1996;335:1206–1212.

Olafsson E, Jones HR, Guay AT, et al. Myopathy of endogenous Cushing's syndrome: a review of the clinical and electromyographic features in 8 patients. *Muscle Nerve* 1994;17:692–693.

Pomares FJ, Canas R, Rodriguez JM, et al. Differences between sporadic and multiple endocrine neoplasia type 2A phaeochromocytoma. *Clin Endocrinol (Oxf)* 1998;48:195–200.

Ten S, New M, et al. Clinical review 130: Addison's disease 2001. *J Clin Endocrinol Metab* 2001;86:2909–2922.

Thomas JE, Rooke ED, Kvale WF. The neurologists's experience with pheochromocytoma: a review of 100 cases. *JAMA* 1966;197:754–758.

Weber KT, Singh KD, et al. Idiopathic intracranial hypertension with primary aldosteronism: report of 2 cases. *Am J Med Sci* 2002;324:45–50.

Werbel SS, Ober KP. Pheochromocytoma: update on diagnosis, localization, and management. *Med Clin North Am* 1995;79:131–153.

Young WF, Jr. Minireview: primary aldosteronism–changing concepts in diagnosis and treatment. *Endocrinology* 2003;144:2208–2213.

Gonads

Allroggen H, Abbott RJ. Cerebral venous sinus thrombosis. *Postgrad Med J* 2000;76:12–15.

Bousser MG, Kittner SJ. Oral contraceptives and stroke. *Cephalalgia* 2000;20:183–189.

Boyle CA. Management of menstrual migraine. *Neurology* 1999;53(Suppl 1):S14–18.

Foldvary N. Treatment issues for women with epilepsy. *Neurol Clin* 2001;19:409–425.

Schipper H. Neurology of sex steroids and oral contraceptives. *Neurol Clin* 1986;4:721–752.

Schwartzhaus JD, Currie J, Jaffe MJ, et al. Neurologic findings in men with isolated hypogonadotropic hypogonadism. *Neurology* 1989;39:223–226.

Shumaker SA, Legault C, Rapp SR, et al. Estrogen plus progestin and the incidence of dementia and mild cognitive impairment in postmenopausal women: the Women's Health Initiative Memory Study: a randomized controlled trial. *JAMA* 2003;289:2651–2662.

Somerville BW. Estrogen withdrawal migraine. I. Duration of exposure required and attempted prophylaxis by premenstrual estrogen administration. *Neurology* 1975;25:239–244.

Somerville BW. Estrogen withdrawal migraine. II. Attempted prophylaxis by continuous estradiol administration. *Neurology* 1975;25:245–250.

Tang MX, Jacobs D, Stern Y, et al. Effect of oestrogen during menopause on risk and age at onset of Alzheimer's disease. *Lancet* 1996;348:429–432.

Chapter 147

Hematologic and Related Diseases

Robert W. Pratt, David Adams, and Casilda Balmaceda

ERYTHROCYTE DISORDERS

Sickle Cell Disease

Sickle cell disease is an autosomal recessively inherited disorder resulting from homozygosity for sickle hemoglobin (hemoglobin S, or HbS). It is prevalent in people of African descent; 1 in 600 African Americans in the United States is homozygous for HbS (SS). A substitution of glutamic acid with valine in the β-globin subunit of hemoglobin leads to the diverse and often devastating complications of sickle cell disease. Normal hemoglobin is exceptionally soluble, but sickle hemoglobin, when deoxygenated, aggregates into large polymers. The resulting red blood cell becomes stiff and distorted in contrast to the pliant normal erythrocyte. Sickled red cells tend to adhere to the vessel wall. Vaso-occlusive disorders affect the kidney, bone, lung, liver, heart, spleen, peripheral nerves, and brain. Neurologic complications include ischemic stroke, intracranial hemorrhage, seizures, CNS infections, retinopathy, myelopathy, sensorineural hearing loss, and neuropathy. Other common sickle genotypes, such as sickle cell-hemoglobin C (SC) disease and the sickle-β-thalassemia syndromes, also have neurologic sequelae.

After infection, ischemic stroke is the second leading cause of death. Cerebral infarcts appear at a mean age of 8 years; by age 45, one-fourth of all patients with SS disease will have had an ischemic stroke. In the Cooperative Study of Sickle Cell Disease, the incidence of first ischemic stroke was 0.70 per 100 patient years in the United States among children between ages 2 and 5 years, 0.51 between 6 and 9 years, 0.24 between 10 and 19 years, and 0.04 between 20 and 29 years. The incidence of stroke is much lower in patients with sickle cell-hemoglobin C (SC) disease and the sickle-β-thalassemias. The incidence of strokes in patients with sickle cell trait does not exceed that of the general population.

Risk factors for cerebral infarct include prior TIA, low hemoglobin content, frequent acute chest syndrome episodes or one within the last 2 weeks, and high systolic blood pressure. Genetic modifiers also influence susceptibility to stroke. Recurrent strokes occur more frequently in younger patients (6.4 per 100 patient years before age 20 and 1.6 per 100 patient years after age 20.

Strokes occur because of both large and small vessel disease. Mechanisms of infarction include occlusion or stenosis of large intracranial arteries (most commonly the intracranial internal carotid and middle cerebral arteries), sludging and occlusion of small vessels by the rigid red cells, and flow-related hemodynamic injury to the arterial endothelium. SS red cells have a sticky surface and attach more readily than normal cells to the endothelium.

Histopathologically, vascular damage includes segmental thickening caused by intimal proliferation of fibroblasts and smooth muscle. Many infarcts occur in watershed distributions, a combination of occlusion, anemia hemodynamic insufficiency, and border zone hypoperfusion. Transcranial Doppler ultrasonography (TCD) can assess the risk of stroke in patients with sickle cell disease. Cerebral arterial blood flow velocity is inversely related to arterial diameter, and high velocity is correlated with stenosis on angiography and subsequent stroke. In the Stroke Prevention Trial in Sickle Cell Anemia (STOP trial), 130 children with no history of stroke but with high blood flow velocities were randomized to either observation or prophylactic transfusions with a goal of reducing the amount of sickle hemoglobin to less than 30% of total hemoglobin.

The incidence of recurrent stroke in patients receiving transfusion therapy is 10%, compared with 46% to 90% without transfusion. Ultimately, the benefits of long-term transfusion in preventing a first or recurrent stroke must be weighed against the complications of transfusions, including autoimmunity, infection, and iron overload. Alternatives include increasing the concentration of hemoglobin F with hydroxyurea and bone marrow transplantation.

Hemorrhagic strokes account for one-third of all strokes in sickle cell disease. The period of lowest risk for cerebral infarcts (ages 20 to 29 years) is the period of highest risk for hemorrhagic stroke. Decreased hemoglobin concentration and high steady state leukocyte count are the major risk factors for hemorrhagic stroke. Subarachnoid hemorrhage is more common in children, whereas intraparenchymal hemorrhage is seen in adults.

Subarachnoid hemorrhage (SAH) follows rupture of an aneurysm. Forty-five percent of patients have multiple aneurysms, which are located at the bifurcation points of large vessels, at the site of endothelial injury and hyperplasia. This damage to the vessel wall integrity presumably leads to aneurysmal dilatation and rupture. Treatment of SAH in sickle cell disease is the same as SAH management in other people, including angiography to identify the source of the bleed, clipping or coiling of the aneurysm, hydration, and prevention or treatment of vasospasm and hydrocephalus.

A *moyamoyalike* disease accounts for almost one-third of all intracranial hemorrhages in sickle cell disease. Severe stenosis or occlusion of the arteries at the base of the brain induces a fragile collateral circulation that gives a "puff of smoke" appearance on angiography. These thinwalled collaterals develop microaneurysms and frequently cause hemorrhage into the basal ganglia and periventricular region. Ischemic strokes also occur. Different surgical techniques have been used for moyamoya, including anastomosis of the superficial temporal artery to the middle cerebral artery. If the temporal artery is too narrow, another bypass procedure is encephalomyosynangiosis (laying the temporalis muscle over the surface of the brain to encourage new anastomoses) or encephaloduroarteriosynangiosis (anastomosing the superficial temporal artery to an incision in the dura).

MRI reveals asymptomatic (silent) infarcts in 10% to 20% of children. In one study, PET was abnormal in six of ten SS children with no history of neurologic events and no abnormality on neurologic examination.

Headache seems common in sickle cell patients, but there are no epidemiologic data to confirm this. Cerebral blood flow is higher in sickle cell disease patients with headache than without, and headache often improves after transfusion.

Epilepsy is more common in sickle cell patients than in the general population, affecting 6% to 12% of patients. Seizures may accompany strokes or meningitis and may be precipitated by dehydration or by commonly used medications such as meperidine. Meningitis is seen primarily in infants and young children. Streptococcal pneumonia with hematologic spread is the most frequent cause. The rapid administration of antibiotics and the conjugate vaccines for *S. pneumoniae* and *H. influenza* has greatly reduced the incidence of meningitis.

Eye manifestations of sickle cell disease include proliferative retinopathy, retinal artery occlusion, and retinal detachment and hemorrhage. Myelopathy is rare but may follow spinal cord infarction or cord compression from epidural abscess or tumorlike extramedullary hematopoiesis. Sensorineural hearing loss is attributed to cochlear ischemia. Peripheral nervous system involvement is unusual; a mononeuropathy, single or multiplex, from nerve infarction, is possible. Finally, peripheral neuropathy from lead intoxication, nitrous oxide anesthesia, and sodium cyanate treatment have been reported.

Thalassemia

β-Thalassemia is an inherited hemoglobin disorder caused by defective synthesis of the β-globin chain, which results in chronic hemolytic anemia. Occurring in people of Mediterranean or Asian descent, the disorder is rapidly fatal if left untreated. Treatment is with hypertransfusion and iron chelation therapy. Clinical manifestations include hepatosplenomegaly, growth retardation, skin changes, bony abnormalities (Fig. 147.1) and high-output heart failure. Transient dizziness and visual blurring are seen in up to 20%. These symptoms typically occur between transfusions and improve when the anemia is ameliorated. Headaches and seizures are seen in 13%. Twenty percent develop a mild peripheral, mainly motor, neuropathy in the second decade of life. Stroke is a rare complication. Both intracranial hemorrhage and cerebral thrombosis have been reported, with coagulopathy owing to liver dysfunction, cardiac abnormalities such as atrial fibrillation and ventricular dysfunction, and thrombocytosis from splenectomy as possible underlying causes. A pseudoxanthoma elasticumlike clinical syndrome, with skin, ocular, and vascular abnormalities, leading to intracranial hemorrhages and cardiac complications, predisposing to thrombotic strokes, is also encountered. Spinal cord and cauda equina compression from extramedullary hematopoiesis have been successfully treated by surgery, hypertransfusion, and radiation. Extramedullary hematopoietic tissue may also lead to vision loss by compression of the optic nerve or chiasm.

Polycythemia

Polycythemia, an abnormal increase in the number of circulating erythrocytes, may occur with the myeloproliferative disorder *polycythemia vera*; secondary etiologies include causes of chronic hypoxemia, such as chronic pulmonary disease, high altitude, sleep apnea, or a right-to-left cardiac shunt. Rarely, erythropoietin-producing neoplasms, including hemangioblastoma, hepatocellular carcinoma, or renal cell carcinoma, may induce the increased red cell mass. Both thrombocytosis (increased number of platelets) and a platelet disorder that leads to a bleeding diathesis may also be seen.

Polycythemia causes hyperviscosity of the blood, leading to accelerated atherosclerosis and thrombosis in both large and small vessels. In polycythemia vera, transient ischemic attacks and ischemic strokes account for 70% of arterial thrombotic events. Cerebral venous thrombosis is a rare complication. Low-dose aspirin (100 milligrams daily) therapy safely and effectively reduces the risk of strokes in these patients. Headache, tinnitus, dizziness, visual disturbances, cognitive impairment, and limb pain or paresthesias may be caused by hyperviscosity; these symptoms often recede when the red blood cell count is lowered by phlebotomy or chemotherapy. Many patients have clinical or electrophysiologic signs of a predominantly sensory axonal polyneuropathy.

Polycythemia vera also leads to *erythromelalgia*, which is characterized by painfully hot, red extremities. Symptoms are more often prominent in the legs than the arms and hands; autonomic small-fiber dysfunction may be responsible. Response to various treatments has been poor,

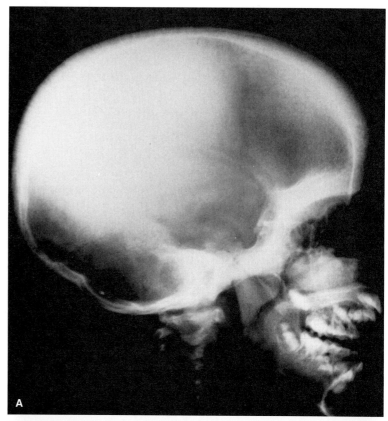

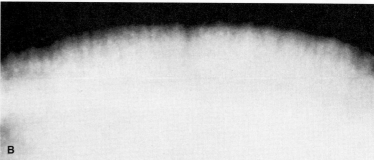

FIGURE 147.1. Skull in chronic hemolytic anemia (thalassemia). **A.** Thickening of vault. **B.** Magnified view of "hair-on-end" appearance as a result of extramedullary hematopoiesis in the widened diploic space. (Courtesy of Dr. William H. McAlister.)

but the condition remits spontaneously in one-third of patients.

PLATELET DISORDERS

Essential Thrombocytosis (Thrombocythemia)

Essential thrombocytosis is an acquired myeloproliferative disorder characterized by a high platelet count, splenomegaly, platelet dysfunction, and a predisposition to both hemorrhage and thrombosis involving the arterial and venous circulations. The specific criteria to make the diagnosis are consistently elevated platelet count of >600,000/μL, megakaryocytic hyperplasia in the bone marrow, normal iron stores, absence of increased erythrocyte mass, absence of the Philadelphia chromosome, a myelodysplastic disorder or myeloid metaplasia, and no cause of a reactive thrombocytosis. Onset is typically after age 50.

Neurologic manifestations occur in 30% of patients with essential thrombocytosis, including headache, paresthesias, TIA, and seizures. These problems are seen at onset or with hematologic relapse. Bleeding complications are seen paradoxically at very high platelet counts (1,500,000/μL). The platelet count should be checked in all patients with ischemic episodes and in those with headaches, visual symptoms, or paresthesias.

Age, a previous thrombotic event, and long duration of thrombocytosis are risk factors for thrombosis. Therapy is aimed at lowering the platelet count. Hydroxyurea, a myelosuppresive agent, is used with low-dose aspirin to prevent strokes in high-risk patients (defined as having an age older than 60 years and a history of a previous thrombotic event). High platelet counts may aggravate platelet dysfunction, leading to controversy about the risk/benefit of low-dose aspirin in preventing thrombosis in asymptomatic patients. Interferon-alpha and anagrelide are both effective in lowering platelet counts, but their efficacy in reducing clinical complications remains unknown. Platelet pheresis is recommended after a serious thromboembolic event.

Thrombotic Thrombocytopenic Purpura

Thrombotic thrombocytopenic purpura (TTP) is characterized by thrombocytopenia, microangiopathic hemolytic anemia, fever, renal abnormalities, and neurologic manifestations. The peak incidence is at age 40, with a 2:1 female-to-male predominance. When promptly recognized and treated, the mortality rate ranges from 10% to 20%. Up to one-third of survivors have infrequent relapses. Some cases may follow an identifiable cause, such as HIV infection, pregnancy, systemic lupus erythematosus, or drug therapy. TTP rarely follows use of clopidogrel, ticlopidine quinine, mitomycin C, or cyclosporine.

Fluctuating neurologic symptoms, usually lasting less than 48 hours, occur in 70% of patients. Headache, confusion, and stupor are the most common and lead to focal neurologic signs, seizures, coma or death. The fluctuating stupor of TTP has been ascribed to microvascular occlusive disease (see below), but nonconvulsive status epilepticus occurs and EEG monitoring can be considered. Hemiparesis tends to improve more readily than mental status; neurologic symptoms are permanent in a few survivors.

Pathophysiologically, immunoglobulin G (IgG) autoantibodies are active against a metalloprotease that normally cleaves large multimers of von Willebrand factor (vWF), a procoagulant produced by vascular endothelium. Systemic endothelial cell injury can lead to excessive release of these extra large vWF multimers. Reduced vWF multimer breakdown leads to platelet microthrombi that characterize the syndrome pathologically. Typical neurohistopathologic changes show hyaline thrombotic occlusion of the microvascular circulation, without inflammation, leading to small infarcts and petechial hemorrhages (Fig. 147.2). These thrombi consist primarily of platelets and vWF.

A variety of brain lesions may be seen on neuroimaging. MRI may show a reversible posterior leukoencephalopathy syndrome. Normal head CT, even in the presence of substantial neurologic dysfunction clinically, suggests the possibility of full clinical recovery in 70% of patients. If CT findings are abnormal, death or permanent neurologic disorder follows in 80%. CSF is usually normal except for elevated protein content.

Plasma exchange with fresh frozen plasma infusion is the treatment of choice for TTP. If response is incomplete, steroids may be added. High-dose plasma infusion (25–30 mL/kg per day) may have a role as emergency treatment while plasma exchange is arranged. A randomized, controlled trial showed no difference in efficacy between whole plasma and cryoprecipitate-poor plasma.

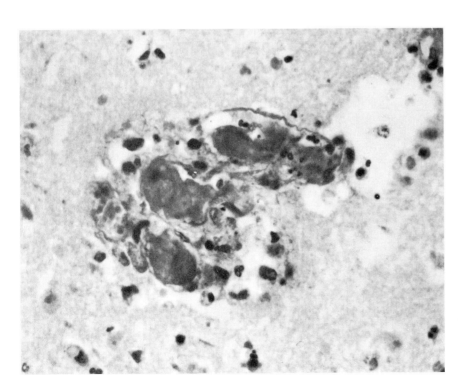

FIGURE 147.2. Thrombotic thrombocytopenic purpura. Occlusion of small cerebral vessels by amorphous hyaline material. (Courtesy of Dr. Abner Wolf.)

Therapy with cryosupernatant plasma must be supplemented by the occasional use of whole plasma to prevent deficiencies of fibrinogen and factor VIII. Successful treatments with IVIG and chemotherapeutic immunosuppressants have also been reported. Platelet transfusion may worsen or induce neurologic and renal dysfunction, presumably because of new or expanding thrombi as the infused platelets are consumed. There is little evidence that heparin is beneficial; however, because vWF causes platelet aggregation by activating GP IIb/IIIa platelet receptors for fibrinogen, platelet GP IIb/IIIa receptor inhibitors such as abciximab and tirofiban might prove useful but await adequate clinical trials. Dialysis is used to treat the renal dysfunction. Death from neurologic complications in TTP is not as common as from other organ failure.

Heparin-Induced Thrombocytopenia

Heparin-induced thrombocytopenia (HIT) is an immune-mediated disorder typically occurring 5 or more days after initiation of therapy in a patient not previously exposed to heparin. The pathogenic IgG immunoglobulin binds a heparin/platelet factor 4 complex, causing platelet activation. This prothrombotic state is characterized by a 50% or greater decrease in platelet count. Spontaneous bleeding is unusual, as the degree of thrombocytopenia is seldom severe. Among 200 patients receiving unfractionated heparin, there was a 2.5% rate of HIT and a 2% rate of HIT-associated thrombosis. Heparin-induced antibodies were found in 29.4% of stroke patients versus 11.2% with other conditions. Heparin therapy should be discontinued immediately and warfarin withheld until platelets recover to avoid venous limb gangrene. Low molecular weight heparin must also be avoided because of possible cross-reactivity. Danaparoid, a heparinoid mixture of anticoagulant glycosaminoglycans, inhibits fibrin formation and is an effective alternative to heparin, as are the direct thrombin inhibitors lepirudin and argatroban. Heparin-associated thrombosis may *precede* thrombocytopenia, so HIT has to be considered in heparin-treated patients with cerebral ischemia, cerebral venous thrombosis, or a transient confusional state, *whether or not the platelet count is decreased*.

BLOOD CELL DYSCRASIAS

Leukemia

All forms of leukemia may lead to decreased production of normal blood cells in the bone marrow, indirectly resulting in hemorrhage from thrombocytopenia, infections from ineffective or immature leukocytes, and fatigue and lightheadedness from anemia. With markedly elevated white blood counts ($>150,000/mm^3$), *leukostasis* may occlude cerebral blood vessels. Furthermore, leukemic blasts can infiltrate the arteriole endothelial walls to cause hemorrhage. Patients at risk for CNS leukostasis are treated with emergency leukapheresis to lower the blast count. Leukemic nodules may also predispose to intracerebral hemorrhage, which may be fatal.

Direct CNS manifestations of leukemia depend on the specific cell type involved. In *acute myelogenous leukemias*, CNS involvement is uncommonly the first manifestation. Patients at risk for CNS symptoms include those with high circulating blast counts and the monocytic M4 subtype. The M4 Eo variant in particular, with eosinophilia and the inv(16)(p13q22) inversion of chromosome 16, is commonly associated with leptomeningeal and intracerebral lesions. Patients may be asymptomatic, complain of headaches, or have symptoms related to a cranial nerve palsy. The optic, trigeminal, and facial nerves are most commonly involved, along with the retina; in one series, almost two-thirds of adults newly diagnosed with AML had retinal or optic nerve involvement. Unless CNS symptoms require therapy, lumbar puncture is deferred until the peripheral blood is cleared of blast cells to avoid possible CNS seeding. Acute myelogenous leukemias may also affect the CNS in the form of a *chloroma* (or *granulocytic sarcoma*), a local collection of blast cells that appears green because of myeloperoxidase produced by the myeloid cells. Chloromas may be seen 1 year before the overt onset of acute leukemia, originating in subperiosteal sites in bone and characteristically causing unilateral or bilateral exophthalmos simulating orbital lymphoma. Other sites include the cranial and facial bones, commonly causing facial palsy, and the spinal epidural space, causing paraplegia. A handful of cases of cerebral intraparenchymal chloromas have been reported, usually in women, and after a period of complete remission; radiation therapy is the treatment of choice.

Acute lymphocytic leukemia (ALL) involves the CNS in 5% to 10% of patients at time of diagnosis, often without symptoms. Without prophylactic chemotherapy, however, most patients will develop CNS disease. Risk factors for CNS involvement include a high lymphocyte count, T-ALL phenotype, and L3 (Burkitt) morphology. Leukemic cells invade the meninges; tumor spreads from the bone marrow centripetally along arachnoid veins, giving rise to leptomeningeal metastases. The infiltrate spreads along the arachnoid into the Virchow-Robin spaces, secondarily affecting the adventitia of arterioles. With leptomeningeal seeding, the CSF cytology is invariably abnormal. As with meningeal involvement by carcinoma, all levels of the CNS are affected, with cranial nerve signs (III, IV, VI, and VII), seizures, cognitive deficit, or hydrocephalus. Uncommon syndromes with leukemic infiltration include hypothalamic infiltration with *hyperphagia* and *obesity* or diabetes insipidus.

The prognosis for acute leukemia was poor before 1960, when therapy was first directed to the eradication of leptomeningeal metastasis. The CNS is a sanctuary because most systemic antileukemic chemotherapy does not achieve CSF levels high enough to eradicate tumor cells. Surviving leukemia cells in the CSF may re-enter the marrow and re-establish the disease. All patients now receive intrathecal chemotherapy, either methotrexate alone or combined with cytarabine and prednisone. Seizures and leukoencephalopathy are recognized side effects. CNS radiation is added for patients with clinical CNS involvement at any time, and sometimes prophylactically in patients with high-risk ALL. Cranial irradiation puts patients at later risk for neuropsychologic decline and leukoencephalopathy. Bone marrow transplantation in patients with leukemia may be complicated by post-transplant leukoencephalopathy.

In contrast, chronic leukemia rarely affects the CNS. When *chronic myelogenous leukemia* enters into blast crisis, leptomeningeal metastases may occur. *Chronic lymphocytic leukemia* (CLL) is common but only exceptionally invades the meninges or brain, most often with late-stage disease.

Plasma Cell Dyscrasias

Several conditions, both neoplastic and non-neoplastic, are characterized by the appearance of monoclonal gamma globulins (M proteins) in the serum. The monoclonal proteins are produced by cells of B-cell lineage, and the associated *plasma cell dyscrasias* include multiple myeloma, Waldenström macroglobulinemia (with IgM paraprotein), and amyloidosis.

If monoclonal gammopathy is the only manifestation, this is termed *monoclonal gammopathy of unknown significance* (MGUS). MGUS may persist asymptomatically for years or decades. In 20% of patients, a plasma cell dyscrasia or one of the lymphoproliferative diseases (CLL, lymphoma) later appears. Differentiation of MGUS from more serious disease depends on bone marrow examination, urinary excretion of light chains (Bence-Jones protein), and survey for bone lesions.

Peripheral neuropathy is a common neurologic manifestation of MGUS. In most cases, the paraprotein is immunoglobulin M (IgM) and less commonly IgG or immunoglobulin A (IgA). In about half of the patients with IgM neuropathy, the monoclonal protein has antibody activity against *myelin-associated glycoprotein* and results in a demyelinating peripheral neuropathy. These patients show large-fiber sensory loss and late-onset distal limb weakness. Some patients with a sensory axonal neuropathy have IgM antibodies that recognize axonal sulfatides or chondroitin sulfate. The role of the M protein in the pathogenesis of these syndromes is debated, but experimentally antibodies to myelin-associated glycoprotein can induce peripheral nerve demyelination.

In myeloma, the protein is usually IgG or less commonly IgA. The most frequent neurologic complication is thoracic or lumbosacral radiculopathy, resulting from nerve compression by a vertebral lesion or collapsed bone. Spinal cord compression develops when myeloma extends from the vertebral marrow into the epidural space. Spinal cord compression occurs from an extramedullary *plasmacytoma* in 5% of patients. Emergent treatment of cord compression with high-dose steroids and radiotherapy is mandatory. Surgery is reserved for diagnostic purposes or in the setting of radiotherapy failure. Intracranial plasmacytomas are usually extensions of myeloma skull lesions. Characteristic multiple osteolytic lesions are seen on radiographs of the skull and other bones (Fig. 147.3). Leptomeningeal invasion is also seen with myeloma. Peripheral neuropathy is uncommon and usually associated with axonal degeneration and amyloidosis. One unusual multisystem disease is POEMS (*p*olyneuropathy, *o*rganomegaly, *e*ndocrinopathy, *M* protein, and *s*kin changes), which is associated with osteosclerotic myeloma or plasmacytoma. The M protein is usually IgG or IgA, invariably associated with a lambda light chain. Surgical removal of the plasmacytoma may reverse the neuropathy.

Patients with *Waldenström macroglobulinemia* (WM), a malignant B-cell proliferation leading to an IgM monoclonal gammopathy, note asthenia, fatigue, weight loss, and bleeding. The most common neurologic complication is a sensorimotor peripheral neuropathy. Anti-myelin-associated glycoprotein (MAG) antibodies are found in about half of these patients. Other autoantibodies, such as anti-GM1 ganglioside and asialo-GM1 ganglioside antibodies, may be found. Peripheral nerve biopsy may show myelin degeneration, cellular infiltration of the nerve, IgM deposits on the myelin sheath, or myelin degeneration.

A *hyperviscosity syndrome* with IgM paraproteinemia is associated with headache, blurred vision, tinnitus, vertigo, ataxia, and a depressed level of consciousness leading to coma. Strokes may occur. Funduscopic exam may show papilledema and dilated, segmented "sausage link" retinal veins. Clinical manifestations are rarely attributable to hyperviscosity if serum viscosity is <4 centipoises. Serum viscosity can be reduced by chemotherapy or by plasmapheresis to lower the paraprotein concentration.

The *Bing-Neel syndrome* refers to Waldenström disease with CNS symptoms of infiltrative origin and either diffuse or focal manifestations. The diffuse form is characterized by personality change or altered alertness and is caused by a mainly periventricular and leptomeningeal plasma cell infiltration; seizures and focal neurologic deficits come from the formation of a mass of lymphoplasmacytic cells.

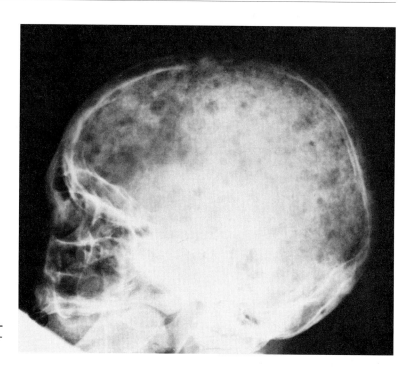

FIGURE 147.3. Multiple myeloma. Myriads of osteolytic lesions. (Courtesy of Dr. Lowell G. Lubic.)

The neuropathies are treated with immunosuppressive drugs, IVIG therapy, or plasmapheresis.

Myelofibrosis

Extramedullary hematopoiesis often accompanies myelofibrosis or polycythemia vera and may cause extradural spinal cord compression, cerebral compression by calvarial-based intracranial masses, or orbital lesions with exophthalmos. The neurologic signs are usually painless and develop insidiously. The syndrome occurs more frequently after splenectomy and responds to radiotherapy.

COAGULATION DISORDERS

Hematologic disorders or coagulopathies may be responsible for stroke in 4% to 17% of young patients and 1% of all patients with ischemic stroke. The role of prothrombotic disorders in older stroke patients is not known. Most prothrombotic disorders are associated with venous thrombosis in unusual sites (mesentery, sagittal sinus), but arterial thrombosis, mainly in the carotid artery, has been described. An inherited thrombophilia is present in 24% to 37% of all patients with a deep vein thrombosis, compared with about 10% in the normal population. Women with hereditary prothrombotic conditions using oral contraception are at a threefold to fourfold risk of cerebral sinus thrombosis. Cerebral thrombosis can occur without systemic manifestations. A hematologic abnormality is attributed a causal role in stroke if the abnormality persists months after the event or is seen in other family members.

Antithrombin Deficiency

Antithrombin (AT), formerly known as antithrombin III, is a plasma glycoprotein synthesized by the liver and endothelial cells. It is an inhibitor of thrombin and other activated clotting factors. AT is required for the anticoagulant action of heparin, which acts by increasing the inhibitory properties of AT. AT activity is measured by its ability to inactivate factor Xa or thrombin. Heparin accelerates this interaction.

Deficiency of AT is inherited or acquired, with a prevalence of 1 in 250 to 500 in the general population. Among patients with a first thrombotic event, the prevalence of hereditary AT deficiency is 0.5% to 1 percent, being less common than factor V Leiden, the prothrombin gene mutation, or protein S or protein C deficiency. There are two types of familial AT deficiency. Type I accounts for about 90% of inherited cases; both antigen level and functional activity of AT are decreased. In type II, levels are normal, but there is dysfunction of AT. The disease is inherited in an autosomal-dominant fashion, affecting both sexes equally. Penetrance is variable. The most common manifestation is leg thrombosis and pulmonary embolus. In heterozygotic individuals, symptomatic thrombosis increases after the age of 15, and by age 55 it is estimated to occur in 85% of gene carriers. More than half of the thrombotic episodes occur with triggering events: pregnancy, surgery, infection, or oral contraceptive use. It is an isolated event in 42%. Cerebral venous thrombosis is the most common neurologic manifestation. Arterial thrombosis may occur, but is not characteristic of AT deficiency. For homozygotes, venous thrombosis is usually seen during the first year of life. Clues to diagnosis are family history of thromboembolism, thrombosis during pregnancy, resistance to heparin therapy, or unusual sites of thrombosis (brain, mesentery).

There are several causes of acquired AT deficiency. Decreased synthesis is seen with liver cirrhosis. Drug-induced AT deficiency occurs with l-asparaginase, heparin, or oral contraceptives containing estrogen. Increased excretion in protein-losing enteropathy, inflammatory bowel disease, or nephrotic syndrome results in low AT levels. Accelerated consumption in disseminated intravascular coagulopathy (DIC) or after major surgery can lead to AT deficiency. Acute thrombosis by itself transiently reduces AT levels. Testing for AT deficiency should not be performed while the patient is receiving heparin, to avoid false-positive results.

AT deficiency is resistant to anticoagulation with heparin. AT concentrate is given to deficient patients with a thrombotic event or at times of maximal risk, such as surgery or delivery. After a thrombotic event, lifelong warfarin therapy is indicated. The value of prophylactic anticoagulation for all carriers during high-risk events is debated.

Protein S Deficiency

Protein S is a vitamin K–dependent plasma protein synthesized in the liver. It facilitates the binding of protein C to the platelet membrane, acting as a nonenzymatic cofactor for the anticoagulant activity of activated protein C. Only 40% of protein S is in a free form; the rest is in an inactive form, bound to C4-binding protein. C4-binding protein levels are elevated during acute inflammation or stress, increasing the inactivation of protein S and thus the risk of thrombosis. The complex of proteins C and S inhibits the clotting cascade. Protein S deficiency can be acquired or congenital, inherited predominantly as autosomal dominant with partial expressivity.

The prevalence of familial protein S deficiency is estimated at 0.03% to 0.13%; among patients with a first venous thrombotic event, 7.3% were found to have protein S deficiency. The lifetime risk of thrombosis is 8.5 times that of the normal population. Acquired deficiency is caused by pregnancy, oral contraceptives, liver dysfunction, vitamin K deficiency, warfarin therapy, nephrotic syndrome, HIV infection, or L-asparaginase chemotherapy.

Thrombosis may affect either arteries or veins, but there is no conclusive evidence that protein S deficiency is a risk factor for arterial thrombosis. Measurement of the free protein S concentration is the most sensitive and specific method of diagnosis; testing must be conducted in the absence of oral anticoagulation. Most patients with protein S deficiency and stroke are given anticoagulation therapy.

Prophylactic anticoagulation is not advocated for asymptomatic protein S deficiency.

Protein C Deficiency

Protein C is a serine protease and an important inhibitor of plasma coagulation. Similar to protein S, its synthesis by the liver depends on vitamin K. Protein C in the plasma is inactive; it is activated by a thrombin–thrombomodulin complex when clotting is initiated at the endothelial surface. Protein S enhances the activity of protein C. Once activated, protein C inactivates factors Va and VIIIa, inhibiting coagulation and enhancing fibrinolytic activity. Deficiency can be inherited or acquired. The trait is autosomal dominant with incomplete penetrance. The prevalence of heterozygous protein C deficiency is 1 per 200 to 500 in the general population. Homozygous individuals develop *purpura fulminans* and severe thrombotic complications in the neonatal period. Most heterozygotes are asymptomatic until the third decade of life. The lifetime risk of developing thrombosis in heterozygotes is 7.3 times more than the general population. Sixty percent have recurrent venous thrombosis. Asymptomatic family members may have subnormal protein C levels.

Cerebral venous thrombosis has been linked to inherited protein C deficiency, usually with a second risk factor such as oral contraceptives or smoking. Protein C deficiency has not been demonstrated to be a risk for arterial thrombosis; strokes are usually attributed to venous thrombosis. Acquired protein C deficiency may occur with liver disease, vitamin K malabsorption or warfarin therapy, infections and sepsis, disseminated intravascular coagulation, or with malignancy or chemotherapy.

In the absence of a cause of an acquired protein C deficiency, a level <55% of normal probably indicates a genetic abnormality. Anticoagulation with heparin or warfarin is recommended only for clinical thrombosis and not for those with asymptomatic subnormal levels. *Warfarin necrosis* of skin and subcutaneous tissues, particularly breast and adipose tissue, may be seen in patients 2 to 5 days into treatment and has been attributed to a transient hypercoagulable state. Protein C deficiency may be associated with homocystinuria, which itself can lead to thrombosis.

Factor V Leiden and Prothrombin G20210A Mutations

Factor V Leiden is the most common known genetic risk factor for thrombosis. A mutation of the factor V gene causing replacement of arginine 506 by glycine results in factor Va resistance to degradation by activated protein C. The resultant imbalance between procoagulant and anticoagulant factors predisposes to venous thrombosis. The incidence of heterozygous factor V Leiden is 1% to 8.5%, depending on the ethnicity and geographic location of the population studied. The prevalence is highest in Greece, Sweden, and Lebanon; the mutation has not been found in African Blacks, Chinese, or Japanese populations. Homozygotes constitute 1% of all patients with the factor V Leiden mutation.

Deep venous thrombosis is the most common clinical manifestation. Cerebral vein thrombosis occurs with increased frequency in heterozygotes. The mutation may also be a risk for recurrent pregnancy loss. Stroke risk has not been shown to be increased in adults with factor V Leiden. The lifetime risk of thrombosis in heterozygotes is 2.2 times that of the normal population. Despite this increase, there is no increased mortality. Use of oral contraceptives by heterozygotes increases the relative risk of thrombosis greater than 30 times that of women without the mutation who were not taking oral contraceptives.

Prothrombin is a vitamin K–dependent protein synthesized in the liver and is the precursor to thrombin. The prothrombin G20210A mutation results in a 30% higher serum prothrombin level than normal controls. This gene mutation is present in 1% to 6% of the White population; it is almost never encountered in nonwhites. It is uncertain whether the prothrombin G20210A mutation, which is associated with an increased risk of venous thrombosis, confers an increased risk of arterial stroke in young patients. Older people have no increased risk. Spinal cord infarction may occur in young women who smoke cigarettes, take an oral contraceptive, and have the prothrombin G20210A mutation. Factor V Leiden may coexist with the prothrombin 20210A allele and also with hereditary deficiencies of AT, protein C, and protein S, increasing the risk of thrombotic events.

Hereditary Abnormalities of Fibrinolysis

There are four inherited abnormalities of fibrinolysis. *Plasminogen* deficiency is inherited as an autosomal dominant trait. *Tissue plasminogen activator* deficiency has been associated with thrombosis in isolated families. Hemorrhage and thrombosis have been seen in patients with *dysfibrinogenemia*. *Factor XII* deficiency is an autosomal recessively inherited condition, in which patients have elevated activated partial thromboplastin time. Risk of venous thrombosis and stroke are theoretically raised owing to reduced plasma fibrinolytic activity. The role of these conditions in venous thrombosis and stroke is uncertain.

Autoantibodies

Antiphospholipid antibodies, encompassing the *lupus anticoagulant* and *anticardiolipin antibodies*, are the most common acquired defects associated with thrombosis. Most, but not all, case-control studies have linked

antiphospholipid antibodies with vascular thrombo-occlusive events. Most prospective studies similarly associate antiphospholipid antibodies and first stroke. However, in a major study, the presence of antiphospholipid antibodies among patients with stroke did not predict a subsequent stroke or a better response to either aspirin or warfarin therapy.

Other manifestations of the antiphospholipid antibody syndrome include fetal loss, thrombocytopenia, and livedo reticularis. Recurrent events are common. Other neurologic manifestations of antiphospholipid antibodies include cerebral venous sinus thrombosis, dementia, and chorea. The presence of a lupus anticoagulant should be suspected if the activated partial thromboplastin time (and prothrombin time in some cases) is prolonged and fails to correct with mixing studies.

Paroxysmal Nocturnal Hemoglobinuria

This clonal myelodysplastic syndrome is characterized by the absence of glycosylphosphatidylinositol, which anchors proteins to the cell surface. Patients are prone to hepatic vein and sagittal sinus thrombosis and may have hemolytic anemia, cytopenia, and headache.

Hemophilia

Twenty-five percent of hemorrhagic deaths in hemophilia are a result of intracranial bleeding, often without known trauma. Bleeding may be subdural, epidural, intracerebral, or intraspinal. Among 2,500 patients followed for 10 years, the incidence of intracranial bleeding was 3%, with a 34% mortality rate; 47% of survivors had residual mental retardation, motor impairment, or seizures. Treatment with factor concentrate should not be delayed for diagnostic procedures if there is a clinical suspicion of intracranial bleeding. Spontaneous spinal epidural hematoma or hematomyelia are rare complications. Peripheral neuropathies may follow intraneural bleeding or nerve compression by hematomas.

CEREBROVASCULAR COMPLICATIONS OF CANCER

At autopsy, as many as 15% of patients with systemic malignancy have evidence of cerebrovascular disease. Cancers cause vascular complications by several indirect or direct mechanisms.

In 1865, Trousseau described an association between venous thromboembolism and cancer. The following year, he himself was stricken with a deep venous thrombosis of the leg and correctly self-diagnosed an occult stomach cancer. The Trousseau syndrome, as it is now known, is characterized by end organ damage from venous thrombosis, arterial thrombosis, and nonbacterial thrombotic endocarditis with sterile platelet-fibrin heart valve vegetations. These vegetations are the most common cause of cerebral infarction in patients with systemic malignancy. Most patients have disseminated malignancy and multiple strokes with ischemic or hemorrhagic infarctions in different vascular territories, often preceded by TIAs. The lesions are differentiated from brain metastases by CT or MRI. The most commonly associated tumors are mucin-producing adenocarcinomas of the gastrointestinal or hepatobiliary tracts. Emboli to other organs (pulmonary embolism, limb arterial emboli, or myocardial infarction) may call attention to the diagnosis, especially in patients with neurologic symptoms. The presence of coagulopathy has not been ascertained. Therapy is directed toward eradication of the primary tumor; the role of anticoagulation is unsettled.

Tumor emboli uncommonly cause cerebral infarction, usually with atrial myxoma or lung carcinoma. Neoplastic angioendotheliomatosis was formerly attributed to tumor emboli or diffuse spread of endothelial cells with stroke-like symptoms, but neoplastic angioendotheliomatosis is a systemic lymphoma with intravascular dissemination (see Chapter 57).

Coagulation disorders may be owing to the underlying tumor, chemotherapy, or radiotherapy. Coagulopathy is often seen with hepatic metastases and depletion of coagulation factors. Many chemotherapeutic agents depress stem cell function to cause thrombocytopenia. Colony-stimulating factors stimulate leukocyte production and permit more intensive chemotherapy, but thrombocytopenia may require platelet transfusions. Spontaneous intraparenchymal or subarachnoid hemorrhage may occur when the platelet count is <20,000/mm^3, a common problem in the cancer patient with sepsis. The combination of coagulopathy and thrombocytopenia, often seen with leukemia, predisposes to cerebral hemorrhage. In contrast, subdural hemorrhage is less common than parenchymal or subarachnoid hemorrhage in patients with coagulopathy or thrombocytopenia and occurs more frequently in the presence of dural metastases from carcinoma of breast, lung, or prostate.

Even with normal coagulation and platelet function, some metastatic tumors (melanoma, lung carcinoma, choriocarcinoma, and hypernephroma) are likely to cause hemorrhage into a tumor. With gliomas, the likelihood of intratumor hemorrhage increases with increasing grade of malignancy. To avert intratumor hemorrhage, patients with known primary or metastatic brain tumors should receive platelet transfusions if the count falls to <20,000/mm^3, and coagulation functions should be maintained with transfusions of fresh frozen plasma. Intracranial or subarachnoid hemorrhage may result from rupture of a neoplastic (oncotic) aneurysm caused by atrial myxoma or direct destruction of arterial walls as a result of invasion by a metastatic lung carcinoma, choriocarcinoma, or glioblastoma.

DIC is readily detected in its acute fulminant form when patients bleed profusely after venipuncture and have intracranial hemorrhage. Acute promyelocytic leukemia is associated with fulminant DIC, probably owing to release of granules from leukemic cells. A more indolent form of DIC may also cause neurologic manifestations. Autopsy examinations reveal evidence of thrombosis in situ, that is, intravascular coagulation. In contrast to nonbacterial thrombotic endocarditis, in which multifocal neurologic signs predominate, the main neurologic manifestation of DIC is diffuse encephalopathy. The diagnosis of chronic DIC is difficult but should be considered if the level of fibrin split products is elevated. Heparin anticoagulation is a logical but unproven therapy.

Occlusion of the superior sagittal sinus may follow direct spread of tumor to the dura. The cardinal symptoms of venous sinus thrombosis include headache secondary to increased intracranial pressure and seizures. It may also be a nonmetastatic complication, presumably caused by coagulopathy. The diagnosis is made by MRI with MR venogram (MRV). Conventional MRI shows loss of the typical signal flow void in the superior sagittal sinus at the site of the thrombosis. MRV is limited by in-plane signal loss that mimics thrombosis; it is necessary to review the source data in such cases. Heparin therapy is frequently beneficial but must be monitored, particularly if there is hemorrhagic cortical infarction. Leptomeningeal metastasis infrequently produces TIA or infarction by compromising vessels near the meningeal infiltrate.

Radiation-induced vasculopathy of the carotid artery may be delayed for years after radiation therapy for tumors of the head or neck. Symptoms of TIAs or infarction point to the involved vessel, and angiography reveals intimal irregularity. Radiotherapy may accelerate atherosclerosis, and appropriate patients benefit from endarterectomy.

OTHER DISORDERS

Idiopathic Hypereosinophilic Syndrome

Hypereosinophilia has been associated with allergies, parasitic infections, Hodgkin and T-cell lymphomas, and vasculitis. When eosinophilia (>1,500/mm^3) persists for more than 6 months without an apparent underlying cause, with evidence of tissue damage by eosinophils, the disorder is termed the idiopathic hypereosinophilic syndrome (IHES). The pathogenesis may be related to T-cell overexpression of cytokines, particularly interleukin-5. Eosinophils contain a number of granule proteins that damage tissue, including the eosinophil-derived neurotoxin that can cause Purkinje cell degeneration, ataxia, and paralysis in experimental animals. Multiple organs are affected, including the heart (endomyocardial fibrosis), skin, lungs, and spleen, and less commonly the eyes, liver, and gastrointestinal tract. Peripheral neuropathy is the most common neurologic complication. The CNS is affected in 15% of cases, usually as encephalopathy, TIA, or stroke. Behavioral changes, confusion, memory loss, ataxia, or upper motor neuron signs may be the first manifestation. Cerebral embolism is attributed to the cardiac disorder and responds poorly to anticoagulation. Steroids and hydroxyurea are the mainstay of therapy for the eosinophilic syndrome. However, in one reported case, the patient continued to deteriorate after treatment with intravenous methylprednisolone that resulted in normalization of the eosinophil count and cardiac enzymes. Autopsy demonstrated multiple ischemic strokes of different ages with diffuse platelet and fibrin thrombi in small caliber cerebral arterioles, consistent with a progressive hypercoagulable state, without evident intraluminal or intraparenchymal eosinophils. There was no cardiac lesion to suggest that occlusion of the small vessels in the brain was a result of thromboembolism. This case illustrates that eosinophil-induced hypercoagulability may progress despite effective treatment of the eosinophilia itself and suggests that in selected cases of IHES, antithrombotic therapy and treatments to suppress cytokine-and interleukin-mediated hypercoagulability may be necessary.

Langerhans Cell Histiocytosis

Langerhans cells are bone marrow-derived dendritic antigen-presenting cells of the immune system. They are identified immunohistochemically by staining positive for CD1a and S-100 protein. Electron microscopy demonstrates Birbeck granules, 200- to 400-nm membranous cytoplasmic structures shaped like tennis rackets. Birbeck granules contain "langerin," a protein that identifies Langerhans cells immunohistochemically. The term Langerhans Cell Histiocytosis (LCH) refers to a group of conditions that result from abnormal proliferation and infiltration of these Langerhans cells. Because the underlying cell type has been revealed in these conditions, the historical terms histiocytosis X, eosinophilic granuloma, Hand-Schüller-Christian disease, Letterer-Siwe disease, and diffuse reticuloendotheliosis are now obsolete. Instead, different manifestations of LCH are best described as single, multifocal, or diffuse organ involvement.

LCH is most commonly seen in children between 1 and 4 years of age. However, symptoms may begin as late as age 60. The incidence of LCH in children is three to five cases per million. Bone, skin, liver, spleen, lymph nodes, bone marrow, lungs, orbits, oral cavity and teeth, ears, and the CNS may be involved (Fig. 147.4). Skull lesions may extend to compress the dura. Diabetes insipidus from hypothalamic–pituitary axis involvement is most common in children and young adults; panhypopituitarism

may emerge. Periorbital mass lesions may cause proptosis, optic nerve compression, or a cavernous sinus syndrome. Cerebral mass lesions or choroid plexus lesions may lead to obstructive hydrocephalus. Diffuse infiltration of the cerebellum causing ataxia, visual symptoms, and behavioral and cognitive dysfunction have all been described. Treatment options include surgery, radiation therapy, chemotherapy, and steroids.

Neurolymphomatosis

In 1934, Lhermitte and Trelles described lymphomatous infiltration of peripheral nerves or neurolymphomatosis. Of more than 40 histologically proven cases reported subsequently, most have had non-Hodgkin lymphoma with progressive sensorimotor peripheral neuropathy. Some also had cranial neuropathy (45%), bowel or bladder incontinence (25%), gait ataxia (18%), or mental change (13%). The CSF protein content was >100 mg/dL in 57% of patients, and 70% had lymphocytic CSF pleocytosis. CSF cytology was abnormal in 33%. Electrodiagnostic studies show axonal neuropathy, mixed, or pure demyelinating neuropathy. Sural nerve biopsy shows equal numbers of patients with purely axonal degeneration or demyelinating lesions. MRI may be useful in identifying appropriate biopsy sites. At postmortem examination, there is often β-lymphocytic infiltration of leptomeninges, dorsal root ganglia, and spinal roots. The histopathologic pattern is indistinguishable from that of primary leptomeningeal lymphoma. Neurolymphomatosis is readily differentiated from the polyclonal T-cell infiltration in human immunodeficiency virus–associated diffuse infiltrative lymphocytosis syndrome. The neurologic disorder sometimes improves with corticosteroids, chemotherapy, or radiation therapy.

Angiocentric Immunoproliferative Lesions

These disorders are discussed in Chapter 57 (Lymphoma).

Chediak-Higashi Syndrome

This rare autosomal-recessive disorder is characterized by partial oculocutaneous albinism, severe immunologic defects, a bleeding diathesis, and progressive neurologic dysfunction. Mutation of the CHS1 gene on chromosome 1q42 q44 appears to result in defective transport of intracellular proteins, producing giant lysosomal granules in granule-containing cells, including neutrophils, monocytes, hepatocytes, and renal tubular cells. The granules are easily recognized on a peripheral blood smear. Impaired neutrophil function and defective T-cell and natural killer cell cytotoxicity predispose to infections that lead to

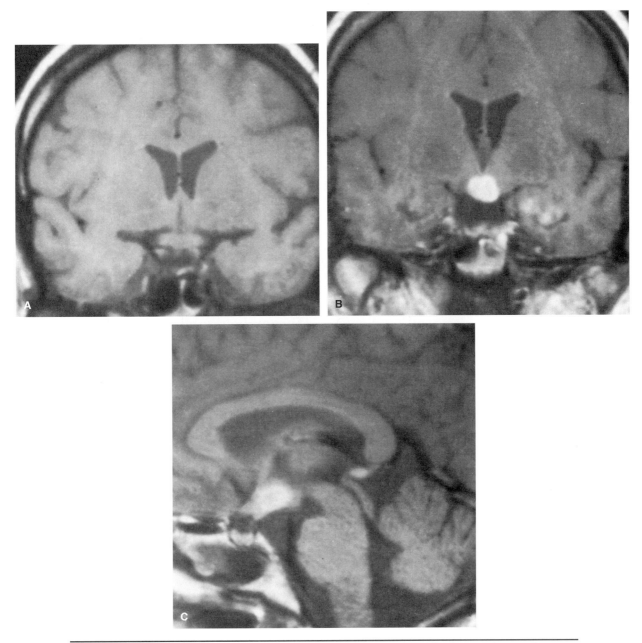

FIGURE 147.4. Eosinophilic granuloma of optic chiasm. **A.** T1-weighted coronal MRI shows enlargement of optic chiasm. **B and C.** T1-weighted coronal and sagittal MRIs after gadolinium enhancement demonstrate focal enhancing nodule involving optic chiasm and hypothalamus, consistent with known eosinophilic granuloma. Incidentally noted are several small enhancing lesions in left temporal lobe (an unusual site for eosinophilic granuloma). (Courtesy of Dr. S. Chan and Dr. S. K. Hilal.)

death, usually within the first decade of life. Neurologic syndromes include a spinocerebellar disorder, peripheral neuropathy, and light-induced nystagmus. The neurologic symptoms may be associated with neuronal or Schwann cell inclusions or by lymphohistiocytic infiltration of peripheral nerves. CT brain findings include diffuse atrophy and decreased periventricular density. Bone marrow transplant is a potentially curative avenue for therapy.

SUGGESTED READINGS

Sickle Cell

Abboud MR, Cure J, Granger S, et al. Magnetic resonance angiography in children with sickle cell disease and abnormal transcranial Doppler ultrasonography findings enrolled in the STOP study. *Blood* 2004;103:2822–2826.

Adams RJ, Brambilla DJ, Granger S, et al. STOP study. Stroke and conversion to high risk in children screened with transcranial

Doppler ultrasound during the STOP study. *Blood* 2004;103:3689–3694.

Adams RJ, McKie VC, Hsu L, et al. Prevention of a first stroke by transfusions in children with sickle cell anemia and abnormal results on transcranial Doppler ultrasonography. *N Engl J Med* 1998;339:5–11.

Earley CJ, Kittner SJ, Feeser BR, et al. Stroke in children and sickle-cell disease: Baltimore-Washington Cooperative Young Stroke Study. *Neurology* 1998;51:169–176.

Fabian R, Peters B. Neurological complications of hemoglobin SC disease. *Arch Neurol* 1984;41:289–292.

Fryer RH, Anderson RC, Chiriboga CA, et al. Sickle cell anemia with moyamoya disease: outcomes after EDAS procedure. *Pediatr Neurol* 2003;29(Aug):124–130.

Hart RG, Kanter MC. Hematologic disorders and ischemic stroke. A selective review. *Stroke* 1990;21:1111–1121.

Liu JE, Gzesh DJ, Ballas SK. The spectrum of epilepsy in sickle cell anemia. *J Neurol Sci* 1994;123:6–10.

Moser FG, Miller ST, Bello JA, et al. The spectrum of brain MR abnormalities in sickle-cell disease: a report from the Cooperative Study of Sickle Cell Disease. *AJNR* 1996;17:965–972.

Ohene-Frempong K, Weiner SJ, Sleeper LA, et al. Cerebrovascular accidents in sickle cell disease: rates and risk factors. *Blood* 1998;91:288–294.

Prengler M, Pavlakis SG, Prohovnik I, et al. Sickle cell disease: the neurological complications. *Ann Neurol* 2002;52:543–552.

Preul MC, Cendes F, Just N, et al. Intracranial aneurysms and sickle cell anemia: multiplicity and propensity for the vertebrobasilar territory. *Neurosurgery* 1998;42:971–977.

Reyes M. Subcortical cerebral infarctions in sickle cell trait. *J Neurol Neurosurg Psychiatry* 1989;52:516–518.

Sloan MA, Alexandrov AV, Tegeler CH, et al; Therapeutics and Technology Assessment Subcommittee of the American Academy of Neurology. Assessment: transcranial Doppler ultrasonography: report of the Therapeutics and Technology Assessment Subcommittee of the American Academy of Neurology. *Neurology* 2004;62:1468–1481.

Steen RG, Hankins GM, Xiong X, et al. Prospective brain imaging evaluation of children with sickle cell trait: initial observations. *Radiology* 2003;228:208–215.

Wang WC, Langston JW, Steen RG, et al. Abnormalities of the central nervous system in very young children with sickle cell anemia. *J Pediatr* 1998;132:994–998.

Thalassemia

Aessopos A, Farmakis D, Karagiorga M, et al. Pseudoxanthoma elasticum lesions and cardiac complications as contributing factors for strokes in beta-thalassemia patients. *Stroke* 1997;28:2421–2424.

Aessopos A, Farmakis D, Loukopoulos D. Elastic tissue abnormalities resembling pseudoxanthoma elasticum in beta thalassemia and the sickling syndromes. *Blood* 2002;199:30–35.

Chehal A, Aoun E, Koussa S, et al. Hypertransfusion: a successful method of treatment in thalassemia intermedia patients with spinal cord compression secondary to extramedullary hematopoiesis. *Spine* 2003;28:E245–249.

Kaufmann T, Coleman M, Giardina P, et al. The role of radiation therapy in the management of hematopoietic neurologic complications in thalassemia. *Acta Haematol* 1991;85:156–159.

Logothetis J, Constantoulakis M, Economidou J, et al. Thalassemia major (homozygous beta-thalassemia). A survey of 138 cases with emphasis on neurologic and muscular aspects. *Neurology* 1972;22:294–304.

Papanastasiou DA, Papanicolaou D, Magiakou AM, et al. Peripheral neuropathy in patients with beta-thalassemia. *J Neurol Neurosurg Psychiatry* 1991;54:997–1000.

Salehi SA, Koski T, Ondra SL. Spinal cord compression in beta-thalassemia: case report and review of the literature. *Spinal Cord* 2004;42:117–123.

Zafeiriou DI, Prengler M, Gombakis N, et al. Central nervous system abnormalities in asymptomatic young patients with Sbeta-thalassemia. *Ann Neurol* 2004;55:835–839.

Polycythemia

Davis MD. Erthromelalgia. *Mayo Clinic Proc* 2004;79:298.

Gruppo Italiano Studio Policitemia. Polycythemia vera: the natural history of 1213 patients followed for 20 years. *Ann Intern Med* 1995;123:656–664.

Landolfi R, Marchioli R, Kutti J, et al.; European Collaboration on Low-Dose Aspirin in Polycythemia Vera Investigators. Efficacy and safety of low-dose aspirin in polycythemia vera. *N Engl J Med* 2004;350:114–124.

Masmas TN, Jacobsen EC, Rasch L, et al. Spinal cord compression due to extramedullary hematopoiesis in polycythemia vera. *Am J Hematol* 2003;73:297–298.

Newton LK. Neurologic complications of polycythemia and their impact on therapy. *Oncology* 1990;4:59–64.

So CC, Ho LC. Polycythemia secondary to cerebellar hemangioblastoma. *Am J Hematol* 2002;71:346–347.

Tefferi A. Polycythemia vera: a comprehensive review and clinical recommendations. *Mayo Clin Proc* 2003;78:174–194.

Yiannikas C, McLeod JG, Walsh JC. Peripheral neuropathy associated with polycythemia vera. *Neurology* 1983;33:139–143.

Essential Thrombocytosis (Thrombocythemia)

Kesler A, Ellis MH, Manor Y, et al. Neurological complications of essential thrombocytosis (ET). *Acta Neurol Scand* 2000;102:299–302.

Koudstaal PJ, Koudstaal A. Neurologic and visual symptoms in essential thrombocythemia: efficacy of low-dose aspirin. *Semin Thromb Hemost* 1997;23:365–370.

Mitus AJ, Tiziano B, Shulman LN, et al. Hemostatic complications in young patients with essential thrombocythemia. *Am J Med* 1990;88:371–375.

Thrombotic Thrombocytopenic Purpura

Allford SL, Machin SJ. Current understanding of the pathophysiology of thrombotic thrombocytopenic purpura. *J Clin Pathol* 2000;53:497–501.

Bakshi R, Shaikh ZA, Bates VE, et al. Thrombotic thrombocytopenic purpura: brain CT and MRI findings in 12 patients. *Neurology* 1999;52:1285–1288.

Bennett CL, Weinberg PD, Rozenberg-Ben-Dror K, et al. Thrombotic thrombocytopenic purpura associated with ticlopidine. A review of 60 cases. *Ann Intern Med* 1998;128:541–544.

Meloni G, Proia A, Antonini G, et al. Thrombotic thrombocytopenic purpura: prospective neurologic, neuroimaging and neurophysiologic evaluation. *Haematologica* 2001;86:1194–1199.

Tsai HM, Lian EC. Antibodies to von Willebrand factor-cleaving protease in acute thrombotic thrombocytopenic purpura. *N Engl J Med* 1998;339:1585–1594.

Yarranton H, Machin SJ. An update on the pathogenesis and management of acquired thrombotic thrombocytopenic purpura. *Curr Op Neurol* 2003;16:367–373.

Heparin-Induced Thrombocytopenia

Harbrecht U, Bastians B, Kredteck A, et al. Heparin-induced thrombocytopenia in neurologic disease treated with unfractionated heparin. *Neurology* 2004;62:657–659.

Hirsh J, Heddle N, Kelton JG. Treatment of heparin-induced thrombocytopenia: a critical review. *Arch Int Med* 2004;164:361–369.

LaMonte MP, Brown PM, Hursting MJ. Stroke in patients with heparin-induced thrombocytopenia and the effect of argatroban therapy. *Crit Care Med* 2004;32:976–980.

Myelofibrosis

Horwood E, Dowson H, Gupta R, et al. Myelofibrosis presenting as spinal cord compression. *J Clin Pathol* 2003;56:154–156.

Landolfi R, Colosimo CJ, De Candia E, et al. Meningeal hematopoiesis causing exophthalmos and hemiparesis in myelofibrosis: effect of radiotherapy. *Cancer* 1988;62:2346–2349.

Masmas TN, Jacobsen EC, Rasch L, et al. Spinal cord compression due to extramedullary hematopoiesis in polycythemia vera. *Am J Hematol* 2003;73:297–298.

Leukemia

Cramer SC, Glaspy JA, Efird JT, et al. Chronic lymphocytic leukemia and the central nervous system: a clinical and pathological study. *Neurology* 1996;46:19–25.

Demopoulos A, DeAngelis LM. Neurologic complications of leukemia. *Curr Opin Neurol* 2002;15:691–699.

Holmes R, Keating MJ, Cork A, et al. A unique pattern of central nervous system leukemia in acute myelomonocytic leukemia associated with inv(16)(p13q22). *Blood* 1985;65:1071–1078.

McCarthy LJ. Leukostasis thrombi. *JAMA* 1985;254:613.

Nathan PC, Maze R, Spiegler B, et al. CNS-directed therapy in young children with T-lineage acute lymphoblastic leukemia: high-dose methotrexate versus cranial irradiation. *Pediatr Blood Cancer* 2004;42(Jan):24–29.

Pinkel D, Woo S. Prevention and treatment of meningeal leukemia in children. *Blood* 1994;84:355–366.

Saarinen-Pihkala UM, Gustafsson G, Carlsen N, et al. Outcome of children with high-risk acute lymphoblastic leukemia (HR-ALL): Nordic results on an intensive regimen with restricted central nervous system irradiation. *Pediatr Blood Cancer* 2004;42(Jan):8–23.

Plasma Cell Dyscrasias

Delauche-Cavallier MC, Laredo JD, Wybier M, et al. Solitary plasmacytoma of the spine. *Cancer* 1988;61:1707–1714.

Delgado J, Canales MA, Garcia B, et al. Radiation therapy and combination of cladribine, cyclophosphamide, and prednisone as treatment of Bing-Neel syndrome: case report and review of the literature. *Am J Hematol* 2002;69:127–131.

Dispenzieri A, Kyle RA, Lacy MQ, et al. POEMS syndrome: definitions and long-term outcome. *Blood* 2003;101:2496–2506.

Gordon PH, Rowland LP, Younger DS, et al. Lymphoproliferative disorders and motor neuron disease: an update. *Neurology* 1997;48:1671–1678.

Kelly JJ Jr, Kyle RA, Miles JM, et al. Osteosclerotic myeloma and peripheral neuropathy. *Neurology* 1983;33:202–210.

Latov N. Pathogenesis and therapy of neuropathies associated with monoclonal gammopathies. *Ann Neurol* 1995;37(Suppl 1):S32–S42.

Nobile-Orazio E, Barbieri S, Baldini L, et al. Peripheral neuropathy in monoclonal gammopathy of undetermined significance: prevalence and immunopathogenetic studies. *Acta Neurol Scand* 1992;85:383–390.

Ropper AH, Gorson KC. Neuropathies associated with paraproteinemia. *N Engl J Med* 1998;338:1601–1607.

Schey S. Osteosclerotic myeloma and "POEMS" syndrome. *Blood Rev* 1996;10:75–80.

Sherman WH, Olarte MR, McKiernan G, et al. Plasma exchange treatment of peripheral neuropathy associated with plasma cell dyscrasia. *J Neurol Neurosurg Psychiatry* 1984;47:813–819.

Disorders of Coagulation

Antiphospholipid Antibodies in Stroke Study (APASS) Group. Anticardiolipin antibodies are an independent risk factor for first ischemic stroke. *Neurology* 1993;43:2069–2073.

de Bruijn SF, Stam J, Koopman MM, et al. Case-control study of risk of cerebral sinus thrombosis in oral contraceptive users and in [correction of who are] carriers of hereditary prothrombotic conditions The Cerebral Venous Sinus Thrombosis Study Group. *BMJ* 1998;316:589–592. Erratum in: *BMJ* 1998;316:822.

De Stefano V, Chiusolo P, Paciaroni K, et al. Prothrombin G20210A mutant genotype is a risk factor for cerebrovascular ischemic disease in young patients. *Blood* 1998;91:3562–3565.

Grewal RP, Goldberg MA. Stroke in protein C deficiency. *Am J Med* 1990;89:538–539.

Hankey GJ, Eikelboom JW, van Bockxmeer FM, et al. Inherited thrombophilia in ischemic stroke and its pathogenic subtypes. *Stroke* 2001;32:1793–1799.

Harris M, Exner T, Rickard K, et al. Multiple cerebral thrombosis in Fletcher factor (prekallikrein) deficiency: a case report. *Am J Hematol* 1985;19:387–393.

Hathaway WE. Clinical aspects of antithrombin III deficiency. *Semin Hematol* 1991;28:19–23.

Heijboer H, Brandjes DP, Buller HR, et al. Deficiencies of coagulation-inhibiting and fibrinolytic proteins in outpatients with deep vein thrombosis. *NEJM* 1990;323:1512.

Israel S, Seshia S. Childhood stroke associated with protein C or S deficiency. *J Pediatr* 1987;111:562–564.

Jorens PG, Hermans CR, Haber I, et al. Acquired protein C and S deficiency, inflammatory bowel disease and cerebral arterial thrombosis. *Blut* 1990;61:307–310.

Kohler J, Kasper J, Witt I, et al. Ischemic stroke due to protein C deficiency. *Stroke* 1990;21:1077–1080.

Kwaan HC. Protein C and protein S. *Semin Thromb Hemost* 1989;15:353–355.

Lee MK, Ng SC. Cerebral venous thrombosis associated with antithrombin III deficiency. *Aust N Z J Med* 1991;21:772–773.

Leone G, Graham JA, Daly HM, et al. Antithrombin III deficiency and cerebrovascular accidents in young adults. *J Clin Pathol* 1992;45:921–922.

Levine SR, Brey RL, Tilley BC; APASS Investigators. Antiphospholipid antibodies and subsequent thrombo-occlusive events in patients with ischemic stroke. *JAMA* 2004;291:576–584.

Levine SR, Brey RL, Sawaya KL, et al. Recurrent stroke and thrombo-occlusive events in the phospholipid syndrome. *Ann Neurol* 1995;38:119–124.

Martinez HR, Rangel-Guerra R, Marfil LJ. Ischemic stroke due to deficiency of coagulation inhibitors. Report of 10 young adults. *Stroke* 1993;24:19–45.

Mateo J, Oliver A, Borrell M, et al. Laboratory evaluation and clinical characteristics of 2,132 consecutive unselected patients with venous thromboembolism–results of the Spanish Multicentric Study on Thrombophilia (EMET-Study). *Thromb Haemost* 1997;77:444–451.

Matsushita K, Kuriyama Y, Sawada T, et al. Cerebral infarction associated with protein C deficiency. *Stroke* 1992;23:108–111.

Mayer S, Sacco R, Hurlet-Jensen A, et al. Free protein S deficiency in acute ischemic stroke. A case-control study. *Stroke* 1993;24:224–227.

Munts AG, van Genderen PJ, Dippel DW, et al. Coagulation disorders in young adults with acute cerebral ischaemia. *J Neurol* 1998;245:21–25.

Prats JM, Garaizar C, Zuazo E, et al. Superior sagittal sinus thrombosis in a child with protein S deficiency. *Neurology* 1992;42:2303–2305.

Pratt CW, Church FC. Antithrombin: structure and function. *Semin Hematol* 1991;28:3–9.

Rich C, Gill JC, Wernick S, et al. An unusual cause of cerebral venous thrombosis in a four-year-old child. *Stroke* 1993;24:603–605.

Ridker PM, Hennekens CH, Lindpaintner K, et al. Mutation in the gene coding for coagulation factor V and the risk of myocardial infarction, stroke, and venous thrombosis in apparently healthy men. *N Engl J Med* 1995;332:912–917.

Shinmyozu K, Ohkatsu Y, Maruyama Y, et al. A case of congenital antithrombin III deficiency complicated by an internal carotid artery occlusion. *Clin Neurol* 1986;26:162–165.

Tait RC, Walker ID, Perry DJ, et al. Prevalence of antithrombin deficiency in the healthy population. *Br J Haematol* 1994;87:106.

Vomberg P, Breederveld C. Cerebral thromboembolism due to antithrombin III deficiency in two children. *Neuropediatrics* 1987;18:42–44.

Cerebrovascular Complications of Cancer

Biller J, Challa VR, Toole JF, et al. Nonbacterial thrombotic endocarditis: a neurologic perspective of clinicopathologic correlations in 99 patients. *Arch Neurol* 1982;39:95–98.

Cestari DM, Weine DM, Panageas KS, et al. Stroke in patients with cancer: incidence and etiology. *Neurology* 2004;62:2025–2030.

Edoute Y, Haim N, Rinkevich D, et al. Cardiac valvular vegetations in cancer patients: a prospective echocardiographic study of 200 patients. *Am J Med* 1997;102:252–258.

Green KB, Silverstein RL. Hypercoagulability in cancer. *Hematol Oncol Clin North Am* 1996;10:499–530.

Hickey WF, Garnick MB, Henderson IC, et al. Primary cerebral venous thrombosis in patients with cancer—a rarely diagnosed paraneoplastic syndrome. *Am J Med* 1982;73:740–750.

Lal G, Brennan TV, Hambleton J, et al. Coagulopathy, marantic endocarditis, and cerebrovascular accidents as paraneoplastic features in medullary thyroid cancer–case report and review of the literature. *Thyroid* 2003;13:601–605.

Murros KE, Toole JF. The effect of radiation on carotid arteries. *Arch Neurol* 1989;46:449.

Samuels MA, King ME, Balis U. Case records of the Massachusetts General Hospital: a 61-year-old man with headache and multiple infarcts. *N Engl J Med* 2002;347:1187–1194.

Singhal AB, Topcuoglu MA, Buonanno FS. Acute ischemic stroke patterns in infective and nonbacterial thrombotic endocarditis: a diffusion-weighted magnetic resonance imaging study. *Stroke* 2002;33:1267–1273.

Hypereosinophilic Syndrome

Brito-Babapulle F. Clonal eosinophilic disorders and the hypereosinophilic syndrome. *Blood Rev* 1997;11:129–145.

Monaco S, Lucci B, Laperchia N, et al. Polyneuropathy in hypereosinophilic syndrome. *Neurology* 1988;38:494–496.

Plotz SG, Simon HU, Darsow U, et al. Use of an anti-interleukin-5 antibody in the hypereosinophilic syndrome with eosinophilic dermatitis. *N Engl J Med* 2003;349:2334–2339.

Roufosse F, Cogan E, Goldman M. The hypereosinophilic syndrome revisited. *Annu Rev Med* 2003;54:169–184.

Sarazin M, Caumes E, Cohen A, et al. Multiple microembolic borderzone brain infarctions and endomyocardial fibrosis in idiopathic hypereosinophilic syndrome and in Schistosoma mansoni infestation. *J Neurol Neurosurg Psychiatry* 2004;75:305–307.

Langerhans Cell Histiocytosis

Grois NG, Favara BE, Mostbeck GH, et al. Central nervous system disease in Langerhans cell histiocytosis. *Hematol Oncol Clin North Am* 1998;12:287–305.

Hurwitz CA, Faquin WC. Case records of the Massachusetts General Hospital: a 15-year-old boy with a retro-orbital mass and impaired vision. *N Engl J Med* 2002;346:513–520.

Ladisch S. Langerhans cell histiocytosis. *Curr Opin Hematol* 1998;5:54–58.

Usmani GN, Westra SJ, Younes S. Case records of the Massachusetts General Hospital: a 14-month-old boy with hepatomegaly, perianal lesions, and a bony lump on the forehead. *N Engl J Med* 2003;348:1692–1701.

van de Warrenburg BP, van der Heijden HF, Pieters G, et al. Langerhans' cell histiocytosis presenting with progressive spinocerebellar ataxia. *J Neurol* 2003;250:1112–1114.

Neurolymphomatosis

Baehring JM, Damek D, Martin EC, et al. Neurolymphomatosis. *Neurooncol* 2003;5(Apr):104–15.

Diaz-Arrastia R, Younger DS, Hair L, et al. Neurolymphomatosis: a clinicopathologic syndrome re-emerges. *Neurology* 1992;42:1136–1141.

Gherardi RK, Chretien F, Delfau-Larue MH, et al. Neuropathy in diffuse infiltrative lymphocytosis syndrome: an HIV neuropathy, not a lymphoma. *Neurology* 1998;50:1041–1044.

Gordon PH, Younger DS. Neurolymphomatosis. *Neurology* 1996;46:1191–1192.

Van den Bent MJ, de Bruin HG, Beun GD, et al. Neurolymphomatosis of the median nerve. *Neurology* 1995;45:1403–1405.

Chediak-Higashi Syndrome

Gordon N, Mullen CA, Tran H, et al. Fludarabine and once-daily intravenous busulfan for allogeneic bone marrow transplantation for Chediak-Higashi syndrome. *J Pediat Hematol/Oncol* 2003;25:824–826.

Misra VP, King RHM, Harding AE, et al. Peripheral neuropathy in the Chediak-Higashi syndrome. *Acta Neuropathol* 1991;81:354–358.

Mottonen M, Lanning M, Baumann P, et al. Chediak-Higashi syndrome: four cases from Northern Finland. *Acta Paediatr* 2003;92:1047–1051.

Spitz RA. Genetic defects in Chediak-Higashi syndrome and the beige mouse. *J Clin Immunol* 1998;18:97–105.

Chapter 148

Hepatic Disease

Neil H. Raskin and Peter Y. Kim

The association between liver disease and neurologic syndromes is well recognized. Alteration in mental status as a result of acute, subacute, or chronic liver failure is *hepatic encephalopathy*. The severity of the encephalopathy can be classified into four stages: mild confusion, lethargy, somnolence, and coma. The often fatal comatose state associated with acute hepatic necrosis is usually attended by striking elevation of serum ammonia content; coma is usually a single event of rapid onset and fulminant course that is characterized by delirium, convulsions, and, occasionally, decerebrate rigidity. The mechanism of this encephalopathy is not clear.

Hepatic encephalopathy usually develops in patients with chronic liver disease when portal hypertension induces an extensive portal collateral circulation; portal venous blood bypasses the detoxification site, which is the liver, and drains directly into the systemic circulation to produce the cerebral intoxication that is properly termed *portal-systemic encephalopathy*. Several examples of portal-systemic encephalopathy have been reported in which the hepatic parenchyma was normal, underlining the anatomic importance of bypassing the liver as the mechanism.

The clinical syndrome resulting from shunting is an episodic encephalopathy comprising admixtures of ataxia, action tremor, dysarthria, sensorial clouding, and asterixis. The episodes are usually reversible, but they may recur. Cerebral morphologic changes are few except for an increase in large Alzheimer type II astrocytes. In a few patients with this disorder, a relentlessly progressing neurologic disorder occurs in addition to the fluctuating intoxication syndrome, including dementia, ataxia, dysarthria, intention tremor, and a choreoathetotic movement. The brains of these patients show zones of pseudolaminar necrosis in cerebral and cerebellar cortex, cavitation and neuronal loss in the basal ganglia and cerebellum, and glycogen-staining inclusions in enlarged astrocytes. This irreversible disorder has been termed *acquired chronic hepatocerebral degeneration*, but it is probably the ultimate morphologic destruction that may result from the chronic metabolic defect that attends portal-systemic shunting.

CLINICAL FEATURES

Thought processes are usually compromised insidiously, although an acute agitated delirium may occasionally usher in the syndrome. Mental dullness and drowsiness are usually the first symptoms; patients yawn frequently and drift off to sleep easily yet remain arousable. Cognitive defects eventually appear. Asterixis almost always accompanies these modest changes of consciousness. This consists of a brief periodic loss of flexion tone best seen in the outstretched hand and can be considered a negative myoclonus. As encephalopathy progresses, bilateral paratonia appears and the stretch reflexes become brisk; bilateral Babinski signs are usually found when obtundation becomes profound. Convulsions are decidedly uncommon in this disorder, in contrast to uremic encephalopathy. Spastic paraparesis may be seen. Decerebrate and decorticate postures and diffuse spasticity of the limbs frequently accompany deeper stages of coma.

In the patient with overt hepatocellular failure with jaundice or ascites, the diagnosis of this disorder is not difficult. When parenchymal liver disease is mild or nonexistent, however, an elevated serum ammonia level or an elevation of CSF glutamine content has high diagnostic sensitivity. However, the concentration of ammonia does not correlate well with progression of the symptoms or the response to treatment. The CSF is otherwise bland. Early in the course of encephalopathy, when the only evidence is seen on neuropsychologic tests, CT may show cortical atrophy, cerebral edema, or normal patterns. MRI usually shows increased signal in the globus pallidus in

T1-weighted studies. Manganese deposition may account for this. Sometimes there is calcification, and there may be abnormalities in the mesencephalon and pons. Cerebral edema is more common in chronic encephalopathy than once believed.

PATHOPHYSIOLOGY

Several substances have been considered possible neurotoxins in portal-systemic encephalopathy. However, ammonia and facilitation of gamma amino butyric acid (GABA) mediated neurotransmission are considered the two most important factors.

Ammonia, a highly neurotoxic substance, is ordinarily converted to urea by the liver; when this detoxification mechanism is bypassed, levels of ammonia in the brain and blood increase. Occasionally, blood ammonia levels are normal or only slightly elevated in the face of full-blown coma. Furthermore, ammonia levels in patients with mild to moderate hepatic encephalopathy are sufficient to induce excitatory responses in electrophysiologic experiments. Infusion of ammonia induces seizures in experimental animals, but in human hepatic encephalopathy, seizures are rarely seen. This is a powerful argument against the implication of ammonia as causal. Ammonia is detoxified in brain astrocytes by conversion to the nontoxic glutamine.

Increased sensitivity to inhibitory neurotransmitters such as GABA may underlie the encephalopathy. This is supported by the clinical observation of impaired consciousness and motor function seen with increased GABA neurotransmission, and animal models of hepatic encephalopathy also show increased GABAergic tone. The GABAergic antagonist, flumazenil, reverses the clinical and electrophysiologic findings of some patients with hepatic encephalopathy. The roles of ammonia and the GABAergic system may combine if high ammonia levels seen in hepatic encephalopathy enhance inhibitory GABAergic neurotransmission.

Dopaminergic systems have also been implicated in the pathophysiology of hepatic encephalopathy. Because levodopa benefited patients in hepatic coma, Fischer and Baldessarini proposed the false neurotransmitter hypothesis to explain the mechanism of this effect. They suggested that amines such as octopamine (or aromatic amino acid precursors tyrosine and phenylalanine), which are derived from protein by gut bacterial action, might escape oxidation by the liver and flood the systemic and cerebral circulations. Octopamine could then replace norepinephrine and dopamine in nerve endings and act as a false neurotransmitter; the accumulation of false neurotransmitters might then account for the encephalopathy, and the amelioration could be achieved by restoring "true" neurotransmitters through an elevation of tissue dopamine levels. L-dopa administration, however, has a powerful peripheral effect, inducing the renal excretion of ammonia and urea; this probably accounts for the beneficial effects of L-dopa in some encephalopathic patients. Furthermore, octopamine concentration in rat brain has been elevated more than 20,000-fold, along with depletion of both norepinephrine and dopamine, without any detectable alteration of consciousness. Although false neurotransmitters do accumulate in portal-systemic encephalopathy, there is little reason to hold them responsible for the encephalopathy.

DIFFERENTIAL DIAGNOSIS

Among the numerous causes of encephalopathy, several affect abusers of alcohol, including acute ethanolic intoxication and delerium tremens, Wernicke encephalopathy, Korsakoff syndrome, drug intoxication, other metabolic disorders (uremia, hyponatremia), and consequences of head injury, such as subdural hematoma. Another consideration is Wilson disease.

TREATMENT

Administration of antibiotics (especially neomycin or metronidazole) decreases the population of intestinal organisms to decrease production of ammonia and other cerebrotoxins. Lactulose is also beneficial for reasons that are not clear, but it lowers colonic pH, increases incorporation of ammonia into bacterial protein, and is a cathartic. The effects of neomycin and lactulose given together seem better than the effects either gives alone.

Although recovery is expected in patients with mild acute encephalopathy, cerebral edema occurs in about 75% of patients in acute coma and may be the cause of death. Intracranial pressure monitoring is often carried out in transplantation centers despite the risk of bleeding. If cerebral perfusion pressure is <40 mm Hg and does not respond to mannitol therapy, transplantation is deemed futile. In some cases of fulminant hepatic failure, emergency hepatectomy has been performed, followed by support with an extracorporeal bioartificial liver and then orthoptic liver transplantation.

NEUROLOGIC COMPLICATIONS OF LIVER TRANSPLANTATION

Neurologic problems arise in 8% to 47% of liver transplant recipients. The complications range from mild encephalopathy to akinetic mutism or coma. Psychiatric syndromes range from mild anxiety or depression to hallucinatory psychosis. Other syndromes include seizures,

▶ **TABLE 148.1** Neurologic Complications of Liver Transplantation

	Adults[a] (n = 40)	Children[b] (n = 24)
Central nervous system		
Seizures	8	9
Cerebrocerebellar syndrome	4	8
Coma	2	0
Cortical blindness	2	0
Delusions, visual hallucinations	2	0
Psychosis without hallucinations	3	0
Headache	3	0
Intracerebral hemorrhage	1	1
Tremor, myoclonus	2	2
Meningitis	0	1
Peripheral nerves		
Brachial plexopathy	2	0
Polyneuropathy	1	0
Partial third nerve palsy	1	0

[a]Thirteen of 40 adults (33%) had one or more neurologic complications.
[b]Eleven of 24 children (46%) had one or more neurologic complications.
Modified from Stein DP, Lederman RJ, Vogt DP, et al. Neurological complications following liver transplantation. *Ann Neurol* 1992;31:644–649; and Garg BP, Walsh LE, Pescovitz MD, et al. Neurologic complications of pediatric liver transplantation. *Pediatr Neurol* 1993;9:44–48.

myoclonus, tremor, cortical blindness, brachial plexopathy, and peripheral neuropathy (Table 148.1). Cerebral hemorrhage is sometimes responsible. Recovery from these disorders is often excellent and has no effect on survival, which is the same for those with or without neurologic syndromes. The acute leukoencephalopathy caused by tacrolimus (FK506) is reversed promptly on withdrawal of the drug. Tacrolimus has also been associated with a demyelinating peripheral neuropathy.

The necessary immunosuppression may lead to the opportunistic infections, and cyclosporine itself is held responsible for some cerebral disorders, possibly including central pontine myelinosis and leukoencephalopathy. Instead of the intravenous administration of cyclosporine, use of an oral formulation has reduced the severity of neurotoxicity. Both cyclosporine and OKT3 may cause seizures, and OKT3 may cause aseptic meningitis.

Epileptiform activity in the electroencephalogram is seen much more often in patients who die than in those who survive. In an autopsy study of 21 patients who had seizures, Estol et al. found combinations of ischemic or hemorrhagic strokes in 18, central pontine myelinosis in 5, and CNS infections in 5. Metabolic abnormalities were also responsible for the seizures in these patients. Graft-versus-host reactions may include polyneuropathy, myasthenia gravis, and polymyositis. Infected donor tissue may transmit cytomegalovirus or Creutzfeldt-Jakob disease.

SUGGESTED READINGS

Hepatic Encephalopathy

Basile AS, Jones EA. Ammonia and GABA-ergic neurotransmission: Interrelated factors in the pathogenesis of hepatic encephalopathy. *Hepatology* 1997;25:1303–1305.

Butterworth RF, Spahr L, Fontaine S, et al. Manganese toxicity, dopaminergic dysfunction and hepatic encephalopathy. *Metab Brain Dis* 1995;10:259–267.

Donovan JP, Schafer DF, Shaw BW, et al. Cerebral oedema and increased intracranial pressure in chronic liver disease. *Lancet* 1998;351:719–721.

Ferenci P, Pappas SC, Munson PJ, et al. Changes in the status of neurotransmitter receptors in a rabbit model of hepatic encephalopathy. *Hepatology* 1984;4:186–191.

Fischer JE, Baldessarini RJ. False neurotransmitters and hepatic failure. *Lancet* 1971;2:75–80.

Haseler LJ, Sibbitt WL Jr, Mojtahedzadeh HN, et al. Proton MR spectroscopic measurement of neurometabolites in hepatic encephalopathy during oral lactulose therapy. *AJNR* 1998;19:1681–1686.

Ichai P, Huguet E, Guettier C, et al. Fulminant hepatitis after grand mal seizures: mechanisms and role of liver transplantation. *Hepatology* 2003;38:443–451.

Jones EA, Weissenborn K. Neurology and the liver. *J Neurol Neurosurg Psychiatry* 1997;63:279–293.

Kjaergard LL, Liu J, Als-Nielsen B, et al. Artificial and bioartificial support systems for acute and acute-on-chronic liver failure: a systematic review. *JAMA* 2003;289:217–222.

Laccetti M, Manes G, Uomo G, et al. Flumazenil in the treatment of acute hepatic encephalopathy in cirrhotic patients: a double blind randomized placebo controlled study. *Dig Liver Dis* 2000;32:335–338.

Lizardi-Cervera J, Almeda P, Guevara L, et al. Hepatic encephalopathy: a review. *Ann Hepatol* 2003;2:122–130.

Lockwood AH, Yap EW, Wong WH. Cerebral ammonia metabolism in patients with severe liver disease and minimal hepatic encephalopathy. *J Cereb Blood Flow Metab* 1991;11:337–341.

Lunzer M, James IM, Weinman J, et al. Treatment of chronic hepatic encephalopathy with levodopa. *Gut* 1974;15:555–561.

Raskin NH, Bredesen D, Ehrenfeld WK, et al. Periodic confusion caused by congenital extrahepatic portacaval shunt. *Neurology* 1984;34:666–669.

Riordan SM, Williams R. Treatment of hepatic encephalopathy. *N Engl J Med* 1997;337:473–479.

Rozga J, Podesta L, LePage E, et al. Control of cerebral oedema by total hepatectomy and extracorporeal liver support in fulminant hepatic failure. *Lancet* 1993;342:898–899.

Shady H, Lieber CS. Blood ammonia levels in relationship to hepatic encephalopathy after propranolol. *Am J Gastroenterol* 1988;83:249–255.

Sherlock S. Chronic portal systemic encephalopathy: update 1987. *Gut* 1987;28:1043–1048.

Summerskill WHJ, Davidson EA, Sherlock S, et al. The neuropsychiatric syndrome associated with hepatic cirrhosis and an extensive portal collateral circulation. *Q J Med* 1956;25:245–266.

Victor M, Adams RD, Cole M. The acquired (non-Wilsonian) type of chronic hepatocerebral degeneration. *Medicine (Baltimore)* 1965;44:345–396.

Zieve L, Doizaki M, Derr RF. Reversal of ammonia coma in rats by L-dopa: a peripheral effect. *Gut* 1979;20:28–32.

Liver Transplantation

Bird GLA, Meadows J, Goka J, et al. Cyclosporin-associated akinetic mutism and extrapyramidal syndrome after liver transplantation. *J Neurol Neurosurg Psychiatry* 1990;53:1068–1071.

Campellone JV, Lacomis D, Kramer DJ, et al. Acute myopathy after liver transplantation. *Neurology* 1998;50:45–53.

De Groen PC, Aksamit AJ, Rakela J, et al. Central nervous system toxicity after liver transplantation: role of cyclosporin and cholesterol. *N Engl J Med* 1987;317:861–866.

Estol CJ, Faris AA, Martinez AJ, et al. Central pontine myelinosis after liver transplantation. *Neurology* 1989;39:493–498.

Estol CJ, Lopez O, Brenner RP, et al. Seizures after liver transplantation: a clinicopathologic study. *Neurology* 1989;39:1297–1301.

Fisher NC, Ruban E, Carey M et al. Late-onset fatal acure leukoencephalopathy in liver transplant recipient. *Lancet* 1997;349:1884–1885.

Garg BP, Walsh LE, Pescovitz MD, et al. Neurologic complications of pediatric liver transplantation. *Pediatr Neurol* 1993;9:44–48.

Small SL, Fukui MB, Bramblett GT, et al. Immunosuppression-induced leukoencephalopathy from tacrolimus (FK506). *Ann Neurol* 1996;40:575–580.

Stein DP, Lederman RJ, Vogt DP, et al. Neurological complications following liver transplantation. *Ann Neurol* 1992;31:644–649.

Torocsik HV, Curless RG, Post J, et al. FK506-induced leukoencephalopathy in children with organ transplants. *Neurology* 1999;52:1497–1500.

Wijdicks EFM, Dahlke LJ, Wiesner RH. Oral cyclosporine decreases severity of neurotoxicity in liver transplant recipients. *Neurology* 1999;52:1708–1710.

Wijdicks EFM, Wiesner RH, Krom RAF. Neurotoxicity in liver transplant recipients with cyclosporine immunosuppression. *Neurology* 1995;45:1962–1964.

Wilson JR, Conwit RA, Eidelman BH, et al. Sensorimotor neuropathy resembling CIDP in patients receiving FK506. *Muscle Nerve* 1994;17:528–532.

Chapter 149

Cerebral Complications of Cardiac Surgery

Mitchell S. V. Elkind and Eric J. Heyer

MAGNITUDE OF THE PROBLEM

Adverse neurologic outcomes are among the most feared and controversial complications after cardiac surgery. Neurologic complications may be divided into acute complications, including stroke and coma, and long-term neurologic and psychiatric problems such as cognitive decline, dementia, and depression. Estimates of the frequency of strokes after coronary artery bypass surgery (CABG) have ranged over an order of magnitude from approximately 0.5% to 5.2%, depending on the population studied, study design, and the methods used to detect the stroke. Patients who suffer stroke after cardiac surgery have a greater mortality, which may be as high as 38%. Valvular surgery and combined valvular and bypass surgery are associated with a higher risk of stroke than CABG alone.

Cognitive decline in the absence of an acute focal insult occurs even more commonly than stroke: a meta-analysis of cohort and interventional trials among coronary artery surgery patients found cognitive deficit on neuropsychologic testing in 22.5% at 2 months after surgery. Consistent with this observation, longitudinal data with repeated testing of a single cohort suggest that about 50% of patients have some cognitive deficit at discharge after surgery, and roughly 25% still have a deficit after 6 months. Cognitive decline was defined as a decrease by at least one standard deviation in performance on at least one of four tests of cognitive function. Late cognitive decline, at 5 years, was found in 42% of patients, a rate much greater than would be expected in similar patients who do not undergo surgery, and was predicted by early cognitive decline.

Controversy surrounds these data, particularly because definitions of cognitive decline differ, and many of these changes are asymptomatic. The functional consequences of these cognitive changes remain uncertain. Among elderly retired people, in particular, mild decrements in cognitive status may be less important than similar changes in younger, working persons. In addition, depression may also follow cardiac surgery, and this may contribute to reversible cognitive dysfunction, although some data suggest that depression and cognitive decline occur independently of each other after surgery.

PATHOPHYSIOLOGY

Strokes after cardiac surgery are generally ischemic infarcts caused by embolization of particulate matter, particularly from an atherosclerotic aorta, during the procedure. Autopsy studies have demonstrated small capillary and arteriolar dilatations (SCADs) in patients dying after CABG, but not in patients dying for other reasons. Moody et al. found these focal dilatations in 90% of patients who died after cardiac surgery on bypass. These SCADs stain for fat and are thought to be secondary to fat microemboli. Air emboli may also occur rarely, either related to bypass or in patients with left ventricular assist devices. In one report, massive fatal infarction of the hemispheres owing to air embolization occurred in a patient with a hole in the membrane separating the blood and air pump chambers of a left ventricular assist device (Fig. 149.1). Because these devices have been approved for treatment of severe and

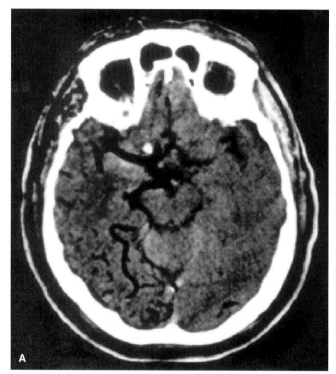
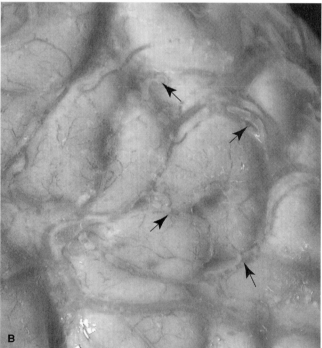

FIGURE 149.1. Massive air embolism in a patient with left ventricular assist device. **A.** CT showing prominent very low-density signal owing to the presence of air in the intravascular space of the brain, with filling and dilatation of the right middle cerebral, posterior communicating, and posterior cerebral arteries. Smaller low-density lesions within brain parenchyma, consistent with air bubbles, are also seen. **B.** Photograph of fresh postmortem brain tissue showing bubbles and columns of air alternating with blood (*black arrows*) in multiple vessels over the surface of the cerebrum. (Reprinted with permission from Elkind MS, Chin SS, Rose EA. Massive air embolism with left ventricular assist device. *Neurology* 2002; 58: 1694). (See color insert).

medically refractory congestive heart failure, neurologists are likely to see more complications.

Air and particulate emboli related to bypass equipment may also contribute to these strokes. The following factors related to the cardiopulmonary bypass apparatus play a role: type of oxygenator, type of cardiopulmonary bypass circuit, body temperature, arterial blood gas management, and use of arterial line filters. Before 1985, cardiopulmonary bypass was achieved with bubble oxygenators that generated particulate or gas bubbles, which could have occluded small cerebral vessels. Capillary membrane oxygenators were substituted to avoid this complication. Arterial line filters also reduce the number of particulate emboli from the cardiopulmonary bypass system.

Transcranial Doppler studies have further demonstrated the importance of microemboli as a cause of neurocognitive sequelae of CABG operations. Postoperatively, carotid Doppler studies demonstrated a mean of 62 emboli for each operation. In open-chamber cardiac operations, carotid and transcranial Doppler studies demonstrated even more cerebrally directed emboli. Times of danger included removal of the aortic side clamp, aortic cannulation, onset of cardiopulmonary bypass, and resumption of ventricular contraction. Emboli and cerebral injuries are even more numerous with aortic disease. Hypoperfusion during bypass is a less common mechanism of adverse neurologic outcome in adults, though it may still play a role in children.

CLINICAL FEATURES

The general imaging appearance of postoperative infarcts from emboli is of a superficial cortical infarction. Most emboli go to the middle cerebral arteries (MCAs), which supply blood to the bulk of the cerebral hemispheres, but other large vessels may also be affected. Approximately 20% of cerebral blood flow goes to the posterior circulation, so as many as one-fifth of infarcts may be expected to occur in these vessels. Not all cerebral infarctions cause weakness; so overreliance on symptoms or signs of hemiparesis may underestimate the frequency of stroke. Common stroke syndromes that do not involve weakness are fluent (Wernicke) aphasia and cortical visual loss. Because the inferior division of the MCA supplies the lateral temporal lobe and parietal lobes, including the Wernicke area, infarcts in that vessel may cause a prosodic, fluent speech with multiple paraphasic errors and poor comprehension, while sparing the motor strip in the frontal lobe.

Emboli traveling up the basilar artery may involve the posterior cerebral arteries bilaterally, causing infarction of both occipital lobes. The resulting "top of the basilar syndrome" may include complete blindness, sometimes with no awareness of the problem by the patient (Anton syndrome). Behavioral abnormalities are common, and memory loss may follow lesions in the medial temporal lobe whereas eye movement abnormalities are caused by midbrain infarcts.

Emboli may be of any size; small emboli to branches of the superior division of the MCA, for example, may cause limited weakness of the hand, particularly fine finger movements, which may be mistaken for a compression neuropathy owing to placement of the patient while under anesthesia. Watershed infarction follows decreased perfusion pressure, especially in vessels already narrowed by intracranial atherosclerosis, and is found in about 25% of the patients. These appear on imaging as more or less broad swaths of infarction over the surface of the brain extending from the frontal to occipital lobes along the borders between the middle cerebral and anterior and posterior cerebral arteries. Infarcts need not be limited to the cortical surface, however, and small deep infarcts owing to embolic obstruction of deep penetrating arterioles may also be seen.

RISK FACTORS FOR NEUROLOGIC COMPLICATIONS AFTER CARDIAC SURGERY

Attempts to identify factors associated with risk of stroke after CABG have produced largely concordant results. Proximal aortic atherosclerosis has been increasingly recognized as the major determinant of stroke and encephalopathy after bypass surgery. A history of prior stroke or TIA is also a predictor of stroke after CABG. Carotid stenosis, similarly, is a predictor of stroke in most, but not all, studies. Women may be at higher risk than men. Although age does not necessarily increase the risk of cardiac complications of heart surgery, it does appear to increase risk of neurologic injury. Nonetheless, emerging data indicate that even among those older than 80 years, the age group expected to be at highest risk of neurologic complications after surgery, most patients have an excellent outcome with resolution of symptoms and improved quality of life. As older patients continue to be referred for cardiac revascularization procedures, therefore, it has become increasingly important to identify factors predictive of neurologic injury and ways to prevent it.

Prospective studies using multivariate regression techniques provide the most robust data on the relation of various risk factors to stroke after surgery. McKhann and others identified five preoperative factors associated with an increased risk of stroke after CABG: age, prior stroke, hypertension, diabetes mellitus, and presence of carotid bruit. The only intraoperative factor of importance was duration of cardiopulmonary bypass. Using these factors in combination, the authors were able to stratify patients into low-, medium-, and high-risk groups for stroke. Roach et al. reviewed data on 2,108 patients undergoing CABG and found a 6.1% incidence of neurologic complications, of which 3.1% could be classified as type I injuries (focal cerebral injury or stupor) and 3% as type II outcomes (cognitive decline or seizures). Not surprisingly, mortality, length of stay, and likelihood of discharge to an institution for long-term care were greater among those who suffered adverse neurologic outcomes. Older age was associated with an increased risk of both types of adverse outcomes, with a 75% increase in risk per decade for type I outcomes and more than a doubling of risk per decade for type II outcomes. Additional risk factors for a type I outcome in multivariate analysis included, in declining order of importance, proximal aortic atherosclerosis, a history of neurologic disease, use of an intra-aortic balloon pump, hypertension, diabetes mellitus, pulmonary disease, and unstable angina. Neurological disease was not carefully defined, and it is unclear whether this included history of dementia as well as stroke. All operations analyzed in this study were elective; neurologic outcomes after urgent or emergent surgery are worse.

INTERVENTIONAL CARDIAC PROCEDURES

Strokes or TIAs after cardiac catheterization are rare, encountered in 0.1% to 0.3% of procedures. Both large and small vessel infarcts may occur. TIAs occur in about 0.2% of angioplasty procedures and rarely in percutaneous balloon valvuloplasty of pulmonary, mitral, and aortic valves. In one series, embolic stroke occurred in 3 of 26 aortic valve procedures and none of 6 mitral procedures. The posterior circulation may be affected more than the carotid territory, with consequent cerebral blindness and visual field defects. About half of the syndromes abate within 48 hours. The episodes are attributed to emboli released by the guidewire or in flushing the catheter in the ascending aorta. Systemic hypotension may be responsible for some. In rare cases, showers of cholesterol emboli from diseased aortic arch cause encephalopathy and strokes, renal infarcts, peripheral occlusive vascular disease, gangrene, and peripheral neuropathy (*cholesterol emboli syndrome*).

CARDIAC TRANSPLANTATION

In the early days of heart transplantation, neurologic complications were seen in 54% of cases, and 20% were fatal. With time, both figures have been much reduced. Because many patients have advanced atherosclerosis, stroke is a major risk, occurring in up to 9%. Other problems include reversible encephalopathy and seizures, sometimes related to medications rather than stroke. Commonly used immunosuppressants, including cyclosporine A, can produce the syndrome of reversible posterior leukoencephalopathy

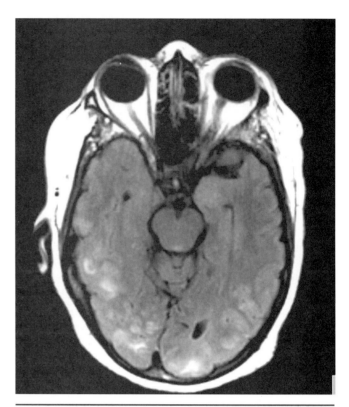

FIGURE 149.2. Reversible posterior leukoencephalopathy secondary to FK506. This 60-year-old woman underwent orthotopic heart transplantation, and approximately 3 months later while taking FK506 developed confusion, headache, and vomiting. The FLAIR MRI shows subcortical white matter hyperintensity in the parieto-occipital regions bilaterally. Her symptoms and MRI fully resolved after changing medications.

that may mimic stroke (Fig. 149.2). Cerebral hemorrhage is rare, linked to anticoagulation or uncontrolled hypertension. Vascular headache is common.

Encephalopathy occurs in about 10% of cases and is attributed to renal or hepatic failure or sepsis. Later, because of the long-term immunosuppression, opportunistic infection becomes a common cause of neurologic disorder; with new antibiotics, the rate has dropped from 15% to 5%. Aspergillus, toxoplasma, cytomegalovirus, herpes zoster, and uncommon organisms may be encountered. The incidence of primary CNS lymphoma is also increased.

PREVENTING NEUROLOGIC COMPLICATIONS AFTER CARDIAC SURGERY

Because aortic arch atherosclerosis is considered the major mechanism responsible for stroke and encephalopathy after cardiac surgery, intraoperative ECG has been recommended as a method for detection of aortic atherosclerosis. Surgeon awareness of significant aortic atheroma may allow a change in technique designed to decrease the risk of embolization. For patients with mobile or protruding plaque, or with aortic plaque >3 mm in thickness, a more proximal cannulation or clamping site may be used, or a fibrillatory arrest approach may be used.

The use of off-pump CABG procedures may also reduce the occurrence of neurologic complications of coronary surgery. The technique remains promising but is unproven. Randomized trials have shown no significant difference between on-pump and off-pump procedures in terms of mortality, quality of life, stroke, or cognitive outcome. Off-pump surgery may lead to a lower rate of long-term graft patency, but it may also be more cost effective.

Intraoperative transcranial Doppler techniques may provide another way of detecting increased risk of cerebral injury. Other methods for monitoring risk have not been successful. Quantitative EEG does not detect impending brain damage, partly because cerebral hypothermia reduces the EEG amplitude. Infrared detection of cerebral oxygenation is beset by technical problems, including contamination of the signal with extracranial blood.

Hypothermia is used as a cerebral protective measure, but there is uncertainty about the optimal temperature to be used (mild hypothermia, 32° to 34°C, versus moderate hypothermia, 28° to 32°C). There is evidence that hyperthermia postoperatively occurs frequently and is harmful. Even normothermia (37°C) is potentially harmful. Maintaining cerebral blood flow by supporting autoregulation also provides sufficient but not excessive flow to support cerebral metabolism. To maintain autoregulation during cardiopulmonary bypass, blood gas values must be kept near normal when measured at 37°C even though the patient may actually be colder. In contrast, correcting the blood gases for the lower temperature would lead to the addition of carbon dioxide to the cardiopulmonary bypass system to normalize the blood gas values at the patient's hypothermic temperature; under those conditions, autoregulation would be lost. Protecting children having cardiac surgery, however, may be best achieved by correcting the blood gases for the lower temperature because childhood injury is not a result of emboli as much as of hypoperfusion. If heparin is bonded to the cardiopulmonary bypass circuit, there is considerably less activation of platelets, white cells, and endothelial cells, resulting in attenuation of coagulation and the inflammatory response. Consequently, less anticoagulation may be required and blood loss decreases. The incidence of cerebral dysfunction may also decrease.

CAROTID SURGERY AND CABG

Because the presence of carotid stenosis predicts a worse outcome after cardiac surgery, carotid endarterectomy prior to heart surgery may reduce the risk. The mean stroke rate after cardiac surgery is as high as 4% among patients with asymptomatic stenosis >50% and increases to approximately 8% among patients with symptomatic stenosis >50%. Among patients with higher degrees of stenosis (>80%, e.g.) the risk may approach 15%. Despite this increase in risk, it remains uncertain what to do about the carotid stenosis. The magnitude of the problem is impressive because many patients with coronary disease also have cerebrovascular disease. Nearly a quarter of patients undergoing elective CABG have moderate carotid stenosis (>50%), and approximately 9% have severe stenosis (>80%). No randomized trial, however, has established that carotid endarterectomy in the neurologically asymptomatic patient prior to cardiac surgery reduces the risk of perioperative stroke or cognitive deterioration.

Options for the patient with combined coronary and cerebrovascular disease include performing (1) cardiac surgery without any carotid surgery, (2) carotid endarterectomy in a separate operation prior to the cardiac surgery, (3) CABG prior to carotid surgery, and (4) a combined operation, with carotid surgery conducted first, followed by cardiac surgery. Several authors have advocated performing carotid surgery prior to CABG in a staged or single procedure on the assumption that correcting the cerebral hemodynamic impairment first will prevent cerebral ischemic complications. However, most strokes occurring with open heart surgery are owing not to hemodynamic impairment but rather to emboli from aortic disruption. The cardiac complication rate of carotid endarterectomy is also significant; the postoperative rate of myocardial infarct (MI) in the North American Symptomatic Carotid Endarterectomy Trial (NASCET) was 0.9%, and the overall stroke or death rate was 5.8%. The MI and mortality rates of endarterectomy are much higher in patients with active cardiac disease. Therefore, although there is intuitive appeal to the approach of correcting the carotid disease prior to the cardiac intervention, there are equally strong theoretical reasons to avoid this approach. Attempts to synthesize the many published series indicate that carotid endarterectomy performed prior to cardiac surgery may reduce the risk of stroke but increase mortality. Combined procedures have no clear benefit in reducing the risk of stroke or mortality and should not be advocated in most patients. Overall, considering the combined risk of stroke and death, there was no benefit to either staged approach over CABG without endarterectomy. This conclusion does not eliminate the potential role of staged procedures in selected subgroups of patients, however.

A rational approach to the problem of the patient with combined coronary artery and carotid disease is to take into account the presence and type of symptoms and the degree of severity of the carotid disease, as well as the severity of the coronary disease. The benefits of carotid surgery for asymptomatic carotid disease are not as clear as they are for symptomatic disease. In the Asymptomatic Carotid Atherosclerosis Study, for example, asymptomatic patients had only a 2% annual risk of stroke. Given the low stroke risk, it seems likely that many of these patients could tolerate cardiac surgery without complications. When patients have both symptomatic coronary and carotid disease, the severity of neurologic symptoms can be considered. For example, medically treated patients with carotid stenosis with transient monocular blindness have a 3-year stroke rate half that of patients with hemispheric TIAs. It may also be important to consider not only the degree of stenosis at the level of the extracranial carotid artery, but also the severity of hemodynamic impairment in the intracerebral vessels. Measurement of cerebrovascular reserve using techniques such as oxygen extraction fraction on PET or carbon dioxide reactivity on transcranial Doppler testing have been used to predict risk of stroke in patients with carotid occlusion or stenosis. There are no reliable, large-scale studies demonstrating the predictive role of these tests for patients undergoing CABG. Nonetheless, a more aggressive approach to correction of the carotid lesion could be entertained in patients with distal hemodynamic impairment who are likely to be at higher risk of stroke.

CONCLUSION

Although investigators continue to debate the relative magnitude and clinical significance of the cognitive changes after CABG, it remains clear that stroke and neurologic dysfunction are among the most important complications of cardiac surgery. Improved methods of prediction and prevention have reduced the occurrence of these complications, but further improvements are sorely needed.

SUGGESTED READINGS

Benavente O, Eliasziw M, Streifler JY, et al. Prognosis after transient monocular blindness associated with carotid-artery stenosis. *N Engl J Med* 2001;345:1084–1090.

Breuer AC, Furlan AJ, Hanson MR, et al. Central nervous system complications of coronary artery bypass graft surgery: prospective analysis of 421 patients. *Stroke* 1983;14:682–687.

Coffey CE, Massey EW, Roberts KB, et al. Natural history of cerebral complications of coronary artery bypass graft surgery. *Neurology* 1983;33:1416–1421.

Das SK, Brow TD, Pepper J. Continuing controversy in the management of concomitant coronary and carotid disease: an overview. *Int J Cardiol* 2000;74:47–65.

Eagle KA, Guyton RA, Davidoff R, et al. ACC/AHA guidelines for coronary artery bypass graft surgery: executive summary and recommendations: a report of the American College of Cardiology/American Heart Association Task Force on Practice Guidelines (Committee to revise the 1991 guidelines for coronary artery bypass graft surgery). *Circulation* 1999;100:1464–1480.

Fruitman DS, MacDougall CE, Ross DB. Cardiac surgery in octogenarians: can elderly patients benefit? Quality of life after cardiac surgery. *Ann Thorac Surg* 1999;68:2129–2135.

Gardner TJ, Horneffer PJ, Manolio TA, et al. Stroke following coronary artery bypass grafting: a ten-year study. *Ann Thorac Surg* 1985;40:574–81.

Gott JP, Thourani VH, Wright CE, et al. Risk neutralization in cardiac operations: detection and treatment of associated carotid disease. *Ann Thorac Surg* 1999;68:850–856.

Grubb RL Jr, Derdeyn CP, Fritsch SM, et al. Importance of hemodynamic factors in the prognosis of symptomatic carotid occlusion. *JAMA* 1998;280:1055–1060.

Heyer EJ. Neurologic assessment and cardiac surgery. *J Cardiothorac Vasc Anesth* 1996;10:99–103.

Heyer EJ, Sharma R, Rampersad A, et al. A controlled prospective study of neuropsychological dysfunction following carotid endarterectomy. *Arch Neurol* 2002:217–22.

Hindman BJ. Emboli, inflammation, and CNS impairment: an overview. *Heart Surg Forum* 2002;5:249–253.

Hogue CW Jr, Murphy SF, Schechtman KB, et al. Risk factors for early or delayed stroke after cardiac surgery. *Circulation* 1999;100: 642–647.

John R, Choudhri AF, Weinberg AD, et al. Multicenter review of preoperative risk factors for stroke after coronary artery bypass grafting. *Ann Thorac Surg* 2000;69:30–35.

Katz ES, Tunick PA, Rusinek H, et al. Protruding aortic atheromas predict stroke in elderly patients undergoing cardiopulmonary bypass: experience with intraoperative transesophageal echocardiography. *J Am Coll Cardiol* 1992;20:70–77.

Khan NE, De Souza A, Mister R, et al. A randomized comparison of off-pump and on-pump multivessel coronary-artery bypass surgery. *N Engl J Med* 2004;350:21–28.

Knipp SC, Matatko N, Wilhelm H, et al. Evaluation of brain injury after coronary artery bypass grafting. A prospective study using neuropsychological assessment and diffusion-weighted magnetic resonance imaging. *Europ J Cardiothorac Surg* 2004;25:791–800.

McKhann GM, Borowicz LM, Goldsborough MA, et al. Depression and cognitive decline after coronary artery bypass grafting. *Lancet* 1997;349:1282–1284.

McKhann GM, Goldsborough MA, Borowicz LM, et al. Predictors of stroke risk in coronary artery bypass patients. *Ann Thorac Surg* 1997;63:516–521.

Menache CC, du Plessis AJ, Wessel DL, et al. Current incidence of acute neurologic complications after open-heart operations in children. *Ann Thorac Surg* 2002:1752–1758.

Moody DM, Bell MA, Chall VR, et al. Emboli occur at the initiation of bypass and during aortic cross-clamping and release brain microemboli during cardiac surgery or aortography. *Ann Neurol* 1990;28: 477–486.

Nathoe HM, van Dijk D, Jansen EW, et al. A comparison of on-pump and off-pump coronary bypass surgery in low-risk patients. *N Engl J Med* 2003;348:394–402.

Newman MF, Kirchner JL, Phillips-Bute B, et al. Longitudinal assessment of neurocognitive function after coronary-artery bypass surgery. *New Engl J Med* 2001;344:395–402.

North American Symptomatic Carotid Endarterectomy Trial Collaborators. Beneficial effect of carotid endarterectomy in symptomatic patients with high-grade carotid stenosis. *N Engl J Med* 1991;325: 445–453.

Parker FB, Marvasti MA, Bove EL. Neurological complications following coronary artery bypass. The role of atherosclerotic emboli. *Thorac Cardiovasc Surg* 1985;33:207–209.

Puskas JD, Winston AD, Wright CE, et al. Stroke after coronary artery operation: incidence, correlates, outcome, and cost. *Ann Thorac Surg* 2000;69:1053–1056.

Riles TS, Kopelman I, Imparato AM. Myocardial infarction following carotid endarterectomy: a review of 683 operations. *Surgery* 1979;85:249–253.

Roach GW, Kanchuger M, Mangano CM, et al. Adverse cerebral outcomes after coronary bypass surgery. *N Engl J Med* 1996;335:1857–1864.

Salasidis GC, Latter DA, Steinmetz OK, et al. Carotid artery duplex scanning in preoperative assessment for coronary artery revascularisation. *J Vasc Surg* 1995;21:154–161.

Schwartz LB, Bridgman AH, Kieffer RW, et al. Asymptomatic carotid stenosis and stroke in patients undergoing cardiopulmonary bypass. *J Vasc Surg* 1995;21:146–153.

Segal AZ, Abernethy WB, Palacios IF, et al. Stroke as a complication of cardiac catheterization: risk factors and clinical features. *Neurology* 2001;56:975–977.

Stamou SC, Hill PC, Dangas G, et al. Stroke after coronary artery bypass: incidence, predictors, and clinical outcome. *Stroke* 2001;32:1508–1513.

Svedjeholm R, Hakanson E, Szabo Z, et al. Neurological injury after surgery for ischemic heart disease: risk factors, outcome and role of metabolic interventions. *Eur J Cardiothorac Surg* 2001;19:611–618.

Thong, WY, Strickler AG. Li S, et al. Hyperthermia in the forty-eight hours after cardiopulmonary bypass. *Anesth Analg* 2002:1489–1495.

Tuman KJ, McCarthy RJ, Najafi H, et al. Differential effects of advanced age on neurological and cardiac risks of coronary artery operations. *J Thorac Cardiovasc Surg* 1992;104:1510–1517.

van Dijk D, Keizer AMA, Diephuis JC, et al. Neurocognitive dysfunction after coronary artery bypass surgery: a systematic review. *J Thorac Cardiovasc Surg* 2000;120:632–639.

van Dijk D, Nierich AP, Jansen EWL, et al. Early outcome after off-pump versus on-pump coronary bypass surgery: results from a randomized study. *Circulation* 2001;104:1761–1766.

Wolman RL, Nussmeier NA, Aggarwal A, et al. Cerebral injury after cardiac surgery: identification of a group at extraordinary risk. *Stroke* 1999;30:514–522.

Youssuf AM, Karanam R, Prendergast T, et al. Combined off-pump myocardial revascularization and carotid endarterectomy: early experience. *Ann Thorac Surg* 2001;72:1542–1545.

Chapter 150

Bone Disease

Roger N. Rosenberg

OSTEITIS DEFORMANS (PAGET DISEASE)

This chronic disease of the adult skeleton is characterized by bowing and irregular flattening of the bones. Any or all skeletal bones may be affected, but the tibia, skull, and pelvis are the most frequent sites. Except for the skeletal deformities and pain, the disease causes disability only when the skull or spine is involved.

Pathology

In affected bones, there is an imbalance between formation and resorption of bone. In most cases, there is a mixture of excessive bone formation and bone destruction. The areas of bone destruction are filled with hyperplastic vascular connective tissue. New bone formation may occur in the destroyed areas in an irregular disorganized manner. The metabolic disturbance is unknown.

Incidence

There is a postmortem incidence of 3% in patients over 40 years of age. Men and women are equally affected. The common age at onset is in the fourth to sixth decades; it is rare before age 30.

Symptoms and Signs

Two types of neurologic symptoms appear: those owing to the abnormalities in bone and those owing to arteriosclerosis, a common accompaniment. The cerebral manifestations that occur with arteriosclerosis are identical to those seen in patients with arteriosclerosis in the absence of Paget disease.

The neurologic defects of osteitis deformans are usually related to pressure on the central nervous system or the nerve roots by the overgrowth of bone. Convulsive seizures, generalized or neuralgic head pain, cranial nerve palsies, and paraplegia occur in a few cases. Deafness caused by pressure on the auditory nerves is the most common symptom; unilateral facial palsy is the next most common symptom. Loss of vision in one eye, visual field defects, or exophthalmos may occur when the sphenoid bone is affected. Compression of the spinal cord is more common than compression of the cerebral substance, which is extremely rare except when there is sarcomatous degeneration of the lesions. Platybasia may occur in advanced cases. Paget disease has been described in a patient with basilar impression and Arnold-Chiari type I malformation.

Laboratory Data

The serum calcium content is normal, and the serum phosphorus is normal or only slightly increased. Serum alkaline phosphatase activity is increased; the level varies with the extent and activity of the process. It may be only slightly elevated when the disease is localized to one or two bones.

Diagnosis

The diagnosis of Paget disease is made from the patient's appearance and the characteristic radiographic changes. Involvement of the skull in advanced cases is manifested by a generalized enlargement of the calvarium, anteroflexion of the head, and depression of the chin on the chest. When the spine is involved, the patient's stature is shortened; the spine is flexed forward, and its mobility is greatly reduced.

Radiographically, the skull shows areas of increased bone density with loss of normal architecture, mingled with areas in which the density of the bone is decreased (Fig. 150.1). The margins of the bones are fuzzy and indistinct. The general appearance is that of an enormous skull with the bones of the vault covered with cotton wool. In advanced cases, there may be a flattening of the base of

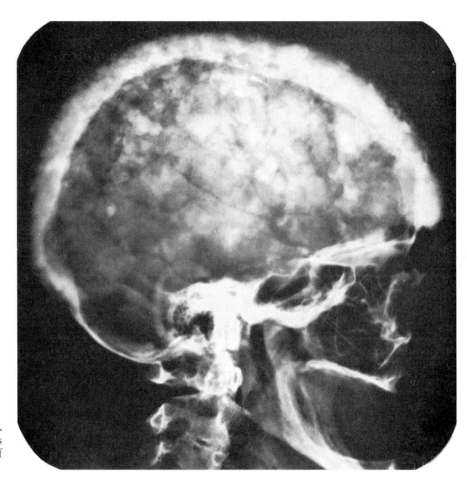

FIGURE 150.1. Osteitis deformans (Paget disease) of the skull. (Courtesy of Dr. Juan Taveras.)

the skull on the cervical vertebrae (*platybasia*) with signs of damage to the lower cranial nerves, medulla, or cerebellum. Both CT and MRI aid diagnosis (Fig. 150.2).

Diagnosis may be difficult if the clinical symptoms are mainly neurologic. In these instances, radiographs of the pelvis and legs or a general survey of the entire skeleton may establish the diagnosis. Rarely, it may be impossible to distinguish monophasic Paget disease of the skull from osteoblastic metastases. Search for a primary neoplasm, particularly in the prostate or biopsy of one of the lesions in the skull may be necessary in those cases.

Course

The course is variable but usually extends over decades. The neurologic lesions seldom lead to serious disability other than deafness, convulsive seizures, or compression of the spinal cord.

Treatment

There is no specific therapy. Calcitonin is given to inhibit the osteolytic process. Salmon calcitonin is given in subcutaneous injections of 50 to 100 units daily. Improvement

of osteolytic lesions and reversal of neurologic manifestations have been noted with long-term therapy. About 25% of the patients develop serum antibodies to salmon calcitonin, sometimes in titers high enough to make the person resistant to the hormonal action of calcitonin; under these circumstances, human calcitonin may be effective.

An alternate therapy is disodium editronate in a dosage of 5.0 mg/kg body weight daily for 6 months. The value of either medical therapy can be evaluated by reduction of serum levels of alkaline phosphatase measured at 4-month intervals and annual radiographs of specific lesions. Decompression of the spinal cord may be indicated for myelopathy secondary to stenosis created by the enlarged vertebrae. Similarly, platybasia may lead to decompression of the posterior fossa.

FIBROUS DYSPLASIA

The skull and the bones in other parts of the body are occasionally involved by a process characterized by small areas of bone destruction or massive sclerotic overgrowth. The clinical picture of fibrous dysplasia is related to the site

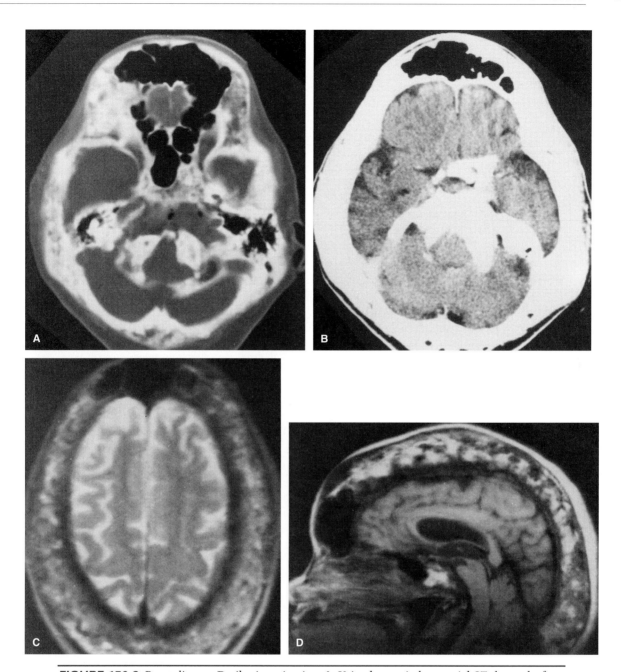

FIGURE 150.2. Paget disease. Basilar invagination. **A.** Using bone windows, axial CT shows the foramen magnum projected within the posterior fossa. Intradiploic calcific density with cotton wool appearance is typical of Paget disease. **B.** Higher section, using soft tissue windows, demonstrates obliteration of basal cisterns and brainstem compression caused by basilar invagination. **C.** Axial T2-weighted MRI shows prominent mottled signal in the diploic space. **D.** Sagittal T1-weighted MRI confirms impingement of brainstem by dens. (Courtesy of Drs. J. A. Bello and S. K. Hilal.)

and extent of the bone overgrowth. Sassin and Rosenberg (1968) described involvement of bones of the skull in 50 cases as follows: frontal, 28; sphenoid, 24; frontal and sphenoid, 18; temporal, 8; facial, 15; parietal, 6; and occipital, 8. Diffuse involvement of the entire skull produces leontiasis ossea, with exophthalmos, optic atrophy, and cranial nerve palsies (Fig. 150.3).

In addition to the disfiguration of the skull in the polyostotic form, symptoms of the monostotic form of the disease include headache, convulsions, exophthalmos, optic atrophy, and deafness. Symptoms may begin at any age, but onset usually occurs in early adult life. The family history is negative, and there is no racial or sexual predominance.

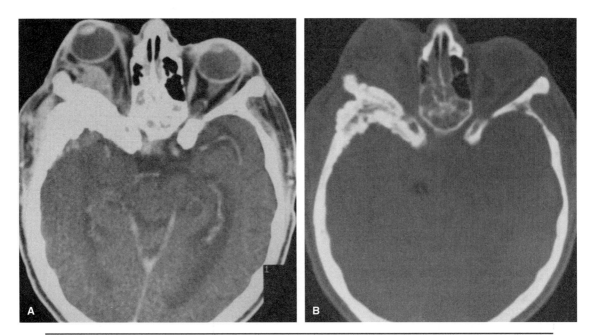

FIGURE 150.3. Fibrous dysplasia. CT. **A.** Axial contrast-enhanced scan shows proptosis on right with abnormal soft tissue enhancement within orbit and middle cranial fossa. **B.** Bone window depicts pronounced thickening of sphenoid bone. (Courtesy of Dr. T. L. Chi.)

A polyostotic form of the disease is characterized by café au lait spots, endocrine dysfunction with precocious puberty in girls, and involvement of the femur (shepherd's crook deformity). Mutations in the Arg201 codon of the Ys G protein subunit have been described in patients with fibrous dysplasia. These Ys G as mutations may be seen in monostotic or polyostotic patients and in the McCune-Albright syndrome that includes multiple endocrinopathies and café au lait lesions with fibrous dysplasia.

The diagnosis is made from the characteristic body configuration of short arms and legs, normal-size trunk, enlargement of the head, and changes in the radiographs of the skeleton (Fig. 150.4). Many affected infants die in the perinatal period, although a normal lifespan is possible for patients with less severe involvement of the bones.

Shunting procedures may be needed for hydrocephalus caused by involvement of the bones at the base of the skull. Laminectomy is indicated for signs of cord compression.

ACHONDROPLASIA

Achondroplasia (*chondrodystrophy*) is the most frequent form of skeletal dysplasia causing dwarfism. It is characterized by short arms and legs, lumbar lordosis, and enlargement of the head caused by mutations in the fibroblast growth factor receptor 3 gene (FGFR3). The disease is rare and is estimated to occur in 15 of one million births in the United States. It is usually inherited as an autosomal-dominant trait.

Symptoms of involvement of the nervous system sometimes develop as a result of hydrocephalus, compression of the medulla and cervical cord at the level of the foramen magnum, compression of the spinal cord by ruptured intervertebral disk, and bone compression of the lower thoracic or lumbar cord. Convulsive seizures, ataxia, and paraplegia are the most common symptoms. Mental development is usually normal.

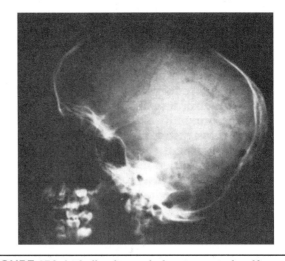

FIGURE 150.4. Skull radiograph showing typical malformation of achondroplasia. The clivus is shortened.

The mutations described in 1994 in the FGFR3 gene at 4p are usually new mutations and result in autosomal-dominant inheritance. The gene product is expressed in cartilage. A frequent FGFR3 mutation is a Gl 138A codon mutation with GGG to AGG or CGG substitutions, resulting in an exchange of glycine at position 380 in the FGFR3 protein to arginine. This mutation results in a gain of negative function, producing an inactive fibroblast growth factor receptor and resultant dwarfism.

ANKYLOSING SPONDYLITIS

This inflammatory disorder affects ligamentous insertions into bones; at first, it usually affects the sacroiliac joints and lumbar spine. In some patients, the entire spine is involved, with ossification of the ligaments and fusion of the vertebra. The spine becomes rigid and susceptible to a variety of disorders that may affect the spinal cord, including fractures and dislocations, atlanto-occipital dislocation, and spinal stenosis. The condition is common, affecting an estimated 1.4% of the general population. It only rarely, however, causes symptoms and signs of myelopathy.

A cauda equina syndrome may appear in patients with long-standing spondylitis. Signs and symptoms are symmetric, with weakness, wasting, and sensory loss in lumbosacral myotomes. Bladder and bowel are commonly affected, and pain may be severe. The mechanism is not clear. Although concomitant arachnoiditis has been suspected as the cause, the syndrome appears late, when there is little evidence that the underlying spondylitis is active. Moreover, there is little inflammation at postmortem examination, which is likely to show chronic fibrosis. There is erosion of posterior bone elements, and, in earlier days, myelography showed enlargement of the caudal sac and prominent diverticulae of the arachnoid. CT shows similar pathology, but MRI is more illuminating, showing nerve root thickening and sometimes enhancement of dura and nerve roots; that pattern suggests inflammation of the arachnoid structures, supporting the earlier theory. Surgery is generally ineffective and has sometimes been deleterious, although there have been rare reports of some relief. Steroid therapy has been similarly without benefit.

ATLANTOAXIAL DISLOCATION

Subluxation of C-1 on C-2 occurs in many conditions that render the odontoid process of C-2 ineffective as a stabilizing post. This occurs most often as a complication of cervical trauma, but also occurs as a congenital malformation (alone or in combination with other anomalies of the cervical spine or cranium) and is seen with disproportionate frequency with Down syndrome, ankylosing spondylitis, and rheumatoid arthritis. It can be demonstrated with plain spine films, CT, or MRI. There is risk of cervical myelopathy or medullary compression, and sudden death has been reported. For symptomatic cases, surgical stabilization is indicated. For asymptomatic cases, there has to be consideration of the risks of surgery against uncertain risks of no surgery. A general recommendation is to consider stabilization or decompression if imaging shows deformation of the neuroaxis, symptomatic or not. A closed reduction and brace immobilization was successfully applied to a patient with traumatic bilateral rotatory dislocation of the atlantoaxial joints.

SUGGESTED READINGS

Osteitis Deformans (Paget Disease)

Boutin RD, Spitz DJ, Newman JS, et al. Complications in Paget disease at MR imaging. *Radiology* 1998:209:641–651.

Chen JR, Rhee RS, Wallach S, et al. Neurologic disturbances in Paget disease of bone: response to calcitonin. *Neurology* 1979:29:448–457.

Davis DP, Bruffey JD, Rosen P. Coccygeal fracture and Paget's disease presenting as acute cauda equina syndrome. *J Emerg Med* 1999;17:251–254.

Douglas DL, Duckworth T, Kanis JA, et al. Spinal cord dysfunction in Paget's disease of bone. Has medical treatment a vascular basis? *J Bone Joint Surg Br* 1981;63B:495–503.

Douglas DL, Kanis JA, Duckworth T, et al. Paget's disease: improvement of spinal cord dysfunction with diphosphate and calcitonin. *Metab Bone Dis Rela tRes* 1981;3:327–335.

Gandolfi A, Brizzi R, Tedesghi F, et al. Fibrosarcoma arising in Paget's disease of the vertebra: review of the literature. *Surg Neural* 1983; 13:72–76.

Ginsberg LE, Elster AD, Moody DM. MRI of Paget disease with temporal bone involvement presenting with sensorineural hearing loss. *J Comput Assist Tomogr* 1992:16:314–316.

Goldhammer V, Braham J, Kosary IZ. Hydrocephalic dementia in Paget's disease of the skull: treatment by ventriculoatrial shunt. *Neurology* 1979;29:513–516.

Hadjipavlou A, Lander P. Paget disease of the spine. *J Bone Joint Surg Am* 1991;73:1376–1381.

Hullar TE, Lustig LR. Paget's disease and fibrous dysplasia. *Otolaryngol Clin North Am* 2003;36:707–732.

lglesias-Osma C. Paget's disease of bone and basilar impression with an Arnold-Chiari type-I malformation. *Ann Med Intern* 1997:14:519–522.

Roberts MC, Kressel HY, Fallon MD, et al. Paget disease: MR imaging findings. *Radiology* 1989:173:341–345.

Szpalski M, Gunzburg R. Lumbar spinal stenosis in the elderly: an overview. *Eur Spine J* 2003;12(Suppl 2):S170–S175.

Wallach S. Treatment of Paget's disease. *Adv Neurol* 1982;27:1–43.

Watts GD, Wymer J, Kovach MJ, et al. Inclusion body myopathy associated with Paget disease of bone and frontotemporal dementia is caused by mutant valosin-containing protein. *Nat Genet* 2004;36:377–381.

Weisz GM. Lumbar spinal canal stenosis in Paget's disease. *Spine* 1983;8:192–198.

Fibrous Dysplasia

Albright F. Polyostotic fibrous dysplasia: a defense of the entity. *J Clin Endocrinol Metab* 1947;7:307–324.

Bhansali A, Sharma BS, Sreenivasulu P, et al. Acromegaly with fibrous dysplasia: McCune-Albright Syndrome–clinical studies in 3 cases and brief review of literature–. *Endocr J* 2003;50:793–799.

Candeliere GA, Roughley PJ, Glorieux FH. Polymerase chain reaction-based technique for the selective enrichment and analysis of mosaic

Arg201 mutations in G alpha S from patients with fibrous dysplasia of bone. *Bone* 1997;21:201–206.

Fitzpatrick KA, Taljanovic MS, Speer DP, et al. Imaging findings of fibrous dysplasia with histopathologic and intraoperative correlation. *AJR Am J Roentgenol* 2004;182:1389–1398.

Katz BJ, Nerad JA. Ophthalmic manifestations of fibrous dysplasia: a disease of children and adults. *Ophthalmology* 1998;105:2207–2215.

Leet AI, Magur E, Lee JS, et al. Fibrous dysplasia in the spine: prevalence of lesions and association with scoliosis. *J Bone Joint Surg Am* 2004;86-A:531–537.

Mohammadi-Araghi H, Haery C. Fibro-osseous lesions of craniofacial bones. The role of imaging. *Radial Clin North Am* 1993;31:121–134.

Saper JR. Disorders of bone and the nervous system: the dysplasias and premature closure syndromes. In: Vinken PJ, Bruyn GW, eds. *Handbook of Clinical Neurology.* New York: Elsevier-North Holland, 1979.

Sassin JF, Rosenberg RN. Neurologic complications of fibrous dysplasia of the skull. *Arch Neurol* 1968;18:363–376.

Selmani Z, Aitasalo K, Ashammakhi N. Fibrous dysplasia of the sphenoid sinus and skull base presents in an adult with localized temporal headache. *J Craniofac Surg* 2004;15:261–263.

Tehranzadeh J, Fung Y, Donahue M, et al. Computed tomography of Paget disease of the skull versus fibrous dysplasia. *Skeletal Radial* 1998;27:664–672.

Achondroplasia

Dandy WF. Hydrocephalus in chondrodystrophy. *Bull Johns Hopkins Hosp* 1921;32:5–10.

Denis JP, Rosenberg HS, Ellsworth CA Jr. Megalocephaly, hydrocephalus and other neurological aspects of achondroplasia. *Brain* 1961;84:427–45.

Duvoisin RC, Yahr MD. Compressive spinal cord and root systems in achondroplastic dwarfs. *Neurology* 1962;12:202–207.

Gollust SE, Thompson RE, Gooding HC, et al. Living with achondroplasia: attitudes toward population screening and correlation with quality of life. *Prenat Diagn* 2003;23:1003–1008.

Haga N. Management of disabilities associated with achondroplasia. *J Orthop Sci* 2004;9:103–107.

Hamarnci N, Hawran S, Biering-Sorensen F. Achondroplasia and spinal cord lesion. Three case reports. *Paraplegia* 1993;31:375–379.

Hecht JT, Butler IJ. Neurologic morbidity associated with achondroplasia. *J Child Neurol* 1990;5:84–97.

Horton WA. Fibroblast growth factor receptor 3 and the human chondrodysplasias. *Curr Opin Pediatr* 1997;9:437–442.

Horton WA, Lunstrum GP. Fibroblast growth factor receptor 3 mutations in achondroplasia and related forms of dwarfism. *Rev Endocr Metab Disord* 2002;3:381–385.

McKusick VA. 1997 Albert Lasker Award for Special Achievement in Medical Science. Observations over 50 years concerning intestinal polyposis, Marfan syndrome, and achondroplasia. *Nat Med* 1997;3:1065–1068.

Shiang R, Thompson LM, Zhu YZ, et al. Mutations in the transmembrane domain of FGFR3 cause the most common genetic form of dwarfism, achondroplasia. *Cell* 1994;78:335–342.

Thomas IT, Frias JL. The prospective management of cervicomedullary compression in achondroplasia. *Birth Defects* 1989;25:83–90.

Thompson NM, Hecht JT, Bohan TP, et al. Neuroanatomic and neuropsychological outcome in school-age children with achondroplasia. *Am J Med Genet* 1999;88:145–153.

Yamanaka Y, Ueda K, Seino Y, et al. Molecular basis for the treatment of achondroplasia. *Horm Res* 2003;60(Suppl 3):60–64.

Ankylosing Spondylitis

Braun J, Sieper J. Biological therapies in the spondyloarthritides–the current state. *Rheumatology (Oxford)* 2004;43:1072–1084.

Bruining K, Weiss K, Zeifer B, et al. Arachnoiditis in the cauda equina syndrome of longstanding ankylosing spondylitis. *J Neuroimag* 1993;3:55–57.

Fox MW, Onofrio BM, Kilgore JE, Neurological complications of ankylosing spondylitis. *J Neurosurg* 1993;78:871–878.

Haywood KL, Garratt AM, Jordan K, et al. Spinal mobility in ankylosing spondylitis: reliability, validity and responsiveness. *Rheumatology (Oxford)* 2004;43:750–757.

Mitchell MJ, Sanoris DJ, Moody D, et al. Cauda equina syndrome complicating ankylosing spondylitis. *Radiology* 1990;175:521–525.

Rowed DW. Management of cervical spinal cord injury in ankylosing spondylitis: intervertebral disc as a cause of cord compression. *J Neurosurg* 1992;77:241–246.

Rubenstein DJ, Alvarez O, Gheirnan B, et al. Cauda equina syndrome complicating ankylosing spondylitis, *J Comput Assist Tomogr* 1989;13:511–513.

Shaw PJ, Allcutt DA, Bates D, et al. Cauda equina syndrome with multiple lumbar arachnoid cysts in ankylosing spondylitis: improvement following surgical therapy. *J Neurol Neurosurg Psychiatry* 1990;53:1076–1079.

Tullous MW, Skerhut HE, Story JL, et al. Cauda equina syndrome of long-lasting ankylosing spondylitis. Case report and review of the literature. *J Neurosurg* 1990;73:441–447.

Zhou H, Buckwalter M, Boni J, et al. Population-based pharmacokinetics of the soluble TNFr etanercept: a clinical study in 43 patients with ankylosing spondylitis compared with post hoc data from patients with rheumatoid arthritis. *Int J Clin Pharmacol Ther* 2004;42:267–276.

Atlantoaxial Dislocation

Braganza SF. Atlantoaxial dislocation. *Pediatr Rev* 2003;24(Mar):106–107.

Crockard HA, Heiman AE, Stevens JM. Progressive myelopathy secondary to odontoid fractures: clinical, radiological, and surgical features. *J Neurosurg* 1993;78:579–586.

Crossman JE, Thompson D, Hayward RD, et al. Recurrent atlantoaxial rotatory fixation in children: a rare complication of a rare condition. Report of four cases. *J Neurosurg Spine* 2004;100:307–311.

Elliott S, Morton RE, Whitelaw RA. Atlantoaxial instability and abnormalities of the odontoid in Down's syndrome. *Arch Dis Child* 1988;63:1484–1489.

Maeda T, Saito T, Harimaya K, et al. Atlantoaxial instability in neck retraction and protrusion positions in patients with rheumatoid arthritis. *Spine* 2004;29:757–762.

Rowland LP, Shapiro JH, Jacobson HG. Neurological syndromes associated with congenital absence of the odontoid process. *Arch Neural Psychiatry* 1958;80:286–291.

Stevens JM, Chong WK, Barber C, et al. A new appraisal of abnormalities of the odontoid process associated with atlantoaxial subluxation and neurological disability. *Brain* 1994;117:133–l48.

Wise JJ, Cheney R, Fischgrund J. Traumatic bilateral rotatory dislocation of the atlanto-axial joints: a case report and review of the literature. *J Spinal Disord* 1997;10:451–453.

Yamashita Y, Takahashi M, Sakamoto Y, et al. Atlantoaxial subluxation, radiography and MRI correlated to myelopathy. *Acta Radiol* 1989;10:135–140.

Chapter 151

Renal Disease

Neil H. Raskin and J. Kirk Roberts

Uremia is the term for a constellation of signs and symptoms in patients with severe azotemia caused by acute or chronic renal failure; symptomatic renal failure is an acceptable definition. The clinical features of the neurologic consequences of renal failure do not correlate well with any single biochemical abnormality, but seem to be related to the rate of development of renal failure. This chapter summarizes the features of uremic encephalopathy and neuropathy and the distinctive neurologic complications of dialysis and renal transplantation.

UREMIC ENCEPHALOPATHY

In uremia, as in other metabolic encephalopathies, there is a continuum of signs of neurologic dysfunction, including dysarthria, instability of gait, asterixis, action tremor, multifocal myoclonus, and sensorial clouding. One or more of these signs may predominate, but fluctuation of clinical signs from day to day is characteristic. The earliest most reliable indication of uremic encephalopathy is sensorial clouding. Patients appear fatigued, preoccupied, and apathetic; they have difficulty concentrating. Obtundation becomes more apparent as perceptual errors, defective memory, and mild confusion become evident. Illusions and perceptions sometimes progress to frank visual hallucinations.

Asterixis is almost always present once sensorial clouding appears: It is most effectively elicited by having the patient hold the arms outstretched in fixed hyperextension at the elbow and wrist, with the fingers spread apart. After a latency of up to 30 seconds, flexion-extension (flapping) of the fingers at the metacarpophalangeal joints and at the wrist appears arrhythmically and at irregular intervals.

Multifocal myoclonus refers to visible twitching of muscles that is sudden, arrhythmic, and asymmetric, involving muscles first in one locus and then in another and affecting chiefly the face and proximal limbs. It is a strong indication of a severe metabolic disturbance and usually does not appear until stupor or coma has supervened. In uremia, asterixis and myoclonus may be so intense that muscles appear to fasciculate, giving rise to the term *uremic twitching*. This form of myoclonus probably signifies cortical irritability;

it is, at times, difficult to distinguish from a multifocal seizure. *Tetany* is commonly associated with myoclonus and other signs of encephalopathy. It may be overt, with spontaneous carpopedal spasms, or latent, manifested by a Trousseau sign. The spasms originate in abnormal peripheral nerve discharges. In uremic patients, tetany does not usually respond to injections of calcium and occurs despite metabolic acidosis (which inhibits hypocalcemic tetany).

The *restless-legs syndrome* occurs in 40% of uremic patients and is probably a symptom of encephalopathy. This syndrome comprises creeping, crawling, prickling, and pruritic sensations deep within the legs. These sensations are almost always worse in the evening; they are relieved by movement of the limbs. Clonazepam, levodopa, dopamine agonists, opioids, and some anticonvulsants are effective in terminating this syndrome.

Alterations in limb tone appear as encephalopathy progresses and brainstem function is compromised. Muscle tone is usually heightened and is sometimes asymmetric. Eventually, decorticate posturing may appear instead of decerebrate attitudes. Focal motor signs are present in about 20% of patients; these signs often clear after hemodialysis.

Convulsions are usually a late manifestation of uremic encephalopathy. In the older literature, convulsions were thought to occur far more often than is now reported; this may have been the result of failing to distinguish hypertensive encephalopathy from uremia, which may coexist. Hypertensive retinopathy and papilledema are major signs that distinguish the two conditions; furthermore, focal signs such as aphasia or cortical blindness are much more common in hypertensive brain disease than in uremia. The treatment of recurring uremic convulsions is not straightforward because the pharmacokinetics of phenytoin are altered in uremic patients. In uremia, plasma protein binding of phenytoin is decreased so much that the unbound fraction of the drug is two to three times more than that found in normal plasma. In uremic patients, however, the volume of distribution of the drug is larger and there is an increased rate of conversion of phenytoin to hydroxylated derivatives, resulting in lower total serum concentrations of the drug for any given dose. This combination of factors allows the physician to administer the usual dosage of phenytoin (300–400 mg daily) to a uremic patient and attain therapeutic unbound levels of the drug despite lower total serum levels (i.e., 5–10 mg/L rather than 10–20 mg/L).

Findings on CT or MRI are usually nonspecific, but may help to exclude other conditions, such as ischemic stroke, intracerebral hemorrhage, subdural hematoma, or hydrocephalus. EEG, like the clinical state, is usually more strikingly abnormal in acute renal failure than in chronic renal failure. The background activity is slow with theta and delta waves more prominent in the frontal regions.

Meningeal signs occur in about 35% of uremic patients; half of those affected have CSF pleocytosis. CSF protein elevations >60 mg/dL occur in 60% of uremic patients; in 20%, the CSF protein exceeds 100 mg/dL. CSF protein content may return to normal immediately after hemodialysis period. The increase in CSF protein is attributed to alteration in the permeability properties of cerebral capillary endothelial cells adjacent to the CSF, which have tight intercellular junctions.

There are no specific pathologic alterations of brain in uremic encephalopathy; cerebral use of oxygen is depressed, as it is in other metabolic encephalopathies, because of a primary interference with synaptic transmission. Depressed cerebral metabolic rate and clinical state usually change together but are probably independent reflections of generally impaired neuronal functions. The profundity of uremic encephalopathy correlates only in a general way, and sometimes poorly, with biochemical abnormalities in the blood. Cerebral acidosis has been suggested as a possible mechanism, but CSF pH is usually normal. Brain calcium is increased by 50% and seems to be owing to excess circulating parathyroid hormone, which is nondialyzable. It is not clear whether calcium changes are related to the cerebral dysfunction.

Rapid clearing of uremic encephalopathy after dialysis suggests that small to moderately sized water-soluble molecules are responsible for symptoms. Excessive accumulation of toxic organic acids overwhelms the normal mechanisms for excluding such compounds from the brain and may be important. These organic acids may block transport systems of the choroid plexus and of glia that normally remove metabolites of some neurotransmitters in brain. Furthermore, a nonspecific increase in cerebral membrane permeability in uremia may permit greater entry into brain of uremic toxins such as the organic acids, which further derange cerebral function.

Erythropoietin is often given to patients on long-term dialysis to correct the anemia. In the process, cognitive functions may improve.

UREMIC NEUROPATHY

Peripheral neuropathy is the most common neurologic consequence of chronic renal failure. It is a distal, symmetric, predominantly axonal, mixed sensorimotor neuropathy affecting the legs more than the arms. It is clinically indistinguishable from the neuropathies of chronic alcohol abuse or diabetes mellitus. The rate of progression, severity, prominence of motor or sensory signs, and prevalence of dysesthesia vary. It is several times more common in men than in women. The symptom of burning feet was considered a common feature of uremic neuropathy, but probably resulted from removal of water-soluble thiamine by hemodialysis, and with near universal B vitamin replacement, this syndrome is now rare.

The rate of progression of uremic neuropathy varies widely; in general, it evolves over several months but may be fulminant. Among most patients who enter chronic hemodialysis programs, the neuropathy stabilizes or improves slowly. Patients with mild neuropathy often recover completely, but those who begin dialysis with severe neuropathy rarely recover even after several years. Lack of improvement or progression of symptoms while on hemodialysis may suggest an alternative diagnosis, such as chronic inflammatory demyelinating polyneuropathy. Patients in chronic renal failure are also more susceptible to drugs that are normally excreted in the urine; for this reason, there may be prolonged paralysis after administration of neuromuscular blocking agents as an aid to endotracheal intubation, and the prolonged paralysis may be mistaken for peripheral neuropathy. An *accelerated neuropathy of renal failure* may progress so rapidly that it is mistaken for the Guillain-Barré syndrome. Mononeuropathies, such as carpal tunnel syndrome, may occur, perhaps owing to an increased susceptibility of at-risk nerves to injury or as a vascular steal phenomenon after arteriovenous fistula. Autonomic dysfunction and cranial neuropathies, particularly visual loss and hearing loss, are seen occasionally.

Successful renal transplantation has a clear, predictable, and beneficial effect on uremic neuropathy. Motor nerve conduction velocities increase within days of transplantation. There is progressive improvement for 6 to 12 months, often with complete recovery, even in patients with severe neuropathy before transplantation.

Pathologically, this neuropathy is usually a primary axonal degeneration with secondary segmental demyelination, probably as a result of a metabolic failure of the perikaryon; there is also a predominantly demyelinating type. Because uremic neuropathy improves with hemodialysis, it seems evident that the neuropathy results from the accumulation of dialyzable metabolites. These substances may be in the "middle molecule" (300–2,000 Da) range; compounds of this size cross dialysis membranes more slowly than smaller molecules such as creatinine and urea, which are the usual measures of chemical control of uremia. Supporting this contention are observations that control of neuropathy in some patients depends on increased hours of dialysis each week (beyond that necessary for chemical control of uremia) and that peritoneal dialysis seems to be associated with a lower incidence of neuropathy. The peritoneal membrane seems to permit passage of some molecules more readily and selectively than the cellophane membrane used in hemodialysis. The transplanted kidney deals effectively with substances of different molecular size; the resulting elimination of middle molecules could explain the invariable improvement of the neuropathy after transplantation.

In experimental uremia, a parathormone-induced increase in calcium in peripheral nerves slows nerve conduction velocity; these changes can be prevented by prior parathyroidectomy. In human uremic patients, circulating parathormone levels correlate inversely with nerve conduction velocity. It seems unlikely, however, that parathormone is involved in uremic neuropathy because the hormone is nondialyzable, and hyperparathyroidism itself is not usually associated with neuropathy.

DIALYSIS DYSEQUILIBRIUM SYNDROME

In this complication of dialysis, symptoms vary from mild headache, nausea, and muscle cramps to, more rarely, obtundation, convulsions, or delirium. The cerebral sequelae are usually seen with rapid dialysis at the outset of a dialysis program; symptoms usually appear toward the third or fourth hour of a dialysis run but occasionally appear 8 to 24 hours later. The syndrome is usually self-limited, subsiding in hours, but delirium may persist for several days. Some patients become exophthalmic because of increased intraocular pressure at the height of the syndrome. Other clinical correlates include increased intracranial pressure, papilledema, and generalized EEG slowing.

The shift of water into brain is probably the proximate cause of dysequilibrium. Rapid reduction of blood solute content cannot be paralleled by brain solutes because of the blood-brain barrier. An osmotic gradient is produced between blood and brain causing movement of water into brain, which results in encephalopathy, cerebral edema, and increased intracranial pressure. MRI may show increased brain volume. The osmotically active substances retained in brain have not yet been identified.

With improvements in dialysis, this syndrome is much less frequent now. Before diagnosing dialysis dysequilibrium, other causes of cerebral symptoms should be excluded.

DIALYSIS DEMENTIA

A distinctive, progressive, usually fatal encephalopathy may occur in patients who are chronically dialyzed for periods that exceed 3 years. The first symptom is usually a stammering, hesitancy of speech, and at times, speech arrest. The speech disorder is intensified during and immediately after dialysis and at first may be seen only during these periods. A thought disturbance is usually evident, and there is a consistent EEG abnormality with bursts of high-voltage slowing in the frontal leads. As the disorder progresses, speech becomes more dysarthric and aphasic; dementia and myoclonic jerks usually become apparent at this time. The other elements of the encepha-

lopathy include delusional thinking, convulsions, asterixis, and occasionally focal neurologic abnormalities. Early in the course, diazepam is effective in lessening myoclonus and seizures and in improving speech; it becomes less effective later. Brain imaging and CSF are usually unremarkable and are most helpful in excluding other causes of encephalopathy. Increased dialysis time and renal transplantation do not seem to alter the course of the disease. No distinctive abnormalities have been found in brain at autopsy.

The geographic variation in the incidence of dialysis dementia suggests a neurotoxin. Aluminum content is consistently elevated in the cerebral gray matter of patients who die from this condition. Municipal water supplies heavily contaminated with aluminum have been linked to the syndrome in epidemiologic studies. The frequency of the disease markedly diminished when aluminum was removed from the water used during dialysis, but did not disappear completely. Another possible source is absorption of aluminum from orally administered phosphate-binding agents that are given to uremic patients. Plasma protein binding of aluminum retards the removal of aluminum during dialysis even when an aluminum-free dialysate is used. Nevertheless, there have been several reports of remission of dialysis dementia when deferoxamine was used to remove aluminum from the diet, from the dialysate, or from the patient. Cerebral aluminum intoxication, still an unconfirmed hypothesis, seems to be the most likely possibility at this time. Brain GABA levels are reduced in numerous regions, but the meaning of this finding is not clear.

NEUROLOGIC COMPLICATIONS OF RENAL TRANSPLANTATION

Renal transplantation is the preferred treatment of end-stage renal disease and, with advances in transplantation medicine, these patients live longer and are more at risk for the adverse consequences of long-term immunosuppression.

Several drugs are used to prevent transplant rejection and each has adverse effects. Of particular interest to the neurologist is the reversible posterior leucoencephalopathy seen in those patients treated with cyclosporine and tacrolimus. Symptoms include headache, visual disturbance, encephalopathy, and seizures. Blood pressure is usually elevated. MRI reveals changes in the white matter, most extensive in the occipital and parietal regions. Complete resolution of the symptoms and the MRI findings usually follows treatment of hypertension and reduction of the dosage of the immunosuppressive medication or changing to an alternative agent.

Stroke, either ischemic or hemorrhagic, is prevalent in renal transplant recipients with a prevalence of nearly 8%. Some of the increased risk may be owing to shared risk factors between stroke patients and end-stage renal disease patients, including hypertension and diabetes mellitus.

The risk that a lymphoma will develop after a transplant is about 35 times greater than normal; this increased risk depends almost entirely on the increased incidence of primary CNS lymphoma. These are almost always B-cell lymphomas developing from immunosuppression-related Epstein-Barr virus (EBV) infection causing lymphocyte proliferation. The tumor usually appears between 5 and 46 months after transplantation. The resulting clinical syndromes include increased intracranial pressure, rapidly evolving focal neurologic signs, or combinations of these. Convulsions are rare. The lymphoma may be multicentric and may involve the meninges. Treatment may include immunosuppression withdrawal, chemotherapy, and radiation.

Infections occur often in transplant patients, and a high index of suspicion must be maintained because the usual inflammatory response may be impaired diminishing the severity of symptoms. New headache or mental changes should lead the clinician to consider brain imaging and lumbar puncture. Viral infections with cytomegalovirus, herpes simplex virus, and Jacob-Creutzfeld (JC) virus can often be diagnosed on CSF with culture or polymerase chain reaction (PCR). Bacterial and tuberculous meningitis are also considerations. Systemic fungal infections are found at autopsy in about 45% of patients who have been treated with renal transplantation and immunosuppression; brain abscess formation occurs in about 35% of these patients. In almost all cases, the primary source of infection is in the lung. Chest radiographs and the presence of fever aid in differentiating fungal brain abscess from brain tumor in recipients of transplants. *Aspergillus* has a unique predilection for dissemination to brain and accounts for most fungal brain abscesses; candida, nocardia, and histoplasma are found in the others. The clinical syndrome resulting from these infections is usually delirium accompanied by seizures. Headache, stiff neck, and focal signs also occur but not commonly. The CSF is often remarkably bland, and brain biopsy may be the only reliable way to establish a diagnosis. The distinction of fungal brain abscess from possibly radiosensitive brain tumor makes it important to consider this procedure.

SUGGESTED READINGS

Bolton CF, Young GB. *Neurological Complications of Renal Disease.* London: Butterworths, 1990.

Bucher SF, Seelos KC, Oertel WH, et al. Cerebral generators involved in the pathogenesis of the restless legs syndrome. *Ann Neurol* 1997;41:639–645.

Burns DJ, Bates D. Neurology and the kidney. *J Neurol Neurosurg Psychiatry* 1998;65:810–21.

Hamed LM, Winward KE, Glaser JS, et al. Optic neuropathy in uremia. *Am J Ophthalmol* 1989;108:30–35.

Healton EB, Brust JCM, Feinfeld DA, et al. Hypertensive encephalopathy and the neurologic manifestations of malignant hypertension. *Neurology* 1982;32:127–132.

Lederman RJ, Henry CF. Progressive dialysis encephalopathy. *Ann Neurol* 1978;4:199–204.

Mattana J, Effiong C, Gooneratne R, et al. Outcome of stroke in patients undergoing hemodialysis. *Arch Intern Med* 1998;158:537–541.

McCarthy JT, Milliner DS, Johnson WJ. Clinical experience with desferrioxamine in dialysis patients with aluminum toxicity. *Q J Med* 1990;74:257–276.

Oliveras A, Roquer J, Puig JM. Stroke in renal transplant patients: epidemiology, predictive risk factors and outcome. *Clin Transplant* 2003;17:1–8.

Pastan S, Bailey J. Dialysis therapy. *N Engl J Med* 1998;338:1428–1437.

Patchell RA. Neurological complications of organ transplantation. *Ann Neurol* 1994;36:688–703.

Raskin NH, Fishman RA. Neurologic disorders in renal failure. *N Engl J Med* 1976;294:143–148, 204–210.

Ropper AH. Accelerated neuropathy of renal failure. *Arch Neurol* 1993;50:536–539.

Russo LS, Beale G, Sandroni S, et al. Aluminum intoxication in undialyzed adults with chronic renal failure. *J Neurol Neurosurg Psychiatry* 1992;55:697–700.

Sidhom OA, Odeh YK, Krumlovsky FA, et al. Low-dose prazosin in patients with muscle cramps during hemodialysis. *Clin Pharm Ther* 1994;56:445–451.

Takaki J, Nishi T, Nangaku M, et al. Clinical and psychological aspects of restless legs syndrome in uremic patients on hemodialysis. *Am J Kidney Dis* 2003;41:833–839.

Vanholder R, De Smet R, Glorieux G, et al. Review on uremic toxins: classification, concentration, and interindividual variability. *Kidney Internat* 2003;63:1934–1943.

Wang HC, Cheng SJ. The syndrome of acute bilateral basal ganglia lesions in diabetic uremic patients. *J Neurol* 2003;250:948–955.

Wills MR, Savory J. Aluminum and chronic renal failure; sources, absorption, transport, and toxicity. *Crit Rev Clin Lab Sci* 1989;27:59–107.

Chapter 152

Respiratory Support for Neurologic Diseases

Stephan A. Mayer and Matthew E. Fink

Many different problems are encountered in a neurologic intensive care unit (ICU); all patients share a common need for meticulous nursing care and cardiorespiratory monitoring to prevent a life-threatening complication. Diagnosis is rarely a problem; the major concern in the ICU is treatment of neurologic disease and the medical complications that determine survival and recovery. Neurologic patients who require ICU treatment frequently have a depressed level of consciousness, impaired airway protection owing to depressed cough and gag reflexes, immobilization and paralysis, or oropharyngeal and respiratory muscle weakness, all of which predispose to pulmonary complications and respiratory failure. In fact, respiratory monitoring and support are the most common reasons for admission of neurologic patients to the ICU.

RESPIRATORY PHYSIOLOGY

Respiratory failure occurs when gas exchange is impaired. The diagnosis of respiratory failure depends on arterial blood gas analysis. $Pao_2 < 60$ mm Hg or $Paco_2 > 50$ mm Hg unequivocally defines respiratory failure. There are warning signs, however, of deteriorating ventilatory function before respiratory failure is overt. Patients with neurologic disease often do not complain of dyspnea. The premonitory signs of mild respiratory failure include somnolence or reduced responsiveness, agitation, confusion, tachycardia, tachypnea, diaphoresis, asterixis, and headache. When muscle weakness is the problem, use of accessory muscles, dysynchronous breathing, and paradoxical respirations (inward movement of the abdomen with inspiration) may be observed. Advanced respiratory failure leads to cyanosis, hypotension, and coma. It is impossible to predict Pao_2 and $Paco_2$ from clinical signs; measurement of arterial blood gases is essential. Normal Pao_2 is a function of age. A healthy 20-year-old breathing room air has a Pao_2 of 90 to 100 mm Hg. With each decade, Pao_2 decreases by 3 mm Hg. Normal $Paco_2$ is 37 to 43 mm Hg and is not affected by age.

Hypoxemia is caused by five conditions: a low inspired oxygen concentration, alveolar hypoventilation, ventilation/perfusion mismatch, intracardiac right-to-left shunting, and impaired oxygen diffusion. Accurate interpretation of Pao_2 requires calculation of the alveolar-arterial (A-a) oxygen tension difference, or *A-a gradient*. Alveolar oxygen tension (PAo_2) can be calculated from the equation $Pao_2 = (Fio_2 \times 713) - (Paco_2/0.8)$, where Fio_2 is the inspired fraction of oxygen (0.21 in room air) and $Paco_2$ is the arterial carbon dioxide tension. The A-a gradient is the difference between the PAo_2 and Pao_2 measured directly via an arterial blood gas.

An A-a gradient exceeding 20 mm Hg usually results from *ventilation/perfusion mismatching*, which in turn comes in two forms. *Dead space ventilation* occurs when ventilated lung segments do not come in contact with pulmonary capillary blood flow; this occurs when the alveolar-capillary interface is destroyed (e.g., emphysema) or when blood flow is reduced (e.g., pulmonary embolism). *Intrapulmonary shunting* occurs when perfused lung segments do not come in contact with ventilated alveoli; this occurs when small airways are occluded (e.g., asthma, chronic bronchitis), when alveoli are filled with fluid (e.g., pulmonary edema, pneumonia), or when alveoli collapse (atelectasis). In most conditions, these two processes occur in combination. Hypoxemia with an A-a gradient <20 mm Hg strongly suggests an extrapulmonary cause of hypoxemia (hypoventilation or a low inspired oxygen concentration).

Hypercapnia is caused by three conditions: increased CO_2 production or inhalation, alveolar hypoventilation, and ventilation/perfusion mismatching with dead space ventilation. Hypoventilation is identified by high $Paco_2$ with a normal A-a gradient. Acute hypercapnia leads to acidosis and cerebral vasodilatation, which in turn can cause a depressed level of consciousness (CO_2 narcosis), aggravation of elevated intracranial pressure, and blunted respiratory drive leading to further hypoventilation.

Pulmonary function testing is the simplest and most reliable way to evaluate respiratory function in patients with neuromuscular respiratory failure (Table 152.1). Arterial blood gases are also important to monitor, but abnormalities (hypoxia and hypercarbia) usually develop later in the cycle of respiratory decompensation and thus are not sensitive for detecting early ventilatory failure. Vital capacity, the volume of exhaled air after maximal inspiration, normally ranges from 40 to 70 mL/kg. Reduction of vital capacity to 30 mL/kg is associated with a weak cough, accumulation of oropharyngeal secretions, atelectasis, and hypoxemia. A vital capacity of 15 mL/kg (1 L in a 70-kg person) is generally considered the level at which intubation is required (Table 152.2). Negative inspiratory pressure, normally >80 cm H_2O, measures the strength of the diaphragm and other muscles of inspiration and generally reflects the ability to maintain normal lung expansion and avoid atelectasis. Positive expiratory force, normally >140 cm H_2O, measures the

▶ **TABLE 152.1 Pulmonary Function Tests in Neuromuscular Respiratory Failure**

	Normal	*Criteria for Intubation and Weaning*	*Criteria for Extubation*
Vital capacity	40–70 mL/kg	15 mL/kg	25 mL/kg
Negative inspiratory pressure	>80 cm H_2O	20 cm H_2O	40 cm H_2O
Positive expiratory pressure	>140 cm H_2O	40 cm H_2O	50 cm H_2O

Adapted from Mayer (1997).

▶ **TABLE 152.2** Criteria for Intubation and Mechanical Ventilation

Respiratory rate > 35/min
Vital capacity < 15 mL/kg
Peak inspiratory pressure < 25 cm H_2O
Pao_2 < 70 mm Hg with maximum oxygen by face mask
$Paco_2$ > 50 mm Hg associated with acidosis (pH < 7.35)
Severe oropharyngeal paresis with inability to protect the airway
These physiologic criteria are intended to serve only as guidelines; treatment decisions must be individualized. As a general rule, intubation in neurologic patients with impending respiratory failure should be performed *before* significant blood gas abnormalities develop.

strength of the muscles of expiration and correlates with strength of cough and the ability to clear secretions from the airway.

The pathophysiology of neuromuscular respiratory failure resembles a vicious cycle. Mild hypoxemia usually precedes hypercapnia because atelectasis (and mild intrapulmonary shunting) is an early development. As weakness progresses, inability to maintain normal lung expansion results in reduced lung compliance and an increase in the work of breathing, which is often further aggravated by a weak cough and inability to clear secretions from the airway. As vital capacity approaches 15 mL/kg, rapid shallow breathing and hypercapnia develop. At this stage, the situation can rapidly and unexpectedly deteriorate once muscle fatigue develops and the patient can no longer compensate with increased respiratory effort.

NEUROLOGIC DISEASES WITH PRIMARY RESPIRATORY DYSFUNCTION

Brainstem Disease

Reticular formation neurons, sensitive to hypoxemia and hypercarbia, are located in the brainstem and may be affected by ischemia, hemorrhage, inflammation, or neoplasms. The medullary center is responsible for initiation and maintenance of spontaneous respirations, whereas the pontine pneumotaxic center helps to coordinate cyclic respirations. Forebrain dysfunction, often from metabolic causes, can lead to Cheyne-Stokes respirations (a cyclic crescendo-decrescendo respiratory pattern with intervening apnea) as burst of respiratory drive becomes dependent on increases in Pco_2. Hypothalamic or midbrain damage, particularly in the setting of brainstem herniation, may cause central neurogenic hyperventilation (low Pco_2 with normal A-a gradient). Lower pontine tegmental damage may lead to apneustic (inspiratory breath holding) or clus-

ter breathing (irregular bursts of rapid breathing alternating with apneic periods). Medullary damage may cause ataxic breathing (irregular pattern with hypoxemia and hypercarbia), gasping, or apnea.

Documentation of apnea in the face of a strong hypercarbic stimulus is an essential component in the diagnosis of brain death. Formal apnea testing requires preoxygenating the patient with 100% oxygen and normalizing the Pco_2 to 40 mm Hg, turning off the ventilator, and allowing the Pco_2 to rise above 55 mm Hg (the Pco_2 will rise 3 to 6 mm Hg per minute). Arterial blood gases are checked at both the beginning and end of the test to confirm the eventual extent of hypercarbia. The physician must stand at the bedside during the apnea test to observe the chest wall and diaphragm to confirm the absence of respiratory muscle movement.

In addition to abnormalities in respiratory rate and pattern and synchronization of diaphragm and intercostal muscles, brainstem damage often alters consciousness and causes paralysis of pharyngeal and laryngeal musculature, predisposing to tracheal aspiration. Patients with severe brainstem dysfunction should undergo endotracheal intubation to prevent respiratory complications.

Brainstem respiratory centers may be depressed (lose responsiveness to CO_2 or O_2) by narcotics or barbiturates, metabolic abnormalities such as hypothyroidism, and by starvation or metabolic alkalosis. Idiopathic primary alveolar hypoventilation and sleep apnea syndrome involve brainstem malfunction. These disorders are easily distinguished from structural brainstem pathology by the lack of associated neurologic signs or imaging abnormalities.

Spinal Cord Disease

The respiratory system is affected depending on the segmental level and severity of the spinal injury. In spinal cord trauma, the most common cause of death is acute respiratory failure owing to apnea, aspiration pneumonia, or pulmonary embolism. The long-term care of a quadriplegic patient heavily depends on the degree of respiratory impairment.

Lower motor neurons that innervate the diaphragm arise from the C-3 to C-5 segments of the spinal cord. A complete lesion at C-3 or higher abolishes both diaphragmatic and intercostal muscle activity, leaving only accessory muscle function. The result is severe hypercapnic respiratory failure, which is fatal without the immediate institution of full ventilatory support. Acute spinal cord lesions at the C-5 to C-6 level produce an immediate fall in vital capacity to 30% of normal. Several months after injury, however, the vital capacity will increase to 50% to 60% of normal. High thoracic lesions will compromise intercostal and abdominal muscles, causing a limitation of inspiratory capacity and active expiration. Midthoracic lesions have little impact on respiratory muscle function because only the abdominal muscles are affected.

Most spinal cord diseases cause respiratory impairment by interrupting the suprasegmental impulses that drive the diaphragm and intercostal muscles. There are two notable exceptions, however: strychnine poisoning and tetanus. Both of these toxins block the inhibitory interneurons within the spinal cord, causing simultaneous increases in the activity of muscles that are normally antagonists. Apnea and respiratory failure can result from intense muscle spasms of the upper airway muscles, diaphragm, and intercostal muscles. In rare cases, severe generalized dystonia can lead to a similar picture.

Motor Neuron Diseases

Amyotrophic lateral sclerosis (ALS) is the main form of motor neuron disease that causes respiratory failure (see Chapter 119). Respiratory failure usually develops late in course of ALS, as the respiratory muscles and strength of cough progressively weaken. If symptoms begin with limb weakness, the disorder may progress to respiratory failure in 2 to 5 years, but occasionally respiratory distress is the first symptom. If oropharyngeal symptoms are prominent, respiratory complications may be caused by recurrent aspiration pneumonitis. Frequent pulmonary function testing can identify patients at risk for respiratory complications. The earliest changes are decreases in maximum inspiratory and expiratory muscle pressures, followed by reduced vital capacity. When vital capacity falls below 30 mL/kg, the ability to cough and maintain lung expansion is impaired, increasing the risk of aspiration pneumonia. Blood gases may show only a compensated respiratory acidosis until the patient is near respiratory arrest.

Peripheral Neuropathies

The Guillain-Barré syndrome, or acute inflammatory demyelinating polyneuropathy, is the prototype neuropathy with respiratory complications (see Chapter 106). Of patients with this syndrome, 20% require tracheal intubation and mechanical ventilation, which can be predicted by a rapidly progressive course, marked oropharyngeal and facial weakness, and prominent dysautonomia. In this subset, there is a 5% mortality rate with the best possible treatment. Most deaths are a result of pulmonary embolism, septic shock, or other medical complications. Some degree of respiratory insufficiency must be expected in all patients with severe disease; therefore, during the 2- to 4-week period of progression, there should be frequent measurements of inspiratory and expiratory pressures and vital capacity. Plasmapheresis or IVIG therapy should be initiated as soon as possible in all Guillain-Barré patients with respiratory muscle weakness.

Disorders of Neuromuscular Transmission

Myasthenia gravis, botulism, and neuromuscular blocking drugs may affect respiratory muscles. Myasthenia gravis almost always affects cranial muscles, causing ptosis, weakness in the ocular and oropharyngeal muscles, and symmetric facial weakness (see Chapter 121). Frequent measurement of inspiratory and expiratory pressures and vital capacity is essential for monitoring ventilatory function in hospitalized patients with myasthenia. Patients with severe dysarthria and dysphagia are at greatest risk for respiratory failure.

Myasthenic crisis is defined as an exacerbation of weakness that requires mechanical ventilation. It occurs in 15% to 20% of patients overall, and one-third of these experience two or more episodes of crisis. As with Guillain-Barré syndrome, mortality is approximately 5%. Infection (usually pneumonia or viral upper respiratory infection) is the most common precipitant (40%), followed by no obvious cause (30%) and aspiration (10%). As a general rule, 25% of patients in crisis can be extubated after 1 week, 50% after 2 weeks, and 75% after 1 month. Plasmapheresis leads to short-term improvement of weakness in 75% of patients and should be performed in all patients unless otherwise contraindicated, although its efficacy for reducing the duration of crisis has not been tested in a randomized controlled trial.

Critical Illness Neuromyopathy

Critical illness neuromyopathy (CINM) refers to a spectrum of acquired neuromuscular syndromes that develop exclusively in ICU patients who require prolonged mechanical ventilation. It is by far the most common form of neuromuscular respiratory failure, but it develops only as a complication of some other illness. CINM presents as generalized weakness and failure to wean from mechanical ventilation. The condition may take the form of an axonal motor neuropathy (sensory involvement is rare), a noninflammatory myopathy characterized by selective loss of thick myosin filaments, or both. Sepsis and multisystem organ failure are risk factors for the neuropathy, and corticosteroid administration or exposure to neuromuscular blocking agents are risk factors for the myopathy. The diagnosis depends on EMG and nerve conduction studies with direct muscle stimulation: because voluntary muscle contraction cannot be performed as part of the EMG exam, demonstration of an absent or low-amplitude compound muscle action potential in response to direct stimulation is usually necessary to diagnose the myopathy. Recovery occurs gradually over weeks to months, and there is no treatment.

Muscle Disease

Muscular dystrophies, myotonic disorders, inflammatory myopathies (e.g., polymyositis), periodic paralyses, metabolic myopathies (especially acid maltase deficiency), endocrine disorders (particularly thyroid disease), infectious myopathies (e.g., influenza or Coxsackie virus infection), mitochondrial myopathies, toxic myopathies, myoglobinuria, and electrolyte disorders (particularly hypophosphatemia and hypokalemia) may cause widespread skeletal muscle weakness leading to respiratory failure.

MANAGEMENT OF RESPIRATORY FAILURE IN NEUROLOGIC DISEASES

Examination

The initial management of the patient with impending neuromuscular respiratory failure is directed toward assessing the adequacy of ventilation and possible need for immediate intubation. The patient's overall comfort level and the rapidity with which the dyspnea has developed are both important. Rapid shallow breathing, with inability to generate adequate tidal volumes, is a danger sign of significant respiratory muscle fatigue. Diaphragmatic strength can be estimated by palpating for normal outward movement of the abdomen with inspiration; with severe weakness, inspiration is associated with spontaneous inward movement of the diaphragm (paradoxical respirations). Ventilatory reserve can be assessed by checking the patient's ability to count from 1 to 20 in a single breath. The strength of the patient's cough should be observed. A wet gurgled voice and pooled oropharyngeal secretions are the best clinical signs of significant dysphagia. When severe, weakness of the glottic and oropharyngeal muscles can lead to stridor, which is indicative of potentially life-threatening upper airway obstruction. Dysphagia is best screened for by asking the patient to sip 3 ounces of water; coughing is diagnostic of aspiration, and if present, oral feedings should be held until swallowing can be formally assessed.

Mechanical Ventilation

Mechanical ventilation is the primary treatment for respiratory failure. The trachea may be intubated orally or nasally; a soft air-filled cuff is then inflated in the trachea to prevent leakage of air around the tube. Indications for endotracheal intubation include physiologic functions (Table 152.2), the rate of respiratory deterioration, and the patient's overall comfort level. Patients should be intubated electively whenever possible; emergency intubation is as-

sociated with an increased risk of adverse outcomes related to prolonged hypoxemia.

In some cases, continuous or bilevel non-invasive positive-pressure ventilation (NPPV) can be delivered with the use of a tight-fitting face mask. Although NPPV has been shown to be helpful for getting patients through a mild episode of respiratory muscle weakness, it is usually ineffective for long periods of time in patients who have oropharyngeal weakness, dysphagia, and a weakened or impaired cough reflex, and should not be used as an alternative to endotracheal intubation.

Positive pressure ventilation may be pressure cycled or volume cycled. Synchronous intermittent mandatory ventilation is the preferred initial mode of ventilation in most patients. With this mode, a predetermined number of volume-cycled positive pressure breaths are delivered per minute. The patient can initiate a spontaneous breath at any time and receive either a volume-assisted breath or an unsupported breath, depending on the phase of the ventilator cycle. Initially, the tidal volume is set at 8 to 10 mL/kg with a respiratory rate of 8 to 12 breaths per minute, and 3 to 5 cm H_2O of positive end-expiratory pressure (PEEP) is maintained to prevent atelectasis. The fraction of inspired air is gradually adjusted downward from 100% until the arterial oxygen saturation is >95%.

Weaning From Mechanical Ventilation

Weaning from the ventilator should be initiated when pulmonary function tests show improvement and when there are no ongoing serious medical complications (Table 152.3). Weaning begins with spontaneous breathing trials in which the ventilator is switched to a mode of ventilation called *pressure support*. In this form of pressure-cycled ventilation, in addition to a constant level of PEEP, each spontaneous breath is supported by supplemental air flow until a predetermined airway pressure is reached. The pressure support level (usually 5–15 cm H_2O) should be adjusted to attain spontaneous tidal volumes of 300 to 500 mL and a comfortable breathing pattern. As an alternative to pressure support ventilation, spontaneous breathing trials can also take the form of T-piece ventilation, in which the patient breathes spontaneously through an open tubing system with oxygen flow-by. Whatever the mode of weaning, an increasing respiratory rate with decreasing

▶ **TABLE 152.3 Criteria for Weaning From Mechanical Ventilation**

Neurologic condition is stable or improving
Vital capacity > 15 mL/kg
Negative inspiratory pressure > 20 mm Hg
Pao$_2$ > 80 mm Hg with 40% oxygen
Patient is free of fever, infection, fluid overload, anemia, gastric distention, or other medical complications

tidal volumes indicates tiring, at which point the weaning trial should be stopped and the patient returned to synchronous intermittent mandatory ventilation for rest overnight. The ability of the patient to tolerate a T tube or continuous positive airway pressure with minimal pressure support (5 cm H_2O) for extended periods, while maintaining a ratio of respiratory rate (breaths/minute) to tidal volume (L) <100, is probably the single best predictor of successful extubation.

Tracheostomy and Long-Term Ventilation

Though clinicians traditionally perform a tracheostomy when mechanical ventilation is required for more that 2 to 3 weeks, this procedure is be performed as soon as possible if it is clear that prolonged support will be necessary. Early tracheostomy is associated with more rapid weaning from mechanical ventilation and shorter ICU stay than a policy of late tracheostomy. Tracheostomy has several advantages over long-term endotracheal intubation, including increased comfort, reduced risk of permanent tracheolaryngeal injury, increased ease of weaning from the ventilator (reduced dead space and less resistance to flow from the endotracheal tube), and improved ability to manage and suction secretions. The latter two considerations are of particular importance when weaning patients with neuromuscular respiratory failure from mechanical ventilation. In some patients with severe persistent oropharyngeal muscle weakness, a tracheostomy is necessary to manage secretions and prevent aspiration, even though respiratory muscle function is adequate.

Some patients require ventilatory support for months or years. Small suitcase- or laptop-sized ventilators are now available for use in the home, and battery-powered portable ventilators can allow wheelchair-bound patients to travel out of the home. In patients with respiratory failure owing to focal brainstem or high cervical cord lesions, an implantable phrenic nerve pacemaker can be used to stimulate diaphragmatic contraction, thus liberating the patient from connection to a machine altogether.

SUGGESTED READINGS

Bach JR, O'Brien J, Krotenberg R, et al. Management of end stage respiratory failure in Duchenne muscular dystrophy. *Muscle Nerve* 1987;10:177–182.

Benditt JO. Management of pulmonary complications in neuromuscular disease. *Phys Med Rehab Clin N Am* 1998;9:167–185.

Bolton CF. Assessment of respiratory function in the intensive care unit. *Can J Neurol Sci* 1994;21:S28–S34.

British Thoracic Society Standards of Care Committee. Non-invasive ventilation in acute respiratory failure. *Thorax* 2002;57:192–211.

Chalela JA. Pearls and pitfalls in the intensive care management of Guillain-Barré syndrome. *Semin Neurol* 2001;21:399–405.

Cohen CA, Zagelbaum G, Gross D, et al. Clinical manifestations of inspiratory muscle fatigue. *Am J Med* 1982;73:308–316.

Howard RS, Wiles CM, Hirsch NP, et al. Respiratory involvement in primary muscle disorders: assessment and management. *Q J Med* 1993;86:175–189.

Koh WY, Lew TWK, Chin NM, et al. Tracheostomy in a neuro-intensive care setting: Indications and timing. *Anaesth Intensive Care* 1997;25:365–368.

Laghi F, Tobin MJ. Disorders of the respiratory muscles. *Am J Resp Crit Care Med* 2003;168:10–48.

Lawn ND, Fletcher DD, Henderson RD, et al. Anticipating mechanical ventilation in Guillain-Barre syndrome. *Arch Neurol* 2001;58:893–898.

MacDuff A, Grant IS. Critical care management of neuromuscular disease, including long-term ventilation. *Curr Op Crit Care* 2003;9:106–112.

Perrin C, Unterborn JN, Ambrosio CD, et al. Pulmonary complications of chronic neuromuscular diseases and their management. *Muscle Nerve* 2004;29:5–27.

Qureshi AI, Suarez JI, Parekh PD, et al. Prediction and timing of tracheostomy in patients with infratentorial lesions requiring mechanical ventilatory support. *Crit Care Med* 2000;28:1383–1387.

Rabinstein AA, Wijdicks EF. Warning signs of imminent respiratory failure in neurological patients. *Semin Neurol* 2003;23:97–104.

Rabinstein A, Wijdicks EF. BiPAP in acute respiratory failure due to myasthenic crisis may prevent intubation. *Neurology* 2002;59:1647–1649.

Thomas CE, Mayer SA, Gungor Y, et al. Myasthenic crisis: clinical features, mortality, complications, and risk factors for prolonged intubation. *Neurology* 1997;48:1253–1260.

Tobin MJ. Mechanical ventilation. *N Engl J Med* 1994;330:1056–1061.

Wijdicks EFM, Borel CO. Respiratory management in acute neurologic illness. *Neurology* 1998;50:11–20.

Yang KL, Tobin MJ. A prospective study of indexes predicting the outcome of trials of weaning from mechanical ventilation. *N Engl J Med* 1991;324:1445–1450.

Yavagal DL, Mayer SA. Respiratory complications of rapidly progressive neuromuscular syndromes: Guillain-Barré syndrome and myasthenia gravis. *Semin Resp Crit Care Med* 2002;23;221–229.

Chapter 153

Paraneoplastic Syndromes

Lisa M. DeAngelis and Lewis P. Rowland

DEFINITION

Neurologic paraneoplastic disorders are caused by indirect damage to central or peripheral nervous system structures from a systemic cancer. They are called *paraneoplastic* because the neurologic disorder is not the result of tumor invasion or metastasis, toxicity from chemotherapy or radiotherapy, malnutrition, or coincidental infection.

▶ **TABLE 153.1**   **Frequency of Associated Tumor with Clinical Syndromes That Are Often Paraneoplastic**

Syndrome[a]	Paraneoplastic (%)
Lambert-Eaton myasthenic syndrome	60
Subacute cerebellar degeneration	50
Opsoclonus/myoclonus (children)	50
Opsoclonus/myoclonus (adults)	20
Subacute sensory neuropathy	20
Myasthenia gravis after age 40 (thymoma)	20
Dermatomyositis after age 40	20
Sensorimotor peripheral neuropathy after age 50	10
Encephalomyelitis	10

[a]Figures are for adults unless age is specifically mentioned; particular tumors are described in text.
Modified from Posner JB. *Neurologic complications of cancer.* Philadelphia: FA Davis, 1995:353–385.

EPIDEMIOLOGY

All neurologic paraneoplastic syndromes are rare, affecting less than 0.1% of patients with cancer. Any cancer may be associated with a paraneoplastic syndrome, but most syndromes are associated with a specific cancer or a particular group of cancers. Most patients with a paraneoplastic syndrome develop neurologic symptoms before the cancer is identified. Frequently the cancer is small enough to elude detection using standard body CT. Body PET is more sensitive for diagnosing small cancers and is the procedure of choice for evaluating patients with presumed paraneoplastic disorders, although even this technique may miss a tumor that later becomes symptomatic or is found only at postmortem examination. Typical clinical syndromes are not associated with cancer in every patient (Table 153.1).

PATHOGENESIS

Most paraneoplastic disorders are probably immune-mediated, marked by the frequent presence of characteristic antibodies against neuronal antigens. These antibodies are useful diagnostically but have not been established as causative in the CNS disorders. In the peripheral neuromuscular disorders of LEMS associated with small cell lung cancer, myasthenia gravis with thymoma, and the anti-MAG peripheral neuropathies with lymphoproliferative disease, the antibodies are pathogenic. These syndromes are discussed in Chapters 106, 121, and 122.

Cancers that cause paraneoplastic syndromes contain antigens that are normally restricted to the nervous system. The host mounts an immune attack against those antigens in the tumor, but the immune response is directed against central or peripheral neural antigens. In some situations (e.g., small cell lung cancer with anti-Hu antibodies), the immune response is associated with more limited disease and better oncologic outcome. In addition to antibodies, antigen-specific cytotoxic T-cells are found in the CSF, and the same T-cells have been identified at autopsy in the nervous system of affected patients.

CLINICAL SYNDROMES

Paraneoplastic Cerebellar Degeneration (PCD)

PCD causes a pancerebellar syndrome with ataxia of gait and limbs, dysarthria, nystagmus, and oscillopsia. Other manifestations are encountered in half of the patients, including bulbar syndromes, corticospinal tract signs, dementia, and peripheral neuropathy. CT and MRI are usually normal, but diffuse hyperintensity of the cerebellum is occasionally seen on T2-weighted MRI, and postgadolinium T1 images rarely reveal enhancement of the folia. As the disease progresses, diffuse cerebellar atrophy develops. Pathology demonstrates loss of Purkinje cells. CSF abnormalities may include modest pleocytosis and high protein content, sometimes with high immunoglobin (IgG) and oligoclonal bands. Associated antibodies may be anti-Yo (with gynecologic cancers), anti-Hu (with small cell lung cancer), anti-Tr or anti-GluR1 with Hodgkin disease, or anti-Ri with cancer of the breast. The nature of these antibodies is discussed later. The differential diagnosis includes viral encephalitis, multiple sclerosis, Creutzfeldt-Jakob disease, alcoholic cerebellar degeneration, and hereditary spinocerebellar atrophy. Treatment is not satisfactory.

Sensory Neuronopathy

Painful paresthesias are the dominant symptoms and progress over weeks to involve all four limbs and occasionally the trunk and face. Paraneoplastic sensory neuronopathy affects all forms of sensation and usually results in a severe sensory ataxia. Motor function is spared or minimally affected. Tendon reflexes are lost and CSF pleocytosis is characteristic. This is usually associated with the anti-Hu antibody and is most commonly associated with small cell lung cancer. Nerve conduction studies show loss of sensory evoked potentials with normal motor functions. Inflammation is seen in the dorsal root ganglia.

Limbic Encephalitis

Personality and mood changes progress rapidly, and within weeks the syndrome is dominated by delirium and dementia with severe memory loss. The disorder may occur alone or with other signs of encephalitis or sensory neuropathy. MRI may show mild enhancement of the medial temporal lobes or increased signal on T_2 or FLAIR images. CSF pleocytosis is characteristic. The anti-Ma2 antibody is characteristically detected in this syndrome when it is associated with testicular cancer. It also occurs in association with the anti-Hu antibody in patients with small cell lung cancer. Pathologic signs of inflammation are limited at first to the limbic and insular cortex, but other gray matter may be affected. The changes include loss of neurons, perivascular infiltration by leukocytes, and microglial proliferation.

Brainstem Encephalitis

Symptoms of brainstem encephalitis are usually part of a more widespread encephalomyelitis occurring in the anti-Hu syndrome, but bulbar symptoms with cranial nerve dysfunction may be the first manifestation. It can also occur as a more isolated syndrome in lung and other cancers associated with the anti-Ma1 antibody. Common findings are oculomotor disorders, including nystagmus and supranuclear vertical gaze palsy, as well as hearing loss, dysarthria, dysphagia, and abnormal respiration. Movement disorders may be prominent.

Opsoclonus-Myoclonus

The term implies chaotic motion of the eyes—arrhythmic, irregular in direction or tempo. The disorder of eye movements is attributed to dysfunction of the pause cells in the paramedian pontine reticular formation. There may be evidence of encephalomyelitis or cerebellar disorder. In children, the disorder is associated with neuroblastoma. In adults, opsoclonus may be part of a complex syndrome with cerebellar signs and encephalomyelitis; it is associated with tumors of several types, usually breast and gynecologic malignancies, and anti-Ri antibodies. However, in both children and adults the opsoclonus-myoclonus is due to cancer in only a minority of patients.

Myelitis

Spinal cord symptoms evolve over days or weeks with clinical evidence of a focal lesion. The CSF may show pleocytosis with high protein content and normal sugar; oligoclonal bands may be present. Myelitis may occur with or without encephalomyelitis. Acute necrotizing myelopathy may be an extreme form of an inflammatory demyelinating myelitis.

Motor Neuron Disease

When cancer and motor neuron disease occur together, it is usually a coincidence of two common illnesses of the elderly. Epidemiologic studies have not shown increased incidence of cancer in amyotrophic lateral sclerosis (ALS) patients. However, there have been reports of patients whose neurologic symptoms disappeared with treatment of the tumor. Also, there have been more than 60 reports of patients with motor neuron and lymphoproliferative diseases. Lower motor neuron signs (amyotrophy), including fasciculation, are seen in combination with paraneoplastic encephalomyelitis with anti-Hu antibodies. A pure upper motor neuron syndrome (primary lateral sclerosis) has been reported in women with breast cancer, but several patients later developed lower motor neuron signs and the disorder became typical of ALS.

Sensorimotor Peripheral Neuropathy

Sensorimotor peripheral neuropathy with or without slow conduction velocity is common after age 50. Among the diverse causes are anti-MAG paraproteinemic peripheral neuropathy associated with Waldenström macroglobulinemia, and paraneoplastic neuropathy. Prominent features may include glove-stocking paresthesias and sensory loss, distal limb weakness, or both. Autonomic failure may be prominent, with disorders of gastrointestinal motility, especially diarrhea or pseudo-obstruction. Cranial symptoms are lacking and the syndrome is slow in evolution; it may respond to immunotherapy, as described in Chapter 106. Vasculitis is found in some acute neuropathies.

Neuromuscular Disorders

The association of myasthenia gravis with thymoma is described in Chapter 121; myasthenia is not known to be associated with other malignancies. LEMS is discussed in Chapter 122. Paraneoplastic neuromyotonia, as described in Chapter 130, is associated most often with thymoma but also with small cell lung cancer or other tumors. The Moersch-Woltman or stiff person syndrome is sometimes associated with cancer of lung or other organs.

Myopathies

About 20% of patients with dermatomyositis starting after age 40 have an associated tumor, which can be of almost any type. Whether there is a higher than expected association of tumor with polymyositis has not been proven. These syndromes are described in Chapters 131 and 132.

LABORATORY DATA

The diagnosis is established by demonstrating a specific antibody in a patient with a characteristic syndrome. MRI is usually normal and may or may not show abnormalities of white or gray matter. Similarly, the CSF may or may not show high CSF protein or pleocytosis, but the CSF sugar content is always normal. The diagnosis of peripheral neuropathy depends in part on the demonstration of conduction abnormalities, and LEMS is virtually defined by the demonstration of an incrementing response to repetitive nerve stimulation, as described in Chapter 122.

Antibodies

Anti-Hu was the first antibody to be identified with small cell lung carcinoma. Like several of the others that followed, it was named after the patient who provided the first serum. It is also called ANNA-1. It is occasionally associated with cancers other than small cell lung cancer such as neuroblastoma or prostate cancer. Anti-Hu is associated with sensory neuronopathy in isolation or as part of an encephalomyelitis syndrome; the neurologic symptoms usually precede discovery of the tumor. Anti-Yo binds to a DNA-binding protein found with cerebellar degeneration in association with a tumor of the ovary, uterus, or breast.

Antiamphiphysin antibodies are seen in patients with breast or small cell lung cancer who have stiff person syndrome. Anti-Ri binds to an RNA-binding protein. The clinical syndrome is ataxia with or without opsoclonus-myoclonus and the tumors are mostly breast and gynecologic cancers. The anti-Ma2 antigen has been found primarily in patients with testicular cancer associated with limbic and brainstem encephalitis. Anti-Tr reacts with Purkinje cells of the cerebellum. The clinical syndrome is primarily a subacute cerebellar disorder, often with dysarthria and nystagmus. The neoplasm is almost always Hodgkin disease. This syndrome usually resolves spontaneously. Anti-VGCC reacts with voltage-gated calcium channel of muscle and is found in patients with LEMS. The antibody is associated exclusively with small cell lung cancer.

TREATMENT

The peripheral disorders of sensorimotor polyneuropathy, LEMS, and myasthenia gravis often respond to IVIG therapy, plasmapheresis, or immunosuppressive drug therapy. The CNS syndromes are refractory to treatment. Corticosteroid therapy is often effective for the opsoclonus-myoclonus syndrome in children. The opsoclonus tends to resolve on its own, but patients are often left with ataxia and cognitive dysfunction. Treatment of the associated tumor may ameliorate the syndrome in adults.

SUGGESTED READINGS

Albert ML, Austin LM, Darnell RB. Detection and treatment of activated T-cells in the cerebrospinal fluid of patients with paraneoplastic cerebellar degeneration. *Ann Neurol* 2000;47:9–17.

Albert ML, Darnell RB. Paraneoplastic neurological degenerations: keys to tumour immunity. *Nat Rev Cancer* 2004;4:36–44.

Antoine JC, Absi L, Honnorat J, et al. Antiamphiphysin antibodies are associated with various paraneoplastic neurological syndromes and tumors. *Arch Neurol* 1999;56:172–177.

Bataller L, Graus F, Saiz A, et al. Clinical outcome in adult onset idiopathic or paraneoplastic opsoclonus-myoclonus. *Brain* 2001;124:437–443.

Bennett JL, Galetta SL, Friedman LP, et al. Neuro-ophthalmologic manifestations of a paraneoplastic syndrome and testicular carcinoma. *Neurology* 1999;52:864–867.

Cooper R, Khakoo Y, Matthay KK, et al. Opsoclonus-myoclonus-ataxia syndrome in neuroblastoma: histopathologic features–a report from the Children's Cancer Group. *Med Pediatr Oncol* 2001;36:623–629.

Croteau D, Owainati A, Dalmau J, et al. Response to cancer therapy in a patient with a paraneoplastic choreiform disorder. *Neurology* 2001;57:719–722.

Dalmau J, Gultekin SH, Posner JB. Paraneoplastic neurologic syndromes: pathogenesis and pathophysiology. *Brain Pathol* 1999;9:275–284.

Darnell JC, Albert ML, Darnell RB. Cdr2, a target antigen of naturally occurring human tumor immunity, is widely expressed in gynecological tumors. *Cancer Res* 2000;60:2136–2139.

Darnell RB. Paraneoplastic neurologic disorders: windows into neuronal function and tumor immunity. *Arch Neurol* 2004;61:30–32.

Darnell RB, Posner JB. Paraneoplastic syndromes involving the nervous system. *N Engl J Med* 2003;349:1543–1554.

Gordon PH, Rowland LP, Younger DS, et al. Lymphoproliferative disorders and motor neuron disease. *Ann Neurol* 1997;48:1671–1678.

Graus F, Keime-Guibert F, Rene R, et al. Anti-Hu associated paraneoplastic encephalomyelitis: analysis of 200 patients. *Brain* 2001;124:1138–1148.

Gultekin SH, Rosenfeld MR, Voltz, R, et al. Paraneoplastic limbic encephalitis: neurological symptoms, immunological findings and tumour association in 50 patients. *Brain* 2000;123:1481–1494.

Hayward K, Jeremy RJ, Jenkins S, et al. Long-term neurobehavioral outcomes in children with neuroblastoma and opsoclonus-myoclonus-ataxia syndrome: relationship to MRI findings and anti-neuronal antibodies. *J Pediatr* 2001;139:552–559.

Lahrmann H, Albrecht G, Drlicek M, et al. Acquired neuromyotonia and peripheral neuropathy in a patient with Hodgkin's disease. *Muscle Nerve* 2001;24:834–838.

Lawn ND, Westmoreland BF, Kiely MJ, et al. Clinical, magnetic resonance imaging, and electroencephalographic findings in paraneoplastic limbic encephalitis. *Mayo Clinic Proc* 2003;78:1363–1368.

Maeda T, Maeda A, Maruyama I, et al. Mechanisms of photoreceptor cell death in cancer-associated retinopathy. *Invest Ophthalmol Vis Sci* 2001;42:705–712.

Musunuru K, Darnell RB. Paraneoplastic neurologic disease antigens: RNA-binding proteins and signaling proteins in neuronal degeneration. *Annu Rev Neurosci* 2001;24:239–262.

Nagashima T, Mizutani Y, Kawahara H, et al. Anti-Hu paraneoplastic syndrome presenting with brainstem-cerebellar symptoms and Lambert-Eaton myasthenic syndrome. *Neuropathology* 2003;23:230–238.

Posner JB. *Neurologic complications of cancer.* Philadelphia: FA Davis, 1995:353–385.

Rosenfeld MR, Eichen JG, Wade DF, et al. Molecular and clinical diversity in paraneoplastic immunity to Ma proteins. *Ann Neurol* 2001;50:339–348.

Smitt PS, Kinoshita A, DeLeeuw B, et al. Paraneoplastic cerebellar ataxia due to autoantibodies against a glutamate receptor. *N Engl J Med* 2000;342:21–27.

Stockton D, Doherty VR, Brewster DH. Risk of cancer in patients with dermatomyositis or polymyositis, and follow-up implications: a Scottish population-based cohort study. *Br J Cancer* 2001;85:41–45.

Thomas L, Kwok Y, Edelman MJ. Management of paraneoplastic syndromes in lung cancer. *Curr Treat Options Oncol* 2004;5:51–62.

Vernino S, Lennon VA. Ion channel and striational antibodies define a continuum of autoimmune neuromuscular hyperexcitability. *Muscle Nerve* 2002;26:702–707.

Vital A. Paraproteinemic neuropathies. *Brain Pathol* 2001;11:399–407.

Voltz R, Carpentier AF, Rosenfeld MR, et al. P/Q type voltage-gated calcium channel antibodies in paraneoplastic disorders of the central nervous system. *Muscle Nerve* 1999;22:119–122.

Wakabyashi K, Horikawa Y, Oyake M, et al. Sporadic motor neuron disease with severe sensory neuronopathy. *Acta Neuropathol* 1998;95:426–430.

Chapter 154

Nutritional Disorders: Malnutrition, Malabsorption, and B$_{12}$ and Other Vitamin Deficiencies

Bradford B. Worrall and Lewis P. Rowland

Many neurologic syndromes are ascribed to lack of vitamins or other essential nutrients. Obesity and caloric excess contribute directly and indirectly to general and neurologic health, especially in the United States and the developed world. Although beyond the scope of this chapter, the wide range of neurologic complications of obesity and dietary excess including ischemic stroke, diabetic neuropathy, and degenerative disease of the spine are covered elsewhere in this text. Treatments for the epidemic of obesity have also led to nutritional disorders and neurologic disease. Malnutrition and malabsorption lead to isolated and multiple nutritional deficiencies with neurologic manifestations.

MALNUTRITION

Malnutrition is still a serious problem throughout the world. In poor countries, dietary deficiency is common. In industrial countries, nutritional syndromes are more

▶ **TABLE 154.1** Neurologic Syndromes Attributed to Nutritional Deficiency

Site of Major Syndrome	Name
Encephalon	Hypocalcemia (lack of vitamin D), tetany, seizures
	Mental retardation (protein-calorie deprivation)
	Cretinism (lack of iodine)
	Wernicke-Korsakoff syndrome (thiamine)
Corpus callosum	Marchiafava-Bignami disease
Optic nerve	Nutritional deficiency optic neuropathy (tobacco-alcohol amblyopia)
Brainstem	Central pontine myelinolysis
Cerebellum	Alcoholic cerebellar degeneration
	Vitamin E deficiency in bowel disease
Spinal cord	Combined system disease (B$_{12}$ deficiency)
	Myeloneuropathy (vitamin E deficiency, copper deficiency)
Peripheral nerves	Beriberi (thiamine), pellagra (nicotinic acid/tryptophan)
	Postgastrectomy (B$_{12}$, thiamine, folate, or polyvitamin)
	Hypophosphatemia (?),
	Tetany (vitamin D deficiency)
Muscle	Myopathy of osteomalacia

likely to be seen in alcohol abusers, in patients with chronic bowel disease, or in patients after some medical treatment that interferes with essential elements of diet (Table 154.1). Diseases of malnutrition may arise if essential nutrients are not provided because the diet is inadequate. The result may be the same if nutrients are lost by vomiting or diarrhea, if there is malabsorption, or if use is impaired at the target organ. Even if acute disorders are corrected, there may be long-term effects; many World War II prisoners continued to have chronic neurologic syndromes long after they had resumed a normal diet.

Maternal malnutrition or nutritional deficiencies may affect the fetus and lead to mental retardation, failure to thrive, or specific neurologic syndromes. Inborn errors of metabolism constitute a family of disorders resulting from the absence of or deficiency in enzymes in specific biochemical pathways. Dietary therapy may be important in the management of some of these disorders to prevent accumulation of toxic substances (as in phenylketonuria) or to amplify the activity of a mutant enzyme (as in vitamin B$_6$-responsive homocystinuria).

Examples of malnutrition syndromes are found in other chapters of this book; a simple listing or table is an oversimplification for two reasons. First, vitamin deficiency is likely to be multiple and to be accompanied by protein-calorie malnutrition, therefore generating complex clinical syndromes. Second, particular deficiency syndromes may target more than one system, making attempts to tabulate

▶ **TABLE 154.2 Neurologic Syndromes Attributed to Dietary Excess**

Syndrome	Condition	Agent
Increased intracranial pressure	Self-medication	Vitamin A
Encephalopathy	Phenylketonuria	Phenylalanine
	Water intoxication	Water
	Hepatic encephalopathy	Protein (and NH₃)
	Ketotic or nonketotic coma	Glucose
Strokes	Hyperlipidemia	Lipid
Peripheral neuropathy	Self-medication	Pyridoxine
Mixed neuropathy/myopathy (eosinophilia-myalgia syndrome)	Insomnia, anxiety; self-medication	Tryptophan, contaminated
Myopathy	Anorexia nervosa, bulimia	Emetine, ipecac
Myoglobinuria	Constipation	Licorice

clinical syndromes and involvement in the neuraxis inherently incomplete. For example, spinal cord syndromes and encephalopathy may be more prominent than peripheral neuropathy in pellagra. In contrast, peripheral neuropathy, optic neuropathy, or dementia may be seen in patients with combined system disease of the spinal cord owing to vitamin B_{12} deficiency. Some neurologic syndromes result from dietary excess (Table 154.2), further complicating the picture.

Alcohol abuse is a major cause of malnutrition and is associated with numerous neurologic syndromes. The pathophysiology may be direct toxicity of ethanol, specific or multiple vitamin deficiencies, or a combination. Alcoholic neuropathy is characterized by a painful, length-dependent sensory or sensorimotor neuropathy. Pain seems to be an invariable feature. In contrast, pure thiamine deficiency neuropathy starts with either weakness or numbness, rapidly subacute progression, and much greater likelihood of hand symptoms. A mixed picture emerges in alcoholic patients with superimposed thiamin deficiency. Other nutritional disturbances associated with chronic alcohol abuse including Wernicke-Korsakoff syndrome are discussed in detail in Chapter 163.

Another common cause of malnutrition in industrialized countries is *anorexia nervosa*. Myopathy can occur in addition to the neuropathy and other syndromes of multiple vitamin deficiency. The clinical picture can be complicated by ingestion of *emetine* to induce vomiting.

An epidemic of *peripheral and optic neuropathy* in Cuba was seen in 1991 after the collapse of support from the Soviet Union and enforcement of an embargo by the United States. As many as 50,000 may have been affected. This combination of disorders had earlier been seen in prisoners of war and other malnourished populations. In Cuba, a few patients had mutations of mitochondrial DNA associated with Leber hereditary optic neuropathy, which may have made them more susceptible to dietary deprivation. Many patients improved with supplemental vita-

min therapy. Viral infection may have been responsible for some cases.

MALABSORPTION

Malabsorption syndromes may arise for any of several reasons (Table 154.3). In patients with these disorders,

▶ **TABLE 154.3 Some Causes of Neurologic Disorder Owing to Malabsorption**

Disorder	Cause
Defective intraluminal hydrolysis	Gastric resection
	Pancreatic insufficiency
	Exclusion or deficiency of bile salts
Primary mucosal cell abnormality	Celiac disease
	Abetalipoproteinemia
Inadequate absorption surface	Massive small gut resection
	Ileal resection or bypass
	Jejunal bypass
	Jejunocolic fistula
	Gastroileostomy
Abnormalities of intestinal wall	Ileojejunitis
	Amyloidosis
	Radiation injury
Lymphatic obstruction and stasis	Lymphoma
	Tuberculosis
Bacterial overgrowth and parasitic infections	Blind loops
	Jejunal diverticula
	Scleroderma
	Whipple disease
	Tropical sprue
	D-Lactic acidosis
Miscellaneous	Diabetic neuropathy
	Hypoparathyroidism
	Hypothyroidism

From Glickman R. In: Wyngaarden JB, Smith LH Jr, eds. *Cecil's Textbook of Medicine.* 16th Ed. Philadelphia: WB Saunders, 1982:678–690.

neurologic abnormalities seem to be disproportionately frequent. Alone or in combination, there may be evidence of myopathy, sensorimotor peripheral neuropathy, degeneration of corticospinal tracts and posterior columns, and cerebellar abnormality. Optic neuritis, atypical pigmentary degeneration of the retina, and dementia are less common signs of malabsorption syndromes.

Initially, the syndromes were attributed to vitamin B_{12} deficiency, which probably accounted for some but not all cases; many patients had normal serum B_{12} levels and did not respond to vitamin B_{12} therapy. Subsequently, there was considerable interest in the relation of the neurologic abnormality to osteomalacia, which often appeared in the same patients. Osteomalacia also accompanied similar neurologic syndromes in patients who had dietary problems other than malabsorption (e.g., lack of sunlight or dietary vitamin D, resistance to vitamin D, renal disease, ingestion of anticonvulsant drugs). Osteomalacia or vitamin D deficiency, however, was hard to prove in some cases, and there was often no response to vitamin D therapy. Recent attention has focused on the lack of vitamin E, which can arise in several different ways: fat malabsorption, cholestatic liver disease, abetalipoproteinemia, and autosomal-recessive absence of the tocopherol transfer protein. In these disorders, ataxia and sensorimotor polyneuropathy are prominent clinical signs and may improve with vitamin E replacement, giving up to 4 g daily of alpha tocopherol.

The main bowel diseases associated with malabsorption and neurologic symptoms are celiac disease and inflammatory bowel disease (Crohn disease or ulcerative colitis). *Celiac disease,* also known as celiac sprue or gluten-sensitive enteropathy, is characterized by the triad of malabsorption, abnormal small bowel mucosa, and intolerance to gluten, a complex of wheat proteins in genetically susceptible individuals (HLA DQ2$^+$ or DQ8$^+$) on exposure to dietary gluten. Gluten sensitivity is best confirmed by biopsy and is supported by the presence of antigliadin, antiendomysial, or anti-tissue transglutaminase autoantibodies. However, up to 8% of the general population may harbor antibodies without gluten sensitivity. Neurologic complications arise from osteomalacic myopathy, B_{12} deficiency with neuropathy or myelopathy, hypokalemia, or hypocalcemia. In some patients, severe ataxia of gait has been related to the gluten sensitivity, with changes in peripheral nerves, posterior columns, and cerebellum.

Both *Crohn disease* and *ulcerative colitis* are associated with increased risk of thromboembolism that may affect other parts of the body but includes arteries and veins of the brain or spinal cord. Neuromuscular disorders are diverse. Peripheral neuropathy is found with Crohn disease for reasons that are uncertain; acute or chronic demyelinating neuropathy is found more often with ulcerative colitis. Myopathy may occur with either disorder, but symp-

▶ **TABLE 154.4 Neurological Complications of Bariatric Surgery**

Syndrome	Mechanism
Wernicke encephalopathy	Thiamin deficiency
Korsakoff syndrome	Thiamin deficiency
Thiamin deficiency neuropathy (dry beriberi)	Thiamin deficiency
Nutritional polyneuropathy	Multivitamin deficiencies
B₁₂ deficiency neuropathy	B₁₂ deficiency
Copper deficiency myelopathy	Copper deficiency
Guillian-Barré syndrome	Inflammatory
Conversion reaction	Psychiatric

Modified from Chang CG, Adams-Huet B, Provost DA. Acute post-gastric reduction surgery (APGARS) neuropathy. *Obes Surg* 2004;14:182–189; Kumar N, McEvoy KM, Ahlskog E. Myelopathy due to copper deficiency following gastrointestinal surgery. *Arch Neurol* 2003;60:1783–1785; and Koike H, Misu K, Hattori N, et al. Postgastrectomy polyneuropathy with thiamine deficiency. *J Neurol Neurosurg Psychiatry* 2001;71:357–362.

tomatic CNS disease is exceptional even though white matter lesions are found by MRI.

Bariatric means treatment of morbid obesity, and bariatric surgery is one of the fastest growing operations in the United States. Most of the numerous procedures involve restricting gastric volume. Neurologic complications are uncommon but myriad in nature and probably result from a combination of malabsorption and hyperemesis (Table 154.4). Patients with extremely rapid weight loss, not taking multivitamin supplementation, or pre-existing nutritional deficiencies are at greatest risk. The incidence of neuropathy in the Acute Post-Gastric Reduction Surgery (APGARS) program was 6/10,000 procedures. Vitamin deficiencies (B_{12}, thiamine, or multivitamin deficiencies) were identified in 40% of the patients with neuropathy, but vitamin supplementation did not always improve symptoms. Neurologic complications of thiamine deficiency after bariatric surgery are widely recognized. Although uncommon, physicians and patients should be aware of these potentially devastating but treatable neurologic complications. Wernicke encephalopathy with altered level of alertness, delirium, and ophthalmoplegia with or without nystagmus and ataxia, Korsakoff syndrome with amnestic dementia, and the sensory motor painful polyneuropathy associated with dry beriberi occur individually or in combination, usually within the first few months following surgery. However, symptoms may commence decades after surgery. After gastric surgery, alcohol abusers may be especially vulnerable to thiamin-related disorders.

Acquired deficiencies of other essential elements following gastric surgery have been suspected. Copper deficiency is extremely rare, may present as a myelopathy or myeloneuropathy, and has been seen in patients after gastrointestinal surgery. These patients have gait difficulty, sensory ataxia, and spasticity. Copper deficiency can also result from idiopathic hyperzincemia, zinc intoxication, or certain chemotherapeutic agents. Whether copper deficiency alone or in combination will prove to be a recognized neurologic complication of gastrointestinal surgery remains unknown.

Malabsorption may occur in other disorders of the stomach and intestine. The major neurologic syndrome of stomach disease results from lack of intrinsic factor and B_{12} deficiency (discussed below). No direct major neurologic consequences of peptic ulcer (other than those that might result from shock after massive hemorrhage) are recognized, but treatment of the ulcer may lead to a neurologic disorder. Antacids may cause a partial malabsorption syndrome. Aluminum containing antacids or phosphate binders can cause encephalopathy, especially in the presence of renal disease. Surgical therapy may cure the ulcer but may also create a neurologic disorder as a result of malabsorption.

Chronic diarrhea from any cause, including malabsorption or abuse of laxatives, may cause hypokalemia with resulting chronic myopathy, acute paralysis, or acute myoglobinuria. Acute hypophosphatemia may arise after fluid and electrolyte resuscitation in chronic alcohol abusers, after treatment of diabetic ketoacidosis, or after hyperalimentation. In these circumstances, limb weakness may simulate Guillain-Barré syndrome, or the acute electrolyte disorder may actually precipitate the neuropathy; seizures and coma may be part of the picture.

In some conditions, diarrhea accompanies but is not thought to cause the neurologic disorder. The combination of diarrhea, orthostatic hypotension, and peripheral neuropathy suggests the possibility of amyloid disease or diabetes mellitus. The combination of chronic diarrhea, arthritis, and dementia or other cerebral disorder suggests *Whipple disease* (see Chapter 35). The disease is often diagnosed only at autopsy because there is no characteristic clinical picture and steatorrhea may be lacking. An unusual sign is *oculomasticatory myorhythmia*, a term that describes rhythmic convergence of the eyes and synchronous contractions of the masticatory muscles. Diagnosis can be made reliably by a polymerase chain reaction test to identify the organism. Recognition is important because although rare, Whipple disease can be cured by treatment with trimethoprim/sulfamethoxazole.

Another unusual syndrome of malabsorption is episodic abnormality of sleep, thirst, hunger, and mood, a combination that suggests a hypothalamic disorder. Other manifestations are episodes of weakness, ataxia, slurred speech, confusion, and nausea. This is attributed to bacterial overgrowth with production of D-lactic acid. D-Lactic acidosis is seen in patients with a short small intestine and an intact colon. Excessive production of D-lactate by abnormal bowel flora overwhelms normal metabolism of D-lactate and leads to an accumulation of this enantiomer in the blood. The condition may be fatal, but oral antibiotic treatment has abolished the syndrome in some patients.

VITAMIN B_{12} (COBALAMIN) DEFICIENCY

History

Although not the first to describe the disorder, in 1849 Thomas Addison made pernicious anemia well known. By the turn of the century, the diagnostic triad was recognized: anemia, neurologic symptoms, and atrophy of the epithelial covering of the tongue. In 1900, Russell, Batten, and Collier introduced the term *combined degeneration of the spinal cord*. The disease was lethal until 1926, when Minot and Murphy used replacement therapy without knowing what had to be replaced; they found that supplementing the diet with liver was therapeutic. Castle administered liver extract parenterally, and in 1948 vitamin B_{12} completely reversed the symptoms. Additionally, the automation of blood counts and measurement of blood vitamin B_{12} levels has made early diagnosis the rule. As a result, the neurologic disorder is now rarely seen in major medical centers of industrialized countries. Although the condition was once thought to affect Nordic people primarily, it is seen in all racial groups. The prevalence of undiagnosed pernicious anemia after age 60 is about 2%. Cobalamin deficiency increases with age; 5% of people 65 to 75 have B_{12} deficiency and 10% of those over 75. Concomitant folate deficiency occurs in about 10% of those with B_{12} deficiency.

Physiology

Cobalamin is synthesized only in specific microorganisms, and animal products are the sole dietary sources for humans. Gastric acid is needed for peptic digestion to release the vitamin from proteins. Achlorhydria of the elderly may suffice to cause B_{12} deficiency, but an intrinsic factor is usually missing as well.

The freed B_{12} is bound by R proteins (R for rapid movement on electrophoresis) and then by gastric intrinsic factor, a glycoprotein produced by gastric parietal cells, which is needed for absorption of B_{12} and which is absent in people with pernicious anemia. The combined intrinsic factor–cobalamin complex is transported across the terminal ileum and binds to transcobalamin, with a half-life of 6 to 9 minutes. The complex enters cells by endocytosis, and the vitamin enters red blood cells in an energy-dependent process.

Cobalamin is converted to adenosyl or methyl coenzymes, which are necessary for normal neural metabolism.

▶ **TABLE 154.5** Causes of Cobalamin Deficiency in 143 Patients

Etiology	No. Patients	Percent
Pernicious anemia		
Proven	95	66.4
Probable	17	11.9
Tropical sprue	8	5.6
Gastric resection	6	4.2
Ileal resection	4	2.8
Jejunal diverticula	3	2.1
Dietary B$_{12}$ malabsorption	3	2.1
Multiple causes	4	2.8
Cause unknown	3	2.1
Total	143	100

Modified from Healton EH, Savage DG, Brust JCM, et al. Neurologic aspects of cobalamin deficiency. *Medicine (Baltimore)* 1991;70:228–245.

If they are missing, abnormal fatty acids may accumulate in myelin or methylating reactions may be defective. A congenital form of methylcobalamin deficiency leads to developmental delay, microcephaly, and seizures, with delayed myelination. Infants breastfed by cobalamin-deficient mothers can develop symptoms within 4 to 8 months—typically failure to thrive, developmental delay, and anemia. The details of B$_{12}$ dependency in the mature nervous system are not well known, and it is not clear why the spinal cord and peripheral nerves are so vulnerable when B$_{12}$ levels are low.

Pathogenesis

About 80% of adult-onset pernicious anemia is attributed to lack of gastric intrinsic factor secondary to atrophic gastritis (Table 154.5). The disorder is thought to be autoimmune in origin because antibodies to gastric parietal cells are found in 90% and antibodies to intrinsic factor occur in up to 76%. The parietal cell antigen is gastric

H$^+$/K$^+$-ATPase. Supporting the view that autoimmunity is important is the frequent association of pernicious anemia with some other autoimmune disease, such as myasthenia gravis, Hashimoto thyroiditis, vitiligo, or the polyglandular deficiencies. In those with normal intrinsic factor, the vitamin is not absorbed because of jejunal diverticulosis, tropical sprue, or loss of the stomach or ileum by surgical resection. Rarely, the vitamin cannot be liberated from dietary animal proteins because peptic digestion is inadequate. Chronic recreational or occupational exposure to nitrous oxide can interfere with cobalamin metabolism and cause neuropathy or combined system disease. Long-term metformin therapy may lead to B$_{12}$ deficiency in 10% to 30% of patients; one cohort study suggested that metformin may play a role in the pathogenesis in up to 6% of patients with B$_{12}$ deficiency. Of those with metformin-associated B$_{12}$ deficiency, approximately 30% had peripheral neuropathy.

Pathology

In the spinal cord, white matter is affected more than gray. Symmetric loss of myelin sheaths occurs more often than axonal loss; changes are most prominent in the posterior and lateral columns (*combined system disease*; Figs. 154.1 and 154.2). The thoracic cord is affected first and then the process extends in either direction. Patchy demyelination may be seen in the frontal white matter (Fig. 154.3).

Clinical Features

Today most patients are probably asymptomatic. If the deficiency persists, symptoms may be those of anemia, neurologic disorder, or other problems such as vitiligo, sore tongue, or prematurely gray hair. Anorexia and weight loss may be prominent.

About 40% of all patients with B$_{12}$ deficiency are said to have some neurologic symptoms or signs, and these

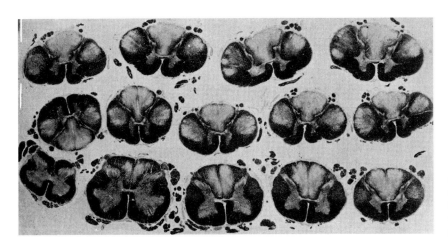

FIGURE 154.1. Subacute combined degeneration. Sections of spinal cord at various levels showing segmental loss of myelin, which is most intense in the dorsal and lateral columns.

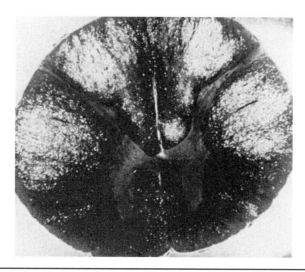

FIGURE 154.2. Subacute combined degeneration. Destruction of myelin predominating in the posterior and lateral columns. Swelling of affected myelin sheaths causes spongy appearance.

are often the first or most prominent manifestations of the disease. Only 20% of patients are younger than age 50; most are over 60. Usually, there are features of both myelopathy and peripheral neuropathy. The most common symptom is acroparesthesia, burning and painful sensations that affect the hands and feet. There may be sensory

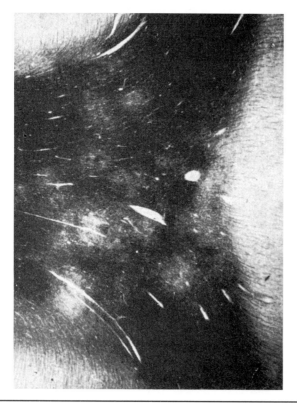

FIGURE 154.3. Subacute combined degeneration. Partial loss of myelin of white matter of frontal lobe. (Courtesy of Dr. L. Roizin.)

ataxia. Memory loss, visual loss (owing to optic neuropathy), orthostatic hypotension, anosmia, impaired taste (dysgeusia), sphincter symptoms, and impotence are other symptoms.

On examination, there is glove-stocking sensory loss, and almost all patients show loss of vibratory sensation and of position sense. The *Romberg sign* is often present; the patient can stand with feet together if the eyes are open but sways and falls on closing the eyes because of the loss of position sense. There may or may not be weakness of limb muscles; the neuropathy is predominantly sensory, but there are upper motor neuron signs: increased tone, impaired alternating movements, and hyperactive tendon jerks, with Babinski and Hoffmann signs. Cognitive loss may be evident as florid dementia or may be manifest only on neuropsychologic tests. Optic atrophy is found in fewer than 1% of patients.

As a measure of the efficacy of modern diagnosis and treatment, even symptomatic patients are usually independent in activities of daily living. Fewer than 10% are restricted to chair or bed.

Diagnosis

The diagnosis rests on demonstration of blood levels of vitamin B_{12} <200 pg/mL, but low normal values (200–350 pg/mL) may be found in people who respond to therapy. Some people with low values are not deficient, and additional tests may be useful. Both methylmalonic acid and homocysteine accumulate when there is impairment of cobalamin-dependent reactions; both metabolites are abnormally increased in serum in more than 99% of patients with true cobalamin deficiency. The *Schilling test*, a measure of the absorption of orally ingested labeled B_{12}, is technically difficult and unreliable because it may be normal in vegetarians and nitrous oxide abusers. Sometimes a therapeutic trial is the only way to determine whether a neurologic syndrome is in fact owing to B_{12} deficiency. MRI may show increased T2-weighted signal and contrast enhancement of the posterior and lateral columns of the spinal cord, with return to normal on treatment. Nerve conduction tests show an axonal sensorimotor neuropathy. Visual, brainstem, and somatosensory evoked responses may be normal or abnormal. CT and MRI of the head may show no abnormality, or there may be cerebral atrophy in patients with dementia.

In patients with neurologic signs, only about 20% show severe anemia. Both the hematocrit and mean corpuscular volume may be normal, although they are the traditional abnormalities. Bone marrow biopsy, however, reliably shows megaloblastic abnormalities. B_{12} deficiency must be considered in any sensorimotor neuropathy, myelopathy, autonomic neuropathy, dementia, or optic neuropathy. Several of these disorders arise in AIDS, but a possible role of B_{12} is doubted.

Folate supplementation can partially mask the hematologic manifestations of B$_{12}$ deficiency. Folate fortification of breads and other grain products was delayed owing to public health concerns. Clinicians must maintain a high index of suspicion in populations at high risk for B$_{12}$ deficiency such as chronic alcoholics. Delays in recognition of B$_{12}$ deficiency with neuropsychiatric sequelae have occurred in patients with sickle cell anemia on folate supplementation.

Treatment

B$_{12}$ is given intramuscularly in a dosage of 1,000 μg daily for the first week, followed by weekly injections for the first month, and then monthly injections for life. Many believe that oral therapy is less reliable largely because absorption without intrinsic factor is inefficient; others have challenged this. Approximately 60% of oral cobalamin is absorbed in the terminal ileum with gastric intrinsic factor; 1% of cobalamin is absorbed in the absence of intrinsic factor. The debate over the effectiveness of oral cobalamin replacement remains unresolved and focuses on many issues including cost, compliance, and patient preference. The development of new B$_{12}$ formulations including nasal spray and sublingual tablets may broaden treatment options, and the efficacy of long-term repletion in patients with B$_{12}$ deficiency using these preparations warrants further study.

After parenteral injection of B$_{12}$, hematologic improvement may be evident within 48 hours, and there is a subjective sense of general improvement. Paresthesias are often the first neurologic symptoms to improve and do so within 2 weeks; corticospinal abnormalities are slower to respond. If there is no response in 3 months, the condition is probably not owing to B$_{12}$ deficiency. About half of the patients are left with some abnormality on examination; the residual disability depends on the duration of symptoms.

SUGGESTED READINGS

General

Keane JR. Neurologic symptoms mistaken for gastrointestinal disease. *Neurology* 1998;50:1189–1190.
Malouf R, Brust JCM. Hypoglycemia: causes, neurological manifestations, and outcome. *Ann Neurol* 1985;17:321–430.
Perkin GD, Murray-Lyon I. Neurology and the gastrointestinal system. *J Neurol Neurosurg Psychiatry* 1998;65:291–300.

Malnutrition and Malabsorption

Albers JW, Nostrant TT, Riggs JE. Neurologic manifestations of gastrointestinal disease. *Neurol Clin* 1989;7:525–548.
Alloway R, Reynolds EH, Spargo E, et al. Neuropathy and myopathy in two patients with anorexia and bulimia nervosa. *J Neurol Neurosurg Psychiatry* 1985;48:1015–1020.

Chin RL, Sander HW, Brannagan TH, et al. Celiac neuropathy. *Neurology* 2003;60:1581–1585.
Cicarelli G, Della Rocca G, Amboni M, et al. Clinical and neurological abnormalities in adult celiac disease. *Neurol Sci* 2003;24:311–317.
Dastur DK, Manghani DK, Osuntokun BO, et al. Neuromuscular and related changes in malnutrition. A review. *J Neurol Sci* 1982;55:207–230.
Gill GV, Bell DR. Persisting nutritional neuropathy amongst former war prisoners. *J Neurol Neurosurg Psychiatry* 1982;45:861–865.
Hadjivassilou M, Grunewald RA, Chattopadhyay AK, et al. Clinical, radiological, neurophysiological, and neuropathological characteristics of gluten ataxia. *Lancet* 1998;352:1582–1585.
Hart PE, Gould SR, MacSweeney JE, et al. Brain white matter lesions in inflammatory bowel disease. *Lancet* 1998;351:1558.
Hedges TR 3rd, Hirano M, Tucker K, et al. Epidemic optic and peripheral neuropathy in Cuba: a unique geopolitical public health problem. *Surv Ophthalmol* 1997;41:341–353.
Hirano M, Cleary JM, Stewart AM, et al. Mitochondrial DNA mutations in an outbreak of optic neuropathy in Cuba. *Neurology* 1994;44:843–845.
Johns DR. Cerebrovascular complications of inflammatory bowel disease. *Am J Gastroenterol* 1991;86:367–370.
Lloyd-Still JD, Tomasi L. Neurovascular and thromboembolic complications of inflammatory bowel disease in childhood. *J Paediatr Gastroenterol Nutr* 1989;9:461–466.
Lossos A, River Y, Eliakim A, et al. Neurologic aspects of inflammatory bowel disease. *Neurology* 1995;45:416–421.
Mitchell JE, Seim HC, Colon E, et al. Medical complications and medical management of bulimia. *Ann Intern Med* 1987;107:71–77.
Palmer EP, Guary AT. Reversible myopathy secondary to abuse of ipecac in patients with major eating disorders. *N Engl J Med* 1985;313:1457–1459.
Patchell RA, Fellows HA, Humphries LL. Neurologic complications of anorexia nervosa. *Acta Neurol Scand* 1994;89:111–116.
Pellecchia MT, Scala R, Filla A, et al. Idiopathic cerebellar ataxia associated with celiac disease: lack of distinctive neurological features. *J Neurol Neurosurg Psychiatry* 1999;66:32–35.
Roman GC. Epidemic neuropathy in Cuba: a public health problem related to the Cuban Democracy Act of the United States. *Neuroepidemiology* 1998;17:111–115.
Schwartz MA, Selhorst JB, Ochs AL, et al. Oculomasticatory myorhythmia: a unique movement disorder occurring in Whipple's disease. *Ann Neurol* 1986;20:677–681.
Smiddy WE, Green WR. Nutritional amblyopia. A histopathologic study with retrospective clinical correlation. *Graefe's Arch Clin Exp Ophthalmol* 1987;225:321–324.

Vitamin E Deficiency

Cavalier L, Ouahchi K, Kayden HJ, et al. Ataxia with isolated vitamin E deficiency: heterogeneity of mutations and phenotypic variability in a large number of families. *Am J Hum Genet* 1998;62:301–310.
Harding AE, Muller DPR, Thomas PK, et al. Spinocerebellar degeneration secondary to chronic intestinal malabsorption: a vitamin E deficiency syndrome. *Ann Neurol* 1982;12:419–424.
Mauro A, Orsi L, Mortara P, et al. Cerebellar syndrome in adult celiac disease with vitamin E deficiency. *Acta Neurol Scand* 1991;84:167–170.
Sitrin MD, Lieberman F, Jensen WE, et al. Vitamin E deficiency and neurologic disease in adults with cystic fibrosis. *Ann Intern Med* 1987;107:51–54.
Sokol RJ. Vitamin E and neurologic deficits. *Adv Pediatr* 1990;37:119–148.

D-Lactic Acidosis

Carr DB, Shih VE, Richter JM, et al. D-lactic acidosis simulating a hypothalamic syndrome after bowel bypass. *Ann Neurol* 1982;11:195–197.

Vella A, Farrugia G. D-Lactic acidosis: pathologic consequence of saprophytism. *Mayo Clin Proc* 1998;73:451–456.

Zhang DL, Jiang ZW, Jiang J, et al. D-lactic acidosis secondary to short bowel syndrome. *Postgrad Med J* 2003;79:110–112.

Neurologic Complications of Bariatric and Other Gastrointestinal Surgery

Chang CG, Adams-Huet B, Provost DA. Acute post-gastric reduction surgery (APGARS) neuropathy. *Obes Surg* 2004;14(Feb):182–189.

Chaves LC, Faintuch J, Kahwage S, et al. A cluster of polyneuropathy and Wernicke-Korsakoff syndrome in a bariatric unit. *Obes Surg* 2003;12:328–334.

Cirignotta F, Manconi M, Mondini S, et al. Wernicke-Korsakoff encephalopathy and polyneuropathy after gastroplasty for morbid obesity. *Arch Neurol* 2000;57:1356–1359.

Koike H, Misu K, Hattori N, et al. Postgastrectomy polyneuropathy with thiamine deficiency. *J Neurol Neurosurg Psychiatry* 2001;71:357–362.

Kumar N, McEvoy KM, Ahlskog E. Myelopathy due to copper deficiency following gastrointestinal surgery. *Arch Neurol* 2003;60:1783–1785.

Vitamin B$_{12}$ Deficiency

Al-Shubali AF, Farah SA, Hussein JM, et al. Axonal and demyelinating neuropathy with reversible proximal conduction block, an unusual feature of vitamin B$_{12}$ deficiency. *Muscle Nerve* 1998;21:1341–1343.

Andres E, Noel E, Goichot B. Metformin-associated vitamin B$_{12}$ Deficiency. *Arch Intern Med* 2002;162:2251–2252.

Anonymous editorial. Still time for rational debate about vitamin B$_{12}$. *Lancet* 1998;351:1523.

Chanarin I, Metz J. Diagnosis of cobalamin deficiency: the old and the new. *Br J Haematol* 1997;97:695–700.

Clarke R, Grimley Evans J, Schneede J, et al. Vitamin B$_{12}$ and folate deficiency in later life. *Age Ageing* 2004;33(Jan):34–41.

Dhar M, Bellevue R, Carmel R. Pernicious anemia with neuropsychiatric dysfunction in a patient with sickle cell anemia treated with folate supplementation. *N Engl J Med* 2003;348:2204–2207.

Elia M. Oral or parenteral therapy for B$_{12}$ deficiency. *Lancet* 1998;352:1721–1722.

Green R, Kinsella LJ. Current concepts in the diagnosis of cobalamin therapy. *Neurology* 1995;45:1435–1440.

Hall CA. Function of vitamin B$_{12}$ in the central nervous system as revealed by congenital defects. *Am J Hematol* 1990;34:121–127.

Healton EH, Savage DG, Brust JCM, et al. Neurologic aspects of cobalamin deficiency. *Medicine (Baltimore)* 1991;70:228–245.

Holloway KL, Alberico AM. Postoperative myelopathy: a preventable complication in patients with B$_{12}$ deficiency. *Neurosurgery* 1990;72:732–736.

Kinsella LJ, Green R. "Anesthesia paresthetica": nitrous oxide-induced cobalamin deficiency. *Neurology* 1995;45:1608–1610.

Layzer RB. Myeloneuropathy after prolonged exposure to nitrous oxide. *Lancet* 1978;2:1227–1230.

Layzer RB, Fishman RA, Schafer JA. Neuropathy following abuse of nitrous oxide. *Neurology* 1978;28:504–506.

Lindenbaum J, Healton EB, Savage DG, et al. Neuropsychiatric disorders caused by cobalamin deficiency in the absence of anemia or macrocytosis. *N Engl J Med* 1988;318:1720–1728.

Lindenbaum J, Savage DG, Stabler SP, et al. Diagnosis of cobalamin deficiency. II. Relative sensitivities of serum cobalamin, methylmalonic acid, and total homocysteine concentrations. *Am J Hematol* 1990;34:99–107.

Lorenzl S, Vogeser M, Muller-Schunk S, et al. Clinically and MRI documented funicular myelosis in a patient with metabolical vitamin B$_{12}$ deficiency but normal vitamin B$_{12}$ serum level. *J Neurol* 2003;250:1010–1011.

Misra UK, Kalita J, Das A. Vitamin B$_{12}$ deficiency neurological syndromes: a clinical, MRI and electrodiagnostic study. *Electromyog Clin Neurophysiol* 2003;43(Jan-Feb):57–64.

Muhammad R, Fernoff P, Rasmussen S, et al. Neurologic impairment in children associated with maternal dietary deficiency of cobalamin–Georgia, 2001. *MMWR* 2003;52:61–64.

Robertson KR, Stern RA, Hall CD, et al. Vitamin B$_{12}$ deficiency and nervous system disease in HIV infection. *Arch Neurol* 1993;50:807–811.

Russell JSR, Batten FE, Collier J. Subacute combined degeneration of the spinal cord. *Brain* 1900;23:39–110.

Saperstein DS, Wolfe GI, Gronseth GS, et al. Challenges in the identification of cobalamin-deficiency polyneuropathy. *Arch Neurol* 2003;60:1296–1301.

Scherer K. Images in clinical medicine. Neurologic manifestations of vitamin B$_{12}$ deficiency. *N Engl J Med* 2003;348:2208.

Sigal SH, Hall CA, Antel JP. Plasma R binder deficiency and neurologic disease. *N Engl J Med* 1987;317:1330–1332.

Stabler SP. Vitamin B$_{12}$ deficiency in older people: improving diagnosis and preventing disability. *J Am Geriatr Soc* 1998;46:1199–1206.

Stojsavljevic N, Levic Z, Drulovic J. 44-month clinical-brain MRI follow-up in a patient with B$_{12}$ deficiency. *Neurology* 1997;49:878–881.

Toh B-H, van Driel IR, Gleeson PA. Pernicious anemia. *N Engl J Med* 1997;337:1441–1448.

Tomkin GH, Hadden DR, Weaver JA, et al. Vitamin-B$_{12}$ status of patients on long-term metformin therapy. *BMJ* 1971;2:685–687.

Victor M, Lear AA. Subacute combined degeneration of the spinal cord. *Am J Med* 1956;20:896–911.

Other Vitamins and Minerals

Brantigan CO. Folate supplementation and the risk of making vitamin B$_{12}$ deficiency. *JAMA* 1997;277:884–885.

Insogna KL, Bordley DR, Caro JF, et al. Osteomalacia and weakness from excessive antacid ingestion. *JAMA* 1980;244:2544–2546.

Koike H, Iijima M, Sugiura M, et al. Alcoholic neuropathy is clinicopathologically distinct from thiamine deficiency neuropathy. *Ann Neurol* 2003;54:19–29.

Kumar N, Crum B, Petersen RC, et al. Copper deficiency myelopathy. *Arch Neurol* 2004;61:762–766.

Parry GJ, Bredsen DE. Sensory neuropathy with low-dose pyridoxine. *Neurology* 1985;35:1466–1468.

Rosenberg M, McCarten JR, Snyder BD, et al. Hypophosphatemia with reversible ataxia and quadriparesis. *Am J Med Sci* 1987;293:261–264.

Schott GD, Wills MR. Muscle weakness in osteomalacia. *Lancet* 1976;1:626–629.

Weintraub MI. Hypophosphatemia mimicking acute Guillain-Barré-Strohl syndrome. A complication of parenteral alimentation. *JAMA* 1980;235:1040–1041.

Chapter 155

Vasculitis Syndromes

*Lewis P. Rowland and
Marcelo R. Olarte*

Several syndromes are commonly linked because they are characterized by a combination of arthritis, rash, and visceral disease. Arthritis is common to all of them and fibrinoid degeneration of blood vessels is common, so they are called *collagen-vascular diseases*. Inflammatory lesions of the blood vessels, however, are the dominant pathologic changes in some syndromes. Periarteritis nodosa was the first vasculitis to be recognized, but the classification of related syndromes depended on autopsy evaluation of histologic changes in the arteries, whether large or small vessels were involved, and which organs were most affected. Similar classifications were applied to clinical diagnosis, but overlap between syndromes and lack of knowledge of etiology or pathogenesis obscured the area. Some of these diseases were attributed to the deposition of circulating immune complexes within vessel walls, and some seemed related to viral infection. With the discovery of antineuronal cytoplasmic autoantibodies (ANCA) and other antibodies, a new classification was adopted by an international consensus conference in 1994 (Table 155.1). An older classification describes syndromes that have characteristic clinical and neurologic manifestations and warrant individual discussion (Table 155.2). Clinical disorders of brain, spinal cord, peripheral nerve, and muscle are prominent in these diseases. All these conditions are said to be rare except for temporal arteritis and polymyalgia rheumatica after age 60 and Kawasaki disease in children.

ANCA tests have had a major impact in clinical practice and in theory, bolstering the view that these diseases are autoimmune in origin. In the United Kingdom, the annual incidence of systemic vasculitis other than temporal arteritis was 42 per million population, and 50% of patients tested positive for ANCA. The antibodies are especially prevalent in Wegener granulomatosis, microscopic polyangiitis, and the Churg-Strauss syndrome. The test depends on immunofluorescence that gives either of two patterns, cytoplasmic ANCA or perinuclear ANCA. The cytoplasmic antigen is a proteinase (PR3-ANCA) and the perinuclear antigen is myeloperoxidase (MPO-ANCA); 90% of patients with Wegener disease have the cytoplasmic PR3-ANCA, and 70% of patients with Churg-Strauss have

the perinuclear MPO-ANCA. However, the missing 10% are important because a negative test does not exclude either diagnosis.

POLYARTERITIS NODOSA

Polyarteritis nodosa or periarteritis nodosa is an inflammatory arteritis that affects small and medium-sized arteritis. It is characterized by nonspecific symptoms commonly associated with an infection or signs and symptoms involving abdominal organs, joints, peripheral nerves, muscle, or the CNS.

Etiology

The cause of periarteritis is unknown; reactions to bacterial or viral infection have been postulated. Association of the disorder with asthma, serum sickness, or drug reactions suggests autoimmunity. Arnold Rich reproduced the lesions in rabbits by repeated injections of horse serum. Immune complexes may play a role; in some cases, immune complexes have been found in vessel walls without vasculitis. Clinical and serologic evidence link some cases to infection with hepatitis B; this form of arteritis may be monophasic with a good prognosis.

Pathology

There is widespread panarteritis. The CNS pathology includes infiltrates in the adventitia and vasa vasorum, polymorphonuclear leukocytes, and eosinophils. Necrosis of the media and elastic membrane may lead to formation of multiple small aneurysms. As these become fibrotic, they may rupture or proliferation of the intima may occlude vessels. Repair and fibrosis of the aneurysms lead to a characteristic beading appearance caused by the nodules.

Incidence

Polyarteritis nodosa is rare, but when it occurs, the CNS is involved in about 25% of cases. Men and women are affected equally. The disease may occur at any age, but more than 50% of cases are in the third or fourth decades of life.

Signs and Symptoms

The onset may be acute or insidious. Fever; malaise; tachycardia; sweating; fleeting edema; weakness and pain in the joints, muscles, or abdomen are common early symptoms (Tables 155.3 and 155.4). Blood pressure may be elevated, and there may be a moderate or severe anemia with leukocytosis.

▶ **TABLE 155.1** Vasculitis Syndromes: Chapel Hill Consensus Criteria

Syndromes	Pathologies
Large-vessel vasculitis	
Giant cell (temporal) arteritis	Granulomatous arteritis of aorta and its major branches; predilection for extracranial branches of carotid artery. Often involves temporal artery; patients older than 50 yr; with polymyalgia rheumatica.
Takeyusu arteritis	Granulomatous arteritis of aorta and major branches; patients younger than age 50.
Medium-sized vessel vasculitis	
Polyarteritis nodosa	Necrotizing inflammation of medium- or small-sized arteries; no glomerulonephritis or vasculitis of arterioles, capillaries, venules.
Kawasaki disease	Arteritis of large, medium-sized, small arteries plus mucocutaneous-lymph node syndrome. Coronary arteries often involved; aorta and veins may be involved; usually in children
Small-vessel vasculitis	
Wegener granulomatosis[a]	Granulomatous inflammation including respiratory tract and necrotizing vasculitis of small-to-medium vessels (capillaries, venules, arterioles, arteries). Necrotizing glomerulonephritis common.
Churg-Strauss syndrome[a]	Eosinophil-rich granulomatous inflammation of respiratory tract and necrotizing vasculitis of small-to-medium-sized vessels; with asthma and eosinophilia.
Microscopic polyangiitis[a]	Necrotizing vasculitis with few or no immune deposits; affects small vessels (capillaries, venules, arterioles). May involve small- and medium-sized arteries. Common features: necrotizing glomerulonephritis and involvement of pulmonary capillaries.
Henoch-Sch$onlein purpura	Vasculitis with IgA-dominant immune deposits on small vessels (capillaries, venules, arterioles). Affects skin, gut, glomeruli plus arthritis or arthralgia.
Essential cryoglobulinemic vasculitis	Vasculitis with immune deposits on small vessels (capillaries, venules, arterioles); cryoglobulins in serum; skin and glomeruli often involved.
Cutaneous leukocytoclastic angiitis	Isolated cutaneous leukocytoclastic angiitis without systemic vasculitis or glomerulonephritis.

[a]Antineuronal cytoplasmic autoantibodies present in most patients with Wegener granulomatosis, Churg-Strauss syndrome, and microscopic polyangiitis. Modified from Jennette et al. (1994) and Jennette and Falk (1997).

Visceral lesions occur in most cases. Kidney involvement is manifest as acute glomerular nephritis. Cutaneous hemorrhages, erythematous eruptions, and tender red subcutaneous nodules may appear in the skin of the trunk or limbs. Gastrointestinal, hepatic, renal, testicular, or cardiac symptoms may develop.

Peripheral neuropathy is the most common neurologic disorder. Periarteritis is probably one of the most common causes of *mononeuritis multiplex*, but there may also be a diffuse sensorimotor peripheral neuropathy. Both forms of neuropathy are attributed to ischemia brought about by the arteritis of nutrient vessels.

Damage to cerebral arteries may lead to thrombosis or hemorrhage; spinal syndromes are exceptional. The most common manifestations of cerebral involvement are headache, convulsions, blurred vision, vertigo, sudden loss of vision in one eye, and confusional states or psychosis.

A disorder characterized by keratitis and deafness in nonsyphilitic individuals is called the *Cogan syndrome*. It occurs predominantly in young adults with negative blood and CSF tests for syphilis and no stigmata of congenital syphilis. The cause of the keratitis and deafness is not known, but in some cases, the syndrome is one feature of polyarteritis nodosa. Symptoms begin suddenly, involving the cornea and both divisions of the eighth nerve. The eye and the eighth nerve are usually involved simultaneously, but there may be weeks or months between their onsets. Involvement of the eighth nerve is usually signaled by nausea, vomiting, tinnitus, and loss of hearing. With progression of the hearing loss to complete deafness, the vestibular symptoms subside.

Laboratory Data

There is a leukocytosis with inconstant eosinophilia. Nontreponemal serologic tests for syphilis may be positive, and there may be positive skin and serologic tests for trichinosis. CSF is normal unless there has been subarachnoid hemorrhage.

Diagnosis

The diagnosis of polyarteritis nodosa should be considered in all patients with an obscure febrile illness with systemic symptoms and chronic peripheral neuropathy. The diagnosis can often be established by biopsy of sural nerve, muscle, or testicle. According to 1990 consensus criteria, the diagnosis is 82% sensitive and 87% specific if there are more than 3 of the following 10 criteria: weight loss (4 kg or more), livedo reticularis, testicular pain or tenderness, myalgia, mononeuritis multiplex or other polyneuropathy, hypertension, azotemia, hepatitis B virus antibody,

▶ **TABLE 155.2 Syndromes Associated with Systemic Vasculitis**

Syndrome	Systemic Manifestations	Laboratory Abnormalities	Neurologic Syndromes
Systemic vasculitis (periarteritis nodosa)	Skin, kidneys, joints, lungs, hypertension; abdominal pain; heart	Serum complement decreased; immune complexes; hepatitis B antigen and antibody rheumatoid factor	Peripheral neuropathy; mononeuritis multiplex; stroke; polymyositis
Wegener granulomatosis	Nose, paranasal sinuses, lungs, other viscera	As above; also increased serum IgE	Peripheral or cranial neuropathy encephalopathy
Churg-Strauss vasculitis	Lungs, other viscera	As above; also eosinophilia	
Temporal arteritis (giant cell arteritis)	Fever, malaise, myalgia, weight loss, claudication of chewing	Increased ESR	Visual loss due to lesions of optic nerve or retina; papilledema; stroke rare
Polymyalgia rheumatica	Fever, malaise; myalgia, weight loss	Increased ESR	None
Cogan syndrome	Interstitial keratitis, aortic insufficiency; occasionally other viscera	Increased ESR; CSF pleocytosis	Vestibular or auditory loss; peripheral neuropathy; stroke; encephalomyelopathy
Takayasu syndrome (aortic arch disease; pulseless disease)	Cataracts, retinal atrophy; cranial muscular wasting; claudication, loss of peripheral pulses; heart	Increased ESR	Stroke; amaurosis fugax; visual loss
Granulomatous angiitis of the brain	None	CSF pleocytosis, increased protein content, normal sugar	Somnolence, confusion; encephalomyelopathy; myeloradiculoneuropathy
Systemic lupus erythematosus	Skin, lungs, kidneys, joints, liver, heart, Raynaud, fever	Leukopenia, multiple autoantibodies, increased ESR; evidence of renal or hepatic disease	Organic psychosis; seizures; chorea; myelopathy; peripheral neuropathy; polymyositis; aseptic meningitis
Systemic sclerosis	Skin, lungs, gastrointestinal tract, kidneys, heart, joints, Raynaud	None characteristic except disordered mobility of esophagus and bowel	Polymyositis
Rheumatoid arthritis	Joints; viscera occasionally	Rheumatoid factor	Polymyositis; mononeuritis multiplex peripheral neuropathy
Dermatomyositis	Skin, by definition; lungs; gastrointestinal tract, rare	Inflammatory cells in muscle	Polymyositis
Mixed connective tissue disease (sclerodermatomyositis?)	Skin lesions of dermatomyositis or scleroderma; joints; Raynaud; lungs; esophagus	Antibody to extractable nuclear ribonucleoprotein	Polymyositis

ESR, erythrocyte sedimentation rate.
From Cupps and Fauci (1982).

arteriographic occlusion of visceral arteries, biopsy evidence of granulocytes in vessel wall.

Course and Prognosis

The prognosis is poor; the 5-year survival rate is about 50%. Death usually occurs because of lesions of the kidneys, other abdominal viscera, or the heart; occasionally, lesions in the brain or peripheral nerves may cause death. The duration of life after symptom onset varies from a few months to several years. Spontaneous heal-ing of the arteritis may occur, with remission of all symptoms and signs, including those of the peripheral neuropathy.

Treatment

There is no specific therapy. Treatment is chiefly supportive, including blood transfusions and symptomatic therapy for associated conditions. Corticosteroids in high doses and immunosuppressive drugs are used together. Cyclophosphamide has been given intravenously in pulses at

▶ **TABLE 155.3** Clinical Features in Patients[a] with Polyarteritis Nodosa

Clinical Manifestation	Percent	No. Patients
Fever	71	460
Weight loss	54	405
Organ system involvement		
Kidney	70	375
Musculoskeletal system	64	301
Arthritis/arthralgia	53	301
Myalgias	31	238
Hypertension	54	356
Peripheral neuropathy	51	495
Gastrointestinal tract	44	507
Abdominal pain	43	122
Nausea/vomiting	40	30
Cholecystitis	17	64
Bleeding	6	205
Bowel perforation	5	64
Bowel infarction	1.4	140
Skin	43	476
Rash/purpura	30	259
Nodules	15	369
Livedo reticularis	4	194
Heart	36	413
Congestive heart failure	12	204
Myocardial infarct	6	64
Pericarditis	4	204
Brain	23	184
Stroke	11	90
Altered mental status	10	90
Seizure	4	90

[a]Mean age of patients was 45; the male-to-female ratio was 2.5:1.
From Cupps TR and Fauci AS (1982).

▶ **TABLE 155.4** Symptoms at Onset in Patients with Polyarteritis Nodosa

Symptoms	Percent of Patients
Malaise/weakness	13
Abdominal pain	12
Leg pain	12
Neurologic signs/symptoms	10
Fever	8
Cough	8
Myalgias	5
Peripheral neuropathy	5
Headache	5
Arthritis/arthralgia	4
Skin involvement	4
Painful arms	4
Painful feet	4

From Cupps TR and Fauci AS (1982).

monthly intervals, and other drugs are also being used. The paucity of patients makes it difficult to do a controlled trial or to offer strict rules for general use. IVIG therapy and plasmapheresis have not gained favor.

TEMPORAL ARTERITIS AND POLYMYALGIA RHEUMATICA (GIANT CELL ARTERITIS) AND TAKAYUSU DISEASE: MEDIUM AND LARGE VESSEL DISEASES.

Temporal arteritis and polymyalgia rheumatica are inextricably linked because they overlap in clinical features, high erythrocyte sedimentation rate (ESR), pathology in the temporal artery and other medium or large vessels (giant cell arteritis), clinical course, and response to steroid therapy. Both affect people older than age 50, and the dominant features include malaise and myalgia. The major differences are the prominent headache and the threat of visual loss in temporal arteritis. However, temporal artery biopsy may be positive in patients who lack the cranial symptoms. It is not clear whether the two syndromes are slightly different manifestations of the same etiology and pathogenesis or whether two separate conditions have overlapping manifestations. Doppler studies may provide a noninvasive mode of diagnosis, but sensitivity and specificity must be assessed.

Giant cell arteritis is a panarteritis, with monocytes penetrating all layers of the artery. Activated T cells and macrophages are seen in the granulomas, and multinucleated giant cells are close to the internal elastic lumina, which may be hyperplasic and occluding the lumen. Four characteristics are clear: First, CD4+ cells are essential. Second, dendritic cells activate the CD4+ cells. Third, cells within the arterial wall respond to the infiltrating T cells. The result is either occlusion or aneurysm. Fourth, genetic susceptibility is determined in part by allelic variants of the class II antigen-presenting HLA molecules. The antigens recognized by the T cells are not known, but infectious agents and drugs have been implicated. In giant cell arteritis, temporal artery biopsies show that dendritic cells in the vessel walls are mature and activated to produce interleukin cytokines and CD86, the receptor needed for interaction with T cells. They continue to activate T cells. In polymyalgia rheumatica, however, temporal arteries show no inflammatory cells and the dendritic cells are mature, producing different cytokines, activation makers. The process involves activation and migration of the dendritic cells with the arterial walls Weyand and Goronzy (2003) explain the complicated molecular immunology involved in inflammation of the vessel wall, granuloma formation, cell damage, and events leading to ischemia.

TEMPORAL ARTERITIS

This syndrome was first described by Horton in 1934. The pathology is similar to that of periarteritis nodosa except that the inflammatory reaction is more severe and there are more multinucleated giant cells in the media (*giant cell arteritis*). It is usually restricted to the temporal artery, but other vessels are sometimes affected. The syndrome occurs after age 50 equally in men and women.

It is said to occur exclusively in Whites and primarily those of Nordic descent. In Sweden, the incidence rate was 18.3 cases per 100,000 inhabitants over age 50. In Italy, the comparable figure was 6.9 per 100,000. The low frequency in African Americans parallels the distribution of HLA-DR4.

Symptoms include headache, which is typically centered on the affected temporal artery but may be more generalized. Systemic symptoms include malaise, fever, anorexia, weight loss, and myalgia. The ESR is almost always >50 mm/hr. The affected temporal artery may be prominent, nodular, tender, and not compressible. Unilateral visual loss, found in 14% to 33% of patients in different series, is attributed to occlusion of the central retinal artery. The disk may appear pale, normal, or swollen with retinal hemorrhages. Ophthalmoparesis may be prominent, but involvement of other cranial nerves is uncommon. Muscle ischemia causes "jaw claudication." Coronary and limb arteries are sometimes affected. Cerebral symptoms are mostly those of cerebral infarction, which is seen in few cases. However, it is also one of the rare forms of *reversible dementia*.

Diagnosis is simple when all typical findings are present. The ESR, however, may not be elevated, and the temporal artery biopsy specimen may be normal in otherwise typical cases. The diagnosis should be considered whenever a person older than 50 begins to have new headaches, unilateral visual loss, or ophthalmoparesis. Diagnosis is then made by the high ESR or typical findings on biopsy, but not necessarily both. Typical abnormalities on temporal artery biopsy are diagnostic because inflammatory cells are not seen at autopsy of control subjects. If the clinical picture includes headache, jaw claudication, and myalgia with high ESR, it is more likely that the biopsy will support the diagnosis, but not always. It is difficult to substantiate the diagnosis if clinical manifestations are not typical and if the ESR or biopsy is normal.

It is now difficult to determine the natural history of periarteritis because the threat of visual loss leads to steroid treatment as soon as the diagnosis is made; it is truly emergency treatment. It is difficult to justify a placebo-controlled trial under these circumstances. However, it is believed that the disease is self-limited, lasting months or a year or two. In the past, when daily prednisone doses were about 60 mg, few patients could stop steroid therapy. In the 1980s, the dose gradually dropped without losing efficacy. The adverse effects of steroid therapy are dose and duration dependent; with standard doses, at least a third of the patients had serious adverse effects of steroids. With maintenance doses of 5 to 10 mg prednisone, the frequency of side effects is much less, and therapy can often be discontinued in 6 to 12 months. In the past decade, the recommended starting dose has dropped from 60 mg daily to 20 to 40 mg daily.

Taylor and Samanta recommend a starting dose of 40 mg daily if there has been no visual loss. They reduce the dose by 10 mg/day each month for 3 months, then from 20 to 10 mg daily over another 3 months, and slower tapering thereafter. If vision is already affected, the dose is 60 to 80 mg daily, and some add 250 mg hydrocortisone intravenously if vision has already been affected; there is no evidence that these higher doses are more effective. In the only controlled trial of steroids and cyclophosphamide, neither was superior.

Early steroid therapy seems to prevent the most feared consequence of temporal arteritis, loss of vision. If therapy is started when one eye is affected, vision in the other eye is protected. If vision has already been lost, chances of recovery are low. Aiello et al. (1993) found that 34 of 245 patients (14%) lost vision; in 32 of them, the visual loss occurred before steroid therapy commenced. In general, it is stated that 30% to 60% of patients lost vision before the era of steroid therapy, which has lowered the incidence of visual loss to 5% to 20%.

Nevertheless, all patients develop Cushing syndrome and 20% to 50% have other serious adverse effects of steroids. It is therefore customary to try to reduce steroid doses by adding an immunosuppressive drug and methotrexate is popular. However, Hoffman et al. (2002) found no benefit from this combination.

The mortality rate is low, and most deaths that do occur are encountered in the first 4 months of the disease.

POLYMYALGIA RHEUMATICA

This condition is defined by the combination of myalgia (especially shoulder pain), malaise, weight loss, fever, and increased ESR in a person older than 50. In many patients, temporal artery biopsy shows the changes of temporal arteritis, even if there is no headache or other symptomatic indication that cranial vessels are affected. The threat of visual loss is lower if there are no cranial symptoms, but the similarities require the same steroid therapy.

The symptoms of polymyalgia rheumatica are nonspecific and could be reproduced by someone with an occult malignant tumor. It becomes a matter of clinical judgment to decide whether there is time for a diagnostic therapeutic trial of steroid therapy (as described for temporal arteritis)

▶ TABLE 155.5 Frequency of Manifestations in Small-Vessel Vasculitis (Percent of Patients)

Organ	Cryoglobulin Vasculitis	Microscopic Polyarteritis	Wegener Granulomatosus	Churg-Strauss Syndrome
Cutaneous	90	40	40	60
Renal	55	90	80	45
Pulmonary	<5	50	90	70
Ear, Nose, Throat	<5	35	90	60
Musculoskeletal	70	60	60	50
Neurologic	40	30	50	70
Gastrointestinal	30	50	50	50

Modified from Jennette and Falk (1997).

with or without search for the possible tumor. The other major consideration in differential diagnosis is *polymyositis*. In polymyalgia, however, there is no limb weakness, serum levels of creatine kinase are normal, and there are no myopathic changes in muscle biopsy or electromyography; if any of these tests gave abnormal results, the syndrome would be indistinguishable from polymyositis.

Treatment is the same as for temporal arteritis, but there may be more consistent symptomatic relief with even smaller doses of prednisolone, 15 to 20 mg daily, dropping to 10 mg daily by 3 months. The long-term outlook is excellent, but there are recurrences in some patients.

A third disease in this class is Takayasu arteritis, a large-vessel disorder that primarily affects the aorta and its branches. Although most reported cases were young women in Asia, it has been seen worldwide and in both sexes. It may be asymptomatic but recognized as pulseless disease before age 30. Systemic symptoms resemble those of polymyalgia rheumatica. Neurologic manifestations arise from renal disease and hypertension or from carotid or vertebral artery occlusion. Aortic valvular disease and congestive heart failure may be prominent. Diagnosis depends on three of six criteria: age under 40; claudication of arms or legs; diminished brachial artery pulse; blood pressure differences in the arms; subclavian bruit; and abnormal arteriogram. Roughly 50% pf patients respond to steroid therapy and half of the others respond to methotrexate or other cytotoxic drugs.

ANTINEURONAL CYTOPLASMIC AUTOANTIBODY-POSITIVE CHURG-STRAUSS SYNDROME AND WEGENER GRANULOMATOSIS

The arterial lesions in these rare syndromes differ from those of periarteritis in that granuloma formation is more prominent, and they may be more necrotizing. There are other differences. For instance, eosinophilia and asthma define the *Churg-Strauss syndrome*. Sensori-

motor neuropathy is seen in about 70% of patients and, sometimes, visual loss. *Microscopic polyangiitis* resembles periarteritis nodosa clinically and neurologically but affects smaller vessels, especially in the kidneys and lungs (Table 155.5).

The advent of tests for ANCA has elaborated the original diagnosis from a simple triad, and the scenario now comprises more acts. First comes allergic rhinitis at about age 28, followed by asthma and eosinophilia at 35. Finally, evidence of vasculitis (Table 155.6) comes at about age 38. PRO3-ANCA tests are positive in the earlier stages in about two-thirds of the patients. Diagnosis can be confirmed by biopsy of any affected tissue, including lung, kidney, or sural nerve.

Leukotriene receptor antagonists (zafirlukast or montelukast) have been used to treat asthma, but there is not yet statistical evidence that these drugs precipitate Churg-Strauss syndrome.

▶ TABLE 155.6 Manifestations of Churg-Strauss Disease

Manifestation	% of 234 Patients
Asthma	100
Eosinophilia	100
Allergic rhinitis	66
Pulmonary infiltrates	57
Cardiac disease	41
Gastrointestinal disease	45
Renal disease	43
Skin nodules	25
Skin purpura	39
Mononeuritis multiplex	72
Musculoskeletal disease	53

Data from Churg A. Recent advances in the diagnosis of Churg-Strauss syndrome. *Mod Pathol* 2001;14:1294–1293; Lanham JG, Elkon KB, Pusey CD, et al. Systemic vasculitis with asthma and eosinophilia: a clinical approach to Churg-Strauss syndrome. *Medicine (Baltimore)* 1984;63:65–81; and Guillevin L, Cohen P, Gayraud M, et al. Churg-Strauss syndrome. Clinical study and long-term follow-up of 96 patients. *Medicine (Baltimore)* 1999;78:26–37.

Wegener granulomatosis has a predilection for the respiratory system and kidneys. According to criteria of the American Academy of Rheumatology, the diagnosis can be made if there are two of the following four criteria: oral ulcers or purulent bloody nasal discharge; abnormal chest film showing nodules, fixed infiltrates, or cavities; microhematuria; and biopsy evidence of granulomatous inflammation in the wall of an artery or perivascular tissue. "Limited" Wegener disease shows the typical pathology but spares lungs and kidney. Ninety percent of typical Wegener patients are ANCA positive; 50% to 80% have the C-ANCA pattern with antiproteinase 3, and 10% to 18% show the P-ANCA pattern with antimyeloperoxidase. Neurologic manifestations, as in other vasculitis syndromes, more often indicate a sensorimotor peripheral neuropathy than a CNS syndrome. The disease was once thought to be uniformly fatal, but survival is reported with steroid and cyclophosphamide or other immunosuppressive drug therapy.

In some patients with polyneuropathy and no signs of systemic disease, nerve biopsy shows arteritis. Again therapeutic recommendations include steroids and cytotoxic drugs.

GRANULOMATOUS ANGIITIS OF THE BRAIN

In one form of granulomatous angiitis, clinical manifestations are restricted to the brain. Thus, this is appropriately called *granulomatous angiitis of the brain* (GAB). In a few cases, the spinal cord is similarly affected, alone or with cerebral lesions. Therefore, the more comprehensive term is granulomatous angiitis of the nervous system (GANS). This disorder is essentially defined by the characteristic histologic lesion, a granulomatous change that includes multinucleated giant cells; it is seen in small or larger named cerebral blood vessels.

Lesions of this nature are found in some patients with clinical evidence of a cerebral infarct ipsilateral to herpes zoster ophthalmicus. Otherwise, there is no clinical clue to the nature of the disease. Some patients have evidence of immunosuppression with sarcoidosis, Hodgkin disease, borreliosis, or AIDS, and about 20 patients had concomitant amyloid angiopathy.

After herpes zoster, the clinical manifestations may be those of an uncomplicated stroke, with severe or mild manifestations in different cases. When there is no evidence of zoster infection, the symptoms include two invariable but nonspecific sets, focal cerebral signs and mental obtundation, which may be preceded by dementia. The course is subacute, so this can be regarded as a progressive encephalopathy.

Characteristically, there is CSF pleocytosis, up to 500 mononuclear cells per high-power field. CSF protein content is usually increased, exceeding 100 mg/dL in 75% of cases, but CSF glucose content is normal.

There has been doubt about the necessity or desirability of brain biopsy for diagnosis. Advocates believe that pathologic proof is needed and that the risks of meningeal biopsy are about 1%. On the other hand, the risks of immunotherapy are much higher and cytotoxic drugs may be given for an erroneous diagnosis. Analyzing 30 biopsies for presumed GANS, Goldstein and associates found that 50% had some other disease. Moreover, angiographic evidence of arteritis is unreliable when positive and is absent in most cases of histologically proven granulomatous angiitis of the brain.

Others contend that a negative biopsy does not exclude the diagnosis and believe that sufficient evidence is given by angiographic beading of arteries. Cases so diagnosed have been treated with cyclophosphamide, and, if the outcome was favorable, the authors concluded that the likely catastrophic outcome had been averted. In autopsy-proven cases, however, the arteriogram is usually normal or shows evidence of an infarct or local tissue swelling but not beading. Moreover, the clinical, arteriographic, and CSF manifestations can be caused by infiltration of meninges by tumor cells or viral infection; beading of cerebral arteries is a nonspecific finding.

These perspectives can be seen in a comparison of series defined by pathologic diagnosis (the neurologist's view) or by cerebral angiography and pathology (the rheumatologist's view; Table 155.7). Neurologists do not consider diagnosis by arteriography reliable, because beading is found in only 10% of pathologically proven cases. Strokes are found in only 15%. In contrast to arteriographic diagnosis, pathologic diagnosis leads to a reasonably consistent picture: encephalopathy (obtundation, cognitive loss); headache; onset over days or weeks, not apoplectic; and CSF protein content >100 mg/dL.

Other problems of diagnosis include subacute bacterial, yeast, or neoplastic meningitis; these conditions are more likely if CSF glucose content is <40 mg/dL, and if the glucose content is normal, CSF cytology is needed. GAB may simulate prion disease by causing severe dementia within a few weeks. Hashimoto encephalopathy produces a similar clinical picture (Chapter 158) but not the brain pathology. If GAB produces a mass lesion, brain biopsy makes the distinction from tumor. The myelopathy of granulomatous arteritis of the nervous system (GANS) is difficult to diagnose in life unless there is concomitant evidence of herpes zoster or sarcoid.

The neurologist's view is that for diagnosis in living patients, GAB can be verified only by a brain biopsy that includes meningeal vessels. In histologically proven cases (without zoster), the outcome in most cases has been fatal within a few years. About half the patients die within 6 weeks, but one-third live longer than 1 year after onset. Treatment with immunosuppressive drugs has not been

▶ **TABLE 155.7   Comparison of Two Concepts of Granulomatosis Angiitis of the Brain: Diagnosis by Histopathology or Arteriography**

	Mode of Diagnosis	
	Pathology[a]	Pathology or Arteriography[b]
Number of patients	78	48
Clinical features		
Onset	"Days or weeks"	"Typically sudden"
Mental changes	61 (78%)	13 (27)
Headache	42 (53%)	28 (58)
Coma	42 (53%)	3 (6)
Focal weakness (hemiparesis)	33 (42%)	17 (35)
Clinical stroke	12 (15%)	
Seizures	18 (23%)	6 (13)
Fever	16 (20%)	5 (10)
Aphasia	10 (12%)	7 (15)
Altered vision	9 (11%)	6 (13)
Quadriparesis or paraparesis (spinal)	8 (10%)	5 (10)
Fatal	68 (87%)	27/38 (71)
CSF examination		
WBC < 3	17/55 (30)	12/40 (30)
3–250	38/55 (69)	28/40 (70)
50–250	24/55 (43)	—
Protein normal	9/55 (16)	12/40 (30)
50–600	39/55 (70)	28/40 (70)
> 100	25/55 (45)	—
CT		
Normal	4/11 (36)	—
Enhancing mass	3/11 (27)	—
Infarct	3/11 (27)	—
Hematoma	1/11 (9)	—
Angiography		
Normal	13/33 (39)	4/31 (13)
Avascular mass	6/33 (18)	—
Diffuse narrowing	5/33 (15)	—
Other abnormality	—	6/31 (19)
Beading	3/33 (9)	20/31 (65)
Brain biopsy		
Normal	4/20 (20)	—
Diagnostic	10/20 (50)	4/14 (29)
Not diagnostic	6/20 (30)	4/14 (29)
Autopsy diagnostic	64/74 (86)	26/48 (54)

[a]Data from Younger et al. (1988).
[b]Data from Calabrese and Mallek (1988).
WBC, white blood cell count.
From Rowland LP. *Merritt's textbook of neurology, update 12.* Philadelphia: Lea & Febiger, 1992.

effective in most proven cases. However, control of GAB has been documented in patients with biopsy-proven GAB who were treated with immunosuppression, died later, and had no autopsy evidence of lingering inflammation; two of those patients also had amyloid angiopathy.

The debate about criteria for diagnosis continues unabated. Some neurosurgeons have joined rheumatologists in believing that "vasculitis" can be diagnosed by arteriography and that it can be as benign as a chronic headache that responds to steroid therapy. Tamargo stated that he relied on angiography only and does not do a brain biopsy; the case he was discussing was one of autopsy-proven GAB. Advocates of biopsy point out that even if the test is negative for GAB, it may show some other diagnosis. With a negative diagnosis, the use of immunosuppressive therapy makes little difference in outcome. Scolding and other European neurologists have documented the inconsistencies of diagnostic approaches and have advocated a prospective study. In the meantime, it seems prudent to rely on biopsy in opting for chronic immunosuppressive therapy.

SYSTEMIC LUPUS ERYTHEMATOSUS

Systemic lupus erythematosus (SLE) is characterized by widespread inflammatory change in the connective tissue (collagen) of the skin and systemic organs. The primary damage is to the subendothelial connective tissue of capillaries, small arteries, and veins; the endocardium; and the synovial and serous membranes.

Etiology and Incidence

The cause is not known, but immune complexes are deposited in small vessels. The initiating event could be a persistent viral infection, but sometimes serologic and clinical manifestations follow soon after the administration of any of 70 drugs, such as procainamide. Although rare, the incidence may be increasing. Most cases begin between ages 20 and 40, but the disease is seen in children. Some 95% of adult patients are women.

Symptoms and Signs

The chief clinical manifestations are prolonged irregular fever, with remissions of variable duration (weeks, months, or even years); erythematous rash; recurrent attacks with evidence of involvement of synovial and serous membranes (polyarthritis, pleuritis, pericarditis); depression of bone marrow function (leukopenia, hypochromic anemia, moderate thrombocytopenia); and, in advanced stages, clinical evidence of vascular alteration in the skin, kidneys, and other viscera.

Neurologic manifestations can be divided into several major categories. One form, affecting up to 25% of

▶ **TABLE 155.8** Neuropsychiatric Manifestations of Systemic Lupus Erythematosus in Finland and Texas

Manifestation	Finland (N = 46) %	Texas (N = 128) %
Stroke, TIA	15	2
Headache	54	57
Mononeuropathy	—	8
Optic neuropathy	7	—
Cranial neuropathy	0	2
Sensorimotor polyneuropathy	28	22
Seizures	9	16
Chorea	1	0
Myasthenia gravis	1	0
Demyelinating disorder	1	0
Psychiatric Disorders	44	—
Anxiety disorder	13	24
Major depression	18	28
Depressive mood disorder	—	19
Mood disorder, manic features	—	3
Mood disorder, mixed features	2	1
Psychosis	—	6
Cognition		
Normal	20	21
Mild impairment	26	43
Moderate impairment	7	30
Severe impairment	4	6

Data from Brey RL, Holliday SL, Saklad AR, et al. Neuropsychiatric syndromes in lupus: prevalence using standardized definitions. Neurology 2002;58:1214–1220; and Ainiala H, Loukkola MA, Peltola J, et al. The prevalence of neuropsychiatric syndromes in systemic lupus erythematosus. Neurology 2001;57:496–500.

all patients with SLE, was originally called *cerebral lupus*, an encephalopathy manifested by seizures, psychosis, dementia, chorea, or cranial nerve disorder. Now, more formal designations are given to NPSLE, which is defined by 19 specific neurologic and psychiatric syndromes (Table 155.8). SLE is one of the few remaining causes of chorea in young women. Other neurologic syndromes are transverse myelopathy, sensorimotor peripheral neuropathy, and polymyositis. These symptoms are often attributed to thrombosis of small vessels or petechial hemorrhages. Microinfarcts may be related to fibrinoid degeneration of small vessels with deposition of antibodies to a platelet membrane glycoprotein. The same neurologic symptoms are encountered in pediatric lupus. Psychiatric disorders and cognitive impairment are also prevalent. One of the most vexing problems is acute psychosis in a patient with lupus who is being treated with large doses of corticosteroids. Is the psychosis a manifestation of the disease or a toxic effect of the treatment?

Seeking an answer to this question, Chau and Mok concluded that hypoalbuminema was most likely responsible, perhaps allowing more serum steroid to be free rather than bound; the person's past psychiatric history was also a factor.

Pathologically, evidence of cerebral vasculitis is meager. The cause of cerebral symptoms is not known, but they are attributed to mixed pathogenesis: antineuronal antibodies of unknown type, microvascular occlusions from vasculitis, antiphospholipid antibodies, and noninflammatory vasculopathy could play a role. Although strokes are a feature of the "antiphospholipid syndrome," there is little evidence they are responsible for cerebral lupus. According to Alfetra et al., patients with neuropsychiatric disorders have higher levels of antiphospholipid abnormalities, but the nature and relatively frequencies do not differ from those who do not have high antibody titers. Antibodies to ribosomal protein P are said to be highly specific for cerebral lupus but are found in only 20% of patients.

Stroke caused by occlusion of large cerebral vessels is distinctly uncommon. In 1994, Mitsias and Levine found only 30 reported cases, and they were owing to diverse mechanisms, including thrombus, dissection, fibromuscular dysplasia, vasculitis, and premature atherosclerosis. The short-term death rate was 40%, and recurrences occurred in 13% of the survivors. Venous sinus thrombosis is also recognized. In general, little information has been provided by brain imaging of any kind, including PET and SPECT.

The cause of cerebral lupus is therefore uncertain. In some cases, cerebral emboli arise from endocarditis or thrombotic thrombocytopenia.

Laboratory Data

In addition to anemia and leukopenia, there is often hematuria or proteinuria, signs of renal damage. Biologic false-positive tests for syphilis may be encountered. The most important diagnostic test is the search for *antinuclear antibodies* (ANA), especially antibodies to double-stranded DNA, which are also used as a measure of activity of the disease. Antibodies to a particular antigen (Sm for Smith) may be found more often in patients with cerebral disease. Although not used these days, phagocytic polymorphonuclear leukocytes (*LE cells*) were found in 80% of all cases. Serum complement levels may be decreased in patients with renal disease; deposits of globulin and complement may be found in renal biopsy specimens. CSF is usually normal, but there may be a modest increase in protein content. For reasons not known, the CSF glucose content is often decreased in SLE patients with myelitis.

Brain CT and MRI show nonspecific changes in cerebral lupus. PET may show lesions in brain in SLE patients with normal MRI; functional abnormality may precede structural abnormality.

Diagnosis

Diagnosis may be difficult. Fever; weight loss; arthritis; anemia; leukopenia; pleuritis; and cardiac, renal, or neurologic symptoms in a young woman should lead to a consideration of SLE. An erythematous rash on the bridge of the nose and the malar eminences in a butterflylike distribution facilitates the diagnosis. ANA is present in 88% of patients and anti–double-stranded DNA in 55%. Other antibodies are anti-Sm, anti-RNP, anti-Ro, and anticardiolipin; all may be helpful in difficult diagnostic problems. Anti-RNP is reportedly positive in 70% of patients with lupus psychosis. Neurologic manifestations are only rarely the first manifestation of SLE, but the diagnosis should be kept in mind when there is an acute encephalopathy in a young woman. Acute psychosis in a woman with known SLE may be owing to the disease or the effects of steroid therapy, which may be difficult to unravel.

Mixed connective tissue disease is an overlap syndrome with features of SLE, systemic sclerosis, and polymyositis. At first, there seemed to be an association with antibodies to ribonucleoprotein, but the specificity disappeared. Also, polymyositis can be a manifestation of any collagen-vascular or vasculitis syndrome, with little specificity. It is primarily systemic sclerosis that overlaps with both SLE and dermatomyositis. For instance, the multisystem disease described in Case Record 24-1995 included polymyositis, with evidence of SLE (rash more like SLE than dermatomyositis and high titer of ANA), and features of systemic sclerosis (esophageal dysmotility, Raynaud phenomenon, and severe lung disease), but no skin lesions of scleroderma. SLE patients may show features of rheumatoid arthritis or Sjögren syndrome. It seems unlikely that mixed connective tissue disease is a unique condition, but the multisystem diseases are a diagnostic and therapeutic challenge.

Course, Prognosis, and Therapy

Cerebral lupus is a medical catastrophe, but the prognosis has improved and the 10-year survival rate is now 80% to 95%. Recommendations include intravenous doses of methylprednisolone (1 g daily for 3 days), followed by low-dose oral prednisolone. Some authorities add intravenous cyclophosphamide in the initial treatment. Other popular drug regimens include cytotoxic drugs and antimalarials. Plasmapheresis and IVIG therapy have not been beneficial. Cases are so few and the disease is so devastating that it has been difficult to carry out a therapeutic trial.

Treatment is equally uncertain for the less-threatening syndromes of peripheral neuropathy, myelitis, or polymyositis. Steroid therapy is the accepted treatment but not established by therapeutic trial. In the long run, death may result from renal failure or infection.

SYSTEMIC SCLEROSIS (SCLERODERMA)

First recognized as *scleroderma* (hard skin), systemic disease was recognized in 1863 when Raynaud described the vasospastic syndrome in a person with the skin disorder. In 1942, cutaneous calcinosis, esophageal dysfunction, and telangiectasia were added to the acronymic CREST for (calcinosis, Raynaud, esophageal, scleroderma, and telangiectasia). Another important systemic complication is pulmonary fibrosis. Formal diagnosis includes the presence of one major criterion (widespread scleroderma) plus at least two the following three: sclerodactyly (skin changes on fingers only), digital finger pad depressions from ischemic lesions, and pulmonary fibrosis. The disorder includes esophageal dysmotility with dysphagia, renal disease owing to a small vessel arteriopathy. The renal disease may cause serious hypertension. Women are affected at least 10 times more often than men, with a peak incidence between ages 30 and 55.

About 15% of the patients have polymyositis. Other neurologic manifestations include migraine, trigeminal sensory neuropathy, transverse myelitis, and sensorimotor axonal neuropathy. Autonomic neuropathy may play a role in the esophageal, gastrointestinal, and bladder symptoms. A localized version (*linear scleroderma* or *en coup de sabre*) may be accompanied by seizures and hemiparesis with MRI or autopsy changes suggesting inflammation. In one patient, the focal signs disappeared with steroid therapy.

Several circulating antibodies have received attention. Anti-RNA polymerase III antibodies are found in 45% of those with generalized disease but not in limited scleroderma. Antitopoisomerase antibodies are found in 30% of generalized and 15% of limited disease. Anticentromere antibodies are found in 70% of those with limited disease or CREST and correlate especially with esophageal disease; these antibodies are useful in excluding other collagen-vascular disease. The role of the antibodies is not known, and only limited information is available about etiology and pathogenesis.

Treatment is not satisfactory, with 5-year survivals about 65%, depending on cardiac, pulmonary, and renal function. D-penicillamine is the most widely used drug with presumed antifibroitc and immunomodulating activity. Other drugs are being evaluated to help the skin and cardiac disorders. Angiotensin-converting enzyme inhibitors are effective in treating the renal disease and may be disease modifying. Epoprostenol helps pulmonary hypertension. Cytotoxic immunosuppressive drugs and bone marrow transplantation may be helpful.

OTHER COLLAGEN-VASCULAR DISEASES

Neurologic syndromes may complicate other collagen-vascular diseases, usually when the systemic disorder is evident. Sometimes, there are characteristic syndromes. For instance, an aggressive polyneuropathy may be seen in patients with rheumatoid arthritis. Some clinicians believe the neuropathy may be precipitated by steroid therapy. Another neurologic syndrome of rheumatoid arthritis is atlantoaxial dislocation with resulting cord compression; the syndrome is attributed to resorption of the odontoid process.

Sjögren syndrome is defined clinically by internationally accepted criteria. There must be at least two of the following: xerostomia (dry mouth), which can be documented by scintigraphy; xerophthalmia (dry eyes); pathologic documentation of abnormality in salivary gland biopsy; or keratoconjunctivitis sicca, as demonstrated by the *Schirmer test* to show decreased tear production. Lip biopsy showing sialoadenitis is important in diagnosis. If the neurologic manifestations dominate, the term *sicca complex* is used. Sensorimotor peripheral neuropathy (primarily sensory or sensorimotor) and polymyositis are the most common neurologic manifestations. Sjögren disease is one of the causes of trigeminal sensory neuropathy. CNS complications are rare, but venous sinus thrombosis, myelopathy, a form of motor neuron disease, or aseptic meningitis are reported. The origin of the neuropathy is not known. Antineuronal antibodies have been found in some cases. Treatment, as usual in these diseases, focuses on steroids in uncontrolled trials.

In Sjögren syndrome, peripheral neuropathy and polymyositis may be prominent. The neuropathy may be primarily sensory and painful; anti-SSA and anti-SSB antibody titers do not correlate with lip biopsies in these patients. Peripheral neuropathy is also seen in more than half the patients with the *idiopathic hypereosinophilic syndrome*, and there may be evidence of vasculitis in the nerve biopsy.

The *Sneddon syndrome* is defined by the combination of livedo reticularis and stroke with occlusive disease of small and medium-sized arteries, with only a few autopsies for guidance; in one report, there was a granulomatous reaction in the meninges; occlusion without inflammation was found with multi-infarct brain disease.

SUGGESTED READINGS

General

Anonymous. Vasculitis—A Medical Dictionary, Bibliography, and Annotated Research Guide to Internet References. San Diego, Icon Health Publications, 2004.
Ball EV, Bridges SL, eds. *Vasculitis*. New York: Oxford University Press, 2002.

Gold R, Fontana A, Zierz S. Therapy of neurological disorders in systemic vasculitis. *Semin Neurol* 2003;23;207–14.
Mendell JR, Kissel JT, Cornblath DR, eds. *Diagnosis and Management of Peripheral Nerve Disorders*. New York: Oxford University Press, 2001.
Olney RK. Neuropathies associated with connective tissue disease. *Semin Neurol* 1998;18:63–72.
Vincent A, Martino G. *Autoantibodies in Neurological Diseases*. Berlin: Springer-Verlag, 2002.

Polyarteritis Nodosa

Bicknell JM, Holland JV. Neurologic manifestations of Cogan syndrome. *Neurology* 1978;28:278–281.
Gayraud M, Guillevin L, Cohen P, et al. Treatment of good-prognosis polyarteritis nodosa and Churg-Strauss syndrome: comparison of steroids and oral or pulse cyclophosphamide in 25 patients. French Cooperative Study Group for Vasculitides. *Br J Rheumatol* 1997;36:1290–1297.
Guillevin L, Cohen P, Marh A, et al. Treatment of polyarteritis nodosa and microscopic polyangiitis with poor prognosis factors: a prospective trial comparing glucocorticoids and six or twelve cyclophosphamide pulses in sixty-five patients. *Arthritis Rheum* 2003; 49(Feb 15):93–100.
Lane SE, Watts RA, Shepstone L, Scott DG. Primary systemic vasculitis: clinical features and mortality. *QJM* 2005 Feb;98(2):97–111.
Lightfoot RW, Michael BA, Bloch DA, et al. The American College of Rheumatology 1990 criteria for the classification of polyarteritis nodosa. *Arthritis Rheum* 1990;33:1088–1093.
Lovelace RE. Mononeuritis multiplex in polyarteritis nodosa. *Neurology* 1964;14:434–442.
Wicki J, Olivieri J, Pizzolato G, et al. Successful treatment of polyarteritis nodosa related to hepatitis B virus with a combination of lamivudine and interferon alpha. *Rheumatology (Oxford)* 1999;38:183–185.

Temporal Arteritis and Polymyalgia Rheumatica (Giant Cell Arteritis)

Aiello PD, Traumann JC, McPhee TJ, et al. Visual prognosis in giant cell arteritis. *Ophthalmology* 1993;100:550–555.
Alwity A, Holden R. One hundred transient monocular central retinal artery occlusions secondary to giant cell arteritis. *Arch Ophthal* 2003;121:1802–1803.
Black A, Rittner HL, Younge BR, et al. Glucocorticoid-mediated repression of cytokine gene transcription in human arteritis-SCID chimeras. *J Clin Invest* 1997;99:2842–2850.
Caselli RJ, Hunder GG, Whisnant JP. Neurologic disease in biopsy-proven giant cell (temporal) arteritis. *Neurology* 1988;38:352–357.
Chui CS, Drya TP, Lessell S. A "negative" temporal artery biopsy, positive for arteritis. *Arch Ophthalmol* 2004;122:1074–1075.
Collins MP, Periquet MI, Mendell JR, et al. Nonsystemic vasculitic neuropathy: insights from a clinical cohort. *Neurology* 2003;61:623–630.
Duhaut P, Pinede L, Bornet H, et al. Biopsy proven and biopsy negative temporal arteritis: differences in clinical spectrum at the onset of the disease. *Ann Rheum Dis* 1999;58:335–341.
Grodum E, Petersen HA. Temporal arteritis with normal erythrocyte sedimentation rate. *J Intern Med* 1990;227:279–280.
Hauser WA, Ferguson RH, Holley KE, et al. Temporal arteritis in Rochester, Minnesota. *Mayo Clin Proc* 1981;46:597–602.
Healy LA. On the epidemiology of polymyalgia rheumatica and temporal arteritis. *J Rheumatol* 1993;20:1639–1640.
Horton BT, Magath TB, Brown GE. Arteritis of the temporal vessels. *Arch Intern Med* 1934;53:400–409.
Hoffman GS, Cid MC, Hellmann DB, et al. A multicenter, randomized, double-blind, placebo-controlled trial of adjuvant methotrexate treatment for giant cell arteritis. *Arthrit Rheum* 2002;46:1309–1318.
Hunder GG, Weyand CM. Sonography in giant-cell arteritis. *N Engl J Med* 1997;337:1385–1386.
Johnston SL, Lock R, Gompels MM. Takayasu arteritis: a review. *J Clin Path* 2002;55:481–486.
Kyle V, Hazleman BL. Stopping steroids in polymyalgia rheumatica and giant cell arteritis. Treatment usually lasts for two to five years. *BMJ* 1990;300:344–345.

Lundberg J, Hedfors E. Restricted dose and duration of corticosteroid treatment in patients with polymyalgia rheumatica and temporal arteritis. *J Rheumatol* 1990;17:1340–1345.

Redlich FC. A new medical diagnosis of Adolf Hitler. Giant cell arteritis-temporal arteritis. *Arch Intern Med* 1993;153:693–697.

Salvarani C, Cantini F, Boiardi L, et al. Polymyalgia rheumatica and giant-cell arteritis. *N Engl J Med* 2002;347:261–271.

Salvarani C, Cantini F, Boiardi L, Hunder GG. Polymyalgia rheumatica. *Best Pract Res Clin Rheumatol* 2004 Oct;18(5):705–722.

Smetana GW, Shmerling RH. Does this patient have temporal arteritis? *JAMA* 2002;287:92–101.

Vilaseca J, Gonzalez A, Cid MC, et al. Clinical usefulness of temporal artery biopsy. *Ann Rheum Dis* 1987;46:282–285.

Weyand CM, Goronzy JJ. Medium- and large-vessel vasculitis. *N Engl J Med* 2003;349:160–169.

ANCA-Positive Vasculitis

Case records of the Massachusetts General Hospital. Case 28-1998. Wegener granulomatosis. *N Engl J Med* 1998;339:755–763.

Case records of the Massachusetts General Hospital. Case 9-1999. Wegener granulomatosis with pachymeningeal granulomatous inflammation. *N Engl J Med* 1998;340:945–953.

Churg A. Recent advances in the diagnosis of Churg-Strauss syndrome. *Mod Pathol* 2001;14:1294–1293.

Green RL, Vayonis AG. Churg-Strauss syndrome after zafirlukast in two patients not receiving systemic steroid treatment. *Lancet* 1999;353:725–726.

Guillevin L, Cohen P, Gayraud M, et al. Churg-Strauss syndrome. Clinical study and long-term follow-up of 96 patients. *Medicine (Baltimore)* 1999;78:26–37.

Jayne D, Rasmussen N, Andrassy K, et al. A randomized trial of maintenance therapy for vasculitis associated with antineutrophil cytoplasmic autoantibodies. *N Engl J Med* 2003;349:36–44.

Lanham JG, Elkon KB, Pusey CD, et al. Systemic vasculitis with asthma and eosinophilia: a clinical approach to Churg-Strauss syndrome. *Medicine (Baltimore)* 1984;63:65–81.

Nishino H, Rubino FA, DeRemee RA, et al. Neurological involvement in Wegener's granulomatosis; analysis of 324 consecutive patients at the Mayo Clinic. *Ann Neurol* 1993;33:4–9.

Williams JM, Kamesh L, Savage CO. Translating basic science into patient therapy for ANCA-associated small vessel vasculitis. *Clin Sci* (Lond) 2005 Feb;108(2):101–112.

Granulomatous Angiitis of the Brain

Alrawi A, Trobe J, Blaivas M, et al. Brain biopsy in primary angiitis of the nervous system. *Neurology* 1999;53:858–860.

Alreshaid AA, Powers WJ. Prognosis of patients with suspected primary CNS angiitis and negative brain biopsy. *Neurology* 2003;61:831–3.

Calabrese LH, Mallek JA. Primary angiitis of the central nervous system. Report of 8 new cases, review of the literature, and proposal for diagnostic criteria. *Medicine (Baltimore)* 1988;67:20–39.

Cupps TR, Moore PM, Fauci AS. Isolated angiitis of the central nervous system. Prospective diagnostic and therapeutic experience. *Am J Med* 1983;74:97–105.

Fountain NB, Lopes MBS. Control of primary angiitis of the CNS associated with cerebral amyloid angiopathy by cyclophosphamide alone. *Neurology* 1999;52:660–662.

Harris KG, Tran DD, Sickels WJ, et al. Diagnosing intracranial vasculitis: the roles of MR and angiography. *AJNR* 1994;15:317–330.

Riemer G, Lamszus K, Zschaber R, et al. Isolated angiitis of the central nervous system: lack of inflammation after long-term treatment. *Neurology* 1999;52:196–199.

Ropper AH, Ayata C, Adelman L. Vasculitis of the spinal cord. *Arch Neurol* 2003;60:1791–1794.

Scolding NJ, Wilson H, Hohlfield R, et al.; EFNS Cerebral Vasculitis Task Force. The recognition, diagnosis and management of cerebral vasculitis: a European survey. *Eur J Neurol* 2002;9:343–347.

Tamargo RJ, Connolly ES, McKhann GM, et al. Clinicopathological reviews: primary angiitis of the central nervous system in association with amyloid angiopathy. *Neurosurgery* 2003;53:136–141.

Wolfenden AB, Teng DC, Marks MP, et al. Angiographically defined primary angiitis of the CNS: is it really benign? *Neurology* 1998;51:183–185.

Younger DS, Hays AP, Brust JCM, et al. Granulomatous angiitis of the brain: an inflammatory reaction of diverse etiology. *Arch Neurol* 1988;45:514–518.

Systemic Lupus Erythematosus

Afeltra A, Garzia P, Mitterhofer AP, et al. Neuropsychiatric lupus syndromes: relationship with antiphospholipid antibodies. *Neurology* 2003;61:108–110.

Ainiala H, Loukkola MA, Peltola J, et al. The prevalence of neuropsychiatric syndromes in systemic lupus erythematosus. *Neurology* 2001;57:496–500.

Brey RL, Holliday SL, Saklad AR, et al. Neuropsychiatric syndromes in lupus: prevalence using standardized definitions. *Neurology* 2002;58:1214–1220.

Case records of the Massachusetts General Hospital. Case 24-1995. Mixed connective tissue disease. *N Engl J Med* 1995;333:369–377.

Devinsky O, Petito CK, Alonso DR. Clinical and neuropathological findings in systemic lupus erythematosus: the role of vasculitis, heart emboli, and thrombotic thrombocytopenic purpura. *Ann Neurol* 1988;23:380–384.

Friedman SD, Stidley CA, Brooks WM, et al. Brain injury and neurometabolic abnormalities in systemic lupus erythematosus. *Radiology* 1998;209:79–84.

Johnson RT, Richardson EP. The neurological manifestations of systemic lupus erythematosus. *Medicine (Baltimore)* 1968;47:337–369.

Levine SR, Brey RL. *Clinical Approach to Antiphospholipid Antibodies.* Boston: Butterworth-Heinemann, 2000.

Mitchell I, Hughes RAC, Maidey M, et al. Cerebral lupus. *Lancet* 1994;343:579–582.

Mukerji B, Hardin JG. Undifferentiated, overlapping, and mixed connective tissue diseases. *Am J Med Sci* 1993;305:114–119.

Penn AS, Rowan AJ. Myelopathy in systemic lupus erythematosus. *Arch Neurol* 1968;18:337–349.

Prockop LD. Myotonia, procaine amide, and lupus-like syndrome. *Arch Neurol* 1966;14:326–330.

Sanna G, Bertolaccini ML, Cuadrado MJ, et al. Neuropsychiatric manifestations in systemic lupus erythematosus: prevalence and association with antiphospholipid antibodies. *J Rheumatol* 2003;30:985–992.

Steinlin MI, Blaser SI, Gilday DL, et al. Neurologic manifestations of pediatric systemic lupus erythematosus. *Pediatr Neurol* 1995;13:191–197.

Trysberg E, Tarkowski A. Cerebral inflammation and degeneration in systemic lupus erythematosus. *Curr Opin Rheumatol* 2004 Sep;16(5):527–533.

Systemic Sclerosis (Scleroderma)

Bertinotti L, Bracci S, Nacci F, et al. The autonomic nervous system in systemic sclerosis. A review. *Clin Rheumatol* 2004;23(Feb);1–5.

Blaszczyk M, Krolicki L, Krasu M, et al. Progressive facial hemiatrophy: central nervous system atrophy and relationship with scleroderma en coup de sabre. *J Rheumatol* 2003;30:1997–2004.

Harris ML, Rosen A. Autoimmunity in scleroderma. *Curr Op Rheum* 2003;15:778–784.

Lin AT, Clements PJ, Furst DE. Update on disease-modifying antirheumatic drugs in the treatment of systemic sclerosis. *Rheum Dis Clinics No Am* 2003;29:409–426.

Poncelet AN, Connolly MK. Peripheral neuropathy in scleroderma. *Muscle Nerve* 2003;28:330–335.

Torabi AM, Patel RK, Wolfe GI, et al. Transverse myelitis in systemic sclerosis. *Arch Neurol* 2004;61:128–128.

Unterberger I, Trinka E, Engelhardt K, et al. Linear scleroderma "en coup de sabre" coexisting with plaque-morphea: neuroradiological manifestation and response to corticosteroids. *J Neurol Neurosurg Psychiatry* 2003;74:661–664.

Sjögren Syndrome and Sicca Complex

Alexander EL, Ranzenbach AJ, Kumar AJ, et al. Anti-Ro(SS-A) autoantibodies in central nervous system disease associated with Sjögren's syndrome (CNS-SS): clinical, neuroimaging, and angiographic correlates. *Neurology* 1994;44:899–908.

Gorson KC, Ropper AH. Positive salivary gland biopsy, Sjögren syndrome, and neuropathy: clinical implications. *Muscle Nerve* 2003;28:553–560.

Kassan SS, Moutsopoulos HM. Clinical manifestations and early diagnosis of Sjogren syndrome. *Arch Int Med* 2004;164:1275–1284.

Katz JS, Houroupian D, Ross MA. Multisystem neuronal involvement and sicca complex: broadening the spectrum of complications. *Muscle Nerve* 1999;22:404–407.

Lafitte C. Neurological manifestations in Sjögren's syndrome. *Arch Neurol* 2000;57:411–413.

Pericot I, Brieva L, Tintore M, et al. Myelopathy in seronegative Sjögren syndrome and/or primary progressive multiple sclerosis. *Multiple Sclerosis* 2003;9:256–259.

Vitali C, Bombardieri S, Moutsopoulos HM, et al. Preliminary criteria for the classification of Sjögren's syndrome. *Arthritis Rheum* 1993;36:340–347.

Wright RA, O'Duffy JD, Rodriguez M. Improvement of myelopathy in Sjögren's syndrome with chlorambucil and prednisone therapy. *Neurology* 1999;52:386–388.

Other Collagen-Vascular Diseases

Cogan DG. Syndrome of nonsyphilitic interstitial keratitis and vestibuloauditory symptoms. *Arch Ophthalmol* 1945;33:144–149.

Hilton DA, Footit D. Neuropathological findings in Sneddon's syndrome. *Neurology* 2003;60:1181–1182.

Kothare SV, Chu CC, VanLandingham K, et al. Migratory leptomeningeal inflammation with relapsing polychondritis. *Neurology* 1998;51:614–617.

Mikulowski P, Wolheim FA, Rotmil P, et al. Sudden death in rheumatoid arthritis with atlanto-axial dislocation. *Acta Med Scand* 1975;198:445–451.

Sundaran MBM, Rajput AH. Nervous system complications of relapsing polychondritis. *Neurology* 1983;33:513–515.

Vollersten RS, Conn DL, Ballard DJ, et al. Rheumatoid vasculitis: survival and associated risk factors. *Medicine (Baltimore)* 1986;65:365–374.

Chapter 156

Hypertrophic Pachymeningitis

John C. M. Brust

Hypertrophic pachymeningitis is an uncommon disorder in which the intracranial or spinal dura mater becomes locally or diffusely thickened and often adherent to the underlying leptomeninges. Inflammation may or may not be present, and etiologies include infections (syphilis, tuberculosis, fungi), autoimmune and vasculitic diseases (Wegener granulomatosis, sarcoidosis, rheumatoid arthritis, Behçet disease, Sjögren syndrome, giant cell arteritis), and malignancy (dural carcinomatosis, skull metastases, histiocytosis, lymphoma). Idiopathic hypertrophic pachymeningitis (IHP) is considered immunologic in origin, possibly part of a continuum that includes Tolosa-Hunt syndrome and orbital pseudotumor.

The most common symptoms of hypertrophic pachymeningitis are chronic headache and cranial neuropathies. Depending on the site of thickening, there may be compression of the optic nerve (which can progress to blindness), cranial nerves passing through the cavernous sinus, or, less often, lower cranial nerves. CNS symptoms include cerebellar ataxia, hemiparesis, altered mentation, seizures, and cervical myelopathy. Hypopituitarism and diabetes insipidus are described. Dural sinus compression can cause increased intracranial pressure or cerebral infarction. In IHP there is often an elevated erythrocyte sedimentation rate, and the CSF examination may reveal lymphocytic pleocytosis and increased protein content. MRI shows gadolinium enhancement that may be linear (resembling what is seen with spontaneous intracranial hypotension) or nodular, the latter involving especially the falx cerebri, the tentorium, and the cavernous sinus. Histopathologically, there is usually lymphocytic, plasma cell, and epithelioid cell infiltration with or without granulomas; vasculitis is rare.

IHP is a progressive disorder, but in most cases headache and neurologic dysfunction improve with high-dose oral corticosteroid therapy. Dural thickening can decrease with treatment, but MRI enhancement usually persists. Relapse may occur when treatment is interrupted, and alternative therapeutic strategies include a pulse intravenous corticosteroid regimen or treatment with methotrexate, azathiaprine, or cyclophosphamide. In some patients, surgical excision of thickened dura may be necessary to prevent irreversible neurologic damage.

SUGGESTED READINGS

Hatano N, Behari S, Nagatani T, et al. Idiopathic hypertrophic cranial pachymeningitis: clinicoradiological spectrum and therapeutic options. *Neurosurgery* 1999;45:1336–1344.

Kupersmith MJ, Martin V, Heller G, et al. Idiopathic hypertrophic pachymeningitis. *Neurology* 2004;62:686–694.

Voller B, Vass K, Wanschitz J, et al. Hypertrophic chronic pachymeningitis as a localized immune process in the craniocervical region. *Neurology* 2001;56:107–109.

Chapter 157

Neurologic Disease During Pregnancy

Alison M. Pack and Martha J. Morrell

Pregnancy and the postpartum period are times of major biologic and social changes. Pregnancy may be associated with alterations in pre-existing neurologic conditions, such as epilepsy or migraine, or herald the emergence of neurologic disorders such as peripheral nerve entrapment or a movement disorder. This chapter addresses the diagnosis, management, and treatment of neurologic disorders arising in or altered by pregnancy.

BIOLOGY OF PREGNANCY

Physiologic changes during pregnancy may influence the expression of neurologic disease and complicate management. Alterations in neuroactive steroid hormones may influence the phenotypic appearance of the disease. Changes in pharmacokinetics, medication compliance, and sleep patterns may make disease management more challenging.

The concentration and type of circulating steroid hormones change during pregnancy. Estrogen production increases. In the nonpregnant state, the main circulating estrogens are estradiol, which is synthesized by ovarian thecal cells, and estrone, which is produced by the extraglandular conversion of androstenedione. Estriol is a peripheral metabolite of estrone and estradiol. In pregnancy, the concentrations of all these estrogens, particularly estriol, increase. As pregnancy progresses, maternal steroids and dihydroisoandrostene from developing fetal adrenal glands are converted principally to estriol. Progesterone production also increases dramatically. These hormonal changes may affect neurologic conditions that are hormone responsive, including migraine, epilepsy, and multiple sclerosis.

Drug pharmacokinetics are affected by the physiologic changes of pregnancy (Table 157.1). Renal blood flow and glomerular filtration increase as a function of increased cardiac output. Plasma volume, extravascular fluid, and adipose tissue increase to create a larger volume of distribution. Serum albumin decreases, which reduces drug binding, increases the free fraction, and increases drug clearance. These pharmacokinetic alterations may affect

TABLE 157.1 Physiologic Changes During Pregnancy

Variable	Change
Extracellular volume	Increases 4–6 L
Plasma volume	Increases 40%
Renal blood flow	Increases 30%–50%
Glomerular filtration rate	Increases 30%–50%
Cardiac output	Increases 30%–50%
Serum albumin	Decreases 20%–30%

Adapted from Silberstein SD. Drug treatment and trials in women. In: Kaplan PW, ed. *Neurologic Disease in Women.* New York: Demos Medical Publishing, 1998:25–44.

drug concentrations and are most important for drugs that are highly protein bound, hepatically metabolized, or renally cleared.

Other events of pregnancy that may compromise management are hyperemesis gravidarum, sleep deprivation, and poor compliance. Hyperemesis gravidarum can make it difficult to maintain adequate concentrations of oral medications. Sleep deprivation aggravates many neurologic conditions and can be a particular problem in the third trimester. Compliance may deteriorate because of a woman's concern that taking medication might harm her baby. Women are often advised by friends, relatives, and even medical personnel to minimize fetal drug exposure. This may lead to skipped doses, reduced doses, or even self-discontinuation of an indicated medication.

EPILEPSY

Each year 20,000 women with epilepsy become pregnant. This number has grown as marriage rates have increased for women with epilepsy, as parenting has become more socially supported, and as the medical management of pregnancy in women with epilepsy has improved.

Seizure frequency may change during pregnancy. In women with preexisting epilepsy, 35% experience an increase in seizure frequency, 55% have no change, and 10% have fewer seizures. Changes responsible for this include changes in sex hormones, antiepileptic drug (AED) metabolism, sleep schedules, and medication compliance. AED concentrations may change. The total AED concentration falls because of an increase in volume of distribution, decreased drug absorption, and increased drug clearance. Although the total concentration decreases, the proportion of unbound or free drug increases because albumin levels and protein binding decline. Therefore, it is necessary to follow the nonprotein-bound drug concentrations for AEDs that are highly protein bound, including carbamazepine (Tegretol), phenytoin sodium (Dilantin), and sodium valproate (Depakene). Dose adjustments should maintain a stable non–protein-bound fraction.

Although lamotrigine (Lamictal) is not highly protein bound, its clearance markedly increases throughout pregnancy. Monitoring of this medication should be performed at least monthly and appropriate adjustments made.

The older AEDs (benzodiazepines, phenytoin, carbamazepine, phenobarbital, and valproate) are teratogenic in humans. Major malformations related to AED exposure include cleft lip and palate, cardiac defects (atrial septal defect, tetralogy of Fallot, ventricular septal defect, coarctation of the aorta, patent ductus arteriosus, and pulmonary stenosis) and urogenital defects. The incidence of major malformations in infants born to mothers with epilepsy taking the older AEDs is 4% to 6%, compared with 2% to 4% for the general population. Neural tube defects (spina bifida and anencephaly) occur in 0.5% to 1% of infants exposed to carbamazepine and 1% to 2% of infants exposed to valproate during the first month of gestation. Minor congenital anomalies associated with AED exposure include facial dysmorphism and digital anomalies, which arise in 6% to 20% of infants exposed to AEDs in utero. This is a twofold increase over the rate in the general population. However, these anomalies are usually subtle and may often be outgrown.

Since 1993, seven new AEDs have been introduced, with little information about effects on the developing fetus. The FDA classifies all of these medications as Category C, indicating that there are no adverse effects in animal studies, but with inadequate information in pregnant women.

A prospective U.S.-based registry gathers information about pregnancy and fetal outcome in women using AEDs (Table 157.2). The registry should be contacted regarding any woman who becomes pregnant while taking AEDs (1-888-233-2334). A European registry includes countries throughout Europe, Asia, and the continent of Australia and prospectively records information about the effects of AEDs as monotherapy on the developing fetus.

Polytherapy is an independent risk factor for teratogenicity. Rates of major malformations are elevated in children exposed to multiple AEDs. A prospective study of pregnant women who took AEDs found that the rate of teratogenicity was higher in children whose mothers took more than one AED.

Several mechanisms have been postulated to explain the teratogenicity of AEDs. Some AEDs may be teratogenic because of free radical intermediates that bind with RNA and disrupt DNA synthesis and organogenesis. Higher concentrations of oxide metabolites increase the risk of fetal malformations. Some AEDs cause folic acid deficiency, which is associated with higher occurrence and recurrence rates of neural tube defects. The AAN and the American College of Obstetric and Gynecologic Physicians (1996) recommend that all women of childbearing age taking AEDs should receive folic acid supplementation of 0.4 to 5.0 mg per day.

In addition to teratogenicity of AEDs, there is growing concern about the impact of AED exposure on neurodevelopment. Retrospective and small prospective studies suggest a negative effect of valproate; children whose mothers took valproate have lower scores on neuropsychologic tests and have more special needs. These studies are limited by retrospective design, size, and inability to control for confounding variables. Larger prospective studies are underway to better identify whether AED exposure affects neurodevelopmental outcome and if certain AEDs have a better profile than others.

Management of epilepsy in women of reproductive age should focus on maintaining effective control of seizures while minimizing fetal exposure to AEDs. This applies to dosage and to number of AEDs. Medication reduction or substitution should be achieved prior to conception. When possible, a long-acting formulation of an AED (e.g., carbamazepine, valproate) should be used to avoid the peak doses seen with shorter-acting AEDs. Altering medication during pregnancy increases the risk of breakthrough seizures and exposes the fetus to an additional AED. The recommended AED management in pregnancy is monotherapy at the lowest effective dose. The drug of choice is the one most likely to be effective and well tolerated. Current information is not sufficient to identify a particular AED as favored in pregnancy. If there is a family history of neural tube defects, an agent other than carbamazepine or valproate might be considered.

Once a woman is pregnant, prenatal diagnostic testing includes a maternal serum α-fetoprotein and a level II (anatomic) ultrasound at 14 to 18 weeks. This combination will identify more than 95% of infants with neural tube defects. In some instances, amniocentesis may be indicated.

AEDs have also been associated with an increased risk for early fetal hemorrhage. This may be owing to an AED-related vitamin K deficiency. Therefore, the AAN recommends vitamin K supplementation (vitamin K_1 at 10 mg/day) for the last month of gestation.

For pregnant women with new-onset seizures, the diagnostic strategy is similar to that for any patient with

▶ **TABLE 157.2 North American Antiepileptic Drug Pregnancy Registry**

This is a prospective registry to gather information on pregnancy and fetal outcome from pregnancies in which the mother has used an antiepileptic drug. Women should contact the registry directly; they will receive information and be requested to provide informed consent.
Genetics and Teratology Unit
14CNY-MGH East
Room 5022A
Charlestown, MA 02129–2000
Telephone: 1-888-233-2334
Web site: neuro-www2.mgh.harvard.edu/aed/registry.nclk

a first-time seizure. The neurologic history and examination can be directed to signs of a specific cause, such as acute intracranial hemorrhage or CNS infection. The evaluation should also screen for hypertension, proteinuria, and edema to exclude eclampsia. Follow-up studies include serologic tests for syphilis and HIV, EEG, and MRI, which is the preferred imaging technique for pregnant women. As in nonpregnant women with a first-time seizure, treatment depends on seizure type and cause.

PRE-ECLAMPSIA AND ECLAMPSIA

Pre-eclampsia and eclampsia are most often seen in young primigravida women and in multiparous women with a change in partner. Pre-eclampsia is a multisystem disorder that is diagnosed clinically by hypertension, proteinuria, and edema. Pre-eclampsia is associated with hepatic and coagulation abnormalities, hypoalbuminemia, increased urate levels, and hemoconcentration. Eclampsia is manifested by seizures, cerebral bleeding, and death. The incidence in Europe and other developed countries is 1 per 2,000. In developing countries, the incidence varies from 1 in 100 to 1 in 1,700. Worldwide, eclampsia probably accounts for 50,000 deaths annually. The main cause of death is pulmonary edema.

Neurologic abnormalities associated with eclampsia include confusion, seizures, cortical blindness, visual-field defects, headaches, and blurred vision. Seizures are most often generalized but may be partial. Cortical blindness and visual-field defects may occur with bilateral occipital lobe involvement.

The differential diagnosis of eclampsia includes subarachnoid hemorrhage and cerebral venous thrombosis. The diagnosis is established by increased blood pressure plus proteinuria, edema, or both. A significant increase in blood pressure is defined as an increase of >15 mm Hg diastolic or 30 mm Hg systolic above baseline measurements obtained before or early in pregnancy. If no early reading is available, a blood pressure of 140/90 mm Hg or higher in late pregnancy is significant.

Neuroimaging, EEG, CSF analysis, and angiography may help in diagnosis. CT is usually normal in eclampsia but may show hypodense regions in areas of cerebral edema. MRI permits better detection of edema in the cortical mantle. During an eclamptic convulsion, the EEG shows spike-and-wave discharges. The CSF is usually normal in preeclampsia. In eclampsia, the CSF protein content is often moderately elevated, and the pressure may be increased. In some patients, angiography shows arterial spasm.

Pathologic examination of eclamptic brains reveals petechial hemorrhages in cortical and subcortical patches. Microscopically, these petechial hemorrhages are ring hemorrhages about capillaries and precapillaries occluded by fibrinoid material. Areas that are predisposed include the parietooccipital and occipital regions.

The most accepted treatment of eclampsia is delivery of the fetus, if possible. Hypertension should be treated with antihypertensive agents. Presently, magnesium sulfate is the first-line treatment for the prevention and treatment of eclamptic seizures. Randomized trials have compared magnesium sulfate and other agents including phenytoin and diazepam, and the results suggest that magnesium sulfate is the agent of choice. An international randomized placebo-controlled trial (MAGPIE trial) compared the use of magnesium sulfate and placebo; magnesium sulfate halved the risk of eclampsia and probably reduced the risk of maternal death. There were no substantive harmful effects to mother or baby in the short-term.

STROKE

Pregnancy is a risk factor for stroke, and the postpartum period is the most vulnerable time. Factors that increase the risk for stroke include pregnancy-related hypertension and cesarean delivery. Presumptive mechanisms include changes in the coagulation and fibrinolytic systems leading to a hypercoagulable state and an increase in viscosity and stasis, which can promote thrombosis. In the postpartum period, the large decrease in blood volume at childbirth, rapid changes in hormone status that alter hemodynamics and coagulation, and the strain of delivery may predispose to a stroke.

Arterial occlusion causes 50% to 80% of ischemic strokes in pregnant women. Cerebral venous thrombosis is the next most common cause. Arterial occlusion occurs primarily in the second and third trimesters, whereas venous thrombosis most often occurs in the postpartum period. Arterial strokes are generally a consequence of identifiable risk factors, including premature atherosclerosis, moyamoya disease, Takayasu arteritis, fibromuscular dysplasia, and primary CNS vasculitis. Hematologic disorders can play an etiologic role in arterial and venous strokes. Such disorders include sickle-cell disease, antiphospholipid syndrome, thrombotic thrombocytopenic purpura, hyperhomocysteinemia, mutations in prothrombin gene, and deficiencies in antithrombin III, protein C, protein S, and factor V Leiden. Other causes are cardiogenic and paradoxic emboli.

The key to early diagnosis is prompt neuroimaging. Typically, CT is obtained first, but if this is negative and clinical suspicion is high, additional studies should be performed, including MRI and cerebral angiography. Treatment of strokes in pregnancy is directed to the specific cause. Heparin does not cross the placenta and is the anticoagulant of choice in pregnancy. However, long-term use (>1 month) is associated with osteoporosis and thrombocytopenia. Warfarin (Coumadin) crosses the placenta and is a known teratogen. It is therefore recommended only for women who cannot tolerate heparin or who have recurrent thromboembolic events. Aspirin complications in pregnancy include teratogenic effects and bleeding in the neonate. However, low-dose aspirin (less than 150 mg) is safe in the second and third trimesters, with no increase in maternal or neonatal adverse effects. Use of low-molecular-weight heparin is safe, and many advocate its use over heparin. Like heparin, low-molecular-weight heparin does not cross the placenta. The risk of bleeding with these compounds is small, and the development of osteoporosis or thrombocytopenia is less likely.

CEREBRAL HEMORRHAGE

The risk of cerebral hemorrhage increases in pregnancy. Cerebral hemorrhage occurs in 1 to 5 pregnancies per 10,000, with an associated mortality of 30% to 40%. Factors that predispose to hemorrhage include physiologic changes of pregnancy such as hypertension, high concentrations of estrogens causing arterial dilation, and increases in cardiac output, blood volume, and venous pressure. Pregnancy-related conditions also increase the risk of hemorrhage. These include eclampsia, metastatic choriocarcinoma, cerebral emboli, and coagulopathies.

Subarachnoid hemorrhage accounts for 50% of all intracranial bleeding in pregnancy and carries a high mortality. Cerebral aneurysms and arteriovenous malformations cause most subarachnoid hemorrhages in pregnancy. Other causes include eclampsia, cocaine use, coagulopathies, ectopic endometriosis, moyamoya disease, and choriocarcinoma. Aneurysmal bleeding usually occurs in older patients in the second and third trimesters. In contrast, hemorrhages from arteriovenous malformations occur in younger women throughout gestation, with the highest risk during labor and the puerperium.

The diagnosis and treatment of subarachnoid hemorrhage and intracerebral hemorrhage in pregnant women are similar to those in nonpregnant patients. Subarachnoid hemorrhage is diagnosed by clinical manifestations and CT. If brain CT is normal and the clinical signs are consistent with intracranial hemorrhage, lumbar puncture should be performed. Once intracranial hemorrhage is detected, follow-up studies include MRI and four-vessel angiography. Noncontrast CT is also the most sensitive means of diagnosing intracerebral hemorrhage. Treatment of these conditions is directed to supporting the mother and fetus and preventing complications. Blood pressure should be carefully monitored, and fetal monitoring is indicated. The specific treatment depends on the etiology of the hemorrhage.

MULTIPLE SCLEROSIS (MS)

MS affects 1 in 10,000 people in Western countries, primarily women in the childbearing years. Prospective studies and other surveys find that the rate of relapse decreases in pregnancy, especially in the third trimester, and increases in the first 3 months postpartum. Long-term disability is not affected. In addition, the outcome of the pregnancy itself is not affected by MS.

The mechanisms responsible for the change in the rate of relapses include humoral and immunologic changes, as seen also in pregnant women with other autoimmune diseases such as rheumatoid arthritis or systemic lupus erythematosus. There is no correlation of relapse rate with the physical stress of childbirth and caring for the newborn, sleep deprivation, type and dose of anesthesia, breastfeeding, or socioeconomic factors.

Many women with relapsing-remitting MS are treated with interferon beta-1b (Betaseron), interferon beta-1a (Avonex), or glatiramer acetate (Copaxone). None of these has been tested formally in pregnant women, and discontinuation of these agents is recommended. In addition, there have been no controlled trials addressing the safety of medication for MS relapses. If a severe relapse does occur with pregnancy, a short course of corticosteroid therapy is recommended. However, neonatal adrenal suppression may follow maternal corticosteroid use, and large prenatal doses in animals caused growth retardation and compromised development of the CNS.

MIGRAINE

Migraine is diagnosed in 18% of women of childbearing years, and 60% to 80% of migraine headaches improve during pregnancy, especially for migraines without aura. Women who had migraine onset at menarche or who have had menstrual migraines are more likely to experience improvement, especially in the first or second trimester. Higher levels of estrogen are probably responsible for this improvement during pregnancy. The subsequent fall in estrogen levels may cause postpartum headaches. It is not known why migraine sometimes starts or becomes worse in pregnancy.

Migraines may also arise during pregnancy. Studies suggest these headaches are more likely to be with aura. If migraine arises in pregnancy, the differential diagnosis must be considered. A new-onset migraine with aura can be a symptom of vasculitis, brain tumor, or occipital arteriovenous malformation. Subarachnoid hemorrhage can cause headache any time during pregnancy or delivery. Other disorders with headache include stroke, cerebral venous thrombosis, eclampsia, pituitary tumor, and choriocarcinoma.

Medication use during pregnancy should be limited. If necessary, acetaminophen, nonsteroidal anti-inflammatory drugs, codeine, or other narcotics may be used; low-dose aspirin may also be given. Antiemetics such as metoclopramide or prochlorperazine may relieve the headache and associated nausea and vomiting. These agents are generally safe and effective. Ergotamine and dihydroergotamine mesylate (DHE 45) should be avoided. The triptans are effective and widely used for the treatment of headache. Limited information is available regarding teratogenic effects. Sumatriptan has been available the longest and is the most widely used. A large increase in birth defects has not been identified with sumatriptan use, but information is insufficient to rule out small increases in birth defects. Therefore, the use of triptans should be approached with caution in pregnancy. For someone with recurrent headaches, a beta-adrenergic blocker, such as propanolol, may be used prophylactically. However, adverse effects including intrauterine growth retardation have been reported with β-adrenergic blockers. Therefore, the choice of medication for migraine in pregnant women should balance the mother's comfort with the least fetal risk.

NEOPLASMS

Brain tumors rarely become symptomatic during pregnancy. The types of tumors arising in pregnancy differ from those in nonpregnant women. Glioma is the most common, followed by meningioma, acoustic neuroma, and then a variety of other tumors, including pituitary tumors. Tumor growth may be exacerbated by pregnancy, especially meningioma. Possible mechanisms include increased blood volume, fluid retention, and stimulation of tumor growth by hormones.

Systemic cancer is unusual in young women and rarely begins during pregnancy. Choriocarcinoma is the only systemic tumor specifically associated with pregnancy. Brain metastases are common in choriocarcinoma; among patients diagnosed with choriocarcinoma, 3% to 20% have brain disease at diagnosis.

Cerebral neoplasms cause headaches, seizures, focal signs, or symptoms of increased intracranial pressure. The seizures may be partial or generalized. Nausea and vomiting in the first trimester can be confused with morning sickness. All women suspected of having a brain tumor should be examined with MRI.

NEUROPATHIES

Women are at an increased risk for peripheral neuropathy during pregnancy and the puerperium. Backache or poorly localized paresthesia is common. At least 50% of pregnant women have back pain. Among the specific rare neuropathies that occur with a higher incidence during pregnancy are carpal tunnel syndrome, facial nerve palsy, meralgia paresthetica, and chronic inflammatory demyelinating polyneuropathy (CIDP).

Carpal tunnel syndrome is the most frequent neuropathy of pregnancy. It usually begins in the third trimester and disappears after delivery; it is attributed to generalized edema. *Bell palsy* appears with a slightly higher frequency during pregnancy, mostly in the third trimester. Prognosis for recovery is excellent and is similar to that in nonpregnant women. Treatment is symptomatic, including protection of the eye. *Meralgia paresthetica*, a sensory neuropathy of the lateral femoral cutaneous nerve of the thigh, is attributed to compression of the nerve under the lateral part of the inguinal ligament. Swelling during pregnancy, increased body weight, and increased lordosis during pregnancy are possible causes. Numbness, burning, tingling, or pain in the lateral thigh suggests the diagnosis. A local anesthetic with or without steroids is usually all that is necessary. Most women improve in the postpartum period. The incidence of *CIDP* is slightly higher during pregnancy. As in nonpregnant women, treatment includes plasmapheresis, IVIG, or steroids.

MYASTHENIA GRAVIS (MG)

Symptoms of MG may increase, improve, or be unchanged during menstruation, pregnancy, or the puerperium. A study of 31 pregnancies in women who were taking therapy before and during conception revealed that 39% had marked improvement, 42% remained unchanged, and 19% worsened.

Treatment of myasthenia during pregnancy includes immunosuppressant drugs, plasmapheresis, and IVIG. Anticholinesterase drugs are also reportedly safe. Thymectomy is deferred until long after delivery. The long-term outcome of MG is not affected by pregnancy. (Myasthenia is also discussed in Chapter 121.)

Neonatal MG affects 12% to 20% of infants born to mothers with MG. The occurrence of neonatal myasthenia gravis does not correlate with maternal disease severity or titer of maternal anticholinesterase receptor antibodies. The symptoms clear within a few weeks.

MOVEMENT DISORDERS

Movement disorders are unusual in young women, but those that specifically occur during pregnancy include the restless leg syndrome, chorea, and drug-induced movement disorders.

The *restless leg syndrome* is probably the most common movement disorder of pregnancy. It is characterized by a crawling, burning, or aching sensation in the calves with an irresistible urge to move the legs. It occurs in 10% to 20% of pregnant women. Iron deficiency has been found in patients with restless leg syndrome, and treatment of iron deficiency in pregnant women has been advocated, but therapeutic trials have yet not been performed. Also, lower folate levels are associated with the restless leg syndrome; and treatment recommendations include folate supplementation. Other treatments include massage, flexion and extension, walking, benzodiazepines, opiates, or levodopa.

Chorea gravidarum occurs in pregnancy (Chapter 110). Treatment is reserved for those with violent and disabling chorea and includes haloperidol or benzodiazepines.

Drugs that block dopamine receptors are often used to treat the nausea and vomiting of pregnancy. These drugs can cause new-onset chorea, tremor, dystonia, or parkinsonism. *Idiopathic Parkinson disease* is uncommon in women younger than 40 years. More common is secondary parkinsonism caused by medication or toxins. There is no definite evidence that Parkinson disease worsens during pregnancy, and there is little information about the toxicity of antiparkinson medications. Successful pregnancies have been reported in women taking levodopa.

SUGGESTED READINGS

Biology of Pregnancy

Harris RZ, Benet LZ, Schwartz JB. Gender effects in pharmacokinetics and pharmacodynamics. *Drugs* 1995;50:222–239.

Neuroendocrinology. In: Speroff L, Glass RH, Kase NG, eds. *Clinical Gynecologic Endocrinology and Fertility*. Baltimore: Williams & Wilkins, 1994:141–182.

Silberstein SD. Drug treatment and trials in women. In: Kaplan PW, ed. *Neurologic Disease in Women*. New York: Demos Medical Publishing, 1998:25–44.

Epilepsy

Adab N, Jacoby A, Smith D, et al. Additional educational needs in children born to mothers with epilepsy. *J Neurol Psychiatry* 2001;70:15–21.

American College of Obstetric and Gynecologic Physicians. Seizure disorders in pregnancy. *ACOG Physicians Educ Bull* 1996;231:1–13.

American Academy of Neurology. Quality Standards Subcommittee. Practice parameter: management issues for women with epilepsy (summary statement). *Neurology* 1998;51:944–8.

Brown JE, Jacobs DR, Hartman TJ, et al. Predictors of red cell folate level in women attempting pregnancy. *JAMA* 1997;277:548–552.

Buehler BA, Delimont D, Van Waes M, et al. Prenatal prediction of risk of the fetal hydantoin syndrome. *N Engl J Med* 1990;322:1567–1572.

Cornelissen M, Steegers-Theunissen R, Kollee L, et al. Increased incidence of neonatal vitamin K deficiency resulting from maternal anticonvulsant therapy. *Am J Obstet Gynecol* 1993;168:923–928.

Czeizel AE, Dudas I. Prevention of the first occurrence of neural-tube defects by periconceptional vitamin supplementation. *N Engl J Med* 1992;327:1832–1835.

Daly LE, Kirke PN, Molloy A, et al. Folate levels and neural tube defects: implications for treatment. *JAMA* 1995;274:1698–1702.

Dansky L, Andermann E, Roseblatt D, et al. Anticonvulsants, folate levels, and pregnancy outcome. *Ann Neurol* 1987;21:176–182.

Finnell RH, Buehler BA, Kerr BM, et al. Clinical and experimental studies linking oxidative metabolism to phenytoin-induced teratogenesis. *Neurology* 1992;42:25–31.

Gaily E, Granstrom ML. Minor anomalies in children of mothers with epilepsy. *Neurology* 1992;42(Suppl 5):128–131.

Gaily E, Kantola-Sorsa E, Hilesmaa V, et al. Normal intelligence in children with prenatal exposure to carbamazepine. *Neurology* 2004;62:28–32.

Gordon N. Folate metabolism and neural tube defects. *Brain Dev* 1995;17:307–311.

Holmes LB, Harvey EA, Coull BA, et al. The teratogenicity of anticonvulsant drugs. *N Engl J Med* 2001;344:1132–1138.

Kaneko S, Otani K, Fukushima Y, et al. Teratogenicity of antiepilepsy drugs: analysis of possible risk factors. *Epilepsia* 1988;29:459–467.

Koch S, Loesche G, Jager-Roman E, et al. Major birth malformations and antiepileptic drugs. *Neurology* 1992;42(Suppl 5):83–88.

Laurence KM, James N, Miller MH, et al. Double-blind, randomised controlled trial of folate before conception to prevent the recurrence of neural tube defects. *BMJ* 1981;282:1509–1511.

Meischenguiser R, D'Giano CH, Ferraro SM. Major malformations in offspring of women with epilepsy. *Neurology* 2003;60:575–579.

Milunsky A, Jick H, Jick SS, et al. Multivitamin/folic acid supplementation in early pregnancy reduces the prevalence of neural tube defects. *JAMA* 1988;262:2847–2852.

Morrell MJ. Seizures and epilepsy in women. In: Kaplan PW, ed. *Neurologic Disease in Women*. New York: Demos Medical Publishing, 1998:189–206.

Mulinare J, Cordero JF, Erickson JD, et al. Periconceptional use of multivitamins and the occurrence of neural tube defects. *JAMA* 1988;260:3141–3145.

Ogawa Y, Kaneko S, Otani K, et al. Serum folic acid levels in epileptic mothers and their relationship to congenital malformations. *Epilepsy Res* 1991;8:75–78.

Omtzigt JGC, Los FJ, Grobee DE, et al. The risk of spina bifida aperta after first-trimester exposure to valproate in a prenatal cohort. *Neurology* 1992;42(Suppl 5):119–125.

Pennell P. Antiepileptic drug pharmacokinetics during pregnancy and lactation. *Neurology* 2003;61:S35–S42.

Prevention of neural tube defects: results of the Medical Research Council Vitamin Study. MRC Vitamin Study Research Group. *Lancet* 1991;338:131–137.

Recommendations for the use of folic acid to reduce the number of cases of spina bifida and other neural tube defects. *MMWR Recomm Rep* 1992;41:1–7.

Richmond JR, Krishnamoorthy P, Andermann E, et al. Epilepsy and pregnancy: an obstetric perspective. *Am J Obstet Gynecol* 2004;190:371–379.

Rosa FW. Spina bifida in infants of women treated with carbamazepine during pregnancy. *N Engl J Med* 1991;324:674–677.

Sabers A, Dam M, A-Rogvi-Hansen B, et al. Epilepsy and pregnancy: lamotrigine as main drug used. *Acta Neurol Scand* 2004;109(Jan):9–13.

Schmidt D, Beck Mannagetta G, Janz D, et al. The effect of pregnancy on the course of epilepsy: a prospective study. In: Janz D, Dam M, Richens A, eds. *Epilepsy, Pregnancy, and the Child*. New York: Raven, 1982:39–49.

Strickler SM, Dansky LV, Miller MA, et al. Genetic predisposition to phenytoin-induced birth defects. *Lancet* 1985;2:746–749.

Thorp JA, Gaston L, Caspers DR, et al. Current concepts and controversies in the use of vitamin K. *Drugs* 1995;49:376–387.

Tomson T, Lindbom U, Ekqvist B, et al. Disposition of carbamazepine and phenytoin in pregnancy. *Epilepsia* 1994;35:131–135.

Tomson T, Lindbom U, Sundqvist A, et al. Red cell folate levels in pregnant epileptic women. *Eur J Clin Pharmacol* 1995;48:305–308.

Vadja FJ, O'brien TJ, Hitchock A, et al. The Australian registry of antiepileptic drugs in pregnancy: experience after 30 months. *J Clin Neurosci* 2003;10:543–549.

Van Allen M, Fraser FC, Dallaire L, et al. Recommendations on the use of folic acid supplementation to prevent the occurrence of neural tube defects. *Can Med Assoc J* 1993;149:1239–1243.

Wegner C, Nau H. Alteration of embryonic folate metabolism by valproic acid during organogenesis: implications for the mechanism of teratogenesis. *Neurology* 1992;42(Suppl 5):17–24.

Werler MM, Shapiro S, Mitchell AA. Periconceptional folic acid exposure and the risk of occurrent neural tube defects. *JAMA* 1993;269:1257–1261.

Yerby M. Management issues for women with epilepsy. *Neurology* 2003;61:S23–S26.

Yerby MS, Friel PN, McCormick K. Pharmacokinetics of anticonvulsants in pregnancy: alterations in protein binding. *Epilepsy Res* 1990;5:223–228.

Zahn CA, Morrell MJ, Collins SD, et al. Management issues for women with epilepsy: a review of the literature. American Academy of Neurology Practice Guidelines. *Neurology* 1998;51:949–56.

Preeclampsia and Eclampsia

Burrows RF, Burrows EA. The feasibility of a control population for a randomized control trial of seizure prophylaxis in the hypertensive disorders of pregnancy. *Am J Obstet Gynecol* 1995;173:929–935.

Dayicioglu V, Sahinoglu Z, Kol E, et al. The use of standard dose of magnesium sulphate in prophylaxis of eclamptic seizures: do body mass index alterations have any effect on success? *Hypertens Pregnancy* 2003;22(3):257–265.

Donaldson JO. Eclampsia. In: Devinsky O, Feldmann E, Hainline B, eds. *Neurological Complications of Pregnancy.* New York: Raven, 1994:25–33.

Hutton JD, James DK, Stirrat GM, et al. Management of severe preeclampsia and eclampsia by UK consultants. *Br J Obstet Gynaecol* 1992;99:554–556.

Lenfant C, Gifford RW, Zuspan FP. Report of the National High Blood Pressure Education Program working group on high blood pressure in pregnancy. *Am J Obstet Gynecol* 1990;163:1691–1712.

Lucas MJ, Leveno KJ, Cunningham FG. A comparison of magnesium sulfate with phenytoin for the prevention of eclampsia. *N Engl J Med* 1995;333:201–205.

Magpie Trial Collaborative Group. Do women with pre-eclampsia, and their babies, benefit from magnesium sulfate? The Magpie Trial: a randomised placebo-controlled trial. *Lancet* 2002;359:1877–1890.

Paternoster DM, Fantinato S, Manganelli F, Nicolini U, Milani M, Girolami A. Recent progress in the therapeutic management of preeclampsia. *Expert Opin Pharmacother* 2004 Nov;5(11):2233–2239.

Repke JT, Friedman SA, Kaplan PW. Prophylaxis of eclamptic seizures: current controversies. *Clin Obstet Gynecol* 1992;35:365–374.

Roberts JM, Redman CWG. Pre-eclampsia: more than pregnancy-induced hypertension. *Lancet* 1993;341:1447–1451.

Sibai BM, Spinnato JA, Watson DL, et al. Eclampsia. IV. Neurological findings and future outcome. *Am J Obstet Gynecol* 1985;152:184–192.

Thomas SV, Somanathan N, Radhakumari R. Interictal EEG changes in eclampsia. *Electroencephalogr Clin Neurophysiol* 1995;94:271–275.

Which anticonvulsant for women with eclampsia? Evidence from the Collaborative Eclampsia Trial. *Lancet* 1995;345:1455–1463. Erratum in: *Lancet* 1995;346:258.

Stroke

Cross JN, Castro PO, Jennett WB. Cerebral strokes associated with pregnancy and the puerperium. *BMJ* 1968;3:214–218.

Gilmore J, Pennell PB, Stern BJ. Medication use during pregnancy for neurologic conditions. *Neurol Clin* 1998;16:189–206.

Jaigobin C, Silver FL. Stroke and pregnancy. *Stroke* 2000;31:2984–2951.

Kittner SJ, Stern BJ, Feeser BR, et al. Pregnancy and the risk of stroke. *N Engl J Med* 1996;335:768–774.

Lamy C, Hamon JB, Coste J, et al., for the French Study Group on Stroke in Pregnancy. Ischemic stroke in young women: Risk of recurrence during subsequent pregnancies. *Neurology* 2000;55:269–274.

Lanska DJ, Kryscio RJ. Risk factors for peripartum and postpartum stroke and intracranial venous thrombosis. *Stroke* 2000;31:1274–1282.

Lanska DJ, Kryscio RJ. Stroke and intracranial venous thrombosis during pregnancy and the puerperium. *Neurology* 1998;51:1622–1628.

Lepercq J, Conard J, Borel-Derlon A, et al. Venous thrombolism during pregnancy: a retrospective study of enoxaparin safety in 624 pregnancies. *BJOG* 2001;108:1134–40.

Mabie WC, DiSessa TG, Crocker LG, Sibai BM, Arheart KL. A longitudinal study of cardiac output in normal human pregnancy. *Am J Obstet Gynecol* 1994;170:849–856.

Mas JL, Lamy C. Stroke in pregnancy and the puerperium. *J Neurol* 1998;245:305–313.

Sephton V, Farquharson RG, Topping J, et al. A longitudinal study of maternal dose response to low molecular weight heparin in pregnancy. *Obstet Gynecol* 2003;101:1307–1311.

Sharshar T, Lamy C, Mas JL. Incidence and cause of strokes associated with pregnancy and the puerperium: a study in public hospitals of Ile de France. Stroke in Pregnancy Study Group. *Stroke* 1995;26:930–936.

Simolke GA, Cox SM, Cunningham FG. Cerebrovascular accidents complicating pregnancy and the puerperium. *Obstet Gynecol* 1991;78:37–42.

Srinivasan K. Cerebral venous thrombosis in pregnancy and the puerperium: a study of 135 patients. *Angiology* 1983;34:731–746.

Turan TN, Stern BJ. Stroke in pregnancy. *Neurol Clin* 2004; Nov;22(4):821–840.

Wiebers D. Ischemic cerebrovascular complications of pregnancy. *Arch Neurol* 1985;42:1106–1113.

Wiebers DO, Whisnant JP. The incidence of stroke among pregnant women in Rochester, Minn, 1955 through 1979. *JAMA* 1985;254:3055–3057.

Wilterdink JL, Feldmann E. Cerebral ischemia. In: Devinsky O, Feldmann E, Hainline B, eds. *Neurological Complications of Pregnancy.* New York: Raven, 1994:1–11.

Witlin AG, Matter F, Sibai BM. Postpartum stroke: a twenty-year experience. *Am J Obstet Gynecol* 2000;183:83–88.

Headache

Bousser MG, Ratinahirana H, Darbois X. Migraine and pregnancy: a prospective study in 703 women after delivery [Abstract]. *Neurology* 1990;40:437.

Callaghan N. The migraine syndrome in pregnancy. *Neurology* 1968;18:197–201.

Chanceller MD, Wroe SJ. Migraine occurring for the first time during pregnancy. *Headache* 1990;30:224–227.

Granella F, Sances G, Zanferrari C, et al. Migraine without aura and reproductive life events: a clinical epidemiological study in 1,300 women. *Headache* 1993;33:385–389.

Lance JW, Anthony M. Some clinical aspects of migraine: a prospective study of 500 patients. *Arch Neurol* 1966;15:356–361.

Loder E. Safety of sumatriptan in pregnancy: a review of the data so far. *CNS Drugs* 2003;17(1):1–7.

Nappi G, Sandrini G, Sances G. Tolerability of the triptans: clinical implications. *Drug Saf* 2003;26(2):93–107.

Sances G, Granella F, Nappi RE, et al. Course of migraine during pregnancy and postpartum: a prospective study. *Cephalgia* 2003;23:197–205.

Scharff L, Marcus DA, Turk DC. Headache during pregnancy and in the postpartum: a prospective study. *Headache* 1997;37:203–210.

Silberstein S. Migraine and pregnancy. *Neurol Clin* 1997;15:209–231.

Silberstein SD. Migraine and pregnancy. *J SGOC* 2000;22:700–707.

Somerville B. A study of migraine in pregnancy. *Neurology* 1972;22:824–828.

Stein GS. Headaches in the first post-partum week and their relationships to migraine. *Headache* 1981;21:201–205.

Welch KMA. Migraine and pregnancy. In: Devinsky O, Feldmann E, Hainline B, eds. *Neurological Complications of Pregnancy.* New York: Raven, 1994:77–82.

Welch KM, Darnley D, Simkins RT. The role of estrogen in migraine: a review and hypothesis. *Cephalalgia* 1984;4:227–236.

Cerebral Hemorrhage

Sharshar T, Lamy C, Mas JL. Incidence and causes of stroke associated with pregnancy and puerperium: a study in public hospitals of Ile de France. Stroke in Pregnancy Study Group. *Stroke* 1995;25:930–936.

Wiebers DO, Whisnant JP. The incidence of stroke among pregnant women in Rochester, Minn, 1955 through 1979. *JAMA* 1985;254:3055–3057.

Wilterdink JL, Feldmann E.Cerebral hemorrhage. In: Devinsky O, Feldmann E, Hainline B, eds. *Neurological Complications of Pregnancy.* New York: Raven, 1994:13–23.

Wong C, Guiliani M, Haley E. Cerebrovascular disease and stroke in women. *Cardiology* 1990;77(Suppl 2):80–90.

Multiple Sclerosis

Abramsky O. Pregnancy and multiple sclerosis. *Ann Neurol* 1994; 36(Suppl):S39–S41.

Bernardi S, Grasso MG, Bertollini R, et al. The influence of pregnancy on relapses in multiple sclerosis: a cohort study. *Acta Neurol Scand* 1991;84:403–406.

Birk K, Ford C, Smeltzer S, et al. The clinical course of multiple sclerosis during pregnancy and the puerperium. *Arch Neurol* 1990;47:738–742.

Birk K, Rudick R. Pregnancy and multiple sclerosis. *Arch Neurol* 1986;43:719–726.

Confavreux C, Hutchinson M, Hours MM, et al. Rate of pregnancy-related relapse in multiple sclerosis. Pregnancy in Multiple Sclerosis Group. *N Engl J Med* 1998;339:285–291.

Cook SD, Troiano R, Bansil S, et al.Multiple sclerosis and pregnancy. In: Devinsky O, Feldmann E, Hainline B, eds. *Neurological Complications of Pregnancy.* New York: Raven, 1994:139–152.

Douglass LH, Jorgensen CL. Pregnancy and multiple sclerosis. *Am J Obstet Gynecol* 1948;55:332–336.

Frith JA, McLeod JG. Pregnancy and multiple sclerosis. *J Neurol Neurosurg Psychiatry* 1988;51:495–498.

Ghezzi A, Caputo D. Pregnancy: a factor influencing the course of multiple sclerosis? *Eur Neurol* 1981;20:115–117.

Hughes MD. Multiple sclerosis and pregnancy. *Neurol Clin* 2004 Nov; 22(4):757–769.

Hutchinson M. Pregnancy in multiple sclerosis. *J Neurol Neurosurg Psychiatry* 1993;56:1043–1045.

Korn-Lubetzki I, Kahana E, Cooper G, et al. Activity of multiple sclerosis during pregnancy and the puerperium. *Ann Neurol* 1984;16:229–231.

Lorenzi AR, Ford HL. Multiple sclerosis and pregnancy. *Postgrad Med* 2002;78:460–464.

Millar JHD, Allison RS, Cheeseman EA, et al. Pregnancy as a factor influencing relapse in disseminated sclerosis. *Brain* 1959;82:417–426.

Nelson LM, Franklin GM, Jones MC. Risk of multiple sclerosis exacerbation during pregnancy and breast-feeding. *JAMA* 1988;259:3441–3443.

Poser CM. MS and postpartum stress [Letter]. *Neurology* 1984;34:704–705.

Poser S, Poser W. Multiple sclerosis and gestation. *Neurology* 1983;33:1422–1427.

Roullet E, Verdier-Taillerfer MH, Amarenco P, et al. Pregnancy and multiple sclerosis: a longitudinal study of 125 remittent patients. *J Neurol Neurosurg Psychiatry* 1993;56:1062–1065.

Sadovnick AD, Ebers GC. Epidemiology of multiple sclerosis: a critical overview. *Can J Neurol Sci* 1993;20:17–29.

Sadovnick AD, Eisen K, Hashimoto SA, et al. Pregnancy and multiple sclerosis: a prospective study. *Arch Neurol* 1994;51:1120–1124.

Schapira K, Poskanzer DC, Newell DJ, et al. Marriage, pregnancy and multiple sclerosis. *Brain* 1996;89:419–428.

Sweeney WJ. Pregnancy and multiple sclerosis. *Am J Obstet Gynecol* 1953;66:124–130.

Thompson DS, Nelson IM, Burns A, et al. The effects of pregnancy in multiple sclerosis: a retrospective study. *Neurology* 1986;36:1097–1099.

Tillman AJB. The effect of pregnancy on multiple sclerosis and its management. *Res Publ Assoc Res Nerv Ment Dis* 1950;28:548–582.

Van Walderveen MAA, Tas MW, Barkhof F, et al. Magnetic resonance evaluation of disease activity during pregnancy in multiple sclerosis. *Neurology* 1994;44:327–329.

Wegmann TG, Lin H, Guilbert L, et al. Bidirectional cytokine interactions in the maternal-fetal relationship: is successful pregnancy a TH2 phenomenon? *Immunol Today* 1993;14:353–356.

Wingerchuk DM, Carter JL. Practical consultations: multiple sclerosis. *Semin Neurol* 2003;23:253–264.

Worthington J, Jones R, Crawford M, et al. Pregnancy and multiple sclerosis: a 3-year prospective study. *J Neurol* 1994;241:228–233.

Neoplasia

DeAngelis LM. Central nervous system neoplasms in pregnancy. In: Devinsky O, Feldmann E, Hainline B, eds. *Neurological Complications of Pregnancy.* New York: Raven, 1994:139–152.

Isla A, Alvarez F, Gonzalez A, et al. Brain tumor and pregnancy. *Obstet Gynecol* 1997;89:19–23.

Picone O, Castaigne V, Ede C, et al. Cerebral metastases of a choriocarcinoma during pregnancy. *Obstet Gynecol* 2003;102:1380–1383.

Tewari KS, Cappuccini F, Asrat T, et al. Obstetric emergencies precipitated by malignant brain tumors. *Am J Obstet Gynecol* 2000;182:1215–1221.

Weinreb HJ. Demyelinating diseases and neoplastic diseases in pregnancy. *Neurol Clin* 1994;12:509–526.

Peripheral Nerve Disorders

Beric A.Peripheral nerve disorders in pregnancy. In: Devinsky O, Feldmann E, Hainline B, eds. *Neurological Complications of Pregnancy.* New York: Raven, 1994:179–192.

Conwit RA, Good JL. Peripheral nerve disease. In: Kaplan PW, ed. *Neurologic Disease in Women.* New York: Demos Medical Publishing, 1998:295–305.

Rosenbaum RB, Donaldson JO. Peripheral nerve and neuromuscular disorders. *Neurol Clin* 1994;12:461–478.

Myasthenia Gravis

Ahisten G, Lefvert AK, Osterman PO, et al. Follow-up study of muscle function in children of mothers with myasthenia gravis during pregnancy. *J Child Neurol* 1992;7:264–269.

Batocchi AP, Majolini L, Evoli A, et al. Course and treatment of myasthenia gravis during pregnancy. *Neurology* 1999;52:447–452.

Ciafaloni E, Massey JM. Myasthenia gravis and pregnancy. *Neurol Clin* 2004 Nov;22(4):771–782.

Eymard B, Vernet der Garabedian B, Berrih Aknin S, et al. Anti-acetylcholine receptor antibodies in neonatal myasthenia gravis: heterogeneity and pathogenic significance. *J Autoimmun* 1991;4:185–195.

Mitchell PJ, Bebbington M. Myasthenia gravis in pregnancy. *Obstet Gynecol* 1992;80:178–181.

Papazian O. Transient neonatal myasthenia gravis. *J Child Neurol* 1992;7 135–141.

Rosenbaum RB, Donaldson JO. Peripheral nerve and neuromuscular disorders. *Neurol Clin* 1994;12:461–478.

Movement Disorders

Earley CJ. Restless legs syndrome. *N Engl J Med* 2003;348:2103–2109.

Golbe LI. Pregnancy and movement disorders. *Neurol Clin* 1994;12:497–508.

Rogers JD, Fahn S. Movement disorders and pregnancy. In: Devinsky O, Feldmann E, Hainline B, eds. *Neurological Complications of Pregnancy.* New York: Raven, 1994:163–178.

Chapter 158

Hashimoto Encephalopathy

Ji Y. Chong

Hashimoto encephalopathy was first described by Lord Brain in 1966. He followed a patient with Hashimoto thyroiditis who later developed recurrent episodes of brain dysfunction. There followed more reports of patients with autoimmune thyroid disease and an encephalopathy that often responded to steroid therapy. Hashimoto encephalopathy became recognized as a syndrome. The bulk of information about the disorder is based on case reports and small case series.

DEFINITION

Hashimoto encephalopathy is a brain disorder in a patient with antithyroid antibodies. Antithyroid antibodies form in the autoimmune condition of Hashimoto thyroiditis. This thyroid disease is characterized by goiter and varying degrees of thyroid dysfunction. Demonstration of thyroid antibodies, either antithyroid peroxidase or antithyroglobulin, is necessary to make the diagnosis of Hashimoto thyroiditis. These antibodies are directed against antigens found only in thyroid tissue and accompany the pathologic findings of lymphocytic infiltration of the thyroid gland.

Although the role of antithyroid antibodies is known in Hashimoto thyroiditis, there is no evidence that the antibodies are pathogenic in the brain. The term *Hashimoto encephalopathy*, therefore, may be misleading, especially because the prevalence of thyroid antibodies may be about 20% in asymptomatic individuals, with higher prevalence in older women.

Multiple autoimmune disorders may occur concurrently. Myasthenia gravis and Hashimoto thyroiditis occur together, but thyroid antibodies are not thought to play a role in myasthenia gravis. Similarly, Hashimoto encephalopathy is probably an autoimmune brain disease in which thyroid antibodies play no role, but some other antibody that causes the brain disease is yet to be discovered. Until the pathophysiology is understood, Hashimoto encephalopathy is defined by two features: the encephalopathy (clouding of consciousness) and high titer of antithyroid antibodies.

TABLE 158.1 Clinical Features of Patients with Hashimoto Encephalopathy

Female	85%
Mean age (yr);	45
Range	9–78
Focal deficit	27%
Seizures	64%
Myoclonus	40%
Psychosis	40%
Relapsing-remitting	55%
High CSF protein content	76%
Abnormal imaging	46%
Abnormal EEG	97%

CLINICAL MANIFESTATIONS

The clinical manifestations are diverse. Patients may have discrete episodes of strokelike events or develop a progressive decline with dementia and psychiatric symptoms. Additional manifestations found in a review of the literature are tremor, seizures, or myoclonus (Table 158.1).

PATHOLOGY

There have been few case reports describing the pathologic findings, which have included: lymphocytic infiltration of leptomeningeal vessels; lymphocytic infiltration of brain parenchymal small arterioles and venules; perivascular cuffs of lymphocytic cells; and spongiform change with gliosis, perivascular mononuclear cells, and parenchymal microglia. In some cases, there were no histologic abnormalities.

PATHOGENESIS

Because of the scarcity of pathologic data, the pathogenesis of Hashimoto encephalopathy is unknown. Some pathologic specimens support an autoimmune mediated process causing lymphocytic infiltration of small blood vessels. This is thought to cause hypoperfusion or cerebral edema. An alternative hypothesis is that an unknown antibody directly affects cortical neurons and causes global cerebral dysfunction. Autoantibodies that have been suggested as pathogenic in Hashimoto encephalopathy include an antineuronal antibody and antibody against α-enolase.

LABORATORY ABNORMALITIES

By definition, antithyroglobulin or antithyroid peroxidase levels are elevated. The plasma antibody titer, however, does not parallel the severity of cerebral symptoms. Patients may also have normal, low, or high levels of TSH and T4. CSF is usually acellular, but the CSF protein concentration is often increased. Systemic markers of inflammation, such as the sedimentation rate or C-reactive protein, or autoimmune markers such as ANA are usually normal.

EEG tracings are almost always abnormal, most commonly showing diffuse slowing. Triphasic waves, photoparoxysmal response, focal sharp waves, and periodic lateralized epileptiform discharges have been described. MRI abnormalities may be seen, but there is no consistent MRI abnormality.

DIFFERENTIAL DIAGNOSIS

The differential diagnosis includes viral encephalitis, toxic or metabolic encephalopathy, and Creutzfeldt-Jakob disease. When infectious and toxic causes are excluded, the response to corticosteroids may be the only distinguishing feature between Hashimoto encephalopathy and Creutzfeldt-Jakob disease. The 14-3-3 protein has been seen in the CSF of patients with Hashimoto encephalopathy, and spongiform change on biopsy has also been reported.

TREATMENT

In general, patients respond well to steroid therapy. In a literature review, 66 patients (96%) improved on treatment with glucocorticoids. However, there has been no formally controlled trial and there is no consensus dose or formulation of steroids. Improvement has followed intravenous as well as oral steroid treatment, and some patients improved without steroids but only treatment of thyroid dysfunction.

SUGGESTED READINGS

Brain L, Jellinek EH, Ball K. Hashimoto's disease and encephalopathy. *Lancet* 1966;2:512–14.

Chong JY, Rowland LP, Utiger R. Hashimoto encephalopathy: syndrome or myth? *Arch Neurol* 2003;60:164–171.

Ferracci F, Bertiato G, Moretto G. Hashimoto's encephalopathy: epidemiologic data and pathogenetic considerations. *J Neurol Sci* 2004;217(Feb 15):165–168.

Josephs KA, Rubino FA, Dickson DW. Nonvasculitic autoimmune inflammatory meningoencephalitis. *Neuropathology* 2004;24:149–152.

Kothbauer-Magreiter I, Sturzenegger M, Komor J, et al. Encephalopathy associated with Hashimoto thyroiditis: diagnosis and treatment. *J Neurol* 1996;243:585–593.

Nolte KW, Unbehaun A, Sieker H, et al. W. Hashimoto encephalopathy: a brainstem vasculitis? *Neurology* 2000;54:769.

Ochi H, Horiuchi I, Araki N, et al. Proteomic analysis of human brain identifies alpha-enolase as a novel autoantigen in Hashimoto's encephalopathy. *FEBS Lett* 2002;528:197–202.

Oide T, Tokuda T, Yazaki M, et al. Anti-neuronal autoantibody in Hashimoto's encephalopathy: neuropathological, immunohistochemical, and biochemical analysis of two patients. *J Neurol Sci* 2004;217:7–12.

Seipelt M, Zerr I, Nau R, et al. Hashimoto's encephalitis as a differential diagnosis of Creutzfeldt-Jakob disease. *J Neurol Neurosurg Psychiatry* 1999;66:172–176.

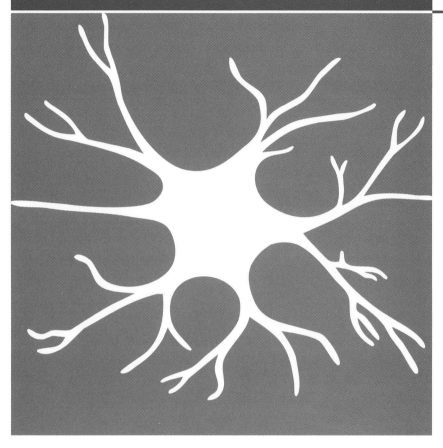

Psychiatry and Neurology

Chapter 159

Mood Disorders

Ralph N. Wharton

Depression: an act of depressing or a state of being depressed: as a (1) a state of feeling sad (2) a psychoneurotic or psychotic disorder marked especially by sadness, inactivity, difficulty with thinking and concentration, a significant increase or decrease in appetite and time spent sleeping, feelings of dejection and hopelessness, and sometimes suicidal thoughts or an attempt to commit suicide.

Merriam-Webster's Medical Dictionary, 2002

EPIDEMIOLOGY AND PUBLIC HEALTH

For hundreds of years, writers, poets, and playwrights have described the psychopathology of depression. Hippocrates attributed the symptoms of melancholia to "black bile." In *The Anatomy of Melancholy*, written by Robert Burton in 1621, he included quotations and poems from Egyptian papyrus documents and early Greek records.

In the 20th century, the incidence of depression increased steadily throughout the world. The incidence increased in every generation, as measured in 20-year epochs in the United States. It is not clear why this should be so; it does not seem to be only the result of more sensitive diagnosis. The data are not confined to suicide and include populations in every industrialized society where the statistics are reliable. It is not known how much of the increase is related to stress in different cultures or to social disruption, genetics, diet, or chronic illness. It also seems impossible to ascertain the role of alcohol, drugs, or family disruptions that include divorce, refugee mobility, and political upheaval.

Depression is called the "common cold of psychiatry" in terms of incidence; but the suicide rate makes it ominous. The public health aspects of major depressive illness are profound, generating needs for patient care and for developing programs to prevent suicide. After hypertensive vascular disease, mood disorders are the second most common cause of visits to internists and general medical practitioners in the United States. Major depression is the leading cause of disability in the United States and worldwide. Depression affects 1 in every 33 children and 1 in every 8 adolescents, according to the National Mental Health Association. In 1998, 18.8 million people were affected.

Internationally, the highest reported incidence is in Chile (29%) and the lowest is Japan (2.6%). The incidence of depression is nearly twice as high in women than in men, and suicide attempts are more numerous in women, but death from suicide is far higher in men. Postpartum depression appears in as many 10% of all deliveries, and some pregnant women commit suicide. Firearms are a risk factor for suicide in any home. According to the Centers for Disease Control and Prevention, suicide is the third leading cause of death in adolescents ages 15 to 19. Between 1980 and 1997, the suicide rate in that group increased by 11%. For those 10 to 14 years old, the suicide rate increased by 109% between 1980 and 1997. The lifetime prevalence in U.S. populations may be around 12% for women and 5% for men.

INDIVIDUALITY

"Words can wound deeper than the sword" to a depressed person. Robert Burton recognized that in 1621. He also thought that "love of learning" and "overmuch study" were risk factors for depression. The "students living a sedentary, solitary life, and free from bodily exercise, with overmuch contemplation" were at increased risk then and now. *The Anatomy of Melancholy* includes descriptions of the "kinds, causes, symptoms, prognostications, and several cures of" depression. The diverse risk factors include medical illness such as malignancy, heart attacks, stroke, diabetes, and menopause, among others. Exogenous factors are sometimes considered reactive or psychosocial and include social rejection, loss of a loved one, or a loved object (e.g., pet, home), loss of a body part (by injury or surgery). The psychologic meaning of the loss may be greater than the actual physical loss. Certainly, loss of income, job, social status, or hope for an important life goal may produce profound mourning. Vulnerability to the sense of loss or injury may bespeak a genetic susceptibility.

Mood disorders are subdivided into depressive disorders, bipolar disease (mania and depression), depression with general medical conditions, and drug (substance)-induced disorders. Each category has specific criteria, differential genetic implication, and likely different pathophysiology. There are also important differences in responses to pharmacotherapy and also to different kinds of cognitive, behavioral, or psychoanalytic psychotherapy. Because the problems differ, we separate the discussions of major depressive disorder (MDD) and bipolar disease (BPD).

DIAGNOSIS OF MAJOR DEPRESSIVE DISORDER (MDD)

By definition, a mood disorder is more than the normal emotional feelings of sadness or loss or a passing state. The primary feature is a profound and sustained alteration in mood that persists for at least 2 weeks. For the diagnosis of depression, clinicians—psychiatrists, psychopharmacologists, or neurologists—use clinical observations that have been validated by consensus-derived mood scales, genetic data, and rating scales (Table 159.1).

Criteria for the diagnosis of depression are given in the *Diagnostic and Statistical Manual of Mental Disorders* (DSM-IV), as follows. Of the nine criteria for MDD, five must be present for at least 2 weeks.

1. Depressed mood—nearly every day;
2. Diminished interest or pleasure in almost all activities;
3. Weight loss without diet (5% or more of body weight);
4. Changes in sleep pattern—insomnia or hypersomnia;
5. Agitation or retardation (slowing of physical activity, speech, and thinking);
6. Fatigue or loss of energy nearly every day;
7. Continuous feelings of worthlessness or excessive or inappropriate guilt;
8. Diminished capacity for concentration or indecisiveness;
9. Recurrent thoughts of death, recurrent suicidal ideas, attempts, or plans.

The diagnosis of MDD is usually not difficult. It is most important to ascertain that the episode has not been precipitated by an underlying medical condition. Also, at least 50 medications and substances of abuse (especially alcohol and sedatives) can cause symptoms indistinguishable from MDD. Adrenal steroid use or abuse can induce either depression or mania. The most important differential diagnosis is discerning unipolar from bipolar depression. Bipolar depression usually has an earlier onset, greater risk of suicide, family history of similarly affected relatives, and more frequent episodes of illness.

Dysthymic disorders, adjustment disorders with depression, depressive personality disorders, seasonal affective disorders, chronic depression, atypical depression, and masked depression are more subtle conditions that

▶ **TABLE 159.1 Hamilton Rating Scale**

1) What's your mood been like this past week?	Depressed Mood (Rate 0–4)
2) How have you been spending your time this past week (when not at work)?	Work and Activities (Rate 0–4)
3) Sometimes people with depression lose interest in sex. This week how has your interest been?	Genital Symptoms (Rate 0–2)
4) How has your appetite been?	Somatic Symptoms Gastrointestinal (Rate 0–2)
5) Have you lost weight since depression began?	Loss of Weight (Rate 0–3)
6) Have you had trouble falling asleep?	Insomnia Early (Rate 0–2)
7) Have you been waking up in the middle of the night?	(Rate 0–2)
8) What time have you been awakening?	Insomnia Late (Rate 0–2)
9) How has your energy been this past week?	Somatic Symptoms General (Rate 0–2)
10) Have you been putting yourself down this week?	Feelings of Guilt (Rate 0–2)
11) Have you had thoughts that life is not worth living?	Suicide (Rate 0–4)
12) Have you been feeling particularly tense?	Anxiety Psychic (Rate 0–4)
13) Have you had any physical symptoms?	Physiological Concomitants of Anxiety (Rate 0–4)
14) Have your thoughts been focused on your physical health or how your body is working?	Hypochondriasis (Rate 0–4)
15) Rating based on observation	Insight vs. Denial (Rate 0–4)
16) Slowness of thought, speech, poor concentration	Retardation (Rate 0–4)
17) Fidgetiness, restlessness	Agitation (Rate 0–4)

A score >14 indicates need for treatment.

meet fewer than the nine criteria. Validation from intimates or family is often necessary. Criteria for these entities are still evolving. Many mildly or moderately depressed people are not good historians. *Dysthymia* literally means ill tempered and refers to chronic depression that is less severe than a major depression. Criteria involve a depressed mood plus two additional symptoms with mild onset. The depressed mood may last most of the day, for more days than not, and may persist for up to 2 years without an episode of major depression.

Biomarkers and Genetics

Twin studies indicate a genetic susceptibility for depression. The overall risk for all mood disorders is three times higher in monozygotic twins than in dizygotic twins. In a study of more than 1000 twin sisters, Kendler addressed the association of anxiety with mood disorders; he found genetic evidence of susceptibility to emotional problems that included depression, anxiety, social phobia, and agoraphobia. However, biomarkers are lacking and classification is still based on symptoms, subjective sensations, self-report, and psychiatric syndromes; chromosomal and other genetic markers are too inconsistent for diagnosis.

Genetic studies have not led to the cloning of any gene. Linkage studies have implicated six genes, suggesting that multiple genes are involved in this example of complex inheritance. A few selected studies illustrate possible progress. First, Caspi et al. studied a gene for the receptor of a transporter of serotonin (HTTLPR) on 17q11.2. Following more than 1,000 children for more than 20 years, they found that. those with one or two copies of the short allele of the 5 HTT promoter polymorphism had more depressive symptoms, more diagnosable depression, and more suicidality in response to stressful life events than others who were homozygous for the long allele. Among the 11% of subjects who had experienced severe maltreatment, homozygous short-allele subjects ran a 63% risk of major depression compared with 30% for the long-allele participants, a significant difference. However, at least 14 distinct receptors for 5 HT and numerous enzymes are involved. That study was one of few tying a specific genetic difference and environmental stressors to a psychiatric disease. No direct paths are likely to be found in single genes causing disease, because many genes probably influence depression and because life stressors are so variable.

Second, linkage has been found for bipolar disease with the promoter of the G-protein receptor kinase (GRK3) and also with one allele of a gene for brain-derived neurotrophic factor (BDNF). Multiple associations imply that strictly Mendelian inheritance is unlikely. Third, gene array expression studies show a decrease in the activity of genes regulating oxidative phosphorylation and also in the activity of mitochondrial proteins in the hippocampus of

bipolar patients. Fourth, bipolar disease may share susceptibility genes with schizophrenia.

The consensus view is that complex inheritance is the problem and has to be solved by better defining phenotypes, analyzing gene–gene interactions, and unraveling gene–environment interactions. Multiple genes of small effect may be involved.

Similar problems are encountered in the genetics of bipolar disease, which is also deemed multigenic. The relative risk of bipolar I disease in first-degree relatives is seven times more than in the general population, and the relative risk in monozygotic twins is more than fifty times greater. However, the age at onset varies in identical twins living in different environments.

Pathophysology

Mood disorders are brain diseases as demonstrated by the efficacy of antidepressant drugs, evidence of genetic susceptibility, reproduction of depression by other drugs, and manifestations of depression in neurodegerative diseases. Nevertheless, just as genetic studies have been tantalizing but limited, so there is no clear understanding of the pathophysiology of mood disorders. Part of the problem is the diversity of clinical manifestations, not only the several types of depression but also differentiating from schizophrenia and the effects of alcohol or substance abuse. Also, there is no animal model, cell culture model, or postmortem pattern of pathology. MRI, fMRI, PET, and MR spectroscopy have given clues to functional abnormalities of the cortex, but confirmation by other studies is lacking. Some strokes seem to cause depression, but there is little consistent evidence from functional studies that particular brain areas are associated with depression, and mania is not often a manifestation of a focal lesion.

Some imaging studies have shown significant reduction in the hippocampal volume of patients with recurrent major depression; the loss is attributed to combinations of stress-induced increases in circulating glucocorticoid levels, decreases in brain-derived neurotrophic factor, and decreases in neurogenesis. The decrease in volume is related to the duration of the depressive episodes, and antidepressants may have neuroprotective effects. Studies of animal stress or people with major stressors (such as chronic child abuse) suggest changes in hippocampal volume.

In mood disorders, sleep is often disrupted, implying that the circadian rhythm of sleep is distorted in the suprachiasmatic nucleus. However, no consistent or characteristic abnormality of sleep has been demonstrated in patients, and sleep deprivation is used as a therapy. Reduction of rapid-eye-movement sleep increases the pressure for this phase of sleep, which seems to be beneficial.

Hen and his associates found that the salutary effects of antidepressant drugs depend on neurogenesis, the formation of new neurons in the brain. In an animal model of depression, they found that blocking neurogenesis also blocked the drug effects. Knockout mice lacking a serotonin receptor do not respond to fluoxetine but do improve with tricyclic antidepressants, which work through norepinephrine. Correspondingly, neurogenesis was active with tricyclics but not with fluoxetine.

For years, the "catechol hypothesis" was a dominant theory, holding that depression resulted from low levels of norepinephrine in the CSF and mania from high levels. That theory has largely passed from the scene because it proved difficult to validate. For instance, in a postmortem study, Young et al. (1994) found no differences in the content of any brain region for norepinephrine, serotonin, or dopamine. Changes in the hypothalamic–pituitary–adrenal system have similarly been difficult to prove.

Perhaps the most popular theory now is a problem in signal transduction, implying problems in the effects of norepinephrine as a neurotransmitter and first messenger that binds to a receptor. There follows activity of G proteins and several second messengers that include adenylate cyclase and nitric oxide.

Finally, the effects of lithium imply a biochemical abnormality in depression. This salt also affects second messengers and may attenuate responses to several neurotransmitter systems. How it functions as a mood stabilizer, modulating both mania and depression, is a matter of much needed research.

Treatment

Lacking a coherent theory of pathogenesis, treatment of depressive syndromes is highly variable, and long-term effects are still to be determined. Diverse drug regimens, alone or with psychotherapy, are still being evaluated.

The consensus of the best clinical judgment for treatment of MDD is a combination of pharmacotherapy and psychotherapy. The choice of treatment depends on availability of treatment and the patient's preference. There is debate about the benefits of specific antidepressant drugs as monotherapy, but the overall response rate is near 80%. A family history of beneficial drug response or previous response to a medication affects selection. The benefits of tricyclic antidepressants (TCAs) are substantial, but side effects may interfere with long-term use; the selective serotonin inhibitors (SSRIs) have fewer initial side effects, but may lose efficacy in time or may have unwanted sexual side effects in 3% to 25% of patients. Dose sensitivity to TCAs varies up to 30-fold; the SSRI drugs have a narrower range, but it is still considerable. Therefore, it is best with most medications to start with a low dose and increase slowly. Full benefit may take up to 3 weeks or even longer.

Because controlled therapeutic trials of psychotherapy are so difficult to devise, it is not possible to compare the benefits of the different forms, such as cognitive, interpersonal, structured, supportive, and emotive techniques. Cognitive and interpersonal therapies may resolve milder depression, but most clinicians use a combination of psychotherapy with psychoactive drugs.

Symptomatic relief with treatment may not result in concomitant improvement in psychosocial function, which may be delayed. Relapses occur in up to 20% patients in 6 months and over 30% in 1 year, according to Keller, and the risk of recurrence increases by 16% with each recurrent episode. Kendler suggested that those with more recurrences tend to become "sensitized" to relapsing symptoms even without external stressful events. The high relapse rates have led to maintenance treatment with drug therapy and prophylactic psychotherapy.

The risk of relapse is also accompanied by risk of mania, which may be spontaneous, therapeutic drug induced, or with substance abuse. With continued use of a mood stabilizer, the risk of antidepressant-induced mania is about 10%. It is not clear whether antidepressants with different mechanisms of action are equally likely to induce mania in different subtypes of depression. Although family history may be unrevealing, there are those individuals who may have a number of depressive episodes prior to an index episode of mania. Once a manic episode appears, treatment choices are quite different.

There is no consensus about a clear end point for the treatment of depression; the physician's judgment or rating scales are used. A 4- to 6-week asymptomatic period is a minimum and predicts there will be no relapse for a first episode. However, treatment for major depressive episode may continue for at least 6 months, especially when overt stressors remain in the environment. Major depression is often resistant, and there are no biomarkers for guidance of treatment. Depression scale measures are limited, and most decisions are necessarily subjective. The indications for long-term maintenance therapy are unclear; if there is symptomatic relapse or incomplete remission within 12 or 18 months, chronic therapy must be considered. Psychosocial stressors in the environment are considerations for long-term prophylaxis. Long-term (up to 3 years) treatment is considered if there have been more than three episodes. There are no lifetime studies to suggest that maintenance must be permanent. Personally, I have followed many patients after age 80. The evidence that TCAs promote neurogenesis in the hypothalamus and prefrontal areas may be an indication to continue drug therapy into late life.

Some clinicians use of diurnal cortisol levels at 8 AM and 4 PM as a measure of stress. However, there are no consensus criteria for response, remission, relapse, or recovery. Efforts have been made to define these terms, but only suicide and suicide attempts are agreed on.

For treatment-refractory subjects, hospital admission is available; patient safety comes first. Requirements or indications for electrical stimulating treatments (ESTs) vary from community to community, and insurance companies have diverse rules for the use of inpatient or outpatient electrical stimulating treatment (EST). Consensus supports the necessity of electroconvulsive therapy (ECT) or hospitalization for people who are actively suicidal—with persistent suicidal ideas. Earlier serious suicide attempts or threats are clear warnings.

ESTs have miniscule risks—approximately 1/50,000—including the risk of anesthetic drug idiosyncrasy or other complication. Treatments have been given in the presence of prior stroke or with clipped aneurysm without complications. There is no substantive evidence for risk of permanent memory loss. Magnetic stimulation and unilateral or focused electric stimulation are being evaluated to limit the transient memory loss while seeking equal efficacy.

Electrical treatment is indicated for patients with the following characteristics:

1. Failure to respond to multiple adequate antidepressant pharmacotherapy trials;
2. Delusional depression;
3. Actively suicidal patients or manic patients so severely agitated that they must be rapidly controlled;
4. Intolerance to side effects or allergies to multiple antidepressants.

Initial unipolar depressive episodes or postpartum depression are sometimes difficult to assess. Certainly the cliché that one postpartum depression means that there will be recurrence with the next pregnancy is not valid. However, a family history of depression leads to consideration of long-term maintenance pharmacotherapy for a woman with postpartum depression. Clinical posttreatment observation, education about the risks of relapse, and advice about likely symptom recurrence are indicated.

Specific Antidepressant Medications

Antidepressant medications (Table 159.2) are classified by molecular structure or by effects on neurotransmitters. Tricyclics, monoamine oxidase inhibitors (MAOIs), and lithium were introduced in the 1960s. In the past two decades, selective serotonin reuptake inhibitors (SSRIs) have become popular, and six are currently available: fluoxetine, sertraline, paroxetine, fluvoxamine, citalopram, and escitalopram. They are clearly not as entirely selective as suggested by the classification scheme, and all affect norepinephrine and dopamine metabolism as well as the kinetics of other drugs; some have antiplatelet activity. Drug reactions occur with all of them.

The purported advantages of the newer SSRIs over the older drugs remain unclear. There are fewer adverse effects

▶ **TABLE 159.2 Antidepressant Medications**

Tricyclic Forms	Dose Range (mg)	SSRI Derivatives	Latest Generation
Amitriptyline (Elavil)	100–250	Fluoxetine (Prozac) 10–60	Venlafaxine (Effexor) 75–375
Imipramine (Tofranil)	150–300	Sertraline (Zoloft) 50–200	
Mirtazapine (Remeron)	15–45		
Nortryptyline (Pamelor)	75–150	Paroxetine (Paxil)10–50	
Nefazodone (Serzone)	200–500		
Doxepin (Sinequan)	100–300	Citalopram (Celexa)10–40	
Trazodone (Desyrel)	200–500		
Clomipramine (Anafranil)	100–350	Escitalopram (Lexapro)10–20	
Buproprion (Wellbutrin)	150–400		
Desipramine (Norpramin)	150–300	Fluvoxamine (Luvox)100–300	

Other considerations: | | **Under study:** | |
Antidepressants / MAOIs — Phenelzine (Nardil) 15–60; Tranylcypromine (Parnate) 30–60. Under study: Lamotrigine (Lamictal), Topiramate (Topamax), Omega-3 fatty acids.

Standard for bipolar patients for acute and chronic illness
Lithium carbonate (Eskalith) 1,200–2,400 mg; blood level 0.6–1.20 mmol/L.
Treatment well established for over 40 yr. Not optimal for rapid cycling disorders.

Adjunctive or in combination for acute mania:
1. Valproic acid (Depakene) 500–1,800 mg; blood level 50–100 mg/L.
2. Carbamazepine (Tegretol) 400–1,200 mg
3. Risperidone (Risperdal) 2–6 mg (no long-term studies yet)
4. Olanzapine (Zyprexa) 10–15 mg (no long-term studies yet)

and cessation of therapy is less frequent in short-term studies, but longer-term studies remain to be done, especially in the elderly.

The dosage for all antidepressants ranges widely. The exquisite vulnerability of most patients makes it wise to start low and increase slowly, particularly after age 60. Protein binding, enzymatic differences, and prior drug exposure impede reliable predictions. Dietary precautions are not needed except for MAOIs and lithium. Drug interactions include anticoagulants and antihypertension drugs.

The SSRIs cause sexual dysfunction in 15% to 30% of men and women alike. When patients ask about alternative schedules, there are several choices: waiting for tolerance to develop to side effects, taking a drug holiday, reducing the dose, switching to another medication, or adding another drug. Another side effect is weight gain, seen in 5% to 10% of patients. Again the choices are few: add an exercise program, add an adjunctive medication, or switch medication.

Lithium can be used in combination with all SSRIs. Monitoring of lithium levels is essential, especially in the first 6 weeks of treatment. Thereafter, monthly, quarterly, or twice-a-year monitoring is adequate unless there are substantial changes in weight.

The newest antidepressant drugs are still finding their places. Lamotrigine (Lamictal) may have a special place in the depression accompanying bipolar disorders. Lamotrigine had been used as an antiepileptic drug but also has antidepressant benefits.

Metabolic differences among patients have been defined with the new drugs, identifying poor, intermediate, extensive, and ultrarapid metabolizers. Some of the differences are attributed to six genetic variants of the drug-metabolizing enzyme P-450. Other enzymes may determine which patients are likely to have a high incidence of side effects.

BIPOLAR DISORDERS

Bipolar disorders (BPD) are separated into types I and II. Type I has a clear manic or psychotic manic episode in addition to major depressive disorders. Type II has a hippomanic episode with one or more major depressive episodes. Hypomania, a state less severe than mania, is defined formally below.

According to the DSM-IV, *mania* is defined as an expansive or irritable mood lasting at least 1 week and also having at least three of the following seven symptoms:

1. Inflated self-esteem or grandiosity;
2. Decreased need for sleep (3 hours or less in 24 hours);
3. More talkative than usual or pressure to continue talking;
4. Flight of ideas or racing thoughts;

5. Distractibility (attention easily drawn to irrelevant stimuli);
6. Psychomotor agitation or marked increase in multiple activities;
7. Excessive involvement in pleasurable activities with high risk for painful consequences, such as buying sprees, sexual indiscretion, or poor business judgment.

Hypomania does not meet the score for mania and is defined by six criteria:

1. A distinct period of expansive or irritable mood lasting throughout at least 4 days;
2. During the period of mood disturbance, at least three of the following persist: inflated self-esteem, decreased need for sleep, more talkative than usual, flight of ideas or racing thought, distractibility, psychomotor agitation, excessive involvement in pleasurable activities that may have painful consequences, such as buying sprees, sexual indiscretions, or foolish business investments.
3. Disturbance in mood and change in functioning as noted by others;
4. No psychotic features;
5. Not owing to a specific substance or medical condition;
6. Associated with unequivocal change that is uncharacteristic of the person when not symptomatic.

Differential Diagnosis of Bipolar Disease

Seasonal affective disorder is a mood disorder related to the greatest seasonal variation in light. It is a major affective disorder in which major depression occurs during fall or winter for at least 2 consecutive years with remission in spring or summer. It is rare and not related to seasonal stressors or external events. It can be treated effectively in some individuals with bright ambient light alone. Remission rates are variable, and some patients prefer medication. There are also those who respond to bright light are not seasonally affected.

Treatment of Bipolar Disease

Treatment of bipolar I manic episodes started with lithium in the early 60s as the treatment of choice, and it is still the most widely used for maintenance therapy. Lithium has been the preferred treatment of bipolar disorder for over 50 years. Its efficacy in preventing suicide is unparalleled, and it has remained the mainstay for treatment and prophylaxis. The international Group for the Study of Lithium followed patients from four countries for >7 years; the suicide rate was 1.5 per 1,000 patient years compared to those who discontinued lithium who had a rate of 7.1 per 1,000 patient years. In another review of 22 studies from 1974 to1998, the suicide rate was seven times less for patients on long-term lithium treatment. Another study of 310 patients found that the rate of all suicide acts rose nearly 14-fold after discontinuing lithium therapy, especially within the first 12 months.

Other mood stabilizers are helpful but also have adverse effects that make them unsuitable for some patients. Lithium cannot be used in patients with renal disease, and it causes hypothyroidism in 10% to 20% of patients; it may produce mild skin reaction, hyperparathyroidism, mild weight gain, or tremor. The mechanism of action of lithium has been uncertain. Glycogen synthase kinase 3 (GSK-3) may be a target. However, like other antidepressants, lithium may affect cellular resilience, neuronal plasticity, or neurogenesis. Lithium protects against the deleterious effects of excess glutamate or deprivation of nerve growth factor. Lithium may also regulate circadian rhythms through the inhibition of GSK-3.

Most initial episodes are not treated by lithium alone because the onset of action is slow. Instead, treatment usually starts with a combination of lithium and either valproate or carbamazepine, which are effective. Maintenance treatment usually combines therapy with multiple medications and psychosocial support.

Therapy is affected by differences in the symptoms of bipolar and unipolar MDD where there may be more somatic symptoms, and also hypersomnia may prevail rather than insomnia. Drug therapy is more like to fail if concomitant substance abuse is accompanied by inadequate social support. The suicide rate in bipolar illness is higher than in any other psychiatric illness, responsible for the death of 10% to 15% of patients and with a 15-fold greater risk of suicide than in the general population.

Both olanzapine (Zyprexa) and risperidone (Risperdal) and ziprasidone (Geodon) may be helpful acutely, but lack the longer-term studies of lithium and valproate. Olanzapine and risperidone provoke weight gains, diabetes, or hypercholesterolemia. Risperidone may cause parkinsonism or tardive dyskinesia.

Long-term treatment with antidepressants in bipolar illness generates an unsolved conundrum. Having seen a patient who had one episode at age 20 (treated with hot and cold packs) and a second episode at age 80, it would have been folly to have given unnecessary medication for 60 years. No data provide reliable guides between the twin hazards of adverse effects and catastrophic drug-induced mania.

Treatment with Other Social Mood Stabilizers

Treatment opportunities for those with mood disorders have expanded in recent years with the appearance and advantages of Internet support groups (ISGs). A patient can get reliable information, maintain anonymity, and find solace day and night all the time. Chat rooms are available around the clock. Walkers in Darkness (www.walkers.org) is a nonprofit organization among many others. According to one research report, patients did not turn to this site in lieu of professional help but as an addition. Most patients discussed their responses with their physicians. The use of the Internet for patients with depression and many other disorders has grown phenomenally in the past years. Although low-quality information is evident, there is a wealth of excellent information from the National Library of Medicine (http://www.medlineplus.gov.depression) and research sites. Sometime in the late 90s, searchers for medical information surpassed porn site hits, which had been the number one use of the Internet. According to one source, Internet users worldwide conducted more than 2.2 million searches during January through March 2003.

MOOD DISORDERS OWING TO NEUROLOGIC CONDITIONS

Epidemiology

Twenty-five percent to 40% of patients with neurologic conditions, including Parkinson disease, Huntington disease, and Alzheimer disease, develop a marked depressive syndrome at some point in the course of the illness, as discussed in related chapters in this book. For all the neurodegenerative diseases, including amyotrophic lateral sclerosis, depression and suicide are not necessarily pathologic considerations.

With systemic disorders that do not directly involve the CNS, the rates of depression differ. For example, up to 60% of patients with Cushing disease develop depression, but those with chronic renal disease fare better; with the advent of transplant therapy, the incidence of depression is 8% to 10%.

Alzheimer Disease

Patients with Alzheimer disease (Chapter 107) frequently develop feelings of worthlessness, tearfulness, apathy, diminished energy, and lack of initiative. Psychiatric manifestations include delusions, hallucinations, transient psychosis, and periods of extreme irritability, agitation, or disinhibition. These episodes are often brief and do not qualify in terms of duration for major depressive disorder. Nevertheless, modest doses of antidepressants may be worthy of a trial. Side effects may be minimal with low doses, and adjustments can be made by family members with clear clinical instructions. Suicide is infrequent (or under-reported) when there is good social and community support.

Huntington Disease

Psychiatric symptoms are almost ubiquitous with Huntington disease (Chapter 109) and may initially present as depressive illness. Depression may antedate the neurologic diagnosis. Suicide and suicide attempts are common. Mania or hypomania has been noted and should be treated with the usual medications but often requiring smaller (one-third to one-half) doses. At times, EST may be life saving.

Parkinson Disease

Depression and depression with dementia occur in almost 25% of patients with Parkinson disease (Chapter 115). The depressive symptoms respond well to low doses of antidepressants including the newer SSRIs. Occasionally SSRI therapy increases the parkinsonism. EST is effective and may improve both the depression and the motor symptoms.

SUGGESTED READINGS

Berns GS, Nemeroff CB. The neurobiology of bipolar disorder. *Am J Hum Genet* 2003;123C:76–84.

Cartwright R, Baehr E, Kirkby J, et al. REM sleep reduction, mood regulation and remission in untreated depression. *Psychiatry Res* 2003;121;159–167.

Caspi A, Sugden K, Moffitt TE, et al. Influence of life stress on depression: moderation by a polymorphism in the 5-HTT gene. *Science* 2003;301:386–389.

Dantzer R, Wollman EE, Yirmiya R. Cytokines, stress, and depression. Conclusions and perspectives. *Adv Exp Med Biol* 1999;461:317–329.

Dean B. The neurobiology of bipolar disorder: findings using human postmortem central nervous system tissue. *Aust N Z J Psychiatry* 2004;38(Mar):135–140.

Devanand DP, Adorno E, Cheng J, et al. Late onset dysthymic disorder and major depression differ from early onset dysthymic disorder and major depression in elderly outpatients. *J Affect Disord* 2004;78(Mar):259–267.

Finnerty M, Levin Z. Acute manic episodes in pregnancy. *Am J Psychiatry* 1996;153:261–263.

Gingrich JA, Ansorge MS. New lessons from knockout mice. The role of serotonin during development and its possible contribution to the origins of neuropsychiatric disorders. *CNS Spectr* 2003;8(Aug):572–577.

Gould TD, Zarate CA, Manji HK. Glycogen synthase kinase-3: a target for novel bipolar disorder treatments. *J Clin Psychiatry* 2004;65(Jan):10–21.

Harris EC, Barraaclough B. Suicide as an outcome for mental disorders. A meta-analysis. *Br J Psychiatry* 1997;170:205–228.

Keller MB. Past, present and future directions for defining optimal treatment outcomes in depression. *JAMA* 2003;289:3152–3160.

Kendler, KS. Major depression and generalized anxiety disorder: same genes, (partly) different environments. *Br J Psychiatry* 1996;168:68–75.

Kendler KS, Thornton LM, Gardner CO. Stressful life events and previous episodes in the etiology of depression. *Am J Psychiatry* 2000;157:1243–1251.

Lenox RH, Hahn CG. Overview of the mechanism of action of lithium on the brain: 50-year update. *J Clin Psychiatry* 2003;61(Suppl 9):5–15.

Lisanby SH, Luber B, Schlaepfer TE, et al. Safety and feasibility of magnetic seizure therapy (MST) in major depression: randomized within-subject comparison with electroconvulsive therapy. *Neuropsychopharmacology* 2003;28:1852–1865.

Merikangas K, Yu K. Genetic epidemiology of bipolar disorder. *Clin Neurosci Res* 2002;27–141.

Merikangas KR, Zhang H, Angst J, et al. Longitudinal trajectories of depression and anxiety in a prospective community study. *Arch Gen Psychiatry* 2003;60:993–1000.

Post RM, Denicoff KD. Presentations of depression in bipolar illness. *Clin Neurosci Res* 2002;2:142–157.

Santarelli L, Saxe M, Gross C, et al. Requirement of hippocampal neurogenesis for the behavioral effects of antidepressants. *Science* 2003;301:805–809.

Solomon DA, Keller MB. Multiple recurrences of major depressive disorder. *Am J Psychiatry* 2000;157:229–233.

Thase ME, Sachs GS. Bipolar depression: pharmacotherapy and related therapeutic strategies. *Biol Psychiatry* 2000;48:558–572.

Vo D, Dunner D. Treatment-resistant bipolar disorder: a comparison of rapid cyclers and nonrapid cyclers. *CNS Spectr* 2003;8:948–952.

Yamaguchi S, Isejima H, et al. Synchronization of cellular clocks in the suprachiasmatic nucleus. *Science* 2003;302:1408–1412.

Young LT, Warch JJ, Kish SJ, et al. Reduced brain 5-HT and elevated turnover and metabolites in bipolar affective disorder. *Biol Psychiatry* 1994;35:121–127.

Chapter 160

Anxiety Disorders

Ralph N. Wharton

DEFINITION

Anxiety can be adaptive or debilitating. Anxiety disorders are the most common of all psychologic disturbances. Community surveys indicate that, in terms of lifetime prevalence, at least 15% of people in the United States have or have had an anxiety disorder. Costs are estimated to be about $82 billion annually, according to the National Foundation for Brain Research. Twin studies suggest heritability in about one-third of cases.

In the earliest Freudian descriptions, the distress was attributed to unexpressed libidinal desires transformed into somatic symptoms as an actual neurosis. Later, it was considered an intrapsychic conflict between id and superego. The origin of instinctual desires that conflicted with society or sexual trauma ended with a physiologic response that generated exaggerated fearfulness, a panic attack, or a generalized anxiety disorder, with agoraphobia or other specific phobias. Finally, Freud thought there were chemical answers.

Anxiety states are stimulated by stressful situations, such as war, rape, or bodily threats. Other stressors may be medications or general medical conditions, but usually the onset is spontaneous, without a clear precipitant in a young adult, sometimes after age 60.

Animal models provide some perspective in understanding the evolution of protective fear as opposed to fearfulness interfering with normal development. Normal fear may have adaptive survival value, including the almost universal recoil from snakes. The transition from normal fear to stress or stress proneness is vague. In animals and humans, chemical signals are produced in response to separation from the mother, called *separation anxiety*, which is novel at a certain age. Unfamiliarity may then produce curiosity or fear. In all species, there is a range of responsive to novelty. The biologic basis of timidity rather than bold exploration is unknown. However, the pathways of withdrawal are known in *Aplysia* and *Drosophila* to involve neurotransmitters—glutamate, γ-aminobutyric acid (GABA) serotonin, norepinephrine, and the corticotrophin-releasing factor. Even after genetic vulnerability is explained, however, environmental determinants will be important.

EPIDEMIOLOGY

Panic attacks occur with similar frequency in most races, more frequently in women than men, at a ratio of 2:1 to 3:1. Panic disorder was not considered a specific entity until the publication of *Diagnostic and Statistical Manual of Mental Disorders*, 3rd edition (DSM III) in 1980, and specific criteria were not developed until the 1987 revised 3rd edition (DSM III-R) was completed.

Currently the prevalence of anxiety states is 7% to 9%. The syndromes include the following: (1) panic disorder, (2) specific phobias and social phobia, (3) post-traumatic stress disorder (PTSD), (4) generalized anxiety disorder (GAD), and (5) obsessive-compulsive disorder (OCD). Some anxiety disorders occur with general medical conditions.

PATHOPHYSIOLOGY

Theories of pathogenesis include chemical, genetic, hormonal, circuitry, psychodynamic, and learning approaches. The sympathetic arousal systems have been most thoroughly studied. Global sympathetic arousal has not been observed, so it cannot be a simple defect in the sympathetic system; epinephrine alone does not explain panic. Extensive evidence indicates that the amygdala plays a major role in fear and anxiety reactions. The hippocampus is part of the neural anxiety network, participating in the consolidation or retrieval of painful memories. Noradrenergic dysregulation may be a factor with changes in receptor sensitivity. A similar explanation has been postulated for benzodiazepine receptor systems, whereas serotonergic drugs are effective in treatment and implicate receptors and projections from

the dorsal raphe, locus ceruleus, and periaqueductal gray.

fMRI studies suggest that neural systems involving unwanted memories are crucial because an active forgetting process suppresses painful memories. Prefrontal cortical and right hippocampal activations predict the magnitude of forgetting. Models of anxiety address circuitry rather than specific transmitter receptors. Conditioned fear involves the amygdala and hippocampus or efferents from amygdala, hippocampus, and brainstem.

SIGNS AND SYMPTOMS

A panic attack is a discrete period of intense fear or discomfort in which four or more of the following clinical manifestations develop abruptly and reach a peak within 10 minutes:

1. Palpitations, pounding heart, awareness of markedly accelerated rate;
2. Sweating;
3. Trembling or shaking;
4. Sensations of shortness of breath, smothering;
5. Choking feelings;
6. Chest pain or discomfort;
7. Nausea or abdominal distress;
8. Feeling unsteady or faint, lightheaded;
9. Derealization (feelings of unreality) or depersonalization (being detached from one's self);
10. Fear of dying;
11. Fear of losing control or going crazy;
12. Paresthesias (numbness or tingling);
13. Chills or hot flashes.

The essential feature of panic disorder is the recurrence of unexpected attacks followed by at least 1 month of persistent concerns about having a repeat attack or significant changes in behavior related to fear of another attack. Panic attacks can occur in the context of social phobia, PTSD, and with or without agoraphobia. Attacks may be cued by special situations, such as the approach of dogs or snakes, or it may be uncued and spontaneous. Some patients become catastrophobic about medical situations, including fear that elevated blood pressure means an immediate stroke or headache means brain tumor. Panic attacks can occur with a major depression. When criteria are met for both panic disorder and another mood or anxiety disorder, both are diagnosed. Many patients self-medicate, generating comorbid substance-related disorders with cannabis, cocaine, or alcohol.

Panic attacks most often appear first between adolescence and the late 30s, but can start after age 45 years. Later-in-life episodes are usually relapses, when new events mimic earlier cued episodes.

DIFFERENTIAL DIAGNOSIS

Medical conditions that may promote similar symptoms include hyperthyroidism, hyperparathyroidism; cardiac arrhythmias; toxic reactions to caffeine, cocaine, amphetamines, marijuana, or alcohol; pheochromocytoma; vestibular malfunction; seizure disorders; or hyperventilation.

TREATMENT

The first widely studied drug treatment for panic attacks was imipramine hydrochloride (Tofranil) in the late 60s. Usually modest doses were adequate, starting as low as 10 mg/day and slowly increasing to 100 mg; rarely, doses up to 300 mg/day were used. The wide range of responsiveness proved to be related to differences between poor and ultrarapid metabolizers, with differences up to 30-fold. Isoenzymes of the enzyme P-450 can be assayed to guide dose adjustments.

Benzodiazepines are widely used and helpful. Alprazolam (Xanax) in divided doses up to 2–4 mg/day, and clonazepam (Klonopin) in the same dose range are both helpful. Dependency, tolerance, and withdrawal risks are modest but real, especially in people with other kinds of dependence and tolerance. Cognitive behavioral treatment in combination with pharmacotherapy is most helpful. However, many British psychiatrists treat successfully with cognitive behavioral approaches alone.

Selective serotonin reuptake inhibitors (SSRIs) have also been useful. Many patients approach treatment with a bias toward one form of treatment or another. For some, psychotherapy is preferred and for others pharmacotherapy offers the most benefit. Clinically, the patient's wishes must always be considered. Three months is usually adequate with a 6-month and then annual follow-up for 2 years. If attacks recur, it is best to re-evaluate the patient rather than permit self-medication long term.

SPECIFIC PHOBIAS AND SOCIAL PHOBIA

Definition

A *phobia* is a specific marked and persistent fear of a clearly discernible circumscribed object or situation, exposure to which evokes an immediate anxiety response that is excessive and/or unreasonable. The duration is at least 6 months. The following are common types:

- Animal: fears cued by animals or insects;
- Natural environment: fears of storms, water, heights, elevators;
- Situational: fear cued by flying, driving, enclosed places;

- Blood-injection-injury: fear of needles, dentist, seeing blood or injury, any invasive bodily procedure; the strong vasovagal response often seen in these individuals is often highly familial.

Epidemiology

The content and prevalence of phobias vary with gender, culture, and ethnicity; the prevalence rate is about 9% with lifetime rates of about 10%. Age at onset varies with the type of phobia. Life events including trauma may elicit the development of a phobia. Repeated parental warnings, observing media events, experiencing a near accident, or being witness to a crash, for example, may result in an airplane or automobile phobia. Relatives with specific phobias are frequently noted. Unlike generalized anxiety disorder, fearfulness is not all pervasive.

Pathophysiology

A strong familial factor for social phobia has been documented in many studies, with perhaps a 10-fold higher risk in avoidant personality disorder or specific social phobia. An underlying neurochemical basis for extreme shyness, however, has not been delineated. Inferences about receptor sensitivity or neurochemical blockade from the responsiveness to pharmacologic treatments have not yet resulted in a clear understanding of etiology. Presumably there is some aberrant response in pathways from hippocampus to amygdala to some prefrontal areas.

Treatment

Specific phobias often go untreated. Desensitization by exposure is unequivocally the best form of treatment whether in groups or individually. Fear of flying and fear of heights have been successfully treated in group therapy. Imaging techniques (i.e., personal imaginations) or 3-D movies are helpful. Some phobic patients are hypnotizable, and hypnotic desensitization can be curative. Pharmacotherapy has had almost no success; small SSRI studies have shown promise, but longer evaluation is necessary. Early life mastery of phobia may relapse late in life and lead to retreatment.

Social Phobia

Social phobia (SP) was defined >20 years ago as a distinct entity. However, it frequently overlaps with other diagnostic entities such as depression, substance abuse, panic disorder, and generalized anxiety. The history may reveal very early onset. Most individuals recognize the unreasonableness and excessiveness of their fear, and fearful situations may be avoided or endured with extreme discomfort.

Twin studies suggest that 30% to 40% is heritable. However, no physiologic or autonomic variables are defined.

Decreased D2 receptors or dopamine transport may be involved.

The earliest treatment involved use of monoamine oxidase inhibitors (MAOIs), now replaced by safer SSRIs with success rates of approximately 60%. Beta-blockers and longer-acting benzodiazepines are helpful. Cognitive behavioral training and restructuring derived from Beck's innovative psychotherapy has proved to be extraordinarily helpful and of long-lasting benefit.

Post-Traumatic Stress Disorder

Stressful situations may often lead to the discovery of new coping capacities; stress may also lead to distress and a sense of traumatization or victimization. Even in the face of actual death, threatened death, or major injury, some people have remarkable coping skills. The incidence of PTSD after the World Trade Center disaster of 9/11/01 was far lower than public health professionals feared.

Definition

A. An individual is exposed to a traumatic event in which both of the following were present:
   1. The person experienced, witnessed, or was confronted with actual or threatened death, serious injury, or a threat to the physical integrity of self or others;
   2. The person's response involved intense fear, helplessness, or horror;
B. The event is persistently re-experienced as:
   1. Recurrent and intrusive distressing recollections of the event, including images, thoughts, and perceptions;
   2. Recurrent dreams of the event;
   3. Acting or feeling as if the event were recurring or hallucinations, flashbacks, illusions;
   4. Intense psychologic distress at exposure to internal or external cues that symbolize or resemble parts of the event;
   5. Intense physiologic reactivity on exposure to external or internal cues that resemble the event;
C. Persistent avoidance of the stimuli associated with the trauma and or numbing of general responsiveness;
D. Persistent symptoms or increased arousal with exaggerated startle response, hypervigilance, difficulty with sleep, outburst of irritability, anger, or both.

The duration of symptoms of B, C, D is for >4 weeks.

Epidemiology

Post-traumatic syndromes have sometimes been found in 30% of victims. However, studies of survivors of the Oklahoma bombing and the 9/11/01 New York Trade Center towers disaster give much lower figures. According to one U.S. study, the overall lifetime prevalence is 1% in the general population; in other countries, the rates may be much higher. Comorbid findings are primarily the affective disorders, often with abuse of marijuana or alcohol.

Pathophysiology

The neurocircuitry disorder in PTSD is an enigma; limbic, paralimbic, and visual areas are involved according to PET studies of traumatic events in nonmilitary subjects. The most constant hormonal finding in PTSD is enhanced suppression of cortisol secretion in response to low-dose dexamethasone. The pattern of suppression suggests enhanced sensitivity of the hypothalamic–pituitary axis as heightened negative feedback. However, this response may be genetically determined rather than a response to the trauma itself. Similarly, findings of reduced hypothalamic volume could explain vulnerability and not the result of illness. Overactivity in the locus ceruleus has been adduced to explain nightmares, flashbacks, and sympathetic overactivity. A family history of PTSD is a risk factor.

Treatment

Time-limited psychotherapies have been studied for treatment, and antidepressant medications including tricyclics, MAOIs, and SSRIs have been used. Most clinicians combine both approaches. Benzodiazepines are not effective.

Psychotherapies include cognitive behavioral and prolonged exposure therapies, cognitive restructuring, supportive counseling, stress inoculation training, and imaginal exposure (in which the patient relives the trauma in imagination and describes it orally in the present tense in a therapy session). The number of sessions can be 9 to 50. Skillful dynamic therapists have dealt successfully with prisoners of war or battlefield trauma.

War veteran studies with MAOIs and imipramine in 8-week trials demonstrated dramatic improvement over placebo. A 12-week multicenter trial of sertraline and a trial of paroxetine demonstrated the efficacy of both drugs, which are approved by the Food and Drug Administration. "Eye movement desensitization and reprocessing" was deemed effective by an international task force.

Obsessive-Compulsive Disorder

Definition

Obsessions are recurrent and persistent thoughts, impulses, or images that are experienced as intrusive and inappropriate and cause marked anxiety or distress. The thoughts and impulses or images are not merely excessive worries about real life problems. The patient attempts to ignore or suppress the thoughts, impulses, or images by substituting other thoughts or images. The patient recognizes that these are products of his or her own mind (not imposed from without as in thought insertion).

Compulsions are repetitive behaviors—hand washing or checking—or mental acts, such as counting or repeating words silently. The person feels driven to perform these acts in response to an obsession or according to some rigid rules. The behaviors are aimed at reducing or preventing distress or preventing a dreaded event. However, these behaviors are not connected in a realistic way with what they are designed to neutralize or prevent, or they are clearly excessive. The subject realizes that the obsessions or compulsions are excessive and that they cause distress by interfering with normal routines, occupation, or social activities.

Pathophysiology

The illness usually begins in adolescence or early adulthood, with a somewhat earlier onset for males (between 6 and 15) than for females (between 20 and 29). The incidence ratio is equal in men and women. The onset is usually gradual with some waxing and waning that may be related to stress. About 15% show gradual and progressive deterioration in occupational and social functioning. A reduction in GABA functioning has been suggested; anxiety is noted in laboratory studies of OCD. Current data suggest a lifetime rate of 2.5%. The molecular basis is not known.

Treatment

OCD is a chronic condition and leads to long-term management; current guidelines recommend pharmacotherapy for at least 1 to 2 years. The starting treatment of choice is either cognitive behavioral management alone or in combination with pharmacotherapy. Studies are needed to determine the optimal duration of treatment. Clomipramine (Anafranil) has the longest and best psychopharmacologic record for OCD. Starting with small doses of 25 mg at bedtime and gradually increasing sometimes up to 300 mg produced benefits in >60% of patients. Slow increments are essential because of modest risks of convulsions. Blood levels may be helpful guides.

Serotonin reuptake inhibitors including fluoxetine (Prozac) 20–60 mg, fluvoxamine (Luvox; 100–300 mg), and sertraline (Zoloft; 50–200 mg) are all widely used. Marks has demonstrated the value of behavioral exposure techniques. Maintenance programs are highly effective in helping patients sustain benefits of treatment for decades. Patients must be motivated to participate in behavioral treatment with drug therapy.

Generalized Anxiety Disorder

Definition

GAD is characterized by apprehension and excessive worry that occur more days than not for at least 6 months and involve several events or activities. This common disorder is often chronic, and 40% of patients report symptoms for more than 5 years. The individual finds it difficult to control the worry, which is associated with three or more of the following six symptoms:

1. Restlessness or feeling keyed up, on edge, or both;
2. Being easily fatigued;
3. Difficulty concentrating or mind going blank;
4. Irritability;
5. Muscle tension;
6. Sleep disturbance (difficulty falling asleep, staying asleep, or restless sleep).

Differential Diagnosis

It is important to rule out substance abuse by history or blood and urine toxicology screen. Medical conditions to be considered are thyroid abnormalities, other endocrinopathies, pneumonia, or occult neoplasms.

Epidemiology

In a community sample, the 1-year prevalence rate was about 3% and lifetime prevalence was 5% in the United States. These reports must be interpreted carefully because criteria have changed since DSM III publication. Comorbidity with personality disorders (as high as 25%) includes dependent, avoidant, or depressive syndromes and makes it difficult to sort out GAD as a distinct entity.

Pathophysiology

Abnormalities in amygdala volumes and heightened cortical activity are evidence that accounts for some of the observed easy arousal and hypervigilance in GAD. The GABA receptor brain complex may be different in these individuals as are decreased benzodiazepine receptor density in peripheral blood cells. However, other (nonbenzodiazepine) receptor sites are also probably involved; recently molecular changes in two antibiotics have been found in early studies to have antianxiety benefits.

Abnormal fear and behavior resembling anxiety are exhibited by mice that lack one of the genes encoding receptors that mediate neurotransmission. At least two critical receptors, particularly serotonin 1A, corticotropin-releasing factor receptor, and some subtype GABA receptors seem to account for and explain some fear circuitry.

Sleep disturbances are recognized and demonstrated in sleep laboratories.

Treatment

Research into different forms of psychotherapy for generalized anxiety disorders is limited. Cognitive therapies appear superior to nondirective or supportive therapies, but there is little information about combined pharmacotherapy and psychotherapy. Relaxation and behavioral anxiety treatments, hypnotherapy, and psychoanalytic therapy have been described. Most patients respond to benzodiazepines. All appear efficacious, with the newer more potent and longer-lasting variants an improvement over the earlier chlordiazepoxide in the 1960s. The risk of physical dependence is not supported by controlled data. Only individuals with alcohol dependence appear to be at risk.

All studies have demonstrated that benzodiazepines are more effective than placebo. It is not definite that any one drug is vastly superior clinically to another. There are differences in rates of absorption, half-life, and patterns of excretion. The cytochrome P-450 enzymes, a superfamily of microsomal drug-metabolizing enzymes, are the most important of those that affect phase 1 of drug metabolism. Alprazolam (Xanax) seems to be the most popular benzodiazepine.

Venlafaxine (Effexor) is a novel structure of an antidepressant that has excellent benefits for generalized anxiety disorder with doses starting at 75 mg/day and increasing up to 225 mg/day. It is generally well tolerated.

The duration of benzodiazepine treatment is not established, although the drugs are used most commonly for acute treatment. Patients with intermittent symptoms can be treated intermittently. Most controlled trials last 6 to 12 weeks. In practice, patients have been maintained on benzodiazepines for 20 years with no adverse effects; blood levels were monitored and stable in a small group. Benzodiazepine treatment has risk for some patients who develop tolerance, loss of beneficial effect, and adverse effects such as paradoxic aggression, impaired memory, poor attention, or psychomotor slowing. Currently no guidelines exist; long-term studies are needed for outcome data.

SUGGESTED READINGS

American Psychiatric Association: *Diagnostic and Statistical Manual of Mental Disorders*. Revised, 4th Ed. Washington, DC: American Psychiatric Association, 2000.

Gelenberg AJ, Lydiard RB, Rudolph RL, et al. Efficacy of venlafaxine extended-release capsules in nondepressed outpatients with generalized anxiety disorder: a 6-month randomized controlled trial. *JAMA* 2000;203:3082–3098.

Hoehn-Saric R, Ninan P, Black DW, et al. Multicenter double-blind comparison of sertraline and desipramine for concurrent obsessive-compulsive and major depressive disorders. *Arch Gen Psychiatry* 2000;57:76–82.

Jenike MA. Clinical practice. Obsessive-compulsive disorder. *N Engl J Med* 2004;350:259–265.

Lader MH. The nature and duration of treatment for GAD. *Acta Psychiatr Scand* 1998;393(Suppl):109–117.

LeDoux J. Fear and the brain: where have we been, and where are we going? *Biol Psychiatry* 1998;44:1229–1238.

Rickels K, Schweizer E. The clinical course and long-term management of generalized anxiety disorder. *J Clin Psychopharmacol* 1990;10(3 Suppl):101S–110S.

Sheehan DV. Venlafaxine extended release (XR) in the treatment of generalized anxiety disorder. *J Clin Psychiatry* 1999;60(Suppl 22):23–28.

Stein DJ. *Clinical Manual of Anxiety Disorders*. Washington, DC: American Psychiatric Publishing, 2004.

Uhl GR, Grow RW. The burden of complex genetics in brain disorders. *Arch Gen Psychiatry* 2004;61:223–229.

Van Ameringen M, Mancini C, Farvolden P, et al. The neurobiology of social phobia: from pharmacotherapy to brain imaging. *Curr Psychiatry Rep* 2000;2:358–366.

Weinberger, DR. Anxiety at the frontier of molecular medicine. *New Engl J Med* 2001;344:1247–1249.

Yehuda R. Post-traumatic stress disorder. *New Eng J Med* 2002;346:108–114.

Chapter 161

Schizophrenia

Arielle D. Stanford, Cheryl Corcoran, and Dolores Malaspina

DEFINITION

Schizophrenia is a severe neuropsychiatric syndrome affecting about 1% of the worldwide population. Symptom onset is usually in late adolescence or early adulthood, whereupon lifelong disability typically ensues. Schizophrenia is defined by characteristic, though nonspecific, abnormalities in the perception of reality, the form and content of thoughts and speech, and emotional deficits, including a disturbed sense of self, social dysfunction, apathy, and peculiar behavior. The term *schizophrenia* literally means "split mind" and refers to the schism between thoughts and emotions that may underlie the break with reality. Schizophrenia should not be confused with a split or multiple personality or with ordinary ambivalence, nor is it synonymous with psychosis. Psychosis, a failure to distinguish between reality and what is created by the mind (e.g., hallucinations, delusions), may be present in many illnesses, both psychiatric and not (see below).

SIGNS AND SYMPTOMS

The symptoms of schizophrenia are often grouped into positive and negative subtypes, although there may be substantive diversity in the pathophysiology of the symptoms within these groups. Positive symptoms include hallucinations and delusions, disorganized thinking or behavior, so denoted because these phenomena occur in addition to usual experiences. Negative symptoms are those that arise from the absence of normal behaviors or experiences, including affective flattening, alogia (impoverished thinking manifested by diminished speech output or content), apathy, avolition (lack of energy and drive,) and social withdrawal. Patients with particularly severe and enduring primary negative symptoms may have a specific form of the illness called *deficit syndrome schizophrenia*. Although positive symptoms and peculiar behavior garner much attention and are frequent reasons for hospital admissions, a stronger relationship to outcome is seen with cognitive deficits and with the negative symptoms, which are less responsive to treatment.

The symptoms of schizophrenia vary among individuals and change with time. Because diverse psychiatric and organic disorders can also resemble schizophrenia, the diagnosis should be based on the course as well as associated features of the illness. The *Diagnostic and Statistical Manual of Mental Disorders*, 4th edition (DSM-IV), diagnostic criteria for schizophrenia require the presence of two or more symptoms (delusions, hallucinations, disorganized speech, grossly disorganized or catatonic behavior, negative symptoms) for 1 month as well as social or occupational dysfunction. The observation period may be <1 month if treatment is effective. Another requirement for diagnosis is continuous evidence for at least 6 months of symptoms or functional impairment, including prodromal (symptoms prior to first psychosis) or residual symptoms (symptoms that remain after an exacerbation).

The duration of symptoms not only alters the diagnosis, but has a considerable impact on prognosis. Those individuals who have symptoms for <6 months have schizophreniform disorder or have brief psychotic episodes if symptomatic for <1 month. Individuals with these proscribed illnesses may have preserved social and occupational functioning and by definition experience a full remission. However, some of these individuals progress to schizophrenia as predicted in part by disrupted social and occupational functioning, blunted affect, absence of severe stressor, absence of mood symptoms, and an insidious onset. The term *psychosis not otherwise specified* (NOS) is reserved for individuals who meet some, but not all, of the criteria for one of the aforementioned disorders, for example, having only one positive symptom with functional impairment for >1 month. Adults with functional impairment and negative symptoms should be considered for a diagnosis of schizoid personality disorder or paranoid or schizotypal personality disorders if only attenuated positive symptoms are present. Personality disorders are persistent and pervasive disturbances that lead to impaired function. Paranoid personality disorders are characterized by suspiciousness, schizoid by social withdrawal, and schizotypal by eccentric behavior.

Any patient with delusions or hallucinations may be described as having a psychosis, but schizophrenia is not diagnosed if there is an identifiable toxic cause, the cause is an underlying medical condition, or the disorder is better defined by another psychiatric condition, such as schizoaffective disorder, mood disorder, substance use, or pervasive developmental disorder. Some positive symptoms were once considered to be indicative of schizophrenia, but can appear in any psychosis. Among these are audible thoughts, hallucinated voices of two or more people arguing or conversing or voices that comment on the patient's actions, and the feeling that one's thoughts are heard by others (thought broadcasting) or are being taken away (thought withdrawal).

COURSE AND ASSOCIATED FEATURES

The psychotic process in schizophrenia typically begins in late adolescence or early adult years and often progresses to a chronic course with substantial deterioration. This process begins with the prodrome, the 6 to 12 months prior to the onset of a first psychotic episode when patients first manifest attenuated psychotic symptoms, change in behavior, or a global decline in function. If the prodrome is short (i.e., the onset of psychosis is abrupt) and if premorbid function was good, prognosis is better. Remission between exacerbations varies. Patients with predominantly negative residual symptoms have a worse prognosis. Women tend to have a later onset and milder symptoms than do men. Underlying sex differences in brain organization may explain these differences, but exposures and gene–environment interactions may vary by sex.

Many schizophrenia patients have abused alcohol or other substances, and there is accumulating evidence that cannabis abuse is an important risk factor for schizophrenia. About 80% of patients smoke tobacco, which may be a form of self-medication to compensate for aberrant dopamine functioning. Independent of cigarette smoking and medication effects, schizophrenia patients show significantly increased medical morbidity and earlier death from cardiovascular disease, diabetes, and other medical conditions. Suicide accounts for approximately 10% of patient deaths. Violence against other individuals by schizophrenia patients is uncommon, although reported cases can be striking and receive much media attention. Predictors of violence include past violent episodes, substance abuse, and male gender (as in nonpsychiatric samples) as well as treatment noncompliance, paranoid delusions, and "command" auditory hallucinations in which voices direct the person's behavior.

ETIOLOGY

Schizophrenia is an etiologically heterogeneous syndrome and not a single disorder. The common schizophrenia phenotype results from a complex pattern of interactions among environmental exposures and genetic mutations and sequence variations, particularly in genes that influence prenatal neurodevelopment. These factors may disrupt neural functioning through diverse pathways. Although a large genetic component had been suspected for over a century, susceptibility genes have been identified only in the last decade. Several of these genes participate in the development, stabilization, or function of synapses, consistent with the theory that glial cells are aberrant in the disease. The list of genes associated with schizophrenia is growing and includes neuregulin 1 (8p21-p12), G72 (13q34), a D-aminoacid oxidase (12q24), and dysbindin (6p22.3). The at-risk haplotypes of these genes may only double the risk of schizophrenia, and most gene carriers do not have the disease. Therefore, these loci are likely to influence risk through epistatic mechanisms, an influence of the genotype at one locus on the effect of a mutation at another locus, or an interaction of nonallelic genes and the impact of environment on genetic expression.

Epidemiologic studies have identified numerous environmental schizophrenia risk factors: prenatal exposure to maternal infection, emotional stress, urban versus rural birth, malnutrition, obstetric complications, and Rh incompatibility. The risk of schizophrenia may be augmented in susceptible individuals by cannabis abuse, adverse childhood environment, major life events, and traumatic brain injury. Schizophrenia risk is linearly related to paternal age at conception and may be tripled for the children of fathers over 45 years of age compared to fathers in their 20s.

Schizophrenia may involve both developmental and degenerative components. According to the neurodevelopmental model, the disease results from an early, probably prenatal, abnormality in neural development. It remains latent or is expressed first as subtle cognitive change or social dysfunction. Many who become ill show subtle nonspecific abnormalities that indicate the presence of pathology long before psychosis commences. These include impairments in verbal memory, gross motor skills, and global attention, as well as social withdrawal and lower intelligence. Enlarged cerebral ventricles at onset, postmortem cellular disarray, and an excess of minor physical anoma-

lies associated with the disease suggest fetal developmental origins. However, the onset of psychosis in premorbidly impaired individuals and the further deterioration in cognition, social capacity, and reduction in neural volume after the onset of disease symptoms provide evidence of an additional degenerative process.

PATHOPHYSIOLOGY

There is no pathognomonic diagnostic clinical finding or laboratory test for schizophrenia. However, group differences are found between schizophrenia patients and healthy individuals that may illuminate key aspects of the pathophysiology. In addition, close examination of more narrowly defined heritable stable features of the disorder, so-called *endophenotypes*, can also shed light on the neurobiologic underpinnings of schizophrenia's diverse clinical manifestations.

Neurotransmitters

Dopamine

The introduction of chlorpromazine, a dopamine receptor antagonist, and its efficacy in treating the psychotic symptoms of schizophrenia led to the development of the dopamine hypothesis by Nobel laureate Arvid Carlsson. To date, all effective antipsychotic medications have antagonistic activity at the dopamine type 2 (D_2) receptor, consistent with the theory that excessive subcortical transmission of dopamine is an integral part of the pathophysiology of psychosis. Imaging studies demonstrate abnormally enhanced release of dopamine in response to amphetamine in patients with schizophrenia. By contrast, *decreased* dopamine activity in the prefrontal cortex may be responsible for the negative symptoms (e.g., flattened affect, alogia, avolition) and cognitive impairment that precede the onset of psychosis. Executive function and working memory are both impaired in schizophrenia and are regulated by the prefrontal cortex. Furthermore, when schizophrenia patients do working memory tasks, the prefrontal cortex shows abnormal activation in PET and functional MRI. Phosphorous MR spectroscopy also shows a deficit of high-energy phosphates in the prefrontal cortex of these individuals.

Glutamate and GABA

Other neurotransmitters may be important in schizophrenia, including glutamate, an excitatory neurotransmitter, and γ-aminobutyric acid (GABA), an inhibitory neurotransmitter. Hallucinogenic substances of abuse, such as phencyclidine (PCP) and ketamine ("Special K"), antagonize glutamate receptors of the *N*-methyl-D-aspartate

(NMDA) type, and in healthy adults, these agents can lead to acute and transient schizophrenialike symptoms, including psychosis, negative symptoms, and cognitive deficits. In contrast, the amino acid glycine, a positive modulator of the NMDA receptor, can partly improve both positive and negative symptoms.

The possibility that schizophrenia is related to hypofunction of NMDA receptors is supported by animal studies. In nonhuman primates, chronic PCP exposure leads not only to negative-type symptoms, but also to prefrontal hypodopaminergic and subcortical hyperdopaminergic activity as seen in humans with schizophrenia. In rodents, mutations in a key subunit of the NMDA receptor lead to reduced expression of NMDA receptors and also to stereotyped and abnormal social behavior that can be attenuated with antipsychotic medication. However, linkages have not been found between schizophrenia and glutamate receptor genes, and postmortem studies have not established any abnormal expression of NMDA receptors in schizophrenia patients.

In contrast, abnormal expression of GABA-related proteins (for synthesis, transport, and uptake) has been found in postmortem studies specifically of patients with schizophrenia, in both prefrontal and temporal cortex. Chandelier cells, a set of prefrontal cortex GABAergic inhibitory neurons that are key to working memory, show decreased expression of GABA-related proteins. Therefore the symptoms of schizophrenia may emerge from a failure of inhibitory activity, resulting in cognitive deficits (impaired focus and attention) and increased sensitivity to stimuli (sensory misperceptions, overvaluing of ideas). Connections between GABA interneurons and glutamatergic cells may explain NMDA receptor hypofunction or may be further aggravated by NMDA hypofunction.

Synaptic Pruning Hypothesis

Neuroimaging studies comparing schizophrenia patients and healthy subjects demonstrate increased size of ventricles, reduced cortical volumes with smaller frontal and temporal lobes, possible thalamic volume reductions, and decreased thickness of the corpus callosum. However, the absence of gliosis in these brain regions in postmortem studies excludes any typical neurodegeneration as a cause of the diminished brain volume. Postmortem studies show cortical thinning with increased cell packing and abnormal cellular patterns without an absolute decrease in the number of neurons. This increased neuronal density, along with low levels of synaptophysin and other synaptic proteins, suggests a glial abnormality in the connections between neurons, including dendrites and synapses. Synaptic reorganization is prominent in adolescence, so abnormalities in this process could explain the usual onset of schizophrenia at that time. Magnetic resonance spectroscopy at the onset of symptoms demonstrates abnormalities in phosphomonoesters and phosphodiesters that are consistent with increased cell membrane turnover.

Neural Circuitry

Functional imaging studies further support the presence of altered neurometabolism, especially prefrontal hypoactivation for cognitive tasks in schizophrenia. Also, abnormalities in cortical and subcortical activation may accompany impaired emotional regulation, memory, executive ability, and other specific symptoms that are attributed to anomalous connectivity in frontal-limbic circuits or failed modulation in cortico-striato-pallido-thalamo-cortical loops by specific neurotransmitter projection systems.

DIFFERENTIAL DIAGNOSIS OF PSYCHOSIS

Psychosis in the Neurology Patient

Psychosis may accompany diverse medical and neurologic disorders and be the first manifestation of the underlying disorder. Although medical and neurologic patients typically have normal premorbid mental function and better insight into their psychotic symptoms, the clinical findings in primary and secondary psychoses are often indistinguishable. In a patient with new-onset psychosis, it is therefore imperative to consider all reversible causes. Urine toxicologic tests for drugs, as well as medical, psychiatric, and family histories, can provide invaluable diagnostic information. Common causes of psychosis in neurologic patients include temporal or limbic seizures, AIDS, neurosyphilis, dementia, and delirium. Substance abuse, withdrawal, and iatrogenic actions are also common causes of reversible psychosis (Table 161.1).

Psychiatric disorders other than schizophrenia may also include psychosis, typically hallucinations, delusions, and thought disorder, such as bipolar disorder, depression, dementia, substance use, acute and chronic post traumatic stress disorders, and mental retardation. Transient psychotic symptoms may also be seen in individuals with personality disorders (e.g., paranoid, schizoid, schizotypal), although with sustained or prominent symptoms a rediagnosis is warranted.

TREATMENT

Antipsychotic Medication

The treatment of schizophrenia has focused primarily on the treatment of psychosis (e.g., hallucinations, delusions). A drastic change occurred in the clinical

▶ **TABLE 161.1** **Differential Diagnosis of Psychosis:**
Medical and Neurologic Disorders

Epilepsy	Temporal lobe epilepsy
Neoplasm	Especially frontal and temporal lobe tumors
Cerebrovascular disease	
Traumatic brain injury	Consider frontal and temporal lobes
Infectious	
AIDS	Progressive multifocal leukoencephalopathy, AIDS dementia, CNS lymphoma, toxoplasmosis, cryptococcal meningitis
Herpes encephalitis	
Neurosyphilis	
Inflammatory	
Metachromatic leukodystrophy	
Systemic lupus erythematosus	
Metabolic	
Acute intermittent porphyria	
B_{12} deficiency	
Delirium	
Homocystinuria	
Pellagra	
Wilson disease	
Degenerative	
Creutzfeldt-Jakob disease	
Frontotemporal dementia	
Huntington disease	
Substance-related	
Alcohol	Delirium tremens
	Hallucinosis
	Wernicke-Korsakoff syndrome
Depressants	Barbiturate withdrawal
Hallucinogens	Lysergic acid diethylamide (LSD), phencyclidine (PCP)
Stimulants	Amphetamines, cocaine
Steroids	For the treatment of MS, lupus, or other diseases
Carbon monoxide poisoning	
Heavy metal poisoning	
Other	
Normal pressure hydrocephalus	

management of psychosis 50 years ago with the introduction of chlorpromazine. Institutions formerly filled with agitated, catatonic, or withdrawn patients suddenly found that some patients could resume function. The efficacy of chlorpromazine and the antipsychotic drugs that followed correlated with antagonism of the dopamine D_2 receptor. The most common medications still used from the first generation of antipsychotic medications include haloperidol, perphenazine, fluphenazine, and chlorpromazine. Common side effects of these medications can include intense psychomotor restlessness (akathisia), parkinsonism,

tardive dyskinesia (TD), extrapyramidal symptoms (EPS), anticholinergic symptoms, prolongation of the QT interval, and the neuroleptic malignant syndrome (discussed in Chapter 130). Hyperprolactinemia from D_2 antagonism is associated with galactorrhea, amenorrhea, gynecomastia, and impotence, and all antipsychotic medications lower the seizure threshold.

In 1989, clozapine was introduced as the first antipsychotic medication to demonstrate superior efficacy to typical antipsychotics. It earned the title of "atypical" antipsychotic for its unique receptor profile, including lower D_2 binding and higher affinity for the serotonin 5-HT_{2A} receptor. Despite this unusual receptor-binding pattern, clozapine has a beneficial therapeutic profile, inducing response in 40% of refractory patients (i.e., patients whose psychotic symptoms were unresponsive to two or more antipsychotic medications). Clozapine has not been associated with TD and rarely with EPS. However, it can have the fatal adverse effect of agranulocytosis in 1% to 2% of patients. Individuals taking this medication must therefore have weekly neutrophil counts. Other important side effects include anticholinergic and antihistaminergic symptoms, hypersalivation, weight gain, and diabetes.

Other antipsychotic medications have been labeled atypical, but would more appropriately be called second-generation antipsychotics: they include risperidone, olanzapine, quetiapine, ziprasidone, and aripiprazole (Table 161.2). With time the frequencies of EPS and TD with risperidone and olanzapine have proved to be similar to the rates of typical antipsychotics. In addition, olanzapine causes weight gain and diabetes, quetiapine and aripiprazole have low rates of extrapyramidal symptoms, and olanzapine and risperidone have demonstrated mood stabilizing effects.

Other Pharmacotherapies

Patients with schizophrenia have high rates of comorbid anxiety and mood disorders. The adjunctive use of anxiolytics, mood stabilizers, and antidepressants is quite common. Such comorbid diagnoses and the further understanding of symptom neurobiology have expanded the pharmacologic possibilities for treating schizophrenia. New receptor research has led to the development of cholinergic, serotonergic and NMDA agonists, and D_4 and sigma antagonists with therapeutic potential.

Nonpharmacologic Therapies

Antipsychotic medications brought about a major change in the management of schizophrenia, but they are symptomatic treatments and do not cure the disease. Although symptoms of psychosis, anxiety, and depression respond

▶ **TABLE 161.2** **Second-Generation Antipsychotics**

Name	Major Receptor Binding Sites	Common Side Effects
Aripiprazole	Partial D2 Agonist	Not well known, little weight gain, low sedation, low EPS
Clozapine	Antagonism of $D_{1,3,4}$, 5-HT_{2A}, α_1, low potency D2	Sedation, dizziness, syncope, tachycardia, hypotension, ECG changes, nausea, hypersalivation, constipation, weight gain, leucopenia, fatigue
Olanzapine	Antagonism of $D_{1,2,4}$, 5-HT_{2A}, α_1, M_{1-5}, and H_1	Somnolence, dry mouth, dizziness, weight gain, constipation, dyspepsia, increased appetite, tremor
Quetiapine	Antagonism of $D_{1,2}$, 5-HT_{2A}, 6, $\alpha_{1,2}$, and H_1	Somnolence, postural hypotension, dizziness (no EPS)
Risperidone	Antagonism of D_2, 5-HT_{2A}, $\alpha_{1,2}$, and H_1, low affinity for β and M	EPS, weight gain, anxiety, nausea, vomiting, erectile dysfunction, hyperprolactinemia, increased pigmentation
Ziprasidone	Antagonism of D_{2-4}, 5-$HT_{1D,2A,2C}$, α_1 and H_1, low affinity for D1, M1, and α_2; Agonism of 5-HT_{1A}	Somnolence, headache, dizziness, nausea, light-headedness, QT prolongation

5-HT, serotonin; $\alpha + \beta$ = adrenergic; D = dopamine; H = histamine; M = muscarine

to pharmacotherapy, the most disabling schizophrenia symptoms rarely improve sufficiently for normal functioning. In particular, negative symptoms (e.g., affect blunting, alogia, avolition), social dysfunction, and cognitive deficits are suboptimally treated by existing interventions and are predictors of an unfavorable outcome. Current studies are examining the efficacy of cognitive behavioral therapy (CBT), social skills training, and other rehabilitation techniques on these symptoms and on quality of life. CBT for schizophrenia indirectly decreases positive and negative symptoms by reducing distress and promoting behavioral changes. Electroconvulsive therapy is successful in some individuals, particularly those with affective symptoms, and some recent trials have demonstrated efficacy of repetitive transcranial magnetic stimulation for auditory hallucinations and negative symptoms.

SUGGESTED READINGS

American Psychiatric Association. *Diagnostic and Statistical Manual of Mental Disorders.* 4th Ed., revised (DSM-IVR). Washington, DC: American Psychiatric Association, 2000.

Carpenter WT. The deficit syndrome. *Am J Psychiatry* 1994;151:327–329.

Dalman C, Allebeck P, Cullberg J, et al. Obstetric complications and the risk of schizophrenia: a longitudinal study of a national birth cohort. *Arch Gen Psychiatry* 1999;56(Mar):234–240.

DeLisi LE, Sakuma M, Tew W, et al. Schizophrenia as a chronic active brain process: a study of progressive brain structural change subsequent to the onset of schizophrenia. *Psychiatry Res* 1997;74(Jul 4):129–140.

Erlenmeyer-Kimling L. Early neurobehavioral deficits as phenotypic indicators of the schizophrenia genotype and predictors of later psychosis. *Am J Med Genet* 2001;105(Jan 8):23–24.

Goff DC, Coyle JT. The emerging role of glutamate in the pathophysiology and treatment of schizophrenia. *Am J Psychiatry* 2001;158:1367–1377.

Gur RE, Turetsky BI, Cowell PE, et al. Temporolimbic volume reductions in schizophrenia. *Arch Gen Psychiatry* 2000;57:769–775.

Laruelle M, Abi-Dargham A, Gil R, et al. Increased dopamine transmission in schizophrenia: relationship to illness phases. *Biol Psychiatry* 1999;46(Jul 1):56–72.

Lewis DA, Pierri JN, Volk DW, et al. Altered GABA neurotransmission and prefrontal cortical dysfunction in schizophrenia. *Biol Psychiatry* 1999;46:616–626.

Malaspina D, Harlap S, Fennig S, et al. Advancing paternal age and the risk of schizophrenia. *Arch Gen Psychiatry* 2001;58(Apr):361–367.

Meltzer HY, Li Z, Kaneda Y, et al. Serotonin receptors: their key role in drugs to treat schizophrenia. *Prog Neuropsychopharmacol Biol Psychiatry* 2003;27:1159–1172.

Mueser KT, McGurk SR. Schizophrenia. *Lancet* 2004;363:2063–2072.

Potkin SG, Alphs L, Hsu C, et al. Predicting suicidal risk in schizophrenic and schizoaffective patients in a prospective two-year trial. *Biol Psychiatry* 2003 Aug15; 54(4):444–452.

Schultz SK, Andreasen NC. Schizophrenia. *Lancet* 1999;353:1425–1430.

Selemon LD, Goldman-Rakic PS. The reduced neuropil hypothesis: a circuit based model of schizophrenia. *Biol Psychiatry* 1999;45:17–25.

Weinberger DR, Egan MF, Bertolino A, et al. Prefrontal neurons and the genetics of schizophrenia. *Biol Psychiatry* 2001;50:825–844.

Chapter 162

▶ Somatoform Disorders

Daniel T. Williams

Somatoform disorders are but one of a group of somatizing disorders that are frequent challenges to neurologists, psychiatrists, and other physicians for differential diagnosis and treatment. The essential features of somatoform disorders are physical symptoms that suggest a general medical condition but are not adequately explained by any general medical disorder, by the direct effects of a substance, or by some other psychiatric disorder. The symptoms must cause clinically meaningful distress or functional impairment. By definition, the symptoms are not intentionally produced, so distinguishing them from factitious disorders and malingering. Furthermore, somatoform disorders differ from "psychologic factors affecting a medical condition" (e.g., stress-induced hypertension) insofar as there is no diagnosable general medical condition that adequately accounts for the physical symptoms.

The physical symptoms usually bring a patient first to a primary care physician or medical specialist, where the crucial task is that of establishing whether a primary organic substrate underlies some or all of the presenting symptoms. If an organic substrate can be ascertained, that, of course, becomes the focus of attention, although a secondary somatoform disorder may coexist and also warrants clinical intervention. If an organic condition is ruled out or if associated indications of emotional stressors are observed and could account for nonphysiologic symptoms, then a crucial medical service is that of facilitating referral to a mental health professional, so that appropriate assessment and treatment can ensue. Several subtypes of somatoform disorder will be briefly described here, followed by differentiation of somatoform disorders from other somatizing disorders.

Conversion disorder connotes the presence of symptoms affecting voluntary motor or sensory function that inappropriately suggest a neurologic or other general medical condition. Psychologic factors are judged to be associated with the symptom, based on the antecedent presence of apparently relevant conflicts or stressors. The symptoms are not intentionally produced, yet cause distress or functional impairment. The symptoms are not limited to pain or sexual dysfunction and are not better accounted for by another psychiatric disorder, such as panic attack, substance abuse, or psychologic factors affecting a medical condition. Insofar as there may be an undiagnosed general medical cause underlying cases of apparent conversion disorder, the diagnosis should be re-evaluated in medical follow-up, especially if the symptoms are not fully alleviated by appropriate psychologic or psychiatric intervention. Undiagnosed or undertreated conversion symptoms in childhood and adolescence may contribute to symptom proliferation and chronicity in later life.

Somatization disorder connotes a pattern of multiple, recurring, clinically important somatic complaints that result in medical treatment or functional impairment. The symptomatic pattern begins before age 30 and persists over several years. In addition to general features of somatoform disorders noted above, the DSM-IVR-TR criteria for psychiatric diagnostic nomenclature stipulate that there must be (a) pain related to at least four sites or functions, (b) at least two gastrointestinal symptoms other than pain, (c) at least one sexual or reproductive symptom other than pain, and (d) at least one symptom other than pain that

suggests a neurologic disorder. A long story of multiple evaluations and treatments with associated morbidity is common, as are coexisting depressive, anxiety and personality disorders.

Somatoform conditions with multiple symptoms that do not fulfill the criteria of somatization disorder are classified as *undifferentiated somatoform disorder* if the duration is 6 months or longer or *somatoform disorder not otherwise specified* if of shorter duration.

In *pain disorder*, the pain must cause functional impairment; psychologic factors are judged to play a major role in the onset, severity, or maintenance of the pain; the pain is not intentionally produced; and it is not better accounted for by another psychiatric disorder. Pain disorder comprises two types. In pain disorder associated with psychologic factors, these factors have a predominant role in the onset, severity, or maintenance of the pain; general medical conditions play no role or a minimal one. In pain disorder associated with both psychologic factors and a general medical condition, both aspects are important. (Pain disorder associated with a general medical condition without major psychologic contributions is not considered a mental disorder.)

Individuals with *hypochondriasis* are preoccupied with fear of having a serious disease based on misinterpreting one or more bodily signs or symptoms. The concern persists despite reassurance that thorough evaluation has not identified a general medical condition to account for the patient's concerns. However, the belief is not of delusional intensity; the patient understands somewhat that the fear and concern may be excessive. The preoccupation causes distress or functional impairment, lasts for at least 6 months, and is not better accounted for by another psychiatric disorder.

Persons with *body dysmorphic disorder* are preoccupied with an imagined defect in appearance. If a slight physical anomaly is present, the individual's concern is markedly excessive. The preoccupation causes distress or functional impairment and is not better accounted for by another mental disorder.

PATHOGENESIS

Hypotheses about the pathogenesis of somatoform disorders have focused on considerations of predisposition, precipitating factors, and perpetuating factors. Predisposition includes personality factors (e.g., internalizing as opposed to externalizing style) and past experiences (e.g., trauma, abuse, or exposure to disabling physical illness in oneself or others) that foster somatization. Limitations of communicative ability may arise from intellectual, emotional, or social constraints and may lead to a "body language expression of distress." Underlying psychiatric or neurologic disorders may also contribute.

Precipitating stressors may involve proximate activation of psychologic conflicts, such as those regarding sexual, aggressive, or dependency issues. Traumatic events, such as those threatening one's physical integrity or self-esteem are frequently cited precipitants. Perpetuating factors include the ways in which the symptom resolves or diminishes the psychologic conflict that gave rise to the symptom (primary gain) and the associated tangible benefits of the symptom (secondary gain).

Somatoform disorders embody dissociative features, insofar as they involve the genesis of somatic symptoms or preoccupations based on psychologic mechanisms that operate outside the individual's conscious awareness. As such, one may conceive that the person is overwhelmed with adversity beyond capacity for effective, conscious processing of the associated affect, leading to a dysfunctional, primitive communication of distress by "somatic metaphor." If an acute somatoform disorder, for instance, a post-traumatic conversion disorder, abates after resolution of a short-term precipitating conflict, the patient may not come to medical attention or may respond expeditiously to supportive reassurance and positive suggestion by a physician. Persistence or exacerbation of somatoform symptoms, however, may require more extensive medical evaluation to rule out medical conditions. Thoroughness and sensitivity by the examining physician facilitate the prospect of successful referral for psychiatric intervention. Attention earlier in the course of somatizing illnesses may diminish the potential for chronic persistence that makes treatment more difficult.

DIFFERENTIAL DIAGNOSIS

The primary task of the neurologist is to evaluate and, if possible, rule out contributory organic illness and to recognize the emotional basis of the disorder so the patient accepts referral for psychiatric diagnosis and treatment. The neurologist may have legitimate clinical impressions regarding the question of conscious versus unconscious intentionality of symptom formation. However, it is generally best to finesse this issue by assuming unconscious etiology, in the interest of protecting the patient's self-esteem and also the therapeutic alliance with both the referring neurologist and the psychiatrist. Premature and flawed confrontation of the patient, alleging presumption of purposeful symptom formation, is guaranteed to alienate the patient, who will then search for a "better" neurologist. If, alternatively, a supportive and successful referral to a mental health professional can be achieved, it becomes the task of the mental health professional to explore psychodynamics, stressors, contingencies of reinforcement, and issues of intentionality relevant to psychiatric differential diagnosis and treatment (Table 162.1).

To avoid the perceived rejection raised by sending the patient to a "shrink," the neurologist might emphasize how stress can generate physical symptoms without a patient's awareness. With this neuropsychiatric perspective, and noting the prospect of continuing collaboration between neurologist and psychiatrist, as well as emphasizing the more favorable prognosis of somatoform disorder than with many neurologic disorders, all can facilitate the patient's acceptance of referral. Furthermore, it is essential to inform the consulting psychiatrist of the detailed neurologic findings, including the level of confidence that a neurologic disorder has been established or excluded. Several follow-up studies of patients with presumptive somatoform disorders indicate that somatoform symptoms may be identified at first, and an undiagnosed physical illness may be identified later. Maintaining collaborative contact and an open mind, both neurologically and psychiatrically as the patient is followed, can minimize medically important errors of diagnostic omission in either domain.

Factitious disorders involve the intentional production of physical or psychologic symptoms owing to a pathologic psychologic need to assume the sick role. Pragmatic incentives for this behavior, such as economic benefit or evasion of legal responsibility, as in malingering, are absent. Numerous medical evaluations and treatments, including hospitalizations and surgical procedures, are often involved. Migration of the patient to many treatment sites may be motivated by the wish to avoid detection of a psychopathologic pattern that would be more likely discerned in a single setting with continuity of care. In factitious disorders, the intense need to be taken care of by duplicitously and intentionally assuming the patient role is frequently associated with severe dependent, histrionic, borderline, and antisocial personality features. As a result, prognosis is generally less favorable than in cases of somatoform disorder. The pattern that emerges can become characteristically chronic, polysymptomatic, and intractable, which has traditionally been called the Munchausen syndrome.

Malingering refers to the intentional production of physical or psychologic symptoms in pursuit of a recognizably pragmatic goal, such as financial gain, avoidance of work or school, evasion of criminal prosecution, or obtaining narcotics. Associated characteristics often include poor cooperation during diagnostic evaluation and treatment, pending litigation, and features of an antisocial personality disorder. Diagnostically, malingering is not classified as a mental disorder, although there may be coexisting psychopathology.

The diagnosis of *psychologic factors affecting a medical condition* requires the documentation of a general medical condition. Psychologic factors adversely affect the medical disorder in one of several ways. Those most pertinent to differential diagnosis from somatoform disorders

▶ **TABLE 162.1 Somatizing Disorders: Defining Characteristics**

	Conscious Intentionality	*Primary Gain*	*Secondary Gain*	*Coexisting Psychopathology*	*Prognosis*
Somatoform disorders	Absent	Repress unacceptable wishes, feelings, or conflicts	Any pragmatic benefits, if present, are secondary	Highly variable: May include affective, anxiety, dissociative, psychotic, developmental, or personality disorders	Highly variable, depending on chronicity, coexisting psychopathology, patient resilience, support network, and treatment
Factitious disorders	Present	Assume the sick role	Generally no significant pragmatic benefits; if present, are secondary	Often includes dependent, histrionic, borderline, or antisocial personality features	Often poor, especially if chronic
Malingering	Present	Pragmatic benefit: financial, legal, drugs	Circumvent authority	Often includes antisocial personality disorder	Symptoms are relinquished only when the goal is either obtained or seen as clearly unobtainable
Psychologic factors affecting a medical condition	Variable	None	Any pragmatic benefits, if present, are secondary	Highly variable	Highly variable, depending on the medical condition, chronicity, patient resilience, support network, and treatment
Undiagnosed medical condition	Absent	None	Any pragmatic benefits, if present, are secondary	Highly variable	Depends on the medical condition and the stage at which diagnosed and treated

include (1) psychologic factors that have been observed to influence the course of the medical condition, or (2) stress-related physiologic responses that precipitate or exacerbate symptoms of the medical condition. Examples include stress-precipitated epileptic seizures or the exacerbation of a parkinsonian tremor by anxiety.

Coexisting psychiatric conditions frequently contribute to the development of, or complicate the treatment of, somatoform disorders. Common examples include affective disorders, anxiety disorders, dissociative disorders, psychotic disorders, developmental disorders, and personality disorders. Specific inquiry should be made not only regarding recent psychosocial stressors and psychiatric symptoms, but also of historically remote, potentially relevant adversities, such as indications of prior physical, sexual, or emotional abuse or neglect, which may be predisposing factors to somatization. Knowledge about relevant psychiatric risk factors often assists in formulating a more effective treatment plan.

TREATMENT

Effective treatment of somatoform disorders requires consideration of the predisposing, precipitating, and perpetuating factors that may have generated the symptoms and then the formulation of a comprehensive plan for sustained remediation. This process presupposes the exploration of an underlying psychiatric or neurologic disorder, of which the patient is often unaware. A combination of treatment modalities is often required: psychotherapeutic inquiry to elucidate and address repressed psychologic conflicts, behavioral advice for the redress of overwhelming environmental stressors and renegotiation of secondary gain of the symptoms, psychopharmacologic intervention for psychobiologic symptoms, and other interventions. Because of these complexities, controlled studies of treatment intervention in this area are sparse, and most of the following treatment options derive from reported clinical experience in open trials.

Psychotherapeutic interventions seek to generate a more effective coping strategy to help the patient deal with preexisting conflicts by a process of emotional and cognitive "restructuring" that allows more effective negotiation of those conflicts without need for maladaptive symptoms. This approach must address as many relevant etiologic variables as possible, preferably with a systems theory perspective that strengthens the patient's capacity to deal with psychologic, biologic, and social variables in the quest for a healthier mode of adaptation. A supportively couched therapeutic alliance, geared to improving the patient's stress management strategies, with regard for the patient's self-esteem, seems to offer a palatable and useful contemporary adaptation of the traditional psychodynamic approach.

Hypnosis is a psychotherapeutic technique that includes the experience of dissociation as an essential ingredient; it can provide a direct modeling experience of the capacity to modify the vulnerability to dissociation under the protective supervision of the therapist. As noted earlier, somatoform disorders inherently embody dissociative features, insofar as they involve the genesis of somatic symptoms or preoccupations based on psychologic mechanisms that operate outside the individual's conscious awareness. *Dissociation* here refers to the intense psychologic absorption with a particular perception that shuts out one's usual critical cognitive processes, presumably based on a neurophysiologic process centered in the reticular formation. An assessment of hypnotizability provides a benign mind–body dissociative experience that constitutes a basis for understanding and experiencing the dissociation that is inherent in conversion symptom formation. Thus, when the patient incorporates the therapist's initial suggestion in hypnotic trance, that the patient's hand will feel light and then it floats upward posthypnotically, apparently without the patient's intent, the patient can observe how a psychologic influence can generate a change in physical sensation and movement, as well as a changed perception of locus of control. This becomes a paradigm to understand how this capacity for dissociation can be both a vulnerability to symptom formation, but also a potential channel for symptom resolution, when restructured with the help of the therapist. Teaching the patient a self-hypnosis format reinforces the confidence-building message of enhanced self-control, associated with suggestions for symptomatic improvement.

Behavior modification strategies offer significant advantages in dealing with those contingencies of reinforcement that contribute to symptom formation and perpetuation. Psychotherapy and positive suggestion have limited motivational traction for many patients unless combined with the alteration of environmental field forces that generated primary and secondary gain benefits that precipitated the symptom formation in the first place.

Physical therapy can be helpful in cases of weakness, fixed postures, or gait abnormalities. The physical therapist provides encouragement, hands-on intervention, and reinforcement for observed improvement. This intervention can provide a face-saving physical format of recovery, which often appeals to patients with difficulty assimilating psychodynamic formulations. Furthermore, physical therapy can be crucial in treating disuse atrophy or contractures that may develop with more persistent somatoform symptoms.

Pharmacotherapy may serve a similar dual biologic and psychologic function with many somatoform disorder patients. Pharmacotherapy is often indicated for coexist-

ing and contributory psychiatric conditions, such as depression, anxiety, or psychosis. The treating neurologist and psychiatrist can realistically and supportively explain how these neuropsychiatric medications can attenuate perturbations of neurotransmitter balance in the brain that are believed to play a central role in many neuropsychiatric conditions, including stress-induced somatoform disorders.

Other potential treatment interventions may include the following: family therapy (to deal with contributory conflicts, abuse, dependency, or enabling issues), intravenous amobarbital infusions (e.g., to evaluate the possible presence of contractures in cases of fixed, dystonic posturing), electroconvulsive therapy (for coexisting treatment-resistant depression or mania), speech therapy (for neuropsychiatric speech problems), or direct environmental intervention (to deal with contributory stressors or secondary gain influences.

With more chronically and severely impaired or resistant patients, such as those with somatization disorder, admission to an inpatient neurology service may help the establishment and patient acceptance of the diagnosis, as well as the initiation of an intensive clinical treatment trial, to be continued on an outpatient basis. For patients with psychosis, indications of suicidal intent or serious self-injury (as in some factitious disorder patients), transfer to an inpatient psychiatry unit may be warranted.

Because malingering is not technically a psychiatric disorder, management, rather than treatment pertains. The important caveat of deferring the articulation of this diagnosis, however, applies not only to the need to carefully rule out both neurologic and psychiatric illness, but also to avoid premature rupture of the treatment relationship that will ensue with its premature communication. Judicious and diplomatic handling of both verbal and written pronouncements is warranted when this diagnosis is suspected.

PROGNOSIS

The prognosis for any patient with a somatizing disorder is influenced by many factors. These include the nature, chronicity, and severity of the underlying psychopathology; the nature, chronicity, and severity of contributory external stressors; the strengths and resilience of the patient; and the effectiveness of the patient's support system, including the appropriateness and comprehensiveness of treatment.

SUGGESTED READINGS

American Psychiatric Association. *Diagnostic and Statistical Manual of Mental Disorders.* 4th Ed., Text revision. Washington, DC: American Psychiatric Association, 2000.

Couprie W, Wijdicks EF, Rooijmans HG, et al. Outcome in conversion disorder: a follow-up study. *J Neurol Neurosurg Psychiatry* 1995;58:750–752.

Crimlisk HL, Bhatia KP, Cope H, et al. Patterns of referral in patients with unexplained medical symptoms. *J Psychosom Res* 2000;49:217–219.

Fahn S, Williams DT, Ford B. Psychogenic movement disorders. In: Noseworthy JH, ed. *Neurological Therapeutics: Principles and Practice, vol 2*. London: Martin Dunitz, 2003:2677–2687.

Hallett M, Fahn S, Jankovic J, et al., eds. *Psychogenic Movement Disorders: Psychobiology and Therapy of a Functional Disorder, Advances in Neurology*. Philadelphia: Lippincott Williams & Wilkins, 2004.

Mace CJ, Trimble MR. Ten year prognosis of conversion disorder. *Br J Psychiatr* 1996;169:282–288.

Moene FC, Landberg EH, Hoogduin KA, et al. Organic syndromes diagnosed as conversion disorder: identification and frequency in a study of 85 patients. *J Psychosom Res* 2000;49:7–12.

Moene FC, Spinhoven P, Hoogduin KA, et al. A randomised clinical trial on the additional effect of hypnosis in a comprehensive treatment programme for in-patients with conversion disorder of the motor type. *Psychother Psychosom* 2002;71:66–76.

Roelofs K, Hoogduin KA, Keijsers GP, et al. Hypnotic susceptibility in patients with conversion disorder. *J Abnorm Psychol* 2002;111:390–395.

Roelofs K, Keijsers GP, Hoogduin KA, et al. Child abuse in patients with conversion disorder. *Am J Psychiatry* 2002;159:1908–1913.

Spiegel D, Maldonado J. Hypnosis. In: Hales R, Yudofsky S, Talbott J, eds. *The American Psychiatric Press Textbook of Psychiatry*. 3rd Ed. Washington, DC: American Psychiatric Press 1999;1243–1274.

Spitzer C, Spelsberg B, Grabe HJ, et al. Dissociative experiences and psychopathology in conversion disorders. *J Psychosom Res* 1999;46:291–294.

Vuilleumier P, Chicerio C, Assal F, et al. Functional neuroanatomical correlates of hysterical sensorimotor loss. *Brain* 2001;124:1077–1090.

Williams D, Fahn S, Ford B, et al. Natural history of neuropsychiatric movement disorders. In: Hallett M, Fahn S, Jankovic J, et al., eds. *Psychogenic Movement Disorders: Psychobiology and Therapy of a Functional Disorder, Advances in Neurology*. Philadelphia: Lippincott Williams & Wilkins, 2004.

Williams DT. Hypnosis. In: Wiener J, Dulcan M, eds. *Textbook of Child & Adolescent Psychiatry*. 3rd Ed. Washington, DC: American Psychiatric Press 2004;1043–1054.

Williams DT. Somatoform disorders, factitious disorders and malingering. In: Noshpitz J, ed. *Handbook of Child and Adolescent Psychiatry, vol 2*. New York: James Wiley & Sons 1997;563–578.

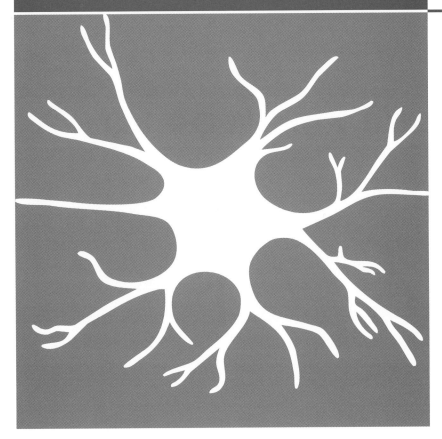

Environmental
Neurology

Chapter 163

Alcoholism

John C. M. Brust

In the United States, 7% of all adults and 19% of adolescents are "problem drinkers": addicted to ethanol or, even if abstinent most of the time, likely to get into trouble when they drink. Ethanol-related deaths exceed 100,000 each year, accounting for 5% of all deaths in the United States. The devastation is direct (from intoxication, addiction, and withdrawal) or indirect (from nutritional deficiency or other ethanol-related diseases).

ETHANOL INTOXICATION

Ethanol acts at many levels of the neuraxis. Although specific ethanol receptors comparable to opioid receptors do not appear to exist, ethanol interacts directly with membrane proteins of a number of neurotransmitter systems, and much of its actions depends on facilitation at inhibitory γ-aminobutyric acid receptors and inhibition at excitatory glutamate receptors.

To obtain a mildly intoxicating blood ethanol concentration (BEC) of 100 mg/dL, a 70-kg person must drink about 50 g (2 oz) of 100% ethanol. Following zero-order kinetics, ethanol is metabolized at about 70 to 150 mg/kg of body weight per hour, with a fall in BEC of 10 to 25 mg/dL per hour. Thus, most adults require 6 hours to metabolize a 50-g dose, and the ingestion of only 8 g of additional ethanol per hour would maintain the BEC at 100 mg/dL.

Symptoms and signs of acute ethanol intoxication are a result of cerebral depression, possibly at first of the reticular formation with cerebral disinhibition and later of the cerebral cortex itself. Manifestations depend not only on the BEC but also on the rate of climb and the person's tolerance, which is related less to increased metabolism than to poorly understood adaptive changes in the brain.

At any BEC, intoxication is more severe when the level is rising than when it is falling, when the level is reached rapidly, and when the level has only recently been achieved. A single BEC determination therefore is not a reliable indicator of drunkenness, and the correlations of Table 163.1 are broad generalizations. Death from respiratory paralysis may occur with a BEC of 400 mg/dL, and survival may occur at 700 mg/dL; a level of 500 mg/dL would be fatal in 50% of individuals.

Low-to-moderate BECs cause slow saccadic eye movements and interrupted jerky pursuit movements that may impair visual acuity. Esophoria and exophoria cause diplopia. With a BEC of 150 to 250 mg/dL, there is increased EEG beta activity ("beta buzz"); higher BECs cause EEG slowing. During sleep, suppression of the rapid eye movement (REM) stage is followed by REM rebound after a few hours.

The term *pathologic intoxication* refers to sudden extreme excitement with irrational or violent behavior after even small doses of ethanol. Episodes are said to last for minutes or hours, followed by sleep and, on awakening, amnesia for the events that took place. Delusions, hallucinations, and homicide may occur during bouts of pathologic intoxication. Some cases might be psychologic dissociative reactions; others may be owing to the kind of paradoxic excitation that sometimes follows barbiturate administration.

▶ **TABLE 163.1 Correlation of Symptoms with Blood Ethanol Concentration (BEC)**

BEC	Symptoms
50–150 mg/dL	Euphoria or dysphoria, shyness or expansiveness, friendliness or argumentativeness
	Impaired concentration, judgment, and sexual inhibitions
150–250 mg/dL	Slurred speech and ataxic gait, diplopia, nausea, tachycardia, drowsiness, or labile mood with sudden bursts of anger or antisocial acts
300 mg/dL	Stupor alternating with combativeness or incoherent speech, heavy breathing, vomiting
400 mg/dL	Coma
500 mg/dL	Respiratory paralysis

The term *alcoholic blackout* refers to amnesia for periods of intoxication, sometimes lasting several hours, even though consciousness at the time did not seem to be disturbed. Although sometimes considered a sign of physiologic dependence, blackouts also occur in occasional drinkers. The amnesia is a direct effect of ethanol on memory encoding.

Acute ethanol poisoning causes more than 1,000 deaths each year in the United States. In stuporous alcoholic patients, subdural hematoma, meningitis, and hypoglycemia are important diagnostic considerations, but it is equally important to remember that ethanol intoxication alone can be fatal.

Blood ethanol causes a rise of blood osmolality, about 22 mOsm/L for every 100 mg/dL of ethanol; however, there are no transmembrane shifts of water, and the hyperosmolarity does not cause symptoms. Ethanol overdose should be considered in any comatose patient whose serum osmolarity is higher than predicted by calculation of the sum of serum sodium, glucose, and urea.

Patients stuporous or comatose from ethanol intoxication are generally managed similarly to those poisoned by other depressant drugs (Table 163.2). Death comes from respiratory depression, and artificial ventilation in an intensive care unit is the mainstay of treatment. Hypovolemia, acid-base or electrolyte imbalance, and abnormal temperature require attention, and if there is any uncertainty about the blood glucose level, 50% glucose is given intravenously, along with parenteral thiamine. Because ethanol is rapidly absorbed, gastric lavage does not help unless other drugs have been ingested. In obstreperous or violent patients, sedatives (including phenothiazines and haloperidol) should be avoided because they may push patients into stupor and respiratory depression. Patients being addressed may appear alert but then lapse into stupor or coma when stimuli are decreased.

▶ **TABLE 163.2** **Treatment of Acute Ethanol Intoxication**

For obstreperous or violent patients
Isolation, calming environment, reassurance–avoid sedatives
Close observation

For stuporous or comatose patients
If hypoventilation, artificial respiration in an intensive care unit
If serum glucose in doubt, intravenous 50% glucose with parenteral thiamine
Careful monitoring of blood pressure; correction of hypovolemia or acid-base imbalance
Consider hemodialysis if patient severely acidotic, deeply comatose, or apneic
Avoid emetics or gastric lavage
Avoid analeptics
Do not forget other possible causes of coma in an alcoholic

In a nonhabitual drinker, a BEC of 400 mg/dL takes 20 hours to return to zero. The only practical agent that might accelerate ethanol metabolism and elimination is fructose, but this causes gastrointestinal upset, lactic acidosis, and osmotic diuresis. (An imidazobenzodiazepine drug has been developed that reverses symptoms of mild-to-moderate ethanol intoxication; it is available for experimental use only.) Hemodialysis or peritoneal dialysis can be used for BECs greater than 600 mg/dL, for severe acidosis, for concurrent ingestion of methanol, ethylene glycol, or other dialyzable drugs, or for severely intoxicated children. Analeptic agents such as ethamivan, caffeine, or amphetamine have no useful role and can cause seizures and cardiac arrhythmia. Although patients are often depleted of magnesium, administration of magnesium sulfate may further depress the sensorium in intoxicated patients. Anecdotal reports describe temporary reversal of ethanol intoxication with naloxone hydrochloride (Narcan).

ETHANOL–DRUG INTERACTIONS

The combination of ethanol with other drugs, often in suicide attempts, causes 2,500 deaths annually, or 13% of all drug-related fatalities. Ethanol is often taken with marijuana, barbiturates, opioids, cocaine, hallucinogens, and inhalants—with varying interactions. Alcoholics often abuse barbiturates, and although ethanol and barbiturates are cross-tolerant, they lower the lethal dose of either alone or when taken acutely in combination. Ethanol with chloral hydrate (Mickey Finn) may be especially dangerous.

Impaired judgment and respiratory depression are also hazards when ethanol is combined with hypnotics, such as methaqualone (Quaalude), sedating antihistamines, antipsychotic agents, and tranquilizers such as meprobamate and benzodiazepines. Hypnotic drugs with long half-lives may cause potentially dangerous incoordination when ethanol is consumed the following day.

The cross-tolerance of ethanol with general anesthetics such as ether, chloroform, or fluorinated agents raises the threshold to sleep induction, but synergistic interaction then increases the depth and length of the anesthetic stage reached. Tricyclic antidepressants do not have a consistent effect; desipramine hydrochloride antagonizes the effects of ethanol, and amitriptyline potentiates them. Ethanol and morphine, repeatedly used, can increase each other's potency, and methadone addicts not only frequently become alcoholic but also then develop a characteristic encephalopathy. Death has followed ethanol taken with propoxyphene hydrochloride. A mild reaction resembling that caused by disulfiram (Antabuse) occurs when patients combine ethanol with sulfonylureas such as tolbutamide (Orinase) or with some antibiotics, including chloramphenicol, griseofulvin, isoniazid, metronidazole, and quinacrine hydrochloride.

> **TABLE 163.3 Ethanol Withdrawal Syndromes**

Early
Tremulousness
Hallucinosis
Seizures

Late
Delirium tremens

ETHANOL DEPENDENCE AND WITHDRAWAL

The term *hangover* refers to the headache, nausea, vomiting, malaise, nervousness, tremulousness, and sweating that can occur in anyone after brief but excessive drinking. Hangover does not imply ethanol addiction, but *ethanol withdrawal* does imply addiction and encompasses several disorders (Table 163.3), which may occur alone or in combination after reduction or cessation of drinking. Severity depends on the length and degree of a particular binge.

Tremulousness, the most common ethanol withdrawal symptom, usually appears in the morning after several days of drinking. It is usually promptly relieved by ethanol, but if drinking cannot continue, tremor becomes more intense, with insomnia, easy startling, agitation, facial and conjunctival flushing, sweating, anorexia, nausea, retching, weakness, tachypnea, tachycardia, and systolic hypertension. Except for inattentiveness and inability to fully recall the events that occurred during the binge, mentation is usually intact. In some patients, tremulousness can persist for weeks or longer.

Perceptual disturbances, with variable insight, occur in about 25% of ethanol-addicted patients and include nightmares, illusions, and hallucinations, which are most often visual but may be auditory, tactile, olfactory, or a combination of these. Imagery includes insects, animals, or people. Hallucinations are usually fragmentary, lasting minutes at a time for several days. Sometimes, however, auditory hallucinations of threatening content last much longer, and occasionally, a persistent state of auditory hallucinosis with paranoid delusions that resembles schizophrenia develops in these patients and may require care in a mental hospital. Repeated bouts of acute auditory hallucinosis may predispose to the chronic form.

Ethanol can precipitate *seizures* in any epileptic; seizures usually occur the morning after weekend or even single-day drinking rather than during inebriation. Alcohol-related seizures affecting alcoholics not otherwise epileptic have traditionally been considered a withdrawal phenomenon, usually occurring within 48 hours of the last drink in persons who have abused ethanol chronically or in binges for months or years. The minimal duration of drinking sufficient to cause seizures is uncertain, but the risk is dose-related, beginning at only 50-g absolute ethanol daily.

Seizures usually occur singly or in a brief cluster; status epilepticus is infrequent. Focal features are present in 25% and do not consistently correlate with evidence of previous head injury or other structural cerebral pathology. Alcohol seizures sometimes accompany tremulousness or hallucinosis, but they may occur in otherwise asymptomatic individuals. Their frequent appearance during active drinking or after more than 1 week of abstinence suggests that mechanisms other than withdrawal play a role in some individuals.

The diagnosis of alcohol-related seizures depends on an accurate history and exclusion of other cerebral lesions. Because reliable follow-up is unlikely, a seizure workup should be done, including CT or MRI and examination of CSF. Fewer than 10% of patients with alcohol-related seizures have spontaneous EEG abnormalities, compared with 50% of those with idiopathic epilepsy. A reported high frequency of electrographic photomyoclonic and photoconvulsant responses during ethanol withdrawal was not borne out by subsequent studies.

In contrast to tremor, hallucinosis, or seizures, which usually occur within 1 or 2 days of abstinence, *delirium tremens* usually begins from 48 to 72 hours after the last drink. Patients with delirium tremens are often hospitalized for other reasons. Delirium tremens may follow withdrawal seizures either before the postictal period has cleared or after 1 or 2 asymptomatic days, but when seizures occur during a bout of delirium tremens, some other diagnosis (e.g., meningitis) should be considered.

Symptoms typically begin and end abruptly, lasting from hours to a few days. There may be alternating periods of confusion and lucidity. Infrequently, relapses may prolong the disorder for a few weeks. Patients are typically agitated, inattentive, and grossly tremulous, with fever, tachycardia, and profuse sweating. They pick at the bed clothes or stare wildly about and intermittently shout at or try to fend off hallucinated people or objects. "Quiet" delirium is infrequent. Mortality is as high as 15%; death is usually owing to other diseases (e.g., pneumonia or cirrhosis), but it may be attributed to unexplained shock, lack of response to therapy, or no apparent cause.

The pathophysiologic basis of ethanol withdrawal in its several forms is probably a combination of glutamate receptor upregulation and γ-aminobutyric acid receptor downregulation. Neuronal excitotoxicity during withdrawal could then set the stage for a kindling pattern of repeated withdrawal episodes, including a lowered seizure threshold.

Treatment of ethanol withdrawal includes prevention or reduction of early symptoms, prevention of delirium tremens, and management of delirium tremens after it starts (Table 163.4). Benzodiazepines, which have cross-tolerance with ethanol, are appropriately given to recently abstinent alcoholics or those with mild early withdrawal

▶ **TABLE 163.4 Treatment of Ethanol Withdrawal**

Prevention or reduction of early symptoms

Diazepam, 5–20 mg, chlordiazepoxide, 25–100 mg, or lorazepam, 1–4 mg, PO or IV, repeated hourly until sedation or mild intoxication. Successive daily doses tapered with resumption of higher dose if withdrawal symptoms recur

Thiamine, 100 mg, and multivitamins, IM or IV

Magnesium, potassium, and calcium replacement as needed

Delirium tremens

Diazepam, 10 mg IV, or lorazepam 2 mg IV or IM, repeated every 5–15 min until calming. Maintenance dose every 1–4 h, PRN

If refractory to benzodiazepines, phenobarbital 260 mg IV repeated in 30 min, PRN

If refractory to phenobarbital, penotobarbital 3–5 mg/kg IV, with endotracheal intubation and repeated doses to produce general anesthesia

Careful attention to fluid and electrolyte balance; several liters of saline per day, or even pressors, may be needed

Cooling blanket or alcohol sponges for high fever

Prevent or correct hypoglycemia

Thiamine and multivitamin replacement

Consider coexisting illness (e.g., liver failure, pancreatitis, meningitis, subdural hematoma)

symptoms. A loading dose may cause symptoms of mild intoxication (calming, dysarthria, ataxia, fine nystagmus); dosage can then be adjusted to avoid both intoxication and tremulousness, and after 1 or 2 days it can be gradually tapered, with reinstitution should withdrawal symptoms reappear. β-adrenergic blocking agents dampen ethanol withdrawal tremor and reportedly decrease agitation and autonomic signs as well, reducing the need for benzodiazepines or other sedatives.

Treating with parenteral ethanol has the disadvantage of a low therapeutic index, and because ethanol is directly toxic to many organs, it should be avoided during hospitalization, even though most patients resume drinking on discharge. Haloperidol and phenothiazines are less likely to prevent hallucinosis or delirium tremens than drugs crosstolerant with ethanol, and they can exacerbate seizures. They are appropriately considered in patients whose only symptoms are hallucinations or in whom hallucinations have outlasted other withdrawal symptoms.

Phenytoin sodium (Dilantin) appears to be of no value in preventing seizures during withdrawal. Parenteral lorazepam given to patients following an ethanol withdrawal seizure reduces the likelihood of recurrence. Status epilepticus during ethanol withdrawal is treated as in other situations; intravenous benzodiazepines have an advantage, compared with phenytoin, of reducing other withdrawal symptoms when the patient awakens. Long-term anticonvulsants in patients with ethanol withdrawal seizures are superfluous; abstainers do not need them, and drinkers do not take them. An epileptic whose seizures are often precipitated by ethanol abuse unfortunately does need treatment, even though compliance is unlikely.

Hypomagnesemia is common during early ethanol withdrawal, and although it may not be the primary cause of symptoms, magnesium sulfate should be given to hypomagnesemic patients. Hypokalemia and hypocalcemia may also be present, and the latter may respond to treatment only when hypomagnesemia is corrected. Parenteral thiamine and multivitamins are given even if there are no clinical signs of depletion.

Delirium tremens, once it appears, cannot be abruptly reversed by any agent, and specific cross-tolerance of a sedative with ethanol is less important in full-blown delirium tremens than in early abstinence. A posenteral benzodiazepine is more effective than other sedatives in rapid calming and has fewer adverse reactions (including apnea) and lower mortality. The required doses might be fatal in a normal person (see Table 163.4), but one cannot predict in any individual patient how high the tolerable dose is. Liver disease decreases the metabolism of benzodiazepines, and patients with cirrhosis are more vulnerable to the depressant effects of sedatives; as delirium tremens clears, hepatic encephalopathy takes its place.

General medical management in delirium tremens is intensive. Although dehydration may be severe enough to cause shock, patients with liver damage may retain sodium and water. Hypokalemia can cause cardiac arrhythmias. Hypoglycemia may be masked, as may other serious coexisting illnesses, such as alcoholic hepatitis, pancreatitis, meningitis, or subdural hematoma. Occasionally encountered during abstinence is either parkinsonism or chorea, which tends to clear over days or weeks. Such movement disorders are presumably related to ethanol effects on striatal dopamine.

WERNICKE-KORSAKOFF SYNDROME

Although they share the same pathology, Wernicke and Korsakoff syndromes are clinically distinct. Wernicke syndrome, when full-blown, consists of mental, eye movement, and gait abnormalities. Korsakoff syndrome is a mental disorder that differs qualitatively from Wernicke syndrome (Table 163.5). Both are the result of thiamine deficiency.

In acute Wernicke syndrome, mental symptoms most often consist of a global confusional state that appears over days or weeks; there is inattentiveness, indifference, decreased spontaneous speech, disorientation, impaired memory, and lethargy. Stupor and coma are unusual, as is selective amnesia. Disordered perception is common; a patient might identify the hospital room as his or her apartment or a bar. In fewer than 10%, mentation is normal.

Abnormal eye movements include nystagmus (horizontal with or without vertical or rotatory components), lateral rectus palsy (bilateral but usually asymmetric), and conjugate gaze palsy (horizontal with or without vertical), progressing to complete external ophthalmoplegia.

▶ **TABLE 163.5** **Major Nutritional Disturbances in Alcoholics**

Disorder	Clinical Features	Deficiency
Wernicke syndrome	Dementia with lethargy, inattentiveness, apathy, and amnesia Ophthalmoparesis Gait ataxia	Thiamine
Korsakoff syndrome	Dementia, mainly amnesia, with or without confabulation	Thiamine
Cerebellar degeneration	Gait ataxia; limb coordination relatively preserved	?
Polyneuropathy	Distal limb sensory loss and weakness; less often autonomic dysfunction	?
Amblyopia	Optic atrophy, decreased visual acuity, central scotomas; total blindness rare	?

Although sluggishness of pupillary reaction is common, total loss of reactivity to light and ptosis are rare. Mental symptoms, including progression to coma, can occur without evident abnormal eye movements in patients with an acute Wernicke syndrome, which sometimes is unexpectedly found at autopsy in patients undiagnosed during life.

Truncal ataxia, present in more than 80% of patients, may prevent standing or walking. Dysarthria and limb ataxia, especially in the arms, are infrequent. Peripheral neuropathy, which occurs to some degree in most patients, may cause weakness sufficient to mask the ataxia. Abnormalities of vestibular caloric testing are common, with gradual improvement, often incomplete, over several months.

Patients with the Wernicke syndrome frequently have signs of nutritional deficiency (e.g., skin changes, tongue redness, cheilosis) or liver disease. Autonomic signs are common. Although beriberi heart disease is rare, acute tachycardia, dyspnea on exertion, and postural hypotension unexplained by hypovolemia are common, and sudden circulatory collapse may follow mild exertion. Hypothermia is less frequent; fever usually indicates infection.

In acute Wernicke syndrome, the EEG may show diffuse slowing or it may be normal. CSF is normal except for occasional mild protein elevation. Elevated blood pyruvate, falling with treatment, is not specific. Decreased blood transketolase (which requires thiamine pyrophosphate as cofactor) more reliably indicates thiamine deficiency.

In most patients, the more purely amnestic syndrome of Korsakoff emerges as the other mental symptoms of Wernicke syndrome respond to treatment. How often Korsakoff syndrome occurs without a background of Wernicke syndrome is disputed and bound up with the question of "alcoholic dementia" (see below). Pathologic changes of Wernicke-Korsakoff are sometimes encountered unexpectedly at autopsy, suggesting the presence of subclinical or atypical forms, including unexplained coma.

The amnesia of Korsakoff syndrome is both anterograde, with inability to retain new information, and retrograde, with rather randomly lost recall for events months or years old. Alertness, attentiveness, and behavior are relatively preserved, but there tends to be a lack of spontaneous speech or activity. Confabulation is not invariable and, if initially present, tends gradually to disappear. Insight is usually impaired, and there may be flagrant anosognosia for the mental disturbance.

The histopathologic lesions of Wernicke-Korsakoff syndrome consist of variable degrees of neuronal, axonal, and myelin loss; prominent blood vessels; reactive microglia, macrophages, and astrocytes; and, infrequently, small hemorrhages. Nerve cells may be relatively preserved in the presence of extensive myelin destruction and gliosis, and astrocytosis may predominate chronically.

Lesions affect the thalamus (especially the dorsomedial nucleus and the medial pulvinar), the hypothalamus (especially the mammillary bodies), the midbrain (especially the oculomotor and periaqueductal areas), and the pons and medulla (especially the abducens and medial vestibular nuclei). Such lesions sometimes produce abnormal signals on MRI, including diffusion weighted. In the anterior-superior vermis of the cerebellum, severe Purkinje cell loss and astrocytosis accompany lesser degrees of neuronal loss and gliosis in the molecular and granular layers.

The traditional view that the memory impairment of Korsakoff syndrome is the result of lesions in the mammillary body has given way to evidence of better correlation with lesions in the dorsomedial or anterior nuclei of the thalamus. The global confusion of Wernicke syndrome can occur without visible thalamic lesions and may be a biochemical disorder. Periaqueductal, oculomotor, or abducens nucleus lesions probably explain ophthalmoparesis. Both cerebellar and vestibular lesions likely contribute to ataxia.

Experimental and clinical evidence ascribes a specific role to thiamine in the Wernicke-Korsakoff syndrome. A genetic influence is implied because only a few alcoholic or otherwise malnourished people are affected, and whites seem more susceptible than blacks.

Untreated Wernicke-Korsakoff syndrome is fatal, and the mortality rate is 10% among treated patients. Concomitant liver failure, infection, or delirium tremens often makes the cause of death unclear. Postural hypotension and tachycardia call for strict bed rest; associated medical problems may require intensive care. The cornerstone of treatment is thiamine, 50–100 mg daily, until a normal diet can be taken; intramuscular or intravenous administration is preferred because thiamine absorption is impaired in chronic alcoholics. Hypomagnesemia may retard improvement after thiamine treatment; magnesium is therefore replaced, along with other vitamins. Protein intake may have to be titrated against the patient's liver status.

With thiamine treatment, the ocular abnormalities (especially abducens and gaze palsies) improve within a few hours and usually resolve within 1 week; in about 35% of patients, horizontal nystagmus persists indefinitely. Global confusion may improve in hours or days and usually resolves within 1 month, leaving Korsakoff amnesia in more than 80%. In <25% of these patients, there is eventual clearing of the memory deficit. Ataxia may improve in a few days, but recovery is complete in <50% of patients, and nearly 35% do not show improvement at all.

ALCOHOLIC CEREBELLAR DEGENERATION

Cerebellar cortical degeneration may occur in nutritionally deficient alcoholics without Wernicke-Korsakoff syndrome (see Table 163.5). Instability of the trunk is the major symptom, often with incoordination of leg movements. Arm ataxia is less prominent; nystagmus and dysarthria are rare. Symptoms evolve in weeks or months and eventually stabilize, sometimes even with continued drinking and poor nutrition. Ataxia without Wernicke disease is less likely to appear abruptly or to improve.

Pathologically, the superior vermis is invariably involved, with nerve cell loss and gliosis in the molecular, granular, and especially the Purkinje cell layers. There may be secondary degeneration of the olives and of the fastigial, emboliform, globose, and vestibular nuclei. Involvement of the cerebellar hemispheric cortex is exceptional and limited to the anterior lobes. Pathologic evidence of Wernicke disease may coexist, even though it is unsuspected clinically. CT and autopsies, moreover, have revealed cerebellar atrophy in alcoholics who were not clinically ataxic.

Although similar cerebellar lesions occur in malnourished nonalcoholics, most patients with alcoholic cerebellar degeneration do not have clinical or pathologic evidence of Wernicke disease. The disorder is probably the result of both nutritional deficiency and ethanol toxicity, perhaps involving glutamate.

ALCOHOLIC POLYNEUROPATHY

Alcoholic polyneuropathy is a sensorimotor disorder that stabilizes or improves with abstinence and an adequate diet (see Table 163.5). Neuropathy is found in most patients with Wernicke-Korsakoff syndrome but more often occurs alone. Paresthesia is usually the first symptom; there may be burning or lancinating pain and exquisite tenderness of the calves or soles. Impaired vibratory sense is usually the earliest sign; proprioception tends to be preserved until other sensory loss is substantial. Loss of ankle jerks is another early sign; eventually, there is diffuse areflexia. Weakness appears at any time and may be severe. Distal leg muscles are affected first, although proximal weakness may be marked. Radiologically demonstrable neuropathic arthropathy of the feet is common, as are skin changes (e.g., thinning, glossiness, reddening, cyanosis, hyperhidrosis). Peripheral autonomic abnormalities are usually less prominent than in diabetic neuropathy but may cause urinary and fecal incontinence, hypotension, hypothermia, cardiac arrhythmia, dysphagia, dysphonia, impaired esophageal peristalsis, altered sweat patterns, or abnormal Valsalva ratio. Pupillary parasympathetic denervation is rare. The CSF is usually normal except for occasional mild elevation of protein content.

Pathologically, there is degeneration of both myelin and axons; it is not certain which occurs first. Clinical and experimental evidence suggests that alcoholic polyneuropathy is both toxic and nutritional in origin. In fact, clinical and pathologic study suggests that pure thiamine deficiency neuropathy (TDN) differs from pure alcoholic neuropathy (ALN); ALN is sensory dominant, slowly progressive, and painful and causes predominantly small fiber axonal loss, whereas TDN is motor dominant and acutely progressive and causes predominantly large-fiber axonal loss.

Peripheral nerve pressure palsies, especially radial and peroneal, are common in alcoholics. Nutritional polyneuropathy may increase the vulnerability of peripheral nerves to compression injury in intoxicated individuals, who tend to sleep deeply in unusual locations and positions. Recovery usually takes days or weeks; splints during this period can prevent contractures.

ALCOHOLIC AMBLYOPIA

Alcoholic amblyopia is a visual impairment that progresses over days or weeks, with development of central or centrocecal scotomas and temporal disc pallor (Table 163.5). Demyelination affects the optic nerves, chiasm, and tracts, with predilection for the maculopapular bundle. Retinal ganglion cell loss is secondary. Although amblyopia improves in patients who receive dietary supplements but continue to smoke and drink ethanol, direct toxicity from ethanol and from compounds in tobacco smoke (perhaps cyanide) could be contributory. Alcoholic amblyopia does not progress to total blindness; it may remain stable without change in drinking or eating habits. Improvement, which is often incomplete, nearly always follows nutritional replacement.

PELLAGRA

Nicotinic acid deficiency in alcoholics causes pellagra, with dermatologic, gastrointestinal, and neurologic symptoms. Altered mentation progresses over hours, days, or weeks to amnesia, delusions, hallucinations, or delirium. Nicotinic acid therapy (plus other vitamins, deficiency of which can be contributory) usually results in prompt improvement.

ALCOHOLIC LIVER DISEASE

Cirrhosis is the sixth leading cause of death in the United States, and nearly all deaths from cirrhosis in people older than 45 years are caused by ethanol. Altered mentation in an alcoholic therefore always raises the possibility of hepatic encephalopathy, which may accompany intoxication, withdrawal, Wernicke syndrome, meningitis, subdural hematoma, hypoglycemia, or other alcohol states. Hepatic encephalopathy is discussed in detail in Chapter 148. Other neurologic disorders encountered in alcoholic cirrhotics include a poorly understood syndrome of altered mentation, myoclonus, and progressive myelopathy following portacaval shunting, as well as acquired chronic hepatocerebral degeneration, a characteristic syndrome of dementia, dysarthria, ataxia, intention tremor, choreoathetosis, muscular rigidity, and asterixis, which usually occurs in patients who have had repeated bouts of hepatic coma. Heavy ethanol use greatly increases the risk for acetaminophen hepatotoxicity and for cirrhosis and hepatocellular carcinoma in patients with hepatitis C infection.

HYPOGLYCEMIA

Metabolism of ethanol by alcohol dehydrogenase and of acetaldehyde by mitochondrial aldehyde dehydrogenase uses nicotinamide adenine dinucleotide (NAD). The resulting elevated NADH-to-NAD ratio impairs gluconeogenesis, and if food is not being eaten and liver glycogen is depleted, there may be severe hypoglycemia with altered behavior, seizures, coma, or focal neurologic deficit. Residual symptoms are common, including dementia. Even after appropriate treatment with intravenous 50% dextrose, these patients require close observation; blood glucose may fall again, with the return of symptoms and possibly permanent brain damage. Ethanol stimulates intestinal release of secretin, which aggravates reactive hypoglycemia, especially in children, by enhancing glucose-stimulated insulin release.

ALCOHOLIC KETOACIDOSIS

In alcoholic ketoacidosis, β-hydroxybutyric acid and lactic acid accumulate in association with heavy drinking. The mechanism relates to starvation, increased lipolysis, and impaired fatty acid oxidation. Typical patients are young binge drinkers who stop drinking when they are overcome by anorexia. Vomiting, dehydration, confusion, obtundation, and hyperventilation ensue. Blood glucose may be normal, low, or moderately elevated, with little or no glycosuria. A large anion gap is accounted for by β-hydroxybutyrate, lactate, and lesser amounts of pyruvate and acetoacetate. Serum insulin levels are low, and serum levels of growth hormone, epinephrine, glucagon, and cortisol are high, but glucose intolerance usually clears without insulin and is not demonstrable on recovery. It is not unusual for patients to have repeated attacks of alcoholic ketoacidosis.

Alcoholics may have other reasons for metabolic acidosis with a large anion gap (e.g., methanol or ethylene glycol poisoning). When β-hydroxybutyrate is the major ketone present, the nitroprusside test (Acetest) may be negative. Treatment includes infusion of glucose (and thiamine), correction of dehydration or hypotension, and replacement of electrolytes such as potassium, magnesium, and phosphate. Small amounts of bicarbonate may be given. Insulin is usually not needed.

INFECTION IN ALCOHOLICS

Alteration of white blood cell function contributes to the alcoholic's predisposition to infection (e.g., bacterial and tuberculous meningitis). Infectious meningitis must always be considered in alcoholics with seizures or altered mental status, even when the clinical picture seems to be that of intoxication, withdrawal, thiamine deficiency, hepatic encephalopathy, hypoglycemia, or other alcoholic disturbances. Alcoholic intoxication is a risk factor for HIV infection.

TRAUMA IN ALCOHOLICS

Thrombocytopenia, a direct effect of ethanol and a consequence of cirrhosis, increases the likelihood of intracranial hematomas after head injury. Abnormalities of clotting factors also increase the possibility of intracranial hematomas. Experimentally, moreover, acute ethanol enhances blood-brain barrier leakage around areas of cerebral trauma. Close observation is essential after even mild head injury in intoxicated patients; an abnormal sensorium must not be dismissed as drunkenness.

ALCOHOL AND CANCER

Independently of tobacco, ethanol in moderate amounts increases the risk of carcinoma of the mouth, esophagus, pharynx, larynx, liver, and, probably, large bowel and breast.

ALCOHOL AND STROKE

As with coronary artery disease, epidemiologic studies suggest that low-to-moderate amounts of ethanol decrease stroke risk, whereas higher amounts increase it. Although reports have been inconsistent, meta-analysis of rigorously designed cohort and case-control studies found a J-shaped association between ethanol consumption and the risk of ischemic stroke and a linear association between ethanol consumption and the risk of hemorrhagic stroke. In the United States, the relationship holds for men and women, for blacks, whites, and Hispanics, and for spirits, beer, and wine. Whether extra risk is temporally associated with binge drinking and whether special benefit is conferred by wine (especially red wine) is less clear. In asymptomatic subjects, moderate ethanol consumption reduces the risk of both carotid atherosclerosis and leukoaraiosis. Ethanol could either prevent or cause stroke by several mechanisms. Acutely and chronically, ethanol causes hypertension. It reportedly lowers blood levels of low-density lipoproteins, raises levels of high-density lipoproteins, decreases fibrinolytic activity, increases or inhibits platelet reactivity, increases or decreases C-reactive protein, dilates or constricts cerebral vessels, and indirectly reduces cerebral blood flow through dehydration. The antioxidant properties of flavenoids in red wine might confer special protection. Alcoholic cardiomyopathy predisposes to embolic stroke.

ALCOHOLIC MYOPATHY

Alcoholic myopathy is of three types. Subclinical myopathy consists of elevated serum creatine kinase levels and electromyographic changes, sometimes with intermittent cramps or weakness. With chronic myopathy, there is progressive proximal weakness. Acute rhabdomyolysis causes sudden severe weakness, muscle pain, swelling, and myoglobinuria with renal shutdown. Ethanol toxicity rather than nutritional deficiency is the likely cause of myopathy, and symptoms sometimes emerge during a binge. Alcoholic cardiomyopathy often coexists. Whether subclinical, chronic, or acute, myopathy improves with abstinence.

CENTRAL PONTINE MYELINOLYSIS AND MARCHIAFAVA-BIGNAMI DISEASE

Central pontine myelinolysis occurs in both alcoholics and nondrinkers and is a consequence of overvigorous correction of hyponatremia. Marchiafava-Bignami disease is nearly always associated with alcoholism (including wine, beer, and whiskey). It is of unknown origin and causes symptoms, including death, that are scarcely explained by the characteristic callosal lesions. Marchiafava-Bignami disease and central pontine myelinolysis are discussed in detail in Chapters 135 and 136, respectively.

ALCOHOLIC DEMENTIA

Whether ethanol, as a direct neurotoxin, can cause progressive mental decline in the absence of nutritional deficiency, brain trauma, or other indirect mechanisms has been controversial for decades. Properly controlled animal studies reveal dose-related impaired learning and neuropathologic changes in hippocampus and other brain regions. Brains of alcoholics without evident nutritional deficiency have reduced volume especially affecting white matter; reports of cortical or hippocampal neuronal loss are less consistent, but neuropathologic changes appear to correlate with memory and other cognitive impairment. A plausible mechanism is inhibition of glutamate neurotransmission with receptor upregulation and rebound excitotoxicity. It is possible that ethanol neurotoxicity and thiamine deficiency are synergistic in this regard.

A number of attempts to identify the safe dose threshold for alcoholic dementia found that low-to-moderate ethanol intake actually reduces the risk for both Alzheimer disease and vascular dementia. A J-shaped curve similar to that describing ethanol and ischemic stroke risk appears to describe ethanol and the risk of dementia as well. Wine, spirits, and beer are each protective; some studies found special benefit in red wine. The mechanism of ethanol's protective effects against nonvascular dementia is uncertain.

FETAL ALCOHOL SYNDROME

Ethanol ingestion during pregnancy causes congenital malformations and delayed psychomotor development. Major clinical features of the fetal alcohol syndrome (FAS) include cerebral dysfunction, growth deficiency, and distinctive facies (Table 163.6); less often, there are abnormalities of the heart, skeleton, urogenital organs, skin, and muscles. Neuropathologic abnormalities include absence or displacement of the corpus callosum, hydrocephalus, cerebellar dysplasia, abnormal neuronal migration, heterotopic cell clusters, and microcephaly. These changes occur independently of other potentially incriminating factors, such as maternal malnutrition, smoking, other drug use, or age. Binge drinking, which may produce high ethanol levels at a critical fetal period, may be more important than chronic ethanol exposure, and early gestation appears to be the most vulnerable period.

Children of alcoholic mothers are often intellectually borderline or retarded without other features of the fetal alcohol syndrome (fetal alcohol effects, FAE); fetal effects

▶ **TABLE 163.6 Clinical Features of Fetal Alcohol Syndrome**

Feature	Majority	Minority
CNS	Mental retardation Microcephaly Hypotonia Poor coordination Hyperactivity	
Impaired growth	Prenatal for length and weight Postnatal for length and weight Diminished adipose tissue	
Abnormal face Eyes	Short palpebral fissures	Ptosis Strabismus Epicanthal folds Myopia Microphthalmia Blepharophimosis Cataracts Retinal pigmentary abnormalities
Nose	Short, upturned Hypoplastic philtrum	
Mouth	Thin vermilion lip borders Retrognathia in infancy Micrognathia or prognathia in adolescence	Prominent lateral palatine ridges Cleft lip or palate Small teeth with faulty enamel
Maxilla	Hypoplastic	
Ears		Posteriorly rotated Poorly formed concha
Skeletal		Pectus excavatum or carinatum Syndactyly, clinodactyly, or campodactyly Limited joint movements Nail hypoplasia Radiolunar synostosis Bifid xiphoid Scoliosis Klippel-Feil anomaly
Cardiac		Septal defects Great vessel anomalies
Cutaneous		Abnormal palmar creases Hemangiomas Infantile hirsutism
Muscular		Diaphragmatic, inguinal, or umbilical hernias Diastasis recti
Urogenital		Labial hypoplasia Hypospadias Small rotated kidneys Hydronephrosis

of ethanol thus cover a broad spectrum. Stillbirth and attention deficit disorder seem especially frequent among offspring of heavy drinkers, and each anomaly of FAS may occur alone or in combination with others. The face of a typical patient with FAS is distinctive and as easily recognized at birth as that of the infant with Down syndrome. Irritability and tremulousness with poor suck reflex and hyperacusis are usually present at birth and last weeks or months. Of these children, 85% perform more than two standard deviations below the mean on tests of mental performance; those who are not grossly retarded rarely have even average mental ability. Older children are often hyperactive and clumsy, and there may be hypotonia or hypertonia. Except for neonatal seizures, epilepsy is not a component of the syndrome.

Ethanol is directly teratogenic to many animals. Proposed mechanisms include apoptosis secondary to blockade of NMDA glutamate receptors during a critical period of synaptogenesis, toxicity to adhesion molecules essential for neuronal migration, and fetal vasospasm and CNS ischemia.

In humans, the risk of alcohol-induced birth defects is established with more than 3 oz of absolute alcohol daily. Below that, the risk is uncertain; a threshold of safety has not been defined. As rates of ethanol use in the United States rose during the 1990s, so did the incidence of FAS. On the basis of data from the United States and France, it was estimated that the combined incidence of FAS and FAE is nearly 1% of all live births. FAE may affect 1% of infants born to women who drink 1 oz of ethanol daily early in pregnancy. More than 30% of the offspring of heavy drinkers are affected by FAS, which thus may be the leading teratogenic cause of mental retardation in the Western world.

TREATMENT OF CHRONIC ALCOHOLISM

The literature on the treatment of alcoholism is voluminous, and strong opinions outweigh scientific data. Not all problem drinkers consume physically addicting quantities of ethanol, no personality type defines an alcoholic, and the relative roles of genetics and social deprivation vary from patient to patient. (Animal and human studies indicate genetic influences in alcoholism, but the association is complex and undoubtedly involves more than one gene.) Of course, such variability of alcoholic populations means that no treatment modality (e.g., psychotherapy, group psychotherapy, family or social network therapy, drug therapy, behavioral [aversion] therapy) or no single therapeutic setting (e.g., general hospital, halfway house, vocational rehabilitation clinic, Alcoholics Anonymous) is appropriate for all. For example, the success rate of Alcoholics Anonymous has been estimated to be 34%.

Use of tranquilizing and sedating drugs is especially controversial because they may lead to switching of dependency or to drug–ethanol interactions. Some clinicians espouse short-term use of these drugs in doses high enough to reduce the psychologic tensions that lead to ethanol use but low enough not to block symptoms of ethanol withdrawal.

Disulfiram inhibits aldehyde dehydrogenase and reduces the rate of oxidation of acetaldehyde, accumulation of which accounts for the symptoms that appear soon after someone taking disulfiram drinks ethanol. Within 5 to 10 minutes, there is warmth and flushing of the face and chest, throbbing headache, dyspnea, nausea, vomiting, sweating, thirst, chest pain, palpitations, hypotension, anxiety, confusion, weakness, vertigo, and blurred vision. The severity and duration of these symptoms depend on the amount of ethanol drunk; a few milliliters can cause mild symptoms followed by drowsiness, sleep, and recovery; severe reactions can last hours or be fatal and require hospital admission, with careful management of hypotension and cardiac arrhythmia.

Taken in the morning, when the urge to drink is least, disulfiram, 0.25–0.5 g daily, does not alter the taste for ethanol and helps only patients who strongly desire to abstain. In the United States, 150,000 to 200,000 patients are maintained on disulfiram, although studies demonstrating long-term benefit lack methodologic rigor. Side effects of disulfiram that are unrelated to ethanol ingestion include drowsiness, psychiatric symptoms, and cardiovascular problems. Paranoia, impaired memory, ataxia, dysarthria, and even major motor seizures may be difficult to distinguish from ethanol effects. So may peripheral neuropathy, which can be fulminant. Hypersensitivity hepatitis also occurs.

Following reports of efficacy in animals and humans, the Food and Drug Administration approved the mu-opioid antagonist naltrexone for treating alcoholism. Subsequent studies, however, showed no benefit.

Acamprosate, a drug that appears to antagonize NMDA receptors, was found to be effective in several clinical trials. As of 2003, it was available in Europe but not the United States.

Other proposed treatments for alcoholism include lithium, serotonin-uptake inhibitors, dopaminergic agonists, opioids, calcium channel blockers, cannabinoid receptor antagonists, γ-hydroxybutyrate, and the Chinese herb kudzu. None is scientifically accredited.

SUGGESTED READINGS

Archibald SK, Fennema-Norestine C, Gamst A, et al. Brain dysmorphology in individuals with severe prenatal alcohol exposure. *Dev Med Child Neurol* 2001;43:148–154.

Brust JCM. Ethanol. In: *Neurological Aspects of Substance Abuse.* Brust JCM, ed. 2nd Ed. Boston: Butterworth-Heinemann, 2004.

Brust JCM. Ethanol. In: Schaumburg HH, Spencer PS, eds. *Experimental and Clinical Neurotoxicology.* 2nd Ed. Baltimore: Williams & Wilkins, 1999:541–557.

Brust JCM. Stroke and substance abuse. In: Mohr JP, Choi D, Grotta J, et al, eds. *Stroke: Pathophysiology, Diagnosis, and Management.* 4th Ed. Philadelphia: WB Saunders, 2004;725–745.

Brust JCM. Wine, flavenoids, and the "water of life." *Neurology* 2002;59:1300–1301.

Caine D, Halliday GM, Kril JJ, et al. Operational criteria for the classification of chronic alcoholics: identification of Wernicke's encephalopathy. *J Neurol Neurosurg Psychiatry* 1997;62:51–60.

Charness ME, Simon RP, Greenberg DA. Ethanol and the nervous system. *N Engl J Med* 1989;321:442–454.

Chu K, Kang DW, Kim HJ, et al. Diffusion-weighted abnormalities in Wernicke encephalopathy: reversible cytotoxic edema? *Arch Neurol* 2002;59:123–127.

Davis KM, Wu J-Y. Role of glutamatergic and GABAergic systems in alcoholism. *J Biomed Sci* 2001;8:7–19.

D'Onofrio G, Rathlev NK, Ulrich AS, et al. Lorazepam for the prevention of recurrent seizures related to alcohol. *N Engl J Med* 1999;340:915–919.

Fernandez-Sola J, Grav Junyent JM, Urbana-Marquez A. Alcoholic myopathies. *Curr Op Neurol* 1996;9:400–405.

Fisch BJ, Hauser WA, Brust JCM, et al. The EEG response to diffuse and patterned photic stimulation during acute untreated alcohol withdrawal. *Neurology* 1989;39:434–436.

Harding A, Halliday G, Caine D, et al. Degeneration of anterior thalamic nuclei differentiates alcoholics with amnesia. *Brain* 2000;123:141–154.

Hughes JC, Cook CC. The efficacy of disulfiram: a review of outcome studies. *Addiction* 1997;92:381–395.

Koike H, Iijima M, Sugiura M, et al. Alcoholic neuropathy is clinicopathologically distinct from thiamine-deficiency neuropathy. *Ann Neurol* 2003;54:19–29.

Kosten TR, O'Connor PG. Management of drug and alcohol withdrawal. *N Engl J Med* 2003;348:1786–1795.

Mukamal KJ, Kuller LH, Fitzpatrick AL, et al. Prospective study of alcohol consumption and the risk of dementia in older adults. *JAMA* 2003;289:1405–1413.

Mukamal KJ, Longstreth WT, Mittleman MA, et al. Alcohol consumption and subclinical findings on magnetic resonance imaging of the brain in older adults. The Cardiovascular Health Study. *Stroke* 2001;32:1939–1946.

Neiman J, Lang AE, Fornazzari L, et al. Movement disorders in alcoholism: a review. *Neurology* 1990;40:741–746.

Ng SKC, Hauser WA, Brust JCM, et al. Alcohol consumption and withdrawal in new-onset seizures. *N Engl J Med* 1988;319:666–673.

O'Connor PG, Schottenfeld RS. Patients with alcohol problems. *N Engl J Med* 1998;338:592–602.

Rehm J, Greenfield TK, Rogers JD. Average volume of alcohol consumption, patterns of drinking, and all-cause mortality: results from the U.S. National Alcohol Survey. *Am J Epidemiol* 2001;153:64–71.

Reynolds K, Lewis LB, Nolan JDL, et al. Alcohol consumption and risk of stroke. A meta-analysis. *JAMA* 2003;289:579–588.

Sacco RL, Elkind M, Baden-Albala B, et al. The protective effect of moderate alcohol consumption on ischemic stroke. *JAMA* 1999;281:53–60.

Sampson PD, Streissguth AP, Bookstein FL, et al. Incidence of fetal alcohol syndrome and prevalence of alcohol-related neurodevelopmental disorder. *Teratology* 1997;56:317–326.

Srisurapanont M, Jarusuraisin N. Opioid antagonists for alcohol dependence. *Cochrane Database Syst Rev* 2002;(2):CD001867.

Thun MJ, Peto R, Lopez AD, et al. Alcohol consumption and mortality among middle-aged and elderly U.S. adults. *N Engl J Med* 1997;24:1705–1714.

Victor M, Adams RD, Collins GH. *The Wernicke-Korsakoff Syndrome.* 2nd Ed. Philadelphia: FA Davis, 1989.

C h a p t e r   1 6 4

Drug Dependence

John C. M. Brust

There are two kinds of drug dependence. *Psychic dependence* leads to craving and drug-seeking behavior. *Physical dependence* produces somatic withdrawal symptoms and signs. Depending on the particular drug and the circumstances of its administration, psychic and physical dependence can coexist or occur alone. *Addiction* is psychic dependence.

In the United States, dependence of one or both types is encountered with a variety of agents, licit and illicit (Table 164.1). Different classes of drugs produce diverse symptoms of intoxication and withdrawal, as well as medical and neurologic complications. Their legal status has little to do with potential harmfulness.

DRUGS OF DEPENDENCE

Opioids

Opioids include agonists (e.g., morphine, heroin, methadone, fentanyl [Sublimaze], meperidine [Demerol], hydromorphone [Dilaudid], codeine, propoxyphene [Darvon]), oxycodone [Oxycontin, Percocet], antagonists (e.g., naloxone [Narcan], naltrexone [ReVia]), nalmefene [Revex], and mixed agonist-antagonists (e.g., pentazocine [Talwin], buprenorphine [Buprenex], butorphanol [Stadol]). At desired levels of intoxication, agonist opioids produce drowsy euphoria, analgesia, cough suppression, miosis, and often nausea, vomiting, sweating, pruritus, hypothermia, postural hypotension, constipation, and decreased libido. Taken parenterally or smoked (often

▶ **TABLE 164.1 Drugs of Dependence**

Opioids
Psychostimulants
Sedatives/hypnotics
Marijuana
Hallucinogens
Inhalants
Phencyclidine
Anticholinergics
Ethanol
Tobacco

in combination with alkaloidal crack cocaine), heroin produces a "rush," a brief ecstatic feeling followed by euphoria and either relaxed "nodding" or garrulous hyperactivity. Overdose causes coma, respiratory depression, and pinpoint (but reactive) pupils. For adults with respiratory depression, treatment consists of respiratory support and naloxone, 2 mg intravenously, repeated as needed up to 20 mg; for those with normal respirations, smaller doses (0.4–0.8 mg) are given to avoid precipitation of withdrawal signs. Naloxone is short acting, and so patients receiving it require admission and close observation.

Opioid agonist withdrawal symptoms include irritability, lacrimation, rhinorrhea, sweating, yawning, mydriasis, myalgia, muscle spasms, piloerection, nausea, vomiting, abdominal cramps, fever, hot flashes, tachycardia, hypertension, and orgasm. In adults, seizures and delirium are not features of opioid withdrawal, which is rarely life threatening and can usually be prevented or treated with methadone, 20 mg once or twice daily. By contrast, untreated opioid withdrawal in newborns is severe, protracted, and often fatal; treatment is with titrated doses of methadone or paregoric. A barbiturate can be added if additional drug withdrawal is suspected or if seizures require treatment. Effective pharmacotherapy for opioid dependence consists of substitution with oral methadone or buprenorphine. Treatment failure is usually attributable to inadequate dosage. Antagonist therapy with naltrexone proved disappointing.

Psychostimulants

Psychostimulants include amphetamines, methamphetamine, methylphenidate (Ritalin), ephedrine, phenylpropanolamine, other anorectics and decongestants, and cocaine (which, in contrast to other psychostimulants, is also a local anesthetic). Desired effects include alert euphoria with increased motor activity and physical endurance. Taken parenterally or smoked as alkaloidal cocaine (crack) or methamphetamine ("ice"), psychostimulants produce a rush clearly distinguishable from that of opioids. With repeated use, there is stereotypic activity progressing to bruxism or other dyskinesias and paranoia progressing to frank hallucinatory psychosis. Overdose causes headache, chest pain, tachycardia, hypertension, flushing, sweating, fever, and excitement. There may be delirium, cardiac arrhythmia, myoclonus, seizures, myoglobinuria, shock, coma, and death. Malignant hyperthermia and disseminated intravascular coagulation are described. Treatment includes benzodiazepine sedation, oxygen, bicarbonate for acidosis, anticonvulsants, cooling, an antihypertensive (preferably an alpha blocker such as phenoxybenzamine or a direct vasodilator such as sodium nitroprusside [Nitropress]), respiratory and blood pressure support, and cardiac monitoring.

Psychostimulant withdrawal produces fatigue, depression, and increased hunger and sleep. Objective signs are few, but depression can require treatment or even hospitalization.

Sedatives

Sedative agents include barbiturates (e.g., phenobarbital, pentobarbital, amobarbital, secobarbital [Seconal]), benzodiazepines (e.g., diazepam [Valium], chlordiazepoxide [Librium], alprazolam [Xanax], lorazepam [Ativan], triazolam [Halcion], flunitrazepam), and miscellaneous products (e.g., glutethimide, ethchlorvynol [Placidyl], methaqualone, zolpidem [Ambien]). Desired effects and overdose both resemble ethanol intoxication, although respiratory depression is much milder with benzodiazepines. Treatment is supportive; for severe benzodiazepine poisoning, there is a specific antagonist, flumazenil (Romazicon). Withdrawal causes tremor and seizures, which can be prevented or treated with titrated doses of a barbiturate or benzodiazepine. Delirium tremens is a medical emergency requiring intensive care.

Gamma-hydroxybutyric acid (GHB), a natural metabolite of gamma-aminobutyric acid, is a popular euphoriant at "rave" parties; so are two of its precursors, gamma-butyrolactone and 1,4-butanediol. Notorious as "date-rape" drugs, these agents are often taken with ethanol, causing sedation and respiratory depression but also agitation, hallucinations, myoclonus, seizures, and coma. Treatment is supportive. Dependence occurs, and withdrawal signs resemble those of other sedatives and ethanol.

Marijuana

Marijuana, from the hemp plant *Cannabis sativa*, contains many cannabinoid compounds, of which the principal psychoactive agent is delta-9-tetrahydrocannabinol. Hashish refers to preparations made from the plant resin, which contains most of the psychoactive cannabinoids. Usually smoked, marijuana produces a relaxed dreamy euphoria, often with jocularity, disinhibition, depersonalization, subjective slowing of time, conjunctival injection, tachycardia, and postural hypotension. High doses cause auditory or visual hallucinations, confusion, and psychosis, but fatal overdose has not been documented. Withdrawal symptoms, other than craving, are minimal; there may be jitteriness, anorexia, and headache. Psychic dependence is common, however.

Hallucinogens

Hallucinogenic plants are used ritualistically or recreationally around the world. In the United States, the most popular agents are the indolealkylamines psilocybin and psilocin (from several mushroom species), the phenylalkylamine mescaline (from the peyote cactus), and the synthetic ergot compound lysergic acid diethylamide (LSD). Several synthetic phenylalkylamines are also available, including 3,4-methylenedioxymethamphetamine (MDMA, "ecstasy"), which has both hallucinogenic and amphetaminelike effects. The acute effects of hallucinogens are perceptual (distortions or hallucinations, usually visual and elaborately formed), psychologic (depersonalization or altered mood), and somatic (dizziness, tremor, and paresthesia). Some users experience paranoia or panic, and some, days to months after use, have flashbacks, the spontaneous recurrence of drug symptoms without taking the drug. High doses of LSD cause hypertension, obtundation, and seizures, but fatalities are usually the result of accidents or suicide. Treatment of overdose consists of a calm environment, reassurance, and, if necessary, a benzodiazepine. Withdrawal symptoms do not occur.

Inhalants

Recreational inhalant use is especially popular among children and adolescents, who sniff a wide variety of products, including aerosols, spot removers, glues, lighter fluid, fire-extinguishing agents, bottled fuel gas, marker pens, paints, and gasoline. Compounds include aliphatic hydrocarbons such as *n*-hexane, aromatic hydrocarbons such as toluene, and halogenated hydrocarbons such as trichloroethylene; in addition, nitrous oxide is sniffed from whipped-cream dispensers and butyl or amyl nitrite from room odorizers. Despite such chemical diversity, desired subjective effects are similar to those of ethanol intoxication. Overdose can cause hallucinations, seizures, and coma; death has resulted from cardiac arrhythmia, accidents, and aspiration of vomitus. Symptoms tend to clear within a few hours, and treatment consists of respiratory and cardiac monitoring. There is no predictable abstinence syndrome other than craving.

Phencyclidine

Developed as an anesthetic, phencyclidine hydrochloride (PCP or "angel dust") was withdrawn because it caused psychosis. As a recreational drug, it is usually smoked. The related agents ketamine and dextromethorphan are also used recreationally. Low doses of PCP cause euphoria or dysphoria and a feeling of numbness; with increasing intoxication, there is agitation, nystagmus, tachycardia, hypertension, fever, sweating, ataxia, paranoid or catatonic psychosis, hallucinations, myoclonus, rhabdomyolysis, seizures, coma, respiratory depression, and death. Treatment includes a calm environment with benzodiazepine sedation and restraints as needed, gastric suctioning, activated charcoal, forced diuresis, cooling, antihypertensives, anticonvulsants, and monitoring of cardiorespiratory and renal function. Neuroleptics, which can aggravate seizures, hypotension, and myoglobinuria, are best avoided. Symptoms can persist for hours or days. Psychic dependence to PCP occurs, but withdrawal signs are infrequent, usually consisting of nervousness, tremor, and upset stomach.

Anticholinergics

The recreational use of anticholinergics includes ingestion of the plant *Datura stramonium*, popular among American adolescents, as well as use of antiparkinson drugs and the tricyclic antidepressant amitriptyline. Intoxication produces decreased sweating, tachycardia, dry mouth, dilated unreactive pupils, and delirium with hallucinations. Severe poisoning causes myoclonus, seizures, coma, and death. Treatment includes intravenous physostigmine salicylate (Antilirium), 0.5 to 3 mg, repeated as needed every 30 minutes to 2 hours, plus gastric lavage, cooling, bladder catheterization, respiratory and cardiovascular monitoring, and, if necessary, anticonvulsants. Neuroleptics, which have anticholinergic activity, are contraindicated. There is no withdrawal syndrome.

TRAUMA

Trauma may be a consequence of a drug's acute effects, for example, automobile and other accidents during marijuana, inhalant, or anticholinergic intoxication; violence in psychostimulant or PCP users; and self-mutilation during hallucinogen psychosis. Trauma among users of illicit drugs, however, is most often the result of the illegal activities necessary to distribute and procure them. Overprescribing of sedatives is a major contributor to falls in the elderly.

INFECTION

Parenteral users of any drug are subject to an array of local and systemic infections, which in turn can affect the nervous system. Hepatitis leads to encephalopathy or hemorrhagic stroke. Cellulitis and pyogenic myositis produce more distant infection, including vertebral osteomyelitis with myelopathy or radiculopathy. Endocarditis, bacterial or fungal, leads to meningitis, cerebral infarction or abscess, and septic or mycotic aneurysm. Tetanus, often severe, affects heroin users, and botulism occurs at injection sites or, among cocaine users, in the nasal sinuses. Malaria has occurred in heroin users from endemic areas.

By 2003, nonhomosexual parenteral drug users composed 26% of AIDS cases reported to the Centers for Disease Control and Prevention; male homosexual drug users accounted for another 6%. In some communities, more than 50% of patients receiving methadone maintenance treatment are seropositive for HIV. Parenteral drug users experience the same neurologic complications of AIDS as do other groups and are particularly susceptible to syphilis and tuberculosis, including drug-resistant forms. Because of promiscuity and associated sexually transmitted diseases, nonparenteral cocaine users are also at increased risk for AIDS. Heroin and cocaine are themselves immunosuppressants (heroin users were vulnerable to unusual fungal infections before the AIDS epidemic), yet their use in HIV-seropositive individuals does not seem to accelerate the development of AIDS.

Progressive myelopathy occurs in parenteral drug users infected with either HTLV-I or HTLV-II.

SEIZURES

Seizures are a feature of withdrawal from sedatives, including, infrequently, benzodiazepines. Methaqualone (no longer legally available in the U.S.) and glutethimide have reportedly caused seizures during intoxication. Opioids lower seizure threshold, but seizures are seldom encountered during heroin overdose. Myoclonus and seizures more often occur in meperidine users, a consequence of the active metabolite normeperidine. Seizures are also frequent in parenteral users of pentazocine combined with the antihistamine tripelennamine ("Ts and blues"). Seizures may occur in cocaine users without other evidence of overdose. In animals, repeated cocaine administration produces seizures in a pattern suggestive of kindling. Amphetamine and other psychostimulants are less epileptogenic than cocaine, but seizures have occurred in users of the over-the-counter anorectic phenylpropanolamine. A case-control study found that marijuana was protective against the development of new-onset seizures. In animal studies, the nonpsychoactive cannabinoid compound cannabidiol is anticonvulsant.

STROKE

Illicit drug users frequently abuse ethanol and tobacco, increasing their risk for ischemic and hemorrhagic stroke. Parenteral drug users are subject to stroke through systemic complications such as hepatitis, endocarditis, and AIDS. Heroin users develop nephropathy with secondary hypertension, uremia, and bleeding. Heroin has also caused stroke in the absence of other evident risk factors, perhaps through immunologic mechanisms. Stroke in injectors of pentazocine combined with tripelennamine resulted from embolism of foreign particulate material passing through secondary pulmonary arteriovenous shunts.

Amphetamine users are prone to intracerebral hemorrhage following acute hypertension and fever. They are also at risk for occlusive stroke secondary to cerebral vasculitis affecting either medium-sized arteries (resembling polyarteritis nodosa) or smaller arteries and veins (resembling hypersensitivity angiitis). Ischemic and hemorrhagic stroke is also a frequent consequence of cocaine use, regardless of route of administration. Over 600 cases have been reported, roughly half hemorrhagic and half ischemic. Most hemorrhagic strokes are prob-

ably consequent to acute surges of hypertension; most ischemic strokes are probably secondary to cocaine's vasoconstrictive actions on cervical and intracranial circulation. Cerebral saccular aneurysms and vascular malformations are often found in patients undergoing angiography for cocaine-related intracranial hemorrhage.

Because of their association with stroke, diet pills and decongestants containing phenylpropanolamine were banned by the Food and Drug Administration. Similar association led to a number of states banning dietary supplements containing ephedra. Intracerebral and subarachnoid hemorrhage are described in MDMA users.

LSD and PCP are vasoconstrictive, and occlusive and hemorrhagic strokes have followed their use. Anecdotal reports also describe ischemic stroke in young marijuana users without other risk factors.

ALTERED MENTATION

Dementia in illicit drug users may be the result of concomitant ethanol abuse, malnutrition, head trauma, or infection. Parenteral drug users are at risk for HIV encephalopathy. Whether the drugs themselves cause lasting cognitive or behavioral change is more difficult to establish, for predrug mental status is nearly always uncertain and many drug users are probably self-medicating pre-existing psychiatric conditions (e.g., cocaine for depression). The weight of evidence is against chronic mental abnormalities secondary to opioids or hallucinogens. Although early reports of a marijuana "antimotivational syndrome" were overstated, more rigorous studies persuasively demonstrate persistent cognitive impairment in heavy marijuana users. Controversy exists over whether psychostimulants predispose to lasting depression or if PCP predisposes to schizophrenia. In animals and humans, methamphetamine damages both dopaminergic and serotonergic nerve terminals, with lasting brain neurotransmitter depletion. MDMA destroys serotonin nerve terminals, and impaired memory and cognition are described in abstinent MDMA users. Cocaine is not neurotoxic, yet chronic users demonstrate cognitive impairment; imaging studies suggest that the cause is widespread cerebral ischemia. Sedatives can cause reversible dementia in the elderly, and their use in small children is associated with delayed learning. Lead encephalopathy is described in gasoline sniffers, and cerebral white matter lesions with dementia are described in toluene sniffers.

FETAL EFFECTS

The effects of illicit drugs on intrauterine development are also difficult to separate from damage secondary to ethanol, tobacco, malnutrition, and inadequate prenatal care or home environment. Infants exposed in utero to heroin have reportedly been small for gestational age, at risk for respiratory distress, and cognitively impaired later in life. Marijuana exposure is associated with decreased birthweight and length and with impaired executive function. Studies of cocaine's fetal effects, including cognitive, are conflicting. A prospective study found diffuse or axial hypertonia more often among cocaine-exposed neonates than controls; this spastic tetraparesis cleared by 24 months of age, and there were no differences in mental or motor development. Animal studies demonstrate that in utero cocaine exposure detrimentally affects learning; if such effects occur in humans, they appear to be small. Gestational exposure to organic solvents increases the risk of major malformations, and animal studies confirm the teratogenicity of toluene and other inhalants.

MISCELLANEOUS EFFECTS

Guillain-Barré-type neuropathy and *brachial* or *lumbosacral plexopathy*, probably immunologic in origin, have been associated with heroin use. (Brachial plexopathy has also resulted from septic aneurysm of the subclavian artery.) Severe sensorimotor polyneuropathy occurs in sniffers of glue containing *n*-hexane. *Myoglobinuria* and renal failure have followed use of heroin, amphetamine, cocaine, and PCP. *Myeloneuropathy* indistinguishable from cobalamin deficiency occurs in nitrous oxide sniffers. Anemia is absent, and serum vitamin B_{12} levels are usually normal. The mechanism is inactivation of the cobalamin-dependent enzyme methionine synthetase. Possibly vascular in origin, acute myelopathy occurs in parenteral heroin users. *Severe irreversible parkinsonism* developed in Californians exposed to a meperidine analog contaminated with 1-methyl-4-phenyl-1,2,3,6-tetrahydropyridine (MPTP), a metabolite of which is toxic to neurons in the substantia nigra. Symptoms respond to levodopa. *Dementia, ataxia, quadriparesis, blindness*, and *death* have occurred in smokers of heroin pyrolysate. Autopsies show spongiform changes in the central nervous system white matter. The responsible toxin has not been identified. *Blindness* developed in a heavy heroin user whose mixture contained quinine; however, it improved when he resumed using a quinine-free preparation. Chronic cocaine users experience *dystonia* and *chorea*, and cocaine can precipitate symptoms in patients with *Tourette syndrome*. Marijuana inhibits luteinizing and follicle-stimulating hormones, causing *reversible impotence* and *sterility* in men and *menstrual irregularity* in women. *Ataxia* and *cerebellar white matter* changes have occurred in toluene sniffers.

SUGGESTED READINGS

Bartzokis G, Beckson M, Lu PH, et al. Age-related brain volume reductions in amphetamine and cocaine addicts and normal controls: implications for addiction research. *Psychiatry Res* 2000;98:93–102.

Bolla KI, Brown K, Eldreth D, et al. Dose-related neurocognitive effects of marijuana use. *Neurology* 2002;59:1337–1343.

Brust JCM. *Neurological Aspects of Substance Abuse.* Brust JCM, ed. 2nd Ed. Boston: Butterworth-Heinemann, 2004.

Brust JCM. Over-the-counter cold remedies and stroke. *Stroke* 2003;34: 1673.

Brust JCM. Stroke and substance abuse. In: Choi DW, Mohr JP, Grotta JC, et al., eds. *Stroke: Pathophysiology, Diagnosis, and Management.* 3rd Ed. Philadelphia: WB Saunders, 2004;724–745.

Cami J, Farré M. Drug addiction. *N Engl J Med* 2003;349:975–986.

Chiriboga CA, Brust JCM, Bateman D, et al. Dose-response effect of fetal cocaine exposure on newborn neurological function. *Pediatrics* 1999;103:79–85.

Eyler FD, Behnke M. Early development of infants exposed to drugs prenatally. *Clin Perinatol* 1999;26:107–150.

Frank DA, Augustyn M, Knight WG, et al. Growth, development, and behavior in early childhood following prenatal cocaine exposure. A systematic review. *JAMA* 2001;285:1613–1625.

Fried PA, Smith AM. A literature review of the consequences of prenatal marijuana exposure. An emerging theme of a deficiency in aspects of executive function. *Neurotoxicol Teratol* 2001;23:1–11.

Gerdeman GL, Partridge JG, Lupica CR, et al. It could be habit forming: drugs of abuse and synaptic plasticity. *Trends Neurosci* 2003;26:184–192.

Kaufman MJ, Levin JM, Ross MH, et al. Cocaine-induced cerebral vasoconstriction detected in humans with magnetic resonance angiography. *JAMA* 1998;279:376–380.

Khattak S, K-Moghtader G, McMartin K, et al. Pregnancy outcome following gestational exposure to organic solvents. A prospective controlled study. *JAMA* 1999;281:1106–1109.

Kosten TR, O'Connor PG. Management of drug and alcohol withdrawal. *N Engl J Med* 2003;348:1786–1795.

Kriegstein AR, Shungu DC, Millar WS, et al. Leukoencephalopathy and raised brain lactate from heroin vapor inhalation ("chasing the dragon"). *Neurology* 1999;53:1765–1773.

Levine SR, Brust JCM, Futrell N, et al. Cerebrovascular complications of the use of the "crack" form of alkaloidal cocaine. *N Engl J Med* 1990;323:699–704.

Lowenstein DH, Massa SM, Rowbotham MC, et al. Acute neurologic and psychiatric complications associated with cocaine abuse. *Am J Med* 1987;83:841–846.

Ng SKC, Brust JCM, Hauser WA, et al. Illicit drug use and the risk of new onset seizures: contrasting effects of heroin, marijuana, and cocaine. *Am J Epidemiol* 1990;132:47–57.

Shekelle PG, Hardy ML, Morton SC, et al. Efficacy and safety of ephedra and ephedrine for weight loss and athletic performance. A meta-analysis. *JAMA* 2003;289:1537–1545.

Sloan MA, Kittner SJ, Feeser BR, et al. Illicit drug-associated ischemic stroke in the Baltimore-Washington Stroke Study. *Neurology* 1998;50:1688–1698.

Volkow ND, Fowler JS, Wang G-J. Role of dopamine in drug reinforcement and addiction in humans: results from imaging studies. *Behav Pharmacol* 2002;13:355–366.

Weiner WJ, Rabinstein A, Lewin B, et al. Cocaine-induced persistent dyskinesias. *Neurology* 2001;56:964–965.

Winberg S, Blaho K, Logan B, et al: Multiple cocaine-induced seizures and corresponding cocaine and metabolite concentrations. *Am J Emerg Med* 1998;16:529–533.

Zakzanis KK, Young DA. Memory impairment in abstinent MDMA ("Ecstasy") users: a longitudinal investigation. *Neurology* 2001;56: 966–969.

Zvosec D, Smith SW, McCutcheon Jr, et al. Adverse events, including death, associated with the use of 1,4-butanediol. *N Engl J Med* 2001;344:87–94.

Chapter 165

Iatrogenic Disease

Louis H. Weimer and
Lewis P. Rowland

The growing number of drugs used to treat human disease and the growing number of invasive procedures used for diagnosis and treatment have generated a new area of neurology. The number and diversity of specific instances are out of the scope of this chapter, but the selected examples given are illustrative (Table 165.1). Observations have been made that medication toxicity plays a direct role in 16% of intensive care unit admissions, 4% of all emergency department visits in one United Kingdom series, and up to 22% of emergency admissions, the majority of which are potentially foreseeable. Neurologic reactions accounted for 20% of all adverse reactions in one study. Symptomatic medicine interactions are also common and a source of preventable admissions, especially in the elderly. Medication toxicity may produce or exacerbate headache, movement disorders, cognitive dysfunction, incoordination, seizures, infections, peripheral neuropathy, and myopathy. Moreover, treatment of systemic illnesses may lead to neurotoxicity, and likewise neurologic treatments can produce systemic toxicity. Moses and Kaden found a 14% incidence of iatrogenic neurologic complications among inpatient neurologic consultations at Johns Hopkins Hospital; however, 27% were unsuspected by the referring physicians.

Further discussion of the listings in Table 165.1 and many others are scattered throughout the book. Even this brief, partial list of the neurologic syndromes requires some perspective. The treatments listed do not cause adverse reactions in most instances. For example, penicillin is high on the list of drugs that cause convulsive encephalopathy, but only a few cases are recorded. Some reactions and risks, however, are more common and accepted to a degree. Examples include a risk of tardive dyskinesia in exchange for suppression of psychosis, levodopa-induced dyskinesia for control of parkinsonism, risk of hemorrhage from anticoagulation or tissue plasminogen activator after stroke and other thrombotic event, and risk of peripheral neuropathy in the treatment of HIV infection and cancer. Drug-induced confusion, ataxia, and cognitive changes are concerns with anticonvulsants and many other drugs. The adverse effects of radiotherapy limit treatment of brain and other tumors and may cause injury to the brain, spinal cord, or peripheral nerves. Control or prevention of neurotoxicity by alternative agents or procedures therefore is highly desirable, but an understanding of the toxic mechanisms involved is needed for rational intervention. Prevention of chemotherapy-induced peripheral neuropathy with neuroprotective agents and neurotrophin gene transfer is one promising example. Neurotoxic mechanisms implicated are highly varied; some are dose dependent and others idiosyncratic; many remain poorly understood. The same is true for the adverse effects of drugs used to treat neurologic disease that may damage other systems (e.g., corticosteroids, immunosuppressive agents, antineoplastic drugs, and IVIG).

It is sometimes difficult to list the rare or questionable side effects of a drug without inappropriately frightening patients or physicians. When considering potential adverse reactions of a treatment, one must carefully consider the relative risks and the benefits expected from the specific drug or procedure and weigh each factor appropriately; patients must understand the trade-offs involved to give truly *informed consent*. The lowest risk and logical option is not always chosen. In some cases, dubious or rare associations appear to override clear benefit against a tangible risk, such as fear of autism from the measles–mumps–rubella vaccination. Alternatively, most iatrogenic complications are not openly discussed and less commonly published, likely in part owing to concerns of litigation and scrutiny. An Institute of Medicine study gathered much media attention in 2000 with a report that projected from 44,000 to 98,000 annual U.S. deaths were a consequence of preventable medical mistakes and laid out a comprehensive strategy to reduce this number; many though were due to systemic health care delivery problems and not direct physician error. However, identification of iatrogenic complications is a critical factor in limiting similar events and is an aspect of medical care quality control.

In some instances, drug reactions have advanced medical knowledge; for example, rabies vaccine neuroparalytic accidents led to the discovery of experimental autoimmune encephalomyelitis, and penicillamine-induced myasthenia gravis led to valuable observations about the idiopathic disease. Medications have been used to analyze the nature of peripheral neuropathies and normal nerve function. Understanding the pathogenesis of some adverse reactions may lead to improved medical care in areas beyond the direct drug involvement.

New syndromes have arisen from these reactions. For instance, *epidural lipomatosis* was first recognized as a complication of steroid therapy, then a consequence of obesity, then an idiopathic disorder, and finally a complication of anabolic steroid abuse. Another example is the *serotonin syndrome*, which is most often caused by use of serotonin-reuptake inhibitors, but is often a result of drug combinations, including neurologic agents such as triptans and selegiline. *Critical illness myopathy*, originally de-

▶ TABLE 165.1 Adverse Neurologic Reactions Due to Drugs or Procedures for Diagnosis or Therapy

Adverse Reaction	Example Treatment or Procedure
Aseptic meningitis	Trimethoprim, sulfadiazine, nonsteroidal antiinflammatory agents, IVIG azathioprine
Basal ganglia syndromes (parkinsonism, tardive dyskinesia, other dyskinesias)	Butyrophenones, levodopa, phenothiazines, reserpine
Brain tumor	Immunosuppression (CNS lymphoma)
	Radiotherapy (meningioma)
Central pontine myelinolysis	Rapid correction of hyponatremia
Encephalopathy	Anticonvulsant drugs, cimetidine, corticosteroids, hemodialysis, insulin (hypoglycemia), lithium, methotrexate, metrizamide, monoamine oxidase inhibitors, overhydration (water intoxication), penicillin, pentazocine, propoxyphene, radiotherapy, vincristine
Leukoencephalopathy	Methotrexate, radiation, vaccines
Malignant neuroleptic syndrome	Neuroleptic drugs
Meningoencephalitis (viral, yeast, toxoplasmosis)	Immunosuppression
Malignant hyperthermia	Succinylcholine, halothane, others
Myopathies and myoglobinuria	Anticonvulsants (with osteomalacia), chloroquine, colchicine, corticosteroids, emetine, hypophosphatemia, ipecac, kaliuretic diuretics (furosemide, thiazides), licorice (glycyrrhizate), statins, penicillamine, zidovudine
Muscle fibrosis	Meperidine, pentazocine injection
Myotonia	Diazacholesterol
Myelopathy	Intrathecal injections, delayed arachnoiditis after myelography, nitrous oxide, radiotherapy, spinal anesthesia, spinal angiography, vaccination
Neuromuscular disorders	
Myasthenia gravis	Antiepileptic drugs, penicillamine
Other neuromuscular blockade	Aminoglycoside antibiotics, succinylcholine
Optic neuropathy	Amiodarone, ethambutol, isoniazid, penicillamine, vincristine
Peripheral neuropathy	Amiodarone, barbiturates (acute porphyria trigger), bortezomib, colchicine, dapsone disulfiram, gold salts, isoniazid, leflunomide, linezolid, metronidazole, nitrofurantoin, nitrous oxide, nucleoside analog agents, phenytoin, platins, pyridoxine (B_6) excess, statins, suramin, tacrolimus, taxoids (paclitaxel, docetaxel), thalidomide, vinca alkaloids
Pseudotumor cerebri	Corticosteroids, nalidixic acid, tetracycline, vitamin A
Serotonin syndrome	Amphetamines, anticoagulants, cerebral angiography and intraarterial interventional therapies, chiropractic neck manipulation, induced hypotension for surgery, insulin-induced hypoglycemia, carotid sinus massage, open heart surgery and cardiopulmonary bypass, oral contraceptives, overcorrection of hypertension, radiotherapy of neck or cranium, thrombolytics
Stroke	

scribed in the setting of steroids and neuromuscular blockade, has led to better understanding of muscle atrophy, catabolism, and loss of excitability mechanisms and an expanded concept of this common clinical phenomenon.

Complications are not limited to medications. Many procedures and interventions generate their own problems, including organ transplantation, cardiovascular surgery and assist devices, neurosurgery, cortical implants, plasmapheresis, pumps for intrathecal drug delivery, shunting of normal pressure hydrocephalus, interventional neuroradiologic and cardiac procedures, anesthesia, and numerous others. Protean complications are too numerous to list and span all areas of neurology. Hospitalization alone carries inherent risk; dangers are magnified in the intensive care unit. Some procedures have remarkably low complication rates, but patients may consider them risky, such as electrodiagnostic studies. Lumbar

puncture (LP) deserves special consideration because it is a prototypical surviving neurologic procedure, performed since 1889. Although headache is a common complication in up to 40%, depending on needle size and type used, more serious complications are quite rare (0.3% in one estimate) despite frequent patient misperceptions. Cerebral herniation is a perennial concern, but even in adults with mass lesions, herniation estimates owing to LP are approximately 1%.

Drugs and procedures are not the only iatrogenic disorders. The actions or inactions of a physician may contribute to patient morbidity. The consequences of misdiagnosis that result in withholding a beneficial treatment or erroneous use of an unnecessary treatment are more critical than ever, given the ever-expanding number of neurologic therapies and ever-increasing complexity of diagnosis.

SUGGESTED READINGS

Al-Shekhlee A, Shapiro BE, Preston DC. Iatrogenic complications and risks of nerve conduction studies and needle electromyography. *Muscle Nerve* 2003;27:517–526.

Atkinson JLD, Sundt TM Jr, Kazmier FJ, et al. Heparin-induced thrombocytopenia and thrombosis in ischemic stroke. *Mayo Clin Proc* 1988; 63:353–361.

Bednall R, McRobbie D, Hicks A. Identification of medication-related attendances at an A & E department. *J Clin Pharm Ther* 2003;28: 41–45.

Bertorini TE. Myoglobinuria, malignant hyperthermia, neuroleptic malignant syndrome and serotonin syndrome. *Neurol Clin* 1997;15:649–671.

Biller J, ed. *Iatrogenic Neurology.* Boston: Buttterworth-Heinemann, 1998.

Brannagan TH 3rd, Nagle KJ, Lange DJ, et al. Complications of intravenous immune globulin treatment in neurologic disease. *Neurology* 1996;47:674–677.

Canbaz S, Turgut N, Halici U, et al. Electrophysiological evaluation of phrenic nerve injury during cardiac surgery—a prospective, controlled, clinical study. *BMC Surg* 2004;4:2.

Caranasos GJ, Stewart RB, Cluff LE. Drug-induced illness leading to hospitalization. *JAMA* 1974;228:713–717.

Ericsson M, Alges G, Schliamser SE. Spinal epidural abscess in adults: review and report of iatrogenic cases. *Scand J Infect Dis* 1990;22:249–257.

Evans RW. Complications of lumbar puncture. *Neurol Clin* 1998;16:83–105.

Fadul CE, Lemann W, Thaler HT, et al. Perforations of the gastrointestinal tract in patients receiving steroids for neurologic disease. *Neurology* 1988;38:348–352.

Fahn S. Welcome news about levodopa, but uncertainty remains. *Ann Neurol* 1998;43:551–554.

Fessler RG, Johnson DL, Brown FD, et al. Epidural lipomatosis in steroid-treated patients. *Spine* 1992;17:183–188.

Gardner DM, Lynd LD. Sumatriptan contraindications and the serotonin syndrome. *Ann Pharmacother* 1998;32:33–38.

Graham GD. Tissue plasminogen activator for acute ischemic stroke in clinical practice: a meta-analysis of safety data. *Stroke* 2003;34:2847–2850.

Graus F, Saiz A, Sierra J, et al. Neurologic complications of autologous and allogeneic bone marrow transplantation in patients with leukemia: a comparative study. *Neurology* 1996;46:1004–1009.

Hunter JM. Adverse effects of neuromuscular blocking drugs. *Br J Anaesthiol* 1987;59:46–60.

Jolles S, Sewell WA, Leighton C. Drug-induced aseptic meningitis: diagnosis and management. *Drug Saf* 2000;22:215–226.

Juurlink DN, Mamdani M, Kopp A, et al. Drug-drug interactions among elderly patients hospitalized for drug toxicity. *JAMA* 2003;289:1652–1658.

Kohn LT, Corrigan J, Donaldson MS, eds. Institute of Medicine Committee on Quality of Health Care in America. *To Err Is Human: Building a Safer Health System.* Washington, DC: National Academy Press, 2000.

Lacomis D, Petrella JT, Giuliani MJ. Causes of neuromuscular weakness in the intensive care unit: a study of 92 patients. *Muscle Nerve* 1998;21:610–617.

Lapsiwala S, Moftakhar R, Badie B. Drug-induced iatrogenic intraparenchymal hemorrhage. *Neurosurg Clin N Am* 2002;13:299–312.

Lee P, Smith I, Piesowicz A, et al. Spastic paraparesis after anaesthesia. *Lancet* 1999;353:554.

Lewis MB, Howdle PD. Neurologic complications of liver transplantation in adults. *Neurology* 2003;61:1174–1178.

Mack EE, Wilson CB. Meningiomas induced by high-dose cranial irradiation. *J Neurosurg* 1993;79:28–31.

Malouf R, Brust JCM. Hypoglycemia: causes, neurological manifestations and outcome. *Ann Neurol* 1985;17:421–430.

Mattle AH, Sieb JP, Rohner M, et al. Nontraumatic spinal epidural and subdural hematomas. *Neurology* 1987;37:1351–1356.

Moses H, Kaden I. Neurologic consultations in a general hospital: spectrum of iatrogenic disease. *Am J Med* 1986;955–958.

Murch S. Separating inflammation from speculation in autism. *Lancet* 2003;362:1498–1499.

Nelson KM, Talbert RL. Drug-related hospital admissions. *Pharmacotherapy* 1996;16:701–707.

Nora LM, Benvenuti RJ. Medicolegal aspects of informed consent. *Neurol Clin* 1998;16:207–216.

Padovan CS, Yousry TA, Schleuning M, et al. Neurological and neuroradiological findings in long-term survivors of allogeneic bone marrow transplantation. *Ann Neurol* 1998;43:627–633.

Rampling R, Symonds P. Radiation myelopathy. *Curr Opin Neurol* 1998; 11:627–632.

Richard IH. Acute, drug-induced, life-threatening neurologic syndromes. *Neurologist* 1998;4:196–210.

Richard IH, Kurlan R, Tanner C, et al. Serotonin syndrome and the combined use of deprenyl and an antidepressant in Parkinson's disease. Parkinson Study Group. *Neurology* 1997;48:1070–1077.

Roughead EE, Gilbert AL, Primrose JG, et al. Drug-related hospital admissions: a review of Australian studies published in 1988–1996. *Med J Aust* 1998;168:405–408.

Schaumberg H, Kaplan J, Windebank A, et al. Sensory neuropathy from pyridoxine abuse: a new megavitamin syndrome. *N Engl J Med* 1983;309:445–448.

Shintani S, Tanaka H, Irifune A, et al. Iatrogenic acute spinal epidural abscess with septic meningitis: MR findings. *Clin Neurol Neurosurg* 1992;94:253–255.

Sieb JP, Gillessen T. Iatrogenic and toxic myopathies. *Muscle Nerve* 2003; 27:142–156.

Steere AC, Taylor E, McHugh GL, et al. The overdiagnosis of Lyme disease. *JAMA* 1993;269:1812–1816.

Sterns RH, Riggs JE, Schochet SS Jr. Osmotic demyelination syndrome following correction of hyponatremia. *N Engl J Med* 1986;314:1535–1542.

Weimer LH. Medication induced peripheral neuropathy. *Curr Neurol Neurosci Rep* 2003;3:86–92.

Wang MS, Davis AA, Culver DG, et al. Calpain inhibition protects against Taxol-induced sensory neuropathy. *Brain* 2004;127:671–679.

Yuen EC, Layzer RB, Weitz SR, et al. Neurologic complications of lumbar epidural anesthesia and analgesia. *Neurology* 1995;45:1795–1801.

Chapter 166

Complications of Cancer Chemotherapy

Lisa M. DeAngelis and Casilda M. Balmaceda

ANTINEOPLASTIC DRUGS

Nervous system toxicity is the second most common cause of dose-limiting toxicity of antineoplastic agents after myelosuppression. It occurs with a wide variety of agents and can result in significant disability. Antitumor chemotherapy may be toxic to both the peripheral and central nervous systems, and several antineoplastic drugs may induce more than one side effect, causing different

▶ **TABLE 166.1** Neurotoxicity of Antineoplastic Drugs

Neurologic Disorder	Drug
Peripheral neuropathy	Carboplatin, cisplatin, cytarabine, docetaxel, etoposide, fludarabine, oxaliplatin, paclitaxel, procarbazine, suramin, vinblastine, vincristine, vinorelbine
Cranial neuropathy	Carmustine, cisplatin (these 2 are with intra-arterial administration only), 5-fluorouracil, vinblastine, vincristine, vinorelbine
Autonomic neuropathy	Vinblastine, vincristine, vinorelbine
Encephalopathy	Asparaginase, busulfan, carmustine, cisplatin, cytarabine, 5-fluorouracil, fludarabine, ifosfamide, methotrexate, procarbazine
Cerebellar syndrome	Cytarabine, 5-fluorouracil, procarbazine
Acute myelopathy	Cytarabine, methotrexate, thiotepa (all with intrathecal administration only)

neurologic disorders (Table 166.1). The incidence of neurotoxicity often depends on dose, route and schedule of administration, patient age and general medical condition, and whether an agent has been combined with other neurotoxic drugs or radiotherapy.

Peripheral Nervous System Toxicity

Vinca Alkaloids

The vinca alkaloids, such as vincristine sulfate and vinblastine sulfate, cause a sensorimotor neuropathy; vincristine is much more likely to cause neuropathy than any other vinca alkaloid. Vincristine binds to tubulin and disrupts microtubules of the mitotic apparatus of cell division, arresting cells in metaphase. The effect on microtubules involved in axoplasmic transport is likely responsible for the axonal neuropathy that develops. The severity of symptoms is related to total dose and duration of therapy. Distal paresthesia is the most common symptom, occurring in almost all patients. Objective sensory loss is rare, but distal weakness is typical. Patients develop impairment of the intrinsic hand muscles and the foot and toe dorsiflexors. Footdrop may develop in some patients, and many have difficulty with fine motor tasks; muscle cramps are seen occasionally. Tendon reflexes are depressed. Paresthesias and weakness improve when dosage is reduced or therapy stopped. Cranial neuropathies rarely occur from vincristine; ptosis, oculomotor paresis, and vocal cord paralysis have been reported. Jaw pain results from trigeminal nerve toxicity; it occurs acutely or within 3 days of drug administration and resolves spontaneously, usually without recurrence with subsequent doses. An autonomic neuropathy may affect the gastrointestinal tract, causing abdominal pain and constipation in about one-third of patients. Paralytic ileus may follow, and prophylactic laxatives should be given to every patient treated with vincristine. Rare manifestations include urinary retention, impotence, and orthostatic hypotension.

Vincristine neurotoxicity may be more severe in patients with older age or pre-existing neuropathy, especially Charcot-Marie-Tooth disease. Patients previously treated with other spindle poisons, such as paclitaxel (Taxol), may not tolerate vincristine. Vinorelbine, a new semisynthetic vinca alkaloid, has less neurotoxicity, but can cause a peripheral neuropathy in patients who have received prior neurotoxic agents.

Platins

Cisplatin causes a dose-dependent, predominantly sensory polyneuropathy. Neuropathy follows a total cumulative dose >300 to 500 mg/M^2, but the symptoms may begin or progress after cisplatin is discontinued. Maximal neurotoxicity may not be seen for several months after the last dose of drug. Symptoms usually improve once therapy is stopped, but recovery may be incomplete and some patients do not recover at all. The dorsal root ganglia are probably the target of damage, followed by the peripheral nerves. Large myelinated fibers are most susceptible; proprioceptive sensory loss may be profound, with marked sensory ataxia. The motor system is spared. Autonomic neuropathy is rare. The adrenocorticotropic hormone analogs, glutathione, and nimodipine may be neuroprotective when given concomitantly, but none of these agents is used in routine clinical practice.

Cisplatin can cause ototoxicity and vestibulopathy. High-frequency hearing loss occurs first, so initial effects are subclinical until patients develop severe hearing impairment; all patients must be followed with audiograms to prevent hearing disability. Hearing loss is a result of toxic effects on cochlear hair cells and may be irreversible. Vestibular neuropathy is much less common and may occur with or without hearing impairment. Intracarotid infusion may cause optic neuropathy or injury to any cranial nerve from VII through XII. The Lhermitte symptom may occur during or shortly after treatment with cisplatin; it resolves completely and spontaneously. It may also occur with spinal cord compression or cervical irradiation. Carboplatin has less severe neurologic toxicity but more pronounced hematologic toxicity. Oxaliplatin has dose-limiting neurotoxicity, producing an acute neuropathy at a dose of 135 mg/M^2; the neuropathy is similar to that seen with cisplatin.

Taxanes

The taxanes, paclitaxel and docetaxel, stabilize microtubules and inhibit cell division. Paclitaxel produces a predominantly axonal sensory neuropathy that may be dose, limiting. After a single dose of 250 mg/M^2 or at lower doses with repeated treatment, 50% to 90% of treated patients are affected, depending on dosing regimens. Early symptoms include distal numbness and tingling; examination reveals loss of tendon reflexes and impaired vibration. Proximal limb weakness and myalgia may occur several days after the drug is given; the weakness is probably neuropathic and not myopathic. Docetaxel causes a similar sensory neuropathy, which may be exacerbated by peripheral edema and skin changes that are a direct cutaneous toxicity of the drug. The combination of a taxane and a platin is more neurotoxic than either medication given alone. Amifostine was ineffective in preventing clinical neuropathy in patients treated with cisplatin and paclitaxel.

Other Agents

Thalidomide causes a peripheral neuropathy. Less frequently, peripheral nerve dysfunction may be caused by other antineoplastic agents, including suramin, cytarabine, procarbazine hydrochloride, and etoposide. Any patient with a pre-existing neuropathy, such as diabetic neuropathy, is more vulnerable to peripheral nervous system toxicity from chemotherapeutic agents.

Central Nervous System Toxicity

Acute CNS Toxicity

CNS toxicity from chemotherapy may be acute, occurring during or within a few days of drug administration, or chronic, occurring weeks to months later. Most chemotherapeutic agents penetrate the blood-brain barrier poorly, so acute neurotoxicity is uncommon. It is characterized by confusion, disorientation, and altered behavior. The patient may have a quiet or agitated delirium. Hallucinations, myoclonus, and seizures are common symptoms.

The agents most frequently responsible are ifosfamide (up to 30% incidence depending on dose), methotrexate (high-dose IV or intrathecal), and procarbazine (<15%). These agents cause an acute encephalopathy that clears with discontinuation of the agent, although reversal is occasionally incomplete after ifosfamide toxicity. Encephalopathy contraindicates further treatment with ifosfamide, but the other agents may be used subsequently af-

ter a patient recovers. 5-Fluorouracil (5-FU) neurotoxicity is rare (<5%) but includes an acute cerebellar syndrome with dysarthria, dysmetria, ataxia, vertigo, and nystagmus. The symptoms usually clear within 1 to 6 weeks after drug withdrawal. An inflammatory leukoencephalopathy with enhancing white matter lesions on MRI may follow combined administration of 5-FU and levamisole hydrochloride. A pancerebellar syndrome may also develop with high-dose cytarabine therapy (usually at a cumulative dose of ≥36 g/M^2 on a 3 g/M^2 every 12 hours schedule), particularly in older patients or those with renal insufficiency. Symptoms often subside within weeks, but permanent disability may occur in some patients. Complications after intrathecal administration of cytarabine include meningismus, seizures, or paraparesis, often with pain and loss of sensation. CNS toxicity is uncommon with vincristine treatment, but encephalopathy, seizures, focal cerebral signs, and cortical blindness have been reported; CNS toxicity from vincristine-induced syndrome of inappropriate secretion of antidiuretic hormone (SIADH) and hyponatremia also occurs.

Methotrexate in conventional doses has little or no neurotoxicity when given intravenously, but high-dose therapy may cause an acute stroke-like encephalopathy. This syndrome usually occurs abruptly several days after the second or third treatment and resolves within days. It is characterized by seizures, confusion, hemiparesis, and aphasia. A vascular etiology has been postulated, perhaps related to the high serum levels of homocysteine that result from methotrexate. Intrathecal methotrexate may induce chemical meningitis in about 10% of patients. Starting a few hours after drug administration; the syndrome includes headache, nausea, vomiting, fever, back pain, dizziness, meningismus, and lethargy. It resolves within a few days and may respond to or be prevented by corticosteroid administration. Transverse myelopathy is a rare acute toxicity of intrathecal methotrexate or any agent. It usually develops within days, and it causes permanent disability.

Chronic CNS Toxicity

Chronic leukoencephalopathy is the most devastating form of neurotoxicity because it is usually irreversible and may be progressive. It is seen most commonly with the antimetabolites, particularly methotrexate. It follows repeated doses of intrathecal or high-dose intravenous drug and rarely occurs after standard doses. It appears months to years after therapy, and young children and older adults are most vulnerable. Methotrexate combined with cranial irradiation has synergistic toxicity, accelerating or enhancing the development of leukoencephalopathy. Symptoms usually start with personality change and progress to a moderate dementia often accompanied by ataxia; it can slowly progress to coma and death. Neuroimaging shows extensive, symmetric white matter hypodensity on CT scan or hyperintensity on FLAIR or T2 MRIs calcification may be observed in children. There is no treatment, although ventriculoperitoneal shunt affords temporary improvement in some patients. A similar chronic encephalopathy may develop after treatment with cytarabine or fludarabine.

Nitrosoureas do not cause CNS toxicity at conventional doses, but encephalopathy is seen after high-dose intravenous or intra-arterial bischloroethylnitrosourea, particularly in patients who have received cranial irradiation; retinopathy may also occur. Carotid artery injection of cisplatin may cause loss of vision or seizures. Drug streaming after intra-arterial infusion may expose local areas of brain to extremely high concentrations of drug, resulting in focal cerebral necrosis from any agent administered in this fashion.

High doses of chemotherapy in conjunction with stem cell support or bone marrow transplantation may result in neurotoxicity that is not seen with conventional doses. This occurs with the alkylating agents busulfan, the nitrosoureas, and thiotepa, as well as with etoposide. Rarely, focal leukoencephalopathy is seen when drug is administered through an Ommaya reservoir into a misplaced catheter. The drug diffuses into the surrounding white matter, causing focal necrosis.

IMMUNOSUPPRESSANT DRUGS

The calcineurin inhibitors, cyclosporine and tacrolimus, frequently cause neurotoxicity. Cyclosporine is an important drug used to prevent organ transplant rejection. It acts by inhibiting interleukin-2 (IL-2) production by T-cells and is successful in suppressing T-cell response to transplantation antigens, thus prolonging graft survival. Neurotoxicity occurs in about 4% (seizures, paresthesias) to 55% (tremors) of patients. Toxicity may occur at therapeutic levels but is more frequent with serum levels >500 ng/mL. Symptoms include headache, tremor, paresthesias, seizures, lethargy, ataxia, and quadriparesis; cortical blindness may also occur. Most symptoms clear with cessation of therapy or dose reduction. Reversible cerebral white matter lesions are seen on CT or MRI, and the occipital lobes are frequently affected. Neurotoxicity may be a direct toxic effect of the drug or related to severe cyclosporine-induced hypertension and hypertensive encephalopathy. Cyclosporine induces activity of the hepatic cytochrome P-450 system. Consequently, hepatic dysfunction or concomitant administration of agents that induce the P-450 system can alter the serum concentrations of cyclosporine. In the circulation, cyclosporine is bound to lipoproteins; a reduction in serum cholesterol to <120 mg/dL may increase free-drug levels and neurotoxicity. Corticosteroids also increase plasma cyclosporine levels.

Tacrolimus has cyclosporine-like activity and is approved for immunosuppression in organ transplantation. Neurotoxicity occurs in 15% or more of patients and is usu-

ally manifested as acute tremor, headache, or insomnia. More serious CNS toxicities include confusion, seizures, psychosis, and hallucinations. A reversible peripheral neuropathy with paresthesias has been reported. Neurologic symptoms begin when the tacrolimus blood level is at a peak and eventually resolve after the dose is reduced or stopped. Tacrolimus-related leukoencephalopathy may cause hyperintense lesions in the parieto-occipital region and centrum semiovale on MRI. Clinical recovery is usually accompanied by reversal of radiographic abnormalities.

OKT3, a powerful immunosuppressive drug, is a monoclonal murine anti–T-cell antibody used to treat acute allograft rejection. Neurologic complications are uncommon, but may develop within hours of administration and include altered mental function, seizures, and lethargy. Contrast-enhancing cerebral lesions may be seen on MRI. Aseptic meningitis, visual loss, and transient sensorineural hearing loss are other adverse effects.

BIOLOGIC RESPONSE MODIFIERS

Cytokines, such as interferons and IL-2, are used as biologic response modifiers to treat cancer. IL-2 causes a capillary leak syndrome that can affect the brain as well as other organs. It can increase brain water content, causing a severe encephalopathy that may be missed because the patient is so ill systemically. Symptoms include seizures, headache, anorexia, depressed level of alertness, and focal neurological signs. Brachial plexopathy is rare. IL-2 encephalopathy is self-limited. Interferons cause a similar spectrum of neurologic toxicity, but the encephalopathy may be irreversible.

HEMATOPOIETIC STEM CELL TRANSPLANTATION

Hematopoietic stem cell transplantation (HSCT) is the accurate term to describe the transfer of bone marrow, peripheral stem cells, or umbilical cord blood from one person to another (allogeneic HSCT) or, after prior procurement and storage, to the same person (autologous HSCT). HSCT is used to treat a wide variety of disorders, mostly neoplastic, but nonmalignant diseases such as aplastic anemia may also be treated with this approach.

Neurologic complications from HSCT are common and occur with greater frequency in patients undergoing allogeneic HSCT because of the need for chronic immunosuppression. Focal processes include infection (0.6%–15%) and cerebrovascular disorders. The most common infections are *Aspergillus fumigatus* and *Toxoplasma gondii* but bacterial abscesses, other fungi and viral infections including herpes simplex encephalitis and progressive multifocal leukoencephalopathy also occur. Stroke is uncommon after HSCT, occurring in about 4% of patients, and may be related to non-bacterial thrombotic endocarditis (NBTE) or CNS angiitis as well as the more common causes. Intracranial hemorrhage has been reported in up to 32% of patients in an autopsy series. Most hemorrhages are subdural hematomas secondary to coagulopathy and thrombocytopenia. Intracerebral hematomas may occur as a consequence of venous sinus thrombosis, aspergillus infection, cyclosporine toxicity, coagulopathy, or a TTP-like syndrome. Subarachnoid hemorrhage is very rare and usually associated with relapsing leukemia.

Drug-induced CNS disorders occur in association with agents used for immunosuppression (see above), which can all cause encephalopathy. However, the incidence of CNS toxicity from cyclosporine, tacrolimus, and OKT3 is ≤5% in HSCT patients, whereas it is much higher in organ transplant recipients. The reason for this is unknown. HSCT patients develop encephalopathy commonly from multiorgan failure and the wide variety of supportive agents necessary in the posttransplant period such as antimicrobial, antiviral, and sedative agents. Leukoencephalopathy without clear cause may develop, particularly in patients who receive cranial radiotherapy as part of total body irradiation administered for their conditioning regimen.

Peripheral nervous system toxicities are seen occasionally in the HSCT patient. Patients may have pre-existing chemotherapy neuropathy. However, acute demyelinating neuropathies, such as Guillain-Barré–like syndromes and chronic forms have been seen. Polymyositis and myasthenia gravis may develop as late complications in patients with chronic graft-versus-host disease. Treatment is similar to that used for idiopathic polymyositis and myasthenia.

SUGGESTED READINGS

Chemotherapy

Peripheral Neurotoxicity

Authier N, Gillet JP, Fialip J, et al. A new animal model of vincristine-induced nociceptive peripheral neuropathy. *Neurotoxicology* 2003;24:797–805.

Bacon M, James K, Zee B. A comparison of the incidence, duration, and degree of the neurologic toxicities of cisplatin-paclitaxel (PT) and cisplatin-cyclophosphamide (PC). *Int J Gynecol Cancer* 2003;13:428–434.

Cavaletti G, Bogliun G, Marzorati L, et al. Grading of chemotherapy-induced peripheral neurotoxicity using the Total Neuropathy Scale. *Neurology* 2003;61:1297–1300.

Chang YW, Yoon HK, Cho JM, et al. Spinal MRI of vincristine neuropathy mimicking Guillain-Barré syndrome. *Pediatr Radiol* 2003;33:791–793.

Chauvenet AR, Shashi V, Selsky C, et al. Pediatric Oncology Group Study. Vincristine-induced neuropathy as the initial presentation of Charcot-Marie-Tooth disease in acute lymphoblastic leukemia: a Pediatric Oncology Group study. *J Pediatr Hematol Oncol* 2003;25:316–320.

Chen YM, Perng RP, Shih JF, et al. A randomised phase II study of weekly paclitaxel or vinorelbine in combination with cisplatin against inoperable non-small-cell lung cancer previously untreated. *Br J Cancer* 2004;90:359–365.

Grothey A. Oxaliplatin-safety profile: neurotoxicity. *Semin Oncol* 2003;30:5–13.

Kuroi K, Shimozuma K. Neurotoxicity of taxanes: symptoms and quality of life assessment. *Breast Cancer* 2004;11:92–99.

Lehky TJ, Leonard GD, Wilson RH, et al. Oxaliplatin-induced neurotoxicity: acute hyperexcitability and chronic neuropathy. *Muscle Nerve* 2004;29:387–392.

Makino H. Treatment and care of neurotoxicity from taxane anticancer agents. *Breast Cancer* 2004;11:100–104.

Moore DH, Donnelly J, McGuire WP, et al.; Gynecologic Oncology Group. Limited access trial using amifostine for protection against cisplatin- and three-hour paclitaxel-induced neurotoxicity: a phase II study of the Gynecologic Oncology Group. *J Clin Oncol* 2003;21:4207–4213.

Morabito A, Fanelli M, Carillio G, et al. Thalidomide prolongs disease stabilization after conventional therapy in patients with recurrent glioblastoma. *Oncol Rep* 2004;11:93–95.

Paccagnella A, Favaretto A, Oniga F, et al.; GSTVP (Gruppo di Studio Tumori Polmonari del Veneto). Cisplatin versus carboplatin in combination with mitomycin and vinblastine in advanced non small cell lung cancer. A multicenter, randomized phase III trial. *Lung Cancer* 2004;43:83–91.

Quasthoff S, Hartung HP. Chemotherapy-induced peripheral neuropathy. *J Neurol* 2002;249:9–17.

Rajkumar SV. Thalidomide in newly diagnosed multiple myeloma and overview experience in smoldering/indolent disease. *Semin Hematol* 2003;40:17–22.

Rose PG, Smrekar M. Improvement of paclitaxel-induced neuropathy by substitution of docetaxel for paclitaxel. *Gynecol Oncol* 2003;91:423–425.

Sathiapalan RK, El-Solh H. Enhanced vincristine neurotoxicity from drug interactions: case report and review of literature. *Pediatr Hematol Oncol* 2001;18:543–546.

Watanabe H, Yamamoto N, Tamura T, et al. Study of paclitaxel and dose escalation of cisplatin in patients with advanced non-small cell lung cancer. *Jpn J Clin Oncol* 2003;33:626–630.

CNS Toxicity

Abrey LE, DeAngelis LM, Yahalom J. Long-term survival in primary CNS lymphoma. *J Clin Oncol* 1998;16:859–863.

Correa DD, DeAngelis LM, Shi W, et al. Cognitive functions in survivors of primary central nervous system lymphoma. *Neurology* 2004;62:548–555.

Dabaja BS, McLaughlin P, Ha CS, et al. Primary central nervous system lymphoma: Phase I evaluation of infusional bromodeoxyuridine with whole brain accelerated fractionation radiation therapy after chemotherapy. *Cancer* 2003;98:1021–1028.

Fliessbach K, Urbach H, Helmstaedter C, et al. Cognitive performance and magnetic resonance imaging findings after high-dose systemic and intraventricular chemotherapy for primary central nervous system lymphoma. *Arch Neurol* 2003;60:563–568.

Keime-Guibert F, Napolitano M, Delattre JY. Neurological complications of radiotherapy and chemotherapy. *J Neurol* 1998;245:695–708.

Kimmel DW, Wijdicks EF, Rodriguez M. Multifocal inflammatory leukoencephalopathy associated with levamisole therapy. *Neurology* 1995;45:374–376.

Kishi S, Griener J, Cheng C, et al. Homocysteine, pharmacogenetics, and neurotoxicity in children with leukemia. *J Clin Oncol* 2003;21:3084–3091.

Lovblad K, Kelkar P, Ozdoba C, et al. Pure methotrexate encephalopathy presenting with seizures: CT and MRI features. *Pediatr Radiol* 1998;28:86–91.

Lyass O, Lossos A, Hubert A, et al. Cisplatin-induced non-convulsive encephalopathy. *Anticancer Drugs* 1998;9:100–104.

Mahoney DH Jr, Shuster JJ, Nitschke R, et al. Acute neurotoxicity in children with B-precursor acute lymphoid leukemia: an association with intermediate-dose intravenous methotrexate and intrathecal triple therapy—a Pediatric Oncology Group study. *J Clin Oncol* 1998;16:1712–1722.

Moore BE, Somers NP, Smith TW. Methotrexate-related nonnecrotizing multifocal axonopathy detected by beta-amyloid precursor protein immunohistochemistry. *Arch Pathol Lab Med* 2002;126:79–81.

Plotkin SR, Wen, PY. Neurologic complications of cancer therapy. *Neurol Clin N Am* 2003;21:279–2318.

Reddick WE, Glass JO, Langston JW, et al. Quantitative MRI assessment of leukoencephalopathy. *Magn Reson Med* 2002;47:912–920.

Sandoval C, Kutscher M, Jayabose S, et al. Neurotoxicity of intrathecal methotrexate: MR imaging findings. *Am J Neuroradiol* 2003;24:1887–1890.

Shuper A, Stark B, Kornreich L, et al. Methotrexate treatment protocols and the central nervous system: significant cure with significant neurotoxicity. *J Child Neurol* 2000;15:573–580.

Verschraegen C, Conrad CA, Hong WK. Subacute encephalopathic toxicity of cisplatin. *Lung Cancer* 1995;13:305–309.

Verstappen CC, Heimans JJ, Hoekman K, et al. Neurotoxic complications of chemotherapy in patients with cancer: clinical signs and optimal management. *Drugs* 2003;63:1549–1563.

Vezmar S, Becker A, Bode U, et al. Biochemical and clinical aspects of methotrexate neurotoxicity. *Chemotherapy* 2003;49:92–104.

Owen RG, Patmore RD, Smith GM, et al. Cytomegalovirus-induced T-cell proliferation and the development of progressive multifocal leucoencephalopathy following bone marrow transplantation. *Br J Haematol* 1995;89:196–198.

Provenzale JM, Graham ML. Reversible leukoencephalopathy associated with graft-versus-host disease: MR findings. *AJNR* 1996;17:1290–1294.

Seong D, Bruner JM, Lee KH, et al. Progressive multifocal leukoencephalopathy after autologous bone marrow transplantation in a patient with chronic myelogenous leukemia. *Clin Infect Dis* 1996;23:402–403.

Snider S, Bashir R, Bierman P. Neurologic complications after high-dose chemotherapy and autologous bone marrow transplantation for Hodgkin's disease. *Neurology* 1994;44:681–684.

Tahsildar HI, Remler BF, Creger RJ, et al. Delayed, transient encephalopathy after marrow transplantation: case reports and MRI findings in four patients. *J Neurooncol* 1996;27:241–250.

IMMUNOSUPPRESSANT DRUGS AND HEMATOPOIETIC STEM CELL TRANSPLANTATION

Chohan R, Vij R, Adkins D, et al. Long-term outcomes of allogeneic stem cell transplant recipients after calcineurin inhibitor-induced neurotoxicity. *Br J Haematol* 2003;123:110–1113.

Devine SM, Newman NJ, Siegel JL, et al. Tacrolimus (FK506)-induced cerebral blindness following bone marrow transplantation. *Bone Marrow Transplant* 1996;18:569–572.

Faraci M, Lanino E, Dini G, et al. Severe neurologic complications after hematopoietic stem cell transplantation in children. *Neurology* 2002;59:1895–1904.

Krouwer HGJ, Wijdicks EFM. Neurologic complications of bone marrow transplantation. *Neurol Clin N Am* 2003;21:319–352.

Patel B, Kerridge I. Cyclosporin neurotoxicity. *Br J Haematol* 2003;123:755.

Pittock SJ, Rabinstein AA, Edwards BS, et al. OKT3 neurotoxicity presenting as akinetic mutism. *Transplantation* 2003;75:1058–1060.

Taque S, Peudenier S, Gie S, et al. Central neurotoxicity of cyclosporine in two children with nephrotic syndrome. *Pediatr Nephrol* 2004;19:276–280.

Tezcan H, Zimmer W, Fenstermaker R, et al. Severe cerebellar swelling and thrombotic purpura associated with FK506. *Bone Marrow Transplant* 1998;21:105–109.

Thaisetthawatkul P, Weinstock A, Kerr SL, et al. Muromonab-CD3-induced neurotoxicity: report of two siblings, one of whom had subsequent cyclosporin-induced neurotoxicity. *J Child Neurol* 2001;16:825–831.

Wong R, Beguelin GZ, de Lima M, et al. Tacrolimus-associated posterior reversible encephalopathy syndrome after allogeneic haematopoietic stem cell transplantation. *Br J Haematol* 2003;122:128–134.

BIOLOGIC RESPONSE MODIFIERS

Anderson BA, Young PV, Kean WF, et al. Polymyositis in chronic graft-versus-host disease. *Arch Neurol* 1982;39:188–190.

Bender CM, Monti EJ, Kerr ME. Potential mechanisms of interferon toxicity. *Cancer Pract* 1996;4:35–39.

Bolger GB, Sullivan KM, Spence AM, et al. Myasthenia gravis after allogeneic bone marrow transplantation: relationship to chronic graft-versus-host disease. *Neurology* 1986;36:1087–1091.

Graus F, Saiz A, Sierra J, et al. Neurologic complications of autologous and allogeneic bone marrow transplantation in patients with leukemia: a comparative study. *Neurology* 1996;46:1004–1009.

Licinio J, Kling MA, Hauser P. Cytokines and brain function: relevance to interferon-alpha-induced mood and cognitive changes. *Semin Oncol* 1998;25:30–38.

Michel M, Vincent F, Sigal R, et al. Cerebral vasculitis after interleukin-2 therapy for renal cell carcinoma. *J Immunother Emphasis Tumor Immunol* 1995;18:124–126.

Chapter 167

Occupational and Environmental Neurotoxicology

Leon D. Prockop and Lewis P. Rowland

Neurotoxicology commands newspaper attention these days. Will chemical terrorism cause catastrophic numbers of deaths and innumerable neurologic sequelae in survivors? Is there a Gulf War syndrome in which exposure to anticholinesterase nerve gases caused amyotrophic lateral sclerosis (ALS)? Are the developing brains of children vulnerable to neurotoxic hazards whereby consequences of early damage may not emerge until advanced age? Are adult behavioral changes a result of subclinical occupational or environmental exposures? Can mercury intoxication result from inhalation of the element from dental amalgams and can that cause autism, Alzheimer disease, or ALS? These questions have been debated in an atmosphere of contentious uncertainty.

In this chapter we focus on the particular clinical syndromes that result from exposure to heavy metals, solvents, and natural neurotoxins (Table 167.1). Clinical diagnosis and laboratory proof of diagnosis are practical issues. Because treatment of neurotoxic damage is mainly symptomatic and supportive, recognition of disease potential and prevention are of paramount importance. We bypass detailed discussion of behavioral effects from chronic

▶ **TABLE 167.1 Neurotoxic Syndromes**

Agent	Occupational or Other Exposure	Syndrome	
		Acute	Chronic
Metals			
Arsenic	Pesticides, pigments, paint, electroplating, seafood, smelter, semiconductors	Encephalopathy	Neuropathy
Lead	Solder, lead shot, illicit whiskey, insecticides, auto body shop, storage battery manufacture, smelter, paint, water pipes, gasoline sniffing	Encephalopathy	Encephalopathy, neuropathy, motor neuron disease-like syndrome
Manganese	Iron industry, welding, mining, smelter, fireworks, fertilizer, dry cell batteries	Encephalopathy	Parkinsonism
Mercury	Thermometers, other gauges; dental office (amalgams); felt hat manufacture Electroplating, photography	Headache, tremor	Neuropathy, encephalopathy with dementia, tremor
Tin	Canning industry, solder, electronics, plastics, fungicides	Delirium	Encephalomyelopathy
Solvents			
Carbon disulfide	Rayon manufacture, preservatives, textiles, rubber cement, varnish, electroplating	Encephalopathy	Neuropathy, parkinsonism
Trichlorethylene	Paints, degreasers, spot removers, decaffeination, dry cleaning, rubber solvents	Narcosis	Encephalopathy, trigeminal neuropathy
Hexacarbons[a]	Paints, paint removers, varnish, degreasers, rapid-drying ink, glues, cleaning agents, glues for making shoes in poorly vented cottage industry, glue sniffing, MNBK in plastics	Narcosis	Neuropathy, encephalopathy, ataxia
Insecticides			
Organophosphates, carbamates	Manufacture, application	Cholinergic syndrome	Ataxia, neuropathy, myelopathy
Carbon monoxide	Accidental or deliberate exposure in motor vehicles, faulty gasoline-fueled heaters	Anoxic encephalopathy	Encephalopathy, delayed neuropsychiatric syndrome
Methyl alcohol	Contaminated illicit whiskey	Retinal blindess	
Recreation abuse			
Nitrous oxide	Dental offices	Encephalopathy	B_{12}-deficient myelopathy
Seafood			
Ciguatera		Sensory neuropathy with temperature inversion	
Shellfish		Acute neuropathy	

[a]Hexacarbons: n-hexane, methyl-n-butyl ketone (MNBK).

low-level exposures as beyond the scope of this chapter. More detailed information is provided in the General section of Suggested Readings.

RECOGNIZING INTOXICATION CLINICALLY

Potential neurotoxins are classified as follows: (1) therapeutic drugs; (2) biologic agents; (3) radiation and electricity; (4) heavy metals; (5) solvents and vapors; (6) insecticides, herbicides, fungicides, and rodenticides; (7) air pollution; (8) food additives; and (9) social poisons. Diagnosis of neurotoxicologic damage requires clinical

thoughtfulness. The history must include the composition and toxicity rating of suspected agents; whether single or mixed substances are involved; host dose exposure; and epidemiology. Additional considerations include the following:

1. Exposure may be acute high dose or chronic low dose;
2. short or long latency may separate exposure and symptoms;
3. pre-existing or coincidental disease may complicate diagnosis;
4. symptoms may be numerous and nonspecific;
5. susceptibility varies in different people, and animal toxicity does not always correlate to that in humans;

6. damage may be reversible or irreversible;
7. a cascade of effects may have secondary and systemic complications as well as psychologic problems;
8. secondary gain, especially in litigious countries, complicates diagnosis;
9. neurologic signs may be absent or subtle within recognized syndromes, such as: peripheral neuropathy, myelopathy, cerebellar damage, movement disorders, or encephalopathy;
10. laboratory data, which might serve as markers of neurotoxic damage, may be normal or only mildly deranged or may be nonspecific despite clear symptoms and signs of neurologic disorder;
11. other possible causes must be excluded (Table 167.2) by considering systemic or metabolic disease and evaluating therapeutic drugs the patient may be taking.

Reliable diagnosis often depends on the recognition of exposure by occupation or recreation, recognition of a specific syndrome, and elimination of other causes. Outbreaks or clusters may be encountered with mild symptoms of glue sniffing or the devastating encephalomyelopathy of Minamata disease in Japan, which was caused by methyl mercury. The circumstances of attempted suicide or fire usually identify carbon monoxide exposure; a motor running in a parked automobile or a faulty gasoline-fueled heater are most often responsible. For the following discussions, the primary at-risk occupations are listed in Table 167.1 and are not repeated in the text. Because of No. 9, a skilled, correctly interpreted neurologic examination is essential. For example, is an examinee's mild difficulty with skilled and rapid successive movements or mild loss of check with rebound just clumsiness within the range of normal, or are they manifestations of cerebellar damage?

Laboratory Evaluation

Sampling of contaminated water, air, or soil provides exposure data. Analysis of blood, hair, and nails provides data about possible heavy metal toxicity. Diagnostic tests may include electrophysiology, neuroimaging, neuropsychology, and biochemical markers. Many become positive only after irreversible damage has occurred; that is, sensitivity is poor. Likewise, specificity may also be poor, except for MRI after carbon monoxide poisoning. EMG and nerve conduction velocity are the most reliable in sensitivity and reproducibility. However, many neurotoxins affect the CNS, not the peripheral nervous system.

Acute Encephalopathy

Syndromes of stupor and coma, confusion, hyperactivity or somnolence, memory impairment, and behavioral change arise from many different disorders, as described in Chapter 1. The acute encephalopathy of lead poisoning affects children; seizures and increased intracranial pressure without a mass lesion may be clues to diagnosis. The circumstances of intoxication may be evident as in glue sniffing or dialysis dementia. Heavy metal intoxication is not encountered frequently among the causes of delirium, but may result from attempted murder by poisoning. The effects of carbon monoxide inhalation include death, prolonged coma, and subsequent dementia, or brief loss of consciousness and prompt recovery.

Chronic Encephalopathy

Dementia, with or without tremor, can arise from occupational exposure to heavy metals. Therefore, when confronted with a patient who may have been poisoned, it may be more important to know the occupational history than to order a sweeping survey of blood and urine. Mercury intoxication may be more often associated with tremor than other exposures, but this is probably not a reliable

▶ **TABLE 167.2** **Clues to the Diagnosis of Intoxications**

Nature of exposure	Occupation with known hazard
	Recreational use of known hazard
	Accidental exposure to hazard
	Dialysis (aluminum)
	Cluster or epidemic of syndrome (seafood, "huffing")
	Dietary exposure to known hazard (seafood)
	Diagnosis of exclusion
	Therapeutic drugs
	Alcohol abuse
	Illicit drug abuse
	Infection
	Systemic disease: renal, pulmonary, calcium, liver, endocrine, electrolytes
	Inherited metabolic diseases
Age of patient	Children—lead encephalopathy
	Adolescents, young adults—sniffing, nitrous oxide
Associated symptoms, signs or laboratory abnormalities	
Lead	Gastrointesinal symptoms: colic, constipation
	Anemia
	Basophilic sippling
	↑ urinary δ-aminolevulinic acid
Thallium	Alopecia
Arsenic	Mees lines (horizontal stratifications of fingernails or leuconychia)
Nitrous oxide	B$_{12}$ deficiency
Specific syndromes	
Optic neuropathy and retinopathy	Methyl alcohol
SMON	Clioquinol
Methyl mercury	Minamata disease
NMBK	Trigeminal neuropathy

NMBK, n-methyl butyl ketone; SMON, subacute myelo-optic neuropathy.

guide. Parkinsonism can appear in workers in manganese smelters if monitoring guidelines are not heeded. Parkinsonism may also follow chronic exposure to carbon disulfide. Chronic encephalopathy is reported in workers and others exposed to solvents, such as volatile organic compounds (VOCs).

Extrapyramidal and Cerebellar Syndromes

VOCs, especially toluene, may cause movement disorders. Carbon monoxide can cause both parkinsonism and cerebellar dysfunction.

Peripheral Neuropathy

Neuropathy may be caused by any heavy metal, almost always the result of occupational exposure. The symptoms are those of any sensorimotor neuropathy with acroparesthesia and distal limb weakness. Toxic optic and autonomic neuropathies seem to be rare. A hallmark of thallium neuropathy is baldness. The neuropathy of organophosphate poisoning may be accompanied by upper motor neuron signs that imply a myelopathy; sometimes the residual signs include those of the lower motor neuron, but the occupational history and sensory loss differentiate the syndrome from motor neuron disease.

Cranial Neuropathy

Trichloroethylene causes a selective sensory neuropathy of the trigeminal nerve; the syndrome is so specific that it was once seriously evaluated as a treatment for idiopathic trigeminal neuralgia. Visual loss from optic neuropathy or retinopathy is a manifestation of methanol toxicity and many therapeutic drugs.

Delayed Effects

A delayed neuropathy has been reported after organophosphate exposure and a delayed neuropsychiatric syndrome after carbon monoxide poisoning. Exposure to pesticides has been implicated in mental retardation and also in Parkinson disease.

HEAVY METAL INTOXICATION

Pathogenesis

The heavy metals have diverse toxic effects on cell nuclei, mitochondria, other organelles, cytoplasmic enzymes, and membrane lipids. Clinical syndromes may result from combinations of these effects that do not readily explain

the real-life disorders or why the assault should affect the CNS in some people, peripheral nerves in others, or both.

Lead provides an example of the complexity. It interferes with the sulfhydryl enzymes of heme biosynthesis, especially δ-aminolevulinic acid dehydratase, coproporphyrin oxidase, and ferrochetalase. As a result of these partial blocks, several metabolites accumulate in blood and urine: δ-aminolevulinic acid, coprophorphyrin III, and zinc protoporphyrin. Other heme-containing enzymes are also affected, including cytochrome P450 in the liver and mitochondrial cytochrome c oxidase. Lead also interferes with calcium-activated enzymes, calcium channels, and Ca^{2+}-ATPase. Lead has similarly multiple and diverse biochemical ill effects on cell metabolism. Sorting out these interactions and their relationship to the clinical syndromes is not a simple task, and there is even less basic information about other neurointoxicants.

Nevertheless, metals and biologic toxins have been used experimentally to analyze the pathogenesis of the neuropathies according to effects on axons, myelin, or Schwann cells.

Specific Clinical Syndromes of Metal Intoxication

Lead

Acute lead encephalopathy in children, attributed to pica or ingestion of flaking lead-containing paint, was first recognized in 1904: however, lead poisoning is among the oldest of occupational diseases and remains a common metal poisoning today. Although acute toxicity is rare, chronic toxicity can cause both central and peripheral effects, the former more common in children and the latter more in adults. Adults with chronic lead exposure yielding blood lead levels of 25 to 60 μg/dL may experience irritability, headache, and depressed mood, with signs of impaired visual-motor dexterity and reaction times. Overt effects—for example, weakness and atrophy of peripheral muscles with wristdrop—occur with long-term levels of 60 or more. Because of links between lead and cognitive dysfunction, behavioral problems, as well as stunted growth in children, the U.S. Centers for Disease Control acted in 1991 to define a childhood blood concentration of 10 μg/dL as a level of concern. Periodic screening of children aged 9 to 36 months is advocated, especially because nonspecific symptoms may emerge: lethargy, anorexia, intermittent abdominal pain with vomiting, or constipation. With blood levels above 80μg/dL, children seem more susceptible than adults to overt lead encephalopathy with delirium, ataxia, seizure, stupor, or coma with associated cerebral edema. In adults, the differential diagnosis includes a flulike viral illness that, like lead poisoning, may present with headache, myalgias, anorexia, nausea, and crampy abdominal pain. However, the symptom complex may evoke a wide differential including: various abdominal conditions, for example, renal colic; collagen-vascular disease; acute intermittent porphria; and others. Lead-induced encephalopathy may resemble acute infectious encephalopathy.

The whole blood lead concentration is the most reliable test because urinary lead levels increase and decrease more rapidly than blood levels in response to changes in lead exposure. The mean whole blood level in adults without exposure to occupational hazards is <5 μg/dL. Standard recommendations now consider levels safe up to 30 μg/dL; some consider a higher limit of 50 μg/dL safe. Workers are monitored closely if levels exceed 40 μg/dL. The upper limit of lead in urine is 150 μg/g creatinine. Peripheral neuropathy is usually accompanied by blood lead levels greater than 70 μg/dL.

Testing blood lead levels is recommended for children with presumed autism, attention deficit disorder, pervasive development disorder, mental retardation, or language problems. A diagnosis of lead intoxication is supported if blood zinc protoporphyrin exceeds 100 μg/dL or if urinary aminolevulinic acid excretion is >15 mg/L. With blood lead levels of 10 μg/dL, the activity of aminolevulinic acid dehydratase is low. At higher lead levels, the activities of coproporphyrinogen oxidase and ferrochetalase are also low. Anemia and basophilic stippling of erythrocytes are characteristic. Nerve conduction velocities are nonspecifically slow in lead and other neuropathies.

Treatment combines decontamination, supportive care, and the judicious use of chelating agents. In diseased individuals, chelation therapy commences with levels of 40 μg/dL. Supportive care may include treatment of increased intracranial pressure by standard use of intravenous mannitol and glucocorticoids, the latter because the pathophysiology of lead encephalopathy involves capillary leak. In patients with lead encephalopathy, calcium disodium edetate, or calcium ethylenediaminetetra-acetic acid (EDTA), should be administered at 30mg/kg every 24 hours. Some advocate initiating chelation with a single dose of dimercaprol (British anti-Lewisite or BAL), 4 to 5 mg/kg deep intramuscularly. Alternatively meso-2, 3-dimercaptosuccinic acid (DMSA or Succimer) is advocated for treatment of moderately severe chronic lead intoxication. Childhood lead exposure carries a risk of long-lasting health impairment, especially with neurocognitive and neurobehavioral sequelae, emphasizing the need for primary prevention and for obtaining occupational and environmental information.

Mercury

The relations between elemental, inorganic, and organic forms of mercury involve transformations from one form to another. Modern epidemics include the Minamata disease from fish contaminated by methyl mercury affecting 2,500 people in Japan; erethism in the hatting industry, which is also called.the "mad hatter" syndrome from mercuric nitrate. About 10,000 tons of mercury are mined per year with 2,000 to 3,000 tons from man-made and natural sources released into the atmosphere per year. Runoff into natural bodies of water occurs as mercury exposures persist. Acute toxicity from elemental mercury may include encephalopathy and seizures, whereas its chronic toxicity includes peripheral sensorimotor neuropathy, dysarthria, and parkinsonism. Subclinical nerve conduction and neuropsychiatric abnormalities have been documented in the modern workplace.

Toxicity from organic mercury differs between short- and long-chain compounds. Organic mercury includes methyl mercury (MeHg), the cause of Minamata disease, and ethyl mercury. Minamata disease produces neuropathologic abnormalities in the cerebral cortex, cerebellum, and peripheral nerves. The short-chain compounds readily enter the CNS. Symptoms of organic mercury toxicity include the following: tremor; ataxia; dysarthria; paresthesias of the hands, feet, and mouth; visual field constriction; erethism; and spasticity. Prenatal exposure to MeHg can cause severe congenital abnormalities such as micrognathia, microcephaly, mental retardation, blindness, and motor deficits. Excessive MeHg intake has been reported in fish-eating communities in Greenland, the Faroe Islands, the Seychelles, the Madeira Basin of the Amazon River, and New Zealand. Several observations indicate that the immature brain is highly susceptible to MeHg toxicity from prenatal maternal exposure.

The 24-hour urine mercury concentration may assess both recent exposure and elimination of tissue burden. The normal blood concentration is less than 10 to 20 μg/L, and the urinary level is less than 20 μg/L. Treatment consists of decontamination and chelation, with established guidelines. If the person is symptomatic, dimercaprol is given intramuscularly 3 to 5 mg/kg every 4 hours for day 1, every 12 hours on day 2, and then once a day for the next 3 days, followed by a 2-day interruption. Other agents are 2,3-dimercaptosuccinic acid and 2,3-dimercapto-propane-1-sulfonate, a water-soluble form of BAL. All agents are somewhat effective for organic and inorganic mercury poisoning.

Prevention of mercury intoxication requires monitoring in high-risk occupations, including dental offices, and correction of inadequate ventilation, avoiding vacuuming of spilled mercury, and removal of workers whose urinary level has increased fourfold or is >50 μg/L.Control of industrial pollution may require major efforts.

Arsenic

Acute arsenic poisoning is a multisystem disaster, with vomiting, bloody diarrhea, myoglobinuria, renal failure, arrhythmias, hypotension, seizures, coma, and death. In survivors, Mees lines on the fingernails and sensorimotor neuropathy appear in 7 to 14 days, sensory symptoms dominate, and weakness is more profound in the legs than in the arms and hands. Slow and incomplete recovery takes years. Nerve conduction velocities are typically slow. Cognition may be impaired in some survivors, depending on the severity of the acute encephalopathy.

Intoxication by inhalation may be acute or chronic. The chronic version is "blackfoot disease" with vascular changes, gangrene, and a less severe peripheral neuropathy. The use of arsenic trioxide to treat leukemia may be followed by arsenic neuropathy.

Arsenic toxicity is a global health problem. It is estimated that tens of millions of people, for example, in Bangladesh, are at risk of excessive arsenic levels from natural geologic sources leaching into aquifers, contaminated drinking water, from mining, and from other industrial processes. Although arsenicosis with resulting cancer in various sites is a major problem, encephalopathy and peripheral neuropathy are also reported. The neuropathy is primarily axonal with secondary demyelination.

The diagnosis of arsenic intoxication is confirmed by urinary levels >75 μg/dL. Hair analysis has been used but is not reliable.

BAL therapy is also used for acute arsenic poisoning. It is most effective before symptoms of neuropathy appear. BAL is considered more effective than penicillamine in treating the chronic neuropathy. Hemodialysis is another treatment for an acute episode.

Thallium

Despite the ban on manufacture of thallium rodenticides in the United States, accidental and suicidal exposures still occur because the poisons are available in other countries. Industrial exposure still occurs. The acute episode is dominated by gastrointestinal symptoms. Paresthesias may be noted soon afterward, but overt signs of neuropathy may take 2 weeks to appear. The encephalopathy may include cognitive impairment and choreoathetosis, myoclonus, or other involuntary movements. The unique clue to diagnosis is alopecia (loss of hair), which begins 1 to 3 weeks after exposure. Neuropathy and dermatitis may be prominent in chronic exposure.

After acute exposure, blood tests are not useful for detecting thallium because the metal is taken up by cells so rapidly that blood levels do not rise. Urinary thallium can be detected by atomic absorption spectrometry. Normal urinary values are 0.3 to 0.8 μg/L. Levels of 200 to 300 are seen in overt poisoning. A provocative test depends on potassium chloride (KCl) which is given orally in a dose of 45 mEq. Potassium displaces thallium from tissue stores, blood levels rise, and urinary content can be followed serially.

Aside from monitoring occupational exposure to thallium, an important preventive measure is protection of children against the ingestion of candylike pellets. Treatment of acute poisoning depends in part on enhancing urinary and fecal excretion of thallium by giving laxatives and using Prussian blue or activated charcoal to retard absorption. Urinary excretion is enhanced by forced diuresis and administration of KCl. Hemodialysis may be effective.

Manganese

George Cotzias, discoverer of the therapeutic value of levodopa in Parkinson disease (PD), followed an unusual path to that achievement. He was a biochemist interested in the role of metals in enzyme activity. Manganese was one such metal, and that took him to an outbreak of parkinsonism in South American miners. At about that time, Hornykewicz identified the lack of dopamine in the substantia nigra of patients with PD. Cotzias successfully pursued the treatment of PD.

Manganese intoxication, still a threat in industrial settings, reproduces the essential motor features of PD but with sufficient clinical and pathologic differences to indicate the conditions are not identical; for instance, exaggerated tendon reflexes and behavioral features occur early in manganese toxicity. The outlook is gloomy, including severe cognitive loss. Responses to levodopa and to chelation therapy are limited.

Aluminum

Dialysis dementia has been attributed to aluminum in the dialysis water and also in ingested phosphate binders used to control blood phosphorus levels. Treatment of the water and avoidance of the binders have decreased the incidence. Encephalopathy, however, has also occurred in uremic patients dialyzed with deionized water and also in some who took the binders without dialysis, implying that abnormal retention of aluminum is a characteristic of uremia.

Paresthesias and weakness were part of "potroom palsy," a complex syndrome in workers in a smelter who were exposed to pots that had not been vented properly. Other manifestations included ataxia, tremor, and memory loss.

Among discarded theories of the pathogenesis of Alzheimer disease is one that related aluminum accumulation in neurofibrillary tangles.

OTHER INTOXICATIONS

Pesticides: Organophosphates and Carbamates

Millions of agriculture workers and amateur gardeners are exposed to these substances. Also exposed are those engaged in their manufacture and those who use or store compounds designed for chemical warfare and/or terrorism. It is estimated that 150,000 to 300,000 people have pesticide-induced illness each year. Popular compounds include malathion, parathion, and others. Most are lipid soluble and readily absorbed after ingestion, inhalation, or application to the skin. They are powerful inhibitors of acetylcholinesterase.

Three clinical stages follow in sequence. First, *acute cholinergic crisis* comprises nicotinic effects (limb weakness, fasciculation, tachycardia) and muscarinic manifestations (miosis, lacrimation, salivation). CNS signs include ataxia, seizures, altered consciousness, and sometimes coma. Second, the *intermediate syndrome* appears 2 to 4 days after exposure. Weakness may be profound, affecting the proximal limbs, cranial muscles, neck flexors, and respiration. Tendon reflexes are lost. The differential diagnosis includes the Guillain-Barré syndrome, periodic paralysis, and myasthenia gravis. Among survivors, recovery may be slow but is the rule. Third, *organophosphate-induced delayed neuropathy* appears 1 to 5 weeks after exposure. The syndrome was first described during the period of Prohibition in the United States when illicit whiskey was made in home stills; 50,000 people consumed "Jamaica ginger" or "Ginger Jake" that was later found to contain triorthocresyl phosphate. Paresthesias and distal leg weakness appeared weeks later. Triorthocresyl phosphate is not an anticholinesterase, but the syndrome was then seen after exposure to cholinergic organophosphates. The disorder has been attributed to inhibition of "neuropathy target esterase," disruption of axonal transport, and a dying back neuropathy. Although paresthesias may be noted, the disorder is dominantly motor. Among survivors, upper motor neuron signs implicate the CNS, which, in combination with profound lower motor neuron signs, may simulate ALS except that there is no progression for years.

Exposure can be documented by levels of the drug or its metabolites in blood or urine. Measurement of red cell or plasma cholinesterase is an indirect marker. In electrodiagnostic studies, there may be a repetitive response to a single nerve stimulus.

The acute disorder is a medical emergency risking death from respiratory paralysis. If the patient has been splashed, clothing must be stripped and the skin washed thoroughly to prevent further absorption. Gastric lavage may be needed. Airway control and ventilation must be ensured and cardiac function monitored. Atropine is the best antidote. Subcutaneous doses of 0.5 to 1.0 mg are given every 15 minutes until an effect is observed in the form of dilated pupils, flushed face, dry mouth, and dry skin with cessation of sweating. To suppress airway secretions, some give intravenous doses up to 2 mg every hour. Glycopyrrolate can be added to atropine.

Oxime therapy is also recommended in seriously ill patients. These compounds reactivate acetylcholinesterase and should be given as soon as possible after exposure by continuous intravenous infusion.

Since 9/11/2001, there has been increasing concern about global terrorism, including the NBCs of nuclear (N), biologic (B), and chemical (C) agents. At least five groups of organophosphorous nerve agents are similar to, but more deadly than, agricultural organophosphate insecticides. Management of survivors of chemical terrorism will include decontamination; ventilation (high resistance airway); antidotes such as. atropine or pralidoxime chloride (phosphotriesterase pralidoxime-2-chloride or 2-PAM); diazepam (for seizures); and intravenous fluids, with other supportive therapy. Subsequently, physicians will manage brain damage caused by the agents or indirectly, for example, from hypoxia and metabolic sequelae. It will be important to separate victims suffering from hysteria or panic. For example, after the 1994 terrorist subway attack in Japan involving phosphonofluoridic acid (sarin), several hundred people were chemically damaged but 5,000 worried people came to health care facilities.

Other related groups of compounds are termed insecticides, including pyrethins, pyrethroids, organochlorines, and N,N diethyl-3-methybenzamide (DEET). All may cause unexplained seizures.

Volatile Organic Compounds (VOC)

Neurologic syndromes to VOCs, also called *solvents*, occur after either occupational or deliberate exposure by inhalation abuse. They include aromatic and aliphatic hydrocarbons, alcohols, esters, ketones, aliphatic nitrates, anesthetic agents, halogenated solvents, and propellants. Aromatic hydrocarbons, especially toluene, produce cerebral and cerebellar damage. Aliphatic hydrocarbons caused outbreaks of peripheral neuropathy in industrial or recreational exposures to *n*-hexane or methyl-*n*-butyl ketone. Paresthesias and weakness appear distally in the legs and only later are the hands affected. Acutely, the syndrome may resemble the Guillain-Barré syndrome, including slow conduction velocity. Alternatively, progression may be slow. Optic neuropathy is rare. The characteristic pathologic change is neurofilamentous axonal swelling and distal axonal degeneration. Effective measures have reduced industrial exposure and eliminated the agents from glues formerly used for sniffing.

Other organic compounds that induce axonal neuropathy by industrial exposure are acrylamide, carbon disulfide, methyl bromide, and triorthocresyl phosphate. Halogenated hydrocarbons are toxic for the CNS by damaging nerve cell membranes and altering neurotransmission; an excitatory phase is rapidly followed by CNS depression. The compounds include chloroform, methylene chloride, and tetrachloroethane. The neurotoxic potential of one substance is sometimes facilitated by others in the same commercial product.

Carbon Monoxide

Carbon monoxide (CO) intoxication is a common cause of neurotoxic damage and death. Deaths averaged 5,600 per year in a recent 10-year period in the United States with 2,700 of these accidental and the rest suicidal. Statistics on nonfatal CO encephalopathy and the delayed CO-induced neuropsychiatric syndrome are imprecise. Accidents are caused predominantly by poorly ventilated gasoline-powered heaters. Toxicity results from tissue hypoxia and direct damage to cellular structures. CO competes with oxygen for binding to hemoglobin. It binds to other proteins including myoglobin and cytochrome c oxidase.

Symptoms may be mild, simulating viral infection, or it may occur with another emergency, smoke inhalation. Nonspecific symptoms may comprise headache, malaise, dizziness, nausea, difficulty concentrating, and dyspnea. More severe exposures can lead to coma and death. In survivors, neurologic symptoms include dementia, cerebellar dysfunction, and parkinsonism. A delayed neuropsychiatric syndrome may follow acute exposure by 3 to 240 days, with cognitive and personality changes and psychotic behavior. This syndrome occurs in 10% to 30% of CO poisonings. Although up to 10% of victims show gross neurologic or psychiatric impairment, more frequent is subtle, persistent neuropsychiatic deficit. CT, MRI, MR spectroscopy, and isotopic imaging can disclose the brain damage. Postmortem findings include multifocal necrosis; myelinopathy with discrete globus pallidus and cortical lesions, and white matter lesions.

Hematologic diagnosis is made by finding high levels of carboxyhemoglobin (COHb). Normal levels are less than 5% in nonsmokers and can be as high as 12% in two-pack-per-day smokers. Although serious toxicity is often associated with levels >25%, neurologic damage is not always directly related to the COHb level. Furthermore, serum levels may have fallen by the time the patient reaches the emergency room such that a normal COHb level does not rule out CO poisoning. Blood taken at the scene by emergency technicians can be used. Measurement of CO in expired air and in the exposure area's ambient air can also be useful. The U.S. government standard for CO prohibits exposure to more than 35 ppm, averaged over an 8-hour workday.

Initial treatment is 100% oxygen by a nonrebreather face mask, which will reduce the elimination half-life of COHb from 4 to 5 hours to 1 to 2 hours. Treatment continues until the COHb levels are below 10%. Most experts advocate hyperbaric oxygen (HBO) for treatment of symptomatic CO poisoning. It enhances elimination of COHb, with an average half-life of 20 minutes at three atmo-

spheres. HBO therapy has been used with increasing frequency, but it is uncertain whether it hastens recovery or reduces the rate of late sequelae. Coma is a clear indication for hyperbaric therapy. Prevention is largely a matter of monitoring equipment such as gas heaters, monitoring workers, and providing public education about the hazards of running a motor vehicle in a closed space.

Nitrous Oxide Myelopathy (Layzer Syndrome)

In 1978, Layzer described 15 patients; 14 were dentists. Thirteen had abused nitrous oxide for 3 months to several years; two patients had been exposed only professionally, working in poorly ventilated offices. Symptoms included early paresthesias, Lhermitte symptoms, ataxia, leg weakness, impotence, and sphincter disturbances. Examination showed signs of sensorimotor polyneuropathy, often with signs implicating the posterior and lateral columns of the spinal cord in a pattern identical to that of subacute combined system disease owing to B_{12} deficiency. Electrodiagnostic tests showed axonal polyneuropathy; CSF examination and other laboratory tests gave normal results. The gas interferes with the action of B_{12}.

Additional cases were reported in abusers of nitrous oxide, and improvement was seen in weeks or months after exposure ceased. Another version of the disorder was seen in people who had hematologic evidence of B_{12} deficiency but were asymptomatic until the neurologic disorder was precipitated by nitrous oxide anesthesia for surgery. MRI shows a characteristic distribution of lesions in the spinal cord.

Scott et al. reproduced the syndrome by maintaining monkeys in an atmosphere of nitrous oxide. If the diet was supplemented with methionine, the disorder was prevented; but in controls, symptoms progressed to a moribund state; the spinal cord and peripheral nerves of the unsupplemented monkeys showed changes of combined degeneration. Inability to resynthesize methionine from homocysteine seemed responsible, and the primary neurologic lesion in human pernicious anemia may also be impaired synthesis of methionine.

Plant and Animal Poisons

Ciguatera poisoning or the *marine neurotoxic syndrome* is the most common nonbacterial form of food poisoning in the United States and Canada. It is caused by eating tropical reef fish that contain several toxins in edible parts; the toxins are thought to arise in dinoflagellates. It is endemic in subtropical regions. Food shipped to other parts of the world spreads the disease. The acute symptoms are gastrointestinal followed by sensory symptoms, paresthesias, and pruritus. *Sensory inversion* describes the peculiarity that cold feels hot and vice versa. Myalgia, fasciculations, areflexia, trismus, and carpopedal spasm may be noted. Respiratory failure is exceptional. Other systems may be involved prominently, including pain on sexual activity.

None of the physical findings is diagnostic, and there are no formal criteria for diagnosis. Most associated toxins open sodium channels, but at least one affects calcium channels. Peripheral nerve conduction velocities are often slow. Bioassays for the ciguatoxins or immunochemical methods are being developed, but none has yet achieved approval by consensus. Treatment is symptomatic.

Shellfish poisoning can result from contamination of mollusks by saxitoxin, which blocks sodium channels. The symptoms are similar to ciguatera but more severe, and respiratory depression is a threat. In the series of De Carvalho et al., cerebellar ataxia was the dominant finding and peripheral nerve conduction was normal. Recovery was rapid in those patients, but among those described by Gessner et al., 3 of 11 patients were treated with mechanical ventilation and one died. Hypertension was also prominent. Binding assays and liquid chromatography identified the toxin in serum and urine. In Japan, the agent of puffer fish poisoning is tetrodotoxin. Treatment of these conditions is symptomatic.

In 1987, an outbreak of severe encephalopathy was traced to ingestion of mussels, and the offending toxin was identified as domoic acid, a glutamate receptor agonist. Other epidemics led to the term *amnesic shellfish poison*.

Many plants contain pharmacologically active substances that cross the blood-brain barrier with resulting delirium, hallucinations, seizures, and sedation. Cicutoxin, a stimulant, from water hemlock may be ingested after mistakenly identifying it as wild carrot or sweet potato. Sedation may follow stimulation. Others, such as andromedotoxin from rhododendron, are depressants. In 1998, 122,578 plant exposures were reported to the American Association of Poison Control Toxic Exposure Surveillance System.

Neurolathyrism is a neurotoxic disease that has caused spastic parparesis in impoverished countries; it is linked to heavy continuous consumption of *Lathyrus* during times of drought or flood. It contains the excitatory amino acid glutamate analog β-oxalylamino-L-alanine (BOAA) which is the major candidate toxin. A similar neurologic picture is attributed to prolonged consumption of the bitter cassava, *Manihot esculenta*. A disease called konzo became prevalent in sub-Saharan Africa when the cassava root was used in times of drought where local prevalence as high as 30 per 1,000 was reported in 1990. Cassava contains a cyanoglucoside linamarin, which is enzymatically converted to cyanide, which then damages neural calls. The clinical picture is a sudden, symmetric, and permanent spastic paraplegia. As in lathyrism, males are predominately affected. Hearing loss, visual impairment, and dysarthria sometimes occur in cassavaism but are not seen in neurolathyrism. Based on epidemiogic criteria, the ALS–parkinsonism–dementia complex in the Western Pacific is an example of environmentally induced neurodegeneration. Some studies linked the use of the neurotoxic seed or seed kernel of *Cycas* spp. and the appearance of the ALS/PD/dementia complex.

Methanol (Methyl Alcohol)

Methanol intoxication is seen in drinkers who take it as a substitute for ethanol. Acute poisoning was dominated by gastrointestinal symptoms, drunkenness, and coma. Severe acidosis results from the conversion of methanol to formaldehyde and formic acid. Viscera and brain show petechial hemorrhages and edema. In the series of Liu et al., the mortality rate was 36%. Coma, seizures, and high methanol concentrations were predictors of poor prognosis. Exposure to large amounts is fatal within 72 hours. Brain CT and MRI may demonstrate signs of diffuse and multifocal damage. Visual loss is attributed to retinal metabolism of methanol (rather than an action of circulating formic acid) because the local oxidation of methanol to formic acid parallels the depletion of retinal adenosine 5′-triphosphate (ATP). Retinal glial cells may be the first target. It has therefore been suggested that inhibitors of aldehyde dehydrogenase could be therapeutic; here it would mean the administration of ethanol to block the first step of the toxic metabolic pathway. For similar reasons, administration of ethanol blocks the metabolism of methanol in the liver, and unchanged toxin is excreted in the urine. 4-Methylpyrazole (fomepizole) has also been used for this purpose. Correction of acidosis and hemodialysis may be used.

Obsolete Epidemics

Many syndromes described here could be eliminated if care were taken to protect the environment. In fact, some epidemics pointed the way to correction. For instance, the outbreak of *subacute myelo-optic neuropathy* was attributed to an oral antiparasitic agent, clioquinol. The resulting peripheral neuropathy and blindness affected an estimated 10,000 people in Japan. The practice has ceased, and there have been no new cases; investigations indicate that the drug is converted to a potent mitochondrial toxin. Another transient outbreak was the *eosinophilia-myalgia syndrome*, which involved skin, muscle, lungs, and blood vessels and axonal neuropathy. The disorder was attributed to a toxic contaminant in the preparation of tryptophan, which was taken as a health supplement. That syndrome has also largely disappeared, but it seems likely that new epidemics will appear as new industries and new health fads arise.

SUGGESTED READINGS

General

Anderson HR, Nielsen JB, Grandjean P. Toxicologic evidence of developmental neurotoxicity of environmental chemicals. *Toxicology* 2000;144(Apr 3):121–127.

Candura SM, Manzo L, Costa LC. Role of occupational neurotoxicants in psychiatric and neurodegenerative disorders. In: Costa LG, Manzo L, eds. *Occupational Neurotoxicology*. Boca Raton, FL: CRC Press, 1998.

Costa LG, Manzo L. *Occupational Neurotoxicology*. Boca Raton, FL: CRC Press, 1998.

Feldman RG. *Occupational and Environmental Neurology*. Philadelphia: Lippincott-Raven, 1999.

Ford MD, Delaney KA, Ling LS, et al. *Clinical Toxicology*. Philadelphia: WB Saunders, 2001.

Goldfrank LR, Flomenbaum NE, Lewin NA, et al. *Goldfrank's Toxicologic Emergencies*. Stamford, CT: Appleton & Lange, 1998.

Greenburg MI, Hamilton R, Phillips SD, et al. *Occupational, Industrial, and Environmental Toxicology*. Philadelphia: Mosby, 2003.

Kales SN, Christiani DC. Current concepts: acute chemical emergencies. *N Engl J Med* 2004;350:800–808.

Prockop LD. Neuroimaging in neurotoxicology. In: Chang LW, Slikker W Sr, eds. *Neurotoxicology Approaches and Methods*. New York: Academic Press, 1995.

Slikker W, Chang W, eds. *Handbook of Developmental Neurotoxicology*. New York: Academic Press, 1998.

Spencer PS, Schaumburg HH, Ludolph A. *Experimental and Clinical Neurotoxicology*. 2nd Ed. New York: Oxford University Press, 1999.

Weiss B. Vulnerability of children and the developing brain to neurotoxic hazards. *Environ Health Perspect* 2000;108(Suppl 3):375–381.

Weiss B, O Donaghue J. *Neurobehavioral Toxicity. Analysis and Intervention*. New York: Raven, 1994.

Aluminum

Alfrey AC, Le Gendre GR, Kaehny WD. The dialysis encephalopathy syndrome: possible aluminum intoxication. *N Engl J Med* 1976;294:184–188.

Cannata JB, Briggs JD, Junor BJR, et al. Aluminum hydroxide intake: real risk of aluminum toxicity. *Br Med J* 1983;286:1937–1938.

Garruto RM, Strong MJ, Yanagihara R. Experimental models of aluminum-induced motor neuron degeneration. *Adv Neurol* 1991;56:327–340.

Longstreth WT Jr, Rosenstock L, Heyer NJ. Potroom palsy?. Neurologic disorders in three aluminum smelter workers. *Arch Intern Med* 1985;145:1972–1975.

Nayak P. Aluminum: impacts and disease. *Eviron Res* 2002;89(Jun):101–115.

Shirabe T, Irie K, Uchida M. Autopsy case of aluminum encephalopathy. *Neuropathology* 2002;22(Sep):206–210.

White DM, Longstreth WT Jr, Rosenstock L, et al. Neurologic syndrome in 25 workers from an aluminum smelting plant. *Arch Intern Med* 1992;152:1443–1448.

Arsenic

Aposhian HV. DMSA and DMPS—water soluble antidotes for heavy metal poisoning. *Annu Rev Pharmacol Toxicol* 1983;23:193–215.

Beckett WS, Moore JL, Keogh JP, et al. Acute encephalopathy due to occupational exposure to arsenic. *Br J Ind Med* 1986;43:66–67.

Gerhardt RE, Crecelius EA, Hudson JB. Moonshine-related arsenic poisoning. *Arch Intern Med* 1980;140:211–213.

Hall AH. Chronic arsenic poisoning. *Toxicol Lett* 2003;128(Mar 10):69–72.

Huang SY, Chang CS, Tang JL, et al. Acute and chronic arsenic poisoning associated with treatment of acute promyelocytic leukemia. *Br J Haematol* 1998;103:1092–1095.

Khan MM, Sakauchi F, Sonoda T, et al. Magnitude of arsenic toxicity in tube-well drinking water in Bangladesh and its adverse effects on human health including cancer: evidence from a review of the literature. *Asian Pac J Cancer Prev* 2003;4(Jan-Mar):7–14.

Ng JC, Wang J, Shraim A. A global health problem caused by arsenic from natural sources. *Chemosphere* 2003;52:1353–1359.

Quecedo E, Samartin O, Ferber MI, et al. Mees lines: a clue for the diagnosis of arsenic poisoning [Letter]. *Arch Dermatol* 1996;132:349–350.

Ratnaike RN. Acute and chronic arsenic toxicity. *Postgrad Med J* 2003;79:391–396.

Lead

Boothby JA, deJesus PV, Rowland LP. Reversible forms of motor neuron disease—lead "neuritis." *Arch Neurol* 1974;31:18–23.

Counter SA, Ortego F, Shannon MW, et al. Succimer (meso-2, 3-dimercaptosuccinic acid (DMSA) treatment of Andean children with environmental lead exposure. *Int J Occup Environ Health* 2003;9(Apr-Jun):164–168.

Davoli CT. *Childhood Lead Poisoning*. Neurobase. La Jolla, CA: Arbor, 1999.

Emory E, Pattillo R, Archibold E, et al. Neurobehavioral effects of low-level lead exposure in human neonates. *Am J Obstet Gynecol* 1999;181(Jul):S2–11.

Kosnett MJ. Lead. In: Ford MD, Delaney KA, Ling LJ, et al., eds. *Clinical Toxicology*. Philadelphia: WB Saunders, 2001:723–736.

Lidsky TI, Schneider JS. Lead neurotoxicity in children: basic mechanisms and clinical correlates. *Brain* 2003;126(Pt 1):5–19.

Marchetti C. Molecular targets of lead in brain neurotoxicity. *Neurotox Res* 2003;5(3):221–236.

Pinkle JL, Brody DJ, Gunter EW, et al. The decline in blood lead levels in the United States. *JAMA* 1994;272:284–291.

Porru S, Alessio L. The use of chelating agents in occupational lead poisoning. *Occup Med* 1996;46:41–48.

Reith DM, O'Regan P, Bailey C, et al. Serious lead poisoning in childhood: still a problem after a century. *J Paediatr Child Health* 2003;39:623–626.

Ryan D, Levy B, Pollack S, et al. Protecting children from lead poisoning and building healthy communities. *Am J Public Health* 1999;89:822–827.

Staudinger KC, Roth VS. Occupational lead poisoning. *Am Fam Physician* 1998;57:719–726, 731–732.

Warren MJ, Cooper JB, Wood SP, et al. Lead poisoning, haem synthesis, and 5-aminolevulinic acid dehydratase. *Trends Biochem Sci* 1998;23:217–221.

Manganese

Aschner M, Aschner JL. Manganese neurotoxicity: cellular effects and blood-brain barrier transport. *Neurosci Behav Rev* 1991;15:333–340.

Chandra SV. Psychiatric illness due to manganese poisoning. *Acta Psychiatr Scand* 1983;303(Suppl):49–54.

Huang C, Chu NS, Lu CS, et al. Long-term progression in chronic manganism: 10 years of follow-up. *Neurology* 1998;50:698–700.

Huang CC, Weng YH, Lu CS, et al. Dopamine transporter binding in chronic manganese intoxication. *J Neurol* 2003;250:1335–1339.

Myers JE, teWaterNaude J, Fourie M, et al. Nervous system effects of occupational manganese exposure on South African manganese mine workers. *Neurotoxicology* 2003;24:649–656.

Schuler P, Oyanguren H, Maturana V, et al. Manganese poisoning. Environmental and medical study at a Chilean mine. *Ind Med Surg* 1957;26:167–173.

Mercury

Adams CR, Ziegler DK, Lin JT. Mercury intoxication simulating amyotrophic lateral sclerosis. *JAMA* 1983;250:642–643.

Albers JW, Kallenbach LR, Fine LJ, et al. Neurologic abnormalities and remote occupational elemental mercury exposure. *Ann Neurol* 1988;24:651–659.

Castoldi AF, Barni S, Turin I, et al. Early acute necrosis, delayed apoptosis and cystoskeletal breakdown in cultured cerebellar granule neurons exposed to methylmercury. *J Neurosci Res* 2000;59:775–787.

Castoldi AF, Coccini T, Manzo L. Neurotoxic and molecular effects of methylmercury in humans. *Rev Environ Health* 2003;18(Jan–Mar): 19–31.

Chiang WK. Mercury. In: Ford MD, Delaney KA, Ling LJ, et al., eds. *Clinical Toxicology*. Philadelphia: WB Saunders, 2001:737–743.

Coccini T, Randine G, Candura SM, et al. Low-level exposure to methylmercury modifies muscarinic cholinergic receptor binding characteristics in rat brain and lymphocytes: physiologic implications and new opportunities in biologic monitoring. *Environ Health Perspect* 2000;108(Jan):29–33.

Eto K. Minamata disease. *Neuropathology* 2000;20(Suppl):S14–17.

Gochfeld M. Cases of mercury exposure, bioavailability, and absorption. *Ecotoxicol Environ Saf* 2003;56(Sep)174–179.

Haley RW, Hom J, Roland PS, et al. Evaluation of neurologic function in Gulf War veterans: a blinded case-control study. *JAMA* 1997;277:259–261.

Hay WJ, Rickards AG, McMenemey WH, et al. Organic mercurial encephalopathy. *J Neurol Neurosurg Psychiatry* 1963;26:199–202.

Kurland LT, Faro SN, Siedler H. Minamata disease. *World Neurol* 1960;1: 370–390.

UNEP Global Mercury Assessment. Retrieved 03/03/2003 from http://www.chem.unep.ch/mercury/report/summaryofthereport.htm.

Thallium

Bank WJ, Pleasure DE, Suzuki K, et al. Thallium poisoning. *Arch Neurol* 1972;26:456–464.

Misra UK, Kalita J, Yadav RK, et al. Thallium poisoning: emphasis on early diagnosis and response to haemodialysis. *Postgrad Med J* 2003;79:103–105.

Nordentoft T, Andersen EB, Mogensen PH. Initial sensorimotor and delayed autonomic neuropathy in acute thallium poisoning. *Neurotoxicology* 1998;19:421–426.

Passarge C, Wieck HH. Thallium polyneuritis. *Fortschr Neurol Psychiatr* 1965;33:477–557.

Rambar AC. Acute thallium poisoning. *JAMA* 1932;98:1372–1373.

Rusyniak DE, Furbee RB, Kirk MA. Thalium and arsenic poisoning in a small midwestern town. *Ann Emerg Med* 2002;39(Mar):307–11.

Shabalina LP, Spiridonova VS. Thallium as an industrial poison (review of literature). *J Hyg Epidemiol Microbiol Immunol* 1979;23:247–255.

Methyl Alcohol

Bennet IL Jr, Cary FM, Mitchell GL, et al. Acute methyl alcohol poisoning: a review based on experience in an outbreak of 323 cases. *Medicine (Baltimore)* 1953;32:431–463.

Burns MJ, Graudins A, Aaron CK, et al. Treatment of methanol poisoning with intravenous 4-methylpyrazole. *Ann Emerg Med* 1997;30:829–832.

Harrop GA Jr, Benedict EM. Acute methyl alcohol poisoning associated with acidosis. *JAMA* 1920;74:25–27.

Liu JJ, Daya MR, Carrasquillo O, et al. Prognostic factors in patients with methanol intoxication. *J Toxicol Clin Toxicol* 1998;36:175–181.

Server A, Hovda KE, Nakstad PH, et al. Conventional and diffusion-weighted MRI in the evaluation of methanol poisoning. *Acta Radiol* 2003;44:691–695.

Volatile Organic Compounds (Solvents)

Allen N, Mendell JR, Billmaier DJ, et al. Toxic polyneuropathy due to methyl n-butyl ketone. *Arch Neurol* 1975;32:209–218.

Griffin JW. *Hexacarbon Neuropathy. Neurobase*. La Jolla, CA: Arbor, 1999.

Juntunen J, Matikainen E, Antti-Poika M, et al. Nervous system effects of long-term occupational exposure to toluene. *Acta Neurol Scand* 1985;72:512–517.

Kamran S, Bakshi R. MRI in chronic toluene abuse: low signal in the cerebral cortex on T2-weighted images. *Neuroradiology* 1998; 40(Aug):519–521.

Prockop LD, Alt M, Tison J. Huffer's neuropathy. *JAMA* 1974;229:1083–1084.

Ramon MF, Ballesteros S, Martinez-Arrieta R, et al. Volatile substance and other drug inhalation in Spain. *J Toxicol Clin Toxicol* 2003; 41:931–936.

Schaumberg HH, Spencer PS. Clinical and experimental studies of distal axonopathy—a frequent form of brain and nerve damage produced by environmental chemical hazards. *Ann N Y Acad Sci* 1979;329: 14–29.

Struwe G. Psychiatric and neurological symptoms in workers occupationally exposed to organic solvents—results of a differential epidemiological study. *Acta Psychiatr Scand* 1983;303(Suppl):100–104.

Organophosphate Insecticides

Aaron C. Organophosphates and carbamate. In: Ford MD, Delaney KA, Ling LJ, et al., eds. *Clinical Toxicology*. Philadelphia: WB Saunders, 2001.

Choi PT, Quinonez LG, Cook DJ, et al. The use of glycopyrrolate in a case of intermediate syndrome following acute organophosphate poisoning. *Can J Anesth* 1998;45:337–340.

Crinnion WJ. Environmental medicine, part 4: pesticides - biologically persistent and ubiquitous toxins. *Altern Med Rev* 2000;5(Oct): 432–47.

De Bleeker J. The intermediate syndrome in organophosphate poisoning: an overview of experimental and clinical observations. *Clin Toxicol* 1995;33:683–686.

de Jager AEJ, van Weerden TW, Houthoff HJ, et al. Polyneuropathy after massive exposure to parathion. *Neurology* 1981;31:603–605.

Di Monte DA. The environment and Parkinson's Disease: is the nigrostriatal system preferentially targeted by neurotoxins?. *Lancet Neurol* 2003;2:531–538.

Ecobichon DJ, Joy RM. *Pesticides and Neurological Diseases*. 2nd Ed. Boca Raton, FL: CRC Press, 1994.

Eriksson P, Talts U. Neonatal exposure to neurotoxic pesticides increases adult susceptibility: a review of current findings. *Neurotoxicology* 2000;21(Feb-Apr):37–47.

Landrigan P. Illness in Gulf War veterans. *JAMA* 1997;277:238–245.

Lotti M, Moretto A, Zoppelari R, et al. Inhibition of lymphocytic neuropathy target esterase predicts the development of organophosphate-induced delayed polyneuropathy. *Arch Toxicol* 1986;59:176–179.

Moretto A, Lotti M. Poisoning by organophosphorus insecticides and sensory neuropathy. *J Neurol Neurosurg Psychiatry* 1998;64:463–468.

Morgan JP, Penovich P. Jamaica ginger paralysis. 47-year follow-up. *Arch Neurol* 1978;35:530–532.

Ohbu S, Yamashina A, Takasu N, et al. Sarin poisoning in Tokyo subway. *South Med J* 1997;90(Jun):587–593.

Salem H. Issues in chemical and biological terrorism. *Intl J Toxicol* 2003;22(Nov-Dec):465–471.

Singh G, Mahajan R, Whig J. The importance of electrodiagnostic studies in acute organophosphate poisoning. *J Neurol Sci* 1998;157:191–200.

Steenland K, Jenkins B, Ames RG, et al. Chronic neurologic sequelae to organophosphate pesticide poisoning. *Am J Public Health* 1994;84: 731–736.

Teke E, Sungurtekin H, Sahiner T, et al. Organophosphate poisoning case with atypical clinical survey and magnetic resonance imaging findings. *J Neurol Neurosurg Psychiatry* 2004;75:936–937.

Thiermann H, Mast U, Klimmeck R, et al. Cholinesterase status, pharmacokinetics, and laboratory findings during obidoxime therapy in organophosphate poisoned patients. *Hum Exp Toxicol* 1997;16:473–480.

Tush GM, Anstead MI. Pralidoxime continuous infusion in the treatment of organophosphorus poisoning. *Ann Pharmacother* 1997;31:441–444.

Wadia RS, Chitra S, Amin RB, et al. Neurological manifestations of organophosphate insecticide poisoning. *J Neurol Neurosurg Psychiatry* 1987;50:1442–1448.

Carbon Monoxide

Abelsohn A, Sanborn MD, Jessiman BJ, et al. Identifying and managing adverse environmental health effects: 6. Carbon monoxide poisoning. *CMAJ* 2002;166:1685–1690.

Choi, IS. Delayed neurologic sequelae in carbon monoxide intoxication. *Arch Neurol* 1983;40(Jul):433–435.

Chu K, Jung KH, Kim HJ, et al. Diffusion-weighted MRI and 99mTc-HMPAO SPECT in delayed relapsing type of carbon monoxide poisoning: evidence of delayed cytotoxic edema. *Eur Neurol* 2004;51(2):98–103.

Ernst A, Zibrak JD. Carbon monoxide poisoning. *N Engl J Med* 1998;339:1603–1608.

Kim JH, Chang KH, Song IC, et al. Delayed encephalopathy of acute carbon monoxide intoxication: diffusivity of cerebral white matter lesions. *AJNR* 2003;24:1592–1597.

Lapresle J, Fardeau M. The central nervous system and carbon monoxide poisoning. II. Anatomical study of brain lesions following intoxication with carbon monoxide (22 cases). *Prog Brain Res* 1967;24:31–74.

Parkinson RB, Hopkins RO, Cleavinger HB, et al. White matter hyperintensities and neuropsychological outcome following carbon monoxide poisoning. *Neurology* 2002;58:1525–1532.

Prockop LD, Naidu K. Brain CT and MRI findings after carbon monoxide toxicity. *J Neuroimag* 1999;9:175–181.

Plant and Animal Poisons

Awada A, Kojan S. Neurological disorders and travel. *Intern J Antimicrobl Agents* 2003;21(Feb):189–192.

Clancy C, Klein schwarz W. Plants: central nervous system toxicity. In: Ford MD, Delaney KA, Ling LJ, et al., eds. *Clinical Toxicology.* Philadelphia: WB Saunders, 2001:909–921.

DeCarvalho M, Jacinto J, Ramos N, et al. Paralytic shellfish poisoning. Clinical and electrophysiological observations. *J Neurol* 1998;2245:551–554.

deHaro L, Pommier P, Valli M. Emergence of imported ciguatera in Europe: report of 18 cases at the Poison Control Centre of Marseille. *J Toxicol Clin Toxicol* 2003;41:927–30.

Gessner BD, Bell P, Doucette GJ, et al. Hypertension and identification of toxin in human urine and serum following a cluster of mussel-associated paralytic shellfish poisoning outbreaks. *Toxicol* 1997;35:711–722.

Getahun H, Lambien F, Vanhoorne M, et al. Food-aid cereals to reduce neurolathyrism related to grass-pea preparations during famine. *Lancet* 2003;362:1775–1776.

Howlett WP, Brubaker GR, Mlingi N, et al. Konzo, an epidemic upper motor neuron disease studied in Tanzania. *Brain* 1990;113(Pt 1):223–235.

Jeffery B, Barlow T, Moizer K, et al. Amnesic shellfish poison. *Food & Chem Toxicol* 2004;42(Apr):545–557.

Perkins RA, Morgan SS. Poisoning, envenomation, and trauma from marine creatures. *Am Fam Phys* 2004;69:885–890.

Ravindranath V. Neurolathyrism: mitochondrial dysfunction in excitotoxicity mediated by L-beta-oxalyl aminoalanine. *Neurochem Int* 2002;40(May):505–509.

Rosling H. Cassava associated neurotoxicity in Africa. In: Volans GN, Smis J, Sullivan FM, et al., eds. *Basic Science of Toxicology.* London: Taylor and Frames, 1990:605–614.

Shaw CA, Wilson JM. Analysis of neurological disease in four dimensions: insight from ALS-PDC epidemiology and animal models. *Neurosci Biobehav Rev* 2003;27(Oct):493–505.

Spencer PS, Schaumberg HH. Lathyrism: a neurotoxic disease. *Neurobehav Toxicol Teratol* 1983;5:625–629.

Sreeja VG, Nagahara N, Li Q, et al. New aspects in pathogenesis of Konzo: neural cell damage directly caused by linamarin contained in cassava. (Manihot esculenta Crantz). *Br J Nutr* 2003;90(Aug):467–472.

Teitelbaum JS, Zatorre RJ, Carpenter S, et al. Neurologic sequelae of domoic acid intoxication due to the ingestion of contaminated mussels. *N Engl J Med* 1990;322:1781–1787.

Yasumoto T, Satake M. Chemistry, etiology and determination methods of ciguatera toxins. *Annu Rev Pharmacol Toxicol* 1988;28:141–161.

Nitrous Oxide

Beltramello A, Puppini G, Cerini R, et al. Subacute combined degeneration of the spinal cord after nitrous oxide anaesthesia: role of magnetic resonance imaging. *J Neurol Neurosurg Psychiatry* 1998;64:563–564.

Flippo TS, Holder WD Jr. Neurologic degeneration associated with nitrous oxide anesthesia in patients with vitamin B_{12} deficiency. *Arch Surg* 1993;128:1391–1395.

Gutmann L, Farrell B, Crosby TW, et al. Nitrous oxide-induced myelopathy-neuropathy: potential for chronic misuse by dentists. *J Am Dent Assoc* 1979;98:58–59.

Hadzic A, Glab K, Sanborn KV, et al. Severe neurologic deficit after nitrous oxide anesthesia. *Anesthesiology* 1995;83:863–866.

Layzer RB. Myeloneuropathy after prolonged exposure to nitrous oxide. *Lancet* 1978;2:1227–1230.

Scott JM, Dinn JJ, Wilson P, et al. Pathogenesis of subacute combined degeneration: a result of methyl group deficiency. *Lancet* 1981;2:334–337.

Obsolete Epidemics

Anonymous. Eosinophilia-Myalgia Syndrome: Review and Reappraisal of Clinical, Epidemiologic and Animal Studies Symposium. *J Rheumatol Suppl* 1996;46:1–110.

Arbiser JL, Kraeft SK, van Leeuwen R, et al. Clioquinol-zinc chelate: a candidate causative agent of subacute myelo-optic neuropathy. *Mol Med* 1998;4:665–670.

Burns SM, Lange DJ, Jaffe IA, et al. Axonal neuropathy in eosinophilia-myalgia syndrome. *Muscle Nerve* 1994;17:293–298.

Emslie-Smith AM, Mayeno AN, Nakano S, et al. 1,1-Ethylidenebis-[tryptophan] induces pathologic alterations in muscle similar to those observed in the eosinophilia-myalgia syndrome. *Neurology* 1994;44:2390–2392.

Martin RW, Duffy J, Engel AG, et al. The clinical spectrum of the eosinophilic-myalgia syndrome associated with L-tryptophan ingestion. *Ann Intern Med* 1990;113:124–134.

Chapter 168

▶ # HIV, Fetal Alcohol and Drug Effects, and the Battered Child

Claudia A. Chiriboga

PEDIATRIC AIDS AND HIV INFECTION

Women and children are the fastest-growing population affected by AIDS and HIV. Most children with AIDS in the United States are infected perinatally. In inner cities, about 2% to 4% of live births are HIV-1 antibody positive. Intravenous drug abuse and sexual contact with HIV-infected partners are the maternal risk factors in >85% of perinatal cases. Most infections occur during the last trimester of pregnancy and time of delivery. Risk factors for vertical transmission are recent maternal HIV seroconversion, high viral load, and maternal AIDS. Premature infants are also at increased risk of infection. Infection may result from exposure to blood and other body fluids at delivery or transmitted in breast milk. Mother-to-child HIV transmission rates range from 14% to 30%; rates decrease to 8% with prenatal and neonatal zidovudine treatment.

Determination of HIV infection in children is complicated because maternal HIV antibody transfers across the placenta and may persist up to age 18 months. HIV-seropositive children are considered HIV infected if they test positive for HIV on two separate occasions by either HIV culture or HIV polymerase chain reaction (PCR) or if they develop AIDS. HIV-seropositive children who do not meet these criteria are considered perinatally exposed, and HIV-seropositive children without AIDS and without laboratory evidence of infection who on testing after age 6 months have negative antibody are seroreverters. The 1994 revised classification system for HIV infection in children has four clinical categories: N, not symptomatic; A, mildly symptomatic; B, moderately symptomatic; and C, severely symptomatic, which includes all AIDS-defining conditions except lymphoid hyperplasia. These clinical categories are further classified immunologically depending on the child's age and absolute CD4 count: no evidence of suppression (>25% of total lymphocytes), moderate suppression (24%–15%), and severe suppression (<15%; Table 168.1). For example, A2 indicates mild signs and symptoms of infection with moderate immunosuppression.

Diagnostic Tests

Because of early testing, most HIV-positive children are identified soon after birth. Viral load (i.e., quantified HIV DNA or RNA PCR) is more sensitive than viral cultures or p24 antigen in identifying HIV infection in asymptomatic newborns and infants. By age 4 to 6 months, >95% of HIV-infected children are identified by a positive PCR. In newborns, a negative PCR test for HIV does not exclude infection, but decreases the risk of HIV infection to 3%. Viral load runs higher in asymptomatic children than in asymptomatic adults. Sustained high viral load in adults predicts progression to AIDS. High viral loads in early infancy predict early onset of symptomatic HIV disease. HIV-1 syncytial-inducing phenotypes are linked to aggressive early symptomatic disease.

Clinical Manifestations

Mild HIV infection includes diarrhea, unexplained persistent fever, lymphadenopathy, and parotitis. Lymphoid interstitial pneumonitis and recurrent bacterial infections are seen in children with AIDS but not in adults. Prior to the advent of antiretroviral therapy, severe manifestations in early infancy, such as progressive encephalopathy or opportunistic infections (e.g., *Pneumocystis carinii*), carried a poor prognosis for survival, but with effective antiretroviral therapy, these disorders are compatible with survival to adulthood.

Mechanism of Action

HIV infection is maintained by viral persistence in helper T lymphocytes and macrophages. HIV strains with tropism for monocyte-derived macrophages have a predilection to infect cerebral vascular endothelium and CNS. Infected macrophages traverse the blood-brain barrier and infect microglial cells; neurons are spared from direct infestation. Nonproductive infection of astrocytes is reported, but infection of other glial cells has not been firmly established. Neuronal dropout is seen as the disease advances, but it is not known how HIV induces neural damage. Postulated mechanisms include release of soluble neurotoxins by HIV-infected macrophages and lymphocytes (e.g., cytokines, quinolinic acid, viral antigens, or undefined viral products), neurotoxin amplification by astrocyte–macrophage interaction, and impaired blood-brain barrier function secondary to HIV-related endothelial damage. These neurotoxins are thought to produce a reversible metabolic encephalopathy that may disappear with effective antiretroviral treatment. Children

▶ **TABLE 168.1**   Immunologic Categories Based on Child's Age-Specific CD4+ T Lymphocyte Count and Percent of Total Lymphocytes

Immunologic Category	< 12 Months		1–5 Years		8–12 Years	
	μl	(%)	μl	(%)	μl	(%)
1. No evidence of suppression	>1500	(>25)	>1000	(>25)	>500	(>25)
2. Moderate suppression	750–1499	(15–24)	500–999	(15–24)	200–499	(15–24)
3. Severe suppression	<750	(<15)	<500	(<15)	<200	(<15)

Adapted from 1994 Revised classification system for human immunodeficiency virus (HIV) infection in children less than 13 years of age. *MMWR Morb Mortal Wkly Rep* 1994;43:RR12.

with HIV encephalopathy who respond to antiretroviral therapy may show nonprogressive corticospinal tract sequelae.

Pathology

Glial nodules and endothelial hyperplasia with calcification, dystrophic calcification, and perivascular mononuclear inflammation are common pathologic findings of subacute encephalitis in HIV-infected brains. The glial nodule comprises a cluster of chronic inflammatory cells in the neurophil and is often associated with multinucleated giant cells that are presumed to arise from coalescent microglia.

HIV Encephalopathy

Two types of encephalopathy are seen in children: progressive and static. The evolution of the progressive encephalopathy may be fulminant, inexorably progressive, or stepwise. Progressive encephalopathy is characterized by loss of developmental milestones, progressive pyramidal tract dysfunction, and acquired microcephaly or impaired brain growth. The static encephalopathy is less well defined, and not all cases may be HIV induced.

The neurologic abnormalities commonly include abnormalities of muscle tone, hyperreflexia, clonus, and impaired head growth. Hypotonia with corticospinal tract dysfunction may be seen in infants early in the course of the encephalopathy and evolves into a spastic diparesis; with newer antiretroviral treatments, progression to a spastic tetraparesis, with or without pseudobulbar palsy, is seldom seen. Ataxia and rigidity are uncommon. Progressive neurologic dysfunction is the first evidence of progression to AIDS in 10% of infected children. There is always evidence of underlying HIV infection, such as immunologic compromise (low CD4 counts) or high viral load, at the time of onset of neurologic symptoms. Many infected children exhibit global developmental delay, regardless of neurologic findings. In young children, motor development is more impaired than mental development.

The incidence of neurologic abnormalities reported in HIV-infected cohorts before the advent of antiretroviral treatments ranged from 15% to 30%. Incidence rates in 2000 after the introduction of combination antiretroviral therapy are less than 2%. Children most at risk are those who have recovered from HIV encephalopathy. Older HIV-infected children may show problems in visual-spatial processing functions and expressive language and may develop AIDS–dementia complex indistinguishable from that described in adults.

HIV-associated myelopathy, polyneuropathy, and myopathy are rare in children. Spinal cord pathology shows demyelinating changes of the corticospinal tracts, vacuolar changes, or myelitis attributable to HIV. Acute inflammatory demyelinating polyneuropathy is a rare complication in pediatric HIV. Low-dose treatment with dideoxyinosine causes a painful sensory neuropathy in less than 10% of patients treated. The neuropathy is dose related and usually reverts with cessation of treatment. A mitochondrial depletion myopathy can be seen in children treated with combination therapy, especially with nucleoside reverse transcript inhibitors that have a high affinity to mitochondrial polymerase gamma (e.g., didanosine).

Focal Manifestations

HIV brain infection is nonfocal and subcortical. Seizures are not common. Focal signs or seizures raise the possibility of neoplasm, strokes, or, less likely, opportunistic infections.

Primary CNS Lymphoma

This is the most common cause of focal cerebral signs in HIV-infected children, found in 3% to 4% of cases. Seizures are reported in about 33% of patients. It may be difficult to differentiate this tumor from toxoplasma brain abscess; diagnosis requires brain biopsy. MRI spectroscopy may prove helpful in distinguishing CNS toxoplasmosis from lymphoma.

Stroke

HIV infection produces inflammation of cerebral vessels, increasing the risk of stroke, which occurs at a rate of 1.3% a year in HIV-infected children. More than 50% of

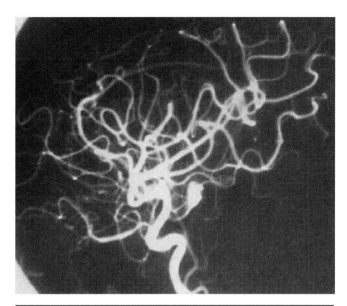

FIGURE 168.1. Fusiform aneurysm in a child with advanced HIV encephalopathy presenting with intraventricular hemorrhage and stroke.

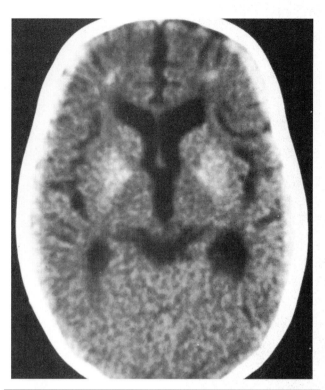

FIGURE 168.2. CT scan of an infant with HIV encephalopathy showing cortical and subcortical atrophy, basal ganglia, and frontal lobe calcifications. (Courtesy of Dr. Ram Kairam.)

strokes are hemorrhagic and occur with thrombocytopenia (especially immune thrombocytopenic purpura) or CNS neoplasia. Nonhemorrhagic stroke and subarachnoid hemorrhage are attributable to an arteriopathy affecting the large vessels of the circle of Willis (fusiform aneurysms) or meninges (Fig. 168.1). HIV-related strokes may be clinically silent, so the true incidence is probably higher. In the setting of stroke, VZV should be excluded as an etiologic agent by CSF PCR, especially when small ER vessels are involved and in eye by an ophthalmologic assessment. Any vasculopathy in HIV-infected patients is presumed to be infectious (either from HIV or varicellazoster virus [VZV]) and should be treated with appropriate antiretroviral and antiviral medications. Steroid medication is not indicated and may result in worsening of vasculopathy.

Opportunistic CNS Infection

Compared to adults, opportunistic CNS infection is infrequent in HIV-infected children, affecting primarily older children and adolescents. Prolonged survival of children with progressive multifocal leukoencephalopathy is possible with antiretroviral medication (e.g., cidofovir) and effective antiretroviral combination therapy that results in immune reconstitution.

Imaging

In children with HIV encephalopathy, atrophy is the most common neuroimaging abnormality (Fig. 168.2). Periventricular or parieto-occipital demyelination can be observed

on MRI (Fig. 168.3). Frontal lobe or basal ganglia enhancement and calcifications are late manifestations of HIV encephalopathy, best seen on CT, and occur primarily in symptomatic infants (Fig. 168.2). HIV-related myelopathy on spinal MRI may show a high signal but is usually normal. Bilateral cerebral lesions may mimic myelopathy and must be excluded with MRI or CT. Lesions of progressive multifocal leukoencephalopathy are commonly located in the parietooccipital or frontal region affecting both periventricular and subcortical white matter. These lesions may be difficult to distinguish from HIV demyelination.

Cerebrospinal Fluid (CSF)

CSF findings are commonly normal in children with HIV infection. In the absence of opportunistic infection, CSF findings in children with progressive encephalopathy are nonspecific, with a lymphocytic pleocytosis and elevated protein content. Intra-blood-brain barrier synthesis of HIV-specific antibody or antigen detection in CSF has not been useful in predicting encephalopathy. CSF viral load, although not routinely available, may prove useful in determining HIV encephalopathy in children, especially in cases of compartmentalization (i.e., a sequestered HIV reservoir in the CNS), in which systemic viral measures do not reflect the level of viral replication in CNS.

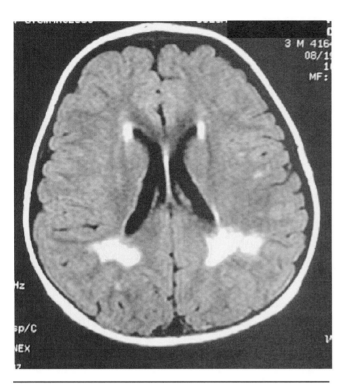

FIGURE 168.3. Parietal occipital demyelination on FLAIR image in a child with advanced HIV encephalopathy and high viral load (RNA HIV = 1.5 million copies/mL).

▶ TABLE 168.2 Fetal Alcohol Syndrome

Typical Features
Prenatal and postnatal growth retardation (weight, length, and/or head size <10th percentile)
Cerebral involvement (neurologic or cognitive impairment, developmental delay)
Dysmorphic features
Microcephaly (head circumference <5th percentile)
Microphthalmia, short palpebral fissures, or both
Poorly developed philtrum
Thin upper lip
Flattening of the maxillary area

Antiretroviral Therapy

Highly active antiretroviral therapies (HAART), consisting of a protease inhibitor (PI) or a non-nucleoside reverse transcriptase inhibitor (NNRTI) administered in combination with nucleoside reverse transcriptase inhibitors (NRTI), has been reported to suppress viral replication, improve immune function, and decrease the likelihood of AIDS-related death as well as diminish rates of HIV encephalopathy. High systemic viral load tends to predict the development of HIV encephalopathy, whereas CD4 count tends to predict HIV disease progression other than HIV encephalopathy.

FETAL ALCOHOL SYNDROME (FAS)

FAS affects children of chronic alcoholic women but also occurs with binge drinking, as defined by five drinks or more on one occasion. Fetal susceptibility to the effects of alcohol is greatest during the first trimester of pregnancy. FAS is characterized by abnormalities of growth, CNS, and facial features; birth defects are common (Table 168.2). FAS rates in the United States are 2 to 4 per 1,000 live births and 2% to 4% among children of alcohol-abusing women. FAS is confined to infants of alcohol-abusing women. Most children with FAS are mildly or moderately retarded, with mean IQ scores of 65 to 70, but intellectual ability varies widely. In families with several affected siblings, the youngest child is usually the most cog-

nitively impaired. Learning disabilities—in particular, difficulty with arithmetic, speech delay, and hyperactivity—are commonly observed.

Less severe alcohol-related effects are associated with wide patterns of drinking. These fetal alcohol effects are probably a lower point on the continuum of alcohol effects on the fetus. Maternal alcohol abuse is associated with increased risk of spontaneous abortions, infant mortality, intrauterine growth retardation, and prematurity. Birth defects are common. Minor or major congenital anomalies occur in about a third of infants born to heavy drinkers, compared with 9% of minor anomalies in infants of women who abstain from alcohol. Decrease of alcohol intake during pregnancy is beneficial to the offspring, reducing rates of growth retardation and dysmorphic features. Heavy alcohol exposure prenatally, but not mild or moderate exposure, has been linked to decrease in IQ scores, hyperactive behavior, attention problems, learning difficulties, and speech disorders.

Postnatal Alcohol Exposure

Alcohol transferred through breast milk impairs motor development but not mental development at age 1 year. Ingestion of alcohol by children may lead to hypoglycemic seizures.

Withdrawal Syndrome

Infants born to women who drink large amounts of alcohol during pregnancy may rarely exhibit signs of withdrawal. Restlessness, agitation, tremulousness, opisthotonus, and seizures are seen shortly after birth and disappear within a few days.

FETAL COCAINE EFFECTS

Although the cocaine epidemic has abated, cocaine is still the most frequent hard drug of abuse in urban centers, whereas methamphetamine is the preferred substance of abuse in rural settings (its effects are similar to cocaine).

Cocaine use during pregnancy has been linked to spontaneous abortion, abruptio placentae, stillbirth, and premature delivery. These events may immediately follow large intakes of cocaine and are attributed to drug-induced vasoconstriction of intrauterine vessels. Women who use cocaine tend to resort to prostitution, increasing risks for syphilis and HIV. They also tend to lack prenatal care, adding to the risks of infant death, low birth weight, and prematurity.

Low birth weight and intrauterine growth retardation are common among cocaine-exposed infants. Fetal brain growth is impaired independently of birth weight or gestational age. Sudden infant death syndrome has also been linked to cocaine exposure in utero.

Neurobehavior

State regulation difficulties are well described among cocaine-exposed newborns. Findings vary from irritability and excitability to decreased organizational response and interactive behavior, even if the exposure to cocaine was limited to the first trimester of pregnancy. Modulation of attention is impaired among cocaine-exposed infants who, unlike unexposed infants, prefer higher rates of stimuli when in a high level of arousal. Exposed infants also show motor and movement abnormalities, including excessive tremor and hypertonia. Dose-response effects of cocaine on state regulation and neurologic findings are reported in newborns. Some studies show no neurobehavioral effects, however.

Strokes

Experimentally, cocaine and its main metabolite, benzoylecgonine, cause vasoconstriction of fetal cerebral vessels. Neonatal stroke and porencephaly have been associated with prenatal cocaine exposure. Some cases may be related to other neonatal stroke risk factors that accompany fetal cocaine exposure, such as abruptio placentae or birth asphyxia. Intraventricular hemorrhage is observed among infants more heavily exposed to cocaine.

Seizures

Focal seizures may occur in cocaine-exposed newborns with strokes. EEGs in cocaine-exposed infants show bursts of sharp waves and spikes that are often multifocal. These findings do not correlate with clinical seizures or neurologic abnormalities and may disappear in 3 to 12 months. Cocaine-exposed premature infants are at increased risk of neonatal seizures. Seizures are rare if there is no stroke.

Malformations

Prenatal cocaine exposure has been linked with urogenital malformations, limb reduction deformities, and intestinal atresia and infarction. Agenesis of the corpus callosum and septo-optic dysplasia have also been noted. These teratogenic effects may result from cocaine-induced vasoconstriction and fetal vascular disruption in early organogenesis.

Neurodevelopmental Impact

In experiment models, prenatal cocaine has been reported to affect serotonin, norepinephrine, and dopaminergic systems. Lower CSF levels of homovanillic acid found in human newborns exposed to cocaine suggest dopaminergic involvement. In infancy, there may be a high incidence of global hypertonia that resolves prior to age 24 months (Table 168.3). Numerous studies in toddlers and school-aged children have failed to show that prenatal cocaine exposure adversely affects cognition, except as mediated through cocaine effects on brain growth. Cocaine-exposed children seem to suffer from an excess of neurobehavioral abnormalities, including irritability, impaired attention, impulsivity, and aggressive behavior.

Cocaine Exposure in Childhood

Passive intoxication with cocaine may be caused by breast-feeding or passive inhalation of free-base cocaine ("crack"). Seizures are the chief manifestation of

▶ **TABLE 168.3 Neurologic Fetal Cocaine Effects and Associations**

Neonatal period	Infancy and childhood
Microcephaly	**Neurologic**
Vascular abnormalities	Hypertonia in infancy
Stroke	**Developmental**
Porencephaly	Language delays
Intraventricular hemorrhage	Semantic delays
Seizures	**Behavioral**
Symptomatic (secondary to vascular complications)	Inattentiveness
	Temperamental differences
?Primary (owing to cocaine or its metabolites)	Impulsivity
	Aggressive behavior
Brain malformations	
Agenesis of corpus callosum	
Septo-optic dysplasia	
Skull defects	
Encephalocele	
Abnormal neurobehavior	
Impaired organizational state	
Depressed sensorium	
Hypertonia	
Coarse tremor	
Irritability/excitable state	

symptomatic intoxication, but intoxication may be unsuspected. Urine toxicology screen to detect illicit substances is indicated in evaluating seizures in infants and children, regardless of socioeconomic status.

Withdrawal Symptoms

There is no evidence of a cocaine-induced withdrawal syndrome. Even with remote prenatal cocaine exposure, cocaine-exposed infants may show hypertonicity and tremor, which are probably cerebral manifestations of fetal cocaine effects.

THE BATTERED CHILD

Child abuse may be physical or psychological. Physical abuse includes skin burns, welts, bruises, bone fractures, head trauma, and failure to thrive. Nonaccidental head trauma is suspected when severity of injury (often intracranial hemorrhage or skull fracture) is not consistent with the history that is given (if known) to explain injury or if the age of the child precludes a self-inflicted accidental injury (e.g. skull fracture in a newborn). Psychologic abuse frequently accompanies physical abuse and may lead to growth, behavioral, and developmental impairments. The shaken baby syndrome, an increasingly recognized form of physical abuse, is characterized by bilateral subdural hematomas or subarachnoid hemorrhage, retinal hemorrhages, and the absence of external signs of trauma. It is seen in infants mostly under age 1 year who are shaken repeatedly and violently. The aggressor, usually a parent, shakes the crying infant until he or she quiets and later denies doing so.

Depressed mental status, seizures, and signs of increased intracranial pressure are common. Neurogenic pulmonary edema may occur rarely. Bilateral retinal hemorrhages, in the absence of a coagulopathy, are the most specific signs of shaken baby syndrome. Hemorrhages may be flame shaped, round and intraretinal, preretinal, or vitreal. The speed with which blood disappears varies by type: Flame-shaped hemorrhage disappears within a few days, but round intraretinal hemorrhage may last 2 weeks. Retinal folds occasionally are seen. A dilated funduscopic examination should be performed quickly in any child with suspected child abuse to identify retinal hemorrhages before they disappear. Glutaric aciduria type I and Menkes disease may rarely mimic shaken baby syndrome.

Shaken baby syndrome should be suspected with sudden infant death syndrome or near-miss sudden infant death syndrome, with sudden lethargy, with seizures of unknown cause, or if there is a discrepancy between the history and the clinical signs. Broken ribs and chest bruises may be seen in infants held by the chest during shaking, and spiral fractures of the long bones or epiphysial separation may be seen in those shaken by the arms or legs. A skeletal survey showing old fractures helps confirm abuse. Brain MRI is helpful in determining the extent of intracranial damage, the severity of which predicts outcome. MRI abnormalities give evidence of the duration of the subdural hematoma; the presence of subdural blood of different ages indicates multiple traumatic events and helps confirm nonaccidental trauma. Infants with shaken baby syndrome may suffer neurologic sequelae, including hydrocephalus, blindness, developmental delay, mental retardation, microcephaly, and spastic tetraparesis.

SUGGESTED READINGS

Bonnier C, Nassogne MC, Saint-Martin C, et al. Neuroimaging of intraparenchymal lesions predicts outcome in shaken baby syndrome. *Pediatrics* 2003;112:808–814.

Burchett SK, Pizzo PA. HIV infection in infants, children, and adolescents. *Pediatr Rev* 2003;24(Jun):186–189.

Caffey J. The whiplash shaken baby syndrome: manual shaking by the extremities with whiplashed-induced intracranial and intraocular bleedings, linked with residual permanent brain damage and mental retardation. *Pediatrics* 1974;54:396–403.

Chiriboga CA. Fetal alcohol and drug effects. *Neurologist* 2003;9(Nov): 267–279.

Chiriboga CA. Neurological complications in HIV infected children and adolescents. In: AIDS Institute Clinical Guidelines—*Criteria for the Medical Care of Children and Adolescents with HIV Infection.* New York Department of Health 2003 http://www.hivguidelines.org/ public_html/center/clinical-guidelines/ped_adolescent_hiv_guidelines/ ped_neuro/ped_neuro.htm. 1994
Revised classification system for human immunodeficiency virus (HIV) infection in children less than 13 years of age. *MMWR Morb Mortal Wkly Rep* 1994;43:RR12.

Mazzoni, P, Chiriboga CA, Millar W, et al. Intracerebral aneurysms in human immunodeficiency virus infection: case report and literature review. *Pediatr Neurol* 2000;23:252–255.

O'Leary CM. Fetal alcohol syndrome: diagnosis, epidemiology, and developmental outcomes. *J Paediatr Child Health* 2004;40(Jan-Feb): 2–7.

Streissguth AP. Fetal alcohol syndrome: early and long-term consequences. *NIDA Res Monogr* 1992;119:126–130.

Chapter 169

Falls in the Elderly

Gary M. Abrams and Lewis P. Rowland

Falls in the elderly are often taken for granted and considered an inevitable consequence of aging. Analysis of the factors that lead to falls, however, indicates that there are strategies for prevention. The problem is certainly serious for individuals, families, and society (Table 169.1).

EPIDEMIOLOGY

More than a third of people age 65 or older fall each year. Five percent to 10% of falls in the elderly result in major injuries, including subdural hematoma and traumatic brain injury. Injury is the sixth leading cause of death after age 65, and most injuries result from a fall. Although people over 65 constitute about 12% of the total population, they account for 74% of all deaths caused by falls. Fatality rates increase with age in both men and women.

The likelihood of admission of an elderly person to a nursing home increases with the number of falls. Most falls occur at home, but the rate of falling is higher in long-term care facilities. Periods of high risk for falling occur during the month after hospital discharge in frail individuals or during episodes of acute illness or exacerbations of chronic conditions. Sensitivity to drugs is another factor. The use of multiple medications, especially psychoactive drugs such as antidepressants, neuroleptics, or benzodiazepines, increases the chances of falling.

THE NEUROLOGY OF FALLS

Few falls seem to be directly related to syncope, drop attacks, TIAs, or overt myopathy. Instead, a propensity to falls is generated by the cumulative impairments of cognitive decline, poor vision, poor balance, and generalized muscle weakness (Table 169.2). In healthy ambulatory individuals, increased volume of cerebral white matter disease as determined by MRI is associated with gait and balance dysfunction. Intuitively, it seems likely that the motor impairment of Parkinson disease or previous stroke would increase falls, as would the impediments of arthritis or postural hypotension.

RISK FACTORS AND ASSESSMENT

The prevalence of risk factors for falling steeply increases after age 70. Thus, all individuals in this age group should be queried about falls, balance, or gait difficulties. They

▶ TABLE 169.1 Falls in the Elderly

Fall rate	33–50% of those >65
Injury owing to falls	5–10% of falls
Proportion of deaths >age 65	33%
Fatalities owing to falls	
Proportion of total population >65	12%
Proportion of all deaths owing to falls, people >65	74%
Site of fatal falls	
Home	60%
Public places	30%
Health care facilities	10%
Fatality rates	
Ages 65–74	8.5 per 100,000
>75	56.7 per 100,000
Proportion of falls resulting in hip fracture in people >65	1%
Annual number of hip fractures in United States	150,000
Cost of hip fractures (1991)	$2.9 billion

Data from Hindmarsh JJ, Estes EF Jr. *Arch Intern Med* 1989;149:2217–2222; Sorock GS. Falls among the elderly: epidemiology and prevention. *Am J Prevent Med* 1988;4:282–288; *CDC MMWR* 1996;45:877–883.

▶ TABLE 169.2 Common Risk Factors for Falls Identified in 16 Studies That Examined Risk Factors

Risk Factor	Significant/Total[a]	Mean RR-OR	Range
Muscle weakness	10/11	4.4	1.5–10.3
History of falls	12/13	3.0	1.7–7.0
Gait deficit	10/12	2.9	1.3–5.6
Balance deficit	8/11	2.9	1.6–5.4
Use of assistive device	8/8	2.6	1.2–4.6
Visual deficit	6/12	2.5	1.6–3.5
Arthritis	3/7	2.4	1.9–2.9
Impaired ADLs	8/9	2.3	1.5–3.1
Depression	3/6	2.2	1.7–2.5
Cognitive impairment	4/11	1.8	1.0–2.3
Age >80 years	5/8	1.7	1.1–2.5

[a]Number of studies with significant odds ratio (retrospective studies) or relative risk ratio (prospective studies) in univariate analysis/total number of studies that included each factor.
Adapted from Guideline for the prevention of falls in older persons. American Geriatrics Society, British Geriatrics Society, and American Academy of Orthopaedic Surgeons Panel on Falls Prevention. *J Am Geriatr Soc* 2001;49:664-72.

should be observed arising from a chair and walking and observed for unsteadiness. Vision can be important in maintaining upright stability and compensating for other risks for falling and should be evaluated. Most falls in the elderly are accidental. Examples include missing the last step on descent, slippery surfaces, poor lighting, unexpected appearance of a child or pet, and poorly fitting shoes.

PREVENTION

In one study, 46% of fallers were repeaters. The first fall led to loss of mobility and loss of confidence, making the next one more likely. A number of interventions have been validated experimentally to prevent falls, including (1) multidisciplinary health and environmental screening to correct falling risk factors, (2) muscle strengthening and balance training at home prescribed by a health professional, (3) home hazard assessment in people with a history of falls, (4) withdrawal of psychotropic medications, (5) cardiac pacing for fallers with cardioinhibitory carotid sinus sensitivity, and (6) tai chi delivered over 15 weeks as a group exercise intervention. Death rates from falls among people age 60 to 85 decreased substantially between 1960 and 1990, primarily owing to improved trauma management.

SUGGESTED READINGS

Avorn J. Depression in the elderly—falls and pitfalls. *N Engl J Med* 1998;339:918–20.

Bloem BR, Steijns JAG, Smits-Engelsman BC. An update on falls. *Curr Opin Neurol* 2003;16(Feb):15–26.

Close J, Ellis M, Hooper R, et al. Prevention of falls in the elderly trial (PROFET): a randomised controlled trial. *Lancet* 1999;353:93–97.

Gill TM, Baker DI, Gottschalk M, et al. A program to prevent functional decline in physically frail, elderly persons who live at home. *N Engl J Med* 2002;347:1068–1074.

Gillespie LD, Gillespie WJ, Robertson MC, et al. Interventions for preventing falls in elderly people (Cochrane Review). In: *The Cochrane Library*, Issue 1, Chichester, UK: John Wiley & Sons. 2004.

Guideline for the prevention of falls in older persons. American Geriatrics Society, British Geriatrics Society, and American Academy of Orthopaedic Surgeons Panel on Falls Prevention. *J Am Geriatr Soc* 2001;49:664–72.

Nutt JG, Marsden CD, Thompson PD. Human walking and higher-level gait disorders, particularly in the elderly. *Neurology* 1993;43:268–279.

Riggs JE. Mortality from accidental falls among the elderly in the United States, 1962–1988: demonstrating the impact of improved trauma management. *J Trauma* 1993;35:212–219.

Saper CB. "All fall down": the mechanism of orthostatic hypotension in multiple systems atrophy and Parkinson's disease. *Ann Neurol* 1998;43:149–151.

Sorock GS. Falls among the elderly: epidemiology and prevention. *Am J Prevent Med* 1988;4:282–288.

Thapa PB, Gideon P, Cost TW, et al. Antidepressants and the risk of falls among nursing home residents. *N Engl J Med* 1998;339:875–882.

Tinetti ME, Speechley M. Prevention of falls in elderly persons. *N Engl J Med* 2003;320:1055–1059.

Whitman GT, Tang Y, Lin A, et al. A prospective study of cerebral white matter abnormalities in older people with gait dysfunction. *Neurology* 2001;57:990–994.

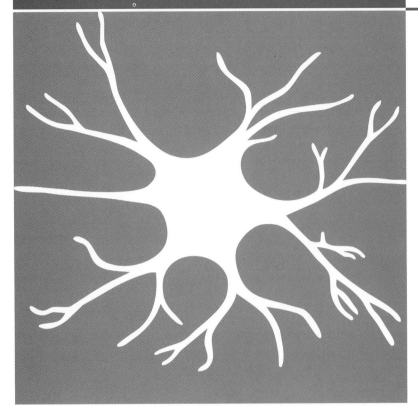

Rehabilitation

Chapter 170

Neurologic Rehabilitation

Laura Lennihan and Glenn M. Seliger

Neurologic disorders commonly cause temporary or permanent impairments that impede simple daily functions and complex intellectual and physical activities. Neurologists play an important role in prescribing rehabilitation therapies to maximize functional recovery. The selection and timing of these therapies make a substantial contribution to optimum quality of life for patient and family despite persistent neurologic impairments. Although it is advisable for rehabilitation to begin soon after a neurologic injury, many people with chronic neurologic conditions have never received adequate rehabilitation therapy. Nevertheless, if they are given proper training and equipment, they may still improve in personal independence, access to the community, and ease with which caregivers assist them. At a time when neurologists are assuming the role of principal care physicians, experience in neurorehabilitation is essential in the management continuum from acute to chronic neurologic disorders.

The World Health Organization Classification of Functioning, Disability and Health defines limitations of body functions, personal activities, and societal participation caused by disease. These definitions provide a structure for understanding the impact of disease on personal independence and integration into society and can help to identify patients who may benefit from rehabilitation. The planning and prescription of a rehabilitation program for a neurologically impaired individual requires characterization of the neurologic disorder in terms of natural history, localization, and extent of nervous system involvement; determination of functional disabilities caused by cognitive and physical impairments; and definition of these disabilities in the context of the patient's physical and social environment. With this information, the type and intensity of rehabilitation therapies can be planned.

Two principal approaches are used together in rehabilitation programs. The first approach is to bypass the neurologic impairment by teaching adaptive techniques using preserved neurologic function. For example, a person with a paralyzed arm can be trained in one-handed techniques using the normal arm. The efficacy of this first approach in improving functional independence and reducing disability is established. The second approach is to facilitate the return of neurologic function. For example, the person with a paralyzed arm is given tasks to practice to improve motor control of that arm. The second approach is the focus of active clinical research. In a primate model, restraint of the normal arm resulting in forced use of the paretic arm after motor cortex injury leads to better functional recovery of the affected arm than when the normal arm is unrestrained. Little functional recovery occurs if the paretic arm is restrained. Small studies in humans similarly support the efficacy of this forced-use paradigm. Gait training on a treadmill with a harness providing partial body weight support is thought to recruit spinal pattern generators for walking. This technique may produce better balance, motor recovery, walking speed, and endurance compared with conventional over-ground gait training with patients bearing their full body weight.

Both quantity and type of training have an impact on functional recovery. Intensive training promotes better recovery, and training that focuses on recovering lost skills, so-called task-specific therapy, is more effective than repetitive strengthening exercises.

Current research on the neurobiology of recovery from CNS injury and the efficacy of treatments to improve the speed and completeness of recovery is relevant to the practice of neurorehabilitation. For example, norepinephrine plays an important role in modulating CNS recovery. In animal models of focal brain injury and in people with strokes, amphetamine administered coincident with physical therapy has resulted in better motor recovery than in placebo-treated subjects. Drugs with central catecholamine antagonist activity, such as haloperidol, prazosin, or clonidine, interfere with motor recovery in animals. Enhancement of activity of the inhibitory neurotransmitter gamma-aminobutyric acid (GABA) by drugs such as diazepam, phenytoin, or phenobarbital also impedes neurologic recovery in animals. In a retrospective study, stroke patients who received either class of drug had poorer motor recovery than those who did not.

Functional outcome is improved by treatment in a comprehensive rehabilitation program. Stroke patients who receive rehabilitation therapies on a stroke rehabilitation unit have better functional outcomes and shorter hospital stays than those treated on a general neurology ward. Similarly, stroke patients admitted to hospital-based intensive rehabilitation programs have better functional recovery and are more likely to return home than those treated in a low-intensity rehabilitation program at a skilled nursing facility.

A comprehensive inpatient neurorehabilitation program requires an interdisciplinary team: physician, physical therapist, occupational therapist, speech therapist, neuropsychologist, social worker, and rehabilitation nurse. The physician, as team leader, defines the type and prognosis of the neurologic disorder; is responsible for coordination of rehabilitation services and setting of realistic treatment goals; and provides medical care, especially for the prevention and treatment of complications of a disabling disorder, for instance, deep vein thrombosis or depression.

The physical therapist's role is to maximize leg function and mobility. The occupational therapist promotes maximum independence in activities of daily living by improving arm function and cognitive skills. The speech therapist characterizes and treats specific language-based cognitive dysfunction and evaluates and treats dysphagia and dysarthria. The neuropsychologist defines cognitive problems and monitors improvement. The rehabilitation nurse, in addition to providing medical nursing care, incorporates skills learned in therapy into the patient's daily routines and institutes treatments to restore sphincter continence. The social worker implements the discharge plan. All team members participate in formulating a discharge plan and in educating and training patient and family in preparation for return home.

OCCUPATIONAL THERAPY

Neurologic injury that interferes with use of the arms and hands can be profoundly disabling. Weakness, loss of sensation, ataxia, abnormal tone, and involuntary movements, alone or in combination, can lead to inability to carry out basic activities of daily living, to drive a car, or to work. Occupational therapy promotes recovery from neurologic injury; prevents permanent disability from complications of temporary neurologic impairments, such as wrist-flexor contractures from a radial nerve palsy; teaches new techniques to perform self-care and other tasks; prescribes equipment to increase use of the impaired arm and hand; and, when the impairment is unilateral, teaches performance of one-handed techniques by the normal arm.

The approach to restoring function to the neurologically impaired arm is determined in part by central or peripheral site of injury. For example, treatment of weakness caused by an upper motor neuron lesion focuses on reestablishing movement at one joint in isolation from movement at other joints; strengthening exercises follow later. Strengthening programs are usually instituted early for peripheral injuries, but it is important not to overwork muscles recovering from a nerve injury because weakness may worsen. Wrist and ankle weights can be used to dampen arm and leg ataxia.

Improving motor skills is only one of the important components in enhancing performance of the activities of daily living, such as dressing, toileting, washing, grooming, feeding, and community skills. Training to overcome visual and perceptual difficulties, unilateral spatial neglect, memory impairment, inattentiveness, and poor safety judgment may also be important. The occupational therapist selects adaptive equipment and trains patient and family to compensate. Advanced programs may include learning special occupational skills or to drive with the left hand and foot.

PHYSICAL THERAPY

Interference with mobility by neurologic disease can be reduced or eliminated by strengthening exercises, gait and balance training, spasticity reduction through stretching or medication, surgical release of shortened tendons, bracing, assistive devices (e.g., cane, walker), and use of a wheelchair. Techniques and orthotics are chosen to maximize safe and independent mobility; to optimize energy efficiency; to prevent decubitus skin ulcers, tendon contractures, and falls; and to enhance motor recovery. Leg and trunk weakness, impaired postural reflexes, ataxia, proprioceptive loss, and hemineglect may all interfere with walking. Even though a person may not be able to walk immediately after neurologic injury, ambulation usually becomes possible through a combination of bracing at the ankle and sometimes the knee and use of a walker or cane. When ambulation is not possible, mobility is attained through training in the use of a wheelchair of the correct size and height, with a special seat to prevent skin breakdown and cushions for trunk support.

DYSPHAGIA THERAPY

Facial, lingual, masticatory, pharyngeal, esophageal, and respiratory muscles participate in swallowing. Neurologic disorders that disturb coordinated contraction of any of these muscles can cause dysphagia and, secondarily, airway obstruction, aspiration pneumonia, and malnutrition. Dysphagia evaluation is indicated for patients who have any of these complications; who report coughing, choking, or nasal regurgitation while eating; who are dysarthric; or who have a disease commonly associated with dysphagia, such as motor neuron disease or myasthenia gravis. This evaluation includes characterization of the neurologic disorder and bedside and fluoroscopic observation of swallowing foods of different consistencies, from thin liquids to chewy meat. Restriction of the diet to consistencies that can be swallowed without aspiration reduces the risk of dysphagia complications. The speech therapist teaches techniques that improve coordinated swallowing and reduce the risk of aspiration, such as tucking the chin before swallowing to close the larynx and open the upper esophagus and swallowing twice after each bite of food to clear the pharynx.

LANGUAGE AND COGNITIVE THERAPIES

Brain injuries that cause behavioral, language, and other cognitive dysfunctions may be focal and discrete or generalized and diffuse. In focal injuries, the neurologic dysfunctions may be restricted, with other brain functions preserved, for instance, Broca aphasia with intact attention, memory, and concentration. In contrast, diffuse injury may affect several areas of cognitive function. The therapeutic approach needs to be tailored to the nature and complexity of the symptoms. The first step in implementing a cognitive rehabilitation program is to define the neurobehavioral impediments and how they interfere with function. For example, a short attention span may prevent participation in group activities such as business meetings, or memory impairment may lead to failure at school.

Speech therapy for aphasia is a specialized part of cognitive rehabilitation. The speech therapist defines receptive and expressive dysfunction and identifies areas of strength and weakness in language. Areas of strength may then be used for compensatory purposes. For instance, if an aphasic patient's written language skills are preserved better than verbal expression, writing may be useful for communication. Training in use of visual imagery as an internal cue may help to overcome the word blocking of Broca aphasia. A picture board may circumvent an expressive language deficit. The use of computer-assisted communication for aphasia is an area of active rehabilitation research. Speech and occupational therapists use treatment strategies for other cognitive deficits, for example visual imagery to create memory cues may improve performance on memory tests; breaking a task into individual steps and then teaching one step at a time helps to overcome constructional problems.

In diffuse or multifocal brain injury that impairs attention and behavior and many aspects of cognition and language, a structured program that permits few distractions is necessary. Speech and occupational therapists collaborate on program development and implementation, and all members of the rehabilitation team contribute. Several strategies may compensate for multiple problems. For example, sensory reduction minimizes distractions by controlling the noise and activity in the environment; development of a rigidly structured daily routine helps to overcome poor planning and organizational skills. Education of patient and family about aphasia and other cognitive problems is essential to reduce frustration with impaired communication, memory, and abnormal behavior.

INCONTINENCE THERAPY

Loss of control of bladder or bowel emptying is a devastating condition and should be addressed by any comprehensive neurorehabilitation program. The cause of impaired emptying or sphincter incompetence, and therefore the treatment, depends on the site of the neural injury. Evaluation includes clinical observations about incontinence and retention; search for non-neurologic factors, such as infection or mechanical problems, particularly urethral obstruction by prostatic enlargement; and cystometrographic measurements of bladder and sphincter functions. The neurorehabilitation nurse plays a crucial role in the treatment of bladder and bowel disorders, including implementation of voiding programs and training patient and family to use urethral catheters.

Incontinence characterized by bladder hyperreflexia, in which the bladder contracts at low urine volumes and voluntary inhibition of bladder contraction and sphincter relaxation fails, commonly complicates cerebral, particularly frontal lobe, injury. Lack of awareness or indifference may impede achievement of continence, but neurologic recovery usually reduces incontinence. Scheduled voiding at 2-hour intervals contributes to regaining continence. Bladder dyssynergia, in which bladder contraction and sphincter relaxation are dissociated and the bladder contracts against a closed sphincter, is usually a consequence of lower brainstem or spinal cord disorders. Bladder emptying, if it occurs at all, is incomplete and occurs at high pressure. Treatment includes bladder antispasmodic drugs and intermittent catheterization. Hydronephrosis and renal failure are potential complications. Peripheral nerve diseases involving the nerves innervating the bladder may cause bladder flaccidity. Bladder emptying, at low pressures, is incomplete, and incontinence occurs between voluntary voiding. Cholinergic agents may improve emptying, but intermittent catheterization is often necessary.

Immobility from any neurologic disorder and loss of cortical control over bowel movements owing to spinal cord injury may cause severe obstipation and even bowel obstruction. Prevention combines a high-fiber diet and stool softeners with laxatives or enemas timed to stimulate evacuation on a regular schedule.

SUGGESTED READINGS

Bennett L, Knowlton GC. Overwork weakness in partially denervated skeletal muscle. *Clin Orthop* 1958;12:22–29.

Dobkin BH. *The Clinical Science of Neurologic Rehabilitation.* Oxford: Oxford University Press, 2003.

Goldstein LB, Matchar DB, Morgenlander JC, et al. Influence of drugs on the recovery of sensorimotor function after stroke. *J Neurol Rehab* 1990;4:137–144.

Good DC, Couch JR, eds. *Handbook of Neurorehabilitation.* New York: Marcel Dekker, 1994.

International Classification of Functioning, Disability and Health. Geneva: World Health Organization, 2001 (http://www3.who.int/icf/icftemplate.cfm).

Kalra L, Dale P, Crome P. Improving stroke rehabilitation: a controlled study. *Stroke* 1993;24:1462–1467.

Kramer AM, Steiner JF, Schlenker RE, et al. Outcomes and costs after hip fracture and stroke. A comparison of rehabilitation settings. *JAMA* 1997;277:396–404.

Selzer ME. Neurological rehabilitation. *Ann Neurol* 1992;32:695–699.

Taub E, Miller NE, Novack TA, et al. Technique to improve chronic motor deficit after stroke. *Arch Phys Med Rehabil* 1993;74:347–354.

Visintin M, Barbeau H, Korner-Bitensky N, et al. A new approach to retrain gait in stroke patients through body weight support and treadmill stimulation. *Stroke* 1998;29:1122–1128.

Walker-Batson D, Smith P, Curtis S, et al. Amphetamine paired with physical therapy accelerates motor recovery after stroke. *Stroke* 1995;26:2254–2259.

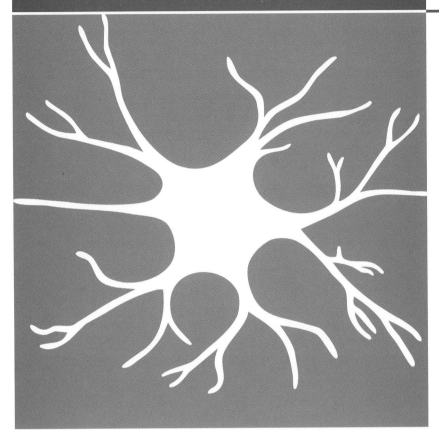

Ethical and Legal Guidelines

Chapter 171

End-of-Life Issues in Neurology

Lewis P. Rowland

Neurologic diseases have been at the center of discussions on issues at the end of life. The American Academy of Neurology has set standards for the determination of cerebral death and for the persistent vegetative state (see Chapter 4). Amyotrophic lateral sclerosis (ALS) and Alzheimer disease have been the focus of debates about assisted suicide. Neurologic intensive care units face the issue of discontinuing mechanical ventilation. Presymptomatic diagnosis is available for incurable conditions like Huntington disease, creating an ethical challenge.

These ethical issues could fill a separate book. Here, we set forth some principles and definitions as an introduction for students and physicians as they learn to deal with the problems. The fundamental ethical and legal guidelines are the basis for actions taken or avoided.

INFORMED CONSENT

One basis for patient autonomy in decision-making is informed consent. A patient may accept or refuse a treatment or diagnostic test after learning about the anticipated benefits and risks and alternative choices. This choice requires access to accurate information about prognosis, which has to be understood by the patient.

ADVANCE DIRECTIVES

Individuals may prepare legal documents that specify their preferences for end-of-life treatments under specific circumstances, and they may also appoint surrogate decision makers if the individual is not competent to make decisions at some future time. Most states recognize living wills as instruments for these advance directives, which usually provide a prohibition against life-sustaining treatments that prolong the dying process if the person is in a terminal condition and can no longer make decisions. A competent person can change the advance directive at any time.

REFUSAL OF LIFE-SUSTAINING TREATMENT

The *doctrine of informed consent* includes the patient's *right to refuse life-sustaining treatment*. Refusal is a decision not to provide consent, without which the physician usually cannot continue treatment. Respect for a *patient's autonomy* does not require acceptance of all decisions; the decision must be based on adequate understanding of the nature and consequences of the choice (*informed consent*) without coercion and with capacity to make a reasoned decision.

The patient's right to consent or refuse is not abrogated when the patient loses the capacity to make decisions. It becomes transferred to a legally authorized *surrogate decision maker*, and the physician must ask the surrogate for consent or refusal on behalf of the patient.

The surrogate must follow the patient's previously expressed wishes as expressed in *advance directives* or other reliable statements. If the patient's expressed wishes have not been explicitly stated, the surrogate must use the *doctrine of substituted judgment*, based on knowledge of the patient's general values and preferences. If the surrogate has no such information, the surrogate must assess the anticipated benefits and burdens, based on the *doctrine of best interest*. This may be problematic, however, because it is not based on the desires of the patient. Despite widely held beliefs to the contrary, it is not necessary to consult legal counsel before withdrawing life-sustaining therapy.

DOUBLE EFFECT

Some actions are morally and ethically acceptable and may have foreseeable but unintended and undesirable outcomes; the morality of the action depends on the morality

1201

of the intended outcome, not the unintended one. According to the American Academy of Neurology Ethics Committee statement on assisted suicide, several conditions must be met: The action to be carried out must be morally or ethically acceptable or at least neutral, the good effect must not depend on the undesired or bad effect, and the good effect must be sufficient to justify the risk of the unintended outcome.

In practice, this principle makes it possible to administer sufficient analgesic and sedative medication to keep a patient comfortable even though the treatment will not prolong life. The principle of *double effect* is the basis of the hospice program.

PALLIATIVE CARE

According to the World Health Organization definition, palliative care is "the active total care of patients whose disease is not responsive to curative treatment, where the control of pain, of other symptoms and of psychological, social, and spiritual problems is paramount, and where the goal is the achievement of the best quality of life for patients and their families." More directly stated, palliative care is "comfort care" or treatment intended to relieve pain and suffering rather than to cure the disease, restore the patient to health, or prolong life at all costs. Oral or parenteral morphine is used in amounts sufficient to control pain and maintain comfort.

A *hospice program* is often the venue for palliative care. This is sometimes carried out in a hospital or separate physical facility but is increasingly a home care program. In the United States, a Medicare Disease-Related Group (DRG) provides reimbursement for the care of patients who are not expected to survive for more than 6 months. However, hospice care is used by only 17% of people who are dying, and three reasons are adduced: First, physicians are uncomfortable about talking with patients about terminal events long enough in advance. Second, it may be difficult to determine precisely the expected time of death. Third, hospices emphasize home care, and family members may not be able to commit the time required or there may be no family members. Most Americans die in hospitals or nursing homes.

Another drawback to the use of home or hospice care is the insensitivity of U.S. physicians to the advance directives of their patients, as detected by the 1995–2000 Study to Understand Prognoses and Preferences for Outcomes and Risks of Treatment (SUPPORT). Fifty percent of the physicians polled did not respect or did not know the advance directives; most do-not-resuscitate (DNR) orders were not written until 24 hours before death; and 40% of the patients had severe pain for several days before death. In a follow-up study, there was no improvement in communication about patients' desires for resuscitation, the time

before death in an intensive care unit, or the incidence or timing of DNR orders, which were not written in 50% of the patients surveyed. Physicians misunderstood the desires of their patients against DNR (80%) or the level of pain.

PHYSICIAN-ASSISTED SUICIDE

As specified by law in the state of Oregon, it is permissible for a physician to prescribe medication to be used by a patient for the purpose of suicide. The physician may not actually administer the drug. This law is restricted to Oregon, and the practice is not legal in any other state.

Neurologic diseases generate problems for this policy. Patients may be incompetent with Alzheimer disease and unable to give consent. Other patients may lose the use of their hands from MS or ALS. Under these circumstances, the patients themselves cannot fill the prescription and take the drug; someone else must assist them physically, which would be euthanasia and specifically banned by the Oregon law.

Many authorities have debated the desirability of assisted suicide. Medical and nursing organizations have uniformly opposed legalization.

TERMINAL SEDATION

The right to forgo treatment includes food and water. Pain or other discomfort can be ameliorated by standard palliative measures that may include sedation to unconsciousness. The patient then dies as a result of the underlying disease, dehydration, or both. It is believed that some form of terminal sedation is applied in up to 40% of deaths in U.S. hospitals. Discontinuing mechanical ventilation in an intensive care unit is another situation that calls for prevention or relief of suffering. Some believe that terminal dehydration has a stronger moral basis than assisted suicide, based as it is on the right to refuse treatment. A physician is morally obligated to honor a competent patient's refusal of food and water but is not obligated by a request for a lethal drug. Nevertheless, detractors consider terminal sedation a form of "slow euthanasia."

EUTHANASIA

If in compliance with a patient's request a physician administers a lethal drug by injection or other means, the act is *euthanasia*, which is illegal in the United States. The public, physicians, and courts have had difficulty separating refusal or discontinuation of therapy, which are legal, from assisted suicide and euthanasia, which are not. The distinction between assisted suicide and euthanasia is the most controversial of all. The Supreme Court concluded that palliative care and terminal sedation are permissible but referred the question of physician-assisted suicide back to legislation by the states.

This issue was highlighted in 2002 when Veldink et al. reported experience in the Netherlands, where euthanasia is legal. Among 279 patients who died of ALS, 17% chose euthanasia and 3% died as a result of physician-assisted suicide. Another 24% received palliative care, "which probably shortened their lives." In an accompanying editorial and correspondence, Ganzini and Block attributed the high rates of assisted death to inadequate palliative care.

AN OVERALL VIEW

The issues discussed here are among the most controversial in modern life. Consensus is not easy to achieve, but views are changing and current practices are likely to change as well. Already, pain control and palliative care have come to the fore and provide effective alternatives to assisted suicide. Documenting the preventive value of palliative care is a challenge for all concerned. Legal changes may be anticipated but do not seem imminent.

SUGGESTED READINGS

Almqvist EW, Block M, Brinkman R, et al. A worldwide assessment of the frequency of suicide, suicide attempts, or psychiatric hospitalization after predictive testing for Huntington disease. *Am J Hum Genet* 1999;64:1293–1304.

American Academy of Neurology Ethics and Humanities Subcommittee. Assisted suicide, euthanasia, and the neurologist. *Neurology* 1998;50:596–598.

American Academy of Neurology Ethics and Humanities Subcommittee. Certain aspects of the care and management of profoundly and irreversibly paralyzed patients with retained consciousness and cognition. *Neurology* 1993;43:222–223.

American Academy of Neurology Ethics and Humanities Subcommittee. Ethical issues in the management of the demented patient. *Neurology* 1996;46:1180–1183.

American Academy of Neurology Ethics and Humanities Subcommittee. Palliative care in neurology. *Neurology* 1996;46:870–872.

American Academy of Neurology Quality Standards Subcommittee. Practice parameter: assessment and management of patients in the persistent vegetative state. *Neurology* 1995;45:1015–1018.

Angell M. The Supreme Court and assisted suicide—the ultimate right. *N Engl J Med* 1997;336:50–53.

Bernat JL. *Ethical Issues in Neurology*. 2nd Ed. Boston: Butterworth-Heinemann, 2002.

Bird TD. Outrageous fortune: the risk of suicide in genetic testing for Huntington disease. *Am J Hum Genet* 1999;64:1289–1292.

Cowan JD, Walsh D. Terminal sedation in palliative medicine—definition and review of the literature. *Support Care Cancer* 2001:9(Sep):401–402.

Doyle D, Hanks GC, Mac Donald N, eds. *Oxford Textbook of Palliative Care* 3rd Ed. New York: Oxford University Press, 2003.

Field MJ, Cassel CK, eds. *Institute of Medicine. Approaching Death: Improving Care at the End of Life*. Washington, DC: National Academy Press, 1997.

Foley KM. Competent care for the dying instead of physician assisted suicide. *N Engl J Med* 1997;336:54–58.

Ganzini L, Block S. Physician-assisted death—a last resort? *N Engl J Med* 2002;346:1663–1665; correspondence, *N Engl J Med* 2002;347:1041–1043.

Ganzini L, Johnston WS, McFarland BH, et al. Attitudes of patients with amyotrophic lateral sclerosis and their care givers toward assisted suicide. *N Engl J Med* 1998;339:967–973.

Gostin LO Deciding life and death in the courtroom: from Quinlan to Cruzan, Glucksberg, and Vacco—a brief history and analysis of constitutional protection of the "right to die." *JAMA* 1997;278:1523–1528.

Lunney JR, Foley KM, Smith TJ, et al., eds. *Describing Death in America: What We Need to Know*. Washington, DC: National Research Council, Institute of Medicine, 2003.

Mayer SA, Kossoff SB. Withdrawal of life support in the neurological intensive care unit. *Neurology* 1999;52:1602–1609.

Medical aspects of the persistent vegetative state (1). Multi-Society Task Force on PVS. *N Engl J Med* 1994;330:1499–1508.

Medical aspects of the persistent vegetative state (2). Multi-Society Task Force on PVS. *N Engl J Med* 1994;330:1572–1579. Erratum in *N Engl J Med* 1995;333:130.

Meier DE, Morrison RS, Cassel CK. Improving palliative care. *Ann Intern Med* 1997;127:223–230.

Miller FG, Meier DE. Voluntary death: a comparison of terminal dehydration and physician-assisted suicide. *Ann Intern Med* 1998;128:559–562.

Morrison RS, Meier DE. Palliative care. *N Engl J Med* 2004;350:2582–2590.

Newton HB, Malkin MG. Ethical issues in neuro-oncology. *Semin Neurol* 1997;17:219–226.

Orentlicher D. The Supreme Court and physician-assisted suicide—rejecting assisted suicide but embracing euthanasia. *N Engl J Med* 1997;337:1236–1239.

Payne SK, Taylor RM. The persistent vegetative state and anencephaly: problematic paradigms for discussing futility and rationing. *Semin Neurol* 1997;17:257–264.

Portenoy RK, Bruera E. *Issues in Palliative Care*. Oxford, UK: Oxford University Press, 2003.

Quill TE. *Caring for Patients at the End of Life*. Oxford, UK: Oxford University Press, 2001.

Quill TE. Dying and decision-making—evolution of end-of-life options. *N Engl J Med* 2004;350:2029–2030.

Quill TE, Lo B, Brock DW. Palliative options of last resort: a comparison of voluntarily stopping eating and drinking, terminal sedation, physician-assisted suicide, and voluntary active euthanasia. *JAMA* 1997;278:2099–2104.

Quill TE, Meier DE, Block SD, et al. The debate over physician-assisted suicide: empirical data and convergent views. *Ann Intern Med* 1998;128:552–558.

Rowland LP. Assisted suicide and alternatives in amyotrophic lateral sclerosis. *N Engl J Med* 1998;339:987–989.

Veldink JH, Wokke JH, van der Wal G, et al. Euthanasia and physician-assisted suicide among patients with amyotrophic lateral sclerosis in the Netherlands. *N Engl J Med* 2002;346:1638–1644.

Note: Page numbers in italic indicate figures; page numbers followed by *t* indicate tables.

A

A-a gradient. *See* Alveolar-arterial gradient
AAMI. *See* Age-associated memory impairment
AB variant, lysosomal/other storage disease of, 622
Abducens nerve injury, cranial/peripheral nerve lesion with, 526–527
Abetalipoproteinemia
  Babinski signs with, 672
  clinical findings on, *672*
  diagnosis of, 672
  laboratory data on, 672
  MTP with, 672
  neurologic abnormalities with, 672
  neurologic syndromes of, 671–673, 674*t*
  pathogenesis of, 672
  symptoms/signs of, 672
  treatment for, 672–673
ABI. *See* Atherothrombotic brain infarction
Abnormal ventilation, coma presentations with, 25*t*
Abscess, CT of, 101
Absence seizures, epilepsy with, 991*t*, 992
Acanthamoeba infections, 257
Acanthocytes, neurologic syndromes with, 671–674, 674*t*
  abetalipoproteinemia in, 671–673, 674*t*
  Bassen-Kornzweig syndrome in, 671–673
  chorea-acanthocytosis in, 673
  hypobetalipoproteinemia in, 673
  Levine-Critchley syndrome in, 673
  McLeod syndrome in, 673–674, 674*t*
  neuroacanthocytosis in, 673, 674*t*
ACD. *See* Apparent diffusion coefficient
Aceruloplasminemia, metal metabolism disorders of, 666–667
Acetylcholine receptor (AChR), myasthenia gravis with, 877–881
Acetylcholinesterase deficiency, myasthenia gravis with, 878
Achondroplasia, *1076*, 1076–1077
  diagnosis of, 1076
  structural malformations of, 590*t*
  symptoms of, 1076
AChR. *See* Acetylcholine receptors
Acoustic nerve injury, cranial/peripheral nerve lesion with, 531
Acquired cerebellar ataxia, 797
Acquired chronic hepatocerebral degeneration, hepatic disease with, 1065
Acquired immunodeficiency syndrome (AIDS), 211–225, 211*t*, 212*t*, 213*t*, 216*t*, *217*, 221*t*, *222*, *223*
  children with, 213
  clinical syndromes associated with, 216–220, 216*t*, *217*
  clinical/laboratory precautions with, 225
  CNS pathogenesis of, 215
  course of, 225
  drug-induced syndromes with, 224–225

epidemiology of, 211–213, 213*t*
etiology of, 213–214
history of, 211
HIV classification and, 211, 211*t*, 212*t*
HIV-related syndromes with, 216–220, 216*t*, *217*
  acute aseptic meningitis as, 216*t*
  acute encephalopathy as, 216*t*
  acute inflammatory demyelinating polyneuropathy as, 216*t*
  ALS as, 219
  autonomic neuropathy as, 216*t*, 219
  Bell palsy as, 216*t*
  cerebellar ataxia as, 216*t*
  cerebrovascular syndromes as, 216*t*
  cranial/peripheral neuropathy as, 216*t*
  dementia as, 216*t*
  leukoencephalitis as, 216*t*, 219
  meningeal pleocytosis as, 216*t*
  myoglobinuria as, 216*t*
  myopathy as, 216*t*, 219, 220
  organic brain syndromes as, 216*t*
  polymyositis as, 216*t*
  seizures as, 216*t*, 219
  transverse myelitis as, 216*t*
neoplasms with, 220–224, 221*t*, *222*, *223*
neurosyphilis and, 241–242
opportunistic infections with, 220–224, 221*t*, *222*, *223*
  focal brain syndromes as, 220
  infectious retinopathy as, 224
  lymphoma as, 223
  movement disorders with, 223–224
  PML with, 220, 223
  spinal cord infection as, 224
  toxoplasmosis as, 220–221, 221*t*, *222*
  viral encephalitis as, 220
pathogenesis of, 214–215
pediatric acquired, 1185–1188, 1186*t*, *1187*, *1188*
  antiretroviral therapy for, 1188
  cerebrospinal fluid with, 1187
  clinical manifestations of, 1185
  CT of, 1187, *1187*
  diagnostic tests for, 1185
  encephalopathy v., 1186
  focal manifestations of, 1186
  HAART for, 1188
  imaging of, 1187, *1187*, *1188*
  MRI of, 1187
  opportunistic central nervous system infection with, 1187
  pathology of, 1186
  primary central nervous system lymphoma with, 1186
  stroke with, 1186–1187, *1187*
polymyositis with, 936
prognosis with, 225
treatment of, 225
Acquired myoglobinuria, 921
Acquired neuropathies, 748–763, *749*, *752*, *754*, *756*
  acromegalic neuropathy as, 754
  alcoholic neuropathy as, 760–761
  amyloid neuropathy as, 753, *754*

brachial neuritis as, 762
carcinoma associated neuropathy as, 753–754
celiac neuropathy as, 755
chronic inflammatory demyelinating polyneuropathy as, 750–751
critical illness polyneuropathy as, 758
cryoglobulinemic neuropathy as, 751–752, *752*
diabetic neuropathy as, 761–762
dietary associated polyneuropathy as, 757–758
diphtheric neuropathy as, 756
Guillain-Barré syndrome as, 748–750, *749*
  course for, 750
  diagnosis/differential diagnosis of, 750
  electrophysiology of, 748, *749*
  etiology of, 748
  incidence of, 748
  laboratory data on, 750
  pathology of, 748, *749*
  prognosis for, 750
  symptoms/signs of, 748
  treatment of, 750
  variants of, 749–750
heavy metal caused neuropathies as, 758–760
  acrylamide monomer in, 759
  arsenic in, 758–759
  dimethylaminopropionitrile in, 759
  lead in, 759
  mercury in, 759
  methylbromide in, 759
  other chemicals in, 759–760
  pyriminil in, 759
  thallium in, 759
  triorthocresyl phosphate in, 759
hepatic disease associated neuropathy as, 755
herpes zoster-related neuropathy as, 757
HIV-related neuropathies as, 756–757
hyperthyroid neuropathy as, 754–755
hypothyroid neuropathy as, 754
idiopathic neuropathy as, 751, 763
IgA monoclonal gammopathies with, 752–753
IgM monoclonal antibodies with, 753
infection associated neuropathy as, 755–757, *756*
leprosy related neuropathy as, 755–756, *756*
Lyme neuropathy as, 762–763
multifocal motor neuropathy as, 751
myeloma with, 752–753
nonmalignant IgG with, 752–753
paraneoplastic neuropathy as, 753–754
sarcoid neuropathy as, 757
sensory neuronopathy/neuropathy as, 751
therapeutic drug caused neuropathies as, 760
uremic neuropathy as, 755
vasculitic neuropathy as, 751–752, *752*

Acromegalic neuropathy, 754
Acromegaly, pituitary endocrine disease of, 1035–1037, *1036, 1037*
Acrylamide monomer, 759
ACTH. *See* Adrenocorticotropic hormone
Action dystonia, 816
Acute akathisia, neuroleptic-induced syndromes with, 849
Acute aseptic meningitis, HIV-related syndromes with, 216t
Acute autonomic neuropathy
    acute cholinergic neuropathy with, 975
    autonomic disorder of, 974–975
    exaggerated orthostatic tachycardia with, 975
    GBS variants of, 750
    management of, 975
    outcome for, 975
    treatment of, 975
Acute brainstem ischemia, MRI with, 106, *107*
Acute cholinergic neuropathy, acute autonomic neuropathy with, 975
Acute disseminated encephalomyelitis (ADEM), 198–200, *200*
    ATM and, 199
    course of, 200
    diagnosis of, 200
    epidemiology of, 199
    etiology of, 198
    laboratory studies on, 200, *200*
    multiple sclerosis v., 954, 957t, 958
    pathogenesis of, 198
    pathology of, 198–199
    prognosis of, 200
    signs/symptoms of, 199
    treatment of, 200
Acute dystonic reactions, neuroleptic-induced syndromes with, 849
Acute encephalopathy
    HIV-related syndromes with, 216t
    occupation/environment neurotoxicology with, 1175
Acute hemorrhagic mass, CT of, 101
Acute inflammatory demyelinating polyneuropathy
    HIV-related syndromes with, 216t
    respiratory dysfunction with, 1085
Acute intermittent porphyria (AIP)
    aminolevulinic acid with, 668
    clinical manifestations of, 669t
    diagnosis of, 670
    differential diagnosis of, 685t
    genetic central nervous disease of, 668–670, 669t, 670t
    incidence of, 669
    laboratory data on, 669–670
    molecular genetics of, 668
    pathogenesis of, 668
    pathology of, 669
    porphobilinogen with, 668
    porphyrin with, 668
    porphyrogenic drugs for, *670*
    protoporphyrinogen oxidase with, 668
    symptoms/signs of, 669, 669t
    treatment of, 670, *670*
    uroporphyrinogen-1 synthase with, 668
    variegate porphyria with, 668
Acute intracerebral hemorrhage, CT scan of, *68*, 69

Acute ischemic brachial neuropathy, radiation injury with, 554
Acute lead encephalopathy, heavy metal intoxication with, 1176
Acute lymphocytic leukemia, blood cell dyscrasias of, 1054
Acute motor axonal neuropathy (AMAN), GBS variants of, 749
Acute motor/sensory axonal neuropathy, GBS variants of, 750
Acute multifocal placoid-pigment epitheliopathy (AMPPE), electrophysiologic vision testing with, 40
Acute pandysautonomia. *See* Acute autonomic neuropathy
Acute purulent meningitis, 139–144, 140t
Acute quadriplegic myopathy (AQM)
    clinical features of, 888t
    corticosteroids causing, 888
    critical-illness polyneuropathy with, 889
    laboratory studies on, 888
    muscle biopsies for, 888–889
    neuromuscular junction disorder of, 888–889, 888t
    nondepolarizing neuromuscular blocking agents causing, 888
Acute sensory neuropathy, GBS variants of, 750
Acute stroke, CT diagnosis of, 75–78
Acute stroke therapy, ESNR with, 118, *119*
Acute symptomatic seizures, epilepsy with, 1000
Acute transverse myelitis (ATM), 199
Acute viral infections, 175–177, 176t
Acute zonal occult outer retinopathy (AZOOR), electrophysiologic vision testing with, 40
ADD. *See* Attention deficit disorder
Addiction, drug dependence with, 1161
Addison disease, 1045
ADEM. *See* Acute disseminated encephalomyelitis
Adenoid cystic carcinoma, 379
Adenoma sebaceum, 724, 725, *725*
Adenovirus infections, 191
Adenyl-succinate deficiency, 587
ADHD. *See* Attention deficit hyperactivity disorder
Adrenal endocrine diseases, 1045–1046, 1046t
    Addison disease with, 1045
    Cushing syndrome with, 1045, 1046t
    hyperadrenalism as, 1045, 1046t
    hypertension with, 1046
    hypoadrenalism as, 1045
    primary hyperadrenalism as, 1045–1046
Adrenocorticotropic hormone (ACTH), pituitary gland tumors with, 421, 423–424
Adrenocorticotropic-hormone function, radiation injury with, 554
Adrenoleukodystrophy (ALD)
    adrenomyeloneuropathy with, 654
    cerebral form of, 655
    dementia resulting from, 779t, 780
    diagnosis of, 656
    differential diagnosis of, 685t, 686t, 687t
    laboratory evaluation of, 656

peroxisomal diseases of, 653t, 654–656, 655t
phenotypes associated with, 655t
structural malformations with, 587
Adult onset primary dystonia, 819–821, *820*
Advance directives, end-of-life issues with, 1201
Advanced-sleep-phase syndrome, 1029
AED. *See* Antiepileptic drugs
Afferent-pupillary defect, Marcus-Gunn syndrome with, 602
AGE. *See* Arterial gas embolism
Age-associated memory impairment (AAMI), dementia diagnosis with, 5
Age-related cognitive change (ARCD), dementia diagnosis with, 5
Agnosia, 12–13
Agrammatism, 9
Agraphia, alexia with, 10
Aicardi syndrome
    differential diagnosis of, 685t
    structural malformations with, 589t
Aicardi-Goutières syndrome, differential diagnosis of, 686t
AIDS. *See* Acquired immunodeficiency syndrome
AIP. *See* Acute intermittent porphyria
Akathisia, 49
    Parkinson disease with, 831
Akinesia, Parkinson disease with, 829
Akinetic mutism, 25
ALA. *See* Aminolevulinic acid
Alcohol, epilepsy with, 1012, 1013t
Alcoholic blackout, ethanol intoxication with, 1152
Alcoholic myopathy, myoglobinuria with, 922
Alcoholic neuropathy, 760–761
Alcoholism, 1151–1160, 1151t, 1152t, 1153t, 1154t, 1155t, 1159t
    amblyopia with, 1156
    cancer with, 1157
    central pontine myelinolysis with, 1158
    cerebellar degeneration with, 1156
    dementia diagnosis with, 5
    dementia with, 1158
    ethanol dependence/withdrawal with, 1153–1154, 1153t, 1154t
    ethanol intoxication with, 1151–1152, 1151t, 1152t
    ethanol-drug interaction with, 1152
    fetal alcohol syndrome with, 1158–1160, 1159t
    hypoglycemia with, 1157
    infection in, 1157
    ketoacidosis with, 1157
    liver disease with, 1157
    Marchiafava-Bignami disease with, 1158
    myopathy with, 1158
    pellagra with, 1157
    polyneuropathy with, 1156
    stroke with, 1158
    trauma in, 1157
    treatment of, 1160
    Wernicke-Korsakoff syndrome with, 1154–1156, 1155t
Alcohol-tobacco amblyopia, cranial/peripheral nerve lesion with, 526

ALD. *See* Adrenoleukodystrophy
Alexander disease
    childhood cerebral degenerations of,
        677–678, *678*
    dementia resulting from, 780
    differential diagnosis of, 686*t*, 687*t*,
        688*t*
Alexia, agraphia with, 10
Alien limb phenomena,
    parkinsonism-plus syndromes
    with, 835
Allelic heterogeneity, DNA diagnostic
    tests with, 136, 136*t*
Allesthesia, neuropathic pain with,
    547
Allodynia
    neuropathic pain with, 547
    pain diagnosis with, 29
Almotriptan, migraine headache treated
    with, 985
Alobar holoprosencephaly, structural
    malformations of, 587
Alpers syndrome, nDNA mutations with,
    708
Alphaviruses, 176*t*, 181
ALS. *See* Amyotrophic lateral sclerosis
Altered mentation, drug dependence
    with, 1164
Aluminum, heavy metal intoxication
    with, 1174*t*, 1178
Alveolar hypoventilation syndrome, sleep
    disorders with, 1026
Alveolar-arterial gradient (A-a gradient),
    respiratory physiology with, 1083
Alzheimer disease, 771–776, *773*, *774*,
    774*t*, 775*t*
    amnestic aphasia with, 11
    brain imaging with, 772
    clinical syndrome of, 771
    CT with, 772
    dementia caused by, 4, 5*t*, 6
    diagnosis of, 771–772
    Down syndrome with, 608
    EEG of, 82
    epidemiology of, 774
    genetic basis of, 774–775, 775*t*
    mood disorders with, 1131
    MRI with, 772
    myoclonus with, 813
    neurologic disorders examination with,
        62
    pathology of, 772–774, *773*, *774*, 774*t*
    Pick disease v., 776
    risk factors for, 775, 775*t*
    tau protein with, 773
    treatment of, 776
    tubulin protein with, 773
AMAN. *See* Acute motor axonal
    neuropathy
Amantadine
    multiple sclerosis treated with, 961
    Parkinson disease drug therapy with,
        837*t*, 838, 839
Amaurosis fugax
    impaired vision with, 42
    transient global amnesia with, 1017
Ambenonium, myasthenia gravis treated
    with, 882
Amblyopia
    alcoholism with, 1156
    ocular motility impairment with, 42
American Spinal Injury Association
    (ASIA), 503

Amino acid metabolism disorders,
    611–618, 615*t*, 616*t*, 617*t*
    Hartnup disease as, 618
    Lowe syndrome as, 618
    maple syrup urine disease as, 614
    other defects of, 615*t*, 616*t*, 617
    phenylketonuria as, 612–614
    sulfur, 614–617, 615*t*
    transport disorders of, 617*t*, 618
Amino acid transport disorders, 617*t*,
    618
    Hartnup disease as, 618
    Lowe syndrome as, 618
Aminoacidurias, differential diagnosis of,
    686*t*
γ-aminobutyric acid (GABA),
    schizophrenia with, 1139–1140
Aminoglycoside antibiotics,
    neuromuscular junction disorders
    induced by, 887
Aminolevulinic acid (ALA), acute
    intermittent porphyria with, 668
Amitriptyline
    migraine headache treated with, 985,
        986*t*
    Parkinson disease drug therapy with,
        837*t*, 840
Amnesia. *See* Anterograde amnesia;
    Transient global amnesia
Amnesic shellfish poisoning,
    occupation/environment
    neurotoxicology with, 1181
Amnestic aphasia, 11
    Alzheimer disease with, 11
    dysnomia and, 11
    primary progressive aphasia with, 11
    Wernicke aphasia with, 11
AMPPE. *See* Acute multifocal
    placoid-pigment epitheliopathy
Amyloid neuropathy, 753, *754*
Amyotrophic lateral sclerosis (ALS)
    autosomal dominant pattern of, 864,
        864*t*
    benign fasciculation and cramps
        syndrome with, 868
    clinical classification of, 866, 866*t*
    clinical manifestations of, 865–866
    Denny-Brown, Foley syndrome with,
        868
    diagnosis of, 866–868
    epidemiology of, 863–864, 864*t*
    Hirayama syndrome with, 867
    HIV-related syndromes with, 219
    laboratory data on, 866
    MMNCB with, 867
    monomelic muscular atrophy with, 867
    motor neuron diseases of, 863–868,
        864*t*, 866*t*
    multiple sclerosis with, 867
    myasthenia gravis with, 867
    occupation/environment
        neurotoxicology with, 1173
    pathogenesis of, 864–865
    postpolio syndrome with, 867
    progressive bulbar palsy with, 866
    pseudobulbar palsy with, 865, 867
    respiratory dysfunction with, 1085
    reversible motor neuron disease with,
        868
    syringomyelia v., 873
    treatment of, 868
ANCL (Adult variant neuronal caroid
    lipofuscinoses). *See* Kufs disease

Andersen syndrome, familial periodic
    paralysis with, 912
Angelman syndrome, 608, 609–610
    DNA maintenance/transcription/
        translation disorders of, 649*t*
    genomic imprinting with, 609
    molecular basis of, 609
Angioblastic meningiomas, 458
Angiography, SAH diagnosis with, 331,
    332
Angioplasty, catheter angiography with,
    109
Animal poisons, occupation/environment
    neurotoxicology with, 1174*t*,
    1180–1181
Ankylosing spondylitis, bone disease of,
    1077
Anorexia nervosa, malnutrition with,
    1092
Antebrachial cutaneous nerves, 536
Antegren. *See* Natalizumab
Antegren, multiple sclerosis treated with,
    960
Anterior ischemic optic neuropathy,
    impaired vision with, 39, *40*
Anterior temporal lobe resection,
    epilepsy treated with, 1008, 1009*t*
Anterior-cord syndrome, spinal injury
    trauma with, 504–505
Anterograde amnesia, transient global
    amnesia with, 1017
Antiamphiphysin, paraneoplastic
    syndromes with, 1090
Antibiotic-induced neuromuscular
    blockade, 887
Antibiotics, head injury trauma with,
    496
Anticardiolipin antibodies, coagulation
    disorders with, 1058
Anticardiolipin antibody syndrome,
    cerebrovascular syndromes of,
    309
Anticholinergic drugs, Parkinson disease
    drug therapy with, 837*t*, 839–840
Anticholinergics, drug dependence with,
    1161*t*, 1163
Anticholinesterase drug therapy,
    myasthenia gravis treated with,
    882
Anticonvulsive drugs
    head injury trauma with, 495
    Krabbe-Weber disease treated with,
        456
    neuropathic pain treated with, 549
    sleep disorders treated with, 1027
    Sturge-Weber disease treated with,
        456
    tumor treatment with, 376–377
Antidepressant medications, 1129–1130,
    1129*t*
Antiepileptic drugs (AED)
    epilepsy treated with, 1001–1006,
        1001*t*, 1002*t*, 1003*t*, *1004*
    neuropathic pain with, 549
    pregnancy with, 1112–1114, 1113*t*
Anti-Hu, paraneoplastic syndromes with,
    1090
Antineoplastic drugs
    cancer chemotherapy complications
        with, 1168–1169, 1169*t*
    central nervous system toxicity with,
        1170–1171
    other agents in, 1170

Antineoplastic drugs (*contd.*)
  peripheral nervous system toxicity
    with, 1169–1170
  platins in, 1169
  taxanes in, 1170
  vinca alkaloids in, 1169
Antineuronal cytoplasmic autoantibody
    (ANCA), vasculitis syndromes
    with, 1104–1105
Antinociceptive agents, neuropathic pain
    treated with, 549
Antiphospholipid syndrome,
    cerebrovascular syndromes of,
    309
Antipsychotic medication, schizophrenia
    with, 1140–1141, 1142*t*
Antiretroviral therapy, pediatric acquired
    HIV/AIDS with, 1188
Antithrombin deficiency, coagulation
    disorders of, 1056–1057
Anxiety disorders, 1132–1137
  animal models of, 1133
  Aplysia with, 1133
  definition of, 1132–1133
  differential diagnosis of, 1134
  Drosophila with, 1133
  epidemiology of, 1133
  generalized anxiety disorder as, 1133,
    1136–1137
  obsessive-compulsive disorder as,
    1133, 1135–1136
  pathophysiology of, 1133
  post-traumatic stress disorder as, 1133,
    1135
  separation, 1133
  signs/symptoms of, 1133
  social phobias of, 1133, 1134–1135
  specific phobias as, 1133, 1134–1135
  treatment of, 1134
AOA. *See* Oculomotor apraxia
Apert syndrome, structural
    malformations with, 589*t*, 594*t*
Aphasia, 8–11
  amnestic, 11
  conduction, 8
  motor, 8, 9–10
  primary progressive, 9
  pure alexia, 9
  pure word deafness, 9
  pure word mutism, 9
  sensory, 8, 10–11
  stroke with, 9
  subcortical motor, 9
  subcortical sensory, 9
  transcortical motor, 9
  transcortical sensory, 8–9
Aplysia, anxiety disorders with, 1133
Apneustic breathing, coma examination
    with, 22
Apomorphine, Parkinson disease drug
    therapy with, 837–838, 837*t*
Apparent diffusion coefficient (ACD),
    MRI with, 75
Applied RF flip angle, 69
Apraxia, 11–12
  ideational dyspraxia as, 11–12
  ideomotor dyspraxia as, 12
  lid opening, Parkinson disease with,
    830
  limb-kinetic dyspraxia as, 11
  senile gait disorders with, 60
Aprosody, Parkinson disease with, 830
AQM. *See* Acute quadriplegic myopathy

Arboviruses infections, 181
  clinical syndromes of, 181
  diagnosis of, 181
  epidemiology of, 181
ARCD. *See* Age-related cognitive change
Arenavirus infections, 190
Argentinian hemorrhagic fever, 190
Arhinencephaly, structural
    malformations of, 587
Arm pain, 30–31
Arnold-Chiari malformations, 596–599,
    597, 598, 599
  diagnosis of, 599
  incidence of, 596–597
  multiple sclerosis v., 956, 957*t*
  obstructive hydrocephalus with, 350
  pathology of, 596
  symptoms/signs of, 598–599
  syringomyelia with, 871, 873
  treatment of, 599
Arsenic, 758–759
  heavy metal intoxication with, 1174*t*,
    1177–1178
Arterial gas embolism (AGE),
    decompression sickness with, 558,
    559
Arterial spin labeling (ASL), MRI with,
    70, 75
Arterial thrombosis
  children's stroke with, *317*, 318–319, *319*
  coagulopathies with, 319
  inflammatory bowel disease with, 319
  malignancies with, 319
  migraine with, 319
  moyamoya syndrome with, 318, *319,
    320*
Arteriovenous malformations (AVM)
  ESNR with, 118–120, *120, 121*
  MRA with, 74
  vascular malformations of, 449–454,
    450, 451, 452, 453
    clinical presentation of, *450, 451, 452,
      452, 453*
    CT scan of, 452, *452*
    diagnosis of, *450, 451, 452, 452, 453*
    left parietal, *450*
    MRA of, 452, 454
    MRI of, 452, *452*
    right temporal, *451*
    risks with, 451
    surgery for, 453–454
    treatment for, 452–454
Arthralgia, polymyositis with, 933
Arthropathy, peripheral neuropathies
    with, 735
Aseptic meningeal reaction, 162
ASIA. *See* American Spinal Injury
    Association
ASL. *See* Arterial spin labeling
Aspartylglucosaminuria, differential
    diagnosis of, 686*t*
Aspartylglycosaminuria, lysosomal/other
    storage diseases of, 638*t*, 639
Aspergillus, renal transplantation
    neurologic complications with,
    1082
Astasia-abasia, gait disorders with, 58
Astatic seizures, epilepsy with, 992
Asterixis, uremic encephalopathy with,
    1079
Astrocytomas, 393–394, 394*t*, 397–400
  biological agents for, 433
  brain-stem gliomas with, 436

cerebellar, 435, *435*
cerebral-hemisphere gliomas with,
    438
chemotherapy for, 398–399, 433, 436
childhood central nervous system
    tumors of, 429–433, 431*t*, 432*t*,
    435–439, *436, 437, 438*
diagnosis of, 431–433, 433*t*
  MRI in, 431, *435, 436*, 436–437
diencephalic gliomas with, 437
EGF with, 429–430
four grads of, 394, 394*t*
glioblastoma multiforme with, 438
low-grade, 399–400
management of, 431–433, 433*t*
optic pathway gliomas with, 437
PDGF with, 429–430
radiation therapy for, 432–433
radiotherapy for, 398
recurrent malignant, 399
spinal cord, 439
surgery for, 398, 431
symptoms of, 430–431
therapy of, 397–399
VEGF with, 438
Asymptomatic neurosyphilis, 238
Ataxia telangiectasia, 784*t*, 786–787, *787*,
    788*t*
  differential diagnosis of, 687*t*, 688*t*
  DNA maintenance/transcription/
    translation disorders of, 649*t*
Ataxia with vitamin E deficiency (AVED),
    784*t*, 787, *787*, 788*t*
Ataxias
  acquired cerebellar, 797
  autosomal-dominant, 784*t*, 789*t*,
    790–796
    dentatorubralpallidoluysian atrophy
      as, 784*t*, 789*t*, 796
    genetic testing for, 796
    Machado-Joseph disease as, 784*t*,
      789*t*, 792–793
    other unmapped cerebellar ataxias
      as, 796
    SCA as, 784*t*, 789*t*, 791–796
  autosomal-recessive, 783–790, 784*t*,
    787, 788*t*
    ataxia telangiectasia as, 784*t*,
      786–787, *787*, 788*t*
    diagnostic evaluation of, 788–790,
      789*t*
    Friedreich ataxia as, 783–786, 784*t*,
      788*t*
    infantile-onset spinocerebellar ataxia
      as, 784*t*, 788, 788*t*
    Marinesco-Sjögren syndrome as,
      784*t*, 788, 788*t*
    MERRF as, 788, 790
    oculomotor apraxia with, 784*t*, 786,
      788*t*
    progressive myoclonus epilepsy as,
      788
    Ramsay Hunt syndrome as, 788
    Unverricht-Lundborg disease as, 788
    vitamin E deficiency with, 784*t*, 787,
      787, 788*t*
    X-linked hereditary ataxias as, 790
  congenital cerebellar, 797
  drug dependence with, 1165
  episodic, 796–797
  hereditary, 783–797, 784*t*, *787*, 788*t*,
    789*t*
    classification of, 783

epidemiology of, 783
management of, 797
paroxysmal, 796–797
sporadic cerebellar, 797
Ataxic breathing, coma examination
with, 22
Ataxic cerebral palsy, motor function
disorders of, 578
Ataxic gait, 58
Atherothrombotic brain infarction (ABI),
stroke treatment with, 324–325
Athetosis, 49, 59
Athetotic dystonia, 49
Atlantoaxial dislocation, bone disease of, 1077
Atlas, structural malformations of, 592
ATM. *See* Acute transverse myelitis
Atonic seizures, epilepsy with, 991*t*, 992
ATRT. *See* Atypical teratoid/rhabdoid
tumor
Attention deficit disorder (ADD)
language disorders with, 582–583
management of, 583
Attention deficit hyperactivity disorder
(ADHD)
language disorders with, 582–583
management of, 583
Attention, neuropsychologic evaluation
tests for, 132
Atypical absence seizures, epilepsy with,
992
Atypical teratoid/rhabdoid tumor (ATRT),
childhood central nervous system
tumors with, 429, 439, 441
Auditory agnosia, 13
Autism
course of, 584
disintegrative disorder with, 584
etiology of, 583
hyperlexia with, 584
language disorders of, 583–585
management of, 584–585
pathology/pathophysiology of, 584
prognosis for, 584
symptoms of, 583–584
Autley-Bixler syndrome, structural
malformations with, 594*t*
Autoantibodies, coagulation disorders of,
1058
Autonomic disorders
acute autonomic neuropathy as,
974–975
autonomic failure as, 971–974, 971*t*,
972*t*, 973*t*
chronic autonomic neuropathies
with, 973
diabetic autonomic neuropathy with,
973
diagnosis of, 973–974, 973*t*
dopamine β-hydroxylase deficiency
with, 972, 972*t*
factors affecting, 971*t*
multiple system atrophy with, 971,
972, 972*t*, 974
parkinsonian syndromes with,
971–973, 972*t*
Shy-Drager syndromes with, 971
familial dysautonomia as, 976–978
biochemical data on, 977
clinical presentation of, 976
diagnosis of, 977
gastroesophageal dysfunction with,
977
laparoscopic surgery for, 977–978

midodrine for, 978
pathological data on, 977
pathophysiology of, 977
prognosis for, 977
treatment of, 977–978
neurogenic orthostatic hypotension as,
971–974, 971*t*, 972*t*, 973*t*
botulism with, 972*t*
chronic autonomic neuropathies
with, 973
diabetic autonomic neuropathy with,
973
diagnosis of, 973–974, 973*t*
dopamine β-hydroxylase deficiency
with, 972, 972*t*
factors affecting, 971*t*
fatal familial insomnia with, 972*t*
Guillain-Barré syndrome with, 972*t*
Holmes-Adie syndrome with, 972*t*
Machado-Joseph disease with, 972*t*
multiple system atrophy with, 971,
972, 972*t*, 974
parkinsonian syndromes with,
971–973, 972*t*
Shy-Drager syndromes with, 971
Sjögren disease with, 972*t*
syringomyelia with, 972*t*
transverse myelitis with, 972*t*
Wernicke-Korsakoff syndrome with,
972*t*
Autonomic neuropathy, HIV-related
syndromes with, 216*t*, 219
Autosomal-dominant ataxias, 784*t*, 789*t*,
790–796
dentatorubralpallidoluysian atrophy
as, 784*t*, 789*t*, 796
genetic testing for, 796
Machado-Joseph disease as, 784*t*, 789*t*,
792–793
other unmapped cerebellar ataxias as,
796
SCA1 as, 784*t*, 789*t*, 791–796
Autosomal-recessive ataxias, 783–790,
784*t*, 787, 788*t*
ataxia telangiectasia as, 784*t*, 786–787,
787, 788*t*
diagnostic evaluation of, 788–790, 789*t*
Friedreich ataxia as, 783–786, 784*t*,
788*t*
clinical expression of, 785
diagnostic testing for, 786
early-onset, 785
genetics of, 784–785
genotype-phenotype correlations
with, 785
laboratory testing for, 786
late-onset, 785
neuropathology of, 785
treatment of, 786
very-late-onset, 785
infantile-onset spinocerebellar ataxia
as, 784*t*, 788, 788*t*
Marinesco-Sjögren syndrome as, 784*t*,
788, 788*t*
MERRF as, 788, 790
oculomotor apraxia with, 784*t*, 786,
788*t*
progressive myoclonus epilepsy as, 788
Ramsay Hunt syndrome as, 788
Unverricht-Lundborg disease as, 788
vitamin E deficiency with, 784*t*, 787,
787, 788*t*
X-linked hereditary ataxias as, 790

AVED. *See* Ataxia with vitamin E
deficiency
AVM. *See* Arteriovenous malformations
Axillary nerve, 534, 534*t*, 536
Axis, structural malformations of, 592
Axonal neuropathy, nerve biopsy and, 129
Axonal shearing injury, head injury
trauma with, 483–484, *485*
AZOOR. *See* Acute zonal occult outer
retinopathy

B
Babinski signs
abetalipoproteinemia with, 672
Moersch-Woltman syndrome with, 928
weak muscles with, 53
Bacterial infections, 139–164, 140*t*, *145,
146, 151, 152, 153*
acute purulent meningitis as, 139–144,
140*t*
aseptic meningeal reaction as, 162
Behçet syndrome as, 160–161
brucellosis as, 160
cerebral subdural empyema as,
148–150
epidural infections as, 148–157, *151,
152, 153*
Escherichia coli with, 139, 143, 151
Hemophilus influenzae meningitis as,
142–143
Hemophilus influenzae with, 139, 140*t*,
142–143
human ehrlichiosis as, 159–160
infective endocarditis as, 154–155
intracranial epidural abscess as, 150,
151
Legionella pneumophila infection as,
163–164
leprosy as, 155–156
meningism as, 163
meningococcal meningitis as, 139–142
Mollaret meningitis as, 161–162
Mycoplasma pneumoniae infection as,
163
Neisseria meningitidis with, 139–142,
140*t*
other acute meningitis as, 143–144
pneumococcal meningitis as, 143
recurrent bacterial meningitis as, 144
rickettsial infections as, 157–160
Rocky Mountain spotted fever as,
157–158
scrub typhus as, 158–159
spinal epidural abscess as, 150–154,
152, 153
staphylococcal meningitis as, 143
streptococcal meningitis as, 143
Streptococcus pneumoniae with, 139, 140*t*,
143
subacute meningitis as, 144–148, *145,
146*
subdural infections as, 148–150
tuberculous meningitis as, *145,*
145–148, *146*
typhus fever as, 158
unknown cause acute purulent
meningitis as, 144
Vogt-Koyanagi-Harada syndrome as,
161
Bacterial toxins, 259–262
botulism as, 261–262
diphtheria as, 259
tetanus as, 259–261

BAEP. *See* Brainstem auditory evoked potentials
Baller-Gerold syndrome, 594*t*
Ballism, 48
Bariatric surgery, malabsorption from, 1093, 1093*t*
Basal ganglia disease, neurologic disorders examination with, 63
Basal-cell nevus syndrome (BCNS), childhood central nervous system tumors with, 428
Basilar artery migraine, seizure with, 18*t*, 19
Basilar impression, structural malformations of, *591*, 591–592
Basilar migraine, 982
  syncope with, 17, 18*t*
Basilar skull fractures, head injury trauma with, 483
Bassen-Kornzweig syndrome
  Babinski signs with, 672
  clinical findings on, *672*
  diagnosis of, 672
  laboratory data on, 672
  MTP with, 672
  neurologic abnormalities with, 672
  neurologic syndromes of, 671–673
  pathogenesis of, 672
  symptoms/signs of, 672
  treatment for, 672–673
BCNS. *See* Basal-cell nevus syndrome
BEC. *See* Blood ethanol concentration
Becker muscular dystrophy (BMD), *898*, 899–901, *900*
  cardiac function with, 901
  diagnosis of, 899
  gene replacement for, 900
  intermediate phenotype with, 899
  manifesting carriers of, 899
  molecular genetics of, 899–900, *900*
  orthopedic measures for, 901
  precautions for, 901
  prednisone therapy for, 900
  pulmonary function with, 901
  rehabilitation for, 901
  supportive management for, 900
  treatment of, 900–901
Behavior modification, somatoform disorders treated with, 1145
Behçet syndrome, 160–161
  course of, 161
  diagnosis of, 161
  etiology of, 160
  laboratory data on, 161
  multiple sclerosis v., 956, 957*t*
  pathology of, 160
  symptoms/signs of, 160–161
  treatment for, 161
Bell palsy
  Cranial/peripheral nerve lesion with, 530
  HIV-related syndromes with, 216*t*
  pregnancy with, 1116
Benign epilepsy syndromes, epilepsy with, 1000–1001
Benign familial neonatal convulsion (BFNC), neonatal seizures with, 570
Benign fasciculation and cramps syndrome, 925
  motor neuron diseases with, 868
Benign focal epilepsy, 993–994

Benign partial epilepsy of childhood, 1001
Benign positional paroxysmal vertigo (BPPV)
  Dix-Hallpike maneuver for, 36
  vertigo/hearing loss caused by, 36–37
Benign rolandic epilepsy, 82*t*
Benign-congenital hypotonia, floppy infant syndrome with, 576
Benserazide, Parkinson disease drug therapy with, 837, 837*t*
Benzerazide, sleep disorders treated with, 1026
Benzodiazepines, sleep disorders treated with, 1027
Beriberi, dietary associated polyneuropathy with, 757
Bethlem myopathy, muscular dystrophy of, 909
BFNC. *See* Benign familial neonatal convulsion
Bibrachial paresis, weak muscles with, 55
Bilharziasis, 247*t*, 249–250, *250*
  clinical manifestations of, 249–250
  diagnosis of, 250
  epidemiology of, 249
  laboratory data on, 250, *250*
  pathology of, 249
  treatment of, 250
Bing-Neel syndrome, blood cell dyscrasias of, 1055
Biochemical assays, muscle biopsy with, 128
Biologic response modifiers, cancer chemotherapy complications with, 1171
BiPAP, 1087
Bipolar disorders
  differential diagnosis of, 1130
  mood disorders as, 1130–1131
  treatment of, 1130–1131
Birth injuries/developmental abnormalities
  developmental disorders of higher cerebral functions as, 579–580, 579*t*, 581*t*
  developmental disorders of motor function as, 576–579, 577*t*
  developmental language disorders as, 580–585
  floppy infant syndrome as, 573–576, 574*t*
  hypoxic-ischemic encephalopathy as, 565–567
  intracranial hemorrhage as, 563
  Laurence-Moon-Biedl syndrome as, 586
  Marcus-Gunn syndrome as, 601–602
  Möbius syndrome as, 602
  neonatal herpes encephalitis as, 567
  neonatal infections as, 567–568
  neonatal meningitis as, 567–568
  neonatal neurology as, 563–571, *564*, 568*t*, *569*, 570*t*
  neonatal seizures as, 568–571, 568*t*, *569*, 570*t*
  parenchymal cerebral hemorrhage as, 563
  periventricular intraventricular hemorrhage as, 563–564, *564*
  periventricular leukomalacia as, 565
  posterior fossa hemorrhage as, 563

primary subarachnoid supratentorial hemorrhage as, 563
  static disorders of brain development as, 576–585, 577*t*, 579*t*, 581*t*
  structural malformations as, 587–599, *588*, 589*t*, 590*t*, *591*, 591*t*, *593*, *594*, 594*t*, *595*, *596*, *597*, *598*, *599*
    achondroplasia as, 590*t*
    adenyl-succinate deficiency with, 587
    adrenoleukodystrophy with, 587
    Aicardi syndrome as, 589*t*
    alobar holoprosencephaly as, 587
    Apert syndrome with, 589*t*, 594*t*
    arhinencephaly as, 587
    Arnold-Chiari, 596–599, *597*, *598*, *599*
    atlas, 592
    Autley-Bixler syndrome with, 594*t*
    axis, 592
    Baller-Gerold syndrome with, 594*t*
    basilar impression as, *591*, 591–592
    brachycephaly with, 593
    Carpenter syndrome with, 594*t*
    cerebral gigantism as, 590*t*
    cervical spine, 589–592, 591*t*
    cervical vertebrae fusion as, 592, *593*
    Cowden disease as, 590*t*
    craniosynostosis as, 592–593, *594*, 594*t*
    cranium bifidum, 593–596, 595*t*, *596*
    Crouzon syndrome with, 594*t*
    dolichocephalic skull with, 593
    Fanconi anemia syndrome with, 589*t*
    FG syndrome as, 590*t*
    fucosidosis as, 590*t*
    glutaric aciduria with, 587
    Greig cephalopolysyndactyly as, 590*t*
    Hurler-Scheie as, 590*t*
    hydrocephalus ex vacuo with, 589
    Kleeblattschädel skull with, 593
    Klippel-Trenaunay-Weber as, 590*t*
    lissencephaly as, 587
    macrocephaly as, 588–589, 590*t*
    Maroteaux-Larny as, 590*t*
    Meckel-Gruber syndrome with, 595
    megalencephaly as, 588–589, 590*t*
    Menkes syndrome with, 587
    Miller-Dieker syndrome with, 589*t*
    mitochondrial respiratory chain as, 590*t*
    mucopolysaccharidosis as, 590*t*
    Neu-Laxova syndrome with, 589*t*
    neural tube closure, 595*t*
    occipital bone, 589–592, 591*t*
    oral-facial digital syndrome with, 589*t*
    osteochondrodysplasia syndrome with, 589*t*
    osteopetrosis as, 590*t*
    Pfeiffer syndrome with, 594*t*
    premature cranial suture closure as, 592–593, *594*, 594*t*
    Proteus syndrome as, 590*t*
    pyruvate-dehydrogenase deficiency with, 587
    Robinow syndrome as, 590*t*
    Ruvalcaba-Myhre syndrome as, 590*t*
    Saethre-Chotzen syndrome with, 594*t*
    scaphocephalic skull with, 593
    Shapiro syndrome with, 589*t*
    Sotos syndrome as, 590*t*
    spina bifida, 593–596, 595*t*, *596*
    spina bifida occulta, 595

trigonocephaly with, 593
   trisomy 9p syndrome as, 590*t*
   Walker-Warburg syndrome with, 595
   XK syndrome with, 589*t*
   Zellweger syndrome with, 587
   subarachnoid hemorrhage as, 563
   supratentorial subdural hemorrhage
      as, 563
Bladder function, spinal injury trauma
   with, 508
Blepharospasm, 820
Blindness, drug dependence with, 1165
Blinking tics, dystonia with, 820
Blood cell dyscrasias, 1054–1056, *1056*
   acute lymphocytic leukemia as, 1054
   Bing-Neel syndrome as, 1055
   chronic leukemia as, 1055
   CLL as, 1055
   extramedullary hematopoiesis as, 1056
   hyperphagia with, 1054
   hyperviscosity syndrome as, 1055
   leukemia as, 1054–1055
   leukostasis as, 1054
   lymphoproliferative diseases as, 1055
   MGUS as, 1055
   myelin-associated glycoprotein with,
      1055
   myelofibrosis with, 1056
   myelogenous leukemia as, 1055
   myeloma with, 1055
   obesity with, 1055
   plasma cell dyscrasias as, 1055–1056,
      1056
   plasmacytoma as, 1055
   Waldenström macroglobulinemia as,
      1055
Blood element abnormalities,
   cerebrovascular syndromes of, 311
Blood ethanol concentration (BEC),
   ethanol intoxication with,
   1151–1152, 1151*t*
Blood-oxygen-level-dependent method
   (BOLD), MRI with, 75
BMD. *See* Becker muscular dystrophy
Body dysmorphic disorder, somatoform
   disorders as, 1143
BOLD. *See* Blood-oxygen-level-dependent
   method
Bolivian hemorrhagic fever, 190
Bolus-tracking method, MRI with, 74
Bone disease, 1073–1077, *1074, 1075, 1076*
   achondroplasia as, *1076,* 1076–1077
   ankylosing spondylitis as, 1077
   atlantoaxial dislocation as, 1077
   chondrodystrophy as, *1076,* 1076–1077
   fibrous dysplasia as, 1074–1076, *1076*
   osteitis deformans as, 1073–1074, *1074,*
      1075
   Paget disease as, 1073–1074, *1074, 1075*
Bone health, epilepsy with, 1007
Botulism, 261–262
   Clostridium botulinum toxin with, 886
   course of, 262
   diagnosis of, 262
   neuromuscular junction disorder from,
      886–887
   orthostatic hypotension with, 972*t*
   pathogenesis of, 261
   respiratory dysfunction with, 1085
   symptoms/signs of, 261–262
   treatment of, 262
Bourneville disease. *See* Tuberous
   sclerosis complex

Bowel training, spinal injury trauma
   influencing, 508
BPPV. *See* Benign positional paroxysmal
   vertigo
Brachial amyotrophy, syringomyelia
   with, 871
Brachial cutaneous nerves, 536
Brachial neuritis, 762
Brachial plexopathy
   drug dependence with, 1165
   radiation injury with, 554
Brachial plexus, 533–536, *534,* 534*t*
Brachycephaly, structural malformations
   with, 593
Bradyphrenia, Parkinson disease with,
   831
Brain abscess
   diagnostic tests for, 171–172, *172*
   etiology of, 168–169
   focal infections of, 168–173, *169, 170,*
      172
   incidence of, 170
   pathology of, 169, *169, 170*
   prognosis for, 173
   symptoms/signs of, 170–171
   treatment of, 172–173
Brain death, criteria for determination
   of, 27*t*–28*t,* 28
Brain edema, 357–360, 358*t*
   cellular (cytotoxic), 357–358, 358*t*
   fulminant hepatic encephalopathy
      with, 358
   glucocorticoids for, 359–360
   granulocytic, 359
   hydrocephalic, 358*t,* 359
   interstitial, 358*t,* 359
   ischemic, 358
   osmotherapy for, 360
   other therapy for, 360
   therapeutic considerations for, 359
   vasogenic, 357, 358*t*
Brain infraction
   cardiac embolism with, 282, 282*t*
   cerebrovascular disease with, 278–284,
      279, 280, 281, 281*t,* 282*t, 283, 284t*
   cryptogenic infraction in, 284
   large-vessel atherosclerotic infraction
      in, 281, *281,* 281*t*
   small vessel lacunar infarction in,
      282–284, *283,* 284*t*
Brain metastasis, 459
   chemotherapy for, 463–464
   clinical evaluation of, 460
   clinical findings on, 460, *460*
   CT of, 460, 461
   differential diagnosis for, 461
   imaging of, 460, *461*
   lymphoma with, 407
   MRI of, 460, 461, *461*
   pathophysiology of, 461–462
   radiotherapy for, 462
   stereotactic radiosurgery for, 462, *463*
   surgery for, 462–463
   treatment of, 462–464
   WBRT for, 462, *463*
Brain tumor headache, paroxysmal
   disorder of, 989
Brainstem auditory evoked potentials
   (BAEP), 85–87, *86, 87*
   neurologic disorders with, 86–87, *87*
Brainstem disease
   neurologic disorders examination with, 62
   respiratory dysfunction with, 1084

Brainstem encephalitis, paraneoplastic
   syndrome of, 1089
Brain-stem gliomas, astrocytomas with,
   436
Brainstem infarction, MRI showing, 106,
   107
Breathy dysphonia, dystonia with, 820
Broca aphasia, 9
   language disorders of, 581
Bromide, myasthenia gravis treated with,
   882
Bromocriptine, Parkinson disease drug
   therapy with, 837, 837*t*
Brown-Séquard syndrome
   spinal injury trauma with, 504–505
   spinal tumors with, 471, 477
Brucellosis, 160
Bunyaviruses, 176*t,* 181
Burned out Ménière disease, 1019
Burr-hole, head injury trauma surgery
   with, 493

C
CABG. *See* Coronary artery bypass graft
CADASIL. *See* Cerebral autosomal-
   dominant arteriopathy with
   subcortical infarcts and
   leukoencephalopathy
   stroke genetics with, 307
CAE. *See* Complete audiologic evaluation
Cafe au lait spots
   neurofibromatosis with, 713, 714,
      715
   tuberous sclerosis complex with, 726
California encephalitis, 185
   diagnosis of, 185
   epidemiology of, 185
   incidence of, 185
   symptoms of, 185
CAMP. *See* Compound motor nerve action
   potential
Canavan disease
   childhood cerebral degenerations of,
      675–676, *676*
   CT of, 675, *676*
   diagnosis of, 676
   differential diagnosis of, 685*t,* 686*t,*
      687*t,* 688*t*
   MRI of, 675
Cancer, alcoholism with, 1157
Cancer chemotherapy complications,
   1168–1172, 1169*t*
   antineoplastic drugs with, 1168–1169,
      1169*t*
   biologic response modifiers with, 1171
   central nervous system toxicity with,
      1170–1171
   hematopoietic stem cell
      transplantation with, 1171–1172
   immunosuppressant drugs with, 1171
   peripheral nervous system toxicity
      with, 1169–1170
Candle gutterings, 725, *725*
Carbamates, 1174*t,* 1178–1179
Carbamazepine (Tegretol)
   epilepsy treated with, 1001, 1003,
      1003*t,* 1004
   multiple sclerosis treated with, 961
   sleep disorders with, 1027
Carbidopa
   Parkinson disease drug therapy with,
      837, 837*t*
   sleep disorders treated with, 1026

Carbohydrate metabolism disorders
genetic central nervous diseases of, 641–644, 642t
glycogen storage diseases as, 641–643, 642t
Lafora disease as, 643–644
polyglucosan storage diseases as, 643–644
Carbon monoxide, occupation/environment neurotoxicology with, 1174t, 1180
Carcinoma associated neuropathy, 753–754
Cardiac arrhythmia, vertigo/hearing loss caused by, 37
Cardiac embolism, 282, 282t
Cardiac surgery, cerebral complications of, 1067–1072
CABG with, 1069, 1071–1072
cardiac transplantation with, 1070, 1070
carotid surgery with, 1071–1072
cholesterol emboli syndrome with, 1070
clinical features with, 1069
conclusion to, 1072
hypothermia with, 1071
interventional cardiac procedures with, 1070
pathophysiology with, 1068, 1068–1069
preventing, 1070–1071
problem magnitude with, 1067–1068
risk factors with, 1069–1070
SCAD with, 1068
Cardiac syncope, 14t, 16
Cardiac transplantation, cerebral complications of, 1070, 1070
Cardiogenic emboli, cerebrovascular syndromes of, 311
Carotic occlusive disease, 116
Carotid artery occlusion, transient global amnesia with, 1017
Carotid Revascularization Endarterectomy versus Stent Trial (CREST), endovascular revascularization with, 116
Carotid sinus syncope, 14t, 15
Carotid surgery, cerebral complications of, 1071–1072
Carotid-cavernous fistula, head injury trauma with, 496–497
Carotidynia syndrome
headache with, 46
migraine headache with, 982
Carpal tunnel syndrome, pregnancy with, 1116
Carpenter syndrome, structural malformations with, 594t
Catamenial migraine, gonads endocrine diseases with, 1046
Catamenial seizures, epilepsy with, 1006
Cataplexy, 1027
Catatonia, coma with, 25
Catheter angiography
angioplasty with, 109
intracranial aneurysms with, 109
intracranial atheromatous with, 109
moyamoya stenoses with, 109
neurovascular imaging with, 108–109, 109
superselective microcatheter techniques with, 109

symptomatic vasospasm-induced stenoses with, 109
Cauda equina lesions, 504–505
Cauda equina tumors, 476
Causalgia
neuropathic pain with, 545
pain diagnosis with, 30–31
Cautious gait, 59
Cavernous malformations, 454, 455
Cavernous sinus thrombosis, 339
CBC. See Complete blood count
CBF. See Cerebral blood flow
CBTRUS. See Central Brain Tumor Registry - United States
CBV. See Cerebral blood volume
CCM. See Central core disease
CDG. See Congenital disorder of glycosylation
CECT. See Contrast-enhanced computed tomography
Celiac disease, malabsorption with, 1093
Celiac neuropathy, 755
Central apnea, 1025–1026
Central Brain Tumor Registry - United States (CBTRUS), 371
Central core disease (CCM), congenital muscle disorder of, 916–917, 916t
Central nervous system toxicity, 1170–1171
Central nociception, 546
Central pontine myelinolysis, 965–967, 966
alcoholism with, 1158
cause of, 967
clinical manifestations of, 965
FLAIR with, 965
MRI of, 965–967, 966
myelinolysis with, 965
pathology of, 967
prevention of, 967
Central transtentorial herniation, coma presentations with, 24
Central-cord syndrome, 504–505
Cerebellar astrocytomas, 435, 435
Cerebellar ataxia
HIV-related syndromes with, 216t
thyroid endocrine diseases with, 1039
Cerebellar degeneration, alcoholism with, 1156
Cerebellar disease
gait disorders with, 58
occupation/environment neurotoxicology with, 1176
Cerebellar white matter changes, drug dependence with, 1165
Cerebellopontine angle meningiomas, 392
Cerebellopontine angle tumors, vertigo/hearing loss caused by, 37
Cerebral amyloid angiopathy, cerebrovascular syndromes of, 309
Cerebral aneurysms
ESNR with, 114–116, 115, 116t
ISAT with, 114
ISUIA assessment of, 114
Rankin score for, 114, 116t
Cerebral autosomal-dominant arteriopathy with subcortical infarcts and leukoencephalopathy (CADASIL), vascular dementia as, 778
Cerebral blindness, 41–42
Cerebral blood flow (CBF), MRI with, 107

Cerebral blood volume (CBV), MRI with, 107
Cerebral concussion
head injury trauma with, 483–484, 484t
ICH with, 484
Cerebral disease, neurologic disorders examination with, 62
Cerebral edema
head injury trauma with, 484–485
SAH with, 333, 333
Cerebral embolism in children, 321, 321
Cerebral gigantism, 590t
Cerebral hemorrhage, pregnancy with, 1115
Cerebral infarction, 295–302, 296, 297, 298, 299t, 300, 301t, 302t
CT of, 101, 101–104
EEG of, 81, 83
specific vessel occlusions with, 295–300, 296–298, 299t
anterior cerebral artery in, 297–298, 299t
anterior choroidal artery in, 299–300
internal choroidal artery in, 299t, 300
middle cerebral artery in, 295–297, 299t
posterior cerebral artery in, 298–299, 299t
vertebrobasilar arteries in, 300
syndromes of, 300, 300–302, 301t, 302t
bilateral upper brainstem infarction in, 302
lateral medullary infarction in, 300, 300–301, 301t
lateral pontine infarction in, 301
medial medullary infarction in, 301
medial pontine infarction in, 301
midbrain infarction in, 302
other posterior fossa syndromes in, 301–302
pseudobulbar palsy in, 302
vascular dementia in, 302, 302t
Cerebral lupus, 1107
See also Systemic lupus erythematosus, 1107
Cerebral malaria, 254–255
diagnosis of, 255
laboratory data on, 255
pathology/pathogenesis of, 255
prognosis of, 255
symptoms/signs of, 255
treatment of, 255
Cerebral palsy, 577–579, 577t
ataxic, 578
Davidoff-Dyke-Masson syndrome with, 577
diparesis as, 578
dyskinetic, 578
gait disorders with, 59
hemiplegia as, 577, 577t
hypotonic, 578
Little disease as, 578
management of, 579
mixed, 579
spastic diplegia as, 577t, 578
spastic hemiparesis as, 577, 577t
spastic quadriplegia as, 577t, 578–579
Cerebral perfusion, MRI assessment of, 106
Cerebral perfusion pressure (CPP), head injury trauma with, 493, 494
Cerebral subdural empyema, 148–150
clinical course with, 150

diagnosis of, 149–150
etiology of, 149
incidence of, 149
laboratory data on, 149
pathology of, 149
symptoms/signs of, 149
treatment of, 150
Cerebral veins/sinuses occlusion, 338–342, *340, 341*
cavernous sinus thrombosis as, 339
dural arteriovenous malformations as, 342
lateral sinus thrombosis as, 338–339
other dural sinus thrombosis as, 341–342
superior sagittal sinus thrombosis as, *340,* 340–341, *341*
Cerebral venous thrombosis, 1057
Cerebral/cerebellar hemorrhage, 303–305, 304*t*
Cerebrohepatorenal syndrome. *See* Zellweger syndrome
Cerebro-oculo-facial-skeletal syndrome (COFS), differential diagnosis of, 686*t*
Cerebrospinal fluid (CSF)
blood in, 124–125
cells, 124, *125*
characteristics of, 125–126
glucose in, 126
immunoglobulin in, 126
pigments in, 125
total protein in, 125–126
delirium diagnosis with, 4
diagnostic tests for, 123, 124–126, 125*t*
differential diagnosis of, 124–125
disorders of, 349–367
brain edema as, 357–360, 358*t*
hydrocephalus as, 349–356, *350–354*, 356*t*
hyperosmolar hyperglycemic nonketotic syndrome as, 366–368
idiopathic intracranial hypertension as, 360–364
spontaneous intracranial hypotension as, *364,* 364–365
superficial siderosis of central nervous system as, 365–366, *366*
evaluation of, 477
lumbar puncture and, 123–126, 125*t*
meningitis with, *125*
pediatric acquired HIV/AIDS with, 1187
pressure, 123–124
spinal tumors with, 477
three-tube test with, 124–125
weak muscles examination with, 54
Cerebrospinal fluid fistula, head injury trauma with, 496
Cerebrotendinous xanthomatosis, lysosomal/other storage diseases of, 627*t,* 630
Cerebrovascular disease, 275–293, *276, 277, 279–281,* 281*t,* 282*t, 283,* 284*t, 286–288,* 288*t, 290*
classification of, 278–286, *279–281,* 281*t,* 282*t, 283,* 284*t, 286*
brain infraction in, 278–284, *279–281,* 281*t,* 282*t, 283*
intracranial hemorrhage in, 284–285, *286*
definition of, 275–276
dementia from, 777–778

HIV-related syndromes with, 216*t*
nosology of, 275–276
other syndromes with, 308–311, 310*t*
anticardiolipin antibody syndrome as, 309
antiphospholipid syndrome as, 309
blood element abnormalities as, 311
cardiogenic emboli as, 311
cerebral amyloid angiopathy as, 309
fibromuscular hyperplasia as, 308
Graham syndrome as, 309
hyperhomocysteinemia as, 309
hypertensive encephalopathy as, 308
Lacunar strokes as, 308
lupus anticoagulant syndrome as, 309
multi-infarct dementia as, 309
vascular dementia as, 309
vascular disorders as, 310–311
young adult stroke as, 309–310, 310*t*
pathogenesis of, 278–286, *279–281,* 281*t,* 282*t, 283,* 284*t, 286*
patient examination with, 291–293
general, 291–292
neurological, 292–293
physiology of, 278
stroke epidemiology with, 286–290, *287, 288,* 288*t, 290*
incidence/mortality of, 286–287
stroke determinants in, *287,* 287–290, *288,* 288*t, 290*
vascular anatomy of, *276,* 276–278, *277*
Cerebrovascular neurosyphilis, 238
Cervical carotid stenosis, MRI with, 74
Cervical disc disease, 512–513, *515,* 516*t*
diagnosis of, 512–513
signs/symptoms of, 512
Cervical dystonia, 820
Cervical spine, structural malformations of, 589–592, 591*t*
Cervical spondylotic myelopathy, 517–521, 518*t, 519, 520*
differential diagnosis of, 519–520
incidence of, 517
laboratory data on, 518, *519, 520*
MRI of, 518, *519, 520*
pathology of, 517
symptoms/signs of, 517, 517*t*
treatment of, 520–521
Cervical tumors, 475–476
Cervical vertebrae fusion, structural malformations of, 592, *593*
CFTD. *See* Congenital muscle fiber type disproportion
Charcot joints
peripheral neuropathies with, 735
syringomyelia with, 871
Charcot triad, multiple sclerosis symptoms of, 949
Charcot variant, multiple sclerosis, 958
Charcot-Marie-Tooth disease (CMT), 738–747, 739*t*–740*t,* 741*t, 742*
biology of, 741, *742*
classification of, 738–741, 738*t*
CMT1, 739*t*–740*t,* 741–742
CMT2, 739*t*–740*t,* 742–743
CMT4, 739*t*–740*t,* 743–744
congenital hypomyelination with, 744
course for, 744
Dejerine-Sottas neuropathy with, 738, 744
distal hereditary motor neuropathies with, 745–746

electrophysiology with, 744–745
epidemiology of, 738
gait disorders with, 60
general considerations for, 735
hereditary motor/sensory neuropathy with, 738
hereditary sensory/autonomic neuropathies with, 746
nerve biopsy and, 129
new therapeutic approaches for, 747
outcome for, 744
pathology of, 745
specific genetic types of, 739*t*–740*t,* 741–744
traditional therapies for, 746–747
treatment of, 747
Chédiak-Higashi disease
differential diagnosis of, 686*t,* 687*t,* 688*t*
hematologic disease of, 1060–1061
Chemotherapy. *See also* Cancer chemotherapy complications
astrocytomas in, 433, 436
brain metastasis with, 463–464
medulloblastoma with, 440–441
PCNSL treatment with, 410
pineal cysts with, 419
Cheyne-Stokes respiration
coma examination with, 22
sleep disorder with, 1026
Chiari malformations. *See* Arnold-Chiari malformations
Child abuse, head injury trauma with, 499
Childhood absence epilepsy, 82*t*
Childhood central nervous system tumors, 428–444, 431*t,* 432*t, 433–438, 440, 441, 443*
astrocytomas as, 429–433, *430–431,* 431*t,* 432*t, 435–439, 436, 437, 438*
biological agents in, 433
brain-stem gliomas with, 436
cerebellar, 435, *435*
cerebral-hemisphere gliomas with, 438
chemotherapy for, 433, 436
diagnosis of, 431–433, 433*t*
diencephalic gliomas with, 437
EGF with, 429–430
glioblastoma multiforme with, 438
infratentorial tumors with, 431
management of, 431–433, 433*t*
MRI in, 431, *435, 436,* 436–437
optic pathway gliomas with, 437
Parinaud syndrome with, 431
PDGF with, 429–430
radiation therapy for, 432–433
spinal cord, 439
supratentorial tumors with, 430
surgery for, 431
VEGF with, 438
ATRT with, 429, 439, 441
BCNS with, 428
cardiovascular late effects from, 444
cerebellar development with, 429
developmental biology with, 429
embryonal tumors as, 439–441, *440*
endocrine dysfunction with, 443
ependymomas as, *441,* 441–442
epidemiology of, 428–429
Ewing sarcoma as, 428
germ-cell tumors as, 428, 442
Gorlin syndrome with, 428

Childhood central nervous system
tumors (*contd.*)
late effects of treatment with, 443–444
lymphomas as, 442
medulloblastoma with, 428, 429, 431*t*,
432*t*, 439–441, *440*
melanoma as, 428
meningiomas as, 442–443, *443*
neuroblastoma as, 428
neurocognitive disorders from, 444
neurosensory sequelae from, 444
NF-1/NF-2 with, 428
osteosarcoma as, 428
PNET, 428, 429, 431*t*, 439–441
MRI of, 440
treatment for, 441
quality of life with, 443–444
radiation effects with, 443
rhabdoid tumors as, 439–441
rhabdomyosarcoma as, 428
sonic hedgehog with, 429
tuberous sclerosis with, 428
von Hippel-Lindau disease with, 428
Wilms tumors as, 428
Wnt signaling with, 429
Childhood cerebral degenerations,
675–681, *676, 679,* 680*t,* 681*t*
Alexander disease in, 677–678, *678*
Canavan disease in, 675–676, *676*
Cockayne syndrome in, 678–679
Hallervorden-Spatz disease in, 676–677
infantile neuroaxonal dystrophy in,
676–677
pantothenate kinase-associated
neurodegeneration in, 676–677
Pelizaeus-Merzbacher disease in, 677
Rett syndrome in, 679–680, 679*t,* 680*t*
spongy degeneration of nervous system
in, 675–676, *676*
xeroderma pigmentosum in, 679
Chlorpromazine, schizophrenia with,
1139
Cholestanol disease, lysosomal/other
storage diseases of, 630
Cholesteatomas, 434, *434*
Cholesterol emboli syndrome, 1070
Cholinergic drug therapy, myasthenia
gravis treated with, 882
Chondrodysplasia punctata, differential
diagnosis of, 686*t*
Chondrodystrophic myotonia, congenital
muscle disorder of, 919–920
Chondrodystrophy, *1076,* 1076–1077
Chondroma, 378
Chondrosarcoma, 380
Chordomas, congenital tumors of, 434
Chorea, 807–811, 807*t,* 808*t*
ballism with, 809–810
common causes of, 807*t,* 808*t*
dentatorubralpallidoluysian atrophy,
810
drug dependence with, 1165
gait disorders with, 59
Haw River syndrome, 810
HDL, 810–811
hereditary nonprogressive, 811
involuntary movements as, 48
neuroacantocytosis, 810
other immune, 809
primary antiphospholipid antibody
syndrome, 809
senile, 811
Sydenham, 807–809, 807*t,* 808*t*

complications of, 808
course of, 809
diagnosis of, 808–809, 808*t*
etiology of, 807–808
incidence of, 808
PANDAS with, 808
pathology of, 807–808
prognosis for, 809
symptoms/signs of, 808
treatment of, 809
withdrawal emergent syndrome
with, 808
systemic lupus erythematosus, 809
vascular, 809–810
Chorea gravidarum
gonads endocrine diseases with, 1046
pregnancy with, 1117
Chorea-acanthocytosis, neurologic
syndromes of, 673
Choreoathetosis, 49
Choristomas, pituitary gland tumors
with, 421
Choroid plexus papilloma,
communicating hydrocephalus
with, 352
Choroid-plexus tumors, congenital
tumors of, 434, *435*
Chromosomal diseases, 607–610
Angelman syndrome as, 608, 609–610
Down syndrome as, 607–608
Prader-Willi syndrome as, 608–610
subtelomeric chromosomal anomalies
as, 610
trisomy 21 as, 607–608
22q11 deletion syndrome as, 610
Chronic autonomic neuropathies
orthostatic hypotension with, 973
pure autonomic failure with, 973
Chronic diarrhea, malabsorption with,
1094
Chronic encephalopathy, occupation/
environment neurotoxicology
with, 1175–1176
Chronic fatigue syndrome, weak muscles
with, 52–53
Chronic inflammatory demyelinating
polyneuropathy (CIDP)
acquired neuropathy of, 750–751
multiple sclerosis with, 947
Chronic leukemia, blood cell dyscrasias
of, 1055
Chronic low-back pain, 516–517
Chronic lymphocytic leukemia (CLL),
blood cell dyscrasias of, 1055
Chronic paroxysmal hemicrania,
paroxysmal disorder of, 987
Chronic traumatic encephalopathy, head
injury trauma with, 499
Chronic viral infections, 200–202
Churg-Strauss syndrome, vasculitis
syndrome of, 1104, 1104*t*
Chvostek sign
hypoparathyroidism with, 1042
tetany with, 927
CIDP. *See* Chronic inflammatory
demyelinating polyneuropathy
Ciguatera poisoning,
occupation/environment
neurotoxicology with, 1180
CIM. *See* Critical illness myopathy
CINM. *See* Critical illness neuromyopathy
Circus propagation, neuropathic pain
with, 547

CJD. *See* Creutzfeldt-Jakob disease
Cladribine (Leustatin), multiple sclerosis
treated with, 960
Classic migraine, 981, 982
Classic tardive dyskineasia, 849, 851
Clinodactyly, myositis ossificans with,
938
Clivus meningiomas, *390,* 392
CLL. *See* Chronic lymphocytic leukemia
Clonazepam, sleep disorders treated
with, 1027
Clonic phase, epilepsy with, 991
Clostridium botulinum
botulism with, 886
Floppy infant syndrome with, 575
Clozapine, neuroleptic-induced
syndromes with, 849
Clozaril, neuroleptic-induced syndromes
with, 849
Cluster breathing, coma examination
with, 22
Cluster headache, 45
paroxysmal disorder of, 986–987
clinical features of, 986
pathogenesis of, 986–987
treatment of, 987
CMT. *See* Charcot-Marie-Tooth disease
CMT1, hereditary neuropathies as,
739*t*–740*t,* 741–742
CMT2, 739*t*–740*t,* 742–743
CMT4, 739*t*–740*t,* 743–744
CMV. *See* Cytomegalovirus
CNS viral syndromes, 175–177, 176*t*
diagnosis of, 176–177
laboratory analysis of, 177
pathology/pathogenesis of, 176
treatment of, 177
Coagulation disorders, 1056–1058
anticardiolipin antibodies with, 1058
antithrombin deficiency with,
1056–1057
autoantibodies with, 1058
cerebral venous thrombosis with, 1057
disseminated intravascular
coagulopathy with, 1057
dysfibrinogenemia with, 1058
factor V Leiden with, 1057–1058
factor XII deficiency with, 1058
hemophilia with, 1058
hereditary fibrinolysis abnormalities
with, 1058
lupus anticoagulant with, 1058
paroxysmal nocturnal hemoglobinuria
with, 1058
plasminogen deficiency with, 1058
protein C deficiency with, 1057
protein S deficiency with, 1057
prothrombin G20210A mutations with,
1057–1058
purpura fulminans with, 1057
tissue plasminogen activator deficiency
with, 1058
warfarin, necrosis with, 1057
Coagulation disorders of, anticardiolipin
antibodies with, 1058
Cochlear Ménière disease, 1019
Cockayne syndrome
childhood cerebral degenerations of,
679–680
differential diagnosis of, 686*t,* 687*t,*
688*t*
DNA maintenance/transcription/
translation disorders of, 647*t*

COFS. *See* Cerebro-oculo-facial-skeletal syndrome
Cognitive impairment, radiation injury with, 555
Cognitive therapy, 1197
Coital headache, paroxysmal disorder of, 988
Collagen-vascular diseases. *See* Vasculitis syndromes
Collateral reinnervation, EMG with, 93
Collier sign, ocular motility impairment with, 43
Colloid cysts of third ventricle, congenital tumors of, 435
Color agnosia, 13
Colorado tick fever, 186
Coma, 20–28, *22*, 25*t*, 26*t*, 27*t*–28*t*
  akinetic mutism with, 25
  brain death and, 27*t*–28*t*, 28
  catatonia with, 25
  confusional state v., 21
  CT diagnosis of, 23, 24
  delirium v., 21
  diagnostic procedures for, 21–24, *22*
  diffuse brain disease causing, 24–25, 25*t*, 26*t*
  examination of, 21–23, *22*
    apneustic breathing in, 22
    ataxic breathing in, 22
    Cheyne-Stokes respiration in, 22
    cluster breathing in, 22
    decerebrate rigidity with, 21
    decorticate rigidity with, 21
    doll's-eye maneuver in, 23
    eyelids in, 23
    gegenhalten with, 21
    hyperventilation in, 22, 25*t*
    motor responses in, 21–22
    ocular bobbing in, 23
    Ondine curse in, 22
    paratonia with, 21
    periodic alternating gaze in, 23
    ping-pong gaze in, 23
    pupils in, 22–23
    respiration in, 22, *22*
    Wernicke-Korsakoff syndrome with, 21
  hysteria with, 25
  lethargy v., 20–21
  locked-in syndrome with, 25
  metabolic disorders causing, 24–25, 25*t*, 26*t*
  MRI diagnosis of, 23, 24
  obtundation v., 20–21
  persistent vegetative state with, 26, 28
  presentations of, 24–25
  stupor v., 20–21
  vegetative state with, 25–28, 26*t*
Common migraine, 982
Communicating hydrocephalus, 349, 352–353
  choroid plexus papilloma with, 352
  congenital agenesis of arachnoid villi with, 352
  CSF oversecretion with, 352
  otitic hydrocephalus with, 352
  venous drainage with, 352
Complete audiologic evaluation (CAE)
  hearing loss diagnosis with, 33, 34
  vertigo diagnosis with, 36, 37
Complete blood count (CBC), delirium diagnosis with, 4

Complex partial seizures, epilepsy with, 991, 991*t*
Complex regional pain, pain diagnosis with, 31
Complicated migraine, 981
Compound fractures, head injury trauma with, 483
Compound motor nerve action potential (CAMP)
  nerve conduction studies with, *90*, 90–91
  RNS with, 94–95, *95*
Compressed spectral array (CSA), EEG with, *84*
Compressive optic neuropathy, impaired vision with, 40
Computed tomography (CT). *See also* Single photon emission computed tomography; Stable-xenon computed tomography
  abscess in, 101
  acute hemorrhagic mass in, 101
  acute intracerebral hemorrhage on, *68*, 69
  acute stroke diagnosis with, 75–78
  Alzheimer disease in, 772
  angiography, 67, 72, 76–77
  arteriovenous malformations in, 452, *452*
  brain metastasis in, 460, 461
  Canavan disease, 675, *676*
  cerebral infarct in, 101, *101–104*
  coma diagnosis with, 23, 24
  contrast-enhanced, 70
  dementia diagnosis with, 6
  dermatomyositis in, 931
  diagnostic tests selection of, 67–78, *68*, *71*
  EEG v., 79
  gliomas in, *397*
  head injury trauma diagnosed with, 492
  headache diagnosis with, 45
  hearing loss diagnosis with, 33
  hematoma in, 101
  hemorrhagic infraction in, 101, *101*, *105*
  HOCM, 70
  hydrocephalus in, *350*, *351*, 354–355
  imaging posterior fossa with, 67
  intervertebral disk trauma in, 516
  LOCM, 70
  lumbar spondylosis in, 522, *522*
  meningiomas in, 387
  MIP with, 72
  MRA v., 103
  MTT with, 72
  neurologic disorders examination with, 60, 61, 62
  neurovascular imaging with, 100–104, *101–105*, 113*t*
  nonhemorrhage infarction in, 103
  organic acidurias in, 660
  PCNSL in, 408, *408*
  pediatric acquired HIV/AIDS in, 1187, *1187*
  perfusion, 76–77
  pituitary gland tumors in, 423
  radiation injury in, 552
  SAH diagnosis with, 331, *331*
  spinal injury trauma in, 505–506
  spinal tumors in, 472, 477
  subarachnoid hemorrhage in, 103
  systemic lupus erythematosus in, 1107

TTP with, 72
  tumor examination with, 101, 375–376
  types of, 103–104
  uses of, 70–72
  vertigo diagnosis with, 36
  weak muscles examination with, 54
Computed tomography angiography (CTA), 67, 72, 76–77
Computed tomography perfusion (CTP), 76–77
Concentric sclerosis of Balo, multiple sclerosis with, 958
Concept formation, neuropsychologic evaluation tests for, 132
Conduction aphasia, 8
Confusional arousals, sleep disorders with, 1029
Confusional state, coma v., 21
Congenital agenesis of arachnoid villi, communicating hydrocephalus with, 352
Congenital cerebellar ataxia, 797
Congenital disorder of glycosylation (CDG), DNA maintenance/ transcription/translation disorders of, 648*t*
Congenital facial diplegia, Möbius syndrome with, 602
Congenital hypomyelination, 744
Congenital muscle disorders
  abnormal inclusions of unknown origin with, 918–919
  central core disease in, 916–917, 916*t*
  chondrodystrophic myotonia in, 919–920
  classification of, 916*t*
  confirmation/investigation needed for, 916*t*
  congenital muscle fiber type disproportion in, 918
  congenital myopathies in, 915–919, 916*t*, 917*t*
  cylindrical spiral myopathy in, 919
  desmin-related myopathies in, 916*t*, 918
  fingerprint body myopathy in, 919
  hyaline body myopathy in, 918
  molecular genetics of, 917*t*
  multiminicore myopathy in, 918
  myopathies of, 915–920, 916*t*, 917*t*
  myotonia congenita in, 919
  myotubular myopathy in, 916*t*, 917–918
  nemaline myopathy in, 916*t*, 917
  reducing body myopathy in, 918–919
  Schwartz-Jampel syndrome in, 919–920
  zebra body myopathy in, 919
Congenital muscle fiber type disproportion (CFTD), congenital muscle disorder of, 918
Congenital muscular dystrophy, 896, 909–910, 909*t*
  floppy infant syndrome with, 576
Congenital myasthenia, myasthenia gravis of, 878–879
Congenital myasthenic syndrome, floppy infant syndrome with, 575
Congenital myopathies, 915–919, 916*t*, 917*t*
  abnormal inclusions of unknown origin with, 918–919
  central core disease in, 916–917, 916*t*

Congenital myopathies (*contd.*)
  classification of, 916*t*
  confirmation/investigation needed for, 916*t*
  congenital muscle fiber type disproportion in, 918
  cylindrical spiral myopathy in, 919
  desmin-related myopathies in, 916*t*, 918
  fingerprint body myopathy in, 919
  floppy infant syndrome with, 576
  hyaline body myopathy in, 918
  mitochondrial encephalomyopathies with, 701
  molecular genetics of, 917*t*
  multiminicore myopathy in, 918
  myotubular myopathy in, 916*t*, 917–918
  nemaline myopathy in, 916*t*, 917
  reducing body myopathy in, 918–919
  zebra body myopathy in, 919
Congenital neurosyphilis, 240
Congenital ocular motor apraxia, ocular motility impairment with, 43
Congenital tumors, 433–435, *433–435*
  cholesteatomas as, 434, *434*
  chordomas as, 434
  choroid-plexus tumors as, 434, *435*
  colloid cysts of third ventricle as, 435
  craniopharyngiomas as, 433
  DACI as, 435
  dermoid tumors as, 434
  DIG as, 435
  DNT as, 435
  epidermoids as, 431*t*, 434, *434*
  gangliogliomas as, 431*t*, 435
  PXA as, 435
  teratomas as, 434
Congophilic angiopathy. *See* Cerebral amyloid angiopathy
Connective tissue disorders, IIH with, 362
Construction, neuropsychologic evaluation tests for, 131–132
Continuous positive airway pressure (CPAP), sleep disorders breathing with, 1026
Contracture, muscle cramps/stiffness with, 925
Contrast-enhanced computed tomography (CECT), 70
  Gd-MRI v., 73
Contusion, head injury trauma with, 485–487, *486*
Convexity meningiomas, *389*, 391
Copaxone. *See* Glatiramer acetate
Copropraxia, 49
Cord injury, 535
Coronary artery bypass graft (CABG), cerebral complications of, 1069, 1071–1072
Corpus callosotomy, epilepsy treated with, 1008, 1009*t*
Corpus callosum
  agenesis of, 567, 587, *588*, 589*t*, 590*t*, 594*t*, *598*, *599*
Cortical tremor, myoclonus with, 812
Cortical-basal ganglionic degeneration, parkinsonism-plus syndrome of, 828*t*, 835–836
Corticodentatonigral degeneration, parkinsonism-plus syndromes with, 835

Corticosteroids
  acute quadriplegic myopathy caused by, 888
  multiple sclerosis treated with, 959
  side effects of, 376*t*
  tumor treatment with, 376, 376*t*
Corynebacterium diphtheriae, Floppy infant syndrome with, 575
Cough headache, paroxysmal disorder of, 987–988
Cowden disease, structural malformations of, 590*t*
Coxsackievirus infections, 179–180
  diagnosis of, 180
  signs/symptoms of, 179–180
  treatment of, 180
CPAP. *See* Continuous positive airway pressure
CPP. *See* Cerebral perfusion pressure
Crack cocaine, 310*t*, 1162, 1189
Cramps. *See* Muscle cramps/stiffness
Cranial muscles, weakness of, 55
Cranial nerve injury, head injury trauma with, 497
Cranial neuropathy, occupation/environment neurotoxicology with, 1176
Cranial/peripheral nerve lesion, 523–541, 525*t*, *526*, *534*, 534*t*, *537*, 537*t*, 538*t*, 539*t*
  abducens nerve injury, 526–527
  acoustic nerve injury, 531
  alcohol-tobacco amblyopia with, 526
  Bell palsy with, 530
  clinical manifestations of, 524
  diagnosis of, 524
  facial nerve injury, 529–531
  general principles of, 523
  glossopharyngeal nerve injury, 531–532
  hypoglossal nerve injury, 533
  oculomotor nerve injury, 526–527
  olfactory nerve injury, 524–525
  optic nerve injury, 525–526, 525*t*, *526*
  optic neuritis with, 526, *526*
  orbital myositis with, 527
  orbital pseudotumor with, 527
  pathophysiology of, 523–524
  prognosis for, 524
  spinal accessory nerve injury, 532–533
  Tolosa-Hunt syndrome with, 527
  treatment of, 524
  trigeminal nerve injury, 527–529
  trigeminal neuralgia with, 527–529
  trochlear nerve injury, 526–527
  vagus nerve injury, 532
Cranial/peripheral neuropathy, HIV-related syndromes with, 216*t*
Craniopharyngiomas, congenital tumors of, 433
Craniosynostosis, structural malformations of, 592–593, *594*, 594*t*
Craniotomy, head injury trauma with, 493
Cranium bifidum, structural malformations of, 593–596, 595*t*, *596*
  diagnosis/pathogenesis with, 593–595
  treatment for, 596
CREST. *See* Carotid Revascularization Endarterectomy *versus* Stent Trial
Cretinism, thyroid endocrine diseases with, 1039

Creutzfeldt-Jakob disease (CJD), 264*t*, 265–268, *266*, *267*, 267*t*
  biohazard potential of, 267–268
  course of, 267
  dementia caused by, 5, 5*t*, 6
  dementia resulting from, 778, 778–779
  diagnosis of, 267
  EEG of, 82, 267, *267*
  familial, 778, *778*
  forms of, 778, 778–779
  laboratory data on, 266–267, *267*
  myoclonus with, 813
  new variant, 778, 779
  new variant of, 268
  pathology of, 266, *266*
  prognosis of, 267
  signs/symptoms of, 266, 267*t*
  sporadic, 778, *778*
  transmissibility of, 267–268
Creutzfeldt-Jakob disease, ethnicity with, 61
Critical illness myopathy (CIM)
  clinical features of, 888*t*
  corticosteroids causing, 888
  critical-illness polyneuropathy with, 889
  iatrogenic disease with, 1167
  laboratory studies on, 888
  muscle biopsies for, 888–889
  neuromuscular junction disorder of, 888–889, 888*t*
  nondepolarizing neuromuscular blocking agents causing, 888
Critical illness neuromyopathy (CINM), respiratory dysfunction with, 1085–1086
Critical-illness polyneuropathy, 758
  acute quadriplegic myopathy with, 889
Crohn disease, malabsorption with, 1093
Crossed hemiplegia, weak muscles with, 52
Crouzon syndrome, structural malformations with, 594*t*
Cryoglobulinemic neuropathy, 751–752, *752*
Cryptococcosis, 229–230, *230*
  course of, 229–230
  laboratory data on, 229
  pathogenesis of, 229
  pathology of, 229
  symptoms/signs of, 229
  treatment of, 230
Cryptogenic epilepsy, 992
Cryptogenic infraction, 284
CSF. *See* Cerebrospinal fluid
CT. *See* Computed tomography
CTP. *See* Computed tomography perfusion
Cushing disease
  pituitary endocrine disease of, 1037
  pituitary gland tumors with, 421, 423
Cushing syndrome, adrenal endocrine disease with, 1045, 1046*t*
Cyclophosphamide, multiple sclerosis treated with, 960
Cylert. *See* Pemoline
Cylindrical spiral myopathy, congenital muscle disorder of, 919
Cysticercosis, 247–248, 247*t*, *248*
  diagnosis of, 248, *248*
  incidence of, 247
  laboratory data on, 248, *248*
  pathology of, 247

symptoms/signs of, 247–248
treatment of, 248
Cytomegalovirus (CMV), 196–197, 196*t*
diagnosis of, 196–197
signs/symptoms of, 196–197, 196*t*
treatment of, 196–197
Cytotoxic brain edema, 357–358, 358*t*

D
DAI. *See* Diffuse axonal injury
Dalrymple sign, thyroid endocrine
diseases with, 1040
DAN. *See* Diabetic autonomic neuropathy
Dandy-Walker syndrome, obstructive
hydrocephalus with, 350, *350*
Dantrolene (Dantrium)
multiple sclerosis treated with, 960
Dantrolene, multiple sclerosis treated
with, 960
Davidoff-Dyke-Masson syndrome, motor
function disorders of, 577
Dawson disease, 201–202
Dawson fingers, Gd-MRI with, 73
DCS. *See* Decompression sickness
Dead space ventilation, respiratory
physiology with, 1083
Deafferentation pain, neuropathic pain
with, 545
Death, drug dependence with, 1165
Decerebrate rigidity, coma examination
with, 21
Decompression sickness (DCS), 558–559
Decorticate rigidity, coma examination
with, 21
Deep-vein thrombosis prophylaxis, head
injury trauma with, 496
Dehydration, epilepsy with, 1013*t*
Dejerine-Sottas neuropathy (DSN),
hereditary neuropathies of, 738,
744
Delayed-sleep-phase syndrome, sleep
disorder of, 1028
Delirium
CBC diagnosis of, 4
coma v., 21
CSF analysis of, 4
definition of, 3
dementia v., 3
diagnosis of, 3, 4
hospitalization risk for, 3
management of, 3–4
medications causing, 3–4
toxicology screen of, 4
Delirium tremens, ethanol withdrawal
with, 1153
Dementia
alcoholism with, 1158
Alzheimer disease as, 771–776, *773, 774*,
774*t*, 775*t*
brain imaging with, 772
clinical syndrome of, 771
CT with, 772
diagnosis of, 771–772
epidemiology of, 774
genetic basis of, 774–775, 775*t*
MRI with, 772
pathology of, 772–774, *773, 774*, 774*t*
Pick disease v., 776
risk factors for, 775, 775*t*
tau protein with, 773
treatment of, 776
tubulin protein with, 773
cerebrovascular disease as, 777–778

CT scan in diagnosis of, 6
definition of, 3, 4
delirium v., 3, 4
diagnosis of, 5–7
AAMI in, 5
alcoholism in, 5
ARCD in, 5
CT in, 6
Korsakoff psychosis with, 6
MCI in, 5
MMSE in, 7
MRI in, 6
neurosyphilis in, 6
SPECT in, 6
diseases causing, 4–7, 5*t*
Alzheimer disease as, 4, 5*t*, 6
Creutzfeldt-Jakob disease as, 5, 5*t*, 6
epilepsy as, 5*t*
Huntington disease as, 4, 5*t*, *6*
Kufs disease as, 5
Lewy bodies disease as, 4
olivopontocerebellar atrophy as, 5*t*
Parkinson disease as, 4, 5*t*
Pick disease as, 5*t*
Wilson disease as, 5
drug dependence with, 1165
EEG of, 82
frontotemporal, 776, 776*t*
HIV-related syndromes with, 5, 216*t*
Huntington disease as, 777
infectious diseases resulting in, *778*,
778–779
inherited metabolic diseases resulting
in, 779–780, 779*t*
Lewy body disease as, 776–777
MRI diagnosis of, 6
neuropsychologic evaluation with, 133
Parkinson disease as, 776–777
parkinsonism-plus syndromes of, 828*t*,
836
Pick disease as, 776
vascular diseases resulting in, 777–778
Dementia diagnosis, 5
Demyelinating diseases
central pontine myelinolysis as,
965–967, *966*
cause of, 967
clinical manifestations of, 965
myelinolysis with, 965
pathology of, 967
prevention of, 967
Marchiafava-Bignami disease as, *963*,
963–964, *964*
multiple sclerosis as, 941–961, *944–947*,
948*t*, *949*, 951*t*, *952, 953*, 955*t*, 956*t*,
957*t*
ADEM v., 954, 957*t*, 958
amantadine for, 961
Arnold-Chiari malformation v., 956,
957*t*
Behçet disease v., 956, 957*t*
bladder management for, 960
carbamazepine for, 961
Charcot triad with, 949
Charcot variant, 958
chronic inflammatory demyelinating
polyneuropathy with, 947
cladribine for, 960
concentric sclerosis of Balo with, 958
corticosteroids for, 959
course of, 956–958, 957*t*
CSF gamma globulin changes with,
951*t*, 954

cyclophosphamide for, 960
dantrolene for, 960
definition of, 941
detrusor muscle hyperexcitability
with, 960
diagnosis of, 952*t*, 954, 955*t*
diazepam for, 960
diet therapy for, 961
differential diagnosis of, 954–956,
957*t*
diplopia with, 948–949, 950
epidemiology of, 941–942
etiology of, 942–944
fatigue with, 948*t*, 950, 961
FLAIR of, 951–952
gamma globulin for, 960
genetic susceptibility with, 942
glatiramer acetate for, 959
hemifacial spasm with, 948*t*, 949
hypertrophic neuropathy with, 947
immunology with, 942–943
immunosuppressants for, 960
β-interferons for, 959
internuclear ophthalmoplegia with,
949
intrathecal IgG synthetic rate with,
954
laboratory data on, 951–954, 951*t*,
952, 953
Lhermitte symptom with, 950
limb weakness with, 949
Lyme disease v., 954–955, 957*t*
management of, 958–961
Marburg variant, 956, 958
mitoxantrone for, 959
modafinil for, 961
MRI of, 951–954, 951*t*, *952, 953*, 955,
956
natalizumab for, 960
onset mode of, 950–951, 951*t*
optic neuritis with, 948–949, *949*
other pathogenesis factors with,
943–944
paraneoplastic syndromes v., 956,
957*t*
parasthesias with, 950
pathogenesis of, 942–944
pathology of, 944–947, *944–947*
pemoline for, 961
physical therapy for, 961
polyarteritis nodosa v., 956, 957*t*
primary progressive, 947
prognosis of, 956–958, 957*t*
psychiatric mood disorder with,
950
pupillary abnormalities with, 949
radiculopathy for, 961
relapsing-remitting, 947, 950, 956
Schilder disease with, 958
secondary progressive, 947, 956
sildenafil for, 961
Sjögren syndrome v., 956, 957*t*
SMON v., 956, 957*t*
symptoms/signs of, 947–950, 948*t*,
949
tizanidine for, 961
tolterodine for, 960
Uhthoff phenomenon with, 950
urinary symptoms with, 949
variants of, 958
vasopressin for, 961
viruses with, 943

Denny-Brown, Foley syndrome
  motor neuron diseases with, 868
  muscle cramps/stiffness with, 925
Dentatorubralpallidoluysian atrophy
  chorea of, 810
  myoclonus with, 813
Dentatorubralpallidoluysian atrophy
    (DRPLA)
  autosomal-dominant ataxia of, 784t,
    789t, 796
  Haw River syndrome as, 796
Depressed fracture, head injury trauma
    with, 483
Depression, 1125–1132, 1126t, 1129t
  biomarkers with, 1127
  definition of, 1125
  dysthymia with, 1127
  epidemiology with, 1125
  epilepsy with, 1013–1014
  genetics with, 1127
  Hamilton rating scale with, 1126t
  individuality with, 1125–1126
  MDD diagnosis with, 1126–1127, 1126t
  multiple sclerosis symptoms of, 950
  pathophysiology of, 1127–1128
  public health and, 1125
  specific antidepressant medications for,
    1129–1130, 1129t
  treatment of, 1128–1129
Dermatomyositis
  CT of, 931
  diagnosis of, 930–931
  Gottron sign with, 930
  incidence of, 930
  mixed connective tissue disease with,
    930
  MRI of, 931
  myopathies of, 929–931
  paraneoplastic syndromes associated
    with, 1088t
  pathology/pathogenesis of, 929–930
  perifascicular atrophy with, 930
  plasmapheresis for, 931
  polymyositis v., 932, 934
  prednisone for, 931
  prognosis for, 931
  rash with, 930
  sclerodermatomyositis with, 930
  steroid treatment for, 931
  symptoms/signs of, 930
  treatment of, 931
Dermoid tumors
  benign skull tumors of, 378–379
  congenital tumors of, 434
Desmin-related myopathies (DRM),
    congenital muscle disorders of,
    916t, 918
Desmoplastic astrocytoma of infancy
    (DACI), congenital tumors of, 435
Desmoplastic infantile ganglioglioma
    (DIG), congenital tumors of, 435
Detrol. See Tolterodine
Detrol, multiple sclerosis treated with,
    960
Detrusor muscle hyperexcitability,
    multiple sclerosis with, 960
Developmental abnormalities. See Birth
    injuries/developmental
    abnormalities
Developmental disorders
  higher cerebral function, 579–580,
    579t, 581t
    etiology of, 579–580

global developmental delay in, 579
intelligence measurement for, 580,
  581t
mental deficiency in, 579, 579t, 580
minimal brain damage in, 579
neuropsychologic skills
  measurement for, 580, 581t
retardation in, 579
Revised Vineland Adaptive Behavior
  Scales for, 580
Revised Wechsler Scales for, 580
specific developmental disorders in,
  579
Wechsler Adult Intelligence Scale for,
  580
Wechsler Intelligence Scale for
  Children for, 580
Wechsler Preschool and Primary
  Scale for Children for, 580
language, 580–585
  ADD in, 582–583
  ADHD in, 582–583
  autism in, 583–585
  Broca aphasia in, 581
  dyscalculia in, 582
  dysgraphia in, 582
  dyslexia in, 582
  dysorthographia in, 582
  etiology of, 582
  executive/planning disorders in, 582
  Landau-Kleffner syndrome with, 581
  memory disorders in, 582
  neurologic basis for, 581
  nonverbal learning disabilities in,
    582
  pathophysiology of, 582
  PDD in, 583–585
  reading disability in, 582
  subtypes of, 581–582
  verbal auditory agnosia in, 581
motor function, 576–579, 577t
  ataxic cerebral palsy in, 578
  cerebral palsy in, 577, 577t
  Davidoff-Dyke-Masson syndrome in,
    577
  diparesis in, 578
  dyskinetic cerebral palsy in, 578
  hemiplegia in, 577, 577t
  hypotonic cerebral palsy in, 578
  Little disease in, 578
  minor motor disability in, 577
  mixed cerebral palsy in, 579
  spastic diplegia in, 577t, 578
  spastic hemiparesis in, 577, 577t
  spastic quadriplegia in, 577t, 578–579
Developmental language disorders
    (DLD), 580–585
  ADD in, 582–583
  ADHD in, 582–583
  autism in, 583–585
    course of, 584
    disintegrative disorder with, 584
    etiology of, 583
    hyperlexia with, 584
    management of, 584–585
    pathology/pathophysiology of, 584
    prognosis for, 584
    symptoms of, 583–584
  Broca aphasia in, 581
  dyscalculia in, 582
  dysgraphia in, 582
  dyslexia in, 582
  dysorthographia in, 582

etiology of, 582
executive/planning disorders in, 582
Landau-Kleffner syndrome with, 581
memory disorders in, 582
neurologic basis for, 581
nonverbal learning disabilities in, 582
pathophysiology of, 582
PDD in, 583–585
reading disability in, 582
subtypes of, 581–582
verbal auditory agnosia in, 581
Diabetes insipidus, pituitary endocrine
    disease of, 1037–1038, 1038
Diabetes mellitus (DM), pancreas
    endocrine disease of, 1044
Diabetic autonomic neuropathy (DAN)
  orthostatic hypotension with, 973
  pure autonomic failure with, 973
Diabetic neuropathic cachexia,
    neuropathic pain with, 548
Diabetic neuropathy, 761–762
  generalized polyneuropathies with,
    761–762
  mononeuropathies with, 761
Diagnostic tests
  catheter angiography as, 108–109, 109
  CSF examination as, 123, 124–126, 125t
  CT as, 67–78, 68, 71, 100–104, 101–105,
    113t
  DNA, 134–136, 135t, 136t
  Doppler measurements as, 109–111,
    110, 111, 113t
  EEG as, 79–88, 80–88, 82t
  EMG as, 89, 92–94, 92–95
  EP as, 79, 85–88, 86–88
  ESNR as, 114–122, 115–121
  microbiologic tests as, 126
  MRI as, 67–78, 68, 71, 76–78, 100,
    104–108, 106, 107, 113t
  muscle biopsy as, 127–128
  NCS as, 89–91, 89–92
  nerve biopsy as, 127, 128–129
  neuromuscular transmission tests as,
    89, 94–97, 95–97
  neuropsychologic evaluation as,
    130–134, 131t
  neurovascular imaging as, 100–113,
    101–107, 109–112, 113t
  PET as, 112–113, 113t
  post-synaptic neuromuscular junction
    dysfunction tests as, 95–96, 96
  pre-synaptic neuromuscular junction
    dysfunction tests as, 96
  RNS studies as, 94–95, 95
  serologic tests as, 126
  SFEMG as, 96–97, 97
  skin punch biopsy as, 129
  SPECT as, 112, 112, 113t
  stable-xenon computed tomography as,
    111–112, 113t
  TMS as, 89, 97–100, 99
Dialysis dementia
  heavy metal intoxication with, 1178
  renal disease of, 1081
Dialysis dysequilibrium syndrome, renal
    disease of, 1081
Dialysis, uremic encephalopathy treated
    with, 1080
Diarrhea, malabsorption with, 1094
Diaschisis, coma presentations with, 24
diazepam (Diastat)
  febrile seizures treated with, 1016
  multiple sclerosis treated with, 960

Diet therapy, multiple sclerosis treated with, 961
Dietary associated polyneuropathy, 757–758
    dry/wet beriberi with, 757
    thiamine deficiency with, 757
Diffuse axonal injury (DAI), head injury trauma with, 484, 487
Diffuse plexus injury, 535–536
Diffuse sclerosis, 682–683, *683*
    differential diagnosis of, 683
    myelinoclastic, 683
    transitional sclerosis with, 683
Diffuse slowing, EEG pattern with, 80, *80*
Diffusion-weighted imaging (DWI), MRI with, 67, 70, *71*, 73, 75, 77, 78, 106, 108
DIG. *See* Desmoplastic infantile ganglioglioma
DiMauro syndrome, nDNA mutations with, 706
Dimethylaminopropionitrile, 759
Diparesis, 578
Diphenhydramine, Parkinson disease drug therapy with, 837*t*, 840
Diphtheria, 259
Diphtheric neuropathy, 756
Diplopia
    multiple sclerosis symptoms of, 948–949, *950*
    ocular motility impairment with, 42
Disequilibrium, 34–35
Disseminated intravascular coagulopathy, coagulation disorders of, 1057
Dissociated sensory loss, syringomyelia with, 871
Dix-Hallpike maneuver, 36
Dizziness, 32, 34–38
    ear anatomy and, 32
DLB. *See* Lewy bodies disease
DLD. *See* Developmental language disorders
DM. *See* Diabetes mellitus
DM 1. *See* Myotonic muscular dystrophy
DM 2. *See* Proximal myotonic myopathy
DMD. *See* Duchenne muscular dystrophy
DNA diagnostic tests, 134–136, 135*t*, 136*t*
    allelic affinity with, 136, 136*t*
    allelic heterogeneity with, 136, 136*t*
    gene identification in, 136
    locus heterogeneity with, 136, 136*t*
    multipurpose analysis with, 136
    neurologic disease in, 135*t*
    nomenclature with, 136, 136*t*
DNA maintenance/transcription/ translation disorders, 646–649, 647*t*–649*t*
    Angelman syndrome in, 649*t*
    ataxia telangiectasia in, 649*t*
    CACH in, 648*t*
    cell cycle control in, 646, 649
    Cockayne syndrome in, 647*t*
    COFS in, 647*t*
    congenital disorder of glycosylation in, 648*t*
    DNA maintenance in, 646
    DNA modification in, 646
    DNA transcription in, 646
    DNA translation in, 646
    progeria in, 647*t*
    Rett syndrome in, 648*t*
    Seckel syndrome in, 649*t*

specific disorders in, 647*t*–649*t*, 649
    spinal muscular atrophy in, 648*t*
    trichothiodystrophy in, 647*t*
    xeroderma pigmentosum in, 647*t*
DNT. *See* Dysembryoplastic neuroepithelial tumor
Doctrine of best interest, 1201
Doctrine of substituted judgment, 1201
Dolichocephalic skull, 593
Dolichoectatic aneurysms, SAH and, 336
Doll's-eye maneuver, coma examination with, 23
Domperidone, Parkinson disease drug therapy with, 837, 837*t*
Dopamine agonists
    Parkinson disease drug therapy with, 837, 837*t*, 840
    sleep disorders treated with, 1026
Dopamine β-hydroxylase deficiency, orthostatic hypotension with, 972, 972*t*
Dopamine, schizophrenia with, 1139
Dopa-responsive dystonia (DRD), 821–822, 822*t*
Doppler measurements
    continuous-wave, 109
    extracranial duplex, 109–110, *110*
    intracranial, 110–111, *111*
    neurovascular imaging with, 109–111, *110*, *111*, 113*t*
Dorsal scapular nerve, 533, 534*t*
Double effect, end-of-life issues with, 1201–1202
Down syndrome, 607–608
    Alzheimer disease with, 608
    clinical features of, 607
    cytogenetics with, 608
    floppy infant syndrome with, 575
    management of, 608
    molecular genetics with, 608
    neuropathology of, 608
Downbeating nystagmus, ocular motility impairment with, 44
DRD. *See* Dopa-responsive dystonia
DRM. *See* Desmin-related myopathies
Drop attacks, epilepsy with, 992
Drop metastases, spinal tumors of, 474, *476*
Dropped-head syndrome, weak muscles with, 55
Drosophila, anxiety disorders with, 1133
DRPLA. *See* Dentatorubralpallidoluysian atrophy
Drug dependence, 1161–1165, 1161*t*
    addiction with, 1161
    altered mentation with, 1164
    anticholinergics, 1161*t*, 1163
    ataxia with, 1165
    blindness with, 1165
    brachial plexopathy with, 1165
    cerebellar white matter changes with, 1165
    chorea with, 1165
    death with, 1165
    dementia with, 1165
    dystonia with, 1165
    fetal effects with, 1164–1165
    Guillain-Barré-type neuropathy with, 1165
    hallucinogens, 1161*t*, 1162–1163
    infection with, 1163–1164
    inhalants, 1161*t*, 1163
    lumbosacral plexopathy with, 1165

marijuana, 1161*t*, 1162
    menstrual irregularity with, 1165
    miscellaneous effects with, 1165
    myeloneuropathy with, 1165
    opioids, 1161–1162, 1161*t*
    phencyclidine, 1161*t*, 1163
    physical, 1161
    psychic, 1161
    psychostimulants, 1161*t*, 1162
    quadriparesis with, 1165
    reversible impotence with, 1165
    rhabdomyolysis with, 1165
    sedatives, 1161*t*, 1162
    seizures with, 1164
    severe irreversible parkinsonism with, 1165
    sterility with, 1165
    stroke with, 1164
    Tourette syndrome with, 1165
    trauma with, 1163
Drug therapy, neuropathic pain treated with, 548–549, 549*t*
Drug toxicity, vertigo/hearing loss caused by, 37
Drug-induced myasthenia, myasthenia gravis of, 879
Drug-induced parkinsonism, 828*t*, 834–835
    neuroleptic-induced syndromes with, 849
Drugs, epilepsy with, 1012, 1013*t*
Dry beriberi, dietary associated polyneuropathy with, 757
DSN. *See* Dejerine-Sottas neuropathy
Duchenne muscular dystrophy (DMD), *896*, 898, 898–901, *900*
    cardiac function with, 901
    diagnosis of, 899
    features of, *896*
    gene replacement for, 900
    Gowers sign with, 898, *898*
    intermediate phenotype with, 899
    manifesting carriers of, 899
    molecular genetics of, 899–900, *900*
    orthopedic measures for, 901
    precautions for, 901
    prednisone therapy for, 900
    pulmonary function with, 901
    rehabilitation for, 901
    supportive management for, 900
    treatment of, 900–901
Dural arteriovenous malformations, 342
Dural fistulas, ESNR with, 118–120, *120*, *121*
Dural metastasis, 464, *465*
Dural sinus thrombosis, head injury trauma with, 497
DWI. *See* Diffusion-weighted imaging
Dysarthria, 9
    Parkinson disease with, 830
Dysautonomia
    differential diagnosis of, 685*t*
    spinal injury trauma with, 507
Dyscalculia, language disorders of, 582
Dysembryoplastic neuroepithelial tumor (DNT), 404–405
    congenital tumors of, 435
Dysesthesia, pain diagnosis with, 29
Dysfibrinogenemia, coagulation disorders with, 1058
Dysgenetic syndromes, floppy infant syndrome with, 575
Dysgraphia, language disorders of, 582

Dyskinesia. *See also* Involuntary movements
  dystonia with, 825, 825*t*
  levodopa therapy with, 843–844
Dyskinetic cerebral palsy, motor function disorders of, 578
Dyslexia, language disorders of, 582
Dysnomia, 11
Dysorthographia, language disorders of, 582
Dysphagia therapy, 1196–1197
Dysphasias, 580–585
  ADD in, 582–583
  ADHD in, 582–583
  autism in, 583–585
    course of, 584
    disintegrative disorder with, 584
    etiology of, 583
    hyperlexia with, 584
    management of, 584–585
    pathology/pathophysiology of, 584
    prognosis for, 584
    symptoms of, 583–584
  Broca aphasia in, 581
  dyscalculia in, 582
  dysgraphia in, 582
  dyslexia in, 582
  dysorthographia in, 582
  etiology of, 582
  executive/planning disorders in, 582
  Landau-Kleffner syndrome with, 581
  memory disorders in, 582
  neurologic basis for, 581
  nonverbal learning disabilities in, 582
  pathophysiology of, 582
  PDD in, 583–585
  reading disability in, 582
  subtypes of, 581–582
  verbal auditory agnosia in, 581
Dysphonia, 9
Dyspraxia, 9
Dysprosody, 9
Dysthymia
  MDD with, 1127
  mood disorders with, 1127
Dystonia, 49, 816–826, 816*t*, 817*t*, *818*, *819*, *820*, 822*t*, 823*t*, 824*t*, 825*t*
  action, 816
  adult onset primary, 819–821, *820*
  blepharospasm with, 820
  blinking tics with, 820
  breathy dysphonia with, 820
  cervical dystonia as, 820
  classification of, 816–817, 816*t*, 817*t*
  dopa-responsive, 821–822, 822*t*
  drug dependence with, 1165
  dyskinesia with, 825, 825*t*
  dystonia plus syndromes as, 816*t*, 817, 821–823, 822*t*
  dystonic storm with, 816
  dystonic tremor with, 816
  early onset primary, 819
  focal, 816*t*, 817
  generalized, 816*t*, 817
  hemidystonia, 816*t*, 817
  heredodegenerative, 816*t*, 817, 824–825, 825*t*
  multifocal, 816*t*, 817
  myoclonus, 823
  Oppenheim, *818*, 818–819, *819*, 822*t*
  overflow with, 816
  primary, 816*t*, 817, *818*, 818–821, *819*

  pseudodystonia as, 825, 825*t*
  psychogenic, 824, 824*t*
  rapid-onset, 822–823
  Sandifer syndrome as, 820
  secondary, 816*t*, 817, 823–824, 823*t*, 824*t*
  Segawa disease as, 821–822, 822*t*
  segmental, 816*t*, 817
  spasmodic torticollis as, 820
  spastic dysphonia with, 820
  status dystonicus with, 816
  Tardive, 823–824
  task-specific, 816
  treatment of, 826
  whispering dysphonia with, 820
  writer's cramp with, 820
  wry neck as, 820
Dystonia musculorum deformans, gait disorders with, 59
Dystonia plus syndromes, 816*t*, 817, 821–823, 822*t*
  dopa-responsive dystonia as, 821–822, 822*t*
  myoclonus-dystonia as, 823
  rapid-onset dystonia as, 822–823
Dystonic storm, 816
Dystonic tremor, 816
Dystrophinopathies
  muscle cramps/stiffness with, 925
  Xp21myopathies with, 901
DYT1. *See* Torsion dystonia gene

E

Early infantile epileptogenic encephalopathy (EIEE), neonatal seizures with, 570
Early myoclonic epilepsy (EME), neonatal seizures with, 570
Early onset primary dystonia, 819
Early syphilis, 240–241, 240*t*, 241*t*
Early-delayed syndromes, radiation injury with, 551–552
ECG. *See* Electrocardiogram
Echinococcosis, 247*t*, 248–249
  diagnosis of, 249
  epidemiology of, 248–249
  symptoms/signs of, 249
  treatment of, 249
Echolalia, 49
Echovirus infections, 180
Eclampsia, pregnancy with, 1114
Ecstasy, 1163
ED. *See* Epileptiform discharges
EDMD. *See* Emery-Dreifuss muscular dystrophy
EEG. *See* Electroencephalogram
EGF. *See* Epidermal growth factor
EIEE. *See* Early infantile epileptogenic encephalopathy
Elderly falls, 1191–1192, 1191*t*
  common risk factors for, 1191–1192, 1191*t*
  epidemiology of, 1191
  neurology of, 1191, 1191*t*
  prevention of, 1192
Electrical injury, 557–558
  epidemiology of, 557–558
  pathogenesis of, 557
  pathology of, 557
  symptoms/signs of, 558
  treatment of, 558
Electrocardiogram (ECG), delirium diagnosis with, 4

Electroencephalogram (EEG)
  Alzheimer disease in, 82
  cerebral infections in, *81*, 83
  CJD in, 267, *267*
  clinical utility of, 81–83, *82*, 82*t*, *83*
  coma diagnosis with, 24, 25, 26
  common abnormalities with, *80*, 80–81, *81*
  Creutzfeldt-Jakob disease in, 82
  CSA with, *84*
  CT v., 79
  delirium diagnosis with, 4
  dementia in, 82
  diagnostic tests selection of, 79–88, *80–82*, 82*t*, *83–88*
  epilepsy in, 81–82, *82*, 82*t*, *83*, 83–84, 994, 997, 998
    benign rolandic, 82*t*
    childhood absence, 82*t*
    juvenile myoclonic, 82*t*
    Lennox Gastaut syndrome with, 82*t*
    localization-related, 82*t*
    long-term monitoring of, 83–84
    West syndrome with, 82*t*
  FFT with, 85
  focal brain lesions in, 82–83
  Huntington disease in, 82
  hypoxic-ischemic encephalopathy in, 567
  long-term monitoring of, 83–85, *84*
  MRI v., 79
  neonatal seizures in, 568, *569*
  normal adult, 79–80, *80*
  seizure with, 19, 20
  sleep disorders with, 1022, 1023
  syncope with, 14
  tumor examination with, 375
  weak muscles examination with, 54
Electromyelography (EMG), weak muscles examination with, 54
Electromyography (EMG). *See also* Single-fiber electromyography
  basic concepts of, 92
  collateral reinnervation with, 93
  diagnostic tests selection of, 89, 92–94, *92–95*
  insertional activity with, 92
  interference patterns with, 92, 93, 94, *95*
  motor unit configuration with, 92–93, *93*
  motor unit recruitment with, 92, 93–94
  MUAP with, 92–93, *93*, *94*
  spontaneous activity with, 92, *92*
  thoracic outlet syndrome with, 544
Electronystagmography (ENG), vertigo diagnosis with, 36, 37
Electrooculography (EOG), sleep disorders measured with, 1022, 1023
Electroretinography (ERG), electrophysiologic vision testing with, 40
Elephantiasis neuromatosa, neurofibromatosis with, 715
Eletriptan, migraine headache treated with, 985
Embryonal tumors, childhood central nervous system tumors of, 439–441, *440*
  MRI of, 440
  treatment for, 440–441

EME. *See* Early myoclonic epilepsy
Emery-Dreifuss muscular dystrophy
  (EDMD), 901–902
  distinct manifestations of, 901
  management of, 902
Emetine, 1092
EMG. *See* Electromyelography
Emotion status, neuropsychologic
  evaluation tests for, 132
Empty sella syndrome, pituitary
  endocrine disease of, 1037
En coup de sabre, vasculitis syndrome of,
  1108
En cuirasse, syringomyelia with, 871
Encephalitis lethargica, 204–205
  complications of, 205
  course of, 205
  diagnosis of, 205
  etiology of, 204
  laboratory studies on, 205
  pathology/pathogenesis of, 204
  postencephalitic parkinsonism with,
    835
  signs/symptoms of, 204
Encephalomyelitis, 187–188
  complications with, 187
  diagnosis of, 188
  epidemiology of, 187
  laboratory data on, 187–188
  Moersch-Woltman syndrome with, 928
  paraneoplastic syndromes associated
    with, 1088t
  pathology of, 187
  symptoms of, 187
  treatment of, 188
Encephalomyelitis with rigidity,
  myoclonus with, 813
Encephalopathy, pediatric acquired HIV
  v., 1186
Encephalotrigeminal angiomatosis
  diagnosis of, 720
  genetics of, 718–719
  Klippel-Trenaunay syndrome v., 720
  laboratory data on, 720, 720, 721
  neurocutaneous disorder of, 718–721,
    719, 719t, 720, 721
  Parkes Weber syndrome v., 720
  symptoms/signs of, 719, 719–720, 719t,
    720, 721
    cutaneous, 719, 719
    neurologic, 719
    ophthalmologic, 719–720
  treatment of, 720
End plate AChR lack, myasthenia gravis
  with, 878
Endocrine diseases, 1033–1047,
  1035–1038, 1040–1042, 1042t, 1043t,
  1046t
  adrenal, 1045–1046, 1046t
    Addison disease with, 1045
    Cushing syndrome with, 1045, 1046t
    hyperadrenalism as, 1045, 1046t
    hypertension with, 1046
    hypoadrenalism as, 1045
    primary hyperadrenalism as,
      1045–1046
  gonads, 1046–1047
    catamenial migraine with, 1046
    chorea gravidarum with, 1046
  pancreas, 1043–1044
    diabetes mellitus as, 1044
    hypoglycemia as, 1043–1044
    islet cell adenoma with, 1044

    pancreatic hyperinsulinism with,
      1043
  parathyroid, 1041–1043, 1042, 1042t,
    1043t
    Chvostek sign with, 1042
    Erb sign with, 1042
    hyperparathyroidism as, 1043, 1043t
    hypoparathyroidism as, 1041–1043,
      1042, 1042t
    latent tetany with, 1042
    pseudohypoparathyroidism with,
      1042, 1042
    tetany with, 1042
    Trousseau sign with, 1042
  pituitary, 1033–1039, 1035–1038
    acromegaly as, 1035–1037, 1036, 1037
    Cushing disease as, 1037
    diabetes insipidus as, 1037–1038,
      1038
    empty sella syndrome as, 1037
    excessive adrenocorticotropic
      hormone as, 1037
    excessive growth hormone as,
      1035–1037, 1036, 1037
    excessive secretion of antidiuretic
      hormone as, 1038–1039
    GH-secreting pituitary tumors as,
      1035, 1036
    hyperprolactinemia as, 1034–1035
    hyponatremia with, 1039
    hypopituitarism as, 1033–1034
    natriuresis with, 1039
    pituitary apoplexy as, 1033
    pituitary tumors as, 1034–1035,
      1034t, 1035
    PRL with, 1033, 1034, 1034t
    PRL-secreting adenoma as, 1034
    prolactinoma as, 1034
    Sheehan syndrome as, 1033
    somatostatin with, 1035
  thyroid, 1039–1041, 1040, 1041
    cerebellar ataxia with, 1039
    cretinism with, 1039
    Dalrymple sign with, 1040
    Graves disease as, 1040, 1041
    Graves ophthalmopathy with, 1040
    Hoffmann syndrome with, 1039
    hyperthyroidism as, 1040–1041, 1041
    hypothyroidism as, 1039–1040, 1040
    juvenile myxedema with, 1039
    Kocher-Debré-Sémélaigne syndrome
      with, 1039, 1040
    myoedema with, 1039
    myxedema staggers with, 1039
    thyrotoxic myopathy with, 1041
    thyrotoxic periodic paralysis with,
      1041
Endocrine diseases parathyroid,
  1041–1043, 1042, 1042t, 1043t
Endocrine dysfunction, radiation injury
  with, 554–555
End-of-life issues
  advance directives with, 1201
  doctrine of best interest with, 1201
  doctrine of substituted judgment with,
    1201
  double effect with, 1201–1202
  euthanasia with, 1202–1203
  informed consent with, 1201
  legal guidelines in, 1201–1203
  overall view of, 1203
  palliative care with, 1202
  physician-assisted suicide with, 1202

  refusal of life-sustaining treatment
    with, 1201
  surrogate decision maker with, 1201
  terminal sedation with, 1202
Endolymphatic shunts, Ménière disease
  treated with, 1020–1021
Endoscopic III ventriculostomy (ETV),
  hydrocephalus with, 355
Endovascular revascularization
  carotic occlusive disease with, 116
  CREST with, 116
  extracranial carotid revascularization
    with, 116–117, 117
  intracranial cerebral revascularization
    with, 118, 118t
  stent-angioplasty with, 116–118, 117,
    118t
Endovascular surgical neuroradiology
  (ESNR)
  acute stroke therapy with, 118, 119
  AVM with, 118–120, 120, 121
  cerebral aneurysms with, 114–116, 115,
    116t
    ISAT and, 114
    ISUIA assessment of, 114
    Rankin score for, 114, 116t
  diagnostic tests with, 114–122, 115,
    116t, 117, 118t, 119, 120, 121
  dural fistulas with, 118–120, 120, 121
  percutaneous spinal intervention with,
    120–122
  stent-angioplasty revascularization
    with, 116–118, 117, 118t
    carotic occlusive disease and, 116
    CREST and, 116
    extracranial carotid
      revascularization in, 116–117, 117
    intracranial cerebral
      revascularization in, 118, 118t
    vascular filtration device for, 116
  vertebroplasty with, 120–122
Endovascular therapy, SAH treatment
  with, 334–335
ENG. *See* Electronystagmography
Enterovirus infections, 177–179
  diagnosis of, 179
  epidemiology of, 178
  laboratory data on, 179
  pathology/pathogenesis of, 177–178
  prognosis for, 179
  prophylaxis with, 178
  symptoms of, 178–179
  treatment of, 179
Entrapment neuropathies, pain diagnosis
  with, 30
Environmental neurology
  alcoholism in, 1151–1160, 1151t, 1152t,
    1153t, 1154t, 1155t, 1159t
    amblyopia with, 1156
    cancer with, 1157
    central pontine myelinolysis with,
      1158
    cerebellar degeneration with, 1156
    dementia with, 1158
    ethanol dependence/withdrawal
      with, 1153–1154, 1153t, 1154t
    ethanol intoxication with,
      1151–1152, 1151t, 1152t
    ethanol-drug interaction with, 1152
    fetal alcohol syndrome with,
      1158–1160, 1159t
    hypoglycemia with, 1157
    infection in, 1157

Environmental neurology (*contd.*)
ketoacidosis with, 1157
liver disease with, 1157
Marchiafava-Bignami disease with, 1158
myopathy with, 1158
pellagra with, 1157
polyneuropathy with, 1156
stroke with, 1158
trauma in, 1157
treatment of, 1160
Wernicke-Korsakoff syndrome with, 1154–1156, 1155*t*
cancer chemotherapy complications in, 1168–1172, 1169*t*
antineoplastic drugs with, 1168–1169, 1169*t*
biologic response modifiers with, 1171
central nervous system toxicity with, 1170–1171
hematopoietic stem cell transplantation with, 1171–1172
immunosuppressant drugs with, 1171
peripheral nervous system toxicity with, 1169–1170
drug dependence in, 1161–1165, 1161*t*
addiction with, 1161
altered mentation with, 1164
anticholinergics, 1161*t*, 1163
ataxia with, 1165
blindness with, 1165
brachial plexopathy with, 1165
cerebellar white matter changes with, 1165
chorea with, 1165
death with, 1165
dementia with, 1165
dystonia with, 1165
fetal effects with, 1164–1165
Guillain-Barré-type neuropathy with, 1165
hallucinogens, 1161*t*, 1162–1163
infection with, 1163–1164
inhalants, 1161*t*, 1163
lumbosacral plexopathy with, 1165
marijuana, 1161*t*, 1162
menstrual irregularity with, 1165
miscellaneous effects with, 1165
myeloneuropathy with, 1165
opioids, 1161–1162, 1161*t*
phencyclidine, 1161*t*, 1163
physical, 1161
psychic, 1161
psychostimulants, 1161*t*, 1162
quadriparesis with, 1165
reversible impotence with, 1165
rhabdomyolysis with, 1165
sedatives, 1161*t*, 1162
seizures with, 1164
severe irreversible parkinsonism with, 1165
sterility with, 1165
stroke with, 1164
Tourette syndrome with, 1165
trauma with, 1163
elderly falls in, 1191–1192, 1191*t*
common risk factors for, 1191–1192, 1191*t*
epidemiology of, 1191
neurology of, 1191, 1191*t*
prevention of, 1192

fetal alcohol syndrome in, 1188, 1188*t*
postnatal alcohol exposure with, 1188
typical features of, 1188, 1188*t*
withdrawal syndrome with, 1188
fetal cocaine effects in, 1188–1190, 1189*t*
childhood cocaine exposure and, 1189–1190
malformations from, 1189
neurobehavior of, 1189
neurodevelopmental impact of, 1189, 1189*t*
seizures with, 1189, 1189*t*
strokes with, 1189
withdrawal symptoms with, 1190
iatrogenic disease in, 1166–1167, 1167*t*
critical illness myopathy with, 1166
epidural lipomatosis with, 1166
informed consent with, 1166
serotonin syndrome with, 1166
neurotoxicology of occupation/environment in, 1173–1181, 1174*t*, 1175*t*
acute encephalopathy with, 1175
amnesic shellfish poisoning with, 1181
amyotrophic lateral sclerosis with, 1173
animal poisons with, 1174*t*, 1180–1181
carbamates with, 1174*t*, 1178–1179
carbon monoxide with, 1174*t*, 1180
cerebellar syndromes with, 1176
chronic encephalopathy with, 1175–1176
ciguatera poisoning with, 1180
clinical recognition of, 1174–1176, 1175*t*
cranial neuropathy with, 1176
delayed effects with, 1176
diagnosis of, 1175, 1175*t*
eosinophilia-myalgia syndrome with, 1181
extrapyramidal syndromes with, 1176
Gulf War syndrome with, 1173
heavy metal intoxication with, 1174*t*, 1176–1178
laboratory evaluation of, 1175
Layzer syndrome with, 1180
marine neurotoxic syndrome with, 1180
methanol with, 1174*t*, 1181
methyl alcohol with, 1174*t*, 1181
nitrous oxide myelopathy with, 1180
obsolete epidemics with, 1181
organophosphates with, 1174*t*, 1178–1179
other intoxication with, 1174*t*, 1178–1181
peripheral neuropathy with, 1176
pesticide intoxication with, 1174*t*, 1178–1179
plant poisons with, 1174*t*, 1180–1181
shellfish poisoning with, 1181
signs/symptoms of, 1175, 1175*t*
subacute myelo-optic neuropathy with, 1181
volatile organic compounds with, 1174*t*, 1179–1180
pediatric acquired HIV/AIDS in, 1185–1188, 1186*t*, *1187*, *1188*

antiretroviral therapy for, 1188
cerebrospinal fluid with, 1187
clinical manifestations of, 1185
CT of, 1187, *1187*
diagnostic tests for, 1185
encephalopathy v., 1186
focal manifestations of, 1186
HAART for, 1188
imaging of, 1187, *1187*, *1188*
MRI of, 1187
opportunistic central nervous system infection with, 1187
pathology of, 1186
primary central nervous system lymphoma with, 1186
stroke with, 1186–1187, *1187*
EOG. *See* Electrooculography
Eosinophilia-myalgia syndrome, occupation/environment neurotoxicology with, 1181
Eosinophilic meningitis, 247*t*, 251–252
Eosinophilic myositis, polymyositis v., 935–936
EPC. *See* Epilepsia partialis continua
Ependymomas, 393–394, 394*t*, 403
childhood central nervous system tumors of, *441*, 441–442
prognosis for, 403
two grades of, 394, 394*t*
Ephaptic transmission
neuropathic pain with, 547
pain diagnosis with, 31
Epidermal growth factor (EGF), astrocytomas with, 429–430
Epidermoid tumors, benign skull tumors of, 378–379
Epidermoids, congenital tumors of, 431*t*, 434, *434*
Epidural hematoma, head injury trauma with, 488–489, *489*
Epidural infections, 148–157, *151–153*
Epidural lipomatosis, iatrogenic disease with, 1166
Epidural spinal cord compression
lymphoma with, 407
spinal tumors with, *472*, 472–473, *473*
Epidural spinal cord metastasis, 467–468
clinical presentation of, 467–468
diagnostic evaluation of, 468
MRI of, 468
pathogenesis of, 467
therapy for, 468
Epilepsia partialis continua (EPC)
epilepsy of, 995
myoclonus with, 812
Epilepsy
active, 995
acute symptomatic seizures with, 1000
age-specific incidence of, 995, *995*
alcohol with, 1012, 1013*t*
anterior temporal lobe resection for, 1008, 1009*t*
antiepileptic drugs for, 1001–1006, 1001*t*, 1002*t*, 1003*t*, *1004*
carbamazepine as, 1001, 1003, 1003*t*, 1004
discontinuing, 1005
dose-related side effects of, 1002, 1002*t*
felbamate as, 1003*t*, 1005
gabapentin as, 1003*t*, 1005
idiosyncratic side effects of, 1002–1003

lamotrigine as, 1001, 1003*t*, 1005
levitiracetam as, 1001, 1003*t*, 1005
oxcarbazepine as, 1003*t*, 1005
pharmacology of, 1003–1004
phenobarbital as, 1003, 1003*t*
phenytoin as, 1001, 1003, 1003*t*,
   1004, *1004*
selection of, 1001, 1001*t*
specific, 1004–1005
tiagabine as, 1003*t*, 1005
topiramate as, 1003*t*, 1005
valproate as, 1001, 1002, 1003*t*, 1005
zonisamide as, 1001, 1003*t*, 1005
benign epilepsy syndromes with,
   1000–1001
benign partial epilepsy of childhood
   with, 1001
benign rolandic, 82*t*
bone health with, 1007
brain imaging for, 998–999, *999*
catamenial seizures with, 1006
childhood absence, 82*t*, 993
childhood benign focal, 992, 992*t*,
   993–994
classification of, 992–993, 992*t*
corpus callosotomy for, 1008, 1009*t*
cryptogenic, 992
dehydration with, 1013*t*
dementia caused by, 5*t*
depression with, 1013–1014
drugs with, 1012, 1013*t*
EEG of, 81–82, *82*, 82*t*, *83*, 83–84, 994,
   997, 998
epidemiology of, *995*, 995–997, 996*t*,
   997*t*
epilepsia partialis continua in, 995
examination of, 997–998, 998*t*
frontal lobe, 994
gene mutations in, 1011–1012, 1012*t*
generalized syndromes of, 993
hemispherectomy for, 1008, 1009*t*
idiopathic, 992
impact seizures with, 995
infantile spasms in, 993
initial diagnostic evaluation of,
   997–999, 998*t*, *999*
juvenile myoclonic, 82*t*, 993
laboratory tests for, 999
Lennox-Gastaut syndrome with, 82*t*,
   992*t*, 993
lesionectomy for, 1008, 1009*t*
liver function tests for, 999
localization-related, 82*t*
localization-related syndromes of,
   993–995
long-term EEG monitoring of, 83–84
long-term monitoring of, 999–1000
medical treatment of, 1000–1006,
   1001*t*, 1002*t*, 1003*t*, *1004*
mesial temporal sclerosis with, 998, *999*
mortality with, 997
MRI for, 998–999, *999*
neonatal seizures with, 570
neuropsychologic evaluation with, 133
noncompliance with, 1012, 1013, 1013*t*
nonlesional cortical resections for,
   1008, 1009*t*
paroxysmal disorder of, 990–1014,
   991*t*, 992*t*, *995*, *996*, 997*t*, 998*t*, *999*,
   1001*t*, 1002*t*, 1003*t*, *1004*, 1010*t*,
   1012*t*, 1013*t*
partial, 1001
patient history for, 997–998, 998*t*

petit mal, 993
polycystic ovary syndrome with, 1007
post-traumatic seizures in, 994–995
pregnancy with, 1006, 1112–1114,
   1113*t*
preoperative evaluation for, 1009
psychosis with, 1013–1014
psychosocial/psychiatric issues with,
   1012–1014, 1013*t*
Rasmussen syndrome in, 995
reproductive endocrine disturbances
   with, 1007
reproductive health issues with,
   1006–1007
resective procedures for, 1008
rolandic, 993, 1001
seizure classification for, 990–992, 991*t*,
   992*t*
   absence seizures in, 991*t*, 992, 1001*t*
   astatic seizures in, 992
   atonic seizures in, 991*t*, 992
   atypical absence seizures in, 992
   clonic phase in, 991
   complex partial seizures in, 991, 991*t*
   drop attacks in, 992
   epileptic cry in, 991
   epileptic prodrome in, 991
   epileptogenic focus in, 991, 991*t*
   focal seizures in, 990, 991, 991*t*
   generalized seizures in, 990,
      991–992, 991*t*, 1001*t*
   generalized tonic-clonic seizures in,
      991, 1001*t*
   grand mal seizures in, 991
   myoclonic seizures in, 991*t*, 992,
      1001*t*
   partial seizures in, 990, 991, 991*t*
   petit mal seizures in, 992
   simple partial seizures in, 991, 991*t*
   tonic phase in, 991
seizure with, 17
sexual dysfunction with, 1007
short-tau inversion recovery MRI of,
   999
sickle cell disease with, 1051
single seizure with, 1000
sleep deprivation with, 1012, 1013*t*
status epilepticus with, 1009–1011,
   1010*t*
   causes of, 1010, 1010*t*
   convulsive, 1009, 1010–1011
   nonconvulsive, 1009, 1011
   treatment protocol for, 1010*t*
stress with, 1013*t*
surgical treatment of, 1007–1009
symptomatic, 992
temporal lobe, 994
trauma with, 1013*t*
vagus nerve stimulation for, 1009
West syndrome with, 82*t*, 992*t*, 993
Epileptic cry, 991
Epileptic myoclonus, 813
Epileptic prodrome, 991
Epileptiform discharges (ED), EEG
   pattern with, 80, 84
Epileptogenic focus, 991, 991*t*
Episodic ataxias, 796–797
   involuntary movements as, 48, 50
Epley maneuver, 1166
Epstein-Barr virus infection, 197
Equine encephalitis, 181–183, *183*
Erb sign, hypoparathyroidism with, 1042
ERG. *See* Electroretinography

Ergonovine, migraine headache treated
   with, 985, 986*t*
Ergotamine, migraine headache treated
   with, 985
Erythrocyte disorders, 1050–1052, *1052*
   erythromelalgia as, 1051
   polycythemia as, 1051–1052
   sickle cell disease as, 1050–1051
   thalassemia as, 1051, *1052*
Erythrocyte sedimentation rate (ESR),
   delirium diagnosis with, 4
Erythromelalgia, erythrocyte disorder of,
   1051
Escherichia coli, 139, 143, 151
ESNR. *See* Endovascular surgical
   neuroradiology
ESR. *See* Erythrocyte sedimentation rate
Essential aliquorrhea. *See* Spontaneous
   intracranial hypotension
Essential congenital hypotonia, floppy
   infant syndrome with, 576
Essential myoclonus, 813
Essential thrombocytosis, platelet
   disorder of, 1052–1053
Essential tremor (ET), 827
Esthesioneuroblastoma, metastasis to
   skull base of, 379, 379*t*
ET. *See* Essential tremor
Ethanol intoxication, 1151–1152, 1151*t*,
   1152*t*
   alcoholic blackout with, 1152
   BEC in, 1151–1152, 1151*t*
   pathologic intoxication and, 1151
   symptoms/signs of, 1151, 1151*t*
Ethanol withdrawal
   alcoholism with, 1153–1154, 1153*t*,
      1154*t*
   delirium tremens in, 1153
   diagnosis of, 1153
   hangover in, 1153
   pathophysiologic basis of, 1153
   perceptual disturbances in, 1153
   seizures in, 1153
   symptoms of, 1153, 1153*t*
   treatment of, 1153–1154, 1154*t*
   tremulousness in, 1153
Ethanol-drug interaction, 1152
Ethical/legal guidelines, end-of-life issues
   in, 1201–1203
   advance directives with, 1201
   doctrine of best interest with, 1201
   doctrine of substituted judgment with,
      1201
   double effect with, 1201–1202
   euthanasia with, 1202–1203
   informed consent with, 1201
   overall view of, 1203
   palliative care with, 1202
   physician-assisted suicide with, 1202
   refusal of life-sustaining treatment
      with, 1201
   surrogate decision maker with, 1201
   terminal sedation with, 1202
Ethnicity
   Creutzfeldt-Jakob disease influenced
      by, 61
   Gaucher disease influenced by, 61
   Marchiafava-Bignami disease
      influenced by, 61
   neurologic disorders examination with,
      61
   sickle cell disease influenced by, 61
   Tay-Sachs disease influenced by, 61

ETV. *See* Endoscopic III ventriculostomy
Euthanasia, end-of-life issues with, 1202–1203
EV 70/EV 71 infections, 180–181
EVOH. *See* Extraventricular obstructive hydrocephalus
Evoked potentials (EP)
  brainstem auditory, 85–87, *86, 87*
  diagnostic tests selection of, 79, 85–88, *86–88*
  motor, 88
  pattern-reversal, 85, *86*
  principles of, 85
  somatosensory, 87–88, *88*
  visual, 85, *86*
Ewing sarcoma, childhood central nervous system tumors of, 428
Excessive adrenocorticotropic hormone, pituitary endocrine disease of, 1037
Excessive growth hormone, 1035–1037, *1036, 1037*
Excessive secretion of antidiuretic hormone, pituitary endocrine disease of, 1038–1039
Executive/planning disorders, language disorders of, 582
Extra-axial hemorrhage, MRI with, 106
Extracranial carotid revascularization, 116–117, *117*
Extradural infections, head injury trauma with, 497
Extramedullary hematopoiesis, blood cell dyscrasias of, 1056
Extramedullary tumors, spinal tumors of, 470–471
Extrapyramidal syndromes, occupation/environment neurotoxicology with, 1176
Extraventricular obstructive hydrocephalus (EVOH), obstructive hydrocephalus with, 349, 352

F
F wave latency, 91, *91*
Fabry disease
  dementia resulting from, 780
  differential diagnosis of, 685*t*, 686*t*, 687*t*, 688*t*
  lysosomal/other storage diseases of, 626, 627*t*
Facial angiofibroma, tuberous sclerosis complex with, 726
Facial migraine, 982
Facial nerve injury, cranial/peripheral nerve lesion with, 529–531
Facial pain, headache with, 46
Facioscapulohumeral muscular dystrophy (FSHD), 896*t*, 902–903
  associated disorders of, 902
  clinical manifestations of, 902
  definition of, 902
  differential diagnosis of, 903
  facial weakness with, 902
  features of, *896*
  laboratory studies on, 902–903
  leg weakness with, 902
  management of, 903
  molecular genetics of, 902
  scapular winging with, 902
  shoulder girdle with, 902

Factor V Leiden, coagulation disorders of, 1057–1058
Factor XII deficiency, coagulation disorders with, 1058
Fahr syndrome, dementia resulting from, 780
Falls in elderly, 1191–1192, 1191*t*
  common risk factors for, 1191–1192, 1191*t*
  epidemiology of, 1191
  neurology of, 1191, 1191*t*
  prevention of, 1192
Familial dilated cardiomyopathy with conduction disease and myopathy, muscular dystrophy of, 908
Familial dysautonomia (FD)
  autonomic disorder of, 976–978
  biochemical data on, 977
  clinical presentation of, 976
  diagnosis of, 977
  gastroesophageal dysfunction with, 977
  laparoscopic surgery for, 977–978
  midodrine for, 978
  pathological data on, 977
  pathophysiology of, 977
  prognosis for, 977
  treatment of, 977–978
Familial periodic paralysis
  Andersen syndrome with, 912
  clinical features of, 912*t*
  course of, 913
  diagnosis of, 913, 913*t*
  high-serum potassium, 912*t*
  hyperkalemic periodic paralysis in, 914, *914*
  hypokalemic periodic potassium in, 912–914, 913*t*
  incidence of, 912–913
  low-serum potassium, 912*t*
  myopathies of, 911–914, 912*t*, 913*t*, *914*
  noninherited forms of, 913*t*
  paramyotonia congenita with, *914*
  paramyotonia with, 912
  pathophysiology of, 914
  symptoms/signs of, 913
  treatment of, 913–914
Familial thalamic dementia. *See* Fatal familial insomnia
Fanconi anemia syndrome, structural malformations with, 589*t*
Farber lipogranulomatosis disease, lysosomal/other storage diseases of, 627*t*, 629
Fasciculation, 925
  amyotrophic lateral sclerosis with, 868
Fast spin-echo (FSE), MRI with, 70, *104*
Fast-channel syndrome, myasthenia gravis with, 878
Fatal familial insomnia
  dementia resulting from, *778, 779*
  orthostatic hypotension with, 972*t*
  sleep disorder of, 1030
Fatal familial insomnia (FFI), 264*t*, 268
Fatigue
  multiple sclerosis symptoms of, 948*t*, 950, 961
  weak muscles with, 52–53
Fazio-Londe syndrome, motor neuron diseases of, 862
FD. *See* Familial dysautonomia
Febrile seizures, 1015–1016
  clinical manifestations of, 1015
  complex, 1015

diagnosis of, 1015
  diazepam for, 1016
  mesial temporal sclerosis with, 1016
  phenobarbital for, 1016
  prognosis for, 1015–1016
  simple, 1015
  treatment of, 1015–1016
Felbamate, epilepsy treatment with, 1003*t*, 1005
Femoral nerve, 539, 540–541
Festination, gait disorders with, 57
Fetal alcohol syndrome
  alcoholism with, 1158–1160, 1159*t*
  environmental neurology, 1188, 1188*t*
  postnatal alcohol exposure with, 1188
  typical features of, 1188, 1188*t*
  withdrawal syndrome with, 1188
Fetal cocaine effects
  childhood cocaine exposure and, 1189–1190
  environmental neurology, 1188–1190, 1189*t*
  malformations from, 1189
  neurobehavior of, 1189
  neurodevelopmental impact of, 1189, 1189*t*
  seizures with, 1189, 1189*t*
  strokes with, 1189
  withdrawal symptoms with, 1190
Fetal dopaminergic tissue implants, Parkinson disease surgery with, 838
Fetal effects, drug dependence with, 1164–1165
FFI. *See* Fatal familial insomnia
FFT. *See* Fourier transforms
FG syndrome, structural malformations of, 590*t*
Fibrodysplasia ossificans, myositis ossificans as, 937
Fibromuscular hyperplasia, cerebrovascular syndromes of, 308
Fibromyalgia, 29
Fibrous dysplasia
  bone disease of, 1074–1076, *1076*
  neoplastic-like lesions affecting skull of, 381, *382*
Fibrous sarcoma, malignant skull tumors of, 380
Fingerprint body myopathy, congenital muscle disorder of, 919
First-pass method, MRI with, 74
Fixation instability, ocular motility impairment with, 44
FLAIR. *See* Fluid inversion recovery technique; Fluid-attenuated inversion recovery
Flaviviruses, 176*t*, 181
Floppy infant syndrome, 573–576, 574*t*
  benign-congenital hypotonia with, 576
  Clostridium botulism with, 575
  congenital muscular dystrophy with, 576
  congenital myasthenic syndrome with, 575
  congenital myopathies with, 576
  Corynebacterium diphtheriae with, 575
  diagnostic considerations for, 573
  Down syndrome with, 575
  dysgenetic syndromes with, 575
  essential congenital hypotonia with, 576
  etiology of, 574

focal neonatal hypotonia with, 574–575
Guillain-Barré syndrome with, 575
histochemically defined myopathies
  with, 576
infantile acid-maltase deficiency with,
  576
infantile botulism with, 575
infantile peripheral neuropathies with,
  575
Lowe syndrome with, 575
metabolic myopathies with, 576
molybdenum cofactor deficiency
  syndrome with, 575
muscular dystrophy with, 576
neuromuscular disorders with,
  575–576
neurotransmitter disorders with, 575
new born conditions with, 573, 574t
poliomyelitis with, 575
Pompe disease with, 576
Prader-Willi syndrome with, 575
Riley-Day syndrome with, 575
Smith-Lemli-Opitz syndrome with, 575
spinal muscular atrophies with, 862
spinal muscular atrophy with, 575
tick paralysis with, 575
Zellweger syndrome with, 575
Floppy-head syndrome, weak muscles
  with, 55
Flow-related enhancement, MRA with, 74
Fluid-attenuated inversion recovery
  (FLAIR)
  central pontine myelinolysis in, 965
  MRI with, 70, 78, *104*, 105, 106
Fluid-attenuated inversion recovery
  (FLAIR), multiple sclerosis in,
  951–952
fMRI. *See* Functional magnetic resonance
  imaging
Focal brain lesions, EEG of, 82–83
Focal brain syndromes, AIDS
  opportunistic infections with, 220
Focal dystonia, 816t, 817
Focal infections, 167–174, *169*, *170*, *172*
  brain abscess as, 168–173, *169*, *170*, *172*
    diagnostic tests for, 171–172, *172*
    etiology of, 168–169
    incidence of, 170
    pathology of, 169, *169*, *170*
    prognosis for, 173
    symptoms/signs of, 170–171
    treatment of, 172–173
  malignant external otitis as, 167–168
    osteomyelitis of skull base with,
      167–168
    Pseudomonas aeruginosa with, 167
  subdural empyema as, 173–174
    lumbar puncture with, 174
Focal muscular atrophies
  Fazio-Londe syndrome as, 862
  motor neuron diseases of, 862–863
Focal neonatal hypotonia, floppy infant
  syndrome with, 574–575
Focal seizures, epilepsy with, 990, 991,
  991t
Focal slowing, EEG pattern with, 80, *80*
Follicle-stimulating hormone (FSH),
  pituitary gland tumors with, 421
Foramen magnum meningiomas, 392
Foramen magnum tumors, spinal tumors
  of, 474–475
Foster Kennedy syndrome, tumors with,
  375

Fourier transforms (FFT), EEG with, 85
Fragile X syndrome, differential
  diagnosis of, 685t
FRDA. *See* Friedreich ataxia
Free sialic acid storage diseases, 637–639
Freezing phenomenon
  levodopa therapy with, 844
  Parkinson disease with, 830
Friedreich ataxia (FRDA), 783–786, 784t,
    788t
  clinical expression of, 785
  diagnostic testing for, 786
  early-onset, 785
  genetics of, 784–785
  genotype-phenotype correlations with,
    785
  laboratory testing for, 786
  late-onset, 785
  neuropathology of, 785
  treatment of, 786
  very-late-onset, 785
Frontal disequilibrium, senile gait
  disorders with, 60
Frontal gait disorder, senile gait disorders
  with, 60
Frontal lobe epilepsy, 994
Frontotemporal dementia, 776, 776t
FSE. *See* Fast spin-echo
FSH. *See* Follicle-stimulating hormone
FSHD. *See* Facioscapulohumeral
  muscular dystrophy
Fucosidosis
  lysosomal/other storage diseases of,
    638t, 639
  structural malformations of, 590t
Fulminant hepatic encephalopathy, brain
  edema with, 358
Functional magnetic resonance imaging
  (fMRI), 74–75
Fungal infections, 228–231, *230*
Fusiform aneurysms, SAH and, 336

G
GAB. *See* Granulomatous angiitis of the
  brain
GABA. *See* γ-aminobutyric acid
Gabapentin (Neurontin)
  epilepsy treatment with, 1003t, 1005
  neuropathic pain treated with, 549
  sleep disorders treated with, 1026–1027
GAD. *See* Generalized anxiety disorder
Gadolinium (Gd), 70
Gadolinium-enhanced MRI (Gd-MRI), 70
  appropriate utilization of, 74
  CECT v., 73
  Dawson fingers in, 73
  indications for, 73
Gait disorders, 56–60
  astasia-abasia with, 58
  ataxic gait as, 58
  athetosis with, 59
  cerebellar disease with, 58
  cerebral palsy with, 59
  Charcot-Marie-Tooth disease with, 60
  chorea with, 59
  dystonia musculorum deformans with,
    59
  examination of, 56–57
  festination with, 57
  Gowers sign with, 59
  hemiparesis with, 57
  hypotonia with, 58
  lower motor neuron disorders with, 60

marche à petits pas with, 57
muscular dystrophy with, 59
normal bipedal locomotion and, 56
paraparesis with, 57
Parkinson disease with, 56, 57–58
psychogenic, 58–59
Romberg sign with, 58
scissors gait as, 57
senile, 59–60
sensory ataxia with, 58
titubation with, 58
vertigo diagnosis with, 36
Galactosemia, differential diagnosis of,
  686t
Galactosialidosis
  differential diagnosis of, 686t, 687t
  lysosomal/other storage diseases of,
    637, 638t
Gamma globulin (IgG), multiple sclerosis
  treated with, 960
Gangliocytomas, 404
Gangliogliomas, 404
  congenital tumors of, 431t, 435
Gastric stress ulcer prophylaxis, head
  injury trauma with, 496
Gaucher disease
  adult form of, 627t, 628
  adult neuronopathic form of, 627t, 628
  dementia resulting from, 779t, 780
  differential diagnosis of, 687t, 691t
  ethnicity with, 61
  infantile neuronopathic form of, 627t,
    628
  juvenile neuronopathic form of, 627t,
    628
  lysosomal/other storage diseases of,
    626–628, 627t
GBS. *See* Guillain-Barré syndrome
Gd. *See* Gadolinium
Gd-MRI. *See* Gadolinium-enhanced MRI
Gegenhalten, coma examination with, 21
Gender, neurologic disorders
  examination with, 61
Gene identification, DNA diagnostic tests
  with, 136
Gene replacement, Duchenne muscular
  dystrophy with, 900
Generalized anxiety disorder (GAD)
  anxiety disorder of, 1133, 1136–1137
  definition of, 1136
  differential diagnosis of, 1136
  epidemiology of, 1136
  pathophysiology of, 1136–1137
  treatment of, 1137
Generalized dystonia, 816t, 817
Generalized periodic sharp waves, EEG
  pattern with, 81
Generalized seizures, epilepsy with, 990,
  991–992, 991t
Generalized tonic-clonic seizures,
  epilepsy with, 991
Genetic central nervous diseases
  acute intermittent porphyria as,
    668–670, 669t, 670t
  aminolevulinic acid with, 668
  clinical manifestations of, 669t
  diagnosis of, 670
  incidence of, 669
  laboratory data on, 669–670
  molecular genetics of, 668
  pathogenesis of, 668
  pathology of, 669
  porphobilinogen with, 668

Genetic central nervous diseases (*contd.*)
  porphyrin with, 668
  porphyrogenic drugs for, *670*
  protoporphyrinogen oxidase with, 668
  symptoms/signs of, 669, 669*t*
  treatment of, *670*, 670
  uroporphyrinogen-1 synthase with, 668
  variegate porphyria with, 668
 amino acid metabolism disorders as, 611–618, 615*t*, 616*t*, 617*t*
  Hartnup disease in, 618
  Lowe syndrome in, 618
  maple syrup urine disease in, 614
  other defects of, 615*t*, 616*t*, 617
  phenylketonuria in, 612–614
  sulfur, 614–617, 615*t*
  transport disorders of, 617*t*, 618
 carbohydrate metabolism disorders as, 641–644, 642*t*
 childhood cerebral degenerations as, 675–681, *676*, *679*, 680*t*, 681*t*
  Alexander disease in, 677–678, *678*
  Canavan disease in, 675–676, *676*
  Cockayne syndrome in, 678–679
  Hallervorden-Spatz disease in, 676–677
  infantile neuroaxonal dystrophy in, 676–677
  pantothenate kinase-associated neurodegeneration in, 676–677
  Pelizaeus-Merzbacher disease in, 677
  Rett syndrome in, 679–680, 679*t*, 680*t*
  spongy degeneration of nervous system in, 675–676, *676*
  xeroderma pigmentosum in, 679
 chromosomal, 607–610
  Angelman syndrome as, 608, 609–610
  Down syndrome as, 607–608
  Prader-Willi syndrome as, 608–610
  subtelomeric chromosomal anomalies as, 610
  trisomy 21 as, 607–608
 differential diagnosis of, *684*, 684–691, 685*t*–687*t*, 688*t*, 690*t*, 691*t*, 889*t*
  acute intermittent porphyria in, 685*t*
  adrenoleukodystrophy in, 685*t*, 686*t*, 687*t*
  age of onset in, 685, 686*t*
  Aicardi syndrome in, 685*t*
  Aicardi-Goutières syndrome in, 686*t*
  Alexander disease in, 686*t*, 687*t*, 688*t*
  aminoacidurias in, 686*t*
  aspartylglucosaminuria in, 685*t*, 686*t*
  ataxia telangiectasia in, 687*t*, 688*t*
  autopsy following, 691
  biopsies in, 689, 691*t*
  Canavan disease in, 685*t*, 686*t*, 687*t*, 688*t*
  Chédiak-Higashi disease in, 686*t*, 687*t*, 688*t*
  chondrodysplasia punctata in, 686*t*
  Cockayne disease in, 686*t*, 687*t*, 688*t*
  COFS in, 686*t*
  developmental curve in, *684*, 685
  dysautonomia in, 685*t*
  electrodiagnosis in, 689, 690*t*
  ethnic background in, 685, 685*t*
  eyes in, 686, 689*t*
  Fabry disease in, 685*t*, 686*t*, 687*t*, 688*t*

  fragile X syndrome in, 685*t*
  galactosemia in, 686*t*
  galactosialidosis in, 686*t*, 687*t*
  Gaucher disease in, 687*t*, 691*t*
  GM gangliosidosis in, 686*t*, 687*t*, 688*t*
  Hallervorden-Spatz disease in, 687*t*, 688*t*
  Hunter syndrome in, 685*t*, 686*t*, 687*t*, 688*t*
  Huntington disease in, 685*t*, 688*t*
  Hurler disease in, 687*t*
  incontinentia pigmenti in, 685*t*
  inheritance pattern in, 685, 685*t*
  Kearns-Sayre syndrome in, 686*t*, 687*t*, 688*t*
  Krabbe disease in, 685*t*, 687*t*, 688*t*
  laboratory tests in, 689, 690*t*
  Lafora disease in, 688*t*, 691*t*
  Leber optic atrophy in, 685*t*
  Leigh syndrome in, 685*t*, 686*t*, 688*t*
  Lesch-Nyhan syndrome in, 685*t*, 686*t*, 687*t*, 688*t*
  leukodystrophy in, 687*t*, 688*t*
  LHON in, 685*t*
  Lowe oculocerebrorenal syndrome in, 685*t*
  Marinesco-Sjögren syndrome in, 686*t*
  MELAS in, 685*t*, 686*t*, 688*t*
  Menkes syndrome in, 685*t*, 686*t*, 687*t*
  MERRF in, 685*t*, 686*t*, 688*t*
  motor signs in, 686, 688*t*
  mucolipidosis in, 685*t*, 688*t*, 691*t*
  mucopolysaccharidoses in, 687*t*, 688*t*, 691*t*
  myoclonus in, 686, 688*t*
  NARP in, 685*t*
  nephrosialidosis in, 686*t*
  neuroaxonal dystrophy in, 686*t*, 687*t*, 688*t*, 691*t*
  neurocutaneous syndrome in, 686*t*
  neurofibromatosis in, 685*t*, 687*t*
  Niemann-Pick disease in, 685*t*, 686*t*, 687*t*, 688*t*, 691*t*
  Norrie disease in, 685*t*
  Online Mendelian Inheritance in Man in, 684
  ornithine transcarbamoylase deficiency in, 685*t*
  Pelizaeus-Merzbacher disease in, 685*t*, 686*t*, 688*t*
  physical examination in, 686, 687*t*–688*t*
  PKAN in, 686*t*, 687*t*
  Pompe disease in, 686*t*, 688*t*
  Prader-Willi syndrome in, 687*t*
  primary generalized dystonia in, 685*t*
  progeria in, 686*t*, 687*t*, 688*t*
  progressive spinal muscular atrophy in, 686*t*
  Refsum disease in, 686*t*, 687*t*, 688*t*
  Rett syndrome in, 685*t*, 686*t*, 687*t*
  Sanfilippo syndrome in, 686*t*, 687*t*, 688*t*
  sialidosis in, 686*t*, 688*t*
  Sjögren-Larsson syndrome in, 686*t*, 687*t*
  sphingolipidoses in, 686*t*
  spinocerebellar ataxias in, 685*t*, 688*t*
  subcortical band heterotopia in, 685*t*
  Tay-Sachs disease in, 685*t*, 687*t*
  trichopoliodystrophy in, 685*t*, 686*t*, 687*t*, 688*t*

  tuberous sclerosis in, 685*t*
  urea cycle disorders in, 686*t*, 687*t*
  von Hippel-Lindau disease in, 685*t*
  Werdnig-Hoffmann disease in, 686*t*
  Wolman disease in, 686*t*
  xeroderma pigmentosum in, 686*t*, 687*t*, 688*t*
  Zellweger syndrome in, 686*t*, 687*t*, 688*t*
 diffuse sclerosis as, 682–683, *683*
  differential diagnosis of, 683
  myelinoclastic, 683
  transitional sclerosis with, 683
 DNA maintenance/transcription/ translation disorders as, 646–649, 647*t*–649*t*
  Angelman syndrome in, 649*t*
  ataxia telangiectasia in, 649*t*
  CACH in, 648*t*
  cell cycle control in, 646, 649
  Cockayne syndrome in, 647*t*
  COFS in, 647*t*
  congenital disorder of glycosylation in, 648*t*
  DNA maintenance in, 646
  DNA modification in, 646
  DNA transcription in, 646
  DNA translation in, 646
  progeria in, 647*t*
  Rett syndrome in, 648*t*
  Seckel syndrome in, 649*t*
  specific disorders in, 647*t*–649*t*, 649
  spinal muscular atrophy in, 648*t*
  trichothiodystrophy in, 647*t*
  xeroderma pigmentosum in, 647*t*
 glucose transporter type I deficiency syndrome as, 644–645, 645*t*
  clinical syndrome of, 644, 645*t*
  CSF glucose values in, 644, 645*t*
  diagnosis of, 645
  features of, 644, 645*t*
  laboratory data on, 644
  lactate values in, 644, 645*t*
  molecular genetics of, 644–645
  pathogenesis of, 644–645
  treatment of, 645
 glucose-6-phosphatase deficiency with, 641
 glycogen storage diseases as, 641–643, 642*t*
 glycogen synthetase deficiency with, 641
 glycogenosis type I with, 641
 hyperammonemia as, 650–652, 650*t*, *651*, 651*t*
  adults with, 652
  differential diagnosis of, 650, 650*t*
  hepatic urea cycle with, 650, 650*t*, 651*t*
  major causes of, 650*t*
  neonatal, 650–652, 650*t*, *651*, 651*t*
  older children with, 652
  valproate-associated, 652
 Lafora disease as, 643–644
 lysosomal/other storage diseases as, 622–640, *623*–*625*, 627*t*–628*t*, 632*t*, *633*, *634*, 635*t*, 638*t*
  AB variant in, 622
  aspartylglycosaminuria in, 638*t*, 639
  cerebrotendinous xanthomatosis in, 627*t*, 630
  cholestanol disease in, 630
  Fabry disease in, 626, 627*t*

Farber lipogranulomatosis disease in, 627t, 629
free sialic acid storage diseases in, 637–639
fucosidosis in, 638t, 639
galactosialidosis in, 637, 638t
Gaucher disease in, 626–628, 627t
globoid-cell leukodystrophy in, 631, 632
GM1-gangliosidoses in, 625–626, 627t
GM2-gangliosidoses in, 622–625, 624, 627t
Haltia-Santavuori disease in, 630–631
hexosaminidase-deficiency diseases in, 622
Hunter syndrome in, 635t, 636
Hurler syndrome in, 634–636, 635t
infantile encephalopathy in, 622–625, 625
infantile Sandhoff diseases in, 622–625
infantile Tay-Sachs diseases in, 622–625, 625
Jansky-Bielschowsky disease in, 631
Krabbe leukodystrophy in, 631, 632
Kufs disease in, 631
leukodystrophies in, 631–634, 632t, 633, 634
lipidoses in, 622, 623
lipid-storage diseases in, 622, 623
α-mannosidosis in, 638t, 639
β-mannosidosis in, 638t, 639
Maroteaux-Lamy syndrome in, 637
metachromatic leukodystrophy in, 631–633, 632t, 633
Morquio syndrome in, 635t, 636–637
mucolipidoses II in, 638t, 639
mucolipidoses III in, 638t, 639
mucolipidoses in, 637–639, 638t
mucolipidoses IV in, 638t, 639–640
mucopolysaccharidoses in, 634–637, 635t
neuronal ceroid lipofuscinoses in, 628t, 630–631
Niemann-Pick disease in, 627t, 628–629
Sanfilippo syndrome in, 635t, 636
sialidosis in, 637, 638t
Spielmeyer-Sjögren disease in, 631
Wolman disease in, 627t, 629–630
metal metabolism disorders as, 660–667, 661t, 662, 663, 663t, 664, 666
aceruloplasminemia in, 666–667
hepatolenticular degeneration in, 660–665, 661t, 662, 663, 663t, 664
kinky hair disease in, 665–666, 666
Menkes disease in, 661t, 665–666, 666
molybdenum cofactor deficiency in, 667
Wilson disease in, 660–665, 661t, 662, 663, 663t, 664
Myoclonus epilepsy with, 643
neurologic syndromes with acanthocytes as, 671–674, 674t
abetalipoproteinemia in, 671–673, 674t
Bassen-Kornzweig syndrome in, 671–673

chorea-acanthocytosis in, 673
hypobetalipoproteinemia in, 673
Levine-Critchley syndrome in, 673
McLeod syndrome in, 673–674, 674t
neuroacanthocytosis in, 673, 674t
organic acidurias as, 658–660, 659t
clinical manifestations of, 658–660
CT for, 660
definition of, 658, 659t
diagnosis of, 658–660
lactic acidemia and, 658
MRI for, 660
neuroimaging for, 660
signs/symptoms of, 658
therapy for, 660
peroxisomal diseases as, 653–657, 653t, 655t
adrenoleukodystrophy in, 653t, 654–656, 655t
Refsum disease in, 653t, 656–657
Zellweger syndrome in, 653–654, 653t, 655t
polyglucosan storage diseases as, 643–644
purine/pyrimidine metabolism disorders as, 620–621, 621t
Lesch-Nyhan syndrome in, 620
other disorders of, 620–621
Schilder disease as, 682–683, 683
differential diagnosis of, 683
myelinoclastic, 683
transitional sclerosis with, 683
Genitofemoral nerve, 540
Germ-cell tumors, 414–415, 414t, 415t
childhood central nervous system tumors of, 428, 442
germinomas, 414–415, 415t
nongerminomatous, 414–415
Germinal matrix (GM), hydrocephalus with hemorrhage of, 350
Germinomas, 414–415, 415t
Gerstmann-Sträussler disease, dementia resulting from, 778, 779
Gerstmann-Sträussler-Scheinker disease (GSS disease), 264t, 268
GH. See Growth hormone
GH-secreting pituitary tumors, Pituitary endocrine disease of, 1035, 1036
Giant cell arteritis
paroxysmal disorder of, 988–989
vasculitis syndrome of, 1102–1103
Gilles de la Tourette syndrome. See Tourette syndrome
Glasgow Coma Scale, head injury trauma with, 490, 490t, 492, 493, 497
Glatiramer acetate (Copaxone), multiple sclerosis treated with, 959
Glioblastoma multiforme, 394t, 397–399
astrocytomas with, 438
chemotherapy for, 398–399
radiotherapy for, 398
surgery for, 398
Gliomas, 393–405, 394t, 396, 397, 401, 403, 404
astrocytoma as, 393–394, 394t, 397–400
clinical features of, 396
CT of, 397
dysembryoplastic neuroepithelial tumor as, 404–405
ependymomas as, 393–394, 394t, 403
epidemiology of, 393
familial conditions with, 395–396
Li Fraumeni syndrome as, 395

neurofibromatosis type 1 as, 395–396
neurofibromatosis type 2 as, 396
Turcot syndrome as, 396
gangliocytomas as, 404
ganglioglioma as, 404
glioblastoma multiforme as, 394t, 397–399
gliomatosis cerebri as, 402–403, 403
imaging of, 396, 396–397, 397
MRI of, 396, 396–397
neuronal glial tumors as, 403–404, 404
neuronal tumors as, 403–404, 404
oligoastrocytomas as, 402
oligodendroglioma as, 393–394, 394t, 400–402, 401
pathology of, 393–395, 394t
PET of, 397
therapy of, 397–402, 401
VEGF with, 395
Gliomatosis cerebri, 402–403, 403
Global developmental delay, higher cerebral function disorders with, 579
Globoid-cell leukodystrophy, lysosomal/other storage diseases of, 631, 632
Glomus jugulare tumors, malignant skull tumors of, 380–381
Glossopharyngeal nerve injury, cranial/peripheral nerve lesion with, 531–532
Glucocorticoids, brain edema treated with, 359–360
Glucose transporter type I deficiency syndrome, 644–645, 645t
clinical syndrome of, 644, 645t
CSF glucose values in, 644, 645t
diagnosis of, 645
features of, 644, 645t
laboratory data on, 644
lactate values in, 644, 645t
molecular genetics of, 644–645
pathogenesis of, 644–645
treatment of, 645
Glutamate, schizophrenia with, 1139–1140
Glutaric aciduria, structural malformations with, 587
Gluteal nerves, 539
Glycogen storage diseases
genetic central nervous diseases of, 641–643, 642t
glucose-6-phosphatase deficiency with, 641
glycogen synthetase deficiency with, 641
glycogenosis type I with, 641
GM. See Germinal matrix
GM-1 gangliosidosis, dementia resulting from, 779t, 780
GM1-gangliosidoses
differential diagnosis of, 686t, 687t, 688t
infantile, 626, 627t
late infantile, 626, 627t
lysosomal/other storage diseases of, 625–626, 627t
GM-2 gangliosidosis, dementia resulting from, 779t, 780
GM2-gangliosidoses, 622–625, 624, 627t

Gonadotropin deficiency, radiation injury with, 554
Gonads endocrine diseases, 1046–1047
    catamenial migraine with, 1046
    chorea gravidarum with, 1046
Gorlin syndrome, 428
Gottron sign, 930
Gowers sign
    Duchenne muscular dystrophy with, 898, *898*
    gait disorders with, 59
Gradient-echo (GRE), MRI with, 69, 70, 74
Graham syndrome, cerebrovascular syndromes of, 309
Grand mal seizures, 991
Granular-cell tumors, pituitary gland tumors with, 421
Granulocytic brain edema, 359
Granulomatous angiitis of the brain (GAB), vasculitis syndrome of, 1105–1106, 1106*t*
Graves disease, thyroid endocrine diseases of, 1040, *1041*
Graves ophthalmopathy, thyroid endocrine diseases with, 1040
GRE. *See* Gradient-echo
Greig cephalopolysyndactyly, structural malformations of, 590*t*
Growth hormone (GH), pituitary tumors secreting, 1035
GSS disease. *See* Gerstmann-Sträussler-Scheinker disease
Guillain-Barré syndrome (GBS), 31
    course for, 750
    diagnosis/differential diagnosis of, 750
    floppy infant syndrome with, 575
    general considerations for, 735
    laboratory data on, 750
    neurologic disorders examination with, 62
    orthostatic hypotension with, 972*t*
    prognosis for, 750
    respiratory dysfunction with, 1085
    treatment of, 750
    variants of, 749–750
    weak muscles with, 54–55
Guillain-Barré-type neuropathy, drug dependence with, 1165
Gulf War syndrome, 1173
Gumma, 239

H

H reflex, 91–92
HAART. *See* Highly active antiretroviral therapies
Hallervorden-Spatz disease
    childhood cerebral degenerations of, 676–677
    dementia resulting from, 780
    differential diagnosis of, 687*t*, 688*t*
Hallpike maneuver, 36
Hallucinogens, drug dependence with, 1161*t*, 1162–1163
Haltia-Santavuori disease (Infantile neuronal ceroid lipofuscinoses), lysosomal/other storage diseases of, 630–631
HAM. *See* HTLV-associated myelopathy; Tropical spastic paraparesis
Hamilton rating scale, MDD in, 1126*t*

Hand-Schüller-Christian disease, malignant skull tumors of, 382
Hangover, ethanol withdrawal with, 1153
Hartnup disease, 618
Hashimoto encephalopathy, 1120–1121, 1120*t*
    clinical manifestations of, 1120, 1120*t*
    definition of, 1120
    differential diagnosis of, 1121
    laboratory abnormalities with, 1120–1121
    pathology of, 1120
    treatment of, 1121
Haw River syndrome, 796
    chorea with, 810
HDL. *See* Huntington-like disease
Head injury trauma, 483–500, 484*t*, 485, 486, 487, 488, 489, 490*t*, 491*t*, 492*t*, 493*t*, 494
    acute complications of, 496–497
    admission to hospital for, 492, 492*t*
    airway with, 495
    antibiotics for, 496
    anticonvulsants for, 495
    autonomic dysfunction with, 484
    axonal shearing injury in, 483–484, 485
    basilar skull fractures in, 483
    birth injuries with, 499
    blood pressure management with, 495
    brain swelling with, 484–485
    burr-hole for, 493
    carotid-cavernous fistula with, 496–497
    cerebral concussion in, 483–484, 484*t*
        ICH with, 484
    cerebral edema in, 484–485
    cerebrospinal fluid fistula with, 496
    child abuse with, 499
    chronic traumatic encephalopathy with, 499
    compound fractures in, 483
    contusion in, 485–487, *486*
    CPP with, 493, *494*
    cranial nerve injury with, 497
    craniotomy for, 493
    CT for, 492
    deep-vein thrombosis prophylaxis with, 496
    depressed fracture in, 483
    diagnosis of, 490–492, 491*t*
    diffuse axonal injury with, 484, 487
    dural sinus thrombosis with, 497
    emergency measures for, 491*t*
    epidemiology of, 483
    epidural hematoma in, 488–489, *489*
    examination for, 491–492
    extradural infections with, 497
    fluid management with, 495
    gastric stress ulcer prophylaxis with, 496
    Glasgow Coma Scale assessment of, 490, 490*t*, 492, 493, 497
    hematoma in, 486–488, *486–488*
    hemorrhage in, 485–487, *486*, 489
    history with, 490–491
    hygromas with, 487
    ICP management for, 493–494, 493*t*, *494*
    ICU management of, 492, 493, 494
    imaging for, 492
    infections with, 497
    initial assessment of, 489–490, 490*t*
    intensive insulin therapy for, 496
    intracerebral abscess with, 497

isotonic fluids with, 495
Kernohan notch with, 487
lacerations in, 486
leptomeningeal cysts with, 499
low/moderate/high risk group with, 492
management of, 492–497, 492*t*, 493*t*, *494*
meningitis with, 497
mortality estimates for, 491*t*
nimodipine for, 495–496
nutrition with, 495
outcomes of, 497–499
parenchymal contusion/hemorrhage in, 485–487, *486*
pathology/pathophysiology of, 483–490, 484*t*, 485, 486, 487, 488, 489, 490*t*, 491*t*
pediatric trauma with, 499
persistent vegetative state with, 498
pneumocephalus with, 496
postconcussion syndrome with, 498
posttraumatic amnesia with, 498
posttraumatic epilepsy with, 498–499
posttraumatic movement disorders with, 499
professional boxing neurology with, 499–500
radiography for, 492
sedation with, 495
seizures with, 498
serial neurologic evaluation for, 494–495
skull fractures in, 483
stabilization of, 489–490, 490*t*
steroids for, 496
subarachnoid hemorrhage in, 489
subdural empyema with, 497
subdural hematoma in, *487*, 487–488, *488*
surgical intervention for, 492–493
temperature management with, 495
thrombosis with, 497
twist-drill for, 493
vascular injury with, 497
ventilation with, 495
Headaches, 45–48, 46*t*
    approach to patient with, 47–48
    brain tumor headache as, 989
    carotidynia with, 46
    chronic paroxysmal hemicrania as, 987
    cluster, 45
    cluster headache as, 986–987
    coital headache as, 988
    cough headache as, 987–988
    CT in diagnosis of, 45
    facial pain with, 46
    general principles on, 46–47, 46*t*
        location in, 45
        pain intensity in, 45
        time-intensity considerations with, 45
    giant cell arteritis as, 988–989
    hemicrania continua as, 987
    ice-pick-like pain with, 45
    idiopathic intracranial hypertension/hypotension as, 989
    jaw claudication with, 46
    lumbar puncture headache as, 989
    migraine headache as, 981–986, *984*, 986*t*
        accompaniments of, 981
        acute treatment for, 985
        almotriptan for, 985

amitriptyline for, 985, 986*t*
with aura, 981, 982
without aura, 981, 982
basilar, 982
carotidynia syndrome as, 982
classic, 981, 982
clinical subtypes of, 981–983
common, 982
complicated, 981
eletriptan for, 985
equivalents of, 981
ergonovine for, 985, 986*t*
ergotamine for, 985
facial, 982
hemicrania and, 981
hemiplegic, 982–983
lower-half headache as, 982
naratriptan for, 985
ophthalmoplegic, 983
paroxysmal disorder of, 981–989, 984, 986*t*
pathogenesis of, 983–984, 984
pharmacologic data on, 984
phenelzine for, 985, 986*t*
prophylactic treatment for, 985–986, 986*t*
propranolol for, 985, 986*t*
rizatriptan for, 985
serotonin receptors with, 984
sumatriptan for, 985
treatment of, 984–986
valproate for, 985, 986*t*
verapamil for, 985, 986*t*
zolmitriptan for, 985
MRI diagnosis of, 45
MRI in diagnosis of, 45
neuralgias with, 46
nocturnal headache as, 988
pain-sensitive head structures with, 46–47
PET in diagnosis of, 47
postconcussion headaches as, 988
studies investigating, 46*t*
SUNCT syndrome as, 987
TMJ with, 47
Hearing loss, 32, 33–34, 36–38
common clinical entities causing, 36–38
BPPV as, 36–37
cardiac arrhythmia as, 37
cerebellopontine angle tumors as, 37
Dix-Hallpike maneuver with, 36
drug toxicity as, 37
Ménière's disease as, 35*t*, 37
perilymphatic fistula as, 37
presbycusis/presbyastasis as, 37–38
vestibular neuritis as, 37
conductive, 33–34
diagnostic testing for, 33, 34
MRI with, 33, 34
sensorineural, 34
Heat cramps, myoglobinuria with, 922
Heat exhaustion, myoglobinuria with, 922
Heat stroke, myoglobinuria with, 922
Heavy metal caused neuropathies, 758–760
acrylamide monomer in, 759
arsenic in, 758–759
dimethylaminopropionitrile in, 759
lead in, 759
mercury in, 759
methylbromide in, 759

other chemicals in, 759–760
pyriminil in, 759
thallium in, 759
triorthocresyl phosphate in, 759
Heavy metal intoxication
acute lead encephalopathy in, 1176
aluminum in, 1174*t*, 1178
arsenic in, 1174*t*, 1177–1178
dialysis dementia in, 1178
lead in, 1174*t*, 1176–1177
manganese in, 1174*t*, 1178
mercury in, 1174*t*, 1177
occupation/environment neurotoxicology with, 1174*t*, 1176–1178
specific syndromes of, 1174*t*, 1176–1178
thallium in, 1174*t*, 1178
Helminthic infection, 246–253, 247*t*, 248, 250
bilharziasis as, 247*t*, 249–250, 250
cysticercosis as, 247–248, 247*t*, 248
echinococcosis as, 247*t*, 248–249
eosinophilic meningitis as, 247*t*, 251–252
hydatid cysts as, 247*t*, 248–249
paragonimiasis as, 247*t*, 250–251
schistosomiasis as, 247*t*, 249–250, 250
strongyloidiasis as, 247*t*, 252–253
trichinosis as, 247*t*, 251
Hemangioblastomas, 458
Hemangioma, benign skull tumors of, 378
Hemangiopericytomas, 458
meninges tumor of, 392
Hematologic diseases, 1050–1061, 1052, 1053, 1056, 1061
blood cell dyscrasias as, 1054–1056, 1056
acute lymphocytic leukemia with, 1054
Bing-Neel syndrome with, 1055
chronic leukemia with, 1055
CLL with, 1055
extramedullary hematopoiesis with, 1056
hyperphagia with, 1054
hyperviscosity syndrome with, 1055
leukemia with, 1054–1055
leukostasis with, 1054
lymphoproliferative diseases with, 1055
MGUS with, 1055
myelin-associated glycoprotein with, 1055
myelofibrosis with, 1056
myelogenous leukemia with, 1055
myeloma with, 1055
obesity with, 1054
plasma cell dyscrasias with, 1055–1056, 1056
plasmacytoma with, 1055
Waldenström macroglobulinemia with, 1055
cerebrovascular complications of cancer as, 1058–1059
coagulation disorders as, 1056–1058
anticardiolipin antibodies with, 1058
antithrombin deficiency with, 1056–1057
autoantibodies with, 1058
cerebral venous thrombosis with, 1057

disseminated intravascular coagulopathy with, 1057
dysfibrinogenemia with, 1058
factor V Leiden with, 1057–1058
factor XII deficiency with, 1058
hemophilia with, 1058
hereditary fibrinolysis abnormalities with, 1058
lupus anticoagulant with, 1058
paroxysmal nocturnal hemoglobinuria with, 1058
plasminogen deficiency with, 1058
protein C deficiency with, 1057
protein S deficiency with, 1057
prothrombin G20210A mutations with, 1057–1058
purpura fulminans with, 1057
tissue plasminogen activator deficiency with, 1058
warfarin, necrosis with, 1057
erythrocyte disorders as, 1050–1052, 1052
erythromelalgia with, 1051
polycythemia with, 1051–1052
sickle cell disease with, 1050–1051
thalassemia with, 1051, 1052
other disorders as, 1059–1061, 1061
Chediak-Higashi syndrome with, 1060–1061
idiopathic hypereosinophilic syndrome with, 1059–1060
Langerhans cell histiocytosis with, 1060, 1061
neurolymphomatosis with, 1060
platelet disorders as, 1052–1054, 1053
essential thrombocytosis with, 1052–1053
heparin-induced thrombocytopenic with, 1054
thrombotic thrombocytopenic purpura with, 1053, 1053–1054
Hematoma
CT of, 101
head injury trauma with, 486–488, 486–488
Hematomyelia, syringomyelia with, 872
Hematopoietic stem cell transplantation (HSCT), cancer chemotherapy complications with, 1171–1172
Hemicrania continua, paroxysmal disorder of, 987
Hemicrania, migraine headache as, 981
Hemidystonia, 816*t*, 817
Hemifacial spasm, multiple sclerosis with, 948*t*, 949
Hemiparesis
gait disorders with, 57
weak muscles with, 53–54
Hemiparkinsonism-hemiatrophy syndrome, 828*t*, 835
Hemiplegia
motor function disorders of, 577, 577*t*
weak muscles with, 52
Hemiplegic migraine, 982–983
Hemispherectomy
epilepsy treated with, 1008, 1009*t*
Krabbe-Weber disease treated with, 456
Sturge-Weber disease treated with, 456
Hemophilia, coagulation disorders of, 1058
Hemophilus influenzae, 139, 140*t*, 142–143
Hemophilus influenzae meningitis, 142–143

Hemorrhage, head injury trauma with, 485–487, *486*, 489
Hemorrhagic infarction
  CT of, 101, *101*, *105*
  MRI showing, *106*
Heparin-induced thrombocytopenic (HIT), platelet disorder of, 1054
Hepatic disease, 1064–1066, 1066*t*
  acquired chronic hepatocerebral degeneration with, 1065
  clinical features of, 1065
  differential diagnosis of, 1066
  hepatic encephalopathy with, 1064
  liver transplantation with, 1066, 1066*t*
  neurologic complications of, 1066, 1066*t*
  neuropathy with, 755
  pathophysiology of, 1065–1066
  portal-systemic encephalopathy with, 1064
  treatment of, 1066
Hepatic encephalopathy, 1064
Hepatic urea cycle, hyperammonemia with, 650, 650*t*, 651*t*
Hepatitis A virus, 180–181
  diagnosis of, 181
  epidemiology of, 180–181
Hepatolenticular degeneration
  diagnosis of, 664–665
  Menkes disease v., 661, 661*t*
  metal metabolism disorders of, 660–665, 661*t*, *662*, *663*, 663*t*, *664*
  MRI for, *664*, 664
  onset of, 663*t*
  pathogenesis/pathology of, 661–662, 661*t*, *662*
  personality disorders with, 663
  rigidity with, 663
  symptoms/signs of, 662–664, *663*, 663*t*, *664*
  tendon reflexes with, 663
  treatment of, 665
Hepatopathy, mitochondrial encephalomyopathies with, 701
Hereditary ataxias, ocular motility impairment with, 43
Hereditary fibrinolysis abnormalities
  coagulation disorders of, 1058
  dysfibrinogenemia with, 1058
  factor XII deficiency with, 1058
  plasminogen deficiency with, 1058
Hereditary motor neuropathies (HMN), 745–746
Hereditary motor/sensory neuropathy (HMSN), 738–747, 739*t*–740*t*, 741*t*, *742*
  biology of, 741, *742*
  classification of, 738–741, 738*t*
  CMT1, 739*t*–740*t*, 741–742
  CMT2, 739*t*–740*t*, 742–743
  CMT4, 739*t*–740*t*, 743–744
  congenital hypomyelination with, 744
  course for, 744
  Dejerine-Sottas neuropathy with, 738, 744
  distal hereditary motor neuropathies with, 745–746
  electrophysiology with, 744–745
  epidemiology of, 738
  hereditary motor/sensory neuropathy with, 738
  hereditary sensory/autonomic neuropathies with, 746

new therapeutic approaches for, 747
outcome for, 744
pathology of, 745
specific genetic types of, 739*t*–740*t*, 741–744
traditional therapies for, 747
treatment of, 747
Hereditary neuropathies, 738–747, 739*t*–740*t*, 741*t*, *742*
  biology of, 741, *742*
  classification of, 738–741, 738*t*
  CMT1, 739*t*–740*t*, 741–742
  CMT2, 739*t*–740*t*, 742–743
  CMT4, 739*t*–740*t*, 743–744
  congenital hypomyelination with, 744
  course for, 744
  Dejerine-Sottas neuropathy with, 738, 744
  distal hereditary motor neuropathies with, 745–746
  electrophysiology with, 744–745
  epidemiology of, 738
  hereditary sensory/autonomic neuropathies with, 746
  new therapeutic approaches for, 747
  outcome for, 744
  pathology of, 745
  specific genetic types of, 739*t*–740*t*, 741–744
  traditional therapies for, 747
  treatment of, 747
Hereditary nonprogressive chorea, 811
Hereditary sensory/autonomic neuropathies (HSAN), 746
Hereditary spastic paraplegia (HSP)
  classification of, 855, 855*t*
  clinical manifestations of, 856
  diagnosis of, 856
  genetics of, 855–856, 855*t*, 856*t*
  laboratory data on, 856
  MRI for, 856
  spinal cord disease of, 855–856, 855*t*, 856*t*
  treatment of, 856
Heredodegenerative dystonia, 816*t*, 817, 824–825, 825*t*
Herpes simplex encephalitis, 191–194, 192*t*, *193*
  diagnosis of, 192–193
  etiology of, 191
  laboratory data on, 192, *193*
  pathogenesis of, 191–192
  pathology of, 192
  prognosis with, 193–194
  signs/symptoms of, 192, 192*t*
  treatment of, 193–194
Herpes zoster, 194–196
  complications of, 195
  diagnosis of, 195
  etiology of, 194
  geniculate herpes with, 195
  incidence of, 194
  laboratory data on, 195
  ophthalmic zoster with, 194–195
  pathology of, 194
  postherpetic neuralgia and, 195–196
  signs/symptoms of, 194
  treatment of, 195
Herpes zoster-related neuropathy, 757
Herpesvirus infections, 191–196, 192*t*, *193*
Hexosaminidase-deficiency diseases, lysosomal/other storage diseases of, 622

HHNS. *See* Hyperosmolar hyperglycemic nonketotic syndrome
HHV-6. *See* Human herpesvirus-6
Hiccups, 300, 377
HIE. *See* Hypoxic-ischemic encephalopathy
Higher cerebral function, developmental disorders of, 579–580, 579*t*, 581*t*
  etiology of, 579–580
  global developmental delay in, 579
  intelligence measurement for, 580, 581*t*
  mental deficiency in, 579, 579*t*, 580
  minimal brain damage in, 579
  neuropsychologic skills measurement for, 580, 581*t*
  retardation in, 579
  Revised Vineland Adaptive Behavior Scales for, 580
  Revised Wechsler Scales for, 580
  specific developmental disorders in, 579
  Wechsler Adult Intelligence Scale for, 580
  Wechsler Intelligence Scale for Children with, 580
  Wechsler Preschool and Primary Scale for Children with, 580
Highly active antiretroviral therapies (HAART), pediatric acquired HIV/AIDS with, 1188
High-osmolar contrast media (HOCM), CT with, 70
High-serum potassium periodic paralysis, 912*t*
Hirayama syndrome, motor neuron diseases with, 867
Histochemical techniques, muscle biopsy with, 128
Histochemically defined myopathies, floppy infant syndrome with, 576
HIT. *See* Heparin-induced thrombocytopenic
HIV. *See* Acquired immunodeficiency syndrome; Human immunodeficiency virus
HIV-related neuropathies, 756–757
HMN. *See* Hereditary motor neuropathies
HMSN. *See* Hereditary motor/sensory neuropathy
HOCM. *See* High-osmolar contrast media
Hoffmann signs, weak muscles with, 53
Hoffmann syndrome, thyroid endocrine diseases with, 1039
Hollenhorst plaques, 42, 294
Holmes-Adie syndrome, orthostatic hypotension with, 972*t*
Homocystinuria, 614–617, 615*t*
  diagnosis of, 617
Homonymous hemianopia, impaired vision with, 41
HoPP. *See* Hypokalemic periodic potassium
Horner syndrome
  ocular motility impairment with, 42
  spinal tumors of, 476
  syringomyelia with, 871
HSAN. *See* Hereditary sensory/autonomic neuropathies
HSCT. *See* Hematopoietic stem cell transplantation
HSP. *See* Hereditary spastic paraplegia
HTLV-associated myelopathy (HAM), 202–203, 856

course of, 203
diagnosis of, 203
epidemiology of, 202–203
etiology of, 202
laboratory studies on, 203
pathology/pathogenesis of, 202
prognosis of, 203
signs/symptoms of, 203
treatment of, 203
HTLV-I. *See* Human T-cell lymphotropic
  virus I
Human ehrlichiosis, 159–160
  course of, 159–160
  diagnosis of, 159
  epidemiology of, 159
  prognosis for, 159–160
  symptoms/signs of, 159
  treatment for, 159–160
Human herpesvirus-6 (HHV-6), 197–198
  complications with, 198
  diagnosis of, 198
  symptoms of, 197
  treatment of, 198
Human immunodeficiency virus (HIV)
  dementia resulting from, 779
  pediatric acquired, 1185–1188, 1186*t*,
    1187, 1188
    antiretroviral therapy for, 1188
    cerebrospinal fluid with, 1187
    clinical manifestations of, 1185
    CT of, 1187, *1187*
    diagnostic tests for, 1185
    encephalopathy v., 1186
    focal manifestations of, 1186
    HAART for, 1188
    imaging of, 1187, *1187, 1188*
    MRI of, 1187
    opportunistic central nervous system
      infection with, 1187
    pathology of, 1186
    primary central nervous system
      lymphoma with, 1186
    stroke with, 1186–1187, *1187*
Human T-cell lymphotropic virus I
  (HTLV-I), 856, 857
Hunter syndrome
  differential diagnosis of, 685*t*, 686*t*,
    687*t*, 688*t*
  lysosomal/other storage diseases of,
    635*t*, 636
Huntington disease
  biochemistry of, 803–804
  choreic movements with, 805
  dementia caused by, 4, 5*t*, 6, 777
  diagnosis of, 806
  differential diagnosis of, 685*t*, 688*t*, 806
  EEG of, 82
  genetics of, 804
  HDL and, 806
  involuntary movements with, 48
  laboratory data on, *805*, 805–806
  mental symptoms of, 805
  movement disorder of, *803*, 803–806,
    805
  neuroleptic-induced syndromes with,
    850
  ocular motility impairment with, 43
  other neurologic manifestations of, 805
  pathology of, 803, *803*
  prevalence of, 804
  symptoms/signs of, 804–805
  tardive dyskinesia with, 806
  treatment of, 806

Huntington-like disease (HDL), 806
  movement disorders of, 810–811
Hurler disease, differential diagnosis of,
  687*t*
Hurler syndrome, lysosomal/other
  storage diseases of, 634–636, 635*t*
Hurler-Scheie malformations, 590*t*
Hyaline body myopathy, congenital
  muscle disorder of, 918
Hydatid cysts, 247*t*, 248–249
  diagnosis of, 249
  epidemiology of, 248–249
  symptoms/signs of, 249
  treatment of, 249
Hydrocephalic brain edema, 358*t*, 359
Hydrocephalus, 349–356, *350–354*, 356*t*
  communicating, 349, 352–353
    choroid plexus papilloma with, 352
    congenital agenesis of arachnoid villi
      with, 352
    CSF oversecretion with, 352
    otitic hydrocephalus with, 352
    venous drainage with, 352
  CT for, 354–355
  endoscopic III ventriculostomy with,
    355
  general clinical data on, 354–356, 356*t*
  germinal matrix hemorrhage with, 350
  intracranial hemorrhage with, 350,
    354, 355
  intraventricular hemorrhage with, 350
  laboratory data on, 354–355
  MRI for, 354–355
  normal pressure, 349, 353–356, 356*t*
  obstructive, 349–352, *350–354*
    Arnold-Chiari malformation with,
      350
    congenital malformations with,
      349–350, *350, 351*
    Dandy-Walker syndrome with, 350,
      350
    developmental lesions with, 349–350,
      350, 351
    EVOH, 349, 352
    IVOH, 349, 352, 355
    mass lesions with, 352, *354*
    postinflammatory/posthemorrhagic,
      350–352, *351–353*
  periventricular hemorrhagic infarction
    with, 350
  prognosis for, 355–356, *356*
  signs/symptoms of, 354
  subarachnoid hemorrhage with,
    332–333, 350
  treatment of, 355–356, *356*
Hydrocephalus ex vacuo, structural
  malformations with, 589
Hydromyelia, syringomyelia with, 871,
  872
Hygromas, head injury trauma with, 487
Hyperadrenalism, adrenal endocrine
  disease of, 1045, 1046*t*
Hyperammonemia, 650–652, 650*t*, *651*,
  651*t*
  adults with, 652
  differential diagnosis of, 650, 650*t*
  hepatic urea cycle with, 650, 650*t*, 651*t*
  major causes of, 650*t*
  neonatal, 650–652, *651*, 651*t*, 662*t*
  older children with, 652
  valproate-associated, 652
Hypercapnia, respiratory physiology
  with, 1083

Hyperekplexia, 50, 51
  Moersch-Woltman syndrome with, 928
  myoclonus with, 814
Hyperhidrosis, muscle cramps/stiffness
  with, 926
Hyperhomocysteinemia, cerebrovascular
  syndromes of, 309
Hyperkalemic periodic paralysis
  myopathies of, 914, *914*
  paramyotonia congenita with, *914*
  pathophysiology of, 914
Hyperosmolar hyperglycemic nonketotic
  syndrome (HHNS), 366–368
  diagnosis of, 367
  treatment of, 367–368
Hyperostosis, neoplastic-like lesions
  affecting skull of, 381
Hyperparathyroidism, parathyroid
  endocrine disease of, 1043, 1043*t*
Hyperphagia, blood cell dyscrasias with,
  1054
Hyperprolactinemia
  pituitary endocrine disease of,
    1034–1035
  radiation injury with, 555
Hypertension, adrenal endocrine disease
  with, 1046
Hypertensive encephalopathy,
  cerebrovascular syndromes of, 308
Hyperthyroid neuropathy, 754–755
Hyperthyroidism, thyroid endocrine
  diseases of, 1040–1041, *1041*
Hypertrophic neuropathy, multiple
  sclerosis with, 947
Hypertrophic pachymeningitis, 1111
Hyperventilation
  coma examination with, 22, 25*t*
  seizure with, 17, 18*t*
  vertigo caused by, 38
Hyperviscosity syndrome, blood cell
  dyscrasias of, 1055
Hypnagogic hallucinations, sleep
  disorder of, 1027
Hypnic jerks, sleep disorders with, 1026
Hypnosis, somatoform disorders treated
  with, 1145
Hypoadrenalism, adrenal endocrine
  disease of, 1045
Hypobetalipoproteinemia, neurologic
  syndromes of, 673
Hypoglossal nerve injury,
  cranial/peripheral nerve lesion
  with, 533
Hypoglycemia
  alcoholism with, 1157
  pancreas endocrine disease of,
    1043–1044
Hypokalemic periodic potassium (HoPP)
  course of, 913
  diagnosis of, 913, 913*t*
  incidence of, 912–913
  myopathies as, 912–914, 913*t*
  noninherited forms of, 913*t*
  symptoms/signs of, 913
  treatment of, 913–914
Hypokinesia, Parkinson disease with, 829
Hypomelanosis of ITO. *See* Incontinentia
  pigmenti achromians
Hypomimia, Parkinson disease with,
  829
Hyponatremia, pituitary endocrine
  disease with, 1039
Hyponeas, sleep disorders with, 1025

Hypoparathyroidism
  Chvostek sign with, 1042
  Erb sign with, 1042
  latent tetany with, 1042
  parathyroid endocrine disease of, 1041–1043, *1042*, 1042*t*
  pseudohypoparathyroidism with, 1042, *1042*
  tetany with, 1042
  Trousseau sign with, 1042
Hypophonia, Parkinson disease with, 830
Hypopituitarism, pituitary endocrine disease of, 1033–1034
Hypotension, head injury trauma with, 489
Hypothermia, cerebral complication prevention with, 1071
Hypothyroid neuropathy, 754
Hypothyroidism, thyroid endocrine diseases of, 1039–1040, *1040*
Hypotonia, gait disorders with, 58
Hypotonic cerebral palsy, motor function disorders of, 578
Hypoxemia, respiratory physiology with, 1083
Hypoxia, head injury trauma with, 489
Hypoxic-ischemic encephalopathy (HIE), 565–567
  EEG of, 567
  incidence of, 565
  laboratory data on, 566–567
  MRI of, 566, 567
  MRS of, 566, 567
  pathology/pathophysiology of, 565–566
  PET of, 566
  prognosis for, 567
  symptoms/signs of, 566
  treatment of, 567
Hysteria, coma with, 25

I

Iatrogenic disease, 1166–1167, 1167*t*
  critical illness myopathy with, 1166
  epidural lipomatosis with, 1166
  informed consent with, 1166
  serotonin syndrome with, 1166
IBM. *See* Inclusion body myositis
Ice-pick-like pain, headache with, 45
ICH. *See* Intracranial hemorrhage
ICU. *See* Intensive Care Unit
Idiopathic autonomic neuropathy, 751
Idiopathic brachial plexitis, 535
Idiopathic epilepsy, 992
Idiopathic hypereosinophilic syndrome (IHES)
  hematologic disease of, 1059–1060
  vasculitis syndrome with, 1109
Idiopathic hypertrophic pachymeningitis (IHP), 1111
Idiopathic insomnia, sleep disorder of, 1024
Idiopathic intracranial hypertension (IIH), 360–364
  clinical manifestations of, 361
  conditions associated with, 360–361
  connective tissue disorders with, 362
  diagnosis of, 363
  drugs leading to, 362
  endocrine disorders with, 362
  hematologic disorders with, 362
  intracranial venous-sinus thrombosis with, 362
  metabolic disorders with, 362

paroxysmal disorder of, 989
  pathophysiology of, 361–362
  pulmonary encephalopathy with, 362
  spinal cord diseases with, 363
  systemic lupus erythematosus with, 362
  toxins leading to, 362
  treatment of, 363–364
  vitamin A with, 362
Idiopathic neuropathy, 763
Idiopathic Parkinson disease, pregnancy with, 1117
IgG. *See* Gamma globulin
IHES. *See* Idiopathic hypereosinophilic syndrome
IHP. *See* Idiopathic hypertrophic pachymeningitis
IICP. *See* Increased Intracranial pressure
IIH. *See* Idiopathic intracranial hypertension
Iliohypogastric nerve, 540
Ilioinguinal nerve, 540
Immunohistochemical stains, muscle biopsy with, 128
Immunologic hypothesis, radiation injury in, 552
Immunosuppressant drugs
  cancer chemotherapy complications with, 1171
  multiple sclerosis treated with, 960
  polymyositis treated with, 936
Impact seizures, epilepsy with, 995
Impaired vision, 38–44, *39–41*
  electrophysiologic testing for, 40, *41*
    AMPPE for, 40
    AZOOR for, 40
    ERG for, 40
    VEP for, 40, *41*
  ocular lesions causing, 38
  ocular motility impairment and, 42–44
    amblyopia with, 42
    Collier sign with, 43
    congenital ocular motor apraxia with, 43
    diplopia with, 42
    downbeating nystagmus with, 44
    fixation instability with, 44
    hereditary ataxias with, 43
    Horner syndrome with, 42
    Huntington disease with, 43
    incomitance with, 42
    internal ophthalmoplegia with, 42
    internuclear ophthalmoplegia with, 43
    jerk nystagmus with, 44
    MLF with, 43
    myasthenia gravis with, 43
    ocular bobbing with, 44
    ocular dysmetria with, 44
    ocular flutter with, 44
    ocular myoclonus with, 44
    OKN with, 43
    one-and-a-half syndrome with, 43
    opsoclonus with, 44
    oscillopsia with, 43
    periodic alternating nystagmus with, 44
    PPRF with, 43
    pursuit system with, 43
    rebound nystagmus with, 44
    saccades with, 42
    saccadic system with, 43

    spasmus nutans with, 44
    sylvian aqueduct syndrome with, 43
    upbeating nystagmus with, 44
    vergence system with, 43
    vertical nystagmus with, 44
    vestibular system with, 43
    Wilson disease with, 43
  optic chiasm lesions causing, *39*, 41
  optic nerve lesions causing, 38–40, *39*, *40*
    anterior ischemic optic neuropathy with, 39, *40*
    compressive optic neuropathy with, 40
    optic nerve infarction with, 39, *40*
    optic neuritis with, 39
    Pulfrich phenomenon with, 39–40
    relative afferent pupillary defect with, 39
    scotoma with, 39, *39*, *41*
    Uhthoff symptom with, 40
  retrochiasmal lesions causing, *39*, 41–42
    cerebral blindness with, 41–42
    homonymous hemianopia with, 41
    macular sparing with, *39*, 41
    optic atrophy with, 41
    retrogeniculate lesions with, 41
    Wernicke hemianopic pupillary phenomenon with, 41
  transient visual effects with, 42
    amaurosis fugax, 42
    phosphenes as, 42
    scintillating homonymous scotoma as, 42
Impotence, drug dependence with, 1165
IMSOP. *See* International Medical Society of Paraplegia
INCL. *See* Haltia-Santavuori disease
Inclusion body myositis (IBM)
  defining features of, 935*t*
  myopathies of, 932, 934–935, 935*t*
  polymyositis v., 932, 934–935
  therapy for, 936
Incomitance, ocular motility impairment with, 42
Incontinence therapy, 1197–1198
Incontinentia pigmenti achromians (IPA)
  clinical manifestations of, 723, *723*
  diagnosis of, 723
  differential diagnosis of, 685*t*
  etiology of, 723
  genetics of, 723
  laboratory data on, 723
  neurocutaneous disorder of, 723
  pathology of, 723
  treatment of, 723
Increased Intracranial pressure (IICP), head injury trauma with, 493–494, 493*t*, *494*
Infantile acid-maltase deficiency, floppy infant syndrome with, 576
Infantile botulism, floppy infant syndrome with, 575
Infantile encephalopathy
  AB variant of, 622
  infantile Sandhoff diseases as, 622–625
  infantile Tay-Sachs diseases as, 622–625, *625*
  lysosomal/other storage diseases of, 622–625, *623*
Infantile neuroaxonal dystrophy, 676–677
  laboratory tests for, 677

Infantile neuronal ceroid lipofuscinoses. *See* Haltia-Santavuori disease
Infantile peripheral neuropathies, floppy infant syndrome with, 575
Infantile spasms, epilepsy with, 993
Infantile-onset spinocerebellar ataxia (IOSCA), 784*t*, 788, 788*t*
Infection
    alcoholism with, 1157
    drug dependence with, 1163–1164
Infection associated neuropathy, 755–757, *756*
Infections of nervous system
    AIDS, 211–225, 211*t*, 212*t*, 213*t*, 216*t*, *217*, 221*t*, *222*, *223*
        children with, 213
        clinical syndromes associated with, 216–220, 216*t*, *217*
        clinical/laboratory precautions with, 225
        CNS pathogenesis of, 215
        course of, 225
        drug-induced syndromes with, 224–225
        epidemiology of, 211–213, 213*t*
        etiology of, 213–214
        history of, 211
        HIV classification and, 211, 211*t*, 212*t*
        HIV-related syndromes with, 216–220, 216*t*, *217*
        neoplasms with, 220–224, 221*t*, *222*, *223*
        opportunistic infections with, 220–224, 221*t*, *222*, *223*
        pathogenesis of, 214–215
        prognosis with, 225
        treatment of, 225
    bacterial, 139–164, 140*t*, *145*, *146*, *151*, *152*, *153*
        acute purulent meningitis as, 139–144, 140*t*
        aseptic meningeal reaction as, 162
        Behçet syndrome as, 160–161
        brucellosis as, 160
        cerebral subdural empyema as, 148–150
        epidural infections as, 148–157, *151–153*
        Escherichia coli with, 139, 143, 151
        Hemophilus influenzae meningitis as, 142–143
        Hemophilus influenzae with, 139, 140*t*, 142–143
        human ehrlichiosis as, 159–160
        infective endocarditis as, 154–155
        intracranial epidural abscess as, 150, *151*
        Legionella pneumophila infection as, 163–164
        leprosy as, 155–156
        meningism as, 163
        meningococcal meningitis as, 139–142
        Mollaret meningitis as, 161–162
        Mycoplasma pneumoniae infection as, 163
        Neisseria meningitidis with, 139–142, 140*t*
        other acute meningitis as, 143–144
        pneumococcal meningitis as, 143
        recurrent bacterial meningitis as, 144
        rickettsial infections as, 156–160
        Rocky Mountain spotted fever as, 157–158
        scrub typhus as, 158–159
        spinal epidural abscess as, 150–154, *152*, *153*
        staphylococcal meningitis as, 143
        streptococcal meningitis as, 143
        Streptococcus pneumoniae with, 139, 140*t*, 143
        subacute meningitis as, 144–148, *145*, *146*
        subdural infections as, 148–150
        tuberculous meningitis as, *145*, 145–148, *146*
        typhus fever as, 158
        unknown cause acute purulent meningitis as, 144
        Vogt-Koyanagi-Harada syndrome as, 161
    bacterial toxins in, 259–262
        botulism as, 261–262
        diphtheria as, 259
        tetanus as, 259–261
    cryptococcosis, 229–230, *230*
    focal, 167–174, *169*, *170*, *172*
        brain abscess as, 168–173, *169*, *170*, *172*
        malignant external otitis as, 167–168
        osteomyelitis of skull base as, 167–168
        Pseudomonas aeruginosa with, 167
        subdural empyema as, 173–174
    fungal, 228–231, *230*
    leptospirosis as, 243–244
    Lyme disease as, 244–246, 245*t*
    mucormycosis, 230–231
    neurosarcoidosis, 232–234, 233*t*
    neurosyphilis as, 235–242, 236*t*, *237*, *239*, 240*t*, 241*t*
        AIDS and, 241–242
        asymptomatic, 238
        cerebrovascular, 238
        classification of, 236*t*
        clinical diagnosis of, 237–238
        clinical syndromes of, 238–240, *239*, 240*t*
        congenital, 240
        definition of, 235, 236*t*
        epidemiology of, 235, 236*t*
        frequency of different forms of, 236*t*
        gumma of, 239
        history of, 235
        meningeal, 238
        meningovascular, 239
        modern diagnostic triad of, 238
        paretic, 239, *239*
        pathology of, 237, *237*
        serology of, 237–238
        tabes dorsalis, 237, *237*, 239–240, 240*t*
        treatment of, 240–241, 240*t*, 241*t*
    parasitic, 246–257, 247*t*, *248*, *250*, *254*
        acanthamoeba infections as, 257
        bilharziasis as, 247*t*, 249–250, *250*
        cerebral malaria as, 254–255
        cysticercosis as, 247–248, 247*t*, *248*
        echinococcosis as, 247*t*, 248–249
        eosinophilic meningitis as, 247*t*, 251–252
        helminthic infection as, 247–253, 247*t*, *248*, *250*
        hydatid cysts as, 247*t*, 248–249
        Naegleria infections as, 256–257
        paragonimiasis as, 247*t*, 250–251
        primary amebic meningoencephalitis as, 256–257
        protozoan infection as, 253–256, *254*
        schistosomiasis as, 247*t*, 249–250, *250*
        strongyloidiasis as, 247*t*, 252–253
        toxoplasmosis as, 253–254, *254*
        trichinosis as, 247*t*, 251
        trypanosomiasis as, 255–256
    Prion diseases in, 264–268, 264*t*, 265*t*, *266*, *267*, 267*t*
        CJD as, 264*t*, 265–268, *266*, *267*, 267*t*
        FFI as, 264*t*, 268
        GSS disease as, 264*t*, 268
        human incidence of, 264–265, 264*t*, *265*
        kuru as, 264*t*, 265
        nvCJD as, 264*t*, 268
        pathology/pathogenesis of, 264
    Reye syndrome in, 262–263
        clinical presentation on, 262–263
        diagnosis of, 263
        pathology/pathogenesis of, 263
        treatment of, 263
    spirochete infections as, 235–246, 236*t*, *237*, *239*, 240*t*, 241*t*, 245*t*
    viral, 175–206, 176*t*, *183*, *189*, 192*t*, *193*, 196*t*, *200*, *204*, *205*
        acute viral infections as, 175–177, 176*t*
        ADEM as, 198–200, *200*
        adenovirus infections as, 191
        alphaviruses as, 176*t*, 181
        arboviruses infections as, 181
        arenavirus infections as, 190
        Argentinian hemorrhagic fever as, 190
        Bolivian hemorrhagic fever as, 190
        bunyaviruses as, 176*t*, 181
        California encephalitis as, 185
        chronic viral infections as, 200–202
        classification of, 175
        CMV as, 196–197, 196*t*
        CNS viral syndromes as, 175–177, 176*t*
        Colorado tick fever as, 186
        coxsackievirus infections as, 179–180
        Dawson disease as, 201–202
        echovirus infections as, 180
        encephalitis lethargica as, 204–205
        encephalomyelitis as, 187–188
        enterovirus infections as, 177–179
        Epstein-Barr virus infection as, 197
        equine encephalitis as, 181–183, *183*
        EV 70/EV 71 infections as, 180–181
        flaviviruses as, 176*t*, 181
        HAM as, 202–203
        hepatitis A virus as, 180–181
        herpes simplex encephalitis as, 191–194, 192*t*, *193*
        herpes zoster as, 194–196
        herpesvirus infections as, 191–196, 192*t*, *193*
        HHV-6 infection as, 197–198
        Japanese encephalitis as, 185
        Junin virus as, 190
        La Crosse encephalitis as, 185
        Lassa fever virus as, 190
        lymphocytic choriomeningitis as, 190
        Machupo virus as, 190
        mumps meningitis as, 187–188

Infections of nervous system,
   viral (contd.)
      myxovirus infections as, 187–188
      picornavirus infections as, 177–179
      PML as, 203–204, *204, 205*
      progressive rubella panencephalitis
         as, 202
      rabies as, 188–190
      reoviruses as, 176*t,* 181
      retrovirus infections as, 202–205,
         204, 205
      rhabdovirus infection as, 188–190
      rubella as, 186–187
      SSPE as, 201–202
      St. Louis encephalitis as, 183–184
      subacute measles encephalitis as, 188
      tick-borne encephalitis as, 186
      TSP as, 202–203
      unclassified enteroviruses as, 180–181
      West Nile virus encephalitis as,
         184–185
   Whipple diseases in, 270–272, 271*t*
Infectious diseases, dementia resulting
      from, 778, 778–779
   Creutzfeldt-Jakob disease in, *778,*
      778–779
   fatal familial insomnia in, *778,* 779
   Gerstmann-Sträussler disease in, *778,*
      779
   HIV in, 779
   kuru in, *778,* 779
   prion-related diseases in, *778,* 778–779
Infectious retinopathy, AIDS
      opportunistic infections with, 224
Infective endocarditis, 154–155
   diagnosis of, 155
   etiology of, 154
   signs/symptoms of, 154–155
   testing for, 155
   treatment of, 155
Inflammatory bowel disease, arterial
      thrombosis with, 319
Informed consent
   end-of-life issues with, 1201
   iatrogenic disease with, 1166
Infratentorial structural lesions, coma
      presentations with, 24
Infundibulomas, pituitary gland tumors
      with, 421
Inhalants, drug dependence with, 1161*t,*
   1163
Inherited metabolic diseases, dementia
      resulting from, 779–780, 779*t*
   adrenoleukodystrophy as, 779*t,* 780
   Alexander disease as, 780
   Fabry disease as, 780
   Fahr syndrome as, 780
   Gaucher disease as, 779*t,* 780
   GM-1 gangliosidosis as, 779*t,* 780
   GM-2 gangliosidosis as, 779*t,* 780
   Hallervorden-Spatz disease as, 780
   Krabbe disease as, 779*t*
   Kufs disease as, 779*t,* 780
   Lafora disease as, 779*t,* 780
   Mast syndrome as, 780
   Metachromatic leukodystrophy as, 779*t*
   mucopolysaccharidosis as, 779*t,* 780
   Niemann-Pick disease as, 779*t,* 780
   Sanfilippo disease as, 780
   Wilson disease as, 779*t,* 780
Insomnia, 1023–1024, 1024*t*
Intellectual ability, neuropsychologic
      evaluation tests for, 130–131, 131*t*

Intelligence measurement, 580, 581*t*
Intelligence quotient (IQ),
      neuropsychologic evaluation tests
      of, 130–131
Intensive care management, SAH
      treatment with, 335, 336*t*
Intensive Care Unit (ICU), head injury
      trauma with, 492, 493, 494
Intensive insulin therapy, head injury
      trauma with, 496
Interference patterns, EMG with, 92, 93,
      94, *95*
β-interferons, multiple sclerosis treated
      with, 959
Internal ophthalmoplegia, ocular motility
      impairment with, 42
International Medical Society of
      Paraplegia (IMSOP), 503
International Study of Unruptured
      Intracranial Aneurysms (ISUIA),
      114
International Subarachnoid Aneurysm
      Trial (ISAT), cerebral aneurysms
      in, 114
Internuclear ophthalmoplegia, ocular
      motility impairment with, 43
Interstitial brain edema, 358*t,* 359
Intervertebral disk trauma, 510–517,
      511*t,* 512*t, 513, 514, 515,* 516*t*
   cervical disc disease as, 512–513, *515,*
      516*t*
   chronic low-back pain as, 516–517
   CT of, 516
   diagnostic features of, 513–516
   imaging of, 516
   incidence of, 511
   lumbar intervertebral disc rupture as,
      511–512, 512*t, 513, 514*
   MRI of, 516
   pathogenesis of, 510–511, 511*t*
   signs/symptoms of, 511
   spinal stenosis with, 510
   syndromes of, 511*t*
   thoracic intervertebral disc rupture as,
      512
   treatment for, 516
Intracerebral abscess, 497
Intracerebral hemorrhage
   cerebral/cerebellar hemorrhage with,
      303–305, 304*t*
   etiologic factors for, 304*t*
   stroke genetics with, 307
   stroke treatment with, 326
Intracranial aneurysms, 329–330, 329*t*
Intracranial atheromatous, catheter
      angiography of, 109
Intracranial cerebral revascularization,
      118, 118*t*
Intracranial epidural abscess, 150, *151*
Intracranial hemorrhage (ICH)
   birth injuries of, 563
   cerebral concussion with, 484
   cerebrovascular disease with, 284–285,
      286
   children's, 321–322, *322*
   clinical presentation of, 285
   hydrocephalus with, 350, 354, 355
   subarachnoid hemorrhage with, 285
Intracranial venous-sinus thrombosis, 362
Intradural tumors, 474, *475, 476*
Intramedullary metastases, 473, *473*
Intramuscular streptomycin, Ménière
      disease treated with, 1021

Intrapulmonary shunting, 1083
Intrathecal IgG synthetic rate, multiple
      sclerosis with, 954
Intratympanic gentamicin, Ménière
      disease treated with, 1021
Intravascular lymphoma, 412
Intravenous Ig therapy (IVIG),
      myasthenia gravis treated with,
      883
Intraventricular hemorrhage (IVH),
      563–564, *564*
   diagnosis of, 564
   hydrocephalus with, 350
   incidence of, 563
   pathology/pathophysiology of, *545,* 563
   prevention of, 564
   prognosis for, 564
   symptoms/signs of, 563–564
Intraventricular meningiomas, 392
Intraventricular obstructive
      hydrocephalus (IVOH), obstructive
      hydrocephalus with, 349, 352, 355
Inversion recovery (IR), MRI with, 69
Involuntary movements
   akathisia, 49
   athetosis, 49
   athetotic dystonia, 49
   ballism, 48
   chorea, 48
   choreoathetosis, 49
   copropraxia, 49
   dystonia, 49
   echolalia, 49
   episodic ataxias, 48, 50
   Huntington disease with, 48
   hyperekplexia, 51
   hyperekplexias, 50
   myoclonus, 48
   orobuccolingual dyskinesia, 49
   palilalia, 49
   paroxysmal dyskinesias, 48, 50
   paroxysmal exertional dyskinesias, 50,
      50*t*
   paroxysmal hypnogenic dyskinesias, 50
   paroxysmal kinesigenic dyskinesias,
      50, 50*t*
   paroxysmal non-kinesigenic
      dyskinesias, 50, 50*t*
   restless legs syndrome with, 49
   stereotypies, 49
   Sydenham chorea, 48
   tics, 49
   tremors, 48
   types of, 48–51, 50*t,* 51*t*
IOSCA. *See* Infantile-onset
      spinocerebellar ataxia
IPA. *See* Incontinentia pigmenti
      achromians
IQ. *See* Intelligence quotient
IR. *See* Inversion recovery
Irregular sleep-wake pattern, sleep
      disorder of, 1029
Isaacs syndrome
   abnormal postures with, 926
   hyperhidrosis with, 926
   liability to cramps with, 926
   manifestations of, 926*t*
   muscle cramps/stiffness with, 925–927,
      926*t*
   myokymia with, 925
   pseudomyotonia with, 926
ISAT. *See* International Subarachnoid
      Aneurysm Trial

Ischemic brain edema, 358
Ischemic paralysis of arm, 536
ISDN. *See* Isosorbide dinitrate
Islet cell adenoma, pancreas endocrine
    disease of, 1044
Isolated gait ignition failure, senile gait
    disorders with, 60
Isosorbide dinitrate (ISDN), neuropathic
    pain treated with, 550
Isotonic fluids, head injury trauma with,
    495
ISUIA. *See* International Study of
    Unruptured Intracranial
    Aneurysms
IVH. *See* Intraventricular hemorrhage
IVIG. *See* Intravenous Ig therapy
IVOH. *See* Intraventricular obstructive
    hydrocephalus

J

Jamaican neuropathy, 856, 857
Jansky-Bielschowsky disease (LINCL),
    lysosomal/other storage diseases
    of, 631
Japanese encephalitis, 185
Jaw claudication, headache with, 46
Jaw winking, Marcus-Gunn syndrome
    with, 601, 602
Jerk nystagmus, ocular motility
    impairment with, 44
JNCL. *See* Spielmeyer-Sjögren disease
Jumping Frenchmen of Maine,
    myoclonus with, 814
Junin virus, 190
Juvenile myoclonic epilepsy, 82*t*, 993
Juvenile myxedema, thyroid endocrine
    diseases with, 1039
Juvenile neuronal ceroid lipofuscinosis.
    See Spielmeyer-Sjögren disease
Juvenile spinal muscular atrophy
    simulating muscular dystrophy. *See*
    Kugelberg-Welander syndrome

K

Kearns-Sayre syndrome (KSS)
    differential diagnosis of, 686*t*, 687*t*,
      688*t*
    laboratory abnormalities with, 699
    mitochondrial encephalomyopathies
      with, 695, 698–699
    molecular genetics with, 698–699
    treatment for, 699
Kennedy disease, motor neuron diseases
    of, 863
Kernohan notch, 487
Ketoacidosis, alcoholism with, 1157
KHD. *See* Kinky hair disease
Kinesia paradoxica, Parkinson disease
    with, 831
Kinky hair disease (KHD)
    diagnosis of, 666
    metal metabolism disorders of,
      665–666, *666*
    MRI of, 666, *666*
    radiograph of, 666
    Wilson disease v., 661, 661*t*
Kleeblattschädel skull, structural
    malformations of, 593
Kleine-Levin syndrome, sleep disorder of,
    1028
Klippel-Trenaunay syndrome,
    encephalotrigeminal angiomatosis
    v., 720

Klippel-Trenaunay-Weber
    malformations, 590*t*
Kocher-Debré-Sémélaigne syndrome,
    thyroid endocrine diseases with,
    1039, *1040*
Konzo, 856
Korsakoff psychosis. *See*
    Wernicke-Korsakoff syndrome
Krabbe disease
    dementia resulting from, 779*t*
    differential diagnosis of, 685*t*, 687*t*,
      688*t*
Krabbe leukodystrophy, lysosomal/other
    storage diseases of, 631, *632*
Krabbe-Weber disease, 455–457,
    455–457
    anticonvulsive drugs for, 456
    clinical presentation of, 456, *456*
    diagnosis of, 456, *456*
    hemispherectomy for, 456
    radiation therapy for, 456
    treatment of, 456
KSS. *See* Kearns-Sayre syndrome
Kufs disease (Adult variant neuronal
    caroid lipofuscinoses)
    dementia caused by, 5
    dementia resulting from, 779*t*,
      780
    lysosomal/other storage diseases of,
      631
Kugelberg-Welander syndrome, motor
    neuron diseases of, 862
Kuru, 264*t*, 265
    dementia resulting from, *778*, 779

L

La Crosse encephalitis, 185
Labyrinthectomy, Ménière disease
    treated with, 1021
Lacerations, head injury trauma with,
    486
Lactic acidemia, organic acidurias and,
    658
Lactic dehydrogenase (LDH), lymphoma
    with, 406
Lacunar strokes, cerebrovascular
    syndromes of, 308
Lafora disease
    dementia resulting from, 779*t*,
      780
    differential diagnosis of, 688*t*, 691*t*
    genetic central nervous diseases of,
      643–644
    myoclonus epilepsy with, 643–644
    myoclonus with, 813
Lambert-Eaton myasthenic syndrome
    (LEMS)
    abnormal voltage-dependent calcium
      channels with, 885
    diagnosis of, 885
    neuromuscular junction disorder of,
      885
    neuromuscular transmission tests
      with, 96
    paraneoplastic syndromes associated
      with, 1088*t*
    treatment of, 885
Lamotrigine
    epilepsy treatment with, 1001, 1003*t*,
      1005
    neuropathic pain treated with, 549
Landau-Kleffner syndrome, language
    disorders with, 581

Langerhans cell histiocytosis (LCH),
    hematologic disease of, 1060, *1061*
Language
    developmental disorders of, 580–585
      ADD in, 582–583
      ADHD in, 582–583
      autism in, 583–585
      Broca aphasia in, 581
      dyscalculia in, 582
      dysgraphia in, 582
      dyslexia in, 582
      dysorthographia in, 582
      etiology of, 582
      executive/planning disorders in,
        582
      Landau-Kleffner syndrome with, 581
      memory disorders in, 582
      neurologic basis for, 581
      nonverbal learning disabilities in,
        582
      pathophysiology of, 582
      pathophysiology with, 582
      PDD in, 583
      reading disability in, 582
      subtypes of, 581–582
      verbal auditory agnosia in, 581
    neuropsychologic evaluation tests for,
      132
Language therapy, 1197
Laparoscopic surgery, familial
    dysautonomia treated with,
    977–978
Large-vessel atherosclerotic infraction,
    281, *281*, 281*t*
Lassa fever virus, 190
Late response, nerve conduction studies
    with, *91*, 91–92
Late-delayed syndromes, radiation injury
    with, 552–555, *553*
Latency, nerve conduction studies with,
    90, 91, *91*
Latent tetany, hypoparathyroidism with,
    1042
Late-onset Friedreich ataxia (LOFA), 785
Lateral cord, 533
Lateral cord injury, 535
Lateral sinus thrombosis, 338–339
Lathyrism, 856, 857
Laurence-Moon-Biedl syndrome, 586
Layzer syndrome, occupation/
    environment neurotoxicology
    with, 1180
LCH. *See* Langerhans cell histiocytosis
LDH. *See* Lactic dehydrogenase
LE cells, systemic lupus erythematosus
    with, 1107
Lead, 759
    heavy metal intoxication with, 1174*t*,
      1176–1177
Learning disability, neuropsychologic
    evaluation with, 133
Leber hereditary optic neuropathy
    (LHON)
    clinical manifestations of, 702–703
    differential diagnosis of, 685*t*, 704
    mitochondrial DNA disorder of,
      702–704, 703*t*
    mitochondrial encephalomyopathies
      with, 696, *696*
    molecular genetics of, 703–704, 703*t*
    mutations associated with, 703*t*
    pathology of, 703–704, 703*t*
    treatment of, 704

Leber optic atrophy, differential diagnosis of, 685*t*
Leg nerve injury, 540–541
Leg pain, 31
Legal guidelines, end-of-life issues in, 1201–1203
  advance directives with, 1201
  doctrine of best interest with, 1201
  doctrine of substituted judgment with, 1201
  double effect with, 1201–1202
  euthanasia with, 1202–1203
  informed consent with, 1201
  overall view of, 1203
  palliative care with, 1202
  physician-assisted suicide with, 1202
  refusal of life-sustaining treatment with, 1201
  surrogate decision maker with, 1201
  terminal sedation with, 1202
Legionella pneumophila infection, 163–164
Leigh syndrome
  differential diagnosis of, 685*t*, 686*t*, 688*t*
  laboratory abnormalities with, 707
  nDNA mutations with, *707*, 707–708, 707*t*
  pathogenesis with, 708
  Wernicke encephalopathy v., 707, 707*t*
LEMS. *See* Lambert-Eaton myasthenic syndrome
Lennox-Gastaut syndrome, epilepsy with, 82*t*, 993
Leprosy, 155–156
  cranial nerves with, 156
Leprosy related neuropathy, 755–756, *756*
Leptomeningeal cysts, head injury trauma with, 499
Leptomeningeal lymphoma, 407
Leptomeningeal metastasis, 464–467, *466, 467*
  diagnosis of, 464–466, *466, 467*
  pathogenesis of, 464
  spinal tumors of, 474
  treatment of, 466–467
Leptospirosis, 243–244
Lesch-Nyhan syndrome, 620
  basic defect of, 620
  diagnosis of, 620
  differential diagnosis of, 685*t*, 686*t*, 687*t*, 688*t*
  neurologic manifestations of, 620
  treatment of, 620
Lesionectomy, epilepsy treated with, 1008, 1009*t*
Lesions of subthalamic nucleus, Parkinson disease surgery with, 838
Lethargy, coma v., 20–21
Leukemia, blood cell dyscrasias of, 1054–1055
Leukodystrophies
  differential diagnosis of, 687*t*, 688*t*
  Krabbe leukodystrophy in, 631, *632*
  lysosomal/other storage diseases of, 631–634, 632*t*, 633, 634
  metachromatic, 631–633, 632*t*, 633
  multiple sulfatase deficiency with, 632*t*, 633
Leukoencephalitis, HIV-related syndromes with, 216*t*, 219
Leukostasis, blood cell dyscrasias of, 1054

Leustatin. *See* Cladribine
Levine-Critchley syndrome, neurologic syndromes of, 673
Levitiracetam, epilepsy treatment with, 1001, 1003*t*, 1005
Levodopa
  Parkinson disease therapy with, 840–844, 842*t*
  sleep disorders treated with, 1026
Lewy bodies disease (DLB), 776–777
  dementia caused by, 4
  Parkinson disease v., 777
LGMD. *See* Limb-girdle muscular dystrophy
LGMD1A, 907*t*, 908
LGMD1B, 907*t*, 908
LGMD1C, 907*t*, 908
LGMD1D-LGMD1F, 907*t*, 908–909
LGMD2A, 906–907, 907*t*
LGMD2B, 907, 907*t*
LGMD2C-LGMD2F, 907*t*, 908
LGMD2J, 907*t*, 908
Lhermitte symptoms
  multiple sclerosis with, 950
  pain diagnosis with, 29
LHON. *See* Leber hereditary optic neuropathy
Li Fraumeni syndrome, gliomas with, 395
Liability to cramps, 926
Lightning injury, 557–558
Limb-girdle muscular dystrophy (LGMD), 905–909, 906*t*, 907*t*
  autosomal-recessive, 906–908, 907*t*, 908–909
    LGMD1A, 907*t*, 908
    LGMD1B, 907*t*, 908
    LGMD1C, 907*t*, 908
    LGMD1D-LGMD1F, 907*t*, 908–909
    LGMD2A, 906–907, 907*t*
    LGMD2B, 907, 907*t*
    LGMD2C-LGMD2F, 907*t*, 908
    LGMD2J, 907*t*, 908
  clinical manifestations of, 906
  conditions simulating, 906*t*
  definition of, 905–906, 906*t*, 907*t*
  history of, 905–906, 906*t*, 907*t*
  molecular genetics with, 906
Limbic encephalitis, paraneoplastic syndrome of, 1089
LINCL. *See* Jansky-Bielschowsky disease
Linear scleroderma, vasculitis syndrome of, 1108
Lipidoses, lysosomal/other storage diseases of, 622, *623*
Lipid-storage diseases, lysosomal/other storage diseases of, 622, *623*
Lissencephaly, structural malformations of, 587
Literal paraphasias, 10
Little disease, Motor function disorders of, 578
Liver disease, alcoholism with, 1157
Liver function tests, epilepsy in, 999
Liver transplantation
  hepatic disease with, 1066, 1066*t*
  neurologic complications of, 1066, 1066*t*
Localization-related epilepsy, 82*t*, 993–995
Locked-in syndrome, coma with, 25
LOCM. *See* Low-osmolar contrast media
Locus heterogeneity, DNA diagnostic tests with, 136, 136*t*

Long thoracic nerve, 533, 534*t*, 536, *537*
Long-latency reflex, 91
Lou Gehrig's disease. *See* Amyotrophic lateral sclerosis
Low back pain, 30
Lowe oculocerebrorenal syndrome, differential diagnosis of, 685*t*
Lowe syndrome
  amino acid metabolism disorder of, 618
  floppy infant syndrome with, 575
Lower body parkinsonism, normal pressure hydrocephalus parkinsonism of, 835
Lower extremity nerve injury, 539–540
  femoral nerve with, 539, 540–541
  genitofemoral nerve with, 540
  gluteal nerves with, 539
  iliohypogastric nerve with, 540
  ilioinguinal nerve with, 540
  lumbar plexus with, 539
  obturator nerve with, 539, 540
  peroneal nerve with, 540, 541
  plantar nerve with, 540
  sacral plexus with, 539–540
  sciatic nerve with, 539–540, 541
  spinal roots with, 539–540
  sural nerve with, 540
  tibial nerve with, 540, 541
Lower motor neuron disorders, 60
Lower radicular syndrome, 535
Lower trunk, 533
Lower-half headache, 982
Low-osmolar contrast media (LOCM), CT with, 70
Low-serum potassium periodic paralysis, 912*t*
LP. *See* Lumber puncture
Luft syndrome, mitochondrial encephalomyopathies with, 695
Lumbar intervertebral disc rupture, 511–512, 512*t*, *513, 514*
  diagnosis of, 512, *514*
  signs/symptoms of, 511–512, 512*t*, *513, 514*
Lumbar plexus, 539
Lumbar puncture headache, paroxysmal disorder of, 989
Lumbar spondylosis, 521–523, *522*
  CT of, 522, *522*
  diagnosis of, 522, *522*
  pathology of, 522
  symptoms/signs of, 522
  treatment of, 522–523
Lumbar tumors, spinal tumors of, 476
Lumber puncture (LP)
  bleeding disorder hazards with, 123
  contraindications for, 123
  CSF cells with, 124, 125*t*
  CSF pressure with, 123–124
  diagnostic tests for, 123–126, 125*t*
  indications for, 123
  SAH diagnosis with, 331
  subdural empyema with, 174
  thrombocytopenia with, 123
Lumbosacral plexopathy
  drug dependence with, 1165
  radiation injury with, 554
Lupus anticoagulant syndrome
  cerebrovascular syndromes of, 309
  coagulation disorders with, 1058
Lyme disease, 244–246, 245*t*
  CSF analysis in, 245, 245*t*

diagnosis of, 245–246, 245*t*
epidemiology of, 244
multiple sclerosis v., 954–955, 957*t*
symptoms/signs of, 244–245
treatment of, 246
Lyme neuropathy, 762–763
Lymphocytic choriomeningitis, 190
Lymphoma, 406–413, *408–410*, 410*t*
AIDS opportunistic infections with,
223
brain metastasis with, 407
childhood central nervous system
tumors of, 442
epidural spinal cord compression with,
407
intravascular, 412
LDH with, 406
leptomeningeal, 407
lymphomatoid granulomatosis,
412–413
metastatic to nervous system of,
406–407
non-Hodgkin, 406–407
primary CNS, 406, 407–412, *408–410*,
410*t*
chemotherapy for, 410
clinical manifestations in, 411
clinical manifestations of, 407
corticosteroids for, 409
CT scan of, 408, *408*
diagnosis in, 411
diagnosis of, 409, 410*t*
epidemiology in, 411
epidemiology of, 407
imaging in, 411
imaging of, 408, *408–410*
immunocompromised patient with,
411–412
MRI of, 408, *409–410*
pathology of, 407–408
pathology/pathogenesis in, 411
patient evaluation for, 410*t*
PET in, 411
prognosis for, 410–411, 412
radiation for, 409–410
SPECT in, 411
surgery for, 409
treatment for, 411–412
treatment of, 409–410
WBRT for, 409–410, 411
Lymphomatoid granulomatosis, 412–413
Lymphoproliferative diseases, blood cell
dyscrasias of, 1055
Lymphorrhages, myasthenia gravis with,
879
Lysosomal/other storage diseases,
622–640, *623–625*, 627*t*–628*t*, 632*t*,
633, 634, 635*t*, 638*t*
AB variant in, 622
aspartylglycosaminuria in, 638*t*, 639
cerebrotendinous xanthomatosis in,
627*t*, 630
cholestanol disease in, 630
Fabry disease in, 626, 627*t*
Farber lipogranulomatosis disease in,
627*t*, 629
free sialic acid storage diseases in,
637–639
fucosidosis in, 638*t*, 639
galactosialidosis in, 637, 638*t*
Gaucher disease in, 626–628, 627*t*
globoid-cell leukodystrophy in, 631, *632*
GM1-gangliosidoses in, 625–626, 627*t*

GM2-gangliosidoses in, 622–625, *624,*
627*t*
Haltia-Santavuori disease in, 630–631
hexosaminidase-deficiency diseases in,
622
Hunter syndrome in, 635*t*, 636
Hurler syndrome in, 634–636, 635*t*
infantile encephalopathy in, 622–625,
625
infantile Sandhoff diseases in, 622–625
infantile Tay-Sachs diseases in,
622–625, *625*
Jansky-Bielschowsky disease in, 631
Krabbe leukodystrophy in, 631, *632*
Kufs disease in, 631
leukodystrophies in, 631–634, 632*t*, *633,*
634
lipidoses in, 622, *623*
lipid-storage diseases in, 622, *623*
α-mannosidosis in, 638*t*, 639
β-mannosidosis in, 638*t*, 639
Maroteaux-Lamy syndrome in, 637
metachromatic leukodystrophy in,
631–633, 632*t*, *633*
Morquio syndrome in, 635*t*, 636–637
mucolipidoses II in, 638*t*, 639
mucolipidoses III in, 638*t*, 639
mucolipidoses in, 637–639, 638*t*
mucolipidoses IV in, 638*t*, 639–640
mucopolysaccharidoses in, 634–637,
635*t*
neuronal ceroid lipofuscinoses in, 628*t*,
630–631
Niemann-Pick disease in, 627*t*,
628–629
Sanfilippo syndrome in, 635*t*, 636
sialidosis in, 637, 638*t*
Spielmeyer-Sjögren disease in, 631
Wolman disease in, 627*t*, 629–630
Lytico-Bodig, Parkinsonism-plus
syndrome of, 828*t*, 836

M

Machado-Joseph disease
autosomal-dominant ataxia of, 784*t*,
789*t*, 792–793
orthostatic hypotension with, 972*t*
Machupo virus, 190
Macroadenomas, pituitary gland tumors
with, 421, *421*
Macrocephaly, structural malformations
of, 588–589, 590*t*
Macular sparing, impaired vision with,
39, 41
Magnetic gait, senile gait disorders with,
60
Magnetic resonance angiography (MRA),
67, 70, 74, 78
arteriovenous malformations in, 452,
454
AVM with, 74
CT v., 103
flow-related enhancement with, 74
MIP with, 74
neurovascular imaging with, 103, 108
pituitary gland tumors with, 423
TIA with, 74
Magnetic resonance imaging (MRI)
ACD with, 75
acute brainstem ischemia on, 106, *107*
acute intracerebral hemorrhage on, *68,*
69
acute stroke diagnosis with, 75–78

Alzheimer disease in, 772
angiography, 67, 70, 74, 78
AVM with, 74
flow-related enhancement with, 74
MIP with, 74
TIA with, 74
arteriovenous malformations in, 452,
452
ASL with, 70, 75
astrocytomas in, 431, *435, 436,* 436–437
BOLD with, 75
bolus-tracking method with, 74
brain metastasis in, 460, 461, *461*
brainstem infarction on, 106, *107*
Canavan disease, 675
CBF with, 107
CBV with, 107
central pontine myelinolysis in,
965–967, *966*
cerebral perfusion assessed with, 106
cervical carotid stenosis with, 74
cervical spondylotic myelopathy in,
518, *519, 520*
coma diagnosis with, 23, 24
dementia diagnosis with, 6
dermatomyositis in, 931
diagnostic tests selection of, 67–78, *68,*
71, 76–78
DWI with, 67, 70, *71,* 73, 75, 77, 78,
106, 108
EEG v., 79
epidural spinal cord metastasis in, 468
epilepsy in, 998–999, *999*
extra-axial hemorrhage on, 106
factors influencing appearance of, 69
applied RF flip angle as, 69
echo time as, 69
gradient time/amplitude/duration as,
69
imaging technique as, 69
pulse sequence as, 69
repetition time as, 69
first-pass method with, 74
FLAIR with, 70, 78, *104,* 105, 106
FSE with, 70, *104*
functional, 74–75
Gd enhancement of, 70
appropriate utilization of, 74
CECT v., 73
Dawson fingers in, 73
indications for, 73
gliomas in, *396,* 396–397
GRE with, 69, 70, 74
headache diagnosis with, 45
hearing loss and, 33, 34
hemorrhagic infarction on, *106*
hepatolenticular degeneration in, 664,
664
hydrocephalus in, *352–354,* 354–355
hypoxic-ischemic encephalopathy in,
566, 567
intervertebral disk trauma in, 516
IR with, 69
medulloblastoma with, 440, *440*
meningiomas in, 387
Menkes disease in, 666, *666*
MRS with, 74, 75, *76,* 107–108
MTT with, 75
MTTP with, 107
multiple sclerosis in, 951–954, 951*t,*
952, 953, 955, *956*
neurologic disorders examination with,
60, 61, 62

Magnetic resonance imaging (MRI) (*contd.*)
neurovascular imaging with, 100, 104–108, *106*, *107*, 113*t*
organic acidurias in, 660
pain diagnosis with, 29, 30
parenchymal hemorrhage on, 106
PC technique with, 74
PCNSL in, 408, *409*, *410*
pediatric acquired HIV/AIDS in, 1187
pineal cysts in, 418
pituitary gland tumors with, 422–423, *423*, *424*
PNET in, 440
primary lateral sclerosis in, 859, 859*t*
PWI with, 67, 70, *71*, 77, 78
radiation injury in, 552, *553*
SE with, 69
spinal cord diseases in, 856
spinal injury trauma in, 505–506
spinal tumors in, 472, 477
spontaneous intracranial hypotension with, 364, *364*
subarachnoid hemorrhage on, 106
Superficial siderosis of central nervous system in, 365, *366*
syringomyelia in, *872*, 872–873
systemic lupus erythematosus in, 1107
TOF method with, 74
TTP with, 75
tumor examination with, 375–376
uses of, 72–73
vertigo diagnosis with, 36, 37
weak muscles examination with, 54
Magnetic resonance spectroscopy (MRS), 74, 75, *76*, 107–108
hypoxic-ischemic encephalopathy in, 566, 567
Main en griffe, syringomyelia with, 871
Main succulente, 871
Maintenance of Wakefulness Test, 1023
Major depressive disorder (MDD)
biomarkers with, 1127
diagnosis of, 1126–1127, 1126*t*
dysthymia with, 1127
genetics with, 1127
Hamilton rating scale for, 1126*t*
pathophysiology of, 1127–1128
specific antidepressant medications for, 1129–1130, 1129*t*
treatment of, 1128–1129
Malabsorption, 1092–1094, 1092*t*, 1093*t*
bariatric surgery with, 1093, 1093*t*
causes of neurologic disorder from, 1092, 1092*t*
celiac disease with, 1093
chronic diarrhea with, 1094
Crohn disease with, 1093
oculomasticatory myorhythmia with, 1094
ulcerative colitis with, 1093
Whipple disease as, 1094
Malignant external otitis, 167–168
osteomyelitis of skull base with, 167–168
Pseudomonas aeruginosa with, 167
Malingering, somatoform disorders with, 1144
Malnutrition, 1091–1092, 1091*t*, 1092*t*
anorexia nervosa as, 1092

emetine for, 1092
peripheral/optic neuropathy with, 1092
tropical myeloneuropathies with, 857
Manganese, heavy metal intoxication with, 1174*t*, 1178
α-mannosidosis, lysosomal/other storage disease of, 638*t*, 639
β-mannosidosis, lysosomal/other storage diseases of, 638*t*, 639
Maple syrup urine disease (MSUD)
amino acid metabolism disorder of, 614
treatment of, 614
Marburg variant, multiple sclerosis, 956, 958
Marche à petits pas, 57
Marchiafava-Bignami disease, *963*, 963–964, *964*
alcoholism with, 1158
course of, 964
diagnosis of, 964
ethnicity with, 61
etiology of, 963
incidence of, 964
pathology of, *963*, 963–964, *964*
symptoms/signs of, 964
treatment of, 964
Marcus-Gunn syndrome, 601–602
Marijuana, 1161*t*, 1162
Marine neurotoxic syndrome, occupation/environment neurotoxicology with, 1180
Marinesco-Sjögren syndrome, 784*t*, 788, 788*t*
differential diagnosis of, 686*t*
Maroteaux-Lamy syndrome, lysosomal/other storage diseases of, 637
Maroteaux-Larny malformations, 590*t*
Masked facies, Parkinson disease with, 829
Mast syndrome, dementia resulting from, 780
Maximum intensity projection (MIP)
CT with, 72
MRA with, 74
MBD. *See* Minimal brain damage
McArdle syndrome, 127, 135*t*, 895, 921
McCune-Albright syndrome, 1076
MCI. *See* Mild cognitive impairment
McLeod syndrome, neurologic syndromes of, 673–674, 674*t*
MDD. *See* Major depressive disorder
MDMA. *See* Ecstasy
Mean transit time (MTT)
CT with, 72
MRA with, 75
Mean transit time or time to peak (MTTP), MRI with, 107
Mechanical ventilation, respiratory support for neurologic diseases with, 1086–1087, 1086*t*
Meckel-Gruber syndrome, structural malformations with, 595
Medial cord, 533
Medial longitudinal fasciculus (MLF), ocular motility impairment with, 43
Median nerve, 534, 534*t*, 537–538, 538*t*
Medical history
neurologic disorders examination with, 60, 62
vertigo diagnosis with, 35

Medulloblastoma, childhood central nervous system tumors of, 428, 429, 431*t*, 432*t*, 439–441, *440*
chemotherapy for, 440–441
MRI of, 440, *440*
radiation therapy for, 440
Megalencephaly, structural malformations of, 588–589, 590*t*
Melanoma, childhood central nervous system tumors of, 428
MELAS. *See* Mitochondrial encephalomyopathy, lactic acidosis, strokelike episodes
Memory
language disorders of, 582
neuropsychologic evaluation tests for, 131, 131*t*
MEN-I. *See* Multiple endocrine neoplasia I
Ménière disease, 1018–1021
burned out, 1019
cochlear, 1019
conservative procedures for, 1020–1021
definitions with, 1018–1019
destructive procedures for, 1021
diagnosis of, 1019–1020
endolymphatic shunts for, 1020–1021
historical review on, 1018
intramuscular streptomycin for, 1021
intratympanic gentamicin for, 1021
introduction to, 1018
labyrinthectomy for, 1021
medical therapy for, 1020
Meniett device for, 1021
surgical therapy for, 1020–1021
tinnitus with, 1018–1019
treatment of, 1020–1021
vertigo with, 1018–1019
vertigo/hearing loss caused by, 35*t*, 37
vestibular neurectomy for, 1021
Meningeal neurosyphilis, 238
Meningeal pleocytosis, HIV-related syndromes with, 216*t*
Meningeal signs, uremic encephalopathy with, 1080
Meningiomas, 386–392, *388–392*, 414*t*, 416
biology of, 386–387
cerebellopontine angle, 392
chemotherapy for, 390–391
childhood central nervous system tumors of, 442–443, *443*
clinical manifestations of, 387
clivus, *390*, 392
convexity, *389*, 391
CT of, 387
etiology of, 386
foramen magnum, 392
hormonal treatment for, 390
imaging of, 387, *388*
intraventricular, 392
medical treatment for, 390–391
olfactory groove, 391
optic-sheath, 392
parasagittal, 391
pathology of, 387
radiation injury with, 555
radiation therapy for, 388–390
specific tumor locations with, *389*, *390*, *391*, 391–392, *392*
sphenoid ridge, 392, *392*

spinal, 392
spinal tumors of, 474
supportive treatment for, 391
surgery for, 388
tentorial, *391*, 392
treatment of, 388–391
tuberculum sellae, 391
VEGF with, 387
Meningism, 163
Meningitis
  CSF with, *125*
  head injury trauma with, 497
Meningococcal meningitis,
    139–142
  complications/sequelae with, 141
  diagnosis of, 141–142
  incidence of, 140
  laboratory data on, 141
  pathogenesis of, 139–140
  pathology of, 140
  prognosis for, 142
  signs of, 141
  symptoms of, 141
  treatment for, 142
Meningovascular neurosyphilis,
    239
Menkes disease, 661*t*, 665–666, *666*
  diagnosis of, 666
  MRI of, 666, *666*
  radiograph of, 666
  Wilson disease v., 661, 661*t*
Menkes syndrome
  differential diagnosis of, 685*t*, 686*t*,
    687*t*
  structural malformations with, 587
Menstrual irregularity, drug dependence
    with, 1165
Mental deficiency, 579, 579*t*, 580
Mental retardation
  subtelomeric chromosomal anomalies
    with, 610
Mental status exam, 7–8, 7*t*
MEP. *See* Motor-evoked potential
Meralgia paresthetica, pregnancy with,
    1116
Mercury, 759
  heavy metal intoxication with, 1174*t*,
    1177
MERRF. *See* Myoclonic epilepsy with red
    ragged fibers
Mesial temporal sclerosis
  epilepsy with, 998, *999*
  febrile seizures with, 1016
Metabolic myopathies, floppy infant
    syndrome with, 576
Metachromatic leukodystrophy, 631–633,
    632*t*, *633*
  adult, 632*t*, 633
  dementia resulting from, 779*t*
  juvenile, 632*t*, 633
  late-infantile, 631–633, 632*t*
Metal metabolism disorders, 660–667,
    661*t*, 662, 663, 663*t*, 664, 666
  aceruloplasminemia in, 666–667
  hepatolenticular degeneration in,
    660–665, 661*t*, 662, 663, 663*t*, 664
  kinky hair disease in, 665–666, *666*
  Menkes disease in, 661*t*, 665–666,
    666
  molybdenum cofactor deficiency in,
    667
  Wilson disease in, 660–665, 661*t*, 662,
    663, 663*t*, 664

Metastasis to skull base
  adenoid cystic carcinoma as, 379
  esthesioneuroblastoma as, 379, 379*t*
  malignant skull tumors as, 379, 379*t*
  nasopharyngeal carcinoma as, 379
  squamous cell carcinoma as, 379
Metastatic tumors, 459–468, *460, 461, 463,*
    465–467
  brain metastasis as, 459
    chemotherapy for, 463–464
    clinical evaluation of, 460
    clinical findings on, 460, *460*
    CT of, 460, 461
    differential diagnosis for, 461
    imaging of, 460, *461*
    MRI of, 460, 461, *461*
    pathophysiology of, 461–462
    radiotherapy for, 462
    stereotactic radiosurgery for, 462, *463*
    surgery for, 462–463
    treatment of, 462–464
    WBRT for, 462, 463
  dural metastasis as, 464, *465*
  epidemiology of, 459
  epidural spinal cord metastasis as,
    467–468
  leptomeningeal metastasis as, 464–467,
    466, 467
Methamphetamine, 1162
Methanol, occupation/environment
    neurotoxicology with, 1174*t*, 1181
Methyl alcohol, occupation/environment
    neurotoxicology with, 1174*t*, 1181
1-methyl-4-pehenyl-1,2,3,6-
    tetrahydropyridine (MPTP),
    parkinsonism with, 828*t*, 835
Methylbromide, 759
MG. *See* Myasthenia gravis
MGUS. *See* Monoclonal gammopathy of
    unknown significance
Microadenomas, pituitary gland tumors
    with, 421, 422, *423*
Microbiologic test, 126
Microdactyly, myositis ossifans with,
    938
Micrographia, Parkinson disease with,
    830
Microscopic polyangiitis, vasculitis
    syndrome of, 1104
Microsomal triglyceride transfer protein
    (MTP), abetalipoproteinemia with,
    672
Microsurgery, spinal tumors treated with,
    479
Middle radicular syndrome, 535
Middle trunk, 533
Midodrine, familial dysautonomia
    treated with, 978
Migraine
  accompaniments of, 981
  acute treatment for, 985
  almotriptan for, 985
  amitriptyline for, 985, 986*t*
  arterial thrombosis with, 319
  with aura, 981, 982
  without aura, 981, 982
  basilar, 982
  carotidynia syndrome as, 982
  classic, 981, 982
  clinical subtypes of, 981–983
  common, 982
  complicated, 981
  eletriptan for, 985

equivalents of, 981
  ergonovine for, 985, 986*t*
  ergotamine for, 985
  facial, 982
  gonads endocrine diseases with,
    1046
  hemicrania and, 981
  hemiplegic, 982–983
  lower-half headache as, 982
  naratriptan for, 985
  ophthalmoplegic, 983
  paroxysmal disorder of, 981–989, *984,*
    986*t*
  pathogenesis of, 983–984, *984*
  pharmacologic data on, 984
  phenelzine for, 985, 986*t*
  pregnancy with, 1115–1116
  prophylactic treatment for, 985–986,
    986*t*
  propranolol for, 985, 986*t*
  rizatriptan for, 985
  seizure with, 18*t*, 19
  serotonin receptors with, 984
  sumatriptan for, 985
  transient global amnesia with, 1017
  treatment of, 984–986
  valproate for, 985, 986*t*
  verapamil for, 985, 986*t*
  zolmitriptan for, 985
Mild cognitive impairment (MCI),
    dementia diagnosis with, 6
Miller-Dieker syndrome, structural
    malformations with, 589*t*
Miller-Fisher syndrome, GBS variants of,
    749–750
Mineralizing microangiopathy, radiation
    injury with, 552
Minimal brain damage (MBD), higher
    cerebral function disorders with,
    579
Mini-mental status exam (MMSE),
    dementia diagnosis with, 7, 7*t*
Minor motor disability, motor function
    disorders of, 577
MIP. *See* Maximum intensity projection
Mitochondrial DNA disorders
  Leber hereditary optic neuropathy as,
    702–704, 703*t*
  mitochondrial encephalomyopathies
    as, 695–701, 695*t*, *696*, 698*t*
  acquired depletion in, 701
  clinical manifestations of, 697–698,
    698*t*, *699*
  congenital myopathy with, 701
  depletion of, 701
  genetic classification of, 695, 695*t*
  genetic principles of, 697–698, 698*t*,
    699
  hepatopathy with, 701
  history of, 695–696, *696*
  infantile myopathy with, 701
  Kearns-Sayre syndrome in, 695, 698
  LHON with, 696, *696*
  Luft syndrome in, 695
  MELAS with, 696, *696*, 700
  MERRF with, 696, *696*, 700–701
  morbidity map of, *696*
  NARP with, 701
  ophthalmoplegia plus with, 695
  pathogenesis of, 697–698, 698*t*, *699*
  progressive external
    ophthalmoplegia in, 698–700, 698*t*
  ragged-red fibers with, 695, 697, *699*

Mitochondrial DNA disorders (*contd.*)
 nDNA mutations as, 705–708, 706*t*, *707*,
  707*t*
  abnormal mitochondrial membrane
   milieu with, 708
  Alpers syndrome with, 708
  citric acid cycle disorder in, 706, 706*t*
  classification of, 705, 706*t*
  DiMauro syndrome with, 706
  fatty acid oxidation disorder in, 706
  impaired mitochondrial transport
   with, 708
  Leigh syndrome with, *707*, 707–708,
   707*t*
  metal metabolism defects in, 706*t*,
   708
  mitochondrial motility defects in,
   706*t*, 708
  PDH complex defects in, 706
  respiratory chain disorder in,
   706–707, 706*t*
  substrate transport disorder in, 706,
   706*t*
  substrate use disorder in, 706, 706*t*
Mitochondrial encephalomyopathies,
  695–701, 695*t*, *696*, 698*t*
 acquired depletion in, 701
 clinical manifestations of, 697–698,
  698*t*, *699*
 congenital myopathy with, 701
 depletion of, 701
 genetic classification of, 695, 695*t*
  heteroplasmy in, 697
  maternal inheritance in, 697
  mitotic segregation in, 697
  polyplasmy in, 697
  threshold effect in, 697
 genetic principles of, 697–698, 698*t*, *699*
 hepatopathy with, 701
 history of, 695–696, *696*
 infantile myopathy with, 701
 Kearns-Sayre syndrome in, 695, 698
 LHON with, 696, *696*
 Luft syndrome in, 695
 MELAS with, 696, *696*, 700
 MERRF with, 696, *696*, 700–701
 morbidity map of, *696*
 NARP with, 701
 ophthalmoplegia plus with, 695
 pathogenesis of, 697–698, 698*t*, *699*
 progressive external ophthalmoplegia
  in, 698–700, 698*t*
 ragged-red fibers with, 695, 697, *699*
Mitochondrial encephalomyopathy, lactic
  acidosis, strokelike episodes
  (MELAS)
 differential diagnosis of, 685*t*, 686*t*,
  688*t*
 mitochondrial encephalomyopathies
  with, 696, *696*, 700
Mitochondrial neurogastrointestinal
  encephalomyopathy (MNGIE)
 laboratory abnormalities in, 700
 molecular genetics in, 700
 progressive external ophthalmoplegia
  with, 700
Mitochondrial respiratory chain,
  structural malformations of,
  590*t*
Mitoxantrone (Novantrone), multiple
  sclerosis treated with, 959
Mixed cerebral palsy, motor function
  disorders of, 579

Mixed connective tissue disease,
  dermatomyositis with, 930
Miyoshi variant myopathy, muscular
  dystrophy of, 910
MLF. *See* Medial longitudinal fasciculus
MMM. *See* Multiminicore myopathy
MMNCB. *See* Multifocal motor
  neuropathy with conduction block
MNGIE. *See* Mitochondrial
  neurogastrointestinal
  encephalomyopathy
Möbius syndrome, 602
 congenital facial diplegia with, 602
Modafinil (Provigil)
 multiple sclerosis treated with, 961
 sleep disorders treated with, 1028
Moersch-Woltman syndrome
 Babinski signs with, 928
 clinical manifestations of, 927–928,
  928*t*
 defining characteristics of, 928*t*
 differential diagnosis of, 928
 encephalomyelitis with, 928
 hyperekplexia with, 928
 laboratory data on, 928
 muscle cramps/stiffness with, 927–928,
  928*t*
 Schwartz-Jampel syndrome v., 928
 startle disease with, 928
 stiff encephalomyelitis with, 928
 stiff limb syndrome with, 928
Mollaret meningitis, 161–162
Molybdenum cofactor deficiency
 floppy infant syndrome with, 575
 metal metabolism disorders of, 667
Monoclonal gammopathy of unknown
  significance (MGUS), blood cell
  dyscrasias of, 1055
Monomelic muscular atrophy, motor
  neuron diseases with, 867
Monomelic paresis, weak muscles with,
  55
Monoplegia, weak muscles with, 52
Monro-Kellie rule, 364
Mood disorders, 1125–1132, 1126*t*,
  1129*t*
 Alzheimer disease with, 1131
 biomarkers with, 1127
 bipolar disorders in, 1130–1131
 dysthymia with, 1127
 epidemiology with, 1125, 1131
 genetics with, 1127
 Hamilton rating scale with, 1126*t*
 Huntington disease with, 1131–1132
 individuality with, 1125–1126
 MDD diagnosis with, 1126–1127, 1126*t*
 multiple sclerosis symptoms of, 950
 neurologic conditions resulting in,
  1131–1132
 Parkinson disease with, 1132
 pathophysiology of, 1127–1128
 public health and, 1125
 social mood stabilizers for, 1131
 specific antidepressant medications for,
  1129–1130, 1129*t*
 treatment of, 1128–1129
Morquio syndrome, lysosomal/other
  storage diseases of, 635*t*, 636–637
Mortality estimates, head injury trauma
  in, 491*t*
Motor aphasia
 agrammatism with, 9
 Broca's aphasia as, 9

classification as, 8
clinical features of, 9–10
 dysarthria with, 9
 dysphonia with, 9
 dyspraxia with, 9
 dysprosody with, 9
 speech dyspraxia with, 9
 telegraphic speech with, 9
 total aphasia with, 9
Motor function, developmental disorders
  of, 576–579, 577*t*
 ataxic cerebral palsy in, 578
 cerebral palsy in, 577, 577*t*
 Davidoff-Dyke-Masson syndrome in,
  577
 diparesis in, 578
 dyskinetic cerebral palsy in, 578
 hemiplegia in, 577, 577*t*
 hypotonic cerebral palsy in, 578
 Little disease in, 578
 minor motor disability in, 577
 mixed cerebral palsy in, 579
 spastic diplegia in, 577*t*, 578
 spastic hemiparesis in, 577, 577*t*
 spastic quadriplegia in, 577*t*, 578–579
Motor nerve conduction studies, 90,
  90–91
 CAMP with, *90*, 90–91
 set up for, *90*
Motor neuron diseases
 adult onset, 863–868, 864*t*, 866*t*
 amyotrophic lateral sclerosis as,
  863–868, 864*t*, 866*t*
 benign fasciculation and cramps
  syndrome with, 868
 classification of, 861, 861*t*
 definitions of, 861, 861*t*
 Denny-Brown, Foley syndrome with,
  868
 Fazio-Londe syndrome as, 862
 focal muscular atrophies as, 862–863
 Hirayama syndrome with, 867
 Kennedy disease as, 863
 Kugelberg-Welander syndrome as, 862
 monomelic muscular atrophy with,
  867
 multifocal motor neuropathy with
  conduction block with, 867
 multiple sclerosis with, 867
 myasthenia gravis with, 867
 paraneoplastic syndrome of, 1089
 postpolio syndrome with, 867
 progressive bulbar palsy as, 866
 pseudobulbar palsy with, 867
 respiratory dysfunction with, 1085
 reversible motor neuron disease with,
  868
 spinal cord diseases of, 861–868, 861*t*,
  864*t*, 866*t*
 spinal muscular atrophies of childhood
  as, 861–862, 861*t*
 Werdnig-Hoffmann syndrome as, 862
 X-linked recessive spinobulbar
  muscular atrophy as, 863, 864*t*
Motor responses, coma examination
  with, 21–22
Motor unit configuration, EMG with,
  92–93, *93*
Motor unit disorders, 893–895, 894*t*
 definitions with, 894–895
 identifying, 893–895, 894*t*
 laboratory data on, 893–894
 muscle biopsy for, 893

muscle cramps/stiffness caused by, 925*t*

serum enzyme determination for, 894, 894*t*

Motor unit recruitment, EMG with, 92, 93–94

Motor-evoked potential (MEP), 88
  TMS with, 98–99

Motor-unit action potential (MUAP)
  EMG with, 92–93, *93*, *94*
  myopathic, 93, *93*
  neurogenic, *93*, *94*

Movement disorders
  AIDS opportunistic infections with, 223–224
  chorea in, 807–811, 807*t*, 808*t*
    ballism with, 809–810
    common causes of, 807*t*, 808*t*
    dentatorubralpallidoluysian atrophy, 810
    Haw River syndrome, 810
    HDL, 810–811
    hereditary nonprogressive, 811
    neuroacantocytosis, 810
    other immune, 809
    primary antiphospholipid antibody syndrome, 809
    senile, 811
    Sydenham, 807–809, 807*t*, 808*t*
    systemic lupus erythematosus, 809
    vascular, 809–810
  dystonia in, 816–826, 816*t*, 817*t*, *818*, *819*, *820*, 822*t*, 823*t*, 824*t*, 825*t*
    action, 816
    adult onset primary, 819–821, *820*
    classification of, 816–817, 816*t*, 817*t*
    dopa-responsive, 821–822, 822*t*
    dyskinesia with, 825, 825*t*
    dystonia plus syndromes as, 816*t*, 817, 821–823, 822*t*
    dystonic storm with, 816
    dystonic tremor with, 816
    early onset primary, 819
    focal, 816*t*, 817
    generalized, 816*t*, 817
    hemidystonia, 816*t*, 817
    heredodegenerative, 816*t*, 817, 824–825, 825*t*
    multifocal, 816*t*, 817
    myoclonus, 823
    Oppenheim, *818*, 818–819, *819*, 822*t*
    overflow with, 816
    primary, 816*t*, 817, *818*, 818–821, *819*
    pseudodystonia as, 825, 825*t*
    psychogenic, 824, 824*t*
    rapid-onset, 822–823
    secondary, 816*t*, 817, 823–824, 823*t*, 824*t*
    Segawa disease as, 821–822, 822*t*
    segmental, 816*t*, 817
    status dystonicus with, 816
    Tardive, 823–824
    task-specific, 816
    treatment of, 826
  essential tremor as, 827
  Huntington disease in, *803*, 803–806, *805*
    biochemistry of, 803–804
    choreic movements with, 805
    diagnosis of, 806
    differential diagnosis of, 806
    genetics of, 804
    HDL and, 806

laboratory data on, *805*, 805–806
    mental symptoms of, 805
    other neurologic manifestations of, 805
    pathology of, 803, *803*
    prevalence of, 804
    symptoms/signs of, 804–805
    tardive dyskinesia with, 806
    treatment of, 806
  myoclonus in, 812–814, 813*t*
    Alzheimer disease with, 813
    classification of, 813, 813*t*
    cortical tremor with, 812
    Creutzfeldt-Jakob disease with, 813
    dentatorubropallidoluysian atrophy with, 813
    encephalomyelitis with rigidity, 813
    epilepsia partialis continua with, 812
    epileptic, 813
    essential, 813
    hyperekplexia with, 814
    jumping Frenchmen of Maine with, 814
    Lafora disease with, 813
    nocturnal, 813
    ocular-palatal-pharyngeal, 813
    opsoclonus with, 813
    opsoclonus-myoclonus syndrome with, 813
    physiologic, 813
    polyminimyoclonus, 813
    propriospinal, 813
    spinal segmental, 813
    symptomatic, 813
  neuroleptic-induced syndromes as, 849–851, 851*t*
    acute akathisia in, 849
    acute dystonic reactions in, 849
    clozapine for, 849
    Clozaril for, 849
    drug-induced parkinsonism in, 849
    Huntington disease in, 850
    neuroleptic malignant syndrome in, 849
    oculogyric crisis in, 849
    olanzapine for, 849
    oral dyskinesia in, 850
    oromandibular dystonia in, 850
    persistent dyskinesia syndromes in, 849
    Risperdal for, 849
    risperidone for, 849
    tardive akathisia in, 850
    withdrawal emergent syndrome in, 849
    Zyprexa for, 849
  Parkinsonism as, 828–845, 828*t*, *829*, 831*t*, 833*t*, 834*t*, 836*t*, 837*t*, 838*t*, 841*t*, 842*t*
    akathisia with, 831
    akinesia with, 829
    alien limb phenomena with, 835
    apraxia of lid opening with, 830
    aprosody with, 830
    behavioral changes with, 844–845
    bradykinesia with, 829, 830
    bradyphrenia with, 831
    classification of, 828, 828*t*
    clinical features of, 829, *829*
    cortical-basal ganglionic degeneration in, 828*t*, 835–836

corticodentatonigral degeneration with, 835
    course of, 845
    dementia syndromes in, 828*t*, 836
    differential diagnosis of, 832–834, 834*t*
    drug therapy for, 837–838, 837*t*
    drug-induced, 828*t*, 834–835
    dysarthria with, 830
    encephalitis lethargica with, 835
    etiology of, 832
    flexed posture with, 829, *829*
    freezing phenomenon with, 830
    genetics of, 832, 833*t*
    hemiparkinsonism-hemiatrophy syndrome as, 828*t*, 835
    hypokinesia with, 829
    hypomimia with, 829
    hypophonia with, 830
    kinesia paradoxica with, 831
    levodopa therapy for, 840–844, 842*t*
    lower body parkinsonism as, 835
    Lytico-Bodig, 828*t*, 836
    masked facies with, 829
    mental changes with, 844–845
    micrographia with, 830
    MPTP induced, 828*t*, 835
    multiple system atrophy in, 828*t*, 836–837, 836*t*
    negative phenomena with, 829
    normal pressure hydrocephalus as, 828*t*, 835
    palilalia with, 830
    Parkinson-dementia-amyotrophic lateral sclerosis complex in, 828*t*, 836
    pathogenesis of, 832
    positive phenomena with, 829
    postencephalitic, 828*t*, 835
    postural reflex loss with, 830
    primary (Parkinson disease), 830–831
    rest tremor with, 829
    restless legs syndrome with, 831
    rigidity with, 829
    secondary, 828*t*, 834–835
    Shy-Drager syndrome in, 828*t*, 836
    sitting en bloc with, 830
    stages of, 838–842, 841*t*
    surgery for, 837*t*, 838, 844
    symptoms/signs of, 831–832, 831*t*
    tachyphemia with, 830
    treatment of, 837
    vascular, 828*t*, 835
    von Economo encephalitis with, 835
  pregnancy with, 1116–1117
  progressive supranuclear palsy as, 846–848, *847*, 848*t*
    diagnosis of, 847–848, 848*t*
    laboratory data on, 847
    pathology of, 846
    subcortical dementia with, 846
    symptoms/signs of, 846–847, *847*
    treatment of, 848
  tardive dyskineasia as, 849–851, 851*t*
    classic, 849, 851
    pathogenesis of, 851
    tardive myoclonus with, 851
    tardive tics with, 851
    tardive tremor with, 851
  Tourette syndrome in, 815

Moyamoya stenoses, catheter angiography of, 109

Moyamoya syndrome
arterial thrombosis with, 318, *319*
children's stroke with, 318, *319*, 320
MPS. *See* Mucopolysaccharidoses
MPTP. *See* 1-methyl-4-pehenyl-1,2,3,6-
tetrahydropyridine
MPTP induced parkinsonism, 828*t*, 835
MRA. *See* Magnetic resonance
angiography
MRI. *See* Magnetic resonance imaging
MS. *See* Multiple sclerosis
MSA. *See* Multiple system atrophy
MSUD. *See* Maple syrup urine disease
MTP. *See* Microsomal triglyceride
transfer protein
MTT. *See* Mean transit time
MTTP. *See* Mean transit time or time to
peak
MUAP. *See* Motor-unit action potential
Mucocele, neoplastic-like lesions
affecting skull of, 381, *382*
Mucolipidoses
Hunter syndrome in, 635*t*, 636
Hurler syndrome in, 634–636, 635*t*
lysosomal/other storage diseases of,
637–639, 638*t*
Maroteaux-Lamy syndrome in, 637
Morquio syndrome in, 635*t*, 636–637
Sanfilippo syndrome in, 635*t*, 636
Mucolipidoses II, lysosomal/other
storage diseases of, 638*t*, 639
Mucolipidoses III, lysosomal/other
storage diseases of, 638*t*, 639
Mucolipidoses IV, lysosomal/other
storage diseases of, 638*t*, 639–640
Mucolipidosis, differential diagnosis of,
685*t*, 688*t*, 691*t*
Mucopolysaccharidoses
differential diagnosis of, 687*t*, 688*t*,
691*t*
lysosomal/other storage diseases of,
634–637, 635*t*
Mucopolysaccharidoses (MPS), 634–637,
635*t*
Mucopolysaccharidosis
dementia resulting from, 779*t*, 780
structural malformations of, 590*t*
Mucormycosis, 230–231
Multifocal dystonia, 816*t*, 817
Multifocal motor neuropathy, 751
Multifocal motor neuropathy with
conduction block (MMNCB),
motor neuron diseases with, 867
Multifocal myoclonus, uremic
encephalopathy with, 1079
Multi-infarct dementia, cerebrovascular
syndromes of, 309
Multiminicore myopathy (MMM),
congenital muscle disorder of, 918
Multiple endocrine neoplasia I (MEN-I),
pituitary gland tumors with, 420
Multiple sclerosis (MS), 941–961, *944–947,*
948*t*, *949,* 951*t*, *952, 953,* 955*t*–957*t*
ADEM v., 954, 957*t*, 958
amantadine for, 961
Arnold-Chiari malformation v., 956,
957*t*
Behçet disease v., 956, 957*t*
bladder management for, 960
carbamazepine for, 961
Charcot variant, 958
chronic inflammatory demyelinating
polyneuropathy with, 947

cladribine for, 960
concentric sclerosis of Balo with, 958
corticosteroids for, 959
course of, 956–958, 957*t*
CSF gamma globulin changes with,
951*t*, 954
cyclophosphamide for, 960
dantrolene for, 960
definition of, 941
detrusor muscle hyperexcitability with,
960
diagnosis of, 952*t*, 954, 955*t*
diazepam for, 960
diet therapy for, 961
differential diagnosis of, 954–956, 957*t*
epidemiology of, 941–942
etiology of, 942–944
fatigue with, 961
FLAIR of, 951–952
gamma globulin for, 960
genetic susceptibility with, 942
immunology in, 942–943
other factors in, 943–944
viruses in, 943
glatiramer acetate for, 959
hypertrophic neuropathy with, 947
immunosuppressants for, 960
incidence of, 941–942
β-interferons for, 959
intrathecal IgG synthetic rate with,
954
laboratory data on, 951–954, 951*t*, *952,
953*
Lyme disease v., 954–955, 957*t*
management of, 958–961
Marburg variant, 956, 958
mitoxantrone for, 959
modafinil for, 961
motor neuron diseases with, 867
MRI of, 951–954, 951*t*, *952, 953, 955,
956*
natalizumab for, 960
onset mode of, 950–951, 951*t*
paraneoplastic syndromes v., 956, 957*t*
pathogenesis of, 942–944
pathology of, *944–947,* 944–947
pemoline for, 961
physical therapy for, 961
polyarteritis nodosa v., 956, 957*t*
pregnancy with, 1115
primary progressive, 947
prognosis of, 956–958, 957*t*
radiculopathy for, 961
relapsing-remitting, 947, 950, 956
Schilder disease with, 958
secondary progressive, 947, 956
sildenafil for, 961
Sjögren syndrome v., 956, 957*t*
SMON v., 956, 957*t*
symptoms/signs of, 947–950, 948*t*, *949*
Charcot triad as, 949
diplopia as, 948–949, 950
fatigue as, 948*t*, 950, 961
hemifacial spasm as, 948*t*, 949
internuclear ophthalmoplegia as, 949
Lhermitte symptom as, 950
limb weakness as, 949
optic neuritis as, 948–949, *949*
parasthesias as, 950
psychiatric mood disorder as, 950
pupillary abnormalities as, 949
Uhthoff phenomenon as, 950
urinary symptoms as, 949

syringomyelia v., 873
tizanidine for, 960
tolterodine for, 960
variants of, 958
vasopressin for, 961
Multiple sleep latency test, sleep
disorders in, 1023
Multiple sulfatase deficiency, 632*t*, 633
Multiple system atrophy (MSA)
orthostatic hypotension with, 971, 972,
972*t*, 974
parkinsonism-plus syndrome of, 828*t*,
836–837, 836*t*
Multisystem atrophy, 267, 797, 1029
Mumps meningitis, 187–188
complications with, 187
diagnosis of, 188
epidemiology of, 187
laboratory data on, 187–188
pathology of, 187
symptoms of, 187
treatment of, 188
Muscle biopsy
biochemical assays with, 128
deciding on, 127
diagnostic tests of, 127–128
histochemical techniques with, 128
immunohistochemical stains with,
128
indications for, 127
motor unit disorders in, 893
polymyositis with, 933–934
routine histology with, 128
skeletal, 127–128
Muscle cramps/stiffness
abnormal postures with, 926
benign fasciculation with cramps and,
925
contracture with, 925
Denny-Brown, Foley syndrome with,
925
hyperhidrosis with, 926
Isaacs syndrome in, 925–927, 926*t*
liability to cramps with, 926
mild dystrophinopathies with, 925
Moersch-Woltman syndrome in,
927–928, 928*t*
motor unit disorders causing, 925*t*
myoadenylate deaminase deficiency
with, 925
myokymia with, 925
myopathies with, 924–928, 925*t*, 926*t*,
928*t*
neuromyotonia in, 925–927, 926*t*
ordinary muscle cramps in, 924–925
pseudomyotonia with, 926
stiff man syndrome in, 927–928,
928*t*
tetany in, 927
Muscle disease, respiratory dysfunction
with, 1086
Muscle spasms, spinal injury trauma
causing, 508
Muscular dystrophy, 895–910, 896*t*, *897,
898, 900, 903,* 906*t*, 907*t*, 909*t*
Becker, *898,* 899–901, *900*
Bethlem myopathy in, 909
classification of, 896–897, 896*t*, *897*
congenital, 896, 909–910, 909*t*
definition of, 895–896
Duchenne, *896, 898,* 898–901, *900*
Emery-Dreifuss, 901–902
facioscapulohumeral, 896*t*, 902–903

familial dilated cardiomyopathy with
conduction disease and myopathy
in, 908
floppy infant syndrome with, 576
gait disorders with, 59
Gower sign with, 898, *898*
laboratory diagnosis of, 897–898
limb-girdle, 905–909, 906*t*, 907*t*
Miyoshi variant myopathy in, 910
myotonia with, 896
myotonic, *896, 903,* 903–904
Nonaka variant myopathy in, 909
oculodistal muscular dystrophies in,
909
proximal myotonic myopathy in, *896,*
903–905
rare dystrophies in, 909
skeletal muscle proteins with, *897*
Welander distal myopathy in, 909
X-linked muscular dyastrophies in, *898,*
898–901, *900*
Xp21myopathies as, 901
Musculocutaneous nerve, 534, 534*t*, 539
Myalgia, polymyositis with, 933
Myasthenia gravis (MG)
abnormal AChR activation kinetics
with, 878
acetylcholine receptor with, 877–881
acetylcholinesterase deficiency with,
878
adult form of, 878
ambenonium for, 882
anticholinesterase drug therapy for, 882
bromide for, 882
cholinergic drug therapy for, 882
congenital myasthenia in, 878–879
diagnosis of, *881,* 881–882
differential diagnosis of, 882
drug-induced myasthenia in, 879
end plate AChR lack with, 878
etiology of, 877–878
exacerbations with, 879
fast-channel syndrome with, 878
incidence of, 879
intravenous Ig therapy for, 883
juvenile form of, 878
laboratory data on, 880–881
lymphorrhages with, 879
motor neuron diseases with, 867
mycophenolate for, 883
neonatal myasthenia in, 878
neostigmine for, 882
neuromuscular junction disorder of,
877–883, *881*
ocular motility impairment with, 43
paraneoplastic syndromes associated
with, 1088*t*
pathogenesis of, 877–878
pathology of, 879
plasmapheresis for, 882
prednisone for, 883
prednisone therapy for, 883
pregnancy with, 1116
pyridostigmine for, 882
remissions with, 879
respiratory dysfunction with, 1085
signs of, 880
slow-channel syndrome with, 878
special forms of, 878–879
symptoms of, 879–880
thymectomy for, 882, 883
treatment of, 882–883
Wilson disease with, 879

Myasthenic crisis, respiratory
dysfunction with, 1085
Mycophenolate, myasthenia gravis
treated with, 883
Mycoplasma pneumoniae infection, 163
Mycotic aneurysm, SAH and, 336–337
Myelin-associated glycoprotein, blood
cell dyscrasias with, 1055
Myelinolysis, central pontine
myelinolysis with, 965
Myelitis, paraneoplastic syndrome with,
1089
Myelofibrosis, blood cell dyscrasias with,
1056
Myelogenous leukemia, blood cell
dyscrasias of, 1055
Myeloma, blood cell dyscrasias with,
1055
Myeloneuropathy, drug dependence with,
1165
Myelotomy, spinal tumors treated with,
479
Myoadenylate deaminase deficiency,
muscle cramps/stiffness with, 925
Myoblastomas, pituitary gland tumors
with, 421
Myoclonic epilepsy with red ragged fibers
(MERRF)
autosomal-recessive ataxias of, 788,
790
differential diagnosis of, 685*t*, 686*t*,
688*t*
mitochondrial encephalomyopathies
with, 696, *696,* 700–701
Myoclonic seizures, epilepsy with, 991*t*,
992
Myoclonus, 48
Alzheimer disease with, 813
classification of, 813, 813*t*
cortical tremor with, 812
Creutzfeldt-Jakob disease with, 813
dentatorubropallidoluysian atrophy
with, 813
encephalomyelitis with rigidity, 813
epilepsia partialis continua with, 812
epileptic, 813
essential, 813
hyperekplexia with, 814
jumping Frenchmen of Maine with,
814
Lafora disease with, 813
movement disorder of, 812–814, 813*t*
nocturnal, 813
ocular-palatal-pharyngeal, 813
opsoclonus with, 813
opsoclonus-myoclonus syndrome with,
813
physiologic, 813
polyminimyoclonus, 813
propriospinal, 813
spinal segmental, 813
symptomatic, 813
Myoclonus epilepsy, Lafora disease with,
643
Myoclonus-dystonia, 823
Myoedema, thyroid endocrine diseases
with, 1039
Myofascial pain, 29
Myoglobinuria, 921–923, 922*t*
acquired, 921
alcoholic myopathy with, 922
classification of, 921, 922*t*
heat cramps with, 922

heat exhaustion with, 922
heat stroke with, 922
HIV-related syndromes with, 216*t*
neuroleptic malignant syndrome with,
921
recurrent, 921
rhabdomyolysis as, 921, 923
ryanodine receptor with, 921
statin myopathy with, 923
Myokymia
muscle cramps/stiffness with, 925
radiation injury with, 554
Myopathies
alcoholism with, 1158
congenital muscle disorders as,
915–920, 916*t*, 917*t*
abnormal inclusions of unknown
origin with, 918–919
central core disease in, 916–917, 916*t*
chondrodystrophic myotonia in,
919–920
classification of, 916*t*
confirmation/investigation needed
for, 916*t*
congenital muscle fiber type
disproportion in, 918
congenital myopathies in, 915–919,
916*t*, 917*t*
cylindrical spiral myopathy in, 919
desmin-related myopathies in, 916*t*,
918
fingerprint body myopathy in, 919
hyaline body myopathy in, 918
molecular genetics of, 917*t*
multiminicore myopathy in, 918
myotonia congenita in, 919
myotubular myopathy in, 916*t*,
917–918
nemaline myopathy in, 916*t*, 917
reducing body myopathy in, 918–919
Schwartz-Jampel syndrome in,
919–920
zebra body myopathy in, 919
dermatomyositis as, 929–931, 932, 934
CT of, 931
diagnosis of, 930–931
Gottron sign with, 930
incidence of, 930
mixed connective tissue disease with,
930
MRI of, 931
pathology/pathogenesis of, 929–930
perifascicular atrophy with, 930
plasmapheresis for, 931
prednisone for, 931
prognosis for, 931
rash with, 930
sclerodermatomyositis with, 930
steroid treatment for, 931
symptoms/signs of, 930
treatment of, 931
familial periodic paralysis as, 911–914,
912*t*, 913*t*, *914*
Andersen syndrome with, 912
clinical features of, 912*t*
course of, 913
diagnosis of, 913, 913*t*
high-serum potassium, 912*t*
hyperkalemic periodic paralysis in,
914, *914*
hypokalemic periodic potassium in,
912–914, 913*t*
incidence of, 912–913

Myopathies
  familial periodic paralysis as (*contd.*)
    low-serum potassium, 912*t*
    noninherited forms of, 913*t*
    paramyotonia congenita with, *914*
    paramyotonia with, 912
    pathophysiology of, 914
    symptoms/signs of, 913
    treatment of, 913–914
  HIV-related syndromes with, 216*t*, 219, 220
  inclusion body myositis as, 932, 934–935, 935*t*
  motor unit disorders as, 893–895, 894*t*
    definitions with, 894–895
    identifying, 893–895, 894*t*
    laboratory data on, 893–894
    muscle biopsy for, 893
    serum enzyme determination for, 894, 894*t*
  muscle cramps/stiffness as, 924–928, 925*t*, 926*t*, 928*t*
    abnormal postures with, 926
    benign fasciculation with cramps and, 925
    contracture with, 925
    Denny-Brown, Foley syndrome with, 925
    hyperhidrosis with, 926
    Isaacs syndrome in, 925–927, 926*t*
    liability to cramps with, 926
    mild dystrophinopathies with, 925
    Moersch-Woltman syndrome in, 927–928, 928*t*
    motor unit disorders causing, 925*t*
    myoadenylate deaminase deficiency with, 925
    myokymia with, 925
    neuromyotonia in, 925–927, 926*t*
    ordinary muscle cramps in, 924–925
    pseudomyotonia with, 926
    stiff man syndrome in, 927–928, 928*t*
    tetany in, 927
  myoglobinuria as, 921–923, 922*t*
    acquired, 921
    alcoholic myopathy with, 922
    classification of, 921, 922*t*
    heat cramps with, 922
    heat exhaustion with, 922
    heat stroke with, 922
    neuroleptic malignant syndrome with, 921
    recurrent, 921
    rhabdomyolysis as, 921, 923
    ryanodine receptor with, 921
    statin myopathy with, 923
  myositis ossificans as, *937*, 937–938
  paraneoplastic syndromes with, 1089
  polymyositis as, 932–936, 934*t*, 935*t*
    AIDS with, 936
    arthralgia with, 933
    clinical manifestations of, 932–933
    definition of, 932
    diagnosis of, 933–934, 934*t*
    differential diagnosis of, 934*t*
    eosinophilic myositis v., 935–936
    immunosuppressive drugs for, 936
    laboratory data on, 933
    muscle biopsy for, 933–934
    myalgia with, 933
    pathogenesis of, 933

    polymyalgia rheumatica with, 936
    Raynaud symptoms with, 933
    steroids for, 936
    therapy for, 936
  progressive muscular dyastrophies as, 895–910, 896*t*, *897*, *898*, *900*, *903*, 906*t*, 907*t*, 909*t*
    Becker, *898*, 899–901, *900*
    Bethlem myopathy in, 909
    classification of, 896–897, 896*t*, *897*
    congenital, 896, 909–910, 909*t*
    definition of, 895–896
    Duchenne, *896*, *898*, 898–901, *900*
    Emery-Dreifuss, 901–902
    facioscapulohumeral, *896*, 902–903
    familial dilated cardiomyopathy with conduction disease and myopathy in, 908
    Gower's sign with, 898, *898*
    laboratory diagnosis of, 897–898
    limb-girdle, 905–909, 906*t*, 907*t*
    Miyoshi variant myopathy in, 910
    myotonia with, 896
    myotonic, *896*, *903*, 903–904
    Nonaka variant myopathy in, 909
    oculodistal muscular dystrophies in, 909
    proximal myotonic, *896*, 903–904
    proximal myotonic myopathy in, *896*, 904–905
    rare dystrophies in, 909
    skeletal muscle proteins with, *897*
    Welander distal myopathy in, 909
    X-linked muscular dyastrophies in, *898*, 898–901, *900*
    Xp21myopathies as, 901
Myositis ossificans
  clinodactyly with, 938
  fibrodysplasia ossificans as, 937
  microdactyly with, 938
  myopathies of, *937*, 937–938
  noggin with, 938
  symptoms of, 937–938
  treatment of, 938
Myotonia, muscular dystrophy with, 896
Myotonic muscular dystrophy (DM 1), *896*, *903*, 903–904
  clinical manifestations of, *903*, 903–904
    cardiac disorder with, 904
    cataracts with, 904
    dysarthria with, 903
    dysphagia with, 903
    endocrinopathy with, 904
    excessive daytime somnolence with, 904
    eye movement impairment with, 903
    gastrointestinal disorder with, 904
    muscle atrophy with, *903*
    myotonia with, 904
    ptosis with, 903
    respiratory difficulties with, 904
  definition of, 903
  diagnosis of, 905
  epidemiology of, 903
  features of, *896*
  genetic counseling for, 905
  laboratory studies on, 905
  management of, 905
  molecular genetics of, 905
  pathophysiology of, 905
Myotubular myopathy, congenital muscle disorder of, 916*t*, 917–918

Myxedema staggers, thyroid endocrine diseases with, 1039
Myxovirus infections, 187–188

N
Naegleria infections, 256–257
Naratriptan, migraine headache treated with, 985
Narcolepsy
  seizure with, 19
  sleep disorder of, 1027, 1028
NARP. *See* Neuropathy, ataxia, retinitis pigmentosa
Nasopharyngeal carcinoma, metastasis to skull base of, 379
Natalizumab (Antegren), multiple sclerosis treated with, 960
Natriuresis, pituitary endocrine disease with, 1039
NCL. *See* Neuronal ceroid lipofuscinoses
NCS. *See* Nerve conduction studies
Neck pain, 29–30
Neck weakness, 55
Neisseria meningitidis, 139–142, 140*t*
Nemaline myopathy, congenital muscle disorder of, 916*t*, 917
Neonatal herpes encephalitis, birth injuries of, 567
Neonatal infections, birth injuries of, 567–568
Neonatal meningitis, birth injuries of, 567–568
Neonatal myasthenia, 878
Neonatal neurology, 563–571, *564*, 568*t*, *569*, 570*t*
  birth injuries of, 563–571, *564*, 568*t*, *569*, 570*t*
  hypoxic-ischemic encephalopathy as, 565–567
    incidence of, 565
    laboratory data on, 566–567
    pathology/pathophysiology of, 565–566
    prognosis for, 567
    symptoms/signs of, 566
    treatment of, 567
  intracranial hemorrhage as, 563
  neonatal herpes encephalitis as, 567
  neonatal infections as, 567–568
  neonatal meningitis as, 567–568
  neonatal seizures as, 568–571, 568*t*, *569*, 570*t*
    BFNC with, 570
    classification of, 568, 568*t*
    EEG patterns of, 568, *569*
    EIEE with, 570
    EME with, 570
    epilepsies with, 570
    etiology of, 568–570
    evaluation of, 570–571
    harmfulness of, 570
    Ohtahara syndrome with, 570
    prognosis in, 572
    treatment of, 570–571
  parenchymal cerebral hemorrhage as, 563
  periventricular intraventricular hemorrhage as, *545*, 563–564, *564*
  periventricular leukomalacia as, 565
  posterior fossa hemorrhage as, 563
  primary subarachnoid supratentorial hemorrhage as, 563

subarachnoid hemorrhage as, 563
supratentorial subdural hemorrhage as, 563
Neonatal seizures, 568–571, 568*t*, 569, 570*t*
  BFNC with, 570
  classification of, 568, 568*t*
  EEG patterns of, 568, *569*
  EIEE with, 570
  EME with, 570
  epilepsies with, 570
  etiology of, 568–570
  evaluation of, 570–571
  harmfulness of, 571
  Ohtahara syndrome with, 570
  prognosis in, 572
  treatment of, 571
Neoplasms, pregnancy with, 1116
Neostigmine, myasthenia gravis treated with, 882
Nephrosialidosis, differential diagnosis of, 686*t*
Nerve biopsy
  axonal neuropathy in, 129
  Charcot-Marie-Tooth disease and, 129
  complications of, 129
  deciding on, 127
  diagnostic tests with, 127, 128–129
  indications for, 128
  peripheral, 128–129
  sural, 129
Nerve conduction studies (NCS)
  conduction block with, 91
  diagnostic tests selection of, *89–91,* 89–92
  F wave latency with, 91, *91*
  H reflex with, 91–92
  late response with, *91,* 91–92
  latency with, 90, 91, *91*
  long-latency reflex with, 91
  motor, *90,* 90–91
  nerve conduction velocity with, 90
  sensory, 89, *89*
Nerve conduction velocity, 90
Nerve-sheath tumors, 382–385, *383–385*
  trigeminal schwannoma as, 385, *385*
  vestibular schwannoma as, *383,* 383–384, *383t, 384*
Neu-Laxova syndrome, structural malformations with, 589*t*
Neural circuitry, schizophrenia with, 1140
Neural tube closure, structural malformations of, 595*t*
Neuralgias
  headache with, 46
  neuropathic pain with, 545
Neuralgic amyotrophy, 30, 535
Neurally mediated reflex syncope, 14–16, 14*t*
Neuroacanthocytosis, neurologic syndromes of, 673, 674*t*
Neuroacantocytosis, chorea of, 810
Neuroaxonal dystrophy, differential diagnosis of, 686*t*, 687*t*, 688*t*, 691*t*
Neuroblastoma, childhood central nervous system tumors of, 428
Neurocognitive disorders, childhood central nervous system tumors with, 444

Neurocutaneous disorders
  encephalotrigeminal angiomatosis as, 718–721, *719,* 719*t, 720, 721*
    diagnosis of, 720
    genetics of, 718–719
    laboratory data on, 720, *720, 721*
    symptoms/signs of, *719,* 719–720, 719*t, 720, 721*
    treatment of, 720
  incontinentia pigmenti achromians as, 722–723, *723*
  neurofibromatosis as, 713–718, *715–717,* 717*t*
    diagnosis of, 717, 717*t*
    genetics of, 713
    incidence of, 713
    merlin gene in, 714
    molecular genetics of, 713–714
    neuropathology of, 714
    pathogenesis of, 713–714
    symptoms/signs of, 714–717, *715–717*
    treatment for, 717–718
  tuberous sclerosis complex as, 724–730, *725–729,* 730*t*
    adenoma sebaceum with, 724, 725, *725*
    cafe au lait spots with, 726
    candle gutterings with, 725, *725*
    course of, 730
    diagnosis of, 729–730, 730*t*
    facial angiofibroma with, 726
    genetics of, 724
    incidence of, 724
    laboratory data on, *728,* 728–729
    pathology/pathogenesis of, 724–726, *725*
    phakomas with, 726
    prognosis for, 730
    renal angiomyolipomas with, 727
    renal lesions with, 727
    shagreen patches with, 726
    symptoms/signs with, 726–728, *727*
    treatment for, 730
    ungual fibroma with, 725–726
Neurocutaneous syndrome, differential diagnosis of, 686*t*
Neurofibromas, 474
Neurofibromatosis (NF), 713–718, *715–717,* 717*t*
  bilateral acoustic neuroma syndrome as, 713
  cafe au lait spots with, 713, 714, *715*
  central, 714
  cutaneous, 714
  diagnosis of, 717, 717*t*
  differential diagnosis of, 685*t*, 687*t*
  elephantiasis neuromatosa with, 715
  genetics of, 713
  incidence of, 713
  merlin gene in, 714
  molecular genetics of, 713–714
  neuropathology of, 714
  pathogenesis of, 713–714
  peripheral, 713, 714
  segmental, 714
  symptoms/signs of, 714–717, *715–717*
    cutaneous, 714, *715*
    miscellaneous, 717
    neurologic, 714–716, *715*
    ocular, 714
    skull/spine/limbs with, *716,* 716–717
  treatment for, 717–718
  von Recklinghausen disease as, 713

Neurofibromatosis type 1 (NF-1)
  childhood central nervous system tumors with, 428
  gliomas with, 395–396
Neurofibromatosis type 2 (NF-2)
  childhood central nervous system tumors with, 428
  gliomas with, 396
Neurogenic cardiac/pulmonary disturbances, SAH with, 334
Neurogenic pain, neuropathic pain with, 545
Neuroleptic malignant syndrome, 849
  myoglobinuria with, 921
Neuroleptic-induced syndromes
  acute akathisia in, 849
  acute dystonic reactions in, 849
  clozapine for, 849
  Clozaril for, 849
  drug-induced parkinsonism in, 849
  Huntington disease in, 850
  movement disorder of, 849–851, 851*t*
  neuroleptic malignant syndrome in, 849
  oculogyric crisis in, 849
  olanzapine for, 849
  oral dyskinesia in, 850
  oromandibular dystonia in, 850
  persistent dyskinesia syndromes in, 849
  Risperdal for, 849
  risperidone for, 849
  tardive akathisia in, 850
  withdrawal emergent syndrome in, 849
  Zyprexa for, 849
Neurologic assessment, spinal injury trauma in, 503–505, *504*
Neurologic disorders
  BAEP with, 86–87, *87*
  CT examination of, 60, 61, 62
  MRI in examination of, 60, 61, 62
  pregnancy with, 1112–1117, 1112*t*, 1113*t*
Neurologic rehabilitation, 1195–1198
  cognitive therapy in, 1197
  dysphagia therapy in, 1196–1197
  incontinence therapy in, 1197–1198
  language therapy in, 1197
  occupational therapy in, 1196
  physical therapy in, 1196
Neurologic syncope, 14, 14*t*
Neurolymphomatosis, hematologic disease of, 1060
Neuroma, neuropathic pain with, 547
Neuromuscular disorders
  floppy infant syndrome with, 575–576
  neurologic disorders examination with, 63
  paraneoplastic syndromes of, 1089
Neuromuscular junction disorders
  acute quadriplegic myopathy as, 888–889, 888*t*
    clinical features of, 888*t*
    corticosteroids causing, 888
    critical-illness polyneuropathy with, 889
    laboratory studies on, 888
    muscle biopsies for, 888–889
    nondepolarizing neuromuscular blocking agents causing, 888
  antibiotic-induced, 887
  botulism as, 886–887
  Clostridium botulinum toxin with, 886

Neuromuscular junction disorders
(*contd.*)
critical illness myopathy as, 888–889,
888*t*
Lambert-Eaton syndrome as, 885
myasthenia gravis as, 877–883, *881*
abnormal AChR activation kinetics
with, 878
acetylcholine receptor with, 877–881
acetylcholinesterase deficiency with,
878
adult form of, 878
ambenonium for, 882
anticholinesterase drug therapy for,
882
bromide for, 882
cholinergic drug therapy for, 882
congenital myasthenia in, 878–879
diagnosis of, *881*, 881–882
differential diagnosis of, 882
drug-induced myasthenia in, 879
end plate AChR lack with, 878
etiology of, 877–878
exacerbations with, 879
fast-channel syndrome with, 878
incidence of, 879
intravenous Ig therapy for, 883
juvenile form of, 878
laboratory data on, 880–881
lymphorrhages with, 879
mycophenolate for, 883
neonatal myasthenia in, 878
neostigmine for, 882
pathogenesis of, 877–878
pathology of, 879
plasmapheresis for, 882
prednisone for, 883
prednisone therapy for, 883
pyridostigmine for, 882
remissions with, 879
signs of, 880
slow-channel syndrome with, 878
special forms of, 878–879
symptoms of, 879–880
thymectomy for, 882, 883
treatment of, 882–883
Wilson disease with, 879
Neuromuscular transmission disorders,
respiratory dysfunction with,
1085
Neuromuscular transmission tests, 89,
94–97, *95–97*
LEMS in, 96
post-synaptic neuromuscular junction
dysfunction tests as, 95–96, *96*
pre-synaptic neuromuscular junction
dysfunction tests as, 96
RNS studies as, 94–95, *95*
SFEMG as, 96–97, *97*
Neuromyotonia
abnormal postures with, 926
hyperhidrosis with, 926
liability to cramps with, 926
manifestations of, 926*t*
muscle cramps/stiffness with, 925–927,
926*t*
myokymia with, 925
pseudomyotonia with, 926
Neuronal ceroid lipofuscinoses (NCL)
adult variant of, 631
Haltia-Santavuori disease type of,
630–631
infantile variant of, 630–631

Jansky-Bielschowsky disease type of,
631
juvenile variant of, 631
Kufs disease type of, 631
late infantile variant of, 631
lysosomal/other storage diseases of,
628*t*, 630–631
Spielmeyer-Sjögren disease in, 631
Neuronal glial tumors, 403–404, *404*
Neuronal tumors, 403–404, *404*
Neuronopathy, GBS variants of, 750
Neurontin. *See* Gabapentin
Neuropathic pain, 29, 545–550, 549*t*
AED for, 549
allesthesia with, 547
allodynia with, 547
anticonvulsants for, 549
antinociceptive agents for, 549
causalgia with, 545
central nociception with, 546
circus propagation with, 547
clinical features of, 548
CPRS with, 545
deafferentation pain with, 545
definitions associated with, 545
diabetic neuropathic cachexia with,
548
drug therapy for, 548–549, 549*t*
ephaptic transmission with, 547
gabapentin for, 549
general treatment principles for, 548
ISDN for, 550
lamotrigine for, 549
neuralgia with, 545
neurogenic pain with, 545
neuroma with, 547
normal processing of pain and,
545–546
other drugs for, 550
painful polyneuropathy with, 545
pathophysiology of, 546–548
peripheral nociception with, 545–546
pharmacologic therapy for, 548–549,
549*t*
reflex sympathetic dystrophy with, 545
selective serotonin reuptake inhibitors
for, 550
surgical therapy for, 548
tramadol hydrochloride for, 549
treatment of, 548–550, 549*t*
tricyclic antidepressants for, 550
venlafaxine for, 550
zonisamide for, 549
Neuropathies, pregnancy with, 1116
Neuropathy, ataxia, retinitis pigmentosa
(NARP)
differential diagnosis of, 685*t*
mitochondrial encephalomyopathies
with, 701
Neuropsychologic evaluation
clinical observation with, 132–133
dementia with, 133
diagnostic tests of, 130–134, 131*t*
epilepsy with, 133
expectations from, 133
learning disability with, 133
medication with, 133
other brain diseases with, 133
psychiatric disorders with, 133
referral issues with, 133
strategy of, 130
tests used in, 130–132, 131*t*
toxic exposure with, 133

Neuropsychologic sequelae, radiation
injury with, 555
Neuropsychologic skills measurement,
higher cerebral function disorders
with, 580, 581*t*
Neuroradiologic abnormalities, radiation
injury with, 552
Neurosarcoidosis, 232–234, 233*t*
course of, 234
diagnosis of, 233–234
epidemiology of, 233
laboratory data on, 233–234
pathology of, 233
presentation signs of, 233, 233*t*
symptoms of, 233, 233*t*
treatment of, 234
Neurosyphilis, 235–242, 236*t*, *237*, *239*,
240*t*, 241*t*
AIDS and, 241–242
classification of, 236*t*
clinical diagnosis of, 237–238
clinical syndromes of, 238–240, *239*,
240*t*
asymptomatic neurosyphilis in, 238
cerebrovascular neurosyphilis in, 238
congenital neurosyphilis in, 240
gumma in, 239
meningeal neurosyphilis in, 238
meningovascular neurosyphilis in,
239
modern diagnostic triad with, 238
paretic neurosyphilis in, 239, *239*
tabes dorsalis with, 237, *237*,
239–240, 240*t*
definition of, 235, 236*t*
dementia diagnosis with, 6
epidemiology of, 235, 236*t*
frequency of different forms of, 236*t*
history of, 235
pathology of, 237, *237*
serology of, 237–238
treatment of, 240–241, 240*t*, 241*t*
diagnostic tests for, 241*t*
early syphilis in, 240–241, 240*t*, 241*t*
Neurotoxicology of
occupation/environment,
1173–1181, 1174*t*, 1175*t*
acute encephalopathy with, 1175
amnesic shellfish poisoning with, 1181
amyotrophic lateral sclerosis with,
1173
animal poisons with, 1174*t*, 1180–1181
carbamates with, 1174*t*, 1178–1179
carbon monoxide with, 1174*t*, 1180
cerebellar syndromes with, 1176
chronic encephalopathy with,
1175–1176
ciguatera poisoning with, 1180
clinical recognition of, 1174–1176,
1175*t*
cranial neuropathy with, 1176
delayed effects with, 1176
diagnosis of, 1175, 1175*t*
eosinophilia-myalgia syndrome with,
1181
extrapyramidal syndromes with, 1176
Gulf War syndrome with, 1173
heavy metal intoxication with, 1174*t*,
1176–1178
acute lead encephalopathy in, 1176
aluminum in, 1174*t*, 1177
arsenic in, 1174*t*, 1177–1178
dialysis dementia in, 1178

lead in, 1174*t*, 1176–1177
manganese in, 1174*t*, 1178
mercury in, 1174*t*, 1177
specific syndromes of, 1174*t*, 1176–1178
thallium in, 1174*t*, 1178
laboratory evaluation of, 1175
Layzer syndrome with, 1180
marine neurotoxic syndrome with, 1180
methanol with, 1174*t*, 1181
methyl alcohol with, 1174*t*, 1181
nitrous oxide myelopathy with, 1180
obsolete epidemics with, 1181
organophosphates with, 1174*t*, 1178–1179
other intoxication with, 1174*t*, 1178–1181
peripheral neuropathy with, 1176
pesticide intoxication with, 1174*t*, 1178–1179
plant poisons with, 1174*t*, 1180–1181
shellfish poisoning with, 1181
signs/symptoms of, 1175, 1175*t*
subacute myelo-optic neuropathy with, 1181
volatile organic compounds with, 1174*t*, 1179–1180
Neurotransmitters, 1139–1140
chlorpromazine and, 1139
dopamine, 1139
floppy infant syndrome with disorders of, 575
GABA, 1139–1140
glutamate, 1139–1140
schizophrenia with, 1139–1140
Neurovascular imaging
catheter angiography as, 108–109, *109*
angioplasty with, 109
intracranial aneurysms with, 109
intracranial atheromatous with, 109
moyamoya stenoses with, 109
superselective microcatheter techniques with, 109
symptomatic vasospasm-induced stenoses with, 109
CT as, 100–104, *101–105*, 113*t*
abscess in, 101
acute hemorrhagic mass in, 101
cerebral infarct in, 101, *101–104*
hematoma in, 101
hemorrhagic infraction in, 101, *101*, *105*
MRA v., 103
nonhemorrhage infarction in, 103
subarachnoid hemorrhage in, 103
tumor in, 101
types of, 103–104
diagnostic tests with, 100–113, *101–107*, *109–112*, 113*t*
Doppler measurements as, 109–111, *110–111*, 113*t*
MRI as, 100 , 104–108, *106*, *107*, 113*t*
PET as, 112–113, 113*t*
plain skull x-ray films v., 100
regional cerebral blood flow in, 111
SPECT as, 112, *112*, 113*t*
stable-xenon computed tomography as, 111–112, 113*t*
New variant Creutzfeldt-Jakob disease (nvCJD), 264*t*, 268
NF-1. *See* Neurofibromatosis type 1
NF-2. *See* Neurofibromatosis type 2

NGGCT. *See* Nongerminomatous germ-cell tumors
NHL. *See* Non-Hodgkin lymphoma
Niemann-Pick disease
dementia resulting from, 779*t*, 780
differential diagnosis of, 685*t*, 686*t*, 687*t*, 688*t*, 691*t*
infantile (type A), 627*t*, 629
juvenile (type B), 627*t*, 629
lysosomal/other storage diseases of, 627*t*, 628–629
type C, 627*t*, 629
Nimodipine, head injury trauma with, 495–496
Nitrous oxide myelopathy, occupation/environment neurotoxicology with, 1180
Nocturnal headache, paroxysmal disorder of, 988
Nocturnal myoclonus, 813
Noggin, myositis ossificans with, 938
Non 24-hour sleep-wake disorder, sleep disorder of, 1029
Nonaka variant myopathy, muscular dystrophy of, 909
Nondepolarizing neuromuscular blocking agents, acute quadriplegic myopathy caused by, 888
Nongerminomatous germ-cell tumors (NGGCT), 414–415
Nonhemorrhage infarction, CT of, 103
Non-Hodgkin lymphoma (NHL), 406–407
Nonlesional cortical resections, epilepsy treated with, 1008, 1009*t*
Non-rapid eye movement (NREM), sleep disorders and, 1029
Nonverbal learning disabilities, language disorders of, 582
Normal pressure hydrocephalus (NPH), 349, 353–356, 356*t*
general clinical data on, 354–356, 356*t*
laboratory data on, 354–355
prognosis for, 355–356, *356*
signs/symptoms of, 354
treatment of, 355–356, *356*
Normal pressure hydrocephalus parkinsonism, 828*t*, 835
lower body parkinsonism as, 835
Norrie disease, differential diagnosis of, 685*t*
Not otherwise specified somatoform disorders, 1143
Novantrone. *See* mitoxantrone
NPH. *See* Normal pressure hydrocephalus
NREM. *See* Non-rapid eye movement
Nuclear deoxyribonucleic acid (nDNA), mutations of
abnormal mitochondrial membrane milieu with, 708
Alpers syndrome with, 708
citric acid cycle disorder in, 706, 706*t*
classification of, 705, 706*t*
DiMauro syndrome with, 706
fatty acid oxidation disorder in, 706
impaired mitochondrial transport with, 708
Leigh syndrome with, *707*, 707–708, 707*t*
metal metabolism defects in, 706*t*, 708
mitochondrial DNA disorders with, 705–708, 706*t*, *707*, 707*t*
mitochondrial motility defects in, 706*t*, 708

PDH complex defects in, 706
respiratory chain disorder in, 706–707, 706*t*
substrate transport disorder in, 706, 706*t*
substrate use disorder in, 706, 706*t*
Nutrition, head injury trauma with, 495
Nutritional deficiency, spinal injury trauma causing, 508
Nutritional deprivation, tropical myeloneuropathies with, 858
Nutritional disorders, 1091–1097, 1091*t*, 1092*t*, 1093*t*, *1095*, 1095*t*, *1096*
dietary excess in, 1092, 1092*t*
malabsorption as, 1092–1094, 1092*t*, 1093*t*
bariatric surgery with, 1093, 1093*t*
causes of neurologic disorder from, 1092, 1092*t*
celiac disease with, 1093
chronic diarrhea with, 1094
Crohn disease with, 1093
oculomasticatory myorhythmia with, 1094
ulcerative colitis with, 1093
Whipple disease as, 1094
malnutrition as, 1091–1092, 1091*t*, 1092*t*
anorexia nervosa as, 1092
emetine for, 1092
peripheral/optic neuropathy with, 1092
neurologic syndromes attributed to, 1091*t*, 1092*t*
vitamin B$_{12}$ deficiency as, 1094–1097, *1095*, 1095*t*, *1096*
clinical features of, 1095–1096
diagnosis of, 1096–1097
history of, 1094
pathogenesis of, 1095, 1095*t*
pathology of, 1095, *1095*, *1096*
physiology of, 1094–1095
Romberg sign with, 1096
treatment of, 1097
Nutritional neuropathy, 856–857
nvCJD. *See* New variant Creutzfeldt-Jakob disease

O

Obesity, blood cell dyscrasias with, 1054
Obsessive-compulsive disorder (OCD)
anxiety disorder of, 1133, 1135–1136
definition of, 1135–1136
pathophysiology of, 1136
treatment of, 1136
Obsolete epidemics, occupation/environment neurotoxicology with, 1181
Obstructive apnea, 1025
Obstructive hydrocephalus, 349–352, *350–354*
Arnold-Chiari malformation with, 350
congenital malformations with, 349–350, *350*, *351*
Dandy-Walker syndrome with, 350, *350*
developmental lesions with, 349–350, *350*, *351*
EVOH, 349, 352
IVOH, 349, 352, 355
mass lesions with, 352, *354*
postinflammatory/posthemorrhagic, 350–352, *351–353*

Obtundation, coma v., 20–21
Obturator nerve, 539, 540
Occipital bone, structural malformations of, 589–592, 591*t*
Occupational therapy, 1196
Occupation/environment neurotoxicology, 1173–1181, 1174*t*, 1175*t*
  acute encephalopathy with, 1175
  amnesic shellfish poisoning with, 1181
  amyotrophic lateral sclerosis with, 1173
  animal poisons with, 1174*t*, 1180–1181
  carbamates with, 1174*t*, 1178–1179
  carbon monoxide with, 1174*t*, 1180
  cerebellar syndromes with, 1176
  chronic encephalopathy with, 1175–1176
  ciguatera poisoning with, 1180
  clinical recognition of, 1174–1176, 1175*t*
  cranial neuropathy with, 1176
  delayed effects with, 1176
  diagnosis of, 1175, 1175*t*
  eosinophilia-myalgia syndrome with, 1181
  extrapyramidal syndromes with, 1176
  Gulf War syndrome with, 1173
  heavy metal intoxication with, 1174*t*, 1176–1178
    acute lead encephalopathy in, 1176
    aluminum in, 1174*t*, 1178
    arsenic in, 1174*t*, 1177–1178
    dialysis dementia in, 1178
    lead in, 1174*t*, 1176–1177
    manganese in, 1174*t*, 1178
    mercury in, 1174*t*, 1177
    specific syndromes of, 1174*t*, 1176–1178
    thallium in, 1174*t*, 1178
  laboratory evaluation of, 1175
  Layzer syndrome with, 1180
  marine neurotoxic syndrome with, 1180
  methanol with, 1174*t*, 1181
  methyl alcohol with, 1174*t*, 1181
  nitrous oxide myelopathy with, 1180
  obsolete epidemics with, 1181
  organophosphates with, 1174*t*, 1178–1179
  other intoxication with, 1174*t*, 1178–1181
  peripheral neuropathy with, 1176
  pesticide intoxication with, 1174*t*, 1178–1179
  plant poisons with, 1174*t*, 1180–1181
  shellfish poisoning with, 1181
  signs/symptoms of, 1175, 1175*t*
  subacute myelo-optic neuropathy with, 1181
  volatile organic compounds with, 1174*t*, 1179–1180
OCD. *See* Obsessive-compulsive disorder
Ocular bobbing
  coma examination with, 23
  ocular motility impairment with, 44
Ocular dysmetria, ocular motility impairment with, 44
Ocular flutter, ocular motility impairment with, 44
Ocular lesions, impaired vision from, 38
Ocular motility impairment
  amblyopia with, 42

Collier sign with, 43
congenital ocular motor apraxia with, 43
diplopia with, 42
downbeating nystagmus with, 44
fixation instability with, 44
hereditary ataxias with, 43
Horner syndrome with, 42
Huntington disease with, 43
impaired vision from, 42–44
incomitance with, 42
internal ophthalmoplegia with, 42
internuclear ophthalmoplegia with, 43
jerk nystagmus with, 44
MLF with, 43
myasthenia gravis with, 43
ocular bobbing with, 44
ocular dysmetria with, 44
ocular flutter with, 44
ocular myoclonus with, 44
OKN with, 43
one-and-a-half syndrome with, 43
opsoclonus with, 44
oscillopsia with, 43
periodic alternating nystagmus with, 44
PPRF with, 43
pursuit system with, 43
rebound nystagmus with, 44
saccades with, 42
saccadic system with, 43
spasmus nutans with, 44
sylvian aqueduct syndrome with, 43
upbeating nystagmus with, 44
vergence system with, 43
vertical nystagmus with, 44
vestibular system with, 43
Wilson disease with, 43
Ocular myoclonus, ocular motility impairment with, 44
Ocular-palatal-pharyngeal myoclonus, 813
Oculocerebrorenal syndrome, 618
Oculodistal muscular dystrophies, 909
Oculogyric crisis, neuroleptic-induced syndromes with, 849
Oculomasticatory myorhythmia, malabsorption with, 1094
Oculomotor apraxia (AOA), autosomal-recessive ataxias of, 784*t*, 786, 788*t*
Oculomotor nerve injury, cranial/peripheral nerve lesion with, 526–527
Oculopharyngeal muscular dystrophy, 698*t*, 908, 935
OH. *See* Orthostatic hypotension
Ohtahara syndrome, neonatal seizures with, 570
OKN. *See* Optokinetic nystagmus
Olanzapine, neuroleptic-induced syndromes with, 849
Olfactory groove meningiomas, 391
Olfactory nerve injury, cranial/peripheral nerve lesion with, 524–525
Oligoastrocytomas, 402
Oligodendroglioma, 393–394, 394*t*, 400–402, *401*
  anaplastic, 400–402, *401*
  low-grade, 402
  therapy of, 400–402, *401*
  two grades of, 394, 394*t*

Olivopontocerebellar atrophy (OPCA), dementia caused by, 5*t*
OMIM. *See* Online Mendelian Inheritance in Man
Ondine curse, Coma examination with, 22
One-and-a-half syndrome, ocular motility impairment with, 43
Online Mendelian Inheritance in Man (OMIM), differential diagnosis with, 684
OPCA. *See* Olivopontocerebellar atrophy
Ophthalmoplegia, multiple sclerosis with, 949
Ophthalmoplegia plus, mitochondrial encephalomyopathies with, 695
Ophthalmoplegic migraine, 983
Opioids, 1161–1162, 1161*t*
Oppenheim dystonia, *818*, 818–819, *819*, 822*t*
Opportunistic central nervous system infection, pediatric acquired HIV/AIDS with, 1187
Opsoclonus
  myoclonus with, 813
  ocular motility impairment with, 44
Opsoclonus-myoclonus syndrome
  myoclonus with, 813
  paraneoplastic syndromes of, 1088*t*
Optic atrophy, impaired vision with, 41
Optic chiasm lesions, impaired vision from, *39*, 41
Optic nerve injury
  cranial/peripheral nerve lesion with, 525–526, 525*t*, *526*
  impaired vision from, 38–40, *39*, *40*
Optic neuritis
  cranial/peripheral nerve lesion with, 526, *526*
  impaired vision with, 39
  multiple sclerosis symptoms of, 948–949, *949*
Optic pathway gliomas, astrocytomas with, 437
Optic-sheath meningiomas, 392
Optokinetic nystagmus (OKN), ocular motility impairment with, 43
Oral dyskinesia, neuroleptic-induced syndromes with, 850
Oral-facial digital syndrome, structural malformations with, 589*t*
Orbital myositis, cranial/peripheral nerve lesion with, 527
Orbital pseudotumor, cranial/peripheral nerve lesion with, 527
Organic acidurias, 658–660, 659*t*
  clinical manifestations of, 658–660
  definition of, 658, 659*t*
  diagnosis of, 658–660
  lactic acidemia and, 658
  neuroimaging for, 660
  signs/symptoms of, 658
  therapy for, 660
Organic brain syndromes, HIV-related syndromes with, 216*t*
Organophosphates, occupation/environment neurotoxicology with, 1174*t*, 1178–1179
Ornithine transcarbamoylase deficiency, differential diagnosis of, 685*t*
Orobuccolingual dyskinesia, 49

Oromandibular dystonia, neuroleptic-induced syndromes with, 850
Orthostatic hypotension (OH)
autonomic disorders of, 971–974, 971*t*, 972*t*, 973*t*
botulism with, 972*t*
chronic autonomic neuropathies with, 973
diabetic autonomic neuropathy with, 973
diagnosis of, 973–974, 973*t*
dopamine β-hydroxylase deficiency with, 972, 972*t*
factors affecting, 971*t*
fatal familial insomnia with, 972*t*
Guillain-Barré syndrome with, 972*t*
syncope and, 14*t*, 16
Orthostatic tachycardia, acute autonomic neuropathy with, 975
Oscillopsia, ocular motility impairment with, 43
Osmotherapy, brain edema treated with, 360
Osteitis deformans, 1073–1074, *1074, 1075*
Osteochondrodysplasia syndrome, structural malformations with, 589*t*
Osteoma, benign skull tumors of, 378, *379*
Osteomyelitis, of skull base, 167–168
Osteopetrosis, structural malformations of, 590*t*
Osteosarcoma
childhood central nervous system tumors of, 428
malignant skull tumors of, 380, *381*
Otitic hydrocephalus, 352
Overflow, dystonia with, 816
Oxcarbazepine, epilepsy treatment with, 1003*t*, 1005

P

PAF. *See* Pure autonomic failure
Paget disease, 1073–1074, *1074, 1075*
neoplastic-like lesions affecting skull of, 381
Pain. *See also* Neuropathic pain
definition of, 545
somatoform disorders as, 1143
spinal injury trauma causing, 509
Pain diagnosis, 29–31
allodynia with, 29
arm, 30–31
causalgia in, 30–31
complex regional pain in, 31
dysesthesia with, 29
entrapment neuropathies in, 30
ephaptic transmission in, 31
fibromyalgia, 29
Guillain-Barré syndrome in, 31
leg pain in, 31
Lhermitte symptoms with, 29
low back, 30
MRI in, 29, 30
myofascial, 29
neck, 29–30
neuralgic amyotrophy in, 30
neuropathic, 29
paresthesia with, 29
pins-and-needles sensation with, 29
radicular pain in, 29

reflex sympathetic dystrophy in, 31
sensory level with, 29
somatic, 29
thoracic outlet syndrome in, 30
Painful polyneuropathy, neuropathic pain with, 545
Pain-sensitive structures in head, 46–47
Paired-pulse TMS, 98
Palilalia, 49
Parkinson disease with, 830
Palliative care, end-of-life issues with, 1202
Pallidotomy, Parkinson disease surgery with, 837*t*, 838
Pancreas endocrine diseases, 1043–1044
diabetes mellitus as, 1044
hypoglycemia as, 1043–1044
islet cell adenoma with, 1044
pancreatic hyperinsulinism with, 1043
Pancreatic hyperinsulinism, pancreas endocrine disease of, 1043
PANDAS. *See* Pediatric autoimmune neuropsychiatric disorders associated with streptococcal infection
Pandysautonomia, GBS variants of, 750
Pantothenate kinase-associated neurodegeneration (PKAN)
childhood cerebral degenerations of, 676–677
differential diagnosis of, 686*t*, 687*t*
Papilledema, tumors with, *374,* 374–375, *375*
Paragonimiasis, 247*t*, 250–251
Paramyotonia congenita, familial periodic paralysis with, *914*
Paraneoplastic cerebellar degeneration, paraneoplastic syndromes of, 1088
Paraneoplastic neuropathy, 753–754
Paraneoplastic syndromes, 1087–1090, 1088*t*
antibodies with, 1090
brainstem encephalitis as, 1089
clinical syndromes of, 1088–1089
definition of, 1087
epidemiology of, 1088, 1088*t*
laboratory data on, 1090
limbic encephalitis as, 1089
motor neuron disease as, 1089
multiple sclerosis v., 956, 957*t*
myelitis as, 1089
myopathies as, 1089
neuromuscular disorders as, 1089
opsoclonus-myoclonus as, 1088*t*
paraneoplastic cerebellar degeneration as, 1088
pathogenesis of, 1088
sensorimotor peripheral neuropathy as, 1089
sensory neuronopathy as, 1088
syndromes associated with, 1088, 1088*t*
dermatomyositis, 1088*t*
encephalomyelitis, 1088*t*
Lambert-Eaton myasthenic, 1088*t*
myasthenia gravis, 1088*t*
sensorimotor peripheral neuropathy, 1088*t*
subacute cerebellar degeneration, 1088*t*
subacute sensory neuropathy, 1088*t*
treatment of, 1090

Paraparesis
gait disorders with, 57
weak muscles with, 54–55
Paraplegia, weak muscles with, 52
Parasagittal meningiomas, 391
Parasitic infections, 246–257, 247*t*, *248, 250, 254*
bilharziasis as, 247*t*, 249–250, *250*
cerebral malaria as, 254–255
cysticercosis as, 247–248, 247*t*, *248*
echinococcosis as, 247*t*, 248–249
eosinophilic meningitis as, 247*t*, 251–252
helminthic infection as, 246–253, 247*t*, *248, 250*
hydatid cysts as, 247*t*, 248–249
paragonimiasis as, 247*t*, 250–251
primary amebic meningoencephalitis as, 256–257
acanthamoeba infections as, 257
Naegleria infections as, 256–257
protozoan infection as, 253–256, *254*
schistosomiasis as, 247*t*, 249–250, *250*
strongyloidiasis as, 247*t*, 252–253
toxoplasmosis as, 253–254, *254*
trichinosis as, 247*t*, 251
trypanosomiasis as, 255–256
Parasomnias, 19
sleep disorders of, 1029
Parasthesias, multiple sclerosis symptoms of, 950
Parathyroid endocrine diseases, 1041–1043, *1042,* 1042*t,* 1043*t*
Chvostek sign with, 1042
Erb sign with, 1042
hyperparathyroidism as, 1043, 1043*t*
hypoparathyroidism as, 1041–1043, *1042,* 1042*t*
latent tetany with, 1042
pseudohypoparathyroidism with, 1042
tetany with, 1042
Trousseau sign with, 1042
Paratonia, coma examination with, 21
Parenchymal cerebral hemorrhage, birth injuries of, 563
Parenchymal contusion, head injury trauma with, 485–487, *486*
Parenchymal hemorrhage, MRI with, 106
Paresis, weak muscles with, 52
Paresthesia
leg pain with, 31
pain diagnosis with, 29–31
Paretic neurosyphilis, 239, *239*
Parinaud syndrome
astrocytomas with, 431
tumors with, 374
Parkes Weber syndrome, encephalotrigeminal angiomatosis v., 720
Parkinson disease, 776–777, 828–845, 828*t,* 829, 831*t,* 833*t*–838*t,* 841*t,* 842*t. See also* Secondary parkinsonism
akathisia with, 831
akinesia with, 829
apraxia of lid opening with, 830
aprosody with, 830
behavioral changes with, 844–845
bradykinesia with, 829, 830
bradyphrenia with, 831
classification of, 828, 828*t*
clinical features of, 829, *829*
course of, 845

Parkinson disease (*contd.*)
dementia caused by, 4, 5*t*
differential diagnosis of, 832–834, 834*t*
drug dependence with, 1165
drug therapy for, 837–838, 837*t*
amantadine in, 837*t*, 838, 839
amitriptyline in, 837*t*, 840
anticholinergic drugs in, 837*t*, 839–840
apomorphine in, 837–838, 837*t*
benserazide in, 837, 837*t*
bromocriptine in, 837, 837*t*
carbidopa in, 837, 837*t*
diphenhydramine in, 837*t*, 840
domperidone in, 837, 837*t*
dopamine agonists in, 837, 837*t*, 840
pergolide in, 837, 837*t*
pramipexole in, 837, 837*t*
ropinirole in, 837, 837*t*
selegiline in, 837*t*, 838, 839
tocopherol in, 837*t*, 839
trihexyphenidyl in, 837*t*, 839
dysarthria with, 830
encephalitis lethargica with, 835
etiology of, 832
flexed posture with, 829, *829*
freezing phenomenon with, 830
gait disorders with, 56, 57–58
genetics of, 832, 833*t*
hypokinesia with, 829
hypomimia with, 829
hypophonia with, 830
kinesia paradoxica with, 831
levodopa therapy for, 840–844, 842*t*
adverse behavioral effects with, 843*t*
dyskinesias with, 843–844
freezing phenomenon with, 844
long term complications of, 842–844, 842*t*
response fluctuations with, 842–843, 842*t*
Lewy body disease v., 777
lower body parkinsonism as, 835
masked facies with, 829
mental changes with, 844–845
micrographia with, 830
mood disorders with, 1132
negative phenomena with, 829
neurologic disorders examination with, 62
neuropathologic changes associated with, 777
orthostatic hypotension with, 16, 971–973, 972*t*
palilalia with, 830
pathogenesis of, 832
positive phenomena with, 829
postural reflex loss with, 830
pregnancy with, 1117
pure autonomic failure with, 971–973, 972*t*
rest tremor with, 829
restless legs syndrome with, 831
rigidity with, 829
sitting en bloc with, 830
stages of, 838–842, 841*t*
early, 838–839
levodopa treatment required, 841–842
symptomatic treatment, 839–841, 841*t*
surgery for, 837*t*, 838, 844

fetal dopaminergic tissue implants in, 838
lesions of subthalamic nucleus in, 838
pallidotomy in, 837*t*, 838
stimulation of subthalamic nucleus in, 838
thalamic stimulation in, 837*t*, 838
thalamotomy in, 837*t*, 838
symptoms/signs of, 831–832, 831*t*
tachyphemia with, 830
treatment of, 837
von Economo encephalitis with, 835
Parkinson-dementia-amyotrophic lateral sclerosis complex, 828*t*, 836
Parkinsonism-plus syndromes
alien limb phenomena with, 835
cortical-basal ganglionic degeneration as, 828*t*, 835–836
corticodentatonigral degeneration with, 835
dementia syndromes as, 828*t*, 836
Lytico-Bodig as, 828*t*, 836
multiple system atrophy as, 828*t*, 836–837, 836*t*
Parkinson-dementia-amyotrophic lateral sclerosis complex as, 828*t*, 836
Shy-Drager syndrome as, 828*t*, 836
Paroxysmal ataxia, 796–797
Paroxysmal disorders
brain tumor headache as, 989
chronic paroxysmal hemicrania as, 987
cluster headache as, 986–987
coital headache as, 988
cough headache as, 987–988
epilepsy as, 990–1014, 991*t*, 992*t*, 995, 996, 997*t*, 998*t*, 999, 1001*t*, 1002*t*, 1003*t*, *1004*, 1010*t*, 1012*t*, 1013*t*
active, 995
acute symptomatic seizures with, 1000
age-specific incidence of, 995, *995*
alcohol with, 1012, 1013*t*
anterior temporal lobe resection for, 1008, 1009*t*
antiepileptic drugs for, 1001–1006, 1001*t*, 1002*t*, 1003*t*, *1004*
benign epilepsy syndromes with, 1000–1001
benign partial epilepsy of childhood with, 1001
bone health with, 1007
brain imaging for, 998–999, *999*
catamenial seizures with, 1006
childhood absence, 993
childhood benign focal, 993–994
corpus callosotomy for, 1008, 1009*t*
dehydration with, 1013*t*
depression with, 1013–1014
drugs with, 1012, 1013*t*
EEG of, 994, 997, 998
epidemiology of, *995*, 995–997, 996*t*, 997*t*
epilepsia partialis continua in, 995
examination of, 997–998, 998*t*
frontal lobe, 994
gene mutations in, 1011–1012, 1012*t*
generalized syndromes of, 993
hemispherectomy for, 1008, 1009*t*
impact seizures with, 995
infantile spasms in, 993

initial diagnostic evaluation of, 997–999, 998*t*, *999*
juvenile myoclonic, 993
laboratory tests for, 999
Lennox-Gastaut syndrome in, 993
lesionectomy for, 1008, 1009*t*
liver function tests for, 999
localization-related syndromes of, 993–995
long-term monitoring of, 999–1000
medical treatment of, 1000–1006, 1001*t*, 1002*t*, 1003*t*, *1004*
mesial temporal sclerosis with, 998, *999*
mortality with, 997
MRI for, 998–999, *999*
noncompliance with, 1012, 1013, 1013*t*
nonlesional cortical resections for, 1008, 1009*t*
partial, 1001
patient history for, 997–998, 998*t*
petit mal, 993
polycystic ovary syndrome with, 1007
post-traumatic seizures in, 994–995
pregnancy with, 1006
preoperative evaluation for, 1009
psychosis with, 1013–1014
psychosocial/psychiatric issues with, 1012–1014, 1013*t*
Rasmussen syndrome in, 995
reproductive endocrine disturbances with, 1007
reproductive health issues with, 1006–1007
resective procedures for, 1008
rolandic, 1001
seizure classification for, 990–992, 991*t*, 992*t*
sexual dysfunction with, 1007
short-tau inversion recovery MRI of, *999*
single seizure with, 1000
sleep deprivation with, 1012, 1013*t*
status epilepticus with, 1009–1011, 1010*t*
stress with, 1013*t*
surgical treatment of, 1007–1009
temporal lobe, 994
trauma with, 1013*t*
vagus nerve stimulation for, 1009
West syndrome in, 993
febrile seizures as, 1015–1016
giant cell arteritis as, 988–989
hemicrania continua as, 987
idiopathic intracranial hypertension/hypotension as, 989
lumbar puncture headache as, 989
Ménière disease as, 1018–1021
burned out, 1019
cochlear, 1019
conservative procedures for, 1020–1021
definitions with, 1018–1019
destructive procedures for, 1021
diagnosis of, 1019–1020
endolymphatic shunts for, 1020–1021
historical review on, 1018
intramuscular streptomycin for, 1021
intratympanic gentamicin for, 1021
introduction to, 1018
labyrinthectomy for, 1021

medical therapy for, 1020
Meniett device for, 1021
surgical therapy for, 1020–1021
tinnitus with, 1018–1019
treatment of, 1020–1021
vertigo with, 1018–1019
vestibular neurectomy for, 1021
migraine/other headaches as, 981–989,
  984, 986t
accompaniments of, 981
acute treatment for, 985
almotriptan for, 985
amitriptyline for, 985, 986t
with aura, 981, 982
without aura, 981, 982
basilar, 982
carotidynia syndrome as, 982
classic, 981, 982
clinical subtypes of, 981–983
common, 982
complicated, 981
eletriptan for, 985
equivalents of, 981
ergonovine for, 985, 986t
ergotamine for, 985
facial, 982
hemicrania and, 981
hemiplegic, 982–983
lower-half headache as, 982
naratriptan for, 985
ophthalmoplegic, 983
pathogenesis of, 983–984, *984*
pharmacologic data on, 984
phenelzine for, 985, 986t
prophylactic treatment for, 985–986,
  986t
propranolol for, 985, 986t
rizatriptan for, 985
serotonin receptors with, 984
sumatriptan for, 985
treatment of, 984–986
valproate for, 985, 986t
verapamil for, 985, 986t
zolmitriptan for, 985
nocturnal headache as, 988
postconcussion headaches as, 988
sleep disorders as, 1022–1030, 1024t
advanced-sleep-phase syndrome in,
  1029
alveolar hypoventilation syndrome
  with, 1026
anticonvulsants for, 1027
benzerazide for, 1026
benzodiazepines for, 1027
carbamazepine for, 1027
carbidopa for, 1026
cataplexy in, 1027
central apnea with, 1025–1026
Cheyne-Stokes breathing with, 1026
clonazepam for, 1027
confusional arousals in, 1029
control dysfunction in, 1027–1028
CPAP with, 1026
delayed-sleep-phase syndrome in,
  1028
diagnostic procedures for, 1023
dopamine agonists for, 1026
EEG with, 1022, 1023
EOG with, 1022, 1023
excessive somnolence in, 1024–1025,
  1024t
eye movement with, 1022–1023
fatal familial insomnia in, 1030

gabapentin for, 1026–1027
hypnagogic hallucinations in,
  1027
hypnic jerks with, 1026
hyponeas with, 1025
idiopathic insomnia in, 1024
insomnia in, 1023–1024, 1024t
irregular sleep-wake pattern in, 1029
Kleine-Levin syndrome in, 1028
levodopa for, 1026
Maintenance of Wakefulness Test
  with, 1023
modafinil for, 1028
movement with, 1026–1027
multiple sleep latency test with, 1023
narcolepsy in, 1027, 1028
neurologic disorders with,
  1029–1030
non 24-hour sleep-wake disorder in,
  1029
NREM, 1022–1023, 1029
obstructive apnea with, 1025
parasomnias in, 1029
periodic limb movements in sleep
  with, 1026
physiology of, 1022–1023
pramipexole for, 1026
recurrent hypersomnia in, 1028
REM, 1022–1023, 1026, 1027,
  1029
REM sleep behavior disorder in,
  1029
respiratory disorders with,
  1025–1026
restless legs syndrome with, 1026
ropinirole for, 1026
sleep apnea with, 1025–1026
sleep misperception state in, 1024
sleep paralysis in, 1027
sleep terrors in, 1029
sleep-wake schedule, 1028–1029
sleepwalking in, 1029
snoring with, 1025
specific, 1023–1030, 1024t
temazepam for, 1027
topiramate for, 1027
transient, 1028
zonisamide for, 1027
SUNCT syndrome as, 987
transient global amnesia as, 1017
Paroxysmal dyskinesias, 48, 50
Paroxysmal exertional dyskinesias, 50,
  50t
Paroxysmal hypnogenic dyskinesias, 50
Paroxysmal kinesigenic dyskinesias, 50,
  50t
Paroxysmal nocturnal hemoglobinuria,
  coagulation disorders of, 1058
Paroxysmal non-kinesigenic dyskinesias,
  50, 50t
Parsonage-Turner syndrome, 535
Partial epilepsy, 1001
Partial seizures, epilepsy with, 990, 991,
  991t
Patent foramen ovale (PFO),
  decompression sickness with, 559
Pattern-reversal visual evoked potentials
  (PRVEP), 85, *86*
PBD. *See* Peroxisome biogenesis disorder
PC technique
  See Phase-contrast technique
PCNSL. *See* Primary CNS lymphoma
PCOS. *See* Polycystic ovary syndrome

PDD. *See* Pervasive developmental
  disorder
PDGF. *See* Platelet derived growth factor
PDH. *See* Pyruvate dehydrogenase
Pectoral nerves, 533, 534t
Pediatric acquired HIV/AIDS, 1185–1188,
  1186t, *1187, 1188*
antiretroviral therapy for, 1188
cerebrospinal fluid with, 1187
clinical manifestations of, 1185
CT of, 1187, *1187*
diagnostic tests for, 1185
encephalopathy v., 1186
focal manifestations of, 1186
HAART for, 1188
imaging of, 1187, *1187, 1188*
MRI of, 1187
opportunistic central nervous system
  infection with, 1187
pathology of, 1186
primary central nervous system
  lymphoma with, 1186
stroke with, 1186–1187, *1187*
Pediatric autoimmune neuropsychiatric
  disorders associated with
  streptococcal infection (PANDAS)
Sydenham chorea with, 808
Tourette syndrome with, 815
Pediatric trauma, head injury trauma
  with, 499
Pelizaeus-Merzbacher disease (PMD)
childhood cerebral degenerations of,
  677
differential diagnosis of, 685t, 686t,
  688t
Pellagra, alcoholism with, 1157
Pemoline (Cylert), multiple sclerosis
  treated with, 961
PEO. *See* Progressive external
  ophthalmoplegia
Perception, neuropsychologic evaluation
  tests for, 132
Percutaneous spinal intervention, ESNR
  with, 120–122
Perfusion-weighted imaging (PWI), MRI
  with, 67, 70, *71*, 77, 78
Pergolide, Parkinson disease drug
  therapy with, 837, 837t
Perifascicular atrophy, dermatomyositis
  with, 930
Perilymphatic fistula, vertigo/hearing loss
  caused by, 37
Periodic alternating gaze, coma
  examination with, 23
Periodic alternating nystagmus, ocular
  motility impairment with, 44
Periodic lateralized epileptiform
  discharges (PLED), EEG pattern
  with, 81, *81,* 83
Periodic limb movements in sleep
  (PLMS), sleep disorder of, 1026
Peripheral nerve biopsy, 128–129
Peripheral nerve disease, neurologic
  disorders examination with, 63
Peripheral nerves, 536–539, 537t, 538t,
  539t
Peripheral nervous system toxicity
cancer chemotherapy complications
  with, 1169–1170
other agents in, 1170
platins in, 1169
taxanes in, 1170
vinca alkaloids in, 1169

Peripheral neuropathies
acquired, 748–763, 749, 752, 754, 756
acromegalic neuropathy as, 754
alcoholic neuropathy as, 760–761
amyloid neuropathy as, 753, 754
brachial neuritis as, 762
carcinoma associated neuropathy as, 753–754
celiac neuropathy as, 755
chronic inflammatory demyelinating polyneuropathy as, 750–751
critical illness polyneuropathy as, 758
cryoglobulinemic neuropathy as, 751–752, 752
diabetic neuropathy as, 761–762
dietary associated polyneuropathy as, 757–758
diphtheric neuropathy as, 756
Guillain-Barré syndrome as, 748–750, 749
heavy metal caused neuropathies as, 758–760
hepatic disease associated neuropathy as, 755
herpes zoster-related neuropathy as, 757
HIV-related neuropathies as, 756–757
hyperthyroid neuropathy as, 754–755
hypothyroid neuropathy as, 754
idiopathic autonomic neuropathy as, 751
idiopathic neuropathy as, 763
IgA monoclonal gammopathies with, 752–753
IgM monoclonal antibodies with, 753
infection associated neuropathy as, 755–757, 756
leprosy related neuropathy as, 755–756, 756
Lyme neuropathy as, 762–763
multifocal motor neuropathy as, 751
myeloma with, 752–753
nonmalignant IgG with, 752–753
paraneoplastic neuropathy as, 753–754
radiation neuropathy as, 762
sarcoid neuropathy as, 757
sensory neuronopathy/neuropathy as, 751
therapeutic drug caused neuropathies as, 760
uremic neuropathy as, 755
vasculitic neuropathy as, 751–752, 752
general considerations for, 735–737, 736t
arthropathy in, 735
Charcot joints in, 735
Charcot-Marie-Tooth disease in, 735
course in, 737
diagnosis in, 736t, 737
ethology in, 736t, 737
Guillain-Barré syndrome in, 735
symptoms/signs in, 735–737
treatment in, 737
hereditary, 738–747, 739t–740t, 741t, 742
biology of, 741, 742
classification of, 738–741, 738t
CMT1, 739t–740t, 741–742
CMT2, 739t–740t, 742–743
CMT4, 739t–740t, 743–744
congenital hypomyelination with, 744
course for, 744
Dejerine-Sottas neuropathy with, 738, 744
distal hereditary motor neuropathies with, 745–746
electrophysiology with, 744–745
epidemiology of, 738
hereditary motor/sensory neuropathy with, 738
hereditary sensory/autonomic neuropathies with, 746
new therapeutic approaches for, 747
outcome for, 744
pathology of, 745
specific genetic types of, 739t–740t, 741–744
traditional therapies for, 747
treatment of, 747
occupation/environment neurotoxicology with, 1176
respiratory dysfunction with, 1085
Peripheral nociception, neuropathic pain with, 545–546
Peripheral-nerve tumors, radiation injury with, 555
Periventricular hemorrhagic infarction (PHI), hydrocephalus with, 350
Periventricular leukomalacia (PVL), 565
pathology of, 565
pathophysiology of, 565
Peroneal nerve, 540, 541
Peroxisomal diseases, 653–657, 653t, 655t
adrenoleukodystrophy in, 652–656, 653t, 655t
peroxisome biogenesis disorder with, 653, 655t
Refsum disease in, 653t, 656–657
rhizomelic chondrodysplasia punctata with, 653
Zellweger syndrome in, 653–654, 653t
Peroxisome biogenesis disorder (PBD), peroxisomal diseases with, 653, 655t
Persistent dyskinesia syndromes, neuroleptic-induced syndromes with, 849
Persistent vegetative state (PVS)
coma with, 26, 28
head injury trauma with, 498
Persistent viral infection, tropical myeloneuropathies with, 857–858
Personality, neuropsychologic evaluation tests for, 132
Pervasive developmental disorder (PDD), language disorders of, 583
Pesticide intoxication, occupation/environment neurotoxicology with, 1174t, 1178–1179
PET. See Positron emission tomography
Petit mal epilepsy, 993
Petit mal seizures, epilepsy with, 992
Pfeiffer syndrome, structural malformations of, 594t
PFO. See Patent foramen ovale
Phakomas, tuberous sclerosis complex with, 726
Pharmacologic therapy
neuropathic pain treated with, 548–549, 549t
somatoform disorders treated with, 1145
Phase-contrast technique (PC technique), MRI with, 74
Phencyclidine, drug dependence with, 1161t, 1163
Phenelzine, migraine headache treated with, 985, 986t
Phenobarbital
epilepsy treatment with, 1003, 1003t
febrile seizures treated with, 1016
Phenylalanine hydroxylase deficiency (PKU)
amino acid metabolism disorder of, 612–614
diagnosis of, 613
pathogenesis/pathology of, 612–614
prognosis for, 614
symptoms/signs of, 612–613
treatment of, 613
Phenylketonuria, 612–614
diagnosis of, 613
pathogenesis/pathology of, 612–614
prognosis for, 614
symptoms/signs of, 612–613
treatment of, 613
Phenytoin, epilepsy treatment with, 1001, 1003, 1003t, 1004, 1004
PHI. See Periventricular hemorrhagic infarction
Phobias, 1133, 1134–1135
definition of, 1134
epidemiology of, 1134
pathophysiology of, 1134
social, 1133, 1134–1135
treatment of, 1134
Phosphenes, impaired vision with, 42
Physical dependence, 1161
Physical therapy, 1196
multiple sclerosis treated with, 961
Physician-assisted suicide, 1202
Physiologic myoclonus, 813
Pick disease, 776
Alzheimer disease v., 776
dementia caused by, 5t
Picornavirus infections, 177–179
diagnosis of, 179
epidemiology of, 178
laboratory data on, 179
pathology/pathogenesis of, 177–178
prognosis for, 179
prophylaxis with, 178
symptoms of, 178–179
treatment of, 179
Pineal cell tumors, 414t, 415
Pineal cysts, 414t, 416, 416–419, 416t, 417, 418, 419
chemotherapy for, 419
diagnosis for, 418
general considerations for, 416, 416–419, 416t, 417, 418, 419
long-term outcome with, 419
MRI for, 418
postoperative staging of, 419, 419
radiotherapy for, 419
surgery for, 417, 418, 418–419
symptoms of, 416, 416–418, 416t
Pineal region tumors, 414–420, 414t, 415, 415t, 416, 416t, 417, 418, 419
germ-cell tumors as, 414–415, 414t, 415t
meningiomas as, 414t, 416
metastasis with, 415–416

miscellaneous tumors of, 414*t*, 416
pineal cell tumors as, 414*t*, 415
pineal cysts as, 414*t*, *416*, 416–419, 416*t*, *417, 418, 419*
    chemotherapy for, 419
    diagnosis for, 418
    general considerations for, *416*, 416–419, 416*t*, *417, 418, 419*
    long-term outcome with, 419
    postoperative staging of, 419, *419*
    radiotherapy for, 419
    surgery for, *417, 418*, 418–419
    symptoms of, *416*, 416–418, 416*t*
pineoblastoma as, 415
pineocytomas as, 415
Pineoblastoma, 415
Pineocytomas, 415
Ping-pong gaze, coma examination with, 23
Pins-and-needles sensation, 29
Pitressin. *See* Vasopressin
Pituitary apoplexy, pituitary endocrine disease of, 1033
Pituitary carcinomas, 421
Pituitary endocrine diseases, 1033–1039, *1035–1038*
    acromegaly as, 1035–1037, *1036, 1037*
    Cushing disease as, 1037
    diabetes insipidus as, 1037–1038, *1038*
    empty sella syndrome as, 1037
    excessive adrenocorticotropic hormone as, 1037
    excessive growth hormone as, 1035–1037, *1036, 1037*
    excessive secretion of antidiuretic hormone as, 1038–1039
    GH-secreting pituitary tumors as, 1035, *1036*
    hyperprolactinemia as, 1034–1035
    hyponatremia with, 1039
    hypopituitarism as, 1033–1034
    natriuresis with, 1039
    pituitary apoplexy as, 1033
    pituitary tumors as, 1034–1035, 1034*t*, *1035*
    PRL with, 1033, 1034, 1034*t*
    PRL-secreting adenoma as, 1034
    prolactinoma as, 1034
    Sheehan syndrome as, 1033
    somatostatin with, 1035
Pituitary gland tumors, 420–427, *421–426*
    ACTH with, 421, 423–424
    choristomas with, 421
    clinical features of, *421*, 421–422, 422*t*
    CT scan of, 423
    Cushing disease with, 421, 423
    differential diagnosis of, 424, *425*
    FSH with, 421
    granular-cell tumors with, 421
    infundibulomas with, 421
    macroadenomas, 421, *421*
    MEN-I with, 420
    microadenomas, 421, 422, *423*
    MRA of, 423
    MRI of, 422–423, *423, 424*
    myoblastomas with, 421
    pathology of, 421
    pituitary carcinomas with, 421
    radiation therapy for, 427
    radiographic features of, 422–424, *423, 424*
    recurrent tumors with, 427
    surgery for, *426*, 426–427

symptoms of, 422, 422*t*
    treatment of, 424–427, *425, 426*
Pituitary tumors, 1034–1035, 1034*t*, *1035*
PKAN. *See* Pantothenate kinase-associated neurodegeneration
PKU. *See* Phenylalanine hydroxylase deficiency
Plain skull x-ray films, neurovascular imaging v., 100
Plant poisons, occupation/environment neurotoxicology with, 1174*t*, 1180–1181
Plantar nerve, 540
Plasma cell dyscrasias, blood cell dyscrasias of, 1055–1056, *1056*
Plasmacytoma, blood cell dyscrasias of, 1055
Plasmapheresis
    dermatomyositis treated with, 931
    myasthenia gravis treated with, 882
Plasminogen deficiency, coagulation disorders with, 1058
Platelet derived growth factor (PDGF), astrocytomas with, 429–430
Platelet disorders, 1052–1054, *1053*
    essential thrombocytosis as, 1052–1053
    heparin-induced thrombocytopenic as, 1054
    thrombotic thrombocytopenic purpura as, *1053*, 1053–1054
Platins, peripheral nervous system toxicity with, 1169
PLED. *See* Periodic lateralized epileptiform discharges
Pleomorphic xanthoastrocytoma (PXA), congenital tumors of, 435
PLMS. *See* Periodic limb movements in sleep
PLS. *See* Primary lateral sclerosis
PMD. *See* Pelizaeus-Merzbacher disease
PME. *See* Progressive myoclonus epilepsy
PML. *See* Progressive multifocal leukoencephalopathy
PNET. *See* Primitive neuroectodermal tumors
Pneumocephalus, head injury trauma with, 496
Pneumococcal meningitis, 143
Poliomyelitis, floppy infant syndrome with, 575
Polyarteritis nodosa
    multiple sclerosis v., 956, 957*t*
    vasculitis syndrome of, 1099–1102, 1102*t*
        clinical features of, 1102*t*
        course of, 1101
        diagnosis of, 1100–1101
        etiology of, 1099
        incidence of, 1099
        laboratory data on, 1100
        pathology of, 1099
        prognosis for, 1101
        signs/symptoms of, 1099–1100, 1102*t*
        treatment of, 1101–1102
Polycystic ovary syndrome (PCOS), epilepsy with, 1007
Polycythemia, erythrocyte disorder of, 1051–1052
Polyglucosan storage diseases, 643–644
Polyminimyoclonus myoclonus, 813
Polymyalgia, vasculitis syndrome of, 1102, 1103–1104

differential diagnosis of, 1104
symptoms of, 1103
Polymyositis
    AIDS with, 936
    arthralgia with, 933
    clinical manifestations of, 932–933
    definition of, 932
    dermatomyositis v., 932, 934
    diagnosis of, 933–934, 934*t*
    differential diagnosis of, 934*t*
    eosinophilic myositis v., 935–936
    HIV-related syndromes with, 216*t*
    immunosuppressive drugs for, 936
    inclusion body myositis v., 932, 934–935
    laboratory data on, 933
    muscle biopsy for, 933–934
    myalgia with, 933
    myopathies of, 932–936, 934*t*, 935*t*
    pathogenesis of, 933
    polymyalgia rheumatica with, 936
    Raynaud symptoms with, 933
    steroids for, 936
    therapy for, 936
Polyneuropathy, alcoholism with, 1156
Pompe disease
    differential diagnosis of, 686*t*, 688*t*
    floppy infant syndrome with, 576
Pontine paramedian reticular formation (PPRF), ocular motility impairment with, 43
Porphobilinogen, acute intermittent porphyria with, 668
Porphyrin, acute intermittent porphyria with, 668
Porphyrogenic drugs, acute intermittent porphyria treated with, *670*
Portal-systemic encephalopathy, hepatic disease with, 1064
Positron emission tomography (PET)
    discussion of, 112–113, 113*t*
    gliomas in, 397
    headache diagnosis with, 47
    hypoxic-ischemic encephalopathy in, 566
    neurovascular imaging with, 112–113, 113*t*
    PCNSL in, 411
    systemic lupus erythematosus in, 1107
    tumors examination with, 376
Postconcussion syndrome
    head injury trauma with, 498
    paroxysmal disorder of, 988
Postencephalitic parkinsonism, 828*t*, 835
    encephalitis lethargica with, 835
    von Economo encephalitis with, 835
Posterior cord, 533
Posterior fossa hemorrhage, birth injuries of, 563
Posterior fossa syndromes, cerebral infarction with, 301–302
Posterior-cord syndrome, 505
Postpolio syndrome, motor neuron diseases with, 867
Post-synaptic neuromuscular junction dysfunction, neuromuscular transmission tests with, 95–96, *96*
Posttraumatic amnesia, 498
Posttraumatic epilepsy, 498–499
Posttraumatic movement disorders, head injury trauma with, 499
Post-traumatic seizures, epilepsy with, 994–995

Post-traumatic stress disorder (PTSD)
anxiety disorder of, 1133, 1135
definition of, 1135
epidemiology of, 1135
pathophysiology of, 1135
treatment of, 1135
Postural reflex loss, Parkinson disease
with, 830
PPMS. *See* Primary progressive multiple
sclerosis
PPRF. *See* Pontine paramedian reticular
formation
Prader-Willi syndrome (PWS), 608–610
differential diagnosis of, 687*t*
floppy infant syndrome with, 575
genomic imprinting with, 609
molecular basis of, 609
Pramipexole
Parkinson disease drug therapy with,
837, 837*t*
sleep disorders treated with, 1026
Praxis, neuropsychologic evaluation tests
for, 132
Prednisone
myasthenia gravis treated with, 883
temporal arteritis treated with, 1103
Prednisone therapy
Duchenne muscular dystrophy with,
900
myasthenia gravis treated with, 883
Pre-eclampsia, pregnancy with, 1114
Pregnancy
AED with, 1112–1114, 1113*t*
Bell palsy with, 1116
biology of, 1112, 1112*t*
carpal tunnel syndrome with, 1116
cerebral hemorrhage with, 1115
chorea gravidarum with, 1117
eclampsia with, 1114
epilepsy with, 1006, 1112–1114, 1113*t*
idiopathic Parkinson disease with,
1117
meralgia paresthetica with, 1116
migraine with, 1115–1116
movement disorders with, 1116–1117
multiple sclerosis with, 1115
myasthenia gravis with, 1116
neoplasms with, 1116
neurologic disease during, 1112–1117,
1112*t*, 1113*t*
neuropathies with, 1116
physiologic changes during, 1112,
1112*t*
pre-eclampsia with, 1114
restless leg syndrome with, 1117
stroke with, 1114–1115
Premature cranial suture closure,
structural malformations of,
592–593, *594*, 594*t*
Presbycusis, vertigo/hearing loss caused
by, 37–38
Pressure sores, spinal injury trauma
causing, 508
Pre-synaptic neuromuscular junction
dysfunction, neuromuscular
transmission tests with, 96
Primary amebic meningoencephalitis,
256–257
acanthamoeba infections as, 257
Naegleria infections as, 256–257
Primary antiphospholipid antibody
syndrome, chorea of, 809
Primary antiphospholipid syndrome, 309

Primary central nervous system
lymphoma, pediatric acquired
HIV/AIDS with, 1186
Primary CNS lymphoma (PCNSL), 406,
407–412, *408–410*, 410*t*
clinical manifestations of, 407
CT scan of, 408, *408*
diagnosis of, 409, 410*t*
epidemiology of, 407
imaging of, 408, *408–410*
immunocompromised patient with,
411–412
MRI of, 408, *409*, *410*
pathology of, 407–408
patient evaluation for, 410*t*
prognosis for, 410–411
treatment of, 409–410
Primary dystonia, 816*t*, 817, *818*,
818–821, *819*
adult onset, 819–821, *820*
blepharospasm with, 820
blinking tics with, 820
breathy dysphonia with, 820
cervical dystonia as, 820
early onset, 819
Oppenheim dystonia as, *818*, 818–819,
819, 822*t*
pathology/pathophysiology of, 821
Sandifer syndrome as, 820
spasmodic torticollis as, 820
spastic dysphonia with, 820
whispering dysphonia with, 820
writer's cramp with, 820
wry neck as, 820
Primary generalized dystonia, differential
diagnosis of, 685*t*
Primary hyperadrenalism, adrenal
endocrine disease of, 1045–1046
Primary intramedullary tumors, spinal
tumors of, 473–474, *474*
Primary lateral sclerosis (PLS)
clinical manifestations of, 858
diagnosis of, 858–859, 859*t*
laboratory data on, 858
MRI for, 859, 859*t*
spinal cord disease of, 858–859, 859*t*
Primary progressive aphasia, 9, 11
Primary progressive multiple sclerosis
(PPMS), 947
Primary subarachnoid supratentorial
hemorrhage, birth injuries of, 563
Primitive neuroectodermal tumors
(PNET), childhood central nervous
system tumors of, 428, 429, 431*t*,
439–441
MRI of, 440
treatment for, 441
Pringle disease. *See* Tuberous sclerosis
complex
Prion diseases, 264–268, 264*t*, 265*t*, *266*,
267, 267*t*
CJD as, 264*t*, 265–268, *266*, *267*, 267*t*
biohazard potential of, 267–268
course of, 267
diagnosis of, 267
EEG of, 267, *267*
laboratory data on, 266–267, *267*
new variant of, 268
pathology of, *266*, 266
prognosis of, 267
signs/symptoms of, 266, 267*t*
transmissibility of, 267–268
FFI as, 264*t*, 268

GSS disease as, 264*t*, 268
human incidence of, 264–265, 264*t*, *265*
kuru as, 264*t*, 265
nvCJD as, 264*t*, 268
pathology/pathogenesis of, 264
Prion-related diseases, 778, 778–779
Creutzfeldt-Jakob disease as, 778,
778–779
fatal familial insomnia as, 778, 779
Gerstmann-Sträussler disease as, 778,
779
kuru as, 778, 779
PRL. *See* Prolactin
PRL-secreting adenoma, pituitary
endocrine disease of, 1034
Professional boxing neurology, head
injury trauma with, 499–500
Progeria
differential diagnosis of, 686*t*, 687*t*,
688*t*
DNA mainte-
nance/transcription/translation
disorders of, 647*t*
Progressive bulbar palsy, motor neuron
diseases of, 866
Progressive external ophthalmoplegia
(PEO)
autosomal dominant, 699–700
classification of, 698*t*
Kearns-Sayre syndrome in, 695,
698–699
maternally inherited, 699
mitochondrial encephalomyopathies
with, 698–700, 698*t*
mitochondrial neurogastrointestinal
encephalomyopathy with, 700
multiple mitochondrial DNA deletions
with, 699–700
sporadic, 698–699
Progressive multifocal
leukoencephalopathy (PML),
203–204, *204*, *205*
AIDS opportunistic infections with,
220, 223
course of, 204
diagnosis of, 203–204, *205*
laboratory data on, 203–204, *205*
pathogenesis of, 204
pathology of, 203–204, *204*
prognosis of, 204
signs/symptoms of, 203
treatment of, 204
Progressive muscular dyastrophies,
895–910, 896*t*, *897*, *898*, *900*, *903*,
906*t*, 907*t*, 909*t*
Becker, *898*, 899–901, *900*
Bethlem myopathy in, 909
classification of, 896–897, 896*t*, *897*
congenital, 896, 909–910, 909*t*
definition of, 895–896
Duchenne, *896*, *898*, 898–901, *900*
Emery-Dreifuss, 901–902
facioscapulohumeral, *896*, 902–903
familial dilated cardiomyopathy with
conduction disease and myopathy
in, 908
Gower sign with, 898, *898*
laboratory diagnosis of, 897–898
limb-girdle, 905–909, 906*t*, 907*t*
Miyoshi variant myopathy in, 910
myotonia with, 896
myotonic, *896*, *903*, 903–904
Nonaka variant myopathy in, 909

oculodistal muscular dystrophies in, 909
proximal myotonic, *896*, 903–904
proximal myotonic myopathy in, *896*,
    904–905
rare dystrophies in, 909
skeletal muscle proteins with, *897*
Welander distal myopathy in, 909
X-linked muscular dyastrophies in, *898*,
    898–901, *900*
Xp21myopathies as, 901
Progressive myoclonus epilepsy (PME),
    autosomal-recessive ataxias, 788
Progressive rubella panencephalitis, 202
diagnosis of, 202
laboratory data on, 202
pathology/pathogenesis of, 202
symptoms of, 202
treatment of, 202
Progressive spinal muscular atrophy,
    differential diagnosis of, 686*t*
Progressive supranuclear palsy (PSP),
    846–848, *847*, 848*t*
diagnosis of, 847–848, 848*t*
laboratory data on, 847
pathology of, 846
subcortical dementia with, 846
symptoms/signs of, 846–847, *847*
treatment of, 848
Prolactin (PRL), pituitary endocrine
    disease with, 1033, 1034, 1034*t*
Prolactinoma, pituitary endocrine
    disease of, 1034
PROMM. *See* Proximal myotonic
    myopathy
Prophylactic treatment, migraine
    headache treated with, 985–986,
    986*t*
Propranolol, migraine headache treated
    with, 985, 986*t*
Propriospinal myoclonus, 813
Prosopagnosia, 13
Protein C deficiency, coagulation
    disorders with, 1057
Protein S deficiency, coagulation
    disorders with, 1057
Proteus syndrome, structural
    malformations of, 590*t*
Prothrombin G20210A mutations,
    coagulation disorders with,
    1057–1058
Protoporphyrinogen oxidase, acute
    intermittent porphyria with, 668
Protozoan infection, 253–256, *254*
cerebral malaria as, 254–255
toxoplasmosis as, 253–254, *254*
trypanosomiasis as, 255–256
Provigil. *See* Modafinil
Proximal myotonic myopathy (DM 2),
    896, 904–905
clinical manifestations of, *903*, 903–904
    cardiac disorder with, 904
    cataracts with, 904
    dysarthria with, 903
    dysphagia with, 903
    endocrinopathy with, 904
    excessive daytime somnolence with,
        904
    eye movement impairment with, 903
    gastrointestinal disorder with, 904
    muscle atrophy with, *903*
    myotonia with, 904
    ptosis with, 903
    respiratory difficulties with, 904

definition of, 903
diagnosis of, 905
epidemiology of, 903
features of, *896*
genetic counseling for, 905
laboratory studies on, 905
management of, 905
molecular genetics of, 905
pathophysiology of, 905
Proximal nerves, *536*, 536–537
PRVEP. *See* Pattern-reversal visual evoked
    potentials
Pseudoaneurysm, 337
Pseudobulbar palsy
cerebral infarction with, 302
motor neuron diseases with, 867
Pseudodystonia, 825, 825*t*
Pseudohypoparathyroidism,
    hypoparathyroidism with, 1042,
    1042
Pseudomonas aeruginosa, malignant
    external otitis from, 167
Pseudoweakness, 53
PSP. *See* Progressive supranuclear palsy
Psychiatric disorders
anxiety as, 1132–1137
    animal models of, 1133
    Aplysia with, 1133
    definition of, 1132–1133
    differential diagnosis of, 1134
    Drosophila with, 1133
    epidemiology of, 1133
    generalized anxiety disorder with,
        1133, 1136–1137
    obsessive-compulsive disorder with,
        1133, 1135–1136
    pathophysiology of, 1133
    post-traumatic stress disorder with,
        1133, 1135
    separation, 1133
    signs/symptoms of, 1133
    social phobias of, 1133, 1134–1135
    specific phobias of, 1133, 1134–1135
    treatment of, 1134
depression as, 1125–1132, 1126*t*, 1129*t*
    biomarkers with, 1127
    definition of, 1125
    dysthymia with, 1127
    epidemiology with, 1125
    genetics with, 1127
    Hamilton rating scale with, 1126*t*
    individuality with, 1125–1126
    MDD diagnosis with, 1126–1127,
        1126*t*
    multiple sclerosis symptoms of,
        950
    pathophysiology of, 1127–1128
    public health and, 1125
    specific antidepressant medications
        for, 1129–1130, 1129*t*
    treatment of, 1128–1129
epilepsy with, 1012–1014, 1013*t*
mood disorders as, 1125–1132, 1126*t*,
    1129*t*
    Alzheimer disease with, 1131
    biomarkers with, 1127
    bipolar disorders in, 1130–1131
    dysthymia with, 1127
    epidemiology with, 1125
    genetics with, 1127
    Hamilton rating scale with, 1126*t*
    Huntington disease with, 1131–1132
    individuality with, 1125–1126

MDD diagnosis with, 1126–1127,
    1126*t*
multiple sclerosis symptoms of, 950
neurologic conditions resulting in,
    1131–1132
Parkinson disease with, 1132
pathophysiology of, 1127–1128
public health and, 1125
social mood stabilizers for, 1131
specific antidepressant medications
    for, 1129–1130, 1129*t*
treatment of, 1128–1129
neuropsychologic evaluation with, 133
psychosis as
    differential diagnosis of, 1140
    medication for, 1140–1141, 1141*t*
    treatment of, 1140–1142, 1141*t*, 1142*t*
schizophrenia as, 1137–1142, 1141*t*,
    1142*t*
    antipsychotic medication for,
        1140–1141, 1142*t*
    associated features with, 1138–1139
    course of, 1138–1139
    definition of, 1137–1138
    differential diagnosis of, 1140
    etiology of, 1139
    neural circuitry with, 1140
    neurotransmitters with, 1139–1140
    nonpharmacologic therapies for,
        1141–1142
    pathophysiology of, 1139–1140
    psychosis with, 1140, 1141*t*
    signs/symptoms of, 1138
    synaptic pruning hypothesis with,
        1140
    treatment of, 1140–1142, 1141*t*, 1142*t*
somatoform disorders as, 1142–1146,
    1145*t*
    behavior modification strategies for,
        1145
    body dysmorphic disorder with, 1143
    coexisting psychologic conditions
        with, 1145
    conversion disorder with, 1143
    differential diagnosis of, 1144–1145,
        1145*t*
    hypnosis for, 1145
    malingering with, 1144
    not otherwise specified, 1143
    other treatment interventions for,
        1145
    pain disorder with, 1143
    pathogenesis of, 1143–1144
    pharmacotherapy for, 1145
    prognosis for, 1145
    psychologic factors affecting medical
        condition, 1144
    psychotherapeutic interventions for,
        1144–1145
    somatization disorder with, 1143
    symptoms of, 1143
    treatment of, 1144–1145
    undifferentiated, 1143
Psychic dependence, 1161
Psychogenic dystonia, 824, 824*t*
Psychogenic gait disorders, 58–59
Psychogenic nonepileptic seizure, 17–19,
    18*t*
Psychologic factors affecting medical
    condition, somatoform disorders
    with, 1144
Psychophysiologic causes, vertigo caused
    by, 38

Psychosis
  differential diagnosis of, 1140
  epilepsy with, 1013–1014
  medication for, 1140–1141, 1141t
  treatment of, 1140–1142, 1141t, 1142t
Psychostimulants, 1161t, 1162
Psychotherapeutic interventions,
    somatoform disorders treated
    with, 1144–1145
PTSD. See Post-traumatic stress disorder
Pulfrich phenomenon, Impaired vision
    with, 39–40
Pulmonary encephalopathy, IIH with, 362
Pulmonary function, spinal injury
    trauma influencing, 507–508
Pulmonary function tests, respiratory
    physiology with, 1083, 1083t
Pure autonomic failure (PAF)
  autonomic disorder of, 971–974, 971t,
    972t, 973t
  chronic autonomic neuropathies with,
    973
  diabetic autonomic neuropathy with,
    973
  diagnosis of, 973–974, 973t
  dopamine β-hydroxylase deficiency
    with, 972, 972t
  factors affecting, 971t
  multiple system atrophy with, 971, 972,
    972t, 974
  parkinsonian syndromes with,
    971–973, 972t
  Shy-Drager syndromes with, 971
Pure word deafness, 9, 13
Pure word mutism, 9
Purine/pyrimidine metabolism disorders,
    620–621, 621t
  Lesch-Nyhan syndrome as, 620
  other disorders of, 620–621
Purpura fulminans, coagulation
    disorders with, 1057
Pursuit system, ocular motility
    impairment with, 43
PVL. See Periventricular leukomalacia
PVS. See Persistent vegetative state
PWI. See Perfusion-weighted imaging
PWS. See Prader-Willi syndrome
PXA. See Pleomorphic
    xanthoastrocytoma
Pyridostigmine, myasthenia gravis
    treated with, 882
Pyriminil, 759
Pyruvate dehydrogenase (PDH), nDNA
    mutations with, 706
Pyruvate-dehydrogenase deficiency,
    structural malformations with, 587

Q
Quadriparesis, drug dependence with,
    1165

R
Rabies, 188–190
  course of, 190
  diagnosis of, 190
  etiology of, 188–189
  incidence of, 189
  laboratory data on, 189
  pathology of, 189
  prognosis of, 190
  symptoms of, 189
  treatment of, 190
Radial nerve, 534, 534t, 536–537

Radiation injury, 551–555, 553
  acute effects of, 551
  acute ischemic brachial neuropathy
    with, 554
  adrenocorticotropic-hormone function
    with, 554
  brachial plexopathy with, 554
  cognitive impairment with, 555
  early effects of, 551
  early-delayed syndromes with, 551–552
  endocrine dysfunction with, 554–555
  gonadotropin deficiency with, 554
  growth hormone function with, 554
  hyperprolactinemia with, 555
  immunologic hypothesis with, 552
  late-delayed syndromes with, 552–555,
    553
  lumbosacral plexopathy with, 554
  mass lesion with, 552
  meningiomas with, 555
  mineralizing microangiopathy with,
    552
  myokymia with, 554
  neuropsychologic sequelae with, 555
  neuroradiologic abnormalities with,
    552
  other complications of, 555
  peripheral-nerve tumors with, 555
  radiation myelopathy with, 553–554
  radiation necrosis with, 552–553, 553
  radiation optic neuropathy with, 555
  radiation-induced plexopathy with, 554
  radiation-induced tumors with, 555
  radiation-induced vasculopathy with,
    554
  rhombencephali with, 551
  sarcomas with, 555
  thyrotropin deficiency with, 554
  transient plexus injury with, 554
  white-matter changes with, 552
Radiation myelopathy, 553–554
Radiation necrosis, 552–553, 553
Radiation neuropathy, 762
Radiation optic neuropathy, 555
Radiation therapy. See also Radiotherapy
  astrocytomas in, 432–433
  ependymomas in, 442
  Krabbe-Weber disease treated with,
    456
  medulloblastoma with, 440
  pituitary gland tumors treatment with,
    427
  Sturge-Weber disease treated with, 456
Radiation-induced plexopathy, 554
Radiation-induced tumors, 555
Radiation-induced vasculopathy, 554
Radicular pain, 29
Radiculopathy, multiple sclerosis treated
    with, 961
Radiculopathy trauma, 510–517, 511t,
    512t, 513, 514, 515, 516t
  cervical disc disease as, 512–513, 515,
    516t
  chronic low-back pain as, 516–517
  diagnostic features of, 513–516
  imaging of, 516
  incidence of, 511
  lumbar intervertebral disc rupture as,
    511–512, 512t, 513, 514
  pathogenesis of, 510–511, 511t
  signs/symptoms of, 511
  spinal stenosis with, 510
  syndromes of, 511t

  thoracic intervertebral disc rupture as,
    512
  treatment for, 516
Radiofrequency (RF), 69
Radiography
  head injury trauma in, 492
  spinal tumors in, 477
Radiotherapy
  brain metastasis with, 462
  pineal cysts with, 419
  spinal tumors treated with, 479
Ragged-red fibers (RRF)
  MERRF with, 788, 790
  mitochondrial encephalomyopathies
    with, 695, 697, 699
RAM. See Tropical spastic paraparesis
Ramsay Hunt syndrome,
    autosomal-recessive ataxias of, 788
Rankin score, cerebral aneurysms with,
    114, 116t
Rapid eye movement (REM), sleep
    disorders and, 1022–1023, 1026,
    1027, 1029
Rapid-onset dystonia, 822–823
Rash, dermatomyositis with, 930
Rasmussen syndrome, epilepsy with, 995
Raynaud symptoms, polymyositis with,
    933
RBD. See REM sleep behavior disorder
RCDP. See Rhizomelic chondrodysplasia
    punctata
Reading disability, language disorders of,
    582
Reasoning, neuropsychologic evaluation
    tests for, 132
Rebleeding, SAH with, 331, 332
Rebound nystagmus, ocular motility
    impairment with, 44
Recurrent bacterial meningitis, 144
Recurrent hypersomnia, sleep disorder
    of, 1028
Recurrent myoglobinuria, 921
Reducing body myopathy, congenital
    muscle disorder of, 918–919
Reflex sympathetic dystrophy
  neuropathic pain with, 545
  pain diagnosis with, 31
Refsum disease
  biochemical defect in, 657
  differential diagnosis of, 686t, 687t,
    688t
  peroxisomal disease of, 653t, 656–657
  symptoms of, 656
  therapy for, 657
Refusal of life-sustaining treatment, 1201
Regional cerebral blood flow,
    neurovascular imaging of, 111
Regional syndromes, spinal tumors as,
    474–476
Rehabilitation, neurologic, 1195–1198
  cognitive therapy in, 1197
  dysphagia therapy in, 1196–1197
  incontinence therapy in, 1197–1198
  language therapy in, 1197
  occupational therapy in, 1196
  physical therapy in, 1196
Relapsing-remitting multiple sclerosis
    (RRMS), 947, 950, 956
Relative afferent pupillary defect,
    impaired vision with, 39
REM. See Rapid eye movement
REM sleep behavior disorder (RBD),
    1029

Renal angiomyolipomas, tuberous sclerosis complex with, 727
Renal disease, 1079–1082
dialysis dementia as, 1081
dialysis dysequilibrium syndrome as, 1081
neurologic complications of renal transplantation as, 1081–1082
aspergillus with, 1082
uremic encephalopathy as, 1079–1080
asterixis with, 1079
dialysis for, 1080
meningeal signs with, 1080
multifocal myoclonus with, 1079
restless-legs syndrome with, 1079
uremic neuropathy as, 1080–1081
accelerated neuropathy of renal failure with, 1080
renal transplantation for, 1080
Renal lesions, tuberous sclerosis complex with, 727
Renal transplantation
neurologic complications of, 1081–1082
aspergillus with, 1082
uremic neuropathy treated with, 1080
Reoviruses, 176t, 181
Repetitive nerve stimulation (RNS), neuromuscular transmission tests with, 94–95, 95
Repetitive transcranial magnetic stimulation (rTMS), TMS and, 98, 99–100
Reproductive endocrine disturbances, epilepsy with, 1007
Respiratory failure, respiratory physiology with, 1083, 1083t
Respiratory support for neurologic diseases, 1082–1087, 1083t, 1084t, 1086t
acute inflammatory demyelinating polyneuropathy in, 1085
ALS in, 1085
botulism in, 1085
brainstem disease in, 1084
critical illness neuromyopathy in, 1085–1086
Guillain-Barré syndrome in, 1085
motor neuron disease in, 1085
muscle disease in, 1086
myasthenia gravis in, 1085
myasthenic crisis in, 1085
neuromuscular transmission disorders in, 1085
peripheral neuropathies in, 1085
primary respiratory disfunction with, 1084–1086
respiratory failure management with, 1086–1087, 1086t
respiratory physiology with, 1082–1084, 1083t, 1084t
alveolar-arterial gradient in, 1083
dead space ventilation in, 1083
hypercapnia in, 1083
hypoxemia in, 1083
intrapulmonary shunting in, 1083
pulmonary function tests in, 1083, 1083t
respiratory failure in, 1083, 1083t
ventilation/perfusion mismatching in, 1083
spinal cord disease in, 1084–1085
Rest tremor, Parkinson disease with, 829

Restless legs syndrome (RLS), 49
Parkinson disease with, 831
pregnancy with, 1117
sleep disorder of, 1026
uremic encephalopathy with, 1079
Retardation, higher cerebral function disorders with, 579
Retrochiasmal lesions, impaired vision from, 39, 41–42
Retrogeniculate lesions, impaired vision with, 41
Retrovirus infections, 202–205, 204, 205
Retrovirus-associated myelopathy. See Tropical spastic paraparesis
Rett syndrome
childhood cerebral degenerations of, 679–680, 679t, 680t
diagnostic criteria for, 679, 679t
differential diagnosis of, 685t, 686t, 687t
DNA maintenance/transcription/translation disorders of, 648t
stages of, 679
variant phenotypes delineated for, 680t
Reversible dementia, temporal arteritis with, 1103
Reversible motor neuron disease, 868
Revised Vineland Adaptive Behavior Scales, higher cerebral function disorders with, 580
Revised Wechsler Scales, higher cerebral function disorders with, 580
Reye syndrome, 262–263
clinical presentation on, 262–263
diagnosis of, 263
pathology/pathogenesis of, 263
treatment of, 263
RF. See Radiofrequency
Rhabdoid tumors, childhood central nervous system tumors of, 439–441
Rhabdomyolysis
drug dependence with, 1165
myoglobinuria as, 921, 923
Rhabdomyosarcoma, childhood central nervous system tumors of, 428
Rhabdovirus infection, 188–190
Rhizomelic chondrodysplasia punctata (RCDP), peroxisomal diseases with, 653
Rhombencephali, radiation injury with, 551
Rickettsial infections, 156–160
Rigidity, Parkinson disease with, 829
Riley-Day syndrome, floppy infant syndrome with, 575
Rinne test, hearing loss diagnosis with, 33
Risperdal, neuroleptic-induced syndromes with, 849
Risperidone, neuroleptic-induced syndromes with, 849
Rizatriptan, migraine headache treated with, 985
RLS. See Restless legs syndrome
RNS. See Repetitive nerve stimulation
Robinow syndrome, structural malformations of, 590t
Rocky Mountain spotted fever, 157–158
course of, 157–158
diagnosis of, 157–158
incidence of, 157
laboratory data on, 157

pathology of, 157
prognosis for, 157–158
symptoms/signs of, 157
treatment for, 158
Rolandic epilepsy, 993, 1001
Romberg sign
gait disorders with, 58
vitamin B_{12} deficiency with, 1096
Ropinirole
Parkinson disease drug therapy with, 837, 837t
sleep disorders treated with, 1026
Routine histology, muscle biopsy with, 128
RRF. See Ragged-red fibers
RRMS. See Relapsing-remitting multiple sclerosis
rTMS. See Repetitive transcranial magnetic stimulation
Rubella, 186–187
diagnosis of, 186
laboratory data on, 186
symptoms of, 186
treatment of, 186–187
Ruvalcaba-Myhre syndrome, structural malformations of, 590t
Ryanodine receptor, myoglobinuria with, 921

S
Saccades, ocular motility impairment with, 42
Saccadic system, 43
Sacral plexus, 539–540
Saethre-Chotzen syndrome, structural malformations with, 594t
Sagging brain, spontaneous intracranial hypotension with, 364, 364
SAH. See Subarachnoid hemorrhage
Sandhoff diseases, lysosomal/other storage diseases of, 622
Sandifer syndrome, dystonia of, 820
Sanfilippo syndrome
dementia resulting from, 780
differential diagnosis of, 686t, 687t, 688t
lysosomal/other storage diseases of, 635t, 636
Sarcoid neuropathy, 757
Sarcoidosis. See Neurosarcoidosis
Sarcomas, radiation injury with, 555
SCA. See Spinocerebellar ataxias
SCA1 (spinocerebellar ataxia), 784t, 789t, 791
SCA2, 784t, 789t, 791–792
SCA3, 784t, 789t, 792–793
SCA4, 784t, 789t, 793
SCA5, 784t, 789t, 793
SCA6, 784t, 789t, 793–794
SCA7, 784t, 789t, 794
SCA8, 784t, 789t, 794
SCA10, 784t, 789t, 794–795
SCA11, 784t, 789t, 795
SCA12, 784t, 789t, 795
SCA13, 784t, 789t, 795
SCA14, 784t, 789t, 795
SCA15, 784t, 789t, 795
SCA16, 784t, 789t, 795
SCA17, 784t, 789t, 795
SCA18, 784t, 789t, 795
SCA19, 784t, 789t, 795
SCA20, 784t, 789t, 796
SCA21, 784t, 789t, 796

SCA22, 784*t*, 789*t*, 795
SCA25, 784*t*, 789*t*, 796
SCAD. *See* Small capillary and arteriolar dilatation
Scaphocephalic skull, structural malformations with, 593
SCD. *See* Sickle cell disease
Schilder disease, 682–683, *683*
  differential diagnosis of, 683
  multiple sclerosis with, 958
  myeloclastic, 683
  transitional sclerosis with, 683
Schirmer test, vasculitis syndrome with, 1109
Schistosomiasis, 247*t*, 249–250, *250*
  clinical manifestations of, 249–250
  diagnosis of, 250
  epidemiology of, 249
  laboratory data on, 250
  pathology of, 249
  treatment of, 250
Schizophrenia
  antipsychotic medication for, 1140–1141, 1142*t*
  associated features with, 1138–1139
  course of, 1138–1139
  definition of, 1137–1138
  differential diagnosis of, 1140
  etiology of, 1139
  neural circuitry with, 1140
  neurotransmitters with, 1139–1140
    chlorpromazine and, 1139
    dopamine, 1139
    GABA, 1139–1140
    glutamate, 1139–1140
  nonpharmacologic therapies for, 1141–1142
  pathophysiology of, 1139–1140
  psychiatric disorder of, 1137–1142, 1141*t*, 1142*t*
  psychosis with, 1140, 1141*t*
  signs/symptoms of, 1138
  synaptic pruning hypothesis with, 1140
  treatment of, 1140–1142, 1141*t*, 1142*t*
Schwannomas, spinal tumors of, 474, *475*
Schwartz-Jampel syndrome
  congenital muscle disorder of, 919–920
  Moersch-Woltman syndrome v., 928
Sciatic nerve, 539–540, 541
Scintillating homonymous scotoma, impaired vision with, 42
Scissors gait, 57
Scleroderma, vasculitis syndrome of, 1108
Sclerodermatomyositis, 930
Scotoma, impaired vision with, 39, *39*, 41
Scrub typhus, 158–159
SE. *See* Spin echo
Seckel syndrome, DNA maintenance/transcription/translation disorders of, 649*t*
Secondary antiphospholipid syndrome, 309
Secondary dystonia, 816*t*, 817, 823–824, 823*t*, 824*t*
  clues suggestive of, 824*t*
  psychogenic dystonia as, 824, 824*t*
  tardive dystonia as, 823–824
Secondary parkinsonism, 828*t*, 834–835
  drug-induced, 828*t*, 834–835
  encephalitis lethargica with, 835
  hemiparkinsonism-hemiatrophy syndrome as, 828*t*, 835

lower body parkinsonism as, 835
  MPTP induced, 828*t*, 835
  normal pressure hydrocephalus as, 828*t*, 835
  postencephalitic, 828*t*, 835
  vascular, 828*t*, 835
  von Economo encephalitis with, 835
Secondary progressive multiple sclerosis (SPMS), 947, 956
Sedatives, drug dependence with, 1161*t*, 1162
Segawa disease, dystonia of, 821–822, 822*t*
Segmental dystonia, 816*t*, 817
Seizures. *See also* Febrile seizures
  basilar artery migraine with, 18*t*, 19
  differential diagnosis of, 18*t*
  drug dependence with, 1164
  EEG with, 19, 20
  epilepsy, 990–992, 991*t*, 992*t*
    absence seizures in, 991*t*, 992
    astatic seizures in, 992
    atonic seizures in, 991*t*, 992
    atypical absence seizures in, 992
    clonic phase in, 991
    complex partial seizures in, 991, 991*t*
    drop attacks in, 992
    epileptic cry in, 991
    epileptic prodrome in, 991
    epileptogenic focus in, 991, 991*t*
    focal seizures in, 990, 991, 991*t*
    generalized seizures in, 990, 991–992, 991*t*
    generalized tonic-clonic seizures in, 991
    grand mal seizures in, 991
    myoclonic seizures in, 991*t*, 992
    partial seizures in, 990, 991, 991*t*
    petit mal seizures in, 992
    simple partial seizures in, 991, 991*t*
    tonic phase in, 991
  epilepsy with, 17
  fetal cocaine effects with, 1189, 1189*t*
  HIV-related syndromes with, 216*t*, 219
  hyperventilation with, 17, 18*t*
  infants with, 17
  migraine with, 18*t*, 19
  narcolepsy with, 19
  panic attacks with, 17, 18*t*
  parasomnia with, 19
  psychogenic nonepileptic, 17–19, 18*t*
  SAH with, 333–334
  sleep disorders with, 18*t*, 19
  somnambulism with, 19
  somniloquy with, 19
  summary on, 20
  syncope v., 15*t*, 18*t*
  TIA with, 18*t*, 19
Selective serotonin reuptake inhibitors (SSRI), neuropathic pain treated with, 550
Selegiline, Parkinson disease drug therapy with, 837*t*, 838, 839
Senile chorea, 811
Senile gait disorders, 59–60
  apraxia of gait as, 60
  cautious gait as, 59
  frontal disequilibrium as, 60
  frontal gait disorder as, 60
  isolated gait ignition failure as, 60
  magnetic gait as, 60
  subcortical disequilibrium as, 59

Sensorimotor peripheral neuropathy, paraneoplastic syndromes associated with, 1088*t*, 1089
Sensory aphasia, 8, 10–11
  alexia with agraphia and, 10
  auditory form of, 10
  literal paraphasias with, 10
  omissions with, 10
  verbal paraphasias with, 10
  visual form of, 10
  Wernicke aphasia as, 10
Sensory ataxia, gait disorders with, 58
Sensory nerve action potential (SNAP), nerve conduction studies with, 89, *89*
Sensory nerve conduction studies, 89, *89*
Sensory neuronopathy, paraneoplastic syndromes of, 1088
Sensory neuronopathy/neuropathy, 751
Serial neurologic evaluation, head injury trauma with, 494–495
Serologic tests, syphilis with, 126
Serotonin receptors, migraine headache with, 984
Serotonin syndrome, iatrogenic disease with, 1166
Serum enzyme, motor unit disorders determined by, 894, 894*t*
Sexual dysfunction, epilepsy with, 1007
Sexual function, spinal injury trauma influencing, 508–509
Shagreen patches, tuberous sclerosis complex with, 726
Shapiro syndrome, structural malformations with, 589*t*
Sheehan syndrome, pituitary endocrine disease of, 1033
Shellfish poisoning, occupation/environment neurotoxicology with, 1181
Shh. *See* Sonic hedgehog
Short-lasting, Unilateral, Neuralgiform Headache (SUNCT) syndrome, paroxysmal disorder of, 987
Short-tau inversion recovery (STIR), epilepsy MRI of, *999*
Shy-Drager syndromes
  orthostatic hypotension with, 971
  Parkinsonism-plus syndrome of, 828*t*, 836
  pure autonomic failure with, 971
Shy-Drager variant, orthostatic hypotension with, 16
Sialidosis
  differential diagnosis of, 686*t*, 688*t*
  lysosomal/other storage diseases of, 637, 638*t*
Sicca complex, vasculitis syndrome with, 1109
Sickle cell disease (SCD)
  children's stroke with, 316, 318
  epilepsy with, 1051
  erythrocyte disorder of, 1050–1051
  ethnicity with, 61
Side effects. *See* Iatrogenic disease
Sildenafil (Viagra), multiple sclerosis treated with, 961
Simple partial seizures, epilepsy with, 991, 991*t*
Single photon emission computed tomography (SPECT)
  dementia diagnosis with, 6

neurovascular imaging with, 112, *112,*
    113*t*
PCNSL in, 411
Single pulse TMS, 98
Single-fiber electromyography (SFEMG)
    jitter with, 96, *97*
    neuromuscular transmission tests
        with, 96–97, *97*
    simulated, 96
    volitional, 96
Sinus pericranii, vascular malformations
    of, 458
Sitting en bloc, Parkinson disease with,
    830
Situational syncope, 14*t*, 15–16
Sjögren syndrome
    multiple sclerosis v., 956, 957*t*
    orthostatic hypotension with, 972*t*
    vasculitis syndrome of, 1109
Sjögren-Larsson syndrome, differential
    diagnosis of, 686*t*, 687*t*
Skeletal muscle biopsy, 127–128
Skeletal muscle proteins, muscular
    dystrophy with, *897*
Skin punch biopsy, diagnostic tests with,
    129
Skull tumors, 378–382, *379, 379t, 380, 381*
    benign, 378–379, *379*
    malignant, 379–381, *379t, 380, 381*
        chondrosarcoma as, 380
        fibrous sarcoma as, 380
        glomus jugulare tumors as, 380–381
        Hand-Schüller-Christian disease as,
            382
        metastasis to skull base as, 379, 379*t*
        osteosarcoma as, 380, *381*
        xanthomatosis as, 382
SLE. *See* Systemic lupus erythematosus
Sleep apnea, 1025–1026
Sleep disorders, 1022–1030, 1024*t*
    advanced-sleep-phase syndrome in,
        1029
    alveolar hypoventilation syndrome
        with, 1026
    anticonvulsants for, 1027
    benzerazide for, 1026
    benzodiazepines for, 1027
    carbamazepine for, 1027
    carbidopa for, 1026
    cataplexy in, 1027
    central apnea with, 1025–1026
    Cheyne-Stokes breathing with, 1026
    clonazepam for, 1027
    confusional arousals in, 1029
    control dysfunction in, 1027–1028
    CPAP with, 1026
    delayed-sleep-phase syndrome in, 1028
    diagnostic procedures for, 1023
    excessive somnolence in, 1024–1025,
        1024*t*
    eye movement with, 1022–1023
    fatal familial insomnia in, 1030
    gabapentin for, 1026–1027
    hypnagogic hallucinations in, 1027
    hypnic jerks with, 1026
    hyponeas with, 1025
    idiopathic insomnia in, 1024
    insomnia in, 1023–1024, 1024*t*
    irregular sleep-wake pattern in, 1029
    Kleine-Levin syndrome in, 1028
    levodopa for, 1026
    Maintenance of Wakefulness Test with,
        1023

modafinil for, 1028
movement with, 1026–1027
multiple sleep latency test with, 1023
narcolepsy in, 1027, 1028
neurologic disorders with, 1029–1030
non 24-hour sleep-wake disorder in,
    1029
NREM with, 1022–1023, 1029
obstructive apnea with, 1025
parasomnias in, 1029
periodic limb movements in sleep with,
    1026
physiology of, 1022–1023
pramipexole for, 1026
recurrent hypersomnia in, 1028
REM, 1022–1023, 1026, 1027, 1029
respiratory disorders with, 1025–1026
restless legs syndrome with, 1026
ropinirole for, 1026
seizure with, 18*t*, 19
sleep apnea with, 1025–1026
sleep misperception state in, 1024
sleep paralysis in, 1027
sleep terrors in, 1029
sleep-wake schedule, 1028–1029
sleepwalking in, 1029
snoring with, 1025
specific, 1023–1030, 1024*t*
temazepam for, 1027
topiramate for, 1027
transient, 1028
zonisamide for, 1027
Sleep misperception state, 1024
Sleep paralysis, 1027
Sleep terrors, 1029
Sleep-wake schedule disorders,
    1028–1029
Sleepwalking, 1029
Slow-channel syndrome, myasthenia
    gravis with, 878
SMA. *See* Spinal muscular atrophies
Small capillary and arteriolar dilatation
    (SCAD), cardiac surgery cerebral
    complications with, 1068
Small vessel lacunar infarction, 282–284,
    283, 284t
Smith-Lemli-Opitz syndrome, floppy
    infant syndrome with, 575
SMN. *See* Survival motor neuron gene
SMON. *See* Subacute myelo-optic neuritis
SNAP. *See* Sensory nerve action potential
Sneddon syndrome, vasculitis syndrome
    of, 1109
Snoring, sleep disorders with, 1025
Social mood stabilizers, 1131
Somatic pain, 29
Somatization disorder, 1143
Somatoform disorders, 1142–1146, 1145*t*
    behavior modification strategies for,
        1145
    body dysmorphic disorder with, 1143
    coexisting psychologic conditions with,
        1145
    conversion disorder with, 1143
    differential diagnosis of, 1144–1145,
        1145*t*
    hypnosis for, 1145
    malingering with, 1144
    not otherwise specified, 1143
    other treatment interventions for, 1145
    pain disorder with, 1143
    pathogenesis of, 1143–1144
    pharmacotherapy for, 1145

prognosis for, 1145
psychologic factors affecting medical
    condition, 1144
psychotherapeutic interventions for,
    1144–1145
somatization disorder with, 1143
symptoms of, 1143
treatment of, 1144–1145
undifferentiated, 1143
Somatosensory evoked potentials
    (SSEP), 87–88, *88*
Somatostatin, pituitary endocrine disease
    with, 1035
Somnambulism, 19
Somniloquy, 19
Somnolence (excessive), sleep disorder
    of, 1024–1025, 1024*t*
Sonic hedgehog (Shh), childhood central
    nervous system tumors with, 429
Sotos syndrome, structural
    malformations of, 590*t*
Spasmodic torticollis, dystonia with, 820
Spasmus nutans, ocular motility
    impairment with, 44
Spastic diplegia, motor function
    disorders of, 577*t*, 578
Spastic dysphonia, 820
Spastic hemiparesis, motor function
    disorders of, 577, 577*t*
Specific phobias, 1133, 1134–1135
Specific sleep disorders, 1023–1030,
    1024*t*
SPECT. *See* Single photon emission
    computed tomography
Sphenoid ridge meningiomas, 392, *392*
Sphingolipidoses, differential diagnosis
    of, 686*t*
Spielmeyer-Sjögren disease (JNCL),
    lysosomal/other storage diseases
    of, 631
Spin echo (SE), MRI with, 69
Spina bifida occulta, structural
    malformations of, 595
Spina bifida, structural malformations
    of, 593–596, 595*t*, *596*
    diagnosis with, 593–595
    pathogenesis with, 593–595
    treatment for, 596
Spinal accessory nerve injury,
    cranial/peripheral nerve lesion
    with, 532–533
Spinal cord
    anatomy of, 342–343, *343*
    hemorrhage of, 345–346
    infractions of, 343–344
    vascular diseases of, 342–346, *343*
    venous disease of, 344–345
Spinal cord astrocytomas, 439
Spinal cord diseases
    hereditary spastic paraplegia as,
        855–856, 855*t*, 856*t*
    motor neuron diseases as, 861–868,
        861*t*, 864*t*, 866*t*
        adult onset, 863–868, 864*t*, 866*t*
        amyotrophic lateral sclerosis in,
            863–868, 864*t*, 866*t*
        benign fasciculation and cramps
            syndrome with, 868
        classification of, 861, 861*t*
        definitions of, 861, 861*t*
        Denny-Brown, Foley syndrome with,
            868
        Fazio-Londe syndrome in, 862

Spinal cord diseases
motor neuron diseases as (*contd.*)
focal muscular atrophies in, 862–863
Hirayama syndrome with, 867
Kennedy disease in, 863
Kugelberg-Welander syndrome in, 862
monomelic muscular atrophy with, 867
multifocal motor neuropathy with conduction block with, 867
multiple sclerosis with, 867
myasthenia gravis with, 867
postpolio syndrome with, 867
progressive bulbar palsy in, 866
pseudobulbar palsy with, 867
reversible motor neuron disease with, 868
spinal muscular atrophies of childhood in, 861–862, 861*t*
Werdnig-Hoffmann syndrome in, 862
X-linked recessive spinobulbar muscular atrophy in, 863, 864*t*
neurologic disorders examination with, 63
primary lateral sclerosis as, 858–859, 859*t*
respiratory dysfunction with, 1084–1085
syringomyelia as, 870–873, *872*
ALS v., 873
Arnold-Chiari malformation with, 871, 873
brachial amyotrophy with, 871
Charcot joints with, 871
clinical manifestations of, 870–871
differential diagnosis of, 873
dissociated sensory loss with, 871
en cuirasse with, 871
hematomyelia with, 872
Horner syndrome with, 871
hydromyelia with, 871, 872
laboratory data on, *872*, 872–873
main en griffe with, 871
main succulente with, 871
MS v., 873
pathology/pathogenesis of, 871–872
syringocephalus with, 871
syringohydromyelia with, 872
treatment of, 873
tropical myeloneuropathies as, 856–858, 857*t*
clinical manifestations of, 856–857
dietary toxins with, 858
etiology of, 857–858
history of, 856–857
Jamaican neuropathy as, 856, 857
konzo as, 856
lathyrism as, 856, 857
malnutrition with, 857
nutritional deprivation with, 858
nutritional neuropathy as, 856–857
other toxins with, 858
pathology of, 856–857
persistent viral infection with, 857–858
prevention of, 858
Strachan syndrome as, 856–857
treatment of, 858
tropical ataxic neuropathy as, 856, 857
tropical spastic paraparesis as, 856, 857, 857*t*

Spinal cord infection, AIDS opportunistic infections with, 224
Spinal epidural abscess, 150–154, *152, 153*
course of, 154
diagnosis of, 152–154
etiology of, 150–151
incidence of, 152
laboratory data on, 152, *152, 153*
pathology of, 151–152
prognosis for, 154
symptoms/signs of, 152
treatment for, 154
Spinal injury trauma, 502–509, 502*t*, *504*
anterior-cord syndrome with, 504–505
ASIA on, 503
bladder function with, 508
bowel training with, 508
Brown-Séquard syndrome with, 504–505
cauda equina lesions with, 504–505
causes of, 502, 502*t*
central-cord syndrome with, 504–505
classification of, 503–505, *504*
clinical patterns of, 504–505
complications with, 507–509
course of, 506
CT for, 505–506
diagnosis of, 505–506
dysautonomia with, 507
etiology of, 502, 502*t*
IMSOP on, 503
mechanism of, 502–503
MRI for, 505–506
muscle spasms with, 508
neurologic assessment of, 503–505, *504*
nutritional deficiency with, 508
pain with, 509
pathology of, 503
posterior-cord syndrome with, 505
pressure sores with, 508
prognosis for, 506
pulmonary function with, 507–508
rehabilitation of, 509
sexual function with, 508–509
spinal-cord concussion with, 505
TENS for, 509
treatment of, 506–507
Spinal meningiomas, 392
Spinal metastases, spinal tumors of, *472*, 472–473, *473*
Spinal muscular atrophies (SMA)
diagnosis of, 863
DNA maintenance/transcription/translation disorders of, 648*t*
facioscapulohumeral form of, 862
floppy infant syndrome with, 575, 862
infantile type I, 862
known biochemical abnormality with, 862–863
Kugelberg-Welander syndrome in, 862
laboratory data on, 862
motor neuron diseases of, 861–862, 861*t*
scapuloperoneal form of, 862
survival motor neuron gene with, 861
treatment of, 862
Werdnig-Hoffmann syndrome in, 862
Spinal roots, 533–536, *534*, 534*t*, 539–540
Spinal segmental myoclonus, 813
Spinal shock, 490
Spinal stenosis, intervertebral disk trauma with, 510

Spinal tumors, 470–479, 470*t*, *471, 472,* 472*t*, *473, 474, 475, 476, 478*
age incidence of, 472*t*
Brown-Séquard syndrome with, 471, 477
cauda equina tumors as, 476
cerebrospinal fluid evaluation for, 477
cervical tumors as, 475–476
conus tumors as, 476
course of, 478
diagnosis of, 476–478
drop metastases as, 474, *476*
epidural spinal cord compression with, *472*, 472–473, *473*
extramedullary tumors as, 470–471
foramen magnum tumors as, 474–475
frequency of, 470, 472*t*
Horner syndrome as, 476
intradural tumors as, 474, *475, 476*
intramedullary metastases as, 473, *473*
leptomeningeal metastasis as, 474
lumbar tumors as, 476
meningiomas as, 474
microsurgery for, 479
myelotomy for, 479
neurofibromas as, 474
pathology of, 470, 470*t*, *471*
primary intramedullary tumors as, 473–474, *474*
prognosis for, 478
radiography for, 477
radiotherapy for, 479
regional syndromes with, 474–476
schwannomas as, 474, *475*
spinal metastases as, *472*, 472–473, *473*
surgery for, 479
symptoms of, 470
thoracic tumors as, 476
treatment of, *478*, 478–479
von Recklinghausen disease with, 477
Spinal-cord concussion, spinal injury trauma with, 505
Spinocerebellar ataxias (SCA), 784*t*, 789*t*, 791–796. *See also* SCA1
differential diagnosis of, 685*t*, 688*t*
Spinocerebellar atrophy, 807*t*, 1088
Spiral CT, 103
SPMS. *See* Secondary progressive multiple sclerosis
Spongy degeneration of nervous system, 675–676, *676*
Spontaneous activity, EMG with, 92, *92*
Spontaneous intracranial hypotension, *364*, 364–365
Monro-Kellie rule with, 364
MRI for, 364, *364*
sagging brain with, 364, *364*
Sporadic cerebellar ataxia, 797
Squamous cell carcinoma, metastasis to skull base of, 379
SSEP. *See* Somatosensory evoked potentials
SSPE. *See* Subacute sclerosing panencephalitis
SSRI. *See* Selective serotonin reuptake inhibitors
St. Louis encephalitis, 183–184
Stable-xenon computed tomography, 103
neurovascular imaging with, 111–112
Stance phase, gait with, 56
Staphylococcal meningitis, 143
Startle disease, Moersch-Woltman syndrome with, 928

Statin myopathy, myoglobinuria with, 923
Status dystonicus, 816
Status epilepticus, 1009–1011, 1010*t*
  causes of, 1010, 1010*t*
  convulsive, 1009, 1010–1011
  nonconvulsive, 1009, 1011
  treatment protocol for, 1010*t*
Stent-angioplasty
  carotic occlusive disease with, 116
  CREST with, 116
  endovascular revascularization with, 116–118, *117*, 118*t*
  ESNR with, 116–118, *117*, 118*t*
  extracranial carotid revascularization with, 116–117, *117*
  intracranial cerebral revascularization with, 118, 118*t*
  vascular filtration device with, 116
Stereotactic radiosurgery, brain metastasis with, 462, *463*
Stereotypies, 49
Sterility, drug dependence with, 1165
Steroid therapy
  dermatomyositis with, 931
  head injury trauma treatment with, 496
  polymyositis treated with, 936
  temporal arteritis treated with, 1103
Stiff encephalomyelitis, Moersch-Woltman syndrome with, 928
Stiff limb syndrome, Moersch-Woltman syndrome with, 928
Stiff man syndrome
  Babinski signs with, 928
  clinical manifestations of, 927–928, 928*t*
  defining characteristics of, 928*t*
  differential diagnosis of, 928
  encephalomyelitis with, 928
  hyperekplexia with, 928
  laboratory data on, 928
  muscle cramps/stiffness with, 927–928, 928*t*
  Schwartz-Jampel syndrome v., 928
  startle disease with, 928
  stiff encephalomyelitis with, 928
  stiff limb syndrome with, 928
Stimulation of subthalamic nucleus, Parkinson disease surgery with, 838
STIR. *See* Short-tau inversion recovery
Storage diseases. *See* Lysosomal/other storage diseases
Strachan syndrome, tropical myeloneuropathies of, 856–857
Streptococcal meningitis, 143
Streptococcus pneumoniae, 139, 140*t*, 143
Striatal necrosis, 688, *696*, 701, 828*t*
Stroke
  alcoholism with, 1158
  aphasia with, 9
  children
    cerebral embolism in, 321, *321*
  children's, 315–322, *316–319*, *321*, *322*
    adult v., 315
    arterial thrombosis with, *317*, 318–319, *319*
    basal occlusion disease with, 320
    clinical evaluation of, 316, 318*t*
    coagulopathies with, 319
    congenital disorder of glycosylation with, 322

    etiology of, 316–318
    extracranial occlusion with, 320
    incidence of, 316, *316*, *317*
    inflammatory bowel disease with, 319
    intracranial hemorrhage with, 321–322, *322*
    laboratory data on, *316–317*, *319*, 319–320
    malignancies with, 319
    metabolic disorders with, 322
    migraine with, 319
    moyamoya syndrome with, 318, *319*, 320
    perforating artery occlusions with, 320
    peripheral leptomeningeal artery occlusions with, 320
    SCD with, 316, 318
    signs/symptoms of, 319
    treatment of, 320–321
  CT diagnosis of, 75–78
  determinants of, *287–288*, 287–290, 288*t*, *290*
    modifiable risk factors with, 288–289, 288*t*
    nonmodifiable risk factors with, 287–288, *288*
    potential risk factors with, 289
  differential diagnosis of, 312–315
    nonvascular disorders in, 313–315
    peeling onion of, 313
    stroke types and, 312–313
  drug dependence with, 1164
  epidemiology, 286–290, *288*, 288*t*, *290*
  frequency of subtypes of, 285–286, *287*
  genetics of, 305–307, *306*
    CADASIL in, 307
    intracerebral hemorrhage in, 307
    subarachnoid hemorrhage in, 307
  ischemic, 305–307, *306*
  outcome for, 289–290, *290*
  pediatric acquired HIV/AIDS with, 1186–1187, *1187*
  pregnancy with, 1114–1115
  prevention of, 327–328
  treatment of, 324–328, 325*t*
    ABI/TIA in, 324–325
    cardiac/aortic origin in, 326
    embolic strokes in, 326
    fixed neurologic defects in, 325–326, 325*t*
    intracerebral hemorrhage in, 326
    rehabilitation in, 326–327
    SAH from congenital/berry aneurysm in, 326–327
  young adult, 309–310, 310*t*
Strokes
  fetal cocaine effects with, 1189
  Lacunar, 308
Strongyloidiasis, 247*t*, 252–253
Structural malformations, 587–599, *588*, 589*t–591t*, *591*, *593*, *594*, 594*t*, 595*t*, *596–599*
  achondroplasia as, 590*t*
  adenyl-succinate deficiency with, 587
  adrenoleukodystrophy with, 587
  Aicardi syndrome with, 589*t*
  alobar holoprosencephaly as, 587
  Apert syndrome with, 589*t*, 594*t*
  arhinencephaly as, 587
  Arnold-Chiari, 596–599, *597–599*

  atlas, 592
  Autley-Bixler syndrome with, 594*t*
  axis, 592
  Baller-Gerold syndrome with, 594*t*
  basilar impression as, *591*, 591–592
  brachycephaly with, 593
  Carpenter syndrome with, 594*t*
  cerebral gigantism as, 590*t*
  cervical spine, 589–592, 591*t*
  cervical vertebrae fusion as, 592, *593*
  Cowden disease as, 590*t*
  craniosynostosis as, 592–593, *594*, 594*t*
  cranium bifidum, 593–596, 595*t*, *596*
  Crouzon syndrome with, 594*t*
  dolichocephalic skull with, 593
  Fanconi anemia syndrome with, 589*t*
  FG syndrome as, 590*t*
  fucosidosis as, 590*t*
  glutaric aciduria with, 587
  Greig cephalopolysyndactyly as, 590*t*
  Hurler-Scheie as, 590*t*
  hydrocephalus ex vacuo with, 589
  Kleeblattschädel skull with, 593
  Klippel-Trenaunay-Weber as, 590*t*
  lissencephaly as, 587
  macrocephaly as, 588–589, 590*t*
  Maroteaux-Larny as, 590*t*
  Meckel-Gruber syndrome with, 595
  megalencephaly as, 588–589, 590*t*
  Menkes syndrome with, 587
  Miller-Dieker syndrome with, 589*t*
  mitochondrial respiratory chain as, 590*t*
  mucopolysaccharidosis as, 590*t*
  Neu-Laxova syndrome with, 589*t*
  neural tube closure, 595*t*
  occipital bone, 589–592, 591*t*
  oral-facial digital syndrome with, 589*t*
  osteochondrodysplasia syndrome with, 589*t*
  osteopetrosis as, 590*t*
  Pfeiffer syndrome with, 594*t*
  premature cranial suture closure as, 592–593, *594*, 594*t*
  Proteus syndrome as, 590*t*
  pyruvate-dehydrogenase deficiency with, 587
  Robinow syndrome as, 590*t*
  Ruvalcaba-Myhre syndrome as, 590*t*
  Saethre-Chotzen syndrome with, 594*t*
  scaphocephalic skull with, 593
  Shapiro syndrome with, 589*t*
  Sotos syndrome as, 590*t*
  spina bifida, 593–596, 595*t*, *596*
  spina bifida occulta, 595
  trigonocephaly with, 593
  trisomy 9p syndrome as, 590*t*
  Walker-Warburg syndrome with, 595
  XK syndrome with, 589*t*
  Zellweger syndrome with, 587
Stupor, coma v., 20–21
Sturge-Weber disease
  anticonvulsive drugs for, 456
  clinical presentation of, 456, *456*
  diagnosis of, 456, *456*
  hemispherectomy for, 456
  radiation therapy for, 456
  treatment of, 456
  vascular malformations of, 455–457, *455–457*

Sturge-Weber-Dimitri syndrome
diagnosis of, 720
genetics of, 718–719
Klippel-Trenaunay syndrome v., 720
laboratory data on, 720, *720, 721*
neurocutaneous disorder of, 718–721,
719, 719t, 720, 721
Parkes Weber syndrome v., 720
symptoms/signs of, *719,* 719–720, *719t,
720, 721*
cutaneous, 719, *719*
neurologic, 719
ophthalmologic, 719–720
treatment of, 720
Subacute cerebellar degeneration,
paraneoplastic syndromes
associated with, 1088t
Subacute measles encephalitis, 188
Subacute meningitis, 144–148, *145, 146*
Subacute myelo-optic neuritis (SMON),
multiple sclerosis v., 956, 957t
Subacute myelo-optic neuropathy,
occupation/environment
neurotoxicology with, 1181
Subacute sclerosing panencephalitis
(SSPE), 201–202
Subacute sensory neuropathy,
paraneoplastic syndromes
associated with, 1088t
Subarachnoid hemorrhage
birth injuries of, 563
head injury trauma with, 489
Subarachnoid hemorrhage (SAH), 285
clinical manifestations of, 330–331,
330t
complications of, 331–334, *332, 333,*
333t
cerebral edema as, 333, *333*
hydrocephalus as, 332–333
neurogenic cardiac/pulmonary
disturbances as, 334
rebleeding as, 331, *332*
seizures as, 333–334
vasospasm as, 332, *332,* 333t
CT of, 103, 331, *331*
diagnostic studies on, 331, *331, 332*
epidemiology of, 329–330, 329t
grading scale for, 330, 330t
hydrocephalus with, 350
MRI with, 106
nonaneurysmal causes of, 329t
other macroscopic aneurysms and,
336–337
dolichoectatic aneurysms as, 336
fusiform aneurysms as, 336
mycotic aneurysm as, 336–337
pseudoaneurysm as, 337
vascular malformations as, 337
outcome after, 335–336
pathology of, 329–330, 329t
signs/symptoms of, 330–331
stroke genetics with, 307
stroke treatment and, 326–327
treatment of, 334–336, 336t
endovascular therapy as, 334–335
intensive care management as, 335,
336t
surgical management as, 334
vascular diseases of, 328–337, 329t,
330t, 331, 332, 333, 333t, 335, 336t
Subclavian steal syndrome, syncope
differential diagnosis with,
17, 18t

Subcortical band heterotopia, differential
diagnosis of, 685t
Subcortical dementia, progressive
supranuclear palsy with, 846
Subcortical disequilibrium, senile gait
disorders with, 59
Subcortical motor aphasia, 9
Subcortical sensory aphasia, 9
Subdural empyema
focal infections of, 173–174
head injury trauma with, 497
lumbar puncture with, 174
treatment of, 174
Subdural hematoma, head injury trauma
with, *487,* 487–488, *488*
Subdural infections, 148–150
Subscapular nerve, 533, 534t
Subtelomeric chromosomal anomalies,
610
chromosomal stability with, 610
mental retardation associated with, 610
telomeres with, 610
22q11 deletion syndrome with, 610
Sulfur amino acid metabolism disorder,
614–617, 615t
diagnosis of, 617
homocystinuria as, 614–617, 615t
Sumatriptan, migraine headache treated
with, 985
SUNCT. *See* Short-lasting, Unilateral,
Neuralgiform Headache
Superficial siderosis of central nervous
system, 365–366, *366*
Superior sagittal sinus thrombosis, *340,*
340–341, *341*
Superselective microcatheter techniques,
catheter angiography with, 109
Suprascapular nerve, 533, 534t, 536–537
Supratentorial structural lesions, coma
presentations with, 24
Supratentorial subdural hemorrhage,
birth injuries of, 563
Supratentorial tumors, astrocytomas
with, 430
Sural nerve, 540
Sural nerve biopsy, 129
Surgery
astrocytomas in, 431
brain metastasis with, 462–463
head injury trauma with, 492–493
neuropathic pain treated with, 548
pineal cysts with, *417, 418,* 418–419
pituitary gland tumors treated with,
426, 426–427
SAH treatment with, 334
spinal tumors treated with, 479
Surrogate decision maker, end-of-life
issues with, 1201
Survival motor neuron gene (SMN),
spinal muscular atrophies with,
861
Susac syndrome, 40
Swing phase, gait with, 56
Sydenham chorea, 807–809, 807t, 808t
complications of, 808
course of, 809
diagnosis of, 808–809, 808t
etiology of, 807–808
incidence of, 808
involuntary movements with, 48
PANDAS with, 808
pathology of, 807–808
prognosis for, 809

symptoms/signs of, 808
treatment of, 809
withdrawal emergent syndrome with,
808
Sylvian aqueduct syndrome, ocular
motility impairment with, 43
Symptomatic epilepsy, 992
Symptomatic myoclonus, 813
Symptomatic vasospasm-induced
stenoses, catheter angiography
of, 109
Symptoms of neurologic disorders
agnosia as, 12–13
amnestic aphasia as, 11
aphasia as, 8–11
apraxia as, 11–12
basilar migraine as, 17, 18t
coma as, 20–28, *22,* 25t–28t
delirium as, 3–4
dementia as, 3, 4–8
dizziness in, 32, 34–38
dyskinesia as, 48–51, 50t, 51t
examination of, 60–63
Alzheimer disease in, 62
basal ganglia disease in, 63
brainstem disease in, 62
cerebral disease in, 62
CT in, 60, 61, 62
duration of disease in, 62
ethnicity in, 61
gender in, 61
Guillain-Barré syndrome in, 62
identifying disorder site in, 62–63
medical history in, 60, 62
MRI in, 60, 61, 62
neuromuscular disorder in, 63
Parkinson's disease in, 62
patient's age in, 61
peripheral nerve disease in, 63
socioeconomic considerations in,
61 62
spinal cord disease in, 63
tempo of disease in, 62
TIA in, 62
gait disorders as, 56–60
headache as, 45–48, 46t
hearing loss in, 32, 33–34, 36–38
ideational dyspraxia as, 11–12
ideomotor dyspraxia as, 12
impaired vision in, 38–44, *39–41*
innervatory dyspraxia as, 11
involuntary movements as, 48–51, 50t,
51t
limb-kinetic dyspraxia as, 11
motor aphasia as, 8, 9–10
pain in, 29–31
paresthesia in, 29–31
seizure as, 17–20, 18t
sensory aphasia as, 8, 10–11
syncope as, 13–17, 14t, 15t, 18t
vertigo in, 34–38
weak muscles as, 52–55
Synaptic pruning hypothesis,
schizophrenia with, 1140
Syncope, 13–17, 14t, 15t, 18t
cardiac, 14t, 16
causes of, 14, 14t
clinical presentation of, 14–16, 15t, 18t
differential diagnosis of, 15t, 17, 18t
basilar migraine in, 17, 18t
epilepsy in, 17
subclavian steal syndrome in, 17, 18t
TIA in, 17, 18t, 19

distinguishing features of, 15*t*
EEG with, 14
morbidity of, 14
neurally mediated reflex, 14–16, 14*t*
  carotid sinus, 14*t*, 15
  situational, 14*t*, 15–16
  vasovagal, 14*t*, 15
neurologic, 14, 14*t*
orthostatic hypotension and, 14*t*, 16
  Parkinson disease with, 16
  Shy-Drager variant of, 16
seizure v., 15*t*
summary on, 20
treatment of, 16–17
Synergistic divergence, Marcus-Gunn
  syndrome with, 601
Synkinesis, 602
Syphilis, serologic tests for, 126
Syringocephalus, 871
Syringohydromyelia, 872
Syringomyelia
  ALS v., 873
  Arnold-Chiari malformation with, 871,
    873
  brachial amyotrophy with, 871
  Charcot joints with, 871
  clinical manifestations of, 870–871
  differential diagnosis of, 873
  dissociated sensory loss with, 871
  en cuirasse with, 871
  hematomyelia with, 872
  Horner syndrome with, 871
  hydromyelia with, 871, 872
  laboratory data on, 872, 872–873
  main en griffe with, 871
  main succulente with, 871
  MRI of, 872, 872–873
  MS v., 873
  orthostatic hypotension with, 972*t*
  pathology/pathogenesis of, 871–872
  spinal cord disease of, 870–873, 872
  syringocephalus with, 871
  syringohydromyelia with, 872
  treatment of, 873
Systemic lupus erythematosus (SLE)
  antinuclear antibodies with, 1107
  cerebral lupus and, 1107
  chorea of, 809
  course of, 1108
  CT of, 1107
  diagnosis of, 1108
  etiology of, 1106
  IIH with, 362
  incidence of, 1106
  laboratory data on, 1107–1108
  LE cells with, 1107
  MRI of, 1107
  PET of, 1107
  prognosis for, 1108
  symptoms/signs of, 1106–1107, 1107*t*
  therapy for, 1108
  vasculitis syndrome of, 1106–1108,
    1107*t*
Systemic sclerosis, vasculitis syndrome
  of, 1108

T
Tabes dorsalis, 237, *237*, 239–240, 240*t*
Tachyphemia, Parkinson disease with,
  830
Tactile agnosia, 13
TAN. *See* Tropical ataxic neuropathy
Tangier disease, 548, 687*t*, 688*t*, 689*t*

Tardive akathisia, neuroleptic-induced
  syndromes with, 850
Tardive dyskineasia, 849–851, 851*t*
  classic, 849, 851
  Huntington disease with, 806
  myoclonus with, 851
  pathogenesis of, 851
  tics with, 851
  tremor with, 851
Tardive dystonia, 823–824
Tardive myoclonus, 851
Tardive tics, 851
Tardive tremor, 851
Task-specific dystonia, 816
Tau protein
  Alzheimer disease with, 773
  degenerative diseases associated with,
    776*t*
Taxanes, peripheral nervous system
  toxicity with, 1170
Tay-Sachs diseases
  differential diagnosis of, 685*t*, 687*t*
  ethnicity with, 61
  lysosomal/other storage diseases of,
    622–625, *625*
TBI. *See* Traumatic brain injury
TCA. *See* Tricyclic antidepressants
Tegretol. *See* Carbamazepine
Telangiectasias, vascular malformations
  of, 455
Telegraphic speech, motor aphasia
  with, 9
Temazepam, sleep disorders treated with,
  1027
Temporal arteritis, 1102–1103
  prednisone for, 1103
  reversible dementia with, 1103
  steroid therapy for, 1103
Temporal lobe epilepsy, 994
Temporomandibular joint (TMJ)
  headache with, 47
  tinnitus with, 32
TENS. *See* Transcutaneous electrical
  neurostimulation
Tentorial meningiomas, *391*, 392
Teratomas, congenital tumors of,
  434
Terminal sedation, end-of-life issues
  with, 1202
TES. *See* Transcranial electrical
  stimulation
Tetanus, 259–261
  course of, 261
  diagnosis of, 260–261
  etiology of, 260
  incidence of, 260
  laboratory data on, 260
  pathogenesis of, 260
  pathology of, 260
  prognosis of, 261
  symptoms of, 260
  treatment of, 261
Tetany
  Chvostek sign with, 927
  clinical manifestations of, 927
  hypoparathyroidism with, 1042
  muscle cramps/stiffness of, 927
  treatment of, 927
  Trousseau sign with, 927
Thalamic stimulation, Parkinson disease
  surgery with, 837*t*, 838
Thalamotomy, Parkinson disease surgery
  with, 837*t*, 838

Thalassemia, erythrocyte disorder of,
  1051, *1052*
Thallium, 759
  heavy metal intoxication with, 1174*t*,
    1178
Therapeutic drug caused neuropathies,
  760
Thiamine deficiency, dietary associated
  polyneuropathy with, 757
Thoracic intervertebral disc rupture,
  512
Thoracic outlet, 533
Thoracic outlet syndrome, 535
  pain diagnosis with, 30
Thoracic outlet syndrome (TOS),
  543–544
  diagnosis of, 544
  disputed form of, 544
  EMG for, 544
  management of, 544
  pathology of, 544
  symptoms/signs of, 544
  true form of, 544
Thoracic tumors, spinal tumors of,
  476
Thoracodorsal nerve, 533, 534*t*
Thrombocytopenia, LP with, 123
Thromboembolism, tumor complications
  of, 377
Thrombosis, head injury trauma with,
  497
Thrombotic thrombocytopenic purpura
  (TTP), platelet disorder of, *1053*,
  1053–1054
Thymectomy, myasthenia gravis with,
  882, 883
Thyroid endocrine diseases, 1039–1041,
  1040, 1041
  cerebellar ataxia with, 1039
  cretinism with, 1039
  Dalrymple sign with, 1040
  Graves disease as, 1040, *1041*
  Graves ophthalmopathy with, 1040
  Hoffmann syndrome with, 1039
  hyperthyroidism as, 1040–1041, *1041*
  hypothyroidism as, 1039–1040, *1040*
  juvenile myxedema with, 1039
  Kocher-Debré-Sémélaigne syndrome
    with, 1039, *1040*
  myoedema with, 1039
  myxedema staggers with, 1039
  thyrotoxic myopathy with, 1041
  thyrotoxic periodic paralysis with,
    1041
Thyrotoxic myopathy, thyroid endocrine
  diseases with, 1041
Thyrotoxic periodic paralysis, thyroid
  endocrine diseases with, 1041
Thyrotropin deficiency, radiation injury
  with, 554
TIA. *See* Transient ischemic attack
Tiagabine, epilepsy treatment with,
  1003*t*, 1005
Tibial nerve, 540, 541
Tick paralysis, floppy infant syndrome
  with, 575
Tick-borne encephalitis, 186
Tics, 49, 851
Time-of-flight method (TOF), MRI with,
  74
Time-to-peak (TTP)
  CT with, 72
  MRI with, 75

Tinnitus, 32–33
  continuous, 32
  Ménière disease with, 1018–1019
  objective, 32
  pulsatile, 32
  subjective, 32
  TMJ syndrome with, 32
Tissue plasminogen activator (tPA), 72,
    118, 325, 325t, 1058, 1166
Tissue plasminogen activator deficiency,
    coagulation disorders with, 1058
Titubation, gait disorders with, 58
Tizanidine (Zanaflex), multiple sclerosis
    treated with, 960
TMJ. *See* Temporomandibular joint
TMS. *See* Transcranial magnetic
    stimulation
Tocopherol, Parkinson disease drug
    therapy with, 837t, 839
TOF. *See* Time-of-flight method
Tolosa-Hunt syndrome, Cranial/
    peripheral nerve lesion with,
    527
Tolterodine (Detrol), multiple sclerosis
    treated with, 960
Tonic phase, epilepsy with, 991
Topiramate
    epilepsy treatment with, 1003t, 1005
    sleep disorders treated with, 1027
Torsion dystonia gene (DYT1), *818,*
    818–819, 819, 822t
Torticollis, 59, 205, 434, 663, 816–818,
    817t, *819,* 820, *820,* 823, 826, 826t,
    948t
TOS. *See* Thoracic outlet syndrome
Tourette syndrome
    drug dependence with, 1165
    movement disorder of, 815
    PANDAS with, 815
Toxicology screen, delirium diagnosis
    with, 4
Toxoplasmosis, 253–254, *254*
    AIDS opportunistic infections with,
    220–221, 221t, *222*
    clinical manifestations of, 253–254
    diagnosis of, 254
    etiology of, 253
    laboratory data on, 253, *253*
    pathology of, 253
    treatment of, 254
tPA. *See* Tissue plasminogen activator
Tracheostomy, respiratory support for
    neurologic diseases with, 1087
Tramadol hydrochloride, neuropathic
    pain treated with, 549
Transcortical motor aphasia, 9
Transcortical sensory aphasia, 8–9
Transcranial electrical stimulation (TES),
    TMS and, 97
Transcranial magnetic stimulation (TMS)
    diagnostic tests with, 89, 97–100, *99*
    MEP with, 98–99
    paired-pulse, 98
    repetitive trains of, 98, 99–100
    silent period with, 98
    single pulse, 98
    TES and, 97
Transcutaneous electrical
    neurostimulation (TENS), spinal
    injury trauma treated with, 509
Transient global amnesia, 1017
    amaurosis fugax with, 1017
    anterograde amnesia with, 1017

carotid artery occlusion with, 1017
    migraine with, 1017
Transient ischemic attack (TIA), 293–294
    diagnosis of, 294
    MRA with, 74
    MRI with, 74
    neurologic disorders examination with,
    62
    significance of, 294
    signs/symptoms of, 294
    stroke treatment with, 324–325
    stroke v., 313
    subclavian steal syndrome with, 293
    syncope differential diagnosis with, 17,
    18t, 19
    transient monocular blindness with,
    294
Transient plexus injury, radiation injury
    with, 554
Transient sleep disorders, 1028
Transient visual effects, impaired vision
    with, 42
Transitional sclerosis, Schilder disease
    with, 683
Transverse myelitis
    HIV-related syndromes with, 216t
    orthostatic hypotension with, 972t
Trauma
    abducens nerve injury, 526–527
    acoustic nerve injury, 531
    alcoholism with, 1157
    cervical spondylotic myelopathy,
    517–521, 518t, *519, 520*
      differential diagnosis of, 519–520
      incidence of, 517
      laboratory data on, 518, *519, 520*
      MRI of, 518, *519, 520*
      pathology of, 517
      symptoms/signs of, 517, 517t
      treatment of, 520–521
    cranial/peripheral nerve lesion,
    523–541, 525t, *526,* 534t, *534t,* 537,
    537t, 538t, 539t
      abducens nerve injury, 526–527
      acoustic nerve injury, 531
      alcohol-tobacco amblyopia with, 526
      Bell palsy with, 530
      clinical manifestations of, 524
      diagnosis of, 524
      facial nerve injury, 529–531
      general principles of, 523
      glossopharyngeal nerve injury,
      531–532
      hypoglossal nerve injury, 533
      oculomotor nerve injury, 526–527
      olfactory nerve injury, 524–525
      optic nerve injury, 525–526, 525t, *526*
      optic neuritis with, 526, *526*
      orbital myositis with, 527
      orbital pseudotumor with, 527
      pathophysiology of, 523–524
      prognosis for, 524
      spinal accessory nerve injury,
      532–533
      Tolosa-Hunt syndrome with, 527
      treatment of, 524
      trigeminal nerve injury, 527–529
      trigeminal neuralgia with, 527–529
      trochlear nerve injury, 526–527
      vagus nerve injury, 532
    decompression sickness, 558–559
    drug dependence with, 1163
    electrical injury, 557–558

epilepsy with, 1013t
facial nerve injury, 529–531
    Bell palsy with, 530
glossopharyngeal nerve injury, 531–532
head injury, 483–500, 484t, *485, 486, 487,*
    488, 489, 490t, 491t, 492t, 493t, *494*
    acute complications of, 496–497
    admission to hospital for, 492, 492t
    airway with, 495
    antibiotics for, 496
    anticonvulsants for, 495
    autonomic dysfunction with, 484
    axonal shearing injury in, 483–484,
    485
    basilar skull fractures in, 483
    birth injuries with, 499
    blood pressure management with,
    495
    brain swelling in, 484–485
    burr-hole for, 493
    carotid-cavernous fistula with,
    496–497
    cerebral concussion in, 483–484, 484t
    cerebral edema in, 484–485
    cerebrospinal fluid fistula with, 496
    child abuse with, 499
    chronic traumatic encephalopathy
    with, 499
    compound fractures in, 483
    contusion in, 485–487, *486*
    CPP with, 493, *494*
    cranial nerve injury with, 497
    craniotomy for, 493
    deep-vein thrombosis prophylaxis
    with, 496
    depressed fractures in, 483
    diagnosis of, 490–492, 491t
    diffuse axonal injury with, 484, 487
    dural sinus thrombosis with, 497
    emergency measures for, 491t
    epidemiology of, 483
    epidural hematoma in, 488–489, *489*
    examination for, 491–492
    extradural infections with, 497
    fluid management with, 495
    gastric stress ulcer prophylaxis with,
    496
    Glasgow Coma Scale with, 490, 490t,
    492, 493, 497
    hematoma in, 486–488, *486–488*
    hemorrhage in, 485–487, *486, 489*
    history with, 490–491
    hygromas with, 487
    hypotension with, 489
    hypoxia with, 489
    ICP management for, 493–494, 493t,
    494
    ICU management of, 492, 493, 494
    imaging for, 492
    infections with, 497
    initial assessment of, 489–490, 490t
    intensive insulin therapy for, 496
    intracerebral abscess with, 497
    isotonic fluids with, 495
    Kernohan notch with, 487
    lacerations in, 486
    leptomeningeal cysts with, 499
    low/moderate/high risk group with,
    492
    management of, 492–497, 492t, 493t,
    494
    meningitis with, 497
    mortality estimates for, 491t

nimodipine for, 495–496
nutrition with, 495
outcomes of, 497–499
parenchymal contusion/hemorrhage
in, 485–487, *486*
pathology/pathophysiology of,
483–490, 484*t*, *485, 486, 487, 488,
489,* 490*t*, 491*t*
pediatric trauma with, 499
persistent vegetative state with, 498
pneumocephalus with, 496
postconcussion syndrome with, 498
posttraumatic amnesia with, 498
posttraumatic epilepsy with, 498–499
posttraumatic movement disorders
with, 499
professional boxing neurology with,
499–500
radiography for, 492
risk stratification with, 490*t*
sedation with, 495
seizures with, 498
serial neurologic evaluation for,
494–495
skull fractures in, 483
spinal shock with, 490
stabilization of, 489–490, 490*t*
steroids for, 496
subarachnoid hemorrhage in, 489
subdural empyema with, 497
subdural hematoma in, *487,* 487–488,
488
surgical intervention for, 492–493
temperature management with, 495
thrombosis with, 497
twist-drill for, 493
vascular injury with, 497
ventilation with, 495
hypoglossal nerve injury, 533
intervertebral disk, 510–517, 511*t*, 512*t*,
513, 514, 515, 516*t*
cervical disc disease as, 512–513, *515,*
516*t*
chronic low-back pain as, 516–517
diagnostic features of, 513–516
imaging of, 516
incidence of, 511
lumbar intervertebral disc rupture
as, 511–512, 512*t, 513, 514*
pathogenesis of, 510–511, 511*t*
signs/symptoms of, 511
spinal stenosis with, 510
syndromes of, 511*t*
thoracic intervertebral disc rupture
as, 512
treatment for, 516
leg nerve injury, 540–541
lightning injury, 557–558
lower extremity nerve injury, 539–540
lumbar spondylosis, 521–523, *522*
neuropathic pain, 545–550, 549*t*
AED for, 549
anticonvulsants for, 549
antinociceptive agents for, 549
causalgia with, 545
central nociception with, 546
clinical features of, 548
CPRS with, 545
deafferentation pain with, 545
definitions associated with, 545
diabetic neuropathic cachexia with,
548
drug therapy for, 548–549, 549*t*

gabapentin for, 549
general treatment principles for, 548
ISDN for, 550
lamotrigine for, 549
neuralgia with, 545
neurogenic pain with, 545
normal processing of pain and,
545–546
other drugs for, 550
painful polyneuropathy with, 545
pathophysiology of, 546–548
peripheral nociception with, 545–546
pharmacologic therapy for, 548–549,
549*t*
reflex sympathetic dystrophy with,
545
selective serotonin reuptake
inhibitors for, 550
surgical therapy for, 548
tramadol hydrochloride for, 549
treatment of, 548–550, 549*t*
tricyclic antidepressants for, 550
venlafaxine for, 550
zonisamide for, 549
oculomotor nerve injury, 526–527
orbital myositis with, 527
orbital pseudotumor with, 527
Tolosa-Hunt syndrome with, 527
olfactory nerve injury, 524–525
optic nerve injury, 525–526, 525*t, 526*
alcohol-tobacco amblyopia as, 526
optic neuritis as, *526,* 526
peripheral nerve injury, 533
radiation injury, 551–555, *553*
acute effects of, 551
acute ischemic brachial neuropathy
with, 554
adrenocorticotropic-hormone
function with, 554
brachial plexopathy with, 554
cognitive impairment with, 555
early effects of, 551
early-delayed syndromes with,
551–552
endocrine dysfunction with, 554–555
gonadotropin deficiency with, 554
growth hormone function with, 554
hyperprolactinemia with, 555
immunologic hypothesis with, 552
late-delayed syndromes with,
552–555, *553*
lumbosacral plexopathy with, 554
mass lesion with, 552
meningiomas with, 555
mineralizing microangiopathy with,
552
myokymia with, 554
neuropsychologic sequelae with, 555
neuroradiologic abnormalities with,
552
other complications of, 555
peripheral-nerve tumors with, 555
radiation myelopathy with, 553–554
radiation necrosis with, 552–553, *553*
radiation optic neuropathy with, 555
radiation-induced plexopathy with,
554
radiation-induced tumors with, 555
radiation-induced vasculopathy
with, 554
rhombencephali with, 551
sarcomas with, 555
thyrotropin deficiency with, 554

transient plexus injury with, 554
white-matter changes with, 552
radiculopathy, 510–517, 511*t,* 512*t, 513,
514, 515,* 516*t*
cervical disc disease as, 512–513, *515,*
516*t*
chronic low-back pain as, 516–517
diagnostic features of, 513–516
imaging of, 516
incidence of, 511
lumbar intervertebral disc rupture
as, 511–512, 512*t, 513, 514*
pathogenesis of, 510–511, 511*t*
signs/symptoms of, 511
spinal stenosis with, 510
syndromes of, 511*t*
thoracic intervertebral disc rupture
as, 512
treatment for, 516
spinal accessory nerve injury, 532–533
spinal injury, 502–509, 502*t, 504*
anterior-cord syndrome with,
504–505
ASIA on, 503
bladder function with, 508
bowel training with, 508
Brown-Séquard syndrome with,
504–505
cauda equina lesions with, 504–505
causes of, 502, 502*t*
central-cord syndrome with, 504–505
classification of, 503–505, *504*
clinical patterns of, 504–505
complications with, 507–509
course of, 506
CT for, 505–506
diagnosis of, 505–506
dysautonomia with, 507
etiology of, 502, 502*t*
IMSOP on, 503
mechanism of, 502–503
MRI for, 505–506
muscle spasms with, 508
neurologic assessment of, 503–505,
504
nutritional deficiency with, 508
pain with, 509
pathology of, 503
posterior-cord syndrome with, 505
pressure sores with, 508
prognosis for, 506
pulmonary function with, 507–508
rehabilitation of, 509
sexual function with, 508–509
spinal-cord concussion with, 505
TENS for, 509
treatment of, 506–507
thoracic outlet syndrome, 543–544
trigeminal nerve injury, 527–529
trochlear nerve injury, 526–527
upper extremity nerve injury, 533–539,
534, 534*t, 537,* 537*t,* 538*t,* 539*t*
antebrachial cutaneous nerves with,
536
axillary nerve with, 534, 534*t,* 536
brachial cutaneous nerves with, 536
brachial plexus in, 533–536, *534,* 534*t*
cord injury with, 535
diffuse plexus injury with, 535–536
dorsal scapular nerve with, 533, 534*t*
idiopathic brachial plexitis with, 535
ischemic paralysis of arm with, 536
lateral cord injury with, 535

Trauma,
  upper extremity nerve injury (*contd.*)
    lateral cord with, 533
    long thoracic nerve with, 533, 534*t*, 536, *537*
    lower radicular syndrome with, 535
    lower trunk with, 533
    medial cord with, 533
    median nerve with, 534, 534*t*, 537–538, 538*t*
    middle radicular syndrome with, 535
    middle trunk with, 533
    musculocutaneous nerve with, 534, 534*t*, 539
    neuralgic amyotrophy with, 535
    Parsonage-Turner syndrome with, 535
    pectoral nerves with, 533, 534*t*
    peripheral nerves with, 536–539, 537*t*, 538*t*, 539*t*
    posterior cord with, 533
    proximal nerves with, *536*, 536–537
    radial nerve with, 534, 534*t*, 536–537
    spinal roots in, 533–536, *534*, 534*t*
    subscapular nerve with, 533, 534*t*
    suprascapular nerve with, 533, 534*t*, 536–537
    thoracic outlet syndrome with, 535
    thoracic outlet with, 533
    thoracodorsal nerve with, 533, 534*t*
    ulnar nerve with, 534, 534*t*, 538–539, 538*t*, 539*t*
    upper radicular syndrome with, 535
    upper trunk with, 533
  vagus nerve injury, 532
Traumatic brain injury (TBI), 483–500, 484*t*, 485, 486, 487, 488, 489, 490*t*, 491*t*, 492*t*, 493*t*, 494
  acute complications of, 496–497
  admission to hospital for, 492, 492*t*
  airway with, 495
  antibiotics for, 496
  anticonvulsants for, 495
  autonomic dysfunction with, 484
  axonal shearing injury in, 483–484, *485*
  basilar skull fractures in, 483
  birth injuries with, 499
  blood pressure management with, 495
  brain swelling in, 484–485
  burr-hole for, 493
  carotid-cavernous fistula with, 496–497
  cerebral concussion in, 483–484, 484*t*
  cerebral edema in, 484–485
  cerebrospinal fluid fistula with, 496
  child abuse with, 499
  chronic traumatic encephalopathy with, 499
  compound fractures in, 483
  contusion in, 485–487, *486*
  CPP with, 493, *494*
  cranial nerve injury with, 497
  craniotomy for, 493
  CT for, 492
  deep-vein thrombosis prophylaxis with, 496
  depressed fracture in, 483
  diagnosis of, 490–492, 491*t*
  diffuse axonal injury with, 484, 487
  dural sinus thrombosis with, 497
  emergency measures for, 491*t*
  epidemiology of, 483
  epidural hematoma in, 488–489, *489*
  examination for, 491–492

extradural infections with, 497
fluid management with, 495
gastric stress ulcer prophylaxis with, 496
hematoma in, 486–488, *486–488*
hemorrhage in, 485–487, *486*, 489
history with, 490–491
hygromas with, 487
ICP management for, 493–494, 493*t*, *494*
ICU management of, 492, 493, 494
imaging for, 492
infections with, 497
initial assessment of, 489–490, 490*t*
  Glasgow Coma Scale in, 490, 490*t*, 492, 493, 497
  hypotension in, 489
  hypoxia in, 489
  risk stratification in, 490*t*
  spinal shock in, 490
intensive insulin therapy for, 496
intracerebral abscess with, 497
isotonic fluids with, 495
Kernohan notch with, 487
lacerations in, 486
leptomeningeal cysts with, 499
low/moderate/high risk group with, 492
management of, 492–497, 492*t*, 493*t*, *494*
meningitis with, 497
mortality estimates for, 491*t*
nimodipine for, 495–496
nutrition with, 495
outcomes of, 497–499
parenchymal contusion/hemorrhage in, 485–487, *486*
pathology/pathophysiology of, 483–490, 484*t*, 485, 486, 487, 488, 489, 490*t*, 491*t*
pediatric trauma with, 499
persistent vegetative state with, 498
pneumocephalus with, 496
postconcussion syndrome with, 498
posttraumatic amnesia with, 498
posttraumatic epilepsy with, 498–499
posttraumatic movement disorders with, 499
professional boxing neurology with, 499–500
radiography for, 492
sedation with, 495
seizures with, 498
serial neurologic evaluation for, 494–495
skull fractures in, 483
stabilization of, 489–490, 490*t*
steroids for, 496
subarachnoid hemorrhage in, 489
subdural empyema with, 497
subdural hematoma in, *487*, 487–488, *488*
surgical intervention for, 492–493
temperature management with, 495
thrombosis with, 497
twist-drill for, 493
vascular injury with, 497
ventilation with, 495
Tremors, 48
Tremulousness, ethanol withdrawal with, 1153
Trichinosis, 247*t*, 251
Trichopoliodystrophy, differential diagnosis of, 685*t*, 686*t*, 687*t*, 688*t*

Trichothiodystrophy, DNA maintenance/transcription/translation disorders of, 647*t*
Tricyclic antidepressants (TCA), neuropathic pain treated with, 550
Trigeminal nerve injury
  cranial/peripheral nerve lesion with, 527–529
  hemifacial spasm with, 529
Trigeminal neuralgia
  cranial/peripheral nerve lesion with, 527–529
  diagnosis of, 528–529
Trigeminal schwannoma, nerve-sheath tumor of, 385, *385*
Trigonocephaly, structural malformations with, 593
Trihexyphenidyl, Parkinson disease drug therapy with, 837*t*, 839
Triorthocresyl phosphate, 759
Triphasic waves, EEG pattern with, 80, *81*, 82
Trisomy 9p syndrome, structural malformations of, 590*t*
Trisomy 21, 607–608
  Alzheimer disease with, 608
  clinical features of, 607
  cytogenetics with, 608
  floppy infant syndrome with, 575
  management of, 608
  molecular genetics with, 608
  neuropathology of, 608
Trochlear nerve, cranial/peripheral nerve lesion with, 526–527
Tropical ataxic neuropathy (TAN), tropical myeloneuropathies of, 856, 857
Tropical myeloneuropathies
  clinical manifestations of, 856–857
  dietary toxins with, 858
  etiology of, 857–858
  history of, 856–857
  Jamaican neuropathy as, 856, 857
  konzo as, 856
  lathyrism as, 856, 857
  malnutrition with, 857
  nutritional deprivation with, 858
  nutritional neuropathy as, 856–857
  other toxins with, 858
  pathology of, 856–857
  persistent viral infection with, 857–858
  prevention of, 858
  spinal cord diseases of, 856–858, 857*t*
  Strachan syndrome as, 856–857
  treatment of, 858
  tropical ataxic neuropathy as, 856, 857
Tropical spastic paraparesis (TSP), 202–203, 856, 857, 857*t*
Trousseau sign
  hypoparathyroidism with, 1042
  tetany with, 927
Trypanosomiasis, 255–256
TSC. *See* Tuberous sclerosis complex
TSP. *See* Tropical spastic paraparesis
TTP. *See* Thrombotic thrombocytopenic purpura; Time-to-peak
Tuberculous meningitis, *145*, 145–148, *146*
  course for, 148
  diagnosis of, 147–148
  incidence of, 147
  pathogenesis of, *145*, 145, *146*
  pathology of, 145–147
  physical findings on, 147

prognosis for, 148
sequelae with, 148
symptoms of, 147
treatment of, 148
Tuberculum sellae meningiomas, 391
Tuberous sclerosis
childhood central nervous system
tumors with, 428
differential diagnosis of, 685*t*
Tuberous sclerosis complex (TSC)
adenoma sebaceum with, 724, 725, *725*
cafe au lait spots with, 726
candle gutterings with, 725, *725*
course of, 730
diagnosis of, 729–730, 730*t*
facial angiofibroma with, 726
genetics of, 724
incidence of, 724
laboratory data on, *728*, 728–729
neurocutaneous disorder of, 724–730,
725–729, 730*t*
pathology/pathogenesis of, 724–726,
725
phakomas with, 726
prognosis for, 730
renal angiomyolipomas with, 727
renal lesions with, 727
shagreen patches with, 726
symptoms/signs with, 726–728, *727*
treatment for, 730
ungual fibroma with, 725–726
Tubulin protein, Alzheimer disease with,
773
Tumors
age-specific incidences rates of, 371,
372
anticonvulsants for, 376–377
benign skull, 378–379, *379*
chondroma as, 378
dermoid tumors as, 378–379
epidermoid tumors as, 378–379
hemangioma as, 378
osteoma as, 378, *379*
other, 379
biology of intracranial neoplasms with,
373
CBTRUS for, 371
childhood central nervous system,
428–444, 431*t*, 432*t*, *433–438*, *440*,
441, *443*
astrocytomas as, 429–433, 431*t*, 432*t*,
435–439, *436*, *437*, *438*
ATRT with, 429, 439, 441
BCNS with, 428
cardiovascular late effects from, 444
cerebellar development with, 429
developmental biology with, 429
ependymomas as, *441*, 441–442
epidemiology of, 428–429
Ewing sarcoma as, 428
germ-cell tumors as, 428, 442
Gorlin syndrome with, 428
late effects of treatment with,
443–444
lymphomas as, 442
medulloblastoma with, 428, 429,
431*t*, 432*t*, 439–441, *440*
melanoma as, 428
meningiomas as, 442–443, *443*
neuroblastoma as, 428
neurocognitive disorders from, 444
neurosensory sequelae from, 444
NF-1/NF-2 with, 428

osteosarcoma as, 428
PNET with, 428, 429, 431*t*, 439–441
quality of life with, 443–444
rhabdoid tumors as, 439–441
rhabdomyosarcoma as, 428
sonic hedgehog with, 429
supratentorial primitive
neuroectodermal tumors as,
439–441
tuberous sclerosis with, 428
von Hippel-Lindau disease with, 428
Wilms tumors as, 428
Wnt signaling with, 429
clinical diagnosis of, 373
complications of, 377
thromboembolism as, 377
congenital, 433–435, *433–435*
cholesteatomas as, 434, *434*
chordomas as, 434
choroid-plexus tumors as, 434, *435*
colloid cysts of third ventricle as, 435
craniopharyngiomas as, 433
DACI as, 435
dermoid tumors as, 434
DIG as, 435
DNT as, 435
epidermoids as, 431*t*, 434, *434*
gangliogliomas as, 431*t*, 435
PXA as, 435
teratomas as, 434
corticosteroids for, 376, 376*t*
CT of, 101
epidemiology of, 371–372, *372*
etiology of, 372–373
general considerations for, 371–377,
372–375, 376*t*
gliomas, 393–405, 394*t*, *396*, *397*, *401*,
403, *404*, 416
astrocytoma as, 393–394, 394*t*,
397–400
clinical features of, 396
CT of, *397*
dysembryoplastic neuroepithelial
tumor as, 404–405
ependymomas as, 393–394, 394*t*, 403
epidemiology of, 393
familial conditions with, 395–396
gangliocytomas as, 404
ganglioglioma as, 404
glioblastoma multiforme as, 394*t*,
397–399
gliomatosis cerebri as, 402–403, *403*
imaging of, *396*, 396–397, *397*
Li Fraumeni syndrome as, 395
MRI of, *396*, 396–397
neurofibromatosis type 1 as, 395–396
neurofibromatosis type 2 as, 396
neuronal glial tumors as, 403–404,
404
neuronal tumors as, 403–404, *404*
oligodendroglioma as, 393–394, 394*t*,
400–402, *401*
pathology of, 393–395, 394*t*
PET of, 397
therapy of, 397–402, *401*
Turcot syndrome as, 396
VEGF with, 395
hemangiopericytomas, 392
laboratory examination of, 375–376
lymphoma, 406–413, *408–410*, 410*t*
brain metastasis with, 407
epidural spinal cord compression
with, 407

intravascular, 412
LDH with, 406
leptomeningeal, 407
lymphomatoid granulomatosis,
412–413
metastatic to nervous system of,
406–407
non-Hodgkin, 406–407
primary CNS, 406, 407–412, *408–410*,
410*t*
malignant skull, 379–381, 379*t*, *380*, *381*
chondrosarcoma as, 380
extension of, 380
fibrous sarcoma as, 380
glomus jugulare tumors as, 380–381
Hand-Schüller-Christian disease as,
382
metastasis to skull base as, 379, 379*t*
osteosarcoma as, 380, *381*
primary, 380, *381*
xanthomatosis as, 382
meninges, 386–392, *388–392*
meningiomas, 386–392, *388–392*
biology of, 386–387
cerebellopontine angle, 392
chemotherapy for, 390–391
clinical manifestations of, 387
clivus, *390*, 392
convexity, *389*, 391
CT of, 387
etiology of, 386
foramen magnum, 392
hormonal treatment for, 390
imaging of, 387, *388*
intraventricular, 392
medical treatment for, 390–391
olfactory groove, 391
optic-sheath, 392
parasagittal, 391
pathology of, 387
radiation therapy for, 388–390
specific tumor locations with, *389*,
390, *391*, 391–392, *392*
sphenoid ridge, 392, *392*
spinal, 392
supportive treatment for, 391
surgery for, 388
tentorial, *391*, 392
treatment of, 388–391
tuberculum sellae, 391
VEGF with, 387
metastatic, 459–468, *460–467*
brain metastasis as, 459
chemotherapy for, 463–464
clinical evaluation of, 460
clinical findings on, 460, *460*
clinical presentation of, 467–468
CT of, 460, *461*
diagnosis of, 464–466, *466*, *467*
diagnostic evaluation of, 468
differential diagnosis for, 461
dural metastasis as, 464, *465*
epidemiology of, 459
epidural spinal cord metastasis as,
467–468
imaging of, 460, *461*
leptomeningeal metastasis as,
464–467, *466*, *467*
MRI of, 460, 461, *461*, 468
pathogenesis of, 464, 467
pathophysiology of, 461–462
radiotherapy for, 462
stereotactic radiosurgery for, 462, *463*

Tumors,
  metastatic (*contd.*)
    surgery for, 462–463
    therapy for, 468
    treatment of, 462–464, 466–467
    WBRT for, 462, 463
  neoplastic-like lesions affecting skull
    and, 381–382, *382*
    fibrous dysplasia as, 381, *382*
    hyperostosis as, 381
    mucocele as, 381, *382*
    Paget disease as, 381
  nerve-sheath, 382–385, *383–385*
    trigeminal schwannoma as, 385, *385*
    vestibular schwannoma as, 383–384,
      383–384
  neuroophthalmologic signs of, *374,*
    374–375, *375*
    Foster Kennedy syndrome as, 375
    papilledema as, *374,* 374–375, *375*
    Parinaud syndrome as, 374
  pineal region, 414–420, 414*t,* *415,* 415*t,*
    416, 416*t,* *417, 418, 419*
    germ-cell tumors as, 414–415, 414*t,*
      415*t*
    germinomas as, 414–415, 415*t*
    meningiomas as, 414*t,* 416
    metastasis with, 415–416
    miscellaneous tumors of, 414*t,*
      415–416
    nongerminomatous as, 414–415
    pineal cell tumors as, 414*t,* 415
    pineal cysts as, 414*t,* *415,* 415*t,* *416,*
      416–419, 416*t,* *417, 418, 419*
    pineoblastoma as, 415
    pineocytomas as, 415
  pituitary gland, 420–427, *421,* 422*t,*
    423–426
    ACTH with, 421, 423–424
    choristomas with, 421
    clinical features of, *421,* 421–422,
      422*t*
    CT scan of, 423
    Cushing disease with, 421, 423
    differential diagnosis of, 424, *425*
    FSH with, 421
    granular-cell tumors with, 421
    infundibulomas with, 421
    macroadenomas, 421, *421*
    MEN-I with, 420
    microadenomas, 421, 422, *423*
    MRA of, 423
    MRI of, 422–423, *423, 424*
    myoblastomas with, 421
    pathology of, 421
    pituitary carcinomas with, 421
    radiation therapy for, 427
    radiographic features of, 422–424,
      423, 424
    recurrent tumors with, 427
    surgery for, *426,* 426–427
    symptoms of, 422, 422*t*
    treatment of, 424–427, *425, 426*
  skull, 378–382, *379,* 379*t,* *380, 381*
  spinal, 470–479, 470*t,* *471, 472,* 472*t,*
    473, 474, 475, 476, 478
    age incidence of, 472*t*
    Brown-Séquard syndrome with, 471,
      477
    cauda equina tumors as, 476
    cerebrospinal fluid evaluation for,
      477
    cervical tumors as, 475–476

    conus tumors as, 476
    course of, 478
    CT of, 477
    diagnosis of, 476–478
    diagnostic imaging of, 477
    differential diagnosis of, 477–478
    drop metastases as, 474, *476*
    epidural spinal cord compression
      with, *472,* 472, *473*
    extramedullary tumors as, 470–471
    foramen magnum tumors as,
      474–475
    frequency of, 470, 472*t*
    Horner syndrome as, 476
    intradural tumors as, 474, *475,* 476
    intramedullary metastases as, 473,
      473
    leptomeningeal metastasis as, 474
    lumbar tumors as, 476
    meningiomas as, 474
    microsurgery for, 479
    MRI of, 477
    myelotomy for, 479
    neurofibromas as, 474
    pathology of, 470, 470*t,* *471*
    primary intramedullary tumors as,
      473–474, *474*
    prognosis for, 478
    radiography for, 477
    radiotherapy for, 479
    regional syndromes with, 474–476
    schwannomas as, 474, *475*
    spinal metastases as, *472,* 472–473,
      473
    surgery for, 479
    symptoms of, 470
    thoracic tumors as, 476
    treatment of, *478,* 478–479
    von Recklinghausen disease with,
      477
  symptomatic management of, 376–377,
    376*t*
  symptoms/signs of, 373–374
  vascular, 449–459, *450–457*
    angioblastic meningiomas as, 458
    clinical presentation of, 458
    diagnosis of, 458
    hemangioblastomas as, 458
    hemangiopericytomas as, 458
    treatment of, 458–459
    von Hippel-Lindau disease with,
      458
Turcot syndrome, gliomas with, 396
22q11 deletion syndrome, 610
Twist-drill, head injury trauma surgery
  with, 493
Typhus fever, 158–159

U

Uhthoff symptom
  Impaired vision with, 40
  multiple sclerosis symptoms of, 950
Ulcerative colitis, malabsorption with,
  1093
Ulnar nerve, 534, 534*t,* 538–539, 538*t,*
  539*t*
Uncal herniation, coma presentations
  with, 24
Unclassified enteroviruses, 180–181
Undifferentiated somatoform disorders,
  1143
Ungual fibroma, tuberous sclerosis
  complex with, 725–726

Unverricht-Lundborg disease,
  autosomal-recessive ataxias of, 788
Upbeating nystagmus, ocular motility
  impairment with, 44
Upper extremity nerve injury, 533–536,
  534, 534*t*
  antebrachial cutaneous nerves with,
    536
  axillary nerve with, 534, 534*t,* 536
  brachial cutaneous nerves with, 536
  brachial plexus in, 533–536, *534,* 534*t*
  cord injury with, 535
  diffuse plexus injury with, 535–536
  dorsal scapular nerve with, 533, 534*t*
  idiopathic brachial plexitis with, 535
  ischemic paralysis of arm with, 536
  lateral cord injury with, 535
  lateral cord with, 533
  long thoracic nerve with, 533, 534*t,*
    536, *537*
  lower radicular syndrome with, 535
  lower trunk with, 533
  medial cord with, 533
  median nerve with, 534, 534*t,* 537–538,
    538*t*
  middle radicular syndrome with, 535
  middle trunk with, 533
  musculocutaneous nerve with, 534,
    534*t,* 539
  neuralgic amyotrophy with, 535
  Parsonage-Turner syndrome with, 535
  pectoral nerves with, 533, 534*t*
  peripheral nerves with, 536–539, 537*t,*
    538*t,* 539*t*
  posterior cord with, 533
  proximal nerves with, *536,* 536–537
  radial nerve with, 534, 534*t,* 536–537
  spinal roots in, 533–536, *534,* 534*t*
  subscapular nerve with, 533, 534*t*
  suprascapular nerve with, 533, 534*t,*
    536–537
  thoracic outlet syndrome with, 535
  thoracic outlet with, 533
  thoracodorsal nerve with, 533, 534*t*
  ulnar nerve with, 534, 534*t,* 538–539,
    538*t,* 539*t*
  upper radicular syndrome with, 535
  upper trunk with, 533
Upper radicular syndrome, 535
Upper trunk, 533
Urea cycle disorders, differential
  diagnosis of, 686*t,* 687*t*
Uremic encephalopathy
  asterixis with, 1079
  dialysis for, 1080
  meningeal signs with, 1080
  multifocal myoclonus with, 1079
  renal disease of, 1079–1080
  restless-legs syndrome with, 1079
Uremic neuropathy, 755
  accelerated neuropathy of renal failure
    with, 1080
  renal disease of, 1080–1081
  renal transplantation for, 1080
Uroporphyrinogen-1 synthase, acute
  intermittent porphyria with, 668

V

VAA. *See* Verbal auditory agnosia
Vagus nerve injury, cranial/peripheral
  nerve lesion with, 532
Vagus nerve stimulation, epilepsy treated
  with, 1009

Valproate
  epilepsy treatment with, 1001, 1002, 1003*t*, 1005
  migraine headache treated with, 985, 986*t*
Valproate therapy, hyperammonemia with, 652
Variegate porphyria, acute intermittent porphyria with, 668
Vascular chorea, 809–810
Vascular dementia, 777–778
  CADASIL as, 778
  cerebral infarction with, 302, 302*t*
  cerebrovascular disease as, 777–778
  cerebrovascular syndromes of, 309
  diagnosis of, 778
Vascular diseases
  CADASIL with, 307
  cerebral infarction as, 295–302, 296–298, 299*t*, 300, 301*t*, 302*t*
    anterior cerebral artery occlusions with, 297–298, 299*t*
    anterior choroidal artery occlusions with, 299–300
    bilateral upper brainstem infarction in, 302
    internal choroidal artery occlusions with, 299*t*, 300
    lateral medullary infarction in, 300, 300–301, 301*t*
    lateral pontine infarction in, 301
    medial medullary infarction in, 301
    medial pontine infarction in, 301
    midbrain infarction in, 302
    middle cerebral artery occlusions with, 295–297, 299*t*
    other posterior fossa syndromes in, 301–302
    posterior cerebral artery occlusions with, 298–299, 299*t*
    pseudobulbar palsy in, 302
    specific vessel occlusions with, 295–300, 296–298, 299*t*
    syndromes of, 300, 300–302, 301*t*, 302*t*
    vascular dementia in, 302, 302*t*
    vertebrobasilar arteries occlusions with, 300
  cerebral veins/sinuses occlusion as, 338–342, 340, 341
    cavernous sinus thrombosis as, 339
    dural arteriovenous malformations as, 342
    lateral sinus thrombosis as, 338–339
    other dural sinus thrombosis as, 341–342
    superior sagittal sinus thrombosis as, 340, 340–341, 341
  cerebral/cerebellar hemorrhage as, 303–305, 304*t*
  cerebrovascular disease as, 275–293, 276, 277, 279–281, 281*t*, 282*t*, 283, 284*t*, 286–288, 288*t*, 290
    classification of, 278–286, 279–281, 281*t*, 282*t*, 283, 284*t*, 286
    definition of, 275–276
    nosology of, 275–276
    pathogenesis of, 278–286, 279–281, 281*t*, 282*t*, 283, 284*t*, 286
    patient examination with, 291–293
    physiology of, 278
    stroke epidemiology with, 286–290, 287, 288, 288*t*, 290

  vascular anatomy of, 276, 276–278, 277
  cerebrovascular syndromes of, 310–311
  children's stroke as, 315–322, 316, 317, 318*t*, 319–322
    adult v., 315
    arterial thrombosis with, 317, 318–319, 319
    basal occlusion disease with, 320
    cerebral embolism in, 321, 321
    clinical evaluation of, 316, 318*t*
    coagulopathies with, 319
    congenital disorder of glycosylation with, 322
    etiology of, 316–318
    extracranial occlusion with, 320
    incidence of, 316, 316, 317
    inflammatory bowel disease with, 319
    intracranial hemorrhage with, 321–322, 322
    laboratory data on, 316, 317, 319, 319–320
    malignancies with, 319
    metabolic disorders with, 322
    migraine with, 319
    moyamoya syndrome with, 318, 319, 320
    perforating artery occlusions with, 320
    peripheral leptomeningeal artery occlusions with, 320
    SCD with, 316, 318
    signs/symptoms of, 319
    treatment of, 320–321
  differential diagnosis of stroke with, 312–315
    nonvascular disorders in, 313–315
    peeling onion of, 313
    stroke types and, 312–313
    TIA v. stroke in, 313
  intracerebral hemorrhage with, 303–305, 304*t*, 307
  ischemic strokes with, 305–307, 306
  other cerebrovascular syndromes with, 308–311, 310*t*
    anticardiolipin antibody syndrome as, 309
    antiphospholipid syndrome as, 309
    blood element abnormalities as, 311
    cardiogenic emboli as, 311
    cerebral amyloid angiopathy as, 309
    fibromuscular hyperplasia as, 308
    Graham syndrome as, 309
    hyperhomocysteinemia as, 309
    hypertensive encephalopathy as, 308
    Lacunar strokes as, 308
    lupus anticoagulant syndrome as, 309
    multi-infarct dementia as, 309
    vascular dementia as, 309
    vascular disorders as, 310–311
    young adult stroke as, 309–310, 310*t*
  spinal cord, 342–346, 343
    spinal cord anatomy with, 342–343, 343
    spinal cord hemorrhage as, 345–346
    spinal cord infarctions as, 343–344
    spinal cord venous disease as, 344–345
  stroke genetics with, 305–307, 306
  stroke prevention with, 327–328
  stroke treatment with, 324–328, 325*t*
    ABI/TIA in, 324–325
    cardiac/aortic origin in, 326
    embolic strokes in, 326

    fixed neurologic defects in, 325–326, 325*t*
    intracerebral hemorrhage in, 326
    rehabilitation in, 326–327
    SAH from congenital/berry aneurysm in, 326–327
  subarachnoid hemorrhage as, 328–337, 329*t*, 330*t*, 331, 332, 333, 333*t*, 335, 336*t*
    angiography of, 331, 332
    cerebral edema with, 333, 333
    clinical manifestations of, 330–331, 330*t*
    complications of, 331–334, 332–333, 333*t*
    CT scan of, 331, 331
    diagnostic studies on, 331, 331, 332
    dolichoectatic aneurysms and, 336
    endovascular therapy for, 334–335
    epidemiology of, 329–330, 329*t*
    fusiform aneurysms and, 336
    grading scale for, 330, 330*t*
    hydrocephalus with, 332–333
    intensive care management for, 335, 336*t*
    lumbar puncture for, 331
    mycotic aneurysm and, 336–337
    neurogenic cardiac/pulmonary disturbances with, 334
    nonaneurysmal causes of, 329*t*
    other macroscopic aneurysms and, 336–337
    outcome after, 335–336
    pathology of, 329–330, 329*t*
    pseudoaneurysm and, 337
    rebleeding with, 331, 332
    seizures with, 333–334
    signs/symptoms of, 330–331
    surgical management for, 334
    treatment of, 334–336, 336*t*
    vascular malformations and, 337
    vasospasm with, 332, 332, 333*t*
  subarachnoid hemorrhage in, 307
  TIA as, 293–294
Vascular endothelial growth factor (VEGF)
  astrocytomas with, 438
  gliomas with, 395
  meningiomas with, 387
Vascular injury, head trauma with, 497
Vascular malformations, 449–458, 450–457
  arteriovenous malformations as, 449–454, 450–453
    clinical presentation of, 450–453, 452
    CT scan of, 452, 452
    diagnosis of, 450–453, 452
    left parietal, 450
    MRA of, 452, 454
    MRI of, 452, 452
    right temporal, 451
    risks with, 451
    surgery for, 453–454
    treatment for, 452–454
  cavernous malformations as, 454, 455
  Krabbe-Weber disease as, 455–457, 455–457
    anticonvulsive drugs for, 456
    clinical presentation of, 456, 456
    diagnosis of, 456, 456
    hemispherectomy for, 456
    radiation therapy for, 456
    treatment of, 456

Vascular malformations (*contd.*)
  SAH and, 337
  sinus pericranii as, 458
  Sturge-Weber disease as, 455–457,
    455–457
  telangiectasias as, 455
  venous malformations as, *453*, 454–455
Vascular parkinsonism, 828*t*, 835
Vascular tumors, 449–459, *450–457*
  von Hippel-Lindau disease with, 458
Vasculitic neuropathy, 751–752, *752*
Vasculitis syndromes, 1099–1109, 1100*t*,
    1101*t*, 1102*t*, 1104*t*, 1106*t*, 1107*t*
  ANCA with, 1104–1105
  Churg-Strauss syndrome as, 1104,
    1104*t*
  en coup de sabre as, 1108
  giant cell arteritis as, 1102–1103
  granulomatous angiitis of the brain as,
    1105–1106, 1106*t*
  linear scleroderma as, 1108
  microscopic polyangiitis as, 1104
  other collagen-vascular diseases as,
    1109
    idiopathic hypereosinophilic
      syndrome with, 1109
    Schirmer test with, 1109
    sicca complex with, 1109
  polyarteritis nodosa as, 1099–1102,
    1102*t*
    clinical features of, 1102*t*
    course of, 1101
    diagnosis of, 1100–1101
    etiology of, 1099
    incidence of, 1099
    laboratory data on, 1100
    pathology of, 1099
    prognosis for, 1101
    signs/symptoms of, 1099–1100, 1102*t*
    symptoms at onset of, 1102*t*
    treatment of, 1101–1102
  polymyalgia as, 1102, 1103–1104
  scleroderma as, 1108
  Sjögren syndrome as, 1109
  Sneddon syndrome as, 1109
  systemic lupus erythematosus as,
    1106–1108, 1107*t*
    antinuclear antibodies with, 1107
    cerebral lupus and, 1107
    course of, 1108
    diagnosis of, 1108
    etiology of, 1106
    incidence of, 1106
    laboratory data on, 1107–1108
    prognosis for, 1108
    symptoms/signs of, 1106–1107, 1107*t*
    therapy for, 1108
  systemic sclerosis as, 1108
  temporal arteritis as, 1102–1103
    prednisone for, 1103
    reversible dementia with, 1103
    steroid therapy for, 1103
  Wegener granulomatosis as, 1104, 1105
Vasogenic brain edema, 357, 358*t*
Vasopressin (Pitressin), multiple sclerosis
    treated with, 961
Vasospasm, SAH with, 332, *332*, 333*t*
Vasovagal syncope, 14*t*, 15
Vegetative state, coma with, 25–28, 26*t*
VEGF. *See* Vascular endothelial growth
    factor
Venlafaxine, neuropathic pain treated
    with, 550

Venous drainage, communicating
    hydrocephalus with, 352
Venous malformations, *453*, 454–455
Ventilation, head injury trauma with, 495
Ventilation/perfusion mismatching,
    respiratory physiology with, 1083
VEP. *See* Visual evoked potentials
Verapamil, migraine headache treated
    with, 985, 986*t*
Verbal auditory agnosia (VAA), language
    disorders of, 581
Verbal paraphasias, 10
Vergence system, ocular motility
    impairment with, 43
Vertebroplasty, ESNR with, 120–122
Vertical nystagmus, ocular motility
    impairment with, 44
Vertigo, 34–38
  common causes of, 35–36, 35*t*
  common clinical entities causing,
    36–38
    BPPV as, 36–37
    cardiac arrhythmia as, 37
    cerebellopontine angle tumors as, 37
    Dix-Hallpike maneuver with, 36
    drug toxicity as, 37
    hyperventilation as, 38
    Ménière's disease as, 35*t*, 37
    perilymphatic fistula as, 37
    presbycusis/presbyastasis as, 37–38
    psychophysiologic causes as, 38
    vestibular neuritis as, 37
  CT in diagnosis of, 36
  definition of, 34
  diagnosis of, 35–36, 35*t*
  Ménière disease with, 1018–1019
  MRI in diagnosis of, 36, 37
  treatment of, 36
Vestibular neurectomy, Ménière disease
    treated with, 1021
Vestibular neuritis, vertigo/hearing loss
    caused by, 37
Vestibular schwannoma, nerve-sheath
    tumor of, *383*, 383–384, 383*t*, *384*
Vestibular system, ocular motility
    impairment with, 43
Viagra. *See* Sildenafil
Vinca alkaloids, peripheral nervous
    system toxicity with, 1169
Viral encephalitis, AIDS opportunistic
    infections with, 220
Viral infections, 175–206, 176*t*, *183*, *189*,
    192t, *193*, 196*t*, *200*, *204*, *205*
  acute viral infections as, 175–177, 176*t*
  ADEM as, 198–200, *200*
  adenovirus infections as, 191
  alphaviruses as, 176*t*, 181
  arboviruses infections as, 181
  arenavirus infections as, 190
  Argentinian hemorrhagic fever as, 190
  Bolivian hemorrhagic fever as, 190
  bunyaviruses as, 176*t*, 181
  California encephalitis as, 185
  chronic viral infections as, 200–202
  classification of, 175
  CMV as, 196–197, 196*t*
  CNS viral syndromes as, 175–177, 176*t*
  Colorado tick fever as, 186
  coxsackievirus infections as, 179–180
  Dawson disease as, 201–202
  echovirus infections as, 180
  encephalitis lethargica as, 204–205
  encephalomyelitis as, 187–188

  enterovirus infections as, 177–179
  Epstein-Barr virus infection as, 197
  equine encephalitis as, 181–183, *183*
  EV 70/EV 71 infections as, 180–181
  flaviviruses as, 176*t*, 181
  HAM as, 202–203
  hepatitis A virus as, 180–181
  herpes simplex encephalitis as,
    191–194, 192*t*, *193*
  herpes zoster as, 194–196
  herpesvirus infections as, 191–196,
    192*t*, *193*
  HHV-6 infection as, 197–198
  Japanese encephalitis as, 185
  Junin virus as, 190
  La Crosse encephalitis as, 185
  Lassa fever virus as, 190
  lymphocytic choriomeningitis as, 190
  Machupo virus as, 190
  mumps meningitis as, 187–188
  myxovirus infections as, 187–188
  picornavirus infections as, 177–179
  PML as, 203–204, *204*, *205*
  progressive rubella panencephalitis as,
    202
  rabies as, 188–190
  reoviruses as, 176*t*, 181
  retrovirus infections as, 202–205, *204*,
    205
  rhabdovirus infection as, 188–190
  rubella as, 186–187
  SSPE as, 201–202
  St. Louis encephalitis as, 183–184
  subacute measles encephalitis as, 188
  tick-borne encephalitis as, 186
  TSP as, 202–203
  unclassified enteroviruses as, 180–181
  West Nile virus encephalitis as,
    184–185
Visual evoked potentials (VEP), 85, *86*
  electrophysiologic vision testing with,
    40, *41*
Vitamin B$_{12}$ deficiency, 1094–1097, *1095*,
    1095*t*, *1096*
  Romberg sign with, 1096
VOC. *See* Volatile organic compounds
Vogt-Koyanagi-Harada syndrome as, 161
Volatile organic compounds (VOC),
    occupation/environment
    neurotoxicology with, 1174*t*,
    1179–1180
Von Economo encephalitis,
    postencephalitic parkinsonism
    with, 835
Von Hippel-Lindau disease
  childhood central nervous system
    tumors with, 428
  differential diagnosis of, 685*t*
  vascular tumors with, 458
Von Recklinghausen disease
  neurofibromatosis as, 713
  spinal tumors with, 477

W

WAIS. *See* Wechsler Adult Intelligence
    Scale
Waldenström macroglobulinemia (WM),
    blood cell dyscrasias of, 1055
Walker-Warburg syndrome, structural
    malformations with, 595
Warfarin, necrosis with, 1057
WBRT. *See* Whole brain radiotherapy
Weak muscles, 52–55

Babinski signs with, 53
bibrachial paresis with, 55
chronic fatigue syndrome with, 52–53
cranial muscles as, 55
crossed hemiplegia with, 52
CSF analysis in examination of, 54
CT examination of, 54
CT in examination of, 54
dropped-head syndrome with, 55
EEG in examination of, 54
EMG in examination of, 54
fatigue with, 52–53
floppy-head syndrome with, 55
Guillain-Barré syndrome with, 54–55
hemiparesis with, 53–54
hemiplegia with, 52
Hoffmann sign with, 53
monomelic paresis with, 55
monoplegia with, 52
MRI examination of, 54
MRI in examination of, 54
neck weakness as, 55
paraparesis with, 54–55
paraplegia with, 52
paresis with, 52
patterns of, 53–55
pseudoweakness and, 53
recognition of, 52–53
Weber test, hearing loss diagnosis with, 33
Wechsler Adult Intelligence Scale (WAIS)
  higher cerebral function disorders with, 580
  neuropsychologic evaluation tests of, 130–131, 131*t*
Wechsler Intelligence Scale for Children (WISC)
  higher cerebral function disorders with, 580
  neuropsychologic evaluation tests of, 130
Wechsler Preschool and Primary Scale for Children (WPPSI), higher cerebral function disorders with, 580
Wegener granulomatosis, vasculitis syndrome of, 1104, 1105
Welander distal myopathy, muscular dystrophy of, 909
Werdnig-Hoffmann disease
  differential diagnosis of, 686*t*
  motor neuron diseases of, 862
Wernicke aphasia, 10
Wernicke aphasia, amnestic aphasia with, 11
Wernicke encephalopathy, Leigh syndrome v., 707, 707*t*
Wernicke hemianopic pupillary phenomenon, Impaired vision with, 41

Wernicke-Korsakoff syndrome
  alcoholism with, 1154–1156, 1155*t*
  coma examination with, 21
  dementia diagnosis with, 6
  orthostatic hypotension with, 972*t*
West Nile virus encephalitis, 184–185
West syndrome. *See also* Tuberous sclerosis complex
  epilepsy of, 993
  epilepsy with, 82*t*
Wet beriberi, dietary associated polyneuropathy with, 757
Whipple diseases, 270–272, 271*t*
  epidemiology of, 270
  laboratory data on, 271
  malabsorption in, 1094
  neurologic manifestations of, 271, 271*t*
  systemic disease with, 270–271
  treatment of, 271–272
Whispering dysphonia, dystonia with, 820
White-matter, radiation injury with, 552
Whole brain radiotherapy (WBRT)
  brain metastasis treated with, 462, 463
  PCNSL treatment with, 409–410, 411
Williams syndrome, 135, 582
Wilms tumors, childhood central nervous system tumors of, 428
Wilson disease
  dementia resulting from, 5, 779*t*, 780
  diagnosis of, 664–665
  Menkes disease v., 661, 661*t*
  metal metabolism disorders of, 660–665, 661*t*, 662, 663, 663*t*, 664
  MRI for, 664, 664
  myasthenia gravis with, 879
  ocular motility impairment with, 43
  onset of, 663*t*
  pathogenesis/pathology of, 661–662, 661*t*, 662
  personality disorders with, 663
  rigidity with, 663
  symptoms/signs of, 662–664, 663, 663*t*, 664
  tendon reflexes with, 663
  treatment of, 665
WISC. *See* Wechsler Intelligence Scale for Children
Withdrawal emergent syndrome
  neuroleptic-induced syndromes with, 849
  Sydenham chorea with, 808
Withdrawal symptoms, fetal cocaine with, 1190
Withdrawal syndrome, fetal alcohol syndrome with, 1188
WM. *See* Waldenström macroglobulinemia
Wnt signaling, childhood central nervous system tumors with, 429

Wolman disease
  differential diagnosis of, 686*t*
  lysosomal/other storage diseases of, 627*t*, 629–630
WPPSI. *See* Wechsler Preschool and Primary Scale for Children
Writer's cramp, dystonia with, 820
Wry neck, 820

X

Xanthomatosis, malignant skull tumors of, 382
Xeroderma pigmentosum (XP)
  childhood cerebral degenerations of, 679
  differential diagnosis of, 686*t*, 687*t*, 688*t*
  DNA maintenance/transcription/translation disorders of, 647*t*
XK syndrome, structural malformations with, 589*t*
X-linked hereditary ataxias, 790
X-linked muscular dyastrophies, 898, 898–901, *900*
X-linked recessive spinobulbar muscular atrophy, motor neuron diseases of, 863, 864*t*
XP. *See* Xeroderma pigmentosum
Xp21 myopathies, 901
  dystrophinopathies with, 901
  non dystrophin-related, 901

Y

Yeast infections. *See* Fungal infections

Z

Zanaflex. *See* Tizanidine
Zebra body myopathy, congenital muscle disorder of, 919
Zellweger syndrome
  differential diagnosis of, 686*t*, 687*t*, 688*t*
  floppy infant syndrome with, 575
  multiple enzymatic pathway dysfunction of, 654
  pathogenesis of, 654
  peroxisomal disease of, 653–654, 653*t*
  structural malformations with, 587
  therapy for, 654
Zolmitriptan, migraine headache treated with, 985
Zonisamide
  epilepsy treatment with, 1001, 1003*t*, 1005
  neuropathic pain treated with, 549
Zonisamide sleep disorders treated with, 1027
Zyprexa, neuroleptic-induced syndromes with, 849